BRADY

11TH EDITION

Emergency Care

BRADY

11TH EDITION

Emergency Care

Daniel Limmer • Michael F. O'Keefe

MEDICAL EDITOR

EDWARD T. DICKINSON, MD, FACEP

LEGACY AUTHORS

HARVEY D. GRANT

ROBERT H. MURRAY, JR.

J. DAVID BERGERON

PEARSON

Prentice Hall

Upper Saddle River, New Jersey 07458

Library of Congress Cataloging-in-Publication Data
Emergency care. — 11th ed. / Daniel Limmer, Michael F. O'Keefe ; medical editor, Edward T. Dickinson ; legacy authors, Harvey D. Grant, Robert H. Murray Jr., J. David Bergeron ; contributors, Jonathan F. Politis, Marc Minkler, Andrew W. Stern.
p. ; cm.
Includes index.
ISBN-13: 978-0-13-500523-1
ISBN-10: 0-13-500523-X
1. Emergency medicine. 2. First aid in illness and injury. 3. Rescue work. 4. Emergency medical personnel. I. Limmer, Daniel. II. O'Keefe, Michael F. III. Dickinson, Edward T.
[DNLM: 1. Emergency Medical Services—methods. 2. Emergencies. 3. Emergency Medical Technicians. 4. Emergency Treatment—methods. WX 215 E483 2009]
RC86.7.B68 2009
616.02'5—dc22
2008024060

Publisher: Julie Levin Alexander
Publisher's Assistant: Regina Bruno
Executive Editor: Marlene McHugh Pratt
Acquisitions Editor: Sladjana Repic
Senior Managing Editor for Development: Lois Berlowitz
Project Manager: Sandra Breuer
Editorial Assistant: Sean Karpowicz
Director of Marketing: Karen Allman
Executive Marketing Manager: Katrin Beacom
Marketing Specialist: Michael Sirinides
Managing Editor for Production: Patrick Walsh
Production Liaison: Faye Gemmellaro
Production Editor: Heather Willison, S4Carlisle Publishing Services
Manufacturing Manager: Ilene Sanford
Manufacturing Buyer: Pat Brown
Senior Design Coordinator: Christopher Weigand
Cover and Interior Design: Delgado and Company, Inc.
Front Cover Image: Shutterstock/Craig Hosterman
Back Cover Image: Getty Images/Mike Powell
Managing Photography Editor: Michal Heron
Photographers: Nathan Eldridge, Michael Gallitelli, Michal Heron, Richard Logan, Stephen Ogilvy
Media Project Manager: Stephen J. Hartner
Media Editor: Joseph Saba
Composition: S4Carlisle Publishing Services
Printer/Binder: Courier/Kendallville
Cover Printer: Phoenix Color

Pearson Education Ltd., London
Pearson Education Australia Pty., Limited
Pearson Education Singapore, Pte. Ltd.
Pearson Education North Asia Ltd., Hong Kong
Pearson Education Canada, Inc.
Pearson Educación de Mexico, S.A. de C.V.
Pearson Education—Japan
Pearson Education Malaysia, Pte. Ltd.
Pearson Education, Upper Saddle River, New Jersey

NOTICE ON CARE PROCEDURES

It is the intent of the authors and publisher that this textbook be used as part of a formal EMT-Basic education program taught by qualified instructors and supervised by a licensed physician. The procedures described in this textbook are based upon consultation with EMT and medical authorities. The authors and publisher have taken care to make certain that these procedures reflect currently accepted clinical practice; however, they cannot be considered absolute recommendations.

The material in this textbook contains the most current information available at the time of publication. However, federal, state, and local guidelines concerning clinical practices, including, without limitation, those governing infection control and universal precautions, change rapidly. The reader should note, therefore, that the new regulations may require changes in some procedures.

It is the responsibility of the reader to familiarize himself or herself with the policies and procedures set by federal, state, and local agencies as well as the institution or agency where the reader is employed. The authors and the publisher of this textbook and the supplements written to accompany it disclaim any liability, loss, or risk resulting directly or indirectly from the suggested procedures and theory, from any undetected errors, or from the reader's misunderstanding of the text. It is the reader's responsibility to stay informed of any new changes or recommendations made by any federal, state, or local agency as well as by his or her employing institution or agency.

NOTICE ON GENDER USAGE

The English language has historically given preference to the male gender. Among many words, the pronouns *he* and *his* are commonly used to describe both genders. Society evolves faster than language, and the male pronouns still predominate in our speech. The authors have made great effort to treat the two genders equally, recognizing that a significant percentage of EMTs are female. However, in some instances, male pronouns may be used to describe both males and females solely for the purpose of brevity. This is not intended to offend any readers of the female gender.

NOTICE RE "STREET SCENES" AND "SCENARIOS"

The names used and situations depicted in the Street Scenes and Scenarios throughout this text are fictitious.

NOTICE ON MEDICATIONS

The authors and the publisher of this book have taken care to make certain that the equipment, doses of drugs, and schedules of treatment, are correct and compatible with the standards generally accepted at the time of publication. Nevertheless, as new information becomes available, changes in treatment and in the use of equipment and drugs become necessary. The reader is advised to carefully consult the instruction and information material included in the page insert of each drug or therapeutic agent, piece of equipment, or device before administration. This advice is especially important when using new or infrequently used drugs. Prehospital care providers are warned that use of any drugs or techniques must be authorized by their Medical Director, in accord with local laws and regulations. The publisher disclaims any liability, loss, injury, or damage incurred as a consequence, directly or indirectly, of the use and application of any of the contents of this book.

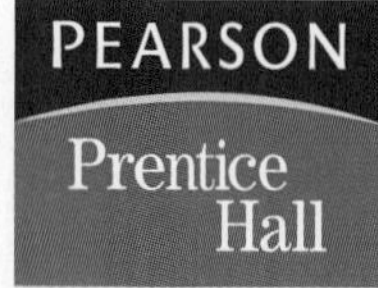

10 9 8 7 6 5
ISBN 13: 978-0-13-500523-1 (paper)
ISBN 10: 0-13-500523-X
10 9 8 7 6 5 4 3
ISBN 13: 978-0-13-500524-8 (case)
ISBN 10: 0-13-500524-8

To the memory of my father, Darwin H. "Punk" Limmer,
1935–2007.

D.L.

To my parents, Mike and Noreen, my first and
best teachers.

M.O'K.

To Debbie, Stephen, and Alex for their endless love
and extraordinary patience throughout this and
many other projects.

E.T.D.

BRIEF CONTENTS

MODULE 1 Preparatory

MODULE 2 Airway

MODULE 3 Patient Assessment

MODULE 4 Medical Emergencies

MODULE 5 Trauma

MODULE 6 Special Patient Populations

MODULE 7 Operations

MODULE 8 Advanced Airway Management

Appendices

DETAILED CONTENTS

MODULE 1 • Preparatory

MODULE 2 • Airway

MODULE 3 • Patient Assessment

Chapter 9 • Vital Signs and SAMPLE History 224

Chapter 10 • Assessment of the Trauma Patient 248

Chapter 11 • Assessment of the Medical Patient 289

Chapter 12 • Ongoing Assessment 306

Chapter 13 • Communications 318

MODULE 4 • Medical Emergencies

Chapter 23 • Behavioral Emergencies 547

Chapter 24 • Obstetrics and Gynecological Emergencies 562

Chapter 25 • Putting It All Together for the Medical Patient 600

MODULE 5 • Trauma

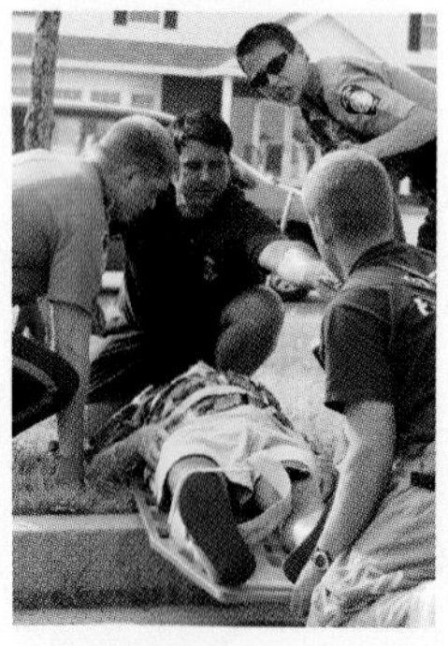

Chapter 26 • Bleeding and Shock 614

Chapter 27 • Soft-Tissue Injuries 642

Chapter 28 • Musculoskeletal Injuries 693

Chapter 29 • Injuries to the Head and Spine 747

Chapter 30 • Putting It All Together for the Trauma Patient 792

MODULE 6 • Special Patient Populations

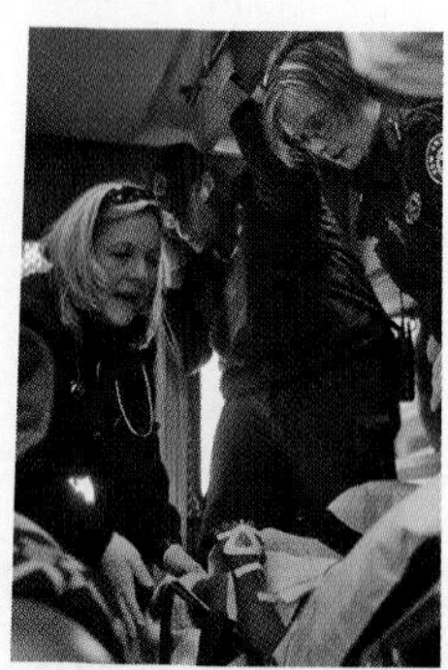

Chapter 31 • Infants and Children 806

Chapter 32 • Patients with Special Needs 864

Chapter 33 • Geriatric Patients 881

MODULE 7 • Operations

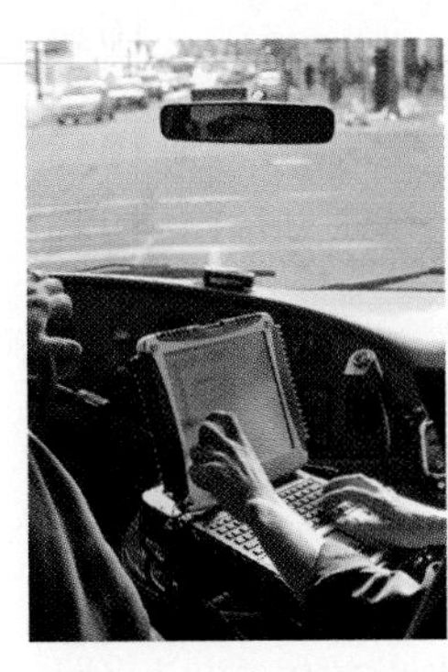

Chapter 34 • Ambulance Operations 900

Chapter 35 • Gaining Access and Rescue Operations 938

Chapter 36 • Special Operations 963

MODULE 8 • Advanced Airway Management

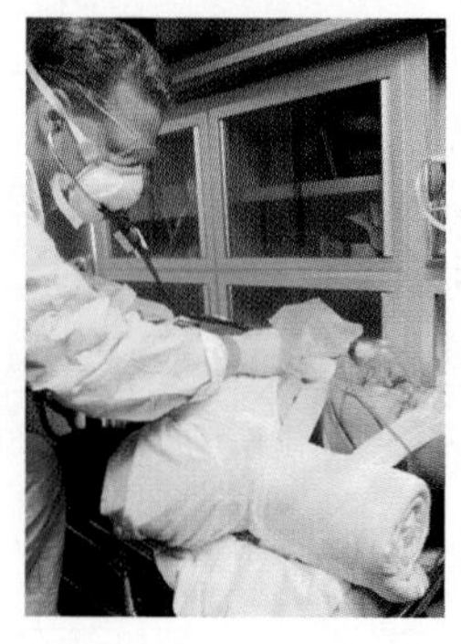

Appendices

Reference Section 1191

NS

Basic Cardiac Life Support Review

PHOTO SCANS

BRADY

IT'S ABOUT PEOPLE

Dear Student:

Thank you for purchasing Brady's *Emergency Care* EMT textbook. The 11th edition is the most recent in a long line of editions that have provided high quality, understandable, and technically accurate material to generations of EMT students. For over 30 years, *Emergency Care* has been the book instructors have chosen to prepare their students for the test...and the field.

This edition has been thoroughly updated to reflect important changes in science and practice. We have also added two new features that reflect the vital impact EMTs have on their patients: Point of View, which tells stories of EMS care from the patient's perspective, and Critical Decision Making, which introduces students to real-life decisions they will face on the street.

Your book is written by real people who have over 80 years of combined EMS experience. Dan Limmer became an EMT-Basic in 1980 and a paramedic in 1981. He actively practices as a paramedic and teaches EMT-B and paramedic courses. Mike O'Keefe is a paramedic. He is the EMS Training Coordinator for the State of Vermont and served as a member of the committee that created the curriculum EMT training is currently based on. Mike is once again helping to shape the future of EMS as the EMT-level content leader for the development of the forthcoming new National EMS Education Standards. Medical Editor Ed Dickinson is an emergency physician with a solid background of EMS field experience. Ed began his career in medicine as an EMT-Paramedic prior to medical school. He has extensive experience in the fire service and has received the prestigious Firehouse Magazine Award for Heroism. He is active as a fire company and paramedic service Medical Director.

We believe that actual practicing authors are critical for a book to provide a practical, street-wise presentation. You want to pass the exam—but you also want to be prepared for the street. *Emergency Care* is the book that provides both.

Our experience has given us perspective in other areas as well. EMS has been a WONDERFUL EXPERIENCE FOR US ALL. Every profession has ups and downs, heartache and triumph. EMS is no different. Patients will be saved, but some patients will be lost. Some calls will be exciting; many will not. What stands out among this mix of calls and patients is that the rewards of EMS are many for those who embrace it. There are lifelong friends with common interests to be made and the ability to affect many people positively, in both large and small ways.

In short, EMS is about people. Welcome. Be safe. Have fun. We wish you well in your education and in the practice of EMS.

Sincerely,

Daniel Limmer   Michael O'Keefe   Edward Dickinson

PREFACE

Emergency Care has set the standard for basic-level EMT training for over 30 years. We strive to stay current with new research and developments in emergency medical services, and this new edition is no exception. We've updated the text to meet 2005 American Heart Association guidelines for CPR and ECC to prepare your students for testing and practice in the year 2008 and beyond.

The foundation of *Emergency* Care is the U.S. DOT 1994 EMT-Basic National Standard Curriculum; everything in the 1994 curriculum is addressed in the text. In the editions since publication of the 1994 curriculum, information has been added in response to changes in research and practice that affect the way prehospital care is delivered. *Emergency Care*, 11th Edition, is the most current reflection of EMS practice today and of what EMS systems and EMTs are actually doing around the country. The caveat "follow local protocols," of course, appears frequently—whenever the equipment or practice described has been adopted in some but not all systems.

In addition, the text and the accompanying CD-ROM were developed taking into account the years of experience that the authors, with the input of countless instructors and students, have had with the DOT curriculum since its publication. The result is a proven text with outstanding readability and a level of detail that more instructors have found appropriate for their classrooms than any other.

The content of the 11th edition is summarized in the following text, with emphasis on "what's new" in each module of this edition.

MODULE 1, PREPARATORY: CHAPTERS 1–5

The first module sets a framework for all the modules that follow by introducing some essential concepts, information, and skills. The EMS system and the role of the basic-level EMT within the system are introduced. Issues of EMT safety and well-being and legal and ethical issues are covered. Basic anatomy and physiology and techniques of safe lifting and moving are also included in this first module.

What's New in the Preparatory Module?

- In Chapter 1, "Introduction to Emergency Medical Care," a section has been added on **forthcoming changes to EMS education standards and levels of certification and training.**
- In Chapter 2, "The Well-Being of the EMT," new sections have been added on **hepatitis C** and **Avian flu** as well as **scene safety at a potential terrorist incident.**
- In Chapter 5, "Lifting and Moving Patients," **automatic power stretchers** and **updated stair chairs** are described and illustrated.

MODULE 2, AIRWAY MANAGEMENT: CHAPTER 6

There is only one chapter in Module 2, but it may be considered the most important module in the text, because no patient will survive without an open airway. Basic airway management techniques that meet newly revised American Heart Association guidelines are covered in detail.

What's New in the Airway Management Module?

- In Chapter 6, "Airway Management," information on the **Venturi mask** has been added.

MODULE 3, PATIENT ASSESSMENT: CHAPTERS 7–14

The ability to perform a thorough and accurate assessment, treat for life-threatening conditions, and initiate transport to the hospital within optimum time limits are the essence of the EMT's job. In this module, all of the steps of the assessment and their application to different types of trauma and medical patients, plus the skills of measuring vital signs, taking a patient history, communication, and documentation, are explained and illustrated.

What's New in the Assessment Module?

- In Chapter 7, "Scene Size-Up," there is an expanded section on **falls.**
- Chapter 9, "Vital Signs and SAMPLE History," includes new information on the **definition and consequences**

of hypertension. The **automatic blood pressure monitor** is introduced, and the pluses and minuses of the new **CO-oximeters** are discussed.
- In Chapter 13, "Communications," expanded cautions are included on **the reliability of cell phone communications.**
- In Chapter 14, "Documentation," **Continuous Quality Improvement (CQI) systems** are discussed.

MODULE 4, MEDICAL EMERGENCIES: CHAPTERS 15–25

The Medical Emergencies module begins with a chapter on pharmacology in which the medications the basic-level EMT can administer or assist with under the 1994 curriculum are introduced. The module continues with chapters on respiratory, cardiac, abdominal, diabetic, allergy, poisoning and overdose, environmental, behavioral, and obstetric/gynecological emergencies. It ends with a chapter on caring for patients with multiple medical complaints.

What's New in the Medical Emergencies Module?

- In Chapter 15, "General Pharmacology," the **table of Medications Patients Often Take has been extensively updated** to remove medications no longer available or recommended and to add medications that have recently come into use.
- In Chapter 19, "Diabetic Emergencies and Altered Mental Status," **blood glucose meters that allow blood to be taken from areas such as the forearm** instead of the finger are described.
- In Chapter 22, "Environmental Emergencies," in accordance with recent World Health Organization and American Heart Association guidelines, **the term *near-drowning* is no longer used. (*Drowning* is used for all such incidents, whether or not the patient survives.)**
- In Chapter 23, "Behavioral Emergencies," information has been added regarding **restraint of a patient when it is necessary in order for the patient to receive medical care.**

MODULE 5, TRAUMA: CHAPTERS 26–30

The Trauma module begins with a chapter on bleeding and shock; continues with chapters on soft-tissue injuries, musculoskeletal injuries, and injuries to the head and spine; and ends with a chapter on caring for multiple-trauma patients.

What's New in the Trauma Module?

- In Chapter 26, "Bleeding and Shock," the terms *golden hour* and *platinum 10 minutes* are deemphasized with greater emphasis placed on the general principle of **improving patient outcomes by limiting time on scene and reducing the time from injury to operating suite.** New information is added on **narrowing pulse pressure as a sign of shock.** There is also new information on the **effects of blood thinner medications** and on **hemostatic agents** used to stop bleeding.
- In Chapter 27, "Soft-Tissue Injuries," more material is included on **specific chest injuries.** A segment on **flail segment** has been added.
- Chapter 29, "Injuries to the Head and Spine," has added a discussion of how **spine immobilization protocols may differ by the patient's age (child, adult, elderly).**

MODULE 6, SPECIAL PATIENT POPULATIONS: CHAPTERS 31–33

Special considerations apply to younger and older patients as well as to patients who rely on advanced medical devices at home. The chapters in this module explore the physical and psychological differences among younger and older patients, as well as patients with special needs, while emphasizing how to serve all of these patients by applying the basics of patient assessment and care that the student has already learned.

What's New in the Special Patient Populations Module?

- Chapter 31, "Infants and Children":
  - Following American Heart Association guidelines, this chapter now addresses only **two age categories: infant (birth to age 1) and child (age 1 to puberty).** (The "child" category was formerly split as ages 1 to 8 and 8 to adult.)
  - Discussion and illustration of the **Pediatric Assessment Triangle** have been updated to conform to the latest American Academy of Pediatrics standards.
  - A new emphasis throughout the chapter is **keeping the ambulance compartment warm** when transporting pediatric patients, who are especially susceptible to hypothermia.
- **Chapter 32, "Patients with Special Needs," is a new chapter** in this edition that concerns patients who rely on advanced medical devices at home. Various types of advanced devices are discussed (respiratory devices, cardiac devices, gastrourinary devices, and central IV catheters) as well as types of physical impairments. Discussions center on how to treat patients for problems not related to their special devices, on how to fix problems with the devices that may occur, and on how to use normal patient assessment and basic life support measures to support patients when their special devices fail.

MODULE 7, OPERATIONS: CHAPTERS 34–37

This module deals with nonmedical operations and special situations, including ambulance operations, motor-vehicle collision rescues, multiple-casualty and hazardous materials incidents, and EMS response to terrorism.

What's New in the Operations Module?

- In Chapter 34, "Ambulance Operations":
  - An expanded discussion is provided of **special kits for the treatment of exposures to specific chemicals and poisons.**
  - An added emphasis is on the **safety of EMTs in the patient compartment** of the ambulance.
  - A new discussion of **helicopter transport of medical patients** (in addition to helicopter transport of trauma and cardiac arrest patients) is added.
- **Chapter 37, "EMS Response to Terrorism,"** has been revised throughout to conform to **National Incident Management System (NIMS) guidelines.**

MODULE 8, ADVANCED AIRWAY MANAGEMENT (ELECTIVE): CHAPTER 38

In some states and regions, basic-level EMTs are trained to perform invasive airway management procedures, including orotracheal intubation and, in children, nasogastric intubation. Module 8 is included as an elective to cover these advanced airway management skills.

What's New in the Advanced Airway Management Module?

- In Chapter 38, "Advanced Airway Management," new information on the **laryngeal mask airway (LMA)** and the **King LT** airway is included.
- Information is included on **esophageal detection devices** and **capnometry** to confirm proper endotracheal tube placement and to provide continual monitoring during transport.

APPENDICES AND BCLS REVIEW

There are four appendices to this textbook, covering advanced life support assist skills, a review of the basic cardiac life support course, a new appendix on the future of EMS education, and a new answer key appendix.

What's New in the Appendices?

- In Appendix A, "ALS Assist Skills," information has been added on **capnometry** and on **alternative placement of ECG electrodes on the extremities** in addition to the traditional chest placement.
- **Appendix B, "Basic Cardiac Life Support Review,"** has been updated to reflect current AHA guidelines.
- **Appendix C, "The Future of EMS Education," is a new appendix** on the past, present, and future of EMS education.
- **Appendix D, "Answer Keys," includes answers for the Critical Decision Making features, Review Questions, Critical Thinking features, and Street Scenes that appear in the chapters.**

Our Goal: Improving Future Training and Education

Some of the best ideas for better training and education methods come from instructors who can tell us what areas of study caused their students the most trouble. Other sound ideas come from practicing EMTs who let us know what problems they faced in the field. We welcome any of your suggestions. If you are an EMS instructor who has an idea on how to improve this book, the companion CD, the Companion Web site, or basic-level EMT training in general, please write to us at:

Brady/Pearson Health Sciences
c/o EMS Editor
Pearson Education
One Lake Street
Upper Saddle River, NJ 07458

If you have access to a computer with a modem, you can also reach us through the following addresses:

danlimmer@mac.com
MikeOKVT@aol.com

Visit Brady's Web Site

http://www.bradybooks.com

If you experience a problem with the companion CD, please write to technical support at **media.support@pearsoned.com** or call 800-677-6337.

ABOUT THE PEOPLE

Content Contributors

Becoming an EMT requires study in a number of content areas ranging from airway to medical and trauma emergencies to pediatrics to rescue. To ensure that each area is covered accurately and in the most up-to-date manner, we have enlisted the help of several expert contributors. We are grateful for the time and energy each has put into his contribution. Contributors to the 11th edition include Jonathan Politis, Andrew Stern, and Marc Minkler.

Jonathan Politis, MA, REMT-P, Chief, Colonie EMS Department, Colonie, New York, contributed the "Gaining Access and Rescue Operations" and the "Special Operations" Chapters. Andrew Stern, MPA, NREMT-P, Senior paramedic and Flight Paramedic, Colonie, New York EMS Department, contributed the "Infants and Children" chapter and also worked tirelessly on the Instructors' Resource manual that accompanies this text. Marc Minkler, REMT-P, CCEMT-P, Portland, Maine, Fire Department, wrote the "Patients with Special Needs" chapter, which appears for the first time in this edition.

We would also like to acknowledge those who have contributed to previous editions of *Emergency Care* including Jeff Dyar, Mike Grill, and Hugh Skerker.

Reviewers

We wish to thank the following reviewers for providing invaluable feedback and suggestions in preparation of the 11th edition of *Emergency Care*.

Christine C. Alvarez, Director
Prehospital Care Programs
LaGuardia Community College, C.U.N.Y.
Long Island City, NY

John L. Beckman, AA, BS, FF/EMT-P Instructor
Affiliated with Addison Fire Protection District
Fire Science Instructor Technology Center
of DuPage, IL

John R. Brophy
EMS Supervisior and EMT–B Instructor
Liberty Health–Jersey City Medical Center EMS
Jersey City, New Jersey

Paul Duckworth, AAT, EMT-P
Augusta Fire Department
Augusta, GA

Eric C. Ganson, EMT, I/D, I.C.
Mayetta, KS

James J. Hasson
Director
EMS Educational Institute
Sharon Regional Health System
Sharon, PA

Sean Kivlehan, NREMT-P
EMS Instructor
St. Vincent's Hospital-Manhattan
New York, NY

Micol Konvicka, NREMT-P, BS
Coordinator
Bulverde, TX

Becky Morris, Director
EMS Department
Trenholm State College
Monotgomery, AL

Jeff Pollakoff MICP (Ret)
EMT Senior Educator
UCLA Center for Prehospital Care
Los Angeles, CA

Frederick H. (Ted) Rogers, BA, NREMT-P
Lead EMT Instructor
St. Petersburg College EMS Program
St. Petersburg, FL

Ryan Sittig, BA, NREMT-P
Avera McKennan School of EMS
Sioux Falls, SD

Al Tompkins, EMT/CIC
SUNY Upstate Medical
Syracuse, NY

Michael L. Wallace, MPA, EMTB, CCEMTP
Captain
Central Jackson Country Fire Protection District
Blue Springs, MO

Brian J. Wilson, BA, NREMT-P
EMS Education Director
Texas Tech School of Medicine, TX

Greg Wommack, EMT-P, AS
Captain
Osceola County Department of Fire/Rescue
and Emergency Medical Services
Kissimmee, FL

We also wish to thank the EMS professionals in the following list who reviewed the 10th edition of *Emergency Care*. They helped to make this program a successful teaching tool.

John L. Beckman, FF/PM
EMS Instructor
Director of Public Education
Lincolnwood Fire Dept.
Lincolnwood, IL

Chris Blaney
Horry-Georgetown Technical College
Myrtle Beach, SC

Joyce S. Bradley
Program Coordinator
Dona Ana Branch Community College
Las Cruces, NM

Mike Buldra, NREMT-P
EMS Program Director
Eastern New Mexico University
Roswell, NM

Richard Criste, BHS, NREMT-P
Chairperson
Emergency Medical Science Dept.
Fayetteville Technical Community College
Volunteer Supervisor Fort Bragg EMS
Fort Bragg, NC

Lyndal M. Curry
Basic Coordinator
University of South Alabama
Mobile, AL

Mark Doerfler, EMT-P
Public Safety Coordinator
Mid-East Ohio Vocational School, Ohio

M. John Dudte, MPA, MICT, I/C
EMS Education
Wichita State University
Wichita, KS

Joseph W. Ferrell, BS, NREMT-P
Iowa Dept. of Public Health
Des Moines, IA

Dwayne A. Gates, MA, BS, EMT-P
Paramedic Program Director
Bossier Parish Community College
Bossier City, LA

Richard J. Harless
Prehospital Care Instructor
Spokane Community College
Spokane, WA

Les Hawthorne, NREMT-P, BA
Adjunct Coordinator
EMT-P Dept.
Southwestern Illinois College
Belleville, IL

Steve Hazelton, EMT-P
Rutland Regional Medical Center
Rutland, VT

Donald Hutchinson, EMT-I,
EMT-B Instructor
Northeastern Technical College
Cheraw, SC

Ken Krupich, NREMT-P
Education Director
Fargo-Moorhead Ambulance Service
Fargo, ND

Robert McGraw, AS, REMT-P
Program Coordinator
Seminole Community College
Sanford, FL

James B. Miller, NREMT-P
U.S. Army EMS Programs Manager
Michael G. Miller, RN, NREMT-P
Creighton University
EMS Education
Omaha, NE

John Mohler, RN, BSN, CCRN, CFRN
REMSA-Care Flight
Reno, NV

Anthony F. Palmisano, BS, MA
EMT Coordinator
Monmouth Medical Center
Long Branch, NJ

Regina K. Pearson, EMT-P
Jackson State Community College
Jackson, TN

Liam Proctor, NREMT-P, CCEMT-P, EMS-I
Advisory Committee
School of EMS Clinic Health Systems
Cleveland, OH

Iggy Rosales, Firefighter/Paramedic
EMS Coordinator
City of Kenner
Louisiana Fire & Rescue Dept.
Kenner, LA

Jose V. Salazar, MPH, NREMT-P
Loudoun County Fire-Rescue
Leesburg, VA

Robert J. Staples, MS, NREMT-P
Daytona Beach Community College
Daytona Beach, FL

Rose Marie Tiernan, NREMT-B
Primary Instructor
Paramus, NJ

Paul Vogt
Hill College EMS Program
Cleburne, TX

Paul A. Werfel, BA, NREMT-P
Stony Brook University, Stony Brook, NY

Cultural Considerations Contributors

Some of the Cultural Considerations features throughout the text are based on information from the following sources:

Andrew, M. M. (1999). Transcultural perspectives in the nursing care of children and adolescents. In M. M. Andrews & J. S. Boyle (Eds.), *Transcultural concepts in nursing care* (3rd ed., pp. 107–159). Philadelphia: Lippinncott.

Gaston-Johansson, F., Albert, M., Fagan, E., & Zimmerman, I. (1990). Similarities in pain descriptions of four different ethnic-culture groups. *Journal of Pain and Symptom Management, 5*(2), 94–100.

Hutchinson, M. K., & Baqi-Aziz, M. (1994). Nursing care of the childrearing Muslim family. *Journal of Obstetric, Gynecologic, and Neonatal Nursing, 23*(9), 767.

Lipson, J. G., Dibble, S. L., & Minarik, P. A., (Eds.). (1996). *Culture and nursing care: A pocket guide*. San Francisco: UCSF Press.

Mattson, S. (2000). Providing culturally competent care: Strategies and approaches for perinatal clients. *AWHONN Lifetimes, 4*(5), 37–39.

Spector, R. E. (2000). *Cultural diversity in health and illness* (5th ed.). Upper Saddle River, NJ: Prentice Hall Health.

Photo Advisors and Sources

All photographs not credited adjacent to the photograph or in the following photo credit section were photographed on assignment for Brady/Prentice Hall, Pearson Education.

Photo Credits for Cultural Considerations Features

Ch. 16, Edward T. Dickinson, MD; Ch. 14, Eastcott/Momatiuk Camp & Associates; Ch. 9 and Ch. 25, Michal Heron; Ch. 37, Richard Levine; Ch. 33, Photo Disc; Ch. 31, Ilene Sanford; Ch. 24, Jules Selmes; Ch. 30, Elaine Sulle/The Image Bank

Module Openers

Module openers 1–7, © Daniel Limmer
Module opener 8, © Corbis

Photo Credits for Point of View Features

Figures 6-2, 35-1, C-4, and C-5, © Daniel Limmer

Technical Advisers

Thanks to the following for providing technical support during the photo shoots for the 11th edition:

Daniel Batsie, NREMT-P, Education Coordinator, Northeast Maine EMS
Judy French, EMT-I
Carl French, CCEMPT-P, FF

Organizations

Thanks to the following organizations for their assistance in creating the photo program for the 11th Edition:

In Kansas, Maine, Missouri, and New York:
Alfred Rescue
Chief Matthew Bors, EMT-B/FF
Alfred, ME

Alfred Fire Department
Chief David Lord, EMT-B/FF
Alfred, ME

BJC Home Care,
St. Louis, MO

BJC Progress West HealthCare Center,
O'Fallon, MO

BJC St. Louis Children's Hospital
St. Louis, MO

Kennebunk Fire and Rescue
Deputy Chief David Cluff, EMT-I
Kennebunk, ME

Lifeflight of Maine
Thomas P. Judge, Executive Director, CCEMT-P
Lewiston, ME

MSA, First Responder,
Lenexa, KS

O'Fallon Fire Protection District,
O'Fallon, MO

Rowles Homes, St. Louis, MO

St. Charles County Ambulance District,
St. Charles, MO

Wells EMS
Susan Hludik, EMS Coordinator, EMT-P
Wells, ME

Wilton Emergency Squad, Inc.,
Wilton, NY

Thank you to the following people who provided locations for our photographs:

Chief Matthew Bors and family
Goodall Regional Wellness Center Staff
Randy and Margaret Kleinrock
Chief David Lord and family
Gary Miller, Miller Ford
Sanford Municipal Airport
Wells EMS, Susan Hludik, EMS Coordinator, EMT-P
West Kennebunk Methodist Church, Reverend Deborah Hanson
Stephanie Limmer
York Hospital/Wells Urgent Care Staff

Thank you to the following people who portrayed patients and EMS providers in our photographs:

In Maine:
Matt Ballou, FF
Eric Beecher, FF/EMT-I
Shira Beecher
Heather Cady, RN, CCEMT-P
Eric Cheney, EMT-B
Jarrett Clarke, EMT-B
Carl French, CCEMT-P, FF
Judy French, EMT-I
Tara LaFrance, FF
Sarah Limmer
Christa Lord
Karen Lord, FF/EMT-B
Kenneth Lovell, FF/EMT-B
Ginny McCarthy and Hattie McCarthy
Robert Munson, FF/EMT-P
Bambi Ouellette, RN
Bryan Piaseczny, FF
Christopher Russell, Police Officer
Dennis Small, EMS Pilot
Captain Brian Smith, Sanford Fire Department
Kenneth Smith
Andy Stevenson, FF/EMT-P
Genie Stevenson
Pete Tilney, CCEMT-P, MS4
Don Wade

In Missouri and New York:
Timothy Bobbitt—Florissant, MO
Nicholas Collins-Feay—Wilton, NY
Albert and Suzanne Kemp—Florissant, MO
Joanna Mezei—Augusta, MO
Rees Remington—St. Charles, MO
Jake Ziegler—Cottleville, MO

Thank you to the following who have provided logistical assistance with photography: Ronald Grondin, Mike Jenkins, Peter Landry, Stephanie Limmer, Hattie McCarthy, Gary Miller, Captain Brian Smith, and Keith Stuart.

Thank you to Boundtree Medical, Grondin Towing, Hartwell Medical, Miller Ford, Nonin Corporation, and Zoll Medical for supplying equipment for the photo shoots.

Model and location coordinator: Judy French, EMT-I
Photo Assistant: Frank Menair
Moulage Technician: Don Wade

ABOUT THE AUTHORS

Daniel Limmer AUTHOR

Began EMS in 1978. Became an EMT in 1980 and a paramedic in 1981.

Enjoys teaching patient assessment and believes critical thinking and decision-making skills are the key to successful clinical practice of EMS.

Works part-time as a freelance photojournalist and is working on a documentary project photographing EMS people and agencies throughout the United States.

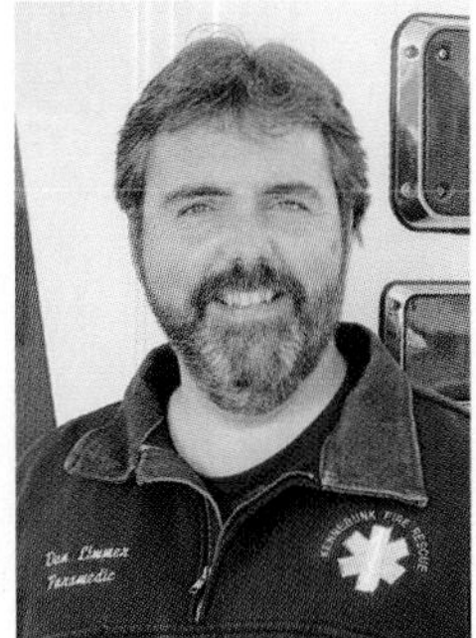

Is an avid blogger. His EMS blog can be seen on www.bradybooks.com.

In addition to his EMS experience, was a dispatcher and police officer in Upstate New York.

Dan lives in Maine. He is married to Stephanie and has two daughters, Sarah and Margo.

Is a Jimmy Buffett fan (Parrothead) who attends at least one concert each year.

Michael F. O'Keefe AUTHOR

EMT Provider Level Leader for National EMS Education Standards.

Expert writer for 1994 revision of EMT-Basic curriculum.

EMS volunteer since college in 1976.

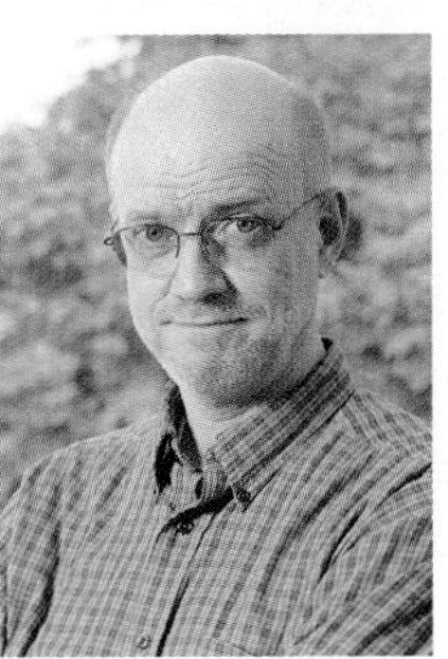

Member of development group for the National EMS *Education Agenda for the Future: A Systems Approach* and *The National EMS Scope of Practice Model.*

Has a special interest in EMS research, and got a master's degree in biostatistics.

Past chairperson of the National Council of State EMS Training Coordinators.

Mike's interests include science fiction, travel, foreign languages, and stained glass.

Edward T. Dickinson MEDICAL EDITOR

In 1985 was the first volunteer firefighter to receive the top award from *Firehouse Magazine* for heroism for the rescue of two elderly women trapped in a house fire.

Is the medical director of the Malvern and Berwyn Fire Companies, and the Haverford Township Paramedics in Pennsylvania.

Has been continuously certified as a National Registry Paramedic since 1983.

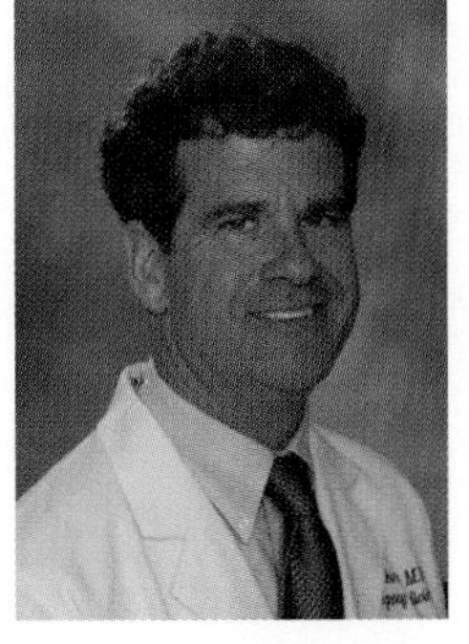

First certified as an EMT in 1979 in Upstate New York.

Has a full-time academic emergency medicine practice at the Hospital of the University of Pennsylvania in Philadelphia.

Has served as medical editor for numerous Brady EMT and First Responder texts.

Ed lives with his wife and two sons in suburban Chester County outside of Philadelphia.

MESSAGE FROM BRADY

Dear Instructor:

Brady, your partner in education, is pleased to present the 11th edition of our best-selling ***Emergency Care***. We continue to offer the high-quality content and innovation that you have come to know and trust. Our mission and message for this 11th edition remains unchanged: **It's About People.** Our commitment to serving the needs of the thousands of people who have used this book to teach and to learn still stands. It continues to be about our authors, reviewers, editors, producers, marketers, and sellers, all with vast experience in both EMS and educational publishing. And most importantly, it's still about the millions of people who have been helped by the efforts of EMTs over the years. We're proud of this association and hope to bring you the best possible education in this edition and many to come.

This is an exciting time to be a part of EMS and EMS education. A new set of Standards will soon replace the DOT curriculum. We also know that our customers have unique and different needs. Not all of you will transition to the Standards at the same time. Your scope of practice and protocols are different, depending on where you work. You teach out of fire houses, ambulance services, or colleges. Your students are 18, 35, and 60. You need tools that enable you to teach and learn in your particular environment. Because of this, we will:

- Continue to strive to create products that are flexible, engaging, and relevant;
- Keep our DOT-curriculum products—such as ***Emergency Care***—current for some time, while at the same time offering new solutions for Standards-based education;
- Offer more ways to assess students' performance;
- Create curricula to assist in the Standards transition;
- Provide the largest and most comprehensive custom solutions in the publishing business.

The following Walkthrough outlines the features found in each chapter. We've retained the tried-and-true and added some new ones based on what we've discovered works in educational publishing. The Walkthrough also provides information on all of our student and instructor supplements, which have been reviewed and updated extensively. We are truly proud to be able to offer you a complete set of resources for education.

As the leading publisher in EMS, we strive to play a positive role in shaping the direction of EMS education. In ***Emergency Care***, we made every effort to serve the rapidly evolving needs of you and your students. We are proud of our tradition of bringing to EMS education the highest standards of writing, development, production, and service that our customers expect and deserve. We feel privileged to be your key partner in your educational mission and hope we can move forward together.

After all, it still is, always has been, and always will be . . . about people.

Sincerely,

Julie Levin Alexander
VP/Publisher

Katrin Beacom
Senior Marketing Manager

Marlene McHugh Pratt
Executive Editor

Thomas Kennally
National Sales Manager

Lois Berlowitz
Managing Editor

Sladjana Repic
Acquisitions Editor

CORE CONCEPTS

The following are core concepts that will be addressed in this chapter:

- How to recognize arterial, venous, and capillary bleeding
- When to use Standard Precautions with a bleeding patient
- Steps for controlling bleeding
- Signs, symptoms, and care of a patient with internal bleeding
- Signs, symptoms, and care of a patient with shock
- How to use the mechanism of injury to identify potential internal injuries

◀ **Core Concepts.** Highlights the key points addressed in each chapter. The topics not only help students anticipate chapter content, but also guide their studies through the textbook and supplements.

KEY TERMS

arterial bleeding, p. 618
brachial artery, p. 625
capillary bleeding, p. 619
cardiogenic shock, p. 632
compensated shock, p. 631
decompensated shock, p. 633
femoral artery, p. 625
hemorrhage, p. 617
hemorrhagic shock, p. 632
hypoperfusion, p. 617
hypovolemic shock, p. 632
irreversible shock, p. 633
neurogenic shock, p. 632
perfusion, p. 617
pressure dressing, p. 621
pressure point, p. 623
shock, p. 617
tourniquet, p. 626
venous bleeding, p. 619

◀ **Key Terms.** Lists important terms found in each chapter, including references to the pages on which the terms first appear.

DOT OBJECTIVES

*KNOWLEDGE AND ATTITUDE

5-1.1 List the structure and function of the circulatory system. (pp. 615–617)

5-1.2 Differentiate between arterial, venous, and capillary bleeding. (p. 618–619)

5-1.3 State methods of emergency medical care of external bleeding. (pp. 621, 623–628) (Scan 26-1, p. 622)

5-1.4 Establish the relationship between Standard Precautions (body substance isolation) and bleeding. (pp. 618, 621, 636)

5-1.5 Establish the relationship between airway management and the trauma patient. (pp. 621, 626, 628, 630, 633, 636)

5-1.6 Establish the relationship between mechanism of injury and internal bleeding. (p. 629–630)

5-1.7 List the signs of internal bleeding. (p. 629–630)

(hypoperfusion). (pp. 633–636) (Scan 26-2, p. 637; Scan 26-3, p. 638)

5-1.11 Explain the sense of urgency to transport patients that are bleeding and show signs of shock (hypoperfusion). (p. 633–634, 636)

*SKILLS

5-1.12 Demonstrate direct pressure as a method of emergency medical care of external bleeding.

5-1.13 Demonstrate the use of diffuse pressure as a method of emergency medical care of external bleeding.

5-1.14 Demonstrate the use of pressure points and tourniquets as a method of emergency medical care of external bleeding.

5-1.15 Demonstrate the care of the patient exhibiting signs and symptoms of internal bleeding.

▲ **DOT Objectives.** Lists the U.S. DOT objectives that form the basis of each chapter, along with references to the page(s) on which the objectives are covered. This list follows the DOT numbering system.

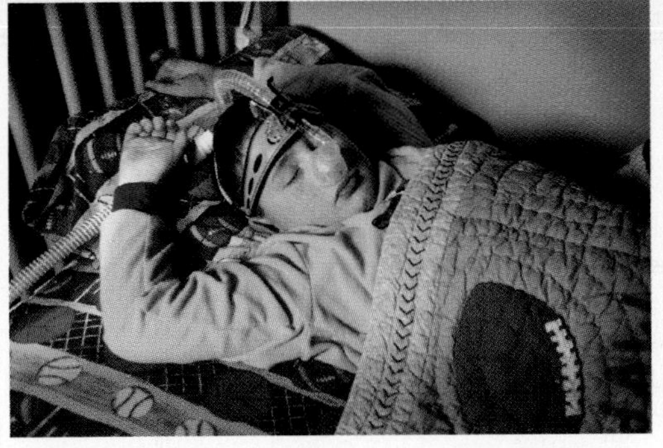

Figure 32-4 • This 9-year-old was thought to have behavior problems but then was diagnosed with sleep apnea. A nasal CPAP machine now helps him sleep through the night. *(© AP Photo/The Herald, Julie Busch)*

◄ **Figures.** Updated illustrations and photos help explain, enhance, and demonstrate key concepts.

continuous positive airway pressure (CPAP) a device that exerts constant pressure through a tube and mask worn by a patient to keep airway passages from collapsing at the end of a breath.

◄ **Running Glossary.** Placed in the margin, directly next to each term's first reference in the text, these definitions help students master new terminology.

PATIENT ASSESSMENT

INTERNAL BLEEDING

Since internal bleeding is not visible, and may not be obvious, you must identify patients who may have internal bleeding by performing a thorough history and physical exam. Suspicion of internal bleeding and estimates of its severity should be based on the mechanism of injury as well as clinical signs and symptoms. If a patient has a mechanism of injury that suggests the possibility of internal bleeding, treat as though the patient has internal bleeding.

Blunt trauma is the leading cause of internal injuries and bleeding. Mechanisms of blunt trauma that may cause internal bleeding include:

- Falls
- Motor-vehicle or motorcycle crashes
- Auto-pedestrian collisions
- Blast injuries

▲ **Patient Assessment/**
◄ **Patient Care.** Describe the assessment and treatment for particular types of patients, disorders, or injuries. The features include important signs and symptoms, as well as key steps of care.

PATIENT CARE

INTERNAL BLEEDING

Care for the patient with internal bleeding centers on the prevention and treatment of shock (hypoperfusion). Definitive treatment for internal bleeding can only take place in the hospital. Patients with suspected internal bleeding must be considered serious and warrant immediate transport to the hospital.

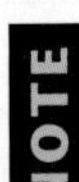

Treatment for internal injuries will cause no harm if it is not needed. But death may be the result of not treating a patient who needs it.

As with all patients, your first priority is the standard ABCs; that is, ensure an open airway, adequate breathing, and circulation. Patients with internal bleeding may deteriorate quickly. Monitor the ABCs and vital signs often. Be prepared to maintain the patient's airway, to provide or assist ventilations, or to administer CPR as needed.

▶ **Tables.** Summarize and condense difficult or complex subjects. Some contain photos to enhance and better explain content.

TABLE 9-1 • Pulse

NORMAL PULSE RATES (BEATS PER MINUTE, AT REST)	
Adult	60 to 100
Infants and Children	
Adolescent 11–14 years	60 to 105
School age 6–10 years	70 to 110
Preschooler 3–5 years	80 to 120
Toddler 1–3 years	80 to 130
Infant 6–12 months	80 to 140
Infant 0–5 months	90 to 140
Newborn	120 to 160

PULSE QUALITY	SIGNIFICANCE/POSSIBLE CAUSES
Rapid, regular, and full	Exertion, fright, fever, high blood pressure, first stage of blood loss
Rapid, regular, and thready	Shock, later stages of blood loss
Slow	Head injury, drugs, some poisons, some heart problems, lack of oxygen in children
No pulse	Cardiac arrest (clinical death)

Infants and Children: A high pulse in an infant or child is not as great a concern as a low pulse. A low pulse may indicate imminent cardiac arrest.

PEDIATRIC NOTE

Infants and children present a special problem when assessing for shock. They have such efficient compensating mechanisms that they can maintain a normal blood pressure until over half of their blood volume is gone. By the time their blood pressure drops, they are already near death. Shock must be considered and cared for early. Do not wait for signs of shock to appear.

◀ **Pediatric/Geriatric Notes.** Help prepare students to deal with these populations by describing special considerations.

▶ **Note.** Facts, figures, and tips that synthesize chapter topics and deal with potentially complicated scenarios, equipment, or populations.

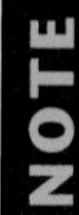

Remember that the tourniquet is used only as a last resort. The tourniquet should be made of wide material that will not cut into the patient's skin. Use a tourniquet only on extremities, and not directly over joints. Once it is applied, do not remove or loosen it.

POINT OF VIEW

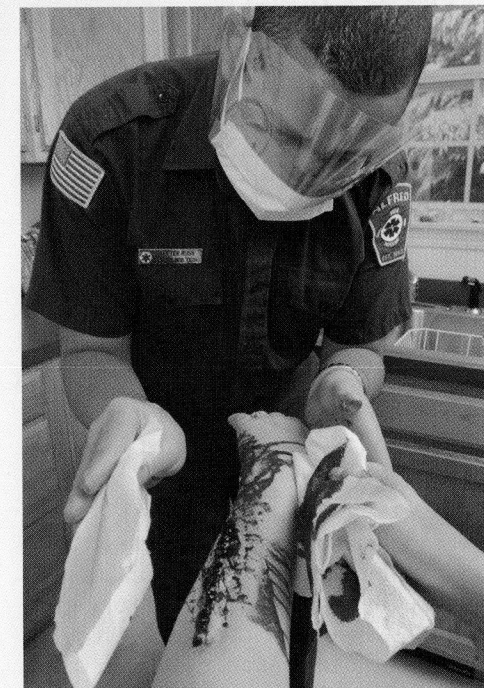

"I remember waiting to see if it would hurt.

"It wasn't the blood. That didn't bother me. I just sat there and waited for the pain. Things were in slow motion. The knife had gone into my forearm. Everyone stopped what they were doing and stared. I grabbed my arm and felt the warm blood drip down over my fingers. But it still didn't seem real.

"I heard someone scream. Someone else called 911. It took me a minute to get my head around what happened. It seemed like only a few seconds had gone by when the EMS people showed up. They put a bandage on my arm and made sure the bleeding had stopped.

"As I look back on it now, I am amazed at how detached I was from the whole thing. I guess some would call that shock.

"And for the record, once I got composed again, it hurt. Oh yes, trust me. It hurt."

▲ **NEW! Point of View.** Tells stories of EMS care from the patient's perspective and includes photos that illustrate the patient's viewpoint.

▼ **Cultural Considerations.** Highlights unique experiences and considerations for providing care to multicultural patients.

Cultural Considerations

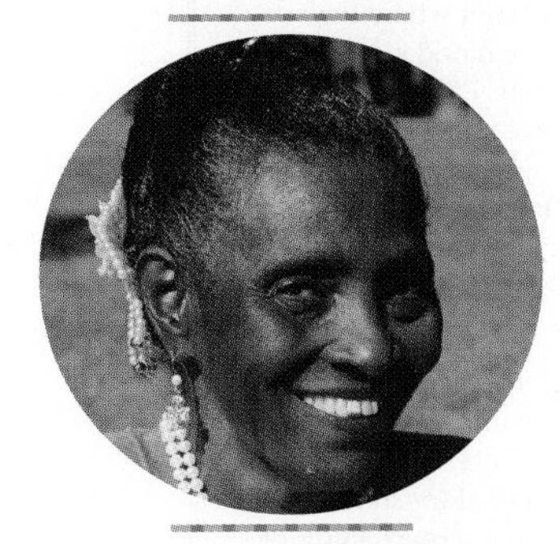

Your patients will, of course, have a wide variety of skin tones. If your patient is dark-skinned, how do you check for pallor or cyanosis—critical signs of the development of shock?

In all patients, skin color is best evaluated where the epidermis (the outer layer of the skin) is thinnest. This includes the fingernails and lips. Open the patient's mouth, or ask him to open it, so that you can examine the color of the mucous membranes inside the mouth. Pull down the patient's lower eyelids and note the color of the conjunctiva (the mucous membrane that lines the eyelids). These are places where pallor or cyanosis will be evident, and these examinations are the same for patients of any skin color.

In dark-skinned patients, you can also check the palms of the hands and soles of the feet, where the skin is lighter, to observe for other colorations such as the yellowish color of jaundice or the small round purplish spots called petechiae that are the result of capillary bleeding. You can also ask the patient or his family if the patient's skin color looks normal, since they may be aware of changes such as an "ashy" look to the skin that would not be obvious to you.

► **NEW! Critical Decision Making.** A scenario-based feature that offers practice in making critical decisions at the scene.

CRITICAL DECISION MAKING: No Pressure, No Problem

Falling blood pressure is a late sign of shock. In the following patients, use material you learned in this chapter to determine if your early decision making would lead you to expedite the call because you suspected shock or if, instead, you believe the patient will likely be stable. You will not be provided a blood pressure—but in each patient you will find enough information to make a proper early decision without a blood pressure reading.

1. Your patient was working on scaffolding that collapsed causing him to fall one story (about 10 feet). He is conscious, is alert but anxious, and complains of pain to the right side of his chest. His pulse is 102 and regular, respirations 26, skin cool and moist, pupils equal and reactive to light.
2. Your patient is found sitting in a bathroom stall at an upscale restaurant. He is pale, sweaty, and leaning against the wall. He tells you he has had a problem with bleeding hemorrhoids recently. There is bright red blood in the toilet bowl. When you stand the patient up to move him to the stretcher, he feels like he is going to pass out.
3. You are called to an assault. A 26-year-old man was struck in the head by his girlfriend. She used a telephone to strike him once in the nose and again in the forehead. The police called you to evaluate a nosebleed. The patient's shirt has blood streaked down it. His nose is oozing blood now. He is alert and oriented. His pulse is 78 strong and regular, respirations 14, skin warm and dry.

◄ **FYI.** Includes material that goes beyond the DOT objectives and broadens students' understanding of individual topics.

F•Y•I

TYPES OF SHOCK

Regardless of the cause, shock is the failure of the circulatory system to provide sufficient blood and oxygen to all the vital tissues of the body. The three major types of shock are hypovolemic shock, cardiogenic shock, and neurogenic shock:

- **Hypovolemic shock.** This is the type of shock most commonly seen by EMTs. When it is caused by uncontrolled bleeding, or hemorrhage, it can be called **hemorrhagic shock.** The bleeding can be internal, external, or a combination of both. Hypovolemic shock may also be caused by burns or crush injuries, where plasma is lost.
- **Cardiogenic shock.** Patients suffering a myocardial infarction, or heart attack, may develop shock from the inadequate pumping of blood by the heart. The strength of the heart's contractions may be decreased because of the damage to the heart muscle. Or the heart's electrical system may be malfunctioning, causing a heartbeat that is too slow, too fast, or irregular. Other cardiac problems, such as congestive heart failure, may also cause shock. Watch for low blood pressure, edema in the feet and ankles, and other signs of heart failure. (Review Chapter 17, "Cardiac Emergencies.")
- **Neurogenic shock.** Shock may result from the uncontrolled dilation of blood vessels due to nerve paralysis caused by spinal cord injuries. While there is no actual blood loss, the dilation of the blood vessels increases the circulatory system's capacity to the point where the available blood can no longer adequately fill it. With sepsis (massive infection) or anaphylactic (severe allergic) reaction, vasodilation may also cause shock. Neurogenic shock is rarely seen in the field.

Keep in mind that, as an EMT, you do not need to diagnose the type of shock. Instead, you must recognize and treat for shock whenever there is a mechanism of injury or signs that indicate the possibility of shock.

▼ **Scans.** Summarize and present key information and step-by-step procedures for easy reference. Medication Scans give students the information they need to help administer medications. Procedure Scans list and describe the steps for performing particular procedures.

SCAN 26-1 • Controlling Bleeding

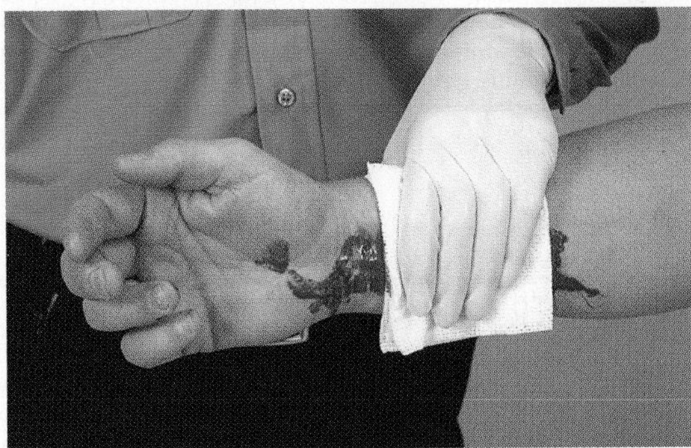

1. Apply direct pressure to a bleeding wound with a gauze pad.

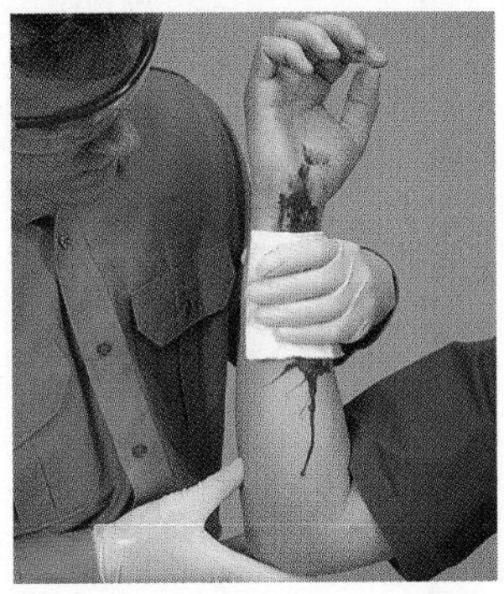

2. Elevate a bleeding extremity above the level of the heart.

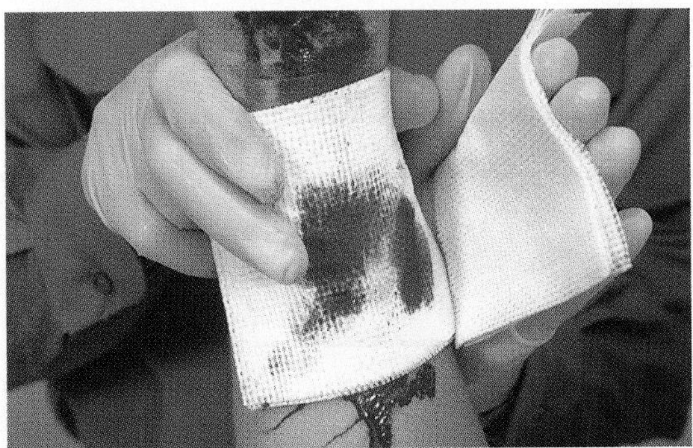

3. If the wound continues to bleed, apply additional dressings over the first one.

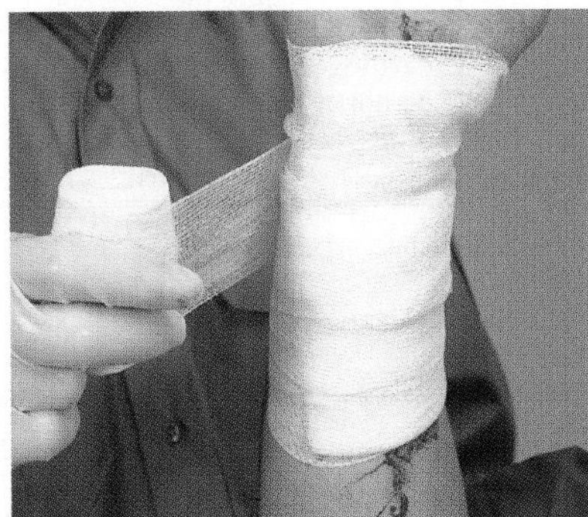

4. Bandage the dressing in place.

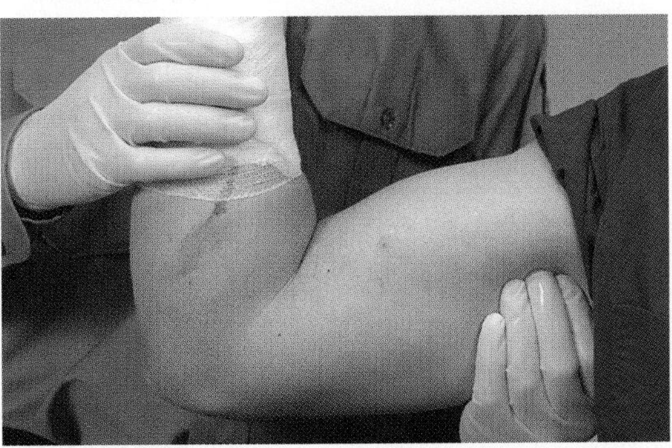

5. If a wound to the arm continues to bleed, apply pressure to the brachial artery, or . . .

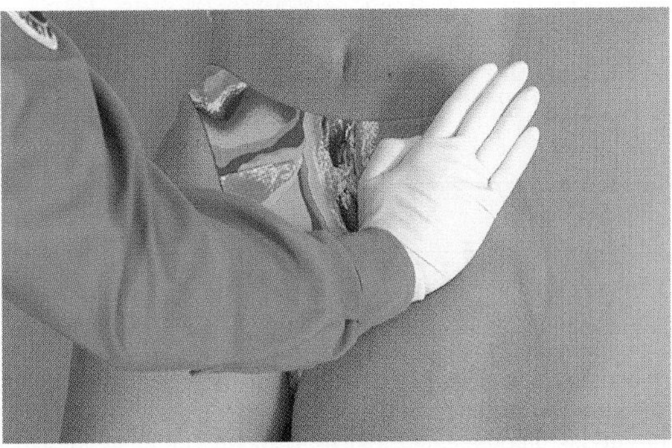

. . . If a wound to the leg continues to bleed, apply pressure to the femoral artery.

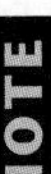

FIRST take Standard Precautions.

▶ **Summary.** Provides students with a concise review of important chapter information.

SUMMARY

Blood loss can be external or internal. External bleeding can be controlled by direct pressure, elevation, and the use of pressure points. Emergency care for internal bleeding is based on the prevention and treatment of shock.

Shock is usually first seen in a patient as restlessness or anxiety. Skin becomes pale, and the pulse and respirations increase. If shock remains uncontrolled, the patient's blood pressure begins to fall. A decrease in blood pressure is a late sign of shock. Signs and symptoms of shock may not be evident early in the call, so treatment based on the mechanism of injury may be life-saving.

Treat shock by airway maintenance; administration of high-concentration oxygen; controlling bleeding; and keeping the patient warm. One of the most important treatments is early recognition of shock and immediate transport to a hospital.

▶ **Key Terms.** All terms that appear in boldface in the chapter are included in the Chapter Review, along with their definitions.

KEY TERMS

arterial bleeding bleeding from an artery, which is characterized by bright red blood and as rapid, profuse, and difficult to control.

brachial (BRAY-ke-al) **artery** the major artery of the upper arm.

capillary bleeding bleeding from capillaries, which is characterized by a slow, oozing flow of blood.

cardiogenic shock shock, or lack of perfusion, brought on not by blood loss, but by inadequate pumping action of the heart. It is often the result of a heart attack or congestive heart failure.

irreversible shock when the body has lost the battle to maintain perfusion to vital organs. Even if adequate vital signs return, the patient may die days later due to organ failure.

neurogenic shock hypoperfusion due to nerve paralysis (sometimes caused by spinal cord injuries) resulting in the dilation of blood vessels that increases the volume of the circulatory system beyond the point where it can be filled.

perfusion the supply of oxygen to and removal of wastes from the cells and tissues of the body as a result of the flow of blood through the capillaries.

REVIEW QUESTIONS

1. Name the three main types of blood vessels, and describe the type of bleeding you would expect to see from each one. (pp. 616–617, 618–619)
2. List the patient care steps for external bleeding control. (p. 621)

◀ **Review Questions.** Ask students to recall information and to apply the principles they've just learned.

CRITICAL THINKING

- A patient has been involved in a motor-vehicle collision. There is considerable damage to his vehicle. The steering column and wheel are badly deformed. The patient complains of a "sore chest." You note no external bleeding. The patient's vital signs are pulse 116, respirations 20, blood pressure 106/70. How would you proceed to assess and care for this patient?

Thinking and Linking

Think back to Chapters 7–12 on scene size-up and patient assessment as well as Chapters 16–25 on medical emergencies. Link information from those chapters with information from this chapter as you consider the following questions:

- You respond to a shopping center parking lot for a motor-vehicle collision. You find an older male patient unresponsive in his vehicle. What facts could you gather at the scene that would help you determine whether the patient's unresponsiveness was caused by trauma and shock or a medical condition?
- What medical conditions can cause shock or present with signs and symptoms similar to shock?

◀ **Critical Thinking.** Asks students to think critically and thoughtfully, applying their new knowledge to more complex subjects. In some chapters, Thinking and Linking Questions also invite students to connect topics learned in multiple chapters.

MEDIA RESOURCES 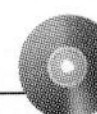

See the Student CD at the back of this book for quizzes, animations, a case study activity, and other features related to this chapter. In particular, take a look at the animation on shock. Also, visit the Companion Website for *Emergency Care* at **www.prenhall.com/limmer**, where you will find additional reinforcement and links to other resources.

▲ **Media Resources.** Refers students to the book's Student CD-ROM and Companion Website, where additional activities and information on the chapter's topics can be found.

Street Scenes

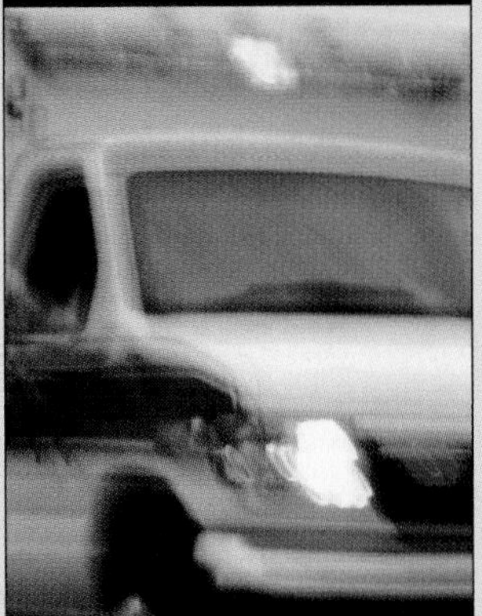

Arnold Johnson likes to do odd jobs around the house. Today's project is to fix a loose shelf in the kitchen. He gets out his ladder and tools and starts to work. As he reaches to hammer his first nail, he loses his footing and falls a few feet, hitting his left side on the corner of the kitchen table. It hurts but he goes back to finish the shelf. After a few minutes, he realizes he is in considerable discomfort. As the pain increases and Arnold starts to feel worse, he knows something is wrong and calls 911. Your ambulance is dispatched with a First Response unit from the fire department, Squad 31, to a 46-year-old male with injuries from a fall. Squad 31 is on scene first, gathering a history and taking a set of vital signs. You arrive about 3 minutes later. Mr. Johnson
a chair and looks anxious.

Street Scene Questions

1. What is the priority for this patient? Does an initial assessment still need to be done?
2. What assessment information do you want to receive from Squad 31?
3. Is the mechanism of injury important information for this patient?

You approach the patient as your partner gets the First Responder information. You notice that Mr. Johnson is pale and seems to have an increased respiratory rate. Your partner gives you the patient history from Squad 31, including their impression that the patient may have broken some ribs. The First Responders report the following vital signs: a thready pulse of 110, respiratory rate of 24 and la-

Street Scenes Sample Documentation

PATIENT NAME: *Arnold Johnson* PATIENT AGE: *46*

CHIEF COMPLAINT: *Tenderness LUQ*

PAST MEDICAL HISTORY: [x] None; [ ] Allergy to ____; [ ] Hypertension; [ ] Stroke; [ ] Seizures; [ ] Diabetes; [ ] COPD; [ ] Cardiac; [ ] Other (List); [ ] Asthma

Current Medications (List): *None*

VITAL SIGNS

TIME	RESP	PULSE	B.P.	MENTAL STATUS	R PUPILS L	SKIN
0922	Rate: 24; [ ] Regular; [ ] Shallow; [x] Labored	Rate: 110; [x] Regular; [ ] Irregular	130/85	[x] Alert; [ ] Voice; [ ] Pain; [ ] Unresp.	R [x] L [x] Normal; Dilated; Constricted; Sluggish; No-Reaction	[ ] Unremarkable; [ ] Cool; [x] Pale; [ ] Warm; [ ] Cyanotic; [x] Moist; [ ] Flushed; [ ] Dry; [ ] Jaundiced
0928	Rate: 28; [ ] Regular; [ ] Shallow; [x] Labored	Rate: 120; [x] Regular; [ ] Irregular	124/80	[ ] Alert; [x] Voice; [ ] Pain; [ ] Unresp.	R [x] L [x] Normal; Dilated; Constricted; Sluggish; No-Reaction	[ ] Unremarkable; [x] Cool; [x] Pale; [ ] Warm; [ ] Cyanotic; [x] Moist; [ ] Flushed; [ ] Dry; [ ] Jaundiced
0935	Rate: 28; [ ] Regular; [ ] Shallow; [x] Labored	Rate: 120; [x] Regular; [ ] Irregular	118/78	[ ] Alert; [x] Voice; [ ] Pain; [ ] Unresp.	R [x] L [x] Normal; Dilated; Constricted; Sluggish; No-Reaction	[ ] Unremarkable; [x] Cool; [x] Pale; [ ] Warm; [ ] Cyanotic; [x] Moist; [ ] Flushed; [ ] Dry; [ ] Jaundiced

NARRATIVE *Our patient states that he fell several feet while standing on a ladder. While falling, he struck his left side on the edge of a protruding kitchen table. Patient denies striking his head, neck, or back. He denies any loss of consciousness. 0922 vital signs were reported by First Responders. Patient is now ashen, respiration has become more rapid and labored, and pulse has become weak and more rapid. Patient has a decreasing level of responsiveness, and is becoming nauseated. Our physical exam reveals a very tender LUQ. Patient placed on 15 LPM via nonrebreather. Monitored and managed patient's body temperature en route to trauma center.*

▲▶ **Street Scenes and Sample Documentation.** Designed to help students integrate all the information they've learned so far. Answers to questions are found inside these real-life "calls." Many chapters also include filled-out Sample Documentation with reports of the Street Scene for that chapter.

STUDENT CD-ROM

The ***Emergency Care*** 11th edition CD-ROM is full of valuable assets, including games and puzzles, multiple-choice quizzes, virtual tours, case-study activities, animations, Hazmat exercises, and much more. A few key components are highlighted here.

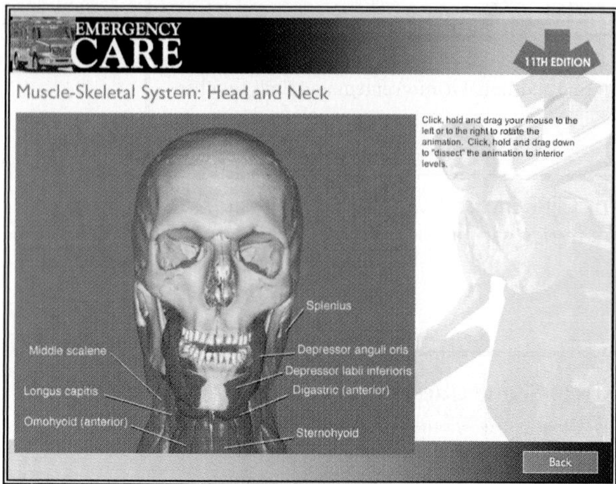

▲ **Virtual Tours.** These 3D animations include a new Brain and Spinal Cord virtual tour and a new animation on cardiovascular disease, with an audio walkthrough. They lead to deeper understanding by helping students to visualize difficult concepts.

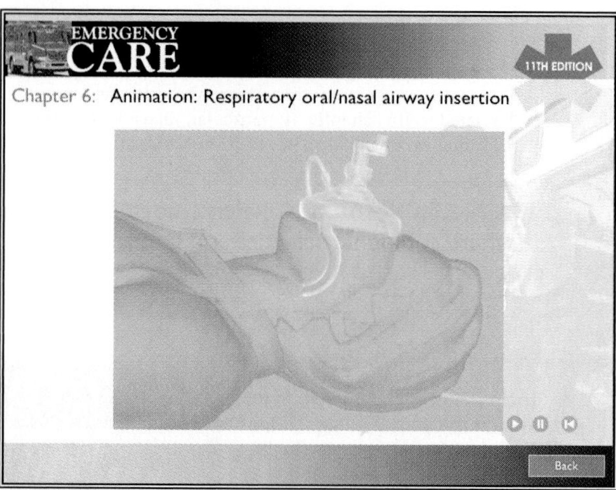

▲ **Animations and Interactives.** Highly visual exercises that enhance and reinforce anatomy, physiology, biology, and specific processes.

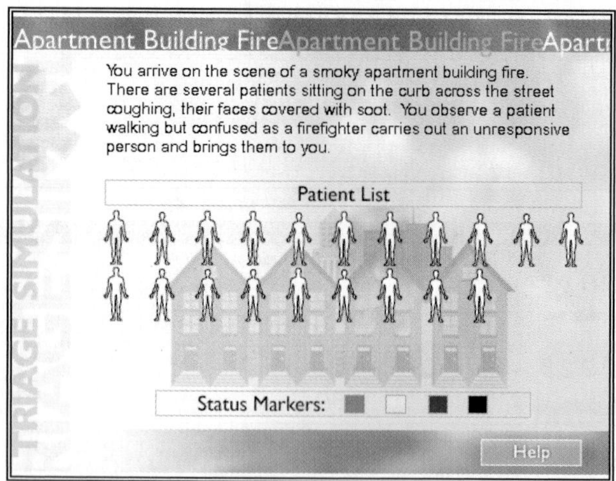

▲ **Triage Simulations.** These simulations test student knowledge of proper triage in MCI scenarios.

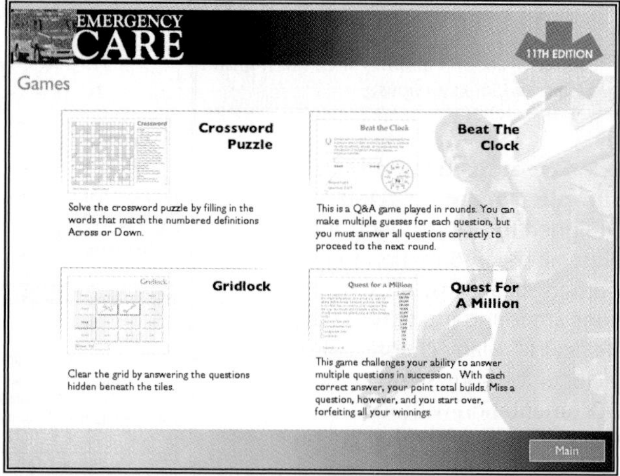

▲ **Games and Puzzles.** Beat the Clock, Crossword Puzzles, Gridlock, and Quest for a Million are games that make learning terminology easy and fun.

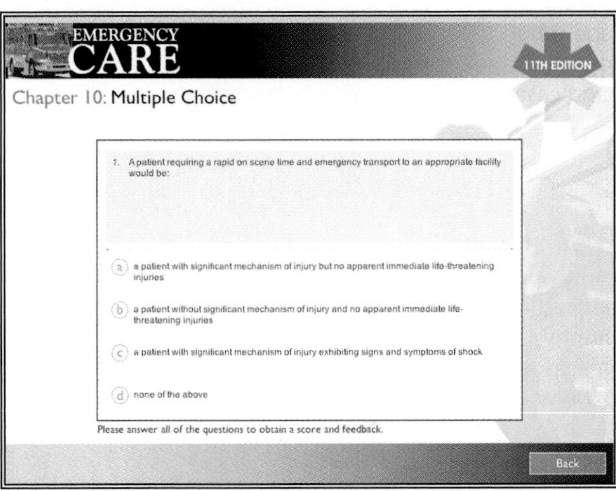

▲ **Quizzes.** Chapter-specific multiple-choice quizzes test and reinforce knowledge.

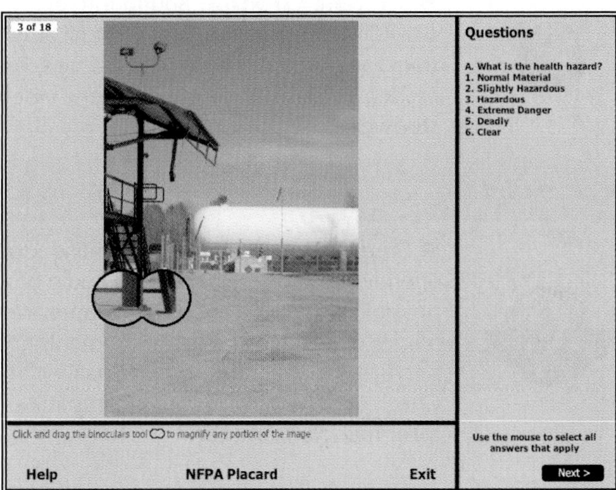

▲ **Hazmat Exercises.** This new interactive exercise aids in the quick and accurate identification of Hazmat place cards.

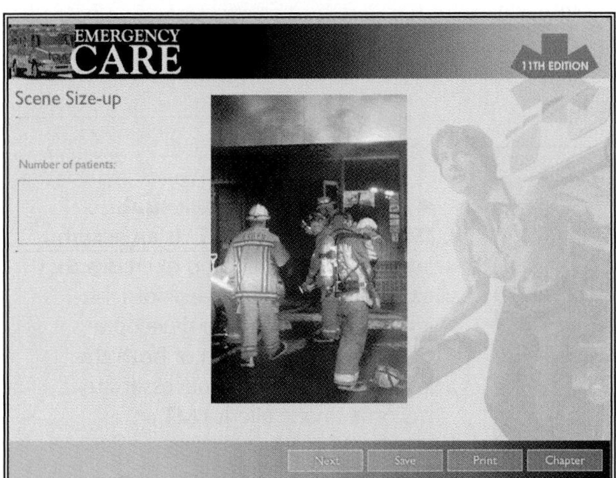

▲ **Scene Size-Up.** Tests students' ability by flashing scenes on screen and asking them to answer questions about number of patients, resources needed, BSI precautions, scene safety, and mechanism of injury.

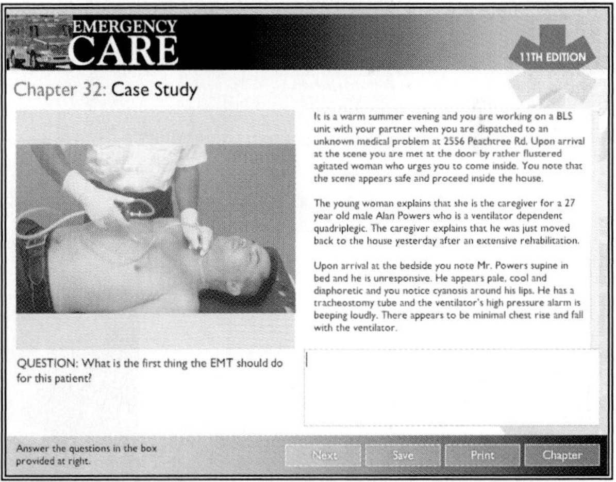

▲ **Case Study.** Scenarios, with questions and rationales throughout, walk students through the critical-thinking process.

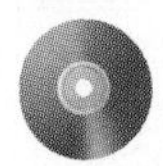

◀ **Student CD-ROM.** Bound into every student textbook, the CD-ROM contains quizzes, a virtual airway tour, triage simulations, animations, games and puzzles, breath sounds, Hazmat exercises, video skills questions, scene video footage, and case-study exercises.

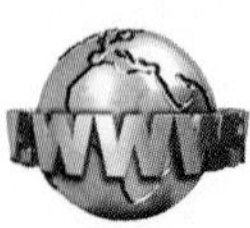

◀ **Companion Website.** An online, open-access self-study tool offering additional assessment, audio glossary, anatomy and physiology labeling exercises, chapter-review questions, summaries of key information, documentation tips, pathophysiology pearls, atlas of injuries, trauma gallery, and real-life anecdotes. Check out ***Emergency Care***'s Companion Website at **www.prenhall.com/limmer.**

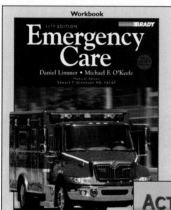

◀ **Workbook.**
ISBN 0-13-500863-8 Contains matching exercises, multiple-choice questions, short-answer questions, street-scene questions, labeling exercises, case studies, case-study questions, references to other resources, and skill performance checklists, all updated for ***Emergency Care***'s 11th edition.

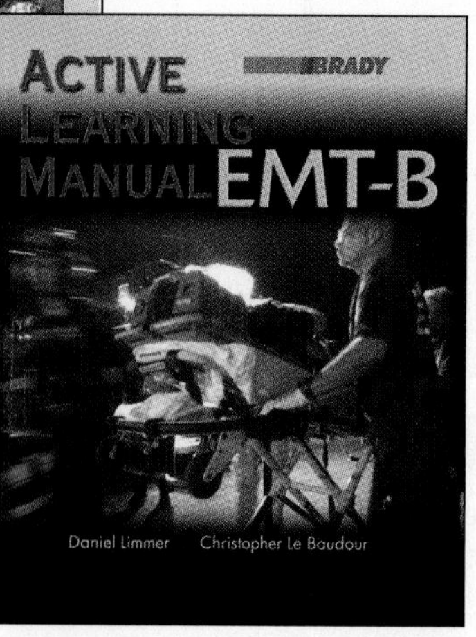

◀ **Active Learning Manual.**
ISBN 0-13-113629-1 Is an accumulation of active-learning exercises that extend beyond the classroom, encouraging students to develop a deeper understanding of both the knowledge and skills necessary to become an excellent EMT.

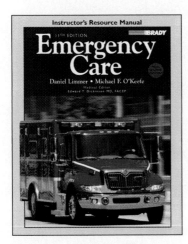

◀ **Instructor's Resource Manual.**
ISBN 0-13-207920-8
This important resource helps instructors utilize and integrate components of ***Emergency Care*** into a unified teaching program. Features include Tips for Program/Classroom Success, suggested course hours, lecture outlines with text/figure and PowerPoint callouts, answers to text review questions, additional case studies and answers, directions for skills demonstrations and practice, assignments, handouts, references to technology support, time/resources needed for each lesson, teaching tips, and additional resources for instructors and students.

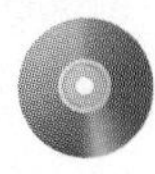

◀ **PowerPoint™ Presentations.**
ISBN 0-13-207924-0
These presentations, which include more than 2,000 customizable slides for classroom use, contain instructor notes to guide presentations. They have been updated to include additional illustrations, photos, and animations. A complete library of all images from the textbook is also provided.

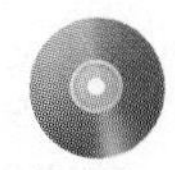

◀ **TestGen.**
ISBN 0-13-207925-9
Thoroughly reviewed and updated, the TestGen contains more than 2,000 exam-style questions, including DOT objectives and page references.

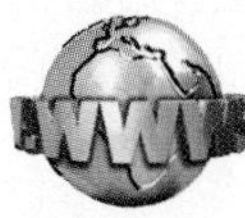

◀ **OneKey.**
A distance learning program to support ***Emergency Care***, it is offered on one of three platforms—CourseCompass, BlackBoard, and WebCT. It includes all instructor resources and Student CD-ROM and Companion Website content. This program, which enables instructors to set up and run online courses, features a course outline, an online gradebook, Weblinks, a discussion board, and a virtual classroom.

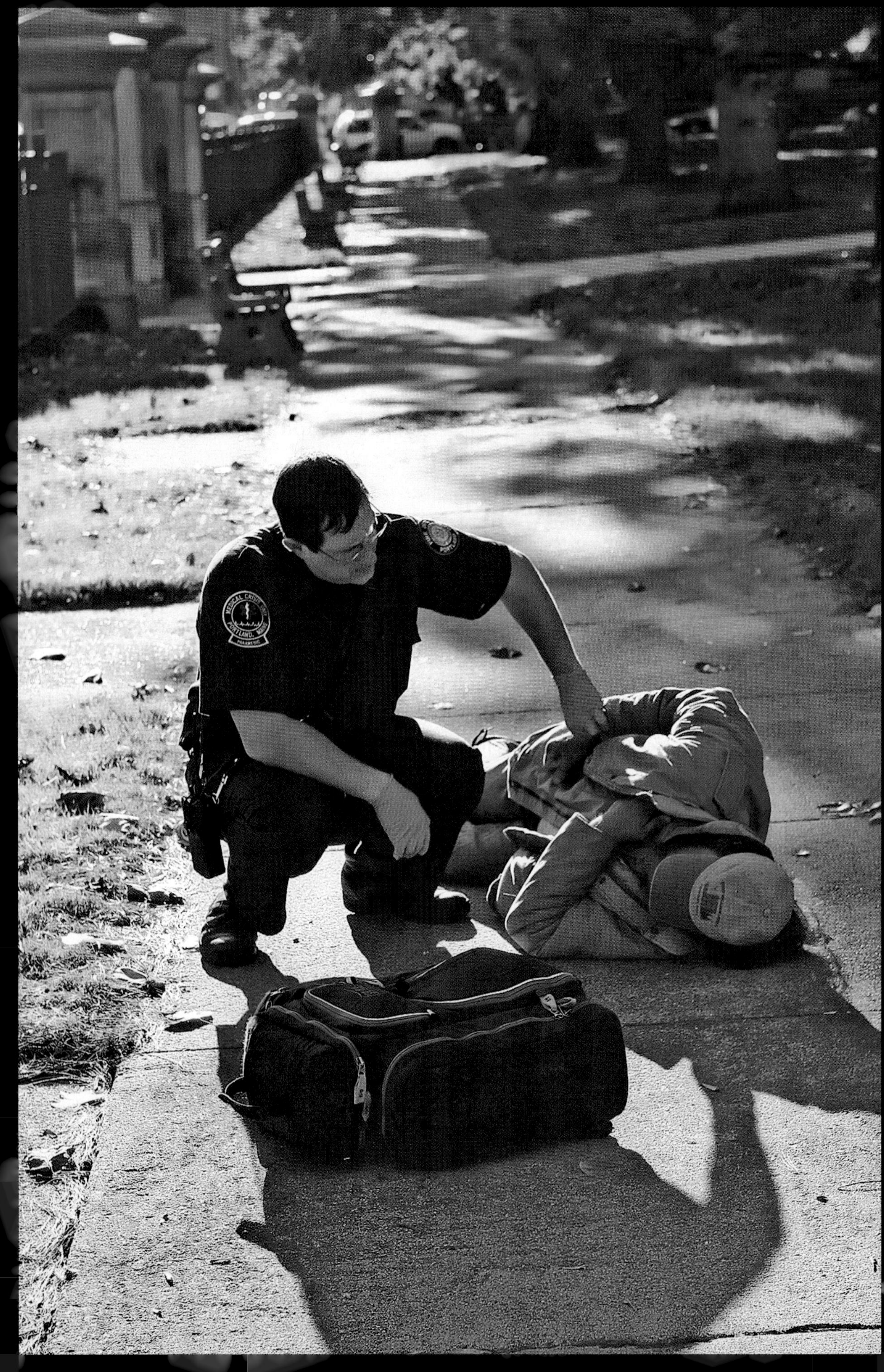
CRISIS
PORTLAND,

MODULE 1

Preparatory

The Preparatory module contains five chapters that introduce some essential concepts, information, and skills you will need as an Emergency Medical Technician.

Chapter 1 overviews the Emergency Medical Services system—the system you will be part of as an Emergency Medical Technician (EMT). Chapter 2 emphasizes that your own safety and well-being are always your first concern (you can't help your patients if you, yourself, become a patient). Chapter 3 discusses legal and ethical issues that you will face as part of your career—such as, "Can I get sued?" and "What is the right thing to do?"

Since most people begin EMT training with little medical knowledge, Chapter 4 provides basic information about the structure and function of the human body. Finally, Chapter 5 explains techniques for lifting and moving without injuring yourself or your patient.

CHAPTER

1

Introduction to Emergency Medical Care

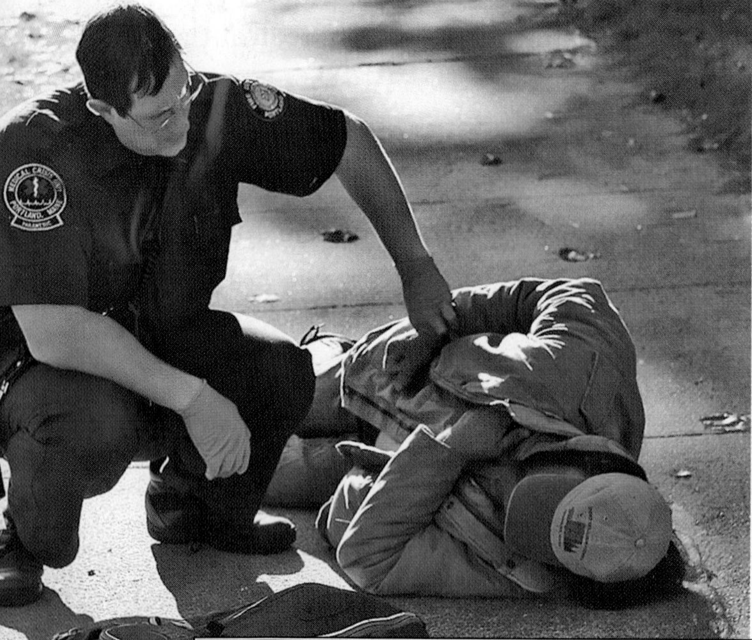

CORE CONCEPTS

The following are core concepts that will be addressed in this chapter:

- The chain of human resources that forms the EMS system
- How the public activates the EMS system
- Your roles and responsibilities as an EMT
- The process of EMS quality improvement (QI)

KEY TERMS

designated agent, p. 17
medical direction, p. 16
Medical Director, p. 16
911 system, p. 8
protocols, p. 17
quality improvement, p. 14
standing orders, p. 17

DOT OBJECTIVES

*KNOWLEDGE AND ATTITUDE

1-1.1 Define Emergency Medical Services (EMS) systems. (pp. 5–9)

1-1.2 Differentiate the roles and responsibilities of the EMT from other prehospital care providers. (pp. 9–10)

1-1.3 Describe the roles and responsibilities related to personal safety. (p. 10)

1-1.4 Discuss the roles and responsibilities of the EMT toward the safety of the crew, the patient, and bystanders. (pp. 10–11)

1-1.5 Define quality improvement, and discuss the EMT's role in the process. (pp. 14–15)

1-1.6 Define medical direction, and discuss the EMT's role in the process. (pp. 16–17)

1-1.7 State the specific statutes and regulations in your state regarding the EMS system. (p. 17)

1-1.8 Assess areas of personal attitude and conduct of the EMT. (p. 12)

1-1.9 Characterize the various methods used to access the EMS system in your community. (pp. 8–9)

When a person is injured or becomes ill, it rarely happens in a hospital with doctors and nurses standing by. In fact, some time usually passes between the onset of the injury or illness and the patient's arrival at the hospital, time in which the patient's condition may deteriorate, time in which the patient may even die. The modern Emergency Medical Services (EMS) system has been developed to provide what is known as *prehospital* or *out-of-hospital* care. Its purpose is to get trained personnel to the patient as quickly as possible and to provide emergency care on the scene, en route to the hospital, and at the hospital. The Emergency Medical Technician (EMT) is a key member of the EMS team.

As you begin to study for a career as an EMT, you will want to answer some basic questions, such as: What is the EMS system? How did it develop? And what will be your role in the system? This chapter will help you begin to answer these questions.

THE EMERGENCY MEDICAL SERVICES SYSTEM

How It Began

In the 1790s, the French began to transport wounded soldiers away from the scene of battle so they could be cared for by physicians. This is the earliest documented emergency medical service. No medical care was provided for the wounded on the battlefield. The idea was simply to carry the victim from the scene to a place where medical care was available.

Other wars inspired similar emergency services. For example, during the American Civil War, Clara Barton began such a service for the wounded and later helped establish the American Red Cross. During World War I, many volunteers joined battlefield ambulance corps. And during the Korean Conflict and the Vietnam War, medical teams produced further advances in field care, many of which led to advances in the civilian sector, including specialized emergency medical centers devoted to the treatment of trauma (injuries).

Non-military ambulance services began in some major American cities in the early 1900s—again as transport services only, offering little or no emergency care. Smaller communities did not develop ambulance services until the late 1940s, after World War II. Often the local undertaker provided a hearse for ambulance transport. Where emergency care was offered along with transport to the hospital, the fire service often was the responsible agency.

The importance of providing hospital-quality care at the emergency scene—that is, beginning care at the scene and continuing it, uninterrupted, during transport to the hospital—soon became apparent. The need to organize systems for such emergency prehospital care and to train personnel to provide it also was recognized.

EMS Today

During the 1960s, the development of the modern EMS system began. In 1966 the National Highway Safety Act charged the United States Department of Transportation (DOT) with developing EMS standards and assisting the states to upgrade the quality of their prehospital emergency care. Most EMT courses today are based on models developed by the DOT.

In 1970, the National Registry of Emergency Medical Technicians was founded to establish professional standards. In 1973, Congress passed the National Emergency Medical Services Systems Act as the cornerstone of a federal effort to implement and improve EMS systems across the United States.

Since then, the states have gained more control over their EMS systems, although the federal government continues to provide guidance and support. For example, the National Highway Traffic Safety Administration (NHTSA) Technical Assistance Program has established an assessment program with a set of standards for EMS systems. The categories and standards set forth by NHTSA, summarized in the following list, will be discussed in more detail throughout this chapter and the rest of this textbook.

- *Regulation and policy.* Each state EMS system must have in place enabling legislation (laws that allow the system to exist), a lead EMS agency, a funding mechanism, regulations, policies, and procedures.
- *Resource management.* There must be centralized coordination of resources so that all victims of trauma or medical emergencies have equal access to basic emergency care and transport by certified personnel, in a licensed and equipped ambulance, to an appropriate facility.
- *Human resources and training.* At a minimum, all transporting prehospital personnel (those who ride the ambulances) should be trained to the EMT level using a standardized curriculum taught by qualified instructors.
- *Transportation.* Safe, reliable ambulance transportation is a critical component. Most patients can be effectively transported by ground ambulances. Other patients require rapid transportation, or transportation from remote areas, by helicopter or airplane.
- *Facilities.* The seriously ill or injured patient must be delivered in a timely manner to the closest appropriate facility.
- *Communications.* There must be an effective communications system, beginning with the universal system access number (911), dispatch-to-ambulance, ambulance-to-ambulance, ambulance-to-hospital, and hospital-to-hospital communications.
- *Public information and education.* EMS personnel may participate in efforts to educate the public about their role in the system, their ability to access the system, and prevention of injuries.
- *Medical direction.* Each EMS system must have a physician as a Medical Director accountable for the activities of EMS personnel within that system. The Medical

Director delegates medical practice to non-physician providers (such as EMTs) and must be involved in all aspects of the patient care system.

- *Trauma systems.* In each state, enabling legislation must exist to develop a trauma system including one or more trauma centers, triage and transfer guidelines for trauma patients, rehabilitation programs, data collection, mandatory autopsies (examination of bodies to determine cause of death), and means for managing and ensuring the quality of the system.
- *Evaluation.* Each state must have a program for evaluating and improving the effectiveness of the EMS system, known as a quality improvement (QI) program, a quality assurance (QA) program, or total quality management (TQM).

With the development of the modern EMS system, the concept of ambulance service as a means merely for transporting the sick and injured passed into oblivion. No longer could ambulance personnel be viewed as people with little more than the strength to lift a patient into and out of an ambulance. The hospital emergency department was extended, through the EMS system, to reach the sick and injured at the emergency scene. "Victims" became patients, receiving prehospital assessment and emergency care from highly trained professionals. The "ambulance attendant" was replaced by the Emergency Medical Technician (EMT).

A current development in some areas is use of the term *out-of-hospital care,* rather than *prehospital care,* as EMS personnel begin to provide primary care for some conditions and in some circumstances without transport to a hospital (Figure 1-1). However, the term *prehospital care* will be used in the remainder of this text.

COMPONENTS OF THE EMS SYSTEM

To understand the EMS system, you must look at it from the patient's viewpoint rather than from that of the EMT (Figure 1-2). For the patient, care begins with the initial phone call to the Emergency Medical Dispatcher (EMD). The EMS system responds to the call for help by sending to the scene available responders, including First Responders, EMTs, and advanced life support providers (EMT-Intermediates and EMT-Paramedics). An ambulance will transport the patient to the hospital.

From the ambulance, the patient is received by the Emergency Department. There the patient receives laboratory tests, diagnosis, and further treatment. The Emergency

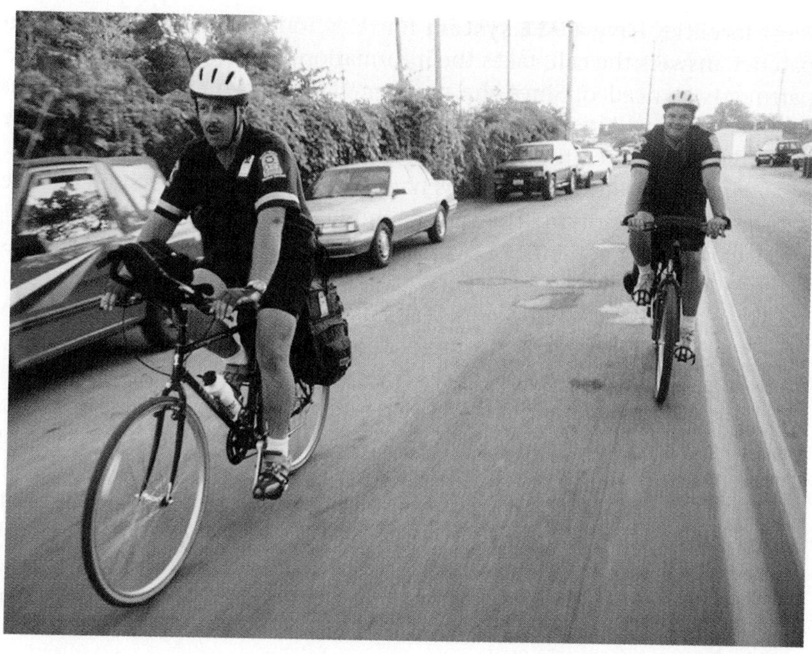

Figure 1-1 • A new method of delivering emergency medical services. *(© Craig Jackson/In the Dark Photography)*

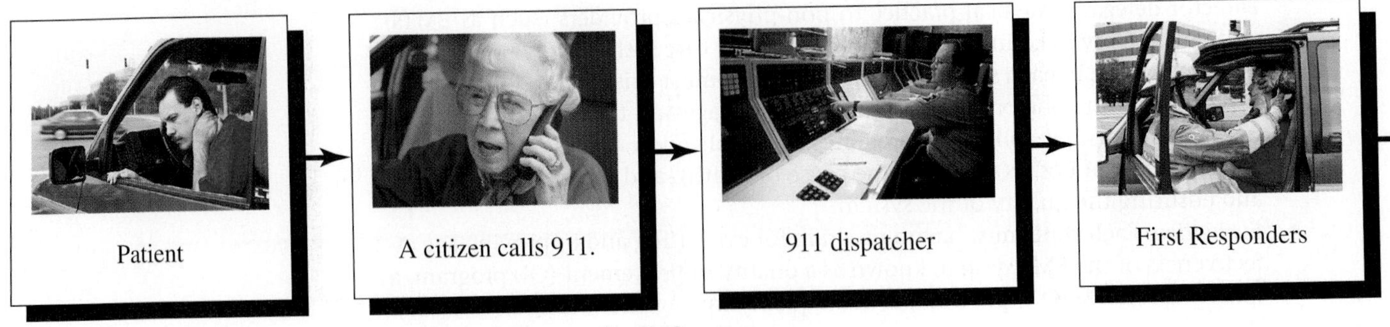

Figure 1-2 • The chain of human resources making up the EMS system.

Department serves as the gateway for the rest of the services offered by the hospital. If a patient is brought to the Emergency Department with serious injuries, care is given to stabilize the patient, and the operating room is readied to provide further life-saving measures.

Some hospitals handle all routine and emergency cases but have a specialty that sets them apart from other hospitals. One specialty hospital is the trauma center. In some hospitals, a surgery team may not be available at all times. In a trauma center, surgery teams are available 24 hours a day.

In addition to trauma centers, there are also hospitals that specialize in the care of certain conditions and patients, such as burn centers, pediatric centers, cardiac centers, stroke centers, and poison control centers.

As an EMT, you will become familiar with the hospital resources available in your area. Many EMS regions have specific criteria for transporting patients with special needs. Choosing the right hospital may actually be a life-saving decision. Of course it is important to weigh the patient's condition against the additional transport time that may be required to take him to a specialized facility. On-line medical direction (discussed later) may be available to help with this decision.

First Responders, EMTs, and dispatchers are key members of the prehospital EMS team. Many others make up the hospital portion of the EMS system. They include physicians, nurses, physician's assistants, respiratory and physical therapists, technicians, aides, and others.

Accessing the EMS System

911 system
a system for telephone access to report emergencies. A dispatcher takes the information and alerts EMS or the fire or police departments as needed. *Enhanced 911* has the additional capability of automatically identifying the caller's phone number and location.

Most localities have a **911 system** for telephone access to report emergencies. A dispatcher answers the call, takes the information, and alerts EMS or the fire or police departments as needed. Since the number 911 is designed to be a national emergency number, there will be a time when someone may dial 911 from any phone in the country and be connected to the appropriate emergency center.

Many communications centers have *enhanced 911*. This system has the capability of automatically identifying the caller's phone number and location. If the phone is disconnected or the patient loses consciousness, the dispatcher will still be able to send emergency personnel to the scene.

There are still a few communities that do not have 911 systems. In these locations, a standard seven-digit telephone number must be dialed to reach ambulance, fire, or police services. Dialing 911 where a 911 system is not in operation will usually connect the caller to an operator who will attempt to route the call to the appropriate dispatch center. This adds an extra step and extra time to the process, so it is important to make sure that the emergency numbers in use in a local area are prominently displayed on all telephones.

Another development in the communication and dispatch portion of the EMS system is the training and certification of EMDs. These specially trained dispatchers not only obtain the appropriate information from callers, they also provide medical instructions for emergency care. These include instructions for CPR, artificial ventilation, bleeding control, and more. Research has consistently pointed to the importance of

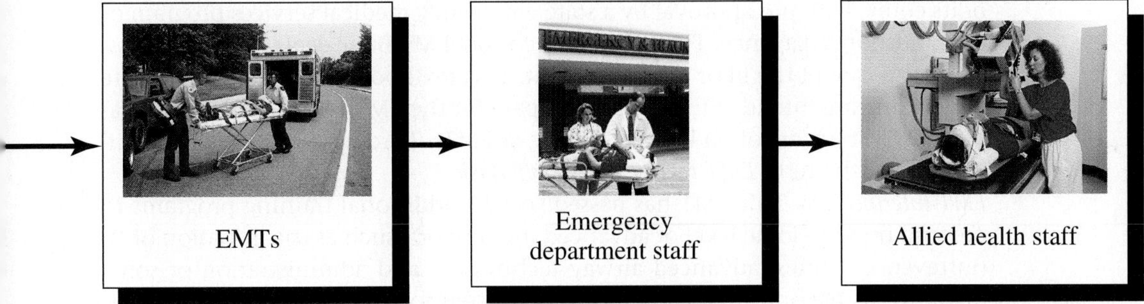

CRITICAL DECISION MAKING: A KEY CONCEPT

Critical decision making is a very important concept. It essentially means that an EMT takes in information from the scene, the patient assessment, and other sources and makes appropriate decisions after synthesizing—or interpreting all of—the information. There are times when the information you obtain initially won't be enough to be a basis for decision making, so you will need to ask more questions and perform additional examinations to get everything you need to make a decision.

It may be difficult to see how this all fits together now. Before long, however, you'll be learning and practicing patient assessment and care. Some examples of critical decision making that will be a part of the assessment and care you will perform include:

1. *Deciding which hospital to transport someone to.* Should you take your patient to the closest hospital or to a more distant specialty hospital?
2. *Deciding whether you should administer a medication to a patient.* Will it help the patient's current condition? Could it make the condition worse?

When you begin to work with more experienced EMTs, you will come across many who are smart and know what to do and how to treat patients (both clinically and personally). These are the EMTs you would want to take care of you or your family should EMS be needed. These EMTs are good critical decision makers.

early access and prompt initiation of emergency care and CPR. The EMD is one example of the EMS system providing emergency care at the earliest possible moment.

Levels of EMS Training

There are four general levels of EMS training and certification (described in the following list). These levels vary from place to place. Your instructor will explain any variations that may exist in your region or state.

- *First Responder.* This level of training is designed for the person who is often first at the scene. Many police officers, firefighters, and industrial health personnel are certified EMS First Responders. The emphasis is on activating the EMS system and providing immediate care for life-threatening injuries, controlling the scene, and preparing for the arrival of the ambulance.
- *EMT-Basic.* In most areas, the EMT-Basic is considered the minimum level of certification for ambulance personnel. Certification as an EMT-Basic requires successful completion of the U.S. DOT's EMT National Standard Training Program

or its equivalent and approval by a state emergency medical services program or other authorized agency. The curriculum for the EMT-Basic deals with the assessment and care of the ill or injured patient. This textbook and the course you are now taking are intended to help you prepare for the EMT-Basic level of certification. EMT-Basics are often known, simply, as EMTs. Throughout this text, we will usually use the term *EMT* rather than *EMT-Basic.*

- *EMT-Intermediate.* This EMT has passed specific additional training programs in order to provide some level of advanced life support, such as the initiation of IV (intravenous) lines, advanced airway techniques, and administration of some medications beyond those the EMT is permitted to administer. In some states, this level includes those EMTs who are given the title of Shock-Trauma Technician or Critical Care Technician.
- *EMT-Paramedic.* Paramedic training includes or equals the U.S. DOT's National Standard Paramedic Curriculum. Paramedics can generally perform relatively invasive field care, including insertion of endotracheal tubes, initiation of IV lines, administration of a variety of medications, interpretation of electrocardiograms, and cardiac defibrillation. Although basic- and intermediate-level EMTs perform some of these kinds of procedures in many areas, the EMT-P may perform such procedures on a more advanced level.

During your career as a certified or licensed EMT there will be changes in the education and practice of EMTs. One of these changes is on the immediate horizon. As of this printing, new education standards are about to be released that will change the training standards and names for some certification levels. Don't worry. The training you are now taking will remain both up-to-date and valid. Your certification or license will remain current when these changes come about. Table 1-1 shows the new titles for EMS education programs. These changes are discussed further in Appendix C.

Roles and Responsibilities of the EMT

As an EMT, you will be responsible for a wide range of activities. In addition to patient assessment and emergency care, your responsibilities will include preparation, a safe response to the scene, safe transportation to the hospital, and transferring the patient to hospital personnel for continuity of care. The following are specific areas of responsibility for the EMT.

- *Personal safety.* It is not possible to help a patient if you are injured before you reach him or while you are providing care, so your first responsibility is to keep yourself safe. Safety concerns include dangers from other human beings, animals, unstable buildings, fires, explosions, and more. Though emergency scenes are usually safe, they also can be unpredictable. You must take care at all times to stay safe.
- *Safety of the crew, patient, and bystanders.* The same dangers you face will also be faced by others at the scene. As a professional, you must be concerned with their safety as well as your own.

TABLE 1-1 • Current and Future Levels of EMS Training

CURRENT LEVELS OF TRAINING	FUTURE LEVELS OF TRAINING
First Responder	Emergency Medical Responder
Emergency Medical Technician-Basic	Emergency Medical Technician
EMT-Intermediate	Advanced EMT
Paramedic	Paramedic

- *Patient assessment.* As an EMT, one of your most important functions will be assessment of your patient, or finding out enough about what is wrong with your patient to be able to provide the appropriate emergency care. Assessment always precedes emergency care.
- *Patient care.* The actual care required for an individual patient may range from simple emotional support to life-saving CPR and defibrillation. Based on your assessment findings, patient care is an action or series of actions that your training will prepare you to take in order to help the patient deal with and survive his illness or injury.
- *Lifting and moving.* Since EMTs are usually involved in transporting patients to the hospital, lifting and moving patients are important tasks. You must perform them without injury to yourself and without aggravating or adding to the patient's existing injuries.
- *Transport.* It is a serious responsibility to operate an ambulance at any time, but even more so when there is a patient on board. Safe operation of the ambulance, as well as securing and caring for the patient in the ambulance, will be important parts of your job as an EMT.
- *Transfer of care.* Upon arrival at the hospital, you will turn the patient over to hospital personnel. You will provide information on the patient's condition, your observations of the scene, and other pertinent data so that there will be continuity in the patient's care. Although this part of patient care comes at the end of the call, it is very important. You must never abandon care of the patient at the hospital until transfer to hospital personnel has been properly completed.
- *Patient advocacy.* As an EMT, you are there for your patient. You are an advocate, the person who speaks up for your patient and pleads his cause. It is your responsibility to address the patient's needs and to bring any of his concerns to the attention of the hospital staff. You will have developed a rapport with the patient during your brief but very important time together, a rapport that gives you an understanding of his condition and needs. As an advocate, you will do your best to transmit this knowledge in order to help the patient continue through the EMS and hospital system. In your role as an advocate you may perform a task as important as reporting information that will enable the hospital staff to save the patient's life—or as simple as making sure a relative of the patient is notified. Acts that may seem minor to you may often provide major comfort to your patient.

EMTs may also be involved in community health initiatives such as injury prevention. The EMT is in a position to observe situations where injuries are possible and help correct them before injuries, or further injuries, are sustained. Hospital personnel do not see the scene and cannot offer this information. An example might be a call to the residence of a senior citizen who has fallen. You make observations about improper railings or slippery throw rugs or shoes and bring this to the attention of the patient and his family. Another place where injury prevention may be beneficial is with children. If you respond to a residence where there are small children and you observe potential for injury (e.g., poisons the child can access or unsafe conditions such as a loose railing) your interventions can make a difference. These community health issues are discussed throughout the book and can be found in the chapters on "Poisoning and Overdose Emergencies" (Chapter 21), "Infants and Children" (Chapter 31), and "Geriatric Patients" (Chapter 33).

Traits of a Good EMT

Certain physical traits and aspects of personality are desirable for an EMT.

Physical Traits

Physically, you should be in good health and fit to carry out your duties. If you are unable to provide needed care because you cannot bend over or catch your breath, then all your training may be worthless to the patient who is in need of your help.

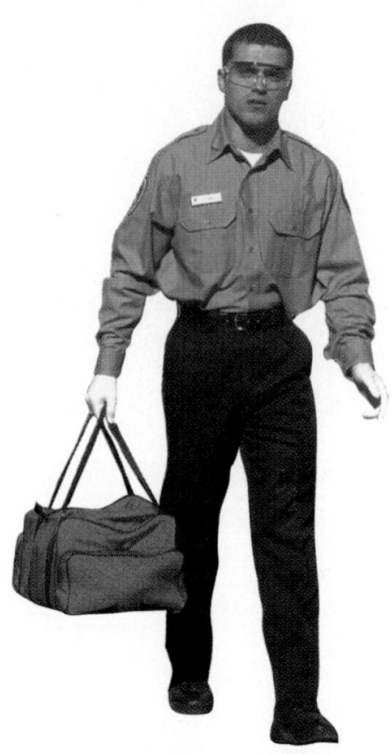

Figure 1-3 • A professional appearance inspires confidence.

You should be able to lift and carry up to 125 pounds. Practice with other EMTs is essential so that you can learn how to carry your share of the combined weight of the patient, stretcher, linens, blankets, and portable oxygen equipment. For such moves, coordination and dexterity are needed, as well as strength. You will have to perform basic rescue procedures, lower stretchers and patients from upper levels, and negotiate fire escapes and stairways while carrying patients.

Your eyesight is very important in performing your EMT duties. Make certain that you can clearly see distant objects as well as those close at hand. Both types of vision are needed for patient assessment, reading labels, controlling emergency scenes, and driving. Should you have any eyesight problems, they must be corrected with prescription eyeglasses or contact lenses.

Be aware of any problems you may have with color vision. Not only is this important to driving, but it could also be critical for patient assessment. Colors seen on the patient's skin, lips, and nail beds often provide valuable clues to the patient's condition.

You should be able to give and receive oral and written instructions and communicate with the patient, bystanders, and other members of the EMS system. Eyesight, hearing, and speech are important to the EMT; thus, any significant problems must be corrected if you are going to be an EMT.

Personal Traits

Good personal traits are very important to the EMT (Figure 1-3). You should be:

- *Pleasant* to inspire confidence and help to calm the sick and injured.
- *Sincere* to be able to convey an understanding of the situation and the patient's feelings.
- *Cooperative* to allow for faster and better care, establish better coordination with other members of the EMS system, and bolster the confidence of patients and bystanders.
- *Resourceful* to be able to adapt a tool or technique to fit an unusual situation.
- *A self-starter* to show initiative and accomplish what must be done without having to depend on someone else to start procedures.
- *Emotionally stable* to help overcome the unpleasant aspects of an emergency so that needed care may be rendered and any uneasy feelings that exist afterward may be resolved.
- *Able to lead* in order to take the steps necessary to control a scene, organize bystanders, deliver emergency care and, when necessary, to take charge.
- *Neat and clean* to promote confidence in both patients and bystanders and to reduce the possibility of contamination.
- *Of good moral character and respectful of others* to allow for trust in situations when the patient cannot protect his own body or valuables and so that all information relayed is truthful and reliable.
- *In control of personal habits* to reduce the possibility of rendering improper care and to prevent patient discomfort. This includes never consuming alcohol within eight hours of duty and not smoking when providing care. (Remember: Smoking can contaminate wounds and is dangerous around oxygen delivery systems.)
- *Controlled in conversation and able to communicate properly* in order to inspire confidence and avoid inappropriate conversation that may upset or anger the patient or bystanders or violate patient confidentiality.
- *Able to listen to others* to be compassionate and empathetic, to be accurate with interviews, and to inspire confidence.
- *Non-judgmental and fair,* treating all patients equally regardless of race, religion, or culture. There are many cultural differences you will encounter among patients. Figure 1-4 highlights one example of the cultures you may encounter in EMS. You will find additional features involving cultural issues throughout the book.

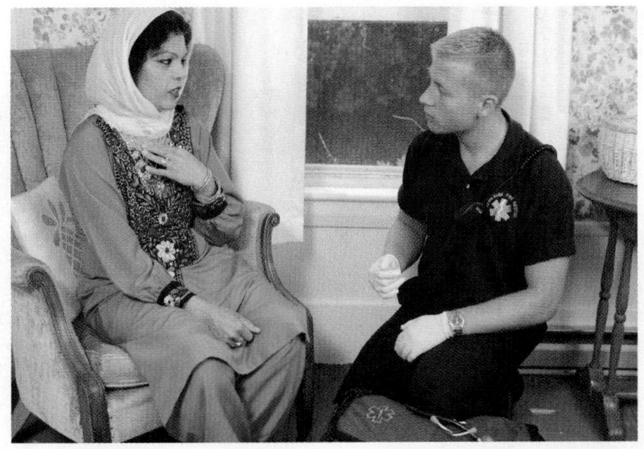

Figure 1-4 • Your patients may come from a wide variety of cultures. As an example, Muslims such as this woman from Afghanistan have standards of modesty that may require examination by an EMT of the same sex.

Education

An EMT must also maintain up-to-date knowledge and skills. Since ongoing research in emergency care causes occasional changes in procedure, some of the information you receive while you are studying to become an EMT will become outdated during your career.

There are many ways to stay current. One way is through refresher training. Most areas require recertification at regular intervals. Refresher courses present material to the EMT who has already been through a full course but needs to receive updated information. Refresher courses, which are usually shorter than original courses, are required at two- to four-year intervals.

Continuing education is another way to stay current. This type of training supplements the EMT's original course. It should not take the place of original training. For example, you may wish to learn more about pediatric or trauma skills or driving techniques. You can obtain this education in conferences and seminars and through lectures, classes, videos, or demonstrations.

It is important for you to realize that training is a constant process that extends long past your original EMT course.

Where Will You Become a Provider?

As an EMT, you will have a wide variety of opportunities to use the skills you will learn in class. EMTs are employed in public and private settings, such as fire departments, ambulance services, and rural/wilderness or urban/industrial settings (Figure 1-5). In fact, many fire departments require their firefighters to be cross-trained as both firefighters and EMTs.

You may be taking this course to volunteer. A large portion of the United States is served by volunteer fire and emergency medical services. Your willingness to participate in training to help others is both necessary for and appreciated by your community.

National Registry of Emergency Medical Technicians

The National Registry of Emergency Medical Technicians (NREMT), as part of its effort to establish and maintain national standards for EMTs, provides registration to First Responders, EMTs, EMT-Intermediates, and EMT-Paramedics. Registration is obtained by successfully completing NREMT practical and computer-based knowledge examinations. Holding an NREMT registration may help in reciprocity (transferring to another state or region). It is usually considered favorably when you apply for employment, even in areas where NREMT registration is not required.

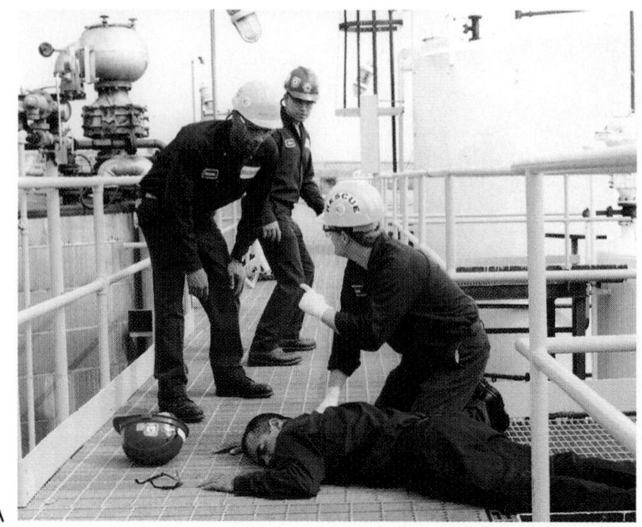

A

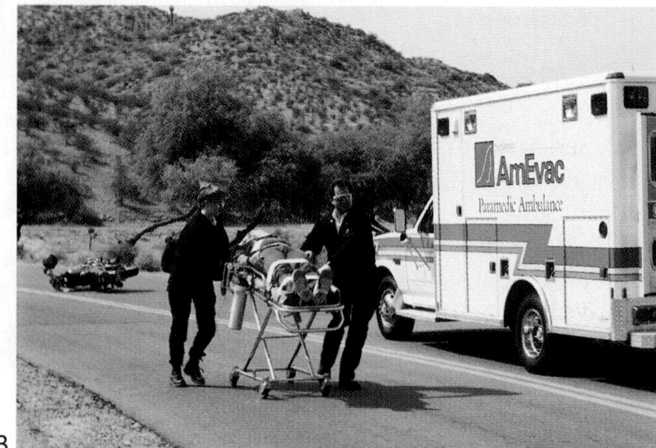

B

Figure 1-5 • There is a wide variety of career opportunities for EMTs, including work in (A) urban/industrial settings and (B) rural/wilderness settings. *(1-5B © Michal Heron Photography)*

Many states use the National Registry examinations as their certification exams. If your state or region does not use the registry exam, ask your instructor how you can sit for the examination. Upon passing the exam and obtaining registry, you will be entitled to wear the NREMT patch (Figure 1-6).

The National Registry is also active in EMS curriculum development and other issues that affect EMS today. For information, contact:

National Registry of Emergency Medical Technicians
6610 Busch Boulevard
P.O. Box 29233
Columbus, OH 43229
614-888-4484
www.nremt.org

Quality Improvement

quality improvement
a process of continuous self-review with the purpose of identifying and correcting aspects of the system that require improvement.

Quality improvement, an important concept in EMS, consists of continuous self-review with the purpose of identifying aspects of the system that require improvement. Once a problem is identified, a plan is developed and implemented to prevent further oc-

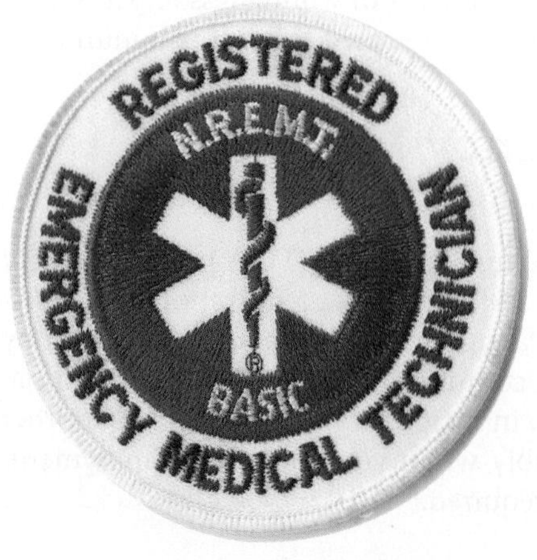

Figure 1-6 • NREMT patch.

currences of the same problem. As implied by the name, quality improvement is designed and performed to ensure that the public receives the highest quality prehospital care.

A sample quality improvement review might go as follows:

> As part of a continuous review of calls, the Quality Improvement (QI) committee has reviewed all of your squad's run reports that involve trauma during one particular month. The committee has noted that the time spent at the scene of serious trauma calls was excessive. (You will learn later that time at the scene of serious trauma should be kept to a minimum, because the injured patient must be transported to the hospital for care that cannot be provided in the field.)
>
> The QI committee has brought this fact to the attention of the Medical Director and the leadership of the ambulance squad. As a result, better protocols have been instituted. Monthly squad training is developed that covers topics such as how to identify serious trauma patients and then requires skill practice to reinforce techniques of trauma care. (Later in the year, the QI committee will review the same criteria to ensure that the extra training has been effective in improving the areas that were found to be deficient.)
>
> During the review, the QI committee has also identified calls during which the crews followed procedures and performed well. A letter has been sent to these EMTs commending them for their efforts.

As an EMT, you will have a role in the quality improvement process. In fact, a dedication to quality can be one of the strongest assets of an EMT. There are several ways you can work toward quality care. These include:

- *Keeping carefully written documentation.* Call reviews are based on the prehospital care reports that you and other crew members write. If a report is incomplete, it is difficult for a QI team to assess the events of a call. If you are ever involved in a lawsuit, an inaccurate or incomplete report may also be a cause for liability. Be sure the reports you write are neat, complete, and accurate.
- *Becoming involved in the quality process.* As you gain experience, you may wish to volunteer for assignment to the QI committee. In addition, quality improvement has a place on every call. An individual ambulance crew can perform a critique after each call to determine things that went well and others that may need improvement. Have another EMT or advanced EMT look over your report before turning it in to ensure that it is accurate and complete.
- *Obtaining feedback from patients and the hospital staff.* This may be done informally or, in some cases, formally. Your organization may send a letter to patients that asks for comments on the care they were given while under your care. Hospital staff may be able to provide information that will help strengthen your caregiving skills.
- *Maintaining your equipment.* It will be difficult to provide quality care with substandard, damaged, or missing equipment. While the ingenuity of EMTs should never be underestimated, it would be impossible to administer oxygen or provide cardiac defibrillation without proper, functional equipment. Check and maintain equipment regularly.
- *Continuing your education.* An EMT who was certified several years ago and has never attended subsequent training will have a problem providing quality care. Seldom-used skills deteriorate without practice. Procedures change. Without some form of regular continuing education, it will be difficult to maintain standards of quality.

Quality improvement is another name for providing the care that you would want to have provided to yourself or a loved one in a time of emergency. That is the best care possible. Maintaining continuous high quality is not easy; it requires constant attention and a sense of pride and obligation. Striving for quality—both in the care you personally give to patients and as a collective part of an ambulance squad—is to uphold the highest standards of the EMS system.

POINT OF VIEW

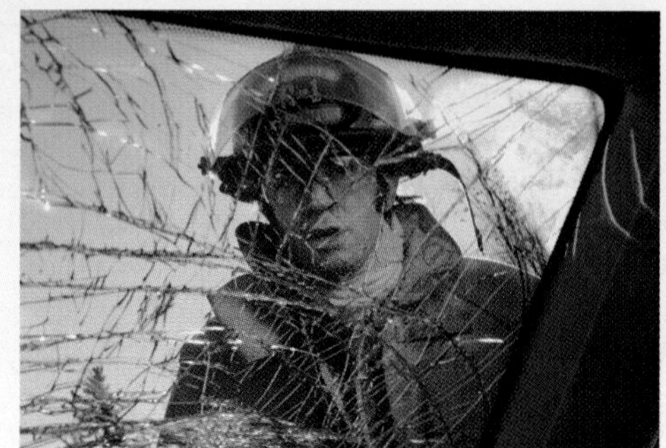

"I was driving along, not a care in the world, when all of a sudden this car pulled out from a side street—and pulled right in front of me. I couldn't brake in time. I couldn't steer in time. The crash made thunder seem like a whisper. I didn't just hear it. I felt it. The next thing I knew I was sitting in my car and it was smoky. I thought it was on fire. Then I noticed the air bag, which must've gone off. People were running up to my window to ask if I was OK. I felt so foggy I didn't even know what to say.

"A fireman came up to my window and asked how I was doing. By then I had a minute to think and compose myself. It felt like I'd cry if I opened my mouth to say anything. The ambulance came in and the EMTs and firefighters worked to get me out of the car. The fireman who came to my window must've climbed into the back seat. I could feel hands alongside my head.

"The collar felt like it was going to choke me. The board was uncomfortable. And everything was so, so loud. But what I remember most, more than the crash or the hospital or the bills, were the kind words the fireman said from behind me. In spite of everything going on that day, his reassuring, kind voice is my best memory from the whole miserable day. It was like an angel being there for me."

As you begin your training as an EMT you will learn many clinical skills. For this patient, you will perform an assessment, immobilize the neck and spine, take vital signs, and transport the patient—perhaps to a trauma center.

You will also provide emotional reassurance and support in this time of crisis. It has been said that you should treat your patients as you would want your family to be treated. This is a good rule.

"Point of View" features like this one will appear throughout the text. Their purpose is to present an emergency from the *patient's* perspective, or point of view, because understanding how the patient feels is a critical element in developing people skills. The clinical skills you learn are vital to your success in becoming an EMT. People skills are essential for you to thrive as an EMT.

Medical Direction

Medical Director a physician who assumes ultimate responsibility for the patient-care aspects of the EMS system.

medical direction oversight of the patient-care aspects of an EMS system by the Medical Director. **Off-line medical direction** consists of standing orders issued by the Medical Director that allow EMTs to give certain medications or perform certain procedures without speaking to the Medical Director or another physician. **On-line medical direction** consists of orders from the on-duty physician given directly to an EMT in the field by radio or telephone.

Each EMS system has a **Medical Director,** a physician who assumes the ultimate responsibility for **medical direction,** or oversight of the patient-care aspects of the EMS system. The Medical Director also oversees training, develops **protocols** (lists of steps for assessment and interventions to be performed in different situations), and is a crucial part of the quality improvement process. An EMT at a basic or advanced level is operating as a **designated agent** of the physician. This means that, as an EMT, your authority to give medications and provide emergency care is actually an extension of the Medical Director's license to practice medicine.

The physician obviously cannot physically be at every call. This is why EMS systems develop **standing orders.** The physician issues a policy or protocol that authorizes EMTs and others to perform particular skills in certain situations. An example may be the administration of glucose. Glucose is very beneficial to certain diabetic patients who are experiencing a medical emergency. The Medical Director issues a standing order that allows EMTs to give glucose in certain circumstances without speaking to the Medical Director or another physician. This kind of "behind the scenes" medical direction is called **off-line medical direction.**

Certain other procedures that are not covered by standing orders or protocols require the EMT to contact the on-duty physician by radio or telephone prior to performing a skill or administering a medication. For example, EMTs carry a medication called "activated charcoal," which is beneficial to many but not all poisoning victims. Prior to administering activated charcoal, you may be required to consult with the on-duty physician. You would use a radio or cell phone from the ambulance to provide patient information to the physician. After receiving your information, the physician would instruct you on how to proceed with care, including whether and how much activated charcoal to give. Orders from the on-duty physician given by radio or phone are called **on-line medical direction.** On-line medical direction may be requested at any time you feel that medical advice would be beneficial to patient care.

Protocols and procedures for on-line and off-line medical direction vary from system to system. Your instructor will inform you what your local policies are. Always follow your local protocols.

protocols
lists of steps, such as assessments and interventions, to be taken in different situations. Protocols are developed by the Medical Director of an EMS system.

designated agent
an EMT or other person authorized by a Medical Director to give medications and provide emergency care. The transfer of such authorization to a designated agent is an extension of the Medical Director's license to practice medicine.

standing orders
a policy or protocol issued by a Medical Director that authorizes EMTs and others to perform particular skills in certain situations.

Special Issues

In the coming weeks and through the chapters that follow in this textbook, you will be studying to become an EMT. As part of your course, your instructor will advise you on local issues and administrative matters, such as a course description, class meeting times, criteria including physical and mental requirements for certification as an EMT, as well as specific statutes and regulations regarding EMS in your state, region, or locality.

The Americans with Disabilities Act (ADA) has set strict guidelines preserving the rights of Americans with disabilities. If you have a disability or have questions about the ADA, ask your instructor for more information.

CHAPTER REVIEW

SUMMARY

The EMS system has been developed to provide prehospital as well as hospital emergency care. The EMS system includes the 911 or other emergency access system, dispatchers, First Responders, EMTs, the hospital emergency department, physicians, nurses, physician's assistants, and other health professionals.

The EMT's responsibilities include safety; patient assessment and care; lifting, moving, and transporting patients; transfer of care; and patient advocacy. An EMT must have certain personal and physical traits to ensure the ability to do the job.

Education (including refresher training and continuing education), quality improvement procedures, and medical direction are all essential to maintaining high standards of EMS care.

KEY TERMS

designated agent an EMT or other person authorized by a Medical Director to give medications and provide emergency care. The transfer of such authorization to a designated agent is an extension of the Medical Director's license to practice medicine.

medical direction oversight of the patient-care aspects of an EMS system by the Medical Director. **Off-line medical direction** consists of standing orders issued by the Medical Director that allow EMTs to give certain medications or perform certain procedures without speaking to the Medical Director or another physician. **On-line medical direction** consists of orders from the on-duty physician given directly to an EMT in the field by radio or telephone.

Medical Director a physician who assumes ultimate responsibility for the patient care aspects of the EMS system.

911 system a system for telephone access to report emergencies. A dispatcher takes the information and alerts EMS or the fire or police departments as needed. *Enhanced 911* has the additional capability of automatically identifying the caller's phone number and location.

protocols lists of steps, such as assessments and interventions, to be taken in different situations. Protocols are developed by the Medical Director of an EMS system.

quality improvement a process of continuous self-review with the purpose of identifying and correcting aspects of the system that require improvement.

standing orders a policy or protocol issued by a Medical Director that authorizes EMTs and others to perform particular skills in certain situations.

REVIEW QUESTIONS

1. What are the components of the Emergency Medical Services system? (pp. 7–8)
2. What are some of the special designations that hospitals may have? List them. Then name the special centers you have in your region. (p. 8)
3. What are the four national levels of EMS training and certification? (pp. 9–10)
4. What are the roles and responsibilities of the EMT? (pp. 10–11)
5. What are desirable personal and physical attributes of the EMT? (pp. 11–12)
6. What is the definition of the term *quality improvement*? (p. 14)
7. What is the difference between on-line and off-line medical direction? (pp. 16–17)

CRITICAL THINKING

- What qualities would you like to see in an EMT who is caring for you? How can you come closer to being this kind of EMT?
- You are devoting a considerable amount of time to becoming an EMT. How do you plan to refresh your knowledge and stay current once you are out of the classroom?

MEDIA RESOURCES 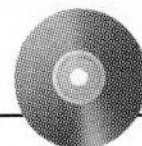

See the Student CD at the back of this book for quizzes, a case study activity, and other features related to this chapter. Also, visit the Companion Website for *Emergency Care* at **www.prenhall.com/limmer**, where you will find additional reinforcement and links to other resources.

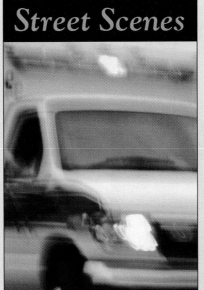

Street Scenes

As a new EMT, you are assigned to Station 2 to ride with Susan Miller, a seasoned EMS veteran with seven years on the job. You have heard that she is a good EMT, and you remember that she helped teach some of your skill sessions. She was a good instructor—patient, understanding, and considerate.

When you arrive at the station, you find out she has been delayed and you will be riding with Chuck Hartley instead. When you are introduced to Chuck, you see that his uniform is unkempt. He tells you to sit until he needs you.

Your first call of the day is a 70-year-old female with abdominal pain. As you approach the ambulance, Chuck tells you to get in the back. He'll let you know when you can help. At the scene, after ensuring scene safety, you both enter the patient's home. Chuck doesn't bother to introduce himself and proceeds to ask the patient, "What's wrong, Hon?" She describes her symptoms. Chuck tells you to put her on a nasal cannula. As you hook up the O_2, Chuck says in a loud voice, "Didn't you learn anything in EMT class? That liter flow rate is too high."

As the patient is being loaded onto the stretcher, she tries to tell Chuck something that she obviously believes is urgent. Chuck tells her that if it's that important, she can tell the doctor at the hospital.

Street Scene Questions

1. What would have been a more appropriate action for Chuck when the shift started?
2. What behavior characteristics of Chuck's would be considered unprofessional?
3. What would you expect from someone providing initial field training?

When you return to the station, Susan Miller has arrived. This time, when you are introduced, you notice that her uniform is pressed and neat. She asks you about your background and when you finished training. She remembers you from class, she says. Then she tells you there are some things you both need to do. "First, let's go to the ambulance and check the equipment. Next, I want to explain how we operate on calls. You need to know what equipment we always take to the patient and responsibilities of the crew members."

Just as you are completing your orientation, a call comes in for a 55-year-old male with chest pain. While en route, Susan briefly goes over the routine that she and her partner use. She asks you to take the automatic defibrillator. When you enter the patient's house, Susan introduces herself and the members of the crew. She asks the patient: "Sir, why did you call 911?" He tells you that he had chest pain but he took a nitroglycerin tablet and now most of the pain is gone. He apologizes for calling.

While you get the vital signs, Susan tells the patient that he did just the right thing by calling EMS. He is reassured and agrees to be transported for further evaluation.

Street Scene Questions

4. What did Susan Miller do that was appropriate and professional?
5. How was Susan's behavior beneficial to you as a new EMT?
6. What personal traits are the professional standards for EMTs?

During the trip to the hospital Susan continues to reassure the patient. In fact, she tells you to talk to the patient about his medical history. When you arrive at the hospital, Susan sees that the oxygen tank is getting low, so she asks you to switch "bottles" before moving the patient, but you forget to turn off the tank being replaced. Susan turns it off, sets it aside, looks you in the eyes, and gives you a smile. You both know that you will not forget the next time.

After the call, Susan gives a short critique and discusses the prehospital care report. When you call back in service, you realize that to be a good EMT you not only need to have good technical skills but, just as important, you also must act as a professional with your patients and with your colleagues.

CHAPTER

The Well-Being of the EMT

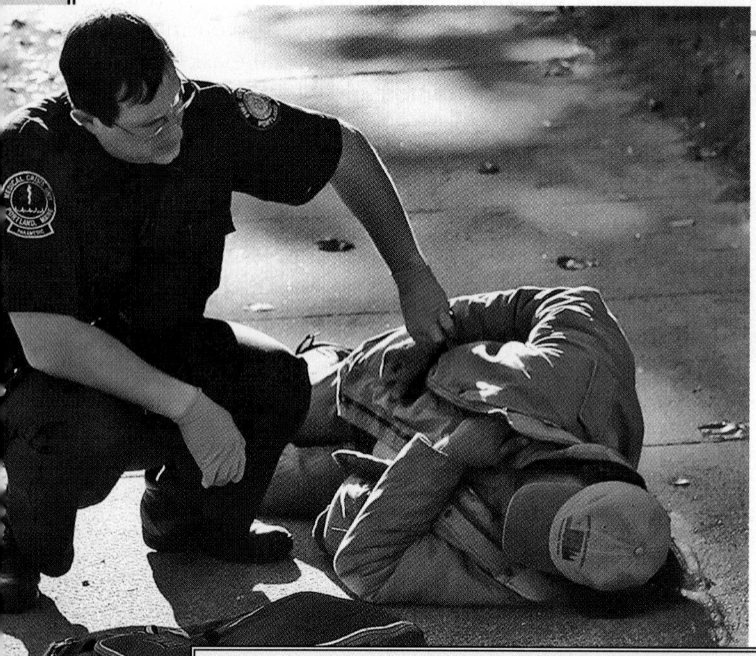

CORE CONCEPTS

The following are core concepts that will be addressed in this chapter:

- Standard Precautions, or how to protect yourself from transmitted diseases
- The impact that dying patients have on you and others
- The kinds of stress caused by involvement in EMS and how they can affect you, your fellow EMTs, and your family and friends
- How to identify potential hazards and maintain scene safety

KEY TERMS

contamination, p. 23
critical incident stress management (CISM), p. 37
decontamination, p. 40
hazardous-material incident, p. 39
multiple-casualty incident (MCI), p. 35
pathogens, p. 21
personal protective equipment (PPE), p. 23
Standard Precautions, p. 22
stress, p. 33

DOT OBJECTIVES

*KNOWLEDGE AND ATTITUDE

1-2.1 List possible emotional reactions that the EMT may experience when faced with trauma, illness, death, and dying. (pp. 33–37)

1-2.2 Discuss the possible reactions that a family member may exhibit when confronted with death and dying. (pp. 38–39)

1-2.3 State the steps in the EMT's approach to the family confronted with death and dying. (pp. 38–39)

1-2.4 State the possible reactions that the family of the EMT may exhibit due to their outside involvement in EMS. (p. 36)

1-2.5 Recognize the signs and symptoms of critical incident stress. (pp. 33–37)

1-2.6 State possible steps the EMT may take to help reduce or alleviate stress. (pp. 37–38)

1-2.7 Explain the need to determine scene safety. (pp. 39–44)

1-2.8 Discuss the importance of body substance isolation (Standard Precautions). (pp. 21–23)

1-2.9 Describe the steps the EMT should take for personal protection from airborne and bloodborne pathogens. (pp. 21–33)

1-2.10 List the personal protective equipment necessary for each of the following situations: (pp. 23–33, 39–44)

- Hazardous materials
- Rescue operations
- Violent scenes
- Crime scenes
- Exposure to bloodborne pathogens
- Exposure to airborne pathogens

1-2.11 Explain the rationale for serving as an advocate for the use of appropriate protective equipment. (p. 26)

*SKILLS

1-2.12 Given a scenario with potential infectious exposure, the EMT will use appropriate personal protective equipment. At the completion of the scenario, the EMT will properly remove and discard the protective garments.

1-2.13 Given the previous scenario, the EMT will complete disinfection/cleaning and all reporting documentation.

Learning how to safeguard your well-being as an EMT is critical. During your EMS career, you will be exposed to all kinds of stress, including that which accompanies death and dying. You will also sometimes be exposed to infectious diseases and dangerous situations.

It is important to use the proper equipment and strategies to help you stay physically safe and emotionally well. *Remember:* If the EMT becomes a patient, he is of little or no use to a patient and even may put other rescuers in jeopardy. Ways to safeguard your well-being include taking Standard Precautions before treating a patient, understanding and dealing with the stress that normally accompanies critical incidents, and ensuring scene safety.

PERSONAL PROTECTION

Standard Precautions

Diseases are caused by **pathogens,** organisms that cause infection, such as viruses and bacteria. Pathogens may be spread through the air or by contact with blood and other body fluids. *Bloodborne pathogens* can be contracted by exposure to the patient's blood and sometimes other body fluids, especially when they come in contact with an open

pathogens
the organisms that cause infection, such as viruses and bacteria.

wound or sore on the EMT's hands, face, or other exposed parts including mucous membranes, such as those in the nose, mouth, or eyes. Even minor breaks in the skin, such as those found around fingernails, can be enough for a pathogen to enter your body. *Airborne pathogens* are spread by tiny droplets sprayed during breathing, coughing, or sneezing. These particles can be absorbed through your eyes or when you inhale.

Since it is impossible for an EMT or other health care professional to identify patients who carry infectious diseases just by looking at them, all body fluids must be considered infectious and appropriate precautions taken for all patients at all times.

Standard Precautions a strict form of infection control that is based on the assumption that all blood and other body fluids are infectious.

Equipment and procedures that protect you from the blood and body fluids of the patient—and the patient from your blood and body fluids—are referred to as **Standard Precautions,** also known as body substance isolation (BSI) precautions or infection control. For each situation you encounter, it is important to apply the appropriate precautions. Taking too few will clearly increase your risk of exposure to disease. Too many can potentially alienate the patient and reduce your effectiveness.

The Occupational Safety and Health Administration (OSHA) has issued strict guidelines about precautions against exposure to bloodborne pathogens. Under the OSHA

CRITICAL DECISION MAKING: STANDARD PRECAUTIONS

While you may be thinking that the most important decisions you will make as an EMT have to do with clinical situations affecting your patient, some of the most important decisions you will make actually have to do with routine things such as Standard Precautions.

Be sure you always carry gloves on your person and have face protection immediately available in kits (e.g., first-in bags) and suction units. Your decision about the level of precautions to take will initially be determined as part of the scene size-up (the first part of the patient assessment process you will learn about in Chapter 8). Take precautions against anything you see *or anything you reasonably expect to encounter.* Some examples include:

1. When called to a motor vehicle collision where you observe broken glass, you should expect broken skin and the potential for contact with blood—even if you don't see wounds. Disposable gloves to protect you from blood as well as heavy-duty gloves to protect you from the broken glass are prudent.
2. When called to a nursing home for an interfacility transfer, you must reach under the patient to move the person to your stretcher. Because of the possibility of contact with urine, feces, or bed sores, you should wear disposable gloves.
3. You are called to a patient with a sprained ankle. There are no open wounds. Guidelines indicate that no precautions are necessary, although many routinely wear gloves on all calls.
4. You are working with an advanced life support crew treating a patient with chest pain. While there are no open wounds, the paramedic started an IV and some blood is present on the patient's forearm from the IV start and a small amount is seen on the IV tubing. Gloves are required.

Your decisions about Standard Precautions do not end at the scene size-up. In fact, you should be alert for changes throughout the call. For example:

5. You are treating a patient with chest pain who suddenly becomes unresponsive. The patient requires suction. In addition to the gloves you may already be wearing you will now need to protect your face from spatter encountered in airway and suction procedures.

guidelines, employers and employees share responsibility for these precautions. Employers must develop a written exposure control plan and must provide emergency care providers with training, immunizations, and proper **personal protective equipment (PPE)** to prevent transmission of disease. (Most volunteer organizations also provide these services for their members.) The employee's responsibility is to participate in the training and to follow the exposure control plan.

personal protective equipment (PPE)
equipment that protects the EMS worker from infection and/or exposure to the dangers of rescue operations.

There is also a requirement for all agencies to have a written policy in place in the event of an exposure to infectious substances. Any contact such as a needle-stick or contact with a potentially infectious fluid must be documented. Refer to your local policy for reporting an exposure incident. Most plans call for baseline testing of the exposed person immediately following the exposure and periodic follow-up testing. Additionally, federal legislation has made it possible for emergency care providers to be notified if a patient with whom they have had potentially infectious contact turns out to be infected by a disease or virus such as tuberculosis (TB), hepatitis B, or HIV (the virus associated with AIDS).

Although deciding on and taking Standard Precautions may seem intimidating—especially if you are just beginning your training—remember that it is possible, by following the proper precautions, to have a long and safe career in EMS free from infection and disease.

Personal Protective Equipment

Protect yourself from all possible routes of **contamination,** or introduction of disease or infectious materials. Follow Standard Precaution guidelines and wear the appropriate personal protective equipment on every call (Figure 2-1).

contamination
the introduction of dangerous chemicals, disease, or infectious materials.

Protective Gloves

Vinyl or other synthetic gloves should be used whenever there is the potential for contact with blood and other body fluids. This includes actions such as controlling bleeding, suctioning, artificial ventilation, and CPR. Make sure that you have the gloves on or available before you come in contact with a patient. Otherwise, you might get distracted and forget the gloves and may accidentally become contaminated. *Be sure to change gloves between patients.*

Most medical equipment and supplies are now latex-free. In many years of using latex in health care—both prehospitally and in the hospital—many patients and providers developed allergies to latex. The gloves you will see in the ambulance are now latex-free as are oxygen delivery devices and other supplies.

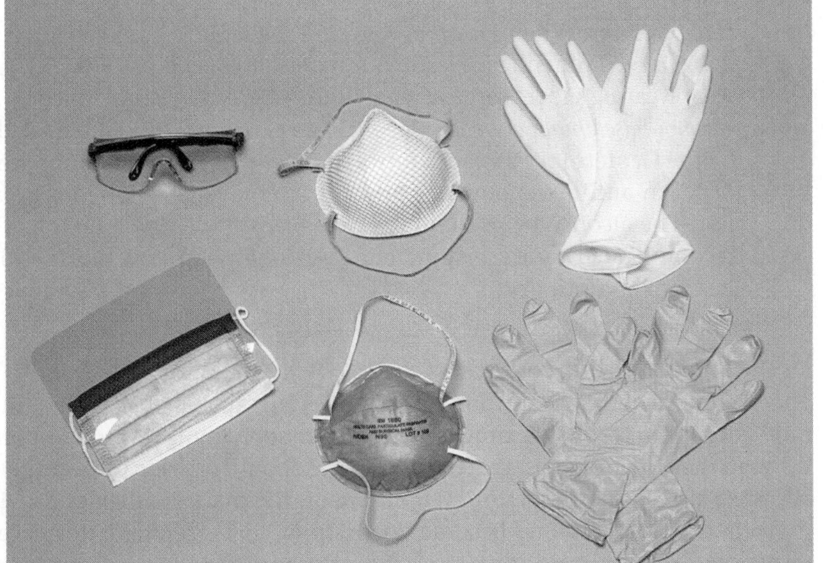

Figure 2-1 • Always wear personal protective equipment to prevent exposure to contagious disease.

POINT OF VIEW

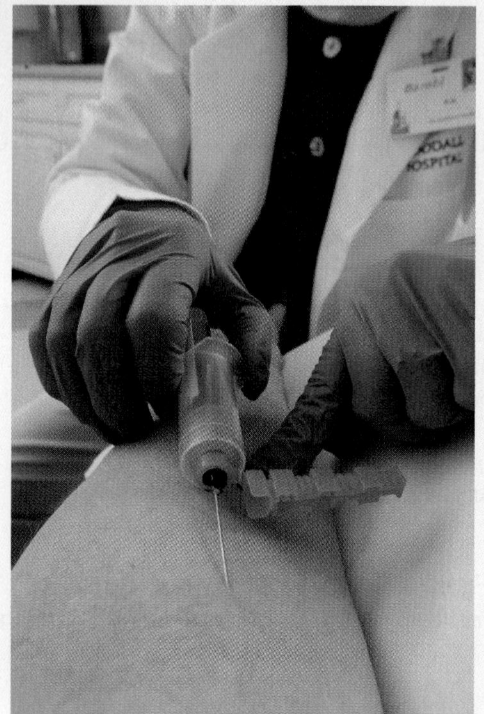

"I consider myself careful. I wear gloves on every call. But here I am getting blood drawn because I had an exposure to a patient's blood.

"I'm really not sure when or how it happened. I guess I put on gloves and then was on auto-pilot. I didn't notice they had a rip in them. Making things worse, I had a cut on my finger. Murphy's Law—the cut was right near the tear in the glove. It didn't even seem like a lot of blood at the scene. I looked at my glove. Saw the tear. Took off the glove and saw the blood on my open skin. My heart sank.

"Now the nurse will draw blood. Then I have to talk with a counselor. I'll get more blood drawn every so often. I already dread waiting to get the results—wondering if I'll get sick.

"Trust me. Never take Standard Precautions lightly. Think about them during the call. If I did, I would've seen that tear in my gloves. And my life would be very different. I'd give anything not to be sitting here right now."

A different type of glove must be worn when you clean the ambulance and soiled equipment. This glove should be heavyweight and tear-resistant. The force and type of movements involved in cleaning can cause lightweight gloves to rip, exposing your hands to contamination.

Hand Washing

Even though you wear gloves when assessing and caring for patients, you must still wash your hands after patient contacts when gloves are removed. There are two methods of hand cleaning. These are:

- *Hand washing.* When soap and water are available, vigorous hand washing (Figure 2-2A) is recommended. Wash your hands after each patient contact (even if you were wearing gloves) and whenever they become visibly soiled.
- *Alcohol-based hand cleaners.* These cleaners (Figure 2-2B) are considered effective by the Centers for Disease Control (CDC)—except when hands are visibly soiled or when anthrax is present—and are often available when soap and water are not. The alcohol helps kill microorganisms. Place the amount of hand cleaner recommended by the manufacturer in one palm and rub it so it covers your hands. Rub until dry.

Eye and Face Protection

The mucous membranes surrounding the eyes are capable of absorbing fluids. Wear eye protection to prevent splashing, spattering, or spraying fluids from entering the body through these membranes. Protective eyewear should provide protection from the front and the sides. Various types of eyewear are on the market. Goggles provide acceptable protection but can fog and become uncomfortable. Goggles are not necessary because acceptable substitutes are available. If you wear prescription eyeglasses, clip-on side pro-

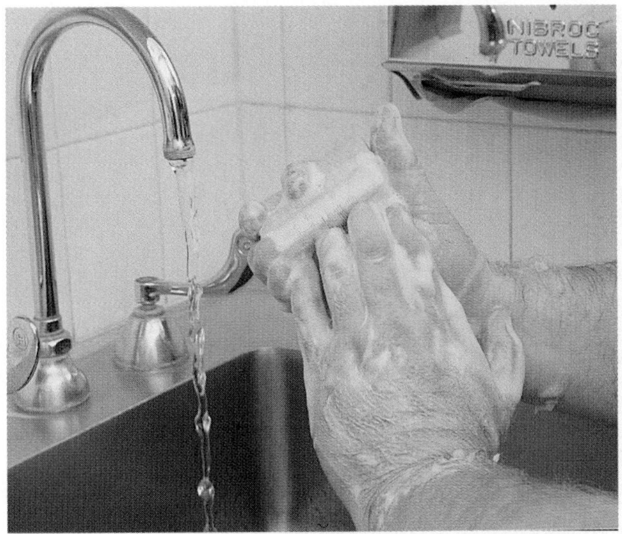

Figure 2-2A • Careful, methodical hand washing is effective in reducing exposure to contagious disease.

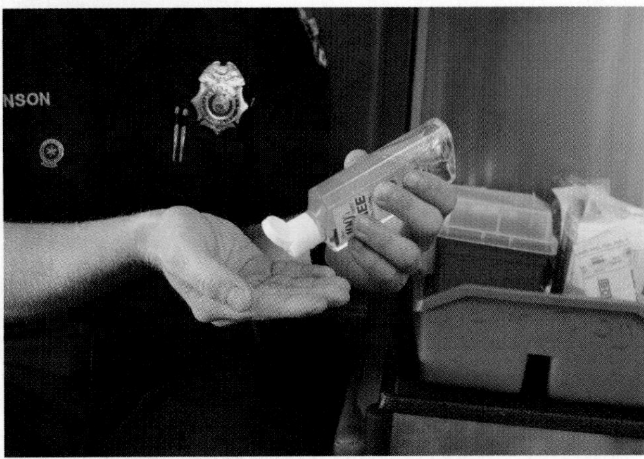

Figure 2-2B • Alcohol-based hand cleaners are effective and often available when soap and water are not.

tectors are available. Some companies offer protective eyewear that resembles eyeglasses. These are much easier than goggles to use and carry, and they do not fog up or cause excessive perspiration.

Masks

In cases where there will be blood or fluid spatter, wear a surgical-type mask. In cases where tuberculosis (a disease that is carried by fine particles in the air) is suspected, an N-95 or a high efficiency particulate air (HEPA) respirator approved by the National Institute for Occupational Safety and Health (NIOSH) is the standard (Figure 2-3). Face shields offer protection of the entire face by use of a mask with an attached see-through shield that covers the eyes (Figure 2-4).

In some jurisdictions, when a patient is suspected of having an infection spread by droplets (such as measles), a surgical-type mask may be placed on the patient if he is alert and cooperative.

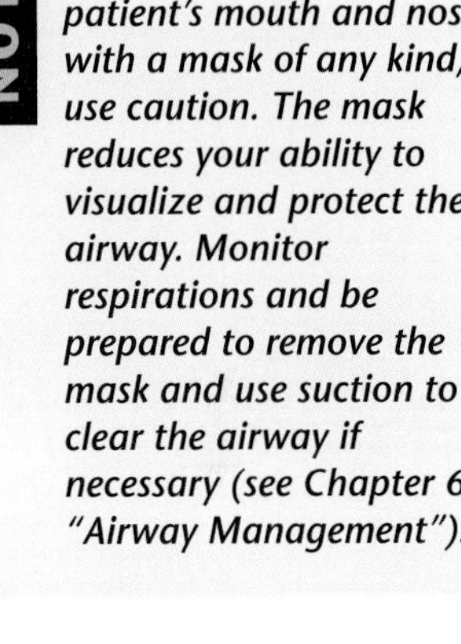

NOTE *When you cover a patient's mouth and nose with a mask of any kind, use caution. The mask reduces your ability to visualize and protect the airway. Monitor respirations and be prepared to remove the mask and use suction to clear the airway if necessary (see Chapter 6, "Airway Management").*

Gowns

A gown is worn to protect clothing and bare skin from spilled or splashed fluids. Arterial (spurting) bleeding is an indication for a gown. Childbirth and patients with multiple

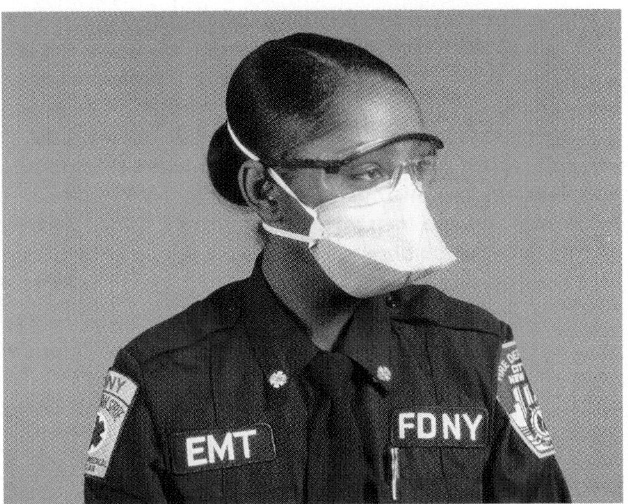

Figure 2-3 • Wear a NIOSH-approved respirator when you suspect a patient may have tuberculosis.

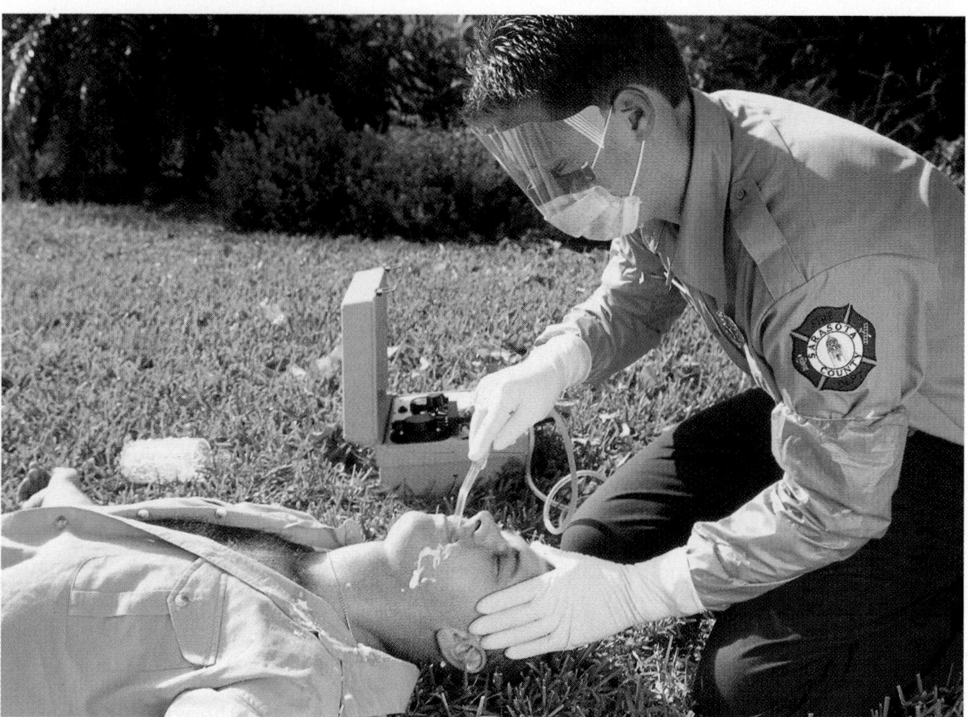

Figure 2-4 • Wear a protective mask and face shield when suctioning a patient.

injuries also often produce considerable amounts of blood. Any situation that would call for the use of a gown would also require gloves, eye protection, and a mask.

It is a good idea not only to use personal protective equipment yourself but also to be an advocate for its use; that is, to encourage members of your crew and others to use appropriate protective equipment. In addition to the moral and ethical obligation to do so, you will be helping to keep your crew in good health.

Always properly remove and discard protective garments after use, carry out disinfection and cleaning operations, and complete all reporting documentation regarding infection control. You will learn more about these procedures in Chapter 34, "Ambulance Operations."

NOTE

When you finish your EMT training and begin in the field, you will observe differences in the methods and levels of Standard Precautions taken by those around you. You will likely notice that some EMTs don gloves and protective eyewear before exiting the ambulance and wear them throughout the call. Others will go through an entire call without even wearing gloves.

In the 1980s an increased emphasis was placed on body substance isolation. Diseases such as AIDS and hepatitis brought a startling reality to the health care professions. As a result, gloves, protective eyewear, and masks were used with increasing frequency. These items were worn as a "precaution," even when not technically necessary.

Today, providers have a more realistic attitude about Standard Precautions. Think back to your last physical examination, for example. Your physician most likely examined your eyes and ears, palpated your abdomen, and performed other examinations without gloves. Why is this? Because it is not necessary to wear gloves if your skin and the skin of your patient is intact. Additionally, wearing gloves while you exit the ambulance, carry equipment, and enter a scene may cause the gloves to rip before you reach the patient, rendering them ineffective.

Common sense should be the rule. To protect yourself from disease:

- *Follow Standard Precautions guidelines as outlined in this chapter and in the rules and policies of your organization.*
- *Always have personal protective equipment immediately available on your person and in your kits.*
- *If in doubt, take Standard Precautions.*

The communicable diseases we are most concerned with are caused by bloodborne and airborne pathogens, such as viruses, bacteria, and other harmful organisms. Bloodborne pathogens are contracted by exposure to an infected patient's blood, especially exposure through breaks in the non-infected person's skin. Airborne pathogens are spread by tiny droplets sprayed when a patient breathes, coughs, or sneezes. These droplets are inhaled or are absorbed through the non-infected person's eyes, mouth, or nose.

Although there are many communicable diseases (Table 2-1), four are of particular concern: hepatitis B, hepatitis C, tuberculosis, and HIV/AIDS.

- **Hepatitis**, an infection that causes an inflammation of the liver, comes in several forms, including hepatitis A, B, C, and other strains. Hepatitis A is acquired primarily through contact with food or water contaminated by stool. The other forms are acquired through contact with blood and other body fluids. The virus that causes hepatitis is especially hardy. Hepatitis B has been found to live for many days in dried blood spills, posing a risk of transmission long after many other viruses would have died. For this reason, it is critical for you to assume that any body fluid in any form, dried or otherwise, is infectious until proven otherwise. Hepatitis B can be deadly. Before hepatitis B vaccine was available, the virus (HBV) killed hundreds of health care workers every year in the United States, more than any other occupationally acquired infectious disease. There is no cure, but an effective vaccine is available. (See "Immunizations" in this chapter.) Today, hepatitis C

F•Y•I

DISEASES OF CONCERN

infects many EMS providers in the same way as hepatitis B, yet there is no vaccine against hepatitis C.
- **Tuberculosis (TB)** is an infection that sometimes settles in the lungs and that in some cases can be fatal. It was thought to be largely eradicated, but in the late 1980s it made a comeback. TB is highly contagious. Unlike many other infectious diseases, it can spread through the air. Health care workers and others can become infected even without any direct contact with a carrier. Because it is impossible for the EMT to determine why a patient has a productive cough, it is safest to assume that it could be the result of TB and that you should take the necessary respiratory precautions. This is especially true in institutions such as nursing homes, correctional facilities, or homeless shelters where there is an increased risk of TB.
- **AIDS (acquired immune deficiency syndrome)** is a set of conditions that result when the immune system has been attacked by HIV (human immunodeficiency virus) and rendered unable to combat certain infections adequately. Although advances are being made in the treatment of HIV/AIDS, no cure has been discovered at the time of publication of this text. However, HIV/AIDS presents far less risk to health care workers than hepatitis and TB, because the virus does not survive well outside the human body. This limits the routes of exposure to direct contact with blood by way of open wounds, intravenous drug use, unprotected sexual contact, or blood transfusions. Puncture wounds into which HIV is introduced, such as with an accidental needle-stick, are also potential routes of infection. However, less than half of 1 percent of such incidents result in infection, according to the U.S. Occupational Safety and Health Administration (OSHA), compared to 30 percent for the hepatitis B virus (HBV). The difference is due to the quantity and strength of HBV compared to HIV.

Hepatitis B, hepatitis C, TB, and HIV/AIDS are the communicable diseases of greatest concern because they are potentially life-threatening. However, there are many communicable diseases to which emergency response and other health care personnel may be exposed. Table 2-1 lists common communicable diseases, their modes of transmission, and their incubation periods (the time between contact and the first appearance of symptoms).

EMERGING DISEASES AND CONDITIONS

Since the prior edition of this book, there have been both worsening of some diseases and discovery of others. West Nile virus, which originally was limited to Europe and Africa, has spread throughout the United States by mosquitoes, causing flu-like symptoms in mild cases and infections of the brain and meninges in severe cases.

continued

F•Y•I

Continued

TABLE 2-1 • Communicable Diseases

DISEASE	MODE OF TRANSMISSION	INCUBATION
AIDS (acquired immune deficiency syndrome)	HIV-infected blood via intravenous drug use, unprotected sexual contact, blood transfusions, or (rarely) accidental needlesticks. Mothers also may pass HIV to their unborn children.	Several months or years
Chicken pox (varicella)	Airborne droplets. Can also be spread by contact with open sores.	11 to 21 days
German measles (rubella)	Airborne droplets. Mothers may pass the disease to unborn children.	10 to 12 days
Hepatitis	Blood, stool, or other body fluids, or contaminated objects.	Weeks to months, depending on type
Meningitis, bacterial	Oral and nasal secretions.	2 to 10 days
Mumps	Droplets of saliva or objects contaminated by saliva.	14 to 24 days
Pneumonia, bacterial and viral	Oral and nasal droplets and secretions.	Several days
Staphylococcal skin infections	Direct contact with infected wounds or sores or with contaminated objects.	Several days
Tuberculosis (TB)	Respiratory secretions, airborne or on contaminated objects.	2 to 6 weeks
Whooping cough (pertussis)	Respiratory secretions or airborne droplets.	6 to 20 days

Severe Acute Respiratory Syndrome (SARS) has caused concern worldwide. SARS appears to be spread through respiratory droplets, by coughing, sneezing, or touching something contaminated and then touching your nose or eyes. It is a respiratory virus with symptoms that include fever, dry cough, and difficulty breathing. Protection against SARS in a patient-care setting includes frequent hand washing and the use of gloves, gowns, eye protection, and an N-95 respirator.

Avian flu is a disease found in poultry that can also affect humans. Outbreaks have been seen in Asia, the Near East, and Africa and have been fatal in about half the reported cases. The virus has not shown to be easily transmissible from human to human. Symptoms include traditional flu-like symptoms that progress to more severe conditions such as pneumonia and acute respiratory distress syndrome. Precautions against this condition are the same as those just listed for SARS.

Interestingly, some diseases are also on the decline. For example, vaccines have significantly reduced the number of cases of chicken pox and epiglottitis in children.

Diseases of concern will change during the time you are an EMT. Your county or state health agencies will issue warnings and advisories on these diseases. You can also look for information from the Centers for Disease Control at **www.cdc.gov.**

INFECTION CONTROL AND THE LAW

Scientists have identified the main culprits in the transmission of many deadly infectious diseases—blood and body fluids. EMTs and other health care workers have been recognized as having a higher-than-usual exposure and, therefore, a higher risk of contracting these unwanted infections.

Congress and federal agencies have responded by taking several steps to ensure the safety of people who are in high-risk positions. In particular, the Occupational Safety and Health Administration (OSHA) of the U.S. Department of Labor and the Centers for Disease Control and Prevention (CDC) of the U.S. Department of Health and Human Services have issued standards and guidelines for the protection of workers whose jobs may expose them to infectious diseases. The Ryan White CARE Act establishes procedures by which emergency response workers may find out if they have been exposed to life-threatening infectious diseases. These legal protections are described in more detail in the next sections.

Occupational Exposure to Bloodborne Pathogens

In 1992, the OSHA standard on bloodborne pathogens took effect. It mandates employers of emergency responders must take certain measures to protect employees who are likely to be exposed to blood and other body fluids. One of the basic principles behind the standard is that infection control is a joint responsibility between employer and employee. The employer must provide training, protective equipment, and vaccinations to employees who are subject to exposure in their jobs. In return, employees must participate in an infection exposure control plan that includes training and proper workplace practices.

Without the active participation of both the employer and the employee, any workplace infection control program is destined to fail. Be sure your system has an active and up-to-date infection exposure control plan and that you and your fellow EMTs follow it carefully at all times. Consult with your state OSHA representative to make sure that specific hazards are identified and corrected.

Contact the U.S. Department of Labor to request the booklet *Occupational Exposure to Bloodborne Pathogens: Precautions for Emergency Responders—OSHA 3106 1998*, an overview of the standard. For details regarding how to develop an infection control plan, request Title 29 Code of Federal Regulation 1910.1030 for the complete text of the standard and all requirements regarding occupational exposure to bloodborne pathogens. Critical elements of the standard are summarized below:

- **Infection exposure control plan.** Each emergency response employer must develop a plan that identifies and documents job classifications and tasks in which there is the possibility of exposure to potentially infectious body fluids. The plan must outline a schedule of how and when the bloodborne pathogen standards will be implemented. It also must include identification of the methods used for communicating hazards to employees, post-exposure evaluation, and follow-up.
- **Adequate education and training.** EMTs must be provided with training that includes general explanations of how diseases are transmitted, uses and limitations of practices that reduce or prevent exposure, and procedures to follow if exposure occurs.
- **Hepatitis B vaccination.** Employers must make the hepatitis B vaccination series available free of charge and at a reasonable time and place.
- **Personal protective equipment.** This equipment must be of a quality that will not permit blood or other infectious materials to pass through or reach an EMT's work clothes, street clothes, undergarments, skin, eyes, mouth, or other mucous membranes. This equipment must be provided by the employer to the EMT at no cost and includes but is not limited to protective gloves, face shields, masks, protective eyewear, gowns, and aprons, plus bag-valve masks, pocket masks, and other ventilation devices.
- **Methods of control.** Engineering controls remove potential infectious disease hazards or separate the EMT from exposure. Examples include pocket masks, disposable airway equipment, and puncture-resistant needle containers. Work practice controls improve the manner in which a task is performed to reduce risk of exposure. Examples include the proper and safe use of personal protective equipment; proper handling, labeling, and disposal of contaminated materials; and proper washing and decontamination practices.
- **Housekeeping.** The EMT and the employer are both responsible for maintaining clean and sanitary conditions of the emergency response vehicles and work sites. Procedures include the proper handling and proper decontamination of work surfaces, equipment, laundry, and other materials.
- **Labeling.** The standard requires labeling of containers used to store, transport, or ship blood and other potentially infectious materials, including the use of the biohazard symbol (Figure 2-5).

Figure 2-5 • The biohazard symbol must be included with warning labels for containers used to ship blood or other potentially infectious materials.

continued

F•Y•I

continued

- **Post-exposure evaluation and follow-up.** EMTs must immediately report suspected exposure incidents—including mucous membrane or broken-skin contact with blood or other potentially infectious materials—that result from the performance of an employee's duties. (See Figure 2-6 for a model plan based on the Ryan White CARE Act, which is described next.)

Ryan White CARE Act

In 1994, the CDC issued the final notice for the Ryan White Comprehensive AIDS Resources Emergency (CARE) Act Regarding Emergency Response Employees. This federal act, which applies to all 50 states, mandates a procedure by which emergency response personnel can seek to find out if they have been exposed to potentially life-threatening diseases while providing patient care. Emergency response personnel referred to in this act include firefighters, law

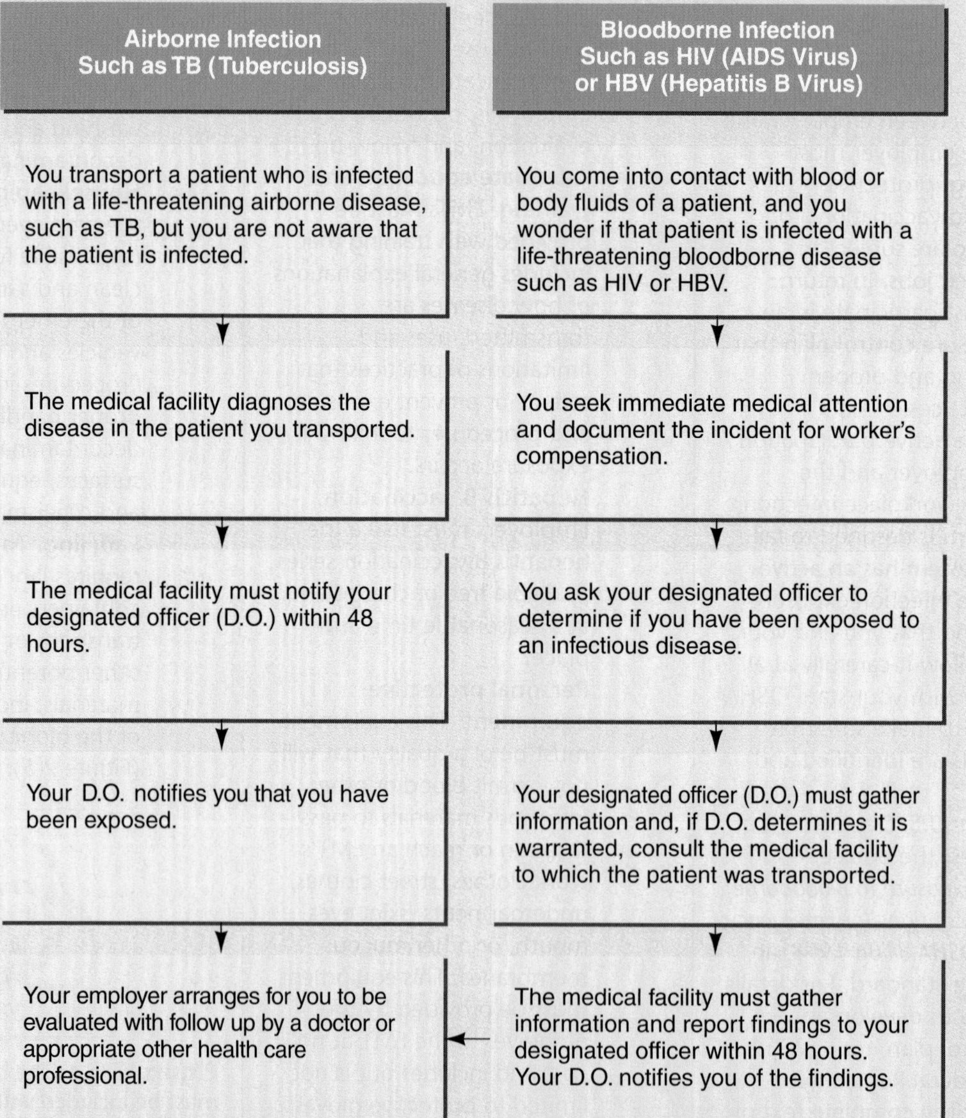

INFECTIOUS DISEASE EXPOSURE PROCEDURE
Airborne Infection Such as TB (Tuberculosis)
Bloodborne Infection Such as HIV (AIDS Virus) or HBV (Hepatitis B Virus)
You transport a patient who is infected with a life-threatening airborne disease, such as TB, but you are not aware that the patient is infected.
You come into contact with blood or body fluids of a patient, and you wonder if that patient is infected with a life-threatening bloodborne disease such as HIV or HBV.
The medical facility diagnoses the disease in the patient you transported.
You seek immediate medical attention and document the incident for worker's compensation.
The medical facility must notify your designated officer (D.O.) within 48 hours.
You ask your designated officer to determine if you have been exposed to an infectious disease.
Your D.O. notifies you that you have been exposed.
Your designated officer (D.O.) must gather information and, if D.O. determines it is warranted, consult the medical facility to which the patient was transported.
Your employer arranges for you to be evaluated with follow up by a doctor or appropriate other health care professional.
The medical facility must gather information and report findings to your designated officer within 48 hours. Your D.O. notifies you of the findings.

Figure 2-6 • Under the Ryan White CARE Act, there is a procedure for finding out and following up if you have been exposed to a life-threatening disease. This act was deauthorized by Congress and is expected to be reinstated in 2009. Other state and federal regulations may apply.

enforcement officers, EMTs, and other individuals such as First Responders who provide emergency aid on behalf of a legally recognized volunteer organization.

CDC has published a list of potentially life-threatening infectious and communicable diseases to which emergency response personnel can be exposed. The list includes airborne diseases such as TB, bloodborne diseases such as hepatitis B and HIV/AIDS, and uncommon or rare diseases such as diphtheria and rabies.

The Ryan White CARE Act requires every state's public health officer to designate an official within every emergency response organization to act as a "designated officer." The designated officer is responsible for gathering facts surrounding possible emergency responder airborne or bloodborne infectious disease exposures. Take time to learn who is the designated officer within your organization.

Two different notification systems for infectious disease exposure are defined in the act:

- **Airborne disease exposure.** You will be notified by your designated officer when you have been exposed to an airborne disease.
- **Bloodborne or other infectious disease exposure.** You may submit a request for a determination as to whether or not you were exposed to bloodborne or other infectious disease.

The difference between the two procedures results from the differences in how an exposure is most likely to be detected. With an airborne disease such as TB, you may not realize that the patient you have cared for and transported was infected. However, a disease like TB will be diagnosed at the hospital. Therefore, the Ryan White CARE Act states that for airborne diseases like TB, the hospital will notify the designated officer, who will notify you.

A bloodborne disease such as hepatitis B or HIV/AIDS may or may not be diagnosed at the hospital, but you will know if you have had contact with a patient's blood or body fluids. If so, you can submit a request to your designated officer who will gather the information necessary to request a determination from the hospital on whether you have been exposed and then will notify you of the result.

In either case, once you have been notified of an exposure, your employer will refer you to a doctor or other health care professional for evaluation and follow-up (Figure 2-7).

Consider how the Ryan White CARE Act would apply in the following example of exposure to an airborne pathogen:

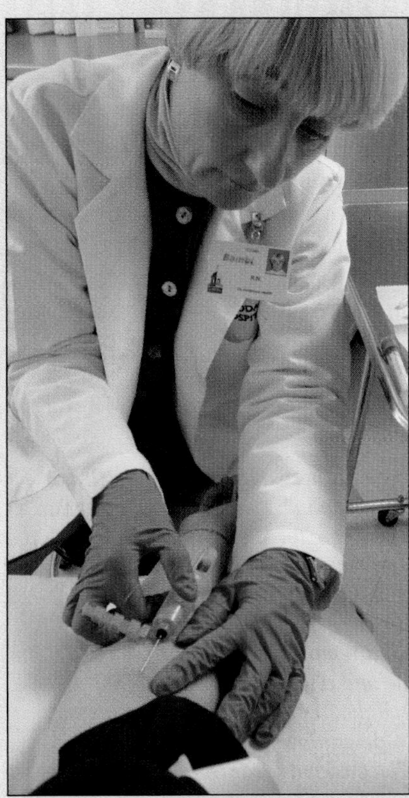

Figure 2-7 • Once you have been notified of an exposure, your employer will refer you to a doctor or other health care professional for evaluation and follow-up.

As an EMT, you treat and transport a patient who complains of weakness, fever, and chronic cough. The next day you receive a phone call from your organization's designated officer, who informs you that you have been exposed to a patient with TB. The designated officer helps you arrange an appointment with a doctor who can determine if you have contracted the disease and arrange for early treatment if you have.

According to CDC guidelines, exposure to airborne pathogens may occur when you share "air space" with a tuberculosis patient. So, if a medical facility diagnoses that patient as having the airborne infectious disease, it must notify the designated officer within 48 hours. The designated officer must then notify the emergency care workers of disease exposure. Finally, the employer must schedule a post-exposure evaluation and follow-up.

Consider a possible exposure to a bloodborne pathogen.

As an EMT, you are called to treat an unconscious woman. Pink, frothy sputum trickles from her mouth. Breathing is labored. A hypodermic needle lies beside her. While you are suctioning the patient, your eye shield slips and fluids from her mouth splash into your eyes. You report the incident immediately after the call is completed. Your designated officer follows up, and you learn that you have not been exposed to a life-threatening bloodborne disease.

Under CDC guidelines, after contact with the blood or body fluids of a patient you have transported, you may submit a request for a determination to your designated officer. The designated officer must then gather information about the possible exposure. If the

continued

F•Y•I

Continued

information indicates a possible exposure, the officer forwards the information to the medical facility where the patient is being treated. If the patient can be identified, medical records are reviewed to determine if the patient has a life-threatening disease. The medical facility then must notify your designated officer of their findings in writing within 48 hours after receiving the officer's request. The designated officer must notify you, and you will be directed by your employer to a health care professional for a post-exposure evaluation and follow-up as appropriate.

It is important to note that the Ryan White CARE Act does not empower hospitals to test patients for bloodborne diseases at the request of the emergency worker or designated officer. Rather, they can only review the patient's medical records to see if evidence of a bloodborne or other disease exists. Thus a patient could be infected, but if the records reveal no testing or known indication of the presence of such an infection, the hospital can only report that "no evidence of bloodborne infection could be detected."

Tuberculosis Compliance Mandate

Thousands of new cases of TB are reported in the United States each year. Hundreds of health care workers have been infected or exposed. Of particular concern is multi-drug resistant TB (MDR-TB), which does not respond to the usual medications. In 1994 CDC issued guidelines for treating a suspected or confirmed TB patient. OSHA has announced it will enforce those guidelines as if they were OSHA rules and will also require employers of health care workers to follow OSHA's respiratory standard (1910.134). This standard describes the selection and proper use of different kinds of respirators including those classified as N-95 or HEPA.

Study the guidelines as summarized in the following text. Learn to recognize situations in which the potential of exposure to TB exists. Those at greatest risk of contracting and transmitting TB are people who have suppressed immune systems, including people with HIV/AIDS and elderly patients such as those living in nursing homes. Patients who have TB may have the following signs and symptoms: productive cough (coughing up mucus or other fluid) and/or coughing up blood, weight loss and loss of appetite, lethargy and weakness, night sweats, and fever. It is safest to assume that any person with a productive cough may be infected with TB.

When the potential exists for exposure to exhaled air of a person with suspected or confirmed TB, OSHA requires that you wear a NIOSH-approved N-95 or high efficiency particulate air (HEPA) respirator. You are required to wear an N-95 or HEPA respirator when you are:

- Caring for patients suspected of having TB. High-risk areas include correctional institutions, homeless shelters, long-term care facilities for the elderly, and drug treatment centers.
- Transporting an individual from such a setting in a closed vehicle. If possible, keep the windows of the ambulance open and set the heating and air conditioning system on the non-recirculating cycle.
- Performing high-risk procedures such as endotracheal suctioning and intubation.

Remember to take all recommended infection control precautions, including hand washing and using personal protective equipment and barrier devices such as pocket masks or bag-valve masks for rescue breathing. Properly dispose of contaminated equipment and materials, and decontaminate all surfaces, clothing, and equipment. ■

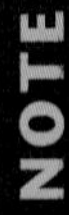

If you are actually exposed to a bloodborne pathogen (e.g., a needlestick or splashing of fluids to a mucous membrane), you must seek medical attention immediately. It is important that you receive care for the wound, obtain baseline blood work including determining hepatitis B immunity, evaluate the need for a tetanus shot, and document the incident for worker's compensation or insurance. You may also be asked to consider taking an antiviral drug or combination of drugs to attempt to counteract the effects of HIV if it is present. This is a personal issue and a very serious decision. It is important to know that current research indicates that waiting 48 hours for the requested Ryan White information to determine if the patient whose blood you were exposed to may be HIV-infected may reduce the effectiveness of the drugs. Even a few hours may make a significant difference in treatment outcome. Do not delay seeking care. Each situation is different. You will wish to seek the advice of the attending physician where you are being treated as well as that of your medical director.

Immunizations

Immunizations against many diseases are available. Most people receive tetanus immunizations either routinely or after certain injuries. There is currently an immunization available to prevent hepatitis B. It will be provided by your EMS agency, usually through a local physician or your Medical Director.

While there is no immunization against tuberculosis used in the United States, the *tuberculin skin test (TST)*, formerly called the purified protein derivative (PPD) test, can detect exposure. EMTs are often given this test during routine or employment screening physicals. If the test determines that you have been exposed to tuberculosis, seek treatment and follow-up from a doctor or other health care professional. EMS workers should be checked for exposure to TB on a regular basis (usually yearly).

Some EMS agencies and medical facilities may require immunizations for measles and other common communicable diseases. Consult your instructor, your Medical Director, or your personal physician for more information on your current status and local protocols for immunizations.

EMOTION AND STRESS

Take a minute to think about the last time you told someone that you felt "stressed out." How did you feel? Did you feel tense, as if every muscle was tight, every nerve on edge? Were your palms sweaty and your stomach in knots? Was your heart pounding and did you have a lump in your throat? Did you have trouble sleeping or always feel exhausted no matter how much sleep you had the previous night? What was going on in your life at that time? Were you preparing for a big exam? Was a family member's illness causing you to worry? Did you feel torn between the demands of family, work, and school? Were you worried about your financial state, wondering how you would cover some large unexpected expense? Were you about to change jobs or were you going through a divorce? How you manage these and other stressors is critical to your well-being.

Physiologic Aspects of Stress

During the Middle Ages and for much of the next 200 or 300 years, people viewed the mind and body as separate entities. In the last third of the twentieth century, however, medical science began to give increasing scrutiny to how the mind and body work together and influence each other. In fact, today it would be hard to find anyone who denies that there is a connection between mind and body or that stress plays a role in illness.

Stress is a widely used term in today's society. It is derived from a word used in the 1600s (*stresse*, a variation of *distresse*), which meant acute anxiety, pain, or sorrow. Today, doctors and psychologists generally define stress as a state of physical and/or psychological arousal to a stimulus. Any stimulus is capable of being a stressor for someone, and stressors vary from individual to individual and from time to time.

stress
a state of physical and/or psychological arousal to a stimulus.

Many agree that stress poses a potential hazard for EMS personnel. However, it is important to recognize that stress is a normal part of life and, when managed appropriately, does not have to pose a threat to your well-being. As an EMT you will be routinely exposed to stress-producing agents or situations. These stressors may be environmental factors (e.g., noise, inclement weather, unstable wreckage), your dealings with other people (e.g., unpleasant family or work relationships, abusive patients or bystanders), or your own self-image or performance expectations (e.g., worry over your expertise at specific skills or guilt over poor patient outcomes).

Ironically these stress-causing factors may be some of the same things that first attracted you to EMS, such as an atypical work environment, an unpredictable but varied work load, dealing with people in crisis, or the opportunity to work somewhat independently. How you manage these stressors is critical to your survival as an EMS provider as well as in life.

Dr. Hans Selye (a Canadian physician and educator who was born in Austria) did a great deal of research in this area and found that the body's response to stress (*general adaptation syndrome*) has three stages.

During the first stage (*alarm reaction*), your sympathetic nervous system increases its activity in what is known as the "fight or flight" syndrome. Your pupils dilate, your heart rate increases, and your bronchial passages dilate. In addition, your blood sugar increases, your digestive system slows, your blood pressure rises, and blood flow to your skeletal muscles increases. At the same time, the endocrine system produces more cortisol, a hormone that influences your metabolism and your immune response. Cortisol is critical to your body's ability to adapt to and cope with stress.

In the second stage (*stage of resistance*), your body systems return to normal functioning. The physiologic effects of sympathetic nervous system stimulation and the excess cortisol are gone. You have adapted to the stimulus and it no longer produces stress for you. You are coping. Many factors contribute to your ability to cope; these include your physical and mental health, education, experiences, and support systems, such as family, friends, and coworkers.

Exhaustion, the third stage of the general adaptation syndrome, occurs when exposure to a stressor is prolonged or the stressor is particularly severe. During this stage, the physiologic effects described by Selye include what he called the stress triad: enlargement (hypertrophy) of the adrenal glands, which produce adrenaline; wasting (atrophy) of lymph nodes; and bleeding gastric ulcers. At this point the individual has lost the ability to resist or adapt to the stressor and may become seriously ill as a consequence. Fortunately, most individuals do not reach this stage.

Types of Stress Reactions

Three types of stress reactions are commonly encountered: acute stress reactions, delayed stress reactions, and cumulative stress reactions. Any of these may occur as a result of a *critical incident*, which is any situation that triggers a strong emotional response. An *acute stress reaction* occurs simultaneously with or shortly after the critical incident. A *delayed stress reaction* (also known as post-traumatic stress disorder) may occur at any time, days to years, following a critical incident. A *cumulative stress reaction* (also known as *burnout*) occurs as a result of prolonged recurring stressors in our work or private lives.

Acute Stress Reaction

Acute stress reactions are often linked to catastrophes, such as a large-scale natural disaster, a plane crash, or a coworker's line-of-duty death or injury. Signs and symptoms of an acute stress reaction will develop simultaneously or within a very short time following the incident. They may involve any one or a combination of the following areas of function: physical, cognitive (the ability to think), emotional, or behavioral. These are signs that this particular situation is overwhelming your usual ability to cope and to perform effectively. It is important to keep in mind that they are ordinary reactions to extraordinary situations. They reflect the process of adapting to challenge. They are normal and are not a sign of weakness or mental illness.

Some of these signs and symptoms require immediate intervention from a physician or mental health professional, while others do not. As a rule, any sign or symptom that indicates an acute medical problem (such as chest pain, difficulty breathing, or abnormal heart rhythms) or an acute psychological problem (such as uncontrollable crying, inappropriate behavior, or a disruption in normal, rational thinking) are the kinds of problems that demand immediate corrective action. These are the same kinds of problems that alert us to a potentially dangerous situation when we see them in a patient, and they should trigger the same response when exhibited by us or our coworkers. Helping people is not just about taking care of your patient; it is also always about taking care of each other and yourself.

As previously mentioned, some signs and symptoms associated with an acute stress reaction may not require intervention. For instance, you may feel nauseated, tremulous, or numb after working a cardiopulmonary arrest, particularly if your patient is close to your age. You may feel confused or have trouble concentrating or difficulty sleeping after working at a particularly bloody crash scene or a prolonged extrication. You may find that you have no appetite for food or cannot get enough to eat. If not too severe or long-lasting, these responses are uncomfortable but probably not dangerous, since they pose no immediate threat to your health, safety, or well-being.

Remember that you are not losing your mind if you exhibit signs and symptoms of stress after a critical incident. You are merely reacting to an extraordinary situation. Remember, too, that there is nothing wrong with you if you do *not* experience any symptoms after such an incident. This, too, is common. In other words, a wide range of responses is normal and to be expected.

Delayed Stress Reaction

Like an acute stress reaction, a delayed stress reaction, also known as *post-traumatic stress disorder (PTSD)*, can be triggered by a specific incident; however, the signs and symptoms may not become evident until days, months, or even years later. This delay in presentation may make it harder to deal with the stress reaction since the individual has seemingly put the incident behind him and moved on with his life. Signs and symptoms may include flashbacks, nightmares, feelings of detachment, irritability, sleep difficulties, or problems with concentration or interpersonal relationships.

It is not uncommon for persons suffering from PTSD to seek solace through drug and alcohol abuse. Because of the delay and the apparent disconnect between the triggering event and the response, the patient with PTSD may not understand what is causing the problems. PTSD requires intervention by a mental health professional.

Cumulative Stress Reaction

Cumulative stress reaction, or burnout, is not triggered by a single critical incident, but instead results from sustained, recurring low-level stressors—possibly in more than one aspect of one's life—and develops over a period of years.

The earliest signs are subtle. They may present as a vague anxiety, progressing to boredom and apathy, and a feeling of emotional exhaustion. If problems are not identified and managed at this point, the progression will continue. Now the individual will develop physical complaints (such as headaches or stomach ailments), significant sleep disturbances, loss of emotional control, irritability, withdrawal from others, and increasing depression. Without appropriate intervention, the person's physical, emotional, and behavioral condition will continue to deteriorate, with manifestations such as migraines, increased smoking or alcohol intake, loss of sexual drive, poor interpersonal relationships, deterioration in work performance, limited self-control, and significant depression.

At its worst, cumulative stress may present as physical illness, uncontrollable emotions, overwhelming physical and emotional fatigue, severe withdrawal, paranoia, or suicidal thoughts. Long-term psychological intervention is critical at this stage if the individual is to recover.

The ultimate key to preventing or managing cumulative stress lies in seeking balance in our lives.

Causes of Stress

Emergencies are stressful by nature. While most EMS calls are considered "routine," some calls seem to have a higher potential for causing excess stress on EMS providers (Figure 2-8). They include the following:

- *Multiple-casualty incidents.* A **multiple-casualty incident (MCI)** is a single incident in which there are multiple patients. Examples range from a motor-vehicle crash in which two drivers and a passenger are injured to a hurricane that causes the injury of hundreds of people.

multiple-casualty incident (MCI)
an emergency involving multiple patients.

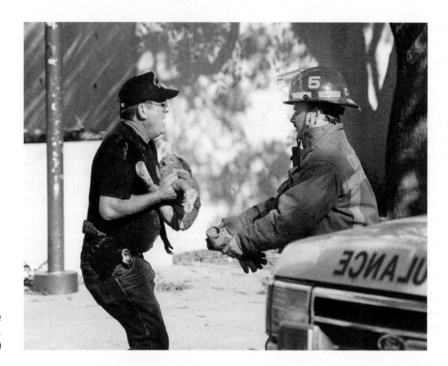

Figure 2-8 • Emergencies are often stressful for EMS providers. *(© Charles H. Porter IV/SYGMA)*

- *Calls involving infants and children.* Involving anything from a serious injury to sudden infant death syndrome (SIDS), these calls are known to be particularly stressful to all health care providers.
- *Severe injuries.* Expect a stress reaction when your call involves injuries that cause major trauma or distortion to the human body. Examples include amputations, deformed bones, deep wounds, and violent death.
- *Abuse and neglect.* Cases of abuse and neglect occur in all social and economic levels of society. You may be called to treat infant, child, adult, or elder abuse victims.
- *Death of a coworker.* A bond is formed among members of the public services. The death of another public-safety worker—even if you do not know that person—can cause a stress response.

Stress may be caused by a single event or it may be the cumulative result of several incidents. Remember that any incident may affect you and your coworkers differently. Two EMTs on the same call may have opposite responses. Try never to make negative judgments about another person's reaction.

Stress may also stem from a combination of factors, including problems in your personal life. One common cause of stress is people who "just don't understand" the job. For example, your EMS organization may require you to work on weekends and holidays. Time spent on call may be frustrating to friends and family members. They may not understand why you cannot participate in certain social activities or why you cannot leave a certain area. You might get frustrated, too, because you cannot plan around the unpredictable nature of emergencies. Then, after a very trying or exciting call, for instance, you may wish to share your feelings with a friend or someone you love. You find instead that the person does not understand your emotions. This can lead to feelings of separation and rejection, which are highly stressful.

Signs and Symptoms of Stress

There are two types of stress: eustress and distress. Eustress is a positive form of stress that helps people work under pressure and respond effectively. Distress is negative. It can happen when the stress of a scene becomes overwhelming. As a result, your response to the emergency will not be effective. Distress also can cause immediate and long-term problems with your health and well-being.

The signs and symptoms of stress include irritability with family, friends, and coworkers; inability to concentrate; changes in daily activities, such as difficulty sleeping or nightmares, loss of appetite, and loss of interest in sexual activity; anxiety; indecisiveness; guilt; isolation; and loss of interest in work.

Dealing with Stress

Lifestyle Changes

There are several ways to deal with stress. They are called *lifestyle changes*:

- *Develop more healthful and positive dietary habits.* Avoid fatty foods and increase your carbohydrate intake. Also reduce your consumption of alcohol and caffeine, which can have negative effects, including an increase in stress and anxiety and disturbance of sleep patterns.
- *Exercise.* When performed safely and properly, exercise helps to "burn off" stress. It also helps you deal with the physical aspects of your responsibilities, such as carrying equipment and performing physically demanding emergency procedures.
- *Devote time to relaxing.* Try relaxation techniques, too. These techniques, which include deep-breathing exercises and meditation, are valuable stress reducers.

In addition to the changes you can make in your personal life to help reduce and prevent stress, there also are changes you can make in your professional life. If you are in an organization with varied shifts and locations, consider requesting a change to a different location that offers a lighter call volume or different types of calls. You may also want to change your shift to one that allows more time with family and friends.

Many types of help are available for EMTs and others experiencing stress. Seek them out. It is not a sign of weakness. Many professionals can help you deal with stress, and much of the care may be covered by health insurance policies or employee assistance programs.

Critical Incident Stress Management

Critical incident stress management (CISM) is a comprehensive system that includes education and resources to both prevent stress and to deal with stress appropriately when it does occur. EMS systems and organizations have different systems for dealing with stress prevention, critical incident stress, and chronic stress, including wellness incentives, professional counseling, and peer support.

critical incident stress management (CISM)
a comprehensive system that includes education and resources to both prevent stress and to deal with stress appropriately when it occurs.

The critical incident stress debriefing (CISD) is a process in which a team of trained peer counselors and mental health professionals meet with rescuers and health care providers who have been involved in a major incident. The meetings are generally held within 24 to 72 hours after the incident. The goal is to assist emergency-care workers in dealing with the stress related to that incident.

The CISD is an open discussion of the feelings experienced during and after the call. Participants are encouraged to talk about any fears or reactions they have had. It is critical that the CISD does not become a method of investigation of the events of the call. Everything discussed at the meetings is confidential and all participants are asked not to disclose information once the meeting is over. Any breach in the confidentiality of the discussion prevents others from sharing information that can help them. After the open discussion, the CISD team offers suggestions on how to deal with and overcome the stress. It is important once again to state that stress after a major incident is normal and should be expected. The CISD process can help to accelerate the recovery process.

Sometimes a "defusing session" is held within the first few hours after a critical incident. While CISD includes all personnel involved in the incident, a defusing session is usually limited to the people who were most directly involved with the most stressful aspects. It provides them an opportunity to vent feelings and receive information before the larger group meets.

After a CISD, follow-up is essential. A member of the peer team should contact all CISD attendees within 24 hours to offer support and referrals. No two emergency-care workers will perceive, experience, or recover from critical incident stress in the same way. The process of overcoming the stress will be different from person to person. Resources must be available immediately as well as long after the incident, including "anniversary dates"—anniversaries of stressful events.

Some criticism exists critical incident stress debriefing. The criticism centers around the need for scientific proof of benefits of the technique as well as ensuring it does not cause more emotional trauma than it prevents. Studies will likely be performed in the future to help answer these questions. Your instructor will be able to provide more information. Comprehensive critical stress management goes beyond the CISD session to include pre-incident stress education, on-scene peer support, one-on-one support, disaster support services, spouse and family support, community outreach programs, and other services such as wellness programs. Remember, stress is a normal and perhaps inevitable response to a critical incident. Learn to recognize the signs and symptoms and find out where to turn for help.

Understanding Reactions to Death and Dying

As an EMT, you will undoubtedly be called to patients who are in various stages of a terminal illness. Understanding what the families and the patients go through can help you deal with the stress they feel as well as your own.

When a patient finds out that he is dying, he goes through emotional stages, each varying in duration and magnitude, sometimes overlapping, and all affecting both the patient and the family.

- *Denial or "Not me."* The patient denies that he is dying. This puts off dealing with the inevitable end of the process.
- *Anger or "Why me?"* The patient becomes angry at his situation. This anger is commonly vented upon family members and EMS personnel.
- *Bargaining or "Okay, but first let me. . . ."* In the mind of the patient bargaining seems to postpone death, even for a short time.
- *Depression or "Okay, but I haven't. . . ."* The patient is sad, depressed, and despairing, often mourning things not accomplished, dreams that will not come true. He retreats into a world of his own, unwilling to communicate with others.
- *Acceptance or "Okay, I'm not afraid."* The patient may come to accept death, although he does not welcome it. Often, the patient may come to accept the situation before family members do. At this stage, the family may need more support than the patient.

Not all patients go through all these stages. Some may seem to be in more than one stage at the same time. Some reactions may not seem to fit any of the described stages. Those who die rapidly are likely not to have such a predictable response to their own mortality. However, a general understanding of the process can help you to communicate with patients and families effectively.

As an EMT, you will also encounter sudden, unexpected death; for example, as a result of a motor-vehicle collision. In cases of sudden death, family members are likely to react with a wide range of emotion.

You can take several steps or approaches in dealing with the patient and family members confronted with death or dying:

- *Recognize the patient's needs.* Treat the patient with respect and do everything you can to preserve the patient's dignity and sense of control. For example, talk directly to the patient. Avoid talking about the patient to family members in the patient's presence as if the patient were incompetent or no longer living. Be sensitive to how the patient seems to want to handle the situation. For example, allow or encourage the patient to share feelings and needs, rather than cutting off such communications because of your own embarrassment or discomfort. Respect the patient's privacy if he does not want to communicate personal feelings.

- *Be tolerant of angry reactions from the patient or family members.* There may be feelings of helpless rage about the death or prospect of death. The anger is not personal. It would be directed at anyone in your position.
- *Listen empathetically.* Although you cannot "fix" the situation, just listening with understanding and patience will be very helpful.
- *Do not falsely reassure.* Avoid saying things like "Everything will be all right," which you, the patient, and the family all know is not true. Offering false reassurance will only be irritating or convey the impression that you do not really understand.
- *Offer as much comfort as you realistically can.* Comfort both the patient and the family. Let them know that you will do everything you can to help or to get them whatever help is available from other sources. Use a gentle tone of voice and a reassuring touch, if appropriate.

SCENE SAFETY

Scene safety is perhaps the most important concept in your EMT training. Unless you stay safe, you will not be able to help your patient and you may suffer serious injury—or die.

Fortunately EMS is safe, especially when care is taken on every call to avoid hazards and danger. Television has given us false information on what the dangers actually are. Based on this you may visualize criminals and drug-crazed people being the most frequent hazard. You may, in fact, see these people. But in most places, these are not the most common EMS hazards.

In a review of EMS provider deaths over the past several years, few EMS providers were killed by violence. Heart attack, motor-vehicle collisions, and air-medical crashes are a greater risk by far. Table 2-2 lists causes of provider deaths for the most recent years available.

The remainder of this chapter will discuss several ways to remain safe in EMS. You will learn more on safety in Chapter 8, "Scene Size-Up."

Hazardous-Material Incidents

Many chemicals are capable of causing death or life-long complications even if they are only briefly inhaled or in contact with a person's body. Many of these materials are commercially transported, often by truck or rail. Such materials are also often stored in warehouses and used in industry. When there is an accident or when containers begin to leak, a **hazardous-material incident** may occur, which will pose serious dangers for you as an EMT as well as for others who are in the vicinity. When you face an emergency involving such materials, remember—you will not be able to help anyone if you are injured. Exercise caution.

hazardous-material incident
the release of a harmful substance into the environment.

TABLE 2-2 • Causes of EMS Provider Deaths

	2004	2005	2006
Air medical crash	17	8	3
Heart attack/medical	3	0	3
Motor vehicle collision	3	10	3
Violence	3	0	0
9/11/2001 complications	0	2	1
Rescue	1	0	1
Other	0	1	0

The primary rule is to maintain a safe distance from the source of the hazardous material. Make sure your ambulance or other emergency vehicle is equipped with binoculars. They will help you identify placards, which are placed on vehicles, structures, and storage containers when they hold hazardous materials (Figure 2-9). These placards use coded colors and identification numbers that are listed in the *Emergency Response Guidebook* developed by the U.S. Department of Transportation, Transport Canada, and the Secretariat of Communications and Transportation of Mexico. This reference book should be placed in every vehicle that responds to or may respond to a hazardous-material incident. It provides important information about the properties of the dangerous substance as well as information on safe distances, emergency care, and suggested procedures in the event of spills or fire. (The *Emergency Response Guidebook* is also available on the internet at **hazmat.dot.gov/pubs/erg/gydebook.htm**.)

Your most important roles at the scene of a hazardous-material incident include recognizing potential problems, taking initial actions for your personal safety and the safety of others, and notifying an appropriately trained hazardous-material response team. Do not take any actions other than those aimed at protecting yourself, patients, and bystanders at the scene. An incorrect action can cause a bigger problem than the one that already exists.

The hazardous-material response team is made up of specially trained technicians who will coordinate the safe approach and resolution of the incident. Each wears a special suit that protects the skin. A self-contained breathing apparatus (SCBA) is also required because of the strong potential for poisonous gases, dust, and fumes at a hazardous-material incident. You will generally not be required to wear personal protective equipment of this sort unless you have been specially trained to be part of a hazardous-material response team. Instead, you will remain at a distance until the team has made the scene safe.

decontamination the removal or cleansing of dangerous chemicals and other dangerous or infectious materials.

As an EMT, you should not be treating patients until after they have undergone **decontamination** (cleansing of dangerous chemicals and other materials). If you take a contaminated patient into your ambulance, it will be considered contaminated and cannot be used again until it is thoroughly decontaminated. Furthermore, should you bring a contaminated patient to the emergency department of a hospital, you could effectively close that hospital down. (See Chapter 36, "Special Operations," for more information on hazardous-material incidents.)

Terrorist Incidents

As an EMT you may be called to respond to a terrorist incident. This incident may be small or large in scale and may include chemical agents, biological agents, radiation,

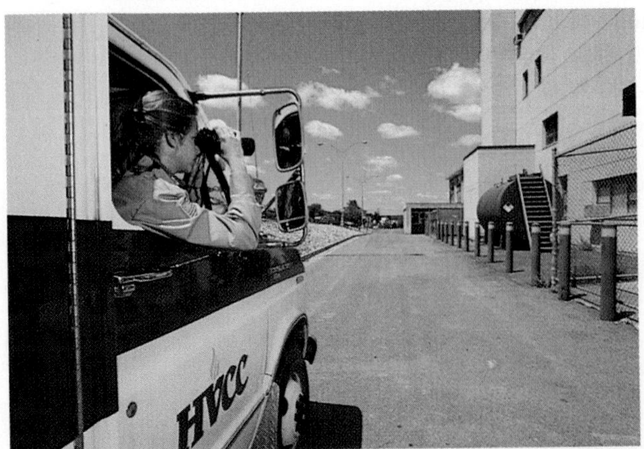

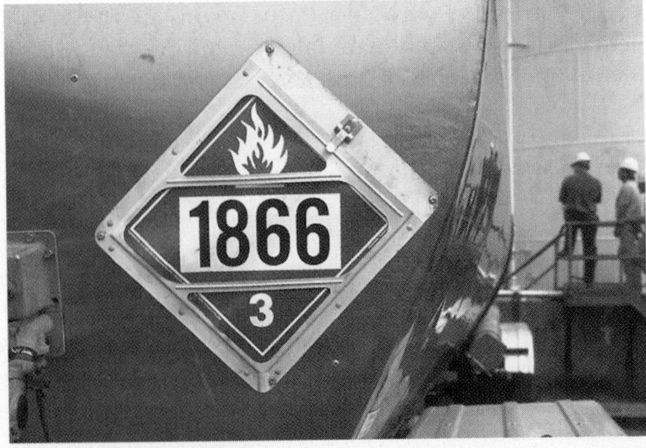

Figure 2-9 • Placards with coded colors and identification numbers must be used on vehicles and containers to identify hazardous materials.

and/or explosive devices. While these topics are covered in other areas of this text—including Chapter 37, "Terrorism and EMS"—it is important to consider this type of incident and its effect on your personal safety in the general context of scene safety.

As part of your initial and subsequent training, you will likely be made aware of any specific threats or targets in your area in addition to any specific protocols relating to potential chemical, biological, nuclear, or explosive incidents.

Rescue Operations

Rescue operations include rescuing or disentangling victims from fires, auto collisions, explosions, electrocutions, and more. As with hazardous materials, it is important to evaluate each situation and ensure that appropriate assistance is requested early in the call. Depending on the emergency, you may need the police, fire department, power company, or other specialized personnel. Never perform acts that you are not properly trained to do. Do your best to secure the scene. Then stand by for the specialists. (You will learn more about rescue operations in Chapter 35, "Gaining Access and Rescue Operations.")

As you work in rescue operations or on patients during a rescue operation, you will need personal protective equipment that includes turnout gear (coat, pants, and boots), protective eyewear, helmet, and puncture-proof gloves.

Violence

As an EMT, you will be called to scenes involving violence. Your first priority—even before patient care—is to be certain that the scene is safe. Dangerous persons or pets, people with weapons, intoxicated people, and others may present problems you are not prepared to handle. Learn to recognize those occasions. If the dispatcher knows that violence is or potentially may be present, he will advise you not to approach the scene until it is safe. The dispatcher may name a certain location where you should wait, or stage, a location that is far enough from the scene to be safe but near enough that you can respond as soon as the scene has been secured. Remember, it is the responsibility of the police to secure a scene and make it safe for you to perform your EMS duties.

Three words sum up the actions required to respond to danger: plan, observe, and react.

Plan

Many EMTs work together to prevent dangerous accidents and know what to do as a team when danger strikes. Scene safety begins long before the actual emergency. Plan to be as safe as possible under all circumstances. Factors to be addressed include the following:

- *Wear safe clothing.* Nonslip shoes and practical clothing will not only help you provide emergency care more efficiently, but they also help you to respond to danger without unnecessary restrictions. For personal protection, have reflective clothing available if you will be near traffic or in areas where it is important for you to be visible. Some EMTs wear body armor (bullet-proof vests) when working in high-risk areas or situations.
- *Prepare your equipment so it is not cumbersome.* You will be carrying your first-response kit into emergencies. If it is too heavy or bulky, it will take your attention away from the careful observation of the scene as you approach and slow you down if retreat becomes necessary. Many practical containers of reasonable size and weight are available.
- *Carry a portable radio whenever possible.* A radio allows you to call for help if you are separated from your vehicle.
- *Decide on safety roles.* If there will be more than one EMT on any call, tasks should be split up. For example, one EMT can obtain vital signs while another applies oxygen. One role that is frequently under-used is that of observer. The EMT directly involved in patient care should always be aware of, but will have trouble

constantly monitoring, the surroundings. The EMT who is not directly involved with patient care will be better able to actively observe for such things as weapons, mechanisms of injury, medications, and other important information.

Observe

Remember that it is always better to prevent a dangerous situation than to deal with one. If you observe or suspect danger, call the police. Do not enter the scene until they have secured it.

Observation begins early in the call. Observe the neighborhood as you look for house or building numbers. As you near the scene, turn off your lights and sirens to avoid broadcasting your arrival and attracting a crowd.

As you approach an emergency scene, notice what is going on. Emergencies are very active events. In situations where you notice an unusual silence, a certain amount of caution is advisable (Figure 2-10). In addition, observe for the following:

- *Violence.* Any indication that violence has occurred or may take place is significant. Signs include broken glass or overturned furniture, arguing, threats, or other violent behavior.
- *Crime scenes.* Try not to disturb a crime scene except as necessary for patient care. Make every effort to preserve evidence. You will learn more about these aspects of emergency care at a crime scene in Chapter 3, "Medical/Legal and Ethical Issues."
- *Alcohol or drug use.* When people are under the influence of alcohol and other drugs, their behavior may be unpredictable. You also may be mistaken for the police because you drove up in a vehicle with lights and sirens.
- *Weapons.* If anyone at the scene (other than the police) is in possession of a weapon, your safety is in danger. Even weapons that are only in view of a hostile person are a potential problem. Remember that almost any item may be used

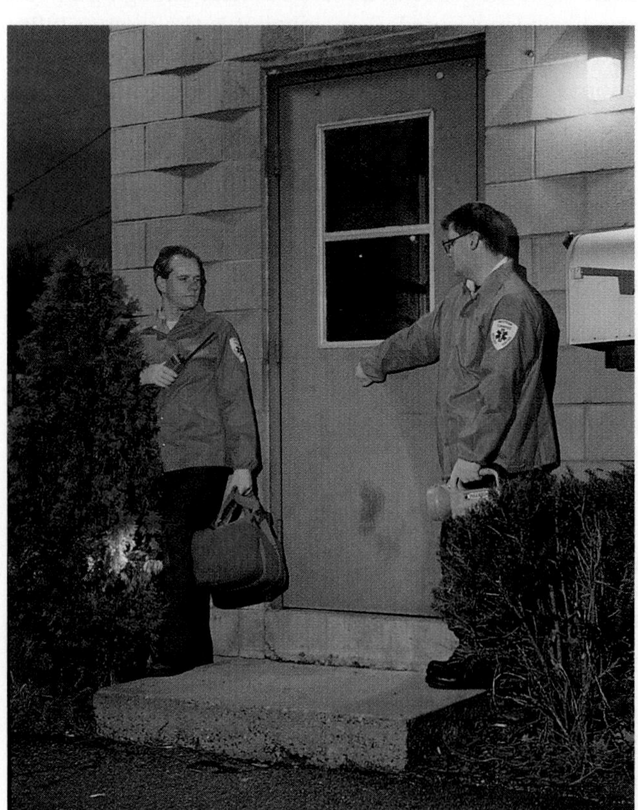

Figure 2-10 • As a safety precaution, do not stand directly in front of a door when knocking or ringing the bell.

as a weapon. Weapons are not limited to knives and guns. If you observe or suspect the presence of any kind of weapon, notify the police immediately.

- *Family members.* Emotional or overwrought family members are often capable of violence or unpredictable behavior. Even though you are there to take care of a loved one, the violence may be directed at you.
- *Bystanders.* Many people gather at the scene of a collision (or anywhere an emergency vehicle parks). Sometimes you will find a bystander or group of bystanders beginning to show aggressive behavior. If this happens, call for the police. In some settings, it may be necessary to place the patient in the ambulance and leave the scene rather than wait for the police.
- *Perpetrators.* A perpetrator of a crime may still be on the scene—in sight or in hiding. Do not enter a crime scene or a scene of violence until police have secured it and told you it is safe to do so.
- *Pets.* While most domestic animals are not dangerous in ordinary circumstances, the presence of an animal at the emergency scene poses problems. Even friendly animals may become defensive when you begin to treat the owner. Animals also can be very distracting, interfere with patient care, and cause falls while you are lifting and moving the patient. No matter what the pet owner says ("He won't hurt you. He's very friendly."), it is usually best to have pets placed securely in another room.

Keep in mind that the vast majority of EMS calls will go by uneventfully. As an EMT, you are a vital part of the EMS system. Nothing in this text is intended to create fear or paranoia. However, when a call does pose some kind of threat, you must be prepared to recognize the subtle and not-so-subtle signs that can warn you before danger strikes.

Reacting to Danger

Observation has provided the critical information needed about the danger. The next step is knowing how to react. The three Rs of reacting to danger are retreat, radio, and reevaluate.

It is not part of your responsibilities as an EMT to subdue a violent person or wrestle a weapon away from anyone. To *retreat* from such dangers is a clear and justified course of action. Note that some ways of retreating are safer than others:

- *Flee.* Get far enough away so you will have time to react should the danger begin to move toward your new position. Place two major obstacles between you and the danger. If the dangerous person gets through one of the obstacles, you have a built-in buffer with the second.
- *Get rid of any cumbersome equipment.* In the event you must flee from the scene, do not get bogged down by your equipment. Discard all of it if this will enhance your ability to get away. Use equipment to your benefit. For example, if you are being pursued, wedge your stretcher in a doorway to slow down the aggressor.
- *Take cover and conceal yourself* (Figure 2-11). Taking cover is finding a position that protects your body from projectiles, such as behind a brick wall. Concealing yourself is hiding your body behind an object that cannot protect you, such as a shrub. Find a position that will both conceal and protect you.

When fleeing danger, your best option is to use distance, cover, and concealment to protect yourself. Do not return to the scene until the police have secured it.

The second R of reacting to danger is *radio.* The portable radio is an important piece of safety equipment. Use it to call for police assistance and to warn other responding units of the danger. Speak into it clearly and slowly. Advise the dispatcher of the exact nature and location of the problem. Specify how many people are involved and whether or not weapons were observed. Remember, the information you have about the scene must be shared as soon as possible to prevent others from encountering the same danger.

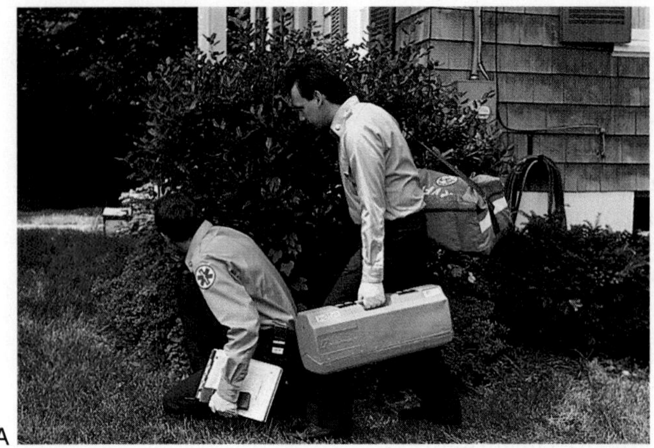

A

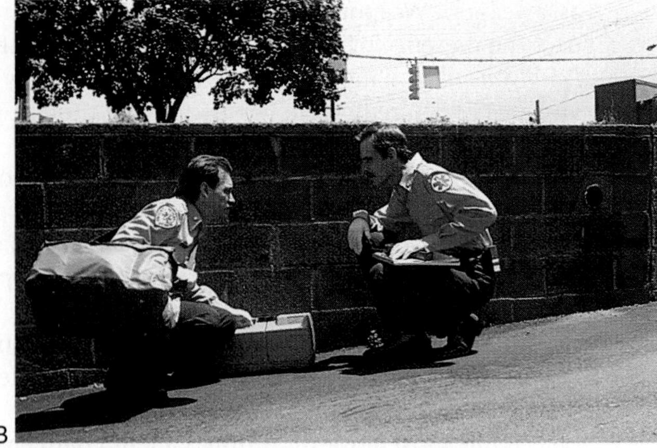

B

Figure 2-11 • (A) Concealing yourself is placing your body behind an object that can hide you from view. (B) Taking cover is finding a position that both hides you and protects your body from projectiles.

Finally, the third R of reacting to danger is *reevaluate*. Do not reenter a scene until it has been secured by the police (Figure 2-12). Even then, be aware that where violence has been, it may begin again. Emergencies are situations packed with stress for families, patients, responders, and bystanders. Maintain a level of alert observation throughout the call. Occasionally you may find weapons or drugs while you are assessing the patient. If that happens, stop what you are doing and radio the police immediately. After the call, document the situation on your run report. Occasionally, the danger may cause delays in reaching the patient. Courts have held this delay acceptable, provided there has been a real and documented danger.

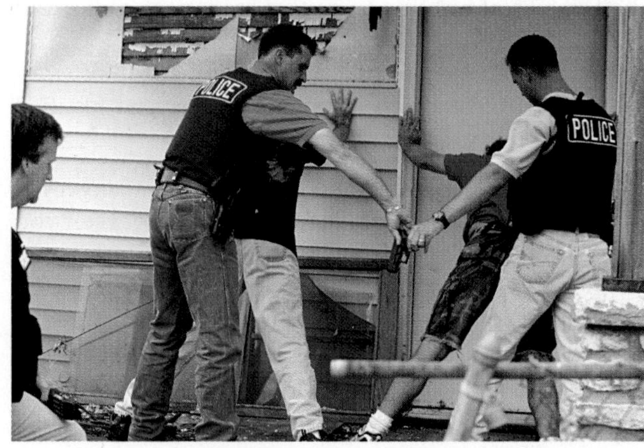

Figure 2-12 • Never enter a scene that is potentially violent until the police have secured it and told you it is safe. *(©Craig Jackson/In the Dark Photography)*

CHAPTER REVIEW

SUMMARY

Safeguarding your well-being as an EMT is critical. One way is to protect yourself from bloodborne and airborne pathogens with the appropriate personal protective equipment (PPE) and other infection-control procedures. Another is to make lifestyle changes that help to reduce the stress associated with treating angry, scared, violent, seriously injured, and ill patients. Finally, you can ensure your personal safety by consistently being alert to the potential for danger at every emergency call.

KEY TERMS

contamination the introduction of dangerous chemicals, disease, or infectious materials.

critical incident stress management (CISM) a comprehensive system that includes education and resources to both prevent stress and to deal with stress appropriately when it occurs.

decontamination the removal or cleansing of dangerous chemicals and other dangerous or infectious materials.

hazardous-material incident the release of a harmful substance into the environment.

multiple-casualty incident (MCI) an emergency involving multiple patients.

pathogens the organisms that cause infection, such as viruses and bacteria.

personal protective equipment (PPE) equipment that protects the EMS worker from infection and/or exposure to the dangers of rescue operations.

Standard Precautions a strict form of infection control that is based on the assumption that all blood and other body fluids are infectious.

stress a state of physical and/or psychological arousal to a stimulus.

REVIEW QUESTIONS

1. Name some of the causes of stress for an EMT and explain some ways the EMT can alleviate job-related stress. (pp. 35–36)
2. Describe the purpose and process of a critical incident stress debriefing (CISD). (pp. 37–38)
3. What are the stages of grief? How should the EMT deal with these emotions? (p. 38)
4. List the types of personal protective equipment used in Standard Precautions. Identify a condition or patient with which each one should be used. (pp. 23–26)

CRITICAL THINKING

- You are called to an unknown emergency at a tavern. As you approach the scene, you see a man lying supine in the parking lot, apparently bleeding profusely. Two other men are scuffling, and one seems to have a gun. What actions must you take?

MEDIA RESOURCES

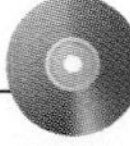

See the Student CD at the back of this book for quizzes, a case study activity, videos, and other features related to this chapter. Also, visit the Companion Website for *Emergency Care* at **www.prenhall.com/limmer**, where you will find additional reinforcement and links to other resources.

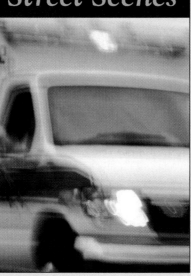

Street Scenes

While you are en route to a motor-vehicle collision, the dispatcher gives your responding ambulance an update. "Ambulance Charlie 7, you have one patient with bad facial injuries." After judging the scene safe to enter, you immediately start to assess the patient. Just as you open the airway and your partner provides oxygen, the paramedic unit arrives and takes over care of the patient.

As you are finishing loading the patient into the back of the paramedic's ambulance, one of them asks where your gloves are. You don't think much of it and start to clean up your equipment. As you get into the ambulance, your partner tells you that not only is it against the ambulance service's standard operating procedure for you not to wear gloves on this type of call, but it is foolish. You reluctantly agree to tell your supervisor.

Later, you enter the supervisor's office, you describe the call, the amount of blood, and then tell her that you did not wear any protective gloves. You also point out that you may have had a partially healed cut on your hand. She tells you that you are out-of-service.

Street Scene Questions

1. Why wear protective gloves on this type of call?
2. What is the impact of an occupational exposure on you, your family, and your fellow EMS workers?
3. What can you expect after exposure?

Your supervisor explains that you need to go to the emergency department for an occupational evaluation. There is a prearrangement with the hospital, and they will have a member of their infection control staff go through your evaluation and counseling.

When you get to the hospital the infection control nurse interviews you and asks many specific questions about the call, your health, and what type of immunizations you have had. She examines your hands for breaks in the skin, and a number are identified. When the interview is over she recommends that you get some baseline blood tests; one is for HIV. All of a sudden you realize how serious this situation is. She recommends that you take some medications, and gives you information on precautions that you need to take when having intimate relations with your spouse. It hits you again how serious this has become.

Street Scene Questions

4. How will stress be a factor in your life for the next few months?
5. How important is hand washing?
6. What type of Standard Precautions should EMTs always be ready to use on all EMS calls?

You try to take your mind off the situation, but you can't. It affects your sleep. You are irritable around your family. When you try to talk to your partner, you find you're too embarrassed.

Quite some time later, the infection control nurse tells you that your latest blood tests are back. They're all negative. A personal tragedy has been avoided. As you start to leave her office, the nurse tells you to remember—gloves and hand washing are very important. With a big smile, you look back and say: "I GET IT!"

CHAPTER

Medical/Legal and Ethical Issues

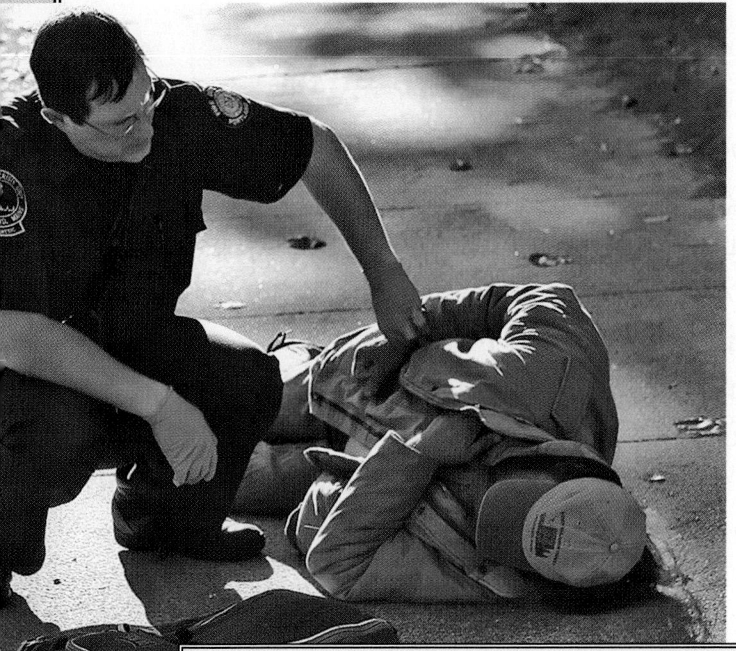

CORE CONCEPTS

The following are core concepts that will be addressed in this chapter:

- The scope of practice of an EMT
- How a patient may consent to or refuse emergency care
- What it means to have a duty to act
- The legal concepts of negligence and abandonment
- The responsibilities of an EMT at a crime scene

KEY TERMS

abandonment, p. 55
advance directive, p. 51
confidentiality, p. 56
consent, p. 49
crime scene, p. 58
do not resuscitate (DNR) order, p. 51
duty to act, p. 55
expressed consent, p. 50
Good Samaritan laws, p. 56
HIPAA, p. 56
implied consent, p. 50
liability, p. 50
negligence, p. 54
organ donor, p. 58
scope of practice, p. 48

DOT OBJECTIVES

*KNOWLEDGE AND ATTITUDE

1-3.1 Define the EMT scope of practice. (p. 48)

1-3.2 Discuss the importance of do not resuscitate (DNR) orders (advance directives) and local or state provisions regarding EMS application. (pp. 51–54)

1-3.3 Define consent and discuss the methods of obtaining consent. (pp. 49–50)

1-3.4 Differentiate between expressed and implied consent. (p. 50)

1-3.5 Explain the role of consent of minors in providing care. (p. 50)

1-3.6 Discuss the implications for the EMT in patient refusal of transport. (pp. 50–51, 52)

1-3.7 Discuss the issues of abandonment, negligence, and battery and their implications to the EMT. (pp. 51, 54–55)

1-3.8 State the conditions necessary for the EMT to have a duty to act. (pp. 55–56)

1-3.9 Explain the importance, necessity, and legality of patient confidentiality. (pp. 56–57)

1-3.10 Discuss the considerations of the EMT in issues of organ retrieval. (pp. 58, 59)

1-3.11 Differentiate the actions that an EMT should take to assist in the preservation of a crime scene. (pp. 58, 60–61)

1-3.12 State the conditions that require an EMT to notify local law enforcement officials. (p. 51)

1-3.13 Explain the role of EMS and the EMT regarding patients with DNR orders. (pp. 51, 53–54)

1-3.14 Explain the rationale for the needs, benefits, and usage of advance directives. (p. 51)

1-3.15 Explain the rationale for the concept of varying degrees of DNR. (p. 53)

Every time you respond to a call, you will be faced with some aspect of medical/legal or medical/ethical issues. The issue may be as simple as making sure that the patient will accept help or as complex as a terminally ill patient who refuses all care. You may also be faced with decisions such as, "Should I stop and help even though I am off duty?" or "Can I get sued if I stop to help outside of my ambulance district?" Understanding of medical, legal, and ethical issues is an essential foundation for all emergency care. This knowledge may also reduce or prevent the legal liability that you may face as a result of calls.

SCOPE OF PRACTICE

scope of practice a set of regulations and ethical considerations that define the scope, or extent and limits, of the EMT's job.

The EMT is governed by many medical, legal, and ethical guidelines. This collective set of regulations and ethical considerations may be referred to as a **scope of practice,** which defines the scope, or extent and limits, of an EMT's job. The skills and medical interventions (what you do to help the patient) the EMT may perform are defined by legislation, which varies from state to state. Sometimes different regions within the same state may have different rules and guidelines for their EMTs.

For example, an EMT in one area may be able to perform certain basic procedures and levels of care. In the adjoining region, EMTs may provide that care and in addition perform special advanced procedures. Your duty is to provide for the well-being of the patient by rendering necessary and legally allowed care as defined under the scope of practice in your area.

Falling within your scope of practice are certain ethical responsibilities. The primary ethical consideration is to make patient care and well-being a priority, even if this requires some personal sacrifice. For example, there may be times when a patient feels cold, even in a hot climate. You may want to turn on the air conditioner in the ambulance, but you refrain out of consideration for your patient. Actions such as this may seem small but mean a lot to the patient.

To be an effective EMT, you must maintain your skills and knowledge. This includes practicing until you have obtained confidence and mastery of the skills. After that, continuing education and recertification are necessary to maintain mastery. Every patient deserves the best care.

Emergency care can be improved on a crew and squad level as well as on an individual level. After a call, constructively critique both yourself and the crew. Accept suggestions from others to improve your skills, communication, and patient outcome. Participation in this kind of mutual critique is part of the process known as *quality improvement*. It should be practiced with the aim of maintaining the standards you would wish to have provided for yourself or someone in your family.

During the rest of this chapter, you will learn about some specific aspects of the scope of practice.

PATIENT CONSENT AND REFUSAL

Consent

Consent, or permission from the patient, is required for any treatment or action by the EMT. Most patients or their families will have called for your assistance and will readily accept it. A simple statement, such as, "I'm Karla Maguire, an EMT from the ambulance. I'd like to help you, okay?" is enough to request consent. Most patients will respond positively. Expressed consent must be obtained from every conscious, mentally competent adult before providing care and transportation.

consent
permission from the patient for care or other action by the EMT.

The principle of consent may seem simple, but it often brings up complex issues in patient care. There are three types of consent: expressed, implied, and consent to treat minors or incompetent patients.

CRITICAL DECISION MAKING: ETHICAL DILEMMAS

Not all critical or difficult decisions you make will be clinical in nature. You may be faced with an ethical dilemma that will test your decision-making skills. For each of the situations listed below describe how you would handle the situation. It may be helpful to list the options available to you in each case and then choose the course you think best.

- You are driving the ambulance to the hospital and listening to the conversation in the back between a paramedic and an EMT. You hear the paramedic say, "Oh, no! I can't believe I just did that. I gave her 10 times the dose I was supposed to." You hear the paramedic ask the EMT not to tell anyone. What do you do?
- You are on the way home from a sporting event. While there you had two drinks. You come across a crash with injury. What do you do?
- A patient tells you that he received the injury you are treating while climbing a fence after being involved in a break-in at a local business. The patient swears he was just the lookout, and if anyone knows he told he may be killed. What do you do?

Expressed Consent

expressed consent consent given by adults who are of legal age and mentally competent to make a rational decision in regard to their medical well-being.

Expressed consent, the consent given by adults who are of legal age and mentally competent to make a rational decision in regard to their medical well-being, must be obtained from all patients who are physically or mentally able to give it. Expressed consent must be *informed consent.* That is, patients must understand the risks associated with the care they will receive. It is not only a legal requirement but also sound emotional care to explain all procedures to the patient.

Implied Consent

In the case of an unconscious patient, consent may be assumed. The law states that rational patients would consent to treatment if they were conscious. This is known as **implied consent.** In this situation, the law allows EMTs and other health care providers to provide treatment, at least until the patient becomes conscious and able to make rational decisions.

implied consent the consent it is presumed a patient or patient's parent or guardian would give if they could, such as for an unconscious patient or a parent who cannot be contacted when care is needed.

Children and Mentally Incompetent Adults

Children and mentally incompetent adults are not legally allowed to provide consent or refuse medical care and transportation. The parents and guardians of these patients have the legal authority to give consent, so it must be obtained before care can be given. There are times, however, when care may be given without this direct consent from a parent or guardian.

In cases of life-threatening illness or injury when a parent or guardian is not present, care may be given based on implied consent. The law provides that it is reasonable to believe that a responsible parent or guardian would consent to care if he were present. In some states, statutes allow emancipated minors—those who are married or of a certain age—to provide consent. Find out the laws where you will practice as an EMT in reference to consent of minors.

When a Patient Refuses Care

You may think that all patients who need medical care will accept it. Most do. However, you will find that some patients who require treatment and transportation to the hospital will refuse care. Many reasons exist for this, including denial, fear, failing to understand the seriousness of the situation, intoxication, and others.

While patients generally have the right to refuse care, it is your responsibility as an EMT to be sure that the patient is fully informed about his situation and the implications of refusing care.

In order for a patient to refuse care or transport, several conditions must be fulfilled:

- *Patient must be legally able to consent.* He must be of legal age or an emancipated minor.
- *Patient must be mentally competent and oriented.* He must not be affected by any disease or condition that would impair judgment. These conditions include unstable vital signs and altered mental status.
- *Patient must be fully informed.* He must understand the risks associated with refusing treatment and/or transport.
- *Patient must sign a "release" form.* Such a form is designed to release the ambulance squad and individuals from **liability** (legal responsibility) arising from the patient's informed refusal.

liability being held legally responsible.

Even carefully following these steps will not guarantee that you will be free from liability if a patient refuses care or transport. Leaving a patient who will not accept care or transport is a leading cause of lawsuits against EMS agencies and providers, even though it was the patient who refused. Occasionally the patient's condition deteriorates to the point of unconsciousness, which leaves the patient unable to summon help, leading to a severely worsened condition or even death.

In addition to the liability factor, there is also an ethical issue. You would undoubtedly feel guilty if a patient was found unconscious or deceased after refusing care and you felt that transportation would have prevented the circumstance.

If in doubt, do everything possible to persuade the patient to accept care and transport. Take all possible actions to persuade a patient who you feel should go to the hospital but refuses. These actions may include:

- *Spend time speaking to the patient.* Use principles of effective communication. It may take reasoning, persistence, "dealing" ("We'll call a neighbor to take care of your cat, but then you go to the hospital"), or other strategies.
- *Inform the patient of the consequences of not going to the hospital,* even if they are not pleasant.
- *Consult medical direction.* If you are in a residence, use the patient's phone to contact medical direction. If the on-line doctor is willing, let him speak to the patient when all else fails.
- *Contact family members to help convince the patient.* Often family members can provide the patient with reasons to go to the hospital. An offer from a loved one to meet the patient at the hospital may be very helpful.
- *Call law enforcement personnel if necessary.* Police may be able to order or "arrest" the patient who refuses care to force him to go to the hospital. This is done under the premise that the patient is temporarily mentally incompetent as demonstrated by refusing care that might save his life.
- *Try to determine why the patient is refusing care.* Often the patient has a fear of the hospital, procedures, prolonged hospitalization, or even death. Refusal to go to the hospital may be a form of denial or unwillingness to accept the idea of being ill. If you identify the cause of the refusal, you may be able to develop a strategy to persuade the patient to accept your care and transportation to the hospital.

Bear in mind, however, that you do not have the right in most cases to force a competent patient to go to the hospital against his will. Subjecting the patient to unwanted care and transport has actually been viewed as assault or battery in court.

If all efforts fail and the patient does not accept your care or transportation, it becomes vital to document the attempts you made—to make your efforts a part of the official record—in order to prevent liability. Write into your records every step you took to persuade the patient to accept care or to go to the hospital. Include the names of any witnesses to your attempts and the patient's refusal. (A sample EMS patient refusal procedures checklist is shown in Figure 3-1.)

In all cases of refusal, you should advise the patient that he should call back at any time if he has a problem or wishes to be cared for or transported. It is advisable to call a relative or neighbor who can stay with the patient in case problems develop. Leave phone stickers with emergency numbers so the patient will be able to call for help if necessary. You should also recommend that the patient or a relative call the family physician to report the incident and arrange for follow-up care. Document all actions you have taken for the patient.

While there may be patients who legitimately refuse care (for minor wounds, unfounded calls, and the like) a patient with any significant medical condition should be transported and seen at a hospital.

Do Not Resuscitate Orders

It will only be a matter of time before you come upon a patient who has a **do not resuscitate (DNR) order** (Figure 3-2). This is a legal document, usually signed by the patient and his physician, which states that the patient has a terminal illness and does not wish to prolong life through resuscitative efforts. A DNR order is called an **advance directive,** because it is written and signed in advance of any event where resuscitation might be undertaken. It is more than the expressed wishes of the patient or family. It is an actual legal document.

do not resuscitate (DNR) order
a legal document, usually signed by the patient and his physician, which states that the patient has a terminal illness and does not wish to prolong life through resuscitative efforts.

advance directive
a DNR order; instructions written in advance of an event.

EMS PATIENT REFUSAL CHECKLIST

PATIENT'S NAME: ______________________ AGE: __________

LOCATION OF CALL: ______________________ DATE: __________

AGENCY INCIDENT #: __________ AGENCY CODE: ______________________

NAME OF PERSON FILLING OUT FORM: ______________________

I. ASSESSMENT OF PATIENT (Check appropriate response for each item)

1. Oriented to: Person? ☐ Yes ☐ No
   Place? ☐ Yes ☐ No
   Time? ☐ Yes ☐ No
   Situation? ☐ Yes ☐ No
2. Altered level of consciousness? ☐ Yes ☐ No
3. Head injury? ☐ Yes ☐ No
4. Alcohol or drug ingestion by exam or history? ☐ Yes ☐ No

II. PATIENT INFORMED (Check appropriate response for each item)

☐ Yes ☐ No Medical treatment/evaluation needed

☐ Yes ☐ No Ambulance transport needed

☐ Yes ☐ No Further harm could result without medical treatment/evaluation

☐ Yes ☐ No Transport by means other than ambulance could be hazardous in light of patient's illness/injury

☐ Yes ☐ No Patient provided with Refusal Information Sheet

☐ Yes ☐ No Patient accepted Refusal Information Sheet

III. DISPOSITION

☐ Refused all EMS assistance

☐ Refused field treatment, but accepted transport

☐ Refused transport, but accepted field treatment

☐ Refused transport to recommended facility

☐ Patient transported by private vehicle to __________

☐ Released in care or custody of self

☐ Released in care or custody of relative or friend

Name: __________ Relationship: __________

☐ Released in custody of law enforcement agency

Agency: __________ Officer: __________

☐ Released in custody of other agency

Agency: __________ Officer: __________

IV. COMMENTS: ______________________

____

____

____

Figure 3-1 • Certain procedures should be followed when a patient refuses care or transport. The checklist is from Spokane County Emergency Medical Services, Washington State.

PREHOSPITAL DO NOT RESUSCITATE ORDERS

ATTENDING PHYSICIAN

In completing this prehospital DNR form, please check part A if no intervention by prehospital personnel is indicated. Please check Part A and options from Part B if specific interventions by prehospital personnel are indicated. To give a valid prehospital DNR order, this form must be completed by the patient's attending physician and must be provided to prehospital personnel.

A) ____________ **Do Not Resuscitate (DNR):**
No Cardiopulmonary Resuscitation or Advanced Cardiac Life Support be performed by prehospital personnel

B) ____________ **Modified Support:**
Prehospital personnel administer the following checked options:

____________ Oxygen administration
____________ Full airway support: intubation, airways, bag/valve/mask
____________ Venipuncture: IV crystalloids and/or blood draw
____________ External cardiac pacing
____________ Cardiopulmonary resuscitation
____________ Cardiac defibrillator
____________ Pneumatic anti-shock garment
____________ Ventilator
____________ ACLS meds
____________ Other interventions/medications (physician specify)

____

Prehospital personnel are informed that (print patient name)____________________ should receive no resuscitation (DNR) or should receive Modified Support as indicated. This directive is medically appropriate and is further documented by a physician's order and a progress note on the patient's permanent medical record. Informed consent from the capacitated patient or the incapacitated patient's legitimate surrogate is documented on the patient's permanent medical record. The DNR order is in full force and effect as of the date indicated below.

Attending Physician's Signature	
Print Attending Physician's Name	Print Patient's Name and Location (Home Address or Health Care Facility)
Attending Physician's Telephone	
Date	Expiration Date (6 Mos from Signature)

Figure 3-2 • Example of a do not resuscitate (DNR) order.

There are varying degrees of DNR orders, expressed through a variety of detailed instructions that may be part of the order. Such an instruction might stipulate, for example, that resuscitation be attempted only if cardiac or respiratory arrest is observed, but not attempted if the patient is found already in arrest (to avoid the possibility of resuscitating a patient who may already have sustained brain damage).

Many states also have laws governing living wills, which are statements signed by the patient, usually regarding use of long-term life-support and comfort measures such as respirators, intravenous feedings, and pain medications. Other states require naming a *proxy*—a person whom the signer of the document names to make health care decisions in case he is unable to make such decisions for himself. Living wills and health

POINT OF VIEW

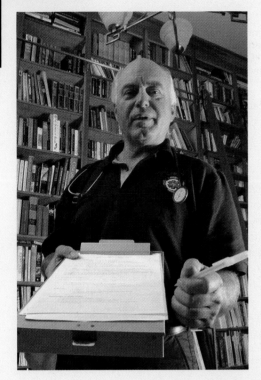

"My wife said I passed out. I don't remember passing out. To be honest, I don't remember much about it at all. I woke up and the ambulance was there. They said they'd take me to the hospital if I wanted. Who wants to go to the hospital? Not me, that's for sure. My parents died in the hospital. My brother died at the hospital. The best thing I could do was stay out of the hospital.

"My wife looked so nervous. She almost convinced me to go. And the boys on the ambulance. No, one was a girl. Nice kids. They put a clipboard in front of me. Wanted me to sign something. Not sure what. I can't hear much anymore anyway. They were telling me all kinds of things in big medical words. At my age what difference does it make anyway?

"So I signed it."

care proxies usually pertain to situations that will occur in the hospital rather than in the prehospital situation.

Become familiar with the laws regarding DNR orders, living wills, and health care proxies for your region or state and the laws and rules governing their implementation. It is important to know the forms and policies before you go to the call, since often the patient is in cardiac arrest (heart and breathing have stopped) or near death. These are stressful times for the family and for you, occasions when the window of time for making a resuscitation decision may be only a few moments.

A legal DNR order prevents unwanted resuscitation and awkward situations. In most cases, the oral requests of a family member are not reason to withhold care. If the family requests you to not resuscitate the patient, and if there are no legal DNR orders available, it is a legal and ethical dilemma that is usually best resolved by providing care. It is better to be criticized or sued for attempting to save a life than for letting a patient die.

OTHER LEGAL ASPECTS

negligence
a finding of failure to act properly in a situation in which there was a duty to act, that needed care as would reasonably be expected of the EMT was not provided, and that harm was caused to the patient as a result.

Negligence

To the layperson, **negligence** means that something that should have been done was not done or was done incorrectly. The legal concept of negligence in emergency care is not that simple. A finding of negligence, or failure to act properly, requires that *all* of the following circumstances be proved:

- The EMT had a duty to the patient (duty to act—see the next section).
- The EMT did not provide the standard of care (committed a breach of duty). This may include the failure to act; that is, he did not provide needed care as would

be expected of an EMT in your locality. Failure to act is a major cause of legal actions against EMS systems or EMTs.
- By not providing the standard of care, the EMT caused harm to the patient. This harm can be physical or psychological.

Negligence is the basis for a large number of lawsuits involving prehospital emergency care. If the previously listed circumstances are proved, the EMT may be required to pay damages if the court considers the harm to the patient to be a loss that requires reimbursement (compensable). The negligent EMT may be required to pay for medical expenses, lost wages (possibly including future earnings), pain and suffering, and various other factors as determined by the court.

Two of the most common and significant causes of lawsuits against EMTs are patient refusal and ambulance collisions (Figure 3-3). In patient refusal situations, EMTs are sued because the patient's condition deteriorated after the ambulance left the scene. This makes it critical to follow your agency's guidelines when a patient refuses care.

Collisions are dangerous in any vehicle. When an ambulance is involved, collisions become serious because of the size and weight of the vehicle, the number of occupants (including the patient), and the nature of emergency driving. It is important to remember that most collisions are preventable. (This is why they are no longer referred to as "accidents.") Emergency driving must be done responsibly.

Lawsuits against EMTs are actually quite rare, especially when compared to the number of calls that are dispatched each day in this country. While liability and negligence should be important considerations, you should not live or work in fear of a lawsuit. When you perform proper care that is within your scope of practice and is properly documented, you will prevent most, if not all, legal problems.

Duty to Act

An EMT in certain situations has a **duty to act,** or an obligation to provide emergency care to a patient. An EMT who is on an ambulance and is dispatched to a call clearly has a duty to act. If there is no threat to safety, the EMT must provide care. This duty to act continues throughout the call.

If an EMT has initiated care, then leaves a patient without ensuring that the patient has been turned over to someone with equal or greater medical training, **abandonment** exists.

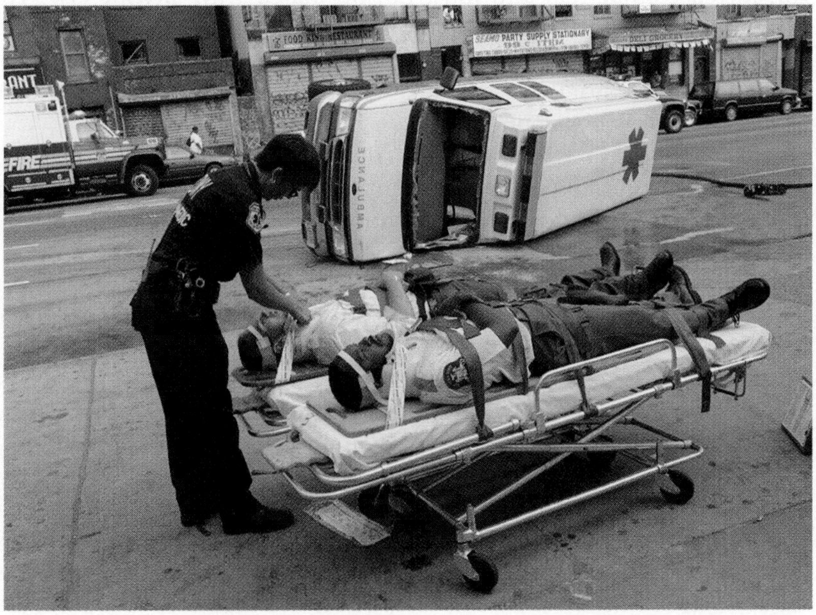

duty to act
an obligation to provide care to a patient.

abandonment
leaving a patient after care has been initiated and before the patient has been transferred to someone with equal or greater medical training.

Figure 3-3 • Ambulance collisions cause injuries and prompt lawsuits. *(© David Handschuh)*

The duty to act is not always clear. It depends on your state and local laws. In many states, an off-duty EMT has no legal obligation to provide care. However, you may feel a moral or ethical obligation to act; for example, if you observe a motor-vehicle collision while off duty. You may feel morally bound to provide care, even if no legal obligation exists. If you are off duty, begin care, and then leave before other trained personnel arrive, you may still be considered to have abandoned the patient.

Other situations are even more confusing. If you are an EMT in an ambulance, but you are out of your jurisdiction, the laws are again often unclear. In general, if you follow your conscience and provide care, you will incur less liability than if you do not act. Always follow your local protocols and laws. Your instructor will provide information about local issues.

Good Samaritan Laws

Good Samaritan laws a series of laws, varying in each state, designed to provide limited legal protection for citizens and some health care personnel when they are administering emergency care.

Good Samaritan laws have been developed in all states to provide immunity to individuals trying to help people in emergencies. Most of these laws will grant immunity from liability if the rescuer acts in good faith to provide care to the level of his training and to the best of his ability. These laws do not prevent someone from initiating a lawsuit, nor will they protect the rescuer from being found liable for acts of gross negligence and other violations of the law.

You must familiarize yourself with the laws that govern your state. Good Samaritan laws may not apply to EMTs in your locality. In some states, the Good Samaritan laws apply only to volunteers. If you are a paid EMT, different laws and regulations may apply.

Some states have specific statutes that authorize, regulate, and protect EMS personnel. Typically, to be protected by such laws, you must be recognized as an EMT in the state where care was provided. Some states have specific licensing and certification requirements that must be met for recognition under Good Samaritan laws.

Confidentiality

When you act as an EMT, you obtain a considerable amount of information about a patient. You also are allowed into homes and other personal areas that are private and contain much information about people.

confidentiality the obligation not to reveal information obtained about a patient except to other health care professionals involved in the patient's care, or under subpoena, or in a court of law, or when the patient has signed a release of confidentiality.

HIPAA the Health Insurance Portability and Accountability Act, a federal law protecting the privacy of patient-specific health care information and providing the patient with control over how this information is used and distributed.

Any information you obtain about a patient's history, condition, or treatment is considered confidential and must not be shared with anyone else. This principle is known as **confidentiality.** Such information may be disclosed only when a written release is signed by the patient. Your organization will have a policy on this. Patient information should not be disclosed based on verbal permission, nor should information be disclosed over the telephone.

However, you may be subpoenaed, or ordered into court by a legal authority, where you may legally disclose patient information (Figure 3-4). If you have a question about the validity of a legal document, contact a supervisor or your agency's attorney for advice.

Patient information also may be shared with other health care professionals who will have a role in the patient's care or in quality improvement. It is appropriate to turn over information about the patient to the nurse and physician at the receiving hospital. This is necessary for continuity in patient care. It may also be necessary and permissible to supply certain patient-care information for insurance billing forms.

While confidentiality has always been a part of health care, newer regulations have given it even greater emphasis. The Health Insurance Portability and Accountability Act **(HIPAA)** has brought significant changes to the record-keeping, storage, access, and discussion of patient-specific medical information. Ambulance services that bill for services (electronically or by employing a service that does this work) are mandated to

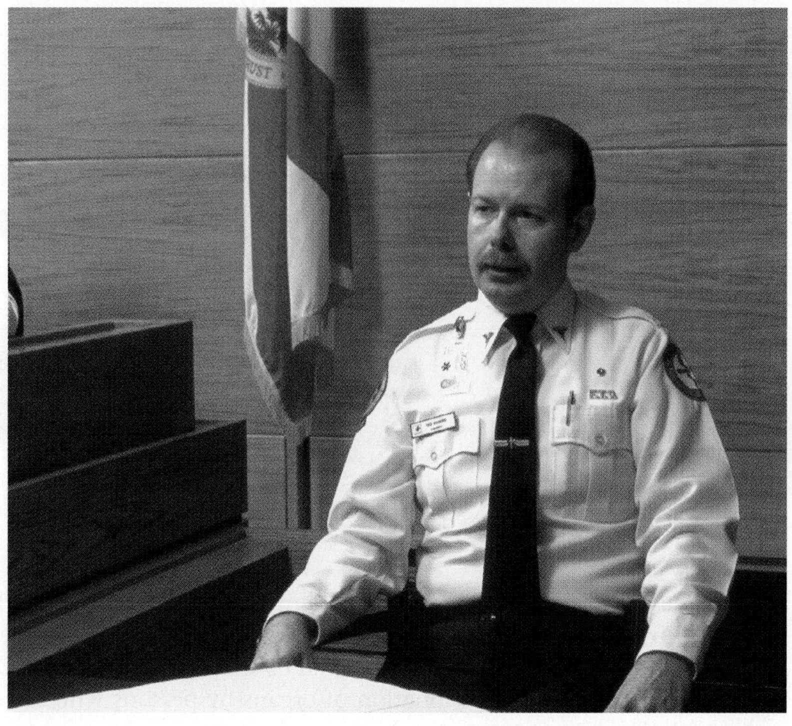

Figure 3-4 • An EMT may be required to testify in court in a variety of legal settings.

have policies, procedures, and training in place to deal with these privacy issues. Table 3-1 summarizes key points about HIPAA and how it will impact your work as an EMT.

Special Situations

A patient may wear a medical identification device (Figure 3-5) to alert EMTs and other health care professionals that he has a particular medical condition. If the patient is found unconscious, the device provides important medical information. The device may be a necklace, bracelet, or card and may indicate a number of conditions including:

- Heart conditions
- Allergies
- Diabetes
- Epilepsy

TABLE 3-1 • Health Insurance Portability and Accountability Act (HIPAA)

When you go through ambulance orientation, or when you begin to work or volunteer, you will likely hear much about HIPAA regulations. These federal regulations are designed to limit access to records by unnecessary personnel as well as to provide the patient the right to review his or her information and have a greater say in its use and distribution. How will this affect you as an EMT?

- You will discuss patient-specific information only with those with whom it is medically necessary to do so.
- Your EMS agency will have specific privacy policies and procedures in place.
- You will get a printed copy of these policies and procedures as will the patients in your care. You will ask your patients to sign a form indicating they have received this information. This form may be combined with your insurance-release form.
- Your EMS agency will have a Privacy Officer to oversee HIPAA issues and deal with the documentation required by law.

Remember that you will be provided information about your agency's specific privacy policies and procedures.

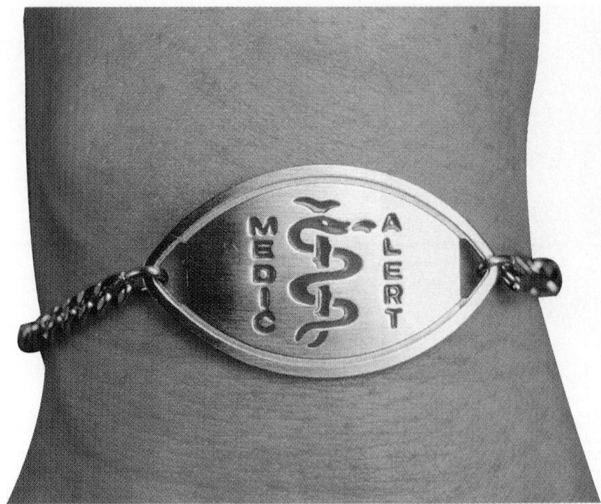

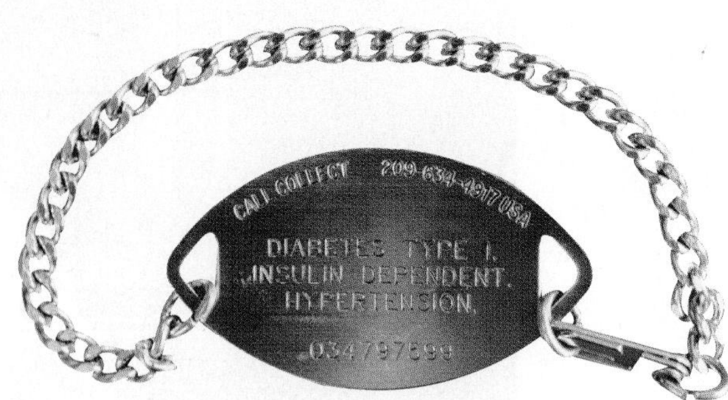

Figure 3-5 • Example of a medical identification device (front and back).

organ donor
a person who has completed a legal document that allows for donation of organs and tissues in the event of death.

You may respond to calls where a patient is critically injured, perhaps near death, and is an **organ donor.** An organ donor is a patient who has completed a legal document that allows for donation of organs and tissues in the event of his death. Many people have benefited from the donation of organs by persons who have completed this paperwork (Figure 3-6).

You may find that the patient is an organ donor when told so by a family member. Often a patient may have an organ donor card on him. The back of the patient's driver's license may also contain an indication that the patient wishes to donate organs upon his death.

The emergency care of a patient who is an organ donor must not differ from the care of a patient who is not a donor. All emergency care measures must be taken. If a patient is recognized as an organ donor, contact medical direction. The on-line physician may order you to perform CPR on a patient when you might normally not resuscitate due to fatal injuries. The oxygen delivered to body cells by CPR will help preserve the organs until they can be harvested for implantation in another person.

Crime Scenes

crime scene
the location where a crime has been committed or any place that evidence relating to a crime may be found.

A **crime scene** is defined as the location where a crime has been committed or any place that evidence relating to a crime may be found. Many crime scenes involve crimes against people. These crimes cause injuries that are often serious. Once police have made the scene safe, the EMT's priority at a crime scene is to provide patient care.

While you are providing care at the crime scene, there are actions that you can take to help preserve evidence. To preserve evidence, you must first know what evidence is, as described in the following list:

- *Condition of the scene.* The way you find the scene is important evidence to the police. Should you arrive first, make a mental note of the exterior of the scene. Remember how you gained access. Doors found ajar, pry marks, and broken windows are signs of danger for you and important evidence for the police. Make a note of whether the lights were on or off and the condition of the TV and radio.
- *The patient.* The patient himself provides valuable information. The position the patient is found in, condition of clothing, and injuries are all valuable pieces of evidence.
- *Fingerprints and footprints.* Fingerprints are perhaps the most familiar kind of evidence. They may be obtained from almost any surface. It is important for you to avoid unnecessarily touching anything at the scene in order to preserve prints. Since you will be wearing gloves at most scenes, you will not leave your

Valley General Hospital
Permission For
Organ Donation/Anatomical Gift
By An Individual Prior To Death

PATIENT IDENTIFICATION PLATE

I, ______________________________ , currently residing at ______________________________

______________________________ , being eighteen (18) years of age or older, do hereby make the following organ donation/anatomical gift to take effect upon my death:

1. I give, if medically acceptable:
   - ☐ My body
   - ☐ Any needed organs or parts
   - ☐ The following organs or parts: ______________________________

     ____

     ____

2. I make this gift to Valley General Hospital or to physicians or institutions designated by them for the following purposes:
   - ☐ Any purpose authorized by law
   - ☐ Transplantation
   - ☐ Therapy
   - ☐ Medical Research and/or Education

3. I acknowledge that I have read this document in its entirety and that I fully understand it and that all blank spaces have either been completed or crossed off prior to my signing.

4. I understand that Valley General Hospital and its authorized designees will rely upon this consent.

______________________________ ______________________________

SIGNATURE DATE | WITNESS TO SIGNATURE (PRINT NAME and ADDRESS BELOW) DATE

____

PRINT NAME

____

ADDRESS

____

TELEPHONE NUMBER

____

WITNESS TO SIGNATURE (PRINT NAME and ADDRESS BELOW) DATE

____

____

Figure 3-6 • Example of an organ donor form.

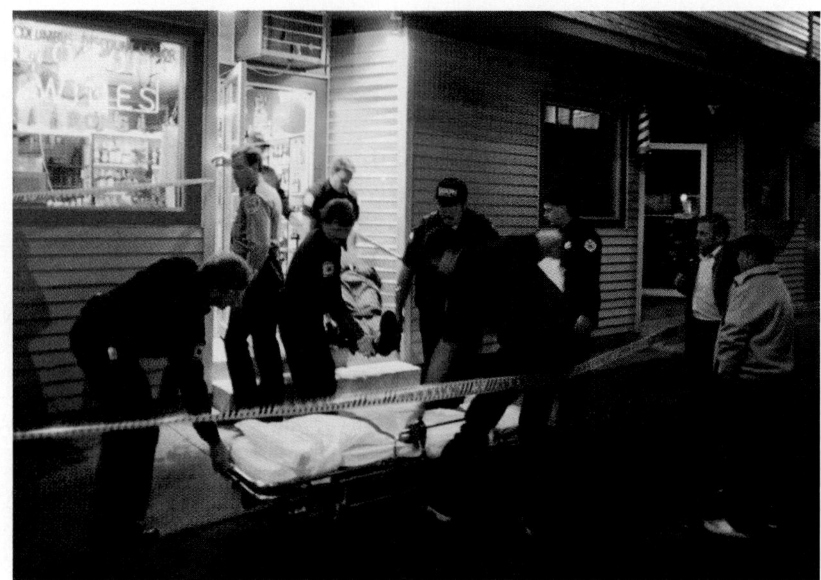

Figure 3-7 • A crime scene. *(© Craig Jackson/In the Dark Photography)*

fingerprints on objects. If you touch these objects, however, even while wearing gloves, you may smudge fingerprints that were left by someone else.

- *Microscopic evidence.* Microscopic evidence is a wide range of evidence that is usually invisible to the naked eye. It consists of small pieces of evidence such as dirt and carpet fibers. To the eye, there may be no way to distinguish one from another. Under the microscope, scientists can develop valuable information. From just a few fibers, the materials and sometimes the brand name of carpets or clothes can be determined. Traces of blood may be enough to determine blood type or to be used for DNA comparison.

To preserve evidence at the crime scene (Figure 3-7), the following actions will be helpful to the police. Remember that your first priority is always patient care.

- *Remember what you touch.* It may be necessary to move the patient or furniture to begin CPR or other patient care. This cannot be avoided, but it is helpful to tell the police what you have touched or moved. Once you leave, if they find furniture moved or blood stains in two locations, they may think that a scuffle took place when in fact it did not. If you are forced to break a window to get to the patient and do not tell the police, they will think that a breaking-and-entering has occurred.
- *Minimize your impact on the scene.* If you are forced to move the patient or furniture to begin care, move as little as possible. Do not wander through the house or go to areas where it is not necessary to go. Avoid using the phone, as this will prevent the police from using the "redial" button to determine who the victim called last. Do not use the bathroom since this may also destroy evidence.
- *Work with the police.* The police may require you to provide a statement about your actions or observations at the scene. While it may not be possible to make notes while patient care is going on, after you arrive at the hospital make notes about your observations and actions at the scene.

You may also wish to critique the scene—both with your crew and, if possible, with the police. Invite a member of your local or state police department to your agency for an in-service drill on crime scenes. Evidence recovery methods and procedures vary from area to area. The police officer who comes to your station will brief you on local procedures.

Interestingly enough, police are often as unfamiliar with EMS procedures as you are with police evidence procedures. The police may ask you to delay your work at the scene so they can take photographs or interview the patient. They may do this because they do not understand—as you will learn in later chapters—that in the case of serious injury, the time that elapses before on-scene care and transport to the hospital must be kept to a minimum for the patient to have the best chance of survival. Education and critiques can be beneficial to both EMTs and police officers.

Special Crimes and Reporting

Many states require EMTs and other health care professionals to report certain types of incidents. Many areas have hotlines for reporting crimes such as child, elder, or domestic abuse. This may be mandatory in your area. Failure to report certain incidents may actually be a crime. There is also a strong moral obligation to report these crimes. Many states offer immunity from liability for people who report incidents such as these in good faith.

Other crimes may also require reports. Violence (such as gunshot wounds or stabbings) and sexual assaults often fall into this category. If you are required by law to report such incidents, you are usually exempt from confidentiality requirements in making these reports.

You may also be required to notify police of other situations, such as cases where restraint may be necessary, intoxicated persons found with injuries, or mentally incompetent people who have been injured.

CHAPTER REVIEW

SUMMARY

Medical, legal, and ethical issues are a part of every EMS call. A number of such issues involve consent, the permission a patient or the patient's parent or guardian gives for care or transport. Consent may be expressed or implied. If a competent patient refuses care or transport, you should make every effort to persuade him, but you cannot force him to accept care or go to the hospital.

Negligence is failing to act properly when you have a duty to act. As an EMT, you have a duty to act whenever you are dispatched on a call. You may have a legal or moral duty to act even when off duty or outside your jurisdiction. Abandonment is leaving a patient after you have initiated care and before you have transferred the patient to a person with equal or higher training. Confidentiality is the obligation not to reveal personal information you obtain about a patient except to other health care professionals involved in the patient's care, under court order or when the patient signs a release. As an EMT, you may be sued or held legally liable on any of these issues. However, EMTs are rarely held liable when they have acted within their scope of practice and have carefully documented the details of the call.

Special situations include patients who are organ donors (care of the patient takes precedence; follow the advice of medical direction) and patients who wear medical identification devices. At a crime scene, care of the patient takes precedence over preservation of evidence, but you should make every effort not to disturb the scene unnecessarily and to report your actions and observations to the police.

KEY TERMS

abandonment leaving a patient after care has been initiated and before the patient has been transferred to someone with equal or greater medical training.

advance directive a DNR order.

confidentiality the obligation not to reveal information obtained about a patient except to other health care professionals involved in the patient's care, or under subpoena, or in a court of law, or when the patient has signed a release of confidentiality.

consent permission from the patient for care or other action by the EMT.

crime scene the location where a crime has been committed or any place that evidence relating to a crime may be found.

do not resuscitate (DNR) order a legal document, usually signed by the patient and his physician, which states that the patient has a terminal illness and does not wish to prolong life through resuscitative efforts.

duty to act an obligation to provide care to a patient.

expressed consent consent given by adults who are of legal age and mentally competent to make a rational decision in regard to their medical well-being.

Good Samaritan laws a series of laws, varying in each state, designed to provide limited legal protection for citizens and some health care personnel when they are administering emergency care.

HIPAA The Health Insurance Portability and Accountability Act, a federal law protecting the privacy of patient-specific health care information and providing the patient with control over how this information is used and distributed.

implied consent the consent it is presumed a patient or patient's parent or guardian would give if they could, such as for an unconscious patient or a parent who cannot be contacted when care is needed.

liability being held legally responsible.

negligence a finding of failure to act properly in a situation in which there was a duty to act, that needed care as would reasonably be expected of the EMT was not provided, and that harm was caused to the patient as a result.

organ donor a person who has completed a legal document that allows for donation of organs and tissues in the event of death.

scope of practice a set of regulations and ethical considerations that define the scope, or extent and limits, of the EMT's job.

REVIEW QUESTIONS

1. Define *scope of practice*, *negligence*, *duty to act*, *abandonment*, and *confidentiality*. (pp. 48, 54, 55, 56)
2. List several steps that must be taken when a patient refuses care or transportation. (pp. 50–51)
3. List several types of evidence and ways you may act to preserve it at a crime scene. (pp. 58, 60–61)

CRITICAL THINKING

- You are called to the scene of a motor-vehicle collision. An 8-year-old child has been struck by a vehicle and fortunately has sustained only slight injuries. Who can give consent for her care? How might you obtain consent?

MEDIA RESOURCES 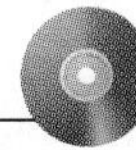

See the Student CD at the back of this book for quizzes, a case study activity, and other features related to this chapter. Also, visit the Companion Website for *Emergency Care* at **www.prenhall.com/limmer**, where you will find additional reinforcement and links to other resources.

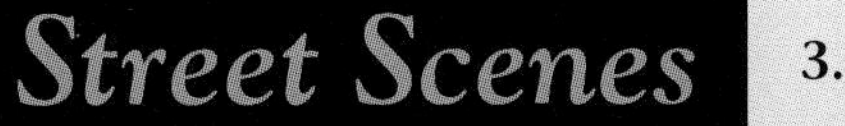

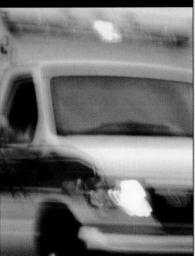

It is a hot summer day when you receive a call for a 37-year-old woman with general body weakness. After your initial assessment, you ask the patient about her medical history. She informs you that she has AIDS. You continue to take vital signs, find it appropriate to provide oxygen, and package her for transport. Your partner makes the radio report to the hospital, and you notice that he makes no reference to AIDS. When you arrive at the hospital, your partner gives the patient report in the hallway leading to the examination room. He provides all the patient information but does not tell the doctor the patient reported she has AIDS until he can do it discreetly in the room. He asks the patient to sign a form that allows release of information for insurance billing and acknowledges receipt of the Notice of Privacy Practices in place at your agency.

Street Scene Questions

1. Was it appropriate not to include the information that the patient has AIDS during the radio report to the hospital?
2. What is the obligation of these EMTs concerning the confidentiality of patient information?
3. Would you have handled the transfer of information differently?

After the call is over, you discuss with your partner issues of confidentiality. He tells you that he felt the fact the patient had AIDS did not need to be part of the radio report. He was concerned that it might breach the patient's confidentiality if it was said over the radio. But your partner was quick to add that AIDS was definitely a pertinent part of the medical history and he made sure it was conveyed in a discreet manner at the hospital.

Street Scene Question

4. Would it be appropriate to tell all the hospital staff so they would know to take infection control precautions?

As you and your partner further discuss the issue, you tell him that alerting the hospital staff so they would know to use infection control precautions would be appropriate. He responds by telling you that all emergency medical personnel, whether EMS or in-hospital, should be taking infection control precautions. However, this should not be a reason for being careless with patient information and possibly breaching a patient's confidentiality.

Street Scene Questions

5. Should the information that this patient has AIDS be shared with other EMS providers in case they get a call for this patient?
6. What are the principles for confidentiality that EMTs should always maintain?

As you pull into the garage, you suggest to your partner that you should alert the other crews about this patient having AIDS. Your partner tells you that this would be a breach of the patient's confidentiality. It would be very inappropriate to do this. He reminds you that patient information is always to be kept confidential unless it needs to be shared for the purpose of giving care. "For example," he says, "the patient's information on the report to the hospital included the fact that she told us she had AIDS. Also, the physician needed to know because it was part of the medical history that we obtained. Unless there is another reason to share this information that I haven't thought of, no one else needs to hear from us that this patient has AIDS. Confidentiality is an EMS standard that pertains to the history, condition, and treatment of all the patients we see." As he gets out of the ambulance at the station, he adds: "Remember, confidentiality is a professional responsibility."

CHAPTER 4

The Human Body

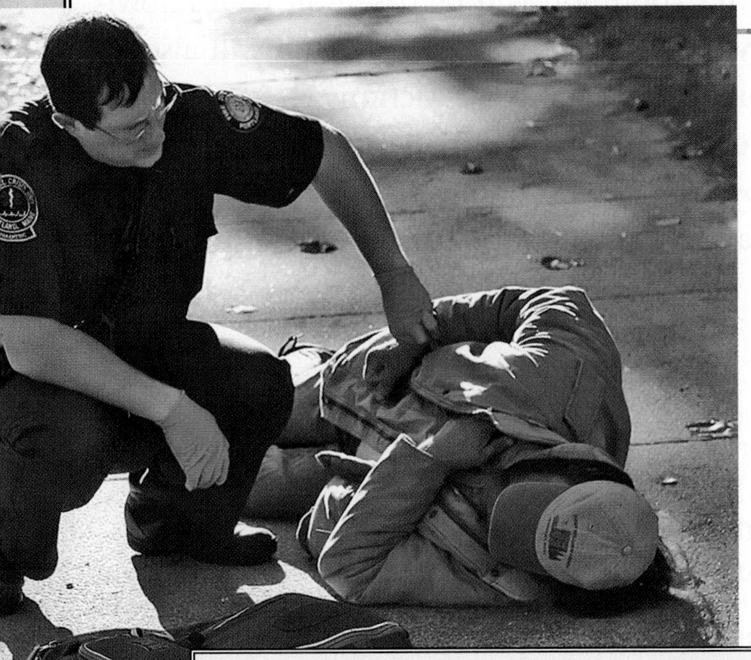

CORE CONCEPTS

The following are core concepts that will be addressed in this chapter:

- The terms used to describe regions of the body
- The terms used for anatomic reference and description
- The structure and function of major body systems

KEY TERMS

anatomical position, p. 66
anatomy, p. 66
anterior, p. 67
cardiovascular system, p. 77
digestive system, p. 85
endocrine system, p. 88
inferior, p. 67
lateral, p. 66
medial, p. 66
mid-axillary line, p. 67
mid-clavicular line, p. 68
midline, p. 66
musculoskeletal system, p. 70
nervous system, p. 83
physiology, p. 66
posterior, p. 67
prone, p. 68
respiratory system, p. 75
supine, p. 68
superior, p. 67

DOT OBJECTIVES

*KNOWLEDGE

1-4.1 Identify the following topographic terms: *medial, lateral, proximal, distal, superior, inferior, anterior, posterior, midline, right and left, mid-clavicular, bilateral, mid-axillary*. (pp. 66–68)

1-4.2 Describe the anatomy and function of the following major body systems: respiratory (pp. 75–77), circulatory (pp. 77–83), musculoskeletal (pp. 70–75), nervous (pp. 83–84), and endocrine. (p. 88) (Scan 4-1, pp. 81–96; Scan 4-2, pp. 97–98)

As an EMT, you will be called when a person has some problem with his body. The problem may be a traumatic injury, or it may be a medical problem such as chest pain. In any case, your assessment of the patient's condition will be based on your knowledge of the **anatomy,** or structure, of the body. You will also be required to know some of the body's functions, referred to as **physiology.** Your knowledge will not only help you assess the patient, it also will allow you to communicate your findings with other EMS personnel and hospital staff accurately and efficiently.

anatomy
the study of body structure.

physiology
the study of body function.

ANATOMICAL TERMS

The body is made up of a number of regions (Figure 4-1). Certain terms are used to describe directions and positions of the body.

Directional Terms

There must be a standardized method of referring to places on the body when describing illness or injury. For this reason, standardized anatomical directional terms are used (Figure 4-2). For example, the directions left and right always refer to the patient's left and right.

All descriptions of the body start with the assumption that the body is in anatomical position, even if the patient is not in that position when found. **Anatomical position** is best described as a person standing, facing forward, with his palms forward (Figure 4-1). The importance of always referring to this standardized position is that all health care providers, anywhere, will use the same anatomical starting point when describing the body and will understand each other's references.

Also, think of the body as if it has been divided into planes. A **plane** is a flat surface, the kind that would be formed if you sliced straight through a department store dummy or an imaginary human body. Cutting through from top to bottom, you could slice the body either into right and left halves or into front and back halves.

The **midline** of the body is created by drawing an imaginary line down the center of the body, passing between the eyes and extending down past the umbilicus (belly button, or navel) (refer again to Figure 4-2). Slicing through the imaginary body at the midline divides the body into right and left halves.

The term **medial** refers to a position closer to the midline, and the term **lateral** refers to a position farther away from the midline. For example, you would say: "The bridge of the nose is medial to the eyes." You also can say that an arm has a medial side (close to the body) and a lateral side (the outer arm, away from the body).

anatomical position
the standard reference position for the body in the study of anatomy. In this position, the body is standing erect, facing the observer, with arms down at the sides and the palms of the hands forward.

plane
a flat surface formed when slicing through a solid object.

midline
an imaginary line drawn down the center of the body, dividing it into right and left halves.

medial
toward the midline of the body.

lateral
to the side, away from the midline of the body.

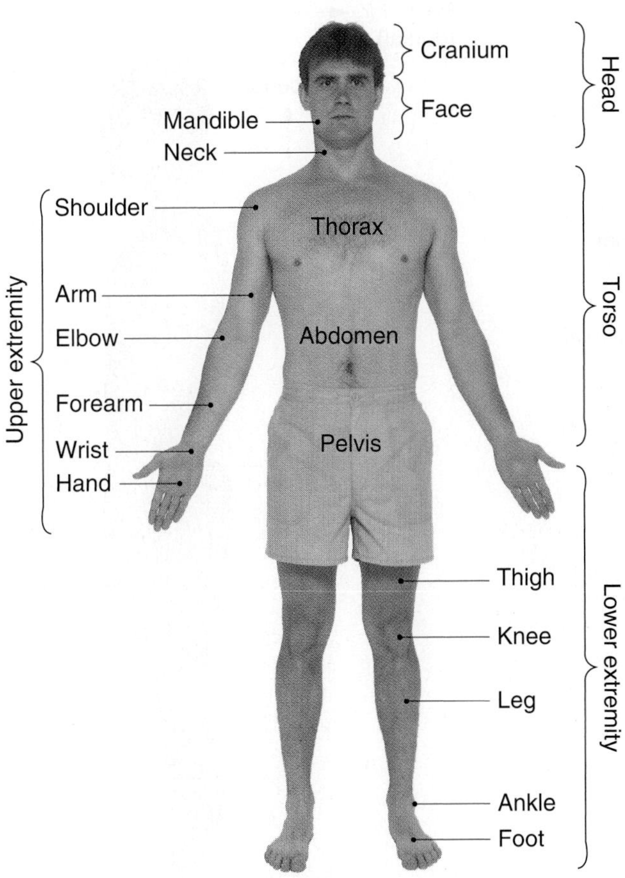

Figure 4-1 • Body regions and anatomical position.

bilateral
on both sides.

mid-axillary (mid-AX-uh-lair-e) **line**
a line drawn vertically from the middle of the armpit to the ankle.

anterior
the front of the body or body part.

posterior
the back of the body or body part.

ventral
referring to the front of the body. A synonym for anterior.

dorsal
referring to the back of the body or the back of the hand or foot. A synonym for posterior.

superior
toward the head (e.g., the chest is superior to the abdomen).

inferior
away from the head; usually compared with another structure that is closer to the head (e.g., the lips are inferior to the nose).

proximal
closer to the torso. *See also* distal.

distal
farther away from the torso. *See also* proximal.

torso
the trunk of the body; the body without the head and the extremities.

palmar
referring to the palm of the hand.

plantar
referring to the sole of the foot.

The term **bilateral** refers to "both sides" of anything. Patients may have diminished lung sounds on both sides when you listen with a stethoscope. This would be reported as, "The patient has diminished lung sounds bilaterally." Or, in a patient with chest pain, you might report that, "The patient has pain in his chest that radiates bilaterally to the shoulders."

The **mid-axillary line** extends vertically from the mid-armpit to the ankle. (The anatomical term for the armpit is axilla, so mid-axillary means "middle of the armpit.") This line divides the body into front and back halves. The term for the front is **anterior.** The term for the back is **posterior.** For example, you would say: "The patient has wounds to the posterior arm and the anterior thigh." A synonym for anterior is **ventral** (referring to the front of the body). A synonym for posterior is **dorsal** (referring to the back of the body or back of the hand or foot).

The terms **superior** and **inferior** refer to vertical, or up-and-down, directions. Superior means above; inferior means below. An example of this would be, "The nose is superior to the mouth."

The terms **proximal** and **distal** are relative terms. Proximal means closer to the **torso** (the trunk of the body, or the body without the head and the extremities). Distal means farther away from the torso. For example, think of an elbow. It is proximal to the hand, because it is closer to the torso than the hand. The elbow also is distal to the shoulder, since the elbow is farther away from the torso than the shoulder. The terms are usually used when describing locations on extremities. For example, to be sure circulation has not been cut off after splinting an arm or leg, you must feel for a distal pulse. This is a pulse found in an extremity, a pulse point that is farther away from the torso than the splint.

Two other terms you may sometimes hear are **palmar** (referring to the palm of the hand) and **plantar** (referring to the sole of the foot).

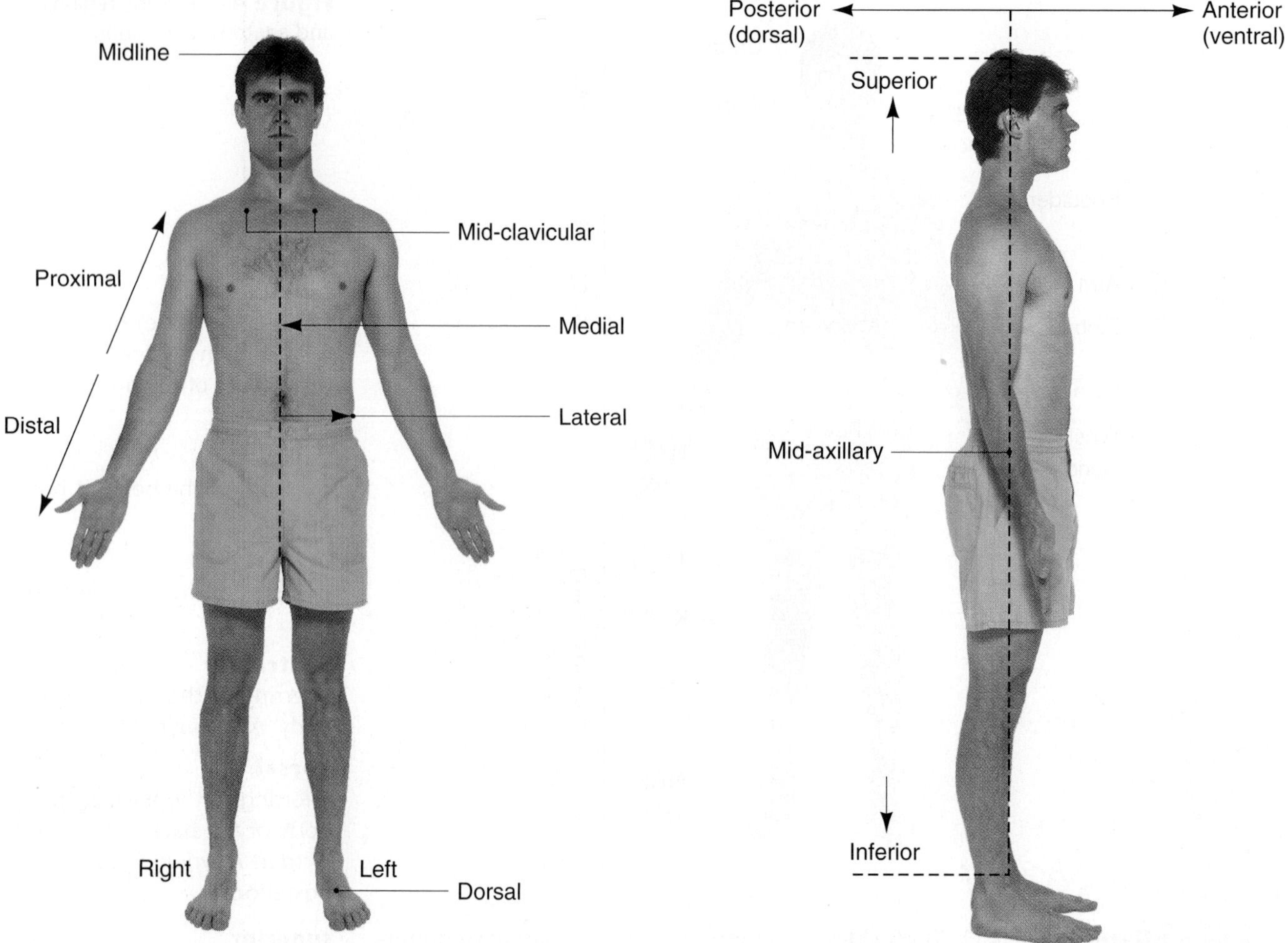

Figure 4-2 • Directional terms.

mid-clavicular (mid-clah-VIK-yuh-ler) **line** the line through the center of each clavicle.

abdominal quadrants four divisions of the abdomen used to pinpoint the location of a pain or injury: the right upper quadrant (RUQ), the left upper quadrant (LUQ), the right lower quadrant (RLQ), and the left lower quadrant (LLQ).

supine lying on the back.

prone lying face down.

recovery position lying on the side. Also called *lateral recumbent position.*

The **mid-clavicular line** runs through the center of a clavicle (collarbone) and the nipple below it. Since there are two clavicles, there are two mid-clavicular lines. When you use a stethoscope to listen for breath sounds, you will place the stethoscope at the mid-clavicular lines to listen to each side of the chest and assess the function of both lungs.

When describing the abdomen, which contains many vital organs, it is helpful to divide it into four parts, or quadrants. This can be done by drawing horizontal and vertical lines through the navel. The **abdominal quadrants** would be the right upper quadrant, the left upper quadrant, the right lower quadrant, and the left lower quadrant (Figure 4-3). These are often abbreviated as, respectively, RUQ, LUQ, RLQ, and LLQ.

Positional Terms

There are five positions for which you will also need to know the names: supine, prone, recovery, Fowler's, and Trendelenburg.

A **supine** patient is lying on his back. A **prone** patient is lying on his abdomen. A person may also be lying on his side, a position traditionally called the **recovery position.** It is the preferred position for any unconscious non-trauma patient, because it is a position in which fluids or vomitus can drain from the mouth and be less likely to be aspirated (inhaled) into the lungs. Because the patient is lying on his side, this position is also called the *lateral recumbent position* (Figure 4-4).

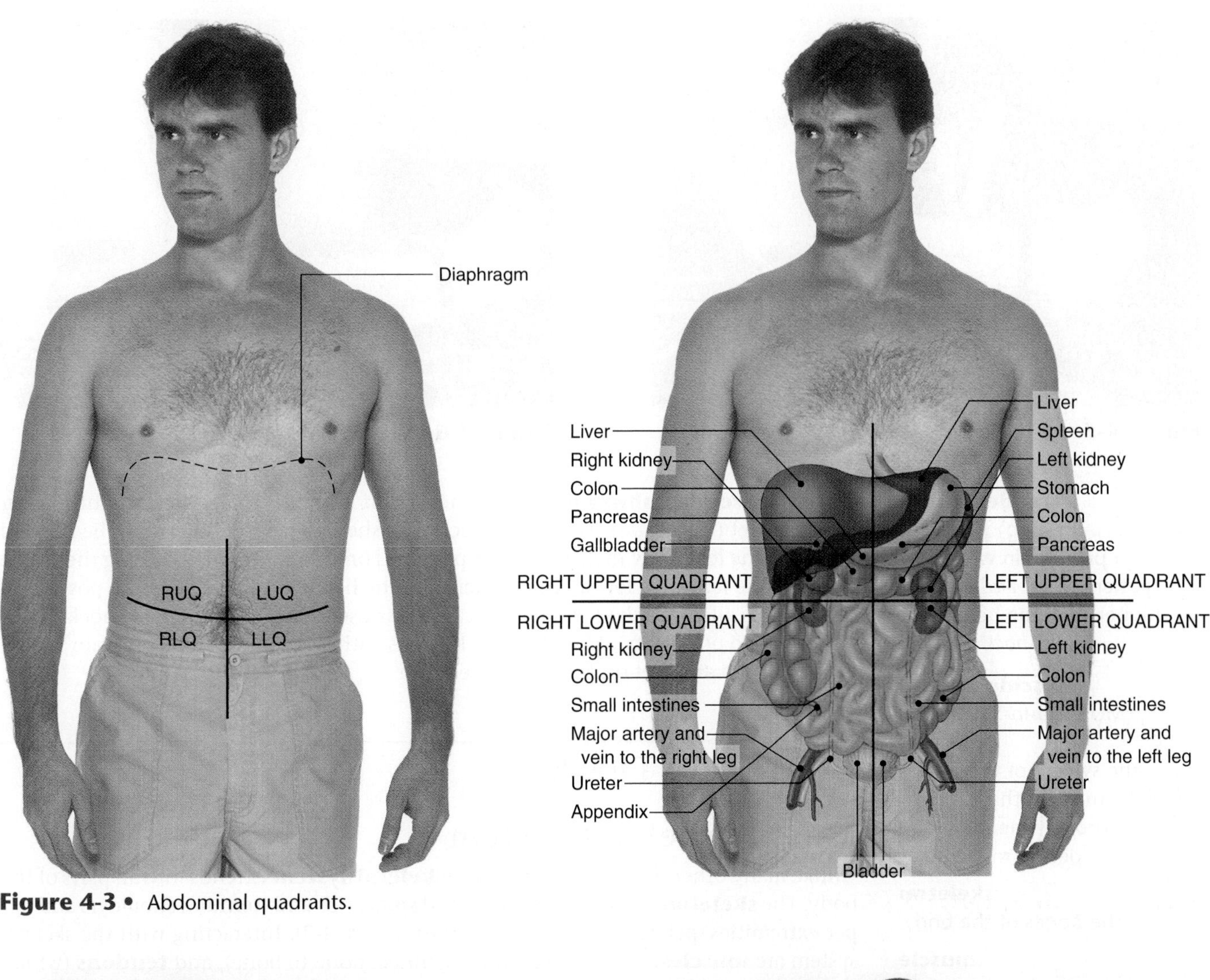

Figure 4-3 • Abdominal quadrants.

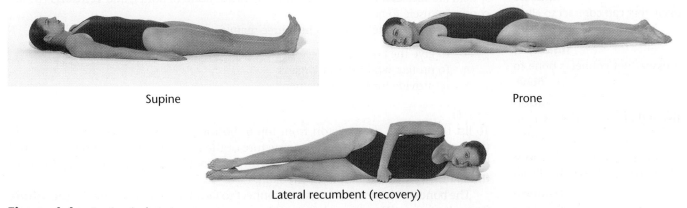

Supine

Prone

Lateral recumbent (recovery)

Figure 4-4 • Anatomical postures.

When patients are transported on a stretcher, there are several positions that they may be placed in. In the **Fowler's position,** the patient is seated. This is usually accomplished by raising the head end of the stretcher so the body is at a 45° to 60° angle. The patient may be sitting straight up or leaning slightly back. If leaning back in a semi-sitting position, this is sometimes called *semi-Fowler's* (Figure 4-5). In a Fowler's position, the legs may be straight out or bent.

Fowler's position
a sitting position.

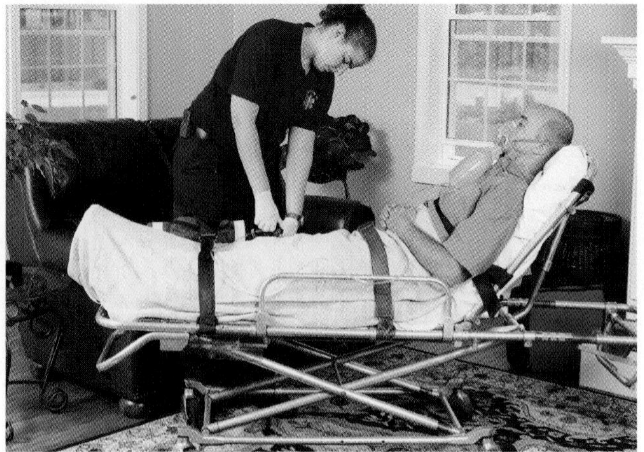

Figure 4-5 • Semi-Fowler's position.

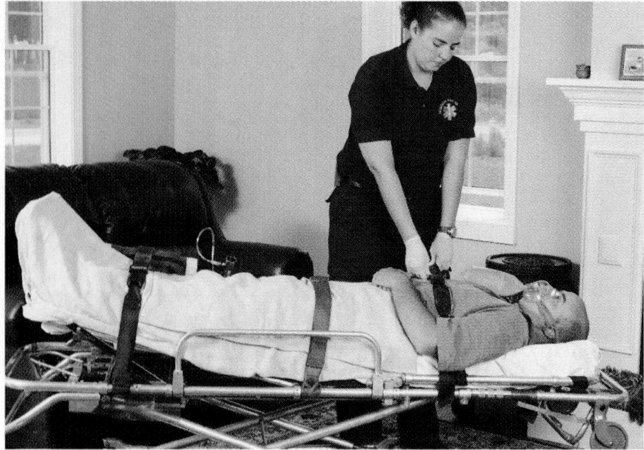

Figure 4-6 • Trendelenburg position.

Trendelenburg (trend-EL-un-berg) **position** a position in which the patient's feet and legs are higher than the head. Also called *shock position.*

musculoskeletal (MUS-kyu-lo-SKEL-e-tal) **system** the system of bones and skeletal muscles that support and protect the body and permit movement.

skeleton the bones of the body.

muscle tissue that can contract to allow movement of a body part.

ligament tissue that connects bone to bone.

tendon tissue that connects muscle to bone.

skull the bony structure of the head.

cranium the top, back, and sides of the skull.

mandible (MAN-di-bul) the lower jaw bone.

maxillae (mak-SIL-e) the two fused bones forming the upper jaw.

nasal (NAY-zul) **bones** the nose bones.

In the **Trendelenburg position,** the patient is lying with the head slightly lower than the feet (Figure 4-6). This may be accomplished by having the patient lie flat and elevating the legs a few inches or, if the patient is on a spine board, by tilting the whole board so the legs are a few inches higher than the head. The Trendelenburg position is sometimes called the *shock position,* because it is used to treat patients in shock (those who have no possibility of head injury. Patients with head injuries must remain supine with the head and feet on the same level).

BODY SYSTEMS

Musculoskeletal System

Unlike many other systems, the **musculoskeletal system** extends into all parts of the body. The **skeleton** consists of the skull and spine, ribs and sternum, shoulders and upper extremities, pelvis and lower extremities (Figure 4-7). Interacting with the skeletal system are **muscles, ligaments** (which connect bone to bone), and **tendons** (which connect muscle to bone).

The musculoskeletal system has three main functions:

- To give the body shape
- To protect vital internal organs
- To provide for body movement

Skull

To list the parts of the skeleton from top to bottom, you would begin with the skull (Figure 4-8). The **skull** is the bony structure of the head. A main function of the skull is to enclose and protect the brain. The **cranium** consists of the top, back, and sides of the skull. The face is the front of the skull.

The bones of the anterior cranium connect to facial bones, including the **mandible** (lower jaw), **maxillae** (fused bones of the upper jaw), and the **nasal bone** (which provides some of the structure of the nose). These bones form the facial structures. Some of these structures consist of multiple bones, such as the **orbits,** which surround the eyes, and the **zygomatic arches,** which form the structures of the cheeks.

Spinal Column

The spinal column is an essential part of the anatomy. Not only does it provide structure and support for the body, it also houses and protects the spinal cord.

The spinal column (also referred to simply as the spine) consists of 33 **vertebrae,** the separate bones of the spine. Like building blocks, vertebrae are stacked one upon

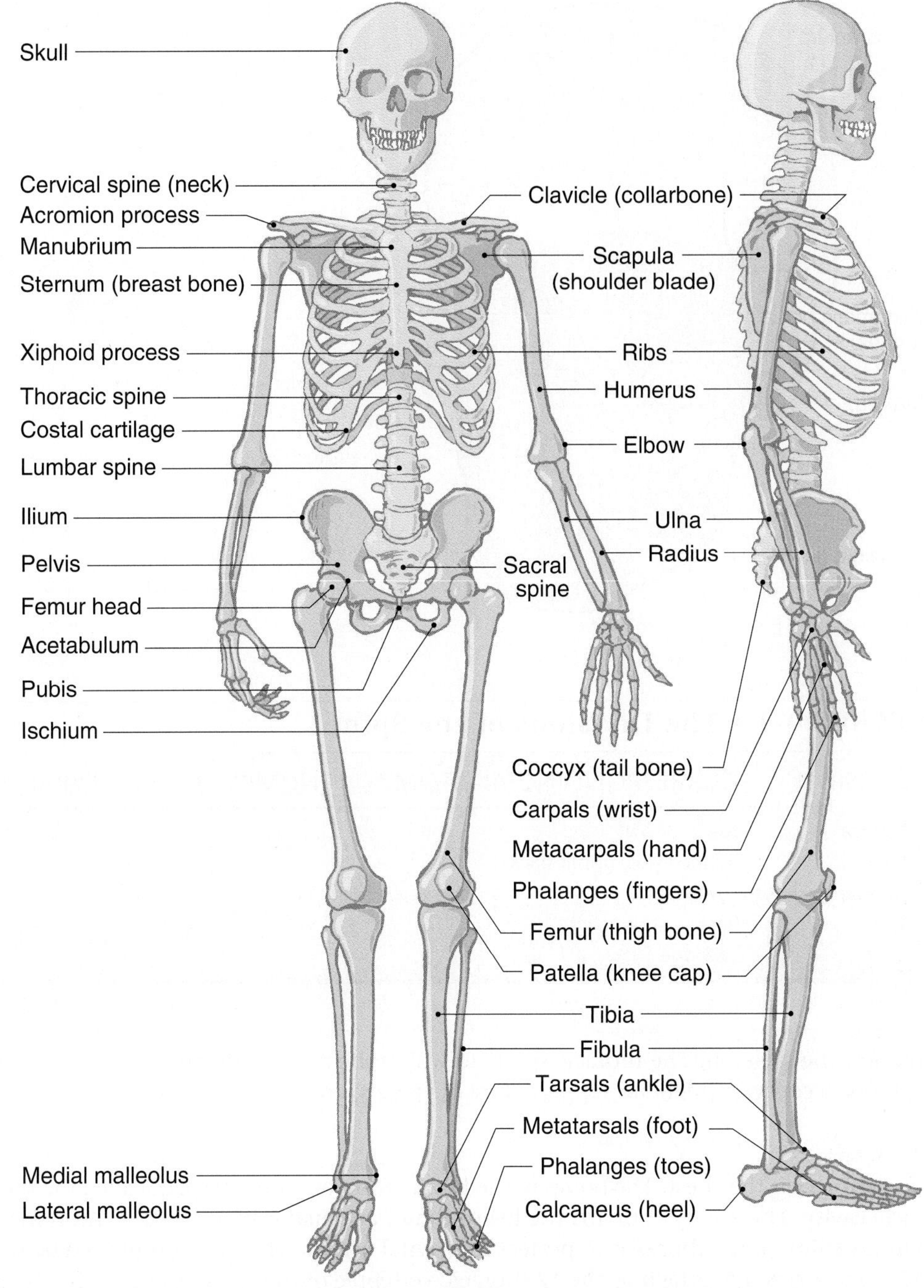

Figure 4-7 • The skeleton.

the other to form the spinal column. Vertebrae are open in the middle, somewhat like donuts, creating a hollow center for the spinal cord. Since the spinal cord is essential for movement, sensation, and vital functions, injuries to the spine have the potential to damage the cord, possibly resulting in paralysis or death. For this reason, you will see references throughout this text to "taking spinal precautions" for some patients.

The five divisions of the spine are listed in Table 4-1 and shown in Figure 4-9.

The anatomy of the body allows some vertebrae to be injured more easily than others. Since the head is large and heavy, resting on the slender neck, incidents such as car crashes may cause the head to whip back and forth or strike an object such as the windshield. This frequently causes injuries to the cervical spine. An injury to the spinal cord at this level may be fatal because control of the muscles of breathing, such as the diaphragm and the muscles between the ribs, arise from the spinal cord in the cervical region. The lumbar region is also subject to injury because it is not supported by other

orbits
the bony structures around the eyes; the eye sockets.

zygomatic (ZI-go-MAT-ik) **arches**
form the structure of the cheeks.

vertebrae (VER-te-bray)
the 33 bones of the spinal column.

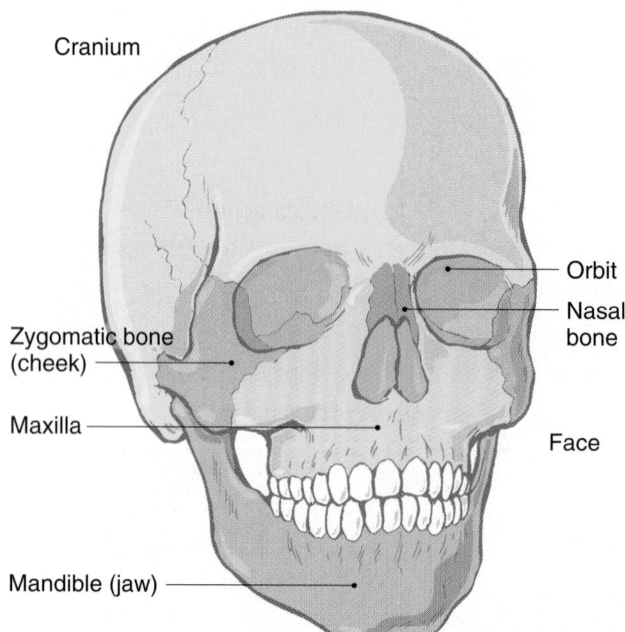

Figure 4-8 • The skull consists of the cranium and face.

thorax (THOR-ax) the chest.

sternum (STER-num) the breastbone.

manubrium (man-OO-bre-um) the superior portion of the sternum.

xiphoid (ZI-foid) **process** the inferior portion of the sternum.

pelvis the basin-shaped bony structure that supports the spine and is the point of proximal attachment for the lower extremities.

ilium (IL-e-um) the superior and widest portion of the pelvis.

ischium (ISH-e-um) the lower, posterior portions of the pelvis.

pubis (PYOO-bis) the medial anterior portion of the pelvis.

acetabulum (AS-uh-TAB-yuh-lum) the pelvic socket into which the ball at the proximal end of the femur fits to form the hip joint.

TABLE 4-1 • The Divisions of the Spine

DIVISION	CORRESPONDING ANATOMY	NUMBER OF VERTEBRAE
Cervical	Neck	7
Thoracic	Thorax, ribs, upper back	12
Lumbar	Lower back	5
Sacral	Back wall of pelvis	5
Coccyx	Tailbone	4

parts of the skeleton. The thoracic spine, to which the ribs are attached, and the sacral spine and coccyx, which are supported by the pelvis, are less easily injured.

Thorax

The **thorax** is the chest. The bones of the thorax form an internal space called the thoracic cavity. This cavity contains the heart, lungs, and major blood vessels. An important function of the thorax is to protect these vital organs. This is accomplished by the 12 pairs of ribs that attach to the 12 thoracic vertebrae of the spine. In the front, 10 of these pairs of ribs are attached to the **sternum** (breastbone) and two are called floating ribs since they have no anterior attachment. You will remember the sternum from your CPR training. This flat bone is divided into three sections: the **manubrium** (superior portion), the body (center portion), and the **xiphoid process** (inferior tip).

Pelvis

The **pelvis** is commonly referred to as the hip, although the hip is actually the joint where the femur (thigh bone) and pelvis join. The pelvis contains bones that are fused together. The **ilium** is the superior bone that contains the iliac crest, which is the wide bony wing that can be felt near the waist. The **ischium** is the inferior, posterior portion of the pelvis. The **pubis** is formed by the joining of the bones of the anterior pubis. The pelvis is joined posteriorly to the sacral spine.

The hip joint consists of the **acetabulum** (the socket of the hip joint) and the ball at the proximal end of the femur.

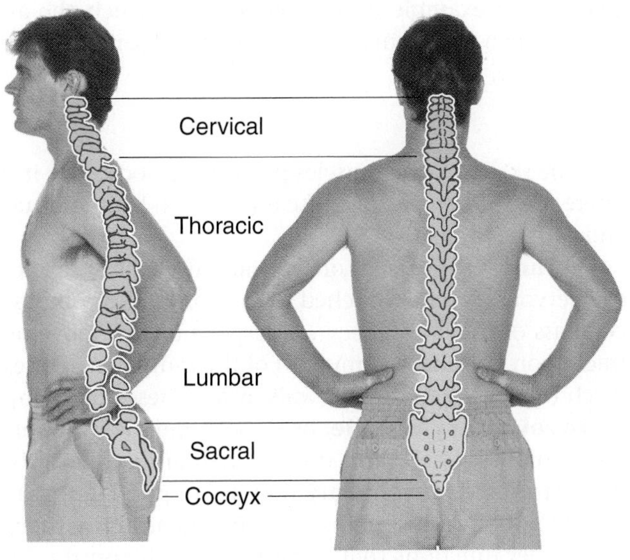

Figure 4-9 • The five divisions of the spine.

Lower Extremities

The pelvis and hip joint, described previously, may be considered part of the lower extremities. Moving downward from the hip, the large thigh bone is the **femur.** Progressing down the leg, the **patella,** or kneecap, sits anterior to the knee joint. The knee connects with the femur superiorly and with the bones of the lower leg, the tibia and fibula, inferiorly. The **tibia** is the medial and larger bone of the lower leg, also referred to as the shin bone. The **fibula** is the lateral and smaller bone of the lower leg.

The ankle connects the tibia and fibula with the foot. Two distinct landmarks are the **lateral malleolus** (at the lower end of the fibula) and the **medial malleolus** (at the lower end of the tibia). These are the protrusions that you see on the lateral and medial aspects of your ankles. The ankle consists of bones called **tarsals.** The foot bones are called **metatarsals.** The heel bone is called the **calcaneus.** The toe bones are the **phalanges.**

Upper Extremities

Each shoulder consists of several bones: the clavicle, the scapula, and the proximal humerus. The **clavicle,** or collarbone, is located anteriorly. The **scapula,** or shoulder blade, is located posteriorly. The **acromion process** of the scapula is the highest portion of the shoulder. It forms the **acromioclavicular joint** with the clavicle and is a frequent area of shoulder injury.

The upper arm and forearm consist of three bones connected at the elbow. The bone between the shoulder and the elbow is the **humerus.** The **radius** and **ulna** are the two bones between the elbow and the hand. The radius is the lateral bone of the forearm. It is always aligned with the thumb. (The radial pulse is taken over the radius.) The ulna is the medial forearm bone.

The wrist consists of several bones called **carpals.** The bones of the hand are the **metacarpals.** The finger bones, like the toe bones, are called *phalanges*.

By this point in the chapter, you are realizing the importance of anatomical terms such as *superior, inferior, medial, lateral, anterior,* and *posterior.* These terms will be used throughout the text, and you will need to use them correctly to properly document and report your patient's injuries and complaints.

Joints

Joints are formed when bones connect to other bones. There are several types of joints, including ball-and-socket joints and hinge joints. The hip is an example of a ball-and-socket joint, in which the ball of the femur rotates in a round socket in the pelvis. The

femur (FEE-mer)
the large bone of the thigh.

patella (pah-TEL-uh)
the kneecap.

tibia (TIB-e-uh)
the medial and larger bone of the lower leg.

fibula (FIB-yuh-luh)
the lateral and smaller bone of the lower leg.

malleolus (mal-E-o-lus)
protrusion on the side of the ankle. The *lateral malleolus,* at the lower end of the fibula, is seen on the outer ankle; the *medial malleolus,* at the lower end of the tibia, is seen on the inner ankle.

tarsals (TAR-sulz)
the ankle bones.

metatarsals (MET-uh-TAR-sulz)
the foot bones.

calcaneus (kal-KAY-ne-us)
the heel bone.

phalanges (fuh-LAN-jiz)
the toe bones and finger bones.

clavicle (KLAV-i-kul)
the collarbone.

scapula (SKAP-yuh-luh)
the shoulder blade.

acromion (ah-KRO-me-on) **process** the highest portion of the shoulder.

acromioclavicular (ah-KRO-me-o-klav-IK-yuh-ler) **joint** the joint where the acromion and the clavicle meet.

humerus (HYU-mer-us) the bone of the upper arm, between the shoulder and the elbow.

radius (RAY-de-us) the lateral bone of the forearm.

ulna (UL-nah) the medial bone of the forearm.

carpals (KAR-pulz) the wrist bones.

metacarpals (MET-uh-KAR-pulz) the hand bones.

joint the point where two bones come together.

voluntary muscle muscle that can be consciously controlled.

involuntary muscle muscle that responds automatically to brain signals but cannot be consciously controlled.

cardiac muscle specialized involuntary muscle found only in the heart.

elbow is an example of a hinge joint in which the angle between the humerus and ulna—which are connected by ligaments—bends and straightens, as the name suggests, like a hinge.

Muscles

Like the skeleton, the muscles protect the body, give it shape, and allow for movement. There are three types of muscle (Figure 4-10): voluntary muscle, involuntary muscle, and cardiac muscle.

Voluntary muscle, or skeletal muscle, is under conscious control of the brain via the nervous system. Attached to the bones, the voluntary muscles form the major muscle mass of the body. They are responsible for movement. Voluntary muscle can contract upon voluntary command of the individual. For example, if you want to, you can reach to pick up an item or walk away. These are examples of voluntary muscle use.

Involuntary muscle, or smooth muscle, is found in the gastrointestinal system, lungs, blood vessels, and urinary system and controls the flow of materials through these structures. Involuntary muscles respond automatically to orders from the brain. You do not have to consciously think about using them to breathe, digest food, or perform other functions that occur under their control. In fact, we have no direct control over involuntary muscles. Involuntary muscles do respond to stimuli such as stretching, heat, and cold.

Cardiac muscle, a specialized form of involuntary muscle, is found only in the heart. Cardiac muscle is extremely sensitive to decreased oxygen supply and can toler-

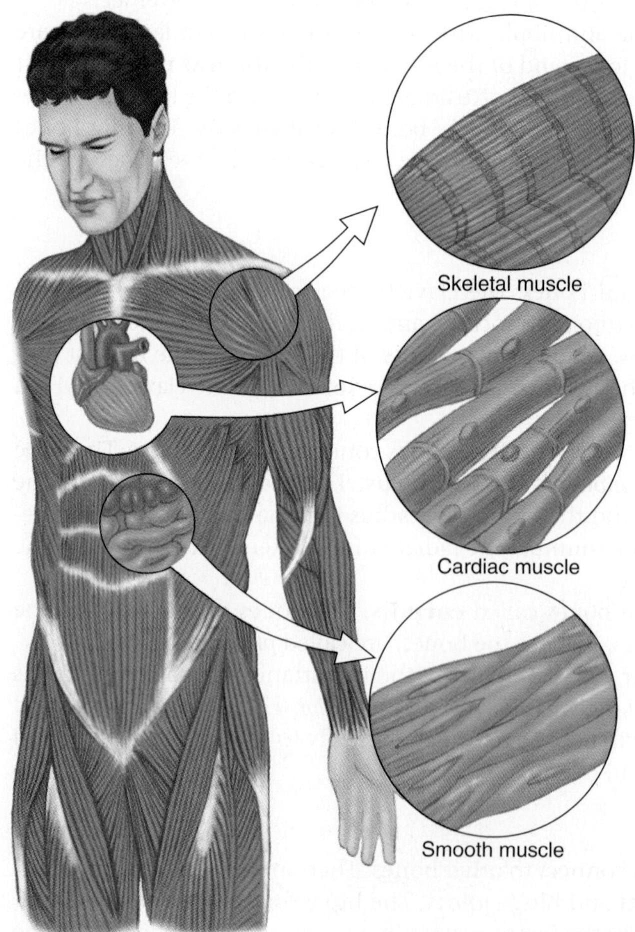

Figure 4-10 • Three types of muscle.

ate interruption of blood supply only for very short periods. The heart muscle has its own blood supply through the coronary artery system.

The heart also has a property called **automaticity.** This means that the heart has the ability to generate and conduct electrical impulses on its own. The heartbeat (contraction) is controlled by these electrical impulses.

automaticity (AW-to-muh-TISS-it-e) the ability of the heart to generate and conduct electrical impulses on its own.

Respiratory System

The purpose of the **respiratory system** is to move oxygen (O_2) into the bloodstream through inhalation and pick up carbon dioxide (CO_2) to be excreted through exhalation. To review the anatomy (structure) of the respiratory system, follow the path of air through the system from the mouth and nose to its final destination in the bloodstream.

respiratory (RES-pir-ah-tor-e) **system** the system of nose, mouth, throat, lungs, and muscles that brings oxygen into the body and expels carbon dioxide.

Respiratory Anatomy

A number of structures make up the respiratory system (Figure 4-11). Air enters the body through the mouth and nose. It moves through the **oropharynx** (the area directly posterior to the mouth) and the **nasopharynx** (the area directly posterior to the nose). The **pharynx** is the area that includes both the oropharynx and the nasopharynx.

oropharynx (OR-o-FAIR-inks) the area directly posterior to the mouth.

nasopharynx (NAY-zo-FAIR-inks) the area directly posterior to the nose.

pharynx (FAIR-inks) the area directly posterior to the mouth and nose. It is made up of the oropharynx and the nasopharynx.

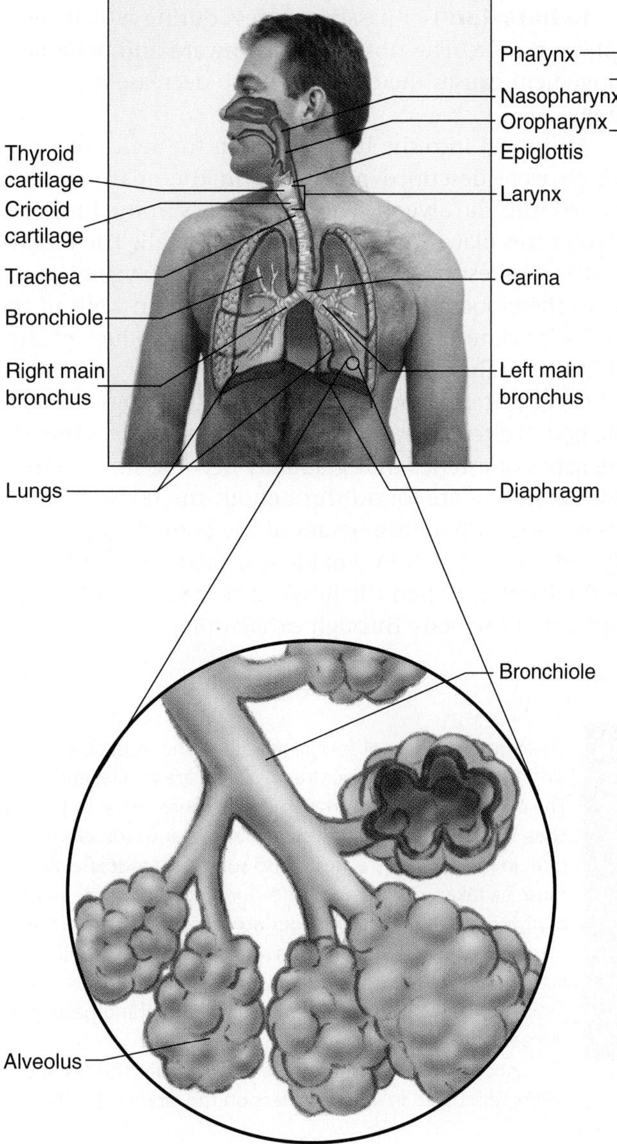

Figure 4-11 • The respiratory system.

epiglottis (EP-i-GLOT-is) a leaf-shaped structure that prevents food and foreign matter from entering the trachea.

larynx (LAIR-inks) the voice box.

cricoid (KRIK-oid) **cartilage** the ring-shaped structure that forms the lower portion of the larynx.

trachea (TRAY-ke-uh) the "windpipe"; the structure that connects the pharynx to the lungs.

lungs the organs where exchange of atmospheric oxygen and waste carbon dioxide take place.

bronchi (BRONG-ki) the two large sets of branches that come off the trachea and enter the lungs. There are right and left bronchi. *Singular* bronchus.

alveoli (al-VE-o-li) the microscopic sacs of the lungs where gas exchange with the bloodstream takes place.

diaphragm (DI-uh-fram) the muscular structure that divides the chest cavity from the abdominal cavity. A major muscle of respiration.

inhalation (IN-huh-LAY-shun) an active process in which the intercostal (rib) muscles and the diaphragm contract, expanding the size of the chest cavity and causing air to flow into the lungs.

exhalation (EX-huh-LAY-shun) a passive process in which the intercostal (rib) muscles and the diaphragm relax, causing the chest cavity to decrease in size and air to flow out of the lungs.

Air then proceeds on a path toward the lungs. A leaf-shaped structure called the **epiglottis** closes to prevent foods and foreign objects from entering the trachea during swallowing. The **larynx,** also known as the voice box, contains the vocal cords. The **cricoid cartilage** is a ring-shaped structure that forms the lower portion of the larynx.

The **trachea,** or windpipe, is the tube that carries inhaled air from the larynx down toward the **lungs.** At the level of the lungs, the trachea splits (bifurcates) into two branches called the **bronchi.** One "mainstem" bronchus goes to each lung. Inside each lung, the bronchi continue to branch and split (the branches are called *bronchioles*) and the air passages get smaller and smaller. Eventually, each branch ends at a group of alveoli. The **alveoli** are the small sacs within the lungs where gas exchange takes place with the bloodstream.

The **diaphragm** is the muscular structure that divides the chest cavity from the abdominal cavity. During a normal respiratory cycle, the diaphragm and other parts of the body work together to allow the body to inhale and exhale. The role of the diaphragm and other muscles in the respiratory cycle is described next.

Respiratory Physiology

Inhalation is an active process. The intercostal (rib) muscles and the diaphragm contract. The diaphragm lowers, and the ribs move upward and outward. This expands the size of the chest cavity, causing air to flow into the lungs.

Exhalation is a passive process during which the intercostal muscles and the diaphragm relax. The ribs move downward and inward, while the diaphragm rises. This movement causes the chest cavity to decrease in size and causes air to flow out of the lungs.

Air moves into the lungs through the series of air passages (known as the airway), which were described previously in the anatomy section. During inhalation, air is moved into the alveoli. These small sacs in the lungs are where gas exchange with the blood takes place. The alveoli are very small. The blood vessels that pass by the alveoli are the smallest type of vessel, capillaries. Oxygen is transferred from the air in the alveoli to the bloodstream through the very thin walls of the alveoli and the capillaries. At the same time carbon dioxide, a waste product of the body's cells, moves from the bloodstream into the alveoli.

Oxygenated blood is carried from the lungs to the heart so it can be pumped into the body's circulatory system. As the blood leaves the heart, it travels through a branching series of arteries that gradually become smaller and smaller until they are capillaries. Capillaries are found throughout the body. Through the capillary walls, gases are exchanged with all the tissues of the body. Oxygen carried by the blood is given up to the cells. Waste carbon dioxide is picked up from the cells and returned through veins to the heart and then the lungs, where it moves from the bloodstream into the alveoli and out of the body through exhalation.

PEDIATRIC NOTE

There are a number of special aspects of the respiratory anatomy of infants and children (Figure 4-12). In general, all structures in a child are smaller and more easily obstructed than in an adult. Their tongues take up proportionally more space in the pharynx than do an adult's. The trachea is relatively narrower than in adults and, therefore, more easily obstructed by swelling or foreign matter. The trachea is also softer and more flexible in infants and children, so more care must be taken during any procedure when pressure might be placed on the neck, such as in applying a cervical collar or during procedures to place a tube in the trachea. The cricoid cartilage is less developed and less rigid in infants and children. Because the chest wall is softer, infants and children tend to rely more on the diaphragm when they are having breathing difficulty. This causes a visible "seesaw" breathing pattern in which the chest and abdomen alternate movement.

Special procedures that take into account the respiratory anatomy of infants and children will be discussed in later chapters on the airway and the respiratory system.

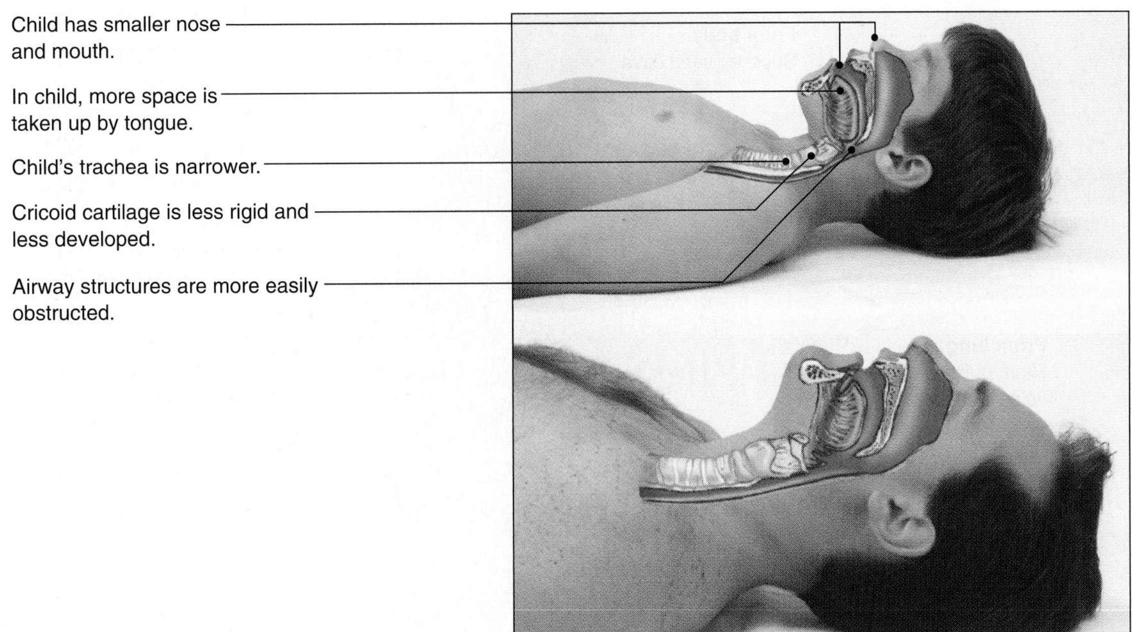

Child has smaller nose and mouth.
In child, more space is taken up by tongue.
Child's trachea is narrower.
Cricoid cartilage is less rigid and less developed.
Airway structures are more easily obstructed.

Figure 4-12 • Comparison of child and adult respiratory anatomy.

This exchange of gases, both in the lungs and at the body's cells, is critical to support life.

Breathing (the process of inhaling and exhaling air) may be classified as adequate or inadequate. Simply stated, adequate breathing is sufficient to support life. Inadequate breathing is not. Adequate and inadequate breathing, and how you as an EMT should assess and care for breathing problems, will be discussed in detail in Chapter 16, "Respiratory Emergencies."

Cardiovascular System

The **cardiovascular system** consists of the heart and the blood vessels through which blood is circulated throughout the body. It is also called the **circulatory system.**

Anatomy of the Heart

The human heart is a muscular organ about the size of your fist, located in the center of the thoracic cavity (Figure 4-13). The heart has four chambers: two upper chambers called **atria** and two lower chambers called **ventricles.**

The atria both contract at the same time. When they contract, blood is forced into the heart's lower chambers, the ventricles. Both ventricles contract simultaneously to pump the blood out of the heart. The path the blood takes on its journey through the body is as follows: right atrium to right ventricle to lungs to left atrium to left ventricle to body, then back to the right atrium to start its journey all over again. This path of the circulatory system is described in a little more detail in the following list:

- *Right atrium.* The **venae cavae** (the superior vena cava and the inferior vena cava) are the two large veins that return blood to the heart. The right atrium receives this blood and, upon contraction, sends it to the right ventricle.
- *Right ventricle.* The right ventricle receives blood from the chamber above it, the right atrium. When the right ventricle contracts, it pumps this blood out to the lungs via the pulmonary arteries. Remember, this blood is very low in oxygen and is carrying waste carbon dioxide that was picked up as the blood circulated through the body. While this blood is in the lungs, the carbon dioxide is excreted (taken out of the blood and when the person exhales, carried out of the body),

cardiovascular (KAR-de-o-VAS-kyu-ler) **system** the system made up of the heart (cardio) and the blood vessels (vascular); the circulatory system.

circulatory system *See* cardiovascular system.

atria (AY-tree-ah) the two upper chambers of the heart. There is a right atrium (which receives unoxygenated blood returning from the body) and a left atrium (which receives oxygenated blood returning from the lungs).

ventricles (VEN-tri-kulz) the two lower chambers of the heart. There is a right ventricle (which sends oxygen-poor blood to the lungs) and a left ventricle (which sends oxygen-rich blood to the body).

venae cavae (VE-ne KA-ve) the *superior vena cava* and the *inferior vena cava.* These two major veins return blood from the body to the right atrium. (Venae cavae is plural, vena cava singular.)

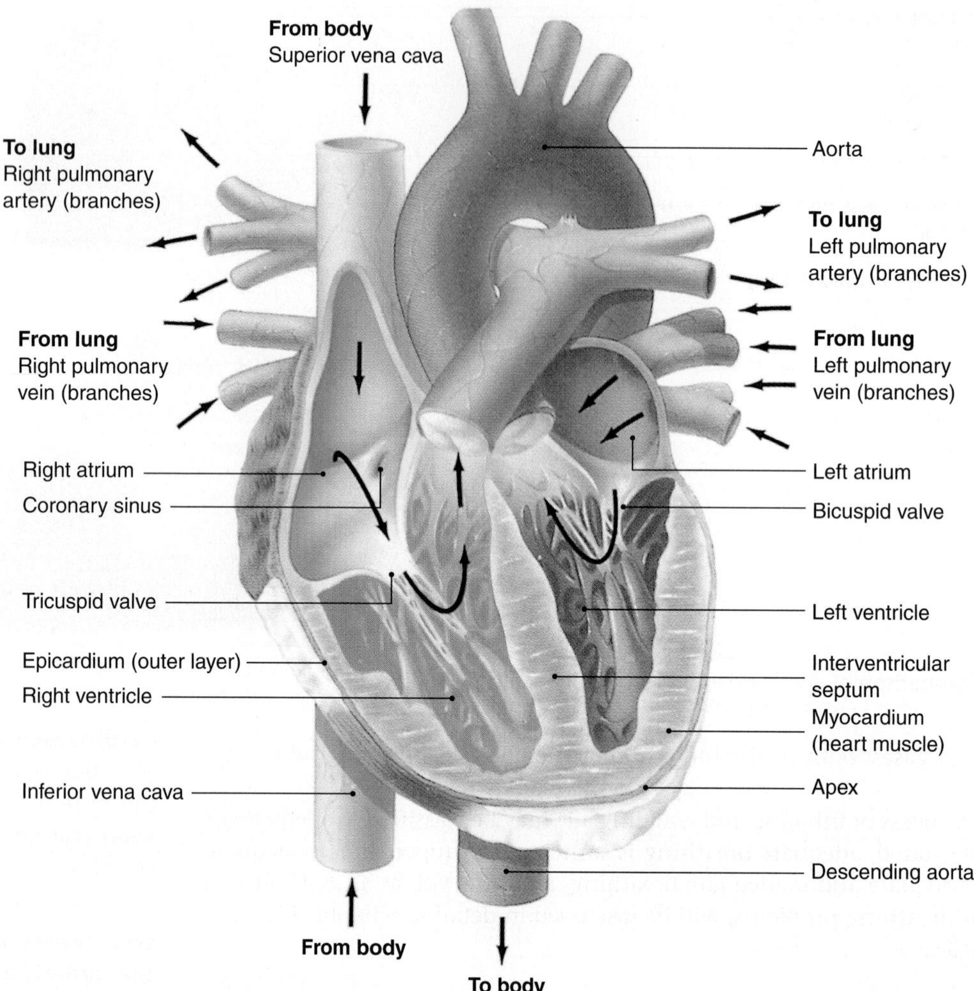

Figure 4-13 • Cross-section of the heart.

and oxygen is obtained (taken into the blood from air the person has inhaled). The oxygen-rich blood is now returned to the left atrium via the pulmonary veins.

- *Left atrium.* The left atrium receives the oxygen-rich blood from the lungs. When it contracts, it sends this blood to the left ventricle.
- *Left ventricle.* The left ventricle receives oxygen-rich blood from the chamber above it, the left atrium. When it contracts, it pumps this blood into the aorta, the body's largest artery, for distribution to the entire body. Since the blood must reach all parts of the body, the left ventricle is the most muscular and strongest part of the heart.

valve
a structure that opens and closes to permit the flow of a fluid in only one direction.

Between each atrium and ventricle is a one-way **valve** to prevent blood in the ventricle from being forced back up into the atrium when the ventricle contracts. The pulmonary artery has a one-way valve so that blood in the artery does not return to the right ventricle. The aorta also has a one-way valve to prevent backflow to the left ventricle. This system of one-way valves keeps the blood moving in the correct direction along the path of circulation.

cardiac conduction system
a system of specialized muscle tissues which conduct electrical impulses that stimulate the heart to beat.

The contraction, or beating, of the heart is an automatic, involuntary process. The heart has its own natural "pacemaker" and a system of specialized muscle tissues that conduct electrical impulses that stimulate the heart to beat. This network is called the **cardiac conduction system** (Figure 4-14). Regulation of rate, rhythm, and force of heartbeat comes, in part, from the cardiac control centers of the brain. Nerve impulses from these centers are sent to the pacemaker and conduction system of the heart. These

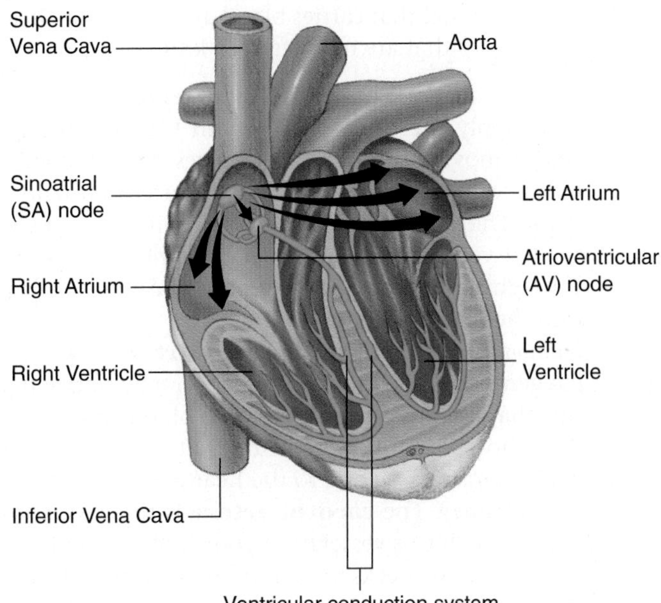

Figure 4-14 • The cardiac conduction system.

nerve impulses and chemicals (epinephrine, for example) released into the blood control the heart's rate and strength of contractions.

Circulation of the Blood

When the blood leaves the heart, it travels throughout the body through several types of blood vessels. Blood vessels are described by their function, location, and whether they carry blood away from or to the heart.

POINT OF VIEW

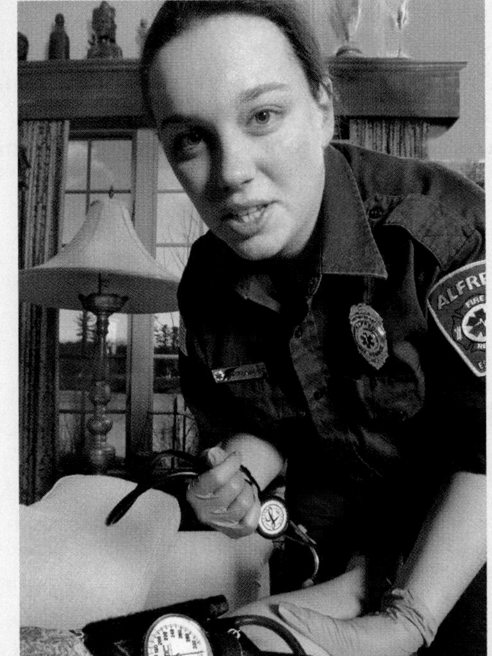

"I got a little dizzy and fell down. It happens at my age. My visiting nurse called the EMTs. They are very nice. Sometimes they talk to the nurse like I am not there. That's probably because of all the medical terms.

"When they talk with me they use words I don't understand. They asked me if I was on beta-something and if I took abra cabra tripto something. Can't they just look at my pills? Or use words I understand? Then they asked me about cardio something and hypo something.

"They were such nice people. They smiled at me even while they had that blasted blood pressure thing wrapped around my arm. But I'll be damned if I knew what they were talking about."

artery
any blood vessel carrying blood away from the heart.

coronary (KOR-o-nar-e) **arteries**
blood vessels that supply the muscle of the heart (myocardium).

aorta (ay-OR-tah)
the largest artery in the body. It transports blood from the left ventricle to begin systemic circulation.

pulmonary (PUL-mo-nar-e) **arteries**
the vessels that carry blood from the right ventricle of the heart to the lungs.

carotid (kah-ROT-id) **arteries**
the large neck arteries, one on each side of the neck, that carry blood from the heart to the head.

femoral (FEM-o-ral) **artery**
the major artery supplying the leg.

brachial artery
artery of the upper arm; the site of the pulse checked during infant CPR.

radial artery
artery of the lower arm. It is felt when taking the pulse at the wrist.

posterior tibial (TIB-ee-ul) **artery**
artery supplying the foot, behind the medial ankle.

dorsalis pedis (dor-SAL-is PEED-is) **artery**
artery supplying the foot, lateral to the large tendon of the big toe.

The kind of vessel that carries blood away from the heart is called an **artery.** There are several arteries that are important to know:

- *Coronary arteries.* The **coronary arteries** (Figure 4-15) branch off from the aorta and supply the heart muscle with blood. Although the heart has blood constantly moving through it, it receives its own blood supply from the coronary arteries. Damage or blockage to these arteries usually results in chest pain.
- *Aorta.* The **aorta** is the largest artery in the body. It begins at its attachment to the left ventricle, travels superiorly, then arches inferiorly in front of the spine through the thoracic and abdominal cavities. At the level of the navel, it splits into the iliac arteries.
- *Pulmonary artery.* The **pulmonary artery** begins at the right ventricle. It carries oxygen-poor blood to the lungs. You may notice that this is an exception to the rule that arteries carry oxygen-rich blood, and veins carry oxygen-poor blood. It does, however, follow the rule that arteries carry blood away from the heart while veins carry blood to the heart.
- *Carotid artery.* The **carotid artery** is the major artery of the neck. You will be familiar with this vessel from your CPR class. It is the artery that is palpated during CPR pulse checks for adults and children. It carries the main supply of blood for the head. There is a carotid artery on each side of the neck. Never palpate both at the same time because of the danger of interrupting the supply of blood to the brain.
- *Femoral artery.* The **femoral artery** is the major artery of the thigh. You can relate the name "femoral" to the bone in the thigh, the femur. Pulsations for this artery can be felt in the crease between the abdomen and the groin. This artery is the major source of blood supply to the thigh and leg.
- *Brachial artery.* The **brachial artery** is in the upper arm. It is the pulse checked during infant CPR. Its pulse can be felt anteriorly in the crease over the elbow and along the medial aspect of the upper arm. It is also the artery that is used when determining blood pressure with a blood pressure cuff and a stethoscope.
- *Radial artery.* This artery travels through and supplies the lower arm. The **radial artery** is the artery felt when taking a pulse at the thumb side of the wrist. Again, you can relate the name "radial" to the radius, a bone in the forearm which the radial artery is near.
- *Posterior tibial artery.* This artery is often used when determining the circulatory status of the lower extremity. The **posterior tibial artery** may be palpated on the posterior aspect of the medial malleolus.
- *Dorsalis pedis artery.* The **dorsalis pedis artery** lies on the top (dorsal portion) of the foot, lateral to the large tendon of the big toe.

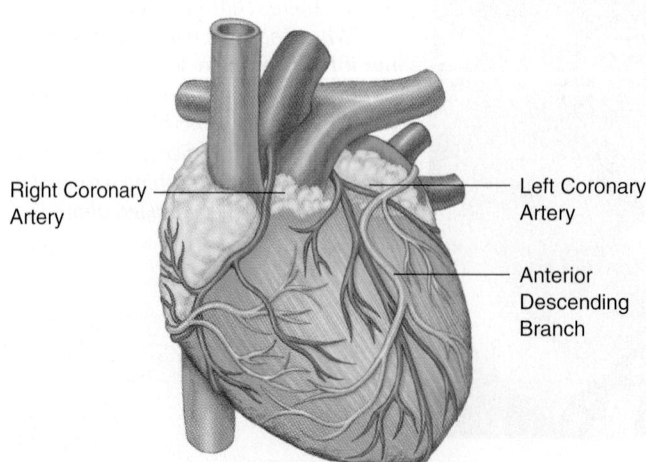

Figure 4-15 • The coronary arteries.

Arteries begin with large vessels, like the aorta. They gradually branch to smaller and smaller vessels. The smallest branch of an artery is called an **arteriole.** These small vessels lead to the capillaries. **Capillaries** are tiny blood vessels found throughout the body. As explained earlier, the capillaries are where gases, nutrients, and waste products are exchanged between the body's cells and the bloodstream. From the capillaries the blood begins its return journey to the heart by entering the smallest veins. One of these small veins is called a **venule** (Figure 4-16).

The kind of vessel that carries the blood from the capillaries back to the heart is called a **vein.** Remember that the blood flow from the heart started in the largest arteries and moved into smaller and smaller arteries until it reached the capillaries. The blood takes an opposite course through the veins. The blood travels from the smaller to the larger vessels on its return trip to the heart. Immediately after leaving the capillaries, the blood enters venules, the smallest veins. From the venules, the veins get gradually larger, eventually reaching the venae cavae.

There are two *venae cavae.* The superior vena cava collects blood that is returned from the head and upper body. The inferior vena cava collects blood from the portions of the body below the heart. The superior and inferior venae cavae meet to return blood to the right atrium, where the process of circulation begins again.

The **pulmonary vein** carries oxygenated blood from the lungs to the left atrium of the heart. This is an exception to the rule that veins carry oxygen-poor blood. It does follow the rule that arteries carry blood away from the heart while veins return blood to the heart.

arteriole (ar-TE-re-ol)
the smallest kind of artery.

capillary (KAP-i-lair-e)
a thin-walled, microscopic blood vessel where the oxygen/carbon dioxide and nutrient/waste exchange with the body's cells takes place.

venule (VEN-yul)
the smallest kind of vein.

vein
any blood vessel returning blood to the heart.

pulmonary veins
the vessels that carry oxygenated blood from the lungs to the left atrium of the heart.

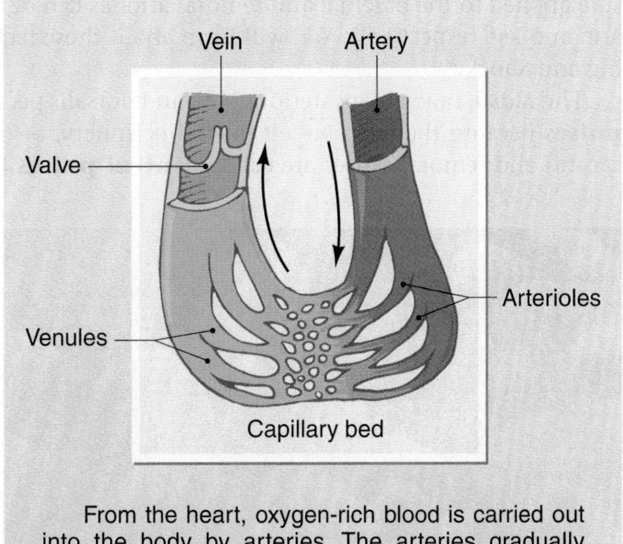

From the heart, oxygen-rich blood is carried out into the body by arteries. The arteries gradually branch into smaller arteries called arterioles. The arterioles gradually branch into tiny vessels called capillaries.

In the capillaries, the blood gives up oxygen and nutrients, which move through the thin walls of the capillaries into the body's cells. At the same time, carbon dioxide and other wastes move in the opposite direction, from the cells and through the capillary walls, to be picked up by the blood.

On its return journey to the heart, the oxygen-poor blood, now carrying carbon dioxide and other wastes, flows from the capillaries into small veins called venules which gradually merge into larger veins.

Figure 4-16 • Arteries, capillaries, and veins.

Composition of the Blood

plasma (PLAZ-mah) the fluid portion of the blood.

red blood cells components of the blood. They carry oxygen to and carbon dioxide away from the cells.

white blood cells components of the blood. They produce substances that help the body fight infection.

platelets components of the blood; membrane-enclosed fragments of specialized cells.

pulse the rhythmic beats caused as waves of blood move through and expand the arteries.

peripheral pulses the radial, brachial, posterior tibial, and dorsalis pedis pulses, which can be felt at peripheral (outlying) points of the body.

central pulses the carotid and femoral pulses, which can be felt in the central part of the body.

The blood is made up of several components: plasma, red and white blood cells, and platelets (Figure 4-17).

- *Plasma.* **Plasma** is a watery, salty fluid that makes up over half the volume of the blood. The red and white blood cells and platelets are carried in the plasma.
- *Red blood cells.* **Red blood cells** are also called *RBCs, erythrocytes,* or *red corpuscles*. Their primary function is to carry oxygen to the tissues and carbon dioxide away from the tissues. These cells also provide the red color to the blood.
- *White blood cells.* **White blood cells** are also called *WBCs, leukocytes,* or *white corpuscles*. They are involved in destroying microorganisms (germs) and producing substances called antibodies, which help the body resist infection.
- *Platelets.* **Platelets** are membrane-enclosed fragments of specialized cells. When these fragments are activated, they release chemical factors needed to form blood clots.

Pulse

A **pulse** is formed when the left ventricle contracts, sending a wave of blood through the arteries. The pulse is felt by compressing an artery over a bone. This allows you to feel the wave of blood, or pulse, as it comes through the artery.

Earlier in this chapter, several arteries were named. Among them were the primary arteries where a pulse is taken for vital signs or CPR: the carotid, brachial, and radial arteries. You will also use the pulses at the ankles and feet (posterior tibial and dorsalis pedis) to check for adequate circulation to the lower extremities.

The points where a pulse can be felt may also be used for control of bleeding. Pressure applied to the brachial and femoral arteries can be used to control bleeding to the arm and leg, respectively. You will learn about these techniques in Chapter 26, "Bleeding and Shock."

The radial, brachial, posterior tibial, and dorsalis pedis pulses are called **peripheral pulses** because they can be felt on the periphery, or outer reaches, of the body. The carotid and femoral pulses are called **central pulses** because they can be felt in the

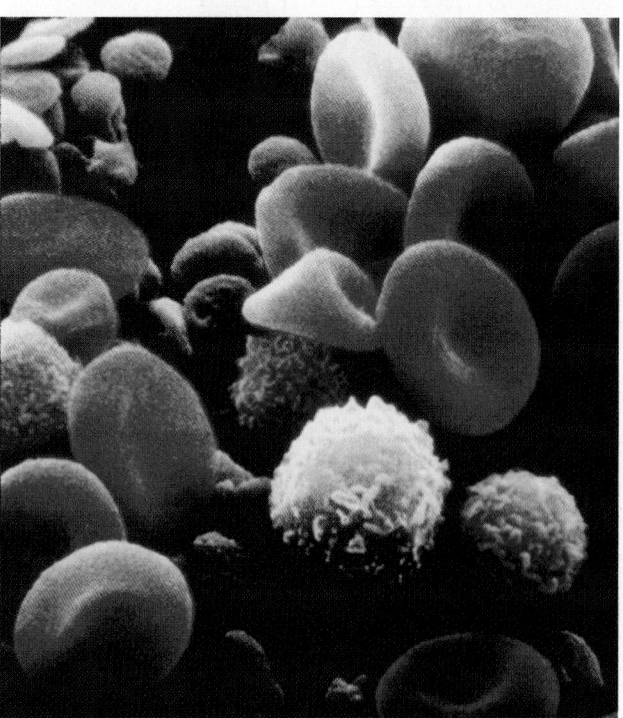

Figure 4-17 • Blood consists of plasma, red and white blood cells, and platelets. *(© Ken Edward/Science Source/Photo Researchers, Inc.)*

central part of the body. Because they are larger vessels closer to the heart, the carotid and femoral pulses can be felt even when peripheral pulses are too weak to be felt.

Providing chest compressions during CPR is dangerous if the heart is beating, however weakly. This is why the carotid pulse, rather than a peripheral pulse, is used to determine pulselessness, the sign that CPR compressions should begin. If a peripheral pulse site were felt when the heartbeat was weak but still present, the EMT might make an incorrect and potentially harmful decision to begin CPR.

Blood Pressure

The force blood exerts against the walls of blood vessels is known as **blood pressure.** Usually, arterial blood pressure (pressure in an artery) is measured.

Each time the left ventricle of the heart contracts, it forces blood out into circulation. The pressure created in the arteries by this blood is called the **systolic blood pressure.** When the left ventricle of the heart is relaxed and refilling, the pressure remaining in the arteries is called the **diastolic blood pressure.** The systolic pressure is reported first, the diastolic second, as in "120 over 80," which is written as "120/80."

Perfusion

The movement of blood through the heart and blood vessels is called circulation. In healthy individuals, circulation is adequate. That is, there is enough blood within the system and there is a means to pump and deliver it to all parts of the body efficiently (Figure 4-18). The adequate supply of oxygen and nutrients to the organs and tissues of the body, with the removal of waste products, is called **perfusion.**

Hypoperfusion (inadequate perfusion), also known as **shock,** is a serious condition. With hypoperfusion, there is inadequate circulation of blood through one or more organs or structures. Blood is not reaching and filling all the capillary networks of the body, which means that oxygen will not be delivered to, and waste products will not be removed from, all the body's tissues. Hypoperfusion can lead to death. It is important to understand what hypoperfusion is, how it occurs, and how to recognize it. This will be discussed in more depth in Chapter 26, "Bleeding and Shock."

Nervous System

The **nervous system** (Figure 4-19), the system of brain, spinal cord, and nerves, transmits impulses and governs sensation, movement, and thought, and controls the body's voluntary and involuntary activity. It consists of the central and peripheral nervous systems.

The **central nervous system** is composed of the brain and the spinal cord. The brain could be likened to a powerful computer that receives information from the body and, in turn, sends impulses to different areas of the body to respond to the changes in and outside the body. The spinal cord rests within the spinal column and stretches from the brain to the lumbar vertebrae. Nerves branch from each part of the cord and reach throughout the body.

The **peripheral nervous system** consists of two types of nerves: sensory and motor. The sensory nerves pick up information from throughout the body and transmit it to the spinal cord and brain. If you touch something hot, your sensory nerves transmit this to the brain so action may be taken. The motor nerves carry messages from the brain to the body. In the example given previously, the brain would send a message to the part of the body that has just touched the hot item to pull away.

The **autonomic nervous system** is the division of the peripheral nervous system that controls involuntary motor functions and affects such things as digestion and heart rate.

blood pressure
the pressure caused by blood exerting force against the walls of blood vessels. Usually arterial blood pressure (the pressure in an artery) is measured. *See also* diastolic blood pressure and systolic blood pressure.

systolic (sis-TOL-ik) **blood pressure**
the pressure created in the arteries when the left ventricle contracts and forces blood out into circulation.

diastolic (di-as-TOL-ik) **blood pressure**
the pressure in the arteries when the left ventricle is refilling.

perfusion
the supply of oxygen to and removal of wastes from the cells and tissues of the body as a result of the flow of blood through the capillaries.

hypoperfusion
inadequate perfusion of the cells and tissues of the body caused by insufficient flow of blood through the capillaries. *See also* perfusion.

shock
See hypoperfusion.

nervous system
the system of brain, spinal cord, and nerves that govern sensation, movement, and thought.

central nervous system (CNS)
the brain and spinal cord.

peripheral nervous system (PNS)
the nerves that enter and leave the spinal cord and travel between the brain and organs without passing through the spinal cord.

autonomic (AW-to-NOM-ik) **nervous system**
the division of the peripheral nervous system that controls involuntary motor functions.

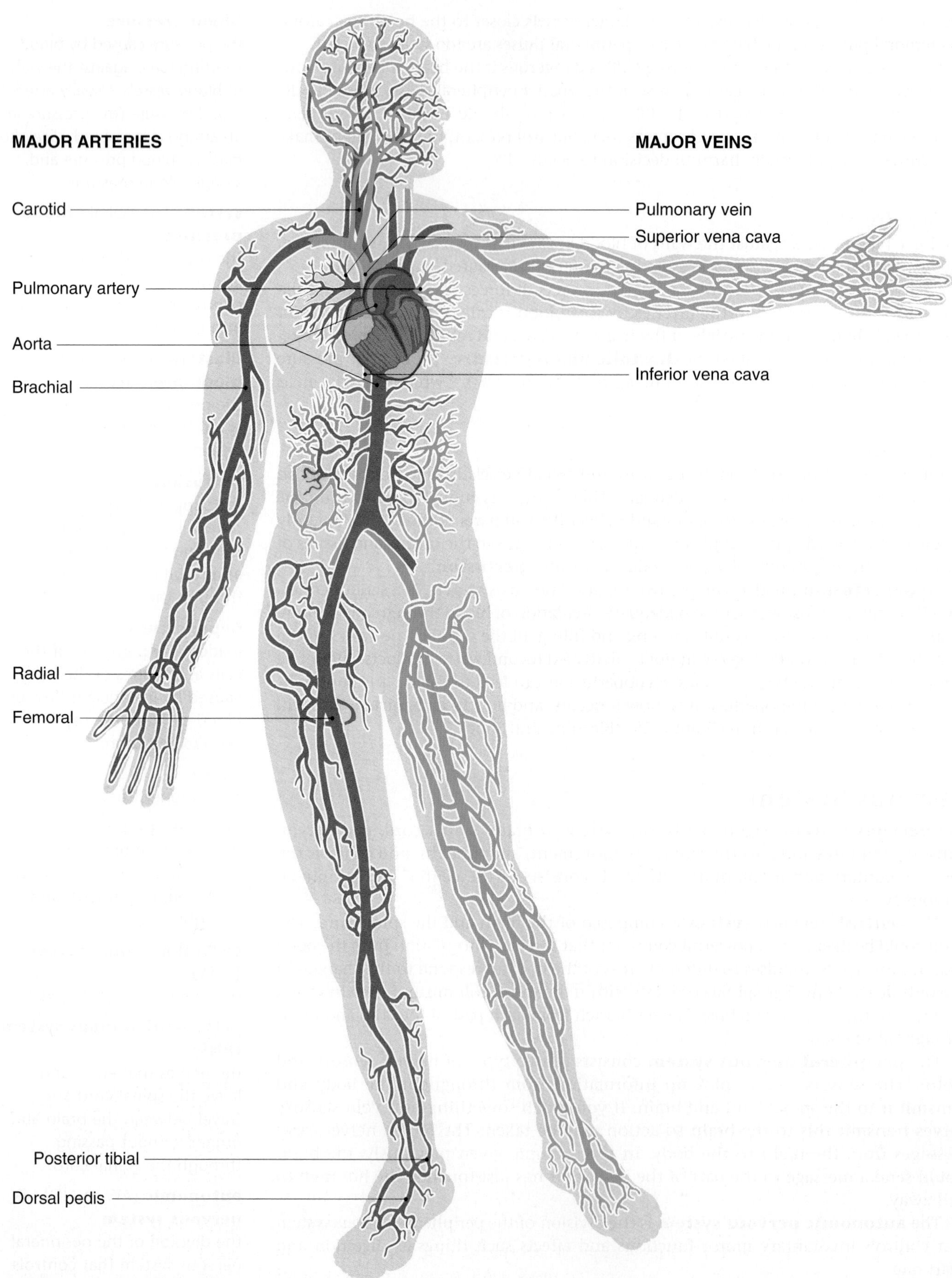

Figure 4-18 • The circulatory system.

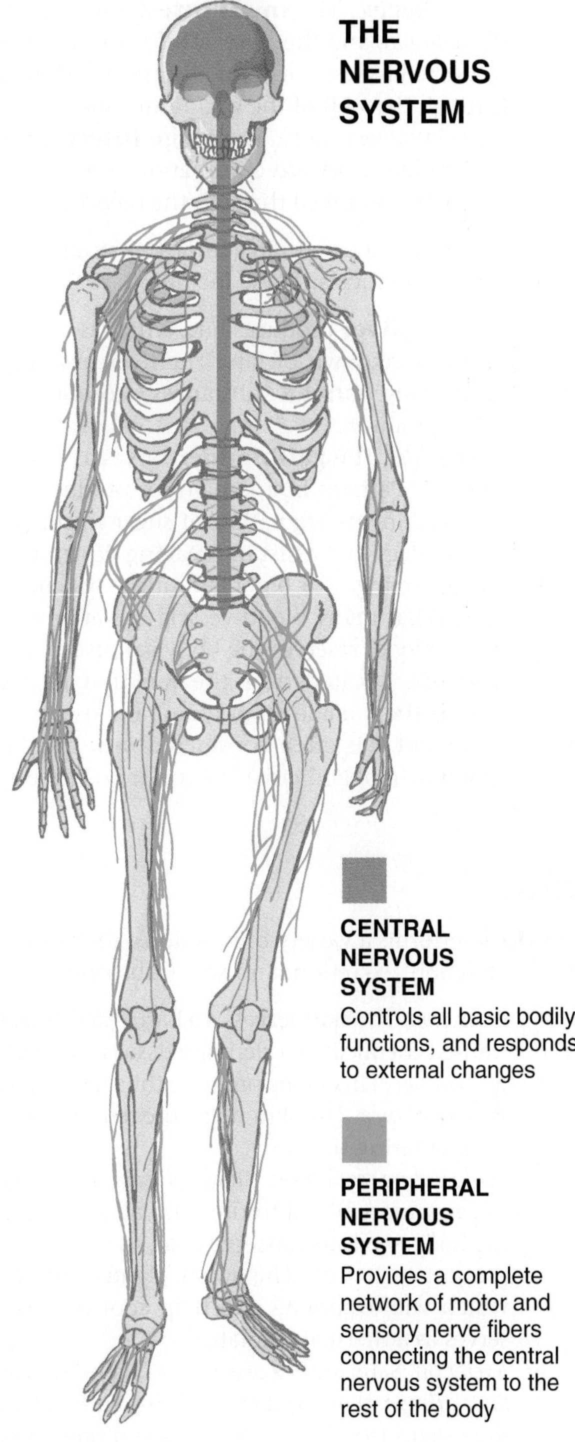
THE
NERVOUS
SYSTEM
CENTRAL
NERVOUS
SYSTEM
Controls all basic bodily functions, and responds to external changes
PERIPHERAL
NERVOUS
SYSTEM
Provides a complete network of motor and sensory nerve fibers connecting the central nervous system to the rest of the body

Figure 4-19 • The nervous system.

Digestive System

The **digestive system** is the system by which food travels through the body and is digested, or broken down into absorbable forms. The abdomen contains the organs of digestion. Food enters the mouth and is broken down by both saliva and chewing. The food passes from the mouth through the oropharynx and into the esophagus, where it is transported to the stomach. Except for the mouth and the esophagus, all of the organs of digestion are contained in the abdominal cavity. These organs include:

- *Stomach.* The **stomach** is a hollow organ that expands as it fills with food. In the stomach, acidic gastric juices begin to break food down into components that the body will be able to convert into energy.

digestive system
system by which food travels through the body and is digested, or broken down into absorbable forms.

stomach
muscular sac between the esophagus and the small intestine where digestion of food begins.

small intestine
the muscular tube between the stomach and the large intestine, divided into the duodenum, the jejunum, and the ileum, which receives partially digested food from the stomach and continues digestion. Nutrients are absorbed by the body through its walls.

large intestine
the muscular tube that removes water from waste products received from the small intestine and removes anything not absorbed by the body toward excretion from the body.

liver
the largest internal organ of the body, produces bile to assist in breakdown of fats and assists in the metabolism of various substances in the body.

gallbladder
a sac on the underside of the liver that stores bile produced by the liver.

pancreas
a gland located behind the stomach that produces insulin and juices that assist in digestion of food in the duodenum of the small intestine.

spleen
an organ located in the left upper quadrant of the abdomen that acts as a blood filtration system and a reservoir for reserves of blood.

appendix
a small tube located near the junction of the small and large intestines in the right lower quadrant of the abdomen, the function of which is not well understood. Its inflammation, called *appendicitis*, is a common cause of abdominal pain.

- *Small intestine.* The **small intestine** is divided into three parts: the *duodenum*, the *jejunum*, and the *ileum*. This organ receives food from the stomach and continues to break it down for absorption. These nutrients are absorbed by the body through the wall of the small intestine.
- *Large intestine (colon).* The **large intestine** removes water from waste products as they move toward elimination from the body. Anything not absorbed from this point is moved through the colon and excreted as feces.

Several organs located outside of the stomach–intestines continuum assist in the food breakdown process. These include:

- *Liver.* The **liver** produces bile, which is excreted into the small intestine to assist in the breakdown of fats. The liver has many additional functions, including detoxifying harmful substances, storing sugar, and assisting in production of blood products.
- *Gallbladder.* The **gallbladder** serves as a storage system for bile from the liver.
- *Pancreas.* Perhaps best known for production of the hormone insulin, which is involved in the regulation of sugar in the bloodstream, the **pancreas** also secretes juices that assist in breaking down proteins, carbohydrates, and fat.
- *Spleen.* Acting as a blood filtration system, the **spleen** filters out older blood cells. It has many blood vessels and at any given time holds significant quantities of blood, reserves the body can use in case of significant blood loss.
- *Appendix.* Located near the junction of the small and large intestines, the **appendix** is made up of lymphatic tissue. Its exact function is not well understood, but it is often considered with the digestive system because an infected appendix (appendicitis) is a common cause of abdominal pain.

Skin

The **skin** performs a variety of functions, including protection, water balance, temperature regulation, excretion, and shock absorption.

- *Protection.* The skin serves as a barrier to keep out microorganisms, debris, and unwanted chemicals. Underlying tissues and organs are protected from environmental contact. This helps preserve the chemical balance of body fluids and tissues.
- *Water balance.* The skin helps prevent water loss and stops environmental water from entering the body.
- *Temperature regulation.* Blood vessels in the skin can dilate (increase in diameter) to carry more blood to the skin, allowing heat to radiate from the body. When the body needs to conserve heat, these vessels constrict (decrease in diameter) to prevent heat loss. The sweat glands found in the skin produce perspiration, which will evaporate and help cool the body. The fat that is part of the skin serves as a thermal insulator.
- *Excretion.* Salts and excess water can be released through the skin.
- *Shock (impact) absorption.* The skin and its layers of fat help protect the underlying organs from minor impacts and pressures.

The skin has three major layers: the epidermis, dermis, and subcutaneous layer (Figure 4-20). The outer layer of the skin is called the **epidermis.** It is composed of four layers (strata) everywhere except at the palms of the hands and soles of the feet. These two regions have five skin layers. The outermost layers of the epidermis are composed of dead cells, which are rubbed off or sloughed off and replaced. The pigment granules of the skin and living cells are found in the deeper layers. The cells of the innermost layer actively divide, replacing the dead cells of the outer layers. Note that the epidermis contains no blood vessels or nerves. Except for certain types of burns and injuries due to cold, injuries of the epidermis present few problems in EMT-level care.

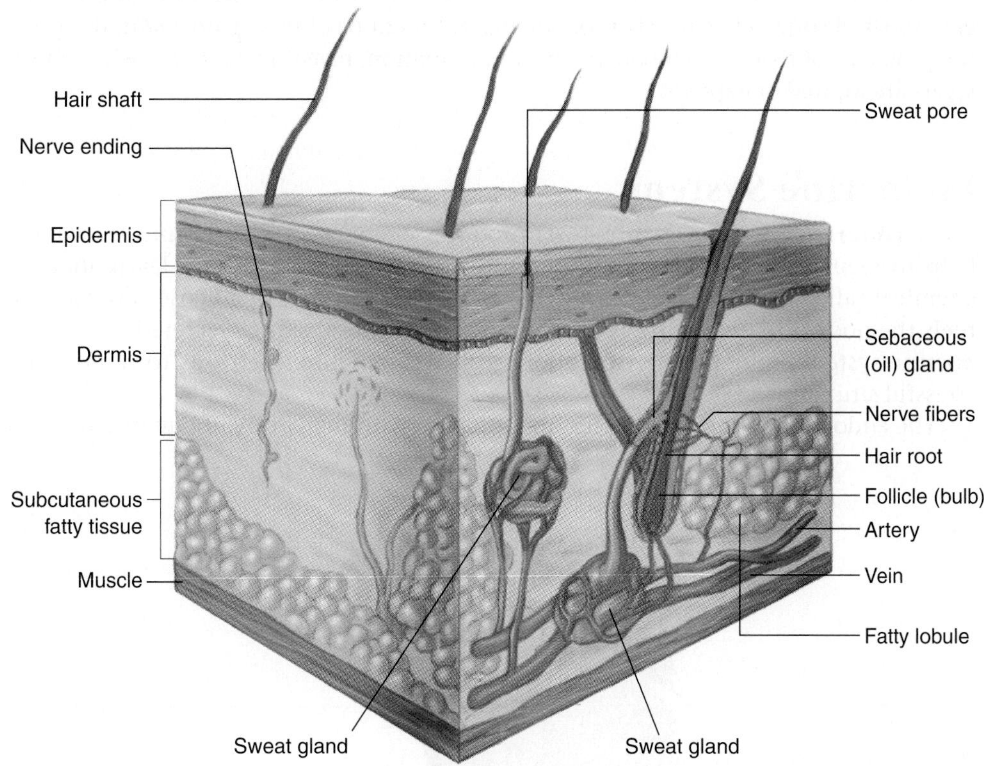

Figure 4-20 • The layers of the skin.

The layer of skin below the epidermis is the **dermis,** which is rich with blood vessels, nerves, and specialized structures such as sweat glands, sebaceous (oil) glands, and hair follicles. Specialized nerve endings are also found in the dermis. They are involved with the senses of touch, cold, heat, and pain. Once the dermis is opened to the outside world, contamination and infection become major problems. These wounds can be serious, accompanied by profuse bleeding and intense pain.

skin
the layer of tissue between the body and the external environment.

epidermis (ep-i-DER-mis)
the outer layer of skin.

dermis (DER-mis)
the inner (second) layer of skin, rich in blood vessels and nerves, found beneath the epidermis.

CRITICAL DECISION MAKING: Identifying Possible Areas of Injury

Your knowledge of anatomy is a critical foundation for making solid clinical decisions in the field. For each of the patients listed below identify what organ or body system may be involved in that patient's complaint. This exercise requires no knowledge of diseases or conditions—just the anatomy of the body.

- Your patient falls in an icy parking lot. She tries to catch herself and breaks the bones of the arm just above the wrist. What are these bones called?
- Your patient was the driver of a car that was hit in a "T-bone," or side impact, crash. He was the driver. He complains of pain in the left upper abdominal quadrant. What organ is located in this area that can cause severe internal bleeding?
- Your patient was riding a motorcycle and was thrown over the handlebars in a crash. She has broken the large bone in her right thigh. What bone is this, and would you expect blood loss from the fracture?

subcutaneous (SUB-ku-TAY-ne-us) **layers** the layers of fat and soft tissues found below the dermis.

endocrine (EN-do-krin) **system** system of glands that produce chemicals called hormones that help to regulate many body activities and functions.

insulin (IN-suh-lin) a hormone produced by the pancreas or taken as a medication by many diabetics.

epinephrine (EP-uh-NEF-rin) a hormone produced by the body. As a medication, it dilates respiratory passages and is used to relieve severe allergic reactions.

The layers of fat and soft tissue below the dermis are called the **subcutaneous layers.** Shock absorption and insulation are major functions of this layer. Again, there are the problems of tissue and bloodstream contamination, bleeding, and pain when these layers are injured or exposed.

Endocrine System

The **endocrine system** (Figure 4-21) produces chemicals called hormones, which help to regulate many body activities and functions. You will later learn about a chemical called **insulin,** a hormone that is critical in the use of glucose, a sugar that fuels the body. **Epinephrine** is another example of a substance secreted by the endocrine system. Epinephrine (sometimes called adrenaline) helps us to respond to stressful situations.

The endocrine system is complex and interacts with many other body systems.

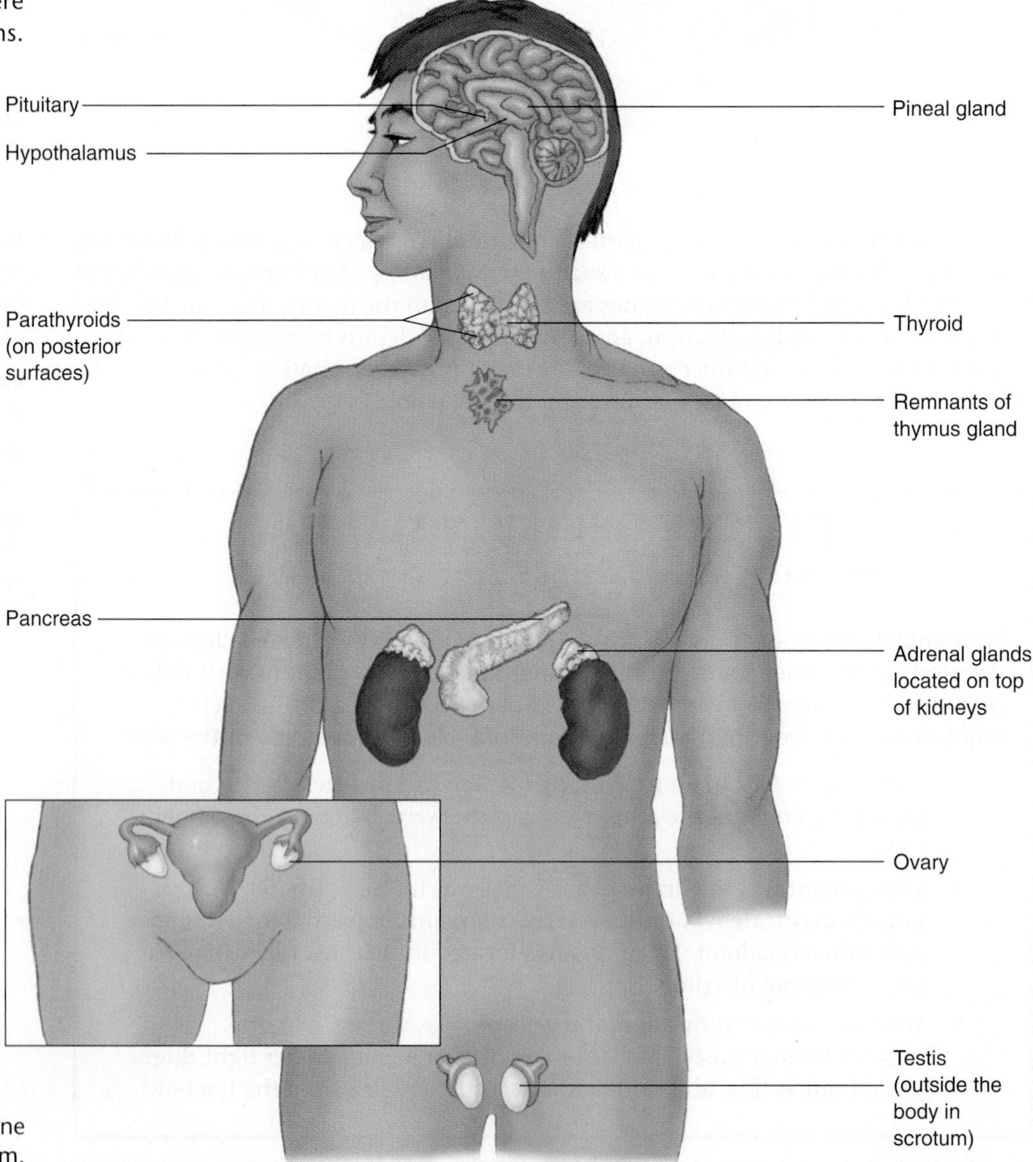

Figure 4-21 • The endocrine system.

F•Y•I

LOCATING BODY ORGANS AND STRUCTURES

As an EMT, you will find it useful to understand the position of the body's major organs and structures. There are two ways to help locate organs and structures of the body. The first is visualizing, or being able to picture, organs and structures inside the body as you look at the external body. The second is topography, or external landmarks such as notches, joints, and "bumps" on bones. Some external landmarks are obvious (e.g., the navel, the nipples), some you know by other names but will have to learn the medical terms (e.g., the "Adam's apple," which is properly called the thyroid cartilage), and some will probably be new to you (e.g., the xiphoid process). It is important to learn where internal organs and structures are in relation to these landmarks, which you can easily see or feel from outside the body.

Scan 4-1 shows the positions of major organs and systems. Scan 4-2 shows the positions of major landmarks on the outer body (topography) and skeletal structures within the body. ■

SCAN 4-1 • Major Body Organs

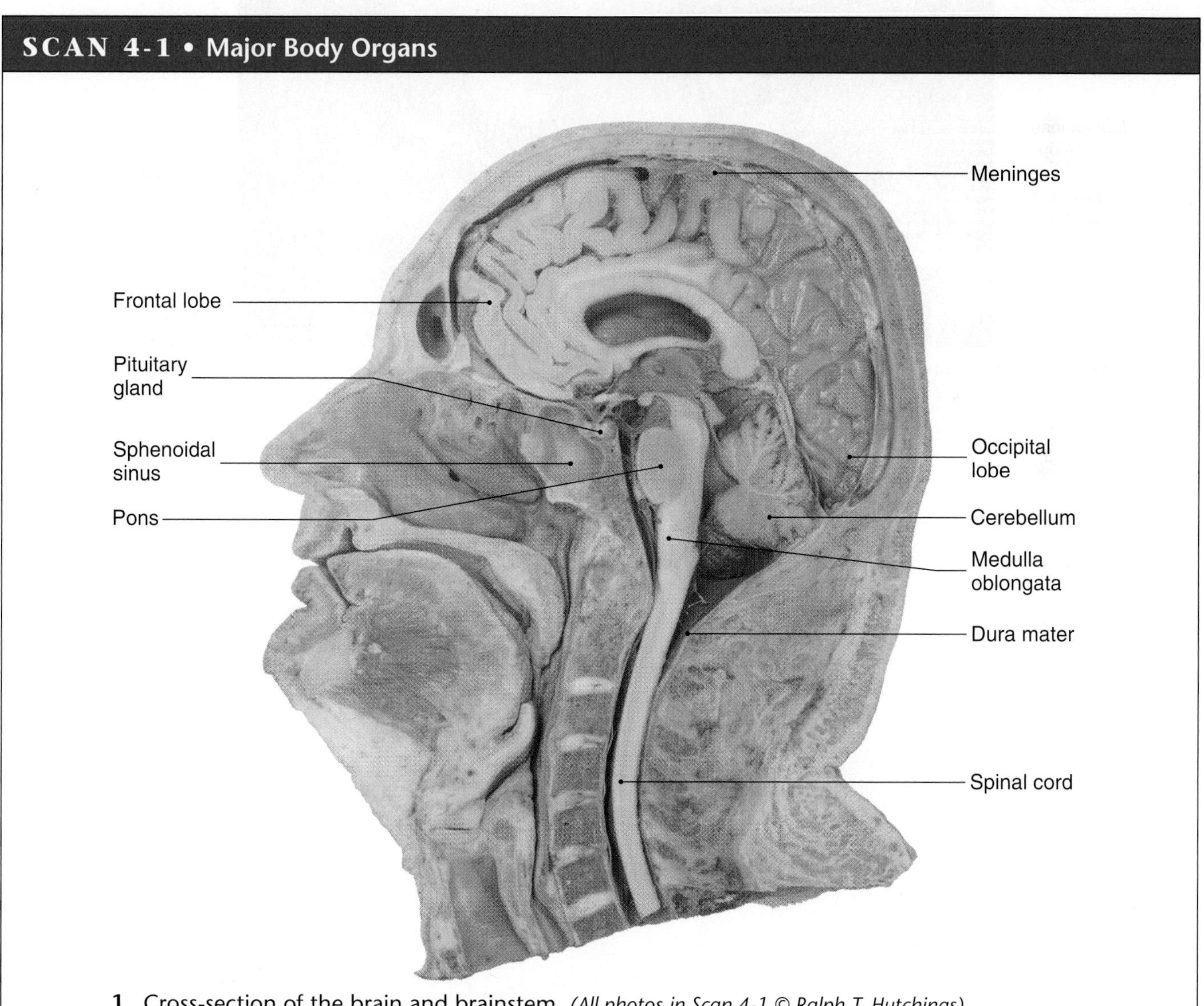

1. Cross-section of the brain and brainstem. *(All photos in Scan 4-1 © Ralph T. Hutchings)*

continued

SCAN 4-1 • (Continued)

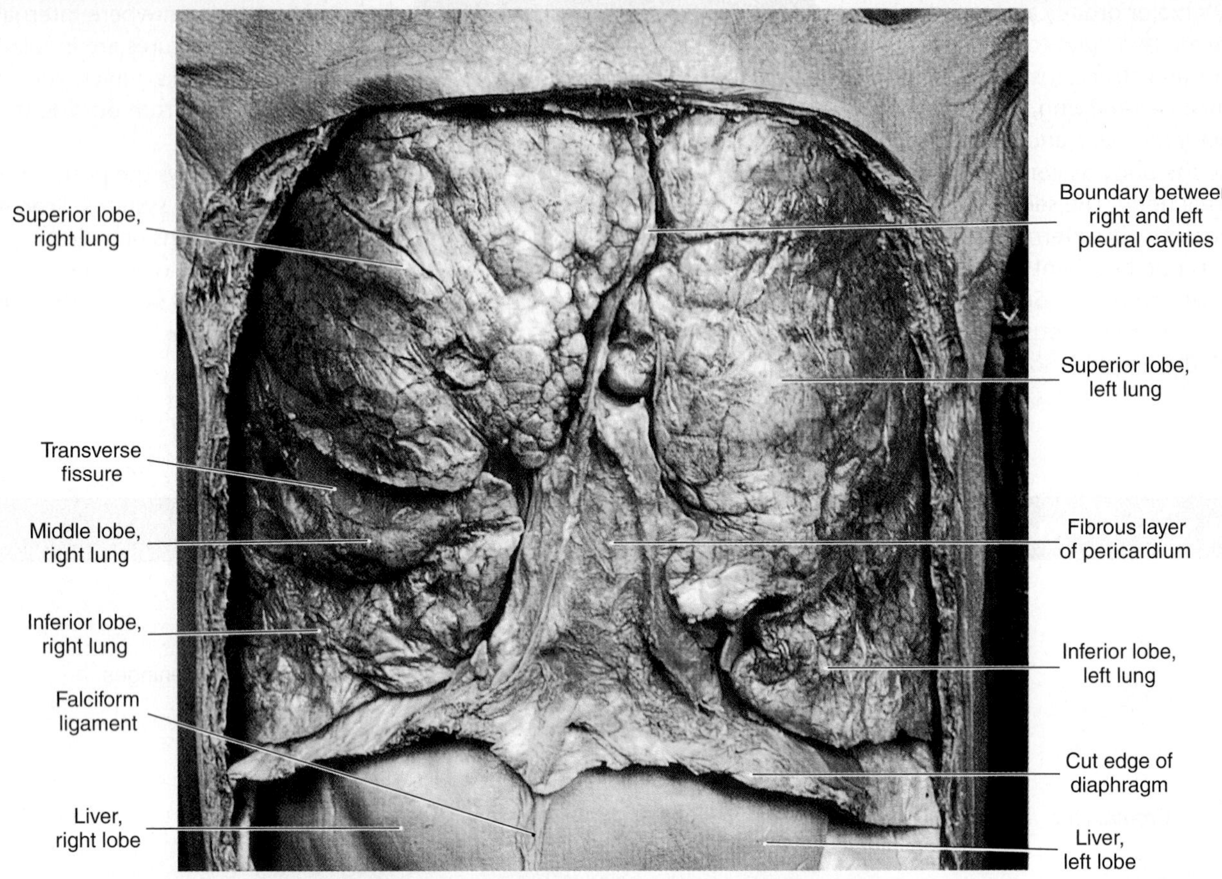

2. The thoracic cavity.

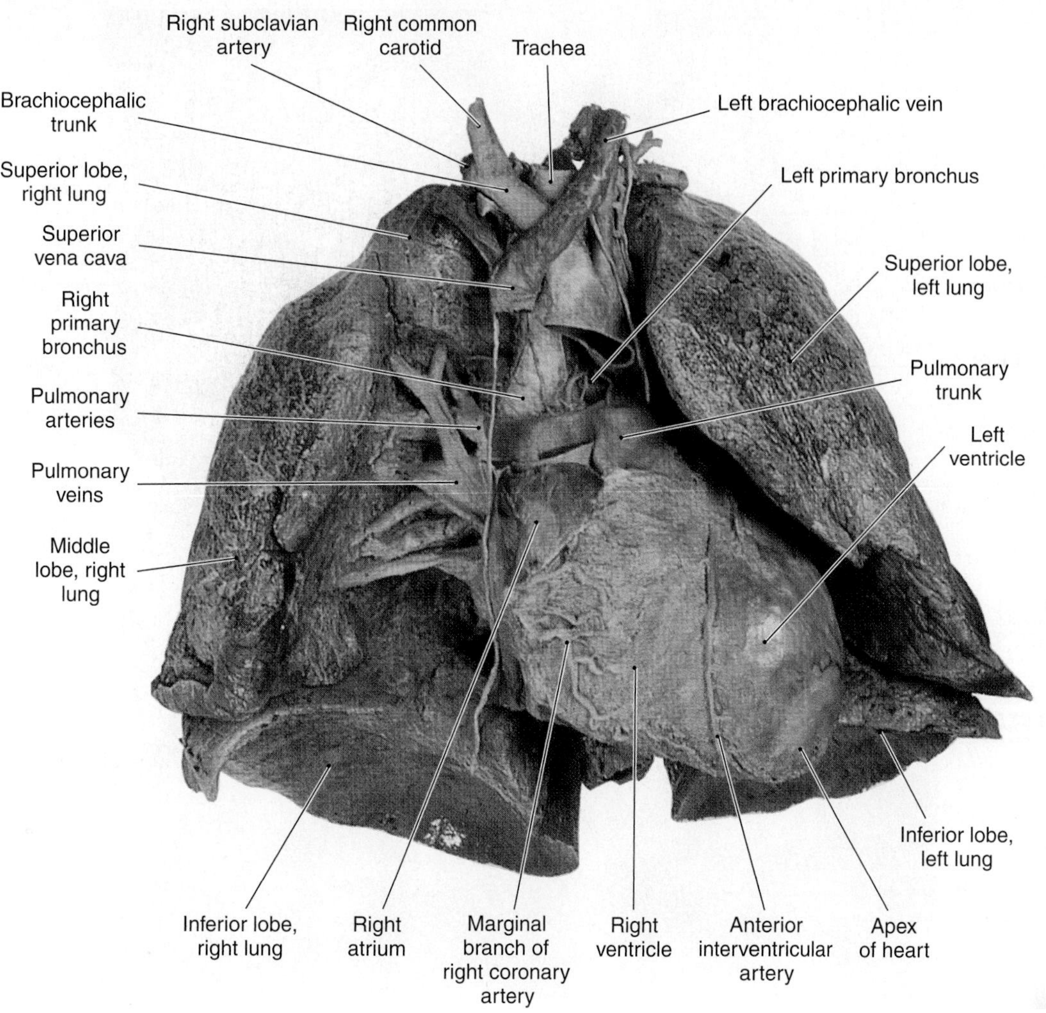
Right subclavian artery
Right common carotid
Trachea
Brachiocephalic trunk
Left brachiocephalic vein
Superior lobe, right lung
Left primary bronchus
Superior vena cava
Superior lobe, left lung
Right primary bronchus
Pulmonary trunk
Pulmonary arteries
Left ventricle
Pulmonary veins
Middle lobe, right lung
Inferior lobe, left lung
Inferior lobe, right lung
Right atrium
Marginal branch of right coronary artery
Right ventricle
Anterior interventricular artery
Apex of heart

3. Lungs, heart, and great vessels.

continued

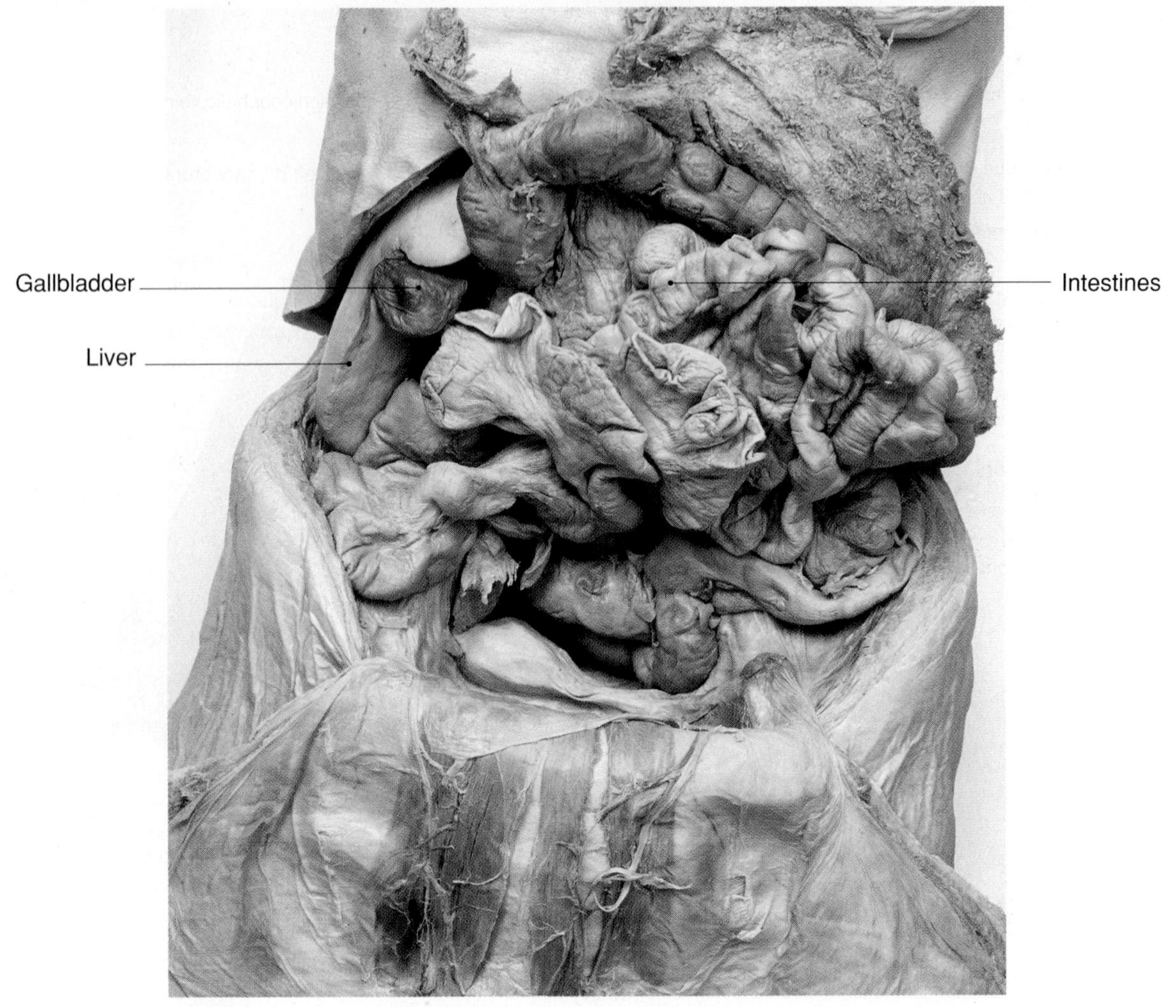

4. Abdominal cavity.

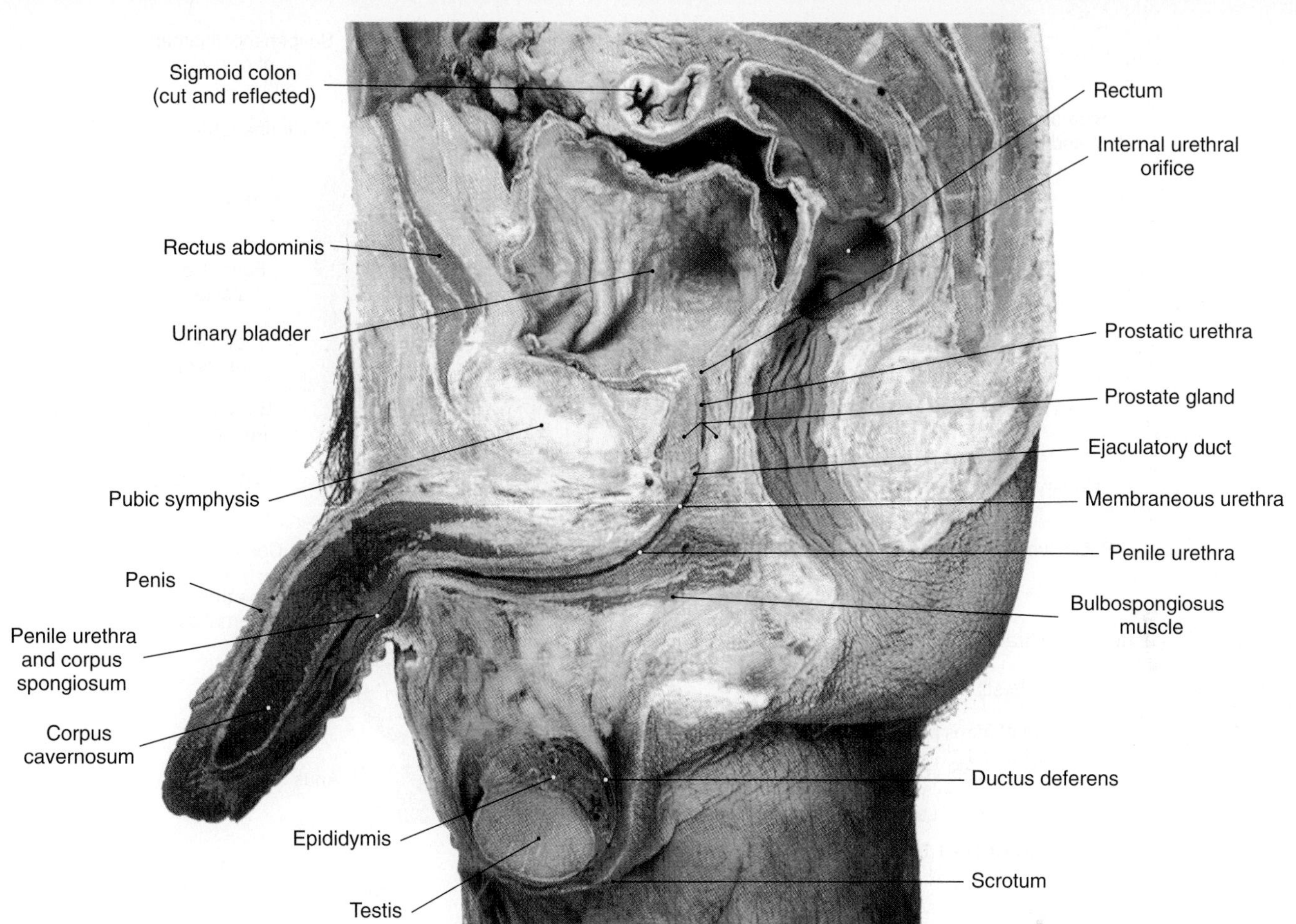

5. Cross-section of the male reproductive system.

continued

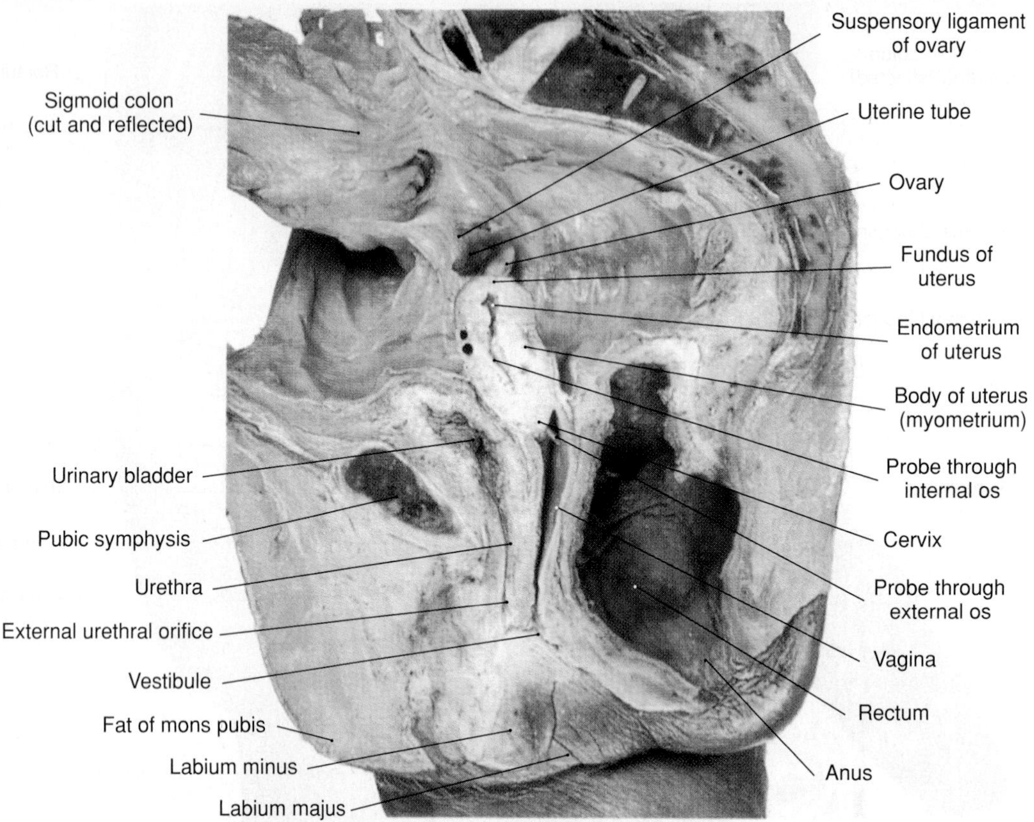

6. Cross-section of the female reproductive system.

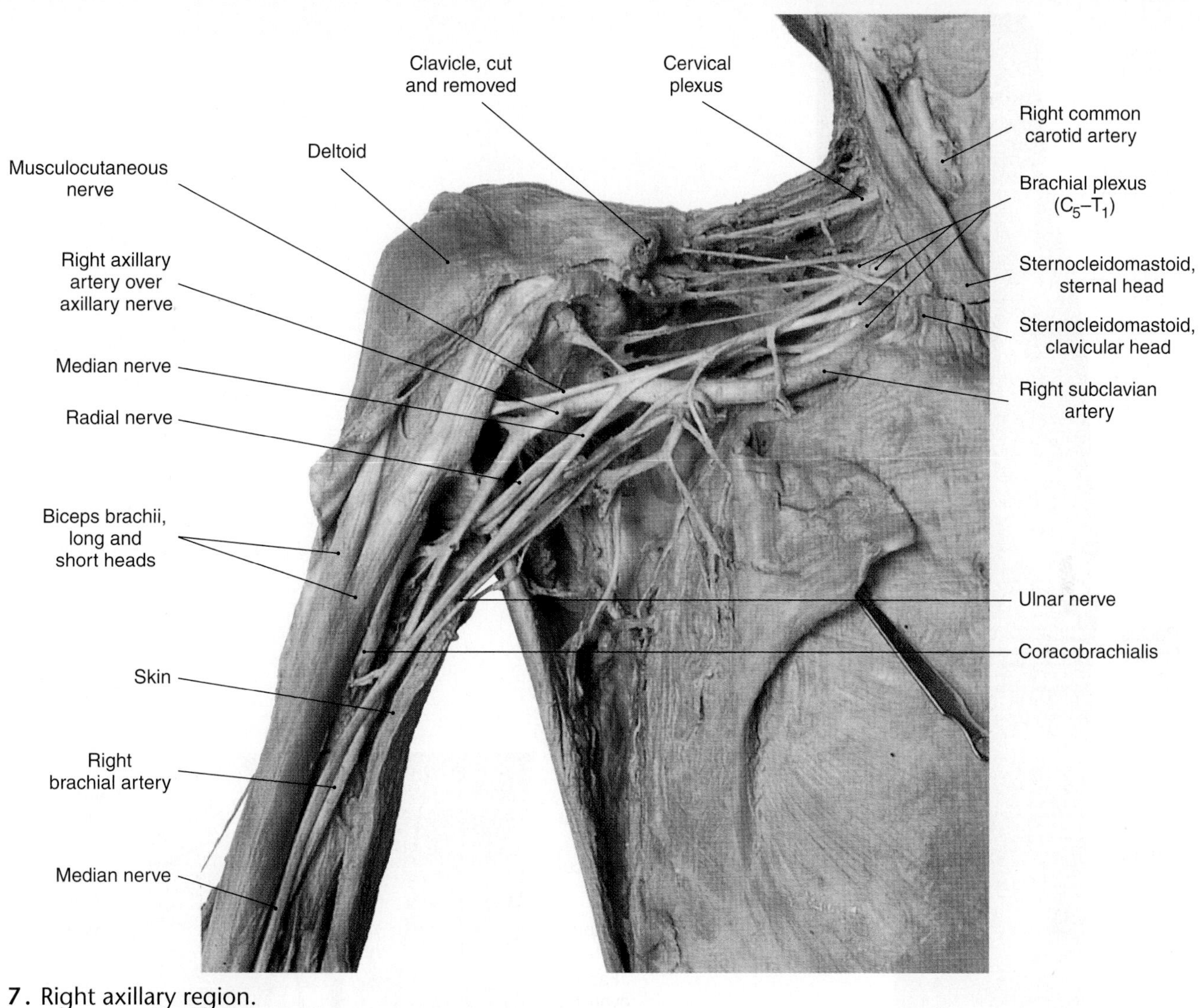

Clavicle, cut and removed
Cervical plexus
Right common carotid artery
Deltoid
Musculocutaneous nerve
Brachial plexus (C_5–T_1)
Right axillary artery over axillary nerve
Sternocleidomastoid, sternal head
Sternocleidomastoid, clavicular head
Median nerve
Right subclavian artery
Radial nerve
Biceps brachii, long and short heads
Ulnar nerve
Coracobrachialis
Skin
Right brachial artery
Median nerve

7. Right axillary region.

continued

SCAN 4-1 • (Continued)

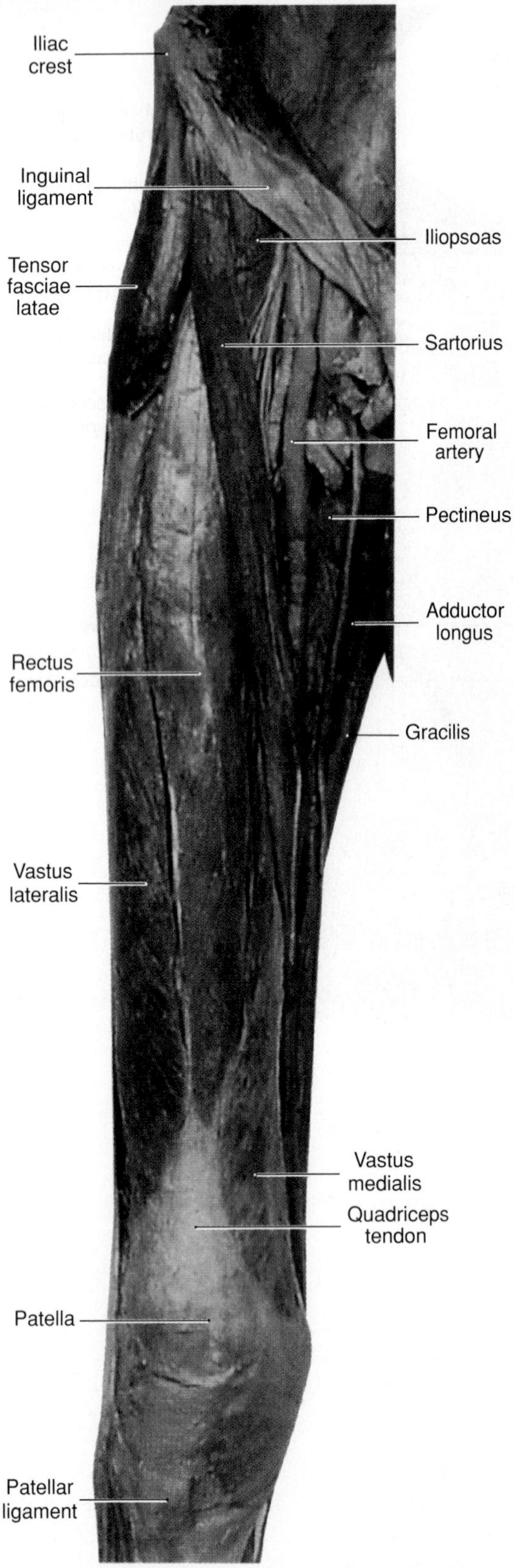

8. Muscles of the lower extremity.

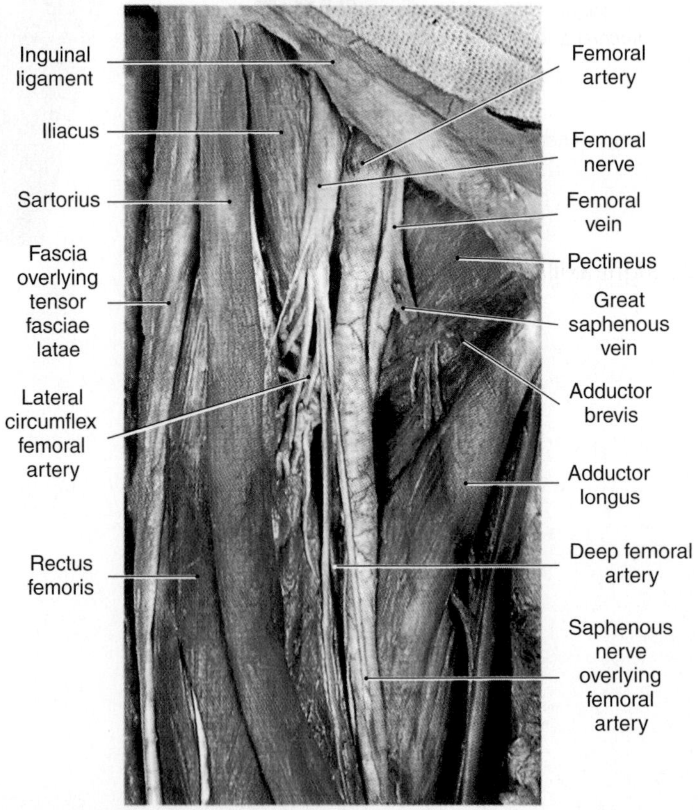

9. Major blood vessels of the thigh.

SCAN 4-2 • Topography and Skeleton

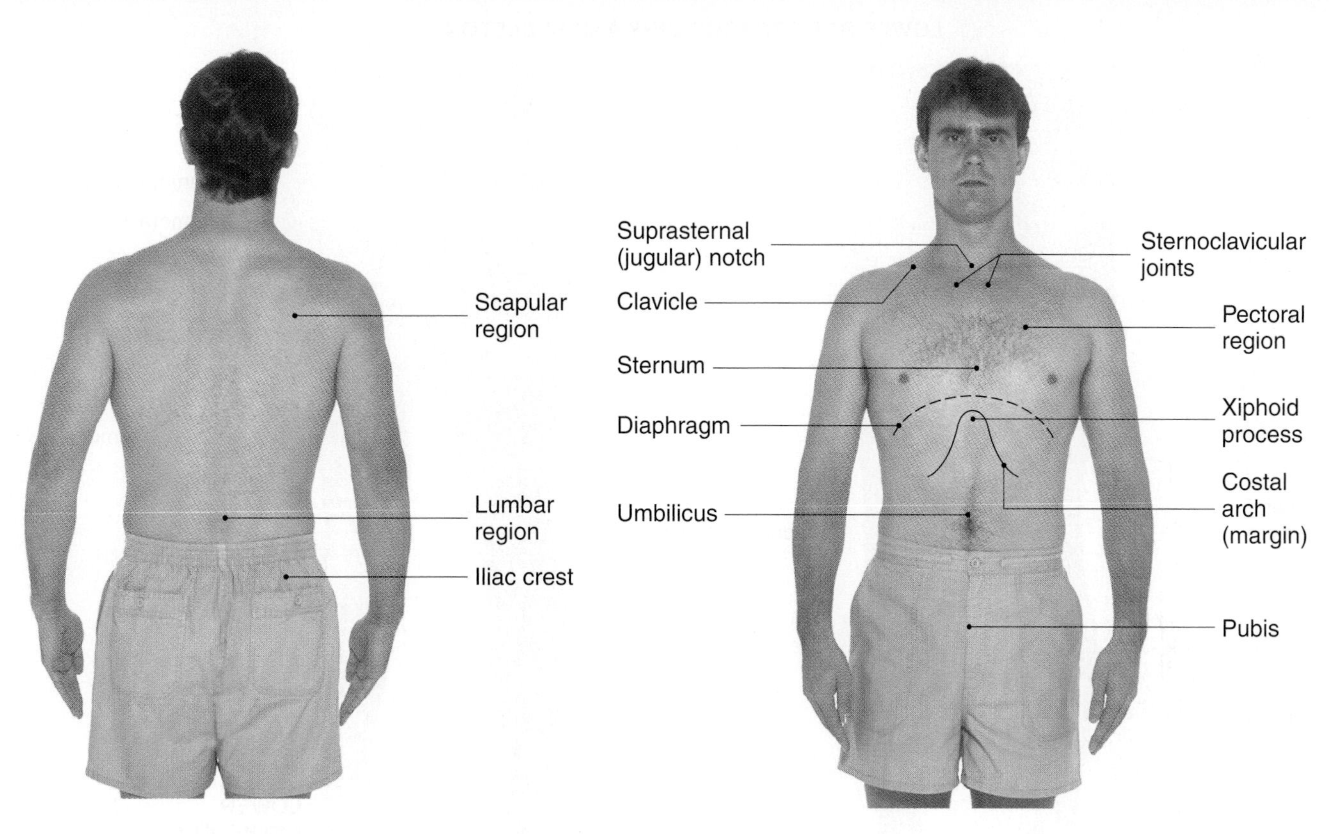

HEAD AND NECK TOPOGRAPHY

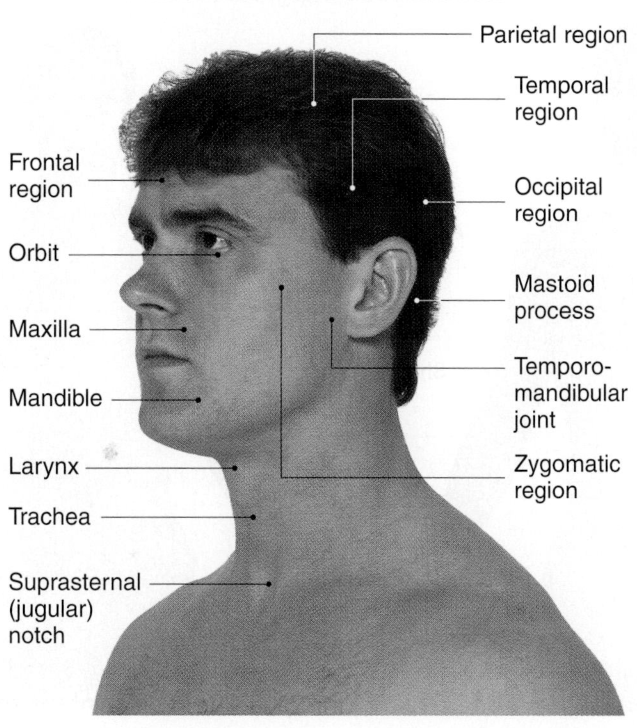

continued

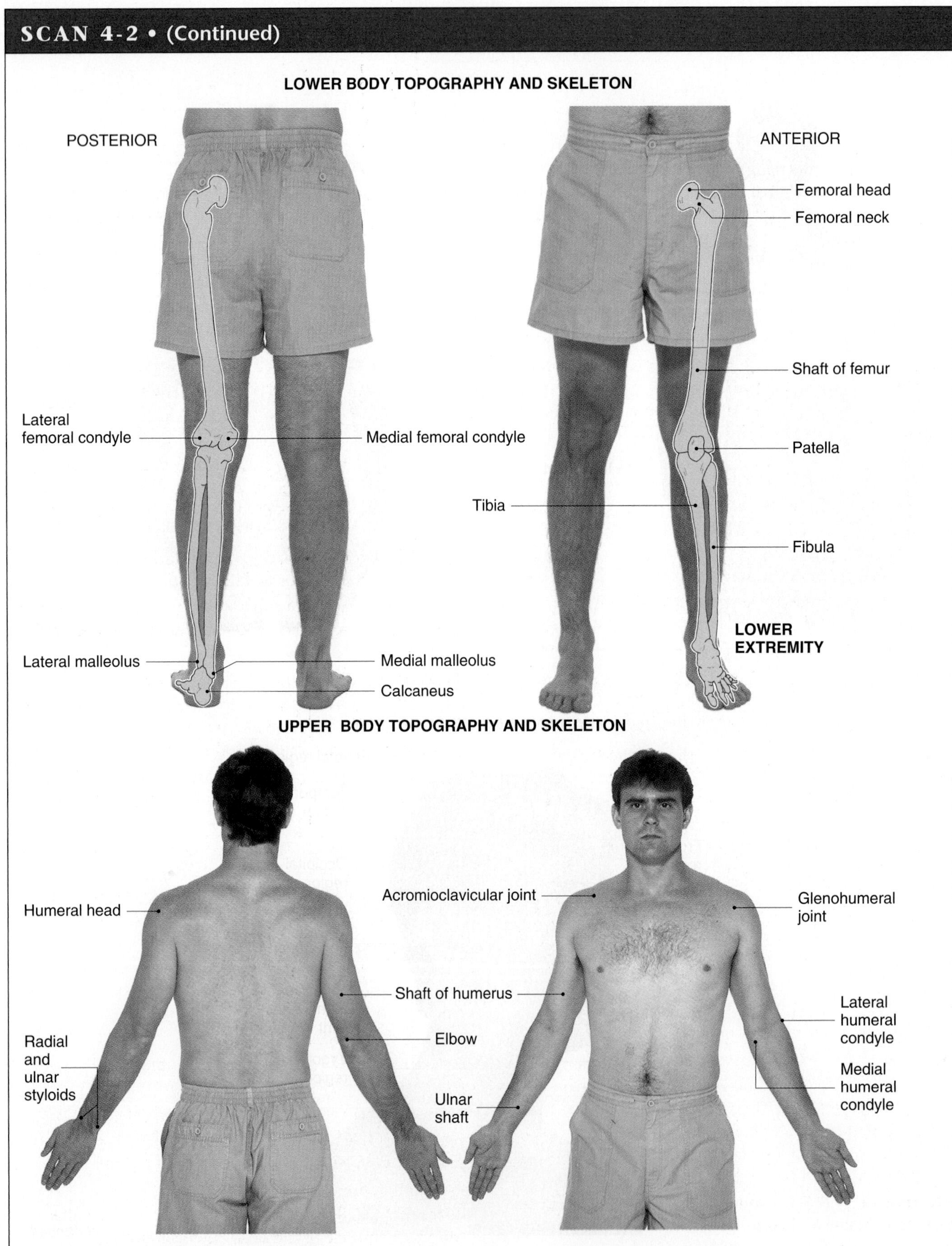
LOWER BODY TOPOGRAPHY AND SKELETON
POSTERIOR
ANTERIOR
Femoral head
Femoral neck
Shaft of femur
Lateral femoral condyle
Medial femoral condyle
Patella
Tibia
Fibula
LOWER EXTREMITY
Lateral malleolus
Medial malleolus
Calcaneus
UPPER BODY TOPOGRAPHY AND SKELETON
Humeral head
Acromioclavicular joint
Glenohumeral joint
Shaft of humerus
Lateral humeral condyle
Radial and ulnar styloids
Elbow
Medial humeral condyle
Ulnar shaft

CHAPTER REVIEW

SUMMARY

As an EMT, your knowledge of the anatomy, or structure, of the body and the functions, or physiology, of the body will be important in allowing you to assess your patient and communicate your findings with other EMS personnel and hospital staff accurately and efficiently.

Major body systems with which you should be familiar include the musculoskeletal system, respiratory system, cardiovascular system, nervous system, digestive system, the skin, and endocrine system.

KEY TERMS

abdominal quadrants four divisions of the abdomen used to pinpoint the location of a pain or injury: the right upper quadrant (RUQ), the left upper quadrant (LUQ), the right lower quadrant (RLQ), and the left lower quadrant (LLQ).

acetabulum (AS-uh-TAB-yuh-lum) the pelvic socket into which the ball at the proximal end of the femur fits to form the hip joint.

acromioclavicular (ah-KRO-me-o-klav-IK-yuh-ler) **joint** the joint where the acromion and the clavicle meet.

acromion (ah-KRO-me-on) **process** the highest portion of the shoulder.

alveoli (al-VE-o-li) the microscopic sacs of the lungs where gas exchange with the bloodstream takes place.

anatomical position the standard reference position for the body in the study of anatomy. In this position, the body is standing erect, facing the observer, with arms down at the sides and the palms of the hands forward.

anatomy the study of body structure.

anterior the front of the body or body part.

aorta (ay-OR-tah) the largest artery in the body. It transports blood from the left ventricle to begin systemic circulation.

appendix a small tube located near the junction of the small and large intestines in the right lower quadrant of the abdomen, the function of which is not well understood. Its inflammation, called appendicitis, is a common cause of abdominal pain.

arteriole (ar-TE-re-ol) the smallest kind of artery.

artery any blood vessel carrying blood away from the heart.

atria (AY-tree-ah) the two upper chambers of the heart. There is a right atrium (which receives unoxygenated blood returning from the body) and a left atrium (which receives oxygenated blood returning from the lungs).

automaticity (AW-to-muh-TISS-it-e) the ability of the heart to generate and conduct electrical impulses on its own.

autonomic (AW-to-NOM-ik) **nervous system** the division of the peripheral nervous system that controls involuntary motor functions.

bilateral on both sides.

blood pressure the pressure caused by blood exerting force against the walls of blood vessels. Usually arterial blood pressure (the pressure in an artery) is measured. diastolic blood pressure and systolic blood pressure.

brachial artery artery of the upper arm; the site of the pulse checked during infant CPR.

bronchi (BRONG-ki) the two large sets of branches that come off the trachea and enter the lungs. There are right and left bronchi. *Singular* bronchus.

calcaneus (kal-KAY-ne-us) the heel bone.

capillary (KAP-i-lair-e) a thin-walled, microscopic blood vessel where the oxygen/carbon dioxide and nutrient/waste exchange with the body's cells takes place.

cardiac conduction system a system of specialized muscle tissues which conduct electrical impulses that stimulate the heart to beat.

cardiac muscle specialized involuntary muscle found only in the heart.

cardiovascular (KAR-de-o-VAS-kyu-ler) **system** the system made up of the heart (cardio) and the blood vessels (vascular); the circulatory system.

carotid (kah-ROT-id) **arteries** the large neck arteries, one on each side of the neck, that carry blood from the heart to the head.

carpals (KAR-pulz) the wrist bones.

central nervous system (CNS) the brain and spinal cord.

central pulses the carotid and femoral pulses, which can be felt in the central part of the body.

circulatory system *See* cardiovascular system.

clavicle (KLAV-i-kul) the collarbone.

coronary (KOR-o-nar-e) **arteries** blood vessels that supply the muscle of the heart (myocardium).

cranium the top, back, and sides of the skull.

cricoid (KRIK-oid) **cartilage** the ring-shaped structure that forms the lower portion of the larynx.

dermis (DER-mis) the inner (second) layer of skin, rich in blood vessels and nerves, found beneath the epidermis.

diaphragm (DI-uh-fram) the muscular structure that divides the chest cavity from the abdominal cavity. A major muscle of respiration.

diastolic (di-as-TOL-ik) **blood pressure** the pressure in the arteries when the left ventricle is refilling.

digestive system system by which food travels through the body and is digested, or broken down into absorbable forms.

distal farther away from the torso. *See also* proximal.

dorsal referring to the back of the body or the back of the hand or foot. A synonym for posterior.

dorsalis pedis (dor-SAL-is PEED-is) **artery** artery supplying the foot, lateral to the large tendon of the big toe.

endocrine (EN-do-krin) **system** system of glands that produce chemicals called hormones that help to regulate many body activities and functions.

epidermis (ep-i-DER-mis) the outer layer of skin.

epiglottis (EP-i-GLOT-is) a leaf-shaped structure that prevents food and foreign matter from entering the trachea.

epinephrine (EP-uh-NEF-rin) a hormone produced by the body. As a medication, it dilates respiratory passages and is used to relieve severe allergic reactions.

exhalation (EX-huh-LAY-shun) a passive process in which the intercostal (rib) muscles and the diaphragm relax, causing the chest cavity to decrease in size and air to flow out of the lungs.

femoral (FEM-o-ral) **artery** the major artery supplying the leg.

femur (FEE-mer) the large bone of the thigh.

fibula (FIB-yuh-luh) the lateral and smaller bone of the lower leg.

Fowler's position a sitting position.

gallbladder a sac on the underside of the liver that stores bile produced by the liver.

humerus (HYU-mer-us) the bone of the upper arm, between the shoulder and the elbow.

hypoperfusion inadequate perfusion of the cells and tissues of the body caused by insufficient flow of blood through the capillaries. *See also* perfusion.

ilium (IL-e-um) the superior and widest portion of the pelvis.

inferior away from the head; usually compared with another structure that is closer to the head (e.g., the lips are inferior to the nose).

inhalation (IN-huh-LAY-shun) an active process in which the intercostal (rib) muscles and the diaphragm contract, expanding the size of the chest cavity and causing air to flow into the lungs.

insulin (IN-suh-lin) a hormone produced by the pancreas or taken as a medication by many diabetics.

involuntary muscle muscle that responds automatically to brain signals but cannot be consciously controlled.

ischium (ISH-e-um) the lower, posterior portions of the pelvis.

joint the point where two bones come together.

large intestine the muscular tube that removes water from waste products received from the small intestine and removes anything not absorbed by the body toward excretion from the body.

larynx (LAIR-inks) the voice box.

lateral to the side, away from the midline of the body.

ligament tissue that connects bone to bone.

liver the largest organ of the body, produces bile to assist in breakdown of fats and assists in the metabolism of various substances in the body.

lungs the organs where exchange of atmospheric oxygen and waste carbon dioxide take place.

malleolus (mal-E-o-lus) protrusion on the side of the ankle. The *lateral malleolus*, at the lower end of the fibula, is seen on the outer ankle; the *medial malleolus*, at the lower end of the tibia, is seen on the inner ankle.

mandible (MAN-di-bul) the lower jaw bone.

manubrium (man-OO-bre-um) the superior portion of the sternum.

maxillae (mak-SIL-e) the two fused bones forming the upper jaw.

medial toward the midline of the body.

metacarpals (MET-uh-KAR-pulz) the hand bones.

metatarsals (MET-uh-TAR-sulz) the foot bones.

mid-axillary (mid-AX-uh-lair-e) **line** a line drawn vertically from the middle of the armpit to the ankle.

mid-clavicular (mid-clah-VIK-yuh-ler) **line** the line through the center of each clavicle.

midline an imaginary line drawn down the center of the body, dividing it into right and left halves.

muscle tissue that can contract to allow movement of a body part.

musculoskeletal (MUS-kyu-lo-SKEL-e-tal) **system** the system of bones and skeletal muscles that support and protect the body and permit movement.

nasal (NAY-zul) **bones** the nose bones.

nasopharynx (NAY-zo-FAIR-inks) the area directly posterior to the nose.

nervous system the system of brain, spinal cord, and nerves that govern sensation, movement, and thought.

orbits the bony structures around the eyes; the eye sockets.

oropharynx (OR-o-FAIR-inks) the area directly posterior to the mouth.

palmar referring to the palm of the hand.

pancreas a gland located behind the stomach that produces insulin and juices that assist in digestion of food in the duodenum of the small intestine.

patella (pah-TEL-uh) the kneecap.

pelvis the basin-shaped bony structure that supports the spine and is the point of proximal attachment for the lower extremities.

perfusion the supply of oxygen to and removal of wastes from the cells and tissues of the body as a result of the flow of blood through the capillaries.

peripheral nervous system (PNS) the nerves that enter and leave the spinal cord and travel between the brain and organs without passing through the spinal cord.

peripheral pulses the radial, brachial, posterior tibial, and dorsalis pedis pulses, which can be felt at peripheral (outlying) points of the body.

phalanges (fuh-LAN-jiz) the toe bones and finger bones.

pharynx (FAIR-inks) the area directly posterior to the mouth and nose. It is made up of the oropharynx and the nasopharynx.

physiology the study of body function.

plane a flat surface formed when slicing through a solid object.

plantar referring to the sole of the foot.

plasma (PLAZ-mah) the fluid portion of the blood.

platelets components of the blood; membrane-enclosed fragments of specialized cells.

posterior the back of the body or body part.

posterior tibial (TIB-ee-ul) **artery** artery supplying the foot, behind the medial ankle.

prone lying face down.

proximal closer to the torso. *See also* distal.

pubis (PYOO-bis) the medial anterior portion of the pelvis.

pulmonary (PUL-mo-nar-e) **arteries** the vessels that carry blood from the right ventricle of the heart to the lungs.

pulmonary veins the vessels that carry oxygenated blood from the lungs to the left atrium of the heart.

pulse the rhythmic beats caused as waves of blood move through and expand the arteries.

radial artery artery of the lower arm. It is felt when taking the pulse at the wrist.

radius (RAY-de-us) the lateral bone of the forearm.

recovery position lying on the side. Also called *lateral recumbent position.*

red blood cells components of the blood. They carry oxygen to and carbon dioxide away from the cells.

respiratory (RES-pir-ah-tor-e) **system** the system of nose, mouth, throat, lungs, and muscles that brings oxygen into the body and expels carbon dioxide.

scapula (SKAP-yuh-luh) the shoulder blade.

shock *See* hypoperfusion.

skeleton the bones of the body.

skin the layer of tissue between the body and the external environment.

skull the bony structure of the head.

small intestine the muscular tube between the stomach and the large intestine, divided into the duodenum, the jejunum, and the ileum, which receives partially digested food from the stomach and continues digestion. Nutrients are absorbed by the body through its walls.

spleen an organ located in the left upper quadrant of the abdomen that acts as a blood filtration system and a reservoir for reserves of blood.

sternum (STER-num) the breastbone.

stomach muscular sac between the esophagus and the small intestine where digestion of food begins.

subcutaneous (SUB-ku-TAY-ne-us) **layers** the layers of fat and soft tissues found below the dermis.

superior toward the head (e.g., the chest is superior to the abdomen).

supine lying on the back.

systolic (sis-TOL-ik) **blood pressure** the pressure created in the arteries when the left ventricle contracts and forces blood out into circulation.

tarsals (TAR-sulz) the ankle bones.

tendon tissue that connects muscle to bone.

thorax (THOR-ax) the chest.

tibia (TIB-e-uh) the medial and larger bone of the lower leg.

torso the trunk of the body; the body without the head and the extremities.

trachea (TRAY-ke-uh) the "windpipe"; the structure that connects the pharynx to the lungs.

Trendelenburg (trend-EL-un-berg) **position** a position in which the patient's feet and legs are higher than the head. Also called *shock position.*

ulna (UL-nah) the medial bone of the forearm.

valve a structure that opens and closes to permit the flow of a fluid in only one direction.

vein any blood vessel returning blood to the heart.

venae cavae (VE-ne KA-ve) the superior vena cava and the inferior vena cava. These two major veins return blood from the body to the right atrium. (Venae cavae is plural, vena cava singular.)

ventral referring to the front of the body. A synonym for anterior.

ventricles (VEN-tri-kulz) the two lower chambers of the heart. There is a right ventricle (which sends oxygen-poor blood to the lungs) and a left ventricle (which sends oxygen-rich blood to the body).

venule (VEN-yul) the smallest kind of vein.

vertebrae (VER-te-bray) the 33 bones of the spinal column.

voluntary muscle muscle that can be consciously controlled.

white blood cells components of the blood. They produce substances that help the body fight infection.

xiphoid (ZI-foid) **process** the inferior portion of the sternum.

zygomatic (ZI-go-MAT-ik) **arches** form the structure of the cheeks.

REVIEW QUESTIONS

1. Define the following anatomical terms (pp. 66–68):

medial	lateral
anterior	posterior
mid-clavicular	distal

2. List the three functions of the musculoskeletal system. (p. 70)
3. Name the five divisions of the spine and describe the location of each. (pp. 71, 72, 73)
4. Describe the physical processes of inhalation and exhalation. (p. 76)
5. List four places a peripheral pulse may be felt. (p. 82)
6. Describe the central nervous system and peripheral nervous system. (pp. 83, 85)
7. List three functions of the skin. (p. 86)

CRITICAL THINKING

- As an EMT, you are called to respond to a teenage boy who has taken a hard fall from his dirt bike. He has a deep gash on the outside of his left arm about halfway between the shoulder and the elbow and another on the inside of his right arm just above the wrist. His left leg is bent at a funny angle about halfway between hip and knee, and when you cut away his pants leg, you see a bone sticking out of a wound on the front side. You take the necessary on-scene assessment and care steps and are on the way to the hospital in the ambulance. How do you describe your patient's injuries over the radio to the hospital staff?

MEDIA RESOURCES 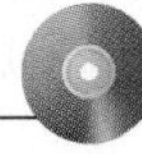

See the Student CD at the back of this book for quizzes, a case study activity, animations, and other features related to this chapter. In particular, take a look at the Virtual Airway Tour, the 3D animations of the respiratory system and the circulatory and nervous systems of the extremities, and the animations of anatomical movements. Also, visit the Companion Website for *Emergency Care* at **www.prenhall.com/limmer,** where you will find additional reinforcement and links to other resources.

Street Scenes

"Respond to Elm Street near the intersection on Central Avenue for a report of a motor-vehicle crash. Third-party call from a passerby on a cell phone. The time is now 1505 hours." Your response time is relatively fast, and you arrive before the dispatcher can provide any additional information. As you approach the scene, you see that two vehicles are involved in the crash. It appears the truck rear-ended the four-door sedan. A police officer has already taken charge of traffic control. You ask him, "How many patients?" and are told there are three. You find an open area to place the ambulance. Once assured that the scene is safe, you begin your assessment.

The driver of the truck is walking around the scene. The other vehicle had two occupants—a mother and her son, who was belted in the back seat. The mother is tending to the child who appears to be unresponsive. It doesn't look as if the impact speed was great, but the child hit his head fairly hard on the arm rest and you can still see the dent. A First Response unit is also on scene and they tell you they will check on the driver of the truck. You turn your attention to the child.

The mother tells you she is fine. "Just take care of Peter. He's only 6 years old." You get into the vehicle next to the child and hear that he has snoring respirations. You remember that the tongue is the most likely cause, so you manually stabilize the head and neck to prevent any further injury to his head and cervical spine. As you do so, you push Peter's jaw forward to move the tongue in the direction of the mandible. It works, and the snoring sound stops. Your partner prepares for extrication to the backboard.

Street Scene Questions

1. As you assess your young patient, how does his anatomy impact on the process?
2. What should you be alert to when examining the child's abdomen?

Before rotating Peter onto the backboard, you apply a cervical collar. Then you rotate him onto the board. Remembering that a child's head is larger in proportion to the rest of the body than an adult's, you place a folded towel under Peter's shoulders in order to keep his head in a neutral position with the airway open. Your partner calls out to Peter to see if his mental status has changed. Peter responds to painful stimuli only.

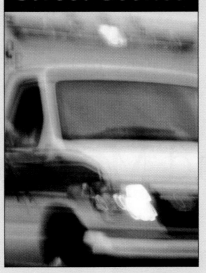

Once Peter has been moved into the ambulance, you perform a head-to-toe exam. When you get to the abdomen, you palpate all four quadrants and observe a bruise, probably caused by the lap portion of the seat belt. Peter reacts as if in pain when you touch the left upper quadrant, and you think that his spleen may have been injured.

En route to the hospital, you find the patient is breathing at a rate of 32 and has a pulse of 150. You call out to Peter, and this time he responds to your voice.

Street Scene Questions

3. What are the significant findings based on the assessment and your knowledge of the human body?
4. Do you have any concerns about additional injuries to this patient? If so, what are they?

You take another set of vital signs and find that Peter has an increase in pulse and respiration rates. You perform an ongoing assessment and find there is still pain in the upper left quadrant of the abdomen. As you run your hands over the patient's back, you are concerned by apparent pain in the lumbar region of the spine, which may have been caused by the force of the crash.

Your partner tells you the ETA to the hospital is 10 minutes and notifies emergency department personnel by radio. The transmission gives an overview of the injuries and the vital signs, noting the change in the last 10 minutes. He mentions how the patient's mental status has changed and describes the abdominal and lumbar pain and location.

When the patient is being wheeled into the trauma room, they do a quick assessment and check the abdomen. The emergency department physician tells you that because of assessment findings given in the radio report, she has a surgeon on the way to check Peter.

"Good job!" she adds.

CHAPTER

Lifting and Moving Patients

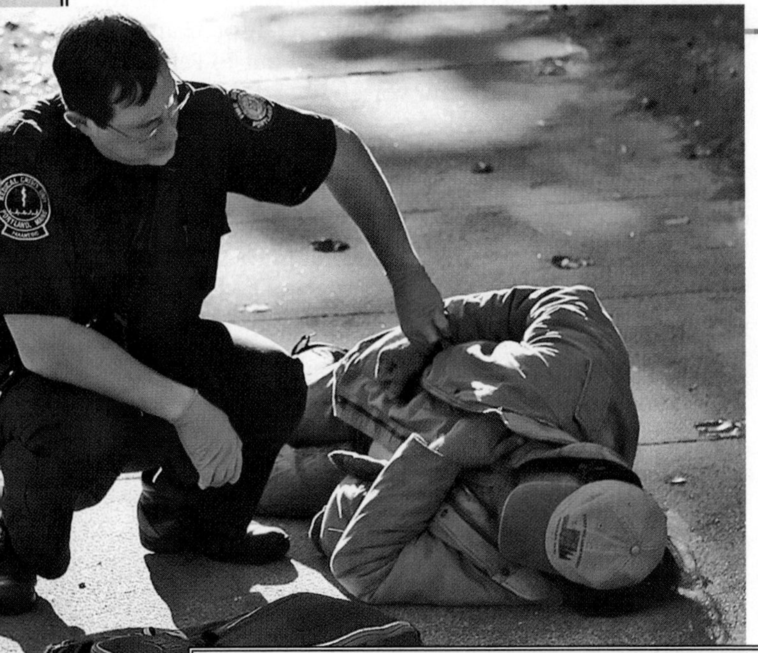

CORE CONCEPTS

The following are core concepts that will be addressed in this chapter:

- How using body mechanics to lift and move patients can help prevent injury
- When it is proper to move a patient, and how to do so safely
- The various devices used to immobilize, move, and carry patients

KEY TERMS

body mechanics, p. 106
direct carry, p. 123
direct ground lift, p. 123
draw-sheet method, p. 123
extremity lift, p. 123
power grip, p. 107
power lift, p. 107

DOT OBJECTIVES

*KNOWLEDGE AND ATTITUDE

1-6.1 Define body mechanics. (p. 106)

1-6.2 Discuss the guidelines and safety precautions that need to be followed when lifting a patient. (pp. 106–108)

1-6.3 Describe the safe lifting of cots and stretchers. (pp. 112–119)

1-6.4 Describe the guidelines and safety precautions for carrying patients and/or equipment. (p. 106)

1-6.5 Discuss one-handed carrying techniques. (p. 106)

1-6.6 Describe correct and safe carrying procedures on stairs. (pp. 117–119)

1-6.7 State the guidelines for reaching and their application. (p. 108)

1-6.8 Describe correct reaching for log rolls. (p. 109)

1-6.9 State the guidelines for pushing and pulling. (p. 108)

1-6.10 Discuss the general considerations of moving patients. (p. 106)

1-6.11 State three situations that may require the use of an emergency move. (pp. 108–109) (Scan 5-1, p. 110; Scan 5-2, p. 111; Scan 5-3, p. 112)

1-6.12 Identify the following patient-carrying devices: (Scan 5-4, p. 113; Scan 5-5, pp. 115–116; Scan 5-6, pp. 120–122)

- wheeled ambulance stretcher
- portable ambulance stretcher
- stair chair
- scoop stretcher
- long spine board
- basket stretcher
- flexible stretcher

1-6.13 Explain the rationale for properly lifting and moving patients. (p. 106) (Scan 5-7, pp. 124–126; Scan 5-8, p. 128)

*SKILLS

1-6.14 Working with a partner, prepare each of the following devices for use, transfer a patient to the device, properly position the patient on the device, move the device to the ambulance, and load the patient into the ambulance:

- wheeled ambulance stretcher
- portable ambulance stretcher
- stair chair
- scoop stretcher
- long spine board
- basket stretcher
- flexible stretcher

1-6.15 Working with a partner, demonstrate techniques for the transfer of a patient from an ambulance stretcher to a hospital stretcher.

Speed is a major objective on many of the calls you will make as an EMT. At certain dangerous scenes, for example, you must rapidly move the patient to a safe place. When the patient has a life-threatening medical problem or a serious injury, getting him to the hospital quickly can mean the difference between life and death.

Doing things fast, however, can mean doing them wrong. You can be so focused on the need to hurry as you lift and carry the patient that you make careless moves. These can injure your patient. They can also injure you. Back injuries are serious and have the potential to end an EMS career as well as cause life-long problems. With the proper techniques, however, you can lift and move patients safely. Proper lifting and moving must be practiced on every call.

PROTECTING YOURSELF: BODY MECHANICS

body mechanics the proper use of the body to facilitate lifting and moving and prevent injury.

Body mechanics refers to the proper use of your body to prevent injury and to facilitate lifting and moving. Consider the following before lifting any patient:

- *The object.* What is the weight of the object? Will you require additional help in lifting?
- *Your limitations.* What are your physical characteristics? Do you (or your partner) have any physical limitations that would make lifting difficult? While it may not always be possible to arrange, EMTs of similar strength and height can lift and carry together more easily.
- *Communication.* Make a plan. Then communicate the plan for lifting and carrying to your partner. Continue to communicate throughout the process to make the move comfortable for the patient and safe for the EMTs.

When it comes time to do the lifting, there are rules that must be followed to prevent injury. These include:

- *Position your feet properly.* They should be on a firm, level surface and positioned shoulder-width apart.
- *Use your legs.* Do not use your back to do the lifting.
- *Never turn or twist.* Attempts to make any other moves while you are lifting are a major cause of injury.
- *Do not compensate when lifting with one hand.* Avoid leaning to either side. Keep your back straight and locked.
- *Keep the weight close to your body, or as close as possible.* This allows you to use your legs rather than your back while lifting. The farther the weight is from your body, the greater your chance of injury.
- *Use a stair chair when carrying a patient on stairs whenever possible.* Keep your back straight. Flex your knees and lean forward from the hips, not the waist. If you are walking backward down stairs, ask a helper to steady your back (Figure 5-1).

There are many kinds of patient-carrying devices, including stretchers, backboards, and stair chairs. (Specifics are offered later in this chapter.) When possible, it is almost

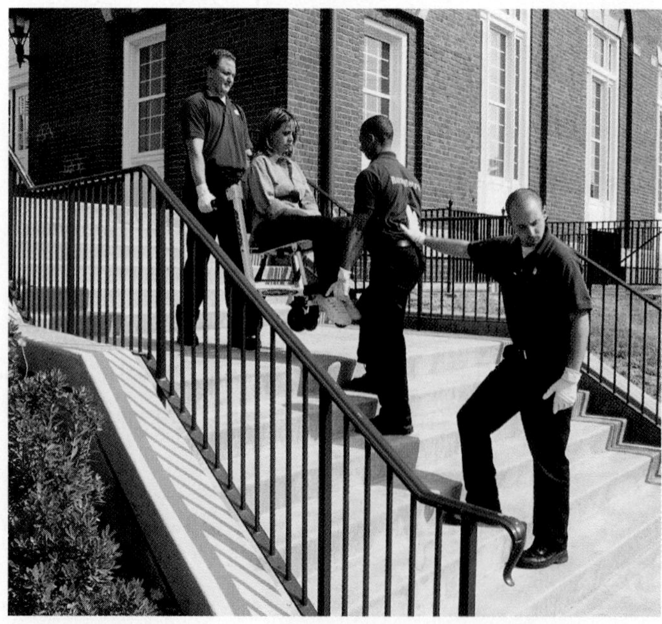

Figure 5-1 • Moving a stair chair down steps.

always safer, as well as more efficient, to move patients over distances on a wheeled device such as a wheeled stretcher or a stair chair. These devices allow the patient to be rolled along instead of carried.

When lifting a patient-carrying device, it is best to use an even number of people. For a stretcher or backboard, one EMT lifts from the end near the patient's head, the other from the feet. If there are four rescuers available, one person can take each corner of a stretcher or board. If there are only three people available, however, never allow the third person to assist by lifting one side. This can cause the device to be thrown off balance, resulting in the stretcher tipping over and injuring the patient.

To prevent injury when lifting a patient-carrying device, the general rules of body mechanics mentioned earlier apply. Two more methods also can help to prevent injury. The first is the **power lift** (Figure 5-2A), so named because it is used by power weight lifters. It is also known as the *squat-lift* position. In this position, you will squat rather than bend at the waist, and you will keep the weight close to your body, even straddling it if possible. When rising, your feet should be a comfortable distance apart, flat on the ground, with the weight primarily on the balls of the feet or just behind them. Your back should be locked-in. Be sure to raise your upper body before your hips. When you are lowering a patient, use the reverse order of this procedure.

The second method is the **power grip** (Figure 5-2B). Remember that your hands are often the only portion of your body actually in contact with the object you are lifting, making your grip a very important element in the process. As great an area of your fingers and palms as possible should be in contact with the object. All of your fingers should be bent at the same angle. When possible, keep your hands at least 10 inches apart.

power lift
a lift from a squatting position with weight to be lifted close to the body, feet apart and flat on the ground, body weight on or just behind balls of feet, back locked in. The upper body is raised before the hips. Also called the *squat-lift position.*

power grip
gripping with as much hand surface as possible in contact with the object being lifted, all fingers bent at the same angle, hands at least 10 inches apart.

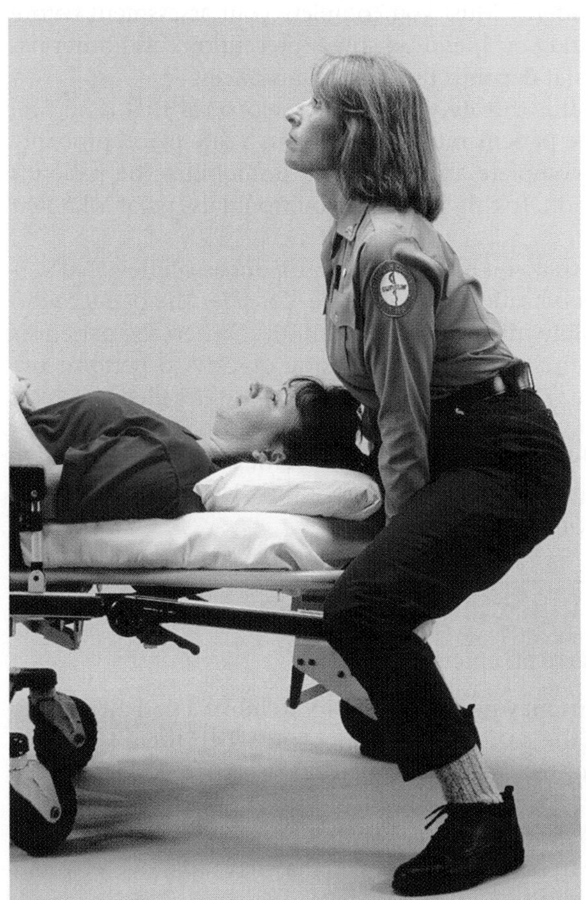
A

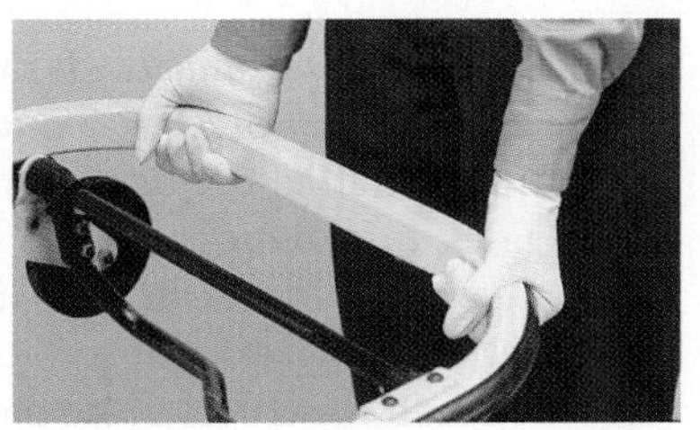
B

Figure 5-2 • (A) The power lift and (B) the power grip.

There are situations in which you will find yourself reaching for patients or using a considerable amount of effort to push and pull a weight. These are moves that must be performed carefully to prevent injury. In general:

When reaching:

- Keep your back in a locked-in position.
- Avoid twisting while reaching.
- Avoid reaching more than 15 to 20 inches in front of your body.
- Avoid prolonged reaching when strenuous effort is required.

When pushing or pulling:

- Push, rather than pull, whenever possible.
- Keep your back locked-in.
- Keep the line of pull through the center of your body by bending your knees.
- Keep the weight close to your body.
- If the weight is below your waist level, push or pull from a kneeling position.
- Avoid pushing or pulling overhead.
- Keep your elbows bent and arms close to your sides.

PROTECTING YOUR PATIENT: EMERGENCY, URGENT, AND NON-URGENT MOVES

How quickly should you move a patient? Must you complete your assessment before moving him? How much time should you spend on spinal precautions and other patient safety measures? The answer is: it depends on the circumstances.

If the patient is in a building that is threatening to collapse or a car that is on fire, speed is the overriding concern. The patient must be moved to a safe place, probably before you have time to begin or complete an assessment, immobilize the patient's spine, or move a stretcher into position. In this situation, you would use what is known as an *emergency move*.

Sometimes the situation is such that you have time to carry out an abbreviated version of assessment and spinal immobilization. For example, consider the patient who has been trapped in wreckage, possibly incurring serious injuries. When the patient is extricated, you would place him on a spine board, working quickly to perform the proper assessments and patient care. That move to the spine board is called an *urgent move*.

Most of the time, you will be able to complete your on-scene assessment and care procedures and then move the patient onto a stretcher or other device in the normal way. This would be called a *non-urgent move*.

Emergency Moves

Three situations may require the use of an emergency move:

- *The scene is hazardous.* Hazards may make it necessary to move a patient quickly in order to protect you and the patient. This may occur when there is uncontrolled traffic, fire or threat of fire, possible explosions, electrical hazards, toxic gases, or radiation.
- *Care of life-threatening conditions requires repositioning.* You may have to move a patient to a hard, flat surface to provide CPR, or you may have to move a patient to reach life-threatening bleeding.

- *You must reach other patients.* When there are patients at the scene requiring care for life-threatening problems, you may have to move another patient to access them.

The greatest danger to the patient in an emergency move is that a spine injury may be aggravated. Since the move must be made immediately to protect the patient's life, full spinal precautions will not be possible. So to minimize or prevent aggravation of the injury, *move the patient in the direction of the long axis of the body when possible.* The long axis is the line that runs down the center of the body from the top of the head and along the spine.

There are several rapid moves called drags. In this type of move, the patient is dragged by the clothes, the feet, the shoulders, or a blanket. These moves are reserved only for emergencies, because they do not provide protection for the neck and spine. Most commonly, a long-axis drag is made from the area of the shoulders. This causes the remainder of the body to fall into its natural anatomical position, with the spine and all limbs in normal alignment.

Drags and other emergency moves known as carries and assists are illustrated in Scans 5-1, 5-2, and 5-3.

Urgent Moves

Urgent moves are required when the patient must be moved quickly for treatment of an immediate threat to life. But unlike emergency moves, urgent moves are performed with precautions for spinal injury. Examples in which urgent moves may be required include the following:

- *The required treatment can only be performed if the patient is moved.* A patient must be moved in order to support inadequate breathing or to treat for shock or altered mental status.
- *Factors at the scene cause patient decline.* If a patient is rapidly declining because of heat or cold, for example, he may have to be moved.

Moving a patient onto a long spine board, also called a *backboard,* is an urgent move used when there is an immediate threat to life and suspicion of spine injury. If the patient is supine on the ground, a log-roll maneuver must be performed to move him onto his side. The spine board is then placed next to the patient's body, and he is log-rolled back onto the board. After the patient is secured and immobilized on the spine board, the board and patient are lifted together onto a stretcher and loaded into the ambulance. (When reaching across the patient to perform a log roll, remember the principles of body mechanics: Keep your back straight, lean from the hips, and use your shoulder muscles to help with the roll. See Figure 5-3.) Log rolls and immobilization on a long spine board will be discussed in Chapter 29, "Injuries to the Head and Spine."

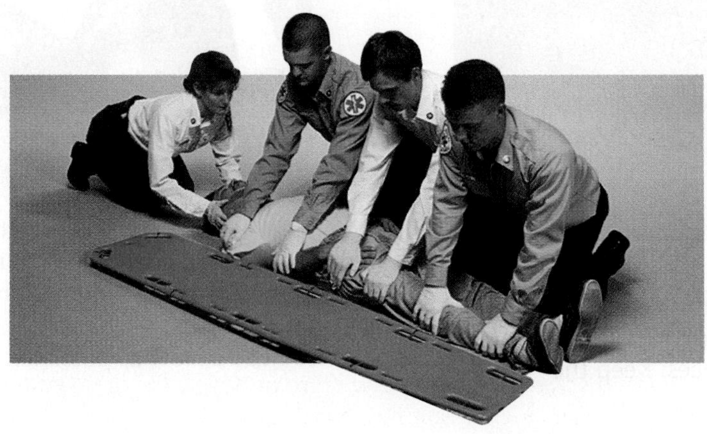

Figure 5-3 • When doing a log roll, keep your back straight, lean from the hips, and use your shoulder muscles.

SCAN 5-1 • Emergency Moves, One-Rescuer Drags

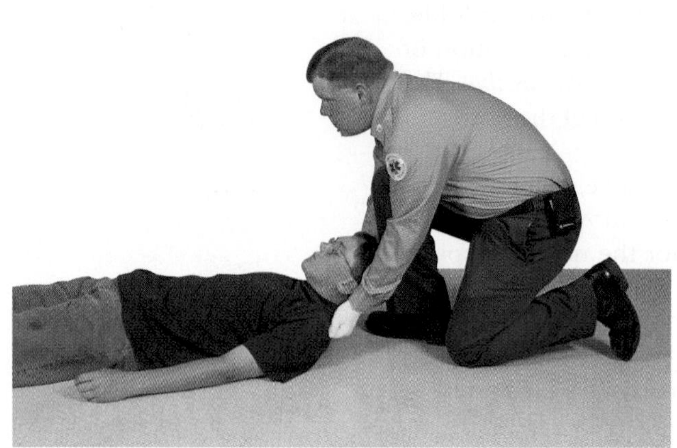

CLOTHES DRAG.

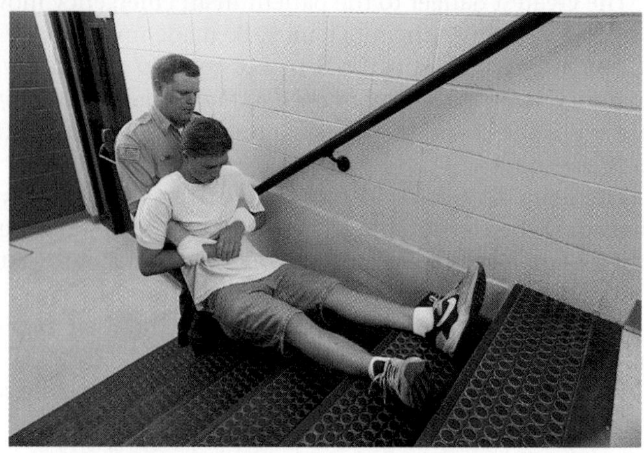

INCLINE DRAG. *Always* head first.

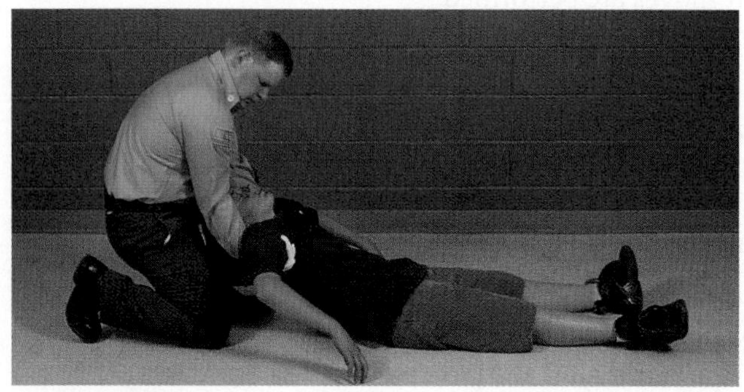

SHOULDER DRAG.

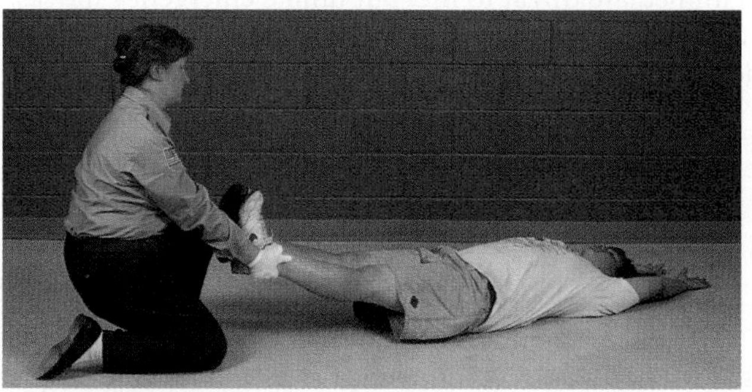

FOOT DRAG. Do not bump the patient's head.

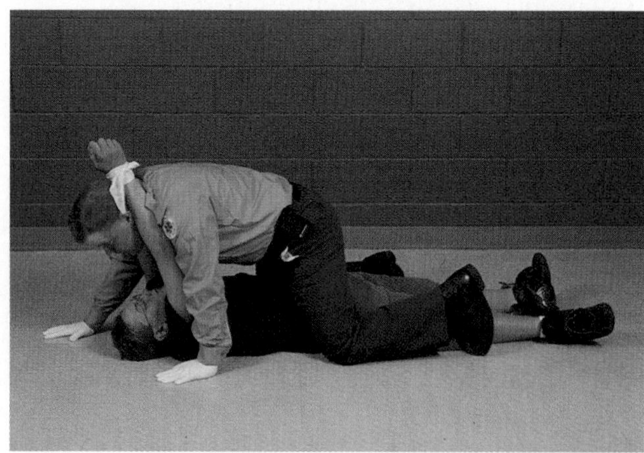

FIREFIGHTER'S DRAG. Place patient on his back and tie his hands together. Straddle him, crouch, and pass your head through his trussed arms. Raise your body, and crawl on your hands and knees. Keep the patient's head as low as possible.

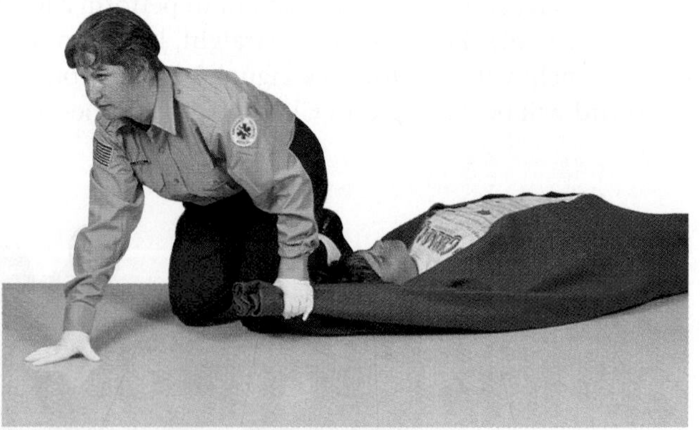

BLANKET DRAG. Gather half of the blanket material up against the patient's side. Roll him toward your knees, place the blanket under him, and gently roll him onto the blanket. During the drag, keep the patient's head as low as possible.

SCAN 5-2 • Emergency Moves, One Rescuer

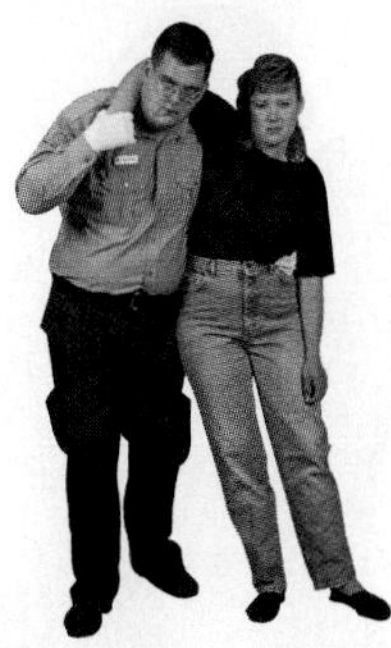

ONE-RESCUER ASSIST. Place patient's arm around your neck, grasping her hand in yours. Place your other arm around the patient's waist. Help patient walk to safety. Be prepared to change movement technique if level of danger increases. Be sure to communicate with patient about obstacles, uneven terrain, and so on.

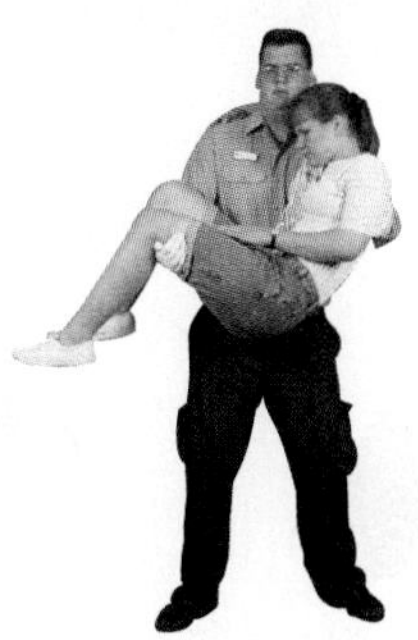

CRADLE CARRY. Place one arm across patient's back with your hand under her arm. Place your other arm under her knees and lift. If patient is conscious, have her place her near arm over your shoulder. NOTE: This carry places a lot of weight on the carrier's back. It is usually appropriate only for very light patients.

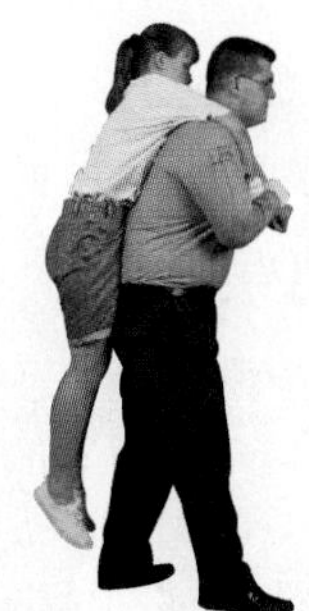

PACK STRAP CARRY. Have patient stand. Turn your back to her, bringing her arms over your shoulders to cross your chest. Keep her arms as straight as possible, her armpits over your shoulders. Hold patient's wrists, bend, and pull her onto your back.

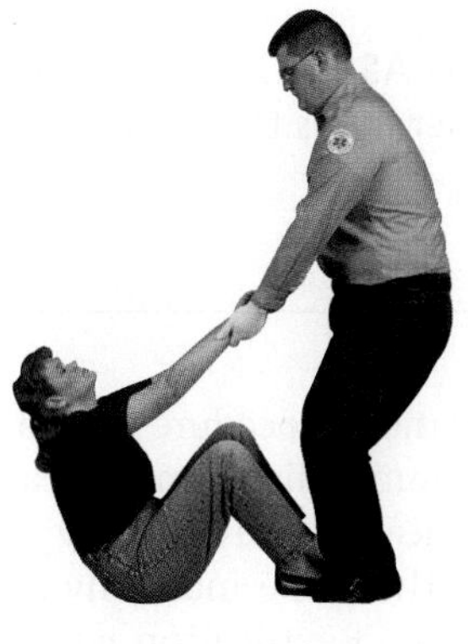

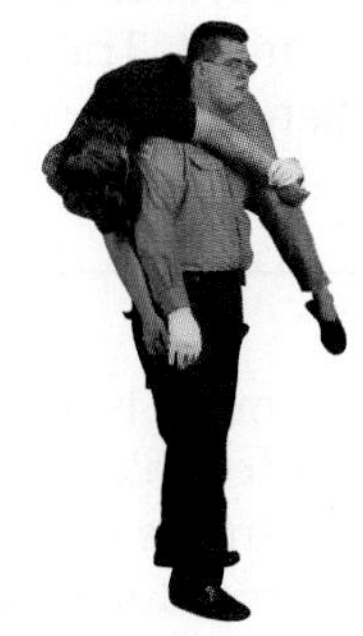

FIREFIGHTER'S CARRY. Place your feet against her feet and pull patient toward you. Bend at waist and flex knees. Duck and pull her across your shoulder, keeping hold of one of her wrists. Use your free arm to reach between her legs and grasp her thigh. Weight of patient falls onto your shoulders. Stand up. Transfer your grip on thigh to patient's wrist.

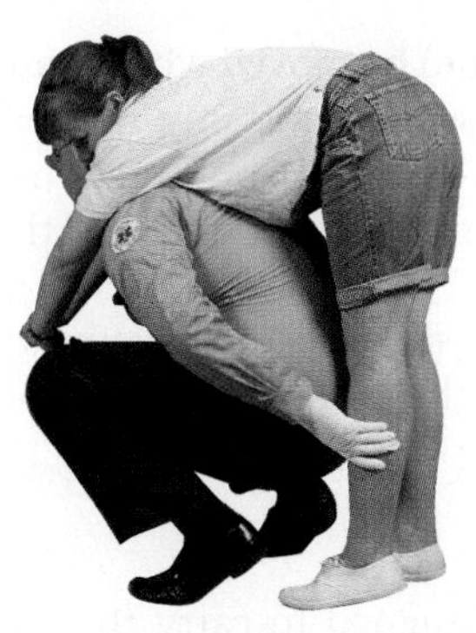

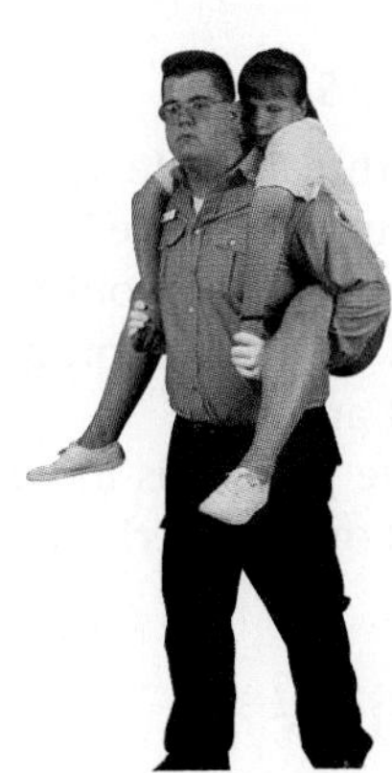

PIGGY BACK CARRY. Assist the patient to stand. Place her arms over your shoulder so they cross your chest. Bend over and lift patient. While she holds on with her arms, crouch and grasp each leg. Use a lifting motion to move her onto your back. Pass your forearms under her knees and grasp her wrists.

SCAN 5-3 • Emergency Moves, Two Rescuers

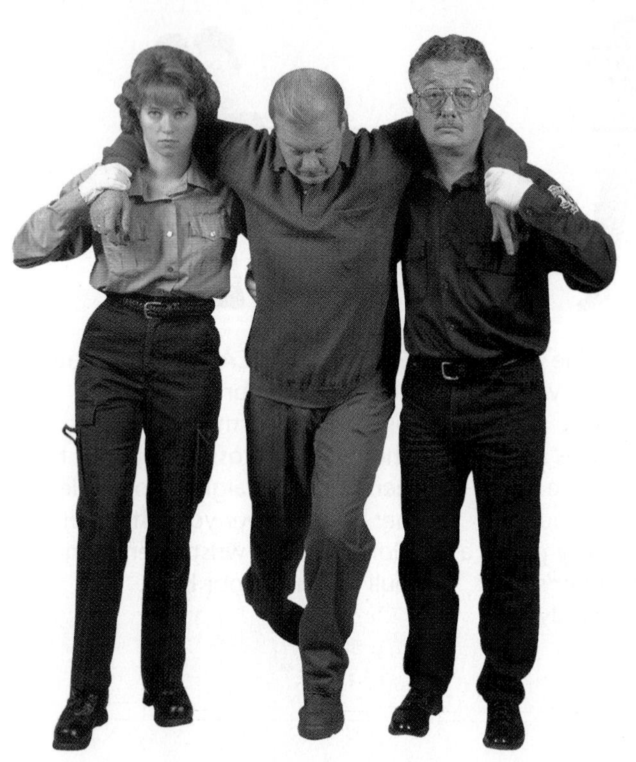

TWO-RESCUER ASSIST. Patient's arms are placed around shoulders of both rescuers. They each grip a hand, place their free arms around patient's waist, and then help him walk to safety.

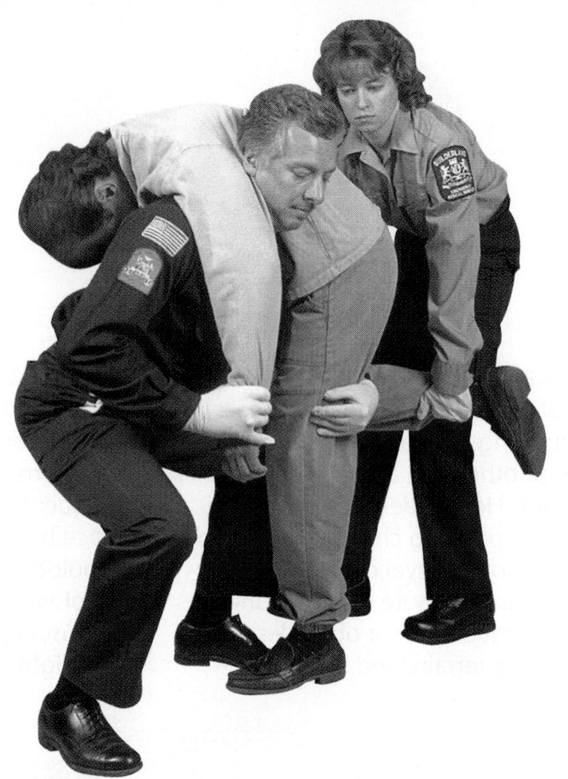

FIREFIGHTER'S CARRY WITH ASSIST. Have someone lift patient. The second rescuer helps to position patient.

Another example of an urgent move is the rapid extrication procedure from a vehicle. If the patient has critical injuries, taking the time to immobilize him with a short backboard or vest while he is still in the car may cause a deadly delay. During a rapid extrication, EMTs use a quicker procedure: they stabilize the spine manually as they move the patient from the car onto a long spine board. Rapid extrication will be discussed in Chapter 29, "Injuries to the Head and Spine."

Non-Urgent Moves

When there is no immediate threat to life, the patient should be moved when ready for transportation, using a non-urgent move. On-scene assessment and any needed on-scene treatments, such as splinting, should be completed first. Non-urgent moves should be carried out in such a way as to prevent injury or additional injury to the patient and to avoid discomfort and pain.

In a non-urgent move, the patient is moved from the site of on-scene assessment and treatment (perhaps a bed or sofa, perhaps the floor or the ground outdoors) onto a patient-carrying device.

Patient-Carrying Devices

A patient-carrying device is a stretcher or other device designed to carry the patient safely to the ambulance and/or to the hospital. Devices described on the following pages are pictured in Scan 5-4.

SCAN 5-4 • Patient-Carrying Devices

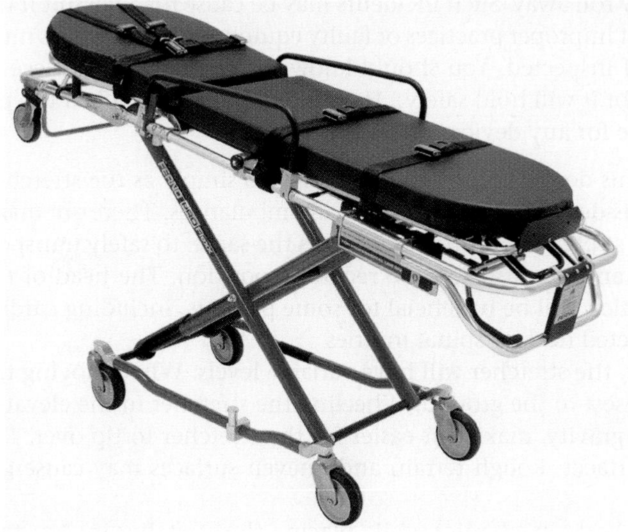

Wheeled ambulance stretcher. *(© Ferno Corporation)*

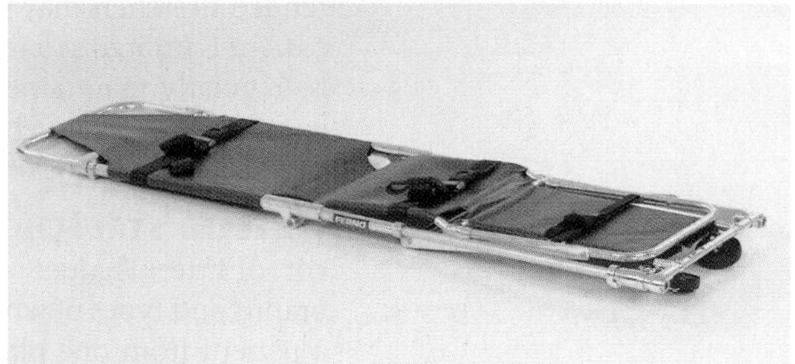

Portable stretcher.

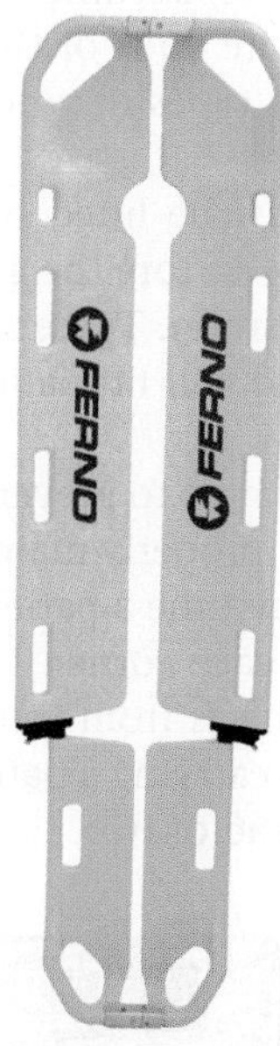

Scoop (orthopedic) stretcher. *(© Ferno Corporation)*

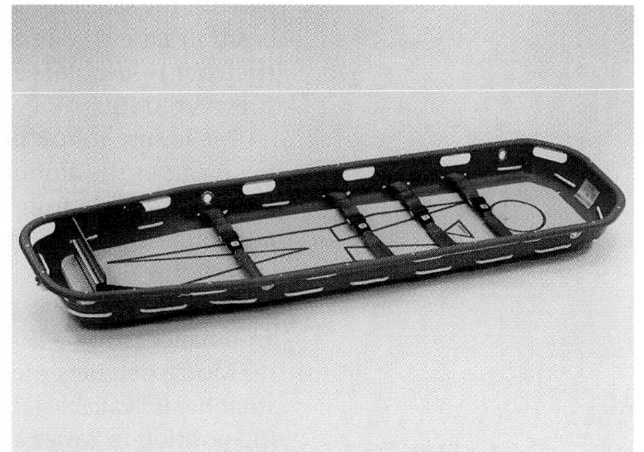

Basket stretcher. *(© Ferno Corporation)*

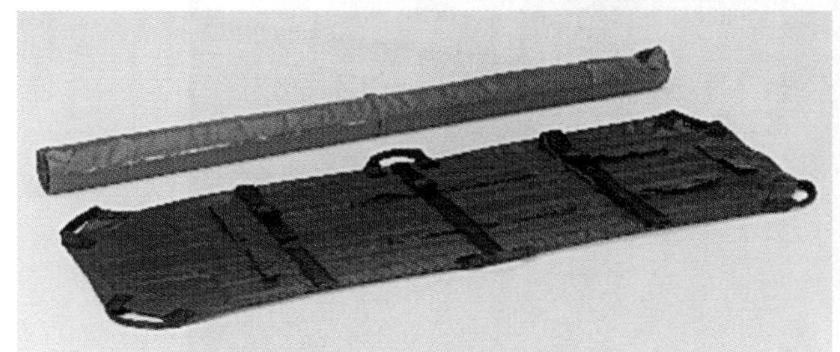

Flexible stretcher.

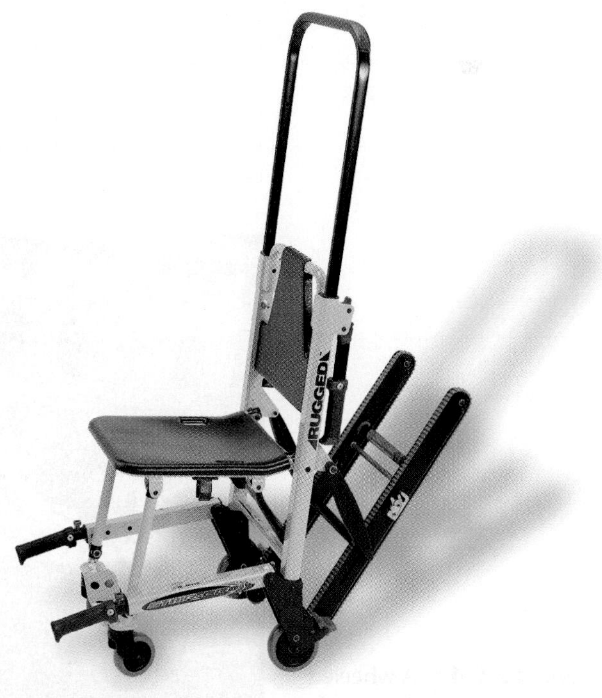

Stair chair. *(Stryker)*

Patient-carrying devices are mechanical devices, and all EMTs must be familiar with how to use them. Errors in use of these devices may result in injuries to the patient and to you. For example, a stretcher that is not locked in position may collapse, and untended stretchers may simply roll away. Such incidents may be cause for a lawsuit if the patient is injured as a result of improper practices or faulty equipment. The devices must be regularly maintained and inspected. You should know the rating of each piece of equipment (how much weight it will hold safely). Have alternatives available if the patient is too heavy or too large for any device.

WHEELED STRETCHER This device is commonly referred to simply as the stretcher, cot, or litter (Figure 5-4). This device is in the back of all ambulances. There are many brands and types of wheeled stretcher, but their purpose is the same: to safely transport a patient from one place to another, usually in a reclining position. The head of the stretcher can be elevated, which will be beneficial for some patients, including cardiac patients, who have no suspected neck or spinal injuries.

Depending on the model, the stretcher will have variable levels. When moving the patient, the safest level is closest to the ground. Wheeling the stretcher in the elevated position raises the center of gravity, making it easier for the stretcher to tip over. The stretcher is ideal for level surfaces. Rough terrain and uneven surfaces may cause the stretcher to tip.

Make sure to use proper body mechanics while placing the stretcher into or taking it out of the ambulance. Proper body mechanics are also important while wheeling the stretcher from place to place. Remember, as discussed earlier in the chapter, odd numbers of EMTs may cause the stretcher to become off-balance. When the stretcher is lifted, two EMTs should lift at opposite ends of the stretcher—head and foot. Scan 5-5 shows procedures for loading two types of wheeled stretcher into an ambulance.

Most stretchers are manual. That is, they must be lifted by EMTs. A new power stretcher is available (Figure 5-5) that will lift a patient from the ground level to the loading position or lower a patient from the raised position. These stretchers use a battery-powered hydraulic system that manufacturers state will lift patients on 20 consecutive runs and will lift patients up to 700 pounds.

While these power stretchers will undoubtedly help to prevent back injuries, it is vital to follow the manufacturer's guidelines for use, properly maintain the stretcher, and use safe techniques as discussed in this chapter any time a patient is on your stretcher.

A stretcher can be carried by four EMTs, one at each corner. This method can be useful on rough terrain because it helps keep the wheels from touching the ground and provides greater stability. It is also beneficial when carrying a patient a long distance because it divides the weight among four EMTs instead of two.

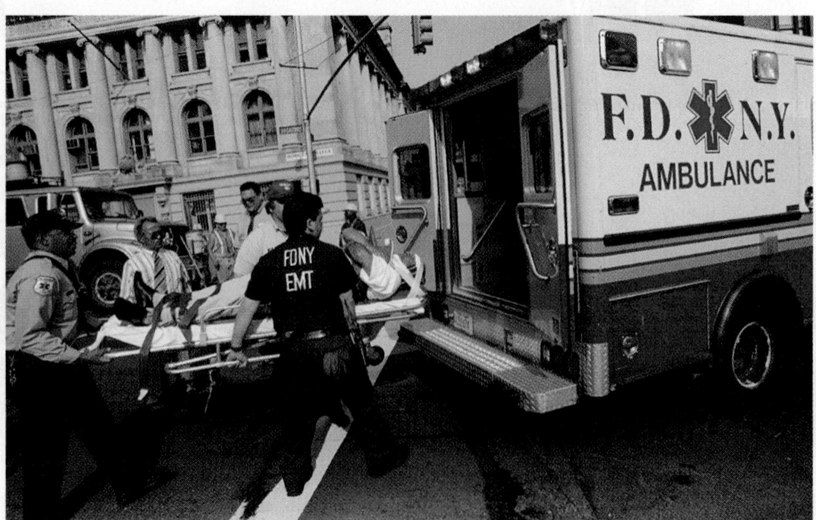

Figure 5-4 • A wheeled stretcher is carried on every ambulance. *(© David Handshuh)*

SCAN 5-5 • Loading the Wheeled Stretcher into the Ambulance

SELF-LOADING STRETCHER

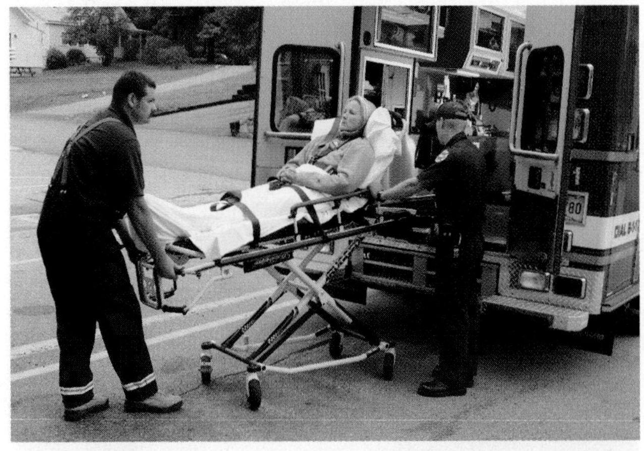

1. Position the wheels closest to the patient's head securely on the inside floor of the ambulance.

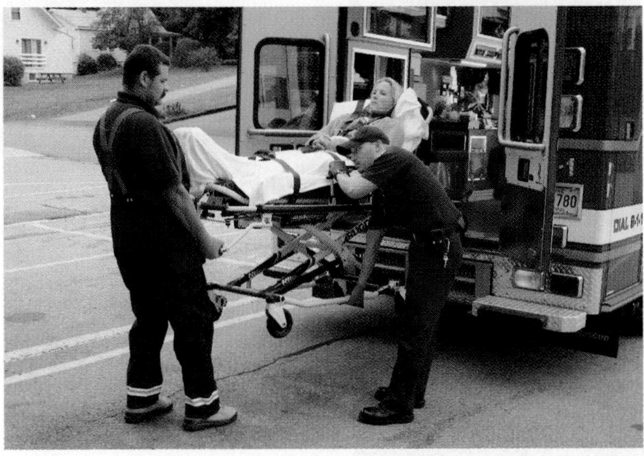

2. Once the wheels are securely on the ambulance floor, rescuer at rear of stretcher activates the lever to release the wheels. (This may require a slight lift to get weight off the wheels.) The second rescuer should guide the collapsing carriage, if necessary.

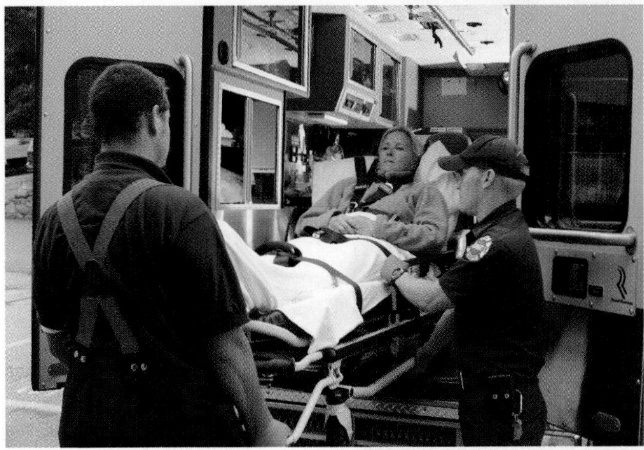

3. Move the stretcher into the securing device and secure the stretcher in front and rear.

continued

SCAN 5-5 • (Continued)

STANDARD STRETCHER

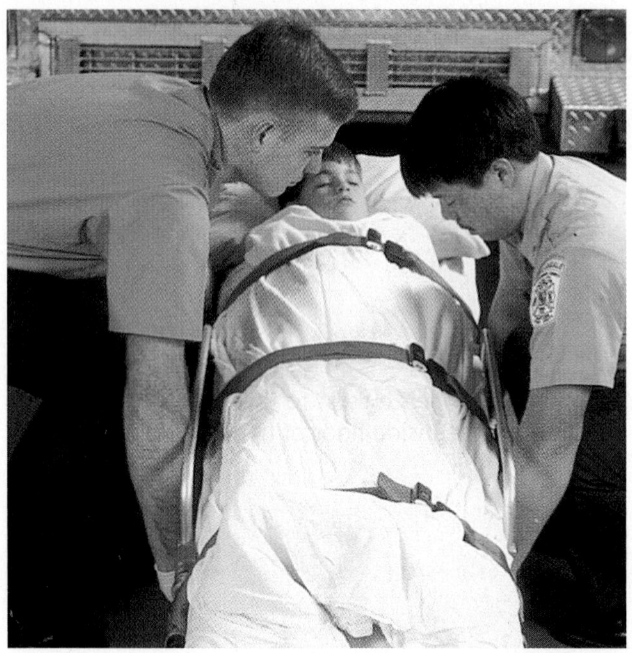

1. After you have moved the stretcher as close to the ambulance as possible, lock it in its lowest level. Then position yourselves on opposite sides, bend at the knees, and grasp the lower bar of the stretcher frame.

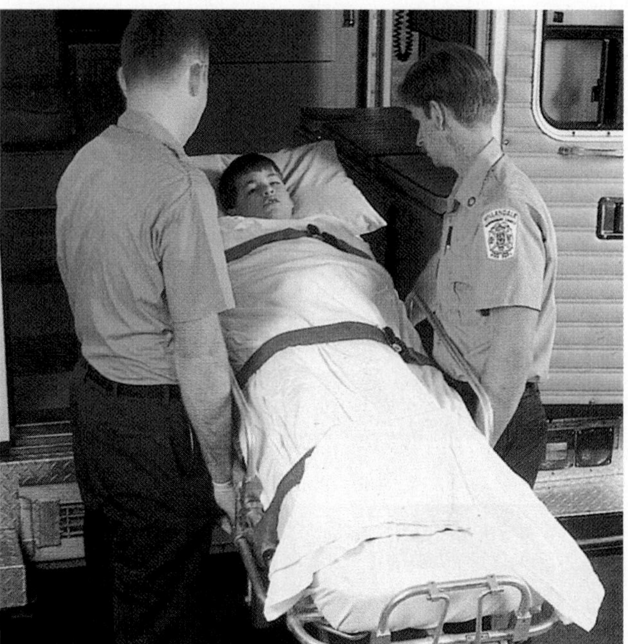

2. Come to a full standing position with your backs straight. Take small sideways steps to move the stretcher into the ambulance.

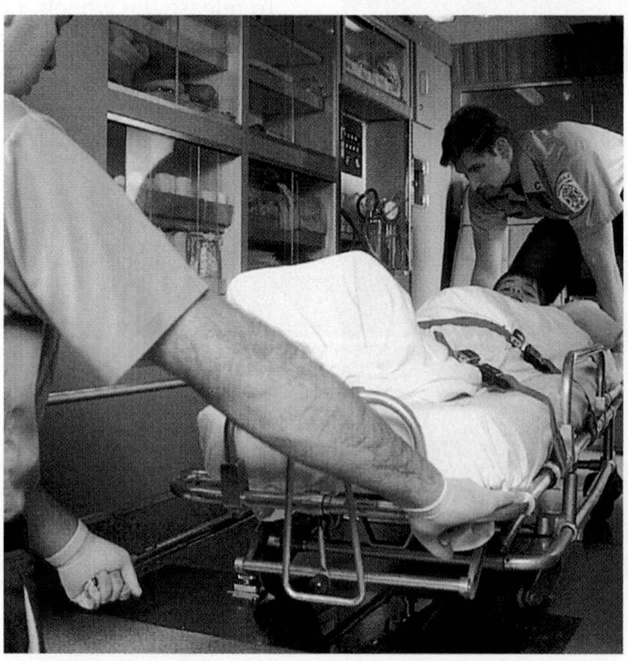

3. Move the stretcher into the securing device, and engage both forward and rear catches.

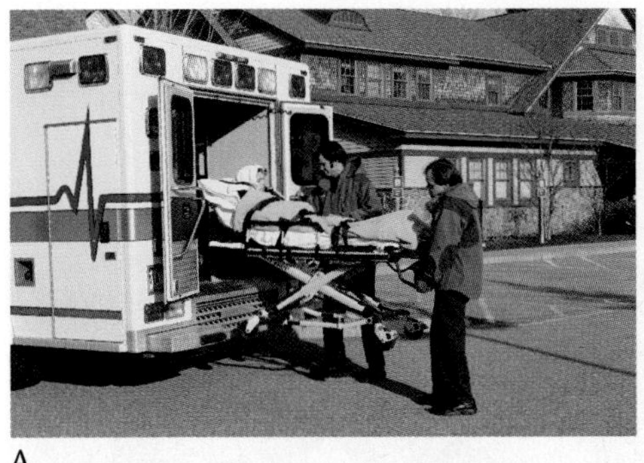
A

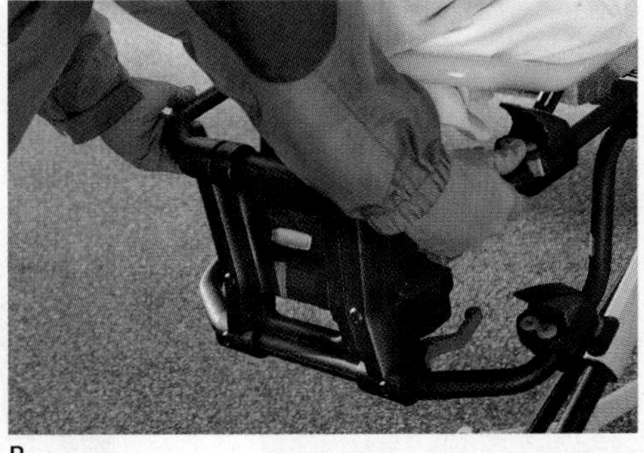
B

Figure 5-5 • (A) A power stretcher will lift a patient from ground level to loading position or lower a patient from the raised position. (B) These stretchers are operated by a battery-powered hydraulic system.

The patient will stay on the stretcher during transport to the hospital. Make sure that the stretcher is always used in accordance with manufacturer's recommendations. Secure the patient to the stretcher before lifting or moving. After placing the patient into the ambulance, secure the stretcher to the ambulance. Ambulances have installed hardware for keeping the stretcher secured while the ambulance is moving. Failure to secure the stretcher properly will cause it to shift during transit, causing an unsafe condition for the EMTs as well as the patient.

STAIR CHAIR The stair chair has many benefits for moving patients from the scene to the stretcher. The first benefit, as the name implies, is that it is excellent for use on stairs. Large stretchers often cannot be carried around tight corners and up or down narrow staircases. The stair chair transports the patient in a sitting position, which greatly reduces the length of patient and device, allowing the EMT to maneuver around corners and through narrow spaces. It also has a set of wheels that allow the device to be rolled like a wheelchair over flat surfaces, lessening the strain on the EMT.

Another type of stair chair has come into wide use in EMS. This chair has wheels to roll the patient along a floor or level ground but also has a tracklike system that allows EMTs to gently slide the patient down a staircase instead of lifting him (Figure 5-6). The patient's weight increases the friction along the track, which helps to control the rate of descent.

As with older stair chair models, two rescuers are necessary and a third as a spotter is preferred when available. Indications and contraindications for this stair chair are the same as for older models.

As with all devices in this chapter, there are times when the stair chair should be used and times when it should not. The device is often ideal for patients with difficulty breathing. (You will learn about this in Chapter 16, "Respiratory Emergencies.") These

POINT OF VIEW

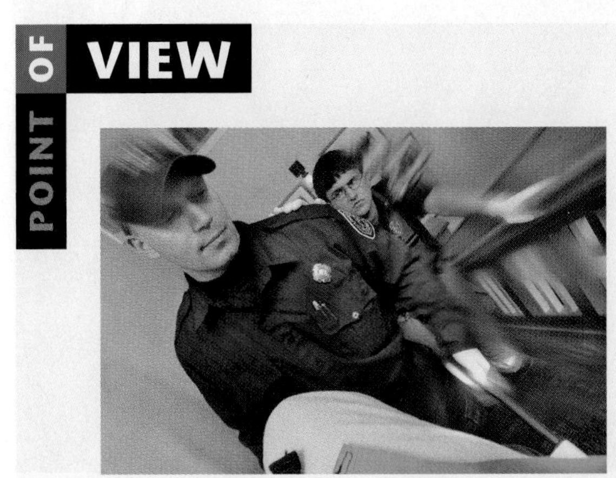

"I just wanted to ask, 'Have you ever dropped anyone before?'

"I really thought I could just walk down the stairs but they said no. They put me in that chair, strapped me in, and off we went.

"'Are you sure it isn't better for me to walk down?' They told me the chair had treads—like a tank—and it wouldn't be a problem. Problem for whom?

"I remember feeling like I should be holding on to something so I kept trying to grab the railing to help. Or maybe to save myself. They were very polite but were getting frustrated when I kept trying to grab.

"Maybe they don't know what it is like to be on stairs with absolutely no control. It was almost as scary as not being able to breathe."

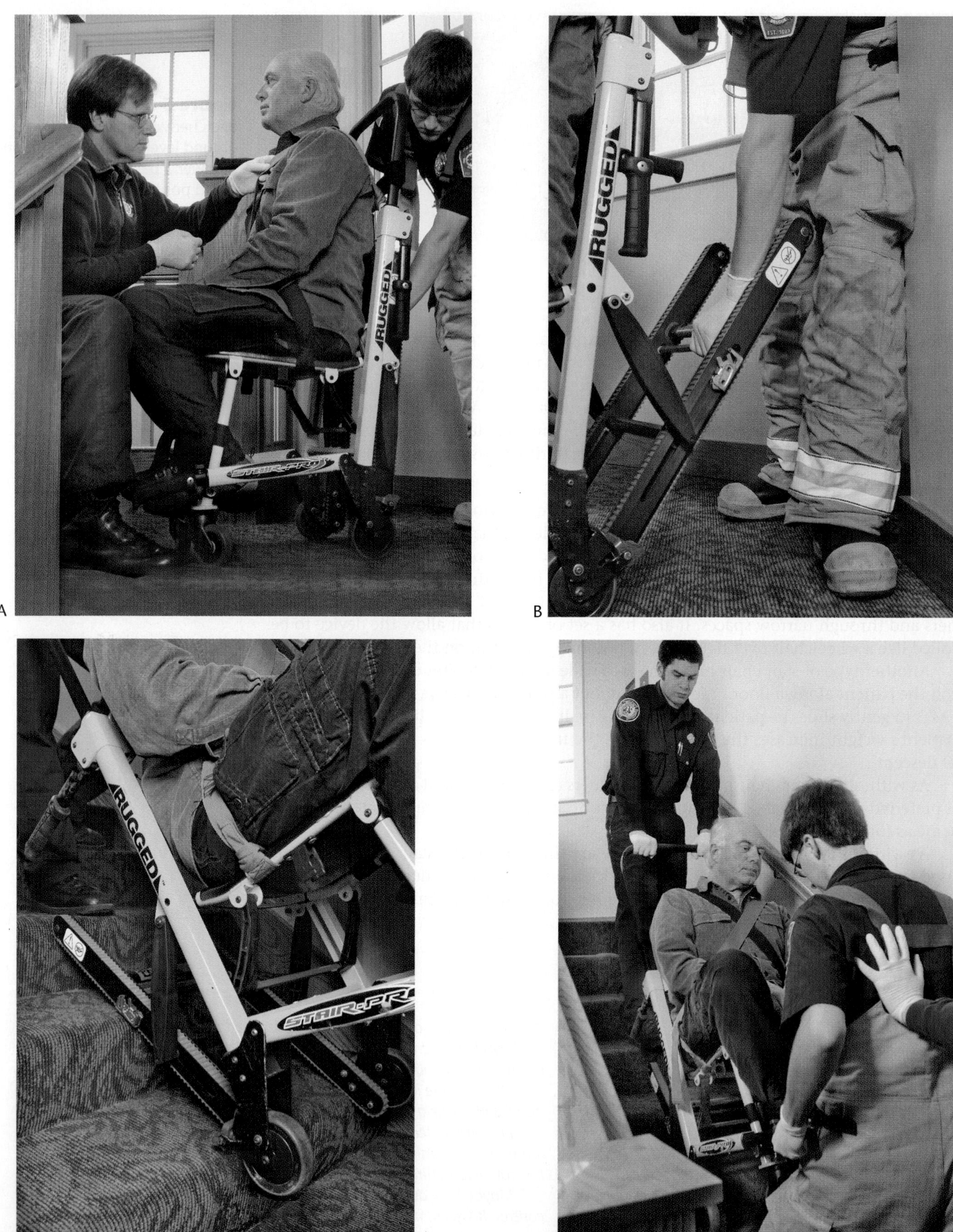

Figure 5-6 • (A) A modern stair chair has wheels to roll the patient along a floor or level ground. (B) It also has a track that can be lowered that (C and D) allows EMTs to gently slide the patient down a staircase.

patients usually find that they must sit up to breathe more easily, which the stair chair allows them to do. The stair chair must not be used for patients with neck or spine injury, because these patients must be immobilized supine on a backboard to prevent further injury.

SPINE BOARDS There are two types of spine boards, or backboards: short and long (Scan 5-6). They are used for patients who are found lying down or standing and who must be immobilized. These devices are available in traditional wood as well as in plastics that resist splintering. (Splintered boards absorb body fluids, which may harbor infection.)

Short spine boards are used primarily for removing patients from vehicles when a neck or spine injury is suspected. A short spine board can slide between the patient's back and seat back. Once secured to the short spine board and wearing a rigid cervical collar, the patient can be moved from a sitting position in the vehicle to a supine position on a long spine board. Often, a vest-type extrication device is used in place of a short spine board. (You will learn more about extrication using short spine boards and vests in Chapter 29, "Injuries to the Head and Spine.")

OTHER TYPES OF STRETCHERS The portable stretcher, or folding stretcher, may be beneficial in multiple-casualty incidents (incidents with many patients). These stretchers may be canvas, aluminum, or heavy plastic and usually fold or collapse.

The *scoop stretcher*, or orthopedic stretcher, splits into two pieces vertically, allowing the patient to be "scooped" by pushing the halves together under him. The scoop stretcher does not offer any support directly under the spine, so it is not recommended for patients with suspected spinal injury. Follow your local protocols on the use of this device.

A *basket stretcher*, or Stokes stretcher, can be used to move a patient from one level to another or over rough terrain. The basket should be lined with a blanket before positioning the patient.

A *flexible stretcher*, or Reeves stretcher, is made of canvas or rubberized or other flexible material, often with wooden slats sewn into pockets and three carrying handles on each side. Because of its flexibility, it can be useful in restricted areas or narrow hallways.

Many services now use a *vacuum mattress* when transporting patients (Figure 5-7). The patient is placed on the device and air is withdrawn by means of a pump. The mattress then becomes rigid and conforming, padding voids naturally for greater comfort. Vacuum mattresses reduce some of the discomfort associated with rigid backboards. In later chapters, you will see vacuum splints that use the same principle.

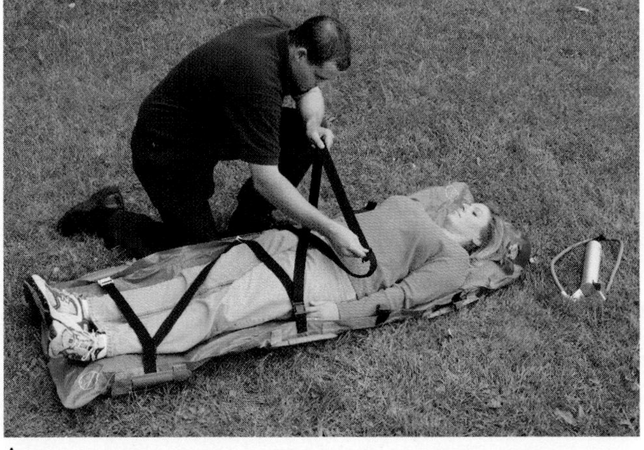

A

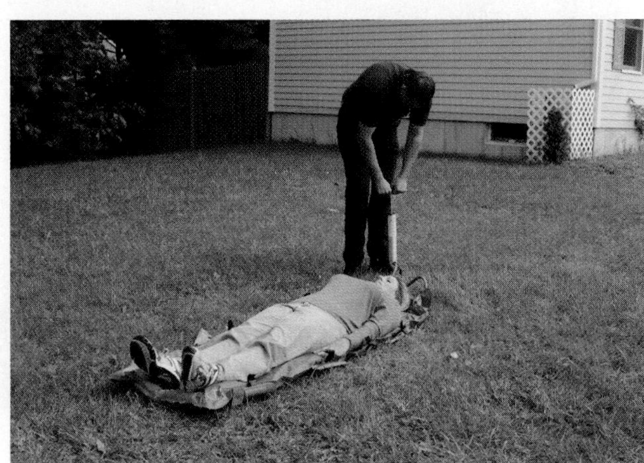

B

Figure 5-7 • (A) A vacuum mattress may be used to transport a patient. (B) When the patient is placed on the device and air is withdrawn, the mattress becomes rigid and conforming, automatically padding voids.

SCAN 5-6 • Patient Immobilizing Devices

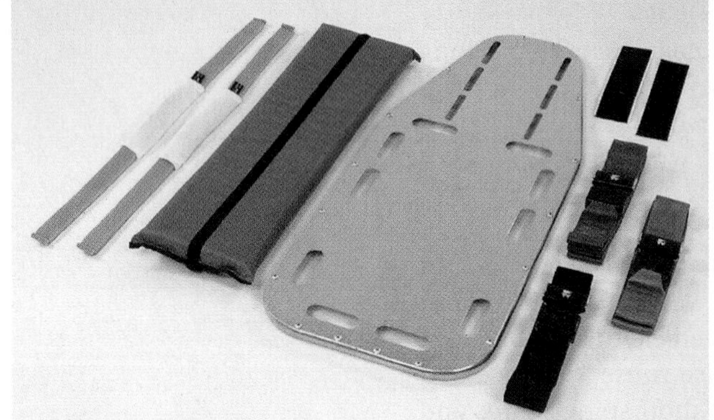

Short spine board.

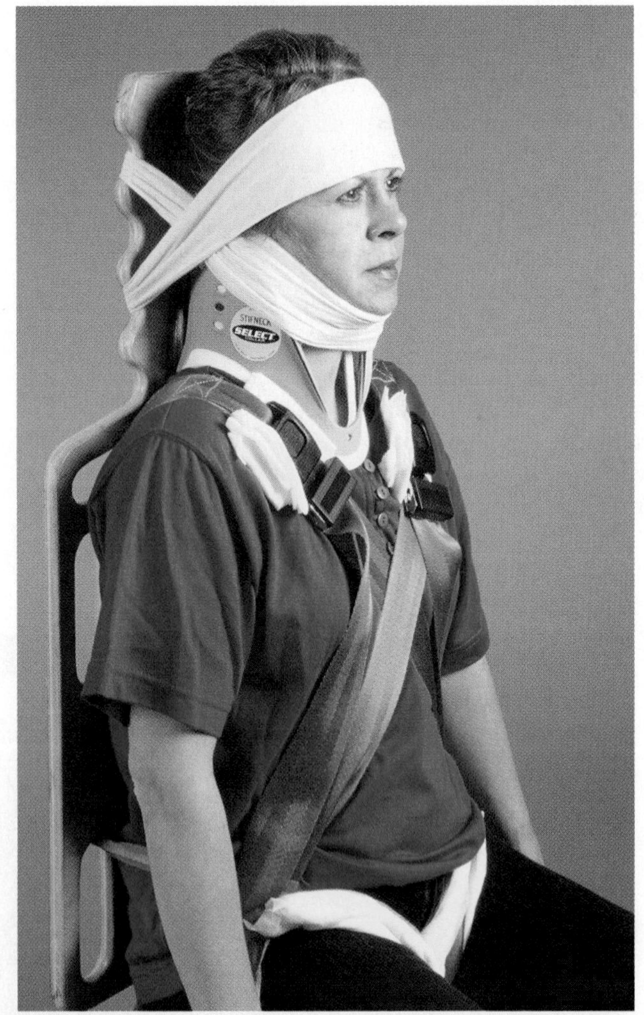

Side view.

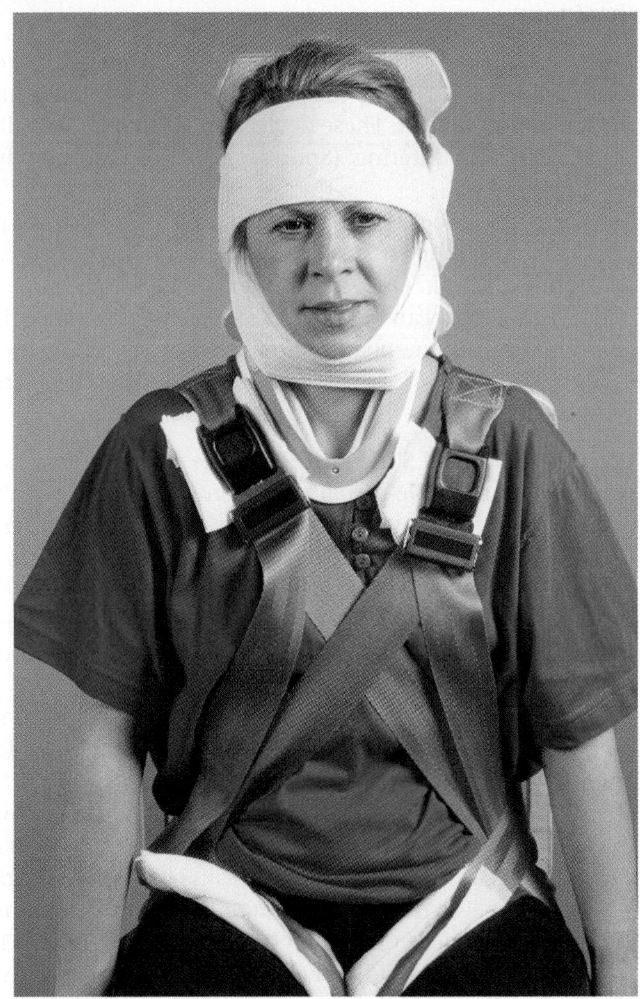

Patient properly secured to short spine board, front view.

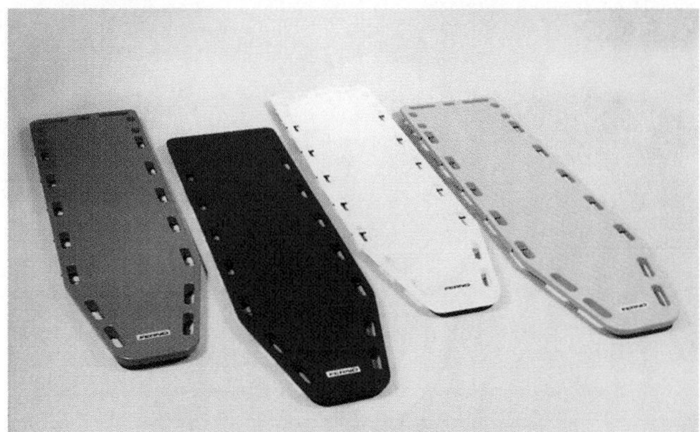

Long spine board.

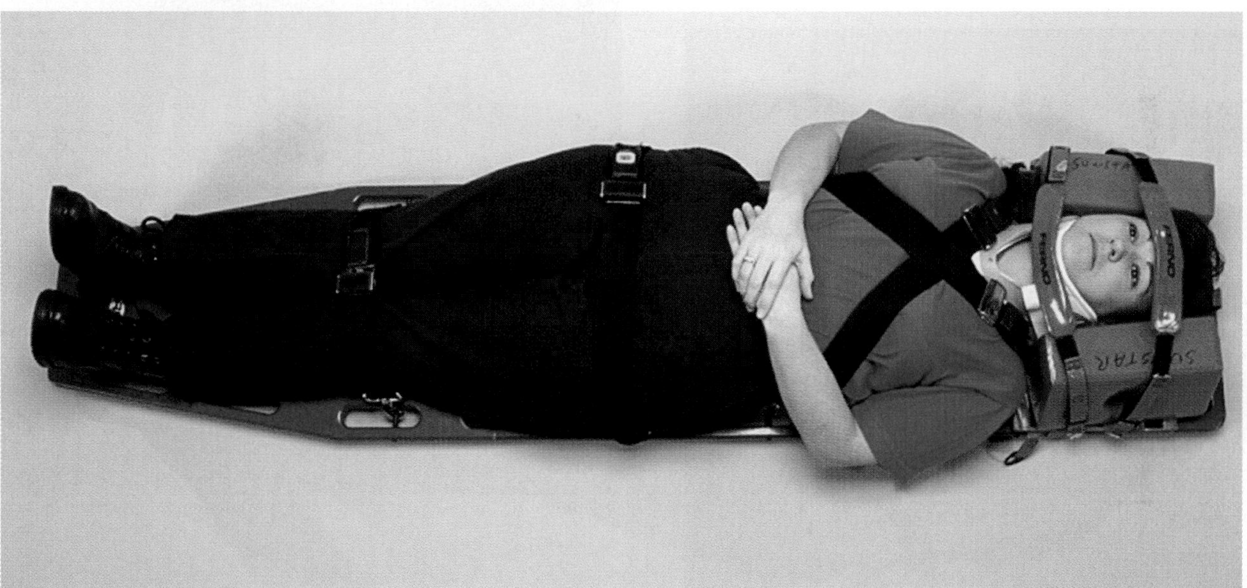

Patient properly secured to long spine board.

continued

SCAN 5-6 • (Continued)

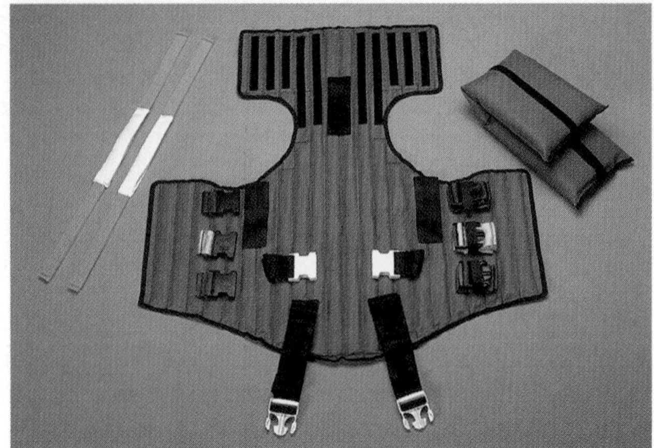

Vest-type extrication device.

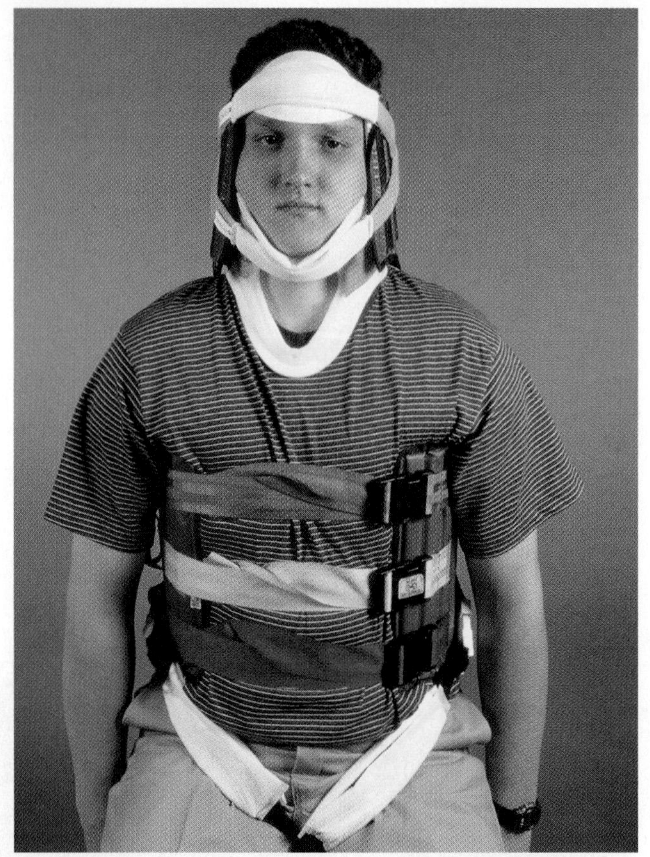

Patient properly secured to vest-type extrication device, front view.

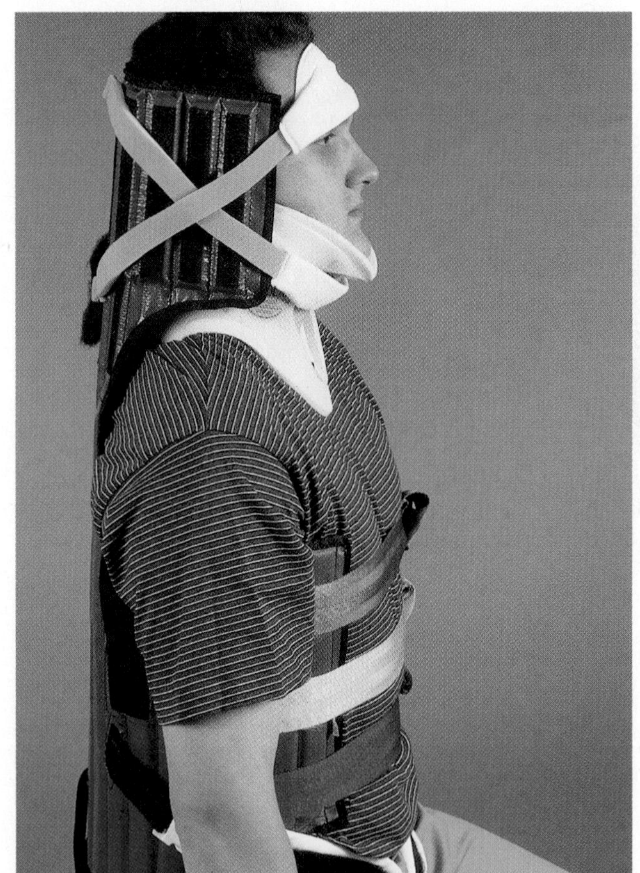

Side view.

CRITICAL DECISION MAKING:
Choosing a Patient-Carrying Device

Lifting and moving patients requires more than just muscles. Decisions made in patient transportation have a significant impact on the patient's condition—and the EMTs' well-being. For each of the following patients, choose a carrying device to get the patient from the scene to the ambulance stretcher:

- A patient complaining of severe respiratory distress who is in an upstairs back bedroom.
- A patient thrown from an ATV several hundred yards into the woods.
- A patient who fell down several stairs from the back deck to the concrete landing. He complains of neck and back pain.
- An unresponsive medical patient found down a narrow hallway on the first floor.

Moving Patients onto Carrying Devices

There are several ways to move a patient onto a carrying device. Choose a move based on the position the patient is in when it is time to move him to a carrying device and whether or not the patient is suspected of having a spine injury.

PATIENT WITH SUSPECTED SPINE INJURY A patient with suspected spine injury must have his head, neck, and spine immobilized before being moved. Perform manual stabilization, place a rigid cervical collar, and maintain manual stabilization until the patient is immobilized to a spine board. If he is seated in a vehicle, you will next immobilize him with a short spine board or vest and then on a long spine board (unless it is an urgent situation and you substitute the rapid extrication procedure described earlier under "Urgent Moves").

If the patient is lying down or standing, move him directly to a long spine board. The long spine board will then be placed on a wheeled ambulance stretcher for transport to the hospital. (You will learn more about manual stabilization in Chapter 8, "Initial Assessment," about cervical collars; in Chapter 10, "Assessment of the Trauma Patient;" and about immobilization for possible spine injury in Chapter 29, "Injuries to the Head and Spine.")

Remember that immobilization is mandatory for any patient who has any possibility of a spine injury.

PATIENT WITH NO SUSPECTED SPINE INJURY The extremity lift, direct ground lift, draw-sheet method, and direct carry, described in the following list, are methods of moving a patient to a stretcher. All are appropriate only for a patient with no suspected spine injury. See Scan 5-7 for pictures and detailed descriptions of these methods:

- An **extremity lift** is used to carry a patient with no suspected spine or extremity injuries to a stretcher or a stair chair. It can be used to lift a patient from the ground or from a sitting position.
- A **direct ground lift** is performed when a patient with no suspected spine injury needs to be lifted from the ground to a stretcher.
- The **draw-sheet method** is one of two methods (along with the direct carry method) that is performed during transfers between hospitals and nursing homes, or when a patient must be moved from a bed at home to a stretcher. It is used for a patient with no suspected spine injury.
- A **direct carry** is performed to move a patient with no suspected spine injury from a bed or from a bed-level position to a stretcher.

extremity lift
a method of lifting and carrying a patient during which one rescuer slips hands under the patient's armpits and grasps the wrists, while another rescuer grasps the patient's knees.

direct ground lift
a method of lifting and carrying a patient from ground level to a stretcher in which two or more rescuers kneel, curl the patient to their chests, stand, then reverse the process to lower the patient to the stretcher.

draw-sheet method
a method of transferring a patient from bed to stretcher by grasping and pulling the loosened bottom sheet of the bed.

direct carry
a method of transferring a patient from bed to stretcher, during which two or more rescuers curl the patient to their chests, then reverse the process to lower the patient to the stretcher.

SCAN 5-7 • Non-Urgent Moves, No Suspected Spine Injury

EXTREMITY CARRY

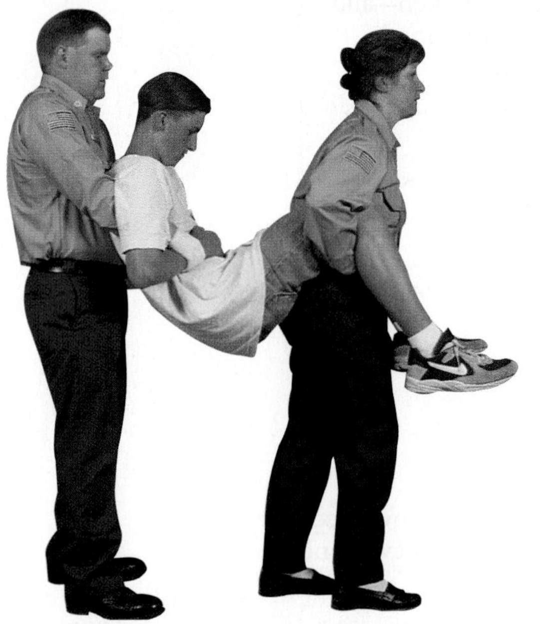

The extremity carry may be used as an emergency move or a non-urgent move for patients with no suspected spine injury.

Place patient on his back with knees flexed. Kneel at patient's head. Place your hands under his shoulders. Second EMT kneels at patient's feet, grasps patient's wrists, and lifts patient forward. At the same time, slip your arms under patient's armpits and grasp his wrists. Second EMT can grasp patient's knees while facing or facing away from patient. Direct second EMT, so you both move to a crouch and then stand at the same time. Move as a unit when carrying a patient.

If patient is found sitting, crouch and slip your arms under patient's armpits and grasp his wrists. Second EMT crouches, then grasps patient's knees. Lift patient as a unit.

DRAW-SHEET METHOD

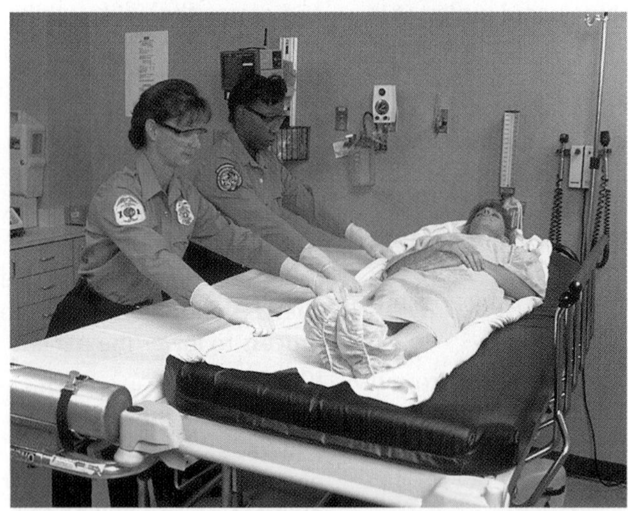

1. Loosen bottom sheet of bed and roll it from both sides toward patient. Place stretcher, rails lowered, parallel to bed and touching side of bed. EMTs use their bodies and feet to lock the stretcher against the bed.

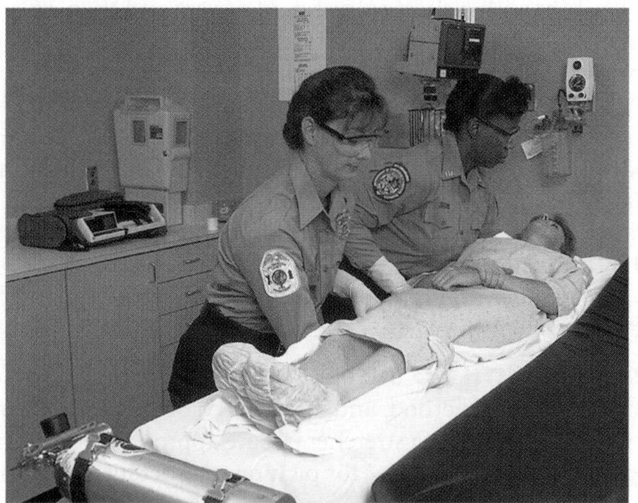

2. EMTs pull on draw sheet to move patient to side of bed. Both use one hand to support patient while they reach under him to grasp draw sheet. Then they simultaneously draw patient onto the stretcher.

DIRECT GROUND LIFT

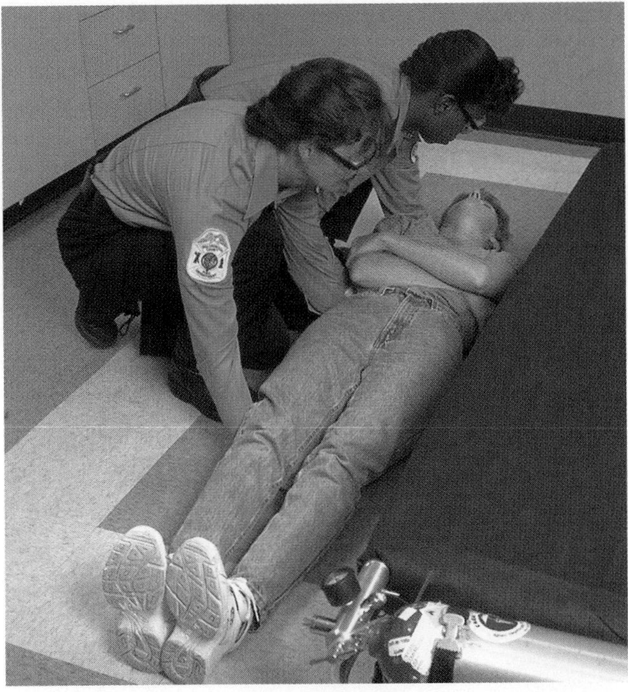

1. Stretcher is set in its lowest position and placed on the opposite side of patient. EMTs face patient, drop to one knee and, if possible, place patient's arms on his chest. Head-end EMT cradles patient's head and neck by sliding one arm under the neck to grasp shoulder, the other arm under patient's back. The foot-end EMT slides one arm under patient's knees and other arm under patient above buttocks.

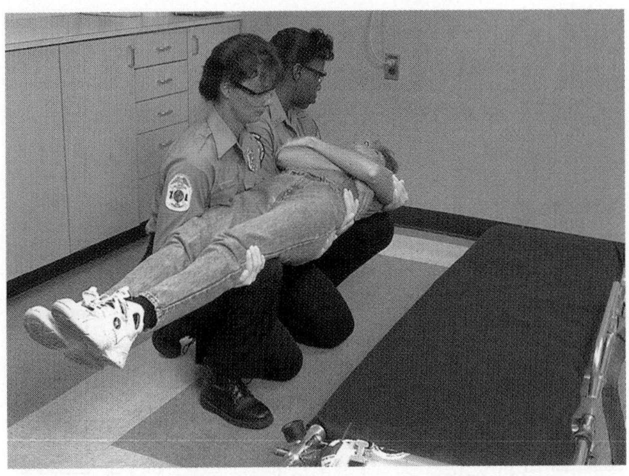

2. On signal, the EMTs lift patient to their knees.

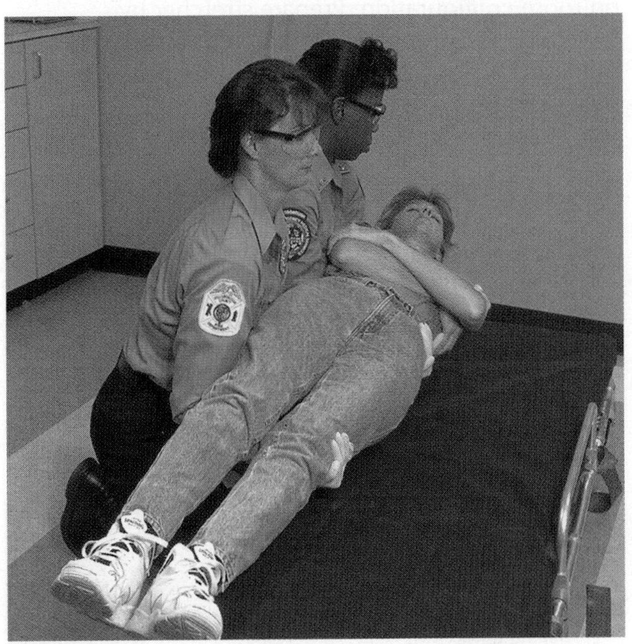

3. On signal, the EMTs stand and carry patient to stretcher, drop to one knee, and roll forward to place him onto mattress.

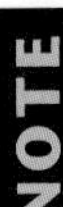

NOTE

If a third rescuer is available, he should place both arms under patient's waist while the other two slide their arms up to the mid back or down to the buttocks, as appropriate.

continued

SCAN 5-7 • (Continued)

DIRECT CARRY

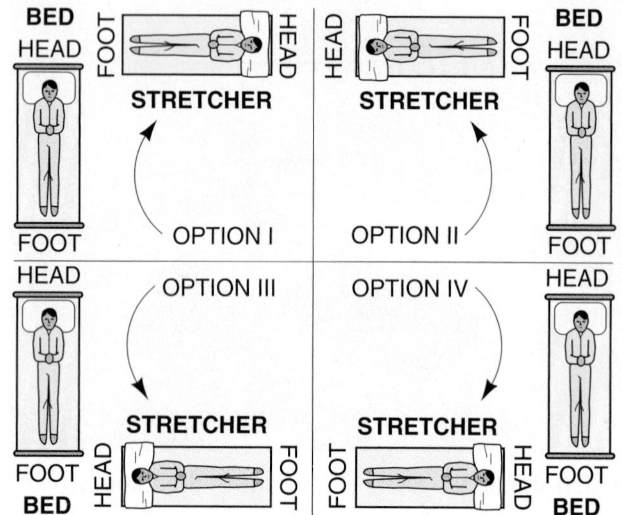

Stretcher is placed at 90° angle to bed, depending on room configuration. Prepare stretcher by lowering rails, unbuckling straps, and removing other items. Both EMTs stand between stretcher and bed, facing patient.

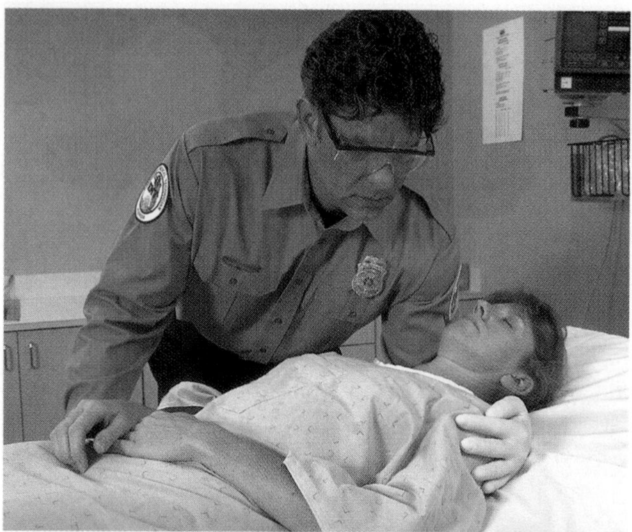

1. Head-end EMT cradles patient's head and neck by sliding one arm under patient's neck to grasp shoulder.

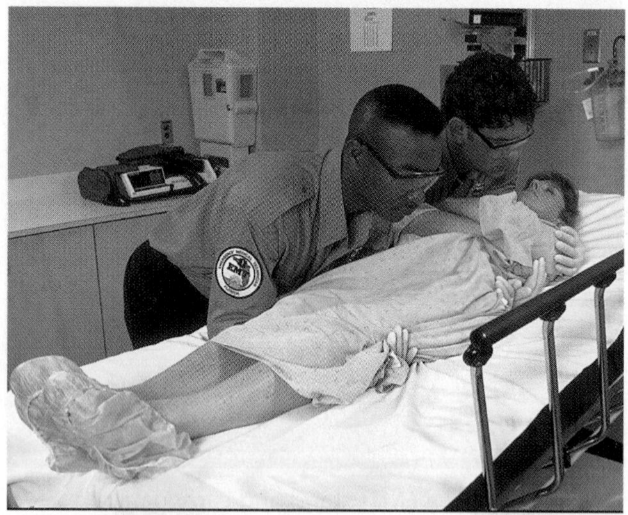

2. Foot-end EMT slides hand under patient's hip and lifts slightly. Head-end EMT slides other arm under patient's back. Foot-end EMT places arms under patient's hips and calves.

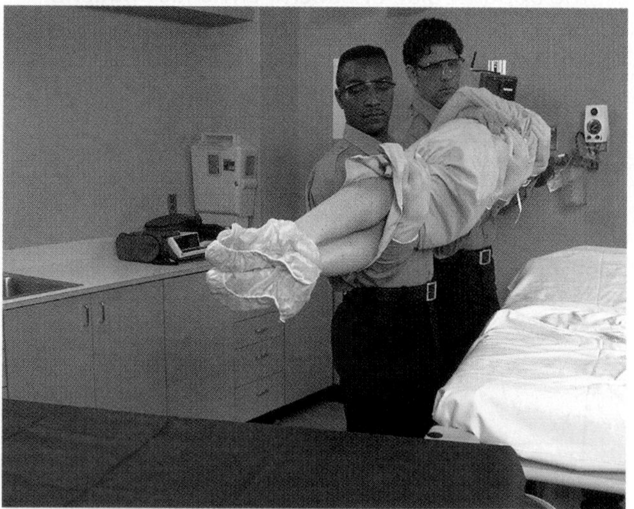

3. EMTs slide patient to edge of bed and bend toward her with their knees slightly bent. They lift and curl patient to their chests and return to a standing position. They rotate, then slide patient gently onto stretcher.

Patient Positioning

Positioning the patient during transfer to the ambulance and during transportation is a very important part of your care. Lifting, moving, and transport must be performed as an integral part of your total patient-care plan. The position in which the patient is transported depends on his medical condition and the device best designed to help this condition.

Unresponsive patients with no suspected spine injury should be placed in the recovery position (Figure 5-8). The patient should be on his side to aid drainage from his mouth and, if he vomits, to help prevent his breathing the vomitus into his lungs. This can be accomplished on a wheeled stretcher. You should avoid transporting the unresponsive patient in a chair-type device since the airway cannot be properly maintained.

Many patients who have no suspected spine injuries may be transported in a position of comfort. This includes many patients with medical complaints such as chest pain, nausea, or difficulty breathing. In this situation, allow the patient to choose a position he feels comfortable in. Breathing is often aided by raising the back of the stretcher so that the patient is in a semi-sitting position, also called Fowler's or semi-Fowler's position (Figure 5-9). The position must be safe and not prohibit the proper use of any transportation device. The position of comfort must be used cautiously in case the patient vomits. Always monitor the patient's airway and level of responsiveness. Place the patient in the recovery position at the first sign of a decreased level of responsiveness.

If any patient has a suspected neck or spine injury, he must be placed on a long backboard. Patients with spinal injuries who are found in a sitting position, such as in a vehicle, should first be secured to a short backboard to prevent injuries while being moved.

Patients in shock for any reason require treatment for that condition (see Chapter 26, "Bleeding and Shock"). If there is no possibility of head or spine injury, elevate the patient's legs 8 to 12 inches. Do not risk harm to a spine-injured patient. For a patient with possible spinal injury, in general, you should elevate the foot end of the backboard 8 to 12 inches so that the patient's entire body is inclined with the head 8 to 12 inches lower than the feet. This is often called the Trendelenburg position (Figure 5-10).

Transferring the Patient to a Hospital Stretcher

When you arrive at the hospital, you will move the patient from the ambulance stretcher to the hospital stretcher. You will probably use a modified draw-sheet method to transfer the patient (Scan 5-8).

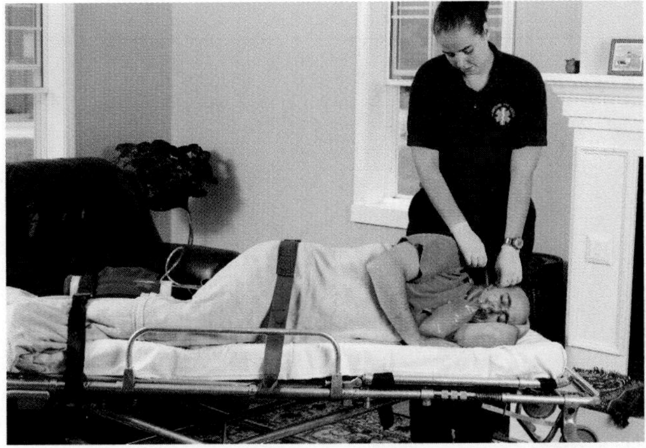

Figure 5-8 • A patient in the recovery position.

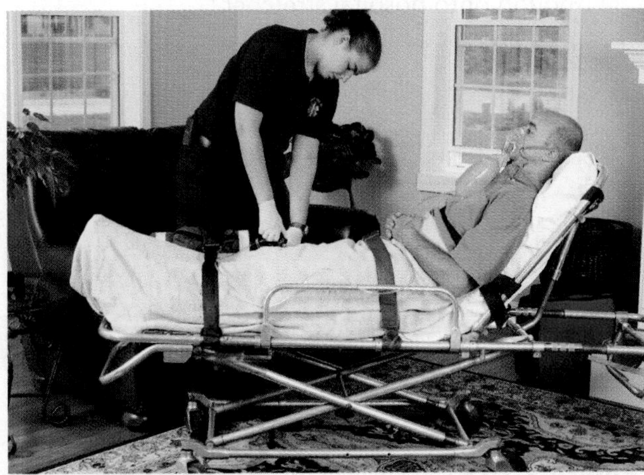

Figure 5-9 • For many patients, the position of comfort is a semi-sitting position.

SCAN 5-8 • Transfer to a Hospital Stretcher

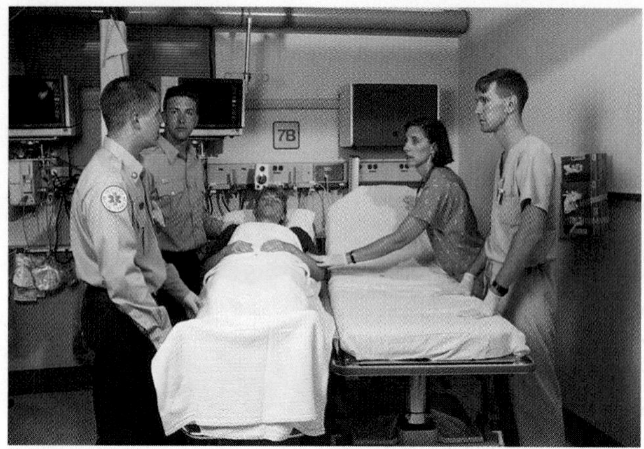

1. Position raised ambulance cot next to hospital stretcher. Hospital personnel then adjust stretcher (raise or lower the head) to receive patient.

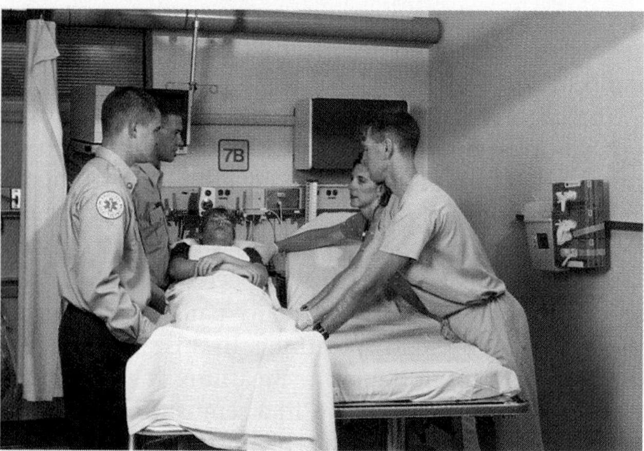

2. You and hospital personnel gather the sheet on either side of the patient and pull it taut in order to transfer the patient securely.

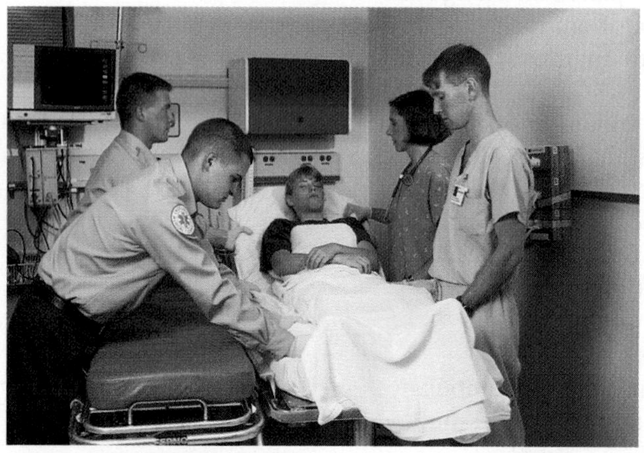

3. Holding the gathered sheet at support points near patient's shoulders, mid torso, hips, and knees, you and hospital personnel slide patient in one motion onto hospital stretcher.

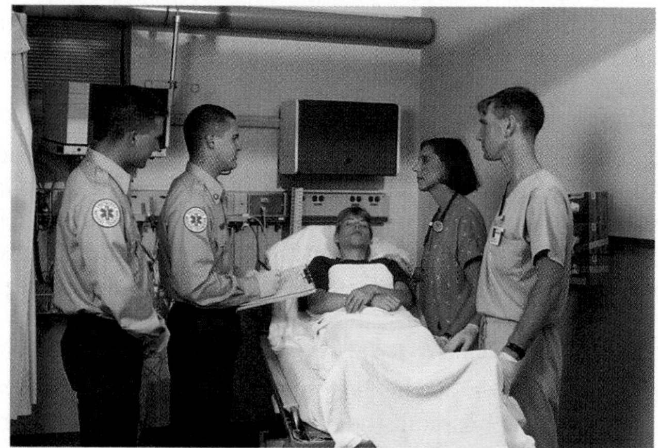

4. Make sure patient is centered on stretcher and stretcher rails are raised before turning him over to emergency department staff.

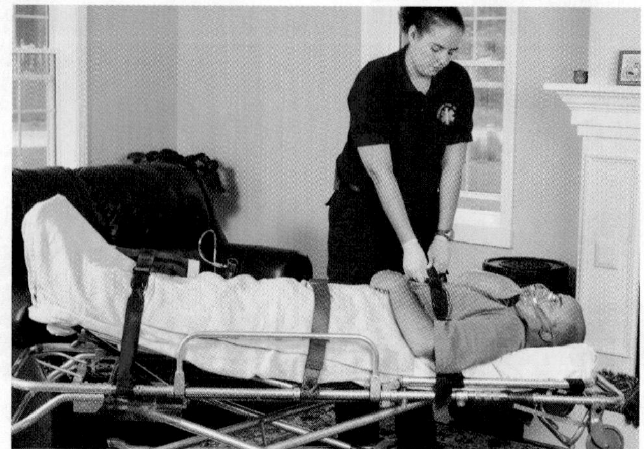

Figure 5-10 • For a patient in shock, raise the legs 8 to 12 inches when appropriate.

CHAPTER REVIEW

SUMMARY

Lifting and moving patients is a task that requires planning, proper equipment, and careful attention to body mechanics in order to prevent injury to your patient and to yourself. While some may feel that this task is only secondary to patient care, it is actually a critical part.

Emergency moves are those that may aggravate spine injuries and, therefore, are reserved for life-threatening situations. Urgent moves are used when the patient must be moved quickly but there is time to provide quick, temporary spinal stabilization. Non-urgent moves are normal ways of moving a patient to a stretcher after performing a complete on-scene assessment and completing any needed spinal stabilization and immobilization.

Positioning the patient for transport should take into account the patient's comfort, medical needs, and safety. Remember the importance of correct lifting and moving techniques on every call. Protect your patient and protect yourself from injury to maintain a long and positive EMS experience.

KEY TERMS

body mechanics the proper use of the body to facilitate lifting and moving and prevent injury.

direct carry a method of transferring a patient from bed to stretcher, during which two or more rescuers curl the patient to their chests, then reverse the process to lower the patient to the stretcher.

direct ground lift a method of lifting and carrying a patient from ground level to a stretcher in which two or more rescuers kneel, curl the patient to their chests, stand, then reverse the process to lower the patient to the stretcher.

draw-sheet method a method of transferring a patient from bed to stretcher by grasping and pulling the loosened bottom sheet of the bed.

extremity lift a method of lifting and carrying a patient during which one rescuer slips hands under the patient's armpits and grasps the wrists, while another rescuer grasps the patient's knees.

power grip gripping with as much hand surface as possible in contact with the object being lifted, all fingers bent at the same angle, hands at least 10 inches apart.

power lift a lift from a squatting position with weight to be lifted close to the body, feet apart and flat on the ground, body weight on or just behind balls of feet, back locked in. The upper body is raised before the hips. Also called the *squat-lift position.*

REVIEW QUESTIONS

1. Define the term *body mechanics*. Then describe several principles of body mechanics related to safe lifting and moving. (p. 106)
2. List several situations that may require an emergency move of a patient. (pp. 108–109)
3. Describe several lifts and drags. (pp. 109, 110–112)
4. Define a long-axis drag and explain its importance. (p. 109)

CRITICAL THINKING

For each of the following patients, use the knowledge gained in this chapter to identify the appropriate procedure or device for lifting and moving that patient:

- A patient who has fallen 18 feet and has suspected spinal injuries
- A patient with chest pain (with no spine injury) who lives on the fifth floor of a building with no elevator
- A patient who is found in an environment with a risk of immediate explosion

MEDIA RESOURCES 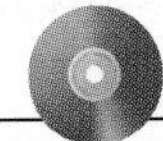

See the Student CD at the back of this book for quizzes, a case study activity, and other features related to this chapter. Also, visit the Companion Website for *Emergency Care* at **www.prenhall.com/limmer**, where you will find additional reinforcement and links to other resources.

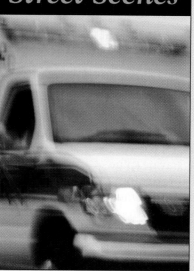

Street Scenes

You are having a discussion with a group of your EMS colleagues about the role of the EMT. You focus on direct patient care and the need to do thorough assessments. Another person argues that EMS focuses on doing airway, breathing, and circulation care really well. Kim, an EMT who has been doing EMS for more time than anyone else in the room, says that EMTs must know how to do all those things well "but don't forget that moving and transporting patients is significant, too." When you hear that, you silently disagree. "That's really not an important part of patient care," you say.

Well, the discussion ends—at least for you—when dispatch sends you and your partner to a single-occupant motor-vehicle crash. When you reach the scene, the police tell you that the patient is conscious and alert but is complaining of neck pain, that the crash appears to be low impact with significant front-end damage, and that the patient was wearing a lap belt only.

You introduce yourself to the patient, who is still sitting in the driver's seat of her car, and begin your assessment. The patient states that she ran into a parked car. At impact, her head hit the steering wheel, but she denies any loss of consciousness. You continue with the initial assessment and determine the patient is alert and having no difficulty breathing. No signs of bleeding are observed.

Street Scene Questions

1. What device should be used to remove the patient from the vehicle?
2. What patient-care issues are important when using an extrication device?
3. What is the next thing to consider when actually moving the patient from the vehicle?

Your local protocol requires that a patient with this mechanism of injury—a car crash resulting in the head impacting the steering wheel—gets a cervical collar and a short immobilization device. Your partner, who has been stabilizing the patient's head and neck since shortly after making contact, asks the First Responder unit from the fire department for assistance and suggests to you that a quick neuro exam should be done to check for pulses, motor function, and sensation in all extremities. After the neuro exam, you size a cervical collar and apply it to the patient. You ask the patient if it is causing any additional pain, and she responds that it is uncomfortable but "no additional pain." Next, while your partner still maintains manual stabilization, you position a vest-type extrication device behind her. As you tighten the straps to secure it in place, you ask if it is causing any difficulty with breathing. The patient responds again, "No." You then perform another quick neuro exam. Once completed, the long backboard is positioned and the patient is rotated onto it, with head and neck stabilization still being maintained. The patient is then lowered to the ground.

Street Scene Questions

4. What emergency-care equipment was used for this patient? Why?
5. What is the next step before moving this patient again?
6. What other safety considerations should be considered when moving the long board to the wheeled stretcher?

After the patient is properly secured to the long board, the head immobilizer is positioned, applied, and secured. You continue to talk to the patient to make sure her level of responsiveness has not changed and no breathing difficulty has developed. Another quick neuro exam is performed, with the patient having pulses, movement, and sensation in all four extremities.

The long board needs to be carried about 30 feet to the stretcher, so you and your partner decide to have someone on each corner of the long board. This will provide stability and all EMS personnel can be facing forward. The move is uneventful, and after placing the stretcher in the ambulance, you recheck the stretcher locking device. During transport to the hospital, you take the patient's vital signs and obtain a patient history. At the hospital, the stretcher is moved from the ambulance and raised onto its wheels. You take the patient to an examination room in the emergency department and, with assistance, you move the long board to the hospital gurney.

After the call, you return to the station. The folks are still in the ready room having the same discussion about the role of an EMT. You pipe in and say, "You know, after this last call, I have to agree with Kim. EMS has a lot to do with knowing how to properly, effectively, and safely move patients."

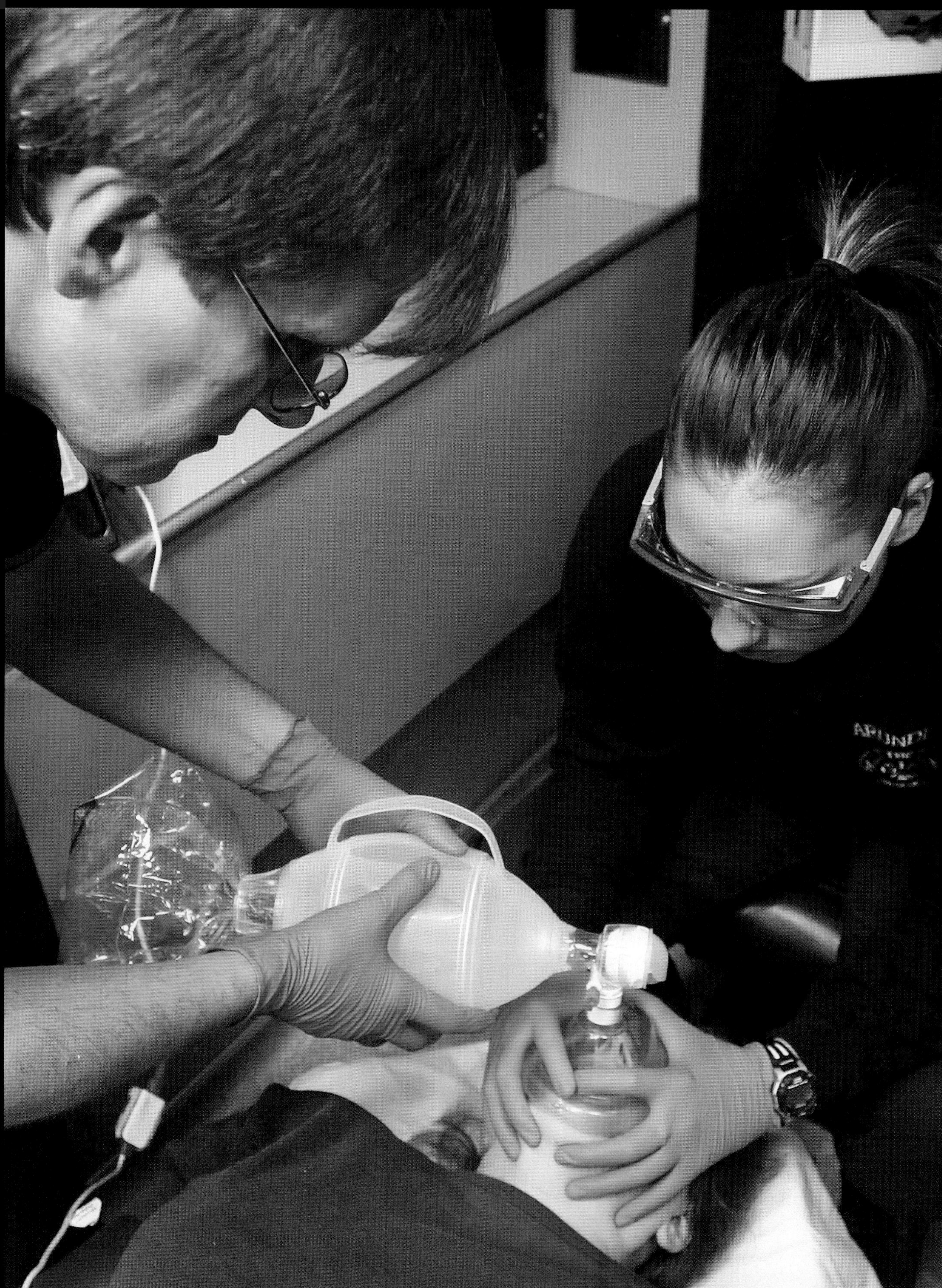

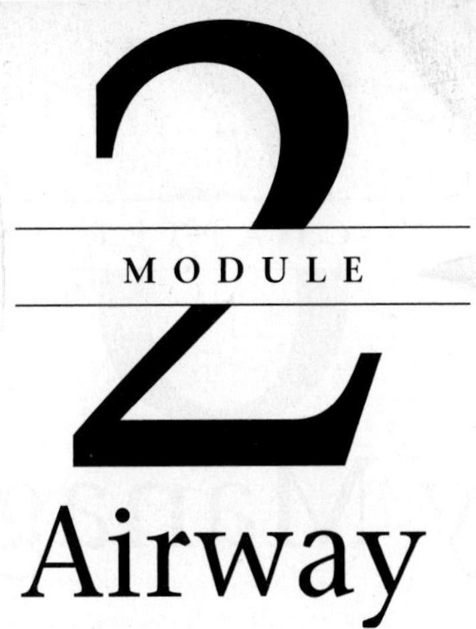

MODULE

Airway

Even though there is only one chapter in this module, it may be the most important module in this textbook. No patient will survive without an open airway!

You will begin assessment of any patient by evaluating the airway. However, keep in mind that airway assessment and care must continue throughout the entire time you spend with a patient. This module will describe the use of devices and skills to improve the patient's airway and oxygen intake. These include oral and nasal airway adjuncts, suction, oxygen administration, and more. This module also covers ways to ventilate a patient who is not breathing or is breathing inadequately—with emphasis on how to tell if a patient is or is not breathing adequately.

Obtaining the knowledge and skills presented in this module may surely mean the difference between life and death for many patients you will treat in the field.

CHAPTER 6

Airway Management

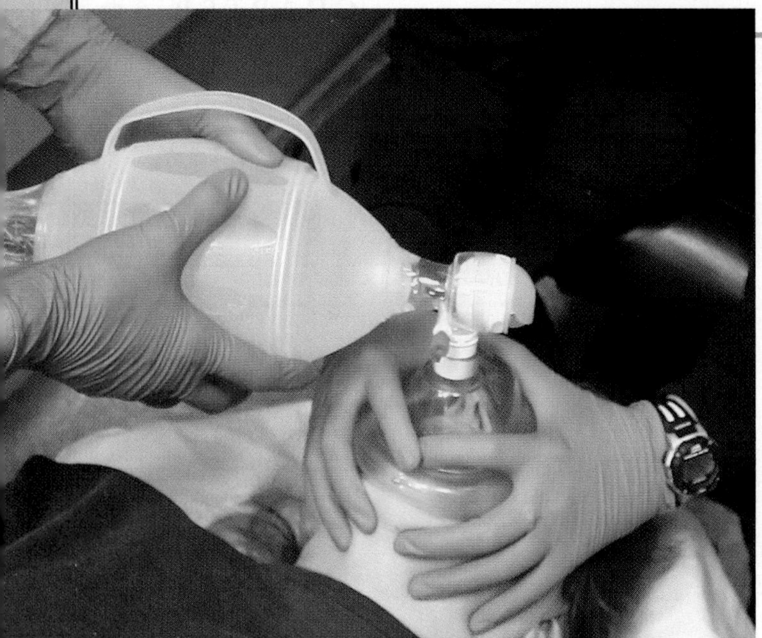

CORE CONCEPTS

The following are core concepts that will be addressed in this chapter:

- Anatomy and physiology of the respiratory system
- How to recognize adequate and inadequate breathing
- How to open an airway, maintain an open airway, and ventilate a patient
- Principles and techniques of oxygen administration
- Principles and techniques of suctioning

KEY TERMS

artificial ventilation, p. 146
cyanosis, p. 142
dead space, p. 141
gag reflex, p. 158
head-tilt, chin-lift maneuver, p. 145
hypoxia, p. 167
jaw-thrust maneuver, p. 145
minute volume, p. 138
positive pressure ventilation, p. 146
respiration, p. 136
respiratory arrest, p. 138
respiratory distress, p. 137
respiratory failure, p. 137
stoma, p. 154
suctioning, p. 162
ventilation, p. 146

DOT OBJECTIVES

*KNOWLEDGE AND ATTITUDE

2-1.1 Name and label the major structures of the respiratory system on a diagram. (pp. 136–137)
2-1.2 List the signs of adequate breathing. (pp. 129–133)
2-1.3 List the signs of inadequate breathing. (pp. 129–133)
2-1.4 Describe the steps in performing the head-tilt, chin-lift. (p. 145)
2-1.5 Relate mechanism of injury to opening the airway. (pp. 143–146)
2-1.6 Describe the steps in performing the jaw-thrust. (pp. 145–146)
2-1.7 State the importance of having a suction unit ready for immediate use when providing emergency care. (p. 163)
2-1.8 Describe the techniques of suctioning. (pp. 165, 167) (Scan 6-4, p. 166)
2-1.9 Describe how to artificially ventilate a patient with a pocket mask. (pp. 148–150)
2-1.10 Describe the steps in performing the skill of artificially ventilating a patient with a bag-valve mask while using the jaw-thrust. (pp. 150–154)
2-1.11 List the parts of a bag-valve-mask system. (p. 150)
2-1.12 Describe the steps in performing the skill of artificially ventilating a patient with a bag-valve mask for one and two rescuers. (pp. 151–154)
2-1.13 Describe the signs of adequate artificial ventilation using the bag-valve mask. (p. 147)
2-1.14 Describe the signs of inadequate artificial ventilation using the bag-valve mask. (p. 147)
2-1.15 Describe the steps in artificially ventilating a patient with a flow-restricted, oxygen-powered ventilation device. (pp. 155–156)
2-1.16 List the steps in performing the actions taken when providing mouth-to-mouth and mouth-to-stoma artificial ventilation. (pp. 146, 154–155)
2-1.17 Describe how to measure and insert an oropharyngeal (oral) airway. (pp. 158–159) (Scan 6-2, pp. 160–161)
2-1.18 Describe how to measure and insert a nasopharyngeal (nasal) airway. (pp. 159–161) (Scan 6-3, p. 162)
2-1.19 Define the components of an oxygen delivery system. (pp. 168–172) (Scan 6-5, pp. 174–176, Scan 6-6, pp. 176–178)
2-1.20 Identify a nonrebreather face mask and state the oxygen flow requirements needed for its use. (pp. 178–179)
2-1.21 Describe the indications for using a nasal cannula versus a nonrebreather face mask. (pp. 178–179)
2-1.22 Identify a nasal cannula and state the flow requirements needed for its use. (pp. 178–179)
2-1.23 Explain the rationale for basic life support artificial ventilation and airway protective skills taking priority over most other basic life support skills. (pp. 135–136)
2-1.24 Explain the rationale for providing adequate oxygenation through high inspired oxygen concentrations to patients who, in the past, may have received low concentrations. (p. 172–175)

*SKILLS

2-1.25 Demonstrate the steps in performing the head-tilt, chin-lift.
2-1.26 Demonstrate the steps in performing the jaw-thrust.
2-1.27 Demonstrate the techniques of suctioning.
2-1.28 Demonstrate the steps in providing mouth-to-mouth artificial ventilation with body substance isolation (barrier shields).
2-1.29 Demonstrate how to use a pocket mask to artificially ventilate a patient.
2-1.30 Demonstrate the assembly of a bag-valve-mask unit.
2-1.31 Demonstrate the steps in performing the skill of artificially ventilating a patient with a bag-valve mask for one and two rescuers.
2-1.32 Demonstrate the steps in performing the skill of artificially ventilating a patient with a bag-valve mask while using the jaw thrust.
2-1.33 Demonstrate artificial ventilation of a patient with a flow-restricted, oxygen-powered ventilation device.
2-1.34 Demonstrate how to artificially ventilate a patient with a stoma.
2-1.35 Demonstrate how to insert an oropharyngeal (oral) airway.
2-1.36 Demonstrate how to insert a nasopharyngeal (nasal) airway.
2-1.37 Demonstrate the correct operation of oxygen tanks and regulators.
2-1.38 Demonstrate the use of a nonrebreather face mask and state the oxygen flow requirements needed for its use.
2-1.39 Demonstrate the use of a nasal cannula and state the flow requirements for its use.
2-1.40 Demonstrate how to artificially ventilate the infant and child patient.
2-1.41 Demonstrate oxygen administration for the infant and child patient.

The cells of the human body must have oxygen to survive. The reason the ABCs—airway, breathing, and circulation—are so important is that they are the means by which oxygen is brought into the body and carried to the cells. If the airway (the passageways that lead from the mouth and nose to the lungs) is not open, air cannot get into the lungs. If the patient is unable to breathe, air does not get into the body even if the airway is open. If the heart is not pumping blood through the lungs to pick up oxygen and circulate it to the cells of the body, an open airway and the ability to breathe are of no use. (In fact, breathing and heartbeat are so dependent on each other that if breathing stops first, the heartbeat will stop very soon, or if the heartbeat stops first, breathing will stop almost at once.)

EMT training puts a great deal of emphasis on the airway because it is so easy and so common for a patient's airway to become occluded (blocked). It is also easy to forget to monitor the patient's airway in the midst of an emergency when so many other details demand the EMT's attention.

The EMT's chief responsibilities (although not the only ones) are to immediately find and correct life-threatening problems—airway, breathing, and circulation problems—and to get the patient to the hospital. As a prerequisite to your EMT course, you took a CPR course, which included providing rescue breathing, performing cardiopulmonary resuscitation (CPR), and treating airway obstructions in infants, children, and adults. You can review these topics by reading Appendix B, "Basic Cardiac Life Support Review," in the back of this book.

In this chapter, you will learn additional EMT-level skills that relate to the airway, artificial ventilation, and oxygen therapy.

RESPIRATION

respiration breathing.

Another word for breathing is **respiration.** You learned about the respiratory system in Chapter 4, "The Human Body." In preparation for this chapter, you should review the following structures of the respiratory system and be able to label them on a blank diagram of the respiratory system (Figure 6-1):

- Nose
- Mouth
- Pharynx
- Oropharynx
- Nasopharynx
- Uvula
- Epiglottis
- Larynx (voice box)
- Cricoid cartilage
- Trachea
- Carina

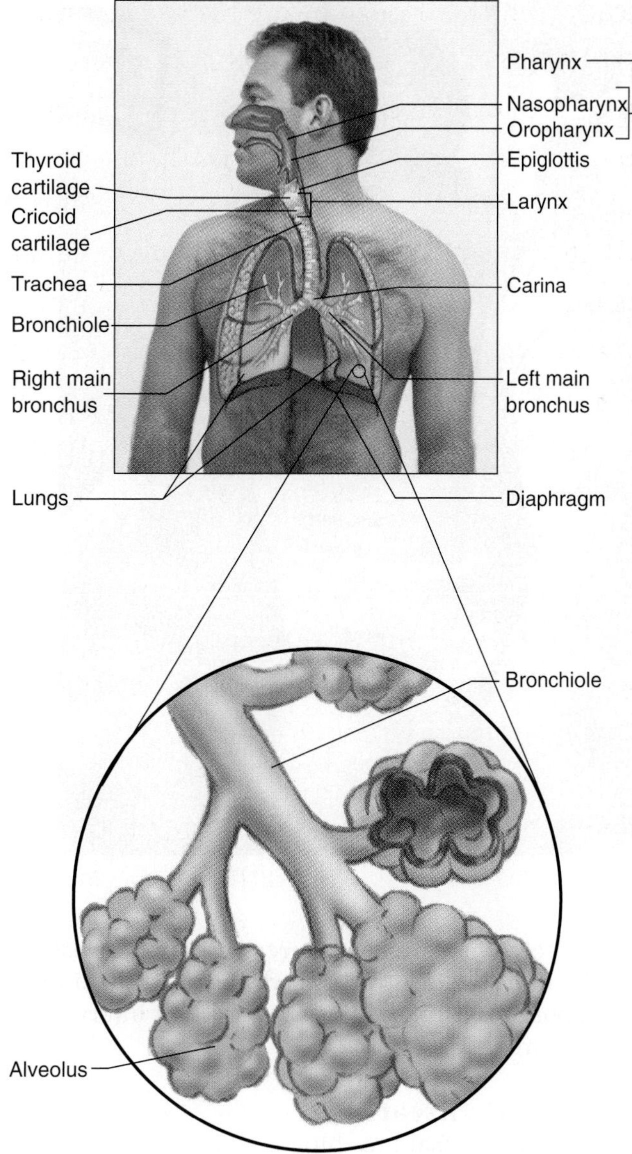

Figure 6-1 • The respiratory system.

- Bronchi (right and left mainstem bronchus)
- Bronchioles
- Lungs
- Alveoli (alveolar sacs)
- Diaphragm

Also review how oxygen and carbon dioxide are exchanged between the alveoli and capillaries in the lungs, and between the capillaries and the cells throughout the body.

Adequate and Inadequate Breathing

The respiratory system's function is to enable the body to inhale (breathe in) oxygen, which is then used by all the cells and organs in the body, and to exhale (breathe out) carbon dioxide, the major waste product of respiration. If either of these vital functions is disrupted, then the patient is likely to develop the sensation of shortness of breath, or **respiratory distress,** and be at risk for respiratory failure.

Simply stated, **respiratory failure** is the reduction of breathing to the point where oxygen intake is not sufficient to support life (Figure 6-2). When breathing stops

respiratory distress increased work of breathing; a sensation of shortness of breath.

respiratory failure the reduction of breathing to the point where oxygen intake is not sufficient to support life.

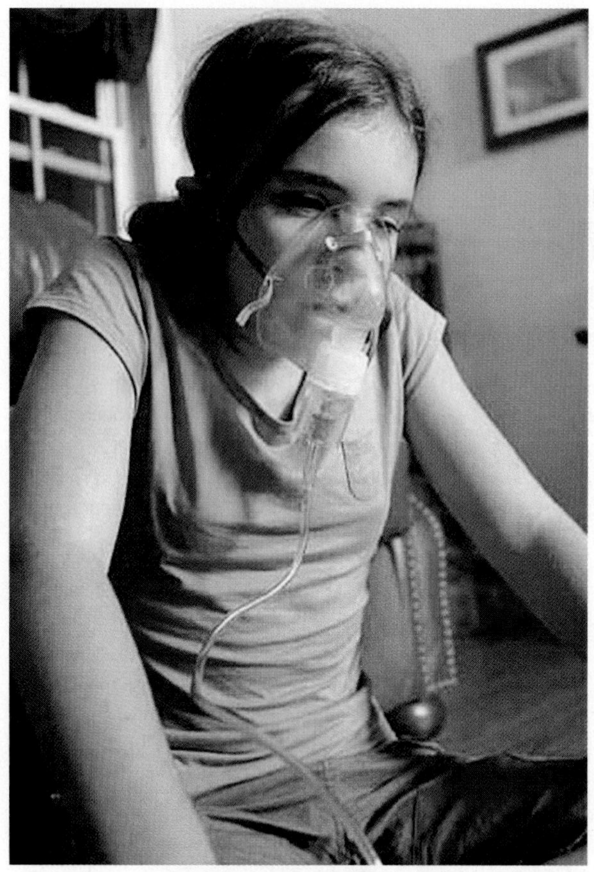

Figure 6-2 • Respiratory distress usually involves accessory muscle use and increased work of breathing. Severe or prolonged respiratory distress can proceed to respiratory failure and inadequate ventilation when the body can no longer work so hard to breathe. In this case you will see a reduced level of responsiveness or an appearance of tiring, shallow ventilations, and other signs of inadequate breathing. *(© Dan Limmer)*

respiratory arrest when breathing completely stops.

completely, the patient is in **respiratory arrest.** Respiratory arrest can develop during heart attack, stroke, airway obstruction, drowning, electrocution, drug overdose, poisoning, brain injury, severe chest injury, suffocation, or prolonged respiratory failure.

Inadequate Breathing

When you note that breathing is absent you will, of course, provide artificial ventilation to the patient. However, there is a time before respiration ceases totally when the patient may show some signs of breathing, although these breathing efforts are not enough to support life. That is, if the patient continues to breathe in this manner, he will eventually develop respiratory arrest and die. This is called inadequate breathing. Either the *rate of breathing* or the *depth of breathing* (or both) falls outside of normal ranges. Recognizing inadequate breathing requires both keen assessment skills and prompt action (Table 6-1). Identifying this condition and providing ventilation to an inadequately breathing patient may actually keep him alive and breathing—where he would have stopped breathing and died without your intervention. (Figure 6-3).

If a patient were breathing four times per minute, it would be pretty clear that the patient required action, since the normal ventilatory rate is at least 12 times per minute. But what if a patient is breathing 40 times per minute, when the normal range is 12 to 20? Is this also a problem? The answer is yes.

minute volume the amount of air breathed in during each respiration multiplied by the number of breaths per minute.

While it might seem that more is better, rapid respirations are often shallow. When this happens, even though more breaths move in and out, the **minute volume** is less. Minute volume is the amount of air per breath multiplied by the number of breaths per minute. If an adult were breathing 12 times per minute and each breath took in 500 mL of air, the patient's minute volume would be 6,000 mL (or 6 liters) of air per minute.

12 breaths per minute × 500 mL of air per breath = 6,000 mL per minute

TABLE 6-1 • Respiratory Conditions with Appropriate Interventions

CONDITION	SIGNS	EMT INTERVENTION	
Adequate breathing Patient is breathing adequately but needs supplemental oxygen due to a medical or traumatic condition	• Rate and depth of breathing are adequate • No abnormal breath sounds • Air moves freely in and out of the chest • Skin color normal	Oxygen by **nonrebreather mask** or **nasal cannula**	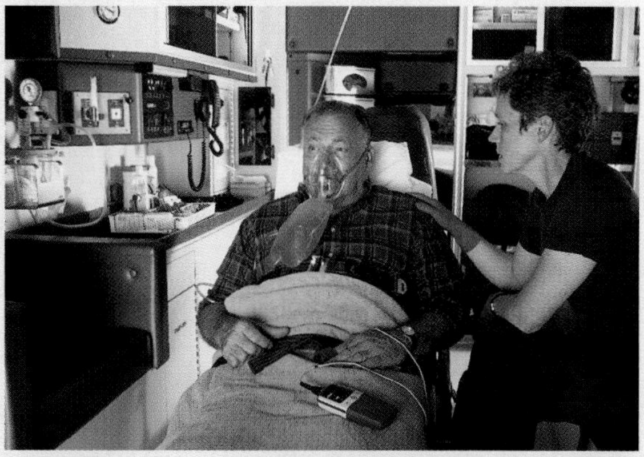
Inadequate breathing Patient is moving some air in and out but it is slow or shallow and not enough to live.	• Patient has some breathing but not enough to live • Rate and/or depth outside of normal limits • Shallow ventilations • Diminished or absent breath sounds • Noises such as crowing, stridor, snoring, gurgling, or gasping • Blue (cyanosis) or gray skin color • Decreased minute volume	Assisted ventilations (air forced into the lungs under pressure) with a **pocket face mask, bag-valve mask,** or **FROPVD.** See chapter text about adjusting rates for rapid or slow breathing. *Note: A nonrebreather mask requires adequate breathing to pull oxygen into the lungs. It DOES NOT provide ventilation to a patient who is not breathing or who is breathing inadequately.*	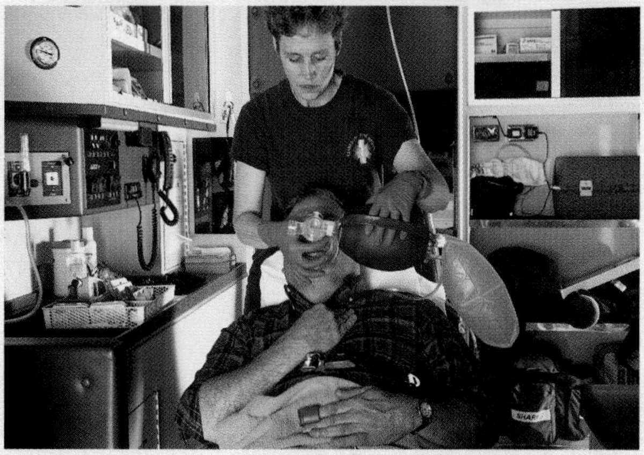
Patient is not breathing at all	• No chest rise • No evidence of air being moved from the mouth or nose • No breath sounds	Artificial ventilations with a **pocket face mask, bag-valve mask, FROPVD,** or **ATV** at 10–12/minute for an adult and 20/minute for an infant or child. *Note: DO NOT use oxygen-powered ventilation devices on infants or children.*	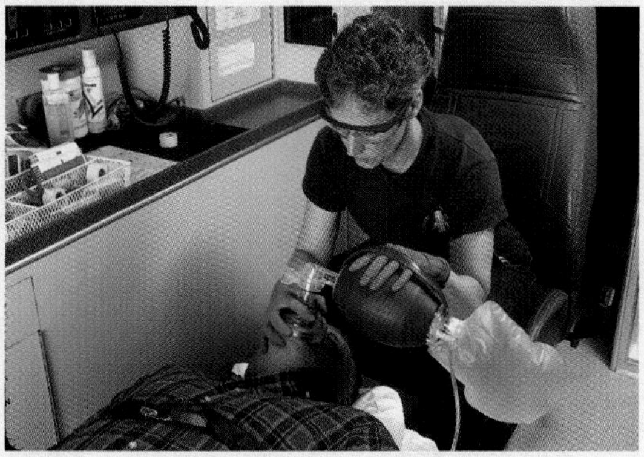

Unfortunately, not all of this inhaled air gets used in the transfer of oxygen from the lungs into the blood and the transfer of carbon dioxide from the blood to the lungs. As you learned in Chapter 4, "The Human Body," air enters the lungs through the trachea and moves through the bronchi (and then the bronchioles, the smaller branches from the bronchi), ending up in the small air sacs called alveoli. Oxygen and carbon dioxide

PATIENT'S CONDITION	WHEN AND HOW TO INTERVENE
Adequate breathing: Speaks full sentences; alert and calm	**Nonrebreather mask or nasal cannula**
Increasing respiratory distress: Visibly short of breath; Speaking 3–4 word sentences; Increasing anxiety	**Nonrebreather mask**
Severe respiratory distress: Speaking only 1–2 word sentences; Very diaphoretic (sweaty); Severe anxiety	**Assisted ventilations** Pocket face mask (PFM), bag-valve mask (BVM), or flow-restricted, oxygen-powered ventilation device (FROPVD) Assist the patient's own ventilations, adjusting the rate for rapid or slow breathing
Continues to deteriorate: Sleepy with head-bobbing; Becomes unarousable	
Respiratory arrest: No breathing	**Artificial ventilation** Pocket face mask (PFM), bag-valve mask (BVM), or flow-restricted, oxygen-powered ventilation device (FROPV) Assisted ventilations at 12/minute for an adult or 20/minute for a child or infant

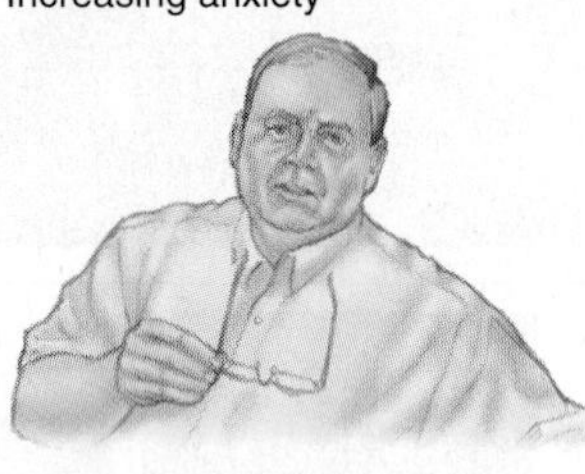

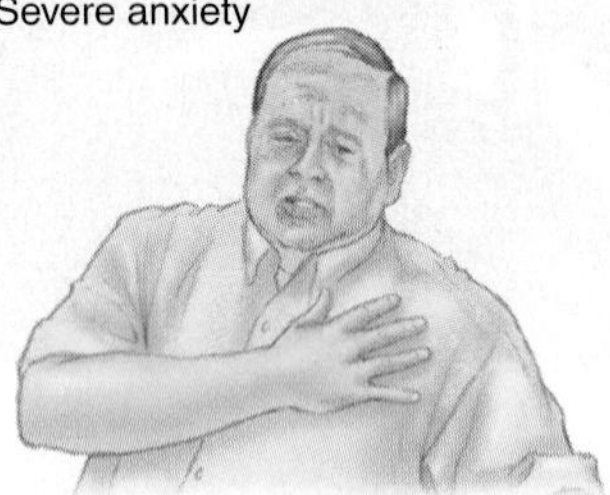

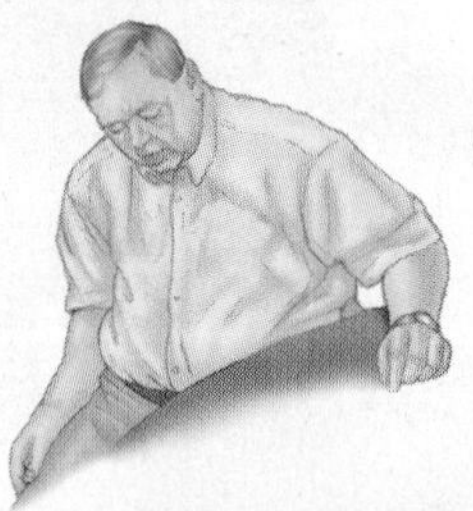

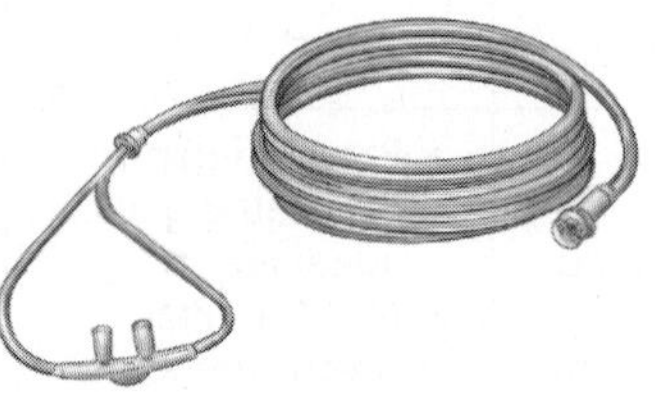

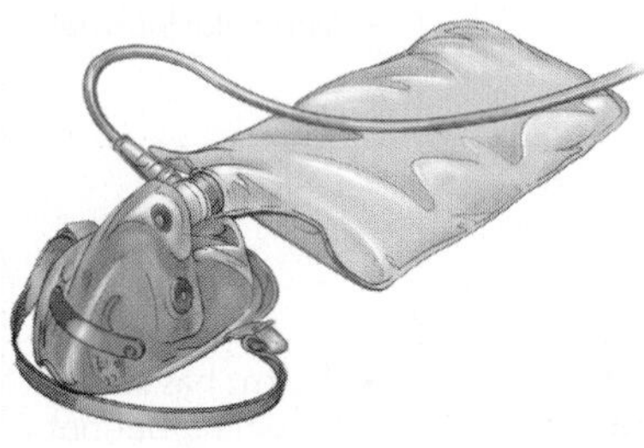

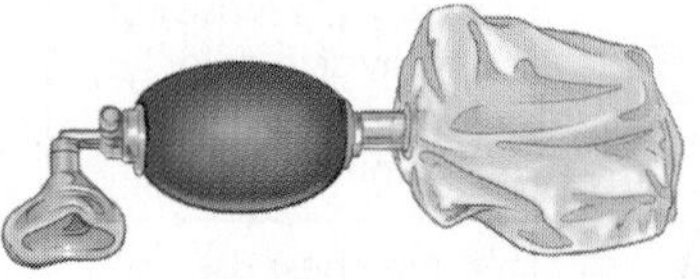

Key decision-making point:

Recognize inadequate breathing before respiratory arrest develops.

Assist ventilations before they stop altogether!

Figure 6-3 • Along the continuum from normal, adequate breathing to no breathing at all, there are milestones where an EMT should apply a nonrebreather mask or switch to positive pressure ventilation with a pocket face mask, BVM, or FROPVD for assisting the patient's own ventilations or providing artificial ventilation. It is essential to recognize the need for assisted ventilations, even before severe respiratory distress develops.

are exchanged only in the alveoli, not in the other parts of the lungs. This means that all the oxygen in the inhaled air that rests in the trachea, the bronchi, and the bronchioles—the air that does not reach the alveoli—does not get transferred into the blood and, therefore, does not get to the body cells.

These areas of the lungs outside the alveoli are known as anatomic **dead space.** About 30 percent of inhaled air rests in this dead space. For discussion and calculation of dead space, we will estimate this volume at 150 mL of dead space per breath. This means that of the 500 mL taken in during each breath, only 350 mL (500 mL – 150 mL dead space = 350) gets to the alveoli to exchange oxygen and carbon dioxide. While depth and rate of breathing may change, the amount of dead space does not. This dead space has a significant effect on how adequate the breathing actually is—especially when the respirations are very slow, very rapid, or very shallow. Figure 6-4A illustrates dead space in the lungs. Figure 6-4B gives several examples of minute volume, dead space, and how they affect adequacy of ventilations.

dead space
areas of the lungs outside the alveoli where gas exchange with the blood does not take place.

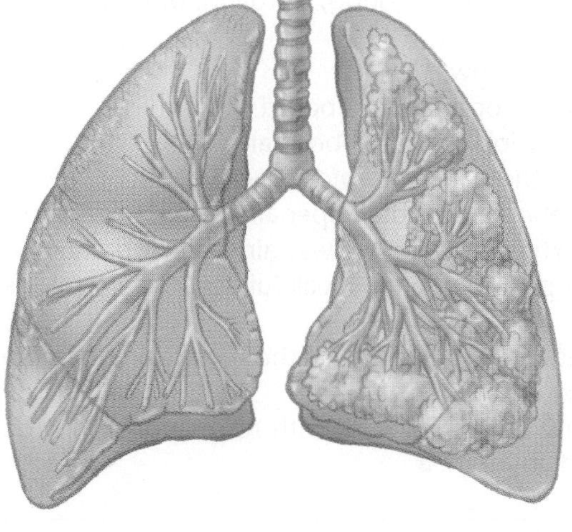

A

MINUTE VOLUME

minute volume = mL of air per breath × breaths per minute
dead space = est 150 mL

EFFECTS OF MINUTE VOLUME AND DEAD SPACE ON RESPIRATION

Not all of the air breathed in reaches the alveoli to be available for gas exchange with the blood. An estimated 150 mL of the air taken in with each breath remains trapped in the "dead space" (the bronchi and bronchioles—see Figure 6-4a) and never reaches the alveoli.

To calculate the effect on respiration (the amount available for gas exchange) air in the dead space must be subtracted from the total air breathed in. The formula would be:

minute volume (mL/breath× breaths/min)
minus **dead space volume** (150 mL × breaths/min)
= **minute volume reaching the alveoli**

Examples:

Normal Breathing:
Minute volume: 500 mL × 12 breaths/minute = 6000 mL/minute
Minus dead space volume: 150 mL × 12 breaths/minute = 1800 mL/minute
Minute volume reaching alveoli = 4200 mL/minute: **adequate**

Shallow Breathing at a Normal Rate:
Minute volume: 250 mL × 12 breaths/minute = 3000 mL/minute
Minus dead space volume: 150 mL × 12 breaths/minute = 1800 mL/minute
Minute volume reaching alveoli = 1200 mL/minute: **inadequate**

Shallow Breathing at a Faster Rate:
Minute volume: 250 mL × 24 breaths/minute = 6000 mL/minute
Minus dead space volume: 150 mL × 24 breaths/minute = 3600 mL/minute
Minute volume reaching alveoli = 2400 mL/minute: **inadequate**

Shallow Breathing at a Rapid Rate:
Note: as respirations become more rapid they often become more shallow (less volume)
Minute volume: 200 mL × 36 breaths/minute = 7200 mL/minute
Minus dead space volume: 150 mL × 36 breaths/minute = 5400 mL/minute
Minute volume reaching alveoli = 1800 mL/minute: **inadequate**

B

Figure 6-4 • (A) Dead space, areas of the lungs that contain inhaled air outside the alveoli. (B) Effect of minute volume and dead space on respiration: Even though the respiratory rate increases, ventilations are often inadequate due to the shallow depth of breathing and the dramatic effect of dead space in the lungs.

PATIENT ASSESSMENT

BREATHING ADEQUACY

As an EMT, you must be able to determine whether or not a patient is breathing adequately so that you can properly manage the airway and breathing.

SIGNS OF ADEQUATE BREATHING

To determine signs of adequate breathing, you should:

- *Look* for adequate and equal expansion of both sides of the chest when the patient inhales.
- *Listen* for air entering and leaving the nose, mouth, and chest. The breath sounds (when auscultated, or listened to, with a stethoscope) should be present and equal on both sides of the chest. The sounds from the mouth and nose should be typically free of gurgling, gasping, crowing, wheezing, snoring, and stridor (harsh, high-pitched sound during inhalation).
- *Feel* for air moving out of the nose or mouth.
- Check for typical skin coloration. There should be no blue or gray colorations.
- Note the rate, rhythm, quality, and depth of breathing typical for a person at rest (Table 6-2).

SIGNS OF INADEQUATE BREATHING

Signs of inadequate breathing include the following:

- Chest movements are absent, minimal, or uneven.
- Movement associated with breathing is limited to the abdomen (abdominal breathing).
- No air can be felt or heard at the nose or mouth, or the amount of air exchanged is below normal.
- Breath sounds are diminished or absent.
- Noises such as wheezing, crowing, stridor, snoring, gurgling, or gasping are heard during breathing.
- Rate of breathing is too rapid or too slow.
- Breathing is very shallow, very deep, or appears labored.
- The patient's skin, lips, tongue, ear lobes, or nail beds are blue or gray. This condition is called **cyanosis,** and the patient is said to be cyanotic.
- Inspirations are prolonged (indicating a possible upper airway obstruction) or expirations are prolonged (indicating a possible lower airway obstruction).
- Patient is unable to speak, or the patient cannot speak full sentences because of shortness of breath.
- In children, there may be retractions (a pulling in of the muscles) above the clavicles and between and below the ribs.
- Nasal flaring (widening of the nostrils of the nose with respirations) may be present, especially in infants and children. ■

cyanosis (SIGH-uh-NO-sis) a blue or gray color resulting from lack of oxygen in the body.

TABLE 6-2 • Adequate Breathing

NORMAL RATES	QUALITY
Adult—12–20 per minute Child—15–30 per minute Infant—25–50 per minute	Breath sounds—present and equal Chest expansion—adequate and equal Minimum effort
RHYTHM	**DEPTH**
Regular	Adequate

PATIENT CARE

INADEQUATE BREATHING

When the patient's signs indicate inadequate breathing or no breathing (respiratory failure or respiratory arrest), a life-threatening condition exists and prompt action must be taken. The principal procedures to treat life-threatening respiratory problems are:

- Opening and maintaining the airway
- Providing artificial ventilation to the nonbreathing patient and the patient with inadequate breathing
- Providing supplemental oxygen to the breathing patient
- Suctioning as needed

These procedures are discussed next and on the following pages. ■

OPENING THE AIRWAY

The **airway** is the passageway by which air enters or leaves the body. The structures of the airway are the nose, mouth, pharynx, larynx, trachea, bronchi, and lungs.

airway
the passageway by which air enters or leaves the body. The structures of the airway are the nose, mouth, pharynx, larynx, trachea, bronchi, and lungs.

The procedures for airway evaluation, opening the airway, and artificial ventilation are best carried out with the patient lying supine (flat on his back). Often you will find a patient already supine in bed. You can perform airway procedures with the patient in this position. Scan 6-1 illustrates the technique for positioning a patient found lying on the floor or ground. Patients who are found in positions other than supine or on the ground should be moved to a supine position on the floor or stretcher for evaluation and treatment.

Any movement of a trauma (injured) patient before immobilization of the head and spine can produce serious injury to the spinal cord. If injury is suspected, protect the head and neck as you position the patient. Airway and breathing, however, have priority over protection of the spine and must be ensured as quickly as possible. If the trauma patient must be moved in order to open the airway or to provide ventilations, you will probably not have time to provide immobilization with a cervical collar or head immobilization device on a stretcher but, instead, will provide as much manual stabilization as possible.

Use the following as indications that head, neck, or spinal injury may have occurred, especially when the patient is unconscious and cannot tell you what happened:

- Mechanism of injury is one that can cause head, neck, or spine injury. For example, a patient who is found on the ground near a ladder or stairs may have such injuries. Motor-vehicle collisions are another common cause of head, neck, and spine injuries.
- Any injury at or above the level of the shoulders indicates that head, neck, or spine injuries may also be present.
- Family or bystanders may tell you that an injury to the head, neck, or spine has occurred, or they may give you information that leads you to suspect it.

As an EMT you must open and maintain the airway in any patient who cannot do so for himself. This includes patients who have an altered mental status (including unconsciousness) or who are in respiratory or cardiac arrest. This is called maintaining a **patent airway.** A patent airway is one that is open and clear and will remain open and clear. Insertion of an oral or nasal airway and suctioning may be required to maintain a patent airway.

patent airway
an airway (passage from nose or mouth to lungs) that is open and clear and will remain open and clear, without interference to the passage of air into and out of the body.

SCAN 6-1 • Positioning the Patient for Basic Life Support

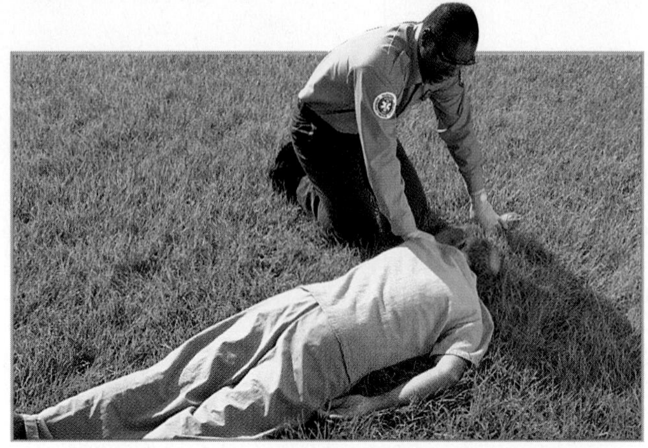

1. Straighten the legs and position the closer arm above the patient's head.

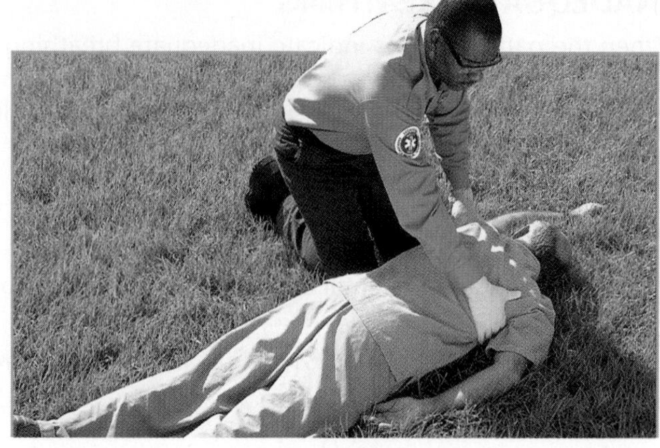

2. Then grasp under the distant armpit.

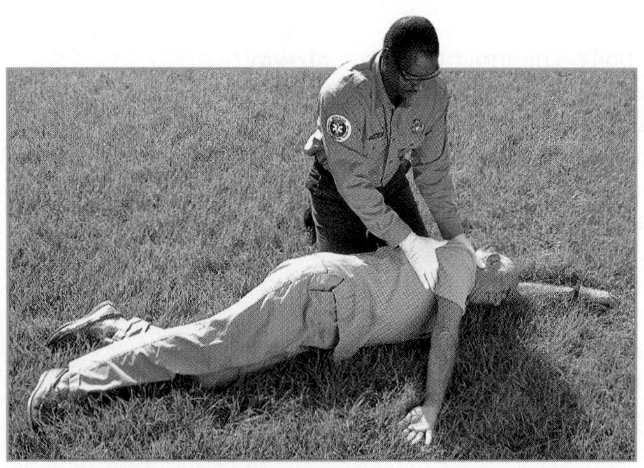

3. Cradle the head and neck, and move the patient as a unit onto his side.

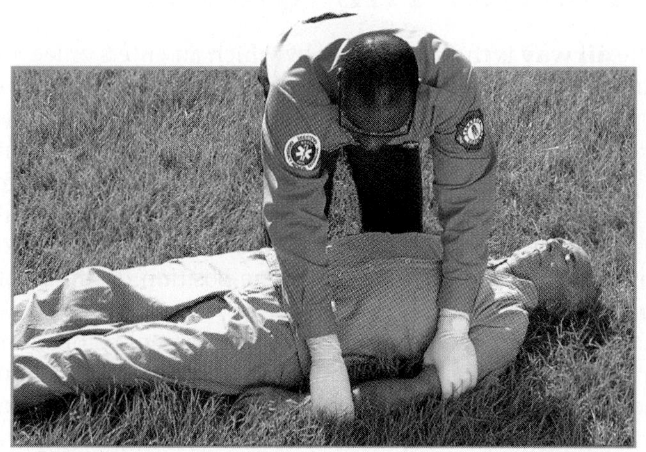

4. Move the patient onto his back and reposition the extended arm.

NOTE ***This maneuver is used when the rescuer must act alone.***

Most airway problems are caused by the tongue. As the head flexes forward, the tongue may slide into the airway, causing an obstruction. If the patient is unconscious, the tongue loses muscle tone and muscles of the lower jaw relax. Since the tongue is attached to the lower jaw, the risk of airway obstruction by the tongue is even greater during unconsciousness. The basic procedures for opening the airway help to correct the position of the tongue.

Two procedures are commonly recommended for opening the airway: the head-tilt, chin-lift maneuver and the jaw-thrust maneuver, the latter being recommended when head, neck, or spine injury is suspected.

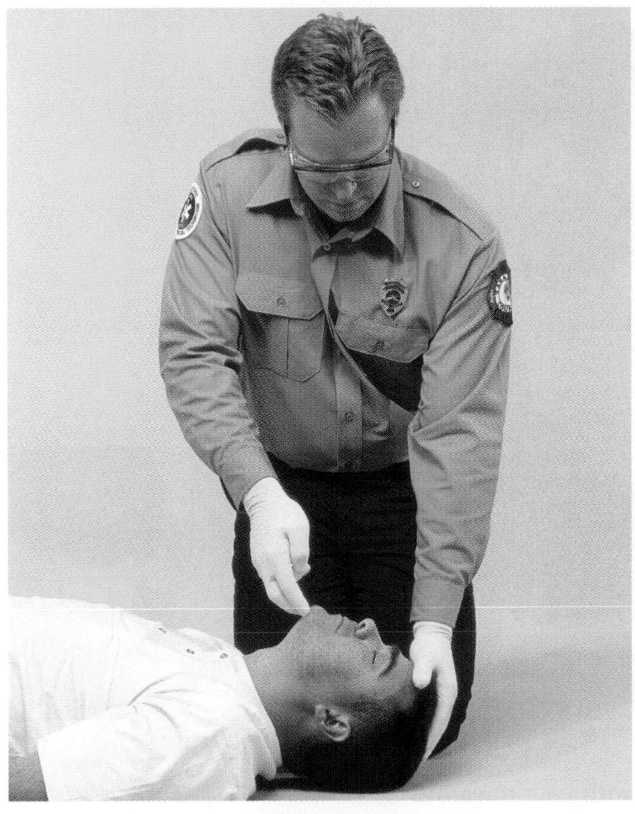

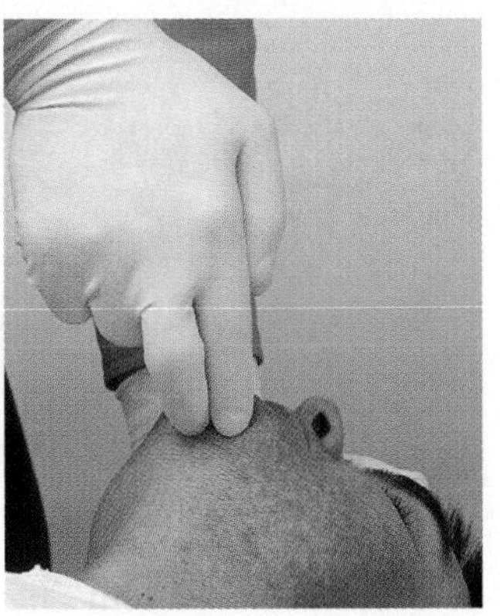

Figure 6-5 • Head-tilt, chin-lift maneuver, side view. Inset shows EMT's fingertips under the bony area at the center of the patient's lower jaw.

head-tilt, chin-lift maneuver
a means of correcting blockage of the airway by the tongue by tilting the head back and lifting the chin. Used when no trauma, or injury, is suspected.

NOTE *If any indication of head, neck, or spine injury is present, do not use the head-tilt, chin-lift maneuver. (Use the jaw-thrust maneuver instead.) Remember that any unconscious and many conscious trauma patients may be suspected of having an injury to the head, neck, or spine.*

Head-Tilt, Chin-Lift Maneuver

The **head-tilt, chin-lift maneuver** (Figure 6-5) provides for the maximum opening of the airway. It is useful on patients who are in need of assistance in maintaining an airway or breathing. It is one of the best methods for correcting obstructions caused by the tongue.

To perform the head-tilt, chin-lift maneuver, follow these steps:

1. Once the patient is supine, place one hand on the forehead and place the fingertips of the other hand under the bony area at the center of the patient's lower jaw.
2. Tilt the head by applying gentle pressure to the patient's forehead.
3. Use your fingertips to lift the chin and to support the lower jaw. Move the jaw forward to a point where the lower teeth are almost touching the upper teeth. Do not compress the soft tissues under the lower jaw, which can obstruct the airway.
4. Do not allow the patient's mouth to be closed. To provide an adequate opening at the mouth, you may need to use the thumb of the hand supporting the chin to pull back the patient's lower lip. Do not insert your thumb into the patient's mouth (to avoid being bitten).

jaw-thrust maneuver
a means of correcting blockage of the airway by moving the jaw forward without tilting the head or neck. Used when trauma, or injury, is suspected to open the airway without causing further injury to the spinal cord in the neck.

NOTE *The jaw-thrust maneuver is the only recommended procedure for unconscious patients with possible head, neck, or spine injury or unknown mechanism of injury.*

NOTE *The purpose of the jaw-thrust maneuver is to open the airway without moving the head or neck.*

Jaw-Thrust Maneuver

The **jaw-thrust maneuver** (Figure 6-6) is most commonly used to open the airway of an unconscious patient with suspected head, neck, or spine injury or unknown mechanism of injury. Follow these steps:

1. Carefully keep the patient's head, neck, and spine aligned, moving him as a unit as you place him in the supine position.
2. Kneel at the top of the patient's head. For long-term comfort it may be helpful to rest your elbows on the same surface as the patient's head.
3. Carefully reach forward and gently place one hand on each side of the patient's lower jaw, at the angles of the jaw below the ears.

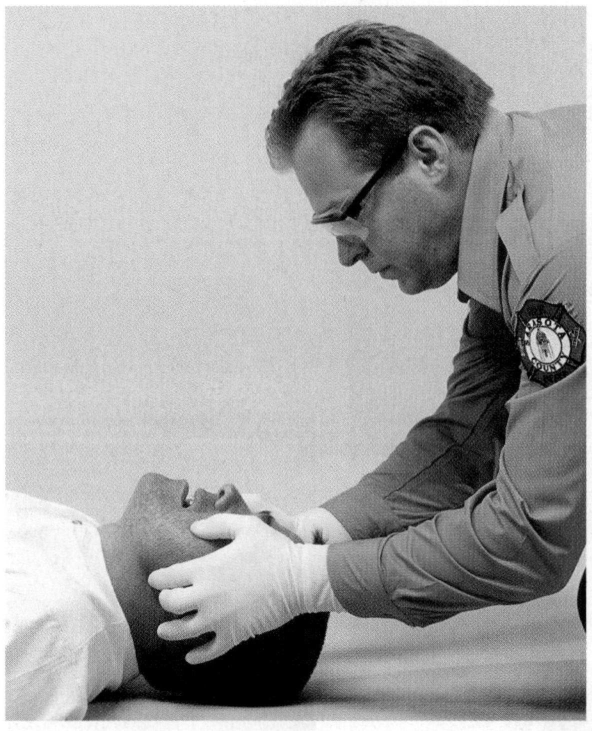

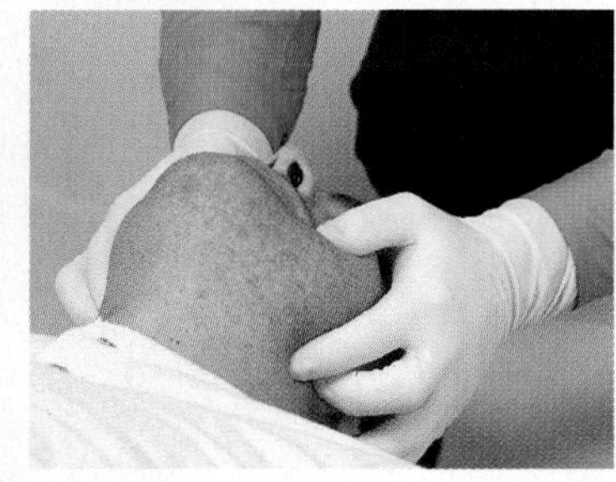

Figure 6-6 • Jaw-thrust maneuver, side view. Inset shows EMT's finger position at angle of the jaw just below the ears.

4. Stabilize the patient's head with your forearms.
5. Using your index fingers, push the angles of the patient's lower jaw forward.
6. You may need to retract the patient's lower lip with your thumb to keep the mouth open.
7. Do not tilt or rotate the patient's head.

In addition to physically opening the airway with the head-tilt, chin-lift or the jaw-thrust maneuver, it is imperative that the airway also be cleared of any secretions, blood, or vomitus. The most effective way to clear the patient's airway is with a wide-bore, rigid-tip Yankauer suction device. *It is crucial that a suction unit be ready for immediate use when opening and maintaining the airway.* The equipment and techniques used for suctioning will be discussed later in this chapter.

TECHNIQUES OF ARTIFICIAL VENTILATION

If you determine that the patient is not breathing or that the respiratory efforts are so minimal that respiratory arrest is imminent, you will have to provide artificial ventilation. **Ventilation** is the breathing in of air or oxygen. **Artificial ventilation,** also called **positive pressure ventilation,** is forcing air or oxygen into the lungs when a patient has stopped breathing or has inadequate breathing. Various techniques are available to you as an EMT with which you can provide artificial ventilations. In order of preference they are:

ventilation
the breathing in of air or oxygen or providing breaths artificially.

artificial ventilation
forcing air or oxygen into the lungs when a patient has stopped breathing or has inadequate breathing. Also called **positive pressure ventilation.**

1. Mouth-to-mask (preferably with high-concentration supplemental oxygen at 15 liters per minute)
2. Two-rescuer bag-valve mask (BVM) (preferably with high-concentration supplemental oxygen at 15 liters per minute)
3. Flow-restricted, oxygen-powered ventilation device
4. One-rescuer bag-valve mask (preferably with high-concentration supplemental oxygen at 15 liters per minute)

No matter what method is used to ventilate the patient, you must ensure that the patient is being ventilated adequately. To determine the signs of *adequate* artificial ventilation, you should:

- Watch the chest rise and fall with each ventilation
- See the patient's heart rate return to normal with artificial ventilation
- Ensure that the rate of ventilation is sufficient—approximately 10–12 per minute in adults, 20 per minute in children, and a minimum of 20 per minute in infants

Inadequate artificial ventilation occurs when:

- The chest does not rise and fall with ventilations
- The patient's heart rate does not return to normal with artificial ventilations
- The rate of ventilation is too fast or too slow

NOTE *Do not ventilate a patient who is vomiting or who has vomitus in his airway. Positive pressure ventilation will force the vomitus into the patient's lungs. Make sure the patient is not actively vomiting and suction any vomitus from the airway before ventilating.*

Techniques used for artificial ventilation should also ensure adequate isolation of the rescuer from the patient's body fluids, including saliva, blood, and vomit. For this reason, mouth-to-mouth ventilation is not recommended unless there is no alternative method of artificial ventilation available. A number of compact barrier devices are available for personal use (Figure 6-7).

As noted earlier, ventilation will also be required on a patient who is breathing but doing so inadequately. This may be due to a very rapid but shallow rate or a very slow rate. In any case, keep in mind that it may be intimidating to ventilate (use a pocket face mask or bag-valve mask on) a patient who is breathing and may even be aware of what you are doing. Follow these guidelines for ventilation of a breathing patient:

NOTE *The skill of assisting a patient's ventilations is difficult to master as it requires careful watching for the chest rise and coordinating delivery of the pocket-mask or BVM ventilation. Fortunately, it is a skill that can be readily practiced in class on other students.*

For a patient with rapid ventilations:

- Carefully assess the adequacy of respirations.
- Explain the procedure to the patient. Calm reassurance and a simple explanation such as, "I'm going to help you breathe," are essential in the awake patient.
- Place the mask (pocket face mask or BVM) over the patient's mouth and nose.
- After sealing the mask on the patient's face, squeeze the bag with the patient's inhalation. Watch as the patient's chest begins to rise and deliver the ventilation with the start of the patient's own inhalation. The goal will be to increase the volume of each breath. Over the next several breaths, adjust the rate so you are ventilating fewer times per minute but with greater volume per breath (increasing the minute volume).

For a patient with slow ventilations:

- Carefully assess the adequacy of respirations.
- Explain the procedure to the patient. Again, calm reassurance and a simple explanation such as, "I'm going to help you breathe," are essential in the awake patient.
- Place the mask (pocket face mask or BVM) over the patient's mouth and nose.
- After sealing the mask on the patient's face, squeeze the bag every time the patient begins to inhale. If the rate is very slow, add ventilations in between the patient's own to obtain a rate of approximately 12 per minute with adequate minute volume.

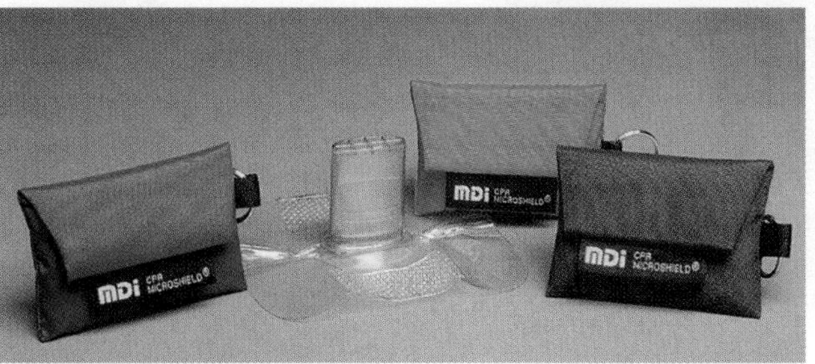

Figure 6-7 • Examples of barrier devices.

Mouth-to-Mask Ventilation

pocket face mask a device, usually with a one-way valve, to aid in artificial ventilation. A rescuer breathes through the valve when the mask is placed over the patient's face. It also acts as a barrier to prevent contact with a patient's breath or body fluids. It can be used with supplemental oxygen when fitted with an oxygen inlet.

Mouth-to-mask ventilation is performed using a **pocket face mask.** The pocket face mask is made of soft, collapsible material and can be carried in your pocket, jacket, or purse (Figure 6-8). Many EMTs purchase their own pocket face masks for workplace or auto first aid kits.

Face masks have important infection control features. Your ventilations (breaths) are delivered through a valve in the mask so that you do not have direct contact with the patient's mouth. Most pocket masks have one-way valves that allow your ventilations to enter but prevent the patient's exhaled air from coming back through the valve and into contact with you (Figure 6-9).

Some pocket masks have oxygen inlets. When high-concentration oxygen is attached to the inlet, an oxygen concentration of approximately 50 percent is delivered. This is significantly better than the 16 percent oxygen concentration (in exhaled air) delivered by mouth-to-mask ventilations without supplemental oxygen.

Most pocket face masks are made of a clear plastic. This is important because you must be able to observe the patient's mouth and nose for vomiting or secretions that need to be suctioned. You also need to observe the color of the lips, an indicator of the patient's respiratory status. Some pocket face masks have a strap that goes around the patient's head. This is helpful during one-rescuer CPR, since it will hold the mask on the patient's face while you are performing chest compressions. However, it does not replace the need for proper hand placement on the mask.

To provide mouth-to-mask ventilation (Table 6-3), follow these steps:

1. Position yourself at the patient's head and open the airway. It may be necessary to clear the airway of obstructions. If necessary, insert an oropharyngeal airway to help keep the patient's airway open (as described later in this chapter).
2. Connect oxygen to the inlet on the mask and run at 15 liters per minute. If oxygen is not immediately available, do not delay mouth-to-mask ventilations.

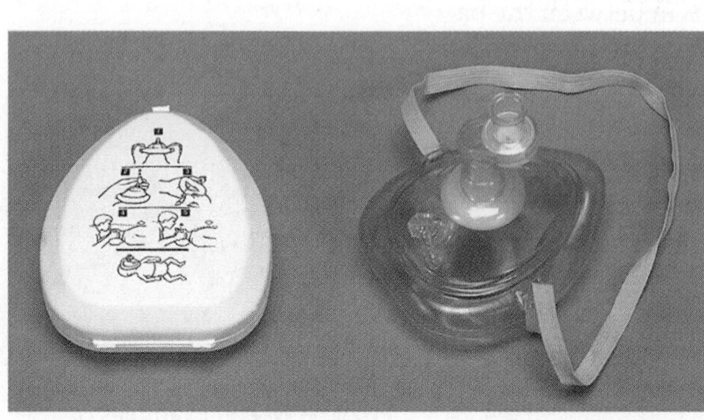

Figure 6-8 • Pocket face mask.

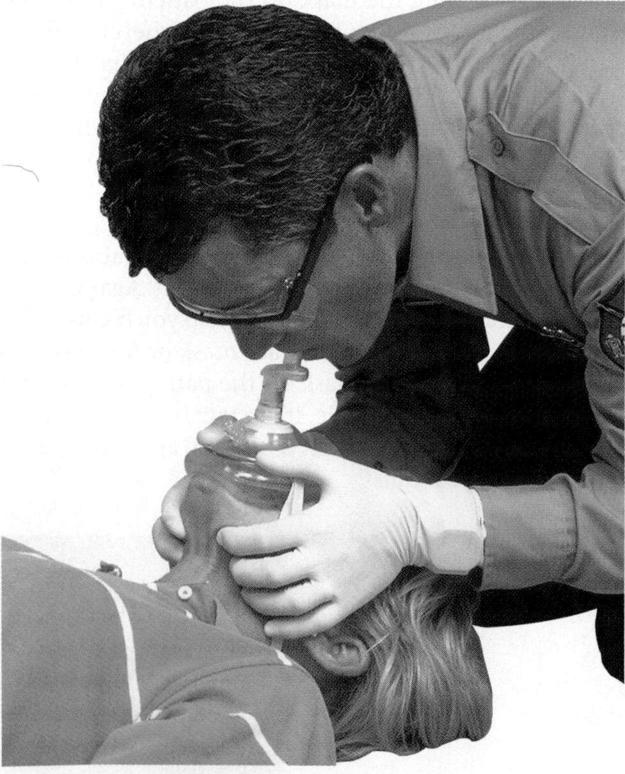

Figure 6-9 • Use only a pocket mask with a one-way valve.

TABLE 6-3 • Use of the Pocket Face Mask

PATIENT	USE OF THE POCKET FACE MASK
Patient <u>without</u> suspected spine injury— EMT at top of patient's head 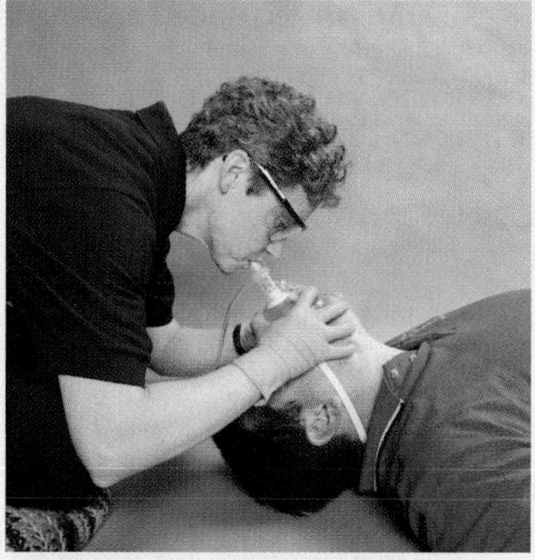	• Position yourself directly above (at the top of) the patient's head. • Apply the mask to the patient. Use the bridge of the nose as a guide for correct position. • Place your thumbs over the top of the mask, your index fingers over the bottom of the mask, and the rest of your fingers under the patient's jaw. • Lift the jaw to the mask as you tilt the patient's head backward and place the remaining fingers under the angle of the jaw. • While lifting the jaw, squeeze the mask with your thumbs to achieve a seal between the mask and the patient's face. • Give breaths into the one-way valve of the mask. Watch for the chest to rise.
Patient <u>without</u> suspected spine injury— Alternative: EMT beside patient's head 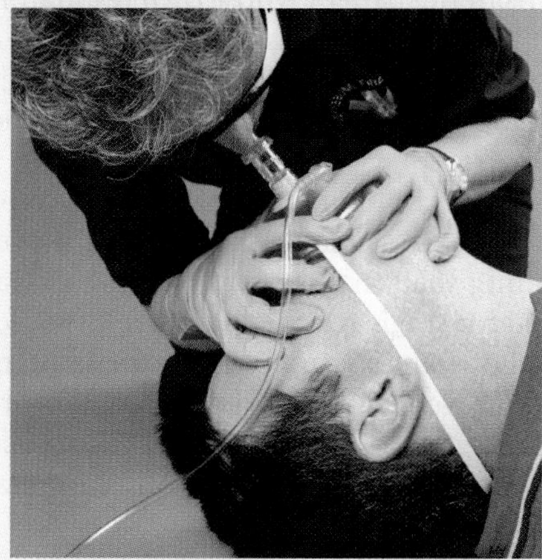	• Position yourself beside the patient's head. • Apply the mask to the patient. Use the bridge of the nose as a guide for correct position. • Seal the mask by placing your index finger and thumb of the hand closer to the top of the patient's head along the top border of the mask. • Place the thumb of the hand closer to the patient's feet on the lower margin of the mask. Place the remaining fingers of this hand along the bony margin of the jaw. • Lift the jaw while performing a head-tilt, chin-lift maneuver. • Compress the outer margins of the mask against the face to obtain a seal. • Give breaths into the one-way valve on the mask. Watch for the chest to rise.
Patient <u>with</u> suspected spine injury— EMT at top of patient's head 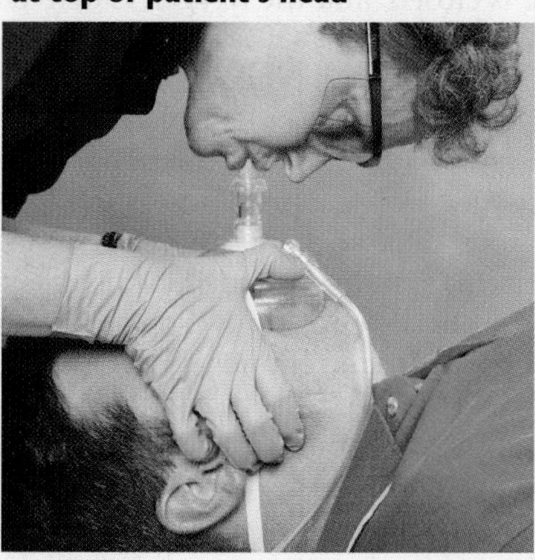	• Position yourself directly above (at the top of) the patient's head. • Apply the mask to the patient. Use the bridge of the nose as a guide for correct position. • Place the thumb sides of your hands along the mask to hold it firmly on the face. • Use your remaining fingers to lift the angle of the jaw. **Do not tilt the head backward.** • While lifting the jaw, squeeze the mask with your thumbs and fingers to achieve a seal. Give breaths into the one-way valve on the mask. Watch for the chest to rise. Note: Factors such as hand size, patient size, or dentures not in place may necessitate modifications in hand position and technique to achieve the necessary tight seal.

3. Position the mask on the patient's face so that the apex (top of the triangle) is over the bridge of the nose and the base is between the lower lip and prominence of the chin. (Center the ventilation port over the patient's mouth.)
4. Hold the mask firmly in place while maintaining head tilt. Use one of these positions or some variation—with the aim of achieving a tight seal:
   - Thumbs over the top of the mask, index fingers over the bottom of the mask, and remaining fingers under the patient's jaw (Table 6-3, top)
   - Thumbs along the side of the mask and remaining fingers under the patient's jaw (Table 6-3, bottom)
5. Take a breath and exhale into the mask port or one-way valve at the top of the mask port. Each ventilation should be delivered over 1 second in adults, infants, and children. Watch for visible chest rise.
6. Remove your mouth from the port and allow for passive exhalation. Continue as you would for mouth-to-mouth ventilations or CPR.

When properly used, the pocket face mask will deliver higher volumes of air to the patient than the bag-valve-mask device.

Bag-Valve Mask

bag-valve mask a handheld device with a face mask and self-refilling bag that can be squeezed to provide artificial ventilations to a patient. It can deliver air from the atmosphere or oxygen from a supplemental oxygen supply system.

The **bag-valve mask** (also called bag mask or bag-mask device) is a handheld ventilation device. It may also be referred to as a bag-valve-mask unit, system, device, resuscitator, or simply BVM. The bag-valve-mask unit can be used to ventilate a nonbreathing patient and is also helpful to assist ventilations in the patient whose own respiratory attempts are not enough to support life, such as a patient in respiratory failure or drug overdose. The BVM also provides an infection-control barrier between you and your patient. The use of the bag-valve mask in the field is often referred to as "bagging" the patient (Table 6-4).

Bag-valve-mask units come in sizes for adults, children, and infants (Figure 6-10). Many different types of bag-valve-mask systems are available; however, all have the same basic parts. The bag must be a self-refilling shell that is easily cleaned and sterilized. (Some bag-valve-mask units are designed for single use and are then disposed of.) The system must have a non-jam valve that allows an oxygen inlet flow of 15 liters per minute. The valve should be nonrebreathing (preventing the patient from rebreathing his own exhalations) and not subject to freezing in cold temperatures. Most systems have a standard 15/22 respiratory fitting to ensure a proper fit with other respiratory equipment, face masks, and endotracheal tubes.

The mechanical workings of a bag-valve-mask device are simple. Oxygen, flowing at 15 liters per minute, is attached to the BVM and enters the reservoir. When the bag is squeezed, the air inlet to the bag is closed, and the oxygen is delivered to the patient.

When the squeeze of the bag is released, a passive expiration by the patient will occur. While the patient exhales, oxygen enters the reservoir to be delivered to the patient the next time the bag is squeezed. BVM systems without a reservoir supply approximately 50 percent oxygen. Systems with an oxygen reservoir provide nearly 100 percent oxygen. The bag itself will hold anywhere from 1,000 to 1,600 milliliters of air. This means that the bag-valve-mask system must be used properly and efficiently.

The most difficult part of delivering BVM artificial ventilations is obtaining an adequate mask seal so that air does not leak in or out around the edges of the mask. It is difficult to maintain the seal with one hand while squeezing the bag with the other, and one-rescuer bag-valve-mask operation is often unsuccessful or inadequate for this reason. Therefore, it is strongly recommended by the American Heart Association that BVM artificial ventilation be performed by two rescuers. In two-rescuer BVM ventilation, one rescuer is assigned to squeeze the bag while the other rescuer uses two hands to maintain a mask seal.

TABLE 6-4 • Use of the Bag-Valve Mask

PATIENT	USE OF THE BAG-VALVE MASK
Patient without suspected spine injury 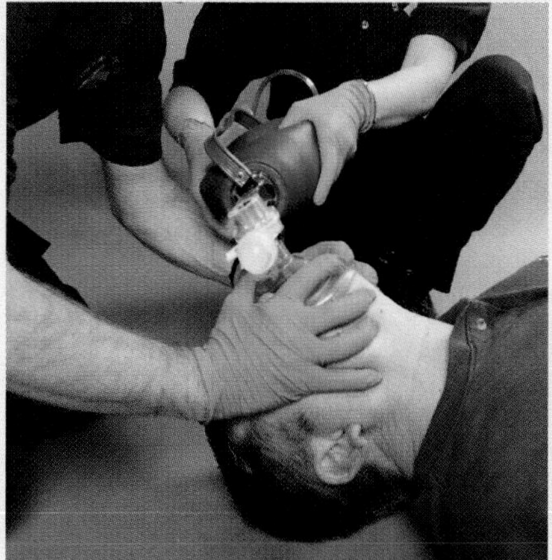	• Open the airway and insert appropriately sized oral or nasal airway (if no gag reflex). • Position your thumbs over the top of the mask, index fingers over the bottom of the mask. • Place the mask over the patient's face. Position the mask over the patient's nose and lower to the chin. (Large, round-style masks are centered first on the mouth.) • Use your middle, ring, and little fingers to bring the jaw up to the mask. • Connect the bag to the mask and have assistant squeeze the bag until the chest rises. • If the chest does not rise and fall, reevaluate head position and mask seal. If unable to ventilate, use another device (e.g., pocket face mask or FROPVD).
Patient with suspected spine injury 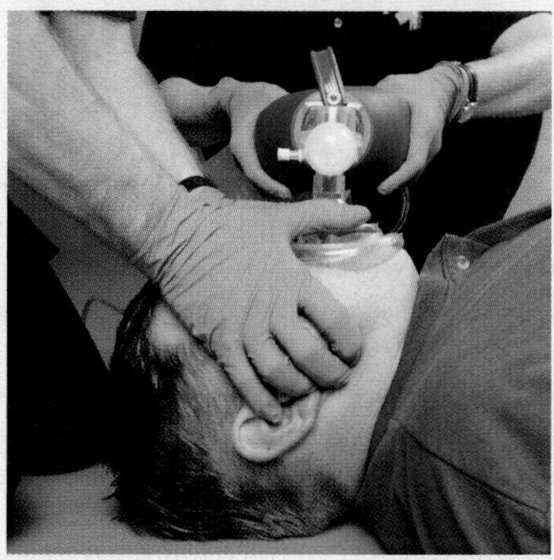	• Open the airway with a jaw thrust and insert an appropriate size airway if no gag reflex. • Have an assistant manually immobilize the head and neck. Immobilization of the head between your knees may be acceptable if no assistance is available. • Place the thumb sides of your hands along the mask to hold it firmly on the face. • Place the mask on the patient's face as previously described. • Use your little and ring fingers to bring the jaw up to the mask without tilting the head or neck. • Have assistant squeeze the bag with two hands until the chest rises. • Continually evaluate ventilations.

NOTE

Many older bag-valve masks have "pop-off" valves, designed to open after certain pressures are obtained. Studies have shown that pop-off valves may prevent adequate ventilations. BVM systems with pop-off valves should be replaced. A BVM system should also have a clear face mask so that you can observe the lips for cyanosis and monitor the airway in case suctioning is needed.

The two-rescuer technique can also be modified so that the jaw-thrust maneuver can be used during BVM ventilations. This technique is to be used when performing BVM ventilation on a patient with a suspected head, neck, or spine injury. Proficiency in this technique requires frequent mannequin practice. To perform BVM ventilation when trauma (injury) is not suspected (Figure 6-11) and when trauma is suspected (Figure 6-12), follow these steps.

Two-Rescuer BVM Ventilation—No Trauma Suspected

1. Open the patient's airway *using the head-tilt, chin-lift maneuver*. Suction and insert an airway adjunct as necessary.

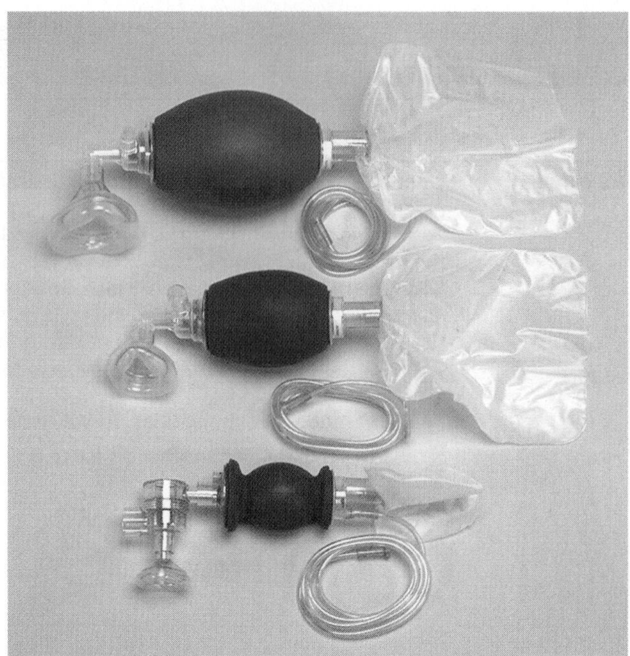

Figure 6-10 • Adult, child, and infant bag-valve-mask units.

2. Select the correct bag-valve mask size (adult, child, or infant).
3. Kneel at the patient's head. Position thumbs over the top half of the mask, index fingers over the bottom half.
4. Place the apex, or top, of the triangular mask over the bridge of the patient's nose. Then lower the mask over the mouth and upper chin. If the mask has a large, round cuff surrounding a ventilation port, center the port over the patient's mouth.
5. Use middle, ring, and little fingers to bring the patient's jaw up to the mask. *Maintain the head-tilt, chin-lift maneuver.*
6. The second rescuer should connect bag to mask, if not already done. While you maintain the mask seal, the second rescuer should squeeze the bag with two hands until the patient's chest rises. The second rescuer should squeeze the bag *once every 5 seconds for an adult, once every 3 seconds for a child or infant.*
7. The second rescuer should release pressure on the bag and let the patient exhale passively. While this occurs the bag is refilling from the oxygen source.

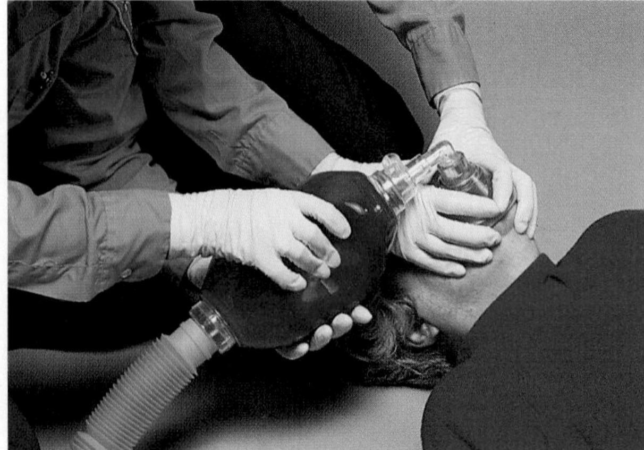

Figure 6-11 • Delivering two-rescuer BVM ventilation when no trauma is suspected in the patient.

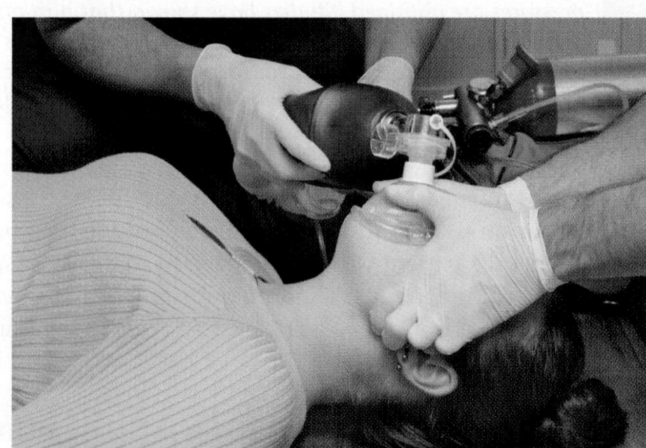

Figure 6-12 • Delivering two-rescuer BVM ventilation while providing manual stabilization of the head and neck when trauma is suspected in the patient.

Two-Rescuer BVM Ventilation—Trauma Suspected

1. Open the patient's airway *using the jaw-thrust maneuver*. Suction and insert an airway adjunct (see later in this chapter) as necessary.
2. Select the correct bag-valve mask size (adult, child, or infant).
3. Kneel at the patient's head. Place thumb sides of your hands along the mask to hold it firmly on the face.
4. Use your remaining fingers to bring the jaw upward, toward the mask, *without tilting the head or neck*.
5. The second rescuer should squeeze the bag to ventilate the patient as previously described for the nontrauma patient.

As noted, use of a bag-valve mask by a single rescuer is the last choice of artificial ventilation procedure—behind use of a pocket face mask with supplemental oxygen, a two-rescuer bag-valve-mask procedure, and use of a flow-restricted, oxygen-powered ventilation device. You should provide ventilations with a one-rescuer bag-valve-mask procedure only when no other options are available. When using the bag-valve-mask device alone you should follow these steps.

One-Rescuer BVM Ventilation

1. Position yourself at the patient's head and establish an open airway. Suction and insert an airway adjunct as necessary.
2. Select the correct size mask for the patient. Position the mask on the patient's face as described previously for the two-rescuer BVM technique.
3. Form a "C" around the ventilation port with thumb and index finger. Use middle, ring, and little fingers under the patient's jaw to hold the jaw to the mask.
4. With your other hand, *squeeze the bag once every 5 seconds. For infants and children, squeeze the bag once every 3 seconds*. The squeeze should be a full one, causing the patient's chest to rise.
5. Release pressure on the bag and let the patient exhale passively. While this occurs the bag is refilling from the oxygen source.

If the chest does not rise and fall during BVM ventilation, you should:

1. Reposition the head.
2. Check for escape of air around the mask and reposition fingers and mask.
3. Check for airway obstruction or obstruction in the BVM system. Re-suction the patient if necessary. Consider insertion of an airway adjunct if not already done.
4. If none of these methods work, use an alternative method of artificial ventilation, such as a pocket mask or a flow-restricted, oxygen-powered ventilation device.

The BVM may also be used during CPR. The bag is squeezed once each time a ventilation is to be delivered. In one-rescuer CPR, it is preferable to use a pocket mask with supplemental oxygen (Figure 6-13) rather than a BVM system. A single rescuer would

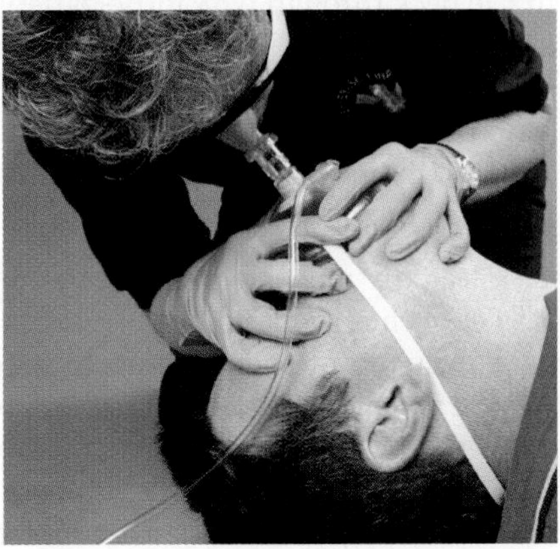

Figure 6-13 • One-rescuer CPR using a pocket face mask with supplemental oxygen. The EMT is beside the patient, from which position chest compressions can also be performed. The strap holds the pocket mask in place while the rescuer switches tasks.

POINT OF VIEW

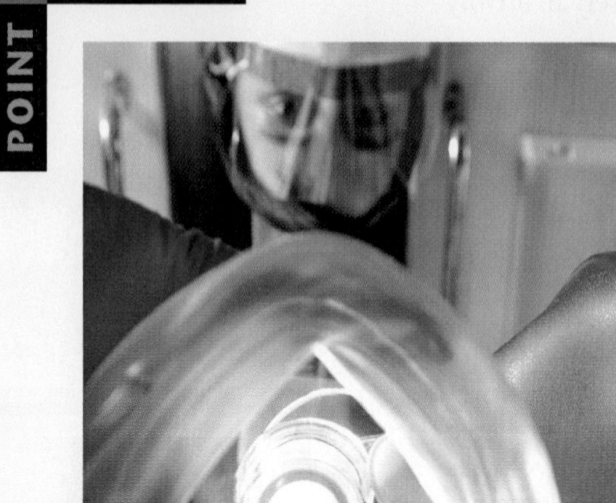

"I still can't tell you why I didn't know it was coming on. I didn't feel right for a few days. Then it hit me. I couldn't move without feeling like I would suffocate. I just couldn't breathe. Couldn't catch my breath. I could tell it was serious when the EMTs came in. It showed in their faces.

"I think I must've started getting even worse, because I remember feeling like I was losing it. I remember them trying to calm me down, but I really felt like I was going to have to be peeled off the ceiling of that ambulance.

"When they tried to put that big mask on my face I felt like it was going to kill me. To take away all my air. I fought it. The EMTs kept calming me and putting that mask on my face. Somehow I calmed down a little and they gave me air or oxygen or something. I made it to the hospital. The doctor told me that the EMTs may have saved my life.

"I appreciate that more than I can say—even if that mask felt pretty intimidating at the time."

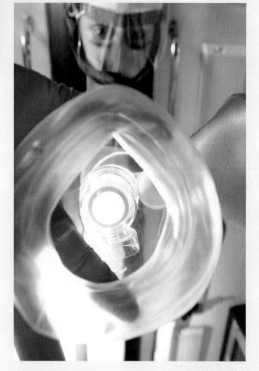

take too much time picking up the BVM and obtaining a face seal each time a ventilation is to be delivered, in addition to the normal difficulty in maintaining a seal with the one-rescuer BVM technique.

NOTE

Bag-valve-mask devices should be completely disassembled and disinfected after each use. Because proper decontamination is often costly and time-consuming, many hospitals and EMS agencies use single-use disposable BVMs.

Artificial Ventilation of a Stoma Breather

stoma
a permanent surgical opening in the neck through which the patient breathes.

The BVM can be used to artificially ventilate patients with a **stoma**, a surgical opening in the neck through which the patient breathes. Patients with stomas who are found to be in severe respiratory distress or respiratory arrest frequently have thick secretions blocking the stoma. It is recommended that you suction the stoma frequently in conjunction with BVM-to-stoma ventilations.

As with other BVM uses, a two-rescuer technique is preferred over a one-rescuer technique. To provide artificial ventilation to a stoma breather using a BVM, follow these steps:

1. Clear any mucus plugs or secretions from the stoma.
2. Leave the head and neck in a neutral position, as it is unnecessary to position the airway prior to ventilations in a stoma breather.
3. Use a pediatric-sized mask to establish a seal around the stoma.
4. Ventilate at the appropriate rate for the patient's age.
5. If unable to artificially ventilate through the stoma, consider sealing the stoma and attempting artificial ventilation through the mouth and nose. (This may work if the

trachea is still connected to the passageways of the mouth, nose, and pharynx. In some cases, however, the trachea has been permanently connected to the neck opening with no remaining connection to the mouth, nose, or pharynx).

Flow-Restricted, Oxygen-Powered Ventilation Device

A **flow-restricted, oxygen-powered ventilation device (FROPVD),** also called a *manually triggered ventilation device,* uses oxygen under pressure to deliver artificial ventilations through a mask placed over the patient's face. This device is similar to the traditional demand-valve resuscitator but includes newer features designed to optimize ventilations and safeguard the patient (Figure 6-14). Recommended features include:

flow-restricted, oxygen-powered ventilation device (FROPVD) a device that uses oxygen under pressure to deliver artificial ventilations. Its trigger is placed so that the rescuer can operate it while still using both hands to maintain a seal on the face mask. It has automatic flow restriction to prevent overdelivery of oxygen to the patient.

- A peak flow rate of 100 percent oxygen at up to 40 liters per minute
- An inspiratory pressure relief valve that opens at approximately 60 cm of water pressure
- An audible alarm when the relief valve is activated
- A rugged design and construction
- A trigger that enables the rescuer to use both hands to maintain a mask seal while triggering the device
- Satisfactory operation in both ordinary and extreme environmental conditions

Follow the same procedures for mask seal as recommended for the BVM (Table 6-5). Trigger the device until the chest rises *and repeat every 5 seconds.* If the chest does not rise, reposition the head, check the mask seal, check for obstructions, and consider the use of an alternative artificial ventilation procedure.

When using the FROPVD on a patient with chest trauma, be especially careful not to over-inflate, as you may actually make the chest injury worse. Also, always make sure the airway is fully opened, and watch the chest rise. Make sure you are not forcing excess air to enter the stomach instead of the lungs, causing gastric distention, which could cause the patient to regurgitate and possibly compromise the airway with stomach contents.

If neck injury is suspected, have an assistant hold the patient's head manually or put a rigid collar or head blocks on the patient to prevent movement. (Using your knees to prevent head movement is sometimes recommended but places you too close to the patient, making it difficult to open the airway and assess chest rise properly.) Bring the jaw up to the mask without tilting the head or neck.

The flow-restricted, oxygen-powered ventilation device should be used only on adults unless you have a child unit and have been given special training in its use by your Medical Director.

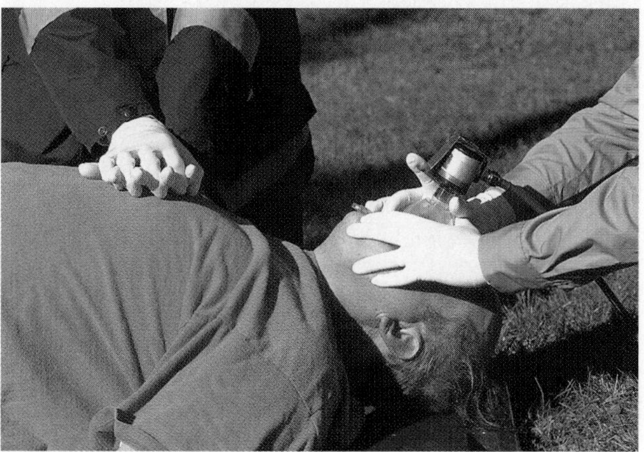

Figure 6-14 • Providing ventilations with a flow-restricted, oxygen-powered ventilation device (FROPVD).

TABLE 6-5 • Use of the Flow-Restricted, Oxygen-Powered Ventilation Device (FROPVD; Manually Triggered Ventilator)

PATIENT	USE OF THE FROPVD
Patient <u>without</u> suspected spine injury 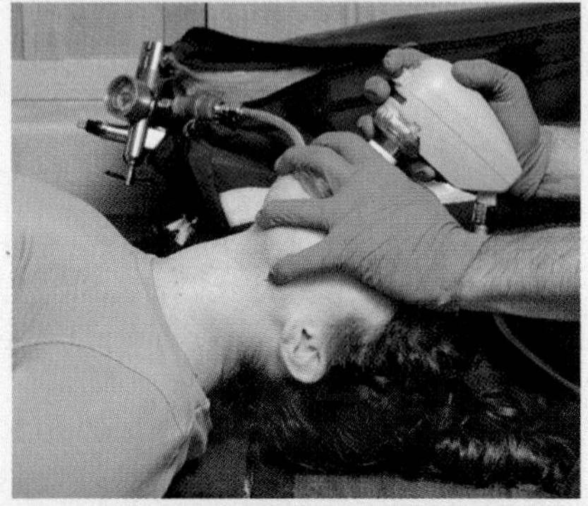	• Open the airway and insert an appropriately sized oral or nasal airway. • Position thumbs over top of mask, index fingers over the bottom half. • Place mask over the face and use the middle, ring, and little fingers to bring the patient's jaw up to the mask. • Trigger the ventilation device until the chest rises. Do not over-inflate. • Reevaluate ventilations frequently.
Patient <u>with</u> suspected spine injury 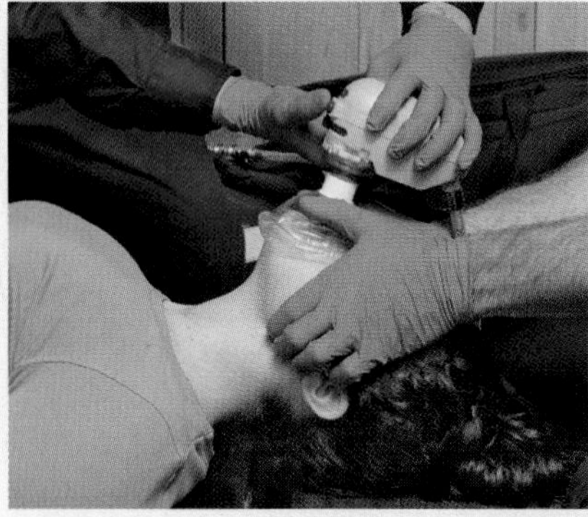	• Open the airway with a jaw thrust and insert appropriate size airway if no gag reflex. • Have an assistant manually immobilize the head and neck. Immobilization of the head between your knees may be acceptable if no assistance is available. • Place the thumb side of your hands along the mask to hold it firmly on the face. • Place the mask on the patient's face as previously described. • Use your remaining fingers to bring the jaw up to the mask without tilting the head or neck. • Trigger the ventilation device until the chest rises. Do not over-inflate. • Monitor ventilations.

Automatic Transport Ventilator

automatic transport ventilator (ATV) a device that provides positive pressure ventilations. It includes settings designed to adjust ventilation rate and volume, is portable, and is easily carried on an ambulance.

The **automatic transport ventilator (ATV)** (Figure 6-15) may be used in EMS to provide positive pressure ventilations to a patient in respiratory arrest. The ATV has settings to adjust ventilation rate and volume. These ventilators are very portable and easily carried on ambulances. When prolonged ventilation is necessary, and when only one rescuer is available to ventilate a patient, the ATV may be beneficial. Caution must

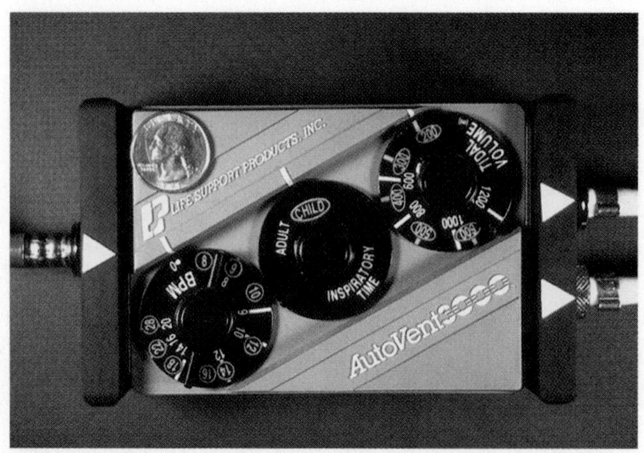

Figure 6-15 • An automatic transport ventilator. The coin is shown for scale. *(© Edward T. Dickinson, MD)*

CRITICAL DECISION MAKING:
OXYGEN OR VENTILATION?

You have learned several methods to administer supplemental oxygen and to provide ventilations to a patient. It has been said that the decision on when to provide supplemental oxygen (e.g., nonrebreather mask or cannula) or to ventilate (e.g., BVM, FROPVD) is one of the most important decisions you will make.

For each of the following patients, decide whether you would administer oxygen or ventilate the patient.

1. A patient who was found on the floor by a relative. He has no pulse or respirations.
2. A 14-year-old patient who has a broken femur. She is alert; pulse 110 strong and regular; respirations 28, rapid and deep.
3. A 64-year-old male with chest pain. He is alert; pulse 56; respirations 18 and normal.
4. A 78-year-old patient with COPD. He has had increasing difficulty breathing over the past few days. He responds verbally but is not oriented. His pulse is 124; respirations 36 and shallow.

be used to be sure the respiratory rate is appropriate for the patient's size and condition. A proper mask seal is required for these devices to effectively deliver a ventilation. For detailed information on automatic transport ventilators see Chapter 38, "Advanced Airway Management."

AIRWAY ADJUNCTS

Once you gain access to a patient and begin your initial assessment, your first course of action is to establish an open airway. The airway must be maintained throughout all care procedures.

The most common impediment to an open airway is the tongue. When a patient becomes unconscious, the muscles relax. The tongue will slide back into the pharynx and obstruct the airway. Even though a head-tilt, chin-lift or jaw-thrust maneuver will help open a patient's airway, the tongue may return to its obstructive position once the maneuver is released. Sometimes even when the head-tilt, chin-lift or jaw-thrust is maintained, the tongue will "fall back" into the pharynx.

Airway adjuncts, devices that aid in maintaining an open airway, may be used early in the treatment of the unresponsive patient and continue throughout your care. There are several types of airway adjuncts. In this chapter, only the devices that are a part of the standard EMT course—those whose main function is to keep the tongue from blocking the airway—will be discussed.

The two most common airway adjuncts for the EMT to use are the **oropharyngeal airway** (or oral airway) and the **nasopharyngeal airway** (or nasal airway). The structure and use of these airways can be understood by analyzing their names. *Oro* refers to the mouth, *naso* the nose, and *pharyngeal* the pharynx. Oropharyngeal airways are inserted into the mouth and help keep the tongue from falling back into the pharynx. Nasopharyngeal airways are inserted through the nose and rest in the pharynx, also helping keep the tongue from becoming an airway obstruction.

oropharyngeal (OR-o-fah-RIN-jul) **airway** a curved device inserted through the patient's mouth into the pharynx to help maintain an open airway.

nasopharyngeal (NAY-zo-fah-RIN-jul) **airway** a flexible breathing tube inserted through the patient's nose into the pharynx to help maintain an open airway.

Rules for Using Airway Adjuncts

Some general rules apply to the use of oropharyngeal and nasopharyngeal airways:

gag reflex vomiting or retching that results when something is placed in the back of the pharynx. This is tied to the swallow reflex.

- Use an airway on all unconscious patients who do not exhibit a **gag reflex.** The gag reflex causes vomiting or retching when something is placed in the pharynx. When a patient is deeply unconscious, the gag reflex usually disappears but may reappear as a patient begins to regain consciousness. A patient with a gag reflex who cannot tolerate an oropharyngeal airway may be able to tolerate a nasopharyngeal airway.
- Open the patient's airway manually before using an adjunct device.
- When inserting the airway, take care not to push the patient's tongue into the pharynx.
- Do not continue inserting the airway if the patient begins to gag. Continue to maintain the airway manually and do not use an adjunct device. If the patient remains unconscious for a prolonged time, you may later attempt to insert an airway to determine if the gag reflex is still present.
- *When an airway adjunct is in place, you must maintain the head-tilt, chin-lift or jaw-thrust maneuver and monitor the airway.*
- When an airway adjunct is in place, you must remain ready to suction the patient's airway to clear secretions as necessary.
- If the patient regains consciousness or develops a gag reflex, remove the airway immediately. Be prepared to suction the patient again.
- Use infection control practices while maintaining the airway. Wear disposable gloves. In airway maintenance, there is a chance of a patient's body fluids coming in contact with your face and eyes. Wear mask and goggles or other protective eyewear to prevent this contact.

Oropharyngeal Airways

Once a patient's airway is opened, an oropharyngeal airway can be inserted to help keep it open. An oropharyngeal airway is a curved device, usually made of plastic, that can be inserted into the patient's mouth. The oropharyngeal airway has a flange that will rest against the patient's lips. The rest of the device holds the tongue as it curves back to the pharynx. The proper use of an oropharyngeal airway greatly reduces the chances of the patient's airway becoming obstructed.

There are standard sizes of oropharyngeal airways (Figure 6-16). Many manufacturers make a complete line, ranging from airways for infants to large adult sizes. An entire set should be carried to allow for quick, proper selection.

The airway adjunct cannot be used effectively unless you select the correct airway size for the patient. An airway of proper size will extend from the corner of the patient's

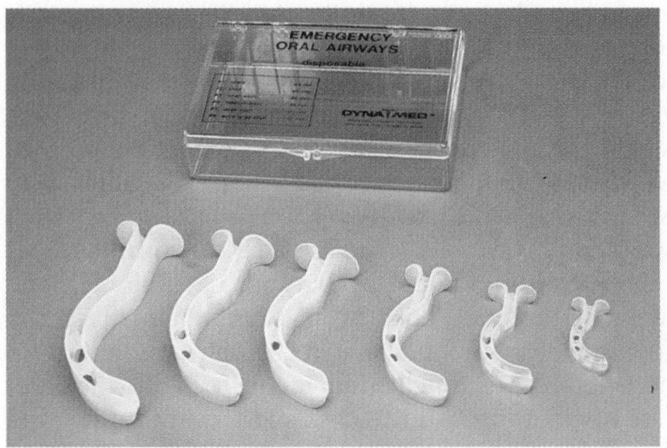

Figure 6-16 • Oropharyngeal airways in various sizes.

mouth to the tip of the earlobe on the same side of the patient's face. An alternative method is to measure from the center of the patient's mouth to the angle of the lower jaw bone. Do not use an airway unless you have measured it against the patient and verified it as being the proper size. If the airway is not the correct size, do not use it on the patient.

To insert an oropharyngeal airway, follow these steps (Scan 6-2):

1. Place the patient on his back. When caring for a medical patient with no indications of spinal injury, the neck may be hyperextended. If there are possible spinal injuries, use the jaw-thrust maneuver, moving the patient no more than necessary to ensure an open airway (the airway takes priority over the spine). Extreme care must be taken.
2. Perform a crossed-finger technique. That is, cross the thumb and forefinger of one hand and place them on the upper and lower teeth at the corner of the patient's mouth. Spread your fingers apart to open the patient's jaws.
3. Position the airway so that its tip is pointing toward the roof of the patient's mouth.
4. Insert the airway and slide it along the roof of the patient's mouth, past the soft tissue hanging down from the back (the uvula), or until you meet resistance against the soft palate. Be certain not to push the patient's tongue back into the pharynx. Any airway insertion is made easier by using a tongue blade (tongue depressor). In a few cases, you may have to use a tongue blade to hold the tongue in place. Watch what you are doing when inserting the airway. This procedure should not be performed by "feel" only.
5. Gently rotate the airway 180 degrees so that the tip is pointing down into the patient's pharynx. This method prevents pushing the tongue back. Alternatively, insert the airway with the tip already pointing "down" toward the patient's pharynx, using a tongue depressor to press the tongue down and forward to avoid obstructing the airway. *This is the preferred method for airway insertion in an infant or child.*
6. Position the patient. Place the nontrauma patient in a maximum head-tilt position. If there are possible spine injuries, maintain cervical stabilization at all times during airway management.
7. Check to see that the flange of the airway is against the patient's lips. If the airway is too long or too short, remove the airway and replace it with the correct size.
8. Place the mask you will use for ventilation over the in-place airway adjunct. If no barrier device is available, provide direct mouth-to-adjunct ventilation just as you would provide mouth-to-mouth ventilation.
9. Monitor the patient closely. If there is a gag reflex, remove the airway adjunct at once by following the anatomical curvature. You do not need to rotate the device when removing it.

NOTE

Some EMS systems allow an oropharyngeal airway to be inserted with the tip pointing to the side of the patient's mouth. The device is then rotated 90 degrees so that its tip is pointing down the patient's pharynx. Use this approach only if it is part of the protocol of your EMS system.

Nasopharyngeal Airways

The nasopharyngeal airway has gained popularity because it often does not stimulate the gag reflex. This allows the nasopharyngeal airway to be used in patients who have a reduced level of responsiveness but still have an intact gag reflex. Other benefits include the fact that it can be used when the teeth are clenched and when there are oral injuries.

Use the soft flexible nasal airway and not the rigid clear plastic airway in the field. The soft ones are less likely to cause soft-tissue damage or bleeding. The typical sizes for adults are 34, 32, 30, and 28 French.

To insert a nasopharyngeal airway, follow these steps (Scan 6-3):

1. Measure the nasopharyngeal airway from the patient's nostril to the earlobe or to the angle of the jaw. Choosing the correct length will ensure an appropriate diameter.
2. Lubricate the outside of the tube with a water-based lubricant before insertion. Do not use a petroleum jelly or any other type of non-water-based lubricant. Such substances can damage the tissue lining of the nasal cavity and the pharynx and increase the risk of infection.
3. Gently push the tip of the nose upward. Keep the patient's head in a neutral position. Most nasopharyngeal airways are designed to be placed in the right nostril. The

SCAN 6-2 • Inserting an Oropharyngeal Airway

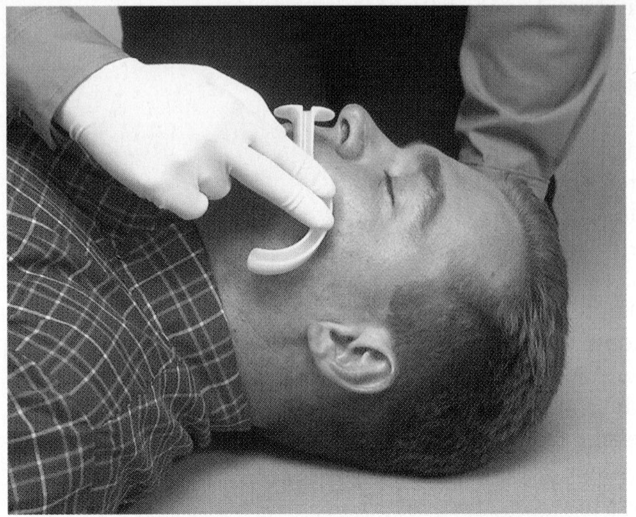

1. Ensure the oropharyngeal airway is the correct size by checking to make sure it either extends from the center of the mouth to the angle of the jaw or . . .

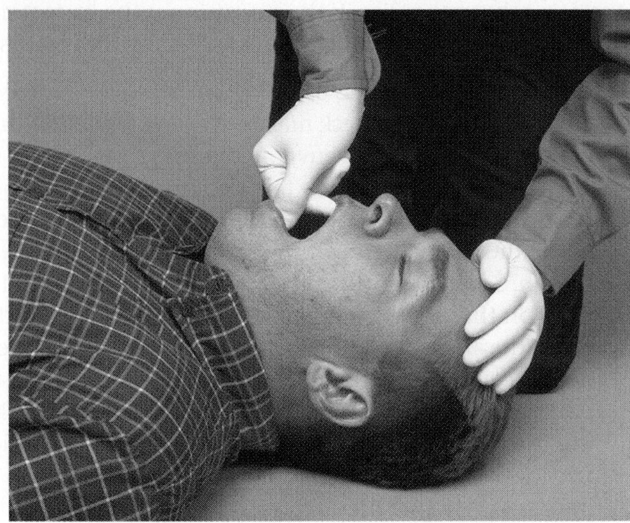

2. Use the crossed-fingers technique to open the patient's mouth.

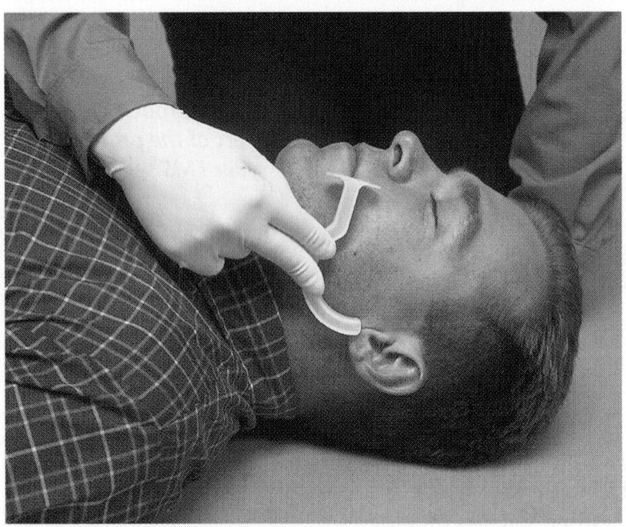

3. Measure from the corner of the patient's mouth to the tip of the earlobe.

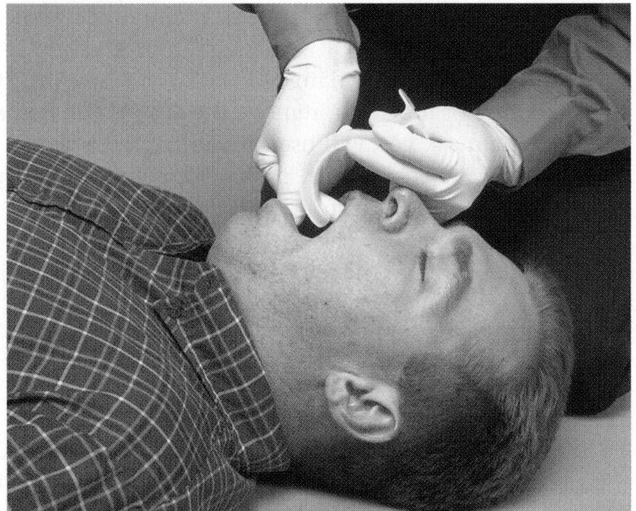

4. Insert the airway with the tip pointing to the roof of the patient's mouth.

bevel (angled portion at the tip) should point toward the base of the nostril or toward the septum (wall that separates the nostrils).

4. Insert the airway into the nostril. Advance the airway until the flange rests firmly against the patient's nostril. Never force a nasopharyngeal airway. If you experience difficulty advancing the airway, pull the tube out and try the other nostril.

Oropharyngeal and nasopharyngeal airways can be a tremendous asset to the EMT when used properly. However, no device can replace the EMT. The proper use of these

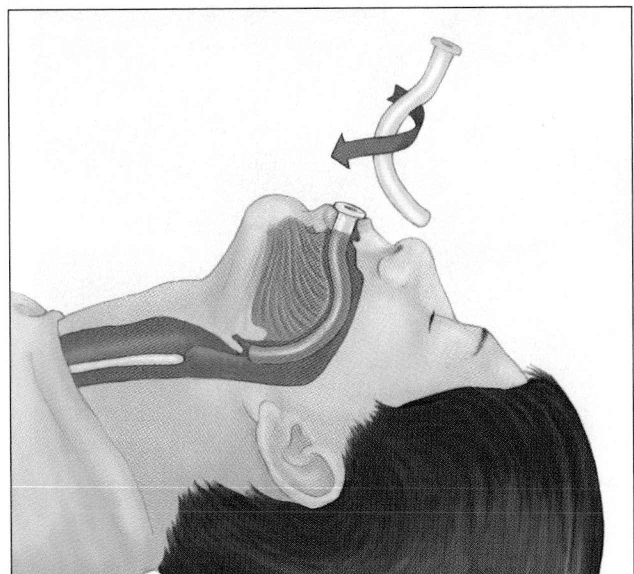

5. Rotate it 180 degrees into position. When the airway is properly positioned, the flange rests against the patient's mouth.

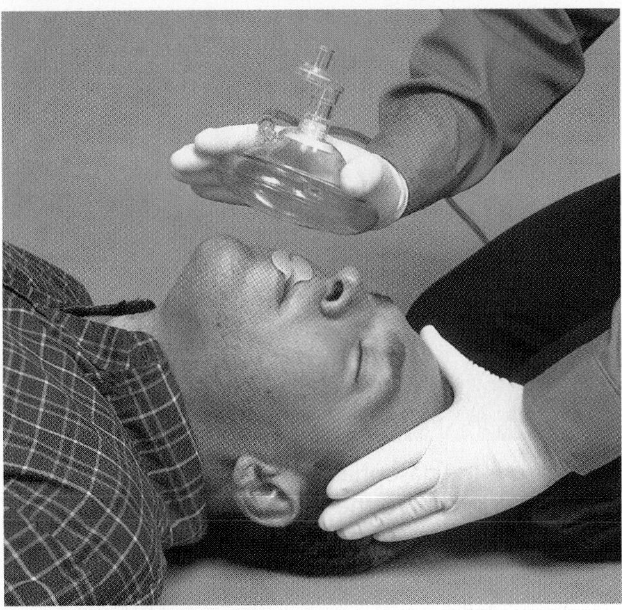

6. After proper insertion, the patient is ready for ventilation.

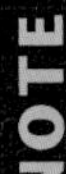

Monitor the patient closely. If there is a gag reflex, remove the airway adjunct at once by following the anatomical curvature. You do not need to rotate the device when removing it.

airways or any other device depends on the appropriate use, good judgment, and adequate monitoring of the patient by the EMT.

Oropharyngeal and nasopharyngeal airways prevent blockage of the upper airway by the tongue. To ensure an open airway to the level of the lungs, it is sometimes necessary to insert an endotracheal (through-the-trachea) tube. Endotracheal intubation is an advanced-life-support procedure that, in some jurisdictions, may be performed by EMTs. The techniques for endotracheal intubation are discussed in Chapter 38, "Advanced Airway Management."

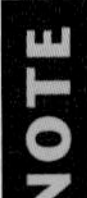

Do not use a nasopharyngeal airway if clear (cerebrospinal) fluid is coming from the nose or ears. This may indicate a skull fracture where the airway would pass.

SCAN 6-3 • Inserting a Nasopharyngeal Airway

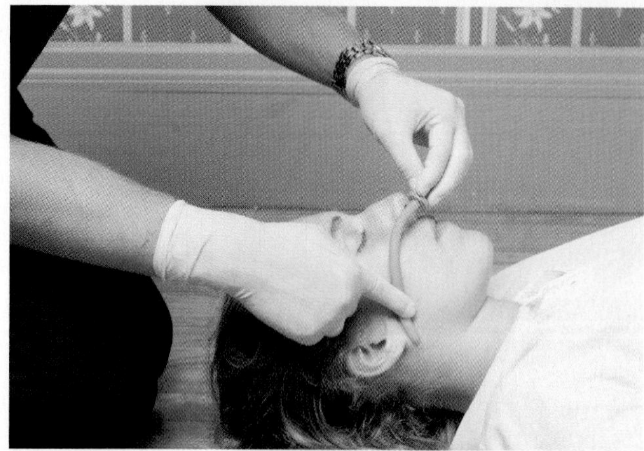

1. Measure the nasopharyngeal airway from the patient's nostril to the earlobe or to the angle of the jaw.

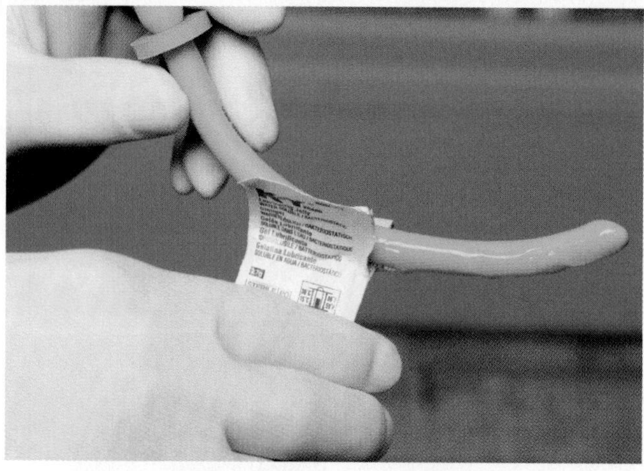

2. Apply a water-based lubricant before insertion.

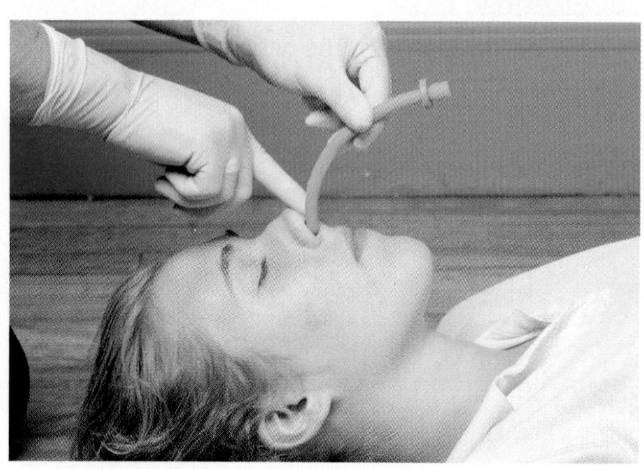

3. Gently push the tip of the nose upward, and insert the airway with the beveled side toward the base of the nostril or toward the septum (wall that separates the nostrils). Insert the airway, advancing it until the flange rests against the nostril.

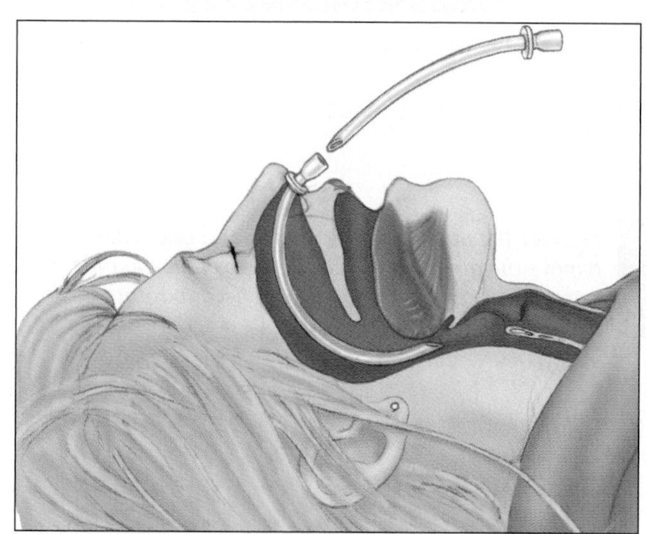

4. Never force a nasopharyngeal airway. If you experience difficulty advancing the airway, pull the tube out and try the other nostril.

SUCTIONING

suctioning (SUK-shun-ing) use of a vacuum device to remove blood, vomitus, and other secretions or foreign materials from the airway.

The patient's airway must be kept clear of foreign materials, blood, vomitus, and other secretions. Materials that are allowed to remain in the airway may be forced into the trachea and eventually into the lungs. This will cause complications ranging from severe pneumonia to complete airway obstruction. **Suctioning** is the method of using a vacuum device to remove such materials. A patient needs to be suctioned immediately whenever a gurgling sound is heard, whether before, during, or after artificial ventilation.

Suctioning Devices

Each suction unit consists of a suction source, a collection container for materials you suction, tubing, and suction tips or catheters. Systems are either mounted in the ambulance or are portable and may be brought to the scene.

Mounted Suction Systems

Many ambulances have a suction unit mounted in the patient compartment (Figure 6-17). These units are usually installed near the head of the stretcher so they are easily used. Mounted systems, often called "on-board" units, create a suctioning vacuum produced by the engine's manifold or an electrical power source. To be effective, suction devices must furnish an air intake of at least 30 liters per minute at the open end of a collection tube. This will occur if the system can generate a vacuum of no less than 300 mmHg (millimeters of mercury) when the collecting tube is clamped.

Portable Suction Units

There are many different types of portable suction units (Figure 6-18). They may be oxygen- or air-powered, electrically powered (by batteries or household current), or manually operated. The requirement for the amount of suction a portable unit must provide is identical to that of the fixed unit (30 liters per minute, 300 mmHg). It is important to have the ability to suction anywhere. Portable suction provides that ability.

Tubing, Tips, and Catheters

For suctioning to be effective, the proper equipment must be used. While a suction unit might be the most powerful available, it will do no good unless used with the proper attachments. Before operating a suction unit, you must have:

- Tubing
- Suction tips
- Suction catheters
- Collection container
- Container of clean or sterile water

The *tubing* attached to a suction unit must be thick-walled, non-kinking, wide-bore tubing. This is because the tubing must not collapse due to the suction, must allow "chunks" of suctioned material to pass, and must not kink, which would reduce the suction. The tubing must be long enough to reach comfortably from suction unit to patient.

Currently, the most popular type of *suction tip* is the rigid pharyngeal tip, also called "Yankauer" or "tonsil sucker" or "tonsil-tip" suction. This rigid device allows you to suction the mouth and pharynx with excellent control over the distal end of the device. It also has a larger bore than flexible catheters. Most successfully used with an unresponsive

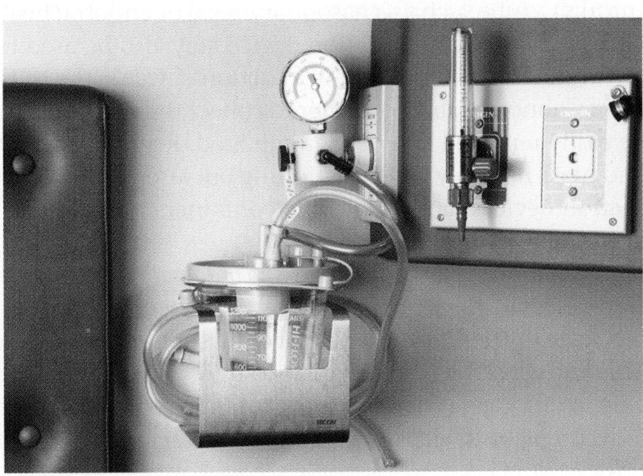

Figure 6-17 • A mounted suction unit installed in the ambulance patient compartment.

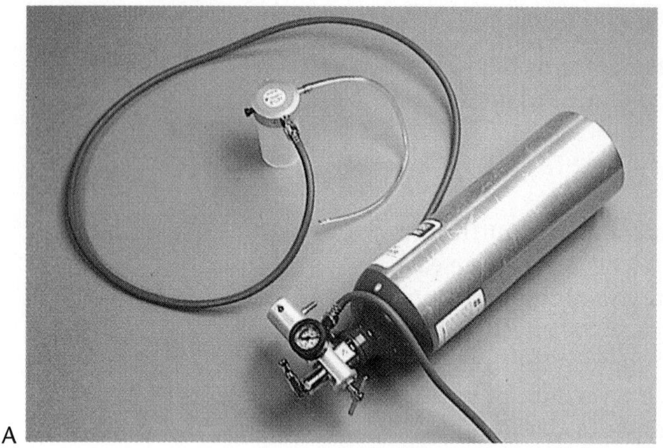
A

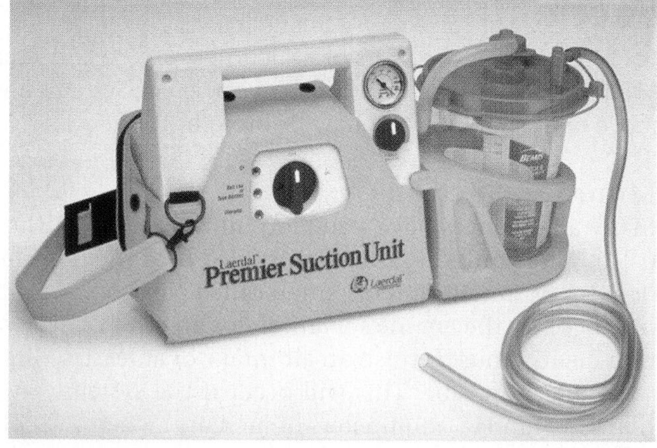

B

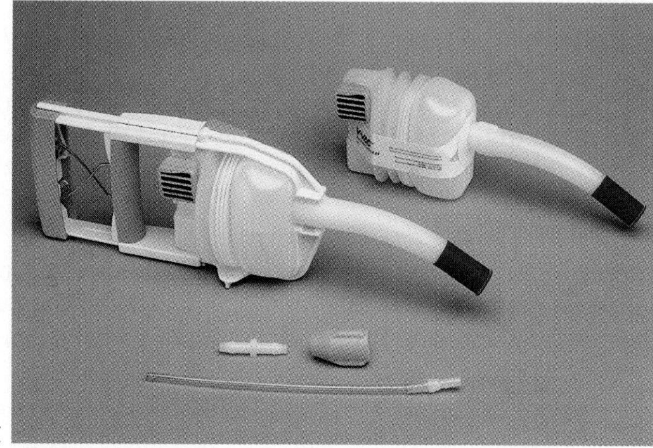
C

Figure 6-18 • (A) Oxygen-powered portable suction unit, (B) battery-powered portable unit, and (C) manually operated unit.

patient, rigid-tip suction must be used with caution especially if the patient is not completely unresponsive or may be regaining consciousness. When the tip is placed into the pharynx, the gag reflex may be activated, producing additional vomiting. It is also possible to stimulate the vagus nerve in the back of the pharynx, which can slow the heart rate. So be careful not to suction more than a few seconds at a time with a rigid tip and never lose sight of the tip.

Suction catheters are flexible plastic tubes. They come in various sizes identified by a number "French." The larger the number, the larger the catheter. A "14 French" catheter is larger than an "8 French" catheter. These catheters are usually not large enough to suction vomitus or thick secretions and may kink. Flexible catheters are designed to be used in situations when a rigid tip cannot be used. For example, a soft catheter can be passed through a tube such as a nasopharyngeal or endotracheal tube or used for suctioning the nasopharynx. (A bulb suction device may also be used to suction nasal passages.)

Another important part of a suction device is the *collection container*. All units should have a nonbreakable container to collect the suctioned materials. These containers must be easily removed and decontaminated. Remember to wear gloves, protective eyewear, and mask not only while suctioning but also while cleaning the equipment. Most newer suction devices have disposable containers to eliminate the time and risks involved in decontamination.

Suction units also must have a *container of clean (preferably sterile) water* nearby. This water is used to clear matter that is partially blocking the tubing. When this partial blockage of the tube occurs, place the suction tip or catheter in the container of water. This will cause a stream of water to flow through the tip and tubing, usually forcing the clog to dislodge. When the tip or tubing becomes clogged with an item that will not dislodge, replace it with a new tip or catheter.

In the event of copious, thick secretions or vomiting, consider removing the rigid tip or catheter and using the large bore, rigid suction tubing. After you are finished, place the standard tip back on for further suctioning.

Techniques of Suctioning

Although there may be some variations in suction technique (a suggested technique is shown in Scan 6-4), a few rules always apply. *The first rule is always use appropriate infection control practices while suctioning.* These practices include the use of protective eyewear, mask, and disposable gloves. Proper suctioning requires you to have your fingers around and sometimes inside the patient's mouth. Disposable gloves prevent contact between the EMT and the patient's bodily fluids. Protective eyewear and mask are also recommended since these fluids might splatter, or the patient may gag or cough, sending droplets to your face, eyes, and mouth.

The second rule is try to limit suctioning to no longer than 15 seconds at a time. This is because prolonged suctioning will cause hypoxia and, potentially, death. If the patient continues to vomit longer than 15 seconds, however, you must still continue to suction. Ventilating foreign matter into the lungs will also cause hypoxia and possible death. In short, suction quickly and efficiently for as short a time as possible.

Patients who need airway control and suctioning are often unconscious and may be in cardiac or respiratory arrest. Oxygen delivery to this patient is very important. During suctioning, the ventilations or other method of oxygen delivery is discontinued to allow for the passage of the suction catheter. To prevent critical delays in oxygen delivery, limit suctioning to a few seconds, then resume ventilations or oxygen delivery.

In a few cases you will preoxygenate a patient before suctioning. This means that you will adequately ventilate the patient with supplemental oxygen before suctioning, because oxygen levels will drop during suctioning; for example, during routine suctioning of an endotracheal tube. If you come upon a patient with vomitus or other materials in his airway, or if a patient vomits suddenly and unexpectedly, you should suction immediately, *without* preoxygenation. In these cases, preoxygenation would force foreign substances into the lungs, which can be fatal.

The third rule for suctioning is place the tip or catheter where you want to begin the suctioning and suction on the way out. Most suction tips and catheters do not produce suction at all times. You have to start the suctioning. The tip or catheter will have an open distal end where the suction is delivered. It will also have an opening, or port, in the proximal portion. When you put your finger over the proximal port, suctioning begins from the distal end.

It is not necessary to measure when using a rigid tip. Rather, you should be sure not to lose sight of the tip when inserting it. However, do measure the suction catheter in a manner similar to an oropharyngeal airway. The length of catheter that should be inserted into the patient's mouth is equal to the distance between the corner of the patient's mouth and earlobe.

Carefully bring the tip of the catheter to the area where suctioning is needed. Never "jab" or force the suction tip into the mouth or pharynx. Then place your finger over the proximal opening to begin the suctioning, and suction as you slowly withdraw the tip from the patient's mouth, moving the tip from side to side.

Suctioning is usually delivered with the patient turned on his side. This allows free secretions to flow from the mouth while suctioning is being delivered. Caution must be used in patients with suspected neck or spine injuries. If the patient is fully and securely immobilized, the entire backboard may be tilted to place the patient on his side. For the patient for whom such injuries are suspected but who is not immobilized, suction the best you can without turning the patient. If all other methods have failed, as a last resort you may turn the patient's body as a unit, attempting to keep the neck and spine in line. Suctioning should not be delayed to immobilize a patient.

SCAN 6-4 • Suctioning Techniques

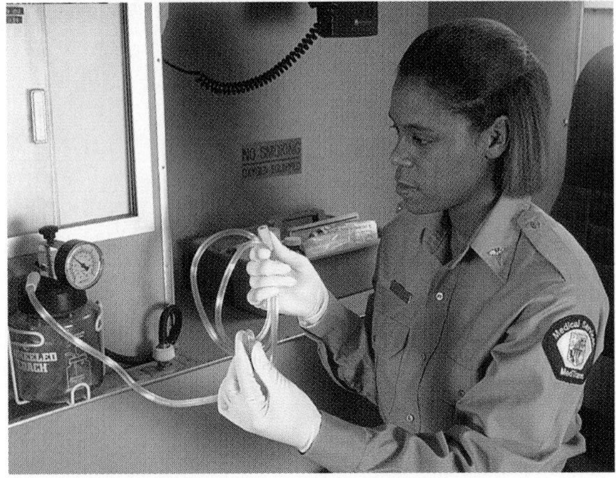

1. Turn the unit on, attach a catheter, and test for suction at the beginning of your shift.

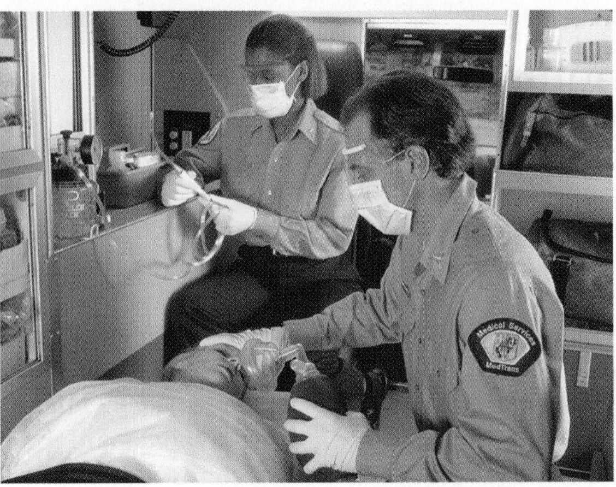

2. Position yourself at the patient's head and turn the patient's head to the side.

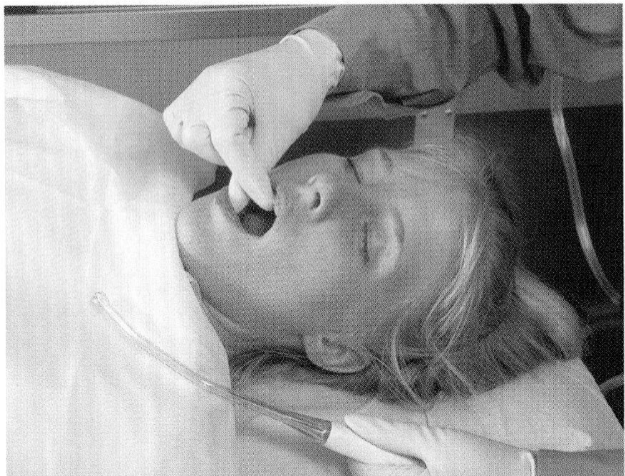

3. Open and clear the patient's mouth.

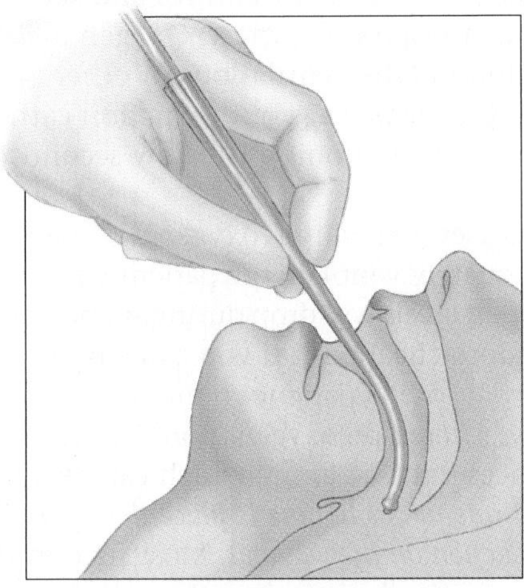

4. Place the convex side of the rigid tip against the roof of the mouth. Insert just to the base of the tongue.

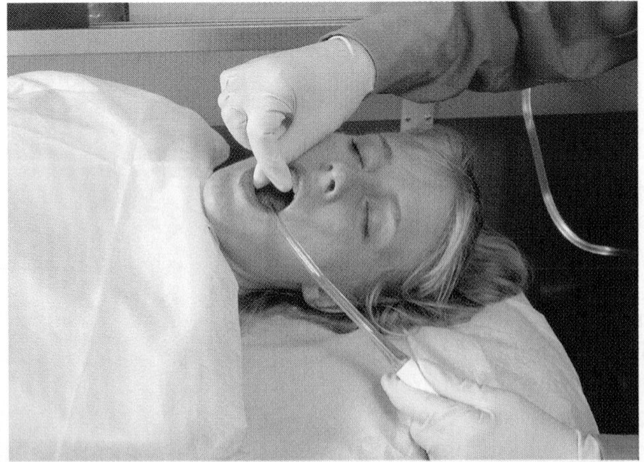

5. Apply suction only after the rigid tip is in place. Do not lose sight of the tip while suctioning. Suction while withdrawing the tip.

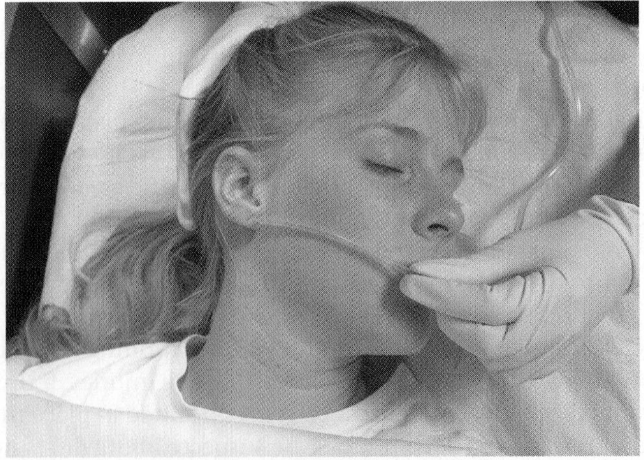

If you are using a flexible catheter, measure it from the patient's earlobe to the corner of the mouth or from the center of the mouth to the angle of the jaw.

The rigid suction tip or flexible catheter should be moved into place carefully and not forced. Rigid suction devices may cause tissue damage and bleeding. Never probe into wounds or attempt to suction away attached tissue with a suction device. Certain skull fractures may actually cause brain tissue to be visible in the pharynx. If this occurs, do not suction near this tissue; limit suctioning to the mouth.

Suction devices may also cause activation of the gag reflex and stimulate vomiting. In a patient who already has secretions that need to be suctioned, vomiting only makes things worse. If you advance a suction catheter or rigid suction tip and the patient begins to gag, withdraw the tip to a position that does not cause gagging and begin suctioning.

These techniques apply to suctioning of the upper airway. Techniques for orotracheal deep suctioning to the level of the lungs—an advanced life support procedure that may be performed by EMTs in some jurisdictions—are discussed in Chapter 38, "Advanced Airway Management."

OXYGEN THERAPY

Importance of Supplemental Oxygen

Oxygen administration is often one of the most important and beneficial treatments an EMT can provide. The atmosphere provides approximately 21 percent oxygen. If a person is without illness or injury, that 21 percent is enough to support normal functioning. However, people EMTs come in contact with are sick or injured and often require supplemental oxygen.

Conditions Requiring Oxygen

Conditions that may require oxygen include:

- *Respiratory or cardiac arrest.* CPR is only 25 to 33 percent as effective as normal circulation. High-concentration oxygen administration provides a better chance of survival for the patient in respiratory or cardiac arrest.
- *Heart attacks and strokes.* These emergencies result from an interruption of blood to the heart or brain. When this occurs, tissues are deprived of oxygen. Providing extra oxygen is extremely important.
- *Shock.* Since shock is the failure of the cardiovascular system to provide sufficient blood to all the vital tissues, all cases of shock reduce the amount of oxygenated blood reaching the tissues. Administration of oxygen helps the blood that does reach the tissues deliver the maximum amount of oxygen.
- *Blood loss.* Whether bleeding is internal or external, there is a reduced amount of circulating blood and red blood cells, so the blood that is circulating needs to be saturated with oxygen.
- *Lung diseases.* The lungs are responsible for turning oxygen over to the blood cells to be delivered to the tissues. When the lungs are not functioning properly, supplemental oxygen helps ensure that the body's tissues receive adequate oxygen.
- *Broken bones, head injuries, and more.* There are very few emergencies where oxygen administration would not be appropriate. All our body's systems work together. An injury in one part may cause shock that affects the rest of the body.

Hypoxia

Hypoxia is an insufficiency in the supply of oxygen to the body's tissues. There are several major causes of hypoxia. Consider the following scenarios:

hypoxia (hi-POK-se-uh) an insufficiency of oxygen in the body's tissues.

- *A patient is trapped in a fire.* The air that the patient breathes contains smoke and reduced amounts of oxygen. Since the patient cannot breathe in enough oxygen, hypoxia develops.

- *A patient has emphysema.* This lung disease decreases the efficiency of the transfer of oxygen between the atmosphere and the body. Since the lungs cannot function properly, hypoxia develops.
- *A patient overdoses on a drug that has a depressing effect on the respiratory system.* The patient's respirations are only 5 per minute. In this case, the victim is not breathing frequently enough to support the body's oxygen needs. Hypoxia develops.
- *A patient has a heart attack.* The lungs function properly by taking atmospheric air and turning it over to the blood for distribution. The damaged heart, however, cannot pump the blood throughout the body, and hypoxia develops.

There are many causes of hypoxia in addition to the examples named, including stroke, shock, and others. The most important thing to know is how to recognize signs of hypoxia so that it may be treated. Hypoxia may be indicated by cyanosis (blue or gray color to the skin). Additionally, when the brain suffers hypoxia, the patient's mental status may deteriorate. Restlessness or confusion may result.

As an EMT your concern will be to prevent hypoxia from developing or becoming worse and, when possible, to reduce the level of hypoxia. This is done with the administration of oxygen.

Oxygen Therapy Equipment

In the field, oxygen equipment must be safe, lightweight, portable, and dependable. Some field oxygen systems are very portable and can be brought almost anywhere. Other systems are installed inside the ambulance so that oxygen can be delivered during transportation to the hospital.

Most oxygen delivery systems (Figure 6-19) contain several items: oxygen cylinders, pressure regulators, and a delivery device (nonrebreather mask or cannula). When the patient is not breathing or is breathing inadequately, additional devices (such as a

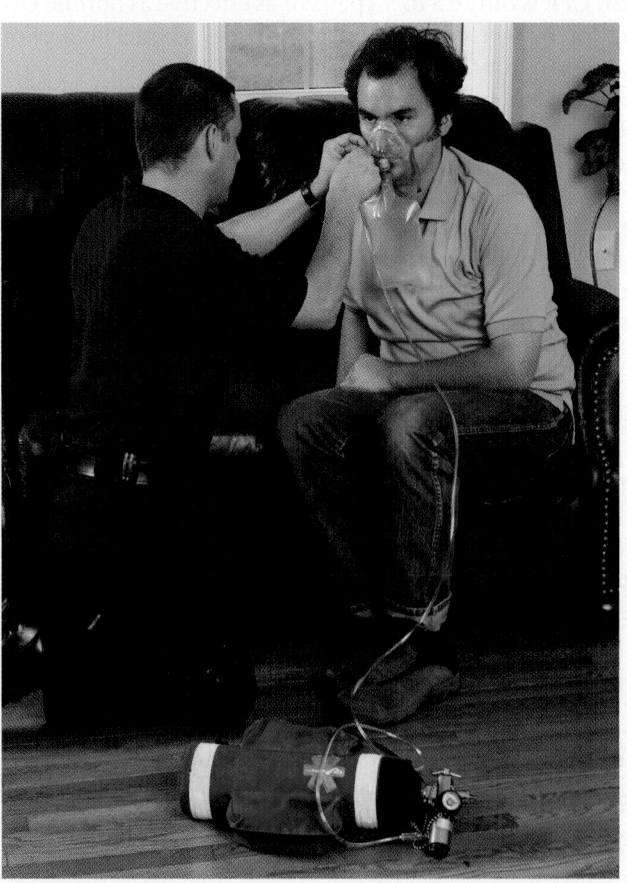

Figure 6-19 • An oxygen delivery system.

pocket mask, bag-valve mask, or positive pressure ventilator) can be used to force oxygen into the patient's lungs.

Oxygen Cylinders

Outside a medical facility, the standard source of oxygen is the **oxygen cylinder,** a seamless steel or lightweight alloy cylinder filled with oxygen under pressure, equal to 2,000 to 2,200 pounds per square inch (psi) when the cylinders are full. Cylinders come in various sizes, identified by letters (Figure 6-20). Those in common use in emergency care include:

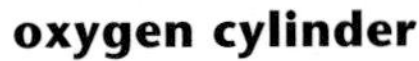
oxygen cylinder
a cylinder filled with oxygen under pressure.

- *D cylinder* contains about 350 liters of oxygen.
- *E cylinder* contains about 625 liters of oxygen.
- *M cylinder* contains about 3,000 liters of oxygen.

Fixed systems on ambulances (commonly called on-board oxygen) include the M cylinder and larger cylinders (Figure 6-21):

- *G cylinder* contains about 5,300 liters of oxygen.
- *H cylinder* contains about 6,900 liters of oxygen.

The *United States Pharmacopoeia* has assigned a color code to distinguish compressed gases. Green and white cylinders have been assigned to all grades of oxygen. Unpainted stainless steel and aluminum cylinders are also used for oxygen. Regardless of the color, always check the label to be certain you are using medical-grade oxygen.

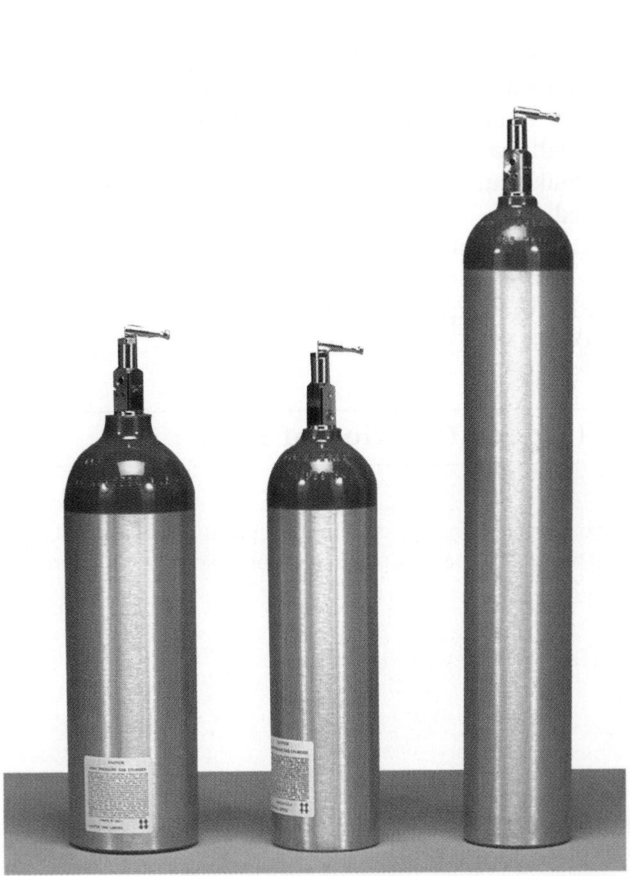

Figure 6-20 • Left to right: jumbo D cylinder, D cylinder, and E cylinder.

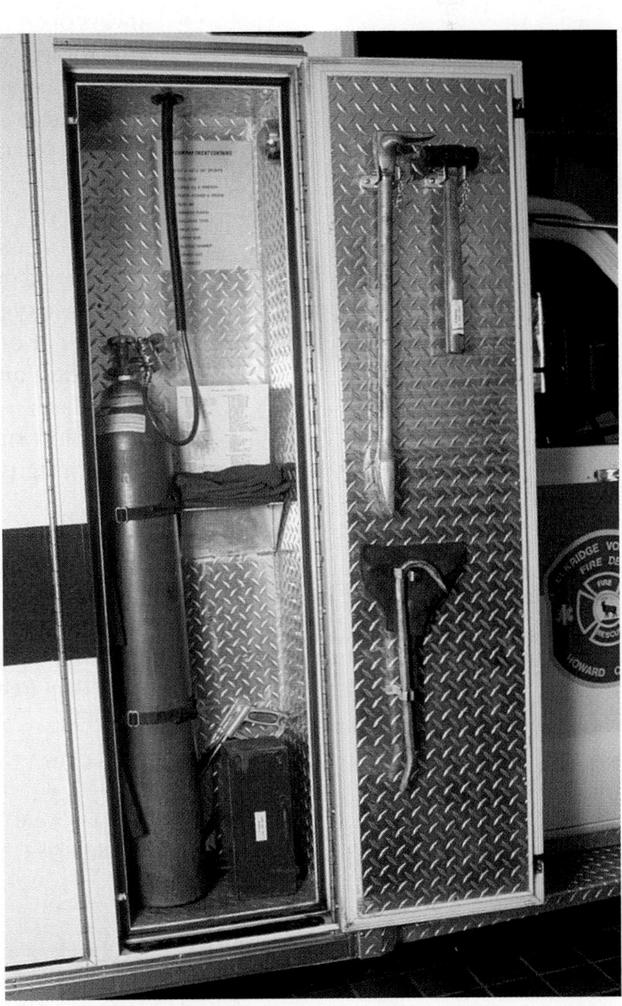

Figure 6-21 • Larger cylinders are used for fixed systems on ambulances.

Part of your duty as an EMT is to make certain that the oxygen cylinders you will use are full and ready before they are needed to provide care. The length of time you can use an oxygen cylinder depends on the pressure in the cylinder and the flow rate. You cannot tell if an oxygen cylinder is full, partially full, or empty by lifting or moving the cylinder. The method of calculating cylinder duration is shown in Table 6-6.

Oxygen cylinders should never be allowed to empty below the safe residual or the tank may be permanently damaged. The safe residual for an oxygen cylinder is when the pressure gauge reads 200 psi or above. Below this point there is not enough oxygen in the cylinder to allow for proper delivery to the patient. Before the cylinder reaches the 200 psi reading, you must switch to a fresh cylinder.

Safety is of prime importance when working with oxygen cylinders. You should:

- *Always* use pressure gauges, regulators, and tubing that are intended for use with oxygen.
- *Always* use nonferrous metal oxygen wrenches for changing gauges and regulators or for adjusting flow rates. Other types of metal tools may produce a spark should they strike against metal objects.
- *Always* ensure that valve seat inserts and gaskets are in good condition. This prevents dangerous leaks. Disposable gaskets on oxygen cylinders should be replaced each time a cylinder change is made.
- *Always* use medical-grade oxygen. Industrial oxygen contains impurities. The cylinder should be labeled "OXYGEN U.S.P." The oxygen must not be more than 5 years old.
- *Always* open the valve of an oxygen cylinder fully, then close it half a turn to prevent someone else from thinking the valve is closed and trying to force it open. The valve does not have to be turned fully to be open for delivery.
- *Always* store reserve oxygen cylinders in a cool, ventilated room, properly secured in place.
- *Always* have oxygen cylinders hydrostatically tested every 5 years. The date a cylinder was last tested is stamped on the cylinder. Some cylinders can be tested every 10 years. These will have a star after the date (e.g., 4M86MM*).
- *Never* drop a cylinder or let it fall against any object. When transporting a patient with an oxygen cylinder, make sure the oxygen cylinder is strapped to the stretcher or otherwise secured.
- *Never* leave an oxygen cylinder standing in an upright position without being secured.
- *Never* allow smoking around oxygen equipment in use. Clearly mark the area of use with signs that read "OXYGEN–NO SMOKING."

TABLE 6-6 • Oxygen Cylinders: Duration of Flow

SIMPLE FORMULA

Gauge pressure in psi (pounds per square inch) minus the safe residual pressure (always 200 psi) times the constant (see following list) divided by the flow rate in liters per minute = duration of flow in minutes.

CYLINDER CONSTANTS

D = 0.16 G = 2.41
E = 0.28 H = 3.14
M = 1.56 K = 3.14

EXAMPLE

Determine the life of an M cylinder that has a pressure of 2,000 psi displayed on the pressure gauge and a flow rate of 10 liters per minute.

$$\frac{(2{,}000 - 200) \times 1.56}{10} = \frac{2{,}808}{10} = 280.8 \text{ minutes}$$

- *Never* use oxygen equipment around an open flame.
- *Never* use grease, oil, or fat-based soaps on devices that will be attached to an oxygen supply cylinder. Take care not to handle these devices when your hands are greasy. Use greaseless tools when making connections.
- *Never* use adhesive tape to protect an oxygen tank outlet or to mark or label any oxygen cylinders or oxygen delivery apparatus. The oxygen can react with the adhesive and debris and cause a fire.
- *Never* try to move an oxygen cylinder by dragging it or rolling it on its side or bottom.

Pressure Regulators

The pressure in an oxygen cylinder (approximately 2,000 psi in a full tank—varying with surrounding temperature) is too high to be delivered to a patient. A **pressure regulator** must be connected to the cylinder to provide a safe working pressure of 30 to 70 psi.

pressure regulator
a device connected to an oxygen cylinder to reduce cylinder pressure to a safe amount for delivery of oxygen to a patient.

On cylinders of the E size or smaller, the pressure regulator is secured to the cylinder valve assembly by a yoke assembly. The yoke is provided with pins that must mate with corresponding holes in the valve assembly. This is called a pin-index safety system. Since the pin position varies for different gases, this system prevents an oxygen delivery system from being connected to a cylinder containing another gas.

Cylinders larger than the E size have a valve assembly with a threaded outlet. The inside and outside diameters of the threaded outlets vary according to the gas in the cylinder. This prevents an oxygen regulator from being connected to a cylinder containing another gas. In other words, a nitrogen regulator cannot be connected to an oxygen cylinder, or vice versa.

Before connecting the pressure regulator to an oxygen supply cylinder, stand to the side of the main valve opening and open (crack) the cylinder valve slightly for just a second to clear dirt and dust out of the delivery port or threaded outlet.

NOTE
You must maintain the regulator inlet filter. It has to be free of damage and clean to prevent contamination of and damage to the regulator.

Flowmeters

A **flowmeter** allows control of the flow of oxygen in liters per minute. It is connected to the pressure regulator. Most services keep the flowmeter permanently attached to the pressure regulator.

flowmeter
a valve that indicates the flow of oxygen in liters per minute.

Three major types of flowmeters are available. For use in the field, the pressure-compensated flowmeter is considered to be superior to the Bourdon gauge flowmeter; however, it is more delicate than the Bourdon gauge and must be operated in an upright position. For these reasons, many EMS systems use the pressure-compensated flowmeter for fixed oxygen systems only.

- *Bourdon gauge flowmeter* (Figure 6-22A). This unit is a pressure gauge calibrated to indicate flow in liters per minute. The meter is fairly inaccurate at low flow rates and has often been criticized as being unstable. However, it is rugged and will operate at any angle. It is a useful gauge for most portable units.

  The major fault with this type of flowmeter is its inability to compensate for back pressure. A partial obstruction (e.g., from kinked tubing) will be reflected in a reading that is higher than the actual flow. The gauge may read 6 liters per minute and only be delivering 1 liter per minute. This type of gauge contains a filter that can become clogged, causing the gauge to read higher than the actual flow. Inspect and change the filter as recommended by the manufacturer.
- *Pressure-compensated flowmeter* (Thorpe tube-type flowmeter, Figure 6-22B). This meter is gravity dependent and must be in an upright position to deliver an accurate reading. The unit has an upright, calibrated glass tube in which there is a ball float. The float rises and falls according to the amount of gas passing through the tube. This type of flowmeter indicates the actual flow at all times, even though there may be a partial obstruction to gas flow (e.g., from a kinked delivery tube). If the tubing collapses, the ball will drop to show the lower delivery rate. This unit is not practical for many portable delivery systems. Recommended use is for larger (M, G, and H) oxygen cylinders.

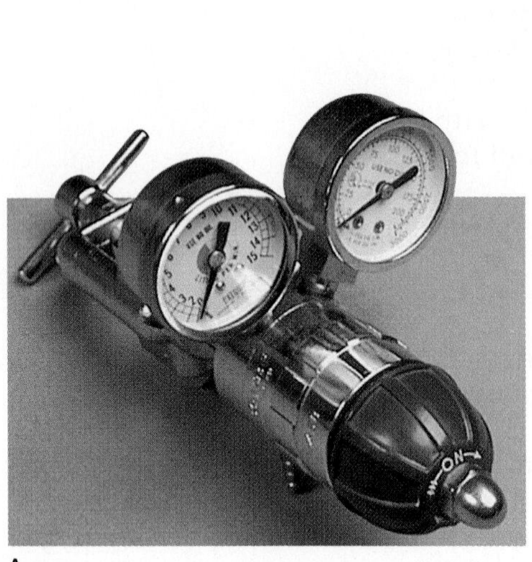

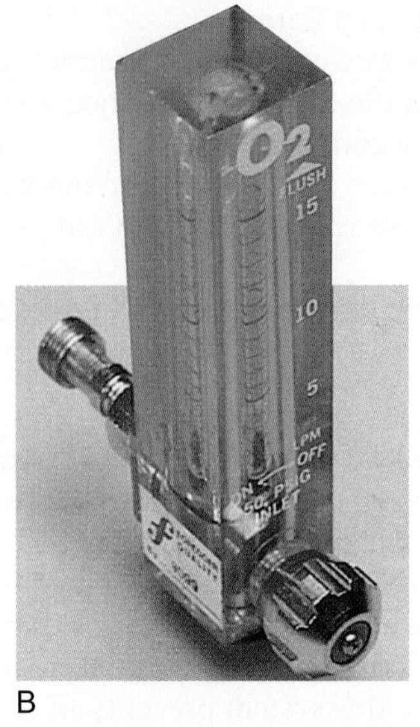

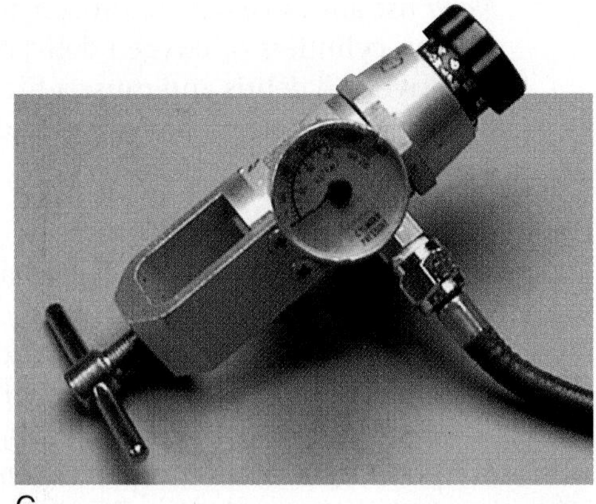

A B C

Figure 6-22 • (A) Bourdon gauge flowmeter (pressure gauge), (B) a pressure-compensated flowmeter, and (C) a constant flow selector valve.

- *Constant flow selector valve* (Figure 6-22C). This type of flowmeter, which is gaining in popularity, has no gauge and allows for the adjustment of flow in liters per minute in stepped increments (2, 4, 6, 8 . . . to 15 liters or more per minute). It can be accurately used with the nasal cannula or nonrebreather mask and with any size oxygen cylinder. It is rugged and will operate at any angle.

When using this type of flowmeter, make certain that it is properly adjusted for the desired flow and monitor it to make certain that it stays properly adjusted. All types of meters should be tested for accuracy as recommended by the manufacturer.

Humidifiers

humidifier
a device connected to the flowmeter to add moisture to the dry oxygen coming from an oxygen cylinder.

A **humidifier** can be connected to the flowmeter to provide moisture to the dry oxygen coming from the supply cylinder (Figure 6-23). Oxygen without humidification can dry out the mucous membranes of the patient's airway and lungs. In most short-term use, the dryness of the oxygen is not a problem; however, the patient is usually more comfortable when given humidified oxygen. This is particularly true if the patient has COPD or is a child.

A humidifier is usually no more than a nonbreakable jar of water attached to the flowmeter. Oxygen passes (bubbles) through the water to become humidified. As with all oxygen delivery equipment, the humidifier must be kept clean. The water reservoir can become a breeding ground for algae, harmful bacteria, and dangerous fungal organisms. Always use fresh water in a clean reservoir for each shift. Sterile single-patient-use humidifiers are available and preferred.

In many EMS systems, humidifiers are no longer used because they are not indicated for short transports and because of the infection risk. The devices may be beneficial on long transports and on certain pediatric patients with signs of inadequate breathing.

Hazards of Oxygen Therapy

Although the benefits of oxygen are great, oxygen must be used carefully. The hazards of oxygen therapy may be grouped into two categories: nonmedical and medical.

Nonmedical hazards are extremely rare and can be avoided totally if oxygen and oxygen equipment are treated properly. They include:

- The oxygen used in emergency care is stored under pressure, usually 2,000 to 2,200 pounds per square inch (psi) or greater in a full cylinder. If the tank is

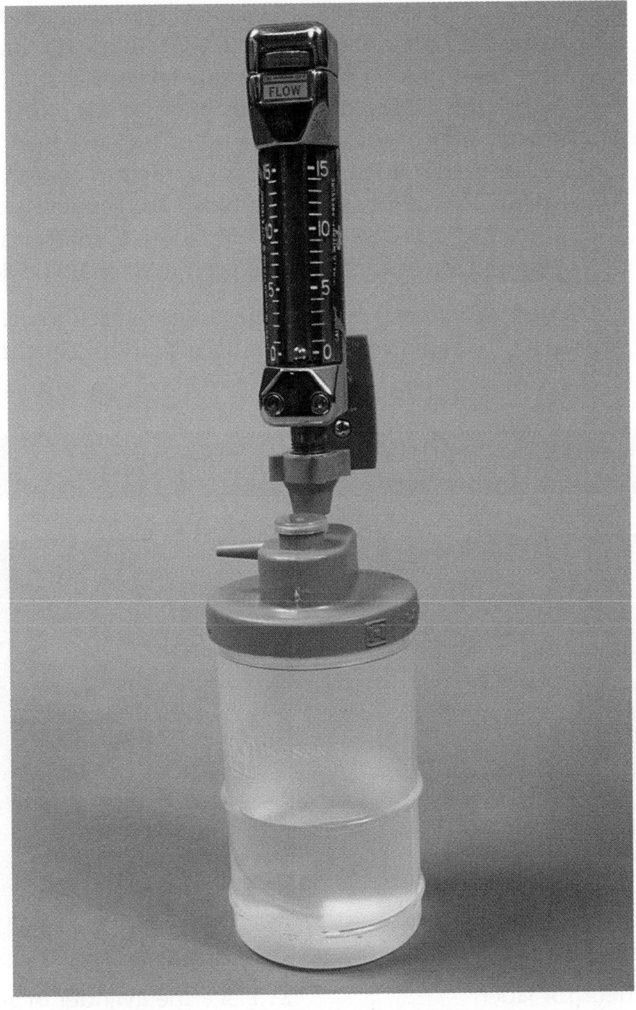

Figure 6-23 • A simple oxygen humidifier.

punctured, or a valve breaks off, the supply tank can become a missile (damaged tanks have been able to penetrate concrete walls). Imagine what would happen in the passenger compartment of an ambulance if such an accident occurred.

- Oxygen supports combustion, causing fire to burn more rapidly. It can saturate towels, sheets, and clothing, greatly increasing the risk of fire.
- Under pressure, oxygen and oil do not mix. When they come into contact, a severe reaction occurs which, for our purposes, can be termed an explosion. This is seldom a problem, but it can easily occur if you lubricate a delivery system or gauge with petroleum products, or allow contact with a petroleum-based adhesive (e.g., adhesive tape).

The medical hazards of oxygen rarely affect the patients treated by the EMT. There are certain patients who, when exposed to high concentrations of oxygen for a prolonged time, may develop negative side effects. These situations are rare in the field:

- *Oxygen toxicity or air sac collapse.* These problems are caused in some patients whose lungs react unfavorably to the presence of oxygen and also may result from too high a concentration of oxygen for too long a period of time. The body reacts to a sensed "overload" of oxygen by reduced lung activity and air sac collapse. Like the other conditions listed here, these are extremely rare in the field.
- *Infant eye damage.* This condition may occur when premature infants are given too much oxygen. These infants may develop scar tissue on the retina of the eye. Oxygen by itself does not cause this condition but it is the result of many factors. Oxygen should never be withheld from any infant with signs of inadequate breathing.

- *Respiratory depression or respiratory arrest.* Patients in the end stage of chronic obstructive pulmonary disease (COPD) may over time lose the normal ability to use the body's blood carbon dioxide levels as a stimulus to breathe. When this occurs, the COPD patient's body may use low blood oxygen as the factor that stimulates him to breathe. Because of this so-called hypoxic drive, EMTs have for years been trained to administer only low concentrations of oxygen to these patients for fear of increasing blood oxygen levels and wiping out their "drive to breathe." It is now widely believed that more harm is done by withholding high-flow, high-concentration oxygen than could be done by administering it.

As an EMT you will probably never see oxygen toxicity or any other adverse conditions that can result from oxygen administration. The time required for such conditions

SCAN 6-5 • Preparing the Oxygen Delivery System

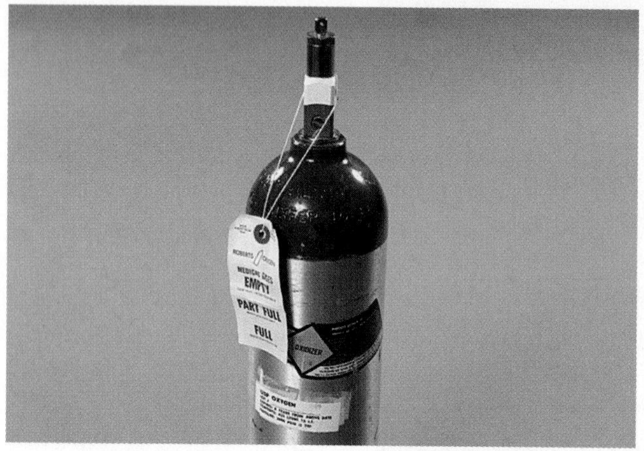

1. Select the desired cylinder. Check for label "Oxygen U.S.P."

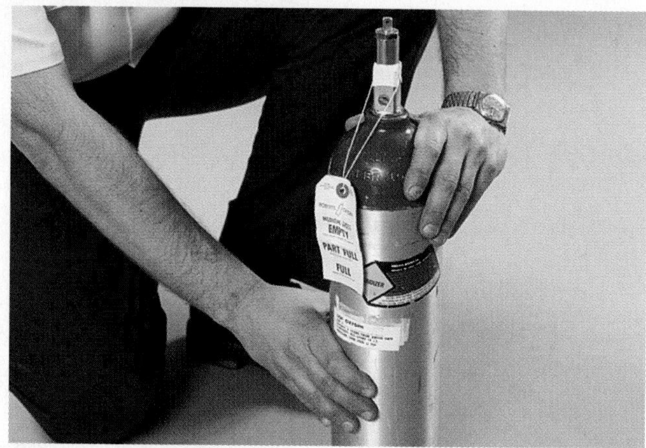

2. Place the cylinder in an upright position and stand to one side.

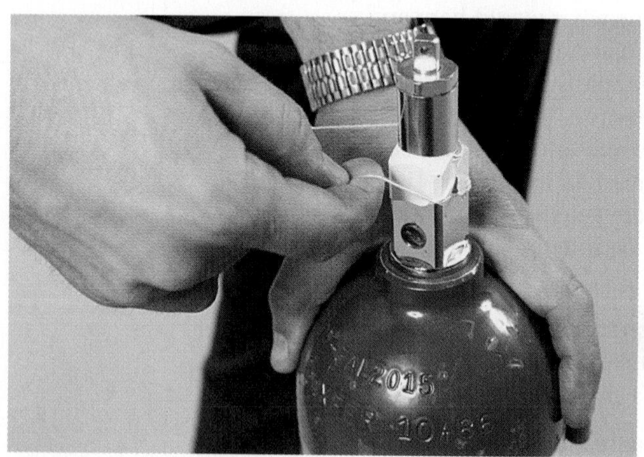

3. Remove the plastic wrapper or cap protecting the cylinder outlet.

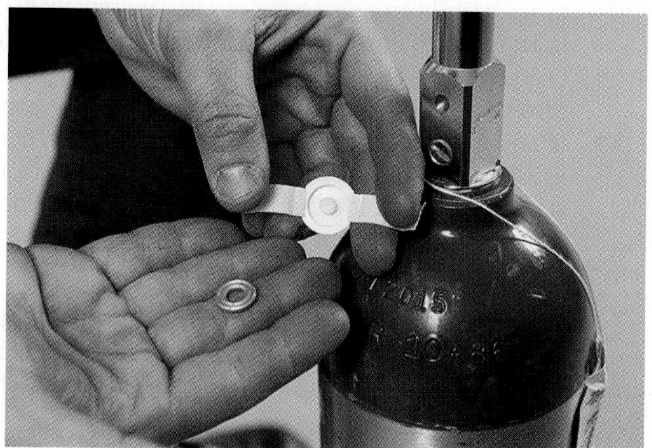

4. Keep the plastic washer (some set-ups).

to develop is too long to cause any problems during emergency care in the field. The bottom line is: *Never withhold oxygen from a patient who needs it!*

Administering Oxygen

Scans 6-5 and 6-6 will take you step by step through the process of preparing the oxygen delivery system, administering oxygen, and discontinuing the administration of oxygen. Do not attempt to learn on your own how to use oxygen delivery systems. You should work with your instructor and follow your instructor's directions for the specific equipment you will be using.

Oxygen is administered to assist in the delivery of artificial ventilations to nonbreathing patients, as was discussed earlier in this chapter under "Techniques of

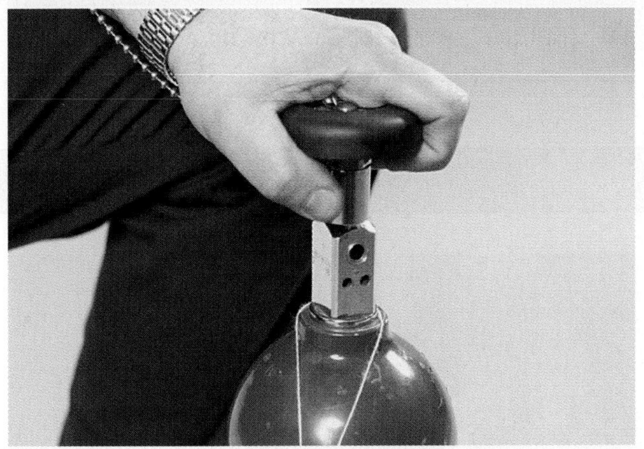

5. "Crack" the main valve for 1 second.

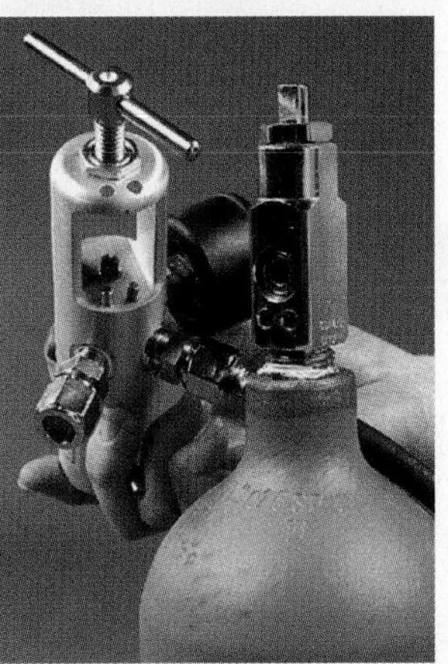

6. Select the correct pressure regulator and flowmeter. Pin yoke is shown on the left, threaded outlet on the right.

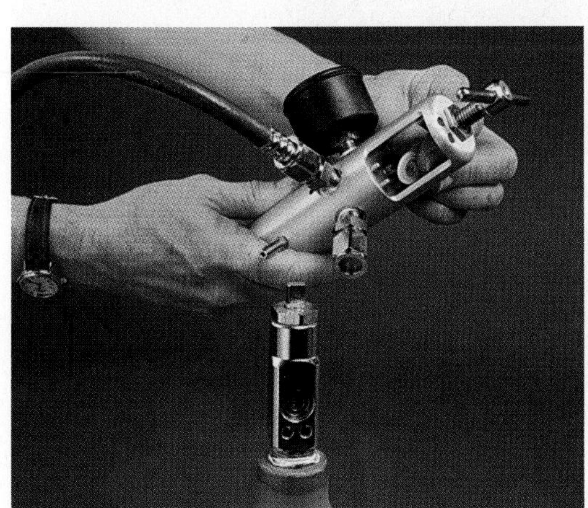

7. Place the cylinder valve gasket on the regulator oxygen port.

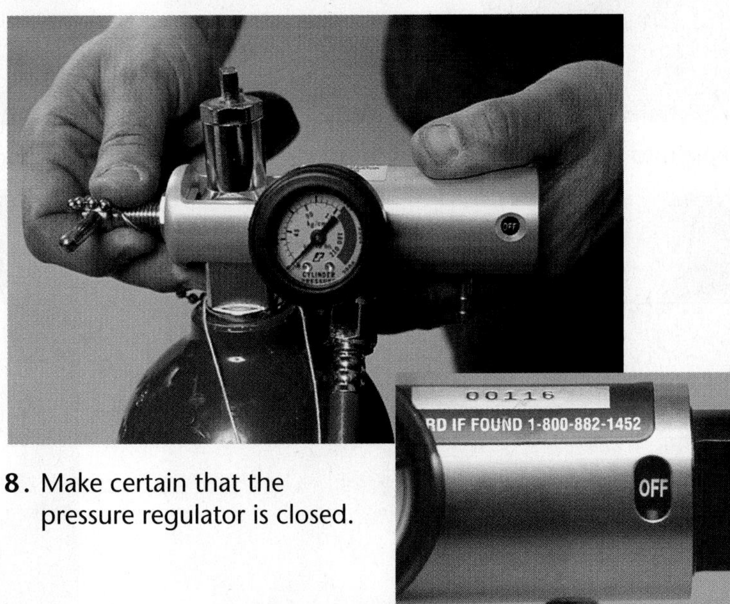

8. Make certain that the pressure regulator is closed.

continued

SCAN 6-5 • (Continued)

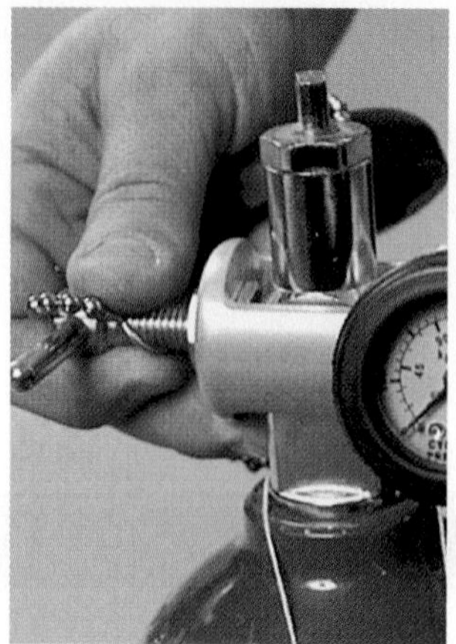

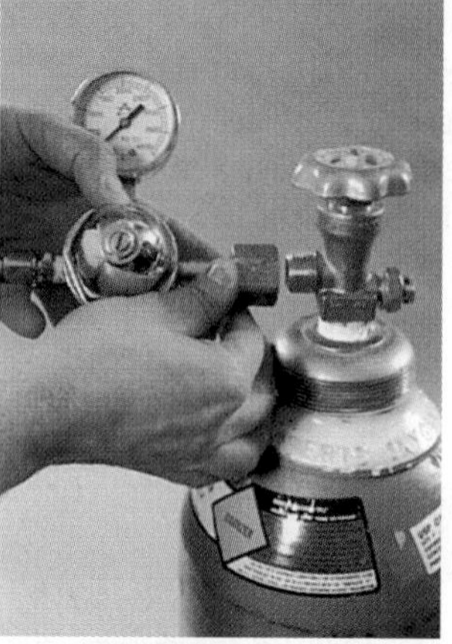

9. Align pins (left), or thread by hand (right).

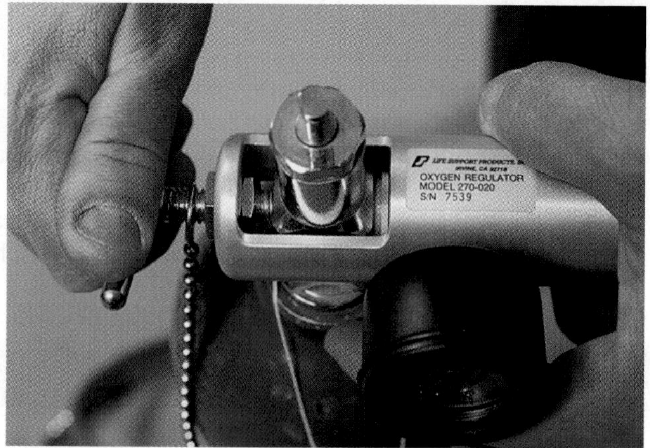

10. Tighten T-screw for pin yoke or . . .

SCAN 6-6 • Administering Oxygen

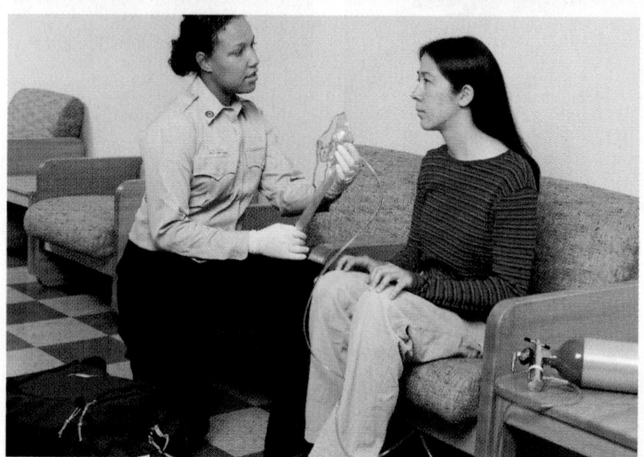

1. Explain to the patient the need for oxygen.

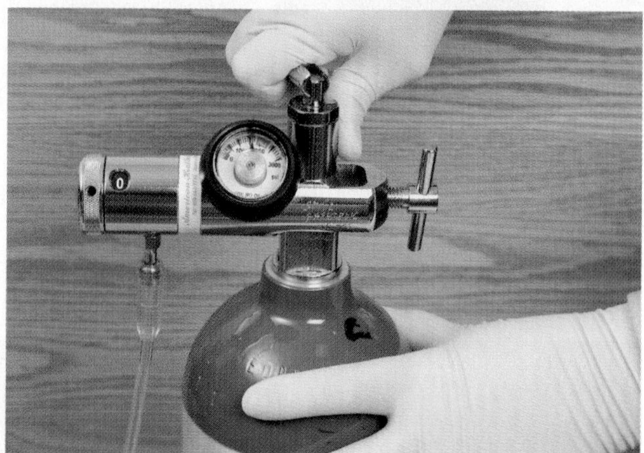

2. Open the main valve and adjust the flowmeter.

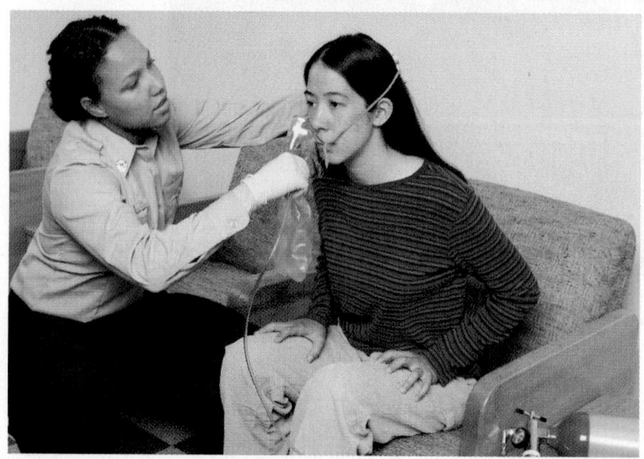

3. Place an oxygen delivery device on the patient.

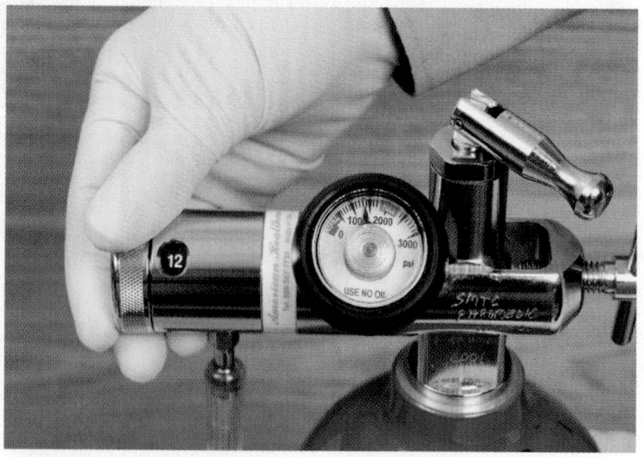

4. Adjust the flowmeter.

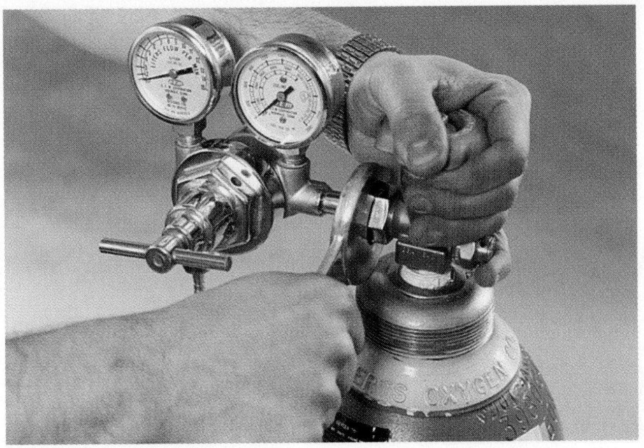

Tighten a threaded outlet with a nonferrous wrench.

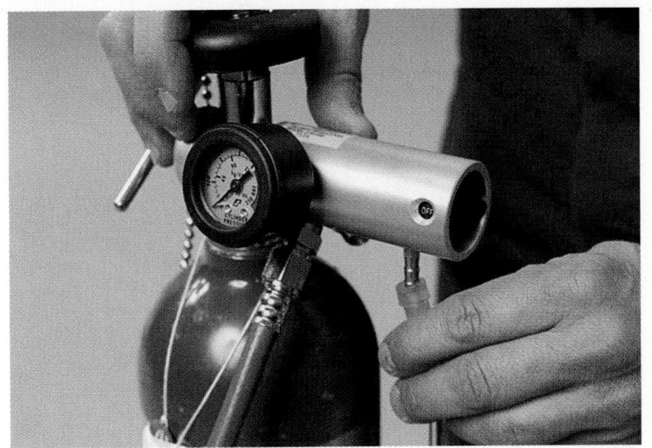

11. Attach tubing and delivery device.

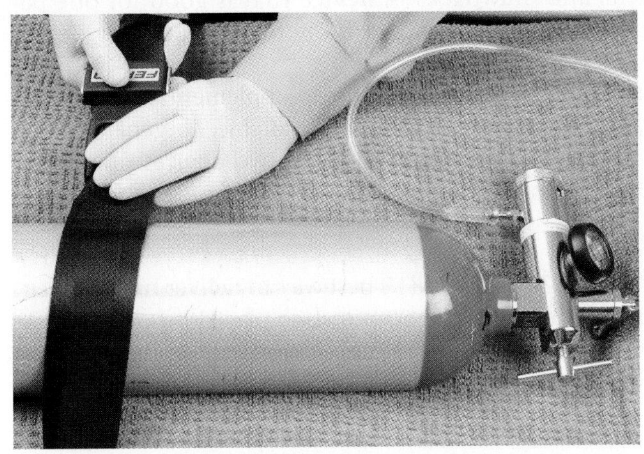

5. Secure the cylinder during transfer.

DISCONTINUING OXYGEN

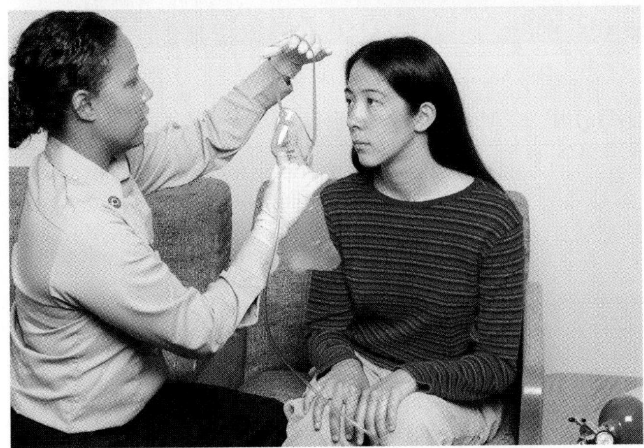

1. Remove the delivery device.

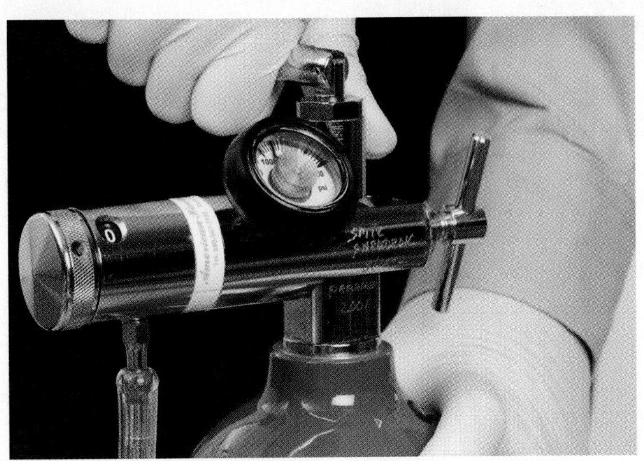

2. Close the main valve.

continued

SCAN 6-6 • (Continued)

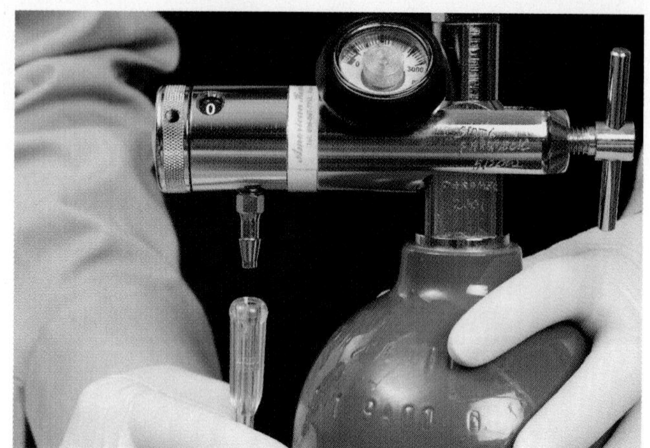

3. Remove the delivery tubing.

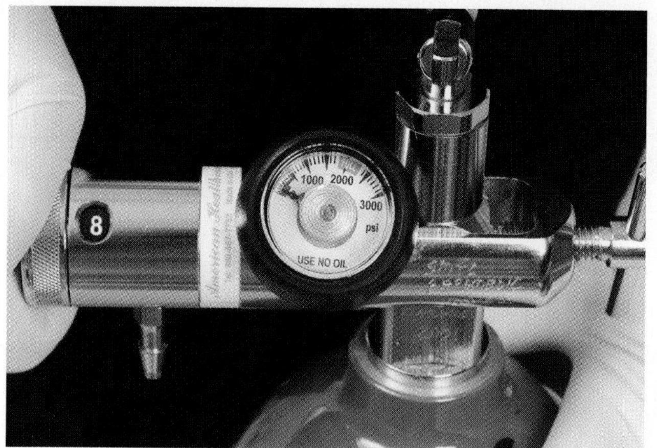

4. Bleed the flowmeter.

Artificial Ventilation." Oxygen is also very commonly administered to breathing patients for a variety of conditions. A number of oxygen-delivery devices and systems are used. Each has benefits and drawbacks. A device that is good for one patient may not be ideal for another. The goal is to use the oxygen-delivery device that is best for each patient.

For the patient who is breathing adequately and requires supplemental oxygen due to potential hypoxia, various oxygen-delivery devices are available. In general, however, the nonrebreather mask and the nasal cannula are the two devices most commonly used by the EMT to provide supplemental oxygen (Table 6-7).

nonrebreather mask
a face mask and reservoir bag device that delivers high concentrations of oxygen. The patient's exhaled air escapes through a valve and is not rebreathed.

Nonrebreather Mask

The **nonrebreather mask** (Figure 6-24) is the EMT's best way to deliver high concentrations of oxygen to a breathing patient. This device must be placed properly on the patient's face to provide the necessary seal to ensure high-concentration delivery. The reservoir bag must be inflated before the mask is placed on the patient's face.

TABLE 6-7 • Oxygen Delivery Devices

DEVICE	FLOW RATE	OXYGEN CONCENTRATION	APPROPRIATE USE
Nonrebreather mask	12–15 liters per minute	80–90 percent	Delivery system of choice for patients with signs of inadequate breathing and patients who are cyanotic, cool, clammy, short of breath, or suffering chest pain, suffering severe injuries, or displaying an altered mental status.
Nasal cannula	1–6 liters per minute	24–44 percent	Appropriate for patients who cannot tolerate a mask.
Venturi mask	Varied, depending on device. Up to 15 liters per minute	24–60 percent	A device used to deliver a specific concentration of oxygen. Device delivers 24–60 percent oxygen, depending on adapter tip and oxygen flow rate.

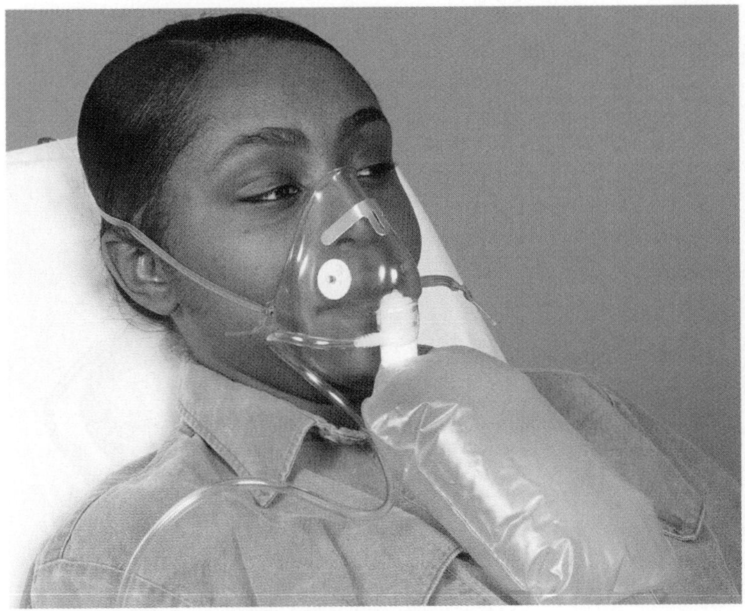

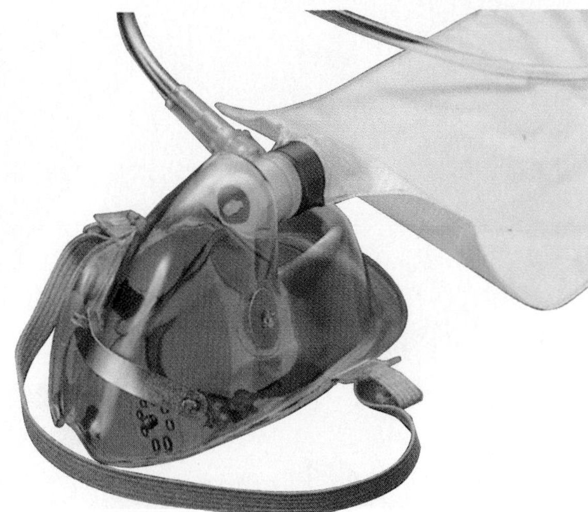

Figure 6-24 • Nonrebreather mask.

To inflate the reservoir bag, use your finger to cover the exhaust port or the connection between the mask and the reservoir. The reservoir must always contain enough oxygen so that it does not deflate by more than one third when the patient takes his deepest inspiration. This can be maintained by the proper flow of oxygen (15 liters per minute). Air exhaled by the patient does not return to the reservoir (is not rebreathed). Instead, it escapes through a flutter valve in the face piece.

This mask will provide concentrations of oxygen ranging from 80 to 100 percent. The minimum flow rate is 8 liters per minute. Depending on the manufacturer and the fit of the mask, the maximum flow can range from 12 to 15 liters per minute. New design features allow for one emergency port in the mask so that the patient can still receive atmospheric air should the oxygen supply fail. This feature keeps the mask from being able to deliver 100 percent oxygen but is a necessary safety feature. The mask is excellent for use in patients with inadequate breathing or who are cyanotic (blue or gray), cool, clammy, short of breath, suffering chest pain, or displaying an altered mental status.

Nonrebreather masks come in different sizes for adults, children, and infants.

Nasal Cannula

A **nasal cannula** (Figure 6-25) provides low concentrations of oxygen (between 24 percent and 44 percent). Oxygen is delivered to the patient by two prongs that rest in the patient's nostrils. The device is usually held to the patient's face by placing the tubing over the patient's ears and securing the slip-loop under the patient's chin.

nasal cannula
(NAY-zul KAN-yuh-luh)
a device that delivers low concentrations of oxygen through two prongs that rest in the patient's nostrils.

Patients who have chest pain, signs of shock, hypoxia, or other more serious problems need a higher concentration than can be provided by a cannula. However, some patients will not tolerate a mask-type delivery device because they feel "suffocated" by the mask. For the patient who refuses to wear an oxygen face mask, the cannula is better than no oxygen at all. The cannula should be used only when a patient will not tolerate a nonrebreather mask.

When a cannula is used, the liters per minute delivered should be no more than 4 to 6. At higher flow rates the cannula begins to feel more uncomfortable, like a windstorm in the nose, and dries out the nasal mucous membranes.

Venturi Mask

A **Venturi mask** (Figure 6-26) delivers specific concentrations of oxygen by mixing oxygen with inhaled air. The Venturi mask package may contain several tips. Each tip

Venturi mask
a face mask and reservoir bag device that delivers specific concentrations of oxygen by mixing oxygen with inhaled air.

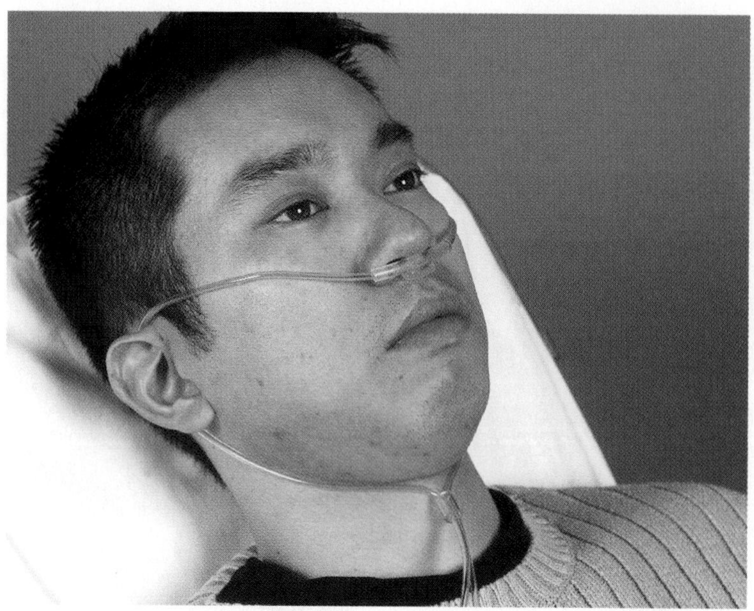

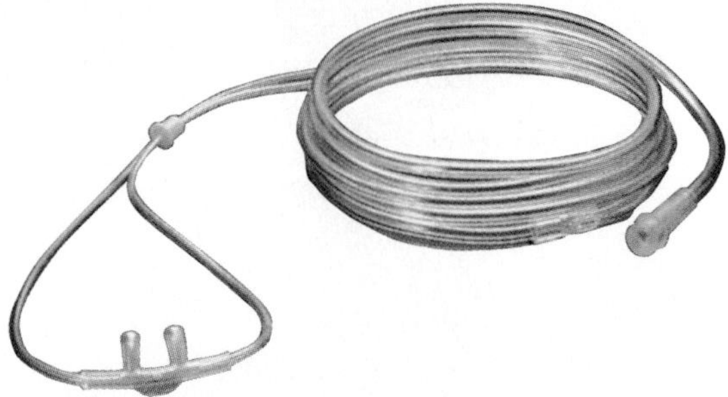

Figure 6-25 • Nasal cannula.

will provide a different concentration of oxygen when used at the flow rate designated on the tip. Some Venturi masks have a set percentage and flow rate while others have an adjustable Venturi port. These devices are most commonly used on patients who have chronic obstructive pulmonary diseases (COPD).

SPECIAL CONSIDERATIONS

There are a number of special considerations in airway management:

- *Facial injuries.* Take extra care with the airway when there have been facial injuries. Because the blood supply to the face is so rich, blunt injuries to the face frequently result in severe swelling or bleeding that may block or partially block the airway. Frequent suctioning may be required. Insertion of an airway adjunct or endotracheal tube may be necessary.
- *Obstructions.* Many suction units are not adequate for removing solid objects like teeth and large particles of food or other foreign objects. These must be removed using manual techniques for clearing airway obstructions, such as abdominal thrusts, chest thrusts, or finger sweeps, which you learned in your basic life support course and which are reviewed in Appendix C, "Basic Cardiac Life Support Review," at the back of this book. You may need to log roll the patient into a supine position to clear the oropharynx manually.

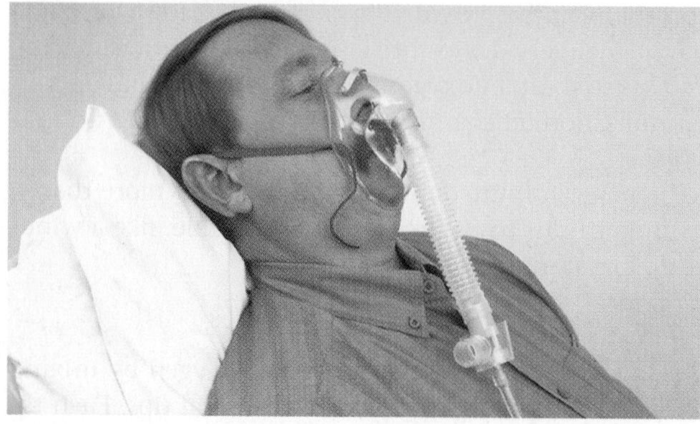

Figure 6-26 • Venturi mask.

- *Dental appliances.* Dentures should ordinarily be left in place during airway procedures. Partial dentures may become dislodged during an emergency. Leave a partial denture in place if possible, but be prepared to remove it if it endangers the airway.

PEDIATRIC NOTE

There are several special considerations that you must take into account when managing the airway of an infant or child (Figure 6-27):

Anatomic Considerations

- The mouth and nose of infants and children are smaller and more easily obstructed than in adults.
- In infants and children, the tongue takes up more space proportionately in the mouth than in adults.
- The trachea (windpipe) is softer and more flexible in infants and children.
- The trachea is narrower and is easily obstructed by swelling.
- The chest wall is softer, and infants and children tend to depend more on their diaphragm for breathing.

Management Considerations

- Open the airway gently. Infants can be placed in a neutral neck position and children only require slight extension of the neck. Do not hyperextend the neck, because it may collapse the trachea.
- When ventilating, avoid excessive pressure and volume. Use only enough to make the chest rise.
- Use properly sized face masks when providing ventilations to ensure a good mask seal.
- Flow-restricted, oxygen-powered ventilation devices are contraindicated (should not be used) in infants and children, unless you have a child unit and have been properly trained in its use.
- Use pediatric-sized nonrebreather masks and nasal cannulas when administering supplemental oxygen.
- Infants and children are prone to gastric distention during ventilations or respiratory distress, which may impair adequate ventilations. (See gastric tube insertion in Chapter 38, "Advanced Airway Management.")
- An oral or nasal airway may be considered when other measures fail to keep the airway open.
- In suctioning infants and children, use a rigid tip but be careful not to touch the back of the airway.

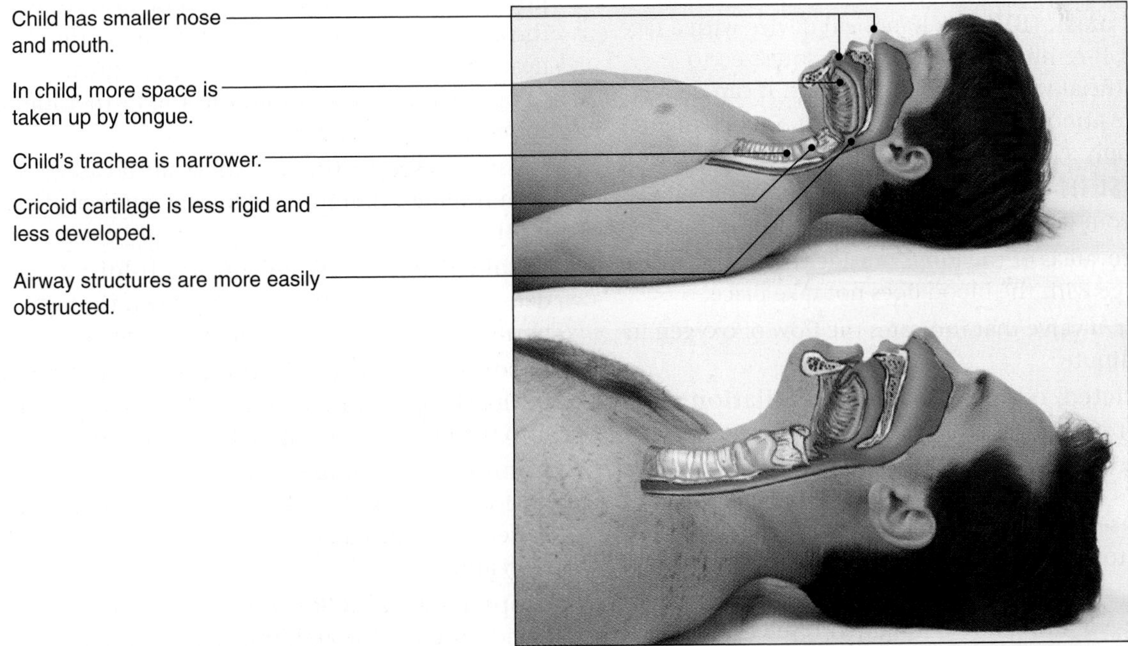
Child has smaller nose and mouth.
In child, more space is taken up by tongue.
Child's trachea is narrower.
Cricoid cartilage is less rigid and less developed.
Airway structures are more easily obstructed.

Figure 6-27 • Comparison of child and adult respiratory passages.

CHAPTER REVIEW

SUMMARY

The airway is the passageway by which air enters the body during respiration, or breathing. A patient cannot survive without an open airway. Maintaining an open airway is the first priority of emergency care.

Respiratory failure is inadequate breathing, breathing that is insufficient to support life. A patient in respiratory failure or respiratory arrest (complete stoppage of breathing) must receive artificial ventilations.

Airway adjuncts—the oropharyngeal and nasopharyngeal airway—can help keep the airway open during artificial ventilation. It may also be necessary to suction the airway or to use manual techniques to remove fluids and solids from the airway before, during, or after artificial ventilation.

Oxygen can be delivered to the nonbreathing patient as a supplement to artificial ventilation. Oxygen can also be administered as therapy to the breathing patient whose breathing is inadequate or who is cyanotic (gray or blue), cool and clammy, short of breath, suffering chest pain, suffering severe injuries, or displaying an altered mental status.

KEY TERMS

airway the passageway by which air enters or leaves the body. The structures of the airway are the nose, mouth, pharynx, larynx, trachea, bronchi, and lungs. *See also* patent airway.

artificial ventilation forcing air or oxygen into the lungs when a patient has stopped breathing or has inadequate breathing. Also called **positive pressure ventilation.**

automatic transport ventilator (ATV) a device that provides positive pressure ventilations. It includes settings designed to adjust ventilation rate and volume, is portable, and is easily carried on an ambulance.

bag-valve mask (BVM) a handheld device with a face mask and self-refilling bag that can be squeezed to provide artificial ventilations to a patient. It can deliver air from the atmosphere or oxygen from a supplemental oxygen supply system.

cyanosis (SIGH-uh-NO-sis) a blue or gray color resulting from lack of oxygen in the body.

dead space areas of the lungs outside the alveoli where gas exchange with the blood does not take place.

flowmeter a valve that indicates the flow of oxygen in liters per minute.

flow-restricted, oxygen-powered ventilation device (FROPVD) a device that uses oxygen under pressure to deliver artificial ventilations. Its trigger is placed so that the rescuer can operate it while still using both hands to maintain a seal on the face mask. It has automatic flow restriction to prevent overdelivery of oxygen to the patient.

gag reflex vomiting or retching that results when something is placed in the back of the pharynx. This is tied to the swallow reflex.

head-tilt, chin-lift maneuver a means of correcting blockage of the airway by the tongue by tilting the head back and lifting the chin. Used when no trauma, or injury, is suspected.

humidifier a device connected to the flowmeter to add moisture to the dry oxygen coming from an oxygen cylinder.

hyperventilate (HI-per-VEN-ti-late) to provide ventilations at a higher rate than normal.

hypoxia (hi-POK-se-uh) an insufficiency of oxygen in the body's tissues.

jaw-thrust maneuver a means of correcting blockage of the airway by moving the jaw forward without tilting the head or neck. Used when trauma, or injury, is suspected to open the airway without causing further injury to the spinal cord in the neck.

minute volume the amount of air breathed in during each respiration multiplied by the number of breaths per minute.

nasal cannula (NAY-zul KAN-yuh-luh) a device that delivers low concentrations of oxygen through two prongs that rest in the patient's nostrils.

nasopharyngeal (NAY-zo-fah-RIN-jul) **airway** a flexible breathing tube inserted through the patient's nose into the pharynx to help maintain an open airway.

nonrebreather mask a face mask and reservoir bag device that delivers high concentrations of oxygen. The patient's exhaled air escapes through a valve and is not rebreathed.

oropharyngeal (OR-o-fah-RIN-jul) **airway** a curved device inserted through the patient's mouth into the pharynx to help maintain an open airway.

oxygen cylinder a cylinder filled with oxygen under pressure.

patent airway an airway (passage from nose or mouth to lungs) that is open and clear and will remain open and clear, without interference to the passage of air into and out of the body.

pocket face mask a device, usually with a one-way valve, to aid in artificial ventilation. A rescuer breathes through the valve when the mask is placed over the patient's face. It also acts as a barrier to prevent contact with a patient's breath or body fluids. It can be used with supplemental oxygen when fitted with an oxygen inlet.

positive pressure ventilation *See* artificial ventilation.

pressure regulator a device connected to an oxygen cylinder to reduce cylinder pressure so it is safe for delivery of oxygen to a patient.

respiration (RES-pir-AY-shun) breathing.

respiratory (RES-pir-uh-tor-e) **arrest** when breathing completely stops.

respiratory distress increased work of breathing; a sensation of shortness of breath.

respiratory failure the reduction of breathing to the point where oxygen intake is not sufficient to support life.

stoma a permanent surgical opening in the neck through which the patient breathes.

suctioning (SUK-shun-ing) use of a vacuum device to remove blood, vomitus, and other secretions or foreign materials from the airway.

ventilation the breathing in of air or oxygen or providing breaths artificially.

Venturi mask a face mask and reservoir bag device that delivers specific concentrations of oxygen by mixing oxygen with inhaled air.

REVIEW QUESTIONS

1. Name the main structures of the airway. (pp. 136–137)
2. Explain why care for the airway is the first priority of emergency care. (pp. 135–136)
3. Name the signs of adequate breathing and of inadequate breathing. (pp. 137–143)
4. Explain when the head-tilt, chin-lift maneuver should be used and when the jaw-thrust maneuver should be used to open the airway—and why. (pp. 145–146)
5. Name the techniques of artificial ventilation in the recommended order of preference. (p. 146)
6. Explain how airway adjuncts and suctioning help in airway management and artificial ventilation. (pp. 157–167)
7. Name patient problems that would benefit from administration of oxygen and explain how to decide whether a nonrebreather mask, or nasal cannula, or Venturi mask should be used to deliver oxygen to a patient. (pp. 167, 178–180)

CRITICAL THINKING

- On arrival at the emergency scene, you find an adult female patient with gurgling sounds in the throat and inadequate breathing slowing to almost nothing. How do you proceed to protect the airway and support the patient's breathing?

Thinking and Linking

Think back to Chapter 5, "Lifting and Moving Patients," and link information from that chapter with information from this chapter, "Airway Management," as you consider the following questions:

- You are treating a patient with a spine injury who is immobilized on a backboard. He begins to vomit. In addition to suctioning, what do you do?
- You are using a pocket mask to ventilate a patient who is breathing inadequately. You are in a bedroom, which is down a narrow hallway. The patient has been placed on a flexible (Reeves) stretcher, and you are ready to move. You will not fit through the door or be able to accompany the patient down the hallway from the side of the stretcher. There is no room at the head, because another EMT will be carrying the stretcher. How do you allow for ventilation while moving the patient to the ambulance?

MEDIA RESOURCES 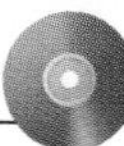

See the Student CD at the back of this book for quizzes, a case study activity, videos and other features related to this chapter. In particular, take a look at the Virtual Airway Tour, the animations of the respiratory system and of oral and nasal airway insertion, and the videos on the nasal cannula and the nonrebreather mask. Also, visit the Companion Website for *Emergency Care* at **www.prenhall.com/limmer**, where you will find additional reinforcement and links to other resources.

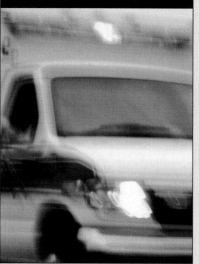

Street Scenes

"Dispatch to ambulance one-five," your radio blurts out. You respond, "Go ahead, Dispatch." Dispatch tells you that you have a priority-one response to a child, age unknown, choking, at 155 Baldwin Street, cross street of Third Avenue. Sonya, your partner, drives, and while en route you make sure that you have a plan. Sonya will take the lead. When she pulls up to the scene, a frantic person is waving his arms. He tells you the child is inside and not breathing.

Street Scene Questions

1. What is your first priority when starting to assess this patient?
2. What type of emergency care should you be prepared to give?
3. What equipment should you have taken into the house to make sure you are properly prepared for this call?

As you enter the house, you immediately see a child about 2 years old, cyanotic, being held by a frantic mother. You take the child and try to open the airway—always your first priority. You hear some air movement, but it appears that the child has an obstruction. The mother tells you he was eating breakfast when he started to cough. After your partner performs a few abdominal thrusts, the child expels a piece of food.

You already have the BVM out with the connective tube attached to the reservoir, so you start to assist ventilations. Your partner takes the child's pulse and reports that it is 60. You both realize that is too low, and you continue ventilating. The child has a gag reflex, so you don't attempt an oropharyngeal airway. You make sure that you have a good airway seal and you squeeze the bag slowly, looking for chest rise. Your partner reminds you to pause between ventilations. You count quietly in order to keep track of the rate.

Street Scene Questions

4. What is the best way to determine if the ventilations are adequate?
5. What additional assessment should be done on this patient?

Your partner comments that there is good chest rise and the child is less cyanotic. "Good technique," she observes. "The pulse rate is now 110." The child starts to get restless and pushes the face mask away. You remove the mask but continue to give oxygen by blow-by. As you package the patient, you reassure the mother. En route to the hospital, you reassess the patient. His color is good, and his pulse rate is 120. He responds well to his mother and calms down quite a bit.

At the hospital, you discuss the call with your partner. She says that it was important to start ventilations quickly. When the heart doesn't get enough oxygen, it will start to slow, so giving 100 percent oxygen is important to bringing the heart rate back up. As you are leaving the emergency department to return to service, the doctor stops you and says the child is doing well.

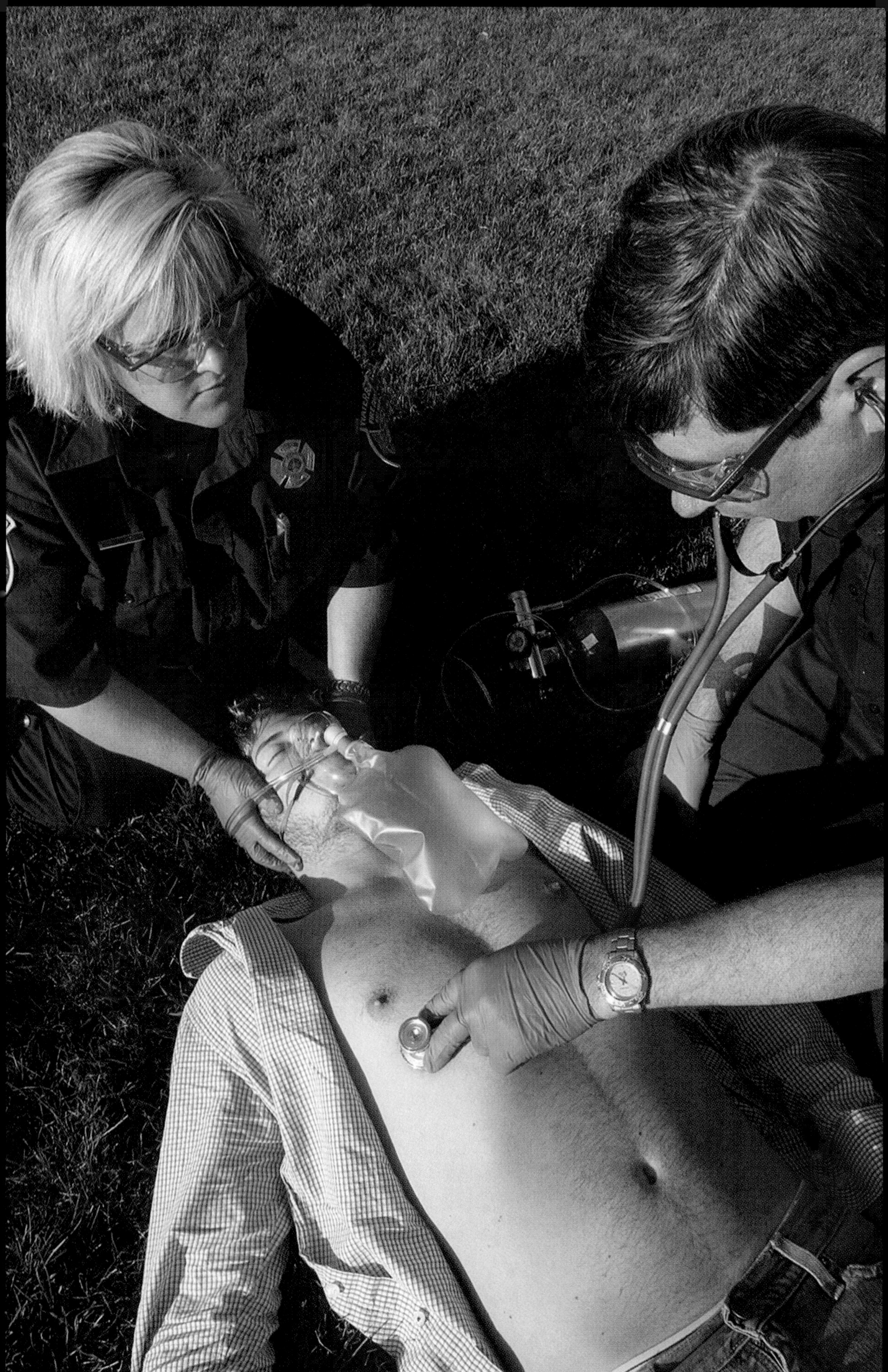

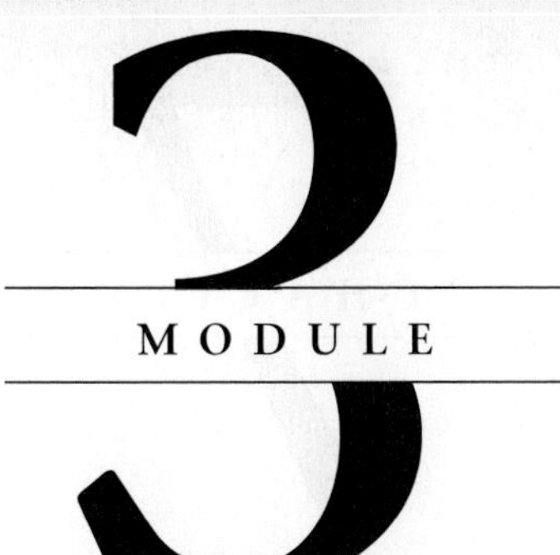

MODULE

Patient Assessment

This module presents the elements of patient assessment. Before you reach a patient, you will perform a scene size-up (Chapter 7) to determine scene safety and evaluate the need for additional resources. When the scene is safe, you must first find and immediately care for any life threats as you perform the initial assessment (Chapter 8).

Next you will measure vital signs and get a patient history (Chapter 9), as well as conduct a physical exam. These steps constitute the *focused history and physical exam.* (Sometimes an additional *detailed physical exam* is also performed.) But these steps are done in a different sequence for trauma patients (Chapter 10) and medical patients (Chapter 11). You will perform *ongoing assessment* en route to the hospital (Chapter 12). Critical skills of communication (Chapter 13) and documentation (Chapter 14) are also covered in this module.

7

CHAPTER

Scene Size-Up

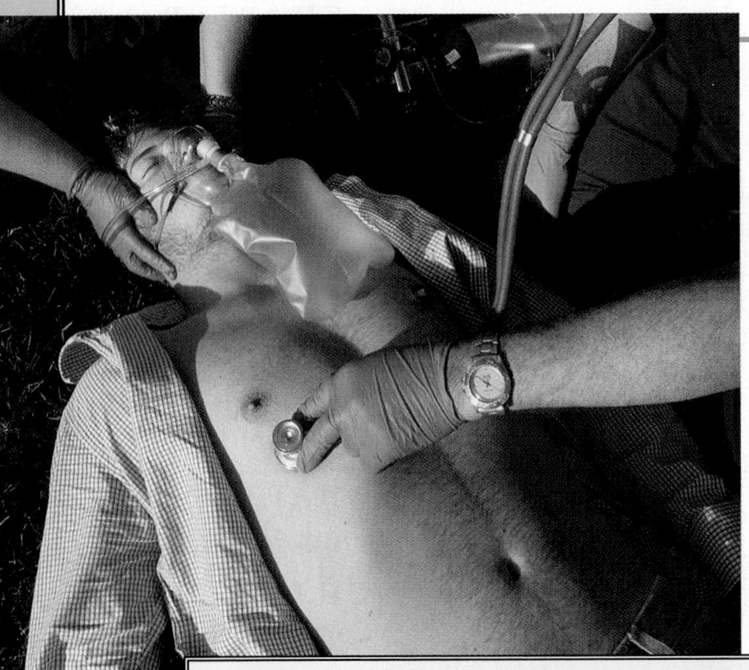

CORE CONCEPTS

The following are core concepts that will be addressed in this chapter:

- How to identify hazards at a scene
- How to determine if a scene is safe to enter
- Mechanism of injury and how it relates to patient condition
- When additional assistance will be needed at a scene

KEY TERMS

blunt-force trauma, p. 203
danger zone, p. 192
index of suspicion, p. 204
mechanism of injury, p. 197
nature of the illness, p. 204
penetrating trauma, p. 202
scene size-up, p. 189

DOT OBJECTIVES

*KNOWLEDGE AND ATTITUDE

3-1.1 Recognize hazards or potential hazards. (pp. 189–192) (Scan 7-1, p. 190)

3-1.2 Describe common hazards found at the scene of a trauma and a medical patient. (pp. 189–194) (Scan 7-2, p. 193)

3-1.3 Determine if the scene is safe to enter. (pp. 190–195)

3-1.4 Discuss common mechanisms of injury or nature of illness. (pp. 197–204) (Scan 7-3, p. 197)

3-1.5 Discuss the reason for identifying the total number of patients at the scene. (pp. 204–205)

3-1.6 Explain the reason for identifying the need for additional help or assistance. (pp. 204–205)

3-1.7 Explain the rationale for crew members to evaluate scene safety prior to entering. (pp. 189–190)

3-1.8 Serve as a model for others, explaining how patient situations affect your evaluation of mechanism of injury or illness. (pp. 197–204)

*SKILLS

3-1.9 Observe various scenarios and identify potential hazards.

Scene size-up sets a foundation for the remainder of the patient assessment process as well as the rest of the call. What potential hazards does this scene present? Do I have the personal protective equipment I may need? What is the likely mechanism of injury or the nature of the patient's illness? Will we need additional assistance? These are questions you will ask as you size up the scene and prepare for the safe and effective care of your patient.

SCENE SIZE-UP

Scene size-up is the first part of the patient assessment process. It begins as you approach the scene, surveying it to determine if there are any threats to your own safety or to the safety of your patients or bystanders, to determine the nature of the call, and to decide if you will need additional help (Scan 7-1).

scene size-up steps taken by an ambulance crew when approaching the scene of an emergency call: checking scene safety, taking Standard Precautions, noting the mechanism of injury or nature of the patient's illness, determining the number of patients, and deciding what, if any, additional resources to call for.

However, scene size-up is not confined to the first part of the assessment process. These considerations should continue throughout the call. Since emergencies are dynamic, always-changing events, you may find, for example, that patients, family members, or bystanders who were not a problem initially become increasingly hostile later in the call or that vehicles or structures that seemed stable suddenly shift and pose a danger.

After your initial scene size-up, you will become more directly involved in patient assessment and care. However, it is a good idea to remember the key size-up elements throughout the call to prevent dangerous surprises later.

You can obtain important information from just a brief survey of the scene. For example, you might see a downed electrical wire at the scene of a vehicle collision, a potentially deadly situation for you as the EMT, your patient, and bystanders. Further observations of the scene are likely to reveal more important information about the mechanism of injury. For example, damage to the steering wheel or windshield would be a strong indicator of potential chest, head, or neck injury caused by driver impact with those surfaces. A deployed air bag would cause you to assess for injuries air bags might cause, especially to an infant or child front-seat passenger (Figure 7-1).

Just as important as your observations will be the actions you take to obtain needed assistance and prevent further injury. For example, if there were two patients at a collision, you would request that a second ambulance be dispatched to the scene—more if

SCAN 7-1 • Scene Size-Up

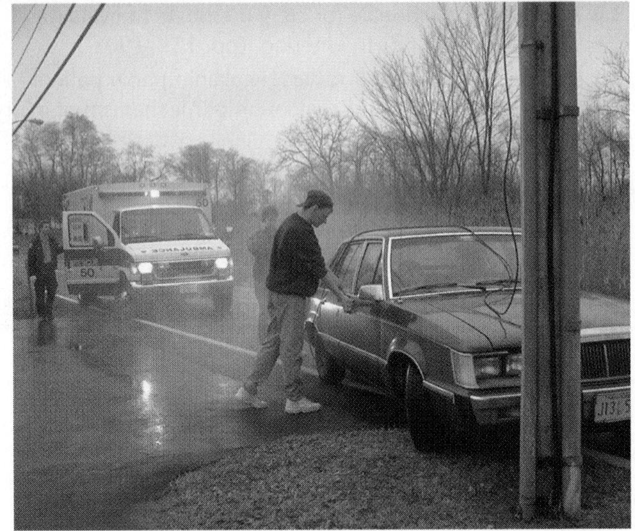

1. Determine scene safety. Look for possible threats to the safety of the crew, patient, and bystanders.

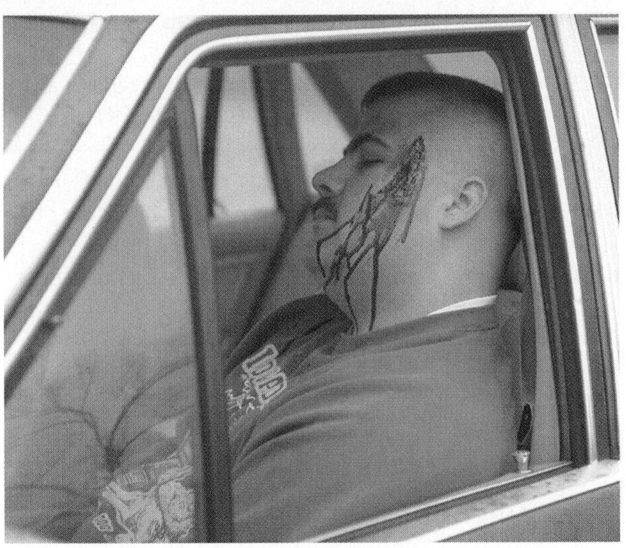

2. Determine the mechanism of injury or the nature of the patient's illness.

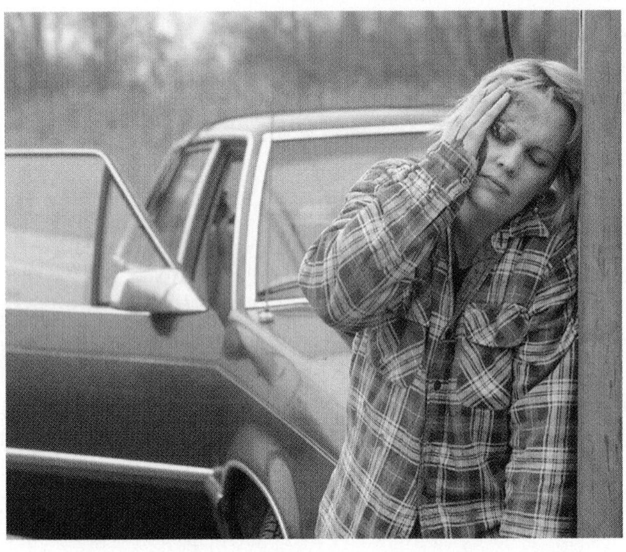

3. Determine the number of patients. Be alert for patients in addition to the first patient you see at the scene.

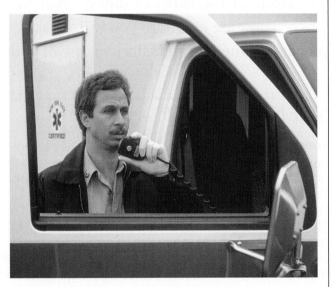

4. Request additional help if necessary.

you discovered that there were additional passengers. If at that scene there also was a downed wire, which poses a danger of fire, you would notify the fire department as well as the power company and the police department. And you would take steps to keep bystanders clear of traffic, the collision, and the patients.

Scene Safety

The only predictable thing about emergencies is that they are often unpredictable and can pose many dangers if you are not careful.

A

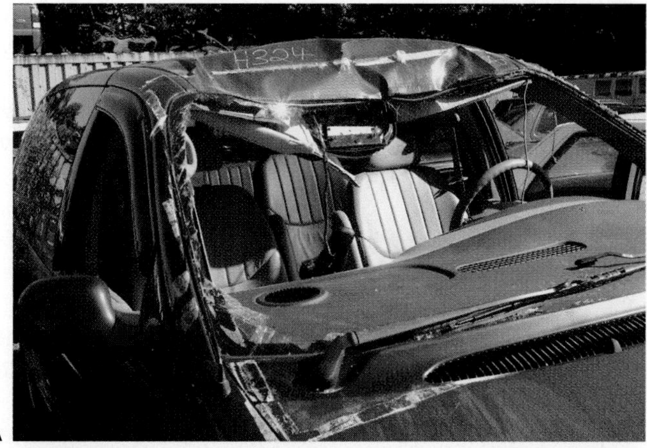

B

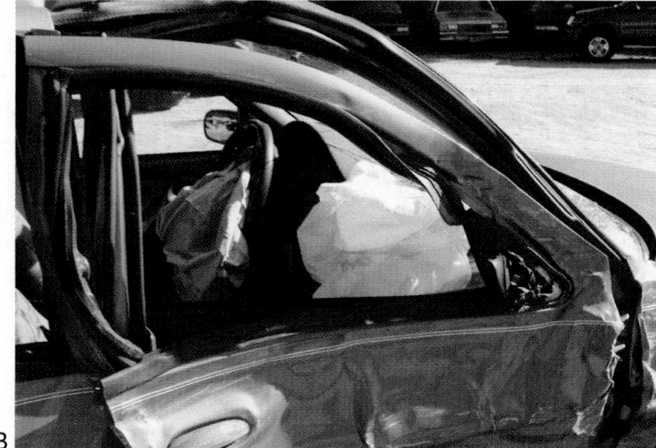

C

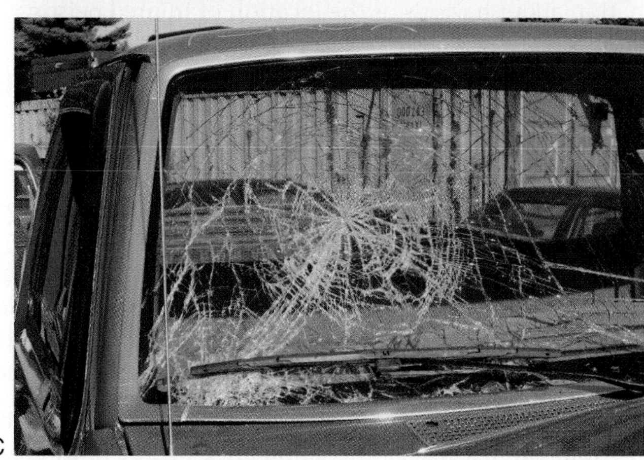

Figure 7-1 • Clues such as (A) exterior damage, (B) a deployed air bag, or (C) a damaged windshield may lead you to suspect certain types of injuries.

Before you arrive on scene, the dispatcher may relay important information to you. A well-trained Emergency Medical Dispatcher (EMD) uses a set of questions to determine information that may affect you directly. For example, if the caller tells the EMD of particular hazards, you could call for additional specialized assistance immediately. You will learn more about the questions an EMD asks in Chapter 34, "Ambulance Operations."

Often you will arrive at a scene where there are police, fire, and even other ambulances already present. In a situation like this, do not assume that the scene is safe or that others have taken care of any hazards. Always perform your own size-up, no matter who arrives first. Scan for scene hazards, infection-control concerns, mechanisms of injury, and number of patients. The scene size-up begins even before the ambulance comes to a stop. Observe the scene while you approach and again before you exit the vehicle.

The following are scene size-up considerations you should keep in mind when you approach a crash or hazardous material emergency:

As you near the collision scene:

- Look and listen for other emergency service units approaching from side streets.
- Look for signs of a collision-related power outage, such as darkened areas which suggest that wires are down at the collision scene.
- Observe traffic flow. If there is no opposing traffic, suspect a blockade at the collision scene.
- Look for smoke in the direction of the collision scene—a sign that fire has resulted from the collision.

When you are within sight of the scene:

- Look for clues to escaped hazardous materials, such as placards, a damaged truck, escaping liquids, fumes, or vapor clouds. If you see anything suspicious, stop the ambulance immediately and consult your hazardous-materials reference book or hazardous-materials team, if one is available. (See more information under "Establishing the Danger Zone.")

- Look for collision victims on or near the road. A person may have been thrown from a vehicle as it careened out of control, or an injured person may have walked away from the wreckage and collapsed on or near the roadway.
- Look for smoke not seen at a distance.
- Look for broken utility poles and downed wires. At night, direct the beam of a spotlight or handlight on poles and wire spans as you approach the scene. Keep in mind that wires may be down several hundred feet from the crash vehicles.
- Be alert for persons walking along the side of the road toward the collision scene. Curious onlookers (excited children in particular) are often oblivious to vehicles approaching from behind.
- Watch for the signals of police officers and other emergency service personnel. They may have information about hazards or the location of injured persons.

As you reach the scene:

- Sniff for odors such as gasoline or diesel fuel or any unusual odor that may signal a hazardous material release.

Establishing the Danger Zone

danger zone the area around the wreckage of a vehicle collision or other incident within which special safety precautions should be taken.

A **danger zone** exists around the wreckage of every vehicle collision, within which special safety precautions must be taken. The size of the zone depends on the nature and severity of collision-produced hazards (Scan 7-2). An ambulance should never be parked within the danger zone. Follow these guidelines in establishing the danger zone:

- *When there are no apparent hazards,* consider the danger zone to extend at least 50 feet in all directions from the wreckage. The ambulance will be away from broken glass and other debris, and it will not impede emergency service personnel who must work in or around the wreckage. When using highway flares to protect the scene, make sure that the person igniting them has been trained in the proper technique.
- *When fuel has been spilled,* consider the danger zone to extend a minimum of 100 feet in all directions from the wreckage. In addition to parking outside the danger zone, park upwind, if possible. (Note the direction of the wind by observing flags, smoke, and so on.) Thus, the ambulance will be out of the path of dense smoke if the fuel ignites. If fuel is flowing away from the wreckage, park uphill as well as upwind. If parking uphill is not possible, position the ambulance as far from the flowing fuel as possible. Avoid gutters, ditches, and gullies that can carry fuel to the ambulance. Do not use flares in areas where fuel has been spilled. Use orange traffic cones during daylight and reflective triangles at night.
- *When a collision vehicle is on fire,* consider the danger zone to extend at least 100 feet in all directions even if the fire appears small and limited to the engine compartment. If fire reaches the vehicle's fuel tank, an explosion could easily damage an ambulance parked closer than 100 feet.
- *When wires are down,* consider the danger zone as the area in which people or vehicles might be contacted by energized wires if the wires pivot around their points of attachment. Even though you may have to carry equipment and stretchers for a considerable distance, the ambulance should be parked at least one full span of wires from the poles to which broken wires are attached.
- *When a hazardous material is involved,* check the *Emergency Response Guidebook (ERG)*—published by the U.S. Department of Transportation, Transport Canada, and the Secretariat of Communications and Transportation of Mexico—for suggestions as to where to park, or ask the Incident Commander to request advice from an agency such as CHEMTREC (Chemical Transportation Emergency

SCAN 7-2 • Establishing the Danger Zone

DANGER

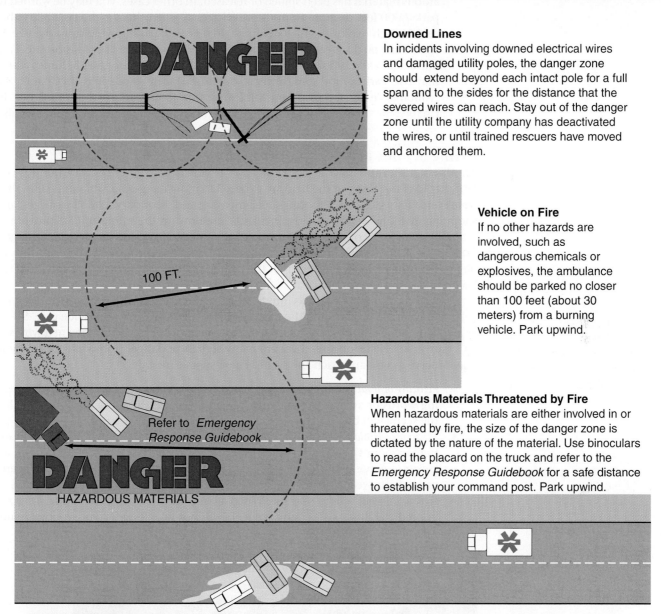

Downed Lines
In incidents involving downed electrical wires and damaged utility poles, the danger zone should extend beyond each intact pole for a full span and to the sides for the distance that the severed wires can reach. Stay out of the danger zone until the utility company has deactivated the wires, or until trained rescuers have moved and anchored them.

100 FT.

Vehicle on Fire
If no other hazards are involved, such as dangerous chemicals or explosives, the ambulance should be parked no closer than 100 feet (about 30 meters) from a burning vehicle. Park upwind.

Refer to *Emergency Response Guidebook*

DANGER
HAZARDOUS MATERIALS

Hazardous Materials Threatened by Fire
When hazardous materials are either involved in or threatened by fire, the size of the danger zone is dictated by the nature of the material. Use binoculars to read the placard on the truck and refer to the *Emergency Response Guidebook* for a safe distance to establish your command post. Park upwind.

Spilled Fuel The ambulance should be parked uphill from flowing fuel. If this is not possible, the vehicle should be parked as far from the fuel flow as possible, avoiding gutters, ditches, and gullies that may carry the spill to the parking site. Remember, your ambulance's catalytic converter is an ignition source over 1000 degrees Fahrenheit.

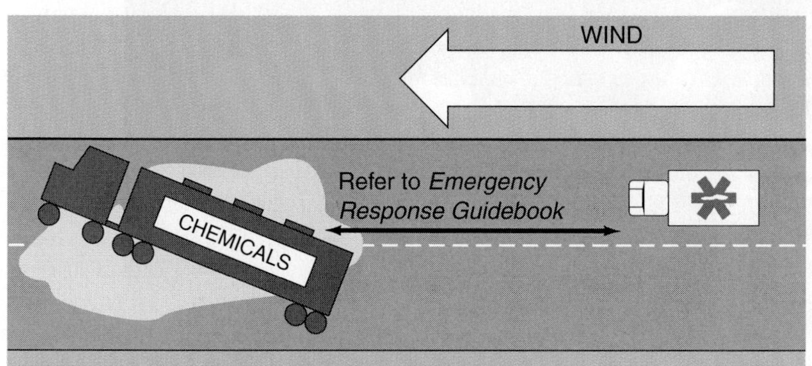

Hazardous Materials
Leaking containers of dangerous chemicals may produce a health as well as a fire hazard. When chemicals have been spilled, whether fumes are evident or not, the ambulance should be parked upwind. If the hazardous material is known, seek advice from experts such as CHEMTREC through the Incident Commander.

Center, Washington, DC, 24-hour hotline 800-424-9300 or 703-527-3887). In some cases you may be able to park 50 feet from the wreckage, as when no hazardous material has been spilled or released. In other cases, you may be warned to park 2,000 feet or more from the wreckage, as when there is the possibility that certain high explosives may detonate. In all cases, park upwind from the wreckage when you discover that a hazardous material is present at a collision site. Park uphill if a liquid is flowing, but on the same level if there are gases or fumes which may rise. Park behind some artificial or natural barrier if possible. (In Chapter 34, "Ambulance Operations," you will learn more about parking the ambulance. In Chapter 36, "Special Operations," you will learn more about hazardous materials.)

Crime Scenes and Acts of Violence

Another significant danger faced by the EMT is violence. Crime risks vary, but it is certain that EMTs working in the field are exposed to more dangerous situations than they were even a few years ago. Shootings at elementary and secondary schools, colleges, and shopping malls, as well as terrorist incidents, are now on the minds of EMS providers.

While a majority of calls go by uneventfully, the EMT must be conscious of dangers from many sources, including other human beings (Figure 7-2). EMTs often envision violence as occurring at bar fights or on the street, but domestic violence (violence in the home) is also a cause for concern.

Protection from violence is as important as protection from the dangers at a vehicle collision. As an EMT, you should never enter a violent situation to provide care. Safety at a violent scene requires a careful size-up as you approach. Just as a downed wire signals danger at a collision site, there are many signals of danger from violence that you may observe as you approach the scene. These signals include:

- *Fighting or loud voices.* If you approach a scene and see or hear fighting, threatening words or actions, or the potential for fighting, there is a good chance that the scene will be a danger to you.
- *Weapons visible or in use.* Any time you observe a weapon, you must use an extreme amount of caution. The weapon may actually be in the hands of an attacker (a grave danger), or simply in sight. Weapons include knives, guns, and martial arts weapons as well as any other items that may be used as weapons.
- *Signs of alcohol or other drug use.* When alcohol or other drugs are in use, a certain unpredictability exists at any scene. It will not take long for you to observe un-

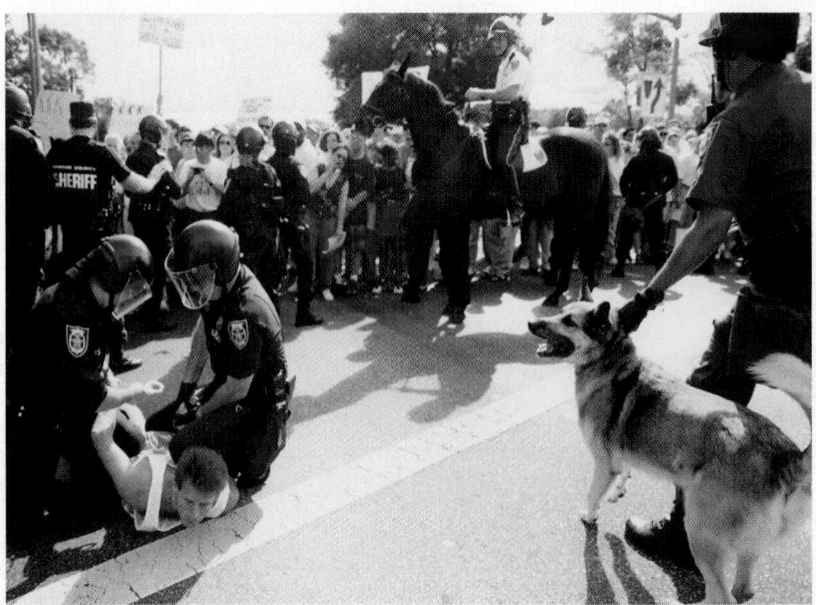

Figure 7-2 • Crowds are a potential source of violence. *(© Craig Jackson/In The Dark Photography)*

usual behavior from a person under the influence of one of these substances. This behavior may result in violence toward emergency personnel at the scene. Additionally, there are hazards associated with the drug culture, such as street violence and the presence of contaminated needles.

- *Unusual silence.* Emergencies are usually active events. A call that is "too quiet" should raise your suspicions. While there may be a good reason for the silence, extra care should be taken.
- *Knowledge of prior violence.* If you or a member of your crew has been to a particular location for calls involving violence in the past, extra caution must be used on subsequent calls to the same location. Neighbors may sometimes volunteer information about previous incidents.

Whether the call is residential or in the street, observe the scene for the signs of danger listed previously and any others you may find (Figure 7-3). This brief danger assessment may be all that is required to prevent harm to you or your crew during the call.

If you observe signs of danger, there are actions that you must take to protect yourself. You learned about these actions in Chapter 2, "The Well-Being of the EMT." To summarize: The specific actions you should take depend on many factors including your local protocols, the type of danger, and the help available to you. In general, you should retreat to a position of safety, call for help, and return only after the scene has been secured by police. Be sure to document the danger and your actions.

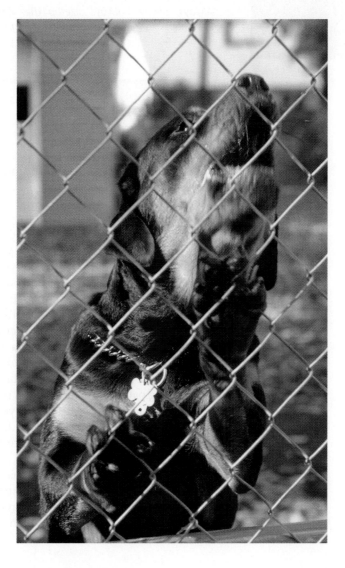

Figure 7-3 • Whether the call is to a residence or to the street, a variety of hazards may be present.

POINT OF VIEW

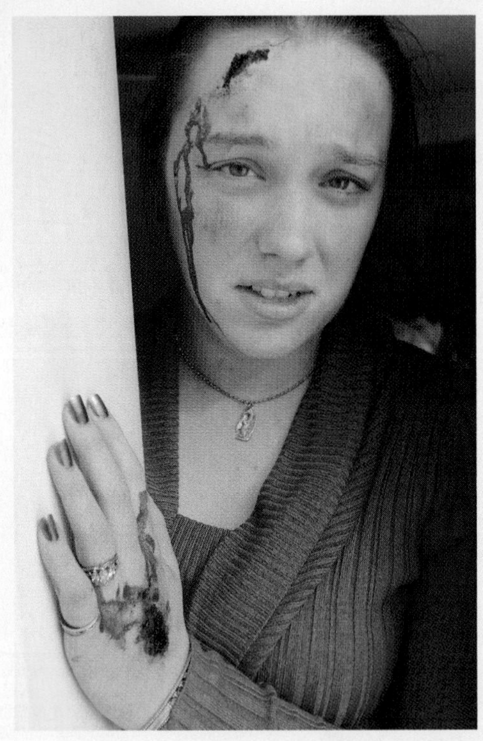

"I am still a relatively new EMT. Everyone always said you never know what you will find when you respond to a call. Well, I found out about this pretty early in my EMS career.

"My crew and I were sent to a 'fall' at a residence in a decent part of town. We pulled up to the house. Everything looked calm—but sometimes you just can't tell from the outside. We went to the door. We stood to the sides of the door like we were trained. We knocked. The woman came to the door and she looked like she had been through a war. I started to move like I was going into the house but she pushed the door closed a bit more and kind of peeked out. My first thought was to say, 'Come on. Let us in. We need to take care of you.' She put her weight behind the door and wouldn't let us in. Then it hit me. She didn't fall. Whatever had happened, she was trying to protect us.

"I asked her to step outside so we could talk but she refused. I motioned for my other crew members to get back to the rig and mouthed, 'Call for help.'

"I felt so helpless. I didn't want her to go back inside, but I was already on borrowed time and should be retreating. 'Come out here. Please!' I urged in a forced whisper. She looked behind her and then shut the door in my face.

"I moved rapidly to the rig, watching my back. We drove out of sight. Two police cruisers came by pretty quickly. I filled them in on what I saw. They went to the scene. About 5 minutes later the dispatcher radioed us to go back in. They had a man in handcuffs. The woman was crying. I'm still not sure whether she was crying because she was hurt or because he was arrested. The look in her eyes was so vacant.

"Always, always, always size-up the scene. I always wonder what would've happened if I wasn't cautious going to that call."

Standard Precautions

As you perform your initial size-up of the scene, there are many important points to consider. One very important aspect of personal protection—and one that you will need long after you have addressed any physical dangers—is Standard Precautions, also called body substance isolation (BSI).

You learned about Standard Precautions in Chapter 2, "The Well-Being of the EMT." To summarize: Body substances include blood, saliva, and any other body fluids or contents. All body substances can carry viruses and bacteria. Your patient's body substances can enter your body through cuts or other openings in your skin. They can also easily enter your body through your eyes, nose, and mouth. You are especially at risk of being infected by a patient's body substances when the patient is bleeding, coughing, or sneezing, or whenever you make direct contact with the patient, as in mouth-to-mouth ventilation. Infection is a two-way street, of course. Your patient can also be infected by you.

For example, at a vehicle collision that is likely to have caused severe injuries with bleeding, all personnel should wear protective gloves and eyewear. Since this potential hazard can be spotted before there is any contact with the patient, everyone should be wearing gloves before beginning patient care. If a patient requires suctioning or spits up blood, this would be another indication for protective eyewear and a mask. Whenever a patient is suspected of having tuberculosis or another disease spread through the air, wear an N-95 or high efficiency particulate air (HEPA) respirator to filter out airborne particles the patient exhales or expels.

A key element of Standard Precautions is always to have personal protective equipment readily available, either on your person or as the first items you encounter when opening a response kit. Remember that taking proper Standard Precautions early in the call and evaluating the need for such precautions throughout the call will prevent needless exposure later on.

SCAN 7-3 • Mechanism of Injury and Affected Areas of the Body

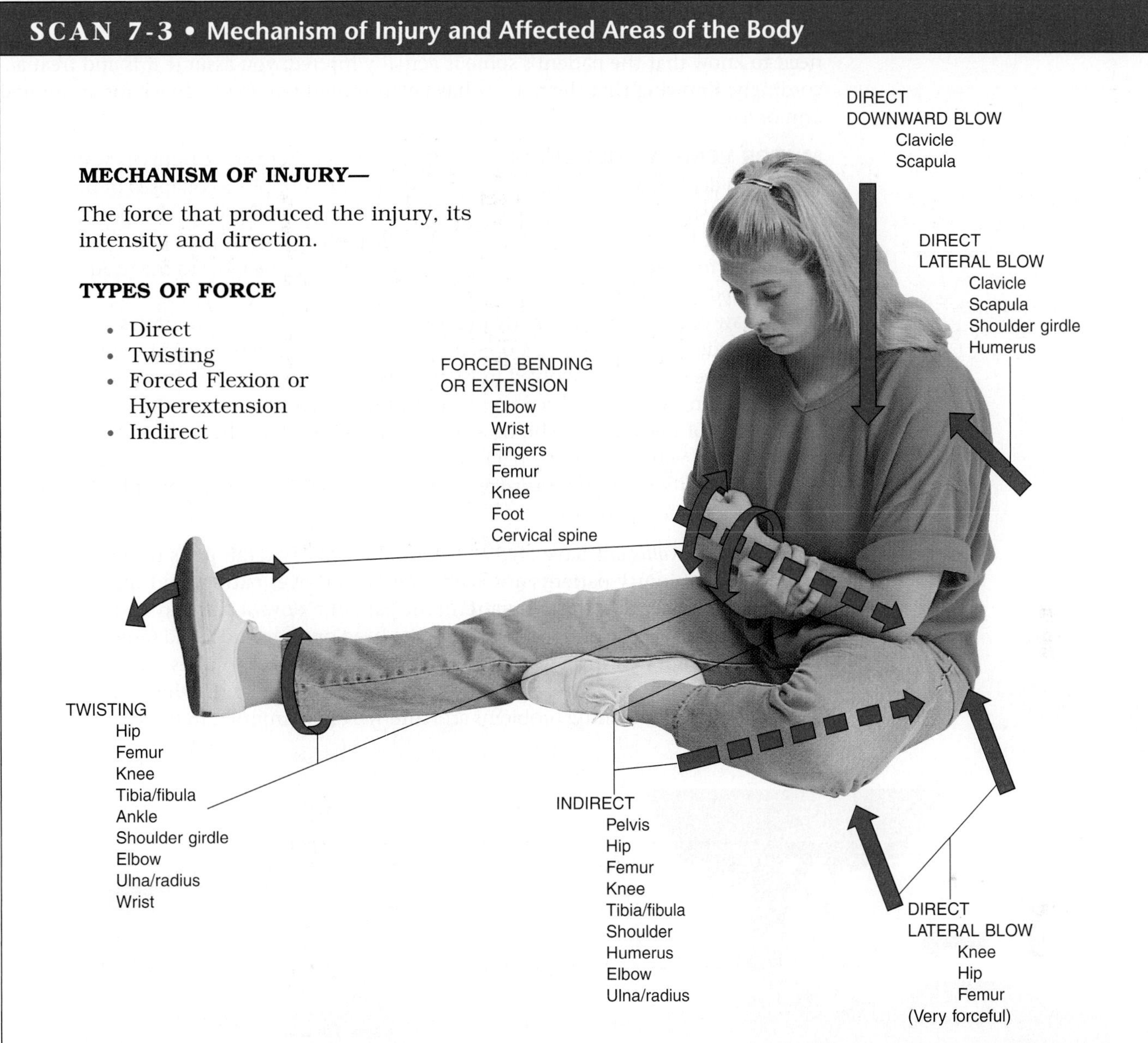

Nature of the Call

After you have ensured scene safety and taken the appropriate Standard Precautions, it is important to determine the nature of the call by identifying the mechanism of injury or the nature of the patient's illness.

Mechanism of Injury

The **mechanism of injury** is what causes an injury (for example, a rapid deceleration causes the knees to strike the dash of a car; a fall on ice causes a twisting force to the ankle) (Scan 7-3).

mechanism of injury a force or forces that may have caused injury.

Certain injuries are considered "common" to particular situations. Injuries to bones and joints are usually associated with falls and vehicle collisions; burns are common to fires and explosions; penetrating soft-tissue injuries can be associated with gunshot wounds, and so on.

Even if you cannot determine the exact injury the patient has sustained, knowing the mechanism of injury may allow you to predict various injury patterns. For example, in many situations you will immobilize the patient's spine because the mechanism of injury, such as a forceful blow, is frequently associated with spinal injury. You do not need to know that the patient's spine is actually injured; you assume it is and treat accordingly. Knowing that the patient has fallen should tell you to check for an injured arm or leg.

MOTOR VEHICLE COLLISIONS Identifying the mechanism of injury is very important when dealing with motor-vehicle collisions. For example, a collapsed or bent steering column suggests that the driver has suffered a chest-wall injury with possible rib or even lung or heart damage. A shattered, blood-spattered windshield points to the likelihood of a forehead or scalp laceration and possibly a severe blow to the head that may have caused a head or spinal injury.

The law of inertia—that a body in motion will remain in motion unless acted upon by an outside force (e.g., being stopped by striking something)—explains why there are actually three collisions involved in each motor-vehicle crash. The first collision is the vehicle striking an object. The second collision is when the body of the patient strikes the interior of the vehicle. The third collision occurs when the organs of the patient strike surfaces within the body (Figure 7-4).

Identifying the type of motor-vehicle collision also provides important information on potential injury patterns:

- *Head-on collisions* have a great potential for injury to all parts of the body. Two types of injury patterns are likely: the up-and-over pattern and the down-and-under pattern. In the first pattern, the patient follows a pathway up and over the steering wheel, commonly striking the head on the windshield (especially when he was not wearing a seat belt), causing head and neck injuries. Additionally, the patient may strike the chest and abdomen on the steering wheel, causing chest injuries or breathing problems and internal organ injuries. In the second pattern,

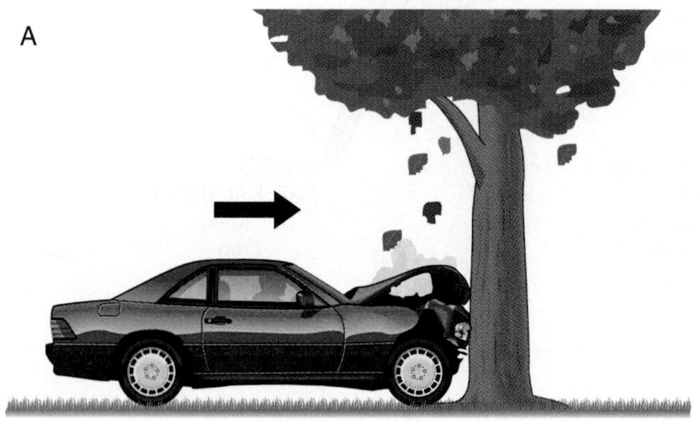

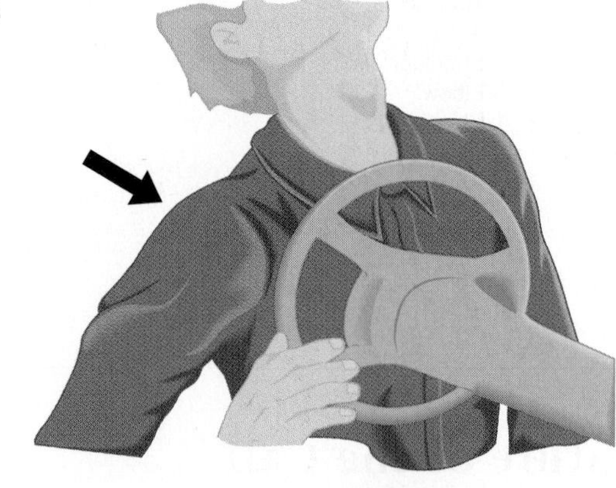

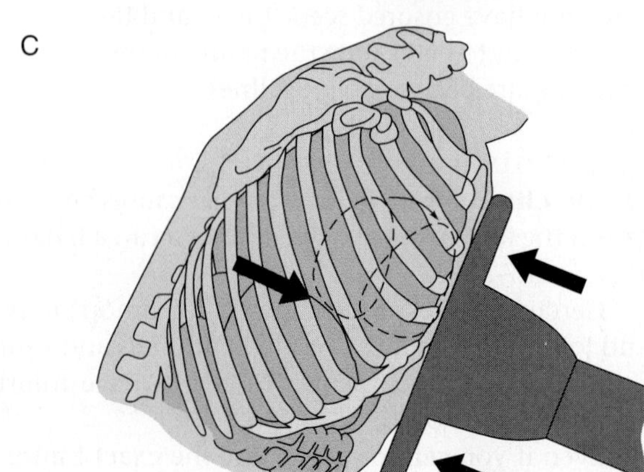

Figure 7-4 • There are three collisions in a motor-vehicle crash: (A) a vehicle collision, when the vehicle strikes an object; (B) a body collision, when the person's body strikes the interior of the vehicle; and (C) an organ collision, when the person's organs strike interior surfaces of the body.

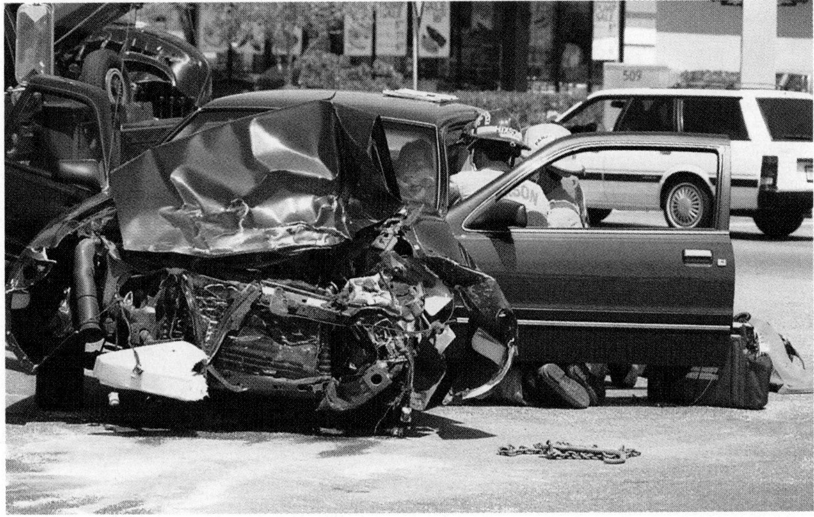

Figure 7-5 • A head-on impact. *(© Eddie M. Sperling)*

the patient's body follows a pathway down and under the steering wheel, typically striking his knees on the dash, causing knee, leg, and hip injuries (Figures 7-5 and 7-6).

- *Rear-end collisions* are common causes of neck and head injuries. The law of inertia states not only that a body in motion will remain in motion unless acted on by an outside force (as discussed earlier), but also that a body at rest will remain at rest unless acted on by an outside force (such as being pushed or jerked). This explains why neck injuries are common in a rear-end collision—the head remains still as the body is pushed violently forward by the seat back, extending the neck backward, if a headrest was not properly placed behind the head (Figures 7-7 and 7-8).
- *Side-impact collisions* (broadside, or "T-Bone") have other injury patterns. The head tends to remain still as the body is pushed laterally, causing injuries to the neck. The head, chest, abdomen, pelvis, and thighs may be struck directly, causing skeletal and internal injuries (Figures 7-9 and 7-10).
- *Rollover collisions* are potentially the most serious because of the potential for multiple impacts. Rollover collisions frequently cause ejection of anyone who is not wearing a seat belt. Expect any type of serious injury pattern (Figures 7-11 and 7-12).

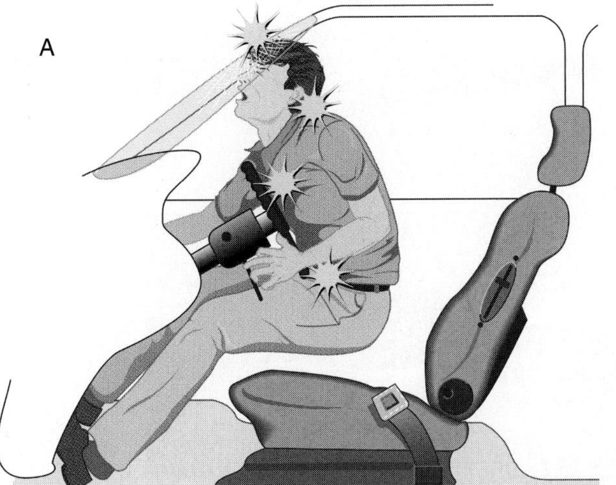

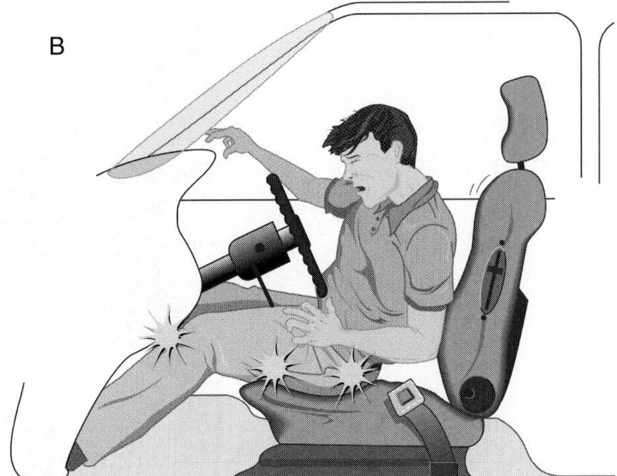

Figure 7-6 • In a head-on collision, an unrestrained person is likely to travel in (A) an up-and-over pathway causing head, neck, chest, and abdominal injuries or in (B) a down-and-under pathway causing hip, knee, and leg injuries.

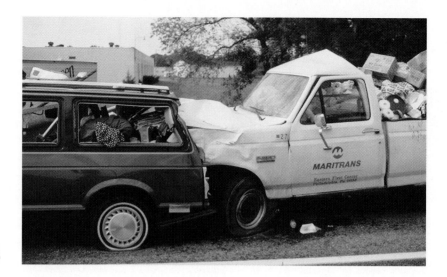

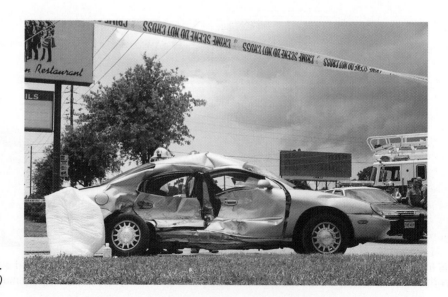

Figure 7-7 • Rear impact.
(© Robert J. Bennet)

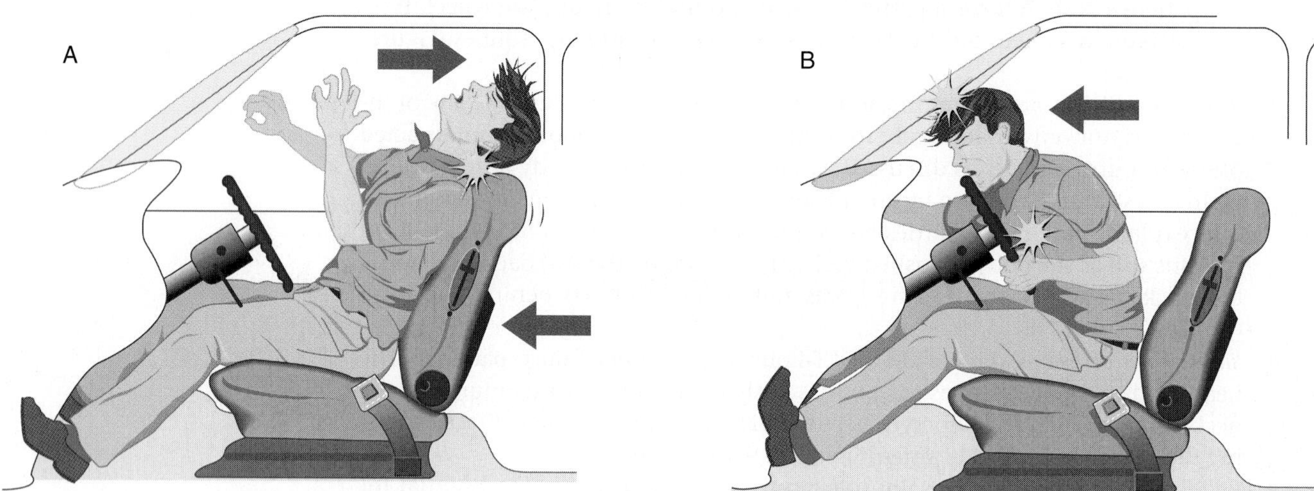

Figure 7-8 • In a rear-end collision, the unrestrained person's head is jerked violently (A) backward and then (B) forward, causing neck, head, and chest injuries.

Figure 7-9 • Side impact.
(© Eddie M. Sperling)

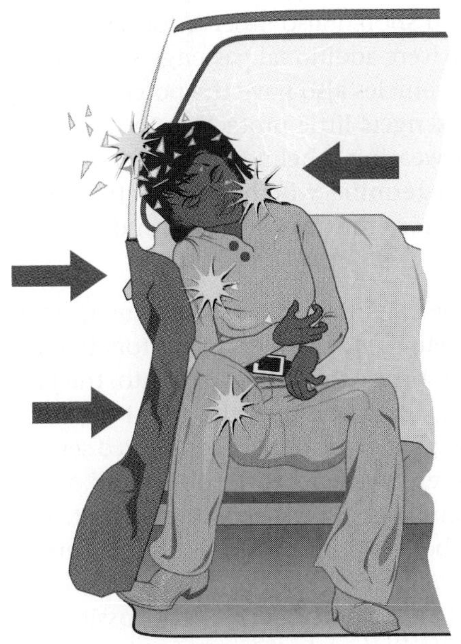

Figure 7-10 • A side-impact collision may cause head and neck injuries as well as injuries to the chest, abdomen, pelvis, and thighs.

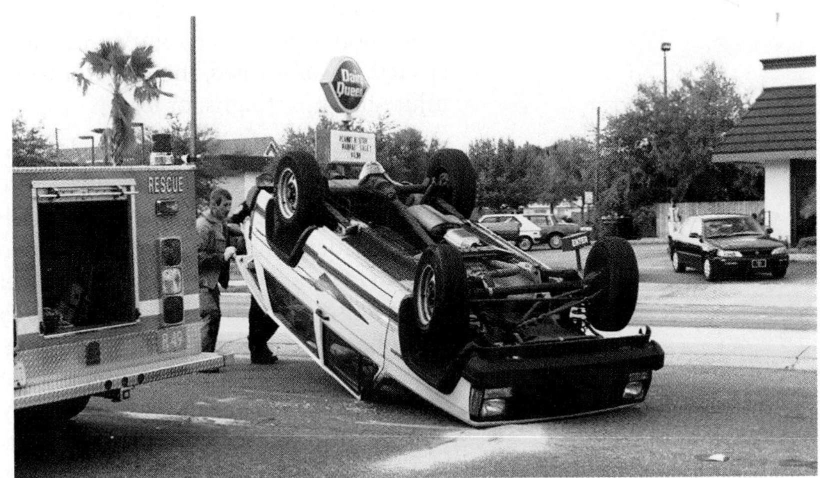

Figure 7-11 • Rollover collision. *(© Eddie M. Sperling)*

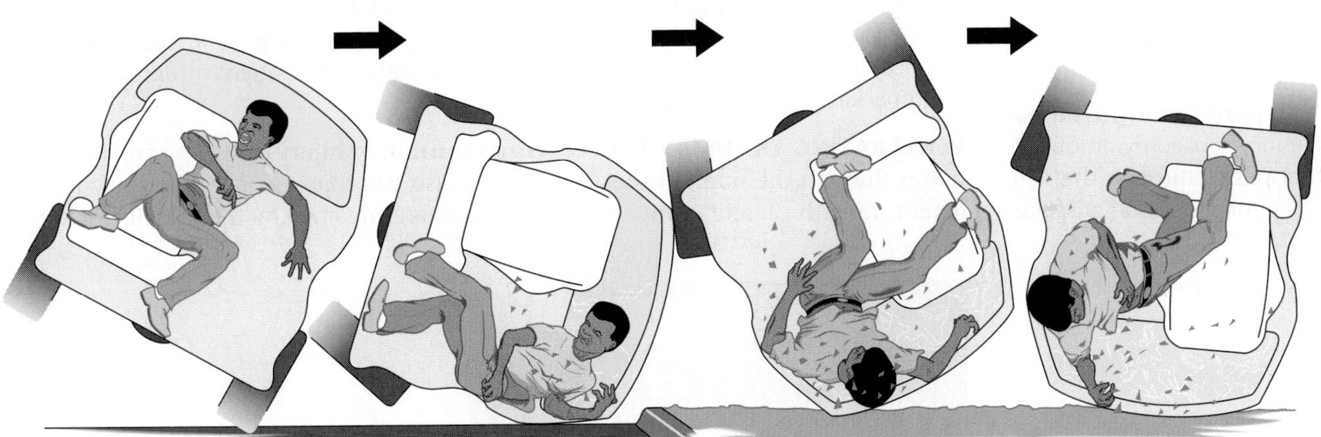

Figure 7-12 • In a rollover collision, the unrestrained person will suffer multiple impacts and possible multiple injuries.

- *Rotational impact collisions* involve cars that are struck, then spin. The initial impact often causes subsequent impacts (the spinning vehicle strikes another vehicle or a tree). As in a rollover collision, this can cause multiple injury patterns.

An important aspect of mechanism of injury determination is to find out where the patient was sitting in the vehicle and if he was wearing lap and shoulder belts. Note any deformities in the steering wheel, dash, pedals, or other structures within the vehicle.

You will often be able to observe important clues regarding mechanism of injury before you even exit the ambulance. At a head-on collision, for instance, you can anticipate up-and-over or down-and-under injury patterns for a driver who remains in his car and multiple injury patterns for a driver who is thrown from his car. For both patients, anticipate external injuries (from the collision of the body with auto interiors and pavement) and internal injuries (from collision of organs with the interior of the body as well as from external blunt-force or penetrating trauma). When a patient appears to have been the driver of a vehicle, look for damage to the windshield, steering wheel, dash, and pedals when you are able to do a close-up inspection. You should also observe for damage to other interior surfaces, which might indicate there were additional passengers/patients.

Injuries involving motorcycles and all-terrain vehicles also have the potential to be serious. These vehicles offer the operator and passengers little protection in the event of collision. Determine whether the patient was wearing a helmet that offered some protection from head injury. Also attempt to determine whether the patient was ejected. In some cases, the operator will be thrown from the bike and strike and severely injure his hips, thighs, or legs.

FALLS Falls are another cause of injury where the extent and pattern of damage may be determined by the characteristics of the fall (Figure 7-13). Important factors to consider are the height from which the patient fell, the surface the patient fell onto, the part of the patient that hit the ground, and anything that interrupts the fall. Falls from heights of greater than three times the height of the patient are usually considered severe.

In falls, injury to the part of the body that comes in contact with the ground or another hard surface is only the beginning of the trauma experienced by the patient. The force is also transmitted to adjoining parts of the body. For example, think of a person who dives head first into a shallow body of water and strikes his head. While the head will be injured, the force travels on to the cervical and thoracic spine, very possibly resulting in severe spinal cord injury and paralysis. Similarly, when a patient jumps from a height and lands squarely on his feet, there is trauma to the feet but also to the ankles, legs, and even the pelvis. Always assess along the path of the energy. It is likely that you will find additional injuries.

The general rule that a fall greater than three times the patient's height is considered to be a severe fall is a reasonable guideline, but it doesn't guarantee a resulting injury (or rule out injury if the fall is less than this distance). It is important to look at all factors at the scene in combination with the patient's complaint, vital signs, and your physical examination findings. When in doubt, assign the patient a high priority for rapid packaging and prompt transport.

penetrating trauma injury caused by an object that passes through the skin or other body tissues.

PENETRATING TRAUMA **Penetrating trauma,** or injury caused by an object that passes through the skin or other body tissue, also has characteristics that may help in determining the extent of injury. These wounds are classified by the velocity, or speed,

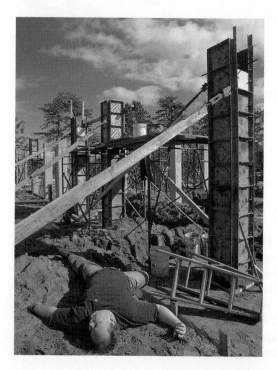

Figure 7-13 • The characteristics of a fall may provide valuable clues to a patient's injuries.

of the item that caused the injury. Low-velocity items are those that are propelled by hand, such as knives. Low-velocity injuries are usually limited to the area that was penetrated. Remember that there can be multiple wounds, or the blade may have been moved inside the patient, so there can be damage to multiple vital organs.

Medium-velocity wounds are usually caused by handguns and shotguns. Some forcefully propelled items such as an arrow launched from a compound bow or a ballistic knife will also cause greater velocities than the same items propelled by hand.

Bullets propelled by a high-powered or assault rifle are at a high velocity. Medium- and high-velocity injuries can cause damage almost anywhere in the body. Bullets cause damage in two ways (Figure 7-14):

- *Damage directly from the projectile.* The bullet itself will damage anything in its path. The damage depends on the size of the bullet, its path, or whether it fragments (breaks up into smaller projectiles), the fragments taking different paths. The path of the bullet once it is inside the body is unpredictable since it may be deflected by bone or other tissue onto a totally different course.
- *Pressure-related damage, or cavitation.* This means that the velocity of the bullet as it enters the body creates a pressure wave that causes a cavity considerably greater than the size of the bullet. This cavity is temporary, but it may damage items in its path.

BLUNT-FORCE TRAUMA **Blunt-force trauma** is injury caused by a blow that strikes the body but does not penetrate the skin or other body tissues (for example, when one is struck by a baseball bat or thrown against a steering wheel). The energy from a blunt-force blow will travel through the body, often causing serious injury to, even rupture of, internal organs and vessels. The resulting compromise of body functions, hemorrhage, or

blunt-force trauma injury caused by a blow that does not penetrate the skin or other body tissues.

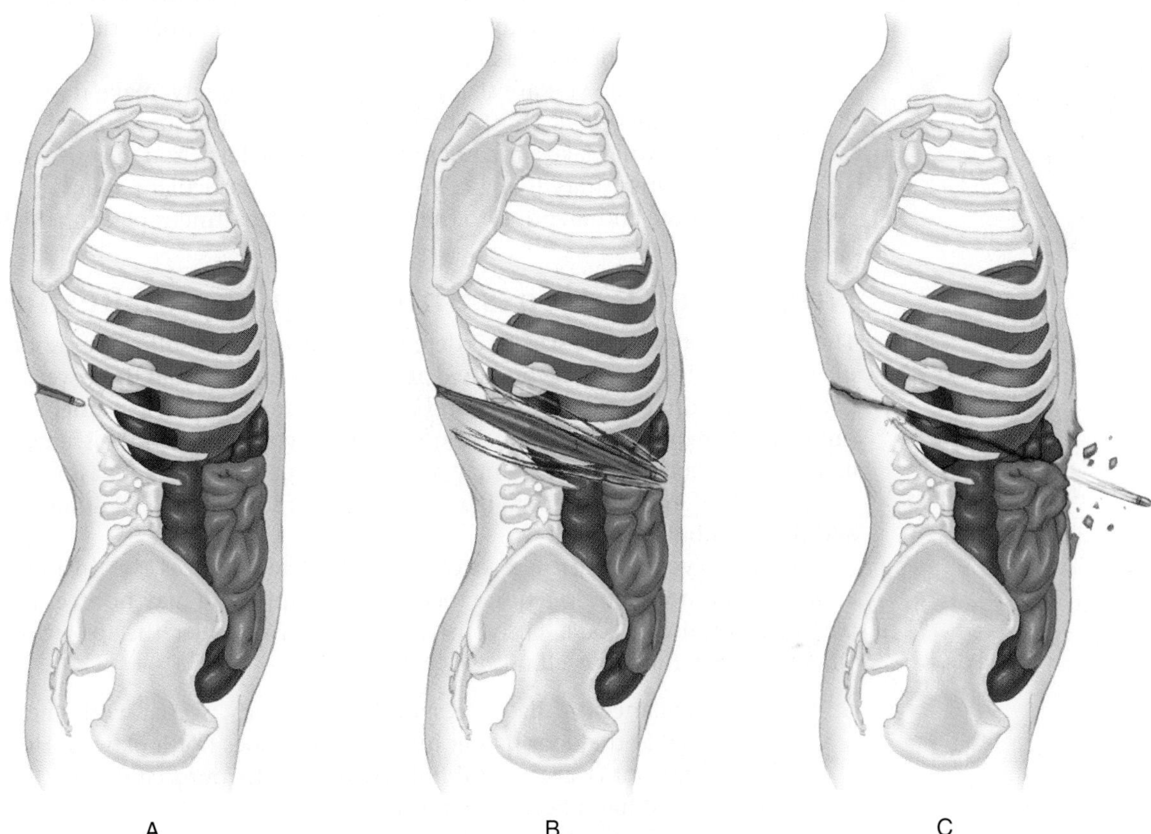

Figure 7-14 • Bullets cause damage in two ways: from the bullet itself (A and C above) and from cavitation, which is the temporary cavity caused by the pressure wave (B).

spillage of organ contents into the body cavity may have more severe consequences for the patient than a penetrating injury. Yet signs of blunt-force trauma are often subtle and easy to overlook. The skin may appear reddened at the site of the blow, but in the prehospital setting the bluish coloration characteristic of a bruise may not have had time to appear. Your main clue that such an injury may exist will often be the presence of a mechanism of injury that could have caused this kind of injury.

Identifying the mechanism of injury will help you, as an EMT, to determine what injuries are possible and to treat these injuries accordingly, even if signs and symptoms are not present. Never assume, based on the mechanism of injury, that there are no injuries. Even very minor collisions may cause injuries.

index of suspicion awareness that there may be injuries.

Maintain a high **index of suspicion**—a keen awareness that there may be injuries—based on the mechanism of injury. Remember to maintain neck and spine stabilization as patient assessment progresses.

Nature of the Illness

nature of the illness what is medically wrong with a patient.

Identifying the **nature of the illness** for a medical patient serves the same purpose as identifying the mechanism of injury for a trauma patient: finding out what is or what may be wrong with the patient. To begin identifying the nature of a patient's illness during the scene size-up, you must scan the entire scene. Information may be obtained from many sources:

- *The patient,* when conscious and oriented, is a prime source of information about his or her condition. Your dealings with the patient will continue throughout the assessment process.
- *Family members or bystanders* can also provide important information, especially for the unconscious patient. Even when the patient is conscious and able to tell you about his condition, however, always consider the information from others who are present. Patients who are disoriented or confused may provide information that is either partially true or even untrue. Use information from all sources to piece the patient assessment "puzzle" together.
- *The scene.* While you are sizing up the scene for safety, make note of other factors that may be clues to the patient's condition. You may observe medications, which you will make a mental note to examine later. You may be struck by dangerous or unsanitary living conditions for this particular patient. This is important to note and mention to the emergency department personnel later.

Number of Patients and Adequacy of Resources

The final part of the scene size-up is determining if you have sufficient resources to handle the call. If, for example, you noted at a two-car collision that there were at least two patients—one driver still in his car and the other thrown to the pavement—you would immediately request an additional ambulance. As you approach the scene, you should actively look for clues that there may be additional patients—other passengers or pedestrians involved in the collision (Figure 7-15)—and if so, you should immediately call for additional ambulances.

Sometimes you may discover a need for additional resources even in a situation that, at first, would not seem to require them. For example, you may not feel that a single-patient medical call could tax your resources, but consider the following scenarios where you may find yourself needing extra help:

- Your ambulance is called to respond to an elderly woman with chest pain. You are greeted at the door by her husband, who does not look well. He denies any complaints but is sweaty and holding his chest. Your first patient tells you that her husband has a heart condition.
- A single patient experiences back pain. This is usually not a reason for additional assistance, but this patient is immobilized on a backboard in a third-floor apartment (no elevator) and weighs 425 pounds.

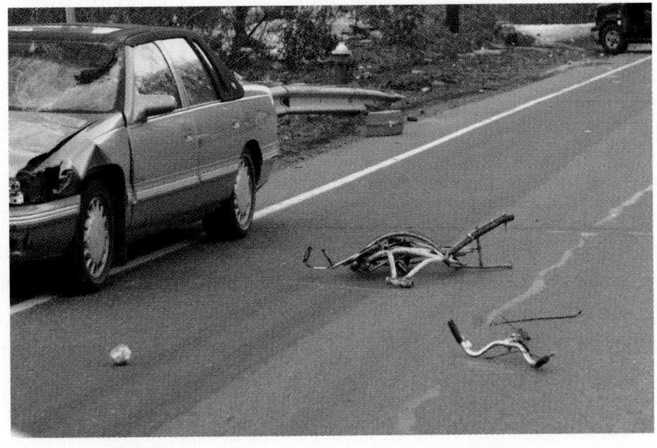

Figure 7-15 • Impact with a pedestrian or cyclist may produce characteristic damage to a vehicle. *(Mark C. Ide)*

- Your ambulance is called for "general weakness." Upon the arrival of you and your partner, two more persons in the same family develop the same flu-like symptoms. You appropriately suspect carbon monoxide poisoning, since they admit that they have been having furnace problems.

In each of these situations, what appeared to be a routine one-patient call actually turned out to be more. An important part of scene size-up is to recognize these situations and call for help immediately. As the call progresses and you get more involved in patient care, it is less likely that you will remember to call for the additional help. It may also be too late when the help arrives if you do not call immediately.

Your response can range from simply calling for another ambulance to care for the ill husband in the first situation, or extra personnel to help move the 425-pound man in the second, to activating a multiple-casualty incident for the family with carbon monoxide poisoning. (You will learn about multiple-casualty incidents in Chapter 36, "Special Operations.") Try to anticipate the maximum numbers of patients and radio for help accordingly. Follow local protocols.

CRITICAL DECISION MAKING:
DETERMINING AREAS OF CONCERN AT THE SCENE

The scene size-up is a vital part of any call. For each of the following scenes determine a few areas of concern you would want to check before proceeding to the patient. Remember each of the components of the scene size-up. You shouldn't try to think of every possibility, only the most likely ones. Practice the critical thinking process of evaluating a scene—something you will do on every call.

1. An 18-wheeler with an enclosed trailer slid off the road into a ditch in an ice storm. The vehicle is in the ditch, leaning to the right.
2. A van and a passenger car collided on an interstate highway.
3. You arrive at an office building and see people running out the front and side doors in a panic. One person appears bloody and is running toward your ambulance.
4. You respond to a residence with the fire department and arrive on scene first. A resident meets you at the end of the driveway and tells you there is a strong smell of natural gas in his house.
5. You respond to a construction site for a fall.

CHAPTER REVIEW

SUMMARY

Scene size-up is the first part of the patient assessment process. It is important during scene size-up to determine what, if any, threats there may be to your own safety and to the safety of others at the scene and to take appropriate Standard Precautions. Next, it is important to determine the nature of the call by identifying the mechanism of injury or the nature of the patient's illness. Finally, you must take into account the number of patients and other factors at the scene to determine if you will need additional help.

KEY TERMS

blunt-force trauma injury caused by a blow that does not penetrate the skin or other body tissues.

danger zone the area around the wreckage of a vehicle collision or other incident within which special safety precautions should be taken.

index of suspicion awareness that there may be injuries.

mechanism of injury a force or forces that may have caused injury.

nature of the illness what is medically wrong with a patient.

penetrating trauma injury caused by an object that passes through the skin or other body tissues.

scene size-up steps taken by an ambulance crew when approaching the scene of an emergency call: checking scene safety, taking Standard Precautions, noting the mechanism of injury or nature of the patient's illness, determining the number of patients, and deciding what, if any, additional resources to call for.

REVIEW QUESTIONS

1. For each of the following dangers, describe actions that must be taken to remain safe at a collision scene. (pp. 191–192)
   - Leaking gasoline
   - Toxic or hazardous material spill
   - Vehicle on fire
   - Downed power lines
2. List several indicators of violence or potential violence at an emergency scene. (pp. 194–195)
3. Describe several situations where it is appropriate to wear disposable gloves. Describe situations where you would additionally wear protective eyewear and mask. Describe situations where you would wear an N-95 or HEPA respirator. (p. 196)
4. Describe common mechanism-of-injury patterns. (pp. 197–204)
5. List sources of information about the nature of a patient's illness. (p. 204)
6. List several medical and trauma situations where you may require additional assistance. (pp. 204–205)

CRITICAL THINKING

- You are called to the scene of a shooting at a fast food restaurant. En route, you plan your scene size-up strategy. What actions do you anticipate taking on arrival?

MEDIA RESOURCES

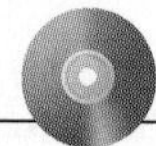

See the Student CD at the back of this book for quizzes, a case study activity, and other features related to this chapter. In particular, try your hand at the Scene Size-Up activity. Also, visit the Companion Website for *Emergency Care* at **www.prenhall.com/limmer**, where you will find additional reinforcement and links to other resources.

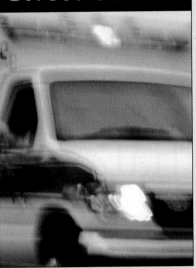

Street Scenes

It is the middle of the night, and you are hoping to get a few hours of sleep. You are just getting relaxed when the monitor activates. "Ambulances Bravo 5 and Delta 2 with heavy rescue to the Avenue A off-ramp for Interstate 55 to the report of a two-vehicle crash."

You are the first EMS responder to arrive, and as you approach the scene, you see both vehicles: one a passenger vehicle, the other a truck with a placard. As you do a scene size-up, you try to get the "big picture." You are concerend about where to stage your ambulance because of traffic, safety of crews, possible gasoline leaking, and not knowing what the placard on the truck identifies. You notify the dispatcher that you are on the scene and request that the Highway Patrol be notified for traffic-control assistance. You find a location upwind about 100 yards from the scene. You place warning markers and flares to alert traffic and to mark the staging area for other responding units. You are putting on your turnout gear with helmet, goggles, and gloves, including a reflective vest, when heavy rescue arrives. You talk with the captain, and he tells you that his crew will stabilize the vehicles and handle the battery disconnects and gasoline leaks. You point out the placard that needs to be checked out.

Street Scene Questions

1. What other scene size-up issues are left to consider?
2. Is this scene now safe or do other precautions need to be taken?
3. What Standard Precautions should be considered?

The crew from heavy rescue approaches the scene, stabilizes the vehicles, and then motions you forward. The Highway Patrol has closed off traffic and the captain from heavy rescue tells you that there is no hazardous material concern. On scene you determine that the drivers were the only occupants of the vehicles. You check one patient and, at the same time, your partner checks the other. Your patient has significant facial cuts and bruises and complains of leg pain. You realize that the extrication gloves you are wearing will not provide the proper Standard Precautions, so you put proper disposable gloves on immediately. After you try unsuccessfully to open the driver's side door next to your patient, you realize that he will require heavy rescue. The captain has already alerted his crew, and they are almost ready to use pry tools. You learn that your partner's patient is conscious and alert with no specific complaints.

Street Scene Questions

4. When the second ambulance arrives, where should it be located in relation to the collision scene?
5. What precautions should you take to protect the patients from any further harm while they are being extricated from the vehicle?
6. How should you plan to make sure that you can safely get the patient from the scene to the ambulance?

As heavy rescue finishes getting their tools ready, you set a protective cloth over your patient. You explain what is being done and stay next to him for reassurance. While this is going on, the second ambulance arrives, parks close to the second collision vehicle, and takes over patient care. Your ambulance is relatively far away, so you ask your partner to bring it closer to prevent having to carry your patient a long distance. This makes packaging the patient for transport safer and easier. The remainder of the call is uneventful, with both patients transported safely to the hospital emergency department.

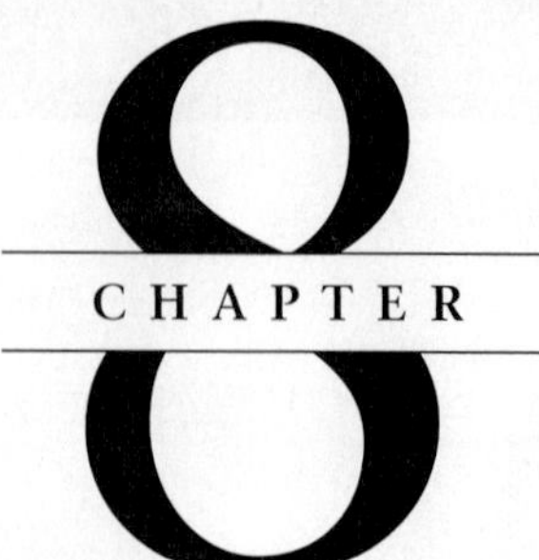

CHAPTER 8

The Initial Assessment

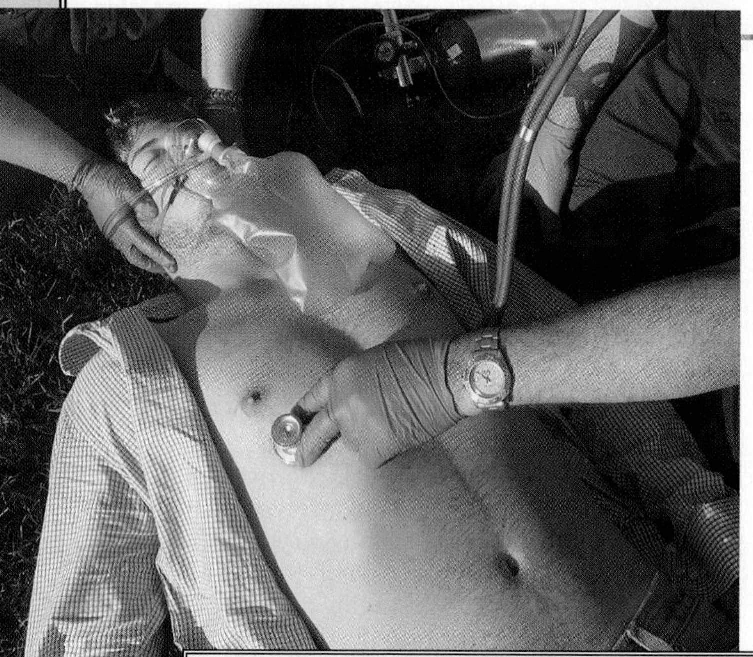

CORE CONCEPTS

The following are core concepts that will be addressed in this chapter:

- The general impression
- Manual stabilization of the spine
- Assessment of mental status using the AVPU scale
- The ABCs as part of the assessment process
- How to make a priority decision

KEY TERMS

ABCs, p. 214
AVPU, p. 213
chief complaint, p. 210
general impression, p. 210
initial assessment, p. 210
interventions, p. 210
mental status, p. 213
priority, p. 215

DOT OBJECTIVES

*KNOWLEDGE AND ATTITUDE

3-2.1 Summarize the reasons for forming a general impression of the patient. (pp. 210, 212)

3-2.2 Discuss methods of assessing altered mental status. (pp. 213–214)

3-2.3 Differentiate between assessing the altered mental status in the adult, child, and infant patient. (pp. 213–214, 216, 219, 221)

3-2.4 Discuss methods of assessing the airway in the adult, child, and infant patient. (pp. 214, 216, 219, 221)

3-2.5 State reasons for management of the cervical spine once the patient has been determined to be a trauma patient. (p. 209) (Scan 8-1, p. 211)

3-2.6 Describe methods used for assessing if a patient is breathing. (pp. 214, 216, 219, 221)

3-2.7 State what care should be provided to the adult, child, and infant patient with adequate breathing. (pp. 214, 216, 219, 221)

3-2.8 State what care should be provided to the adult, child, and infant patient without adequate breathing. (pp. 214, 216, 219, 221)

3-2.9 Differentiate between a patient with adequate and inadequate breathing. (pp. 214, 216)

3-2.10 Distinguish between methods of assessing breathing in the adult, child, and infant patient. (pp. 214, 216, 219, 221)

3-2.11 Compare the methods of providing airway care to the adult, child, and infant patient. (pp. 214, 216, 219, 221)

3-2.12 Describe the methods used to obtain a pulse. (pp. 214, 216, 221)

3-2.13 Differentiate between obtaining a pulse in an adult, child, and infant patient. (pp. 214, 216, 221)

3-2.14 Discuss the need for assessing the patient for external bleeding. (pp. 215, 216, 221)

3-2.15 Describe normal and abnormal findings when assessing skin color. (pp. 214, 216)

3-2.16 Describe normal and abnormal findings when assessing skin temperature. (pp. 214, 216)

3-2.17 Describe normal and abnormal findings when assessing skin condition. (pp. 214, 216)

3-2.18 Describe normal and abnormal findings when assessing skin capillary refill in the infant and child patient. (pp. 216, 219, 221)

3-2.19 Explain the reason for prioritizing a patient for care and transport. (p. 215)

3-2.20 Explain the importance of forming a general impression of the patient. (pp. 210, 212)

3-2.21 Explain the value of performing an initial assessment. (p. 210) (Scan 8-2, pp. 212–213)

*SKILLS

3-2.22 Demonstrate the techniques for assessing mental status.

3-2.23 Demonstrate the techniques for assessing the airway.

3-2.24 Demonstrate the techniques for assessing if the patient is breathing.

3-2.25 Demonstrate the techniques for assessing if the patient has a pulse.

3-2.26 Demonstrate the techniques for assessing the patient for external bleeding.

3-2.27 Demonstrate the techniques for assessing the patient's skin color, temperature, condition, and capillary refill (infants and children only).

3-2.28 Demonstrate the ability to prioritize patients.

For further information on these objectives

Objectives 3-2.4, 6, 7, 8, 9, 10, 11 (airway/breathing)
Objectives 3-2.12, 13 (pulse)
Objective 3-2.14 (external bleeding)
Objectives 3-2.15, 16, 17, 18 (skin/shock)
Objectives 3-2.3, 4, 7, 8, 10, 11, 13, 18 (infants/children)

See these chapters

Chapter 6 "Airway Management"
Chapter 9 "Vital Signs and SAMPLE History"
Chapter 26 "Bleeding and Shock"
Chapter 31 "Infants and Children"

Usually, you will take the time to do a thorough assessment (patient evaluation), transporting your patient to the hospital only after the complete assessment is finished. But if the patient has an immediately life-threatening problem—such as a blocked airway, a stoppage of breathing or heartbeat, or severe bleeding—you must provide emergency care immediately and consider the need to transport the patient without delay. One intervention for any patient with possible spine injury is to apply manual stabilization of the head and spine.

THE INITIAL ASSESSMENT

initial assessment
the first element in assessment of a patient; steps taken for the purpose of discovering and dealing with any life-threatening problems. The six parts of initial assessment are: forming a general impression, assessing mental status, assessing airway, assessing breathing, assessing circulation, and determining the priority of the patient for treatment and transport to the hospital. Also called *primary assessment* or *primary survey.*

The assessment steps to discover and treat any life-threatening problems are called the **initial assessment.** You may also hear EMTs refer to it as the *primary assessment* or *primary survey*. It is always the first element in the total assessment of the patient. The initial assessment has six parts: forming a general impression, assessing mental status (and manually stabilizing the patient's head and neck, when appropriate—Scan 8-1), assessing airway, assessing breathing, assessing circulation (and correcting any immediately life-threatening problems as soon as they were found), and determining patient priority (Scan 8-2).

NOTE

If during the initial assessment you discover any life-threatening condition, you must immediately perform the appropriate **interventions** *(actions to correct those problems).*

interventions
actions taken to correct a patient's problems.

general impression
impression of the patient's condition that is formed on first approaching the patient, based on the patient's environment, chief complaint, and appearance.

chief complaint
in emergency medicine, the reason EMS was called, usually in the patient's own words.

Form a General Impression

Forming a **general impression** helps you to determine how serious the patient's condition is and to set priorities for care and transport. It is based on your immediate assessment of the environment and the patient's chief complaint and appearance (Figure 8-1).

The environment can provide a great deal of information about the patient. It frequently gives clues—to the EMT who looks for them—about the patient's condition and history. One of the most important things it can sometimes tell you is what happened. Is there an overturned ladder, indicating that the patient may have fallen? Has the patient been exposed to a cold outdoor environment for a long time? Or is there no apparent mechanism of injury, leading you to presume that the patient has a medical problem rather than trauma (an injury)? Although the EMT cannot rely completely on the patient's environment to rule out trauma, when combined with the chief complaint (e.g., the patient complaining of symptoms that sound more like a medical problem than an injury), environmental clues become extremely useful.

The **chief complaint** is the reason EMS was called, usually in the patient's own words. It may be as obvious as abdominal pain or as vague as "not feeling good." In any case, it is the patient's description of why you were called.

You form a general impression by looking, listening, and smelling. You look for the patient's age and sex—which are easy to determine once the patient is in sight. You look at the patient's position to see if it indicates an injury, pain, or difficulty in breathing. You listen for sounds like moaning, snoring, or gurgling respirations. You sniff the air to detect any smells like hazardous fumes, urine, feces, vomitus, or decay.

Something that is more difficult to describe than your direct observations but just as important is the feeling or sense you get when you arrive at the scene or encounter

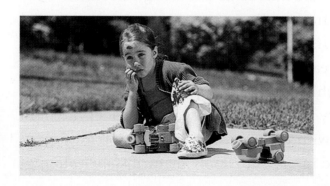

Figure 8-1 • Forming a general impression includes your immediate assessment of the environment and the patient's chief complaint and appearance.

SCAN 8-1 • Manual Stabilization of the Head and Neck

You should apply manual stabilization on first contact with any patient you suspect may have an injury to the spine based on mechanism of injury, or history, or signs and symptoms—that is, to virtually any trauma patient.

When you apply manual stabilization, your object is to hold the patient's head still in a neutral, in-line position. That is, the head should be facing forward and not turned to either side not tilted forward or backward. You must be careful not to pull or twist the patient's head but rather to hold it perfectly still and to remind the patient not to try to move it.

If your patient is in another position (for example, crumpled on his side) or is being moved by other EMS personnel, adapt the technique to the best of your ability to hold the head in a steady position in line with the spine. Some EMS systems have specific guidelines for when to use and when not to use spine immobilization. If this is the case in the system where you work, you should familiarize yourself with the local protocols and follow them.

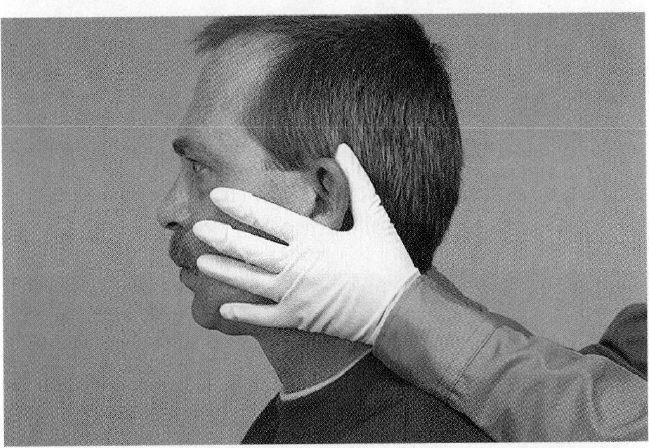

1. When your patient is sitting up, position yourself just behind the patient and hold the head by spreading your fingers over the sides of the head and placing your thumbs behind the ears.

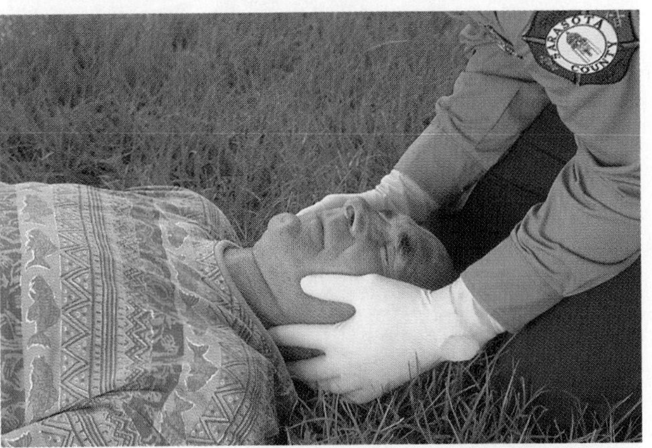

2. When your patient is supine, kneel behind the patient and spread your fingers and thumbs around the sides of the head to hold it steady.

Cultural Considerations

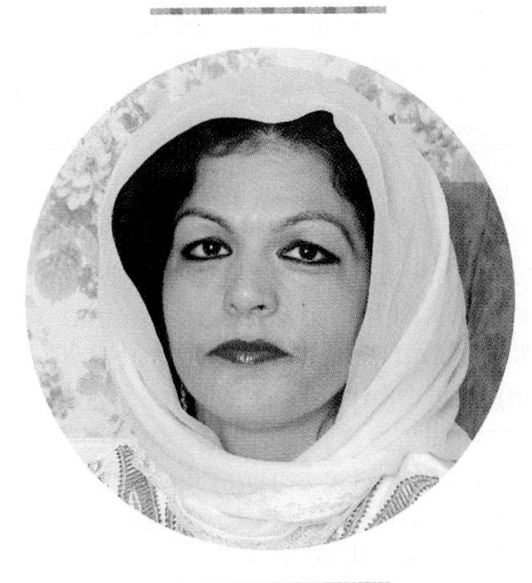

The woman of Afghani origin pictured here, if she were your patient, would share the sensibilities of the majority of Muslim women. Modesty is not only a personal choice, it is a religious obligation for women who practice Islam or are from Islamic cultures. Some Muslim women, when in public, wear head-to-toe coverings that conceal their entire bodies including their faces. Others may show their faces in public but must cover their hair. Even Muslim women who have adopted Western customs and styles of dress may retain a deep sense of modesty that forbids their being touched or their bodies seen by men other than their husbands.

When your patient is a Muslim woman, the assessment should be conducted by a female EMT with care taken to shield the patient from the view of others.

As always, consent to begin assessment and care must be given by the awake and competent patient. When the patient is a Muslim woman, this requirement is even more critical. If possible, there should be witnesses to the consent. Be sure to request consent in very clear language and be sure consent is clearly given. If practical and the patient's condition allows, explain what will be done at every step and allow a moment to be sure the patient agrees to the procedure.

SCAN 8-2 • Performing an Initial Assessment

FIRST TAKE STANDARD PRECAUTIONS

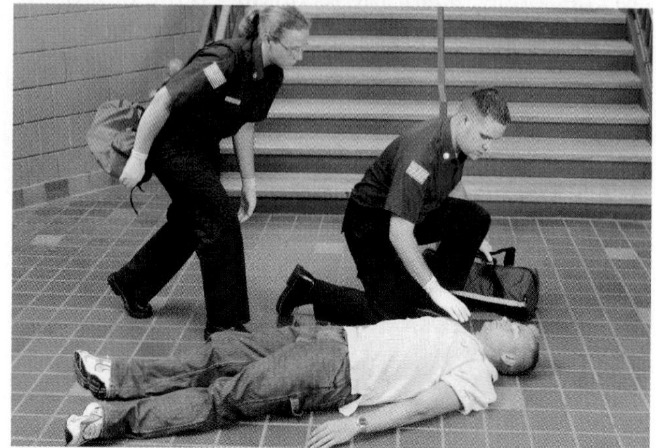

1. Form a general impression of the patient and patient's environment.

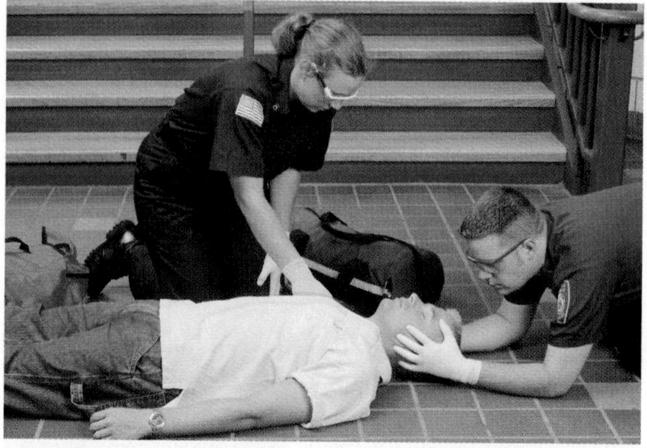

2. Assess patient's mental status. (Intervention: maintain spinal stabilization.)

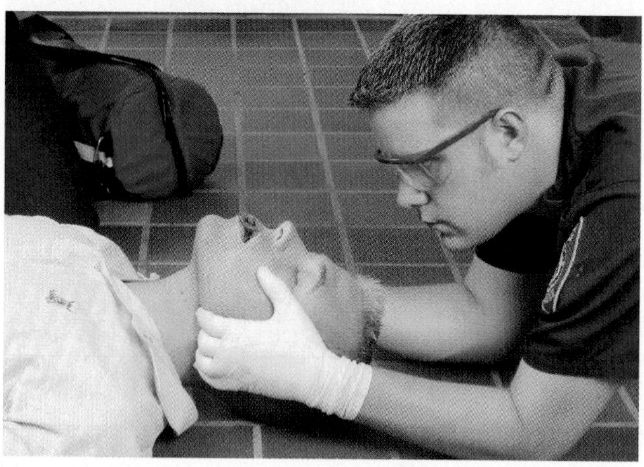

3. Assess airway. (Intervention: Perform appropriate maneuver to open and maintain the airway. If necessary, insert oro- or nasopharyngeal airway.)

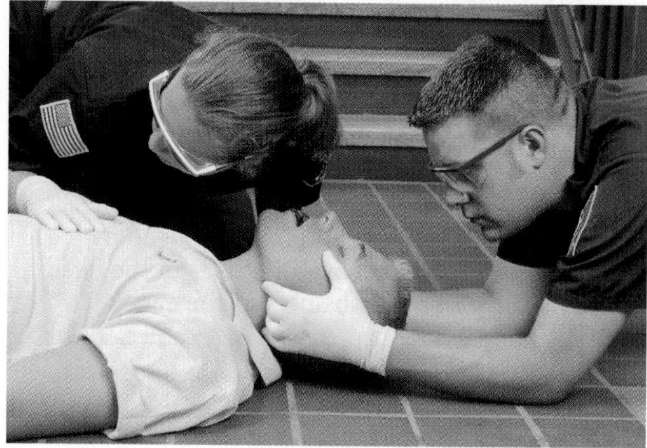

4. Assess breathing. (Interventions: If respiratory arrest or inadequate breathing, ventilate with 100 percent oxygen. If breathing above 24/min, give high-concentration oxygen.)

the patient. You may become anxious when you see a patient who exhibits no outward signs of illness or injury, yet "just doesn't look right" to you. Or you may feel reassured when you are dispatched to a "sick baby," but see that the infant is alert and smiling. After you gain some practice assessing and managing patients, you may develop a "sixth sense" that clues you in to the severity of a patient's condition. This is part of what is called "clinical judgment," or judgment based on experience in observing and treating patients. Some people find it easier than others to cultivate this ability, but even those who have excellent clinical judgment do not depend on it alone. A systematic approach to finding threats to life is the best way to make sure they are not missed.

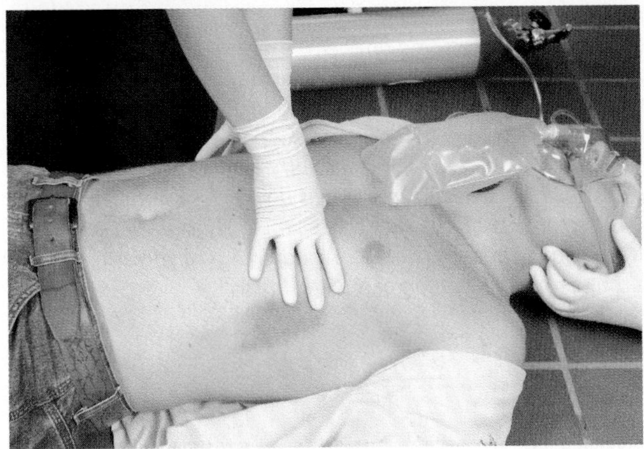

5. Assess for any life-threatening injury. (Interventions as necessary to correct the problem.)

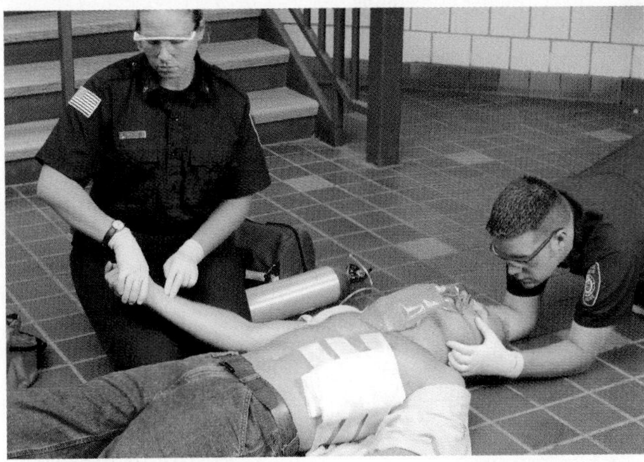

6. Evaluate circulation by taking the patient's pulse and evaluating skin temperature, color, and condition, and assess for bleeding. (Intervention: Control severe bleeding.)

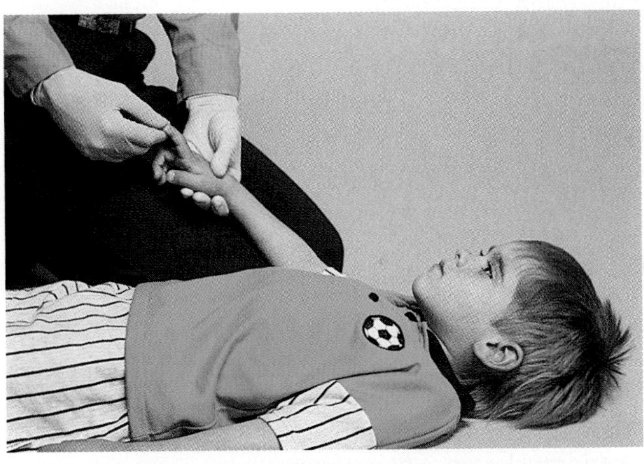

. . . In infants and young children, also assess circulation by testing capillary refill. (Interventions: For indications of poor circulation, treat for shock. If no pulse, perform CPR.)

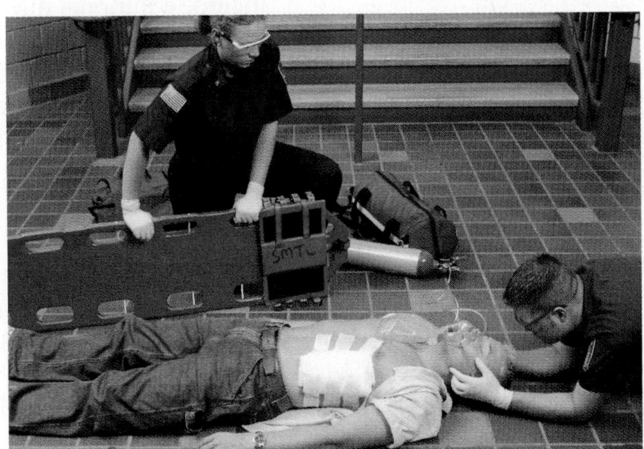

7. Make a decision about the patient's priority for further assessment, interventions, or immediate transport.

Assess Mental Status

Determining the **mental status,** or level of responsiveness, will usually be easy, since most patients are alert and responsive; that is, they are awake and will talk and answer questions sensibly. Some are not awake but will respond to verbal stimuli, such as talking or shouting. At a lower level of responsiveness, the patient will respond only to painful stimuli, such as pinching a toe or rubbing the sternum briskly. The lowest and most serious status is unresponsiveness, when the patient will not respond even to a painful stimulus. An easy way to keep these levels of responsiveness in mind is by remembering the letters **AVPU,** for *alert, verbal response, painful response,* and *unresponsive.*

mental status
level of responsiveness.

AVPU
a memory aid for classifying a patient's level of responsiveness, or mental status. The letters stand for alert, verbal response, painful response, unresponsive.

POINT OF VIEW

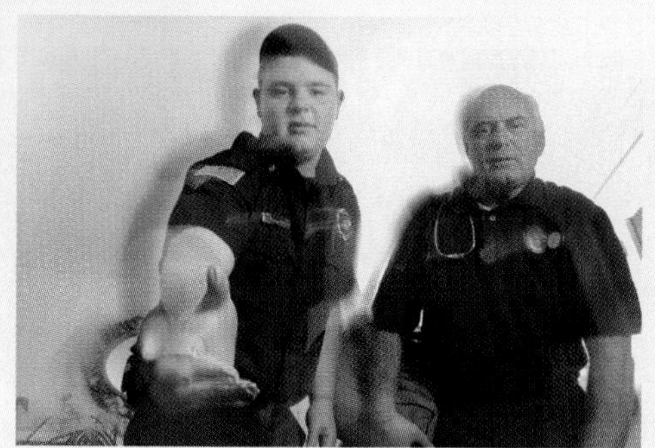

"I thought I'd just lay down for a nap. I wasn't feeling that well. Most everything from then on is really a blur. I remember my wife trying to wake me up. I can't even tell you how much time had passed.

"The next thing I knew here were these two big guys standing over me in dark clothes. I had a hard time focusing on them ... or even hearing them. I know this sounds silly, but it was like everyone on earth was walking through air and I was walking through Jell-O. It took me extra time to do everything—extra time to hear or think do something simple like move my arms. They'd ask me a question, and I couldn't even think about the right answer, and they moved on to the next question. It felt like all I was doing was mumbling.

"All I can say is that it was one of the scariest things I have ever experienced. Turns out my blood sugar was off. I'm glad EMS was there to help, that's for sure, although my recollection of it is still fuzzy."

A patient may be awake but confused. An awake patient's mental status can be described by specifying what he is "oriented to." Most EMS systems document orientation to person, place, and time. A patient who can speak clearly can almost always tell you his name (orientation to person). A few patients are oriented to person, but cannot tell you where they are (orientation to place). Some patients are oriented to person and place but cannot tell you the time, day, or date (orientation to time). A few EMS systems include additional questions to determine orientation.

A depressed mental status may indicate a life-threatening problem such as insufficient oxygen reaching the brain or shock (hypoperfusion). If the level of responsiveness is lower than alert, provide high-concentration oxygen by nonrebreather mask and consider the patient a high transport priority.

Assess the ABCs

ABCs airway, breathing, and circulation.

You will always check the **ABCs**—airway, breathing, and circulation—as you look for life-threatening problems.

If the patient is alert and talking clearly or crying loudly, you know that the airway is open. If the airway is not open or is endangered (the patient is not alert, is supine, or is breathing noisily), take measures to open the airway, such as the jaw-thrust or head-tilt, chin-lift maneuver, suctioning, or insertion of an oropharyngeal or nasopharyngeal airway. If the airway is blocked, perform clearance procedures.

Once an open airway is ensured, assess breathing. If the patient is in respiratory arrest, perform rescue breathing. If he is not alert and his breathing rate is slower than 8 breaths per minute, provide positive pressure ventilations with 100 percent oxygen. If the patient is alert and his breathing is adequate but the rate is faster than 24 breaths per minute, give high-concentration oxygen by nonrebreather mask. If the rate is faster than 24 breaths per minute and his breathing is inadequate, ventilate with 100 percent oxygen using one of the methods you learned in Chapter 6, "Airway Management."

Once any breathing problems are corrected, assess circulation. Begin by taking the patient's pulse. If there is no pulse, perform CPR. Keep in mind, however, that cardiac arrest is not the only possible life-threatening circulation problem. Inadequate circulation and severe blood loss are also life threatening.

To evaluate circulation, assess pulse, skin, and bleeding. If the patient is light-skinned, you can check pulse and skin at the same time. As you take the radial pulse, note whether the skin at the wrist is warm, pink, and dry—indicating good circulation—or pale and clammy (cool and moist)—indicating poor circulation. If your patient is dark-skinned, you can check the color of the lips or nail beds, which should be pink.

Also check for and control severe bleeding. If even one large vessel or several smaller ones are bleeding, a patient can lose enough blood in just a minute or two to die. Quick control of severe external bleeding can be life saving. Transport decisions should take into account the potential for shock resulting from inadequate circulation and blood loss.

Determine Priority

Any life-threatening airway, breathing, or circulation problem must be treated as soon as it is discovered. Once life-threats are under control, you will decide on the patient's **priority** for immediate transport versus further on-scene assessment and care.

priority
the decision regarding the need for immediate transport of the patient versus further assessment and care at the scene.

Most patients do not need immediate transport, but a few do, and you must be able to determine which are which. If any life-threatening problem cannot be controlled or threatens to recur, or if the patient has a depressed level of responsiveness, you may decide that he has an immediate priority for transport to the hospital, with assessment and care continuing en route.

A number of findings indicate a high priority for transport (Table 8-1). These are conditions for which, usually, there is little or no treatment that can be given in the field that will make a difference in how well the patient does. You will learn more about these conditions in later chapters.

Initial assessment steps and interventions are summarized in Table 8-2.

PATIENT CHARACTERISTICS AND INITIAL ASSESSMENT

Patient assessment takes different forms, depending on the following characteristics of the patient:

- Whether the patient has a medical problem or trauma (injury)
- Whether the patient is responsive or unresponsive
- Whether the patient is an adult, a child, or an infant

How can the steps of initial assessment be applied to such varied types of patients? The following scenarios—plus some final paragraphs—will help to show you.

Mr. Schmidt—A Responsive Adult Medical Patient

One afternoon, you are dispatched to "an elderly man whose stomach hurts." Mrs. Schmidt greets you at the door and leads you to her husband.

TABLE 8-1 • High-Priority Conditions
• Poor general impression
• Unresponsive
• Responsive, but not following commands
• Difficulty breathing
• Shock
• Complicated childbirth
• Chest pain with systolic blood pressure less than 100
• Uncontrolled bleeding
• Severe pain anywhere

TABLE 8-2 • Initial Assessment Steps and Interventions

MEDICAL PATIENT		TRAUMA PATIENT	
RESPONSIVE	UNRESPONSIVE	RESPONSIVE	UNRESPONSIVE
1. General impression: Form general impression of patient's condition.	**1. General impression:** Form general impression of patient's condition.	**1. General impression:** Form general impression of patient's condition. Evaluate mechanism of injury. **Intervention:** Manual stabilization of head.	**1. General impression:** Form general impression of patient's condition. Evaluate mechanism of injury. **Intervention:** Manual stabilization of head.
2. Mental Status: AVPU (alert)	**2. Mental Status:** AVPU (responsive only to verbal or painful stimulus or not responsive) **Intervention:** High-concentration oxygen as soon as airway is open.	**2. Mental Status:** AVPU (alert)	**2. Mental Status:** AVPU (responsive only to verbal or painful stimulus or not responsive) **Intervention:** High-concentration oxygen as soon as airway is open.
3. Airway is open.	**3. Airway** is compromised. **Interventions:** Open airway with head-tilt, chin-lift maneuver; consider oro- or nasopharyngeal airway; suction as needed. For foreign body obstruction, use abdominal thrusts or other blockage-clearing technique.	**3. Airway** is open.	**3. Airway** is compromised. **Interventions:** Open airway with jaw thrust; consider oro- or nasopharyngeal airway; suction as needed. For foreign body obstruction, use abdominal thrusts or other blockage-clearing technique.
4. Breathing: Look for rise and fall of chest, listen and feel for rate and depth of breathing. Look for work of breathing (use of accessory muscles, retractions). **Interventions:** If rate is greater than 24, high-concentration oxygen by nonrebreather mask. If breathing becomes inadequate, provide positive pressure ventilations and high-concentration oxygen.	**4. Breathing:** Look for rise and fall of chest, listen and feel for rate and depth of breathing. Look for work of breathing (use of accessory muscles, retractions). **Interventions:** If rate is greater than 24, high-concentration oxygen by nonrebreather mask. Position patient on side. If breathing is inadequate, provide positive pressure ventilations and high-concentration oxygen. If respiratory arrest, perform rescue breathing.	**4. Breathing:** Look for rise and fall of chest, listen and feel for rate and depth of breathing. Look for work of breathing (use of accessory muscles, retractions). **Interventions:** If rate is greater than 24, high-concentration oxygen by nonrebreather mask. If breathing becomes inadequate, provide positive pressure ventilations and high-concentration oxygen.	**4. Breathing:** Look for rise and fall of chest, listen and feel for rate and depth of breathing. Look for work of breathing (use of accessory muscles, retractions). **Interventions:** If rate is greater than 24, high-concentration oxygen by nonrebreather mask. Position patient on side once spinal stability is assured. If breathing is inadequate, provide positive pressure ventilations and high-concentration oxygen. If respiratory arrest, perform rescue breathing.
5. Circulation: Pulse; bleeding; skin color, temperature, condition (capillary refill in infants and children under 6). **Interventions:** Control bleeding. Treat for shock. If cardiac arrest occurs, perform CPR.	**5. Circulation:** Pulse; bleeding; skin color, temperature, condition (capillary refill in infants and children under 6). **Interventions:** Control bleeding. Treat for shock. If cardiac arrest occurs, perform CPR.	**5. Circulation:** Pulse; bleeding; skin color, temperature, condition (capillary refill in infants and children under 6). **Interventions:** Control bleeding. Treat for shock. If cardiac arrest occurs, perform CPR.	**5. Circulation:** Pulse; bleeding; skin color, temperature, condition (capillary refill in infants and children under 6). **Interventions:** Control bleeding. Treat for shock. If cardiac arrest occurs, perform CPR.
6. Priority: A responsive patient's priority depends on chief complaint, status of ABCs, and other factors.	**6. Priority:** An unresponsive patient is automatically a high priority for immediate transport.	**6. Priority:** A responsive patient's priority depends on chief complaint, status of ABCs, and other factors.	**6. Priority:** An unresponsive patient is automatically a high priority for immediate transport.

CRITICAL DECISION MAKING:
DETERMINING PRIORITY

At the end of the initial assessment you will make a priority determination. This determination is a key decision that will affect the rest of your assessment and care. Patients deemed a high priority will receive a streamlined assessment process leading to prompt transport. Patients who are not a high priority will receive their assessment and care at a slower (although not slow) pace. For each patient described here, determine whether that patient should be classified as a high or low priority at the end of the initial assessment.

1. A responsive patient who is sitting up and having difficulty breathing.
2. A man who "passed out" at a wedding and is still unresponsive.
3. A responsive child who got his foot caught in bike spokes and may have broken the foot.
4. A responsive patient who describes severe pain in his abdomen.
5. A patient who only moans (doesn't respond with words or actions) and appears to have ingested alcohol.

General Impression

As you approach the sofa where Mr. Schmidt is sitting, you see that he is an older male who appears ill and in pain. You see nothing around him to suggest that he has been injured. All of this suggests a medical problem rather than an injury.

Mental Status, Airway, Breathing

You introduce yourself by saying, "Hello, Mr. Schmidt. I'm Gerry Jones. I'm an emergency medical technician from the Fairfield Ambulance Service. How can I help you?" "My stomach hurts," he replies. As you ask questions, you note that Mr. Schmidt is alert and answering clearly. The fact that he is speaking in a normal way indicates that his airway is open. You can hear that his breathing is not labored. You look at his chest and note that his breathing is normal in rate and depth.

Circulation

"I'm going to check your pulse," you explain as you reach for his wrist. You quickly assess Mr. Schmidt's circulation by palpating his radial pulse, observing his skin, and looking for bleeding. Although you do not stop to count exactly how fast his pulse is, you can tell that it is normal in rate and strength and regular in rhythm. The skin at his wrist is pink, warm, and dry. No blood is evident anywhere around him.

Priority

With the information you have gathered in just a few seconds, you conclude that Mr. Schmidt has no problems that are likely to kill him in the next few minutes. No immediate life-saving measures are required, and neither is immediate transport to the hospital. You are able, instead, to move ahead with the next steps of your assessment as Mr. Schmidt continues to rest on the sofa.

Mrs. Malone—An Unresponsive Adult Medical Patient

Your dispatcher sends you to an "unconscious" woman. Her daughter says she cannot wake her mother, Mrs. Malone, and leads you to the bedroom.

General Impression

An older woman in nightclothes is lying on her back in bed. Her eyes are closed and she is not moving.

Mental Status

You say loudly, "Mrs. Malone, can you hear me?" In response to your question, she moans a little, so you know she responds to a verbal stimulus. In your report, you will describe both the stimulus (verbal) and the response (moaning). If Mrs. Malone had not responded to verbal stimulus, you would have inflicted a painful stimulus to try to get a response from her.

Airway and Breathing

Because she is lying on her back, Mrs. Malone's airway is threatened by her tongue. Since patients with depressed responsiveness are always at risk for airway problems, you know that you need to be aggressive about opening and maintaining her airway. So even though you haven't heard any sounds indicating partial airway obstruction (like snoring or gurgling), your partner removes the pillow, tilts her head back, and lifts her chin.

Next, you evaluate her breathing by bringing your ear next to her mouth and looking for movement of her chest and abdomen as you listen and feel for the movement of air with your ear. You determine the depth of Mrs. Malone's respirations and if her breathing rate is slow or fast. If you found that her breathing was inadequate, you would ventilate Mrs. Malone with 100 percent oxygen.

Her respirations are in the normal range, but you will give Mrs. Malone high-flow, high-concentration oxygen by nonrebreather mask anyway because her level of responsiveness is depressed. You put in a nasopharyngeal airway and move Mrs. Malone onto her side in order to help protect her airway.

Circulation

Mrs. Malone's pulse is strong, regular, and in the normal range for rate. You look for blood, but find none. The skin at her wrist is cool and dry. Because Mrs. Malone is dark-skinned, you assess for skin color at her lips and nail beds, which are pale. Although the pulse and bleeding check are normal, the pallor and coolness of her skin are slightly abnormal.

Priority

The priority of this patient is high because her mental status is depressed, her airway is at risk, and her skin indicates a circulation problem. You arrange immediate transport to the hospital, planning to continue assessment and care en route.

Clara Diller—A Responsive Child Trauma Patient

You respond to the scene where, the dispatcher says, a child has fallen.

General Impression

As you get out of the ambulance, you see a girl who is about 5 years old sitting on the sidewalk. She is crying and holding a bloody cloth on her knee. The mechanism of injury is apparent: a pair of skates indicates that she has probably taken a tumble while skating.

Mental Status, Airway, and Breathing

When you reach the patient, you kneel next to her and introduce yourself. You ask what happened. She confirms your suspicion that she fell down while trying her new skates. When you ask her, she tells you her name is Clara Diller and that her head and knee hurt. Since she is crying and answers your question easily, you determine that her mental status is alert and her airway is clear.

Because there is a mechanism of injury indicating possible trauma, you explain to her that she should not move her head and that your partner is going to hold her head to help her keep it still. Her breathing is not labored and her respiratory rate and depth are in the normal range.

Circulation

You feel Clara's radial pulse. It is slightly rapid but strong and regular. You look around her and see no blood except on the cloth and on her knee. Since it is hard to tell how much bleeding may be under the cloth, you tell Clara you want to look at her knee. You see a 2-inch laceration which is oozing some blood, so you put the cloth back on and ask the neighbor who takes care of Clara to apply a little pressure to it. When you felt Clara's radial pulse, you noted that her skin is warm, pink, and dry. You also assess her capillary refill by pressing on the end of her fingernail. The color in the nail bed returns to pink in less than 2 seconds, so all indications are that Clara's circulation is good.

Priority

Based on the information you have gathered, you determine that Clara's priority for immediate transport is low. She has no significant mechanism of injury and no immediately life-threatening problems. There is no evidence that she was struck by a car or hit any object other than the sidewalk. However, since the sidewalk is a hard surface and she may have been moving fast, you maintain a high index of suspicion for possible cervical-spine injury. As soon as it is practical, you will apply a cervical collar and immobilize Clara on a backboard.

PEDIATRIC NOTE

Because Clara is a child, several other factors were different in her case than they were for your adult patients, Mr. Schmidt and Mrs. Malone.

Since children are often shy or distrustful of strangers or adults, you made a special effort to gain Clara's trust by kneeling to her level as you talked with her. Responsive children need to have some trust in the EMT. This may take a minute or two, but the general impression will guide you in determining how long to spend developing a rapport with the child.

Infants and children breathe faster than adults and their hearts beat faster, and you kept this in mind when you evaluated Clara's breathing and circulation.

A special part of checking circulation in infants and children is capillary refill. Nail beds are typically pink in healthy, normal people. When the end of the fingernail is gently pressed, it turns white. When the pressure is released, the nail bed turns pink again very quickly, usually in less than 2 seconds. In children, this may help you to evaluate the circulation of blood. In an infant or small child with small nail beds, press the back of the hand or top of the foot instead. Count, "one-one thousand, two-one thousand" or say "capillary refill." If the nail or skin regains its pink color in the time it takes to say one of these, it is probably normal. Abnormal responses include prolonged and absent capillary refill (taking too long to turn pink again, or not turning pink again at all). These usually indicate problems with circulation.

Capillary refill is not a reliable sign for adults, so it is used only in infants and young children. In some adults, it is normal for capillary refill to take longer than 2 seconds, especially in the elderly. Even in infants and young children, it can be affected by factors such as the weather. Cold temperatures will prolong capillary refill. It should be used as one factor to consider in determining the priority of the young patient, but not the only one.

Like adult trauma patients, child and infant trauma patients need to have their heads immobilized in order to prevent injury to the spinal cord.

An infant has an airway that is different from an adult's, so opening an infant's or child's airway means moving the head to a neutral position, not tilting it back the way an adult's airway is opened. The mental status of unresponsive infants is typically checked by talking to the infant and flicking the feet.

You will learn about other considerations in approaching and assessing pediatric patients in Chapter 31, "Infants and Children."

Brian Sawyer—An Unresponsive Adult Trauma Patient

At the scene of a motor-vehicle collision, you go to the aid of a young man who has been thrown from his car.

General Impression

The young man appears to be approximately 25 years old. His eyes are closed and he is not moving. As you approach, you can hear snoring respirations. The mechanism of injury, the collision, and the fact that he is quite a distance from his vehicle are obvious. A police officer who has retrieved the patient's wallet tells you that his name is Brian Sawyer.

Mental Status and Airway

Your partner moves to stabilize Brian's head and the two of you position him on his back. Your partner attends to Brian's airway as you begin to check his mental status. He doesn't respond to your calling his name, and he is unresponsive to a brisk rub of your knuckles on his sternum.

Your partner has started to treat the airway problem you both heard, snoring respirations that mean partial obstruction of the airway. Your partner manually stabilizes the head at the same time that he does a jaw thrust, which relieves the snoring sound. You listen closely and hear no other noises from his airway. If you heard gurgling or saw fluid in Brian's airway, you would suction him.

Breathing and Circulation

To evaluate breathing, you look, listen, and feel. Brian has respirations that appear normal in rate and depth. Because he is unresponsive but with adequate respirations, you decide to give Brian high-concentration oxygen by nonrebreather mask as soon as you finish checking circulation. You select an oropharyngeal airway and insert it, then apply a nonrebreather mask with 15 liters per minute of high-concentration oxygen.

You start to assess circulation by feeling the radial pulse. It is rapid and weak. There is no blood on or near the patient that you can see. His skin is pale, cool, and sweaty.

Priority

The priority you assign Brian is high. He is unresponsive to pain and his rapid, weak pulse and pale, clammy skin are signs of diminished circulation. You will spend as little time on the scene as possible. You plan to monitor his airway, place a cervical collar on him, immobilize him on a backboard, and get him to an appropriate facility quickly. Since you and your partner will both be needed to care for this patient en route to the hospital, you radio for additional personnel to drive the ambulance.

Comparing the Initial Assessments

The four patients—Mr. Schmidt, Mrs. Malone, Clara Diller, and Brian Sawyer—were very different in their characteristics. Notably:

- Mr. Schmidt and Mrs. Malone were medical patients, while Clara Diller and Brian Sawyer had suffered trauma.
- Both Mr. Schmidt and Clara Diller were responsive and neither was a priority for immediate transport. However, both Mrs. Malone and Brian Sawyer had an altered mental status and airway and circulation problems that made them a high priority for immediate transport to the hospital.
- Clara Diller was a child, while the other three patients were adults.

There were a few obvious differences in the initial assessments of these patients. For example, both Clara Diller and Brian Sawyer, as trauma patients, required stabilization and immobilization of the head and spine, while Mr. Schmidt and Mrs. Malone, as medical patients with no evidence of any mechanism of injury, did not. For all four patients, the purpose of the initial assessment was to discover and correct any life-threatening problems. Mrs. Malone and Brian Sawyer had more problems to correct (mainly airway problems), so there were more actions to take, and the initial assessment of these two patients took a little longer than the initial assessment of Mr. Schmidt and Clara Diller.

In spite of these differences, the main thing to note is that the initial assessment steps were the same for all of them: forming a general impression; assessing mental status; checking airway, breathing, and circulation (and correcting any immediately life-threatening problems as soon as they were found); and making a priority decision regarding immediate transport vs. continued on-scene assessment and care.

These steps of the initial assessment must be followed systematically for every patient, no matter if that patient has a medical condition or trauma, is responsive or unresponsive, is an infant, child, or adult—and no matter how mild or serious that patient's condition may seem to be. If these steps are not followed consistently and systematically, it is very possible to overlook and neglect to manage a life-threatening problem.

To consider how the steps of the initial assessment are applied to responsive and unresponsive medical and trauma patients, review Table 8-2. For a summary of how the steps of the initial assessment are applied to adults, children, and infants, see Table 8-3.

TABLE 8-3 • Initial Assessment of Adults, Children, and Infants

	ADULTS	CHILDREN 1–5 YEARS	INFANTS TO 1 YEAR
Mental Status	AVPU: Is patient alert? responsive to verbal stimulus? responsive to painful stimulus? unresponsive? If alert, is patient oriented to person, place, and time?	As for adults.	If not alert, shout as a verbal stimulus, flick feet as a painful stimulus. (Crying would be infant's expected response.)
Airway	Trauma: jaw-thrust. Medical: head-tilt, chin-lift. Both: Consider oro- or nasopharyngeal airway, suctioning.	As for adults, but see Chapter 6 and BCLS Review for special child airway techniques. If performing head-tilt, chin-lift, do so without hyperextending (stretching) the neck.	As for children, but see Chapter 6 and BCLS Review for special infant airway techniques.
Breathing	If respiratory arrest, perform rescue breathing. If depressed mental status and inadequate breathing (slower than 8 per minute), give positive pressure ventilations with 100 percent oxygen. If alert and respirations are more than 24 per minute, give 100 percent oxygen by nonrebreather mask	As for adults, but normal rates for children are faster than for adults. (See Chapter 9 for normal child respiration rates.) Parent may have to hold oxygen mask to reduce child's fear of mask.	As for children, but normal rates for infants. Are faster than for children and adults. (See Chapter 9 for normal infant respiration rates.)
Circulation	Assess skin, radial pulse, bleeding. If cardiac arrest, perform CPR. See Chapter 26 on how to treat for bleeding and shock.	Assess skin, radial pulse, bleeding, capillary refill. See Chapter 9 for normal child pulse rates (faster than for adults). If cardiac arrest, perform CPR. See BCLS Review for child techniques. See Chapter 26 on how to treat for bleeding and shock.	Assess skin, brachial pulse, bleeding, capillary refill. See Chapter 9 for normal child pulse rates (faster than for children and adults). If cardiac arrest, perform CPR. See BCLS Review for special infant techniques. See Chapter 26 on how to treat for bleeding and shock.

CHAPTER REVIEW

SUMMARY

It is essential to assess patients in a systematic way that allows for quickly finding and treating immediate threats to life. This search is called the initial assessment. By forming a general impression; determining mental status; evaluating airway, breathing, and circulation; and determining the patient's priority, you can find and correct the problems that could otherwise end a patient's life in just a few minutes. You will also be able to determine how urgent the patient's need to be transported is and how to conduct the rest of your assessment.

KEY TERMS

ABCs airway, breathing, and circulation.

AVPU a memory aid for classifying a patient's level of responsiveness, or mental status. The letters stand for alert, verbal response, painful response, unresponsive.

chief complaint in emergency medicine, the reason EMS was called, usually in the patient's own words.

general impression impression of the patient's condition that is formed on first approaching the patient, based on the patient's environment, chief complaint, and appearance.

initial assessment the first element in assessment of a patient; steps taken for the purpose of discovering and dealing with any life-threatening problems. The six parts of initial assessment are: forming a general impression, assessing mental status, assessing airway, assessing breathing, assessing circulation, and determining the priority of the patient for treatment and transport to the hospital. Also called *primary assessment* or *primary survey.*

interventions actions taken to correct a patient's problems.

mental status level of responsiveness.

priority the decision regarding the need for immediate transport of the patient versus further assessment and care at the scene.

REVIEW QUESTIONS

1. List factors you will take into account in forming a general impression of a patient. (pp. 210, 212, 216)
2. Explain how to assess a patient's mental status with regard to the AVPU levels of responsiveness. (pp. 212, 213–214, 216, 221)
3. Explain how to assess airway, breathing, and circulation during the initial assessment. Explain the interventions you will take for possible problems with airway, breathing, and circulation. (pp. 212, 214–215, 216, 221)
4. Explain what is meant by the term *priority decision.* (p. 215)
5. Explain what special interventions are required. (pp. 210, 211, 213, 216)
   - if a patient has suffered trauma
   - if a patient is unresponsive

CRITICAL THINKING

Thinking and Linking

Think back to Chapter 6, "Airway Management," and link information from that chapter (regarding oxygen administration and artificial ventilation) with information from this chapter, "The Initial Assessment," as you consider the following situation:

- Your patient, injured in a car crash, is breathing at 6/minute. Would you administer oxygen by nonrebreather mask or provide artificial ventilations? Describe the technique you would use.

MEDIA RESOURCES

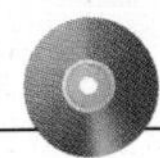

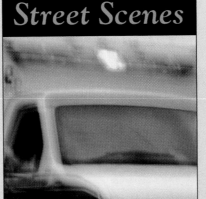

See the Student CD at the back of this book for quizzes, a case study activity, animations, and other features related to this chapter. In particular, look at the case study about conducting an initial assessment at the scene of a vehicle crash and the 3D animations of areas of the human body. Also, visit the Companion Website for *Emergency Care* at **www.prenhall.com/limmer**, where you will find additional reinforcement and links to other resources.

Street Scenes

Your patient is a 78-year-old unconscious male, who was shaving with his electric razor when he fell to the floor. You manually stabilize his head and neck and determine that the patient responds to painful stimuli. You then perform a jaw-thrust maneuver, assess breathing, and find that the patient has snoring respirations. With the help of your partner, you insert an oropharyngeal airway, reassess breathing, and observe labored respirations and cyanosis around the lips. After you give the patient high-concentration oxygen by nonrebreather mask, circulation is assessed. In a minute or so, the patient regains consciousness and his skin color improves. He tells you his name is Danya and explains that he had suddenly felt lightheaded, sat down, and must have passed out. Later, during transport, you keep the patient on oxygen, take another set of vital signs, and gather a patient history.

Street Scene Questions

1. What should be done immediately upon contact with an unconscious patient who has fallen?
2. What are some considerations when opening the airway of an unconscious patient?
3. Using the AVPU scale, what is the level of responsiveness of a patient who responds to you calling out his name?

When you return to quarters, you hope to get a short break, but it's just minutes before you receive a call for a 7-year-old patient reported to be unresponsive at the Mount Hope Elementary School. Upon arrival, you are directed to the athletic field where the coach and school nurse tell you that Joey Sullivan had a seizure for the second time this month. His eyes are closed, he is not moving, and his skin color appears normal. Your partner gets down next to the patient to assess mental status. "Hey, Joey," she calls out. He does not respond. She rubs his sternum briskly with her knuckles. There is still no response. "Unresponsive to pain," she says to you. When she tilts Joey's head back, there is a good deal of saliva visible in his mouth. Suctioning removes it without difficulty, and you administer oxygen to the patient by nonrebreather mask. You turn Joey onto his side and get a complete set of vital signs as your partner gets the stretcher. By the time you place Joey on the stretcher, he is becoming more responsive. Because of his improving mental status, you downgrade his priority and transport him along with the school nurse.

Street Scene Questions

4. Would knowing the cause of Joey's seizures change how you perform his initial assessment?
5. For Joey, what is the best position to prevent airway problems from occurring?
6. How did Joey's priority change during this call?

It isn't long after you leave Joey at the hospital before you are called again. "Ambulance 10, respond to the Traveler's Diner for a person having a heart attack." When you arrive, you find a woman in her mid-forties slumped in a chair. The manager tells you he thinks she is having a heart attack. You assess her airway and breathing and find she is not breathing. You are unable to ventilate her, so you perform an abdominal thrust. This results in expulsion of a piece of meat. Reassessment reveals that she is making shallow, infrequent attempts to breathe, so you ventilate her with high-concentration oxygen. Her pulse is rapid and weak and her skin is cyanotic and sweaty. You transport her immediately as a high-priority patient.

Street Scene Questions

7. What is the value of following a systematic method of assessment for threats to life?
8. How much more assessment is appropriate before you transport this patient?

CHAPTER

Vital Signs and SAMPLE History

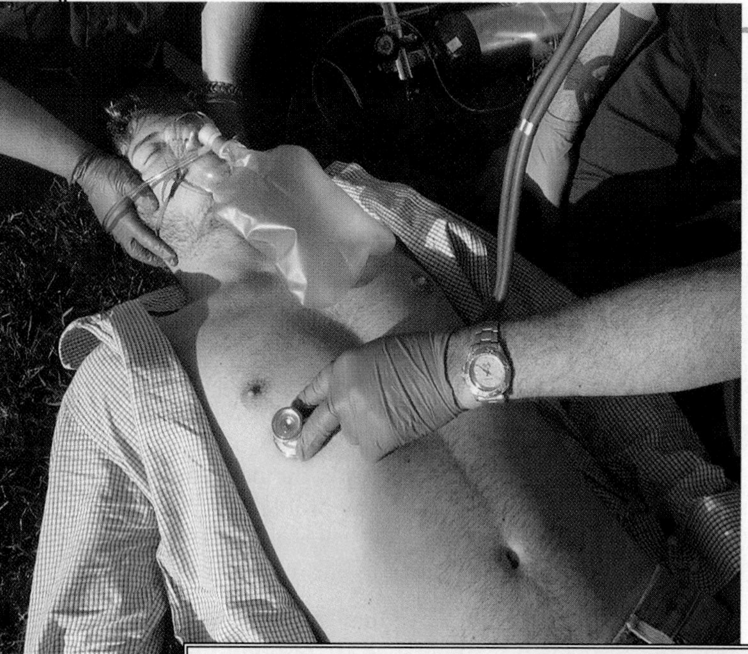

CORE CONCEPTS

The following are core concepts that will be addressed in this chapter:

- How to obtain vital signs, including pulse, respirations, blood pressure, skin, and pupils
- How to obtain an accurate SAMPLE history
- How to document vital signs on a prehospital care report

KEY TERMS

auscultation, p. 236
blood pressure, p. 234
brachial pulse, p. 228
bradycardia, p. 228
carotid pulse, p. 228
constrict, p. 233
diastolic blood pressure, p. 234
dilate, p. 233
oxygen saturation (SpO_2), p. 240
palpation, p. 236
pulse, p. 227
pupil, p. 233
radial pulse, p. 228
reactivity, p. 233
respiration, p. 229
SAMPLE history, p. 242
sign, p. 242
sphygmomanometer, p. 236
symptom, p. 242
systolic blood pressure, p. 234
tachycardia, p. 228
vital signs, p. 226

DOT OBJECTIVES

*KNOWLEDGE AND ATTITUDE

1-5.1 Identify the components of vital signs. (p. 226)

1-5.2 Describe the methods used to obtain a breathing rate. (p. 229)

1-5.3 Identify the attributes that should be obtained when assessing breathing. (pp. 229–231)

1-5.4 Differentiate between shallow, labored, and noisy breathing. (pp. 229–230)

1-5.5 Describe the methods to obtain a pulse rate. (pp. 227–228)

1-5.6 Identify the information obtained when assessing a patient's pulse. (pp. 225–228)

1-5.7 Differentiate between a strong, weak, regular, and irregular pulse. (p. 228)

1-5.8 Describe the methods used to assess skin color, temperature, and condition (capillary refill in infants and children). (pp. 231–233)

1-5.9 Identify the normal and abnormal skin colors. (pp. 231–232)

1-5.10 Differentiate between pale, blue, red, and yellow skin color. (pp. 231–233)

1-5.11 Identify the normal and abnormal skin temperature. (pp. 232–233)

1-5.12 Differentiate between hot, cool, and cold skin temperature. (pp. 232–233)

1-5.13 Identify normal and abnormal skin conditions. (p. 232)

1-5.14 Identify normal and abnormal capillary refill in infants and children. (p. 233)

1-5.15 Describe the methods used to assess the pupils. (pp. 233–234)

1-5.16 Identify normal and abnormal pupil size. (pp. 233–234)

1-5.17 Differentiate between dilated (big) and constricted (small) pupil size. (pp. 233–234)

1-5.18 Differentiate between reactive and nonreactive pupils and equal and unequal pupils. (pp. 233–234)

1-5.19 Describe the methods used to assess blood pressure. (pp. 236–239)

1-5.20 Define systolic pressure. (p. 234)

1-5.21 Define diastolic pressure. (p. 234)

1-5.22 Explain the difference between auscultation and palpation for obtaining a blood pressure. (pp. 236–238)

1-5.23 Identify the components of the SAMPLE history. (p. 242)

1-5.24 Differentiate between a sign and a symptom. (p. 242)

1-5.25 State the importance of accurately reporting and recording the baseline vital signs. (p. 236)

1-5.26 Discuss the need to search for additional medical identification. (p. 242)

1-5.27 Explain the value of performing the baseline vital signs. (p. 236)

1-5.28 Recognize and respond to the feelings patients experience during assessment. (pp. 242–243)

1-5.29 Defend the need for obtaining and recording an accurate set of vital signs. (p. 236)

1-5.30 Explain the rationale of recording additional sets of vital signs. (pp. 236, 238)

1-5.31 Explain the importance of obtaining a SAMPLE history. (p. 242)

*SKILLS

1-5.32 Demonstrate the skills involved in assessment of breathing.

1-5.33 Demonstrate the skills associated with obtaining a pulse.

1-5.34 Demonstrate the skills associated with assessing the skin color, temperature, condition, and capillary refill in infants and children.

1-5.35 Demonstrate the skills associated with assessing the pupils.

1-5.36 Demonstrate the skills associated with obtaining blood pressure.

1-5.37 Demonstrate the skills that should be used to obtain information from the patient, family, or bystanders at the scene.

Following the initial assessment and control of any immediate life threats, you will begin a more thorough assessment of your patient. Two essential elements of this assessment will be measuring vital signs and taking a medical history. Vital signs are measurable things like pulse, blood pressure, and respirations. Because they reflect the patient's condition—and changes in the patient's condition—you will take them early and repeat them often. The medical history includes information about the present medical problem and facts about the patient that existed before the patient needed EMS. This information can affect the treatment you give. It is called a SAMPLE history because the letters in the word SAMPLE stand for elements of the history.

GATHERING THE VITAL SIGNS AND HISTORY

When you begin to assess a patient, some things are obvious or easy to discover. For example, the most important part of patient assessment is the chief complaint, the reason the patient called for EMS. Usually, the patient will tell you what his complaint is. Other parts of assessment that are usually apparent as soon as you see and talk to the patient are age, sex, and general alertness. However, not all your assessment is so obvious or so easy to find out. The vital signs and medical history, for example, are major components of assessment that will take a few minutes to complete.

Vital signs as well as the current and past medical history (SAMPLE history) are gathered on virtually every EMS patient. Occasionally, a patient will be so seriously injured or ill that you are not able to get this information because you are too busy treating immediate threats to life. This is the exception, however. The vast majority of patients you will encounter as an EMT should have an assessment that includes vital sign measurement and SAMPLE history gathering, among other things. If you do not get this information, you may remain unaware of important conditions or trends in patient conditions that require you to provide particular treatments in the field or prompt transport to a hospital.

Where do vital signs and SAMPLE history fit into the sequence of patient assessment? After the initial assessment to find and treat immediate life threats (which was the subject of Chapter 8, "The Initial Assessment") you will conduct a more thorough assessment known as the *focused history and physical exam* (which will be the subject of Chapter 10, "Assessment of the Trauma Patient," and Chapter 11, "Assessment of the Medical Patient"). Vital signs and SAMPLE history will be obtained during the focused history and physical exam. This chapter serves as a preview of these two important procedures.

VITAL SIGNS

vital signs
outward signs of what is going on inside the body, including respiration; pulse; skin color, temperature, and condition (plus capillary refill in infants and children); pupils; and blood pressure.

NOTE: *It is essential that you record all vital signs as you obtain them, along with the time at which you took them.*

Vital signs are outward signs of what is going on inside the body. They include pulse; respiration; skin color, temperature, and condition (plus capillary refill in infants and children); pupils; and blood pressure.

Evaluation of these indicators can give valuable information to the EMT. The first measurements you obtain are called the baseline vital signs. You can gain even more valuable information when you repeat the vital signs and compare them to the baseline measurements. This allows you and other members of the patient's health care team to see trends in the patient's condition and to respond appropriately.

Another sign that gives important information about a patient's condition is mental status. It is not considered one of the vital signs; however, whenever you take the vital signs, you should also assess the patient's mental status. Chapter 8, "The Initial Assessment," described how to evaluate mental status.

Pulse

The pumping action of the heart is normally rhythmic, causing blood to move through the arteries in waves, not smoothly and continuously at the same pressure like water flowing through a pipe. A fingertip held over an artery where it lies close to the body's

CRITICAL DECISION MAKING:
SOLVING ASSESSMENT PROBLEMS

An accurate history and set of vital signs are an important foundation for critical decision making. For each of the common EMS situations that follow, describe how you would solve the problem you are faced with. In some cases, you may think of more than one potential solution.

1. You are trying to count the respiratory rate of a very talkative middle-aged male. Every time you think you're beginning to get an accurate count, he starts talking again.
2. You are about to put a blood pressure cuff on a 40-year-old male when he says that you can't put the cuff on that arm. He is a kidney dialysis patient and says he has a "shunt" in that arm. Because of the small room he is in, you can't get over to his other side.
3. An 80-year-old male is complaining of mild abdominal pain. When you ask him if he has any medical problems, he says no. On the kitchen table you can easily see at least half a dozen prescription bottles.
4. The patient is an unconscious 32-year-old female who was thrown from a car when it flipped over. When you attempt to check the pulse at the patient's wrist, you search and search but can't find it.

surface and crosses over a bone can easily feel the characteristic "beats" as the surging blood causes the artery to expand. What you feel is called the **pulse.** When taking a patient's pulse, you are concerned with two factors: rate and quality (Figure 9-1).

pulse
the rhythmic beats felt as the heart pumps blood through the arteries.

pulse rate
the number of pulse beats per minute.

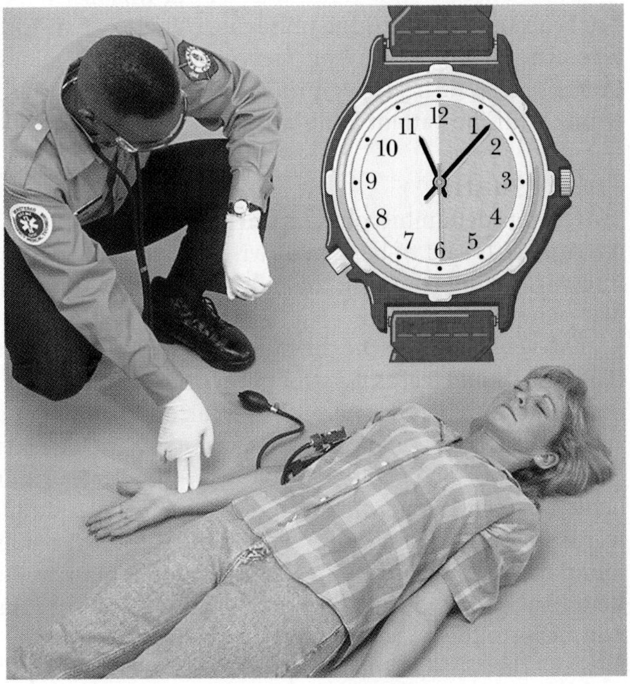

Pulse Rate

The **pulse rate** is the number of beats per minute. The number you get will allow you to decide if the patient's pulse rate is normal, rapid, or slow (Table 9-1).

Figure 9-1 • Assess pulse rate and quality. Count for 30 seconds and multiply by 2.

TABLE 9-1 • Pulse

NORMAL PULSE RATES (BEATS PER MINUTE, AT REST)	
Adult	60 to 100
Infants and Children	
Adolescent 11–14 years	60 to 105
School age 6–10 years	70 to 110
Preschooler 3–5 years	80 to 120
Toddler 1–3 years	80 to 130
Infant 6–12 months	80 to 140
Infant 0–5 months	90 to 140
Newborn	120 to 160

PULSE QUALITY	SIGNIFICANCE/POSSIBLE CAUSES
Rapid, regular, and full	Exertion, fright, fever, high blood pressure, first stage of blood loss
Rapid, regular, and thready	Shock, later stages of blood loss
Slow	Head injury, drugs, some poisons, some heart problems, lack of oxygen in children
No pulse	Cardiac arrest (clinical death)

Infants and Children: A high pulse in an infant or child is not as great a concern as a low pulse. A low pulse may indicate imminent cardiac arrest.

tachycardia (TAK-uh-KAR-de-uh) a rapid pulse; any pulse rate above 100 beats per minute.

bradycardia (BRAY-duh-KAR-de-uh) a slow pulse; any pulse rate below 60 beats per minute.

Pulse rates vary among individuals. Factors such as age, physical condition, degree of exercise just completed, medications or other substances being taken, blood loss, stress, and body temperature all have an influence on the rate. The normal rate for an adult at rest is between 60 and 100 beats per minute. Any pulse rate above 100 beats per minute is rapid, while a rate below 60 beats per minute is slow. A rapid pulse is called **tachycardia.** A slow pulse is called **bradycardia.** An athlete may have a normal at-rest pulse rate between 40 and 50 beats per minute. This is a slow pulse rate, but it is certainly not an indication of poor health. The same pulse rate in a non-athletic or elderly person may indicate a serious condition. You should be concerned about the typical adult whose pulse rate stays above 100 or below 60 beats per minute.

In an emergency, it is not unusual for this rate temporarily to be between 100 and 140 beats per minute. If the pulse rate is higher than 150, or if you take a patient's pulse several times during care on scene and find him maintaining a pulse rate above 120 beats or below 50 beats per minute, consider this a sign that something may be seriously wrong with the patient and transport as soon as possible.

Pulse Quality

pulse quality the rhythm (regular or irregular) and force (strong or weak) of the pulse.

radial (RAY-de-ul) **pulse** the pulse felt at the wrist.

brachial pulse the pulse felt in the upper arm.

carotid (kah-ROT-id) **pulse** the pulse felt along the large carotid artery on either side of the neck.

Two factors determine **pulse quality:** rhythm and force. *Pulse rhythm* reflects regularity. A pulse is said to be regular when intervals between beats are constant. When the intervals are not constant, the pulse is irregular. You should report and document irregular pulse rhythms.

Pulse force refers to the pressure of the pulse wave as it expands the artery. Normally, the pulse should feel as if a strong wave has passed under your fingertips. This is a strong or full pulse. When the pulse feels weak and thin, the patient has a thready pulse.

Many disorders can be related to variations in pulse rate, rhythm, and force (Table 9-1).

Pulse rate and quality can be determined at a number of points throughout the body. During the determination of vital signs, you should initially find a **radial pulse** in patients 1 year of age and older. This is the wrist pulse, named for the radial artery found on the lateral (thumb) side of the forearm. In an infant 1 year old or less, find the **brachial pulse** in the upper arm (Figure 9-2) rather than the radial pulse. If you cannot measure the pulse on one arm, try the pulse of the other arm. When you cannot measure the radial or brachial pulse, use the **carotid pulse,** felt along the large carotid

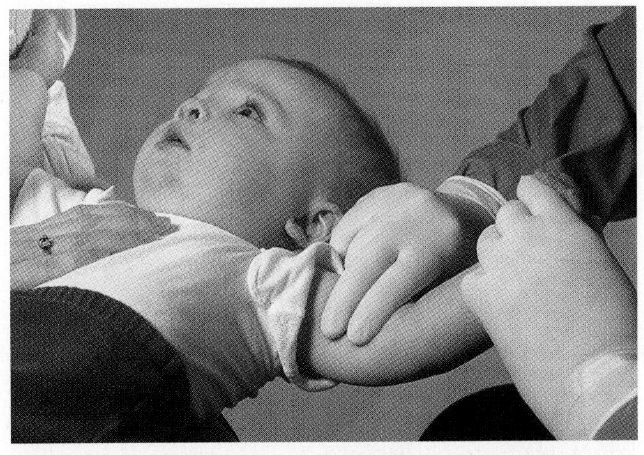

Figure 9-2 • Palpating a brachial pulse in an infant.

artery on either side of the neck, as you learned to do in cardiopulmonary resuscitation (CPR). Be careful when palpating a carotid pulse in a patient. Excessive pressure on the carotid artery can result in slowing of the heart, especially in older patients. If you have difficulty finding the carotid pulse on one side, try the other side, but *do not assess the carotid pulses on both sides at the same time.*

In order to measure a radial pulse, find the pulse site by placing your first three fingers on the thumb side of the patient's wrist just above the crease (toward the shoulder). Do not use your thumb. It has its own pulse that may cause you to measure your own pulse rate. Slide your fingertips toward the thumb side of the patient's wrist, keeping one finger over the crease. Apply moderate pressure to feel the pulse beats. A weak pulse may require applying greater pressure. But take care—if you press too hard you may press the artery shut. Remember: If you experience difficulty, try the patient's other arm.

Count the pulsations for 30 seconds and multiply by 2 to determine the beats per minute. While you are counting, judge the rhythm and force. Record the information: for example, "Pulse 72, regular and full," and the time of determination.

If the pulse rate, rhythm, or force is not normal, continue with your count and observations for a full 60 seconds.

Respiration

The act of breathing is called **respiration.** A single breath is considered to be the complete process of breathing in (called *inhalation* or *inspiration*) followed by breathing out (called *exhalation* or *expiration*). For the determination of vital signs, you are concerned with two factors: rate and quality (Figure 9-3).

respiration (res-puh-RAY-shun) the act of breathing in and breathing out.

Respiratory Rate

The **respiratory rate** is the number of breaths a patient takes in 1 minute (Table 9-2). The rate of respiration is classified as *normal, rapid,* or *slow*. The normal respiration rate for an adult at rest is between 12 and 20 breaths per minute. Keep in mind that age, sex, size, physical conditioning, and emotional state can influence breathing rates. Fear and other emotions experienced during an emergency can cause an increase in respiratory rate. However, if you have an adult patient maintaining a rate above 24 (rapid) or below 8 breaths per minute (slow), you must administer high-concentration oxygen and be prepared to assist ventilations.

respiratory rate the number of breaths taken in 1 minute.

Respiratory Quality

Respiratory quality, the quality of a patient's breathing, may fall into any of four categories: *normal, shallow, labored,* or *noisy*. Normal breathing means that the chest or abdomen moves an average depth with each breath and the patient is not using his accessory muscles (look for pronounced movement of the shoulder, neck, or abdominal

respiratory (RES-puh-ruh-tor-e) **quality** the normal or abnormal (shallow, labored, or noisy) character of breathing.

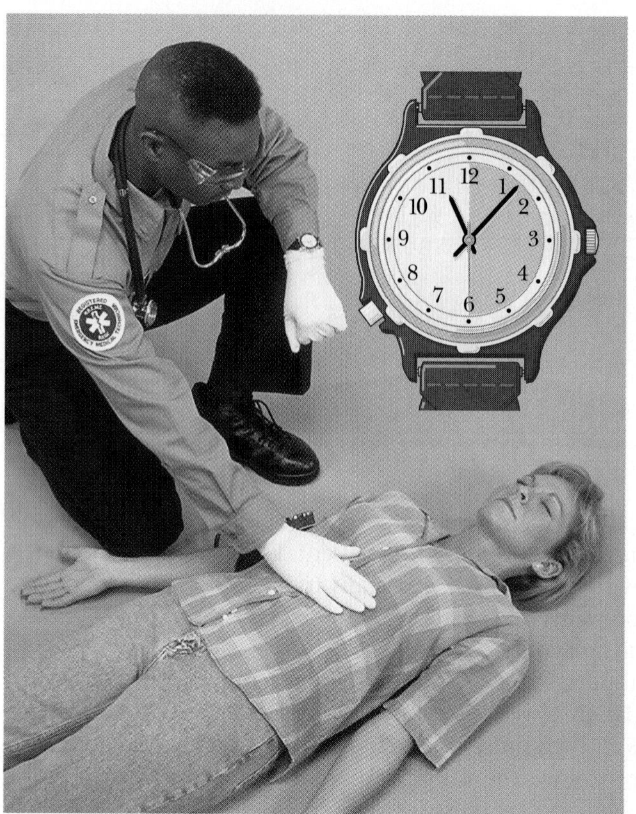

Figure 9-3 • Assess respiration rate and quality. Count for 30 seconds and multiply by 2.

TABLE 9-2 • Respirations

NORMAL RESPIRATORY RATES (BREATHS PER MINUTE, AT REST)	
Adult	12 to 20 Above 24: Serious Below 10: Serious
Infants and Children	
Adolescent 11–14 years	12 to 20
School age 6–10 years	15 to 30
Preschooler 3–5 years	20 to 30
Toddler 1–3 years	20 to 30
Infant 6–12 months	20 to 30
Infant 0–5 months	25 to 40
Newborn	30 to 50
RESPIRATORY SOUNDS	**POSSIBLE CAUSES/INTERVENTIONS**
Snoring	Airway blocked/Open patient's airway; prompt transport
Wheezing	Medical problem such as asthma/Assist patient in taking prescribed medications; prompt transport
Gurgling	Fluids in airway/Suction airway; prompt transport
Crowing (harsh sound when inhaling)	Medical problem that cannot be treated on the scene/ Prompt transport

muscles) to breathe. How can you tell if breathing is normal? Normal depth of respiration is something you can learn to judge by watching healthy people breathe when at rest.

Shallow breathing occurs when there is only slight movement of the chest or abdomen. This is especially serious in the unconscious patient. It is important to look not only at the chest but also at the abdomen when assessing respiration. Many resting people breathe more with their diaphragm (the muscle between the chest and the abdomen) than with their chest muscles.

Labored breathing can be recognized by signs such as an increase in the work of breathing (the patient has to work hard to move air in and out), the use of accessory muscles, nasal flaring (widening of the nostrils on inhalation), and retractions (pulling in) above the collarbones or between the ribs, especially in infants and children. You may also hear stridor (a harsh, high-pitched sound heard on inspiration), grunting on expiration (especially in infants), or gasping.

Noisy breathing is obstructed breathing (when something is blocking the flow of air). Sounds to be concerned about (Table 9-2) include snoring, wheezing, gurgling, and crowing. A patient with snoring respirations needs to have his airway opened. Wheezing may respond to prescribed medication the patient has and that you may be able to assist the patient in taking. Gurgling sounds usually mean that you need to suction the patient's airway. Crowing (a noisy, harsh sound when breathing in) may not respond to any treatment you give. The patient who is crowing needs prompt transport—as do all patients with difficulty breathing.

Respiratory Rhythm

Respiratory rhythm is not important in most of the conscious patients you will see. This is because the regularity of an awake patient's breathing is affected by his speech, mood, and activity, among other things. If you observe irregular respirations in an unconscious patient, however, you should report and document it.

respiratory rhythm the regular or irregular spacing of breaths.

Start counting respirations as soon as you have determined the pulse rate. Many individuals change their breathing rate if they know someone is watching them breathe. For this reason, do not move your hand from the patient's wrist or tell the patient you are counting the respiratory rate. After you have counted pulse beats, immediately begin to watch the patient's chest and abdomen for breathing movements. Count the number of breaths taken by the patient during 30 seconds and multiply by 2 to obtain the breaths per minute. While counting, note the rate, quality, and rhythm of respiration. Record your results; for example, "Respirations are 16, normal, and regular." Record the time of the assessment.

Skin

The color, temperature, and condition of the skin can provide valuable information about your patient's circulation. There are many blood vessels in the skin. Since the skin is not as important to survival as some of the other organs (like the heart and brain), the blood vessels of the skin will receive less blood when a patient has lost a significant amount of blood or the ability to adequately circulate blood. Constriction (growing smaller) of the blood vessels causes the skin to become pale. For this reason, the skin can provide clues to blood loss as well as a variety of other conditions.

The best places to assess skin color in adults are the nail beds, the inside of the cheek, and the inside of the lower eyelids. Tiny blood vessels called capillaries are very close to the surface of the skin in all of these places, so changes in the blood are quickly reflected at these sites. They are also more accurate indicators than other sites in adults with dark complexions. In infants and children, the best places to look are the palms of the hands and the soles of the feet. In patients with dark skin you can check the lips and nail beds.

Ordinarily, the color you see (Table 9-3) in any of these places is pink. Abnormal colors include pale, cyanotic (blue-gray), flushed (red), and jaundiced (yellow). Pale skin frequently indicates poor circulation of blood. A common cause of this in the field is loss of blood. Cyanotic skin is usually a result of not enough oxygen getting to the red blood cells. Flushed skin may be caused by exposure to heat. Jaundice is a yellowish tint to the skin from liver abnormalities. An uncommon skin coloration is mottling, a blotchy appearance that sometimes occurs in patients, especially children and the elderly, who are in shock.

TABLE 9-3 • Skin Color

SKIN COLOR	SIGNIFICANCE/POSSIBLE CAUSES
Pink	Normal in light-skinned patients. Normal at inner eyelids, lips, and nail beds of dark-skinned patients
Pale	Constricted blood vessels possibly resulting from blood loss, shock, hypotension, emotional distress
Cyanotic (blue-gray)	Lack of oxygen in blood cells and tissues resulting from inadequate breathing or heart function
Flushed (red)	Exposure to heat, emotional excitement
Jaundiced (yellow)	Abnormalities of the liver
Mottled (blotchy)	Occasionally in patients with shock

To determine skin temperature (Table 9-4), feel the patient's skin with the back of your hand. A good place to do this is the patient's forehead (Figure 9-4). Note if the skin feels normal (warm), hot, cool, or cold. If the patient's skin seems cold, then further assess by placing the back of your hand on the abdomen beneath the clothing. At the same time, notice the patient's condition—Is the skin dry (normal), moist, or clammy (both cool and moist)? Look for "goose pimples," which are often associated with chills. Many patient problems are exhibited by changes in skin temperature and condition. Continue to be alert for major temperature differences on various parts of the body. For

TABLE 9-4 • Skin Temperature and Condition

SKIN TEMPERATURE/ CONDITION	SIGNIFICANCE/ POSSIBLE CAUSES
Cool, clammy	Sign of shock, anxiety
Cold, moist	Body is losing heat
Cold, dry	Exposure to cold
Hot, dry	High fever, heat exposure
Hot, moist	High fever, heat exposure
"Goose pimples" accompanied by shivering, chattering teeth, blue lips, and pale skin	Chills, communicable disease, exposure to cold, pain, or fear

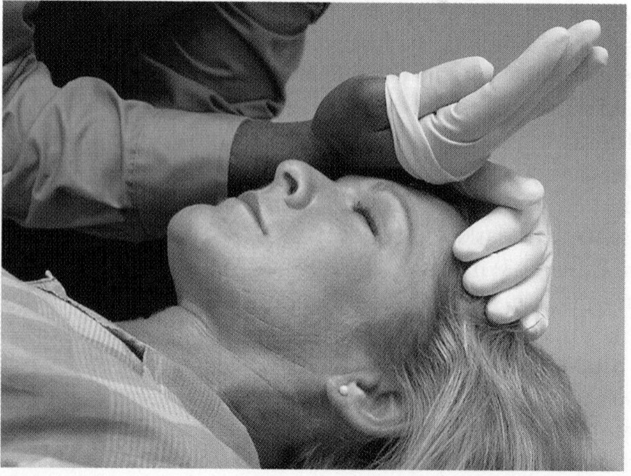

Figure 9-4 • Determining skin temperature.

PEDIATRIC NOTE

In infants and children under 6 years of age, you should also evaluate capillary refill. Press on the nail bed—or the top of the hand or foot—and watch how long it takes for the normal pink color to return after you release it. Normally, this takes no more than 2 seconds. If it takes longer, the patient's blood is probably not circulating well. Abnormal responses include prolonged and absent capillary refill. This sign is not reliable in infants and children who have been exposed to cold temperatures.

example, you may note that the patient's trunk is warm but his left arm feels cold. Such a finding can reveal a problem with circulation.

Pupils

The **pupil** is the black center of the eye. One of the things that cause it to change size is the amount of light entering the eye. When the environment is dim, the pupil will **dilate** (get larger) to allow more light into the eye. When there is a lot of light, it will **constrict** (get smaller). So you will check a patient's pupils by shining a light into them (Figures 9-5 and 9-6). When you check pupils, you should look for three things: size, equality, and **reactivity** (reacting to light by changing size). Under ordinary conditions, pupils are neither large nor small, but midpoint. Dilated pupils are extremely large. In fact, it is usually difficult to tell what color eyes the patient has if his pupils are dilated. Both pupils are normally the same size, and when a light shines into them, they react by constricting. The rate at which they constrict should be equal. Nonreactive (fixed) pupils do not constrict in response to a bright light.

pupil
the black center of the eye.

dilate (DI-late)
get larger.

constrict (kon-STRIKT)
get smaller.

reactivity (re-ak-TIV-uh-te)
in the pupils of the eyes, reacting to light by changing size.

To check the patient's pupils, first note their size before you shine any light into them. Next, cover one eye as you shine a penlight into the other eye. The pupil should constrict when the light is shining into it and enlarge when you remove the light. Repeat with the other eye. You should cover the eye you are not examining because light entering one eye usually affects the size of the pupils in both eyes. When you are examining a patient in direct sunlight or very bright conditions, initially cover both eyes. After a few seconds, uncover one eye and evaluate it. Cover it again and repeat with the other eye.

Pupils that are dilated, constricted to pinpoint size, unequal in size or reactivity, or nonreactive may indicate a variety of conditions (Table 9-5) including drug influence, head injury, or eye injury. Any deviations from normal should be reported and documented.

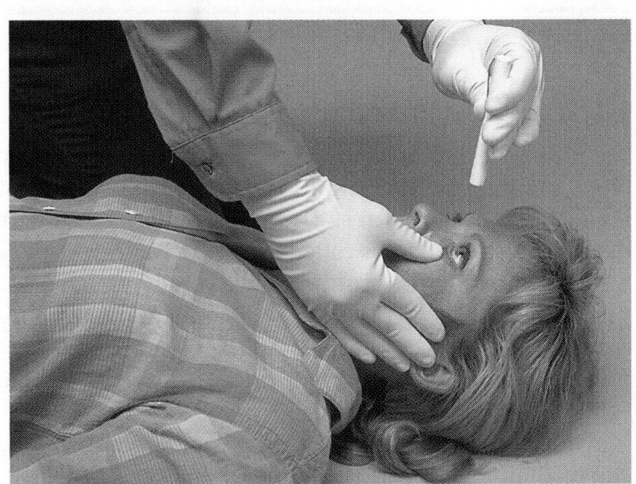

Figure 9-5 • Examining the pupils.

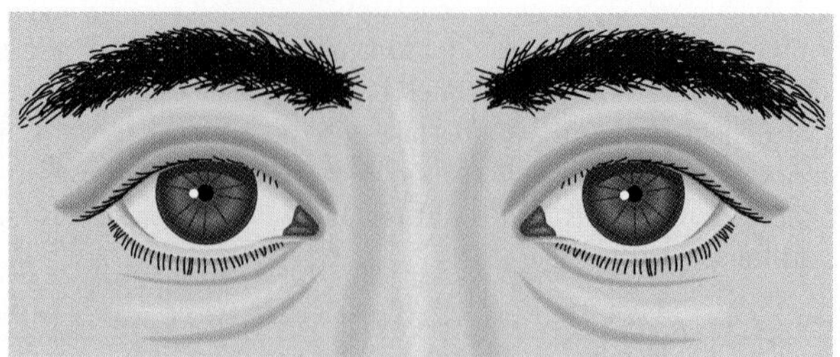
Constricted pupils

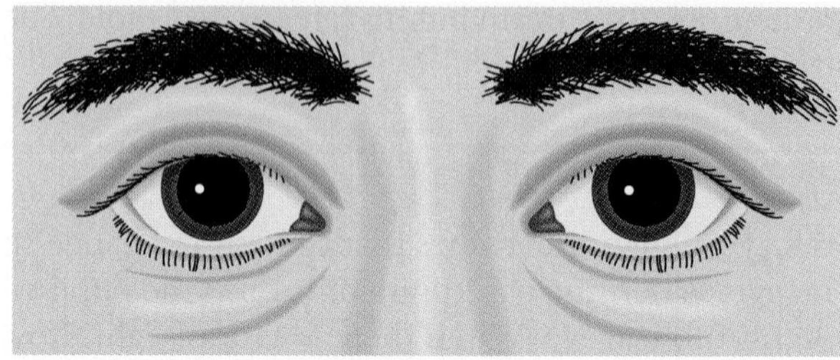
Dilated pupils

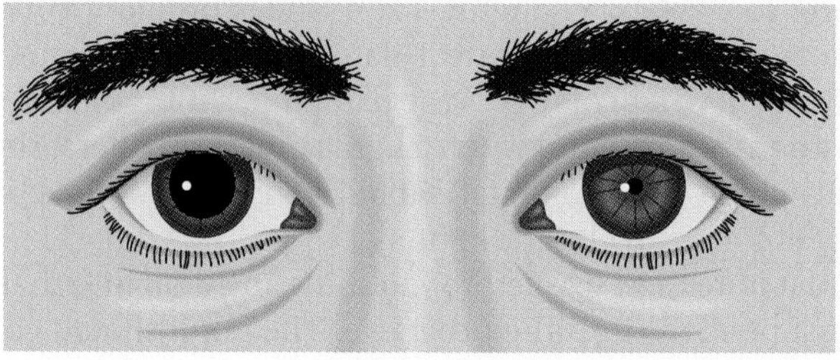
Unequal pupils

Figure 9-6 • Constricted, dilated, and unequal pupils.

TABLE 9-5 • Pupils

PUPIL APPEARANCE	SIGNIFICANCE/POSSIBLE CAUSES
Dilated (larger than normal)	Fright, blood loss, drugs, treatment with prescription eye drops
Constricted (smaller than normal)	Drugs (narcotics), treatment with prescription eye drops
Unequal	Stroke, head injury, eye injury, artificial eye
Lack of reactivity	Drugs, lack of oxygen to brain

blood pressure the force of blood against the walls of the blood vessels.

systolic (sis-TOL-ik) **blood pressure** the pressure created when the heart contracts and forces blood out into the arteries.

diastolic (di-as-TOL-ik) **blood pressure** the pressure remaining in the arteries when the left ventricle of the heart is relaxed and refilling.

Blood Pressure

Each time the ventricle (lower chamber) of the left side of the heart contracts, it forces blood out into the circulation. The force of blood against the walls of the blood vessels is called **blood pressure.** The pressure created when the heart contracts and forces blood into the arteries is called the **systolic blood pressure.** When the left ventricle relaxes and refills, the pressure remaining in the arteries is called the **diastolic blood pressure.** These two pressures indicate the amount of pressure against the walls of the arteries and together are known as the blood pressure. When you take a patient's blood pressure, you report the systolic pressure first, the diastolic second, as "120 over 80," or "120/80."

One blood pressure reading may not be very meaningful. You will need to take several readings over a period of time while care is provided at the scene and during transport. Changes in blood pressure can be very significant. The patient's blood pressure

POINT OF VIEW

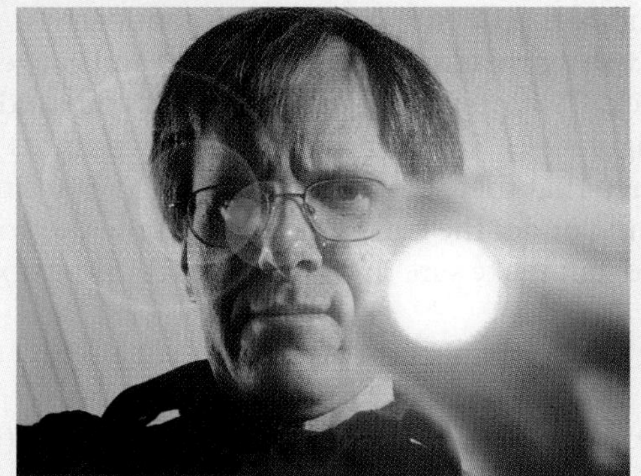

"I have to tell you, people are glad when the ambulance shows up, but it is intimidating as hell. Pardon my language and everything, but I remember when I hit my head and passed out. It was like the cavalry came into my kitchen.

"My sister-in-law is an EMT. She talks about medical things like other people talk about going shopping. Really easy, like something you do every day. But when the EMTs came to my house I was a little intimidated. They started doing this and checking that. It was hard enough to focus after just getting my bell rung. I couldn't even start to answer their questions, and to make things worse they kept shining a flashlight in my eyes.

"On the way to the hospital it got better. Actually, I think my head got clearer and it turns out they were worried about me. Something about 'altered mental status.' Maybe that means I was kind of nuts. We had a nice talk and they told me it was good news that my pupils looked ok (Aha! That's why they were shining that light in my eyes...) and also good news that I was talking with them now.

"I just finally felt like I had some control over what was going on."

may be normal in the early stages of some very serious problems, only to change rapidly in a matter of minutes.

Pulse and respiratory rates vary among individuals, but blood pressure is a little different (Table 9-6). A normal blood pressure is a systolic pressure of no greater than 120 millimeters of mercury (mmHg) and a diastolic pressure of no greater than 80 mmHg. *Millimeters of mercury* refers to the units on the blood pressure gauge. If an adult has a systolic pressure of 140 mmHg or greater or a diastolic pressure of 90 mmHg or greater, the person has hypertension (high blood pressure). Readings between these limits (121 to 139 mmHg systolic and 81 to 89 mmHg diastolic) indicate a condition sometimes called prehypertension. This means the patient is at risk of developing some of the complications of hypertension like heart disease, stroke, or kidney disease.

Serious low blood pressure is generally considered to exist when the systolic pressure falls below 90 mmHg. Many individuals under stress (like that caused by having the ambulance come to their home) will exhibit a temporary rise in blood pressure.

TABLE 9-6 • Blood Pressure

BLOOD PRESSURE NORMAL RANGES	SYSTOLIC	DIASTOLIC
Adults	Less than or equal to 120	Less than or equal to 80
Infants and Children	Approx. 80 + 2* age (yrs)	Approx. 2/3 systolic
Adolescent 11–14 years	Average 114 (88 to 120)	Average 76
School age 6–10 years	Average 105 (80 to 115)	Average 69
Preschooler 3–5 years	Average 99 (78 to 104)	Average 65

BLOOD PRESSURE	SIGNIFICANCE/POSSIBLE CAUSES
High blood pressure	Medical condition, exertion, fright, emotional distress, or excitement
Low blood pressure	Athlete or other person with normally low blood pressure; blood loss; late sign of shock

Infants and Children: Blood pressure is usually not taken on a child under 3 years. In cases of blood loss or shock, a child's blood pressure will remain within normal limits until near the end, then fall swiftly.

sphygmomanometer (SFIG-mo-mah-NOM-uh-ter) the cuff and gauge used to measure blood pressure.

brachial (BRAY-key-al) **artery** the major artery of the arm.

auscultation (os-kul-TAY-shun) listening. A stethoscope is used to auscultate for characteristic sounds.

palpation touching or feeling. A pulse or blood pressure may be palpated with the fingertips.

blood pressure monitor machine that automatically inflates a blood pressure cuff and measures blood pressure.

More than one reading will be necessary to decide if a high or low reading is only temporary. If the blood pressure drops, your patient may be developing shock (however, other signs are usually more important early indicators of shock). Report any major changes in blood pressure to emergency department personnel without delay.

To measure blood pressure with a **sphygmomanometer** (the cuff and gauge), first place the stethoscope around your neck. Position yourself at the patient's side and place the blood pressure cuff on his arm (Figure 9-7). The cuff should cover two-thirds of the upper arm, elbow to shoulder. Be certain that there are no suspected or obvious injuries to this arm. There should be no clothing under the cuff. If you can expose the arm sufficiently by rolling the sleeve up, do so, but make sure that this roll of clothing does not become a constricting band.

Wrap the cuff around the patient's upper arm so that the lower edge of the cuff is about 1 inch above the crease of the elbow. The center of the bladder must be placed over the **brachial artery,** the major artery of the arm. The marker on the cuff (if provided) should indicate where you place the cuff in relation to the artery, but many cuffs do not have markers in the correct location. Tubes entering the bladder are not always in the right location, either. According to the American Heart Association, the only accurate method is to find the bladder center. Apply the cuff so it is secure but not overly tight. You are now ready to begin your determination of the patient's blood pressure.

Three common techniques are used to measure blood pressure with a sphygmomanometer: (1) **auscultation,** when a stethoscope is used to listen for characteristic sounds (Figure 9-8); (2) **palpation,** when the radial pulse or brachial pulse is palpated (felt) with the fingertips (Figure 9-9); and (3) **blood pressure monitor,** when a machine controls inflation of the cuff and detects changes in blood flow in the artery

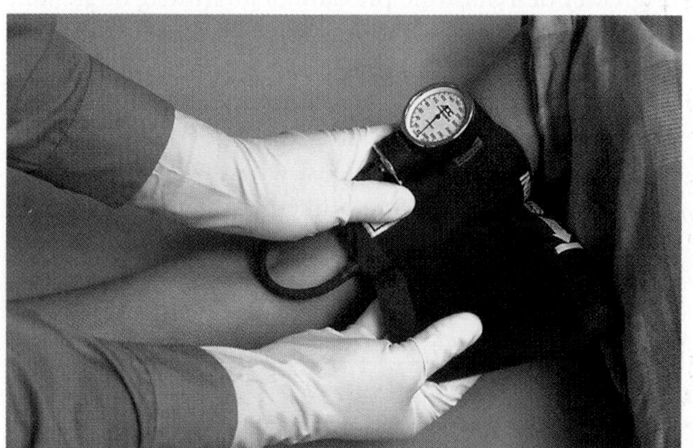

Figure 9-7 • Positioning blood pressure cuff.

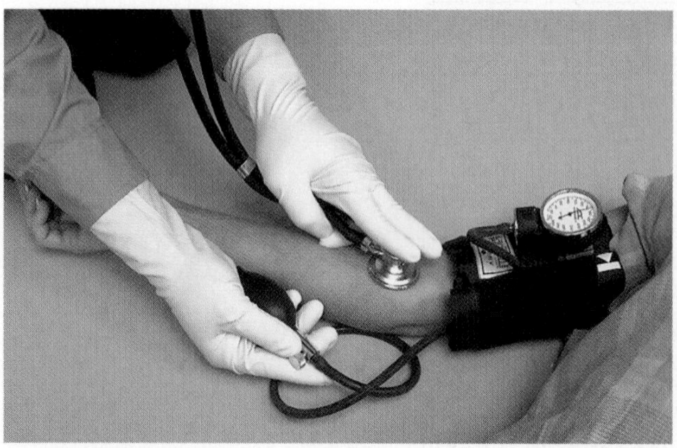

Figure 9-8 • Measuring blood pressure by auscultation.

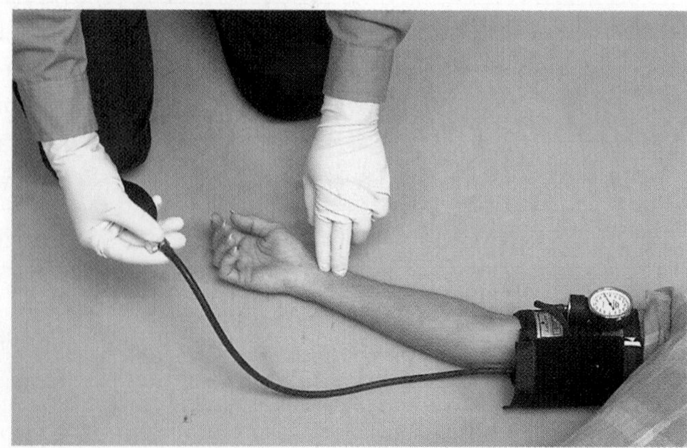

Figure 9-9 • Measuring blood pressure by palpation.

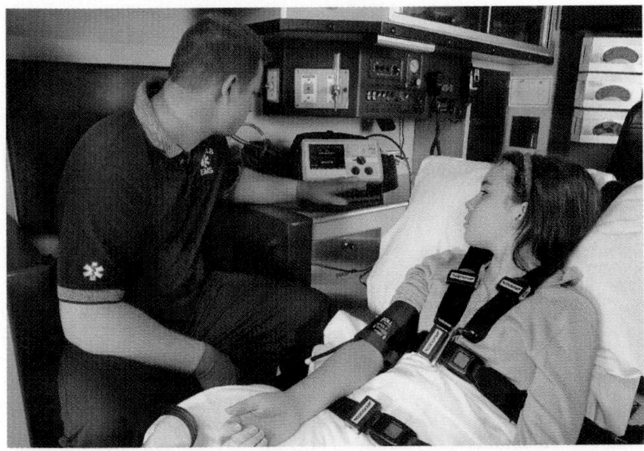

A

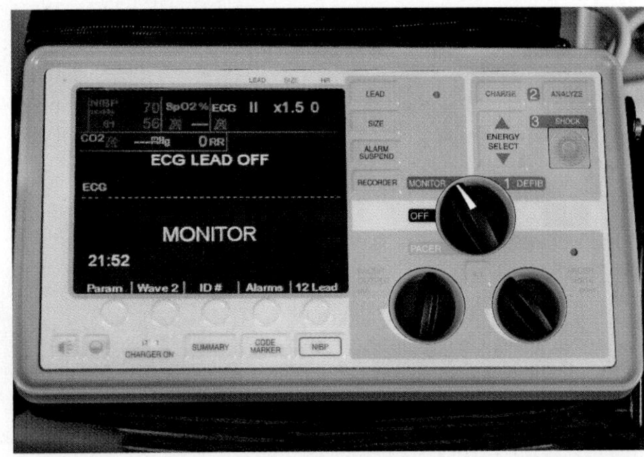

B

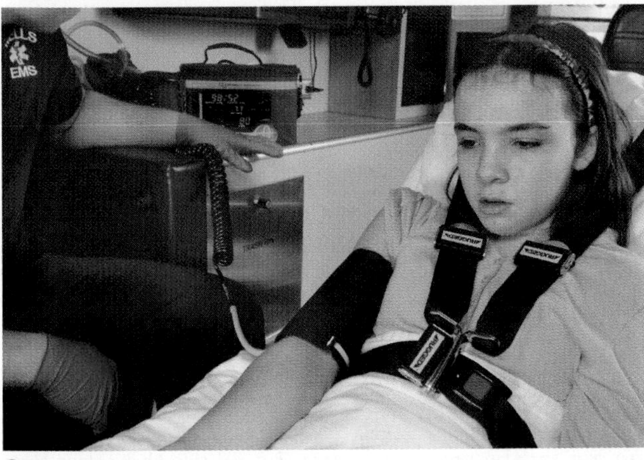

C

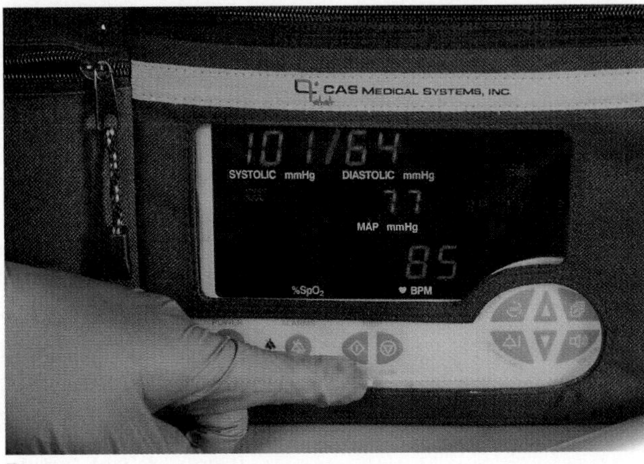

D

Figure 9-10 • (A and B) Automated blood pressure cuff as part of an ECG monitor. (C and D) Stand-alone automated blood pressure cuff.

(Figure 9-10). Palpation is not as accurate as auscultation, since only an approximate systolic pressure can be determined. Palpation is used when there is too much noise around a patient to allow the use of the stethoscope. Blood pressure monitors are improving in quality and many emergency departments and EMS agencies use them.

Determining Blood Pressure by Auscultation

1. *Prepare.* The patient should be seated or lying down. If the patient has not been injured, support his arm at the level of his heart.
2. *Position the cuff and the stethoscope.* Place the cuff snugly around the upper arm so that the bottom of the cuff is just above the elbow. With your fingertips, palpate the brachial artery at the crease of the elbow (Figure 9-11). Place the ear pieces of the stethoscope in your ears (the ear pieces should be pointing forward in the direction of your ear canals). Position the diaphragm of the stethoscope directly over the brachial pulse or over the medial anterior elbow (front of the elbow) if no brachial pulse can be found. Do not place the head of the stethoscope underneath the cuff, since this will give you false readings.
3. *Inflate the cuff.* With the bulb valve (thumb valve) closed, inflate the cuff. As you do so, you soon will be able to hear pulse sounds. Inflate the cuff, watching the gauge. At a certain point, you will no longer hear the brachial pulse. Continue to inflate the cuff until the gauge reads 30 mm higher than the point where the pulse sound disappeared.

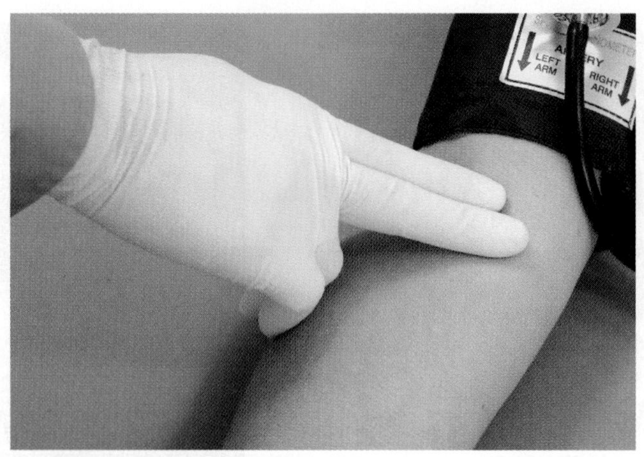

Figure 9-11 • When measuring blood pressure by auscultation, locate the brachial artery by palpation before placing the stethoscope.

4. *Obtain the systolic pressure.* Slowly release air from the cuff by opening the bulb valve, allowing the pressure to fall smoothly at the rate of approximately 5 to 10 mm per second. Listen for the start of clicking or tapping sounds. When you hear the first of these sounds, note the reading on the gauge. This is the systolic pressure.
5. *Obtain the diastolic pressure.* Continue to deflate the cuff, listening for the point at which these distinctive sounds fade. When the sounds turn to dull, muffled thuds, the reading on the gauge is the diastolic pressure. Sometimes you will not be able to hear a change in these sounds. When this happens, the point at which the sounds disappear is the diastolic pressure.
6. *Record measurements.* After obtaining the diastolic pressure, let the cuff deflate rapidly. Record the measurements and the time. For example, "Blood pressure is 140/90 at 1:10 p.m." Blood pressure is reported in even numbers. If a reading falls between two lines on the gauge, use the higher number.

If you are not certain of a reading, repeat the procedure. You should use the other arm or wait 1 minute before re-inflating the cuff. Otherwise, you will tend to obtain an erroneously high reading. If you are still not sure of the reading, try again or get some help. Never make up vital signs!

NOTE

Some patients who have high systolic blood pressures will have the pulse sounds disappear as you deflate the cuff, but reappear as you continue with deflation. When this happens, false readings may be obtained. If you determine a high diastolic reading, wait 1 to 2 minutes and take another reading. As you inflate the cuff, feel for the disappearance of the radial pulse to ensure that you are not measuring a false diastolic pressure. Listen as you deflate the cuff down into the normal range. The diastolic pressure is the reading at which the last clear sound takes place.

Determining Blood Pressure by Palpation

1. *Position the cuff and find the radial pulse.* Apply the cuff as described for auscultation. Then find the radial pulse on the arm to which the cuff has been applied. If a radial pulse cannot be palpated, find the brachial pulse.
2. *Inflate the cuff.* Make certain that the adjustable valve is closed on the bulb and inflate the cuff to a point where you can no longer feel the radial pulse. Note this point on the gauge and continue to inflate the cuff 30 mmHg beyond this point.
3. *Obtain and record the systolic pressure.* Slowly deflate the cuff, noting the reading at which the radial pulse returns. This reading is the patient's systolic pressure. Record your findings as, for example, "blood pressure 140 by palpation" or "140/P" and the time of the determination. (You cannot determine a diastolic reading by palpation.)

Determining Blood Pressure by Blood Pressure Monitor

1. *Position the cuff.* Apply the cuff as described for auscultation.
2. *Inflate the cuff.* Press the button that tells the monitor to begin inflating the cuff.
3. *Obtain and record the blood pressure.* After the monitor has finished deflating the cuff, it will indicate the patient's blood pressure on a screen. If it cannot get a blood pressure, it will tell you. Some monitors will give not only the systolic and diastolic pressures but also the mean arterial pressure (MAP). This is not typically used in prehospital care. Do not let it distract you from the numbers you are seeking.

PEDIATRIC NOTE

Obtain a blood pressure on every patient who is more than 3 years old. Blood pressures on infants and children younger than 3 are difficult to obtain with any accuracy and have little bearing on field management of the patient. You can get more useful information about the condition of an infant or very young child by observing for conditions such as a sick appearance, respiratory distress, or unconsciousness.

Unless medical direction advises otherwise, the first blood pressure you get should be with the auscultation method. Although the quality of blood pressure monitors has been improving, these machines still make errors, and this may be more likely in the prehospital environment. The blood pressure obtained by auscultation is the standard that other blood pressures will be compared to. If a reading from the blood pressure monitor is very different from the auscultated blood pressure, check the blood pressure yourself by auscultation or palpation.

Many blood pressure monitors have timers you can set to take the blood pressure every 5 minutes, every 15 minutes, or at some other interval determined by the operator. This can provide a useful reminder to the EMT when it is time to check the rest of the vital signs again.

It is important that the EMT follow the manufacturer's directions and local medical direction in using an automated blood pressure monitor or any other device used in patient assessment.

Vital signs are usually taken more than once. How frequently they should be repeated depends on the condition of the patient and your interventions. Stable patients need repeat vital signs at least every 15 minutes. Unstable patients need repeat vital signs at least every 5 minutes. Also repeat vital signs after every medical intervention. Record every reading of the vital signs (Figure 9-12).

Oxygen Saturation

EMTs and other health care providers commonly measure the level of oxygen circulating through a patient's blood vessels. A measurement of oxygen saturation is not a vital sign, but many EMS providers incorporate it into their gathering of vital signs. Your EMS system may have specific guidance on when to perform this measurement.

The device that measures oxygen saturation of the blood is called a **pulse oximeter** (Figure 9-13). It sends different colors of light into the tissue at the end of a finger or on an earlobe and measures the amount of light that returns. The machine then determines

pulse oximeter an electronic device for determining the amount of oxygen carried in the blood, known as the oxygen saturation or SpO_2.

Time	Pulse	Respirations	Blood Pressure
1410	88 str, reg	28	132/84
Pupils	**Skin Color**	**Skin Temperature**	**Skin Condition**
Equal ☑ Unequal ☐	Normal ☐	Cold ☐	Moist ☑
Reactive (L) (R)	Pale ☑	Cool ☑	Dry ☐
Nonreactive L R	Cyanotic ☐	Warm ☐	
Dilated ☐	Flushed ☐	Hot ☐	
Normal Size ☑	Jaundiced ☐		
Constricted ☐			

Figure 9-12 • The prehospital care report (run sheet) provides spaces for recording vital signs.

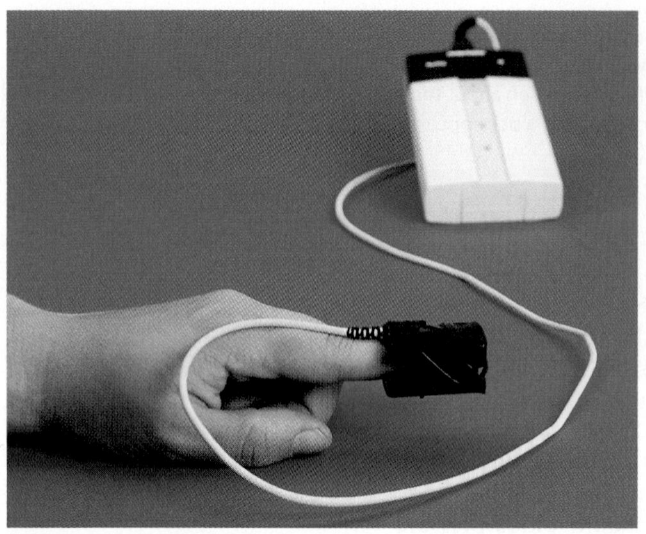

A

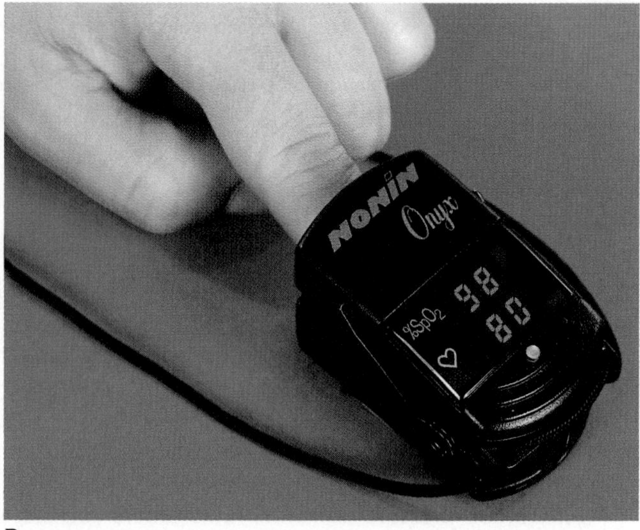

B

Figure 9-13 • (A) A pulse oximeter with sensor applied to the patient's finger. (B) A mini "finger-size" pulse oximeter with all-in-one sensor and read-out display.

oxygen saturation (SpO_2) the ratio of the amount of oxygen present in the blood to the amount that could be carried, expressed as a percentage.

the proportion of oxygen in the blood and displays the **oxygen saturation** percentage, also called the SpO_2.

A different kind of oximeter uses different wavelengths of light that allow it to measure carbon monoxide (CO) as well as oxygen. For this reason, it is sometimes called a CO-oximeter (Figure 9-14). Future versions of this device will very likely be more accurate, less expensive, and easier to use than early models. Interpreting CO-oximeter readings in a particular clinical situation can be challenging, so if you use a CO-oximeter, be sure to follow your local protocols regarding its application and interpretation.

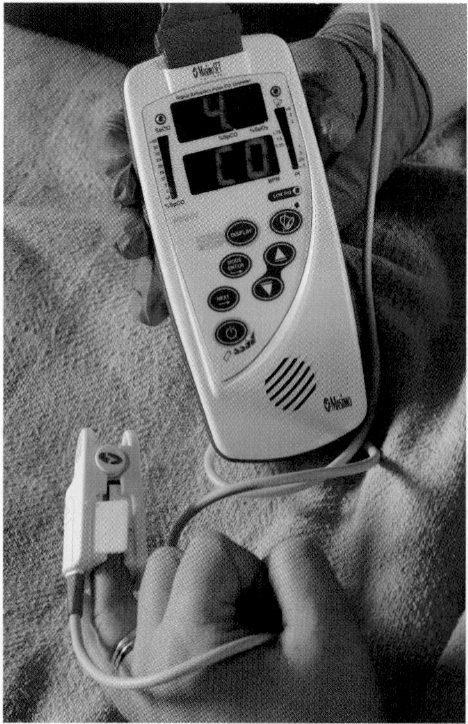

Figure 9-14 • A CO-oximeter detects carbon monoxide as well as oxygen levels in the blood.

When to Use a Pulse Oximeter

If your service has a pulse oximeter, you should have a protocol describing when to use it. Generally, this will include all patients complaining of respiratory problems. When used properly, the device can help you to assess the effectiveness of artificial respirations, oxygen therapy, and bronchodilator (inhaler) therapy. Some services recommend its use in other patients as well. Follow your local protocols.

Interpreting Pulse Oximeter Readings

The oxygen saturation, or SpO_2, is typically 96 to 100 percent in a normal healthy person. A value less than 96 percent may sound good, but that is not really the case. A reading of 91 to 95 percent indicates hypoxia, 86 to 90 percent indicates significant hypoxia, and 85 percent or less indicates severe hypoxia. The lower the oxygen saturation reading you get, the more aggressive your management should be. Any indication of hypoxia is reason to administer high-concentration oxygen by nonrebreather mask. For very low readings, you will need to look at the patient's clinical condition and decide whether to ventilate the patient with high-concentration oxygen. You should try to get the SpO_2 up to at least 96 percent.

The reverse situation is not true; that is, a reading above 96 percent does NOT mean you should withhold oxygen from a patient with signs and symptoms that indicate the need for oxygen.

Cautions

- The oximeter is inaccurate with patients in shock and hypothermic patients (those whose body temperatures have been lowered by exposure to cold) because not enough blood is flowing through the capillaries for the device to get an accurate reading.
- The oximeter will produce falsely high readings in patients with carbon monoxide and certain other uncommon types of poisoning. This is because carbon monoxide binds with hemoglobin in the blood, producing the red color read by the device. Cigarettes produce carbon monoxide, so chronic smokers may have 10 to 15 percent of their hemoglobin bound to carbon monoxide. This means their oxygen saturation readings will be higher than the actual oxygen saturation.
- Excessive movement of the patient can cause inaccurate readings. So can nail polish, if the device is attached to a finger. Carry acetone wipes to quickly remove the nail polish from a patient's fingernail before attaching the oximeter. Anemia, hypovolemia, and certain kinds of poisoning are other potential causes of falsely high oxygen saturation readings.
- The accuracy of the pulse oximeter should be checked regularly, following the manufacturer's recommendations. The batteries used to power the device must be in good condition and the probe needs to be kept clean to get accurate readings.
- Pulse oximetry is most useful in two situations: evaluating the effect of an intervention you have instituted (when you hope the SpO_2 goes up or remains high) and alerting you early to a deterioration in the patient's oxygen saturation (when the SpO_2 starts going down). Like any other device, the pulse oximeter can distract you from the patient. Keep it in its proper place. Remember, the oximeter is just another tool. Do not rely on it solely for indications of the patient's condition. Treat the patient, not the device.

NOTE

Never deprive a patient in respiratory distress of supplemental oxygen while attempting to obtain an accurate pulse oximetry reading. For these patients, providing supplemental oxygen, or even assisting ventilations, is a far more important intervention than documenting their "room air" saturation of oxygen.

Determining Oxygen Saturation

1. Connect the sensor lead to the monitor and clip it onto a fingertip (toe or distal foot in an infant).
2. Turn the device on. After a few seconds the device should display the SpO_2 and heart rate. Make sure the heart rate displayed on the monitor screen is the same as

the patient's pulse rate (which you palpated already). If the heart rate shown on the pulse oximeter does not match the pulse rate that you have determined, it is likely that the oxygen saturation will not be an accurate reading either.

3. If you get a poor signal or "trouble" indicator, try repositioning the sensor on the finger or moving it to a different finger.
4. Once you get an accurate reading, check the oximeter reading every 5 minutes. A convenient time to do this is when you check the patient's vital signs.

SAMPLE HISTORY

sign
an indication of a patient's condition that is objective, or can be observed by another person; an indication that can be seen, heard, smelled, or felt by the EMT or others.

symptom
an indication of a patient's condition that cannot be observed by another person but rather is subjective, or felt and reported by the patient.

SAMPLE history
the present and past medical history of a patient, so called because the elements of the history begin with the letters of the word sample: signs/symptoms, allergies, medications, pertinent past history, last oral intake, events leading to the injury or illness.

An EMT can gain two kinds of information about the patient's present problem: signs and symptoms. A **sign** is objective—something you see, hear, feel, and smell when examining the patient. The vital signs are, of course, signs, as are sweaty skin, staggering, and vomiting, for example. A **symptom** is subjective—an indication you cannot observe but that the patient feels and tells you about. Such things as chest pain, dizziness, and nausea are considered symptoms.

An important part of the information you should gain on all of your patients is information about the present problem (signs and symptoms) plus the past medical history—together called the **SAMPLE history** because the letters in SAMPLE stand for elements of the history: signs and symptoms, allergies, medications, pertinent past history, last oral intake, and events leading to the injury or illness. To obtain the SAMPLE history, ask your patient (or, if the patient is unconscious, ask the family and bystanders) these questions:

- *Signs and symptoms.* What's wrong?
- *Allergies.* Are you allergic to medications, foods, or environmentals? Is there a medical identification tag describing allergies?
- *Medications.* What medications are you currently taking or supposed to be taking (prescription, over-the-counter, or recreational)? Are you on birth control pills? Is there a medical identification tag with the names of medications on it? Do you take any herbal supplements or medications?
- *Pertinent past history.* Have you been having any medical problems? Have you been feeling ill? Have you recently had any surgery or injuries? Have you been seeing a doctor? What is your doctor's name?
- *Last oral intake.* When did you last eat or drink? What did you eat or drink? (Food or liquids can cause symptoms or aggravate a medical condition. Also, if a patient will need to go to surgery, the hospital staff must know when he last had anything to eat or drink, since stomach contents can be vomited while a patient is under anesthesia, which is a very dangerous occurrence.)
- *Events leading to the injury or illness.* What sequence of events led up to today's problem (e.g., the patient passed out, then got into a car crash versus got into car crash and then passed out)?

When conducting a patient interview:

- Position yourself close to the patient. Depending on the patient's situation, kneel or stand close to him. If possible, position yourself so that the sun or bright lights are not at your back. That way the patient will not have to squint to see you. When practical, position yourself so the patient can see your face and it is at a level close to that of the patient's face. This is especially important with children.
- Identify yourself, and reassure the patient. It is important that the patient know he is in competent hands. Maintain eye contact with the patient and state your name, that you are an Emergency Medical Technician, and the organization you represent.

Cultural Considerations

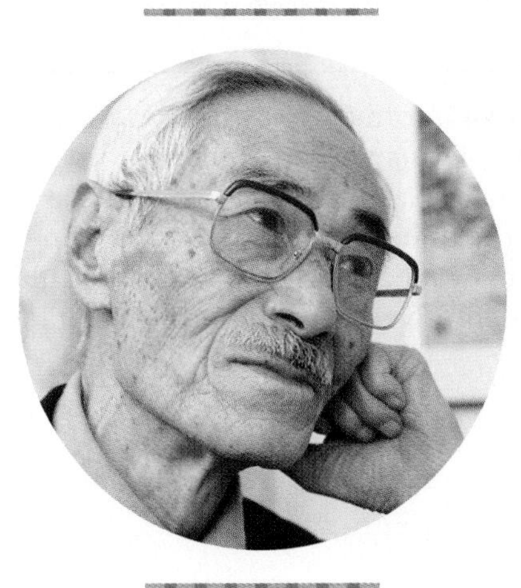

Some cultural groups, particularly Asian cultures, place a premium on being pleasant and accommodating to strangers. When you are conducting the SAMPLE history, you may find that your Asian patient is trying to anticipate the answers he thinks you want to hear and, in an effort to be polite, will answer "yes" even when he doesn't understand the question. This may be especially true of older Asian patients or those who were adults before they moved to a western country.

In this situation, pose open-ended questions that require the patient to volunteer information rather than simply agreeing with your suggestion. Avoid "Do you/did you" questions and try to ask "What/when/how" questions.

For example, instead of asking "Do you feel pain in this area?" ask "What do you feel here?" Instead of asking "Do you have any allergies?" ask "What are you allergic to, if anything?" Instead of asking "Do you take any medications?" ask "What medications do you take?" Instead of asking "Have you felt this way before?" ask "When have you felt this way before?" Instead of asking "Did you get dizzy before you fell?" ask "What do you think made you fall?" Instead of asking "Did you eat lunch today?" ask "When did you last eat something? What did you eat or drink?"

- Speak in your normal voice. When you ask a question, wait for a reply. Work to gain the patient's confidence through calm conversation. Avoid inappropriate remarks like, "Don't worry," and "Everything is all right." The patient knows everything is not all right.
- If you believe it to be appropriate, gently touch the patient's shoulder or rest your hand over his. A simple touch is comforting to most people.
- Learn your patient's name. Once you know it, use it in the rest of your conversations. Children will expect you to use their first names. For adults, use the appropriate Mr., Mrs., Miss, or Ms. unless they introduce themselves by their first name. If you are unsure how to address the patient, ask what he would like you to call him. You need the patient's name for completion of your forms and to give a personal touch that is often very reassuring to the patient. Having the patient's name could prove to be of great importance should he become unconscious and not be carrying any identification.
- Learn your patient's age. This will be needed for reports and communications with the medical facility.

The SAMPLE history gives valuable information about the patient's condition. This will sometimes influence the field management of the patient, but it will more often affect the patient's hospital treatment. If the patient should lose consciousness before arriving at the hospital, he will be unable to give his history. This is one of the most important reasons for the EMT to get this information.

PEDIATRIC NOTE

One of the most important factors that determines the normal range of vital signs is age. Infants and children have faster pulse and respiratory rates and lower blood pressures than adults. Compare the ranges for infants and children with those for adults in the tables in this chapter.

Another way in which infants and children under 6 differ from adults is that capillary refill can be a useful guide to the status of their circulation, which is not generally true of adults.

CHAPTER REVIEW

SUMMARY

As an EMT, you can gain a great deal of information about a patient's condition by taking a complete set of baseline vital signs. These include pulse, respirations, skin, pupils, and blood pressure. (See Tables 9-7, 9-8, and 9-9 for a summary of normal ranges for pulse, respirations, and blood pressure.) These must then be followed by repeat vital signs in order to recognize trends in the patient's condition. How often you repeat the vital signs will depend on the patient's condition.

Another source of information is the SAMPLE history. By determining the signs/symptoms, allergies, medications, pertinent past history, last oral intake, and events leading to the injury or illness, you will gain information that may affect field treatment and will be important to the definitive treatment of the patient at the hospital.

TABLE 9-7 • Pulse, Normal Ranges

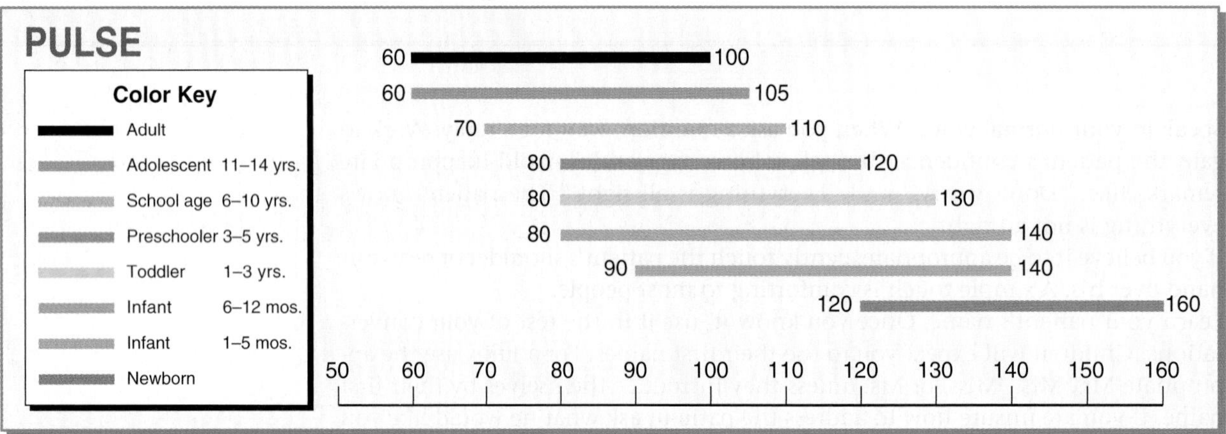

TABLE 9-8 • Respiration, Normal Ranges

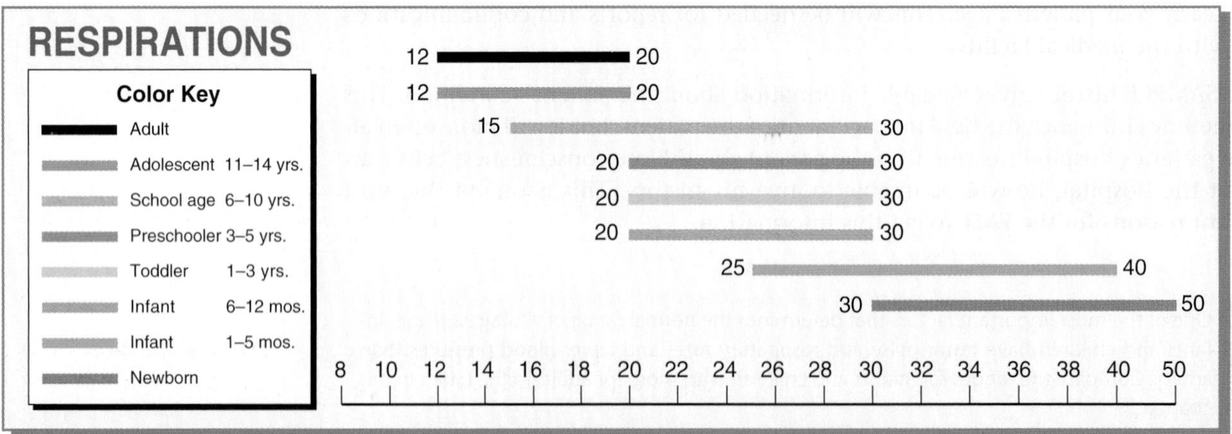

TABLE 9-9 • Blood Pressure, Normal Ranges

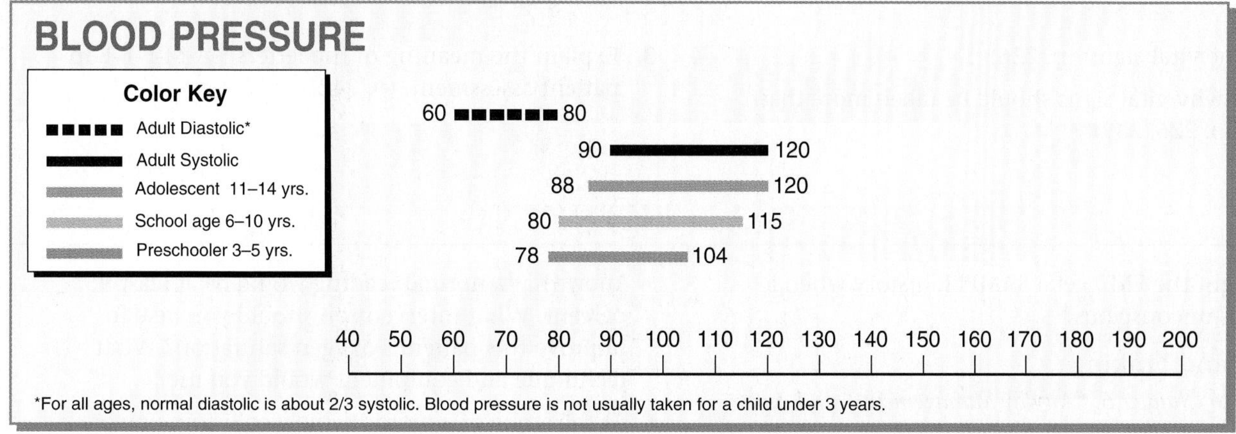

KEY TERMS

auscultation (os-kul-TAY-shun) listening. A stethoscope is used to auscultate for characteristic sounds.

blood pressure the force of blood against the walls of the blood vessels.

blood pressure monitor machine that automatically inflates a blood pressure cuff and measures blood pressure.

brachial (BRAY-key-al) **artery** the major artery of the arm.

brachial pulse the pulse felt in the upper arm.

bradycardia (BRAY-duh-KAR-de-uh) a slow pulse; any pulse rate below 60 beats per minute.

carotid (kah-ROT-id) **pulse** the pulse felt along the large carotid artery on either side of the neck.

constrict (kon-STRIKT) get smaller.

diastolic (di-as-TOL-ik) **blood pressure** the pressure remaining in the arteries when the left ventricle of the heart is relaxed and refilling.

dilate (DI-late) get larger.

oxygen saturation (SpO_2) the ratio of the amount of oxygen present in the blood to the amount that could be carried, expressed as a percentage.

palpation touching or feeling. A pulse or blood pressure may be palpated with the fingertips.

pulse the rhythmic beats felt as the heart pumps blood through the arteries.

pulse oximeter an electronic device for determining the amount of oxygen carried in the blood, known as the oxygen saturation or SpO_2.

pulse quality the rhythm (regular or irregular) and force (strong or weak) of the pulse.

pulse rate the number of pulse beats per minute.

pupil the black center of the eye.

radial (RAY-de-ul) **pulse** the pulse felt at the wrist.

reactivity (re-ak-TIV-uh-te) in the pupils of the eyes, reacting to light by changing size.

respiration (res-puh-RAY-shun) the act of breathing in and breathing out.

respiratory (RES-puh-ruh-tor-e) **quality** the normal or abnormal (shallow, labored, or noisy) character of breathing.

respiratory rate the number of breaths taken in 1 minute.

respiratory rhythm the regular or irregular spacing of breaths.

SAMPLE history the present and past medical history of a patient, so called because the elements of the history begin with the letters of the word sample: signs/symptoms, allergies, medications, pertinent past history, last oral intake, events leading to the injury or illness.

sign an indication of a patient's condition that is objective, or can be observed by another person; an indication that can be seen, heard, smelled, or felt by the EMT or others.

sphygmomanometer (SFIG-mo-mah-NOM-uh-ter) the cuff and gauge used to measure blood pressure.

symptom an indication of a patient's condition that cannot be observed by another person but rather is subjective, or felt and reported by the patient.

systolic (sis-TOL-ik) **blood pressure** the pressure created when the heart contracts and forces blood out into the arteries.

tachycardia (TAK-uh-KAR-de-uh) a rapid pulse; any pulse rate above 100 beats per minute.

vital signs outward signs of what is going on inside the body, including respiration; pulse; skin color, temperature, and condition (plus capillary refill in infants and children); pupils; and blood pressure.

REVIEW QUESTIONS

1. Name the vital signs. (p. 226)
2. Explain why vital signs should be taken more than once. (pp. 226, 239)
3. Explain the meaning of the letters S-A-M-P-L-E in patient assessment. (p. 242)

CRITICAL THINKING

- How might the EMT get a SAMPLE history when a patient is unconscious?

Thinking and Linking

Think back to Chapter 6, "Airway Management," and link information from that chapter (regarding oxygen administration and artificial ventilation) with information from this chapter (regarding oxygen saturation) as you consider the following situations:

- You are assessing a patient who complains of "feeling dizzy." On initial assessment, her breathing appears to be adequate, but when you apply the pulse oximeter during vital signs measurement, you note that her blood oxygen saturation reading is 93 percent. You know that a normal reading would be at least 96 percent. What intervention should you take to improve this patient's oxygen saturation? What technique and equipment would you use?
- At the scene of a motor-vehicle collision, you are caring for a patient with multiple injuries. Because his breathing was obviously inadequate (shallow and rapid), you initiated artificial ventilation with a bag-valve-mask unit. However, a subsequent reading on this pulse oximeter shows his blood oxygen saturation level—even with assisted ventilations—is only 90 percent. What can you do to attempt to improve his oxygen saturation level?

MEDIA RESOURCES 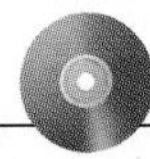

See the Student CD at the back of this book for quizzes, a case study activity, and other features related to this chapter. In particular, read the case study about taking a SAMPLE history and assessing vital signs on an elderly patient to be transported from a nursing home. Also, visit the Companion Website for *Emergency Care* at **www.prenhall.com/limmer**, where you will find additional reinforcement and links to other resources.

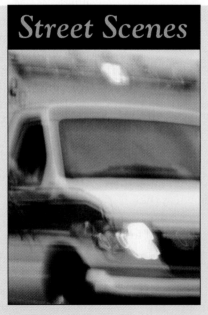

Street Scenes

You are just sitting down to relax when the dispatcher calls to notify you of a 73-year-old female patient with abdominal pain at 19 Oakwood Lane. Before getting to the scene, you and your partner agree that you will do the patient interview and he will assess vital signs. When you arrive, you find the patient sitting at her kitchen table. She tells you her name is Ms. Socorro Alvarez. She says she has stomach pain, "But I don't need to go to the hospital."

As you look at this patient, you find that you aren't confident that this is a good decision. You start to think ABCs and realize that her airway is obviously open and clear, but her breathing seems a little rapid.

Street Scene Questions

1. What is your primary concern for this patient?
2. What vital signs should be taken even if a no transport decision is being considered?
3. Ideally, what should the patient history include?

You tell Ms. Alvarez that if she called EMS, she must be concerned. So you ask her permission to assess her vital signs and ask her a few questions. She consents. "Tell me about the abdominal pain you had today," you ask. She explains that the pain was pretty bad and worse than the pain she had yesterday. "It is a sharp pain," she says. "It got much worse when I had a bowel movement." She tells you that her stools are black and tarry, she hasn't eaten today, and she was cleaning the kitchen when this last "attack" came on.

After your partner takes the patient's vital signs, he tells you that her pulse is 110 and thready, respirations are 28, and blood pressure is 100/70. You ask the patient if she knows her usual blood pressure, and she tells you 150/90.

Street Scene Questions

4. What other patient history information should be obtained?
5. Should you take another set of vital signs?
6. How might you get the patient to rethink her decision not to be transported?

You ask the patient if she is taking any medication. When she hands you two bottles from the kitchen table, you notice that her skin is pale and clammy. You write down the names of the medications and ask if she has any allergies. She tells you she is allergic to penicillin. You tell the patient that you think she really needs to go to the hospital and be seen by a doctor. You explain that her pulse is high and some of the other information she has provided needs to be evaluated. Your partner takes another set of vital signs and reports that the pulse is now 120 and thready. The other vital signs have not changed. Finally, after a bit more talk, the patient gives consent for transport.

You load the patient onto a stretcher and provide oxygen. The transport to the hospital is less than 10 minutes and uneventful. En route, your partner gives the radio report and you obtain another set of vital signs. After you transfer patient care to the emergency department personnel and you are doing your paperwork, you notice a great deal of activity around her. After a while, a woman approaches and tells you that she is Mrs. Alvarez's daughter. "The doctor told me that mama is bleeding internally," she says, "and that she needed immediate medical attention. Thank you."

CHAPTER

10

Assessment of the Trauma Patient

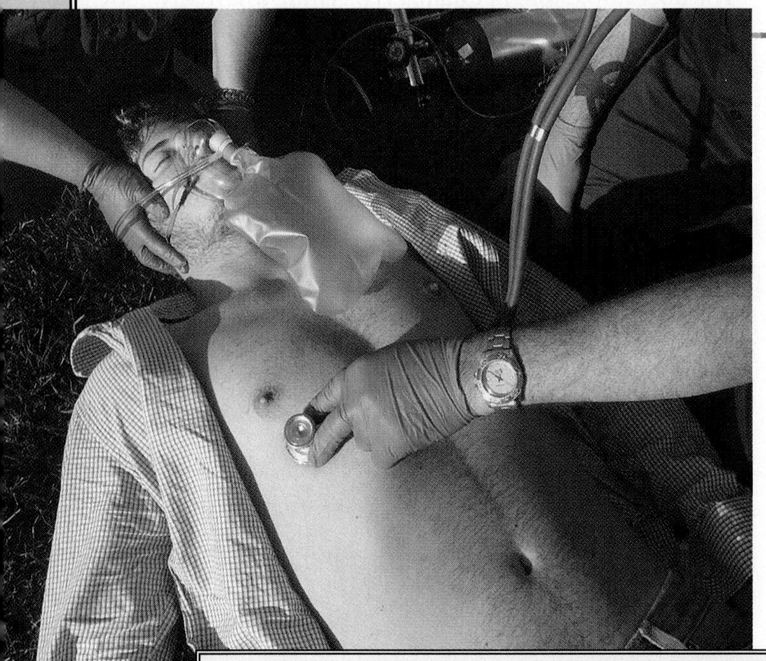

CORE CONCEPTS

The following are core concepts that will be addressed in this chapter:

- The difference between a significant and nonsignificant mechanism of injury
- The difference between patients who need a rapid trauma assessment and patients who need a focused physical exam
- How to perform a focused physical exam for a trauma patient
- How to perform a rapid trauma assessment
- How to perform a detailed physical examination for a trauma patient

KEY TERMS

colostomy, p. 267
crepitation, p. 265
DCAP-BTLS, p. 251
detailed physical exam, p. 273
distention, p. 266
focused history and physical exam, p. 249
ileostomy, p. 267
jugular vein distention (JVD), p. 265
paradoxical motion, p. 266
priapism, p. 268
rapid trauma assessment, p. 265
stoma, p. 265
tracheostomy, p. 265
trauma patient, p. 249

DOT OBJECTIVES

*KNOWLEDGE AND ATTITUDE

3-3.1 Discuss the reasons for reconsideration concerning the mechanism of injury. (pp. 251, 255, 263–264)

3-3.2 State the reasons for performing a rapid trauma assessment. (p. 265)

3-3.3 Recite examples and explain why patients should receive a rapid trauma assessment. (p. 265)

3-3.4 Describe the areas included in the rapid trauma assessment and discuss what should be evaluated. (pp. 265–269, 272) (Scan 10-1, pp. 252–253; Scan 10-3, pp. 260–262; Scan 10-4, p. 268; Scan 10-5, pp. 270–271)

3-3.5 Differentiate when the rapid assessment may be altered in order to provide patient care. (p. 272)

3-3.6 Discuss the reason for performing a focused history and physical exam. (pp. 249–250)

3-3.7 Recognize and respect the feelings that patients might experience during assessment. (pp. 251, 254, 266, 272, 273)

3-5.1 Discuss the components of the detailed physical exam. (pp. 273–274, 278–281) (Scan 10-6, pp. 275–277)

3-5.2 State the areas of the body that are evaluated during the detailed physical exam. (p. 273)

3-5.3 Explain what additional care should be provided while performing the detailed physical exam. (pp. 273–274, 278–281)

3-5.4 Distinguish between the detailed physical exam that is performed on a trauma patient and that of the medical patient. (pp. 260–261)

3-5.5 Explain the rationale for the feelings that these patients might be experiencing. (pp. 251, 254, 266, 272, 273)

*SKILLS

3-3.8 Demonstrate the rapid trauma assessment that should be used to treat a patient based on mechanism of injury.

3-5.6 Demonstrate the skills involved in performing the detailed physical exam.

For the **trauma patient**—especially one whose injuries are serious—time must not be wasted at the scene. This patient needs to get to a hospital as quickly as possible. However, enough time must be spent at the scene to adequately assess the patient and give proper emergency care. How can you strike the right balance between care and speed? The key is focus. Instead of performing a time-consuming, comprehensive assessment on every patient, the EMT focuses in on what is important for this particular patient. This process is known as the focused history and physical exam. En route to the hospital, you may have time to do a more complete patient assessment called the detailed physical exam.

trauma patient
a patient suffering from one or more physical injuries.

FOCUSED HISTORY AND PHYSICAL EXAM FOR THE TRAUMA PATIENT

Immediately following the initial assessment for immediate life threats (which was discussed in Chapter 8, "The Initial Assessment"), you will conduct a **focused history and physical exam,** sometimes referred to as the *secondary assessment* or *secondary survey.* This exam takes a somewhat different path for trauma versus medical patients. In this chapter we will discuss the focused history and physical exam for the trauma patient.

focused history and physical exam
the step of patient assessment that follows the initial assessment.

Remember that *trauma* means "injury." Injuries can range from slight to severe, from a cut finger to a massive wound. Often you will not be able to see the injury or how serious it is, especially if it is internal. Usually, however, you will be able to identify the

TABLE 10-1 • Focused History and Physical Exam—Trauma Patient	
NO SIGNIFICANT MECHANISM OF INJURY	SIGNIFICANT MECHANISM OF INJURY
After scene size-up and initial assessment:	**After scene size-up and initial assessment:**
1. Reconsider the mechanism of injury.	**1.** Reconsider the mechanism of injury.
2. Perform focused physical exam based on chief complaint and mechanism of injury.	**2.** Continue manual stabilization of head and neck.
3. Assess baseline vital signs.	**3.** Consider requesting advanced life support personnel.
4. Obtain a SAMPLE history.	**4.** Reconsider your transport decision.
	5. Reassess mental status.
	6. Perform rapid trauma assessment.
	7. Assess baseline vital signs.
	8. Obtain a SAMPLE history.

mechanism of injury (MOI). If it is significant, you will do the focused history and physical exam differently than if the mechanism of injury is not significant.

The procedures for a trauma patient who does not have a significant mechanism of injury are discussed in the following section. The procedures for a patient who does have a significant mechanism of injury will be discussed later in the chapter. Table 10-1 lists and contrasts the procedures for these two categories of trauma patient.

Trauma Patient with No Significant Mechanism of Injury

The first step of the focused history and physical exam for any trauma patient is to reconsider the mechanism of injury. The main purpose of this is to help you to determine how quickly you must transport the patient. If the patient has no significant mechanism of injury (as listed in Table 10-2) and no immediately life-threatening injuries, you will know that you have time to assess the patient more thoroughly at the scene.

TABLE 10-2 • Significant Mechanisms of Injury
SIGNIFICANT MECHANISMS OF INJURY
Ejection from vehicle
Death in same passenger compartment
Falls of more than 15 feet or three times patient's height
Rollover of vehicle
High-speed vehicle collision
Vehicle-pedestrian collision
Motorcycle crash
Unresponsive or altered mental status
Penetrations of the head, chest, or abdomen (e.g., stab and gunshot wounds)
ADDITIONAL SIGNIFICANT MECHANISMS OF INJURY FOR A CHILD
Falls from more than 10 feet
Bicycle collision
Vehicle in medium speed collision

When the patient has no significant mechanism of injury, the steps of the focused history and physical exam are appropriately simplified. Instead of examining the patient from head to toe, you focus your assessment on just the areas that the patient tells you are painful or that you suspect may be injured because of the mechanism of injury. The assessment will include a physical exam, a set of baseline vital signs, and a SAMPLE history.

Reconsider the Mechanism of Injury

As part of scene size-up and the initial assessment, you will have already evaluated the mechanism of injury. Because the mechanism of injury is so important in determining your next steps, you should now re-evaluate it. Why? When you first arrive on a scene and must take in a lot of information at once, it is easy to miss things. You are looking not only at how the patient was injured, but also for anything that might threaten you or your crew. You also have other concerns on your mind, like whether or not you need to call for help. Combine that with the stress of knowing that you may have a patient with serious injuries and it is easy to see how an EMT can miss important information about the mechanism of injury during the scene size-up.

So once the initial assessment has been completed and all life threats are under control, it is important to reconsider the mechanism of injury so you can reconsider, if necessary, the patient's priority for transport and appropriately tailor further assessment and care.

Determine the Chief Complaint

The chief complaint is what the patient tells you is the matter. For example, one patient may tell you he has cut his finger. Another may complain of pain after twisting his ankle.

Perform a Focused Physical Exam

Your decision on which areas of a patient's body to assess will depend partly on what you can see (e.g., the cut on the patient's finger) and what the patient tells you (the chief complaint, perhaps "My ankle hurts"). But you will not rely just on these obvious signs and symptoms. You will also pay attention to potential injuries the mechanism of injury causes you to suspect. For example, if the patient with the painful ankle suffered his injury by falling down a flight of steps, you should suspect that he may have more than just an ankle injury—including a potential spine injury that would require stabilization and, later, immobilization of the patient's head and spine.

An easy way to remember what you are trying to find is the memory aid **DCAP-BTLS** (Scan 10-1). (You can pronounce it as "Dee-cap, B-T-L-S.") When you assess areas of the patient's body that you suspect may be injured, you will evaluate them in two main ways: by inspecting (looking) and by palpating (feeling). First you will look for contusions, abrasions, punctures, penetrations, burns, and lacerations. Then you will palpate for deformities, tenderness (pain on pressure), and swelling.

DCAP-BTLS
a memory aid to remember deformities, contusions, abrasions, puncture/penetrations, burns, tenderness, lacerations, and swelling—symptoms of injury found by inspection or palpation during patient assessment.

Deformities are just what they sound like, parts of the body that no longer have the normal shape. Common examples are broken or fractured bones that push up the skin over the bone ends. *Contusions* is the medical term for bruises. *Abrasions*, or scrapes, are some of the most common injuries you will see. *Punctures and penetrations* are holes in the body, frequently the result of gunshot wounds and stab wounds. When they are small, they are easy to overlook. *Burns* may be reddened, blistered, or charred-looking areas. *Tenderness* means that an area hurts when pressure is applied on it, as when it is palpated. Pain (which is present even without any pressure) and tenderness frequently, but not always, go together. *Lacerations* are cuts, open wounds that sometimes cause significant blood loss. *Swelling* is a very common result of injured capillaries bleeding under the skin.

In order to find these signs, you will need to expose the patient. This means removing or cutting away clothing in order to see and palpate the area or areas of the body you are assessing. Be sure to tell the patient what you are doing and offer reassurance as necessary. Protect the patient's privacy and take steps to prevent unnecessarily long exposure to cold.

SCAN 10-1 • DCAP-BTLS

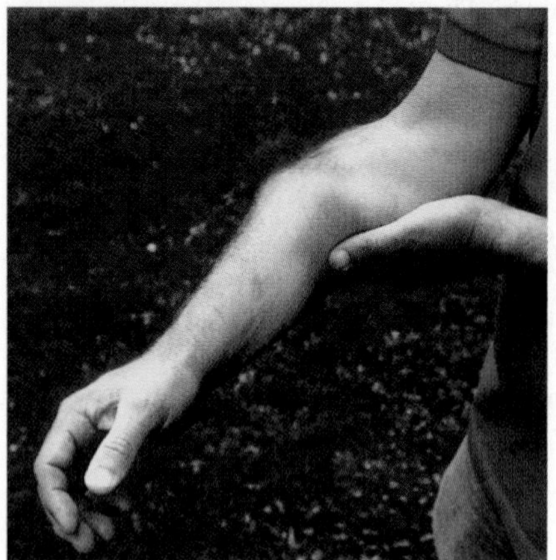
Deformities

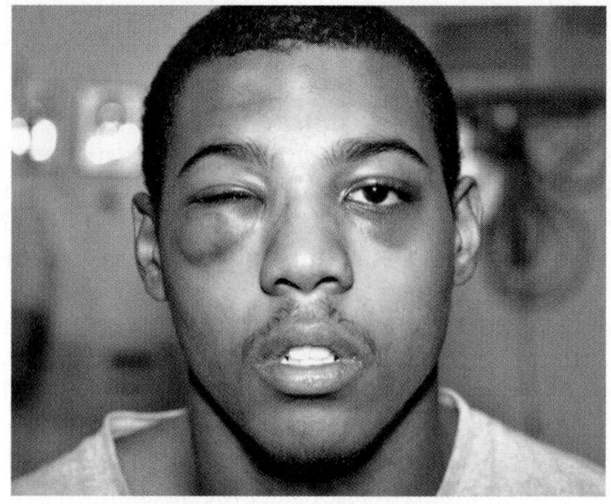
Contusions *(© Edward T. Dickinson, MD)*

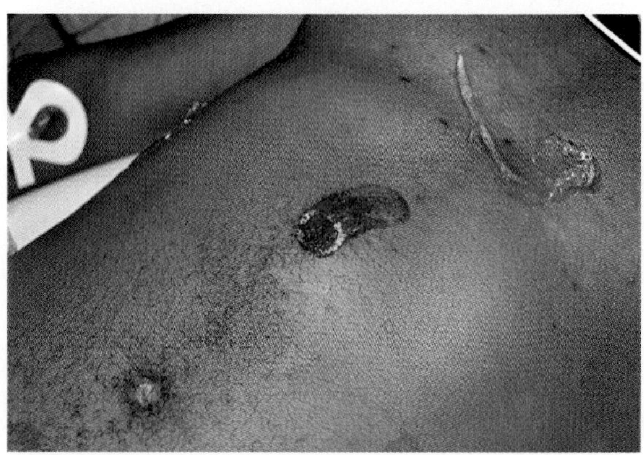
Abrasion *(© Edward T. Dickinson, MD)*

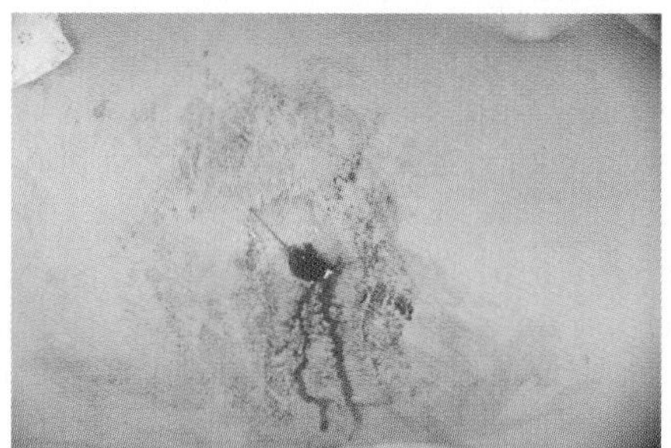
Punctures/Penetrations

When you practice doing a physical exam, you can repeat "DCAP-BTLS" to yourself as you look at each body part, making sure to remember what each letter is prompting you to inspect or palpate. You will also check each part for the special signs and symptoms listed in the "Plus" column of Table 10-3 and described under "Perform a Rapid Trauma Assessment" later in this chapter.

Obtain Baseline Vital Signs and a SAMPLE History

For a trauma patient, first conduct a physical exam to assess injuries. Next, assess baseline vital signs and take a SAMPLE history (Figure 10-1).

Applying a Cervical Collar

Apply a cervical collar to any patient who may have an injury to the spine based on mechanism of injury, history, or signs and symptoms. (Remember that signs are what you observe; symptoms are what the patient tells you he feels.)

When is it appropriate to apply a cervical collar? There is a simple principle you can follow: If the mechanism of injury exerts significant force on the upper body or if there is any soft-tissue damage to the head, face, or neck from trauma (such as a cut or bruise from being thrown against a dashboard), you may then assume that there is a possible

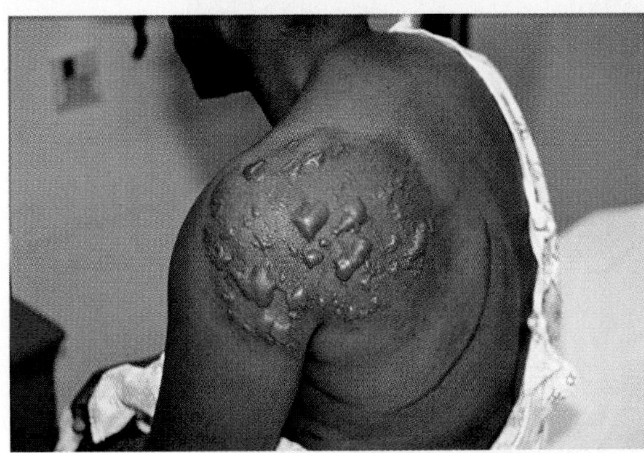

Burns *(© Edward T. Dickinson, MD)*

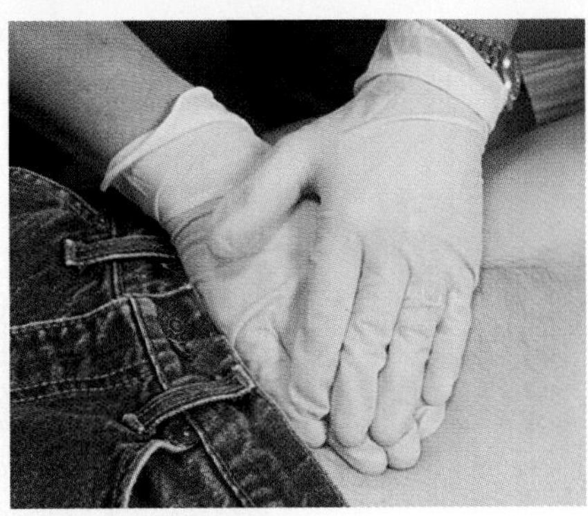

Tenderness

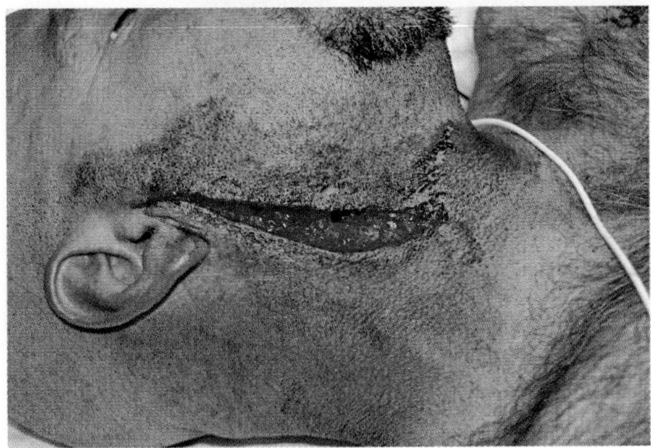

Lacerations *(© Edward T. Dickinson, MD)*

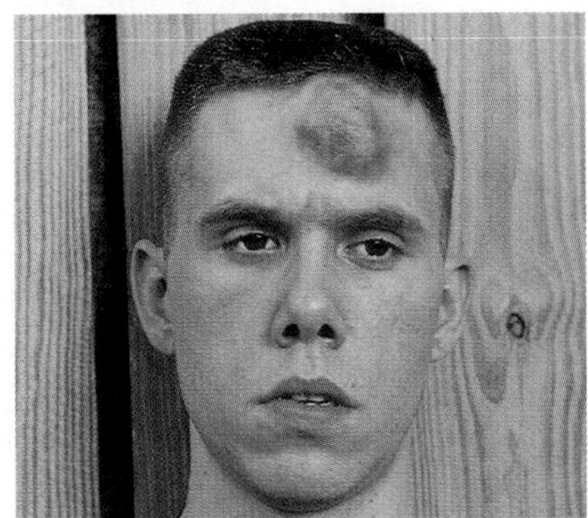

Swelling

TABLE 10-3 • Physical Exam/Trauma Assessment

BODY PART	DCAP-BTLS	PLUS
Head	DCAP-BTLS	Crepitation
Neck	DCAP-BTLS	Jugular vein distention, crepitation
Chest	DCAP-BTLS	Paradoxical motion, crepitation, breath sounds (present, absent, equal)
Abdomen	DCAP-BTLS	Firmness, softness, distention
Pelvis	DCAP-BTLS	Pain tenderness, motion
Extremities	DCAP-BTLS	Distal pulse, motor function, sensation
Posterior	DCAP-BTLS	—

cervical-spine injury. Any blow above the clavicles (collarbones) may damage the cervical spine, as may a fall from a height, even if the patient landed on his feet. If the patient has a depressed level of responsiveness or if injury cannot be ruled out—even if the mechanism of injury is not known—suspect cervical-spine injury. When any of these conditions exists, apply a cervical collar.

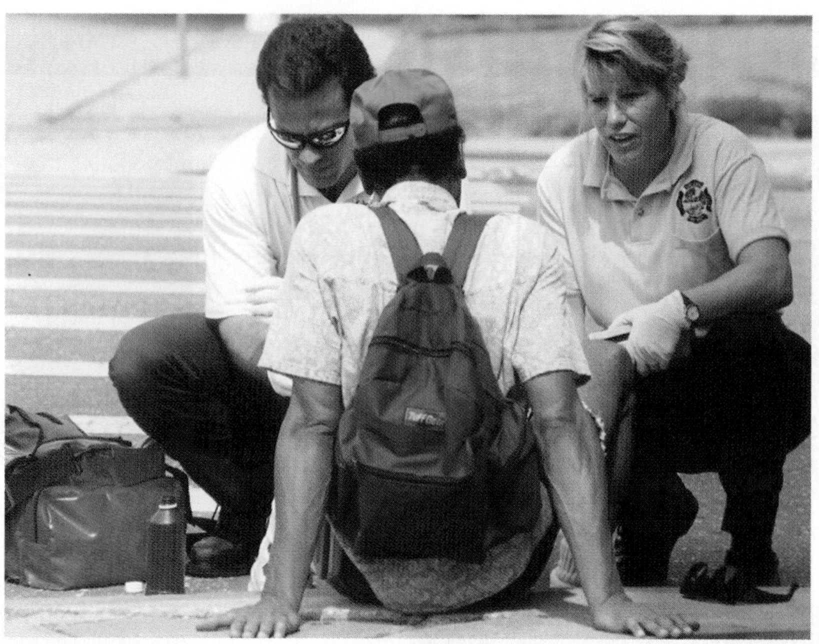

Figure 10-1 • Taking a SAMPLE history. *(© Craig Jackson/In the Dark Photography)*

Several types of cervical-spine immobilization devices are on the market. It is important that you select one that is rigid (stiff, not easily movable) and that is the right size. The traditional soft collar that you occasionally see someone wearing on the street has no role in immobilizing a prehospital patient's cervical spine. A soft collar provides so little restriction of neck motion that you may hear experienced EMTs refer to it as a "neck warmer."

The wrong size immobilization device may actually harm the patient by making breathing more difficult or obstructing the airway. Whatever device is used must not obstruct the airway. If the proper size collar is not available, it is better to place a rolled towel around the neck (to remind the patient not to move his head) and tape the patient's head to the backboard.

The techniques for selecting the right size cervical collar and for applying a cervical collar are presented in Scan 10-2. As you study the scan and practice applying a cervical collar, consider the following:

- Make certain that you have completed the initial assessment and that you have cared for all life-threatening problems before you apply the collar.
- Use the mechanism of injury, level of responsiveness, and location of injuries to determine the need for cervical immobilization. Apply a rigid cervical collar whenever any of these factors leads you to believe that spine injury is a possibility.
- Assess the patient's neck prior to placing the collar. Once the collar is in place, you will not be able to inspect or palpate the back of the neck.
- Reassure the patient. Having a cervical collar applied around your neck can be a constricting and frightening experience. Explain the procedure to the patient.
- Make sure the collar is the right size for the patient. The proper size rigid collar depends more on the length of the patient's neck than on the width. A large patient may not be able to wear a large collar. A small patient with a long neck may need your largest collar. The front height of the collar should fit between the point of the chin and the chest at the suprasternal (jugular) notch—the U-shaped dip where the clavicle and sternum meet. Once in place, the collar should rest on the clavicles and support the lower jaw. It should not stretch the neck (too high), it should not support the chin (too short), and it should not constrict the neck (too tight).
- Remove the patient's necklaces and large earrings before applying the collar.

- Keep the patient's hair out of the way.
- Keep the patient's head in the in-line anatomical position (a neutral position with head facing front, not tilted forward or back or turned to either side) when applying manual stabilization and the collar.
- Cervical collars alone do not provide adequate in-line immobilization. Nor is applying the collar the first step. Whenever there is the possibility of a spine injury, you must manually stabilize the patient's head and neck immediately upon first patient contact, before the collar is applied (as you learned in Chapter 8, "The Initial Assessment"). Continue to manually stabilize the head and neck, both before and after the cervical collar is applied, until the patient is completely immobilized and secured to a backboard. (You learned about immobilization on a backboard in Chapter 5, "Lifting and Moving Patients," and will learn more in Chapter 29, "Injuries to the Head and Spine," and in Chapter 35, "Gaining Access and Rescue Operations.")

Trauma Patient with a Significant Mechanism of Injury

When you have a patient to whom you have assigned a high priority because of problems found in the initial assessment or because of a significant mechanism of injury, you will do all of the following: reconsider the mechanism of injury, continue manual stabilization of the head and neck, consider requesting advanced life support (ALS) personnel, reconsider your transport decision, reassess the patient's mental status, and perform a rapid trauma assessment (Review Table 10-1 and see Scan 10-3).

Note that there are several additional steps for the patient with a significant mechanism of injury as compared to the steps for the patient with no significant mechanism of injury (manual stabilization, ALS request consideration, reconsideration of transport decision, and reassessment of mental status). Also note that instead of a physical exam focused just on the area of injury, the patient with a significant mechanism of injury receives a complete, head-to-toe rapid trauma assessment.

Reconsider the Mechanism of Injury

What is a significant mechanism of injury? Simply put, it is a way of getting hurt that carries a high risk of serious injury. A patient who has been ejected from a vehicle, for example, is several times more likely to have fatal injuries than a patient who has not been ejected. A patient who is in a passenger compartment where another person died can be assumed to have sustained serious injury because of the amount of force that had to have been involved to kill the other person. Review Table 10-2, which lists a number of high-risk situations.

All of these mechanisms involve potentially large forces being exerted on a patient's body. In the case of a motor-vehicle collision, you can gain a great deal of information by walking around the vehicle and looking at all of its outside surfaces. You should also look inside the vehicle, concentrating your attention on the steering wheel, pedals, dashboard, and rear-view mirror. Look for deformities that could have been caused by

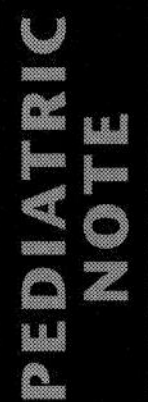

Infants and children are more fragile than adults. This means that a child may sustain the same injury as an adult, but from less force. For this reason, there are additional mechanisms of injury that the EMT needs to consider significant when children and infants are concerned. (Review Table 10-2.)

SCAN 10-2 • Applying a Cervical Collar

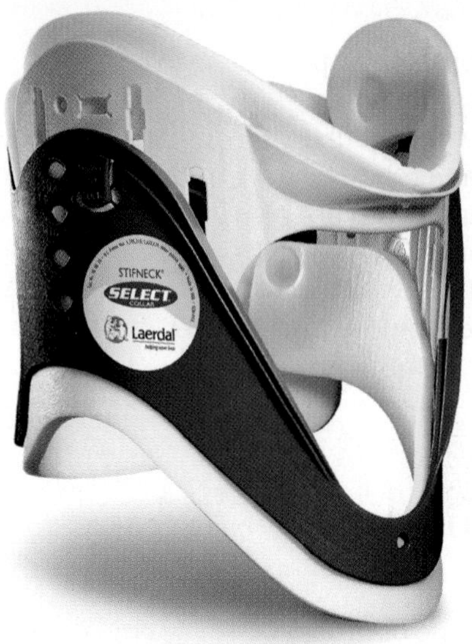

STIFNECK®SELECT™ *(© Laerdal Medical Corporation)*

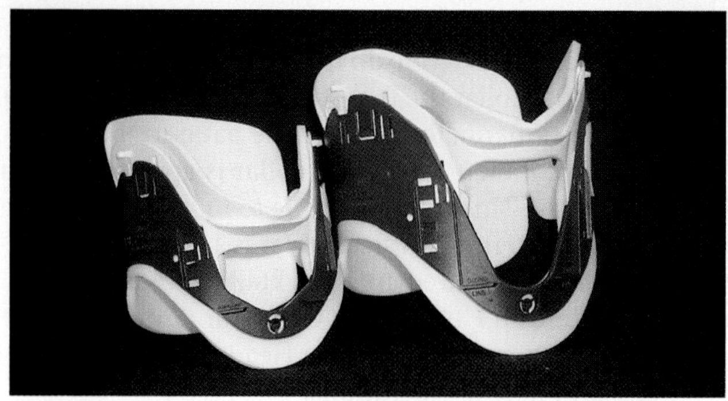

Philadelphia Cervical Collar™ Patriot Adult and Pediatric. *(© Philadelphia Collar Corporation.)*

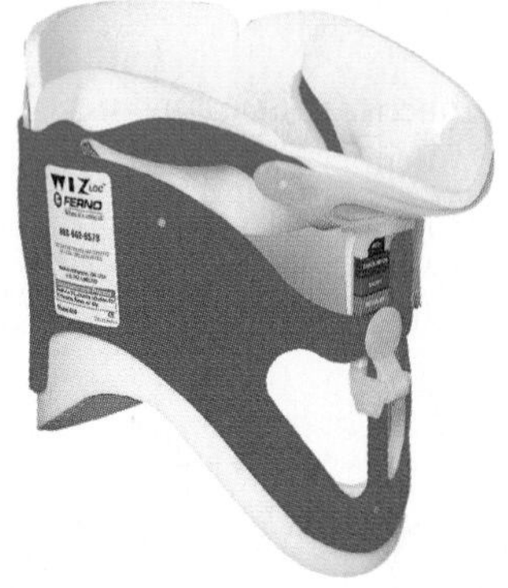

WIZLOC Cervical Collar. *(© Ferno Corporation)*

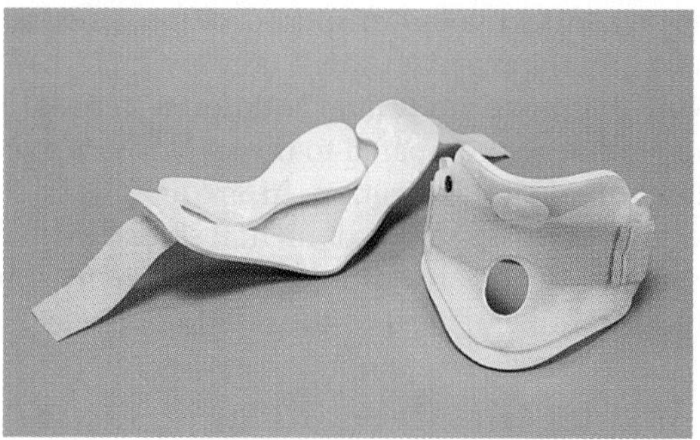

NEC-LOC™ rigid extrication collar, opened. Rigid cervical collars are applied to protect the cervical spine. DO NOT apply a soft collar.

SIZING A CERVICAL COLLAR

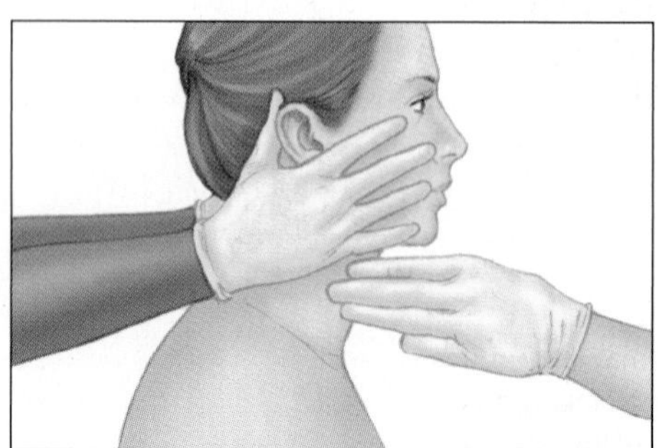

1. Measure the patient's neck.

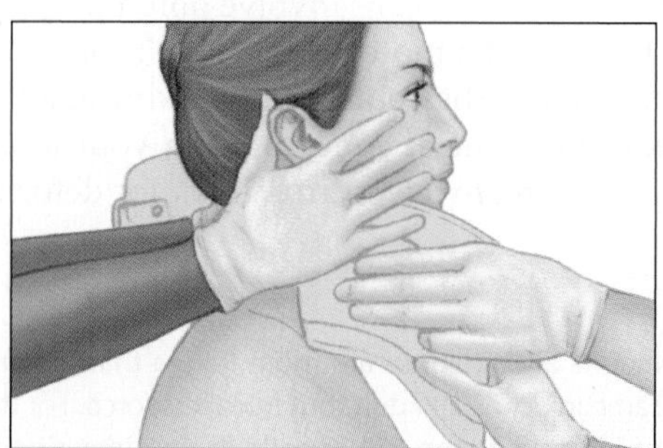

2. Measure the collar. The chin piece should not lift the patient's chin and hyperextend the neck. Make sure the collar is not too small or tight, which would make the collar act as a constricting band.

APPLYING AN ADJUSTABLE COLLAR TO A SEATED PATIENT

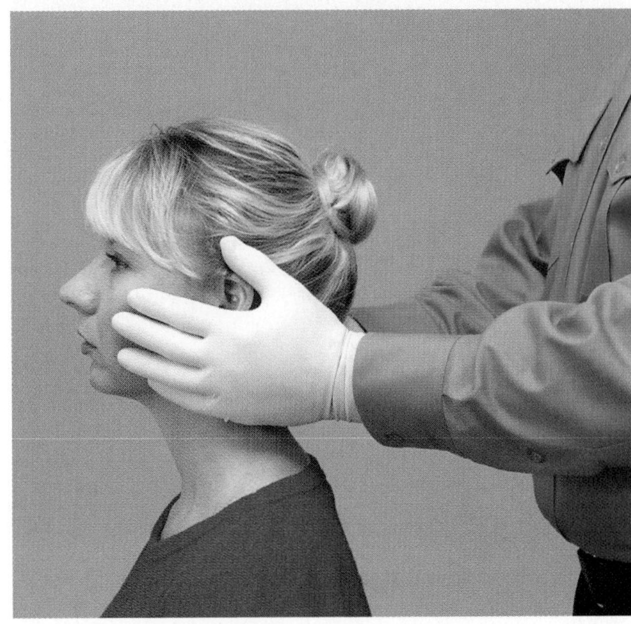

1. Stabilize the head and neck from the rear.

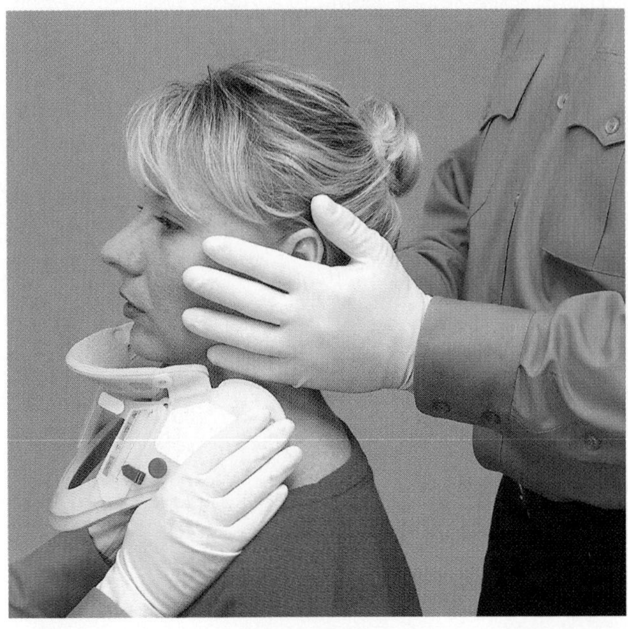

2. Properly angle the collar for placement.

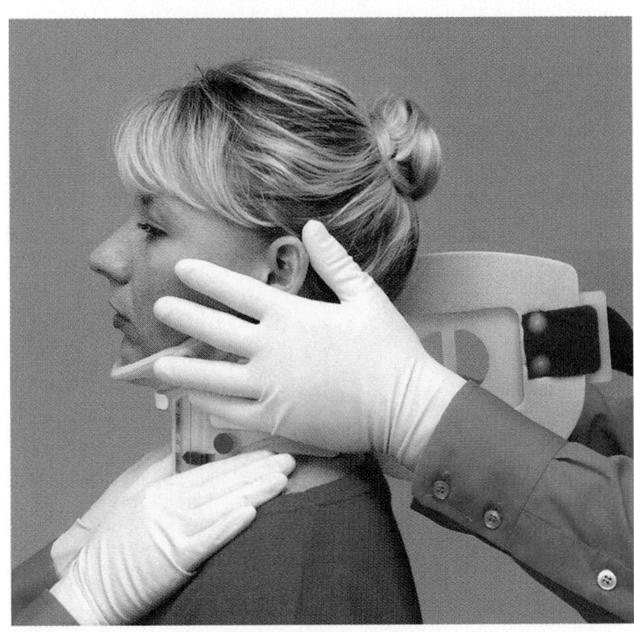

3. Position the collar bottom.

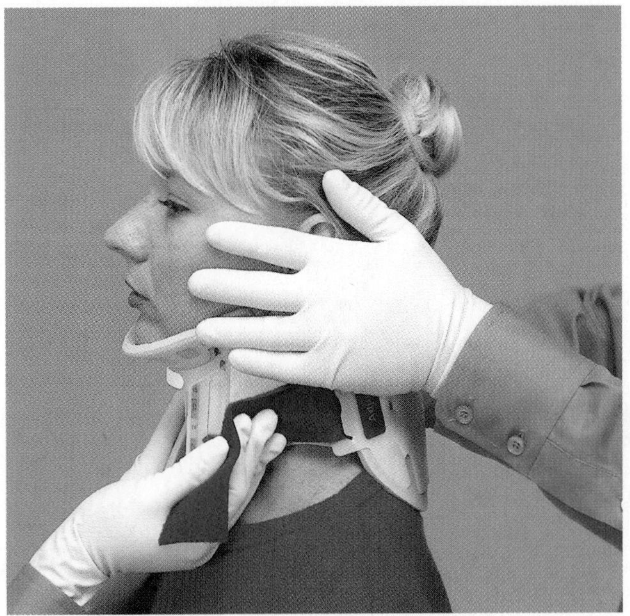

4. Set the collar in place around the neck.

continued

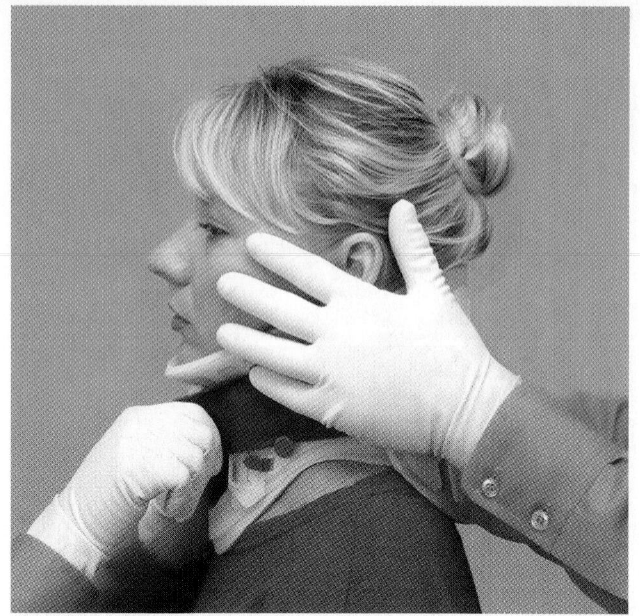

5. Secure the collar.

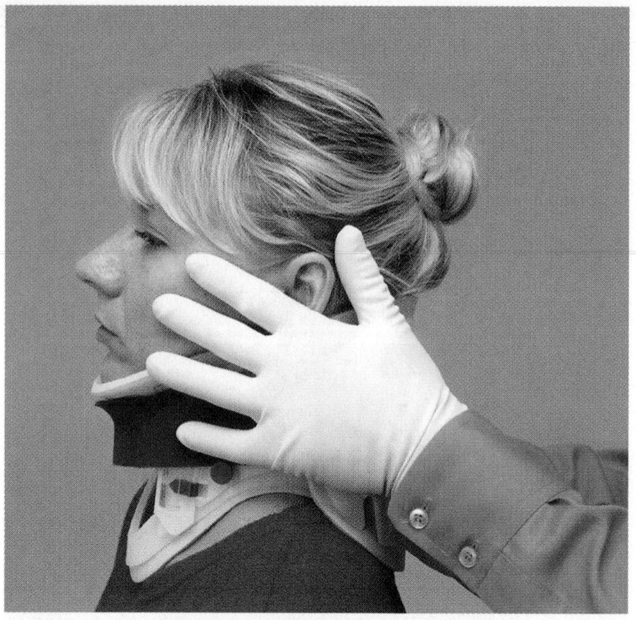

6. Maintain manual stabilization of the head and neck.

APPLYING AN ADJUSTABLE COLLAR TO A SUPINE PATIENT

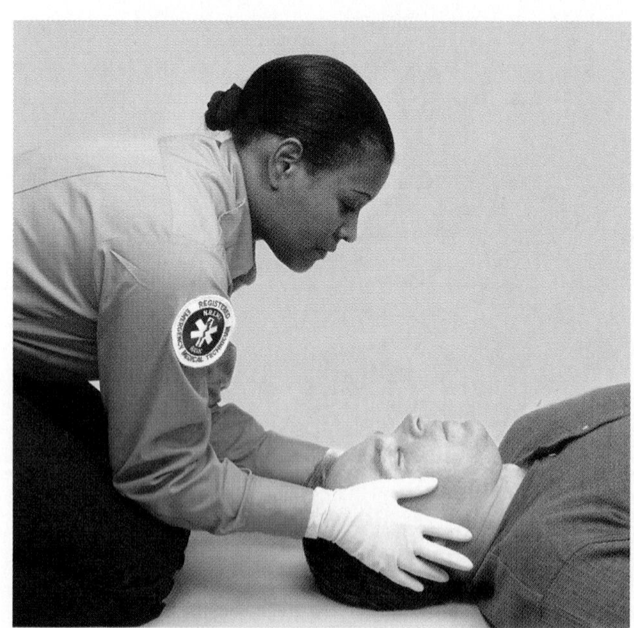

1. Kneel at the patient's head and stabilize the head and neck.

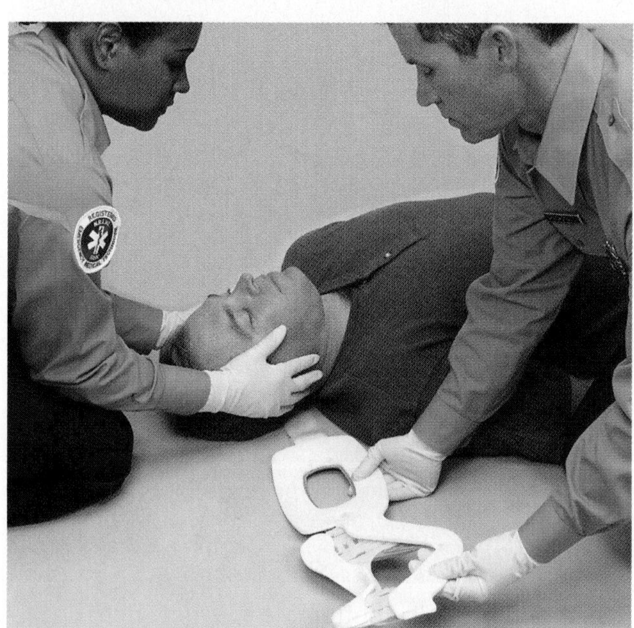

2. Set the collar in place.

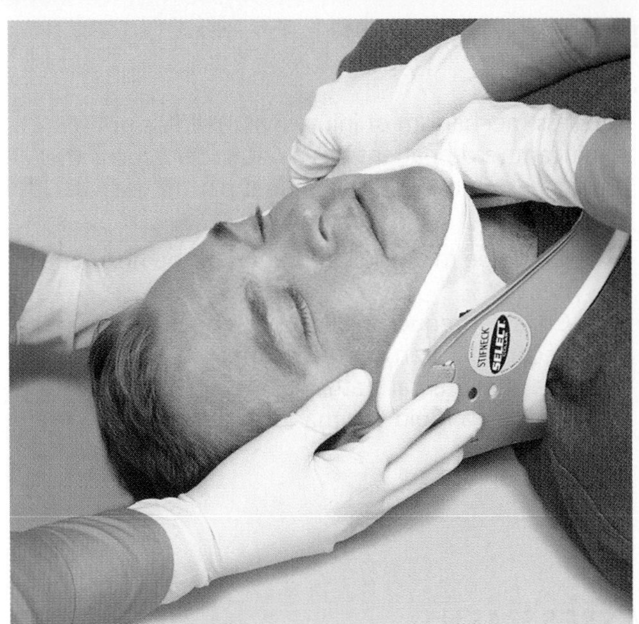

3. Secure the collar.

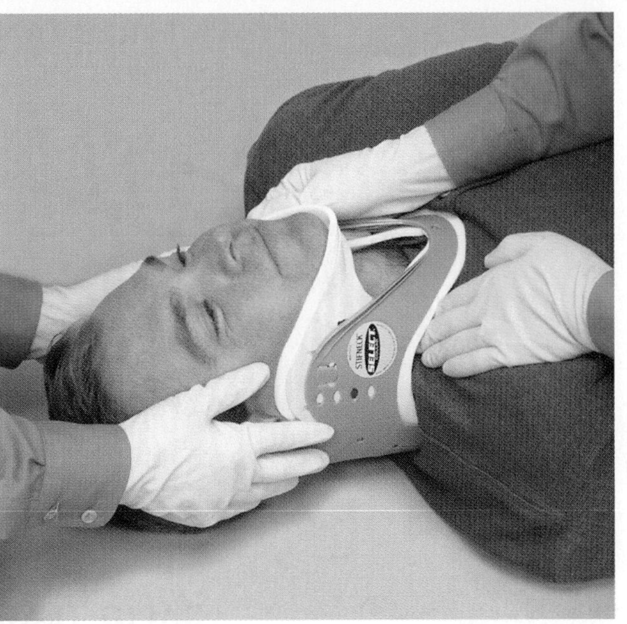

4. Continue to manually stabilize the head and neck.

SCAN 10-3 • Focused History and Physical Exam—Trauma Patient

FIRST TAKE STANDARD PRECAUTIONS

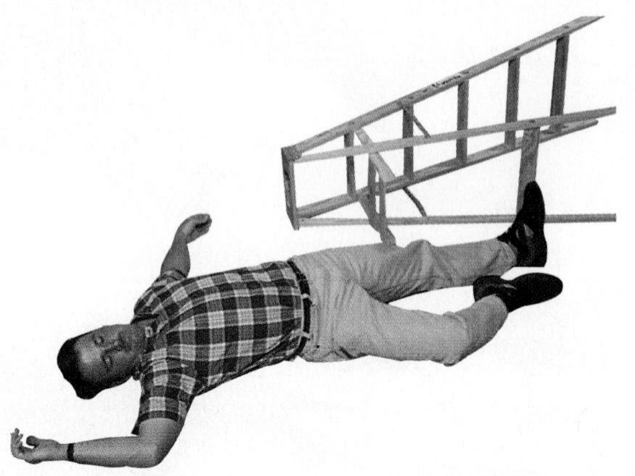

Reassess mechanism of injury (MOI). If it is not significant (e.g., patient has a cut finger), focus the physical exam only on the injured part. If the MOI is significant:

- Continue manual stabilization of the head and neck.
- Consider requesting ALS personnel.
- Reconsider transport decision.
- Reassess mental status.
- Perform a rapid trauma assessment.

RAPID TRAUMA ASSESSMENT

Rapidly assess each part of the body for the following problems (say "Dee-cap B-T-L-S" as a memory prompt):

Deformities	Burns
Contusions	Tenderness
Abrasions	Lacerations
Punctures/Penetrations	Swelling

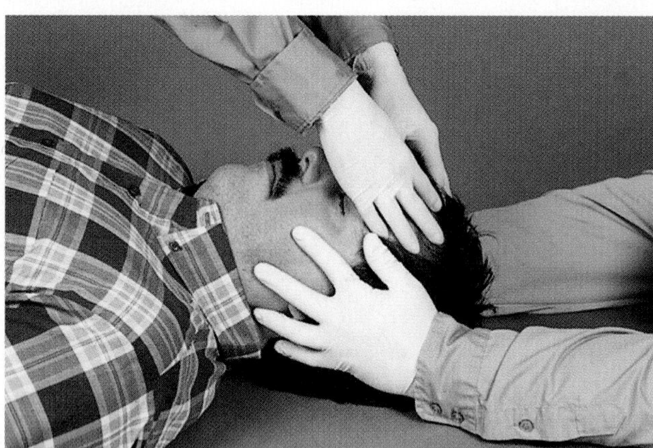

HEAD: DCAP-BTLS plus crepitation.

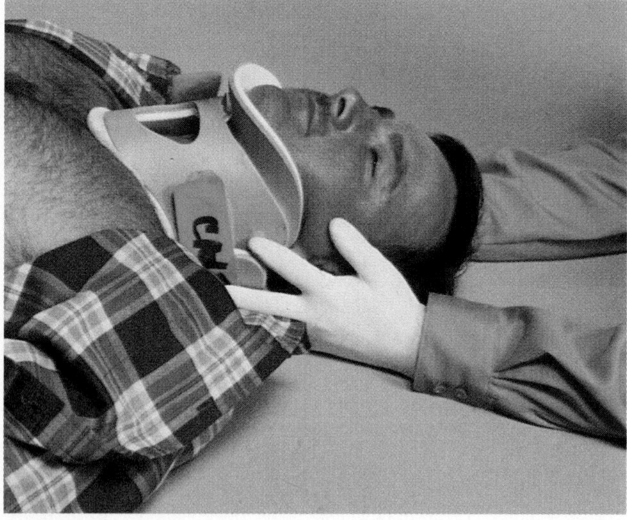

NECK: DCAP-BTLS plus jugular vein distention and crepitation (then apply cervical collar).

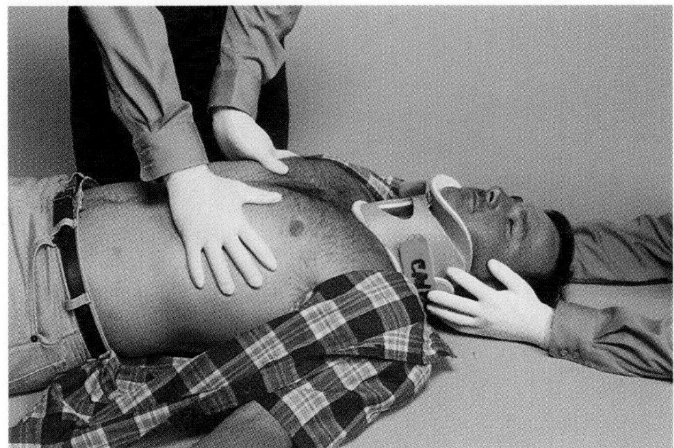

CHEST: DCAP-BTLS plus crepitation, paradoxical motion, and breath sounds (absent, present, equal).

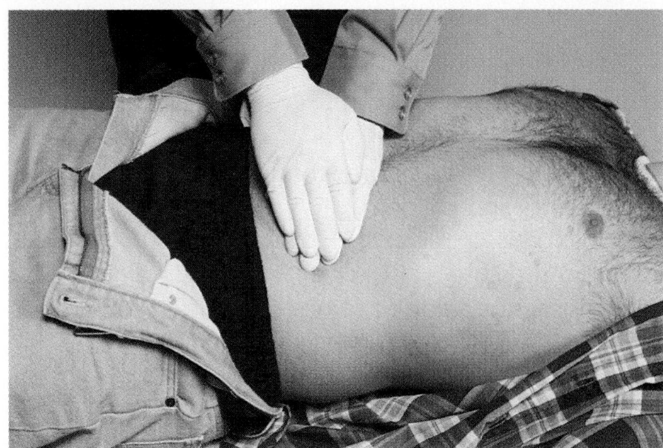

ABDOMEN: DCAP-BTLS plus firm, soft, distended.

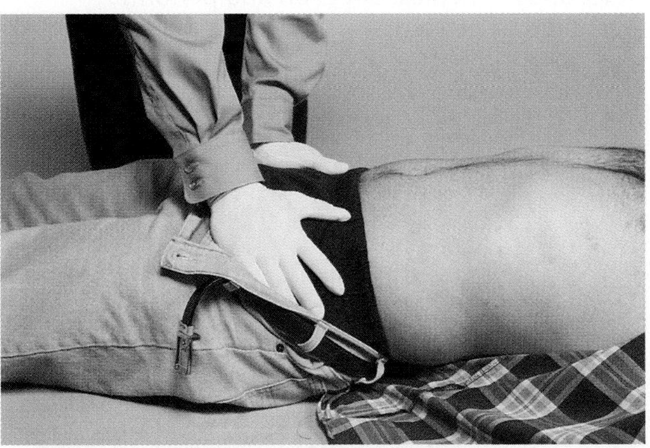

PELVIS: DCAP-BTLS with gentle compression for tenderness or motion.

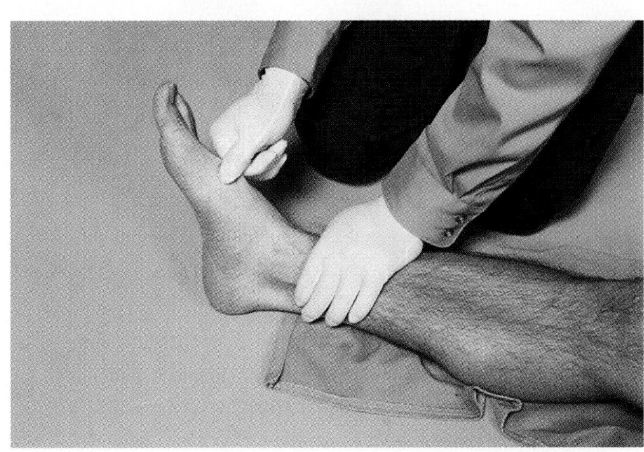

EXTREMITIES: DCAP-BTLS plus distal pulse, motor function, and sensation.

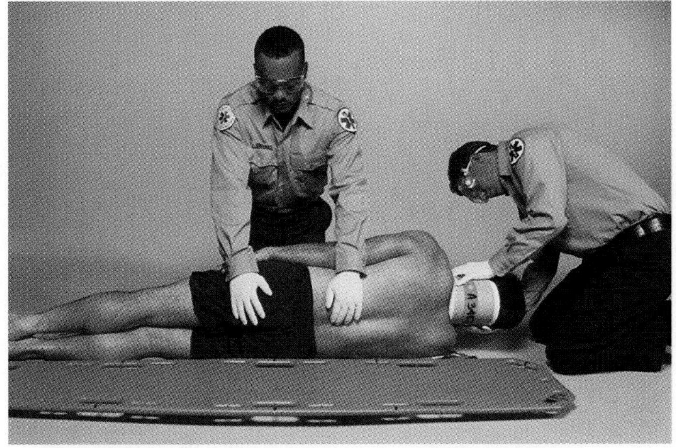

POSTERIOR: DCAP-BTLS. (To examine posterior, roll patient using spinal precautions.)

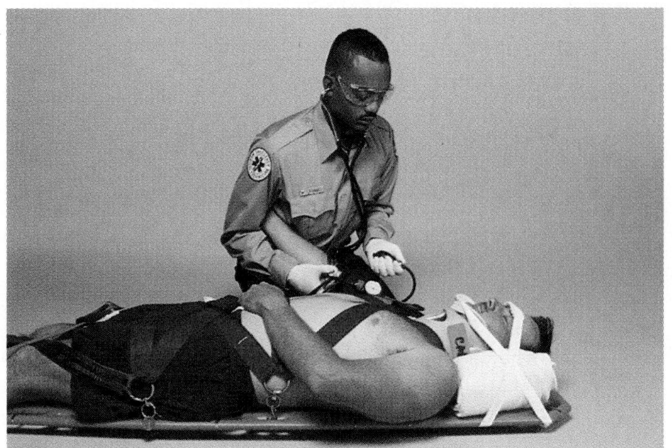

VITAL SIGNS

continued

SCAN 10-3 • (Continued)

VITAL SIGNS

Assess the patient's baseline vital signs:

- Respiration
- Pulse
- Skin color, temperature, condition (capillary refill in infants and children)
- Pupils
- Blood pressure
- Oxygen saturation (if directed by local protocol)

SAMPLE HISTORY

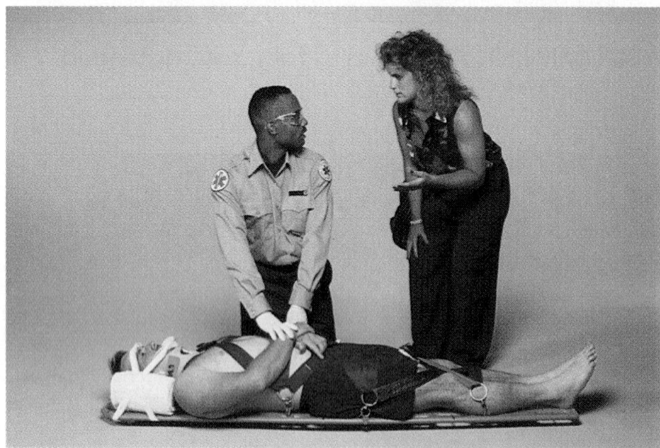

Interview patient or (if patient is unresponsive) interview family and bystanders to get as much information as possible about the patient's problem. Ask about:

Signs and Symptoms
Allergies
Medications
Pertinent past history
Last oral intake
Events leading to problem

INTERVENTIONS AND TRANSPORT

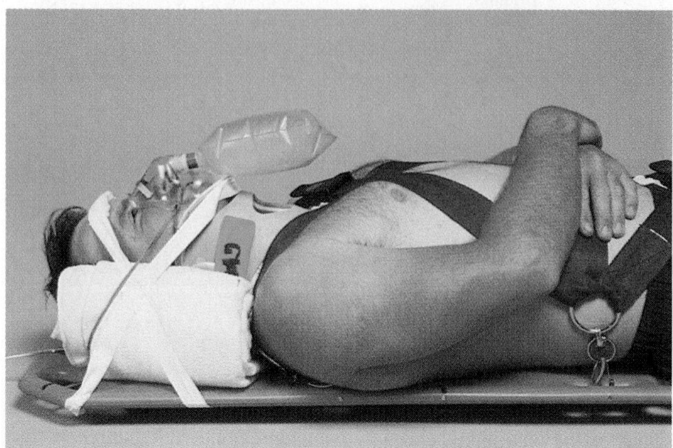

Contact on-line medical direction and perform interventions as needed.

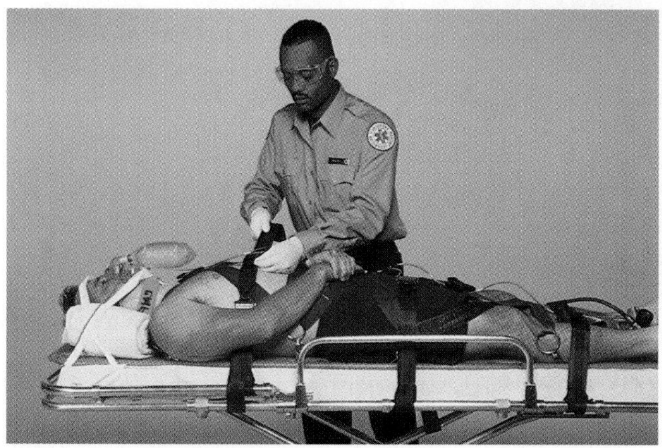

Package and transport the patient.

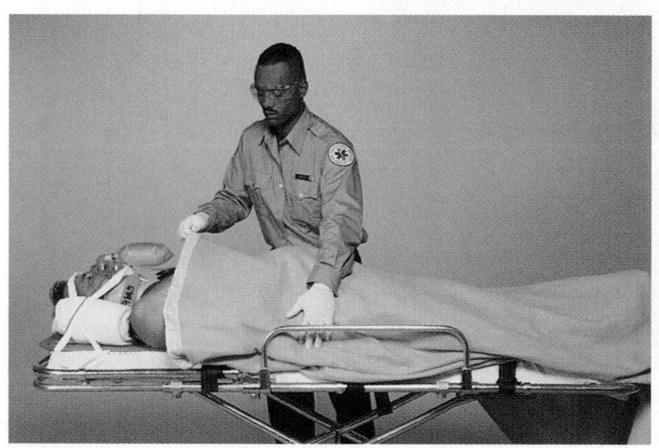

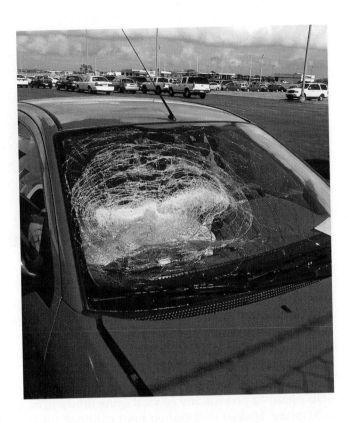

Figure 10-2 • Deformities of the interior of a vehicle may give you clues to potential injuries to the passengers.

a person striking the surface (Figure 10-2). Also look for intrusion of the body of the car into the passenger compartment (i.e., was the car crunched so that the inside is smaller than it used to be?). The preferred way to identify the mechanism of injury is, of course, to do it yourself. If patient care prevents this, you may ask someone else, such as a police officer at the scene, to get the information for you.

Some patients who undergo experiences like those listed in Table 10-2 will escape without serious injury, but many more will not be so lucky. For this reason, you should provide rapid assessment and treatment to any patient with a mechanism of injury listed in Table 10-2.

Although the mechanism of injury can provide a lot of information about the kinds of injuries a patient may have, there is still the possibility that patients will have "hidden injuries." These injuries are considered to be hidden because patients may have no signs or symptoms initially but nevertheless have serious conditions that may become apparent only later.

Seat belt injuries are a good example. There is no doubt that properly used seat belts save lives by preventing drivers and passengers from hitting hard objects inside a vehicle and by preventing them from being ejected. But seat belts can also cause injuries. When patients are in high-velocity collisions, the force of being thrown forward against buckled seat belts will occasionally cause injury to the bowel and other abdominal organs. These injuries may not become apparent for several hours or even days. It is important to realize that even people who were wearing seat belts may have sustained serious injuries.

Air bags may also save lives but do not provide total protection from injury (Figure 10-3). Air bags prevent occupants from going through the windshield and hitting hard objects inside the vehicle. They are most effective when used in combination with seat belts. In a few instances, especially with a small driver or passenger (particularly a child) or when the front seat is pulled far forward, or when a seat belt is not in place to keep the person from being thrown forward, the expanding air bag may cause injury. Also, the driver may sustain an arm injury because of improper positioning of hands on the steering wheel or may sustain a chest injury from hitting the steering wheel after the bag deflates. When inspecting a vehicle in which an air bag has deployed, you should look at the steering wheel. Whenever you see a bent or broken steering wheel, you

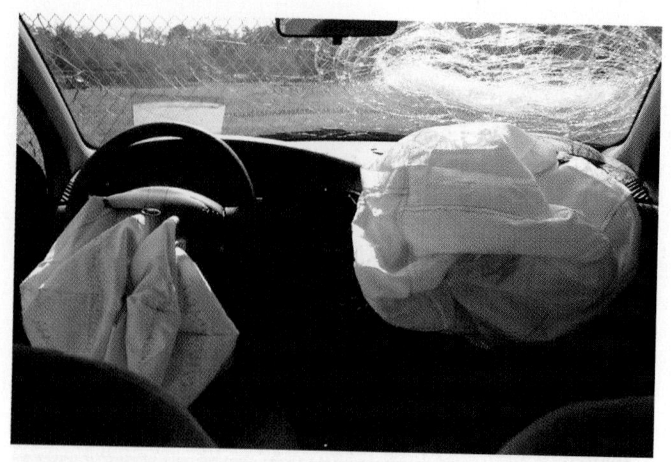

Figure 10-3 • An air bag can prevent injuries, but once deployed, it also can conceal important information about the patient's mechanism of injury. When you see a deployed air bag, remember to "lift and look."

should treat the patient like every other patient who has a significant mechanism of injury. A good way to find this kind of damage is to remember to "lift and look" under the air bag after the patient has been removed from the vehicle.

Continue Spinal Stabilization

During the initial assessment, make sure that someone is manually stabilizing the patient's head to prevent any cervical-spine injury from becoming a paralyzing spinal-cord injury. Manual stabilization must continue throughout the assessment until the patient is fully immobilized on a backboard.

Consider a Request for Advanced Life Support Personnel

Some areas of the country, particularly urban and suburban areas, have advanced life support (ALS) personnel—paramedics who respond with EMTs when they are transporting patients who might benefit from the additional interventions paramedics can provide. If this is the case where you practice as an EMT, you should familiarize yourself with your local protocols. Rural EMTs do not usually have this option, but they may have other means by which to improve the patient's care before arrival at a hospital.

In some areas that are very distant from hospitals, local clinics arrange to provide advanced care to certain kinds of patients. For example, if an ambulance is an hour away from the closest hospital, but a local clinic is only 10 minutes away, the ambulance may be able to stop there with a patient in cardiac arrest. There are limits, though, on what can be done at health care centers like these. Many of them would not be able to provide additional care that is worth a delay in transport for awake trauma patients.

If arrangements like these exist where you work as an EMT, you must be familiar with the types of patients your clinic can help. The arrangements should be in writing in order to reduce confusion and prevent loss of precious time with critical patients. In any case, the patient with serious trauma must ultimately, if at all possible, be transported to a trauma center.

Reconsider Your Transport Decision

Assigning a high priority for transport is appropriate when the patient has a condition for which you cannot provide definitive treatment—treatment that can only be provided at the hospital. As you prepare to do the rapid trauma assessment (described on the following pages), it is a good time to re-evaluate that decision. You will have had a chance to look at the mechanism of injury more closely and, if appropriate, to call for assistance from advanced life support (ALS) personnel at the scene or by intercept en route to the hospital. At this point you should take just a moment to consider again how urgently you need to transport the patient.

Reassess Mental Status

Repeat the AVPU assessment (alert, verbal response, painful response, unresponsive) as described in Chapter 8, "The Initial Assessment." Note whether your patient's mental status is unchanged, improved, or deteriorated. A patient who is less than fully alert or whose mental status is deteriorating is a high priority for transport.

Perform a Rapid Trauma Assessment

A patient with a significant mechanism of injury needs a **rapid trauma assessment.** This requires only a few moments and should be performed at the scene, before loading the patient into the ambulance, even if the patient is a high priority for transport. The care that you provide en route will be based on the results of this rapid assessment, and you will obtain valuable information to relay to the hospital staff so that they can be prepared for your patient.

rapid trauma assessment
a rapid assessment of the head, neck, chest, abdomen, pelvis, extremities, and posterior of the body to detect signs and symptoms of injury.

During the rapid trauma assessment, you will be able to detect injuries that may later threaten life or limb. You may also find life-threatening injuries that you did not find during the initial assessment. When dealing with a responsive patient, you should ask the patient before and during the trauma assessment about any symptoms.

To perform the rapid trauma assessment, you will use your sense of sight to inspect and your sense of touch to palpate different areas of the body. You may also use your sense of hearing to detect abnormal sounds, not just from the airway but also from other areas, such as the sound of broken bones rubbing against each other. You may use your sense of smell, as well, to detect odors like gasoline, urine, feces, or vomitus.

The rapid trauma assessment emphasizes evaluation of the areas of the body where the greatest threats to the patient may be. You will evaluate the patient from head to toe, in the sequence described in the following text.

The signs and symptoms you will assess each area for are summarized in Table 10-3. Remember, however, that this is a quick evaluation, so you will not spend a lot of time on any one area.

RAPID ASSESSMENT OF THE HEAD Assess the head for DCAP-BTLS and also for the sound or feel of broken bones rubbing against each other, known as **crepitation.** Run your gloved fingers through the patient's hair and palpate gently. A good way to check the back of the head in a supine patient is to start with your fingers at the top of the neck and carefully slide them upward toward the top of the patient's head. If there is blood on your gloves, there is an open wound. However, if you do not see any blood on the floor or ground, then you do not need to apply a dressing to the wound right away.

crepitation
(krep-uh-TAY-shun)
the grating sound or feeling of broken bones rubbing together.

RAPID ASSESSMENT OF THE NECK Assess the neck for DCAP-BTLS, crepitation, and **jugular vein distention (JVD).** Jugular vein distention is present when you can see the patient's neck veins bulging. The neck veins are usually not visible when the patient is sitting up. If they are bulging when the patient is upright, it means that blood is backing up in the veins because the heart is not pumping effectively. This could be the result of a tension pneumothorax (air trapped in the chest) or cardiac tamponade (blood filling the sac around the heart). However, it is normal to see bulging of the neck veins when the patient is lying in a horizontal position or with his head down. Flat neck veins in a patient who is lying down may be a sign of blood loss, showing that there is not enough blood to fill them. When you see FLAT neck veins in a FLAT patient, think "blood loss." To summarize, *either* neck veins that are bulging when the patient is sitting up *or* neck veins that are flat when the patient is flat are abnormal and should be noted during the exam.

jugular (JUG-yuh-ler) **vein distention (JVD)**
bulging of the neck veins.

Another thing you might find when assessing the patient's anterior neck is a surgical opening. A **stoma** is a permanent surgical opening in the neck through which the patient breathes. A **tracheostomy** is a surgical incision held open by a metal or plastic tube. If the patient requires artificial ventilation, you may need to provide it through the stoma, as described in Chapter 6, "Airway Management."

You may also find a medical identification medallion on a necklace when assessing the neck. Note the information on the necklace if you find one.

stoma (STO-ma)
a permanent surgical opening in the neck through which the patient breathes.

tracheostomy
(TRAY-ke-OS-to-me)
a surgical incision held open by a metal or plastic tube.

Cultural Considerations

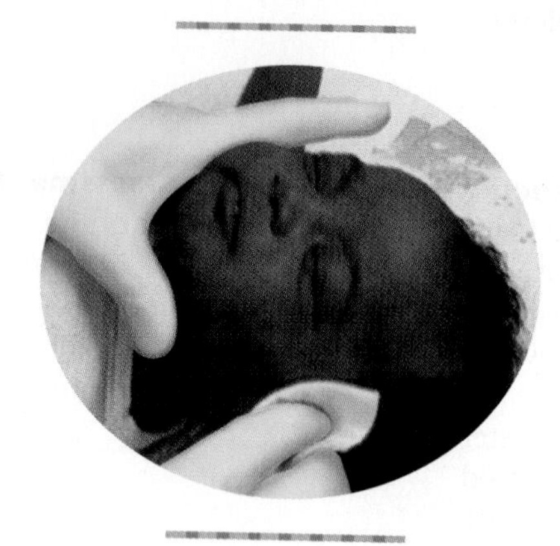

People of different cultures may respond in different ways to aspects of the physical exam. In Southeast Asian cultures, for example, the head is considered a sacred part of the body. Southeast Asians will often be very upset when you touch the patient's head during the physical examination. When your patient is from a Southeast Asian background, be sure to request permission before palpating the head or the face, especially if your patient is a child or an infant.

By contrast, in some Latin American cultures there is a belief that touching the head wards off the "evil eye" or brings good luck. In fact, if you examine a Latin American patient and fail to touch the head, this may be considered bad luck.

APPLICATION OF A CERVICAL COLLAR After you assess the head and neck, size and apply a rigid cervical spine immobilization collar. Use the principles and methods that were described earlier in this chapter and in Scan 10-2.

paradoxical (pair-uh-DOCK-si-kal) **motion** movement of a part of the chest in the opposite direction to the rest of the chest during respiration.

RAPID ASSESSMENT OF THE CHEST Next, assess the chest for DCAP-BTLS, crepitation, breath sounds, and paradoxical motion. **Paradoxical motion,** or movement of part of the chest in the opposite direction from the rest of the chest, is a sign of a serious injury. It usually occurs when a segment of ribs has broken at two ends and is "floating" free of the rest of the rib cage. (This condition is sometimes known as "flail chest.") The opposite motion of the broken section is obvious during respiration, moving inward when the lungs expand with air and outward when the lungs empty (Figure 10-4). Paradoxical motion also indicates that a great deal of force was applied to the patient's chest; in other words, there was a significant mechanism of injury.

You can check for crepitation and paradoxical motion of the chest at the same time. Start by palpating the clavicles (collarbones). Next, gently feel the sternum (breastbone). Position your hands on the sides of the chest and feel for equal expansion of both sides of the chest. During this process you may feel broken bones or floating paradoxical segments.

Palpate the entire rib cage for deformities. Use your hands to apply gentle pressure to the sides of the rib cage. If there is an injured rib and the patient is able to respond, he will tell you that it hurts. Occasionally, you may detect a crackling or crunching sensation under the skin from air that has escaped from its normal passageways. This is called subcutaneous emphysema.

Listen for breath sounds (Scan 10-4) just under the clavicles in the mid-clavicular line and at the bases of the lungs in the mid-axillary line. Notice whether the breath sounds are present and equal. A patient who has breath sounds that are absent or very hard to hear on one side may have a collapsed lung or other serious respiratory injury. There are many other characteristics of breath sounds, but in the trauma patient, presence and equality are the two things to look for at this time.

It is important to remember that when you reach the point of examining the patient's chest in the rapid trauma assessment, you need to expose the chest if you have not already done so. However, keep the weather and the patient's privacy in mind when doing this.

distention (dis-TEN-shun) a condition of being stretched, inflated, or larger than normal.

RAPID ASSESSMENT OF THE ABDOMEN When you assess the abdomen for DCAP-BTLS, also check for firmness, softness, and distention. The term **distention** is another way of saying the abdomen appears larger than normal. One of its causes can be internal bleeding. Whether the abdomen is abnormally distended or not may be a very difficult

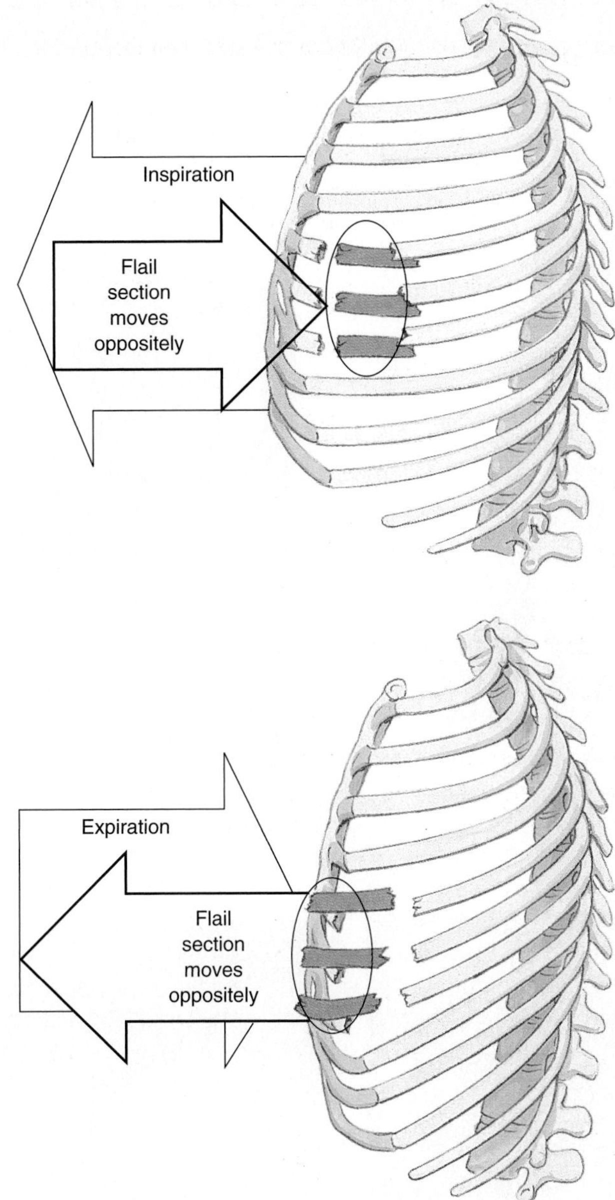

Figure 10-4 • Paradoxical motion.

judgment to make, so do not spend a lot of time on it. You may also see a **colostomy** or **ileostomy** when you inspect the abdomen. This is a surgical opening in the wall of the abdomen with a bag in place to collect excretions from the digestive system. If you see such a bag, leave it in place and be careful not to cut it if you cut clothing away.

Palpate the abdomen by gently pressing down once on each abdominal quadrant. (Picture the abdomen divided into four segments—upper left, upper right, lower left, lower right—and press on each quadrant in turn.) If the patient tells you he has pain in a specific area of the abdomen, palpate that site last. When practical, make sure your hands are warm. Press in on the abdomen with the palm side of your fingers, depressing the surface about 1 inch. Many EMTs prefer to use two hands, one on top of the other at the fingertips. Normally the abdomen is soft. Firmness of the abdomen can be a sign of injury to the organs in the abdomen and internal bleeding.

Another finding you may occasionally come across when palpating a patient's abdomen is a pulsating mass. This may be an enlarged aorta. If you do feel such pulsations, do not press any farther into the abdomen. Doing so could cause further injury to a weakened blood vessel.

colostomy (ko-LOS-to-me) similar to an ileostomy, a surgical opening in the wall of the abdomen with a bag in place to collect excretions from the digestive system.

ileostomy (il-e-OS-to-me) *See* colostomy.

SCAN 10-4 • Assessing Breath Sounds

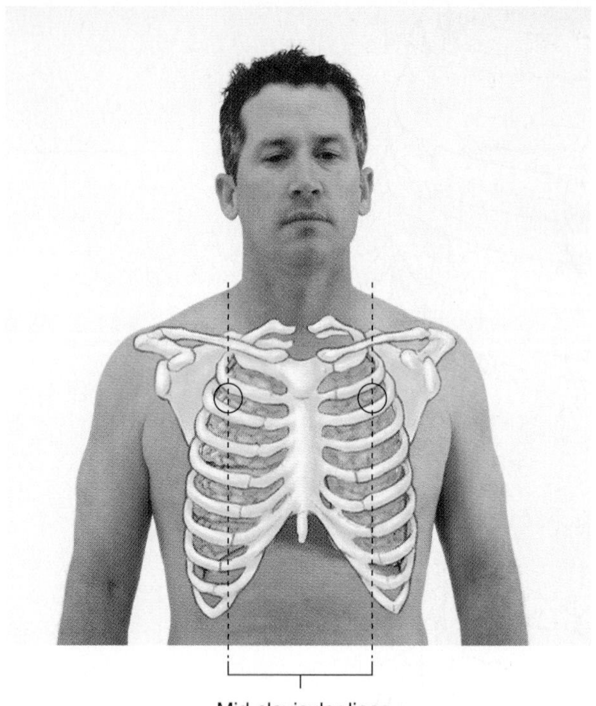

Mid-Clavicular Line

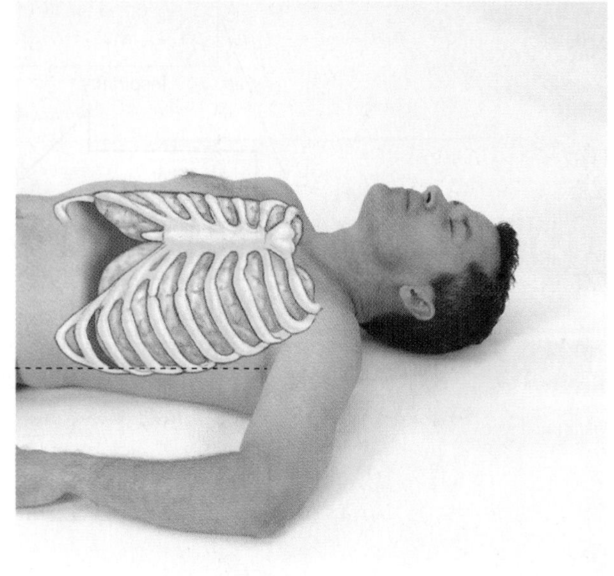

Mid-Axillary Line

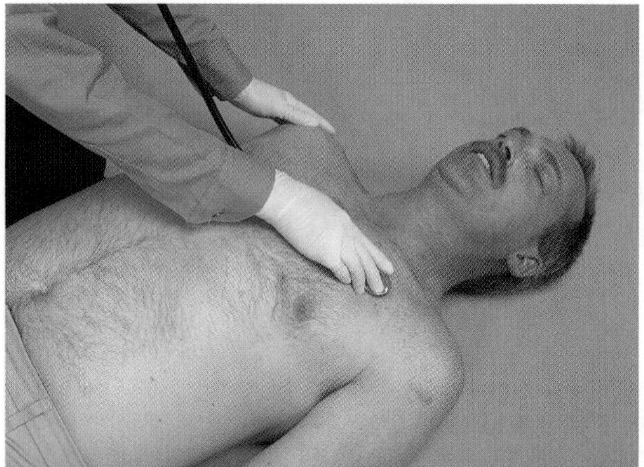

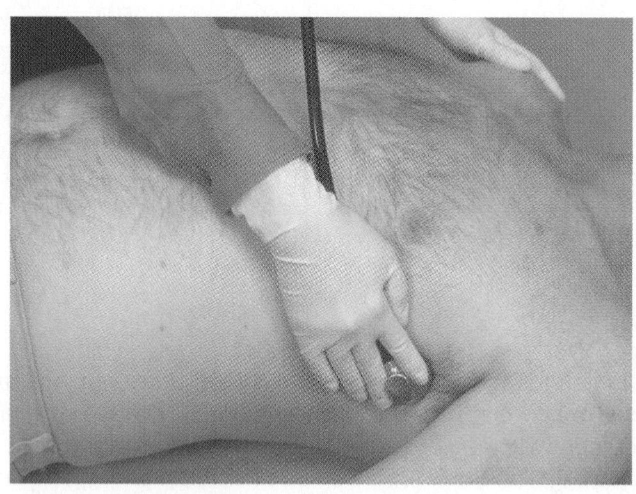

Listen to both sides of the chest. Is air entry present? Absent? Equal on both sides?

priapism (PRY-ah-pizm) persistent erection of the penis that may result from spinal injury and some medical problems.

RAPID ASSESSMENT OF THE PELVIS Next assess the pelvis for DCAP-BTLS. You may observe bleeding or **priapism,** a persistent erection of the penis that can result from spinal cord injury or certain medical problems. If the patient is awake, palpate the pelvis gently, stopping as soon as the patient identifies pain in the pelvis. Consider the complaint of pain as reason enough to treat the patient for an injury to the pelvis. Continuing to palpate or compress the painful pelvis of a conscious patient will not give you any more useful information, but it can produce excruciating pain and, if done too strenuously, may injure the patient.

An unconscious patient, however, cannot tell you if his pelvic area hurts. So you will gently compress the pelvis of the unconscious patient to detect tenderness (if there is enough responsiveness to pain to cause him to flinch or groan) and motion of the bones (indicating instability or broken bones). These signs will help you determine whether you need to treat the unconscious patient for a pelvic injury.

RAPID ASSESSMENT OF THE EXTREMITIES Quickly assess all four extremities for DCAP-BTLS as well as distal pulse, motor function, and sensation—that is, whether a pulse is present, the patient can move his hands and feet, and he has feeling in his hands and feet (Scan 10-5). In a conscious patient, you would touch the patient's hand or foot and ask whether he could feel your touch. If you are not sure whether the patient is telling you the truth, you can ask where on the hand or foot you are touching him. You would also test movement in the extremities of a conscious patient by asking him to squeeze your fingers in his hands and to move his feet against your hands.

If you find a deformity, diminished function, or other indication of injury to an extremity in a patient who is a high priority for transport, you will not splint the extremity at the scene but will treat it en route.

RAPID ASSESSMENT OF THE POSTERIOR BODY AND IMMOBILIZATION ON A BACKBOARD Roll the patient onto his side as a unit (you will learn how to do a log-roll maneuver in Chapter 29, "Injuries to the Head and Spine") and assess the posterior body, inspecting and palpating for DCAP-BTLS in the area of the spine and to the sides of the spine, the buttocks, and the posterior extremities. Meanwhile, have someone slide a backboard next to the patient so that, when you roll the patient back into a supine position, he is on the backboard.

If the patient has shown signs or symptoms of an injury to the pelvis, local protocol may direct placing a pneumatic antishock garment (PASG) on the board before you roll the patient onto it. Local protocol may direct you to place the antishock garment on the backboard for other kinds of trauma, too. (You will learn about the PASG in Chapter 26, "Bleeding and Shock.") A newer method of stabilizing an injured pelvis is forming a pelvic wrap from a folded sheet. (You will learn about how to apply a pelvic wrap in Chapter 28, "Musculoskeletal Injuries.") Become familiar with how local medical direction wishes you to manage these patients.

OBTAIN BASELINE VITAL SIGNS AND A SAMPLE HISTORY Quickly obtain a set of baseline vital signs, as discussed in Chapter 9, "Vital Signs and SAMPLE History." If using a pulse oximeter is part of your assessment, apply it now (or earlier, if your local protocol suggests doing so). If the patient is unresponsive, you will not be able to get a SAMPLE history from him. If there is a friend or family member nearby, that person may be able to give you information about the patient's medical history.

POINT OF VIEW

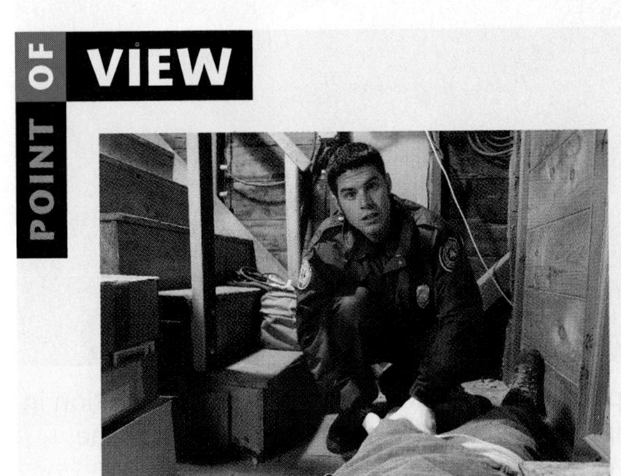

"I was putting some boxes up in the loft in our barn. I must've missed a step. I fell down the first few stairs and felt a 'crack' in my leg. I heard it, but man, I really felt it snap. If that wasn't proof enough, it hurt more than anything I ever felt before. It was broken!

"The EMTs came. They were great, but I gotta tell you, even when they said they'd be careful, they made horrible pain even worse. When the one EMT examined my leg, I thought I was going to jump out of my skin. Any little movement was just so painful.

"They put a splint on and took me to the hospital. I won't even tell you how much the bumps hurt on the ride to the hospital. I don't want to be a complainer, but, well, it hurts to break your leg. Let me tell you."

SCAN 10-5 • Assessing Distal Function

Assess all four extremities for distal pulse, motor function, and sensation. Diminished function may be a sign of injury that has compromised circulation, motor function, or nerve function. Distal function should be checked both before and after any interventions such as splinting, bandaging, and immobilization, and at intervals during transport, to be sure such interventions are not interfering with distal function. If distal function has become compromised, adjust interventions as necessary.

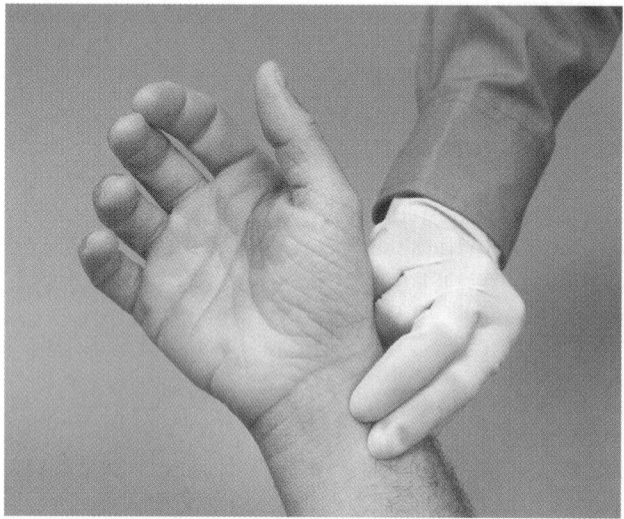

1. Assess distal circulation in the upper extremities by feeling for radial pulses.

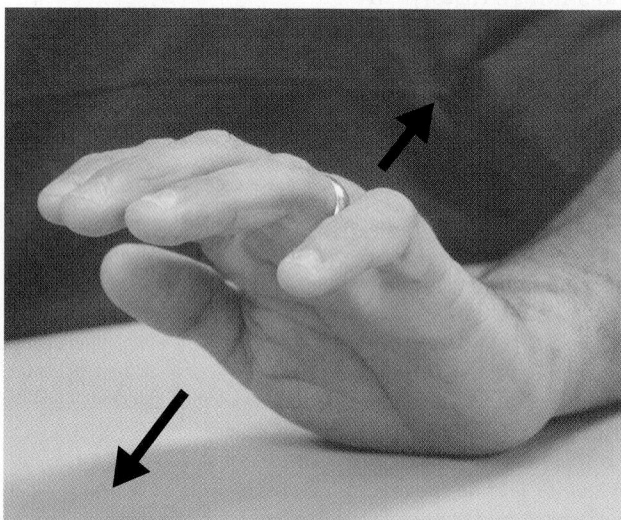

2. Assess distal motor function by checking the patient's ability to move both hands.

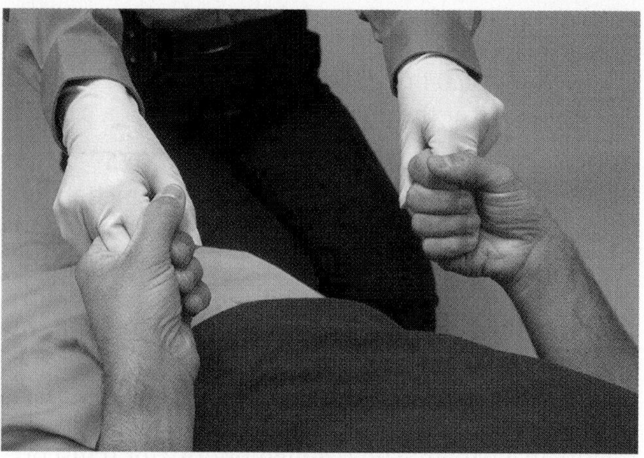

3. Assess strength in the hands by asking the patient to squeeze your fingers.

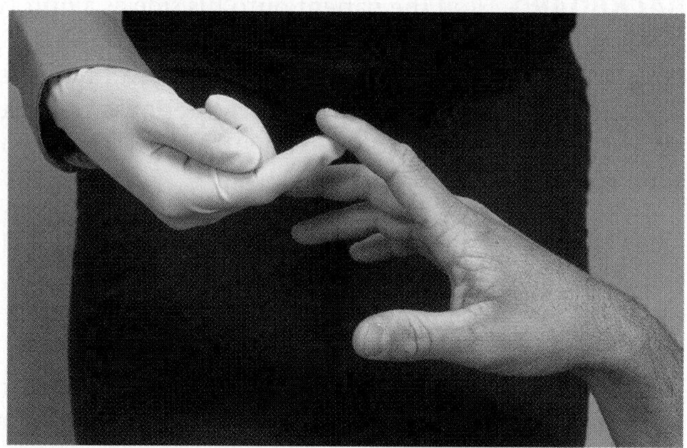

4. Assess distal sensation to the upper extremities by asking the patient, "Which finger am I touching?" (Be sure the patient cannot see which finger.)

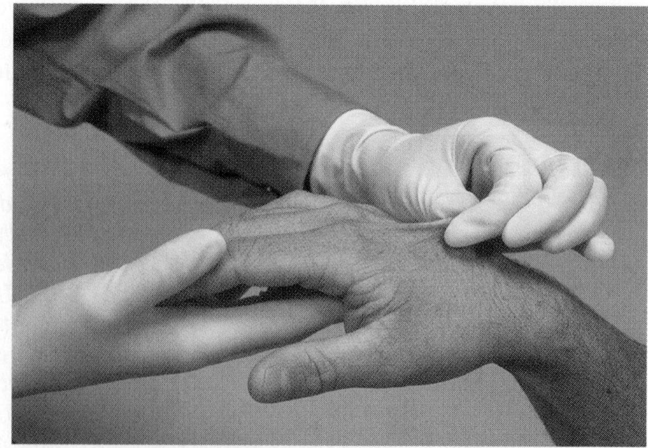

If the patient is unresponsive, check distal sensation in the upper extremities by pinching the back of the hand. Watch and listen for a response.

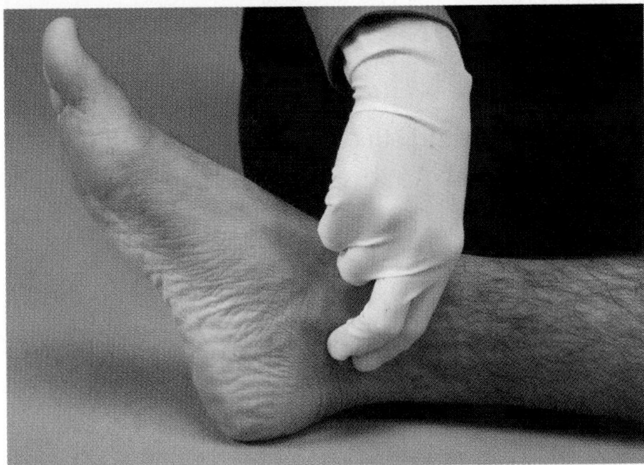

5. Check distal circulation in the lower extremities by feeling the posterior tibial pulse just behind the medial malleolus of the ankle, or . . .

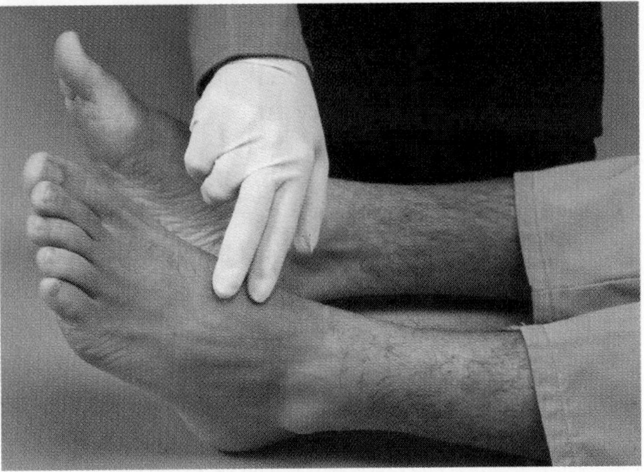

. . . feel the dorsalis pedis pulse at the top of the foot.

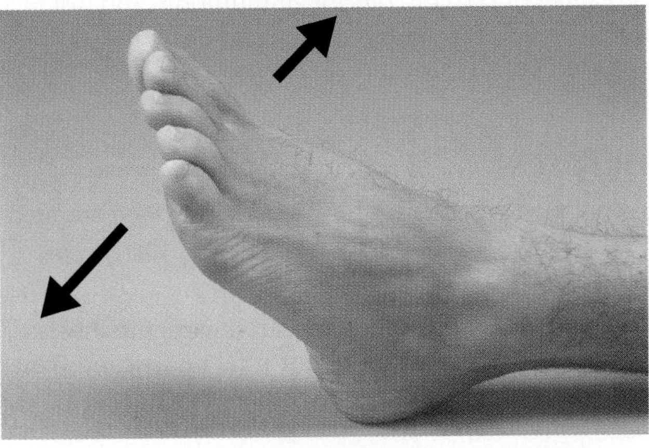

6. Assess distal motor function by checking the patient's ability to move his feet.

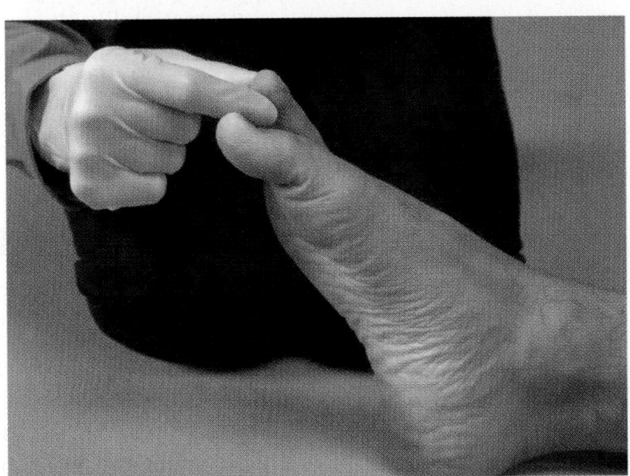

8. Assess distal sensation in the lower extremities by asking the patient, "Which toe am I touching?" (Be sure the patient cannot see which toe.)

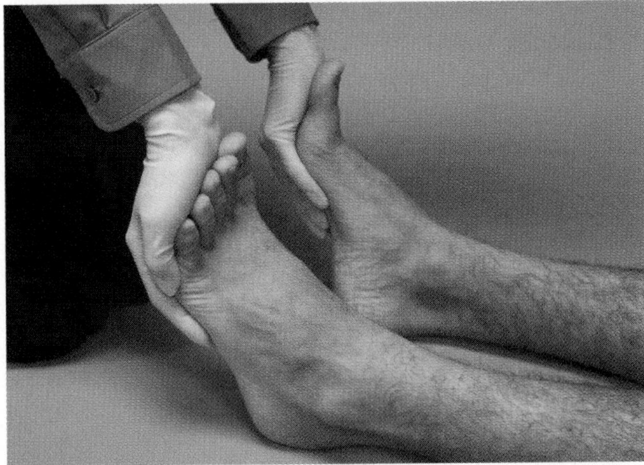

7. Assess strength in the feet and legs by asking the patient to push against your hands.

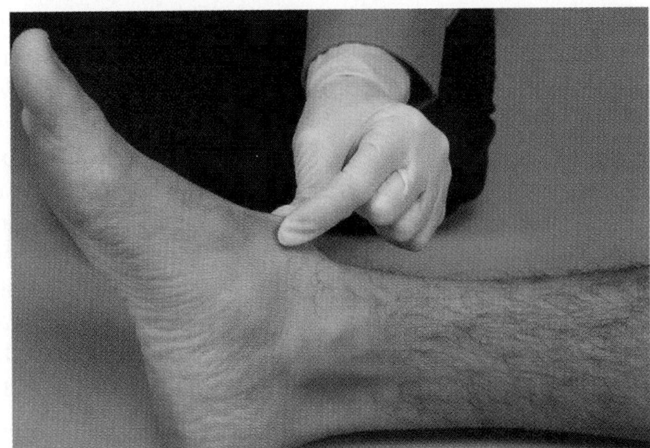

If the patient is unresponsive, check distal sensation in the lower extremities by pinching the top of the foot. Watch and listen for a response.

CRITICAL DECISION MAKING:
RAPID TRAUMA OR FOCUSED EXAM?

For each of the following patients determine if you should perform a rapid trauma exam or a focused exam.

1. Your patient was found ejected from a vehicle in a rollover collision.
2. Your patient tripped and believes he broke his wrist. He complains of no other injuries.
3. Your patient only complains of minor neck pain after a frontal impact accident in which there was considerable damage and airbag deployment.
4. Your patient fell about 6 feet from a tree and believes he broke his ankle. Bystanders tell you he briefly lost consciousness.

In trauma situations, it is good to think of the "S" in SAMPLE as standing for not just "signs and symptoms" but also for "story," or the history of the injury. This means information like the speed of the vehicle, whether seat belts were used, and whether the patient had a loss of consciousness. With patients who have been shot, information you should try to obtain includes the caliber of the gun, type of ammunition, and distance of the gun from the patient when the gun was discharged. When you are treating a patient who has been stabbed, try to find out the size and type of the knife.

Some General Principles

Several important principles to remember when examining a patient, which are mentioned throughout the chapter, are summarized in the following list:

- *Tell the patient what you are going to do.* In particular, let the patient know when there may be pain or discomfort. Stress the importance of the examination and work to build the patient's confidence. Ask the patient if he understands what you are doing, and explain your actions again if needed.
- *Expose any injured area before examining it.* By exposing areas, you can see such things as bruises and puncture wounds. Let the patient know when you must lift, rearrange, or remove any article of clothing. Do all you can to ensure the patient's privacy.
- *Try to maintain eye contact.* Do not turn away while you are talking or while the patient is answering your questions.
- *Assume spinal injury.* Unless you are sure that you are dealing with a patient who does not have a spine injury (e.g., a medical patient with no mechanism of injury or reason to suspect trauma), assume the patient has such injuries. Always assume that the unconscious trauma patient has a spine injury. Manually stabilize the head and neck on first contact with the patient, fit the patient with a properly sized cervical collar as soon as you have examined the head and neck, and fully immobilize the patient to a spine board before transport to the hospital.
- *During the focused physical exam, you may stop or alter the assessment process to provide care that is necessary and appropriate for the priority of the patient.* For a patient who is not a priority for rapid transport, you may pause to bandage a bleeding wound, even if the bleeding is not life threatening, or to splint an injured extremity.
- *During the rapid trauma assessment, apply a cervical collar if spine injury is suspected.* For a patient who is a priority for rapid transport, treatments such as controlling non-life-threatening bleeding or splinting an injured extremity may take place en route to the hospital if time and the patient's condition permit.

PEDIATRIC NOTE

The focused history and physical exam of the pediatric (infant or child) trauma patient is very similar to the focused history and physical exam of the adult patient. One important difference is that you may need to spend more time reassuring children and explaining procedures to them. You will want to kneel or find another way to get on the same level with the child as you speak with him. Young children may be less frightened if you begin your assessment at the toes and work toward the head instead of proceeding in the usual head-to-toe direction. (Assessment of infants and children will be discussed in greater detail in Chapter 31, "Infants and Children.")

A child's airway is narrower than an adult's and more susceptible to being closed. A cervical collar that is too tight can easily constrict a child's airway. A collar that is too high can close the airway by stretching the neck. So it is especially important to choose the correct size cervical collar for a child.

DETAILED PHYSICAL EXAM

The initial assessment and the focused history and physical exam are done rapidly because of the necessity of getting the seriously injured or ill patient into the ambulance and to the hospital without delay. En route to the hospital, you may have time to do a more complete patient assessment known as the **detailed physical exam.** If you are not on a transporting unit and the ambulance has not arrived, you may do the detailed physical exam at the scene.

detailed physical exam an assessment of the head, neck, chest, abdomen, pelvis, extremities, and posterior of the body to detect signs and symptoms of injury. It differs from the rapid trauma assessment only in that it also includes examination of the face, ears, eyes, nose, and mouth during the examination of the head. It may be done less rapidly, and it may be done en route to the hospital after earlier on-scene assessments and interventions are completed.

The purpose of the detailed physical exam is to gather additional information about the patient's injuries and conditions. Some of this information may help you to determine the proper treatment for the patient, and some of the information you gather in the detailed physical exam will assist the emergency department staff.

The detailed physical exam is performed most often on the trauma patient with a significant mechanism of injury, less often on a trauma patient with no significant mechanism of injury, and seldom on a medical patient.

Trauma Patient with a Significant Mechanism of Injury

For a trauma patient who is not responsive or has a significant or unknown mechanism of injury, you will have assessed almost the entire body during the rapid trauma assessment—but very quickly. For this patient, a detailed physical exam may reveal signs or symptoms of injury that you missed or that have changed since the rapid trauma assessment.

Before Beginning the Detailed Physical Exam

It is important to remember that you should perform the detailed physical exam only after you have performed all critical interventions. The best way to ensure this is to repeat your initial assessment before you begin the detailed physical exam. To do this, reassess your general impression of the patient, his mental status, plus airway, breathing, and circulation.

If you are treating a severely injured patient, you may be too busy to begin or complete the detailed physical exam at all. This is not a failure on your part. Your responsibility is to give the patient the best care possible under the difficult conditions found in the field. If you do not do a complete assessment, but you keep a critical patient's airway, breathing, and circulation intact, you have helped the patient far more than if you had done the complete assessment. *Performing a detailed physical exam is always a lower priority than addressing life-threatening problems.* Table 10-4 shows the place of the detailed physical exam among the priorities and sequence of assessment.

TABLE 10-4 • Detailed Physical Exam in the Sequence of Assessment Priorities

1. Scene size-up.
2. Initial assessment and critical interventions for immediately life-threatening problems.
3. Focused history and physical exam, vital signs, plus interventions as needed.
4. Repeat initial assessment for immediately life-threatening problems. Provide critical interventions as needed.
5. Detailed physical exam (time and critical-care needs permitting).
6. Ongoing assessment for life-threatening problems, plus reassessment of vital signs. Provide critical interventions as needed.

Performing the Detailed Physical Exam

If you have not already exposed the patient, you need to do so now. Since you are now in the enclosed ambulance, it is much easier to protect the patient's privacy and protect him from exposure to the environment.

The detailed physical exam will look a lot like the rapid trauma assessment that you did during the focused history and physical exam. You will look for the familiar DCAP-BTLS signs (review Scan 10-1). You will also look for certain additional signs as you examine the head, neck, chest, abdomen, pelvis, extremities, and posterior body. The only areas you will assess in the detailed physical exam that you did not assess during the rapid trauma assessment portion of the focused history and physical exam will be the face, ears, eyes, nose, and mouth (Table 10-5 and Scan 10-6).

TABLE 10-5 • Detailed Physical Exam Compared to Rapid Trauma Assessment

FOCUSED HISTORY AND PHYSICAL EXAM: RAPID TRAUMA ASSESSMENT		DETAILED PHYSICAL EXAM	
Head	DCAP-BTLS + crepitation	Scalp and cranium	DCAP-BTLS + crepitation
		Face	DCAP-BTLS
		Ears	DCAP-BTLS + drainage, bleeding
		Eyes	DCAP-BTLS + discoloration, unequal pupils, foreign bodies, blood in anterior chamber
		Nose	DCAP-BTLS + drainage, bleeding
		Mouth	DCAP-BTLS + loose or broken teeth, objects that could cause obstruction, swelling or laceration of tongue, unusual breath odor, discoloration
Neck	DCAP-BTLS + jugular vein distention, crepitation	Neck	DCAP-BTLS + jugular vein distention, crepitation
Chest	DCAP-BTLS + paradoxical motion, crepitation, breath sounds	Chest	DCAP-BTLS + paradoxical motion, crepitation, breath sounds
Abdomen	DCAP-BTLS + firmness, softness, distention	Abdomen	DCAP-BTLS + firmness, softness, distention
Pelvis	DCAP-BTLS + pain, tenderness, motion	Pelvis	DCAP-BTLS + pain, tenderness, motion
Extremities	DCAP-BTLS + distal pulse, motor function, sensation	Extremities	DCAP-BTLS + distal pulse, motor function, sensation
Posterior	DCAP-BTLS	Posterior	DCAP-BTLS

SCAN 10-6 • Detailed Physical Exam

The detailed physical exam is similar to the rapid trauma assessment—with some important differences:

- The head (scalp, cranium, face, ears, eyes, nose, mouth) is more thoroughly examined.
- The exam usually takes place in the ambulance, en route. Noise and motion may interfere with some procedures.
- Immobilization devices have been applied and you must work around them; for example, examining the ears through holes in the head immobilizer or below head tape, examining the neck through openings in the rigid collar, and examining only as much of the posterior as you can reach.

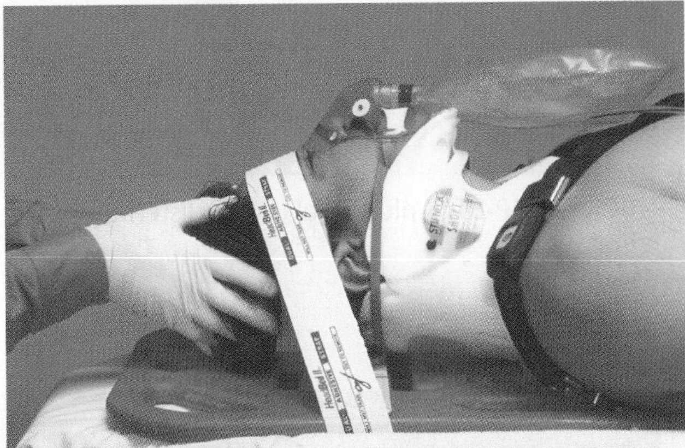

SCALP AND CRANIUM: DCAP-BTLS plus crepitation.

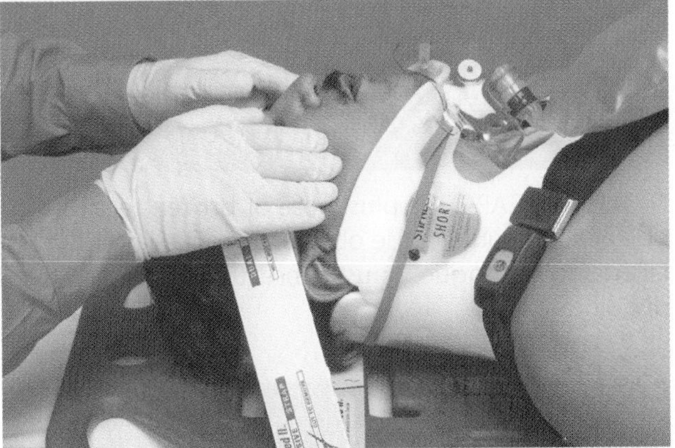

FACE: DCAP-BTLS

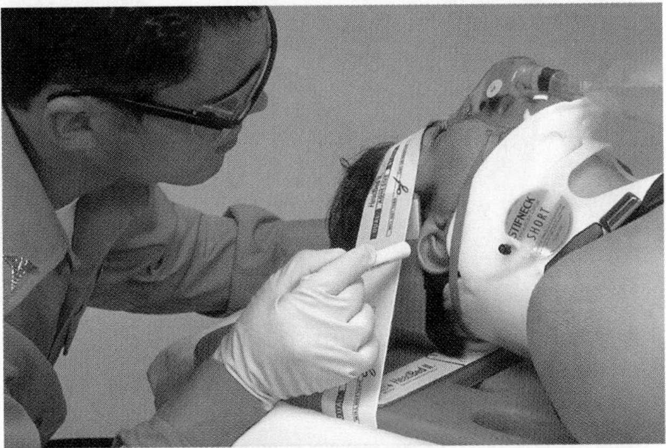

EARS: DCAP-BTLS plus drainage of blood or clear fluid.

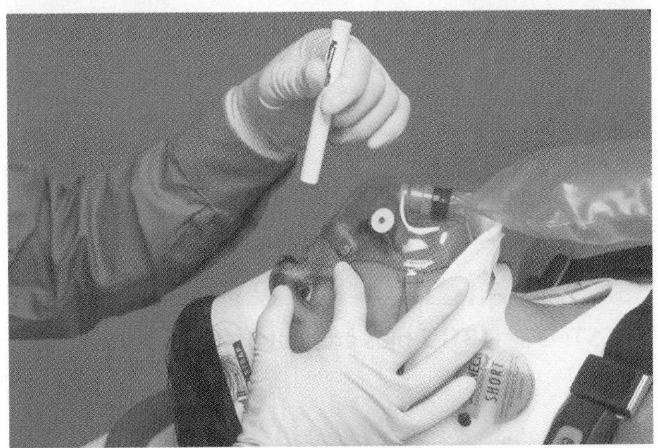

EYES: DCAP-BTLS plus discoloration, unequal pupils, foreign bodies, blood in anterior chamber.

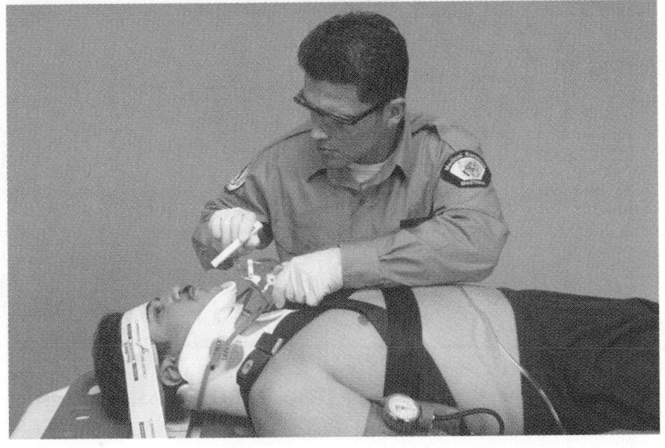

NOSE: DCAP-BTLS plus drainage of blood or clear fluid.

continued

SCAN 10-6 • (Continued)

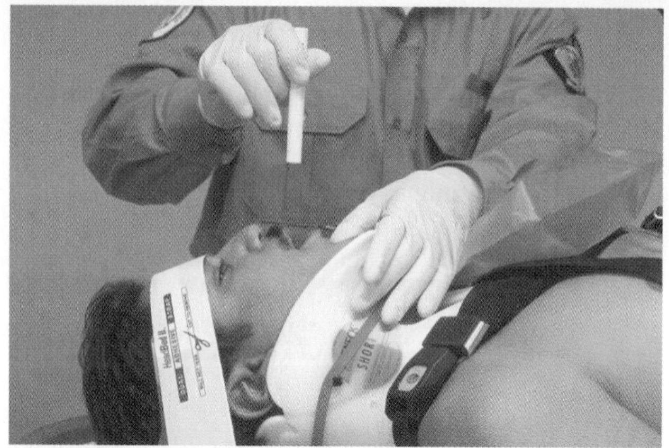

MOUTH: DCAP-BTLS plus loose or broken teeth, objects that could cause obstruction, swelling or laceration of tongue, unusual breath odor, discoloration.

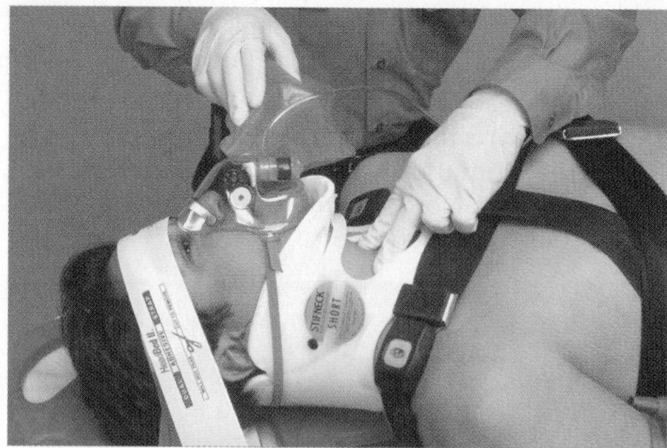

NECK: DCAP-BTLS plus jugular vein distention, crepitation.

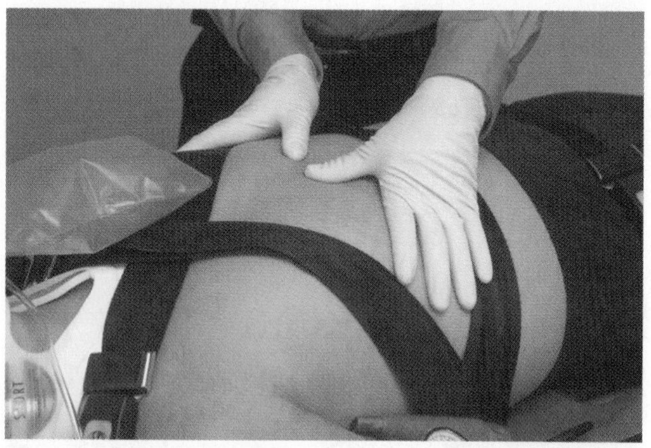

CHEST: DCAP-BTLS plus crepitation, paradoxical motion.

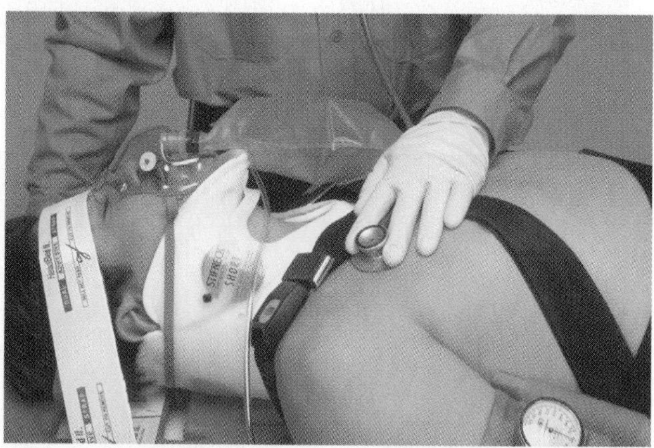

Auscultate chest for breath sounds: presence, absence, and equality.

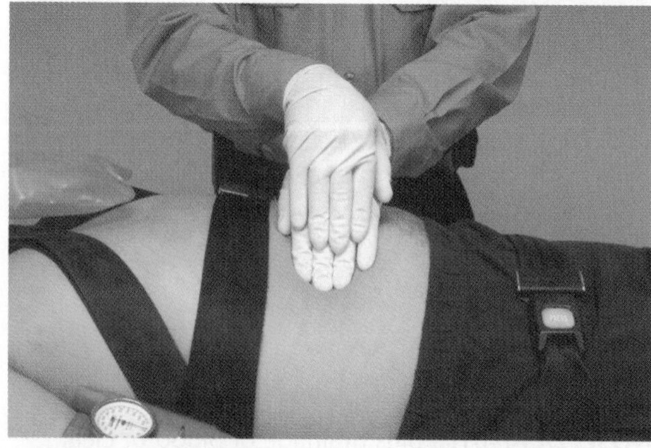

ABDOMEN: DCAP-BTLS plus firmness, softness, distention.

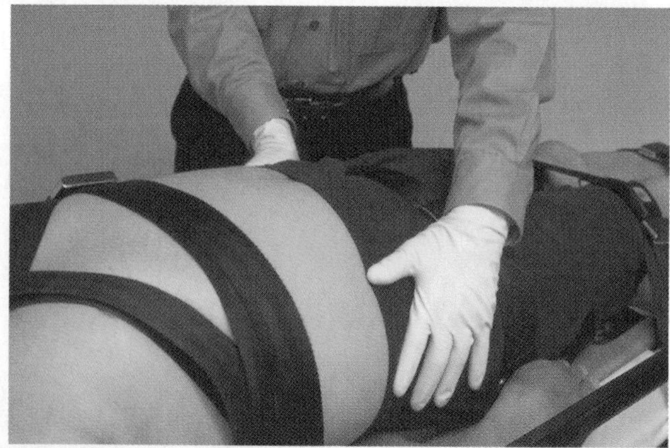

PELVIS: DCAP-BTLS plus pain, tenderness, motion.

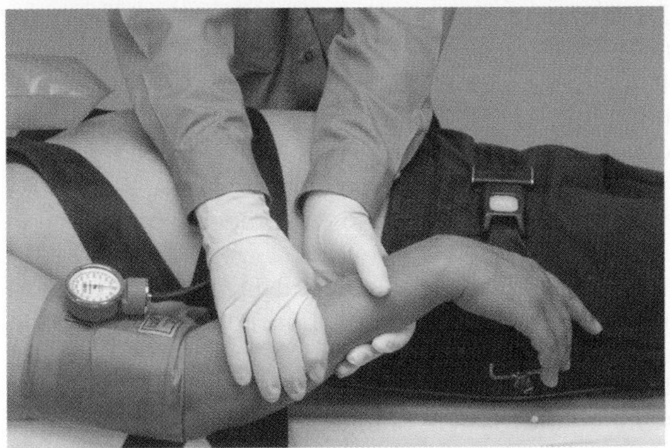

UPPER EXTREMITIES: DCAP-BTLS.

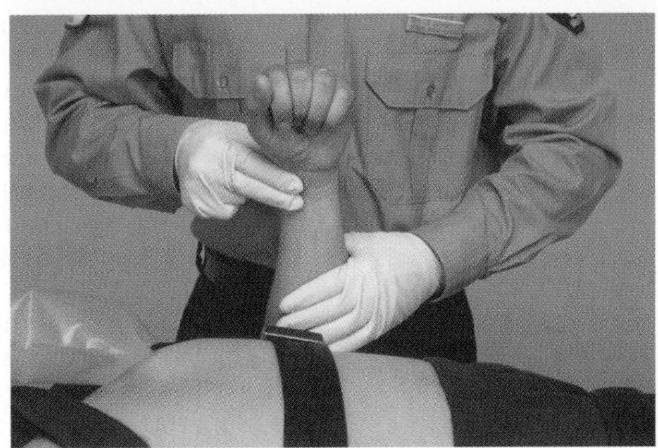

Assess upper extremities for distal pulse, motor function, and sensation.

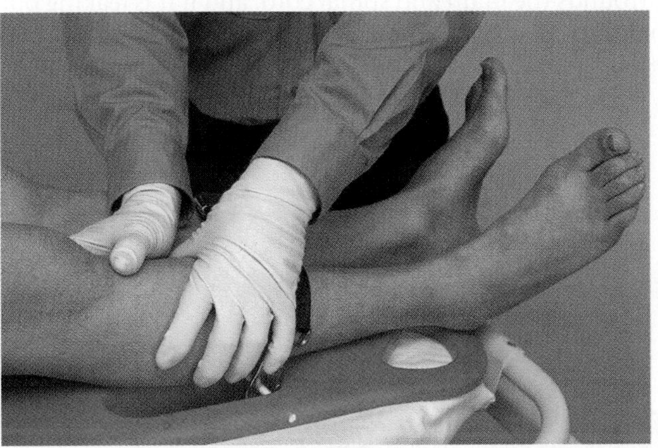

LOWER EXTREMITIES: DCAP-BTLS.

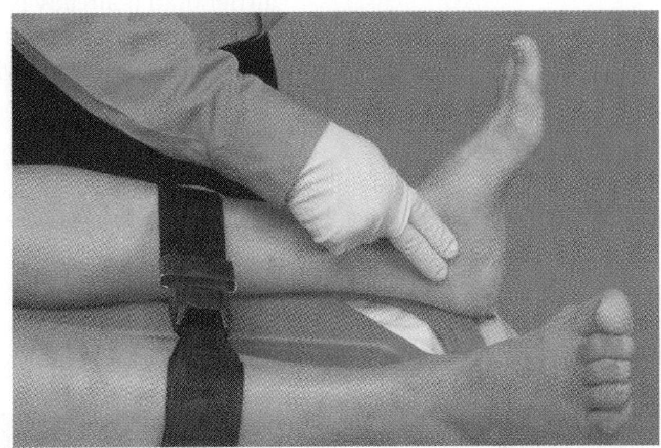

Assess lower extremities for distal pulse, motor function, and sensation.

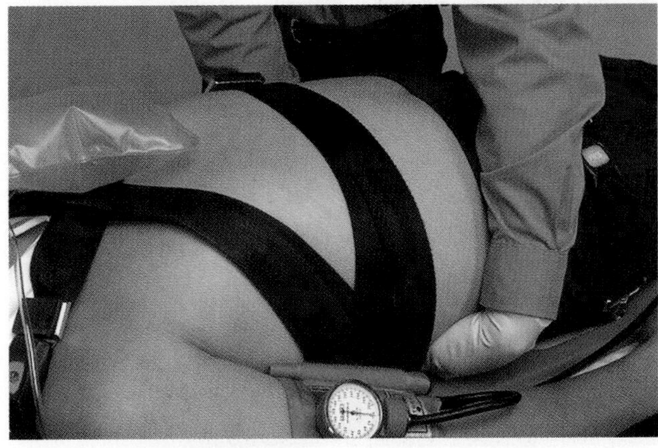

POSTERIOR: DCAP-BTLS.

Gently palpate the cranium for DCAP-BTLS and crepitation and then inspect your gloves for blood. Inspect and palpate the face for DCAP-BTLS by looking and then gently palpating the cheekbones, forehead, and lower jaw. The bones in the face are fragile and may break when subjected to significant forces.

Inspect and palpate the ears, searching for DCAP-BTLS and drainage of blood or other fluid. If found, this is an important piece of information to pass on to the emergency department staff because it may be an indication of injury to the skull (Figure 10-5). Also gently bend each ear forward to look for any bruising. (You can do this if you were careful when you applied the cervical collar to make sure you did not enclose the ears.) A bruise behind the ear of a patient is called Battle's sign and is another important sign of skull injury to tell hospital staff about.

Next assess the eyes, inspecting for the usual DCAP-BTLS and discoloration, unequal pupils, foreign bodies, and blood in the anterior chamber (front) of the eye. Blood in the anterior chamber is not common but, when present, it is a sign that the eye sustained significant force and is bleeding inside (Figure 10-6).

Inspect and palpate the nose for injuries or signs of injury. Look not only for DCAP-BTLS but also for drainage and bleeding.

When assessing the ears and nose, you may find blood or clear fluid draining from them. Blood may be from a laceration of that area or it may be coming from inside the skull. Clear fluid may be just from a runny nose or it may be cerebrospinal fluid (CSF). You should prevent an ear or nose that is draining blood or clear fluid from getting any dirtier than it already is. CSF surrounds the brain and spinal cord, and if it is leaking out then bacteria can get into the brain. Similarly, a wound from inside the skull that is leaking blood can also provide a route for bacteria to get in. Figure 10-7 summarizes signs of brain injury.

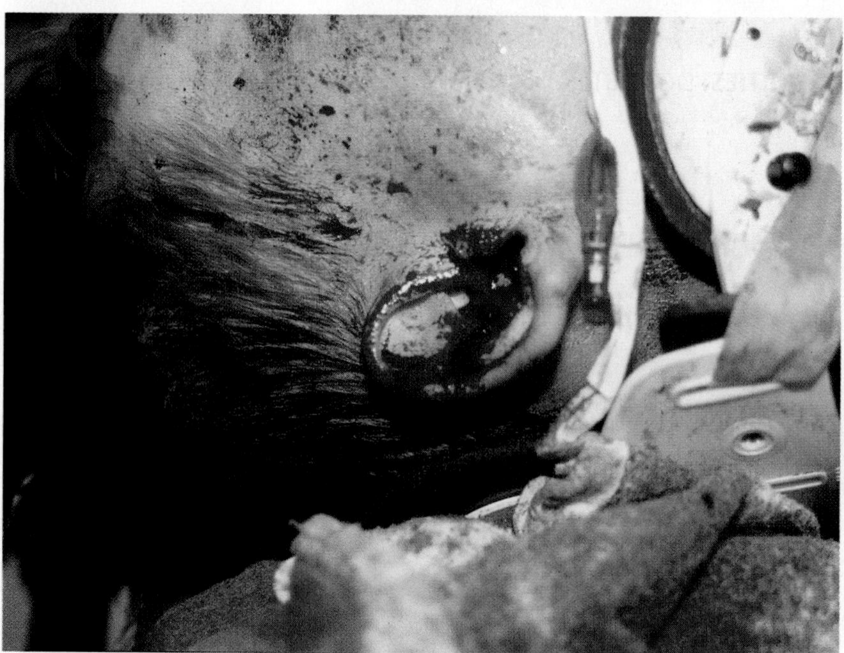

Figure 10-5 • Cerebrospinal fluid draining from the ear of a trauma patient. *(© Edward T. Dickinson, MD)*

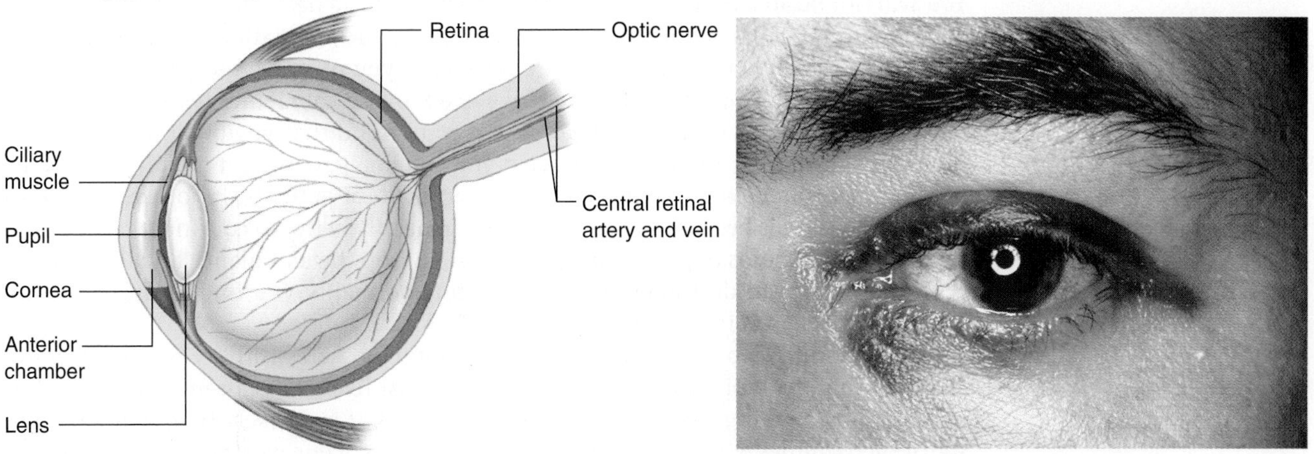

Figure 10-6 • Blood in the anterior chamber of the eye is a sign that the eye has sustained considerable force. (The white ring in the photo is a reflection of the flash.) *(© Western Ophthalmic Hospital/Science Photo Library/Photo Researchers, Inc.)*

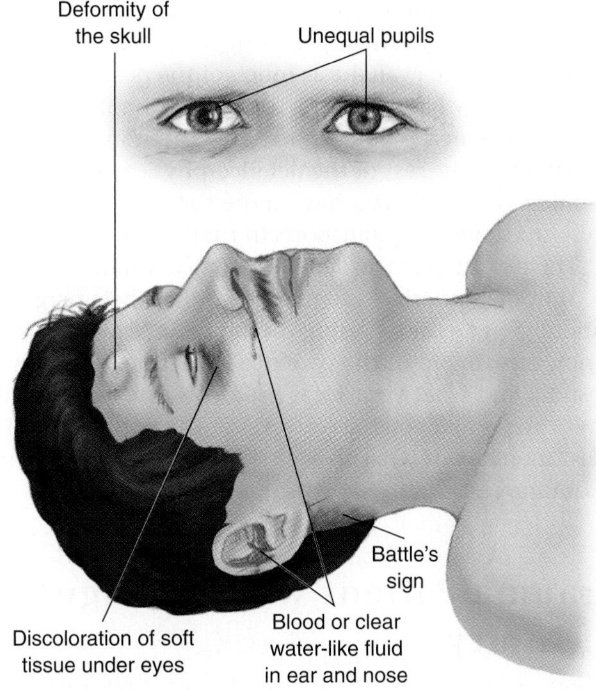

Figure 10-7 • Battle's sign and other signs of brain injury.

Open the mouth and look for DCAP-BTLS, loose or broken teeth, other objects that could cause obstruction, swelling or laceration of the tongue, unusual breath odor, and discoloration. A foreign body like a broken tooth is a potential source of airway obstruction and must be removed as soon as possible from the patient's mouth. The most common unusual breath odor is from alcoholic beverages. Other conditions besides alcohol, though, can cause similar odors.

There are only a few differences in the rest of the exam compared to what you did in the rapid trauma assessment. These differences result from either the different environment (the back of the ambulance) or from the treatment you have already given to the patient (e.g., cervical collar and immobilization on a backboard).

When you assess the neck you will be limited by the cervical collar that you placed on the patient during the focused history and physical exam (rapid trauma assessment).

You will not be able to inspect or palpate the back of the neck, but you will be able to assess for DCAP-BTLS, jugular vein distention (JVD), and crepitation through the openings in the collar. You should make sure the collars you use have these openings.

Reassessing the chest can be a challenge in a moving ambulance because road noise makes breath sounds difficult to hear. Just keep in mind that you are listening for the presence and equality of breath sounds in your trauma patient, not the different kinds of abnormal sounds that are more common in medical patients. If you are unable to hear breath sounds because of road noise, it is generally better to continue transporting the patient to the hospital. It makes little sense to stop the ambulance and delay transport unless you can do something to treat an abnormality you find. Reassess the abdomen and pelvis as in the rapid assessment.

Any deformities or other indications of a musculoskeletal injury to an extremity found during the rapid trauma assessment will most likely have been temporarily immobilized by securing the patient to the spine board. It is unlikely that taking time to splint such injuries would have been appropriate at the scene when rapid transport was a priority. En route to the hospital, if the patient's other injuries are not keeping you too busy, a good time to apply a splint to an injured extremity would be after you perform the detailed physical exam. You will learn splinting techniques in Chapter 28, "Musculoskeletal Injuries."

When it comes to reassessing the posterior body it would, of course, be inappropriate to roll the patient up off the backboard. By having the patient immobilized on a backboard, you are already treating for possible spine injury, so your primary concern at this point is to evaluate as much of the posterior body as you can reach for other injuries that may have been missed earlier. Simply reassess the flanks (sides) and as much of the spinal area as you can touch without moving the patient.

Although the rest of the detailed physical exam is essentially the same as the rapid trauma assessment, you have more time, so you can be more thorough. This is especially true with long transports in rural or wilderness areas.

The final step of the detailed physical exam is to reassess the vital signs.

Your next priority is to make sure that the emergency department is ready for your patient. You do this by using the ambulance radio or cellular phone to notify the emergency department of the patient's condition. Depending on how far you are from the hospital and what your local protocols say, you may do this step before the detailed physical exam. If you have not yet notified the hospital, you should do it now. You will learn more about what to say to hospital personnel and how to say it in Chapter 13, "Communications."

Trauma Patient with No Significant Mechanism of Injury

When caring for a trauma patient who is responsive and has no significant mechanism of injury, you will have focused your assessment on just the areas the patient tells you hurt plus those areas that you suspect may be injured based on the mechanism of injury.

This kind of patient received all the assessment he needed while still at the scene. He does not generally need a detailed physical exam. It is important to keep a high index of suspicion, though. When in doubt, do a detailed physical exam. Be aware of the responsive trauma patient's fear and need for emotional support.

You should perform a detailed physical exam on a trauma patient who has a significant mechanism of injury and on any patient who has an unclear or unknown mechanism of injury. But the detailed physical exam is not meant for medical patients. This is because there are usually few signs an EMT can find in the physical exam of a medical patient that are significant or about which you can or should do anything. Most of the assessment information on medical patients comes from the history and vital signs.

Occasionally, you may come across a patient who could be either medical or trauma, or both. For example, imagine you have responded to an elderly man who is found alone and unconscious, slumped over the steering wheel of his car. The car is off the road and there is no damage to it. Did the patient lose consciousness first and then drive his car off the road, or did he drive off the road and then get knocked out from a blow to the head? The safest and best thing to do for a patient like this is generally to treat him as a trauma patient who gets a rapid trauma assessment and, if there is time, a detailed physical exam—but whenever possible, also get a history from any witnesses you can find.

COMPARING ASSESSMENTS

Following are two scenarios that may help you see the difference between assessment of a trauma patient with a significant mechanism of injury and assessment of a trauma patient with no significant mechanism of injury:

Clara Diller—Responsive Child with No Significant Mechanism of Injury

You have been dispatched to a 5-year-old girl, Clara, who has fallen while skating. She is crying and holding a bloody cloth to her knee. After completing the scene size-up and initial assessment, and deciding that she is not a priority for immediate transport, you begin the focused history and physical exam for a trauma patient.

Mechanism of Injury

The first step of the focused history and physical exam for a trauma patient is to reconsider the mechanism of injury. Therefore, you take a careful look around to be sure that Clara has only fallen down, not suffered a more severe incident like striking a pole or being hit by a car. There is no indication of this, and since a young child trying skates for the first time is unlikely to have been going very fast, even though a sidewalk is a hard surface to fall on, you conclude that Clara has no significant mechanism of injury. So you continue the on-scene assessment.

Chief Complaint

"Where do you hurt, Clara?" you ask her. You are not surprised when she says, "My knee hurts," because you can see that her knee is bleeding. Then she adds, "My head hurts, too." So you know that she may have struck her head. Based on the mechanism of injury—a fall to a hard surface—you suspect that she may have injured her spine as well. So you now focus your assessment according to the chief complaint and mechanism of injury. You focus not on Clara's whole body, but on her head, neck, spine, and knee.

Focused Physical Exam

You look at Clara's head and the back of her neck, searching for injuries such as contusions, abrasions, punctures or penetrations, burns, and lacerations. You find only some swelling on her forehead. Next, you gently press on her head and cervical spine, starting at the top, then moving to the back of her head and going down her neck to the large bump that indicates the lower end of the neck. You find no deformities, tenderness, or swelling. You now determine the proper cervical collar for a child Clara's size. You put it around her neck without moving her head or neck while your partner continues to hold her head.

During the initial assessment, you controlled the bleeding from Clara's knee. Now you tell her, "Clara, I need to lift up that cloth and look underneath. I'm going to feel around your knee, too. If it hurts, you can tell me. Okay?" Clara agrees, and you look at her knee for contusions, abrasions, punctures or penetrations, burns, or lacerations. There is only the laceration you found earlier. It is bleeding very slowly and does not appear to be deep. You palpate the area around the knee. You find no deformities or swelling, but the lateral side of the knee is tender. You place a sterile dressing over the wound in place of the cloth Clara was holding.

Baseline Vital Signs

Next, you assess Clara's vital signs. Her pulse is 104 per minute, strong and regular. She has respirations of 24 per minute. They are normal in depth. You check her skin by looking at the palm of her hand and see that it is pink. You feel it and determine that it is warm and dry. You squeeze the end of her fingernail and find that her capillary refill is normal. After telling Clara what you are going to do, you shine a light into her eyes and find that her pupils are equal and reactive. Again, you tell Clara what to expect before you inflate a pediatric cuff on her arm and find her blood pressure is 90/60.

History

While you are doing the focused exam, you ask Clara for more information. She is 5 years old, she tells you, and very scared because "my mommy told me not to try my new skates till later." The neighbor who takes care of Clara says, "I called Clara's mother at work when I saw her fall." You ask, "Did you see if Clara got knocked out? Even for a moment?" The neighbor tells you Clara did not lose consciousness.

Just now, Clara's mother arrives on scene. You reassure her that Clara seems to have just an injury to her knee and a slight bump on her head. You also explain that you have put a special collar on her just in case she injured her neck and that she will be placed on a spine board for the ride to the hospital.

Clara's mother is a better source of medical information than a 5-year-old, so you interview her for the SAMPLE history. You have already asked Clara what symptoms she has, so you ask her mother if Clara has any allergies or takes any medicines. You also ask about pertinent past history. She tells you that Clara has no allergies, takes no medicines, and is healthy. The neighbor tells you Clara's last food or drink was lunch a couple of hours ago. When you ask her about events leading to the injury, she tells you Clara has been feeling fine and acting normal today.

Detailed Physical Exam and Further Care

You immobilize Clara on a backboard and transport her to the emergency department. Although she has no significant mechanism of injury, there is time on the way to the hospital to do a detailed physical exam. You take special care in examining her head, since she had a bump on her forehead. You discover no new significant findings.

Clara's visit to the hospital is brief. The hospital staff rules out any serious head or spine injury. She gets some ointment and a cartoon bandage for her knee. She talks excitedly about her ambulance ride all the way home.

Brian Sawyer—Unresponsive Adult with Significant Mechanism of Injury

You are caring for a young man who has been thrown to the pavement during a vehicle collision. After completing the scene size-up, you conducted an initial assessment during which you checked Brian's mental status, took steps to correct an airway problem, checked breathing and circulation, and applied high-concentration oxygen. Because your initial assessment revealed that he was unresponsive to pain and showed signs of diminished circulation (rapid, weak pulse and pale, clammy skin), you assigned Brian a high priority for rapid transport and now take just a few moments to conduct a rapid version of the focused history and physical exam for a trauma patient.

Mechanism of Injury

You have no opportunity to take a closer look at the car Brian was in because it is 20 feet away. Instead, you ask a police officer to inspect the car for any deformities that would indicate where Brian might have struck interior surfaces. The officer reports that there are no deformities in the interior of the car. However, the fact that Brian appears to have been thrown from the car is a significant mechanism of injury.

Manual Stabilization of the Head and Neck

Your partner started manual stabilization during the initial assessment. He continues to hold the head and neck in a neutral in-line position and keep the airway open.

Advanced Life Support Request

If you were in an area where paramedics are available to respond, this would be a good time to call them. However, in your area, you do not have this option, so you continue your focused history and physical exam.

Transport Decision

The priority you assigned Brian at the end of your initial assessment was high. After you reconsider the mechanism of injury, you confirm your decision to transport him quickly—just as soon as you complete a rapid focused history and physical exam.

Mental Status

Now you assess Brian's mental status. You determined during the initial assessment that he was unresponsive to pain. You confirm that this is still the case by pinching his shoulder muscle. There is still no response.

Rapid Trauma Assessment

The physical exam you perform on Brian is different from the one you did on Clara. Clara did not have a significant mechanism of injury. She was able to tell you where she hurt, and you were able to focus your exam on just the parts identified by her complaint and mechanism of injury. You examined only her head, neck, and knee. Then you put on a cervical collar and dressed and bandaged her knee.

Brian is unresponsive to pain and cannot tell you what hurts. Even if he could, you would want to give him a more thorough exam because he had a significant mechanism of injury. Being thrown from a car during a collision is likely to produce more than just a localized cut or scrape. Yet, your examination of Brian must be speedy. You must do a more comprehensive exam than you did for Clara, but you must do it rapidly so that you can get Brian into the ambulance and en route to the hospital without delay.

So you now perform a rapid trauma assessment. As you inspect and palpate each part of his body, you look and feel for DCAP-BTLS. In addition, with particular areas of Brian's body, you also look for certain signs. You expose each part of the body as necessary. Your rapid trauma assessment of Brian goes as follows:

- Head. You assess Brian's head for DCAP-BTLS and crepitation (the sound or feel of broken bones rubbing against each other). You find a laceration on the back of his head that is not bleeding.
- Neck. You assess the neck for DCAP-BTLS, crepitation, and bulging or flat neck veins. There is no response from Brian when you palpate along his cervical spine. Brian's neck veins are flat, indicating possible blood loss, but no other abnormalities.

- Stabilization. You now size and apply a cervical collar. Your partner continues to hold manual stabilization as well.
- Chest. Next, you open Brian's shirt and assess his chest for DCAP-BTLS, crepitation, breath sounds, and paradoxical motion (movements of part of the chest in a direction that is different from the rest of the chest). You find no abnormalities.
- Abdomen. When you cut open Brian's trousers and assess his abdomen for DCAP-BTLS, you also check for firmness, softness, and distention. Brian's abdomen is very firm but does not look distended.
- Pelvis. Next, you assess Brian's pelvis for DCAP-BTLS. You find no abnormalities. Since he is not able to complain of any pain in the pelvis, you compress it gently to determine tenderness or motion. You find nothing unusual, except for confirming that his mental status is still such that he does not respond to any pain from compression.
- Extremities. Now you quickly assess all four extremities for DCAP-BTLS, plus distal pulse, motor function, and sensation. You find a deformity in Brian's right lower leg. You do not pause to splint the leg now but will tend to it en route to the hospital. He has weak pulses in all extremities and does not respond to a pinch there. Since he is not responsive, you cannot determine whether he has sensation or motor function.
- Posterior and immobilization. A firefighter has gotten a backboard from your ambulance and places it next to Brian. You and your partner roll Brian onto his side as a unit and cut away his clothing to assess his posterior body, inspecting and palpating for DCAP-BTLS. You find nothing abnormal. The firefighter places the board next to Brian and you roll him back onto the board.

You have been able to conduct the entire assessment in just a few moments. If any life-threatening problem had been discovered before or during the rapid trauma assessment, you would have altered the procedure as needed to allow for treatment of the problem.

Baseline Vital Signs

You quickly assess Brian's baseline vital signs. He has a pulse of 120, regular and weak. His respirations are 20 per minute. His skin is pale, cool, and sweaty. His left pupil is dilated and slow to react (the right pupil reacts normally to light). He has a blood pressure of 130/80. His oxygen saturation is 96 percent.

History

No one is available to give you a SAMPLE history. You did not come across any medical identification bracelet or necklace when you assessed Brian's extremities and neck.

Detailed Physical Exam

Inside the ambulance, before conducting a detailed physical exam on Brian, you first ensure that any critical interventions are performed. You accomplish this by repeating your initial assessment. Your general impression is that he appears to have serious injuries. His mental status is still unresponsive to pain. You are now managing his airway with an oropharyngeal airway and suction. You are giving him high-concentration oxygen, but he is breathing adequately and you do not need to ventilate him. A check of his circulation shows that his radial pulse is still rapid and weak, there is no external bleeding, and his skin is pale, cool, and sweaty.

After you feel certain that Brian's ABCs are under control, you have time to undertake the detailed physical exam. You reassess his head. The main difference from the rapid trauma assessment you did at the scene is that now you pay special attention to several areas you did not evaluate in detail before: the scalp and cranium, face, ears, eyes, nose, and mouth.

You gently palpate Brian's cranium for DCAP-BTLS and crepitation. You inspect your gloves for blood and find none. You assess Brian's face for DCAP-BTLS, gently palpating his cheekbones, forehead, and lower jaw. You inspect and palpate his ears, searching for DCAP-BTLS and drainage. You see a little bit of blood in the left ear. You also gently bend each of his ears forward to look for bruising, but find none.

Next, you assess Brian's eyes, inspecting for the usual DCAP-BTLS and discoloration, unequal pupils, foreign bodies, and blood in the front of the eye. His left pupil is dilated and slow to react. You do not see any blood in the front of his eye or any other abnormalities.

Next, you assess Brian's nose, inspecting and palpating for injuries or signs of injury. In this case, you look not only for DCAP-BTLS, but also for drainage and bleeding. You do not find any.

When you assess his mouth, you open it and look for DCAP-BTLS, loose or broken teeth, other objects that could cause obstruction, swelling or laceration of the tongue, unusual breath odor, and discoloration, even though you looked for these things when you inserted the oropharyngeal airway. You do not find any of these.

You go on to reassess Brian's neck, chest, abdomen, pelvis, extremities, and posterior body as you did during the rapid trauma assessment. You find no changes.

The last step in the detailed physical exam is to repeat Brian's vital signs. You obtain a pulse of 136, regular and weak; respirations of 14 per minute; skin that is still cool, pale, and sweaty; a left pupil that is still dilated and slow to react; and a blood pressure of 100/70—indicating a more rapid pulse, slower respirations, and a lower blood pressure than during the rapid trauma assessment at the scene.

You continue to care for Brian as the ambulance proceeds toward the hospital.

CHAPTER REVIEW

SUMMARY

The focused history and physical exam of the trauma patient takes place immediately after the initial assessment. It starts with a reconsideration of the mechanism of injury. This allows you to determine which path you are going to take in assessing a patient.

The patient without a significant mechanism of injury receives a physical exam focused on areas that the patient complains about and areas that you think may be injured based on the mechanism of injury. It is important to have a high index of suspicion and evaluate any areas that you feel may have been injured. When in doubt, assess it. Next, gather a set of baseline vital signs and a SAMPLE history.

The patient who has a significant mechanism of injury receives a somewhat different assessment. Ensure continued manual stabilization of the head and neck, consider whether to call advanced life support personnel (if available), reconsider how urgently to transport the patient, reassess mental status, and then perform a rapid trauma assessment. In the rapid trauma assessment look for deformities, contusions, abrasions, punctures and penetrations, burns, tenderness, lacerations, and swelling, plus certain additional signs appropriate to the part being assessed (as summarized in Table 10-3). Systematically examine the head, neck, chest, abdomen, pelvis, extremities, and posterior body. After assessing the neck, apply a cervical collar. After completing the physical assessment, immobilize the patient to a spine board and get a baseline set of vital signs and a SAMPLE history.

After you have performed the appropriate critical interventions and transport has begun, the patient may receive a detailed physical exam en route to the hospital.

The detailed physical exam is very similar to the rapid trauma assessment, but it has several differences. A few more areas are assessed (scalp, cranium, face, ears, eyes, nose, and mouth). There is time to be more thorough in the assessment. And the detailed physical exam does not take place before transport unless transport is delayed.

The detailed physical exam is most appropriate for the trauma patient who is unresponsive or has a significant or unknown mechanism of injury. A responsive trauma patient with no significant mechanism of injury will seldom require a detailed physical exam. A detailed physical exam is not appropriate for most medical patients.

KEY TERMS

colostomy (ko-LOS-to-me) similar to an ileostomy, a surgical opening in the wall of the abdomen with a bag in place to collect excretions from the digestive system.

crepitation (krep-uh-TAY-shun) the grating sound or feeling of broken bones rubbing together.

DCAP-BTLS a memory aid to remember deformities, contusions, abrasions, puncture/penetrations, burns, tenderness, lacerations, and swelling—symptoms of injury found by inspection or palpation during patient assessment.

detailed physical exam an assessment of the head, neck, chest, abdomen, pelvis, extremities, and posterior of the body to detect signs and symptoms of injury. It differs from the rapid trauma assessment only in that it also includes examination of the face, ears, eyes, nose, and mouth during the examination of the head; it may be done less rapidly; and it may be done en route to the hospital after earlier on-scene assessments and interventions are completed.

distention (dis-TEN-shun) a condition of being stretched, inflated, or larger than normal.

focused history and physical exam the step of patient assessment that follows the initial assessment.

ileostomy (il-e-OS-to-me) *See* colostomy.

jugular (JUG-yuh-ler) **vein distention (JVD)** bulging of the neck veins.

paradoxical (pair-uh-DOCK-si-kal) **motion** movement of a part of the chest in the opposite direction to the rest of the chest during respiration.

priapism (PRY-ah-pizm) persistent erection of the penis that may result from spinal injury and some medical problems.

rapid trauma assessment a rapid assessment of the head, neck, chest, abdomen, pelvis, extremities, and posterior of the body to detect signs and symptoms of injury.

stoma (STO-ma) a permanent surgical opening in the neck through which the patient breathes.

tracheostomy (tray-ke-OS-to-me) a surgical incision held open by a metal or plastic tube.

trauma patient a patient suffering from one or more physical injuries.

REVIEW QUESTIONS

1. Explain why it is important to reconsider the mechanism of injury at the beginning of the focused history and physical exam of a trauma patient. (pp. 251, 255, 263–264)
2. Explain how the focused history and physical exam of a trauma patient with a significant mechanism of injury differs from that of a trauma patient with no significant mechanism of injury. (pp. 249–251)
3. Name the signs and symptoms for which the letters DCAP-BTLS stand. (p. 251)
4. List the steps of the rapid trauma assessment and describe the kind of patient for whom the rapid trauma assessment is appropriate. (pp. 265–272)
5. What are the additional areas that you assess in the detailed physical exam that you did not evaluate in the rapid trauma assessment? (p. 274)
6. List the areas covered in the detailed physical exam. What do you look and feel for as you assess each of these areas? (pp. 273–281)

CRITICAL THINKING

As an EMT, how would you balance the need for appropriate on-scene assessment and treatment with the need for speed in getting the patient to the hospital in each of the following situations?

- You arrive at the residence to find a patient who explains that he has accidentally cut his finger with a kitchen knife. The cut is bleeding profusely.
- You arrive at a schoolyard to find a girl who bystanders say was shot by a rival gang member. She is lying in a pool of blood but is able to speak to you.
- You are called to respond to a man who has been found unconscious on a sidewalk next to an apartment building in the middle of the night. There were no witnesses to explain what may have happened to him.

Thinking and Linking

Think back to Chapter 7, "Scene Size-Up," and link information from that chapter with information from this chapter, "Assessment of the Trauma Patient," as you consider the following situation:

- You have been dispatched to the scene of a car that struck a light pole. You have gained access to the front seat and are beginning your assessment of an adolescent female who appears to be seriously injured. From the corner of your eye, you suddenly notice that the transformer is starting to spark. What should you do?

MEDIA RESOURCES

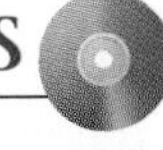

See the Student CD at the back of this book for quizzes, a case study activity, and other features related to this chapter. Also, visit the Companion Website for *Emergency Care* at **www.prenhall.com/limmer**, where you will find additional reinforcement and links to other resources.

Street Scenes

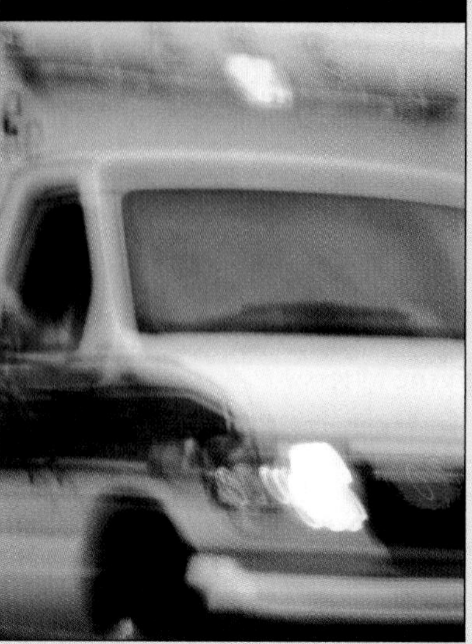

It's Saturday night, and you've been assigned to one of the ambulances that covers downtown, where there is usually some kind of excitement going on. As you sit in quarters, you're listening to the scanner. The police seem to be busy with a variety of calls—disturbances, domestics, and larcenies to name a few. Then you hear on the police frequency: "Dispatch, we need an ambulance ASAP. We have a stabbing here." You don't wait for your pager to activate before you're in the ambulance bay with your partner. The pager follows shortly: "Delta 55, respond to 1512 Broadway, outside, for a stabbing. Police on the scene, and scene is secure."

Your response takes only a few minutes. When you arrive, you see a male in his twenties lying on the sidewalk. "What happened?" you ask him.

"Some punks punched me in the face and threw me into the street when they stole my wallet."

At this point, you tell the patient not to move his head and that you will help by manually stabilizing it. The patient continues: "When I tried to fight them off, they stabbed me in the chest."

The patient's airway is open, but the patient is out of breath and his breathing is rapid and shallow. You check the chest and see the entrance wound. You listen for breath sounds. There is silence on the side of the wound. You put on an occlusive dressing and administer oxygen by nonrebreather mask. You rapidly check for external bleeding.

Street Scene Questions

1. What is the priority of this patient?
2. What should be done next?
3. When should vital signs be taken?

You and your partner agree that this patient needs to be rapidly transported to the trauma center. You are still holding manual stabilization of the patient's head and neck, so your partner gets a backboard and collar. You perform a quick focused physical exam from head to toe. The patient has abrasions on the left cheek, the left wrist is swollen with pain on movement, and there is tenderness in both lower abdominal quadrants. Your partner takes a set of vital signs. You will do the SAMPLE history in the ambulance. You immobilize the patient to the backboard with head immobilizer in place. During this transfer, you check the patient's back for any wound, bleeding, or tenderness.

Once the patient is loaded in the ambulance, your partner starts toward the hospital with red light and siren. The patient is still conscious, but he is having trouble talking in complete sentences. He reports a lot of discomfort. You think there may be pressure building up in his chest because of injury to the lung.

Street Scene Questions

4. What should you do next?
5. What should be done for the detailed physical exam, if there is time before reaching the trauma center?
6. How will DCAP-BTLS help with the assessment?

You are confident that you need to treat the patient's worsening difficulty breathing. You lift the corner of the occlusive dressing and hear some air escape. The patient starts to breathe easier almost immediately. You take another set of vital signs. Then you secure the bandage over the chest wound again, but only on three sides. You turn your attention to the detailed exam, starting at the head, then the chest and abdomen, and finally all four extremities and as much of the back as you can reach. With each location, you use DCAP-BTLS to remind yourself to check for deformities, contusions, abrasions, punctures or penetrations, burns, tenderness, lacerations, and swelling.

The remainder of the transport is uneventful and care is transferred with an updated prehospital care report that includes the latest set of vital signs.

11 CHAPTER

Assessment of the Medical Patient

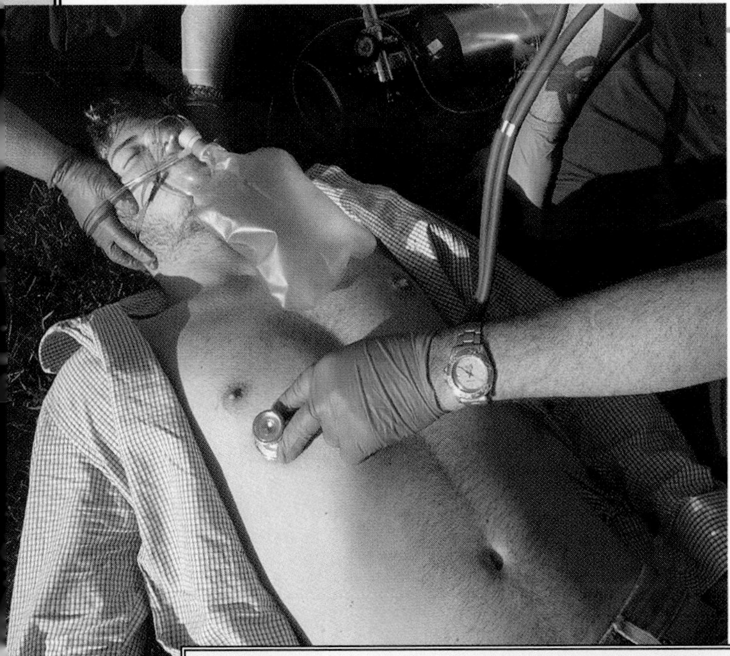

CORE CONCEPTS

The following are core concepts that will be addressed in this chapter:

- How to perform a focused history and physical examination for a medical patient
- The difference between patients who need a rapid physical assessment and patients who need a focused physical exam
- How to obtain a history of the present illness
- How to use the OPQRST mnemonic for history taking

KEY TERMS

medical patient, p. 290 **OPQRST, p. 293**

DOT OBJECTIVES

*KNOWLEDGE AND ATTITUDE

3-4.1 Describe the unique needs for assessing an individual with a specific chief complaint with no known prior history. (p. 294)

3-4.2 Differentiate between the history and physical exam that is performed for responsive patients with no known prior history and responsive patients with a known prior history. (pp. 291, 292–293) (Scan 11-1, pp. 291–292)

3-4.3 Describe the needs for assessing an individual who is unresponsive. (pp. 293, 296, 298–299) (Scan 11-2, p. 297)

3-4.4 Differentiate between the assessment that is performed for a patient who is unresponsive or has an altered mental status and other medical patients requiring assessment. (p. 293)

3-4.5 Attend to the feelings that these patients might be experiencing. (pp. 292, 295)

*SKILLS

3-4.6 Demonstrate the patient assessment skills that should be used to assist a patient who is responsive with no known history.

3-4.7 Demonstrate the patient assessment skills that should be used to assist a patient who is unresponsive or has an altered mental status.

The key to moving from the initial assessment into the focused history and physical exam is reconsideration of the mechanism of injury, as well as of the patient's complaint. If there is a mechanism of injury, you will perform the focused history and physical exam for the trauma patient, which was described in Chapter 10, "Assessment of the Trauma Patient." When the patient has a complaint that is medical in nature, and you have confirmed that there is no significant mechanism of injury, you will perform the focused history and physical exam for the **medical patient**—the subject of this chapter.

medical patient a patient suffering from one or more medical diseases or conditions.

FOCUSED HISTORY AND PHYSICAL EXAM FOR A MEDICAL PATIENT

Responsive Medical Patient

As you learned in Chapter 8, "The Initial Assessment," it makes a great deal of difference in the assessment process whether the patient is responsive or unresponsive. This is especially true of the medical patient. In trauma patients, there are often many external signs of trauma, or injury, but this is not true of a medical condition. The most important source of information about a medical patient's condition is what the patient can tell you. This is why, when the patient is awake and responsive, obtaining the patient's history comes first.

A good example of the kind of patient you will see often is one who is awake and has a medical problem, with no immediately life-threatening problems. After you finish the initial assessment for this patient, perform a focused history and physical exam. This will tell you what you need to know in order to administer the proper treatment.

The focused history and physical exam for a medical patient has four parts: history of the present illness, SAMPLE history, focused physical exam, and baseline vital signs (Scan 11-1 and Table 11-1).

SCAN 11-1 • Focused History and Physical Exam—Responsive Medical Patient

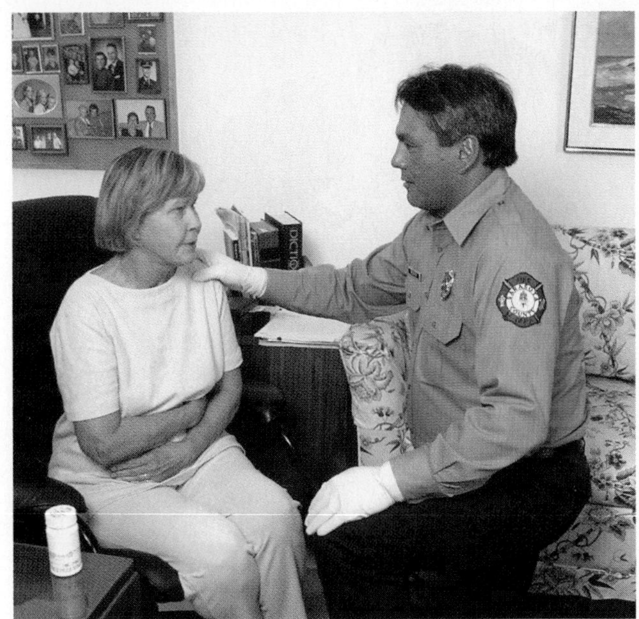

1. **HISTORY OF PRESENT ILLNESS.** Ask the OPQRST questions:
   Onset
   Provokes
   Quality
   Radiation
   Severity
   Time

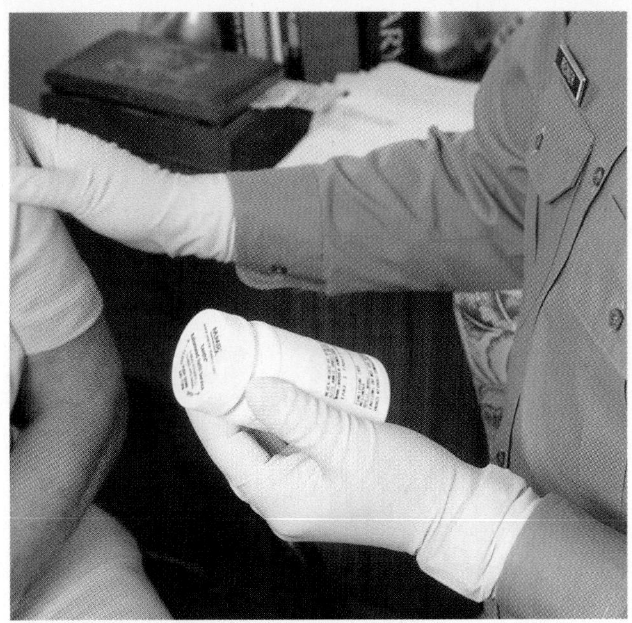

2. **SAMPLE HISTORY.** Ask the SAMPLE questions:
   Signs and symptoms
   Allergies
   Medications
   Pertinent past history
   Last oral intake
   Events leading to the illness

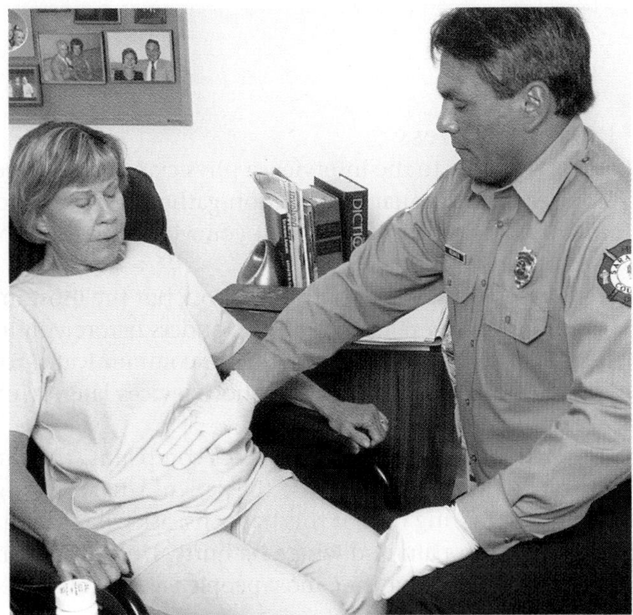

3. **FOCUSED PHYSICAL EXAM.** Perform a quick assessment of the affected body part or system:
   Head
   Neck
   Chest
   Abdomen
   Pelvis
   Extremities
   Posterior

continued

SCAN 11-1 • (Continued)

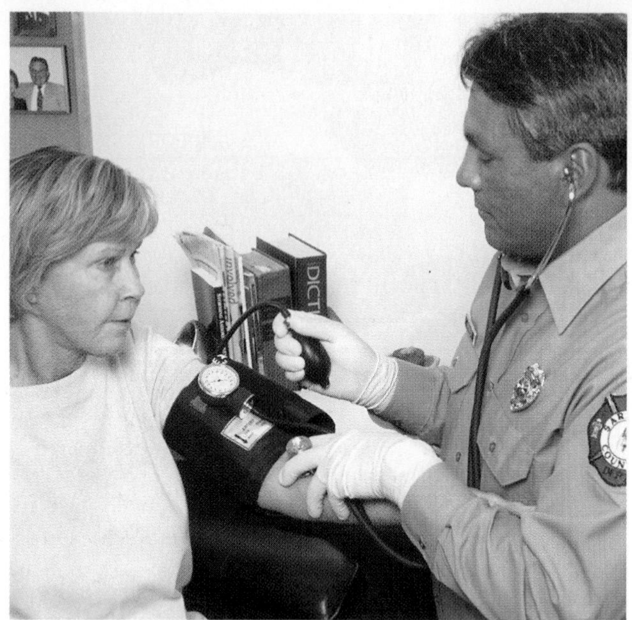

4. **VITAL SIGNS.** Assess the patient's baseline vital signs:
   Respiration
   Pulse
   Skin color, temperature, condition (and capillary refill in infants and children)
   Pupils
   Blood pressure
   Oxygen saturation (if directed by local protocol)

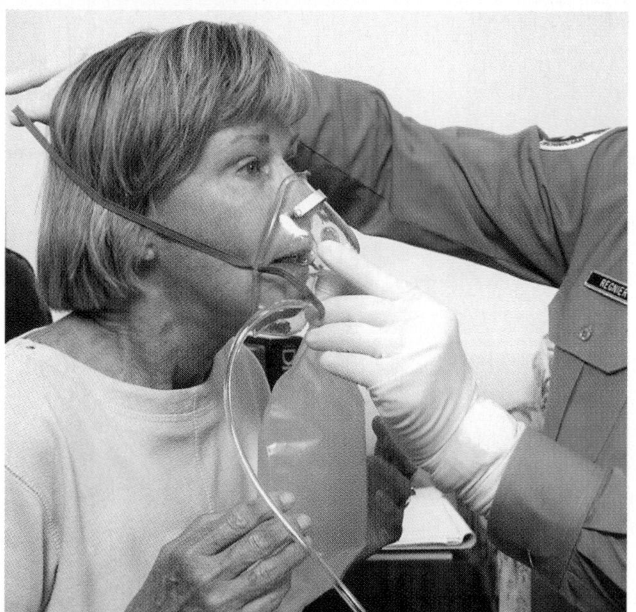

5. **INTERVENTIONS AND TRANSPORT.** Perform interventions as needed and transport the patient. Contact on-line medical direction as needed.

Take a History of the Present Illness

The interview you do with a patient is similar to the interview a physician conducts before a physical examination. It is a conversational information-gathering effort. Not only will you gain needed information from the interview, but you will also reduce the patient's fear and promote cooperation.

Relatives and bystanders may also serve as sources of information, but the most important source is the patient. Do not interview relatives and bystanders before you interview the patient unless the patient is unconscious or unable to communicate. You may gain information from bystanders and medical identification devices later, while you are conducting the physical examination.

One purpose of talking to the patient is to find out his chief complaint, the one thing that seems most seriously wrong to him. When you ask the patient what is wrong, he may tell you that several things are bothering him. If this happens, ask what is bothering him most. Find out if the patient is in pain and where he hurts. Unless the pain of one injury or medical problem masks that of another, most people will be able to tell you of painful areas.

Try to ask open-ended questions, or questions that the patient answers with responses other than "Yes" or "No." For example, do not ask "Is your chest pain dull and crushing?" Ask instead "How would you describe your pain?" In this way, you will avoid

TABLE 11-1 • Focused History and Physical Exam—Medical Patient

RESPONSIVE MEDICAL PATIENT	UNRESPONSIVE MEDICAL PATIENT
1. Gather the history of the present illness (OPQRST) from patient: Onset Provokes Quality Radiation Severity Time	1. Conduct a rapid physical exam: Head Neck Chest Abdomen Pelvis Extremities Posterior
2. Gather a SAMPLE history from the patient: Signs and symptoms Allergies Medications Pertinent past history Last oral intake Events leading to the illness	2. Obtain baseline vital signs: Respirations Pulse Skin Pupils Blood pressure Oxygen saturation*
3. Conduct a focused physical exam (focusing on the area the patient complains about).	3. Gather the history of the present illness (OPQRST) from family or bystanders: Onset Provokes Quality Radiation Severity Time
4. Obtain baseline vital signs: Respirations Pulse Skin Pupils Blood pressure Oxygen saturation*	4. Gather a SAMPLE history from bystanders or family: Signs and symptoms Allergies Medications Pertinent past history Last oral intake Events leading to the illness

*If directed by local protocol
Note: This table shows the general order of steps. You may alter this order in accordance with the situation and the number of EMTs available and when the patient's condition warrants immediate action due to immediate life threats.

giving the patient the impression that you want a particular answer. If the patient says that he cannot describe his pain, you can try giving him several choices: "Is your pain dull, or sharp, or burning?"

An easy way to remember the questions to ask to obtain a history of the present illness is to use the letters **OPQRST:**

OPQRST
a memory device for the questions asked to get a description of the present illness: Onset, Provokes, Quality, Radiation, Severity, Time.

- *Onset.* What were you doing when it started?
- *Provokes.* Can you think of anything that might have triggered this pain?
- *Quality.* Can you describe it for me?
- *Radiation.* Where exactly is the pain? Does it seem to spread anywhere or does it stay right there?
- *Severity.* You look uncomfortable. How bad is the pain? If zero was no pain and 10 was the worst pain you can imagine, what number would you assign to your pain? (Use the system of determining pain severity recommended by local protocols.)
- *Time.* When did the pain start? Has it changed at all since it started?

Take a SAMPLE History

After finding out the patient's age, you should then get the rest of the SAMPLE history (as you learned in Chapter 9, "Vital Signs and SAMPLE History") and the name of his personal physician:

- *Signs/symptoms.* Have you had any other symptoms?
- *Allergies.* Are you allergic to anything?
- *Medications.* What medicines do you take? What do you take those for? Are there any other medicines you are supposed to take, but don't?
- *Pertinent past history.* Do you have any other medical problems? Have you ever had this kind of problem before? Who is your doctor?
- *Last oral intake.* When was the last time you ate or drank anything? What did you eat or drink?
- *Events leading to the illness.* How have you felt today? Anything out of the ordinary?

SPECIFIC CHIEF COMPLAINT/NO KNOWN PRIOR HISTORY Often the patient whose history you are gathering has no known prior history. For example, a patient who complains of breathing difficulty may answer "No" when you ask him if he has ever had this kind of problem before. This and other questions you ask as part of the SAMPLE history may tell you that the patient has not been under treatment for this problem and does not have any medicines on hand for the problem that you might want to assist the patient in taking. You will generally transport this patient to the hospital and provide the information to the emergency department staff.

SPECIFIC CHIEF COMPLAINT/KNOWN PRIOR HISTORY Often, during the SAMPLE history interview, you will learn from your patient that he has a history relating to his chief complaint. Your patient has had this problem or something related to it before and may be under a physician's care for the problem. The patient can tell you what medical condition the current complaint probably relates to. For example, a woman with vaginal bleeding may be pregnant or have just undergone an abortion. A man who suffers a seizure may explain that he has epilepsy. Knowing this history may help you determine what interventions you can take at the scene or en route to the hospital, as well as providing information that you will give to the hospital staff. Chapters that appear

CRITICAL DECISION MAKING:
CHALLENGES IN HISTORY GATHERING

Obtaining a history is a key part of the assessment of the medical patient. Some patients are easier to get a history from than others. Consider what you might say and do to improve your history gathering in the following circumstances:

1. A 79-year-old female keeps talking, saying a lot about things that have nothing to do with the problem you are there for.
2. A 16-year-old female is surrounded by her family. She has abdominal pain that you suspect may be from a pregnancy, but you have not yet asked her if she might be pregnant.
3. A-32-year-old male with diabetes, according to his family, has not eaten lately. He is sometimes combative, sometimes quiet. When you ask him questions, he gives you a vacant stare and says nothing.
4. A 22-year-old male college student, his roommate tells you, has been acting strangely the last few weeks. The patient is now sitting on his bed with his knees drawn up against his chest, rocking back and forth, saying things that don't make sense to you.

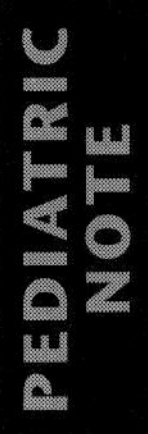
PEDIATRIC NOTE

When gathering a history from a child, be sure to kneel or find another way to get on the same level with the child. Put the OPQRST and SAMPLE questions in simple language the child can understand. Note that much of the history for a child and all of the information for an infant will need to be gathered from the parents, guardian, or other adult caretaker.

later in this book will cover these and other situations and the specific prehospital interventions you can perform.

Three situations involving a known prior history of the medical complaint deserve special mention here. They are different from other medical emergencies because the patient may carry part of the treatment with him, and because the past medical history is essential in determining the prehospital treatment. The three situations are:

- Patient with difficulty breathing who has an inhaler prescribed by his physician
- Patient with chest pain who has nitroglycerin prescribed by his physician
- Patient with an allergic reaction who has an epinephrine auto-injector prescribed by his physician

In each of these cases, the patient has been evaluated by his physician, has been determined to have a condition that can be treated with medication the patient can carry, and has filled a prescription for that medication. You will learn more about these conditions, also, later in this book.

When a medical patient does not have a condition for which you have an intervention, you should generally transport the patient to the hospital. Similarly, when you have a patient with difficulty breathing, chest pain, or an allergic reaction, but the patient does not have his medication or has not received a prescription for a medication, you should generally transport the patient. Note that you will generally transport the patient to the hospital even if he does have medication you can assist him in taking. In fact, you may load the patient into the ambulance and assist him with his medication en route.

Perform a Focused Physical Exam

With responsive medical patients, the EMT's physical exam is usually brief. You will gather most of the important assessment information in this type of patient from the history and vital signs. The physical exam procedure will be the same as you learned for the trauma patient in Chapter 10, "Assessment of the Trauma Patient." For each part of the body you examine, you will inspect and palpate for DCAP-BTLS (deformities, contusions, abrasions, punctures/penetrations, burns, tenderness, lacerations, swelling) plus the information that is specific to each body part. (Review Table 10-3 and Scan 10-1 in Chapter 10.) For the responsive medical patient, focus the exam on the body part that the patient has a complaint about. For example, if the patient complains of abdominal pain, you will inspect and palpate his abdomen.

Obtain Baseline Vital Signs

A complete set of baseline vital signs is essential to the assessment of a medical patient. Later assessments of the vital signs will be compared to the baseline set obtained during the focused history and physical exam to determine trends in the patient's condition. Determine the patient's oxygen saturation if local protocols direct you to do so.

Administer Interventions and Transport the Patient

In later chapters, you will learn when to provide treatment for specific medical conditions. The only treatment you have learned about so far that might be appropriate for a responsive patient is oxygen.

POINT OF VIEW

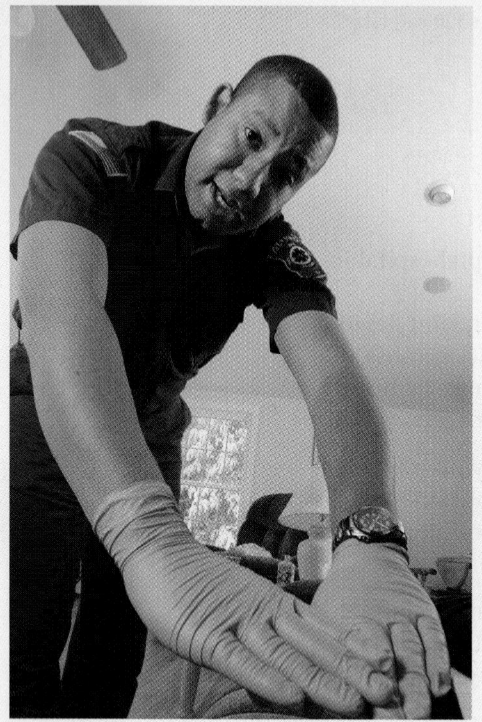

"At first I thought it might be a stomach bug. You know how your belly gets kind of achy? But then it got worse. The pain was strong. And came in waves. I curled up in a ball and asked my husband to call the ambulance. I knew something was really wrong.

"By the time the ambulance got to the house I had vomited. But it still was painful. And it still wasn't the flu. I could tell.

"The EMT was very nice. He asked where it hurt and then pushed on my belly. He was pretty gentle but it hurt anyhow. He also asked me questions. Everything from if I thought I had a fever to if I was pregnant to when I ate last . . . even when I pooped last. He sure was thorough.

"Well, I can look back at it now and laugh . . . now that they took out my appendix and I'm walking around again. But it sure wasn't funny then."

Unresponsive Medical Patient

For an unresponsive medical patient, the sequence of assessment is not the same as for a responsive medical patient. If the patient were responsive, the first step of your focused history and physical exam would be talking with the patient to obtain the history of his present illness and the SAMPLE history, followed by performing the physical exam and gathering the baseline vital signs. For an unresponsive patient, the process is done in reverse (Table 11-1 and Scan 11-2). Since you cannot obtain a history from the patient, you will begin with the physical exam and baseline vital signs. After these procedures, you will gather as much of the patient's history as you can from any bystanders or family members who may be present.

Another difference between the focused history and physical exam for the responsive and the unresponsive patient is the nature of the physical exam. For a responsive patient, you will be able to focus your exam on just the part of the body the patient complains of. Since an unresponsive patient cannot tell you where the problem is, you will need to do a rapid assessment of the entire body.

Perform a Rapid Physical Exam

The physical exam of an unresponsive medical patient will be almost the same as the physical exam for a trauma patient. You will rapidly assess the patient's head, neck, chest, abdomen, pelvis, extremities, and posterior. As you assess each area, you will look for signs of injury such as deformities, contusions, abrasions, penetrations, burns, tenderness, lacerations, and swelling (DCAP-BTLS). Other things to look for in the medical patient include:

- *Neck.* Jugular vein distention, medical identification devices
- *Chest.* Presence and equality of breath sounds
- *Abdomen.* Distention, firmness or rigidity
- *Pelvis.* Incontinence of urine or feces
- *Extremities.* Pulse, motor function, sensation, medical identification devices

SCAN 11-2 • Focused History and Physical Exam—Unresponsive Medical Patient

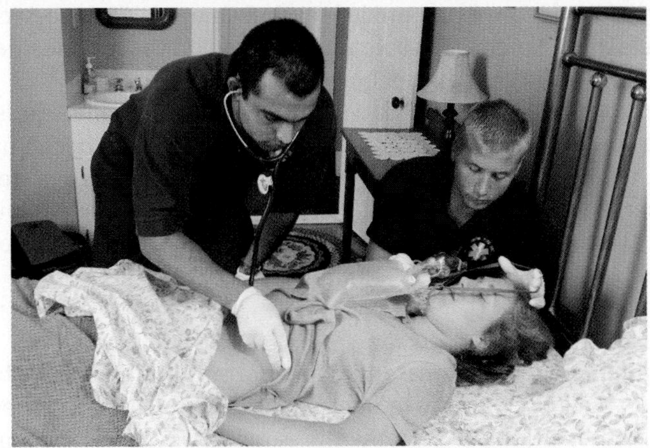

1. **RAPID PHYSICAL EXAM.** Perform a rapid assessment of the entire body:
   Head
   Neck
   Chest
   Abdomen
   Pelvis
   Extremities
   Posterior

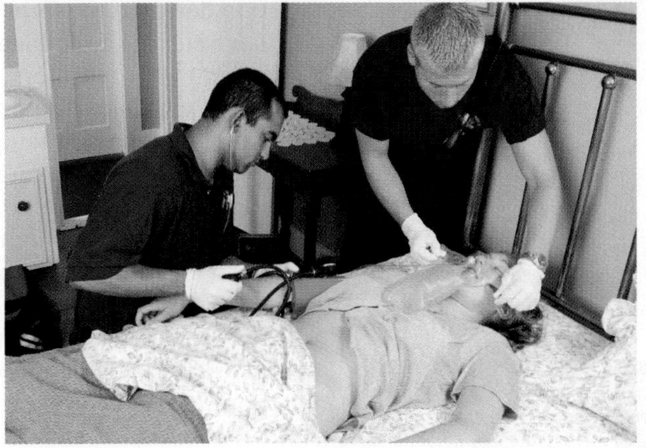

2. **VITAL SIGNS.** Assess the patient's baseline vital signs:
   Respiration
   Pulse
   Skin color, temperature, condition (and capillary refill in infants and children)
   Pupils
   Blood pressure
   Oxygen saturation (if directed by local protocol)

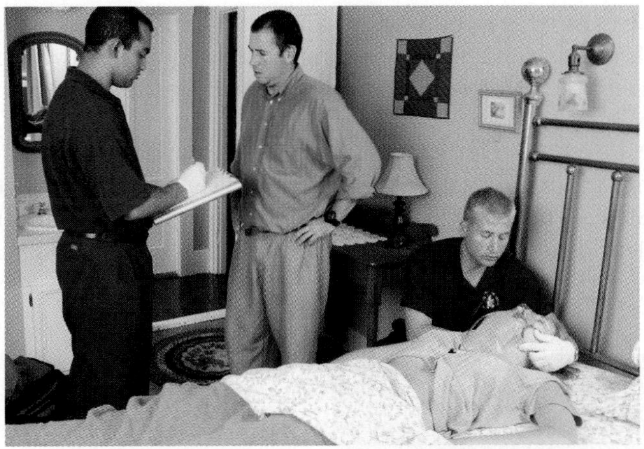

3. **SAMPLE HISTORY.** Interview family and bystanders for information about the present illness (OPQRST) and also the SAMPLE history:
   Signs and symptoms
   Allergies
   Medications
   Pertinent past history
   Last oral intake
   Events leading to the illness

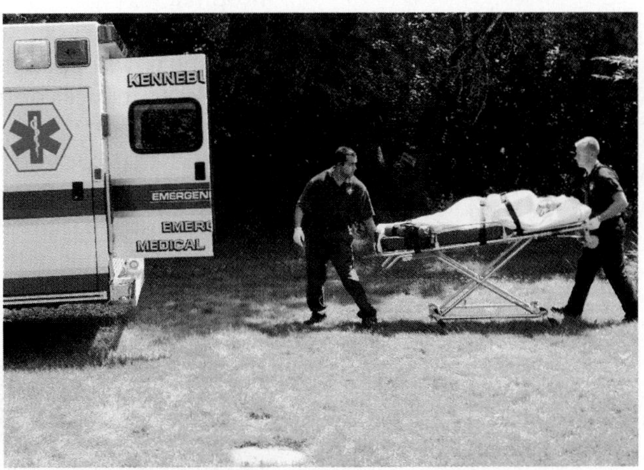

4. **INTERVENTIONS AND TRANSPORT.** Contact on-line medical direction as needed. Perform interventions as needed and transport the patient.

MEDICAL ID DEVICES Medical identification devices can provide important information. One of the most commonly used medical identification devices is the Medic Alert emblem shown in Figure 11-1. Over one million people wear a medical identification device in the form of a necklace or a wrist or ankle bracelet. One side of the device has a Star of Life emblem. The patient's medical problem is engraved on the reverse side, along with a telephone number to call for additional information.

When doing the physical exam, look for necklaces and bracelets or wallet cards. Never assume you know the form of every medical identification device. Check any necklace or bracelet carefully, taking care when moving the patient or any of his extremities. You should alert the emergency department staff when you arrive that the patient is wearing or carrying medical identification and tell them what is on it (diabetes or heart condition, for example).

Obtain Baseline Vital Signs

NOTE

It is easy to forget to check the pupils of a patient who is unresponsive. Try to keep in mind that the most important time to check the pupils is when the patient's eyes are closed!

Assess the patient's pulse, respirations, skin, pupils, and blood pressure and note any abnormalities. Be sure to record your observations so later vital sign assessments can be compared with these baseline observations. Determine the patient's oxygen saturation if you are able to do so (Figure 11-2).

Consider a Request for ALS Personnel

In accordance with local protocols, and if advanced life support personnel are available, consider at this time if the additional services paramedics can provide would benefit your patient.

If you are serving in a rural area or other area where you do not have the option of requesting advanced life support, and if you are very distant from a hospital, there may be a closer local clinic or other health facility that has an arrangement to provide advanced care. Consider if it is worth a delay to stop at such a facility for the special care that may help stabilize your patient before you continue transporting the patient to the hospital.

If arrangements like these exist where you work as an EMT, you must be familiar with the types of patients this facility can help. The arrangements should be in writing in order to reduce confusion and prevent loss of precious time with critical patients.

Take a History of the Present Illness and a SAMPLE History

Since an unresponsive patient cannot talk, you will have to interview bystanders to get as much information as possible. When interviewing bystanders, determine if any are relatives or friends of the patient. They usually have more information to provide about

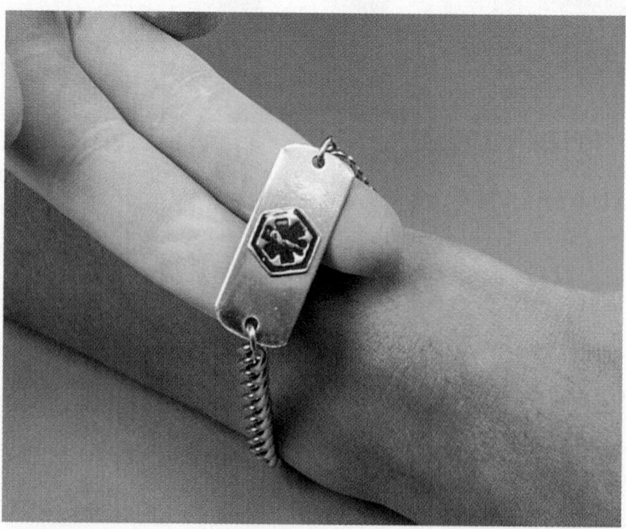

Figure 11-1 • A medical identification device.

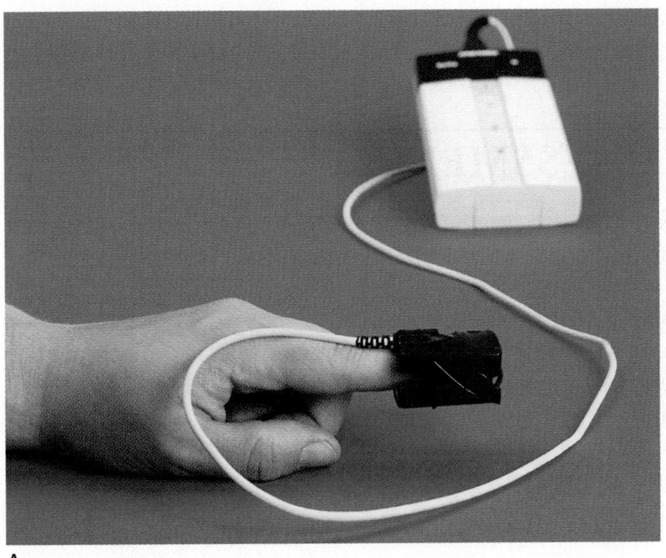

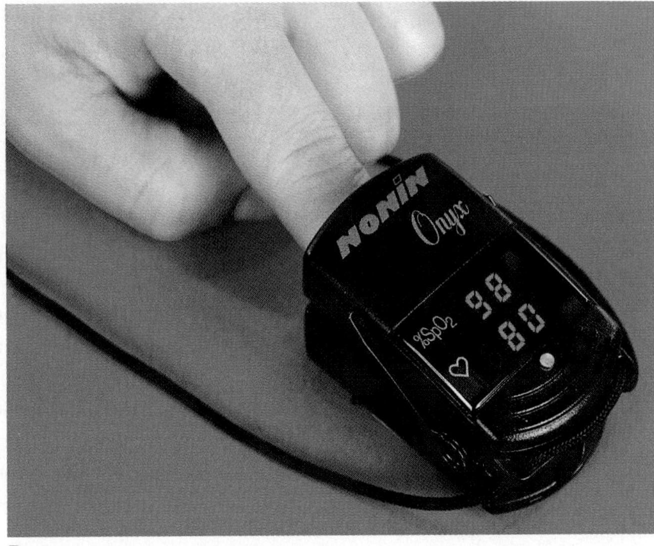

A B

Figure 11-2 • (A) Pulse oximeter applied to the patient's finger. (B) "Mini finger-size" oximeter.

past problems than other bystanders would have. See which of the bystanders saw what happened. When questioning bystanders, you should ask:

- *What is the patient's name?* If the patient is obviously a minor, ask if the parent or guardian is present or if he or she has been contacted.
- *What happened?* You may be told that the patient fell off a ladder, appeared to faint, fell to the ground and began seizing, was hit on the head by a falling object, or other possible clues.
- *Did the bystander see anything else?* For example, was the patient clutching his chest or head before he fell?
- *Did the patient complain of anything before this happened?* You may learn of chest pain, nausea, concern about odors where he was working, or other clues to the problem.
- *Does the patient have any known illnesses or problems?* This may provide you with information about heart problems, alcohol abuse, allergies, or other problems that could cause a change in the patient's condition.
- *Is the patient taking any medications?* Be sure to use the word *medications* or *medicines*. If you say "drugs" or some other term, bystanders may not answer you, thinking that you are asking questions as part of a criminal investigation. In rare cases, you may feel that the bystanders are holding back information because the patient was abusing drugs. Remind them that you are an EMT and you need all the information they can give you so proper care can begin.

While gathering the patient's history, you should also see if there is a "Vial of Life" or similar type of sticker on the main outside door, closest window to the main door, or the refrigerator door. If so, patient information and medications can usually be found in the refrigerator. (The Vial of Life is not used in some regions.)

Administer Interventions and Transport the Patient

There is not usually much information gained from the focused history and physical examination of an unresponsive medical patient that will change treatment in the field. The most important thing to look for is mechanism of injury or signs of injury that would make you suspect a spine injury. Either of these would mean that you need to immobilize the patient's spine. Most of the time, the information you gather in your assessment of unresponsive medical patients will be particularly helpful to the staff in the emergency department. Emergency physicians and nurses depend on EMTs to evaluate the scene carefully and to gather as much useful information as possible that they cannot get in the hospital.

COMPARING ASSESSMENTS

Following are two scenarios that may help you see the difference between assessment of a responsive medical patient and assessment of an unresponsive medical patient.

Mr. Schmidt—Responsive Adult Medical Patient

You have been dispatched to an older man who is complaining of stomach pain. After completing the scene size-up, you conduct the initial assessment. You determine that Mr. Schmidt is alert and that his airway, breathing, and circulation are not compromised. You decide that he is a medical patient with no immediately life-threatening problems and you proceed to the focused history and physical exam for a medical patient.

History

You tell Mr. Schmidt that you need to get some information about his condition. You start by asking him questions that will give you the history of the present illness:

You: When did the pain start, Mr. Schmidt?
Mr. Schmidt: About 2 hours ago.
You: Can you describe it for me?
Mr. Schmidt: It's kind of a burning pain.
You: Has it changed at all since it started?
Mr. Schmidt: It's gotten worse, especially in the last hour.
You: Where exactly is the pain?
Mr. Schmidt: (points to his upper abdomen) Right here.
You: Does it seem to spread anywhere or does it stay right there?
Mr. Schmidt: It just stays right here.
You: What were you doing when it started?
Mr. Schmidt: I was talking with my wife.
You: Can you think of anything that might have triggered this pain?
Mr. Schmidt: No, not really.
You: You look uncomfortable. How bad is the pain?
Mr. Schmidt: Pretty bad. I've never had a pain this bad.
You: If zero was no pain and 10 was the worst pain you can imagine, what number would you assign to your pain?
Mr. Schmidt: Probably a 6.

Now that you have the history of the present illness, you can find out the patient's age and proceed with the rest of the SAMPLE history:

You: How old are you, Mr. Schmidt?
Mr. Schmidt: I'm 68.
You: Have you had any other symptoms?
Mr. Schmidt: Well, I've been sick to my stomach.
You: Do you have any pain in your chest, arms, neck, or shoulders?
Mr. Schmidt: No.
You: Have you vomited?
Mr. Schmidt: No.
You: Have you had any diarrhea?
Mr. Schmidt: No.
You: Are you allergic to anything?
Mr. Schmidt: Just cats.

You: What medicines do you take?
Mr. Schmidt: Ibuprofen and Minipress.
You: What do you take those for?
Mr. Schmidt: I have arthritis and high blood pressure.
You: Do you have any other medical problems?
Mr. Schmidt: No.
You: Have you ever had this kind of problem before?
Mr. Schmidt: No.
You: Who is your doctor?
Mr. Schmidt: Dr. Anderson.
You: When was the last time you ate or drank anything?
Mr. Schmidt: I had dinner about 3 hours ago.
You: How have you felt today? Anything out of the ordinary?
Mr. Schmidt: No, it was a pretty normal day.

Focused Physical Exam

The next step in assessment is a focused physical exam. Since Mr. Schmidt is complaining of abdominal pain, you unbutton his shirt to expose his abdomen so you can inspect and palpate it. His abdomen does not appear distended, but there is some tenderness in both upper quadrants.

Vital Signs

Next, you assess Mr. Schmidt's baseline vital signs. His pulse is 92, regular and full. Respirations are 20 and unlabored. Skin is normal (warm, pink, and dry). Blood pressure is 140/86. Because his complaint is of abdominal pain, which has no direct relationship to the brain, you do not check his pupils.

Together, the initial assessment, history, physical exam, and vital signs did not give you any reason to believe that Mr. Schmidt needed oxygen. (If your protocols had told you to, however, or if you wished, you could have given Mr. Schmidt oxygen. It would not harm him.) Throughout the exam you reassured Mr. Schmidt and tried to calm his fears. Now you move Mr. Schmidt to your stretcher and put him in the position in which he is most comfortable: sitting. You and your partner move him to the ambulance and begin the trip to the hospital.

Mrs. Malone—Unresponsive Adult Medical Patient

You arrive at the home of an older woman whose daughter has reported that she cannot waken her mother. After completing the scene size-up, you conduct the initial assessment. You find that Mrs. Malone only responds to verbal stimulus by moaning. Her airway is endangered because of her depressed level of responsiveness and the fact that she is supine. Your partner performs a head-tilt, chin-lift maneuver to open and protect the airway and you provide high-concentration oxygen by nonrebreather mask. Her circulation is normal. Because of her depressed level of responsiveness and threatened airway, you determine that Mrs. Malone is a high priority for transport to the hospital—but before loading her into the ambulance you will quickly conduct the focused history and physical exam for a medical patient.

Rapid Physical Exam

Because Mrs. Malone is unresponsive, you have no way of knowing what part of her body to focus on. So you do a rapid assessment of her head, neck, chest, abdomen, pelvis, extremities, and posterior in just the same way as you would for an unresponsive trauma patient. As you assess each area of her body, you remove enough clothing to be able to inspect and palpate it, then quickly replace the clothing. You find no abnormalities.

Vital Signs

Your partner finds that Mrs. Malone has a pulse of 92, strong and regular. Her respirations are 20, full and unlabored. Skin is cool and dry. Pupils are equal and reactive. Blood pressure is 160/90. Her oxygen saturation is 98 percent when she is on 15 liters per minute of oxygen by nonrebreather mask. Everything is in the normal range except for her high blood pressure. You note this, but it does not require any action on your part.

You have placed Mrs. Malone in the recovery position, and you now check her airway again. Since you turned her on her side, you have not heard any abnormal sounds from her airway like snoring or gurgling. This, and the fact that she is breathing adequately, means that her airway is open. You check the oxygen and confirm that you are administering oxygen at 15 liters per minute by nonrebreather mask.

History

Because Mrs. Malone has a decreased level of responsiveness and you could not get a history by interviewing her, you need to depend on others to provide as much of this information as possible. The family member who met you at the door is Mrs. Malone's daughter, Florence. You question her to find out what happened and what medical history her mother has.

You: What happened?
Florence: I think she had a convulsion.
You: What happened to make you say that?
Florence: Well, I heard some choking sounds from the room next door, and when I came in her arms and legs were moving around.
You: Was it both arms and both legs?
Florence: Yes, I think so.
You: Was anyone with her when this started?
Florence: No, no one else was home.
You: When did this happen?
Florence: About 10 minutes ago, just before I called 911.
You: How long did you see her arms and legs moving?
Florence: I think it was only about a minute, but it felt like a lot longer when it was happening.
You: Has she ever had anything like this happen before?
Florence: I don't think so, but my mother lives alone, so I'm not sure.
You: How old is your mother?
Florence: She's 60.
You: Is she allergic to anything?
Florence: Not that I know of.
You: Does she take any medicines?
Florence: No, I don't think so.
You: Is she generally healthy?
Florence: Yes, although sometimes she gets migraines.
You: Does she take any medicine for her migraines?
Florence: No, she used to, but she had to stop taking it because it made her feel so tired.
You: When did she stop taking the medicine?
Florence: Oh, that was months ago.
You: Do you know when she last ate?
Florence: We had lunch about four hours ago—just a cheese sandwich and some tomato soup. I was starting to make dinner when this happened.
You: Can you think of anything unusual that happened today that might explain what happened to your mother?
Florence: No, it seemed like a normal day until just a little while ago.

You: I think you were right when you said she had a convulsion, or seizure. What you described sounds a lot like a seizure. We're going to take her to the hospital to be checked by a doctor in the emergency department.
Florence: Thank you. Should I come with you or drive to the hospital myself?
You: You're welcome to come with us, but it might be easier for you to get home if you drive.
Florence: OK. I'll meet you there.
You: Don't follow the ambulance too closely. Take your time and be careful.

Having completed the focused history and physical exam, you move Mrs. Malone to your stretcher and take her to the ambulance for transport to the hospital. You will not do a detailed physical exam en route because there is no reason to suspect injuries of the kind that a detailed physical exam would assess. Since Mrs. Malone is unresponsive, however, you maintain a high index of suspicion and remain ready to do a more detailed exam en route if anything about her condition should change so as to cause you to suspect that she may have been injured.

Mrs. Malone's condition is potentially very serious. At the hospital, she will be scheduled for a series of tests and referred to a specialist.

CHAPTER REVIEW

SUMMARY

The focused history and physical exam of the medical patient takes two forms. You assess the responsive patient by getting a history of the present illness (a fuller description of the chief complaint), and a SAMPLE history, then performing a physical exam of affected parts of the body before getting baseline vital signs. The primary purpose of gathering this information is to determine the proper treatment of the patient.

Since unresponsive medical patients cannot communicate, history gathering will not provide as much useful information. In these patients, it is appropriate to start the assessment with a rapid physical exam. This exam looks almost the same as the trauma patient's rapid assessment. Baseline vital signs come next, and then you interview bystanders, family, and friends to get any history that can be obtained. You may not change any field treatment as a result of the information gathered here, but the results of the assessment may be very important to the emergency department staff.

KEY TERMS

medical patient a patient with one or more medical diseases or conditions.

OPQRST a memory device for the questions asked to get a description of the present illness: Onset, Provokes, Quality, Radiation, Severity, Time.

REVIEW QUESTIONS

1. Explain how and why the focused history and physical exam for a medical patient differs from the focused history and physical exam for a trauma patient. (p. 290)
2. Explain how and why the focused history and physical exam for a responsive medical patient differs from the focused history and physical exam for an unresponsive medical patient. (p. 293)

CRITICAL THINKING

As an EMT, how would you deal with the following situations?

- What questions would you ask to get a history of the present illness from a patient with a chief complaint of chest pain?
- You are trying to get information from the very upset son of an unresponsive man. He is the only available family member. He is so upset that he is having difficulty talking to you. How can you quickly get him to calm down and give you his father's medical history?
- You are interviewing a very pleasant older man. Unfortunately, your assessment is taking a long time because he does not answer your questions and instead starts talking about other things. He lives alone and appears to be lonely. How should you handle this?

Thinking and Linking

Think back to Chapter 7, "Scene Size-Up," and link information from that chapter with information from this chapter, "Assessment of the Medical Patient," as you consider the following situation.

- You are at the home of an elderly man whose wife called 911 because her husband was complaining of chest pain. While assessing your patient, the wife begins to complain of shortness of breath. Now you have two patients. What should you do?

MEDIA RESOURCES

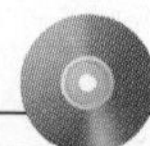

See the Student CD at the back of this book for quizzes, a case study activity, and other features related to this chapter. Also, visit the Companion Website for *Emergency Care* at **www.prenhall.com/limmer**, where you will find additional reinforcement and links to other resources.

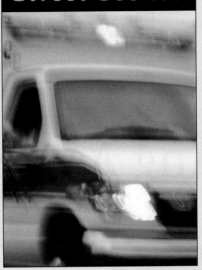

Street Scenes

Just as we sat down to eat lunch, our ambulance was dispatched to a local health club for a 50-year-old female having an asthma attack. Upon arrival, we found the scene to be safe. Taking Standard Precautions, we were directed to the women's locker room where we found our patient sitting on a workout bench.

"Hello. How can we help you today?" I asked. My general impression was of an alert middle-aged woman in moderate respiratory distress.

"Oh, I'm having an asthma attack," she said. I could see her airway was open, but breathing was rapid and moderately labored. I observed no bleeding, found her skin to be normal, and determined her radial pulse to be slightly rapid but strong and regular.

Street Scene Questions

1. What priority is this patient?
2. What are the next steps in the management of this patient?

Satisfied there were no life threats for which I had to provide immediate intervention, I determined this patient's priority to be medium in severity with the potential to get worse.

"What's your name?" I asked. She told me her name was Andrea.

"What were you doing when the difficulty breathing started?" I asked. It turned out she had been exercising on the treadmill. I noted she spoke in complete sentences and did not have to stop every few words to catch her breath. I asked Juan, my partner, to begin administering oxygen by way of a nonrebreather mask. While Juan was doing that, I continued my examination.

Street Scene Questions

3. What part of the focused history and physical exam should follow next?
4. What signs or symptoms would you look for to determine if the patient was getting better or worse?

"What do you think caused your shortness of breath?" I asked. She told me that she's had a mild case of asthma for about 10 years and that it was exercise induced. I asked how long she had been having trouble breathing with this episode. "About 10 minutes," she said.

I knew that many asthmatics carry their own medication for asthma, so I asked what medications she was taking. "I have an inhaler, but I left it at home. I think it's called Al Butterball or something like that." I asked her if it was "albuterol" and she nodded her head.

Meanwhile, Juan had placed the oxygen mask on Andrea's face. I asked if she was allergic to anything and she shook her head no. While I listened to lung sounds, Juan obtained baseline vitals. I noted that the lung sounds were equal but noisy, like a whistling sound. Juan informed me that her pulse was 120 and regular; skin was warm and dry; respirations were 24 and slightly labored; and her blood pressure was 130/70. Her oxygen saturation was 96 percent.

Andrea accepted our offer to transport her to the emergency department, so we put her on the stretcher in her position of comfort, sitting up. During the short trip to the hospital, I used the radio to inform the emergency department of our patient's condition and treatment, took another set of vital signs, and reassessed the patient. She appeared to be a little better, but her breathing was still slightly labored and a little noisy. She did not have any of the signs that would have made me think she was getting worse, things like retractions above the clavicles and between the ribs, the ability to speak only a few words at a time, and cyanosis, particularly of the lips and nailbeds. After we transferred Andrea to the care of the emergency department staff, we returned to service.

CHAPTER 12

Ongoing Assessment

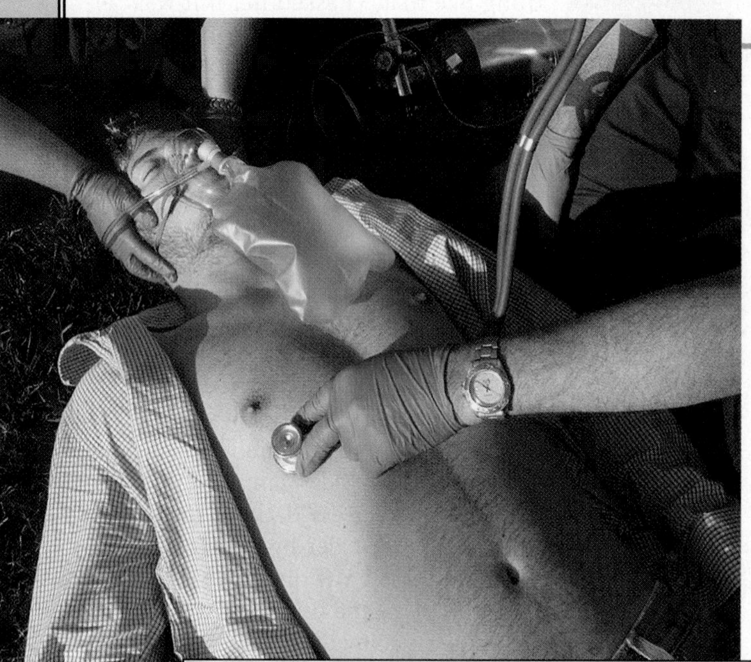

CORE CONCEPTS

The following are core concepts that will be addressed in this chapter:

- How to perform an ongoing assessment
- The significance of changes in vital signs over time
- The difference in ongoing assessments for stable versus unstable patients

KEY TERMS

ongoing assessment, p. 308

trending, p. 310

DOT OBJECTIVES

*KNOWLEDGE AND ATTITUDE

3-6.1 Discuss the reasons for repeating the initial assessment as part of the ongoing assessment. (pp. 308–309)

3-6.2 Describe the components of the ongoing assessment. (pp. 308–310) (Scan 12-1, p. 308)

3-6.3 Describe trending of assessment components. (pp. 310–311)

3-6.4 Explain the value of performing an ongoing assessment. (p. 307)

3-6.5 Recognize and respect the feelings that patients might experience during assessment. (pp. 307, 309)

3-6.6 Explain the value of trending assessment components to other health professionals who assume care of the patient. (p. 311)

*SKILLS

3-6.7 Demonstrate the skills involved in performing the ongoing assessment.

An appropriate assessment at the scene and en route to the hospital allows you to detect and treat injuries and illnesses. Your job does not stop there, though. The patient's condition can change, either gradually or suddenly. You will be able to detect these changes by performing a series of steps called the ongoing assessment.

ONGOING ASSESSMENT

It is important to observe and re-observe your patient, not only to determine his condition when you first see him, but also to detect any changes. The patient may exhibit an obvious change like loss of consciousness or more subtle differences such as restlessness, anxiety, or sweating. These may indicate a change in blood circulation. Some patients may take a turn for the worse before they reach the hospital, although this is uncommon, or you may see patient improvement, possibly in response to interventions you perform.

You will perform the ongoing assessment on every patient after you have finished performing life-saving interventions and, often, after you have done the detailed physical exam. Sometimes you may skip doing a detailed physical exam because you are too busy taking care of life-threatening problems, or for a medical or noncritical trauma patient for whom the detailed physical exam would not yield useful information. *The ongoing assessment, however, must never be skipped except when life-saving interventions prevent doing it.* Even in the latter situation, one partner can often perform the ongoing assessment while the other continues life-saving care.

Throughout the assessment procedures that take place on the way to the hospital, remember to explain to a conscious patient what you are doing, to talk in a reassuring tone, and to consider the patient's feelings, such as anxiety or embarrassment.

PEDIATRIC NOTE

Remember to keep eye contact with a conscious child, staying as much as possible on the child's level, and explaining what you are doing in a quiet and reassuring voice.

SCAN 12-1 • Ongoing Assessment

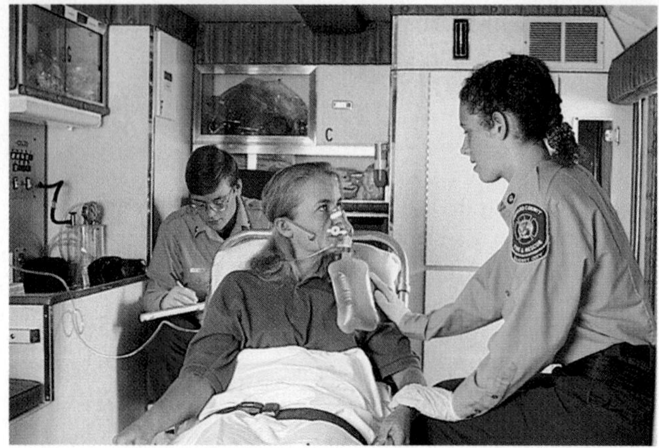
1. Repeat the initial assessment.

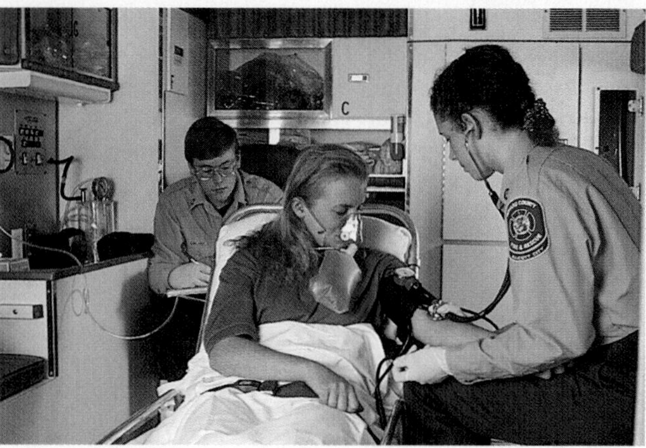
2. Reassess and record vital signs.

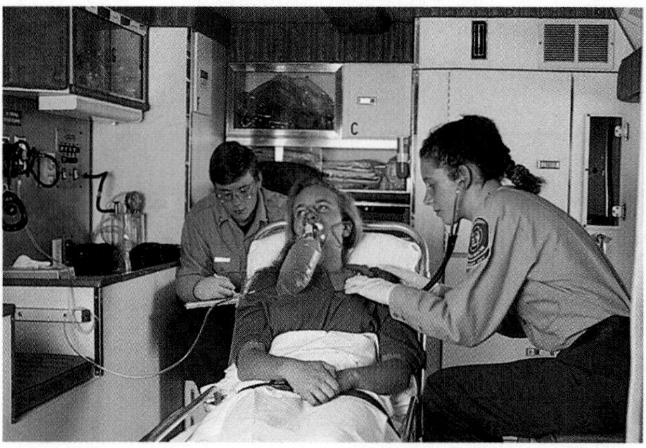
3. Repeat the focused assessment.

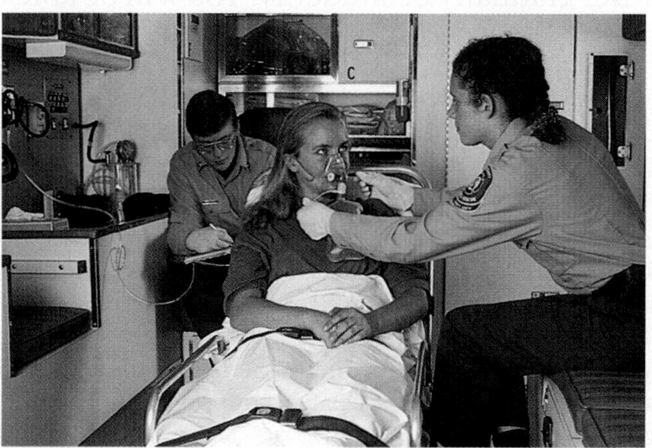
4. Check interventions.

Components of the Ongoing Assessment

ongoing assessment a procedure for detecting changes in a patient's condition. It involves four steps: repeating the initial assessment, repeating and recording vital signs, repeating the focused assessment, and checking interventions.

During the **ongoing assessment,** you will repeat key elements of assessment procedures you have already performed. You will repeat the initial assessment (to check for life-threatening problems), reassess vital signs, repeat the focused assessment related to the patient's specific complaint or injuries, and check any interventions you have performed (see Scan 12-1).

Repeat the Initial Assessment

Begin the ongoing assessment by repeating the initial assessment to recheck for life-threatening problems:

- Reassess mental status.
- Maintain an open airway.
- Monitor breathing for rate and quality.
- Reassess the pulse for rate and quality.
- Monitor skin color and temperature.
- Re-establish patient priorities.

Remember, life-threatening problems that were not present or were brought under control during the initial assessment may develop or redevelop before the patient

PEDIATRIC NOTE

The mental status of an unresponsive child or infant can be checked by shouting (verbal stimulus) or flicking the feet (painful stimulus). Crying would be an expected response from a child with an adequate mental status.

When reassessing the circulation of a young child or infant, do not forget to check capillary refill. Remember that when you press on a nail bed and then release the pressure, the pink color should return in less than 2 seconds. Counting "one-one thousand, two-one thousand" or saying "capillary refill" takes about 2 seconds, so the pink color should return before you finish saying either of these. In small children who have very small nail beds, press on the top of a hand or foot to check capillary refill.

reaches the hospital. For example, the mental status of the patient who was responsive and alert may begin to deteriorate—a significant trend and worrisome sign. The airway that was open may become occluded, the patient who was breathing adequately on his own may now require respiratory support, and other signs—such as a rapid pulse, cool skin, and pallor—may indicate the onset of shock. Life threats must be continually watched and managed immediately when discovered.

Reassess and Record Vital Signs

During the focused history and physical exam, you took and recorded a set of baseline vital signs: pulse, respiration, skin, pupils, and blood pressure. During the ongoing assessment, you will reassess and record the vital signs, comparing the results with the earlier baseline measurements and any other vital sign measurements you may have taken (for example, during the detailed physical exam, if you conducted one). Evaluate oxygen saturation in accordance with local protocol.

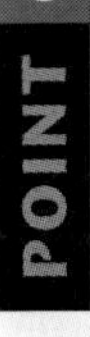

POINT OF VIEW

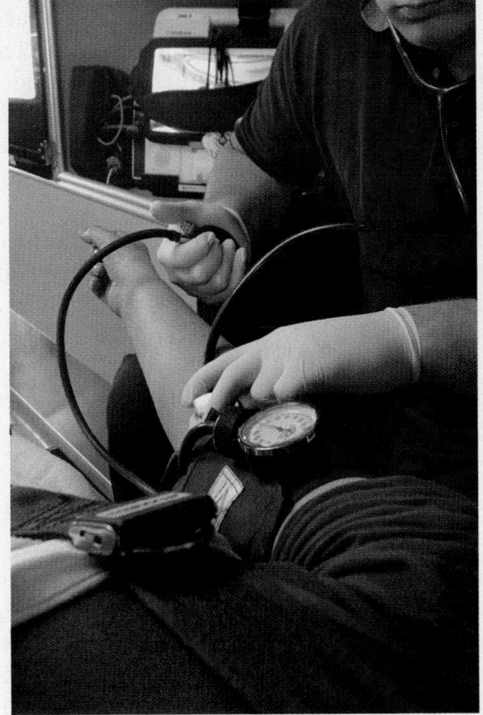

"Do you know what I hate? I hate when a medical person does a test and doesn't tell you what the result is.

"The EMTs were polite and knew what they were doing, but I really wish they would have told me what my blood pressure was. And my pulse. They take it, write it down, talk about it, but they don't tell me what it is.

"I take mine at home and write it down so my doctor can see how I am doing between appointments. I've had high blood pressure for years. I was going to ask but they were so busy. I didn't want to bother them."

It is especially important to record each vital sign measurement as soon as you obtain it. In this way, you will not need to worry about remembering the different numbers you get for pulse rate, blood pressure, and respiratory rate. When you have more than one set of vital signs, it becomes even easier to forget them if you have not written them down. Another reason to document your ongoing assessment is so that you can see trends in the patient's condition, which we will discuss later in this chapter.

Repeat the Focused Assessment

You may find many changes as you repeat the physical exam. For example, a chest injury may become apparent as muscles get tired and you see paradoxical motion that was not present or noticeable when you first assessed the patient (paradoxical motion is present when a part of the chest goes in as the patient inhales and goes out as the patient exhales, opposite to the motion of the rest of the chest). The abdomen may become distended, a sign that you are especially likely to see if you have a long transport. As you learn more about specific injuries and illnesses in later chapters, you will learn more signs to look for in your ongoing assessment.

Check Interventions

Whenever you check the interventions that you have performed for a patient, try to take a fresh look at the patient. Attempt to see the patient as though you had never seen him before. This may help you to evaluate the adequacy of your interventions more objectively and to adjust them as necessary. Always do the following:

- Ensure adequacy of oxygen delivery and artificial ventilation.
- Ensure management of bleeding.
- Ensure adequacy of other interventions.

The fact that you put the patient on oxygen initially does not prevent the tank from running out later, or the tubing from becoming kinked or disconnected. A good habit to develop is to check the entire path of the oxygen from the tank to the patient. This means looking at the regulator on the tank and confirming that it has sufficient oxygen and that the flowmeter is set to the proper flow. Make sure that the tube is firmly connected to the regulator. Follow the tubing and make sure there are no kinks that would prevent the flow of oxygen. Look at the mask. Make sure the tubing is connected to it, and that it is the proper mask, a nonrebreather (sometimes simple or rebreather masks are accidentally stocked in an ambulance). Confirm that the mask is snug on the patient's face and that the nonrebreather bag does not completely deflate when the patient inhales. Increase the flow rate if it does. With practice, this sequence of steps will take just a few seconds.

Wounds that stopped bleeding can start bleeding again, so it is important to check them as part of the ongoing assessment. Check any bandage you have applied and make sure it is dry with no blood seeping through. When an unbandaged wound is in a location where you cannot see it, gently palpate it with gloved hands and check your gloves for blood.

Also be sure to check other interventions, such as cervical collars, backboard straps, and splints. Any of these can slip and need adjustment.

trending
changes in a patient's condition over time, such as slowing respirations or rising pulse rate, that may show improvement or deterioration, and that can be shown by documenting repeated assessments.

Observing Trends

Because ongoing assessment is a means of determining **trending** (changes over time) in the patient's condition, you will need to repeat the ongoing assessment steps frequently. Be sure to record your findings and compare them to earlier findings. It is important to notice and document any changes or trends. In later chapters, you will learn about specific trends to look for in patients' vital signs. For example, when you reach

CRITICAL DECISION MAKING:
Trending Vital Signs

Observing a trend in vital signs is more valuable than getting an individual set of vitals. Observing trends is essential for making accurate decisions such as transport destination and whether ALS may be necessary. Look at the following sets of vital signs for three patients and determine the trend for each patient.

1. A 32-year-old male fell about 15 feet from a roof and has multiple injuries. His vital signs have been:

Time	Pulse	BP	Resp	Skin
2140	88	120/90	20, shallow	Pale but dry
2155	84	100/80	18, shallow	Pale but dry
2200	80	90/60	16, full	Pale but dry

How would you describe the trend of his vital signs: deteriorating, essentially unchanged, returning to normal, or not possible to determine?

2. A 64-year-old female fell to the floor and is complaining of hip pain. Her vital signs have been:

Time	Pulse	BP	Resp	Skin
1330	108	160/90	24, shallow	Pale but dry
1345	112	150/90	20, shallow	Pale but dry
1350	96	140/80	20, full	Pale but dry

How would you describe the trend of her vital signs: deteriorating, essentially unchanged, returning to normal, or not possible to determine?

3. A 19-year-old female injured her left ankle and lower leg in a soccer game. Her vital signs have been:

Time	Pulse	BP	Resp	Skin
1922	108	126/96	20, shallow	Pale and sweaty
1930	116	110/80	22, shallow	Pale and sweaty
1935	124	90/70	22, full	Pale and sweaty

How would you describe the trend of her vital signs: deteriorating, essentially unchanged, returning to normal, or not possible to determine?

Chapter 26, "Bleeding and Shock," you will learn about trends in the pulse rate and blood pressure as signs of shock.

Based on your findings, you may need to institute new treatments or adjust treatments you have already started. Your findings, in particular any trends you have noted, will also be important information for the hospital staff and will let them know if the patient's condition is improving or deteriorating.

Ongoing Assessment for Stable and Unstable Patients

The patient's condition, as well as the length of time you spend with the patient, will determine just how often you will conduct the ongoing assessment. The more serious the patient's condition, the more often you will do it. The recommended intervals are as follows:

- Every 15 minutes for a stable patient, such as a patient who is alert, has vital signs in the normal range, and has no serious injury
- Every 5 minutes for an unstable patient, such as a patient who has an altered mental status; difficulty with airway, breathing, or circulation, including severe blood loss; or a significant mechanism of injury

Whenever you believe there may have been a change in the patient's condition, repeat at least the initial assessment. In this way, you will detect signs of life-threatening conditions as soon as possible. When in doubt, repeat the ongoing assessment every 5 minutes or as frequently as possible (Figure 12-1).

COMPARING ASSESSMENTS

Following are two scenarios that may help you see the difference between an ongoing assessment of a responsive medical patient and assessment of an unresponsive trauma patient.

Mr. Schmidt—Responsive Adult Medical Patient

You have been dispatched to an older man who is complaining of stomach pain. You complete the scene size-up and initial assessment. You determine that there is no mechanism of injury, that Mr. Schmidt is alert, and that his airway, breathing, and circulation are not compromised. Since he is alert and has no immediate life threats, he is not a priority for immediate transport. You conduct the focused history and physical exam, discovering that Mr. Schmidt is suffering a burning pain localized to his upper abdomen that started about 2 hours ago and is getting worse. He reports no history of any similar disorder. The physical exam reveals some tenderness in the upper quadrants but no distention. His vital signs are normal. You load him into the ambulance for transport to the hospital, placing him in a position he finds comfortable, sitting up. Deciding that a detailed physical exam will not be useful, you proceed with ongoing assessment en route.

Ongoing Assessment—Stable Medical Patient

To begin the ongoing assessment, you repeat the initial assessment to check for any immediately life-threatening problems. You get a general impression of an

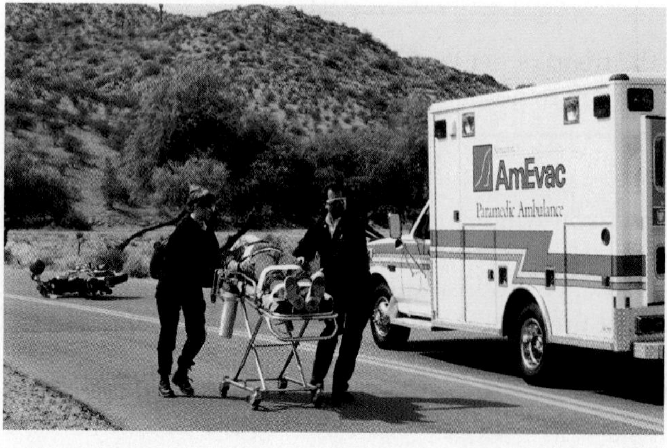

Figure 12-1 • In rural EMS, long transport distances and times may dictate the need for many ongoing assessments—at least every 15 minutes for a stable patient, at least every 5 minutes for an unstable patient. *(© Michal Heron Photography)*

older man who is in discomfort. By talking to him, you confirm that his mental status is alert and his airway and breathing are adequate. You check circulation by feeling his radial pulse and looking for external bleeding. His radial pulse is normal in rate and strength and regular in rhythm. The skin at his wrist is warm, pink, and dry. You do not see any blood around him. You conclude that Mr. Schmidt's condition has not changed and he is still not a high priority patient.

Next, you repeat and record the vital signs. Mr. Schmidt has a pulse of 88, regular and full, respirations 20 and unlabored, skin normal (warm, pink, and dry), and blood pressure 134/88. His pulse and blood pressure are somewhat lower than when you assessed them during the focused history and physical exam, but well within normal ranges, probably indicating that he is somewhat calmer than before. You record your new findings.

Now you repeat the focused history and physical exam. When you ask Mr. Schmidt about his abdominal pain, he tells you there has been no change. He is still a little nauseated, but does not feel as though he will vomit. Nevertheless, you anticipate that he may vomit, so you keep a basin nearby. You very gently palpate his abdomen again. He reports no change in the amount of tenderness present, and you find no firmness or distention.

Next, you check interventions you have performed. In Mr. Schmidt's case, the only intervention that was appropriate was positioning. You ask Mr. Schmidt whether you can make him more comfortable, but he says he is fine sitting up.

The trip to the hospital takes about 20 minutes, so 15 minutes after you leave the scene, you repeat the ongoing assessment and find no changes in Mr. Schmidt's condition.

At the hospital, after you drop off another patient, you see Mr. Schmidt as he is leaving the emergency department. He tells you the doctor diagnosed a probable ulcer, gave him a prescription for medication, and advised him to follow up for further tests with Dr. Anderson, his regular physician.

Brian Sawyer—Unresponsive Adult Trauma Patient

You have responded to a collision in which Brian, the driver, was thrown from his car. You complete the scene size-up and initial assessment, determining that there is a significant mechanism of injury and that Brian is unresponsive with a compromised airway. Your partner stabilizes Brian's spine and performs a jaw-thrust maneuver. You insert an oral airway and administer high-concentration oxygen. You assign Brian a high priority for transport and quickly complete the rapid trauma assessment, finding a head laceration, flat neck veins, and a deformity to his right leg. You apply a cervical collar during the rapid trauma assessment. As soon as the assessment is finished, you immobilize Brian to a backboard, load him into the ambulance, and conduct a detailed physical exam en route, making no further significant findings. You then proceed immediately to the ongoing assessment.

Ongoing Assessment—Unstable Trauma Patient

You and your partner both need to be with this critically injured patient on the way to the hospital. Fortunately during your initial assessment, when you realized how seriously injured Brian might be, you asked dispatch to send another qualified driver so the two of you could continue to work on Brian en route to the hospital. In accordance with your local protocol, you told the driver to drive to the closest hospital able to provide quality trauma care.

You start the ongoing assessment by repeating the initial assessment to check for life-threatening problems. First you reassess Brian's mental status. When he does not respond to your shouting his name, you pinch his shoulder. There is no response. You re-evaluate his airway by putting your ear next to his mouth and listening for abnormal sounds like snoring, gurgling, or stridor. There is a little bit of gurgling, so you suction his mouth. When you listen again, you hear no more abnormal sounds. You also look in Brian's mouth. You see nothing that could cause his airway to become obstructed. Next, you look at Brian's breathing. It is now slow (approximately 8 per minute) and shallow, so you get the flow-restricted, oxygen-powered ventilation device for your partner, who starts to ventilate Brian at a rate of 12 per minute. Brian's pulse is rapid and weak. His skin is still pale, cool, and sweaty. You reconfirm that Brian is a high-priority patient. In fact, his condition is even more serious than before, because you now need to assist his ventilations.

The next step in the ongoing assessment is to repeat and record vital signs. Brian has a pulse of 132, regular and weak, respirations of 8 and shallow, and a blood pressure of 100 by palpation. As you record these findings, you note that his pulse and blood pressure have not changed from your earlier readings, but—as you noted when repeating the initial assessment of respiration—his breathing has now slowed to a dangerous level that requires assisted ventilations.

Next you repeat the rapid trauma assessment. You palpate the laceration on the back of Brian's head and check your gloves but find no fresh blood. The deformity to his right leg is temporarily stabilized by his immobilization on the backboard. You find no additional injuries.

Finally, you check the interventions you performed for Brian. You confirm that oxygen is running into the flow-restricted, oxygen-powered ventilation device and that Brian's chest is rising with each ventilation. There is no bleeding to control. Now you check the other interventions: the cervical collar, straps, and long backboard. The collar is the right size and is in the right place (sometimes cervical collars can slip). The straps are snug, and Brian has not moved on the board. You find time now to splint his injured leg.

During the ride to the hospital, you repeat your ongoing assessment every 5 minutes (performing any needed interventions), recording your findings and noting any trends in his condition.

The importance of the ongoing assessment became clear in Brian's case. Unlike Mr. Schmidt, the medical patient whose condition improved somewhat during the trip to the hospital, Brian took a turn for the worse. Because you closely re-evaluated his airway, you discovered that he had some fluid in his pharynx (which caused the gurgling sound), and so you suctioned him. His respiratory rate had decreased to the point where his breathing was inadequate, and so your partner began to assist his ventilations with a flow-restricted, oxygen-powered ventilation device.

The value of looking at trends also became apparent. If you look at Brian's vital signs (Table 12-1), you can see that his respiratory rate was decreasing, a bad sign in an unresponsive patient. During the course of Brian's recovery, your Quality Improvement officer checks with hospital personnel from time to time to see how he's doing. You are told that the quick work you and your partner did in opening Brian's airway and assisting his ventilations have prevented any brain damage that might have occurred. Brian is transferred to the rehabilitation institute and, after several months, returns to work.

TABLE 12-1 • Vital Sign Trends for Brian Sawyer

ASSESSMENT STEP	PULSE	RESPIRATIONS	BLOOD PRESSURE
Focused history/physical exam	120, regular and weak	20 and normal	130/80
Detailed physical exam	136, regular and weak	14 and normal	100/70
Ongoing assessment	132, regular and weak	8 and shallow	100/P (by palpation)

CHAPTER REVIEW

SUMMARY

The ongoing assessment is the last step in your assessment of a patient. You will repeat it at least every 15 minutes for a stable patient and at least every 5 minutes for an unstable patient. This means repeating the initial assessment, vital signs, focused assessment, and checking the interventions you performed for the patient. Interventions you need to check include oxygen, bleeding, spine immobilization, and splints.

KEY TERMS

ongoing assessment a procedure for detecting changes in a patient's condition. It involves four steps: repeating the initial assessment, repeating and recording vital signs, repeating the focused assessment, and checking interventions.

trending changes in a patient's condition over time, such as slowing respirations or rising pulse rate, that may show improvement or deterioration, and that can be shown by documenting repeated assessments.

REVIEW QUESTIONS

1. Name the four steps of the ongoing assessment and list what assessments you will make during each step. (p. 308)
2. Explain the value of recording, or documenting, your assessment findings, and explain the meaning of the term *trending*. (pp. 310–311)

CRITICAL THINKING

What do you need to do if your ongoing assessment turns up one of these findings?

- Gurgling respirations
- Bag on nonrebreather mask collapses completely when the patient inhales
- Snoring respirations

MEDIA RESOURCES 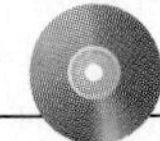

See the Student CD at the back of this book for quizzes, a case study activity and other features related to this chapter. Also, visit the Companion Website for *Emergency Care* at **www.prenhall.com/limmer**, where you will find additional reinforcement and links to other resources.

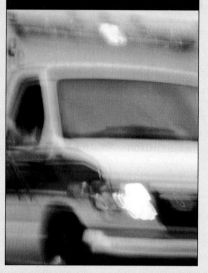

Street Scenes

We received a call for an elderly woman with a possible stroke. After taking the appropriate Standard Precautions, we ensured scene safety and entered the house. An older man, identifying himself as the patient's husband, met us at the door. As he led us to the kitchen, he explained that he had come home after being out for a while and found his wife unable to stand up. When we reached the kitchen, we found Althea Stokes sitting in a chair.

My general impression was of an elderly woman who appeared awake but was slumped onto her left side. As I introduced myself, I noticed the patient's eyes were open and she appeared awake, but her speech was slow and slurred. She did not appear to be in pain. A small amount of saliva was drooling onto her blouse. Her airway was open (at least for the moment); breathing appeared normal and unlabored; there was no sign of bleeding; and her radial pulse was strong, slightly rapid, and very irregular. I assigned Mrs. Stokes a medium priority as a medical patient. In our BLS system, calling for advanced life support is not an option.

Street Scene Questions

1. How does the patient's mental status affect the way you maintain the patient's airway?
2. What questions should you ask the patient and her husband?

We wiped the saliva away from the patient's mouth and considered how to maintain her airway. If she should lose consciousness, we should be prepared to suction. In the meantime, we made a mental note to keep an eye on further potential threats to her airway.

Since the patient was having difficulty speaking, I got most of the focused history from Mr. Stokes. His 82-year-old wife is usually alert and very active, he informed us. She was fine when he left about 4 hours ago, but when he came home, she was slumped over in the chair and couldn't seem to move her left arm and leg. When I asked Mrs. Stokes if she was having any pain or difficulty breathing, she slowly responded with slurred speech, "No, I'm not." As my partner gathered vital signs, I looked at the patient more carefully. The right side of her face seemed to be drooping, especially her cheek and upper eyelid. When I asked her to hold her arms out in front of her, she picked up her right arm, but could barely move her left one. When I asked her to smile, only the left side of her face moved. Her pupils were equal and reactive to light. Her vital signs were pulse 92 and irregular, blood pressure 180/96, respirations 20 and unlabored.

According to Mr. Stokes, the only medical problem his wife had was high blood pressure, for which she takes just one medication, Vasotec. She had no allergies to medications. She was a patient of Dr. Newman and had not been hospitalized recently.

Because her brain might not be getting enough oxygen, we gave her 12 liters per minute by nonrebreather mask even though she had an oxygen saturation of 98 percent. We took special care to put Mrs. Stokes on her left side on the stretcher so she would be able to still move her right arm and saliva would not obstruct her airway.

Street Scene Question

3. How should you perform an ongoing assessment on this patient?

En route, we contacted the receiving hospital and reported on the patient's condition and treatment. I repeated her vital signs and this time got a pulse of 88 and irregular, blood pressure 170 by palpation, and respirations of 22 and unlabored. When I asked the patient how she felt now, she replied in a clear voice, "Why, much better, young man." Surprised at this sudden improvement, I proceeded to assess her again. She could now hold both arms up in front of her with her eyes closed. When she smiled, there was no longer any sign of a deficit. Cheered up by this turn of events, I confirmed that her husband's version of events was accurate. I also learned that Mrs. Stokes had led an interesting life, having been a history teacher for 40 years.

About 5 minutes after this improvement, I noticed that the patient seemed to be having trouble speaking again. When I asked her to hold her arms out in front of her, she was able to pick both of them up, but her left arm drifted off and fell down. Her smile barely showed her teeth. When I asked her to repeat the phrase, "The sky is blue in Cincinnati," she could get only the first few words out and only with great difficulty. Concerned about these changes in the patient's condition, I called the hospital again and advised them of the developments.

When we arrived at the emergency department a few minutes later, Mrs. Stokes' condition had not changed again. The nurse undressed her and the emergency physician assessed her as we prepared the ambulance for the next call and completed our patient care report. Just as I was finishing the report, the doctor came out of the patient's room. "Well, I'm glad you brought this patient here," he said. "She's not a candidate for clot-busting drugs, but since this is a teaching hospital, we can offer Mrs. Stokes the opportunity to participate in a research project evaluating a new experimental treatment for stroke."

"Do you think she's really having a stroke? Her condition kept changing, getting better and then getting worse again," I asked.

Knowing that understanding the manifestations of a disease in a patient is an important part of Quality Improvement, the doctor told us, "We often see changes in the condition of stroke patients in the first few hours of the episode. It can make assessment a real challenge. I'm glad you were able to detect the changes and let us know about them."

With a new appreciation for the value of an ongoing assessment, we returned to our service area, ready for another call.

CHAPTER 13

Communications

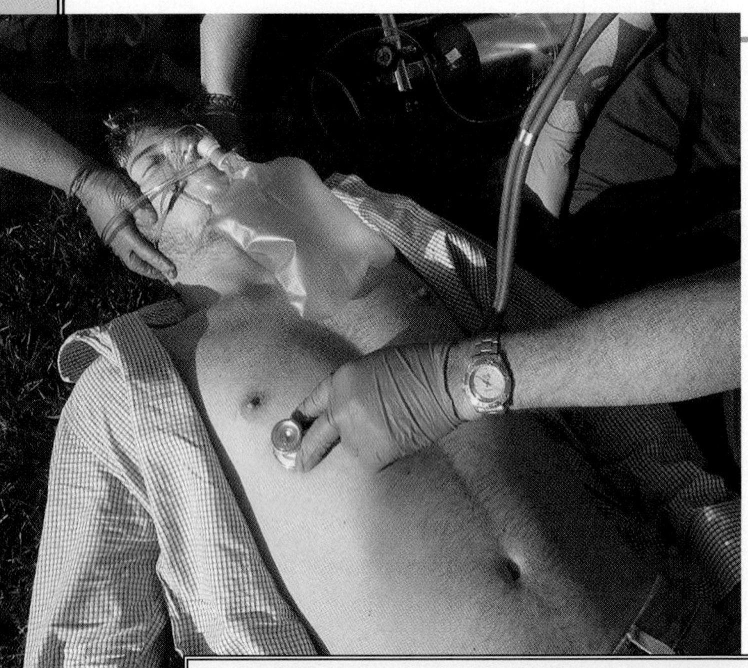

CORE CONCEPTS

The following are core concepts that will be addressed in this chapter:

- Communication skills used when interacting with the patient
- Radio procedures used at various stages of the EMS call
- Delivery and format of a radio report to the hospital
- Delivery and format of a verbal handoff report

KEY TERMS

base station, p. 320
cell phone, p. 320
mobile radio, p. 320
portable radio, p. 320
repeater, p. 320
watt, p. 320

DOT OBJECTIVES

*KNOWLEDGE AND ATTITUDE

3-7.1 List the proper methods of initiating and terminating a radio call. (pp. 321–323)

3-7.2 State the proper sequence for delivery of patient information. (pp. 323–324)

3-7.3 Explain the importance of effective communication of patient information in the verbal report. (p. 326)

3-7.4 Identify the essential components of the verbal report. (p. 326)

3-7.5 Describe the attributes for increasing effectiveness and efficiency of verbal communications. (pp. 326–329)

3-7.6 State legal aspects to consider in verbal communication. (pp. 321, 322)

3-7.7 Discuss the communication skills that should be used to interact with the patient. (pp. 326–329)

3-7.8 Discuss the communication skills that should be used to interact with the family, bystanders, and individuals from other agencies while providing patient care, and the difference between skills used to interact with the patient and those used to interact with others. (pp. 326–329)

3-7.9 List the correct radio procedures in the following phases of a typical call (pp. 321–323):
- To the scene
- At the scene
- To the facility
- At the facility
- To the station
- At the station

3-7.10 Explain the rationale for providing efficient and effective radio communications and patient reports. (pp. 321–323)

*SKILLS

3-7.11 Perform a simulated, organized, concise radio transmission.

3-7.12 Perform an organized, concise patient report that would be given to the staff at a receiving facility.

3-7.13 Perform a brief, organized report that would be given to an ALS provider arriving at an incident scene at which the EMT was already providing care.

You will learn about three types of communication in this chapter: radio communication, the verbal report at the hospital, and interpersonal communication. As the name implies, radio communication is conducted by radio. Technology has allowed the use of cell phones and other equipment to be used where radio transmissions were previously the only choice. The verbal report is your chance to convey information about your patient directly to the hospital personnel who will be taking over his care. Interpersonal communications are important in dealing with other EMTs, the patient, family and bystanders, medical direction, and other members of the EMS system.

COMMUNICATIONS SYSTEMS AND RADIO COMMUNICATION

Radio equipment is often taken for granted since it is now so common (Figure 13-1). However, the development of radio links between dispatchers, mobile units, and hospitals has been one of the key contributors to improvement in EMS over the years. Imagine if you had to call the dispatcher by phone every few minutes to see if there is a call! Without radio transmissions from ambulances, hospitals would be unable to prepare for the arrival of patients, as they do now.

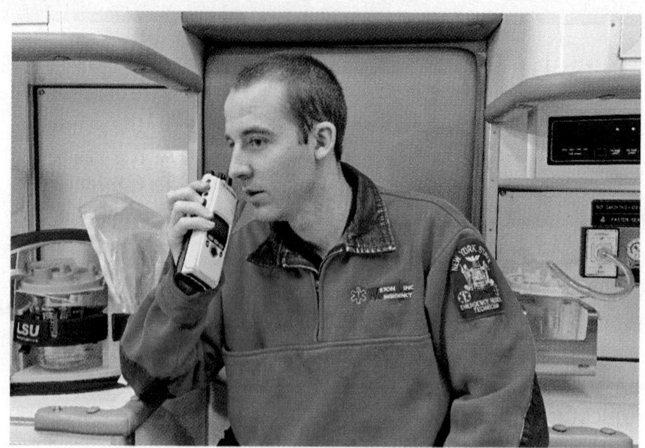

Figure 13-1 • Communication from the ambulance can be by radio or cell phone. *(© Ray Kemp/911 Imaging)*

Communications Systems

There are a number of components to any radio or communications system: base stations, mobile radios, portable radios, repeaters, cell phones, and other devices.

base station
a two-way radio at a fixed site such as a hospital or dispatch center.

mobile radio
a two-way radio that is used or affixed in a vehicle.

watt
the unit of measurement of the output power of a radio.

portable radio
a handheld two-way radio.

repeater
a device that picks up signals from lower-power radio units, such as mobile and portable radios, and retransmits them at a higher power. It allows low-power radio signals to be transmitted over longer distances.

cell phone
a phone that transmits through the air instead of over wires so that the phone can be transported and used over a wide area.

- **Base stations** are two-way radios that are at a fixed site such as a hospital or dispatch center.
- **Mobile radios** are two-way radios that are used or affixed in a vehicle. Most are actually mounted inside the vehicle. These devices have lower transmitting power than base stations. The unit used to measure output power of radios is the **watt.** The output of a mobile radio is generally 20–50 watts with a range of 10–15 miles.
- **Portable radios** are handheld two-way radios with an output of 1–5 watts. This type of radio is important because it will allow you to be in touch with the dispatcher, medical direction, and other members of the EMS system while you are away from the ambulance.
- **Repeaters** are devices that are used when transmissions must be carried over a long distance. Repeaters may be in ambulances or placed in various areas around an EMS system. The repeater picks up signals from lower-power units, such as mobile and portable radios, and re-transmits them at a higher power. The re-transmission is done on another frequency (Figure 13-2).
- **Cell phones** are phones that transmit through the air instead of over wires so that the phones can be transported and used over a wide area. These devices are widely available and extremely popular. In many areas where the distances or expense is too great to set up a conventional EMS radio system, cell phones allow EMS communications through an already established commercial system. Cell phones are not always a solution to the problem of radio communication because a cell phone needs to be able to reach a cell tower or site. As the number of cell towers increases, the ability to use these devices should improve.

New technology is developing almost constantly. Microwave radio transmissions are used in some areas. In others, radio communications are carried via phone lines for part of the signal's journey from one point to another. Digital radio equipment permits transmission of some standard messages, such as ambulance identification or arrival at the scene, by punching a key. The messages are transmitted in a condensed form that helps keep busy frequencies less crowded.

Since radios are so important to EMS today, many systems have back-up radios. This means that in the event of power failure or malfunction, another option is available. If the base station fails, there may be a back-up radio or alternative power supply available. If the mobile radio in your ambulance malfunctions, portable radios or phones may be used in its place.

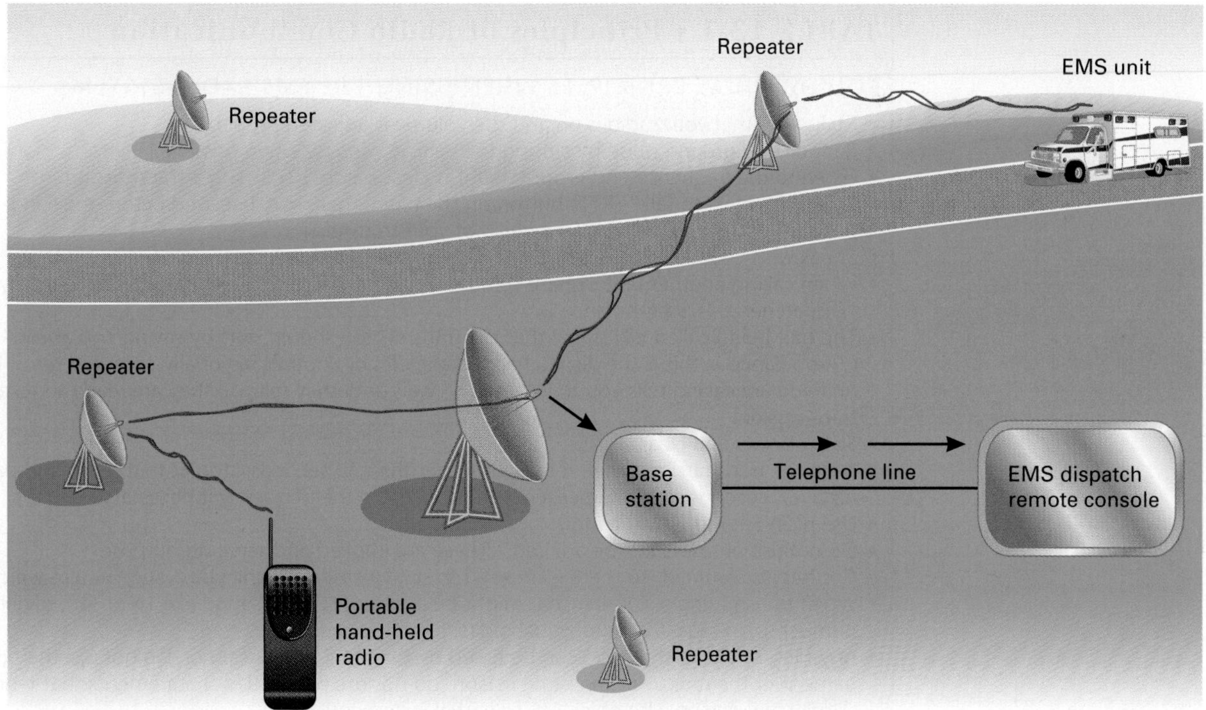

Figure 13-2 • Example of an EMS communication system using repeaters.

Note that radio systems require preventive maintenance and repair, just as the ambulance and your EMS equipment do. Radio equipment must be treated with care on a daily basis and not mishandled.

Radio Communication

EMS is just one of many public services that use radio communication. To maintain order on the airwaves, the Federal Communications Commission (FCC) assigns and licenses radio frequencies. This is to prevent two or more agencies from trying to use the same frequency and interfering with each other's communications. There are also strict rules about interfering with emergency radio traffic and prohibiting profanities or offensive language.

Some general rules for radio transmissions should always be followed. These rules prevent delays and allow all persons to use the frequencies. There may be some minor variations within your EMS system, but always keep in mind the principles shown in Table 13-1.

Radio Transmissions throughout the Call

When the Emergency Medical Dispatcher (EMD) receives the initial call for help, the call most often comes via telephone but may also be radioed from another agency, such as the police. After proper information is obtained, the units are dispatched. The following is a sample flow of information between the dispatcher and units in the field. You are the EMT on ambulance number 6:

Dispatcher: Ambulance 6 . . .
You: Ambulance 6. Go ahead.
Dispatcher: Ambulance 6, respond to 1243 Magnolia Boulevard—that's one-two-four-three Magnolia Boulevard—for an assault. The police are en route. Stand by at the corner of Magnolia and Third until the police report the scene secure.
You: Ambulance 6 received that. Will stand by at Magnolia and Third.

TABLE 13-1 • Principles of Radio Communication

FOLLOW THESE PRINCIPLES WHEN USING THE EMS RADIO SYSTEM:

- Make sure that your radio is on and the volume is adjusted properly.
- Reduce background noise by closing the vehicle window when possible.
- Listen to the frequency and ensure that it is clear before beginning a transmission.
- Press the "press to talk" (PTT) button on the radio, then wait 1 second before speaking. This prevents cutting off the first few words of your transmission.
- Speak with your lips about 2 to 3 inches from the microphone.
- When calling another unit or base station, use their unit number or name, followed by yours. "Dispatcher, this is Ambulance 2."
- The unit being called will signal that the transmission should start by saying "go ahead" ("Ambulance 2, this is the dispatcher. Go ahead") or another regionally accepted term. If the unit you are calling tells you to "stand by," wait until they tell you they are ready to take your transmission.
- Speak slowly and clearly.
- Keep the transmissions brief. If it takes longer than 30 seconds, stop at that point and pause for a few seconds so that emergency traffic can use the frequency if necessary.
- Use plain English. Avoid codes.
- Do not use phrases like "be advised." These are implied and serve no purpose.
- Courtesy is assumed, so there is no need to say "please," "thank you," and "you're welcome."
- When transmitting a number that might be unclear (15 may sound like 16 or 50), give the number, then repeat the individual digits. Say "15, one-five."
- Anything said over the radio can be heard by the public on a scanner. Do not use the patient's name over the radio. For the same reason, do not use profanities or statements that tend to slander any person. Use objective, impartial statements.
- Use "we" instead of "I." As an EMT, you will rarely be acting alone.
- "Affirmative" and "negative" are preferred over "yes" and "no" because the latter are difficult to hear.
- Give assessment information about your patient, but avoid offering a diagnosis of the patient's problem. For example, say "Patient complains of chest pain," but not "Probably having a heart attack."
- After transmitting, say "Over." Wait for acknowledgment that the person to whom you were speaking heard your message.
- Avoid slang or abbreviations that are not authorized.
- Use EMS frequencies only for authorized EMS communication.

Without a prompt and efficient receipt and dispatch of information, the ambulance could easily be sent to the wrong location. In this situation, the dispatcher also relayed important safety information. Since the call was for an assault, the dispatcher "staged" the ambulance, or ordered it to stand by, until the scene is safe.

You respond to the assigned location, reporting your arrival to the dispatcher:

You: Dispatcher, Ambulance 6 is arriving at the staging area.
Dispatcher: Message received, Ambulance 6. I will advise you when the scene is secure.

Most scenes are safe. However, in this case the dispatcher has decided, from the nature of the call and other information he was able to obtain, that it is not. Police arrive at the scene and separate the parties involved in the assault. The police radio the dispatcher and advise that the scene is secure. The next transmission is to your ambulance:

Dispatcher: Ambulance 6, the police report that the scene is secure. Respond in.
You: Message received by Ambulance 6. (You drive two blocks to the scene and report to the dispatcher.) Dispatcher, Ambulance 6 is at the scene.
Dispatcher: Ambulance 6 at the scene (gives the time on the 24-hour clock) at 1310 hours.

The dispatcher records all the times from the time of the original call, the time dispatched, at the staging area, and finally at the scene. Should this case go to court, the records of the dispatch center, your care report, and the dispatch audio tape of the call may be subpoenaed. Unless there is a need for medical direction or assistance from the scene, the next call will be when you are en route to the hospital:

You: Dispatcher, Ambulance 6 is en route to Mercy Hospital with one patient.
Dispatcher: Ambulance 6 en route to Mercy Hospital at 1323 hours.

You will call the hospital via radio or phone to advise them of the status of your patient and the estimated time of arrival (ETA). When arriving at the hospital, you again advise the dispatcher:

You: Ambulance 6 is arriving at Mercy Hospital.
Dispatcher: Ambulance 6 at Mercy at 1334 hours.

You will note that the dispatcher gives the time after most transmissions. This will allow you to record times if they are required on your patient care record. The dispatcher also usually acknowledges by briefly repeating the message to ensure that he has acknowledged the right unit. If two units happened to transmit at exactly the same time and the dispatcher simply acknowledged a transmission, both units would think that the dispatcher heard them when, actually, only one unit was able to get through.

After turning the patient over to the hospital staff and preparing the ambulance for the next run, you will advise the dispatcher that you are leaving the hospital. You may also find it part of your local procedure to advise the dispatcher when you are back in your district or area and when you are back in quarters (the station or ambulance garage).

A majority of these transmissions were made between the mobile radio within the ambulance and the dispatcher at a base station. Remember, when you have one available, bring your portable radio with you whenever you leave the ambulance. You may need to call for assistance during scene size-up if hazards or multiple patients are found, and the portable radio allows you to do that without running back to the ambulance to make the call on the fixed unit.

Medical Radio Reports

Reports must be made to medical personnel as part of almost every call. These reports may be by radio, verbally (in person), or in writing. The radio report is specifically structured to present pertinent facts about the patient without telling more detail than necessary. Too much detail ties up the radio frequency and takes up the time of hospital personnel.

In an effort to protect patient privacy, some hospitals encourage EMTs to use the telephone at the patient's house or a cell phone en route to the emergency department rather than the radio. Follow your local protocols.

Experienced EMTs often try to "paint a picture" of the patient in words. This requires knowledge of radio procedure and practice. If you have a critical patient, your radio report should make that clear. This can be done by describing the chief complaint, injuries, vital signs, treatments, and mechanism of injury. Even with critical patients you must keep a clear, steady tone to your voice. Resist the urge to talk fast or appear excited as it will prevent effective communication.

A medical radio report has 12 parts (Table 13-2). The following example, broken into its individual parts, shows a report you might make to the hospital:

1. **Unit identification and level of provider**
   Memorial Hospital, this is Community BLS Ambulance 6 en route to your location . . .
2. **Estimated time of arrival**
   . . . with a 15-minute ETA.
3. **Patient's age and sex**
   We are transporting a 68-year-old male patient . . .
4. **Chief complaint**
   . . . who complains of pain in his abdomen.
5. **Brief, pertinent history of the present illness**
   Onset of pain was 2 hours ago and is accompanied by slight nausea.

TABLE 13-2 • Radio Medical Report

TWELVE PARTS OF A RADIO MEDICAL REPORT
1. Unit identification and level of provider
2. Estimated time of arrival
3. Patient's age and sex
4. Chief complaint
5. Brief, pertinent history of the present illness
6. Major past illnesses
7. Mental status
8. Baseline vital signs
9. Pertinent findings of the physical exam
10. Emergency medical care given
11. Response to emergency medical care
12. Contact medical direction if required or if you have questions

6. **Major past illnesses**
   The patient has a history of high blood pressure and arthritis.
7. **Mental status**
   He is alert and oriented, never lost consciousness.
8. **Baseline vital signs**
   His vital signs are pulse 88 regular and full, respirations 20 and unlabored, skin normal, and blood pressure 134 over 88; SpO_2 is 98 percent.
9. **Pertinent findings of the physical exam**
   Our exam revealed tenderness in both upper abdominal quadrants. They did not appear rigid.
10. **Emergency medical care given**
    For care, we have placed him in a position of comfort.
11. **Response to emergency medical care**
    The level of pain has not changed during our care. Mental status has remained unchanged. Vital signs are basically unchanged.
12. **Contact medical direction if required or if you have questions**
    Does medical direction have any orders?

After giving this information, you will continue with ongoing assessment of the patient en route to the hospital. Additional vital signs will be taken, there may be changes in the patient's condition, or you may discover new information about the patient, particularly on long transports. In some systems, you should radio this additional information to the hospital in a follow-up radio call while en route (follow local protocols).

When medical direction is contacted, orders may be given to the EMT. The on-line physician may order you to assist in administering the patient's own medication, or order the administration of a medication you carry on the ambulance, or give other orders. In any case, the communication between you and medical direction must be clear and concise to avoid misinterpretations that can inadvertently harm the patient. For example, a patient may have a medication for chest pain called nitroglycerin. This medication, as you will learn in Chapter 15, "General Pharmacology," is one that you may assist the patient in taking (according to local protocols). The medication should be given only if the patient's blood pressure is above a certain level. If there is a misunderstanding between you and the physician and this medication is ordered improperly, harm may come to the patient.

To avoid misunderstanding and miscommunication, use the following guidelines when communicating with medical direction:

- Give the information to medical direction clearly and accurately. Speak slowly and clearly. The orders of the physician will be based on what you report.
- After receiving an order for a medication or procedure, repeat the order word for word. You may also ask to do a procedure or give a medication and be denied by medical direction. Repeat this also.
- If an order is unclear, ask the physician to repeat it. After you have a clear understanding of the order, repeat it back to the physician.
- If an order appears to be inappropriate, question the physician. There may have been a misunderstanding. Your questioning may prevent the inappropriate administration of a medication. If the physician verifies the order, he may explain to you why he has given you that particular order.

CRITICAL DECISION MAKING: COMMUNICATIONS CHALLENGES

Communication may take various forms in EMS: for example, written, face-to-face verbal, or by radio. Make your decisions based on the scenarios below.

1. You are en route to a call of unknown nature for an elderly patient. First responders arrived at the scene about 5 minutes ago and you are still 10 minutes from the scene. Dispatch has not called you on the radio with an update on the patient's condition. What are some of the reasons why this might be the case? How should you proceed?
2. A 17-year-old male drank a large amount of alcohol and then "passed out," according to his friends, who called 911. When you arrive, you find the patient initially unresponsive to painful stimuli, then a few minutes later able to slur some words when you ask him questions. A few minutes after that, he withdraws when you apply a painful stimulus. How should you describe his mental status to the hospital while you are en route?
3. You are at the scene of a two-car motor vehicle collision and would like to give the local hospital some warning that you will be transporting a severely injured patient in a few minutes. Unfortunately, when you try to call the hospital on the radio, they are unable to understand what you are saying. How should you proceed?
4. You have just arrived at the scene of a 34-year-old diabetic male who is "out of it," according to what the caller told dispatch. One of his friends, trying to be helpful, tells you that he thinks the patient is "conscious but unresponsive." Confused as to what this might mean, you proceed to the patient and find him sitting in a chair, staring straight ahead, not saying anything. When you ask him a question, he doesn't answer and doesn't even look at you. When you pinch his arm, he looks down at his arm but doesn't respond in any other way. How can you describe this patient's mental status in a way that will give the hospital an accurate impression of what is going on? Hint: Describe what you observe instead of trying to attach labels to this patient.

THE VERBAL REPORT

At the hospital, you will give a written report on your patient to hospital personnel. (See Chapter 14, "Documentation.") However, it will take some time to complete your written report, so the first information you give to hospital personnel will be your verbal report.

As you transfer your patient to the care of the hospital staff, introduce the patient by name. Then summarize the same kind of information you gave over the radio, pointing out any information that is updated or different from your last radio report. Include the following in your verbal report:

- Chief complaint
- History that was not given previously
- Additional treatment given en route
- Additional vital signs taken en route

INTERPERSONAL COMMUNICATION

While communication between two or more human beings is a skill that you have learned over the years, many people still do not communicate as well as they could. Communicating with patients and others who are in crisis is even more difficult. While interpersonal communication could be presented as a course in itself, the following guidelines will help when dealing with patients, families, friends, and bystanders:

- *Use eye contact.* Make frequent eye contact with your patient. It shows that you are interested in your patient and that you are attentive. Failure to make eye contact signals that you feel uneasy around the patient. (If your patient is avoiding eye contact, consider that in some cultures eye contact is considered rude. You may want to match your behavior to the patient's in this situation.)
- *Be aware of your position and body language.* Your positioning in respect to the patient is important. If you are higher than the patient, you may appear intimidating. If possible, position yourself at or below the patient's eye level (Figure 13-3). This will be less threatening to the patient. Body language is also important.

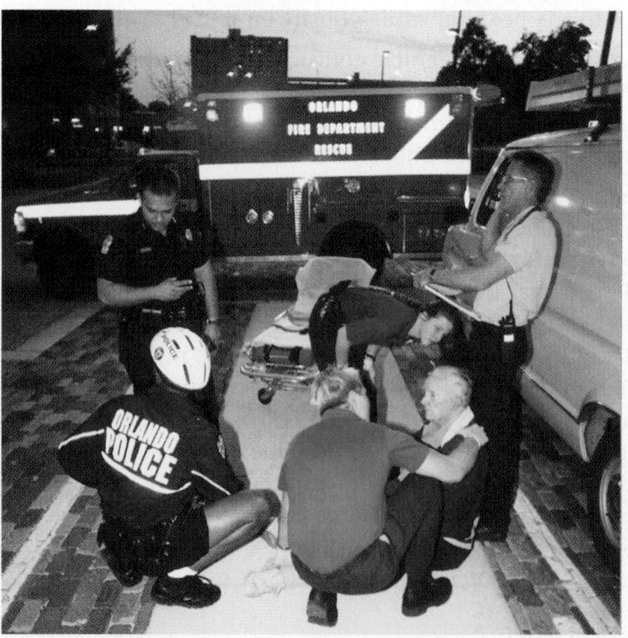

Figure 13-3 • Position yourself at or below the patient's eye level to be less intimidating and to aid communication. *(© Craig Jackson/In the Dark Photography)*

Standing with your arms crossed or not directly facing the patient (a closed stance) sends a signal to the patient that you are not interested. Use a more open stance (arms down, facing the patient), when it can be done safely, to communicate a warmer attitude.

A closed or more serious stance may sometimes be beneficial, however, when you need to calm or direct bystanders at the scene. Standing above a patient may convey authority and can be done to gain control when necessary.

Watch the patient's body language to see how your communication with him is going. If the patient uses a closed stance, your communication efforts may not be working.

- *Use language the patient can understand.* Speak slowly and clearly. Do not use medical or other terms that the patient will not understand. Explain procedures before they are performed, to prevent anxiety.
- *Be honest.* Honesty is important. You will frequently be asked questions that you will not have the answer to: "Is my leg broken?" "Am I having a heart attack?" At other times you will know the answer to the question, but it is not pleasant: "Will it hurt when you put that splint on?" If the answer is yes, tell the truth. Explain that you will do it as gently as possible to reduce pain, but some pain may be experienced. It is much worse to lie to the patient and have him find out that you were not being truthful. This will erode the patient's confidence in you as well as in other EMTs and medical personnel the patient may meet later on.
- *Use the patient's proper name.* Especially with senior citizens and other adults, do not assume familiarity. As a general rule, call patients as they introduce themselves to you. If a person many years older than you introduces himself as William Harris, it might be best to call him Mr. Harris as a sign of respect. Immediately calling him "Bill" when he clearly stated his name was "William" would be disrespectful. If, after you call him "Mr. Harris," he says "Please call me Bill," you have shown respect and can then use the less formal name. If in doubt, ask what the patient would like to be called.
- *Listen.* If you ask the patient a question, get an answer, then have to ask again, it will show the patient that you were not listening. If you are not listening, the patient will feel that you are not interested in what he has to say, or that you just don't care. If you ask a question, wait for the answer. Then write it down so you will not forget.

If a person has a mental disability or is hard of hearing, speak slowly and clearly. Do not talk down to the patient. If the patient has a hearing disability, he may read lips. In any case, seeing your lips may help him understand what you are saying. Therefore, be sure that a deaf or hearing-impaired person can see your mouth when you talk.

Remember that a person who is blind or has a visual deficit can usually hear, so do not give in to the temptation to speak to him loudly or unnaturally. For the visually impaired person, you will want to take extra effort to explain anything that is happening that he cannot see.

You may also find people who do not speak the same language as you. In this case, use an interpreter (for example, a family member or friend who speaks both languages) or a manual that provides translations. You may also find that your communications center or medical direction has someone available who speaks the patient's language.

The elderly are a rapidly growing segment of the population who often need EMS care. These older patients may have medical problems simply because of their age. They may also be more prone to falls and serious injury from trauma due to the condition of their bones and body systems.

Many elderly patients are well oriented and physically able. Others, however, may have problems with hearing, sight, or orientation that have come on with age. These patients may seem confused or simply find it difficult to communicate. In spite of their sensory limitations, of course, these patients still have needs and feelings. They deserve patience, kindness, and understanding—along with proper emergency care (Figure 13-4).

POINT OF VIEW

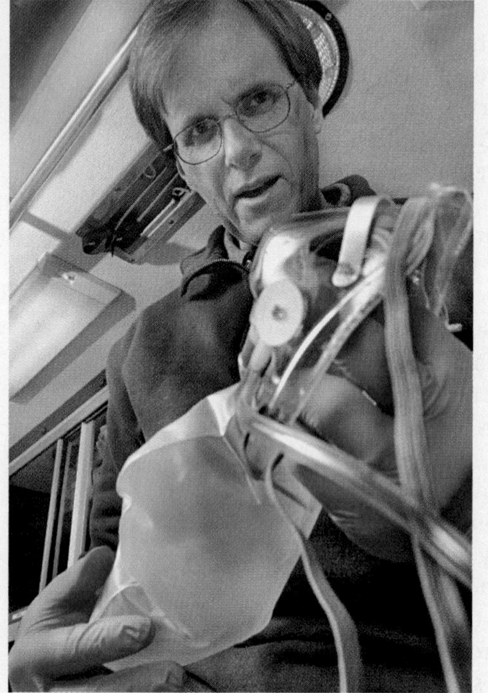

"Unless you have been in an ambulance, I'm not sure you'd know how scary it is. I remember the only time I was in an ambulance. I had passed out waiting for a ride home from work. I came to just as the ambulance got there.

"First they are standing over you. Then they are doing tests. Then they want to put this mask on your face. It smells like plastic, and quite frankly I thought it would smother me. If it wasn't for the EMT with the calmest voice I ever heard I think I would've totally freaked out. I mean totally. Looking back I don't even remember what he said but I just remember feeling I would be all right. He was so reassuring. He had a way of talking that was better than Valium.

"If he was selling something I would've bought one. He was good."

PEDIATRIC NOTE

Since children sometimes can be difficult to assess and communicate with, it is often best to involve the parents of the child when communicating. Two rules of communication are critically important to children:

- Always come down to the child's level (Figure 13-5). Never stand above a child, as you will literally tower over the child and appear very intimidating. Crouching down reduces the size difference and greatly improves communication. If the child is not critically ill, you might even take the time to sit on the floor and get slightly below the child in the beginning.
- Children often sense lies even faster than adults. It is important to tell the truth to children. Remember, you may be the first contact from the EMS system that the child has ever had. Work to make it positive.

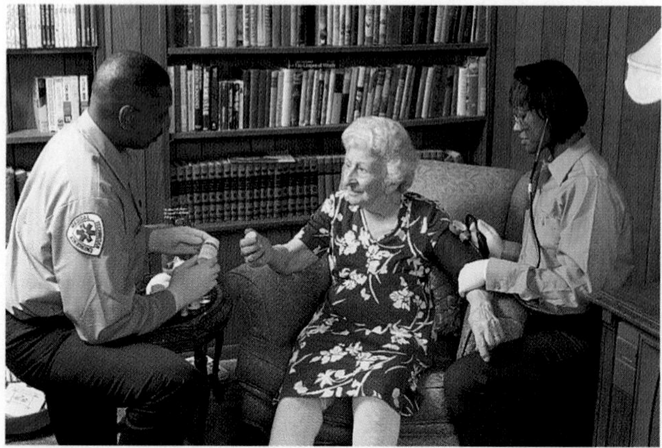

Figure 13-4 • Be considerate of the elderly patient.

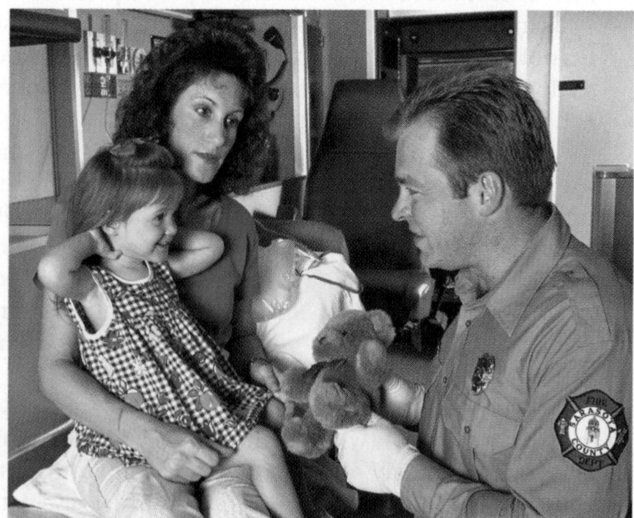

Figure 13-5 • Stay at a child's eye level or lower.

CHAPTER REVIEW

SUMMARY

Communication is not as tangible a skill as putting on a splint or taking a pulse, but it is a very important part of every call. Communication may be face to face with people—hospital personnel, other EMTs, patients, family, bystanders, and others. Radio communication is important as your link to the dispatcher and medical direction. Use communication by any means or method carefully and accurately.

KEY TERMS

base station a two-way radio at a fixed site such as a hospital or dispatch center.

cell phone a phone that transmits through the air instead of over wires so that the phone can be transported and used over a wide area.

mobile radio a two-way radio that is used or affixed in a vehicle.

portable radio a handheld two-way radio.

repeater a device that picks up signals from lower-power radio units, such as mobile and portable radios, and retransmits them at a higher power. It allows low-power radio signals to be transmitted over longer distances.

watt the unit of measurement of the output power of a radio.

REVIEW QUESTIONS

1. List several guidelines for proper use of the EMS radio system. (p. 322)
2. List the steps of a medical radio report and describe the communication that may be necessary during each part. (pp. 323–324)
3. List several guidelines for effective interpersonal communication with patients. (pp. 326–328)

CRITICAL THINKING

The following information, describing a patient, is in random order. Organize the information and present a medical radio report as if you were radioing the hospital.

Chest pain radiating to the shoulder
56 years old
Oxygen applied at 15 liters per minute via nonrebreather
Alert and oriented
Female
Came on 20 minutes ago while mowing the lawn
History of high blood pressure and diabetes
ETA 20 minutes
Pulse 86, respirations 22, skin cool and moist, blood pressure 110/66, SpO_2 96 percent
Oxygen relieved the pain slightly
Denies difficulty breathing
You are requesting orders from medical direction
You are on Community BLS Ambulance 4
Lung sounds equal on both sides
Placed in a position of comfort

MEDIA RESOURCES

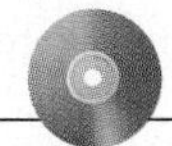

See the Student CD at the back of this book for quizzes, a case study, and other features related to this chapter. Also, visit the Companion Website for *Emergency Care* at **www.prenhall.com/limmer**, where you will find additional reinforcement and links to other resources.

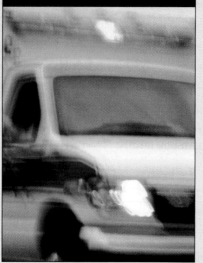

Street Scenes

You are just about to leave the hospital emergency department after your last run, when the dispatcher calls on the portable radio. You answer: "Go ahead, dispatch. This is Ambulance 40." Unfortunately, your radio will not transmit out of the hospital, so you call the communications center by telephone. The dispatcher informs you of a 911 call from a cell phone reporting someone trapped in a vehicle on the side of the road near mile marker 21 on Route 15. The sheriff and a fire department First Response unit with extrication equipment have been dispatched. Your response time is approximately 15 minutes.

While en route, you receive a transmission from the dispatcher that the deputy sheriff reports only one patient who is trapped and unresponsive. You are now 10 minutes from the scene and the next transmission that you hear is the First Response unit arriving on scene.

Street Scene Questions

1. What type of scene safety information do you want to know from the sheriff's deputy?
2. Should you contact the First Responders or wait until they contact you?
3. What patient information would be helpful to know?

You radio the dispatcher and request that he contact the deputy sheriff on the scene to find out what the best access is and where you can stage the ambulance. As you finish this transmission, you hear: "Ambulance 40, this is Fire Rescue 8 at the scene." You acknowledge, and they provide you with the following information: "Patient is unconscious with an open airway, breathing is 24 and labored, pulse is 120, pale and diaphoretic, with possible head and chest trauma. His SpO_2 is 89 percent. He was wearing a seat belt but no air bag deployment. He needs to be extricated which should take about 10 minutes. Consider rapid extrication to a backboard. A cervical collar is already in place."

You are now 4 minutes from the scene and the dispatcher notifies you that you should approach using the northbound lane, which has been blocked off. In addition, Fire Rescue 8 has identified a safe location to stage the ambulance close to the crash site. As you approach the scene, you are advised that a helicopter has been requested for transport to the trauma center.

Street Scene Questions

4. What information should be provided to the incident commander upon arrival?
5. What type of coordinated effort between Ambulance 40 and Fire Rescue 8 should be done to ensure the best care?
6. What information about both the patient's condition and the landing zone need to be relayed to the helicopter?

As you pull up to the scene, you are directed to an area about 30 feet from the crashed vehicle. The extrication is underway. You approach the incident commander who tells you that the helicopter is 15 minutes from the scene and he is having a landing zone prepared. You are advised to work with Fire Rescue 8 to provide patient care and oversee rapid extrication to a backboard when freed.

You identify yourself to the fire captain and ask what equipment is needed. He tells you that access to the patient will be gained in a matter of minutes and he thinks that rapid extrication would be most appropriate. He has two firefighters available to help with boarding the patient. He asks if you think the plan will work and for any suggestions. You tell him the plan sounds good.

While your partner is getting the needed equipment, you get additional patient information and ask what is the best way to access the patient. You reassess the patient and convey the information to the helicopter, which is making its landing approach.

You agree with your partner and the crew from Fire Rescue 8 on who will do what to stabilize the patient's head and neck and to rotate the patient onto the backboard. The procedure goes quickly and smoothly. You reassess the patient and obtain a new set of vital signs. The flight medics are now next to the patient, and you update them on patient status. You assist with care and loading onto the helicopter. As the helicopter lifts off, you think how well this call went and realize that communication among all the emergency providers made a significant difference.

CHAPTER

14

Documentation

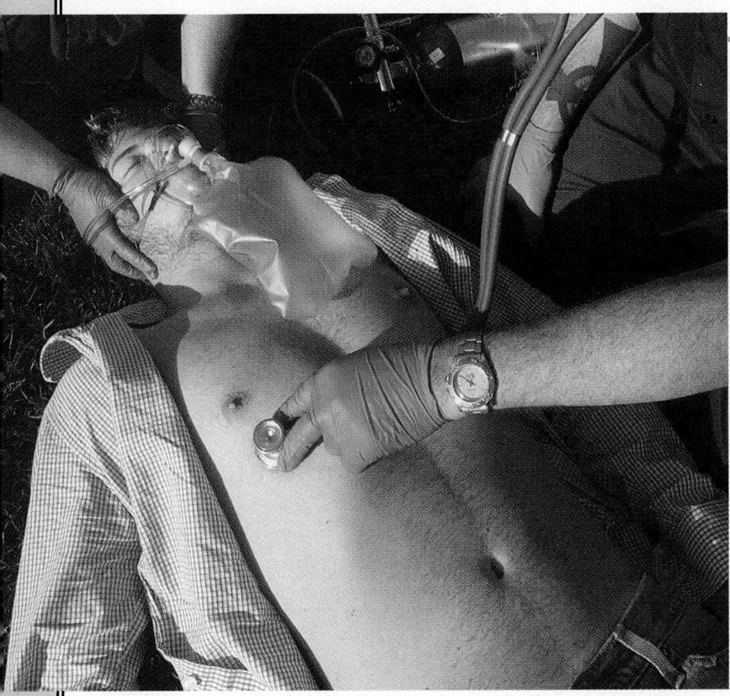

CORE CONCEPTS

The following are core concepts that will be addressed in this chapter:

- Components and procedures for the written run report
- Legal aspects and benefits of documentation
- Documentation concerns in patient refusal

DOT OBJECTIVES

*KNOWLEDGE AND ATTITUDE

3-8.1 Explain the components of the written report and list the information that should be included in the written report. (pp. 336–341)

3-8.2 Identify the various sections of the written report. (pp. 336–341)

3-8.3 Describe what information is required in each section of the prehospital care report and how it should be entered. (pp. 336–341)

3-8.4 Define the special considerations concerning patient refusal. (pp. 342–345)

3-8.5 Describe the legal implications associated with the written report. (pp. 332, 336, 341–346)

3-8.6 Discuss all state and/or local record and reporting requirements. (pp. 346–349)

3-8.7 Explain the rationale for patient care documentation. (pp. 332, 335–336)

3-8.8 Explain the rationale for the EMS system gathering data. (pp. 332, 335–336)

3-8.9 Explain the rationale for using medical terminology correctly. (p. 341)

3-8.10 Explain the rationale for using an accurate and synchronous clock so that information can be used in trending. (pp. 337–338)

*SKILLS

3-8.11 Complete a prehospital care report.

Documentation is an important part of the patient care process and lasts long after the call. The report you write will become a part of the patient's permanent hospital record. As records of your agency, your reports and those written by other EMTs become a valuable source for research on trends in emergency medical care and a guide for continuing education and quality improvement. A report you have written may be used as evidence in a legal case. Documentation has short-term benefits as well. Noting vital signs and patient history will help you remember important facts about the patient during the course of the call.

PREHOSPITAL CARE REPORT

The record that you produce during a call is called a *prehospital care report* or, informally, a PCR. Your region or service may use a different name for the same kind of document, such as trip sheet, run report, or another name.

Prehospital care reports vary from system to system and state to state. While the information that is required to complete each is relatively similar, the method used to record the data may be somewhat different. *Written reports* are those that have portions with narrative areas, areas to record vital signs in written number form, and check boxes (Figure 14-1). *Computerized reports* are those that are completed by shading boxes to record data and then scanned for easy data storage and evaluation. In order to be scanned correctly, each box must be filled in completely with no stray marks (Figure 14-2).

A recent development in prehospital care reports is *direct data entry*. This can take several forms. An electronic clipboard is a computer in a clipboard format. The computer is able to recognize handwriting and convert it to computer text. The data are stored and eventually downloaded to a larger computer. The computers, also called pen-based computers, may be attached to printers at receiving hospitals to print out a hard copy of the report for the emergency department staff. Some EMS agencies use laptop computers or personal digital assistants (PDAs) in the ambulance (Figure 14-3). They allow the EMT to enter information about a call directly into a database. Still another

MAINE EMS **PRESS DOWN, YOU ARE MAKING THREE COPIES.**

RUN REPORT # 746118	Mo. Day Year	M T W Th F S Sun	SERVICE NAME	SERVICE NO.	VEHICLE NO.	ALS ☐ Performed ☐ Back-up called	SERVICE RUN NO.

NAME

BILLING INFORMATION

STREET OR R.F.D.

CITY/TOWN STATE ZIP

AGE/DATE OF BIRTH ☐ Male ☐ Female PHONE

INCIDENT LOCATION: ADDRESS CITY/TOWN

TRANSPORTED TO: TREATING/FAMILY PHYSICIAN

CREW LICENSE NUMBERS

TRANSPORTATION/COMMUNICATIONS PROBLEMS

☐ Medical
☐ Cardiac
☐ Poisoning/OD
☐ Respiratory
☐ Behavioral
☐ Diabetic
☐ Seizure
☐ CVA
☐ OB/Gyn
☐ Other ________

☐ Trauma
☐ Multi-Systems Trauma
☐ Head
☐ Spinal
☐ Burn
☐ Soft Tissue Injury
☐ Fractures
☐ Other ________

☐ Code 99

R	L	LUNG SOUNDS
☐	☐	CLEAR
☐	☐	ABSENT
☐	☐	DECREASED
☐	☐	RALES
☐	☐	WHEEZE
☐	☐	STRIDOR

TYPE OF RUN
☐ Emergency Transport
☐ Routine Transfer
☐ Emergency Transfer
☐ No Transport
☐ Refused Transport

TIME	CODE		ODOMETER
		Call Received	
		Enroute	
		At Scene	
		From Scene	
		At Destination	
		In Service	

☐ MEDICATIONS ☐ ALLERGIES

CHIEF COMPLAINT:

TIME	PULSE	RESP	BP	PUPILLARY RESPONSE	SKIN	VERBAL RESPONSE	MOTOR RESPONSE	EYE-OPENING RESPONSE	CAPILLARY REFILL
			/			5 4 3 2 1	6 5 4 3 2 1	4 3 2 1	☐ Normal ☐ None ☐ Delayed
			/			5 4 3 2 1	6 5 4 3 2 1	4 3 2 1	☐ Normal ☐ None ☐ Delayed
			/			5 4 3 2 1	6 5 4 3 2 1	4 3 2 1	☐ Normal ☐ None ☐ Delayed

☐ MVA ☐ Concern AOB/ETOH SEAT BELTS: ☐ Used ☐ Not Used ☐ N/A ☐ Helmet Used

MUTUAL AID: Assisted/Assisted by Service # ________ Time Called: ________

PATIENT'S SUSPECTED PROBLEM: 746118

☐ Medication Administered ☐ Defib Lic.# ________ MEDICAL CONTROL ☐ Written Order/Protocol ☐ Verbal Order/Protocol

☐ Monitor ☐ Chest Decomp IV Total Attempts ☐ SUC LIC.# ________ ☐ UNSUC LIC.# ________

☐ Pacing ☐ Caricothyrotomy

EOA Total Attempts ☐ SUC LIC.# ________ ☐ UNSUC LIC.# ________

ET Total Attempts ☐ SUC LIC.# ________ ☐ UNSUC LIC.# ________

Cleared Airway	Extrication
Artificial Respiration/BVM	Cervical Immobilization
Oropharyngeal Airway	KED/Short Board
Nasopharyngeal Airway	Long Board
CPR–Time:	Restraints
Bystander CPR	Traction Splinting
AED	General Splinting
Suction	Cold Application
Oxygen–LPMin ___ ☐ Nasal ☐ Mask	MAST Inflated
Pulse Oximetry	
Autovent	

LIC #	EKG RHYTHM	TIME	MEDS/DEFIB/C-VERT	DOSE W/S	ROUTE

NAME OF E.D. TREATING PHYSICIAN SIGNATURE OF CREW MEMBER IN CHARGE COPY 1 HOSPITAL

Figure 14-1 • Example of a prehospital care report with fill-in boxes and a narrative space.

Do Not Staple or Fold

AGENCY CODE | UNIT # | UNIT TYPE: AMBULANCE, RESCUE, OTHER

DATE: Jan, Feb, Mar, Apr, May, Jun, Jul, Aug, Sep, Oct, Nov, Dec | DAY | YR: 91, 92, 93, 94, 95

PERSONNEL INFORMATION: ATTENDANT #1 | ATTENDANT #2 | ATTENDANT #3 (F, B, P, N, O, RPT)

RESPONSE/TRANSPORT MODE: To Scene: (2) Non-Emerg, (3) Emergency; From Scene: (2) Non-Emerg, (3) Emergency

RESPONSE OUTCOME: Transported By This Unit; Care Transfer/Another Unit; Cancelled Enroute; Cancelled On Scene; False Call/No Patient Found; Dead on Scene; Refused Treatment; Treated, Refused Transport; P.O.V.; Standby; Unknown; Other

CALL RECEIVED | ENROUTE | ARRIVE SCENE | DEPART SCENE | ARRIVE HOSPITAL | RETURN TO SERVICE (MILITARY TIME)

INCIDENT LOCATION: Residence; Interstate; Highway; Street/Road.; Public Access; Industrial/Off.; HMO/Clinic/Doctors Office; Hospital; Other ______

DISPATCH/INCIDENT TYPE: Abdominal Pain; Asphyxiation/Choke; Chest Pain; Diff. Breathing; Drowning; Heat/Cold Problems; Ill Person; OB/GYN; OD/Poison; Person Down/Unconsc.; Psych/Behavioral; Seizures; Other Medical; MVA; MVA - Motorcycle; MVA - Ped/Bike; Assault; Assault - Sexual; Bite/Sting; Burn/Elect.; Fall; Person Trapped; Stab/Gunshot; Other Trauma; Standby; InterFacility Transfer

SUSPECTED MEDICAL ILLNESS: None; Abdom. Pain; Airway Obstr; Allergic React; Cancer Compli; Cardiac Arrest; Cardiac Sympt.; Chest Pain; Childbirth; COPD; Diabetes Comp.; Drug Reaction; Heat/Cold Problems; Inhalation; OB/GYN; OD/Poison; Psych/Behv; Resp. Arrest; Resp. Dist; Seizures; Stroke; Syncope; Unconscious; Other; P=Primary S=Secondary

INJURY SITE/TYPE: None; Amputate; Bite/Sting; Blunt-Major; Burn/Elec; Frac/Disloc.; Penetrate; Soft-Closed; Soft-Open — Head; Face; Eye; Neck; Chest; Back; Upper Ext; Abdomen; Pelvis; Lower Ext

MECHANISM OF INJURY: Flail Chest; Burns 10+%/face/arwy; Fall 20+ feet; Speed 40+ mph; 20+ speed change; Deformity 20+"; Intrusion 12+"; Rollover; Ejection; Death same MV; Pedest.vs. MV 5+mph; Pedst. thrown/run over; Mtcycle 20+mph/sep.; Extrication > 15 min.

GLASGOW COMA SCALE: EYES: (4) Spontaneous; (3) To Voice; (2) To Pain; (1) Unresponsive. VERBAL: (5) Oriented; (4) Confused; (3) Inappropriate; (2) Garbled; (1) None. MOTOR: (6) Obeys Comm.; (5) Pain-Local.; (4) Pain-Withdraws; (3) Pain-Flexion; (2) Pain-Extends; (1) None

PRIOR AID: None; CPR; Extricate; Wound Mgt. — Fire; Police; 1st Resp.; Rescue; Bystander

THIS PATIENT LOCATION/PROTECTION: Driver; Front Pass; Rear Pass; Other; Unknown; Shlder/Lap Belt; Shoulder Belt; Lap Belt; Safety Seat; Helmet; Not Used; Not Available; Unknown; Airbag (Deployed) Yes

SEX: (F) (M) | AGE | INITIAL VITAL SIGNS: Unable to Take; Not Taken; Pt. Refused — SYSTOLIC; DIASTOLIC; PULSE; RESP; PUPILS L R (N, D, C, NR)

This Patient Resident of: City; County; Arizona; Out of State; Unknown — Months; Apprx.

BLS TREATMENT: Assessment; C-Spine Precautions; Oxygen; CPR; Crisis Intervention; Defibrillation (AUTO); Extrication; Fracture Stabilize; Hemorrhage Control; Ipecac/Charcoal Admin.; MAST Application; MAST Inflation; Monitor IV; Oral Care/Airway; Oral Glucose; Restraints Applied; Suction; Traction Splint; Wound Management; Other ______ (A1 A2 A3 O)

CPR INFORMATION: Time: Minutes <4 4-10 >10 Unk — Arrest to CPR; Arrest to Defib; Arrest to ALS; Witnessed Arrest? (Y) (N) Unk; Pulse/Rhythm Restored? (Y) (N); Traumatic Cardiac Arrest? (Y) (N)

ALS TREATMENT: Cardiac Monitoring; Cardioversion; Cricothyroidotomy; Defibrillation; EOA; Intubation - Nasal; Intubation - Oral; IV-Central; IV-Peripheral; Medication Admin; NG Tube; Needle Thoracostomy; Phlebotomy; SVN; Other ______ (A1 A2 A3 O)

ATTEMPTS: IV; ET; OTH (1) (2) (3) (U)

MEDICATIONS: Albuterol; Aminoph.; Atropine 1/10; Atropine 8/20; Bretylium; Calcium Chl.; D50; Diazepam; Diphenhydram.; Dopamine; Epi 1:1000; Epi 1:10,000; Furosemide; Isoetharine; Isoproterenol; Lidocaine-Bolus; Lidocaine Drip; Methylprednisone; Morphine; Naloxone; Nifedipine; Nitrostat. Tab.; Nitrous Oxide; Oxytocin; Phenobarbital; Sodium Bicarbonate; Thiamine; Verapamil; Other ______; HAZMAT

EKG INITIAL/LAST: Nrml Sinus; Sinus Tach; Sinus Brady; Asystole; AV Block; Atrial Fib; Atrial Flut; EMD; Junctional; Paced; SV Tach; Vent Tach; Vent Fib; Other; PVC's

IV TYPE/RATE: TKO; Bolus; Wide; Other — D5W; Normal Saline; Ringers Lact.; Other

LINES: # Peripheral; # Central

MEDICAL CONTROL: First; Hospital — Radio/Good; Radio/Poor; Protocol; Telephone; Radio/Phone Patch; Cellular; Phys On-Scene; None Required; Unable

ORDERS BY: Protocol; Standing; Verbal

PT. RECEIVED BY | RESEARCH CODE

PATIENT DISPOSITION: Improved; Worsened; Unchanged; Died in ER

MISCELLANEOUS: If Multiple Pts On Scene, How Many? (2) (3) (4) (5) (6) (7) (8) 9+; If Transport to Level 1 Receiving Facility, Due to: Pt. Condition; Mechanism

PLEASE DO NOT MARK IN THIS AREA — 2002094

EMS FIRST CARE FORM - ARIZONA DEPARTMENT OF HEALTH SERVICES — Return to State EMS Office

SCANTRON® FORM NO. F-3087-EMS 0792-C 671-5 4 3 2 1

© 1992 EMS DATA SYSTEMS

Figure 14-2 • Example of a prehospital care report that is scannable by computer.

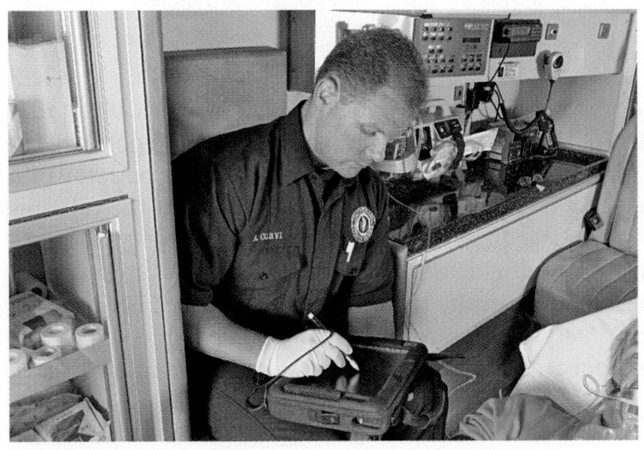

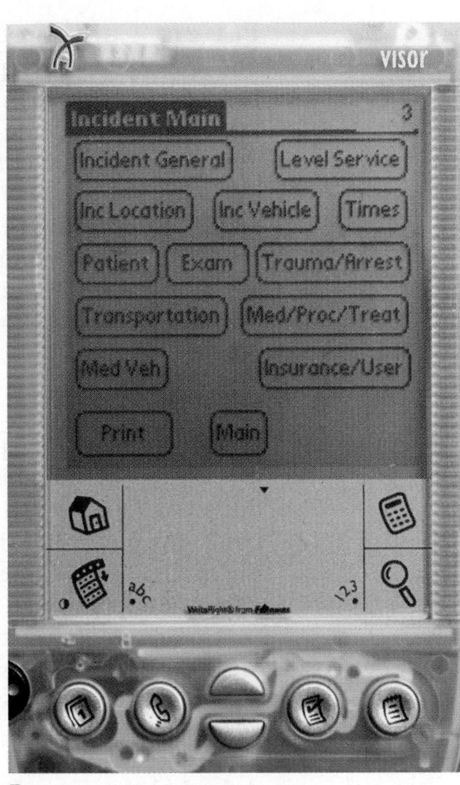

A B

Figure 14-3 • Direct data devices as documentation tools: (A) a pen-based computer, (B) a PDA.

variation is the web-based approach. With this increasingly popular method, the EMT signs on to a secure web site and enters the data through a keyboard.

When possible, it is a good idea to complete the PCR while you are still at the receiving facility with fresh memory of the call (Figure 14-4).

Functions of the Prehospital Care Report

The prehospital care report has many functions. It is the record of patient care, serves as a legal document, provides information for administrative functions, aids education and research, and contributes to quality improvement. These functions are discussed in the following paragraphs.

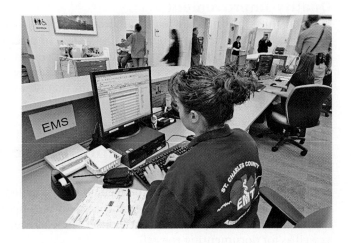

Figure 14-4 • An EMT completes her prehospital care report, using a computer in the receiving hospital ED. *(© Ray Kemp/911 Imaging)*

Patient Care Record

The prehospital care report conveys important information about the patient to members of the EMS system and beyond. Although you provide a verbal report to the hospital staff before you leave the patient, your written record allows emergency department personnel to see the status of the patient when you arrived on scene, the care you gave, and how the patient's status may have changed during your care. An example of this would be the emergency department staff looking back at your original set of vital signs to compare the patient's current condition with the patient's condition when he was first found at the scene.

A copy of the prehospital care report becomes part of the patient's permanent hospital record.

Legal Document

The prehospital care report also serves as a legal document, which may be called for at any legal proceeding resulting from the call. The person who wrote the report will ordinarily go to court with the form. If the patient was the victim or perpetrator of a crime, the report and the writer may be called into court to testify about the call during criminal proceedings. Civil law proceedings for negligence in injuries (e.g., a patient falls in a shopping mall and sues) are another reason that your report may be examined.

Unfortunately, there may be a time when the report is being examined because you are the subject of a lawsuit. Fortunately, this is rare and usually preventable, but in this case too, the report in which you documented the circumstances and the care you gave will be very important.

Administrative Purposes

Depending on the service you belong to, you may have to obtain insurance and billing information from the patient or patient's family. This may be recorded on your prehospital care report, on a separate form, or on both.

Education and Research

Your report may be examined later as part of a research project. Analysis of statistics compiled from prehospital care reports can reveal patterns and trends in EMS management and care. For example, analysts may see instances in which response time could be improved or ways of scheduling and deploying units to prepare for busy areas and times. Statistics also may justify a request for additional resources.

Prehospital care reports can help management keep track of each EMT's experience and skills. Extra practice may be scheduled during continuing education sessions for skills that the reports reveal are underutilized, for instance. When an unusual or uncommon type of call has taken place, the prehospital care report may be used for demonstration of how to document such a case after it is stripped of data that might identify the patient.

Quality Improvement

Most organizations have a Quality Improvement (QI)—or Quality Assurance (QA) or Continuous Quality Improvement (CQI)—system in place by which calls are routinely reviewed for conformity to current medical and organizational standards. Examination of prehospital care reports is one major way of conducting this review. At times, QI evaluations reveal excellent care by an EMT team that deserves special recognition and a "pat on the back."

Elements of the Prehospital Care Report

Data Elements

Each individual box in the prehospital care report is called a *data element.* While some elements may seem insignificant, each is actually an important part of the report and the description of the patient and response. These elements are necessary for research as well as for documenting the call.

POINT OF VIEW

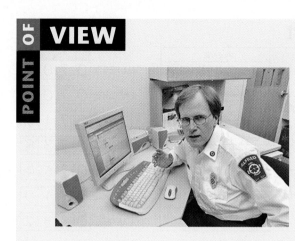

"I remember the day I found out the right way to do documentation.

"I turned in a run report one evening. When I came in to work the next day the chief called me in. He wasn't happy. And, looking back, he had reason not to be. It wasn't my best work. I had listened to my partner. He has been around for 25 years. He told me to just put down a couple of sentences and the vitals. Said it was a 'no brainer.'

"Now I know that if I got sued it would've looked bad. But the thing that really got me is when the chief told me it looked like I was doing a poor job. I know I took good care of that patient. And I even helped contact her family on the cell phone so someone would be at the hospital for her.

"I don't want a bad report to go to the QI committee—or to court—but most important I am proud of what I do. The chief made me realize my reports should reflect that pride. And believe me, now they do."

To aid in research across many states and regions, the U.S. Department of Transportation has developed a *minimum data set*. These are the minimum elements recommended to be included in all prehospital care reports nationwide. There is also a standardized definition of what each element means. Over a period of time, it is hoped, the minimum data set will be widely adopted. The minimum data set is briefly summarized in Table 14-1.

The prehospital care report can be broken down into several sections, each containing different types of information. The sections include run data, patient data, check boxes, and the narrative section.

Run Data

This section includes the agency name, unit number, date, times, run or call number, and crew members' names, licensure levels, and numbers (Figure 14-5). Times recorded must be accurate and synchronous (by clocks or watches that show the same time). Be sure to use the time as given by the dispatcher when noting times on your report. Unless your watch or the ambulance clock displays exactly the same time as the dispatch center, the times on your report will not match. There may be a difference of several minutes between the time displayed on your watch and the dispatch center's official time.

TABLE 14-1 • Minimum Data Set

PATIENT INFORMATION

Gathered at the time of the EMT's initial contact with a patient upon arrival at the scene, following all interventions, and upon arrival at medical facility:

- Chief complaint
- Level of responsiveness (AVPU)—mental status
- Systolic blood pressure for patients greater than 3 years old
- Skin perfusion (capillary refill) for patients less than 6 years old
- Skin color and temperature
- Pulse rate
- Respiratory rate and effort

ADMINISTRATIVE INFORMATION

- Time of incident report
- Time unit notified
- Time of arrival of patient
- Time unit left scene
- Time of arrival at destination
- Time of transfer of care

Prehospital Care Report

		MILEAGE	
Agency Name	ARLINGTON RESCUE	END	24496
Dispatch Information	CARDIAC	BEGIN	24476
Call Location	124 CYPRUS ST 2nd FLOOR	TOTAL	00020
CHECK ONE	☑ Residence ☐ Health Facility ☐ Farm ☐ Indus. Facility ☐ Other Work Loc. ☐ Roadway ☐ Recreational ☐ Other	LOCATION CODE	0124

CALL TYPE AS REC'D	MECHANISM OF INJURY	
☑ Emergency	☐ MVA (✓ seat belt used → N/A)	☐ Knife
☐ Non-Emergency	☐ Fall of ____ feet	☐ Machinery
☐ Stand-by	☐ Unarmed assault	☐ ______
	☐ GSW	

USE MILITARY TIMES	
CALL REC'D	0705
ENROUTE	0707
ARRIVED AT SCENE	0719
FROM SCENE	0738
AT DESTIN	0754
IN SERVICE	0810
IN QUARTERS	0832

Figure 14-5 • One section of a prehospital care report contains run data.

This time difference may seem insignificant but is actually very important in such areas as determining how long a patient has been in cardiac arrest, trends in patient condition, or measurement of system efficiency in response times.

Patient Data

This section contains information about the patient, the patient's condition throughout the call, and the care given to the patient (Figure 14-6). This is the major portion of your report. Specifically, it contains:

- Patient's name, address, date of birth, age, sex
- Billing and insurance information (in many jurisdictions)
- Nature of the call
- Mechanism of injury
- Location where the patient was found
- Treatment administered before arrival of the EMT (by bystanders, First Responders)
- Signs and symptoms, baseline and subsequent vital signs
- SAMPLE history
- Care administered and the effect that the care had on the patient (e.g., improved, no change)
- Changes in condition throughout the call

Check Boxes

Many prehospital care reports have check boxes for many data elements. This can be an efficient way to document parts of the call. In some cases, you will write a number or a few words into a short blank (Figure 14-7).

CHIEF COMPLAINT
"MY CHEST HURTS"
PAST MEDICAL HISTORY
☐ None
☒ Allergy to ASPIRIN
☐ Hypertension ☐ Stroke
☐ Seizures ☐ Diabetes
☐ COPD ☑ Cardiac
☐ Other (List) ☐ Asthma
Current Medications (List) CARDIZEM

VITAL SIGNS TIME	RESP	PULSE	B.P.	LEVEL OF CONSCIOUSNESS	R PUPILS L	SKIN
0724	Rate: 18 ☒ Regular ☐ Shallow ☐ Labored	Rate: 88 ☐ Regular ☒ Irregular	148/88	☑ Alert ☐ Voice ☐ Pain ☐ Unresp.	☑ Normal ☑ ☐ Dilated ☐ ☐ Constricted ☐ ☐ Sluggish ☐ ☐ No-Reaction ☐	☐ Unremarkable ☑ Cool ☑ Pale ☐ Warm ☐ Cyanotic ☐ Moist ☐ Flushed ☐ Dry ☐ Jaundiced
0730	Rate: 18 ☒ Regular ☐ Shallow ☐ Labored	Rate: 84 ☐ Regular ☒ Irregular	144/86	☑ Alert ☐ Voice ☐ Pain ☐ Unresp.	☑ Normal ☑ ☐ Dilated ☐ ☐ Constricted ☐ ☐ Sluggish ☐ ☐ No-Reaction ☐	☐ Unremarkable ☑ Cool ☑ Pale ☐ Warm ☐ Cyanotic ☐ Moist ☐ Flushed ☐ Dry ☐ Jaundiced
0745	Rate: 20 ☒ Regular ☐ Shallow ☐ Labored	Rate: 88 ☐ Regular ☒ Irregular	144/86	☑ Alert ☐ Voice ☐ Pain ☐ Unresp.	☑ Normal ☑ ☐ Dilated ☐ ☐ Constricted ☐ ☐ Sluggish ☐ ☐ No-Reaction ☐	☐ Unremarkable ☑ Cool ☑ Pale ☐ Warm ☐ Cyanotic ☐ Moist ☐ Flushed ☐ Dry ☐ Jaundiced

Figure 14-6 • One section of a prehospital care report is devoted to patient data.

TREATMENT GIVEN

- [x] Moved to ambulance on stretcher/backboard
- [ ] Moved to ambulance on stair chair
- [ ] Walked to ambulance
- [ ] Airway Cleared
- [ ] Oral/Nasal Airway
- [ ] Esophageal Obturator Airway/Esophageal Gastric Tube Airway (EOA/EGTA)
- [ ] Endotracheal Tube (E/T)
- [x] Oxygen Administered @ 15 L.P.M., Method NON-REBREATHER MASK
- [ ] Suction Used
- [ ] Artificial Ventilation Method ______
- [ ] C.P.R. in progress on arrival by: ☐ Citizen ☐ PD/FD/Other First Responder ☐ Other
- [ ] C.P.R. Started @ Time ▶ ____ Time from Arrest Until C.P.R. ▶ ____ Minutes
- [ ] Bleeding/Hemorrhage Controlled (Method Used: ______)
- [ ] Spinal Immobilization Neck and Back
- [ ] Limb Immobilized by ☐ Fixation ☐ Traction
- [ ] (Heat) or (Cold) Applied
- [ ] Restraints Applied, Type ______
- [ ] Baby Delivered @ Time ______ In County ______ ☐ Alive ☐ Stillborn ☐ Male ☐ Female
- [ ] Transported in Trendelenburg position
- [ ] Transported in left lateral recumbent position
- [x] Transported with head elevated
- [ ] Other ______

Figure 14-7 • Most prehospital care reports have check boxes for some data elements.

Narrative

The narrative section of a prehospital care report is less structured than the fill-in blanks and check-box sections. It provides space to write information about the patient that cannot fit into fill-in blanks or check-off boxes (Figure 14-8).

Experienced EMTs consider a good prehospital care report as one that "paints a picture" of their patient. The report, as mentioned previously, is read by many people and is a vital part of the patient's record. When hospital personnel or your quality improvement team reads your report, it should tell the patient's story fully and appropriately.

Remember, you were there throughout the call and are familiar with the patient, his chief complaint, and the care you gave. The people who read your report will have no prior knowledge of the call or the patient. It is imperative that you provide complete, accurate, and pertinent information about your patient and present the information in a logical order. The following guidelines will help you prepare narrative portions of your prehospital care reports:

- *Include both objective and pertinent subjective information.* Objective statements are those that are observable, measurable, or verifiable, such as, "The patient has a swollen, deformed extremity." This is backed up by your visual observation. Or an objective statement might be, "The patient's blood pressure was 110/80," based on a measurement you took. Or it might be "Patient uses a prescribed inhaler," a verifiable fact provided by the patient.

  Subjective information is information from an individual point of view. It may be provided by the patient as a symptom ("I feel dizzy"). It also may be provided by the EMT, such as your general impression of the patient ("Patient appears to have difficulty breathing"). Avoid subjective statements that are merely opinions, beyond your level of training or scope of practice ("I do not believe that the leg is broken" or "Patient is probably having a heart attack"), or are irrelevant ("Patient's daughter was rude").

NARRATIVE THE PATIENT DEVELOPED A SUDDEN ONSET OF CHEST PAIN WHILE WATCHING TV. THE PAIN IS SUBSTERNAL, CRUSHING, AND RADIATES TO THE LEFT SHOULDER AND ARM. THE PATIENT STATES THAT THIS PAIN IS "EXACTLY THE SAME AS WHEN I HAD A HEART ATTACK 2 YEARS AGO." HE DENIES LOSS OF CONSCIOUSNESS OR DIFFICULTY BREATHING....

Figure 14-8 • The narrative portion of a prehospital care report provides space to write information that will not fit into check-off boxes or fill-in blanks.

Cultural Considerations

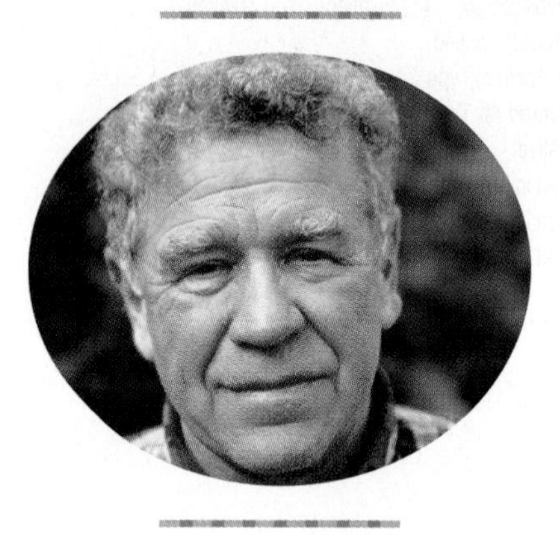

In the course of your EMS career, you are bound to encounter people of cultures and beliefs that are different from your own. Rather than closing your mind and thinking, privately, "Why can't they do . . . think . . . be . . . the 'right' way" (that is, like you), adopt the attitude of being interested in how other people live and think and consider it an opportunity to expand your horizons. Keep in mind that, whether or not you personally agree with your patient, you owe that patient respect.

A receptive attitude can improve your documentation skills. Instead of anticipating what the patient is thinking and feeling—and writing it down that way—develop the habit of drawing the patient out. For example, you may inadvertently do or say something that your patient finds offensive. If the patient gives you a funny look, instead of dismissing it, ask the patient what is on his mind. His answer may surprise you, and this may lead to a more honest and insightful narrative report.

It may also increase your patient's feeling of being listened to and respected. In turn, this will help to shrink the cultural differences between you and to improve the therapeutic relationship between you and your patient.

Prehospital care reports are designed to be factual documents. Use objective statements whenever possible and only pertinent subjective statements. If you record something you did not observe yourself, put it in quotation marks (e.g., A bystander stated that "the patient passed out at the wheel before crashing"). Placing a statement in quotation marks and identifying the source lets readers of the report know where the information came from.

The chief complaint is another piece of information that is usually given in quotes. If a patient is conscious and oriented, he will usually tell you why he or someone else called you ("My chest hurts"). If the patient is not conscious or oriented, the person who called EMS may provide the chief complaint (She said he "felt faint and then passed out"). Since the chief complaint is in someone else's words, it should be placed in quotes.

In documenting your assessment procedures, remember to document important observations about the scene, such as suicide notes, weapons, and any other facts that would be important for patient care but not available to the emergency department personnel.

NOTE *The simple fact that there is no pain or complaint of difficulty does not mean that the patient should not be treated. If the patient's medical condition or if the mechanism of injury so indicates, treat the patient despite absence of pain or other symptoms.*

- *Include pertinent negatives.* These are examination findings that are negative (things that are not true), but are important to note. For example, if a patient has chest pain, you will ask that patient if he has difficulty breathing. If the patient says he does not have difficulty in breathing, that is an important piece of negative information. On your prehospital care report, you would note "the patient denies difficulty breathing." Negative information often applies to trauma patients. For example, if the mechanism of injury indicates that there may be an injury to the arm but the patient says he feels no pain, you would note "the patient denies pain in right arm." Documenting pertinent negatives lets other medical professionals know that you thought to examine these areas and that the findings were negative. Not documenting them might leave the reader wondering if this area was explored at all.
- *Avoid radio codes and nonstandard abbreviations.* Codes you may use on the radio may not be familiar to hospital personnel, so do not use them in written documentation. Abbreviations, when used properly, make writing efficient and accurate, but nonstandard abbreviations will cause confusion and possibly lead to errors in patient care.
- *Write legibly and use correct spelling.* A prehospital care report will have absolutely no value if it cannot be read, so take the time to make your handwriting readable. Unclear writing, misread by others, may cause errors that could harm the patient. Additionally, your QI team will be unable to read the report for review,

and it will have no value for research or training. Spelling is also important. If you cannot properly spell a word, look it up (many ambulances and emergency departments have medical dictionaries) or use another word.

- *Use medical terminology correctly.* Be sure that any medical terms you use are used correctly. If you are not sure of the meaning of a term, look it up in a medical dictionary or use everyday language to describe the condition instead. Careless use of medical terms could make your report unclear or cause a misunderstanding that might result in harm to the patient.
- *If it's not written down, you didn't do it.* This is a statement that you will most likely hear from your instructor and experienced EMTs in the field. It explains an important concept of EMS documentation. Make sure that you document all your interventions thoroughly. If you did not document them, it will appear as if they were never performed when the call is later reviewed.

The most important function of the prehospital care report is to present an accurate representation of the patient's condition throughout the call, the patient's history and vital signs, treatments performed, and changes or lack of changes in the patient's condition following treatments.

SPECIAL DOCUMENTATION ISSUES

Legal Issues

There are several legal issues pertaining to prehospital care reports and other documents you may be asked to complete. These include issues of confidentiality, patient refusals, falsification, and error correction.

CRITICAL DECISION MAKING: CHOOSING HOW AND WHAT TO DOCUMENT

Documentation is an important and challenging duty of the EMT. The documentation you produce may be looked at years later in criminal and civil cases—as well as being reviewed by your QI committee. You will need to make decisions about how and what you document . . . as you will see in the questions that follow.

1. After the police secure the scene, you treat a man and woman who apparently had a dispute. Neither sustained any life-threatening injuries, so you have time to gather more information at the scene. Even though you and your partner evaluate them in different rooms, they are still angry and trading insults. The boyfriend claims she is a two-timing slut who has syphilis and chlamydia. The girlfriend claims he is an alcoholic and a drug addict. How much of this should you document on the PCR? How should you phrase any information you obtained in this way?
2. Three years from now, you receive a notice to appear for a deposition regarding a call you had a long time ago. So much time has passed that you don't remember the call. Are you allowed to look at the PCR before you go? Why or why not?
3. When you treat a 3-year-old girl for an arm injury, you suspect she has been abused. How do the privacy rules of HIPAA affect what you may and should do with regard to reporting this situation to the authorities?

Confidentiality

The prehospital care report itself and the information it contains are strictly confidential. The information must not be discussed with or distributed to unauthorized persons. The Health Insurance Portability and Accountability Act (HIPAA) requires ambulance services that are covered by the law to take certain steps to safeguard patient confidentiality (Figure 14-9). This typically includes placing completed PCRs into a locked box. HIPAA, state, and local regulations will indicate to whom the information may be distributed. Obviously, the receiving hospital must receive patient care information so they can treat the patient properly. Most reports have a copy that will be left at the hospital. Confidentiality has been discussed in Chapter 3, "Medical/Legal and Ethical Issues."

Patient Refusals

Chapter 3, "Medical/Legal and Ethical Issues," discussed the issue of liability when patients refuse treatment. It is one of the foremost causes of liability for EMTs and their EMS systems. Chapter 3 presented several suggestions on what to do when a patient refuses care or transportation.

Document all actions you take to persuade the patient to go to the hospital. Additionally, you will have to make notes on the patient's competency, or his ability to make an informed, rational decision on his medical needs. If the patient was not capable of making this determination for any reason—including age, intoxication (alcohol and/or other drugs), mental competency, or as a result of the patient's medical condition—actions you took to protect the patient must also be documented. The patient must be informed of the potential results of not going to the hospital or of refusing your care.

The fact that a patient refuses transport to a hospital does not mean that you should not perform an assessment. If the patient greets you with a statement such as, "I don't know why my daughter called, because I'm not going anywhere," you may still be able to persuade the patient to get "checked out." Perform as much of a physical exam as possible, including vital signs. Document all of your findings and emergency care given on the prehospital care report. This information will be important to give to medical direction when you talk to them. Be sure to consult medical direction, according to your local protocols, whenever there is a patient refusal.

Most EMS agencies have a refusal-of-care form to use in the event that you have done your best to persuade the patient to accept care or transport and the patient still refuses. This form may be part of either the prehospital care report or a separate document. You should make sure the patient reads and signs this form (Figure 14-10). It is rare that a patient will refuse to sign the form, but if he does, be sure to document this, as well, and note the names of witnesses to the refusal. If possible, when a patient refuses

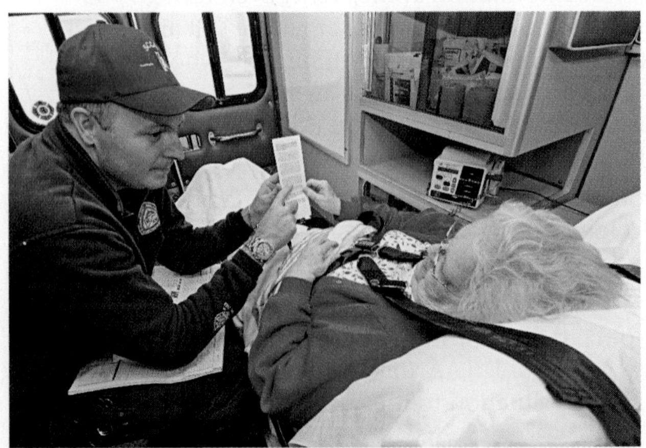

Figure 14-9 • An EMT explains a HIPAA privacy information leaflet with a patient. *(© Ray Kemp/911 Imaging)*

GUIDELINES

REFUSAL INFORMATION SHEET

PLEASE READ AND KEEP THIS FORM!

This form has been given to you because you have refused treatment and/or transport by Emergency Medical Services (EMS). Your health and safety are our primary concern, so even though you have decided not to accept our advice, please remember the following:

1) The evaluation and/or treatment provided to you by the EMS providers is not a substitute for medical evaluation and treatment by a doctor. We advise you to get medical evaluation and treatment.

2) Your condition may not seem as bad to you as it actually is. Without treatment, your condition or problem could become worse. If you are planning to get medical treatment, a decision to refuse treatment or transport by EMS may result in a delay which could make your condition or problem worse.

3) Medical evaluation and/or treatment may be obtained by calling your doctor, if you have one, or by going to any hospital Emergency Department in this area, all of which are staffed 24 hours a day by Emergency Physicians. You may be seen at these Emergency Departments without an appointment.

4) If you change your mind or your condition becomes worse and you decide to accept treatment and transport by Emergency Medical Services, please do not hesitate to call us back. We will do our best to help you.

5) DON'T WAIT! When medical treatment is needed, it is usually better to get it right away.

I have received a copy of this information sheet.

PATIENT SIGNATURE: ____________________ DATE: ______

WITNESS SIGNATURE: ____________________ DATE: ______

AGENCY INCIDENT #: ______________ AGENCY CODE: ______

NAME OF PERSON FILLING OUT FORM: ____________________

G 11A

Figure 14-10 • Example of a refusal information sheet.

to sign a refusal form, get the witnesses to sign a statement confirming that the patient has refused care or transport.

You should also include information about the patient refusal in the narrative section of the prehospital care report. Figure 14-11 shows a sample documentation of a patient refusal that might go into the narrative portion of the prehospital care report.

You will note that the narrative shown in Figure 14-11 contains many points of information, including pertinent negatives. The report states that the patient "denies" chest pain or difficulty in breathing. Statements from the patient's daughter are noted as to the source: "according to her daughter . . ." and "The daughter denies seeing any seizure activity."

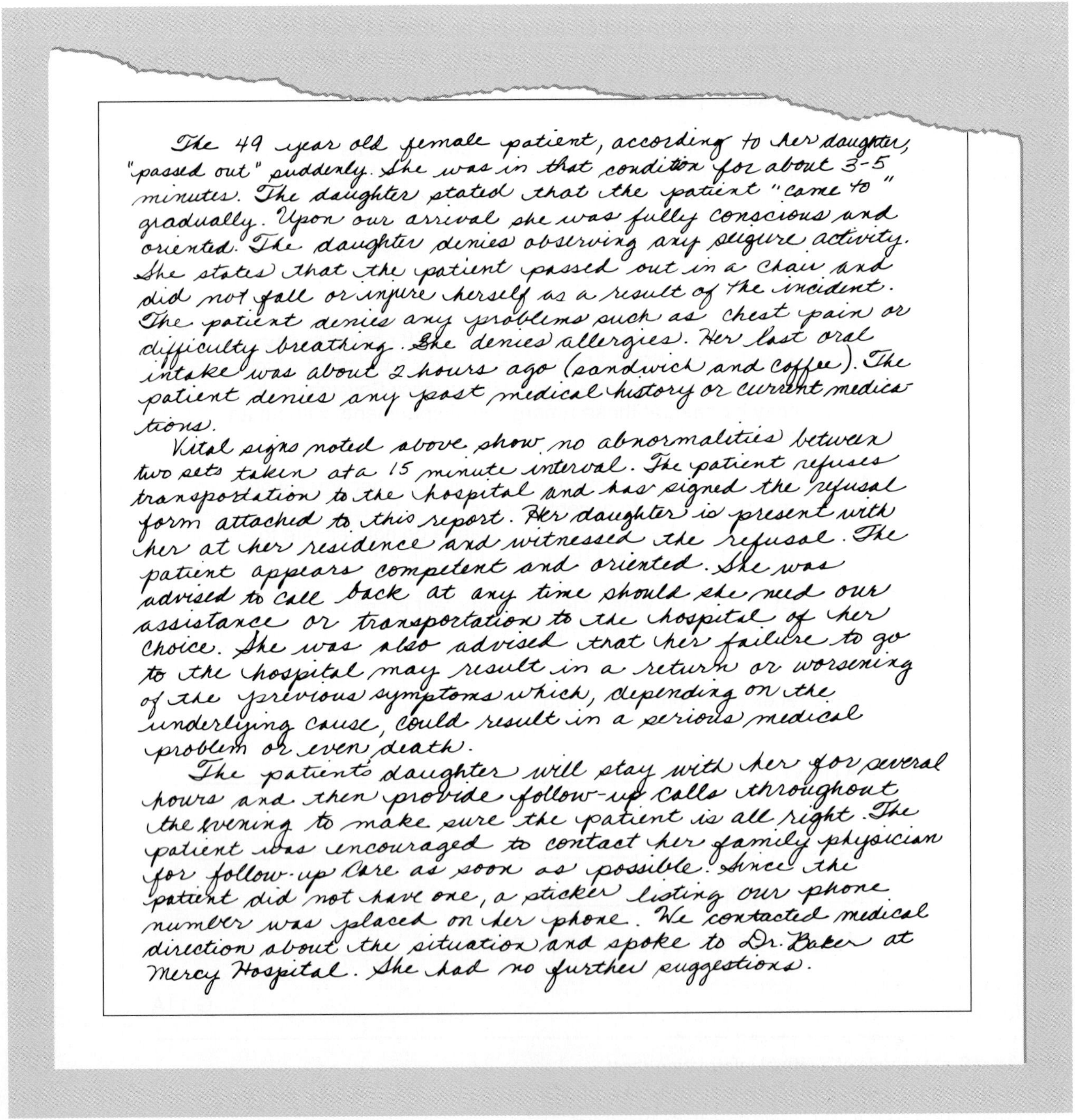

The 49 year old female patient, according to her daughter, "passed out" suddenly. She was in that condition for about 3-5 minutes. The daughter stated that the patient "came to" gradually. Upon our arrival she was fully conscious and oriented. The daughter denies observing any seizure activity. She states that the patient passed out in a chair and did not fall or injure herself as a result of the incident. The patient denies any problems such as chest pain or difficulty breathing. She denies allergies. Her last oral intake was about 2 hours ago (sandwich and coffee). The patient denies any past medical history or current medications.

Vital signs noted above show no abnormalities between two sets taken at a 15 minute interval. The patient refuses transportation to the hospital and has signed the refusal form attached to this report. Her daughter is present with her at her residence and witnessed the refusal. The patient appears competent and oriented. She was advised to call back at any time should she need our assistance or transportation to the hospital of her choice. She was also advised that her failure to go to the hospital may result in a return or worsening of the previous symptoms which, depending on the underlying cause, could result in a serious medical problem or even death.

The patients daughter will stay with her for several hours and then provide follow-up calls throughout the evening to make sure the patient is all right. The patient was encouraged to contact her family physician for follow-up care as soon as possible. Since the patient did not have one, a sticker listing our phone number was placed on her phone. We contacted medical direction about the situation and spoke to Dr. Baker at Mercy Hospital. She had no further suggestions.

Figure 14-11 • Document a patient refusal of care thoroughly in the narrative portion of the prehospital care report.

Before you leave the patient who has refused care or transport, be sure to make alternative care suggestions, such as encouraging him to seek care from a doctor, and document them. Try to be sure that a responsible family member or friend remains with the patient. Make sure that person also understands that the patient should seek care. Never convey the impression that you are annoyed about being called to the scene "for nothing." Make certain the patient understands that if his condition worsens or if he changes his mind, he can call EMS and you or another EMT team will gladly come back.

Falsification

Prehospital care reports document the information obtained and the care rendered during the call. False entries or misrepresentations on a report are usually intended to cover up serious flaws in assessment or in care. However, falsification may actually make the problem look worse when it is uncovered.

Two types of errors may be committed during a call: omission and commission. Errors of omission are those in which an important part of the assessment or care was left out. An example is oxygen. If a patient is experiencing chest pain, oxygen is an appropriate treatment. If it is overlooked for any reason, never write that oxygen was administered when it was not.

Occasionally, because of events during transport to a hospital, an EMT may only be able to get one set of vital signs. Never be tempted to write down an extra set of vital signs when none were taken. Just don't do it! Document only the vital signs that were taken. If there is a reason why you have only taken one set, document the reason (e.g., "The patient became combative and disoriented en route, preventing a second set of vital signs.").

Errors of commission are actions performed on the patient that are wrong or improper. An example of this is incorrect administration of medication. There are certain medications that you will be able to administer or assist the patient in administering to himself. This is a great responsibility. If a medication was administered when it was not indicated, it is important to tell medical direction and document the incident on the prehospital care report. Failure to document exactly what happened may have a negative effect on the patient's care. The hospital may think that the patient's condition is due to some other cause. In other situations, the hospital may readminister the medication, not realizing that it had already been given.

Document the situation surrounding any error of omission or commission and explain exactly what happened. Document what was done to correct the situation, including advising medical direction and verbally notifying hospital personnel.

Falsification or misrepresentation on a prehospital care report leads to poor patient care because the facts were not documented, and hospital personnel may be misled about the patient's condition and the care he received. Falsification or misrepresentation may also lead to the suspension or revocation of your certification or license as an EMT.

You will avoid falsifications if you follow this rule: Write everything important that did happen and nothing that didn't.

Correction of Errors

Prehospital care reports are not always written in ideal circumstances. You may even find yourself being dispatched to another call before you finish writing up your last one. In situations such as this, you may inadvertently write incorrect information on the report.

Any time there is incorrect information on the report, it must be corrected. If the report is still intact (all copies attached and not yet distributed), draw a single horizontal line through the error, initial it, then write the correct information beside it (Figure 14-12). Do not completely cross out the error or obliterate it. This may be looked on by others as an attempt to cover up a mistake in patient care.

If the error is discovered at a later date, after the report has been submitted, draw a single line through the error, mark the area with your initials and the date, and add the correct information to the end of the report or on a separate note. This should be done in a different color ink when possible so the change will be obvious. Copies of the report

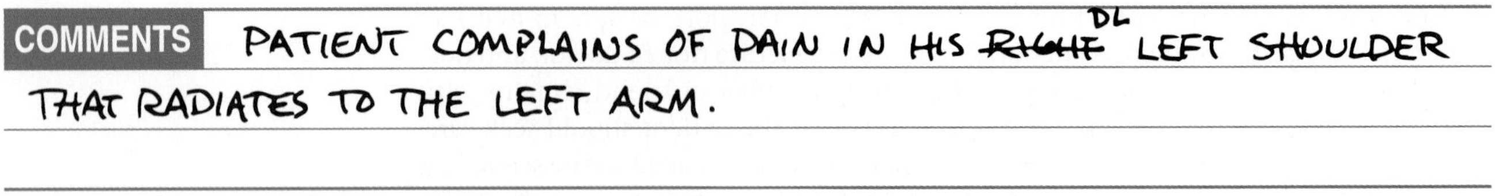

COMMENTS PATIENT COMPLAINS OF PAIN IN HIS ~~RIGHT~~ DL LEFT SHOULDER THAT RADIATES TO THE LEFT ARM.

Figure 14-12 • Cross out an error with a single line and initial the change.

may have already been distributed to other agencies, your Quality Improvement committee, insurance companies, or attorneys, and a corrected copy may need to be sent. Make sure that you place the date on the changes so the most recent copy is identifiable. If information has been omitted and you wish to add it, be sure also to date this information and place your initials by the added information. If you have a direct data entry system instead of the traditional paper forms, follow your agency's procedures for correction of errors.

Special Situations

Multiple-Casualty Incidents

An incident in which there are many patients or injuries—such as a multiple-vehicle collision, a major fire, or a plane crash—causes many logistical problems for an EMS system. Documentation of information for each individual patient may be difficult. A patient in a multiple-casualty incident (MCI) will probably be moved from one treatment area to another at the scene and then receive transport to a hospital. Possibly patients will be transported to several different hospitals. It is very important to keep the information with the patient as he moves through the system. This is often done through the use of a triage tag (Figure 14-13). This tag is affixed to the patient and used to record chief complaint and injuries, vital signs, and treatments given. At a point later in the emergency, the tag will be used to complete a traditional prehospital care report.

When completing a prehospital care report for a patient involved in a multiple-casualty incident, it will not be possible to provide the detail that you would normally provide for a single-patient call. This is an understandable consequence of the MCI. Your region or agency may have requirements for what information must be completed on the report during an MCI.

Special Situation Reports

Many states use a supplemental form for advanced life support (ALS) calls or additional documentation for calls that were complex or involved (Figure 14-14).

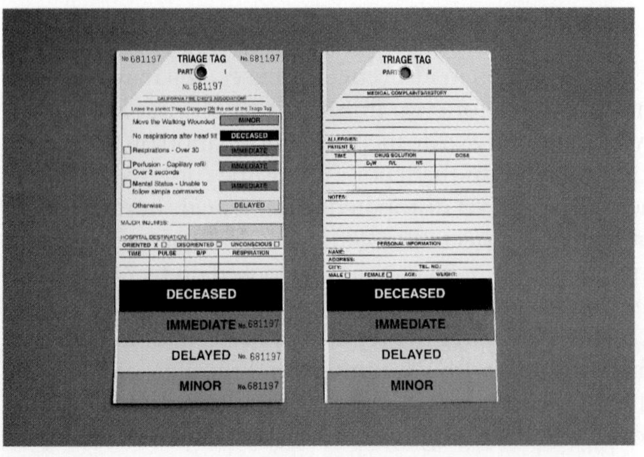

Figure 14-13 • During a multiple-casualty incident, triage tags are used to document information for each patient.

USE BALL POINT PEN ONLY.

CONTINUATION FORM for the Prehospital Care Report

Press Down Firmly. You're Making 4 Copies.

M D Y DATE	RUN NO.	AGENCY CODE	VEH. ID

Name	Agency Name	Enter PCR ID# (Top Center of PCR)
ADDITIONAL HISTORY & PHYSICAL EXAM FINDINGS		Weight in Kilograms

R BREATH SOUNDS L	NECK VEINS	EDEMA	ABDOMEN
☐ Normal ☐	☐ Normal	☐ Pedal	☐ Normal
☐ Decreased ☐	☐ Distended	☐ Sacral	☐ Tender
☐ Absent ☐	TRACHEAL SHIFT	☐ Ascites	☐ Rigid
☐ Rales ☐	R L	☐ Other	☐ Distended
☐ Rhonchi ☐	☐ ☐		☐ Other
☐ Wheezes ☐			

SERIAL VITAL SIGNS, EKG, RHYTHMS, MEDICATIONS AND TREATMENT

TIME	RESP.	PULSE	B.P.	LEVEL OF CONSCIOUSNESS	EKG RHYTHMS	DEFIBRILLATION CARDIOVERSION	MEDICATIONS	DOSE	ROUTE
	Rate: ☐ Regular ☐ Shallow ☐ Labored	Rate: ☐ Regular ☐ Irregular		☐ **A**lert ☐ **V**oice ☐ **P**ain ☐ **U**nresp.	☐ NSR ☐ Brady ☐ Asystole ☐ IVR ☐ V. Fib. ☐ V. Tach. ☐ PVC ☐ SVT ☐ Other____		☐ Epinephrine ☐ Dopamine ☐ Naloxone ☐ Atropine ☐ Sodium Bicarb. ☐ Bretylium ☐ Dextrose ☐ Isoproterenol ☐ Nitroglycerin ☐ Lidocaine ☐ Lasix ☐ Other____		☐ IV ☐ ET ☐ IM ☐ SL ☐ SQ ☐ PO ☐ Nebulizer
	Rate: ☐ Regular ☐ Shallow ☐ Labored	Rate: ☐ Regular ☐ Irregular		☐ **A**lert ☐ **V**oice ☐ **P**ain ☐ **U**nresp.	☐ NSR ☐ Brady ☐ Asystole ☐ IVR ☐ V. Fib. ☐ V. Tach. ☐ PVC ☐ SVT ☐ Other____		☐ Epinephrine ☐ Dopamine ☐ Naloxone ☐ Atropine ☐ Sodium Bicarb. ☐ Bretylium ☐ Dextrose ☐ Isoproterenol ☐ Nitroglycerin ☐ Lidocaine ☐ Lasix ☐ Other____		☐ IV ☐ ET ☐ IM ☐ SL ☐ SQ ☐ PO ☐ Nebulizer
	Rate: ☐ Regular ☐ Shallow ☐ Labored	Rate: ☐ Regular ☐ Irregular		☐ **A**lert ☐ **V**oice ☐ **P**ain ☐ **U**nresp.	☐ NSR ☐ Brady ☐ Asystole ☐ IVR ☐ V. Fib. ☐ V. Tach. ☐ PVC ☐ SVT ☐ Other____		☐ Epinephrine ☐ Dopamine ☐ Naloxone ☐ Atropine ☐ Sodium Bicarb. ☐ Bretylium ☐ Dextrose ☐ Isoproterenol ☐ Nitroglycerin ☐ Lidocaine ☐ Lasix ☐ Other____		☐ IV ☐ ET ☐ IM ☐ SL ☐ SQ ☐ PO ☐ Nebulizer
	Rate: ☐ Regular ☐ Shallow ☐ Labored	Rate: ☐ Regular ☐ Irregular		☐ **A**lert ☐ **V**oice ☐ **P**ain ☐ **U**nresp.	☐ NSR ☐ Brady ☐ Asystole ☐ IVR ☐ V. Fib. ☐ V. Tach. ☐ PVC ☐ SVT ☐ Other____		☐ Epinephrine ☐ Dopamine ☐ Naloxone ☐ Atropine ☐ Sodium Bicarb. ☐ Bretylium ☐ Dextrose ☐ Isoproterenol ☐ Nitroglycerin ☐ Lidocaine ☐ Lasix ☐ Other____		☐ IV ☐ ET ☐ IM ☐ SL ☐ SQ ☐ PO ☐ Nebulizer
	Rate: ☐ Regular ☐ Shallow ☐ Labored	Rate: ☐ Regular ☐ Irregular		☐ **A**lert ☐ **V**oice ☐ **P**ain ☐ **U**nresp.	☐ NSR ☐ Brady ☐ Asystole ☐ IVR ☐ V. Fib. ☐ V. Tach. ☐ PVC ☐ SVT ☐ Other____		☐ Epinephrine ☐ Dopamine ☐ Naloxone ☐ Atropine ☐ Sodium Bicarb. ☐ Bretylium ☐ Dextrose ☐ Isoproterenol ☐ Nitroglycerin ☐ Lidocaine ☐ Lasix ☐ Other____		☐ IV ☐ ET ☐ IM ☐ SL ☐ SQ ☐ PO ☐ Nebulizer
	Rate: ☐ Regular ☐ Shallow ☐ Labored	Rate: ☐ Regular ☐ Irregular		☐ **A**lert ☐ **V**oice ☐ **P**ain ☐ **U**nresp.	☐ NSR ☐ Brady ☐ Asystole ☐ IVR ☐ V. Fib. ☐ V. Tach. ☐ PVC ☐ SVT ☐ Other____		☐ Epinephrine ☐ Dopamine ☐ Naloxone ☐ Atropine ☐ Sodium Bicarb. ☐ Bretylium ☐ Dextrose ☐ Isoproterenol ☐ Nitroglycerin ☐ Lidocaine ☐ Lasix ☐ Other____		☐ IV ☐ ET ☐ IM ☐ SL ☐ SQ ☐ PO ☐ Nebulizer
	Rate: ☐ Regular ☐ Shallow ☐ Labored	Rate: ☐ Regular ☐ Irregular		☐ **A**lert ☐ **V**oice ☐ **P**ain ☐ **U**nresp.	☐ NSR ☐ Brady ☐ Asystole ☐ IVR ☐ V. Fib. ☐ V. Tach. ☐ PVC ☐ SVT ☐ Other____		☐ Epinephrine ☐ Dopamine ☐ Naloxone ☐ Atropine ☐ Sodium Bicarb. ☐ Bretylium ☐ Dextrose ☐ Isoproterenol ☐ Nitroglycerin ☐ Lidocaine ☐ Lasix ☐ Other____		☐ IV ☐ ET ☐ IM ☐ SL ☐ SQ ☐ PO ☐ Nebulizer

COMMENTS:

MEDICAL FACILITY CONTACTED

CREW	ADDITIONAL NAME — CREW	ADDITIONAL NAME — CREW	ADDITIONAL NAME — CREW	ADDITIONAL NAME — CREW
	☐ EMS-FR ☐ EMT ☐ AEMT #	☐ EMS-FR ☐ EMT ☐ AEMT #	☐ EMS-FR ☐ EMT ☐ AEMT #	☐ EMS-FR ☐ EMT ☐ AEMT #

EMS 100A (11/86) provided by NYS-EMS PROGRAM

AGENCY COPY/**WHITE** HOSPITAL PATIENT RECORD COPY/**PINK** RESEARCH COPY/**BLUE** EXTRA SERVICE COPY/**GREEN**

PAGE ______ OF ______

Figure 14-14 • Example of a supplemental form.

Special Incident Report

Town of Colonie
Department of Emergency Medical Services

EMERGENCY MEDICAL SERVICES
TOWN OF COLONIE

Date of Incident: ______________________ **Time:** ____________ **REMO #:** ____________

Town Run #: ________ **Reported by:** ______________________ **Zone:** ________

Type of Incident: ☐ MCI ☐ Rescue ☐ Personnel Matter ☐ Injury ☐ Accident with an EMS vehicle
☐ Infectious Disease Exposure ☐ Scene Conflict ☐ Other ____________

Total # of Patients: ☐ #P-1: ____ ☐ #P-2: ____ ☐ #P-3: ____ ☐ #P-0: ____
Elapsed Scene Time: *(First unit arrival to last unit to hospital)* ____________
Total Time of Incident: ____________

Describe the Incident Below:
Attach any additional documentation such as news clipppings and the pre-hospital care report.
Attach additional sheets if necessary.

Signature: ______________________ **Date:** ____________

Office Use Only
This incident relates to: ☐ Day Operation: TOT ☐ Night Operations: TOT: ☐ Administration: TOT:

Disposition: ______________________

Date:

Notifications/Copies: ☐ Director ☐ Deputy Director ☐ Supervisors
☐ Deputy Supervisors ☐ Senior Medics ☐ Zone Coordinator(s)
☐ Other ____________ Zone: ☐ 2 ☐ 3 ☐ 4

Figure 14-15 • Example of a special incident report.

Your activities as an EMT may also take you to some unusual situations that will require documentation on a form other than a prehospital care report. Such forms are usually specific to a local agency rather than mandated statewide (Figure 14-15). Some examples of situations that might require this kind of special report include:

- Exposure to infectious disease
- Injury to yourself or another EMT
- Hazardous or unsafe scenes to which other crews should be alerted
- Referrals to social service agencies for elderly or other patients in need of home care
- Mandatory reports for child or elderly abuse

This list is not all-inclusive. If there is any situation that requires extra documentation, the special report form may be the place to note it. It is important to remain accurate and objective when filling out this type of report, especially in an unusual or emotional situation. Follow local guidelines for the documentation of confidential information in these reports and for distribution of copies to appropriate agencies or persons.

CHAPTER REVIEW

SUMMARY

Documentation is an important skill. A properly completed prehospital care report, or PCR, provides important patient care and medical information about your patient. This form will become a permanent record in the patient's hospital chart as well as in the files of your agency. It may be used to help determine future treatments or as a legal document in a court proceeding. Your report will also be vital in charting trends, research, and quality improvement. Your report should "paint a picture" of your patient and his condition, accurately describing your contact with the patient throughout the call.

REVIEW QUESTIONS

1. Explain the term *minimum data set* and why it is important. (p. 337)
2. Explain what is meant by "objective" and "subjective" information in the narrative portion of the prehospital care report. Explain what is meant by "a pertinent negative." (pp. 339–341)
3. Explain how spelling and the use of codes, abbreviations, and medical terms relate to writing a clear and accurate narrative report. (pp. 340–341)
4. List some important steps to take and information to include when documenting a patient refusal. (pp. 342–344)
5. Describe some possible consequences of falsifying information on a prehospital care report. (p. 345)
6. Describe how to properly correct an error in a prehospital care report. (pp. 345–346)

CRITICAL THINKING

- Write a narrative report for a call you have been on. If you have not yet been on an ambulance, write a report that describes an injury or illness that has happened to you or a family member. If a prehospital care report form is available, complete the whole form, including the check-off or fill-in boxes as well as the narrative portion.

Thinking and Linking

Think back to Chapter 9, "Vital Signs and SAMPLE History," and link information from that chapter with information from this chapter, "Documentation," as you consider the following situation:

- Five minutes before arrival, you obtain a pulse of 108 on your critically injured patient. As you are writing up your prehospital care report, your partner tells you that just as you arrived, he was taking the patient's pulse and got a rate of 59. You are slightly stunned. How could the patient's pulse have dropped from 108 to 59? Then common sense kicks in. "You forgot to multiply by 2," you tell him. "The pulse must have been 118." How did you figure out that the rate of 59 had not been multiplied by 2? What is the reason for multiplying by 2?

MEDIA RESOURCES 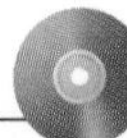

See the Student CD at the back of this book for quizzes, a case study, and other features related to this chapter. Also, visit the Companion Website for *Emergency Care* at **www.prenhall.com/limmer**, where you will find additional reinforcement and links to other resources.

Street Scenes

You and your partner have just finished a call involving a motor-vehicle crash with two vehicles. It was the first call of the day, just after you had checked out the ambulance but before you had time for breakfast. It is now 9:30 a.m. and you are sitting at a desk in the emergency department doing the prehospital care report. Although the patient didn't seem to be hurt badly, he had been complaining of lower back pain. Based on the patient complaint and the patient assessment, you decided to do a full immobilization.

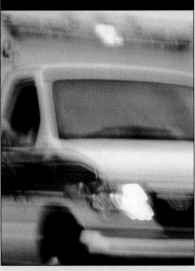

Street Scene Question

1. What information is important to include in the prehospital care report?

Although your partner is hurrying you, you write a very complete and thorough prehospital care report. You detail the patient's pulses, motor function, and sensation in all extremities before and after immobilization, including the fact that you observed the patient had difficulty moving his left foot and that it felt numb. The patient also told you that he was wearing only a lap-style seat belt at the time of the crash, and that he had a considerable amount of pain. He had not moved from the vehicle prior to the arrival of EMS.

Street Scene Questions

2. What is the importance of doing an accurate and thorough prehospital care report?
3. Should you have your partner read and comment on the prehospital care report before considering it complete?
4. What are the ramifications of having a prehospital care report in the hospital record that is different from the original copy on file with your EMS agency?

After writing your prehospital care report, your partner reviews it and a copy is left at the hospital for inclusion with the hospital chart. You manage to make it to breakfast, and you put this call behind you.

A few months later the director of your ambulance service stops you and asks if you remember this call. You think for a moment but only have a vague recollection. He informs you that the patient has started a lawsuit and claims that he sustained damage as the result of prehospital care. The prehospital care report has been reviewed by the ambulance service's lawyer, who believes that it will be a very good defense and the case will probably be dismissed. The director lets you read a copy of the prehospital care report, and as you read it, you start to remember the call. You had forgotten about the patient's complaint of pain and other symptoms.

As he walks away, the director tells you that good documentation will make all the difference in how this case gets decided. This is very different from a case he had a few years ago when an EMT changed the service's copy of the PCR after he left a copy at the hospital. The lawyer for the plaintiff noticed the discrepancies and made things very difficult for the service.

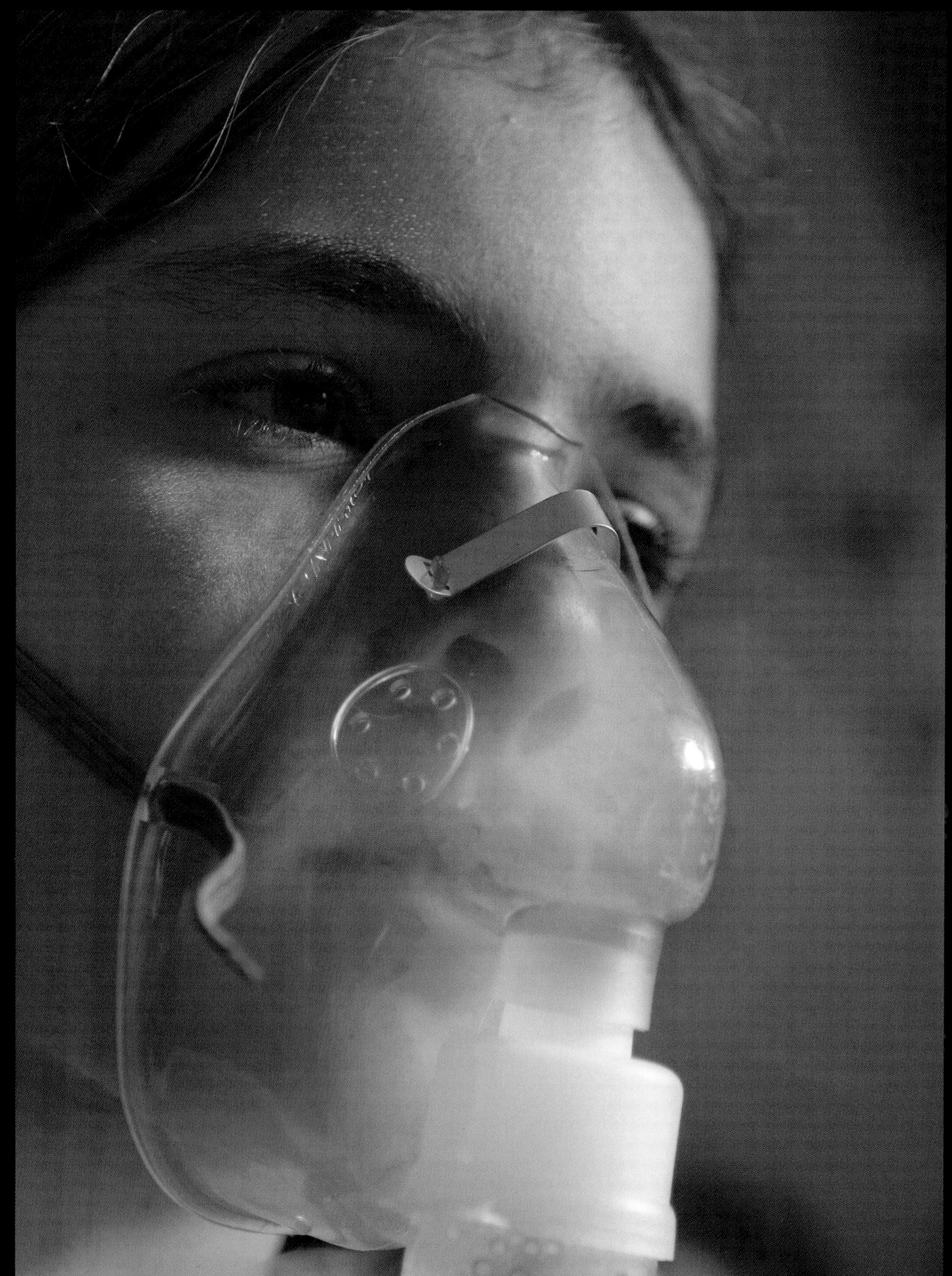

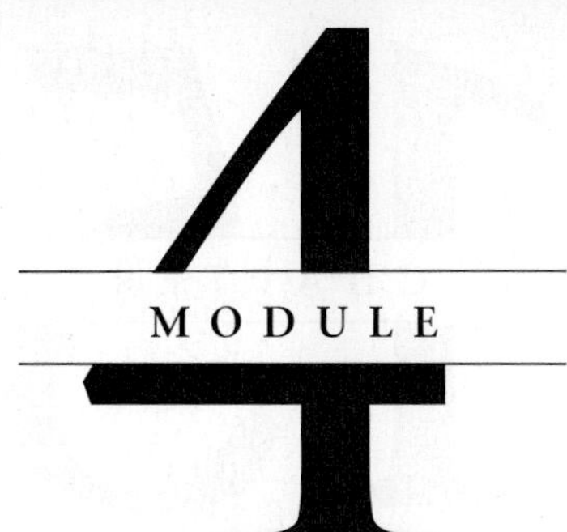

Medical Emergencies

Medical emergencies are usually caused by a disease or malfunction within the body. This module begins with a chapter on pharmacology (Chapter 15), or the study of drugs and medicines, focusing on the drugs EMTs are permitted to administer or help administer.

The remaining chapters focus on types of medical emergencies that commonly prompt emergency calls to EMS, including respiratory emergencies (Chapter 16), cardiac emergencies (Chapter 17), abdominal emergencies (Chapter 18), diabetic and altered mental status including seizures and stroke (Chapter 19), allergic reactions (Chapter 20), poisoning and overdose (Chapter 21), environmental emergencies including heat, cold, bites and stings, and drowning (Chapter 22), behavioral emergencies including suicide attempts (Chapter 23), and obstetrics, or childbirth, and gynecological emergencies (Chapter 24) with a final overview (Chapter 25).

CHAPTER 15

General Pharmacology

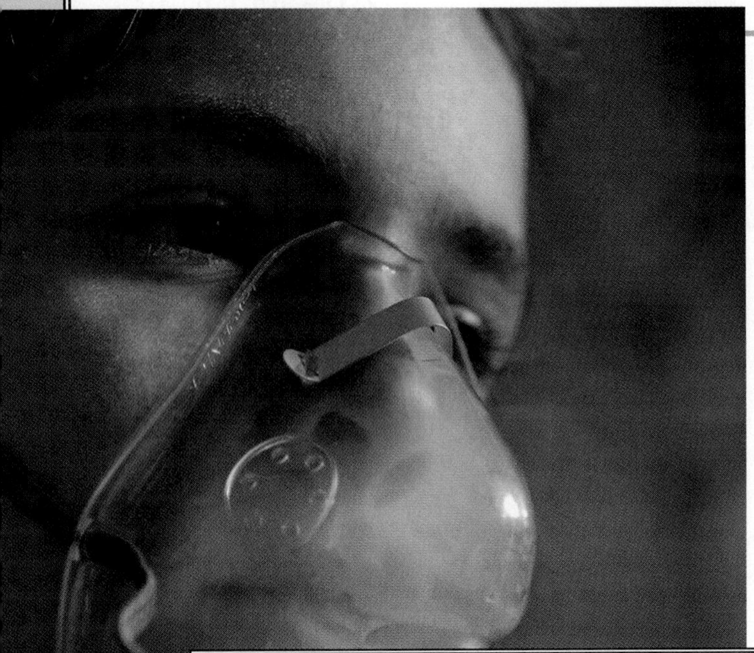

CORE CONCEPTS

The following are core concepts that will be addressed in this chapter:

- Which medications may be carried by the EMT and which medications the EMT may help administer to patients
- What to consider when administering any medication
- The role of medical direction in medication administration

KEY TERMS

activated charcoal, p. 355
contraindications, p. 360
epinephrine, p. 359
indications, p. 360
inhaler, p. 357
nitroglycerin, p. 358
oral glucose, p. 355
oxygen, p. 356
pharmacology, p. 355
side effect, p. 360

DOT OBJECTIVES

*KNOWLEDGE AND ATTITUDE

4-1.1 Identify which medications will be carried on the unit. (pp. 355–357)

4-1.2 State the medications carried on the unit by the generic name. (pp. 355–357)

4-1.3 Identify the medications which the EMT-Basic may assist the patient with administering. (pp. 357–359)

4-1.4 State the medications the EMT-Basic can assist the patient with by the generic name. (pp. 357–359)

4-1.5 Discuss the forms in which the medications may be found. (p. 360)

4-1.6 Explain the rationale for the administration of medications. (pp. 355–360)

*SKILLS

4-1.7 Demonstrate general steps for assisting patient with self-administration of medications.

4-1.8 Read the labels and inspect each type of medication.

The study of drugs—their sources, characteristics, and effects—is called **pharmacology.** Note that although EMS personnel use the terms *medications* and *drugs* interchangeably, the public often associates the word *drugs* with illegal or abused substances. When dealing with the public, therefore, use the terms *medicines* or *medications*.

pharmacology (FARM-uh-KOL-uh-je) the study of drugs, their sources, characteristics, and effects.

This chapter introduces the medications carried by the EMT on the ambulance, as well as prescribed medications the EMT may assist the patient in taking with approval from medical direction. You will learn the forms of medications your patients may be taking as well as the names for common types of medications and why they are used.

MEDICATIONS EMTS CAN ADMINISTER

You will be able to administer or assist with six medications in the field: activated charcoal, oral glucose, oxygen, prescribed inhalers, nitroglycerin, and epinephrine auto-injectors. The information that follows is a brief introduction to each of these drugs.

Medications on the Ambulance

As an EMT, you will carry activated charcoal, oral glucose, and oxygen on the ambulance. Under specific circumstances that will be described later, you will be able to administer these medications to patients.

Activated Charcoal

Activated charcoal is a powder prepared from charred wood, usually premixed with water to form a slurry for use in the field (Figure 15-1). It is used to treat a poisoning or overdose when a substance is swallowed and is in the patient's digestive tract. Activated charcoal will adsorb some poisons (bind them to the surfaces of the charcoal) and help prevent them from being absorbed by the body. The procedure for administering activated charcoal will be found in Chapter 21, "Poisoning and Overdose Emergencies."

activated charcoal a powder, usually premixed with water, that will adsorb some poisons and help prevent them from being absorbed by the body.

Oral Glucose

Glucose is a kind of sugar. **Oral glucose** is a form of glucose that can be taken by mouth as a treatment for a conscious patient (who is able to swallow) with an altered mental status and a history of diabetes. The brain is very sensitive to low levels of sugar, which

oral glucose (GLU-kos) a form of glucose (a kind of sugar) given by mouth to treat an awake patient (who is able to swallow) with an altered mental status and a history of diabetes.

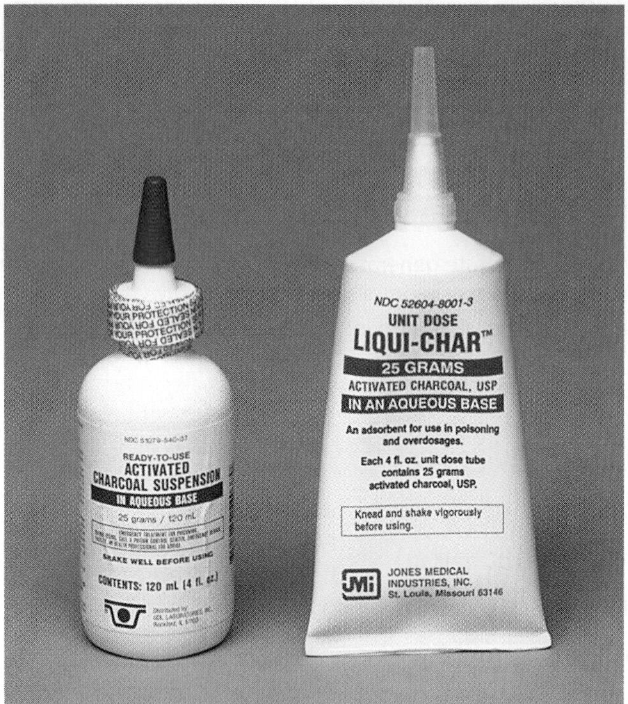

Figure 15-1 • Activated charcoal is often used in poisoning cases.

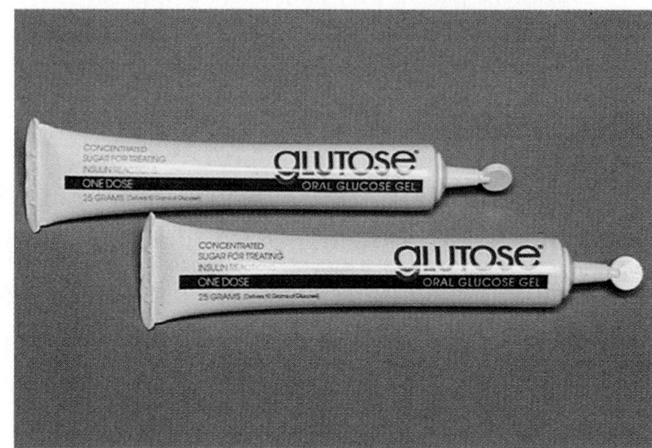

Figure 15-2 • Oral glucose may help a patient with diabetes.

can be caused by poorly managed diabetes, and this can be a cause of the altered mental status. Oral glucose usually comes as a tube of gel (Figure 15-2) that you can apply to a tongue depressor and place between the patient's cheek and gum or under the tongue. This allows the patient to swallow the glucose so it can be easily absorbed into the digestive tract and bloodstream, which carries it to the brain. This action may begin to reverse the patient's potentially life-threatening condition. The procedure for administering oral glucose will be found in Chapter 19, "Diabetic Emergencies and Altered Mental Status."

Oxygen

oxygen
a gas commonly found in the atmosphere. Pure oxygen is used as a drug to treat any patient whose medical or traumatic condition may cause him to be hypoxic, or low in oxygen.

Oxygen is a gas commonly found in the atmosphere. Pure oxygen is used as a drug to treat any patient whose medical or traumatic condition causes him to be hypoxic (low in oxygen) or in danger of becoming hypoxic (Figure 15-3). Throughout this text, you have learned—and will continue to learn—many situations in which a patient should

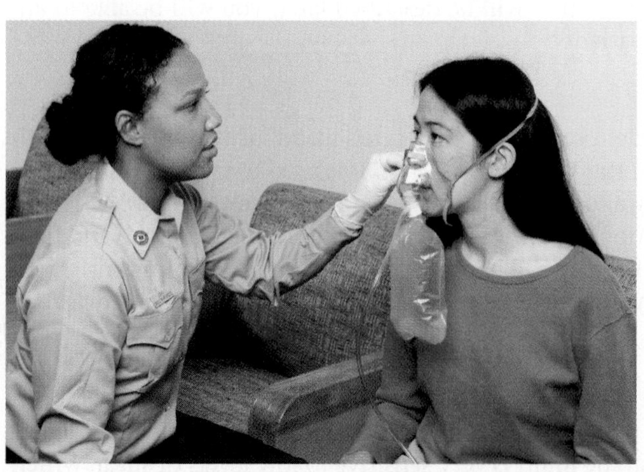

Figure 15-3 • Oxygen is a powerful drug.

POINT OF VIEW

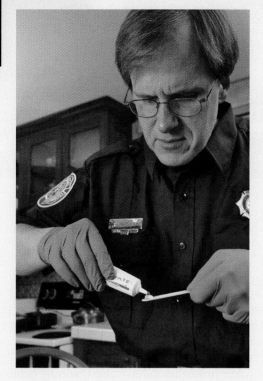

"I woke up and checked my blood sugar. It was a little higher than I expected. I ate a light breakfast and took a few extra units of insulin as my endocrinologist explained for me to do.

"The next thing I know my husband was looking very concerned. Then the ambulance showed up. I remember the EMTs being there, but I couldn't make out what they were saying. I remember wanting so much to talk to them but the words weren't coming out right.

"I saw the sugar. They put it in my mouth on the tongue blade. I am not sure how long it took. I was pretty out of it. But suddenly the world was again in focus—like someone adjusted the camera lens and everything was clear.

"I saw the EMTs smiling at me. My husband still had a worried look. But I was OK. I could think and talk and function again. I must have taken too much insulin or read the meter wrong. Thank goodness for the EMTs—and for that sugar."

be given oxygen. Specific methods of administering oxygen are explained in Chapter 6, "Airway Management."

Prescribed Medications

The three medications described next—prescribed inhaler, nitroglycerin, and epinephrine auto-injector—are drugs that you, as an EMT, may assist the patient in taking if they have been prescribed for the patient by a physician.

Prescribed Inhalers

Patients can carry various medications to help them through a period of difficulty breathing. Most often patients with diseases like asthma, emphysema, or chronic bronchitis carry a "bronchodilator," a medication designed to enlarge constricted bronchial tubes, making breathing easier. Many of these medications can be carried in an **inhaler,** which contains an aerosol form of a medication the patient can spray directly into his airway (Figure 15-4). Examples of these medications include: albuterol, Ventolin, Proventil, and Volmax.

inhaler
a spray device with a mouthpiece that contains an aerosol form of a medication that a patient can spray into his airway.

Since many bronchodilators also have an effect on the heart, an increased heart rate and patient jitteriness are common side effects of treatment.

Be sure to determine that the inhaler is actually the patient's and not that of a family member or bystander. You may need to have permission from medical direction to help a patient self-administer a prescribed inhaler. This permission from medical direction may come by phone or radio, or there may be a standing medical order that permits you to assist a patient with this kind of medication. *Always comply with the protocols of your EMS system.* More details on the use of a prescribed inhaler will be found in Chapter 16, "Respiratory Emergencies."

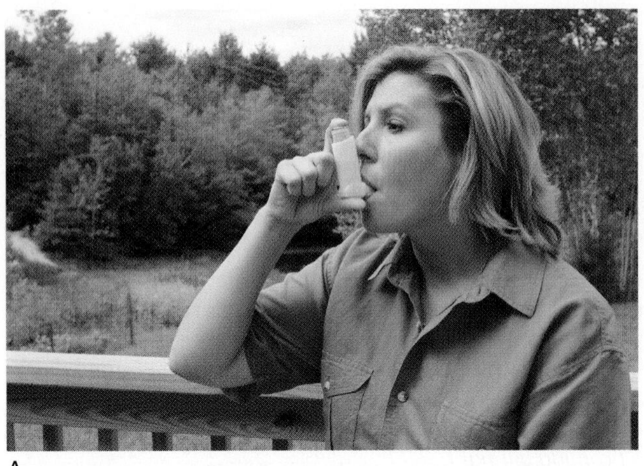

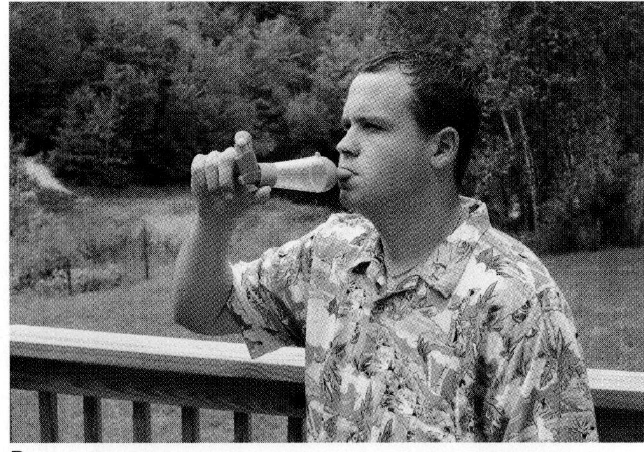

Figure 15-4 • (A) A prescribed inhaler may help a patient who has respiratory problems. (B) A spacer attached to the inhaler helps the patient by allowing the medication to be released into the spacer where it remains airborne for a time so the patient can inhale it without feeling rushed—as he would be if inhaling it directly, without the spacer.

Nitroglycerin

nitroglycerin (NYE-tro-GLIS-uh-rin) a drug that helps to dilate the coronary vessels that supply the heart muscle with blood.

Many patients with problems such as recurrent chest pain or a history of heart attack carry **nitroglycerin** pills or spray. Nitroglycerin (Figure 15-5) is a drug that helps to dilate the coronary vessels, which supply the heart muscle with blood. It is often called just "nitro." A common trade name is Nitrostat.

This drug is taken by the patient when he begins to have chest pain he believes to be cardiac in origin. It is not uncommon for EMTs to treat patients who have already taken a nitroglycerin pill or who are carrying a bottle of nitroglycerin tablets and have not thought to try one. (Many patients are instructed by their physician to take up to three nitroglycerin pills for their chest pain and, if the chest pain persists, to call EMS.)

Be sure to determine that the nitroglycerin is actually the patient's and not that of a family member or bystander. Also determine whether the patient has recently taken anything to treat erectile dysfunction, such as Viagra (sildenafil), Levitra (vardenafil), or similar medication. If so, he should not also take nitroglycerin because of the possibility of serious negative interaction.

Since nitro causes a dilation of blood vessels, a drop in the patient's blood pressure is always a potential side effect of administration. If this should occur, you may also need to lay the patient down and raise his legs as you recontact medical direction for advice.

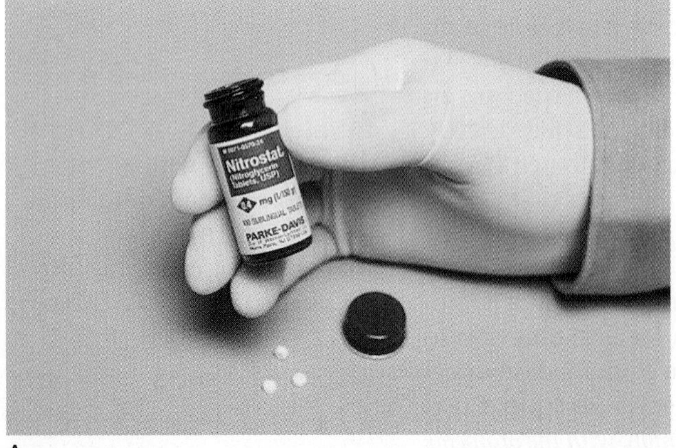

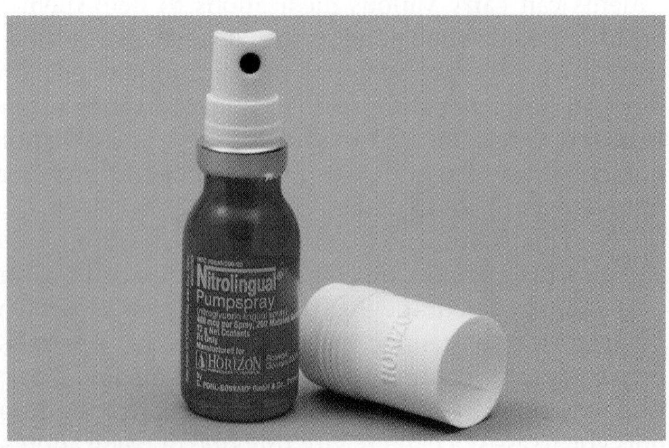

Figure 15-5 • Nitroglycerin is often prescribed for chest pain. Forms of nitroglycerin include (A) tablets or (B) a spray.

You may need to seek permission from medical direction by phone or radio, or there may be a standing medical order that permits you to assist a patient with nitroglycerin administration. *Always comply with the protocols of your EMS system.* More information on assisting a patient in taking nitroglycerin will be found in Chapter 17, "Cardiac Emergencies."

Epinephrine Auto-Injectors

When a patient is highly allergic to something like shellfish, penicillin, or a bee sting, he may have a very severe reaction that may cause life-threatening changes in the airway and circulation. The reaction can be reversed by using **epinephrine,** a medication that will help to constrict the blood vessels and relax airway passages.

epinephrine (ep-uh-NEF-rin) a drug that helps to constrict the blood vessels and relax passages of the airway. It may be used to counter a severe allergic reaction.

Because severe allergic reactions may reach a life-threatening stage in a very short time, epinephrine must be administered quickly. Many patients who are prone to severe allergic reactions carry an epinephrine auto-injector (Figure 15-6). This is a syringe with a spring-loaded needle that will release and inject epinephrine into the muscle when the auto-injector is pushed against the thigh. Epi-Pen® is the trade name of a commonly carried epinephrine auto-injector. Twinject® is the trade name of an auto-injector that contains two doses of epinephrine. If you need to assist a patient with the use of an epinephrine auto-injector, be sure to determine that the auto-injector is actually the patient's and not that of someone else.

Since epinephrine has a potent effect on the heart and vascular system, increased heart rate and blood pressure commonly occur after its administration to the patient.

You may need to seek permission from medical direction by phone or radio, or there may be a standing medical order that permits you to assist a patient with an epinephrine auto-injector. *Always comply with the protocols of your EMS system.* More information on assisting a patient in using an epinephrine auto-injector will be found in Chapter 20, "Allergic Reactions."

NOTE

An increasing number of states are expanding the scope of practice to allow the basic-level EMT to carry and use an epinephrine auto-injector to treat life threatening allergic reactions. The authority to administer epinephrine to the patient, rather than to assist a patient in the use of his own auto-injector, is normally granted by the Medical Director only after the EMT has received additional education and testing.

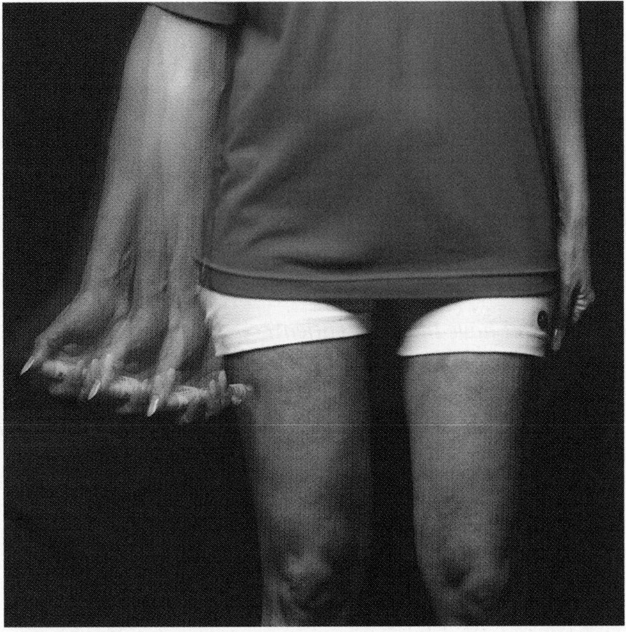

Figure 15-6 • An epinephrine auto-injector can reverse a severe allergic reaction.

GENERAL INFORMATION ABOUT MEDICATIONS

Drug Names

Every drug or medication is listed in the *U.S. Pharmacopoeia* (USP), which is a comprehensive government publication. Each drug is listed by its generic name (a general name that is not the brand name of any manufacturer). However, each drug actually has at least three names: the chemical name, the generic name, and one or more trade (brand) names given the drug by various manufacturers. For example, *epinephrine* is a generic drug name. Its chemical name is B-(3, 4 dihydroxyphenyl)-a-methylaminoethanol. (Chemical names are technical formulas used only by scientists or manufacturers.) As mentioned earlier, Epi-Pen® is the trade name of an epinephrine auto-injector.

What You Need to Know When Giving a Medication

indications
specific signs or circumstances under which it is appropriate to administer a drug to a patient.

contraindications
(KON-truh-in-duh-KAY-shunz) specific signs or circumstances under which it is not appropriate and may be harmful to administer a drug to a patient.

side effect
any action of a drug other than the desired action.

Every drug has **indications,** or specific signs, symptoms, or circumstances under which it is appropriate to administer the drug to a patient. For example, nitroglycerin is indicated when a patient has chest pain or squeezing, dull pressure. Each drug also has **contraindications,** or specific signs, symptoms, or circumstances under which it is not appropriate, and may be harmful, to administer the drug to the patient. For example, nitroglycerin is contraindicated (should not be given) if the patient has low blood pressure, because nitroglycerin, in dilating the arteries, causes a slight drop in the systolic blood pressure. As noted earlier, nitroglycerin is also contraindicated if the patient has recently taken Viagra or a similar medication because of possible serious negative interactions.

A **side effect** is any action of a drug other than the desired actions. Some side effects are predictable, like the drop in blood pressure from nitroglycerin. If you were not aware of the side effect of a drop in blood pressure and gave the drug to a patient who started out with low blood pressure, the results could be devastating. The patient's blood pressure might "bottom out"—which is definitely not a desirable effect for a cardiac patient.

Medications come in many different forms. A few examples are:

- Compressed powders or tablets, such as nitroglycerin pills
- Liquids for injection, such as the epinephrine in an auto-injector
- Gels, such as the paste in a tube of oral glucose
- Suspensions, such as the thick slurry of activated charcoal in water
- Fine powder for inhalation, such as that in a prescribed inhaler
- Gases for inhalation, such as oxygen
- Sublingual (under-the-tongue) sprays such as a nitroglycerin spray
- Liquid that is vaporized, such as a fixed-dose nebulizer

Before administering a drug to any patient, confirm the order and write it down. Then check the "four rights" by asking yourself the following questions as you select the medication and confirm that it is not expired:

- *Do I have the right patient?*
- *Is this the right medication?*
- *Is this the right dose?* Generally, a dose is given in milligrams.
- *Am I giving this medication by the right route of administration?*

The route by which the drug is administered affects the rate that the medication enters the bloodstream and arrives at its target organ to achieve its desired effect. Routes of administration include:

- Oral, or swallowed
- Sublingual, or dissolved under the tongue

It would be impossible to learn and carry around in your head all the types of medications you might discover your patients are taking. However, the medications a patient is taking may be a clue to a pre-existing medical condition or, if improperly used, a cause of the patient's current problem. For example, a patient who is taking antihypertensives and antidiabetics might also be taking or misusing other medications that can contribute to an altered mental status—perhaps Dilantin to control seizures, codeine for pain, or Inderal for a heart rhythm disorder. Some medications that may be prescribed to a patient for daily use in managing a respiratory condition (one example would be beclomethasone, another would be Advair, Figure 15-7) should not be used to reverse an acute attack or to alleviate breathing difficulty.

It is a good idea to have a resource from which you can find out additional information about a patient's medications en route to the hospital. Many ambulances

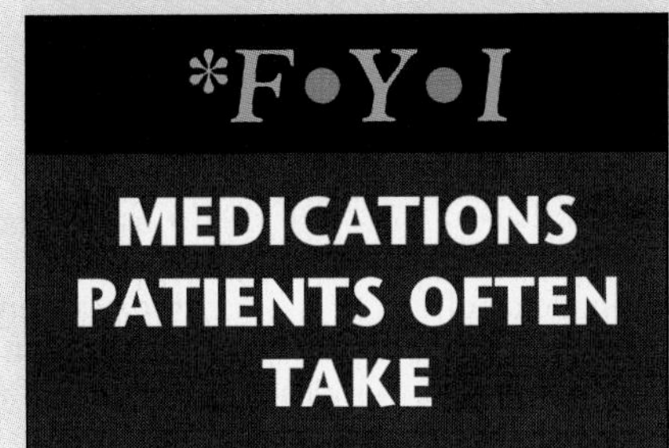

carry a *Physician's Desk Reference,* or *PDR,* for this purpose. Most EMTs carry, or have available to them, a pocket guide that contains useful information such as commonly used abbreviations. These pocket guides usually list the most commonly prescribed medications along with the general category of that medication to help you understand what the medication may be used for. A high-tech version of this guide is available that can be carried on a personal digital assistant (PDA). This approach has the advantages of often being more comprehensive than the paper version and more easily updated over the Internet. Several PDA-compatible programs are available, some of them at very little cost. However, remember that your main purpose in finding out what medications the patient is taking is not to make a diagnosis but to report this information to medical direction and hospital personnel.

Table 15-1 lists the seven most common categories of medications you will find in the field that are relevant to patient care, with a few examples of medications in each category. Table 15-2 lists some common herbal agents patients sometimes take. A sizable number of people use these preparations, but they do not always think of them as medications that they should tell you about when you ask them what medications they take. Some of these agents have powerful effects, both intended and unintended, and should be recorded on the prehospital care report. Many also have interactions with prescription or over-the-counter medications. There are many other drugs and drug categories in addition to those listed in the table.

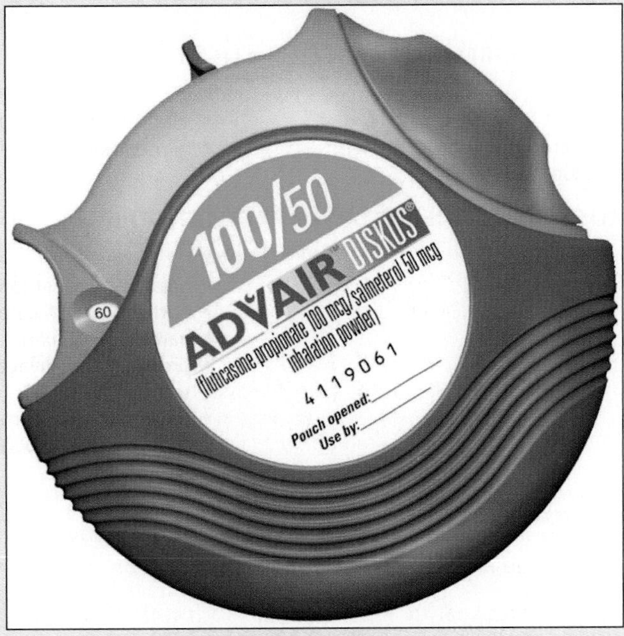

Figure 15-7 • Advair is a medication that may be prescribed to a patient for daily management of a respiratory disease. It should not be used for emergency treatment of an acute attack or breathing difficulty. *(© GlaxoSmithKline)*

TABLE 15-1 • Medications Patients Often Take

ANALGESICS: DRUGS PRESCRIBED FOR PAIN RELIEF

- propoxyphene (Darvon)
- nalbuphine (Nubain)
- morphine (Astramorph PF, Duramorph, MS Contin, Roxanol)
- acetaminophen (Anacin-3, Panadol, Tempra, Tylenol)
- ibuprofen (Actiprofen, Advil, Excedrin IS, Motrin, Novoprofen, Nuprin)
- aspirin (Ecotrin, Emprin)
- codeine
- oxycodone (OxyContin)
- naproxen (Naprosyn)
- indomethacin (Indocin)

ANTIDYSRHYTHMICS: DRUGS PRESCRIBED FOR HEART RHYTHM DISORDERS

- digoxin (Lanoxin)
- propranolol (Inderal)
- verapamil (Calan, Calan SR, Isoptin, Isoptin SR, Verelan)
- procainamide (Procan SR, Promine, Pronestyl)
- disopyramide (Norpace)
- carvedilol (Coreg)
- metoprolol (Lopressor, Toprol XL)

ANTICONVULSANTS: DRUGS PRESCRIBED FOR PREVENTION AND CONTROL OF SEIZURES

- carbamazepine (Epitol, Tegretol)
- phenytoin (Dilantin)
- primidone (Mysoline)
- phenobarbital (Phenobarbital, Phenobarbital Sodium, Solfoton)
- valproic acid (Depakene)
- lamotrigine (Lamictal)
- topiramate (Topamax)
- ethosuximide (Zarontin)
- gabapentin (Neurontin)

ANTIHYPERTENSIVES: DRUGS PRESCRIBED TO REDUCE HIGH BLOOD PRESSURE

- captopril (Capoten)
- clonidine (Catapres)
- guanabenz (Wytensin)
- hydralazine (Apresoline, Hydralazine HCL)
- hydrochlorothiazide (Esidrix, HydroDiuril, Oretic)
- methyldopa (Aldomet)
- nifedipine (Adalat, Adalat CC, Procardia)
- prazosin (Minipress)

BRONCHODILATORS: DRUGS THAT RELAX THE SMOOTH MUSCLES OF THE BRONCHIAL TUBES. THESE MEDICATIONS PROVIDE RELIEF OF BRONCHIAL ASTHMA AND ALLERGIES AFFECTING THE RESPIRATORY SYSTEM

- albuterol (Proventil, Ventolin, Volmax)
- isoetharine (Bronkometer, Bronkosol)
- metaproterenol (Alupent, Metaproterenol Sulfate, Metaprel)
- terbutaline (Brethaire, Brethine, Bricanyl)
- ipratropium (Atrovent)
- salmeterol (Serevent)
- albuterol/ipratropium (Combivent, DuoNeb)
- montelukast (Singulair)
- zafirlukast (Accolate)

ANTIDIABETIC AGENTS: DRUGS PRESCRIBED TO DIABETIC PATIENTS TO CONTROL HYPERGLYCEMIA (HIGH BLOOD SUGAR)

- glipizide (Glucotrol)
- glyburide (DiaBeta, Glynase PresTab, Micronase)
- insulin (Humulin, Novolin, NPH, Humalog)
- metformin (Glucophage)
- glimepiride (Amaryl)

ANTIDEPRESSANT AGENTS: DRUGS PRESCRIBED TO HELP REGULATE THE EMOTIONAL ACTIVITY OF THE PATIENT TO MINIMIZE THE PEAKS AND VALLEYS IN THEIR PSYCHOLOGICAL AND EMOTIONAL STATE

- amitriptyline (Elavil)
- amoxapine
- bupropion (Wellbutrin)
- clomipramine (Anafranil)
- venlafaxine (Effexor)
- escitalopram (Lexapro)
- fluoxetine (Prozac)
- imipramine (Tofranil, Tripamine)
- nefazodone (Serzone)
- nortriptyline (Aventyl, Pamelor)
- paroxetine (Paxil)
- protriptyline (Vivactil)
- sertraline (Zoloft)
- trimipramine (Surmontil)
- citalopram (Celexa)

Note: Generic names are lowercase. Trade names are capitalized.

TABLE 15-2 • Herbal Agents and What They Are Sometimes Used For

HERBAL AGENT	SOMETIMES USED FOR
Gingko or gingkobiloba	Dementia, poor circulation to the legs, ringing in the ears
St. John's wort	Depression
Echinacea	Prevention and treatment of common cold
Garlic	High cholesterol
Ginger root	Nausea and vomiting
Saw palmetto	Swollen prostate
Hawthorn leaf or flower	Heart failure
Evening primrose oil	Premenstrual syndrome
Feverfew leaf	Migraine prevention
Kava kava	Anxiety
Valerian root	Insomnia

- Inhaled, or breathed into the lungs, usually in tiny aerosol particles as from an inhaler or as a gas such as oxygen
- Intravenous, or injected into a vein
- Intramuscular, or injected into a muscle
- Subcutaneous, or injected under the skin
- Endotracheal, or sprayed directly into a tube inserted into the trachea

After any medication is given to a patient, it is important that you reassess the patient to see how the drug has affected him. Obtain another set of vital signs and compare them to the vital signs that you took before administering the medication. Ongoing patient assessment should include an evaluation of the changes in the patient's condition and vital signs after administration of medication. Be sure to document the patient's response to each drug intervention. For example, "The patient's respiratory distress decreased after 5 minutes of high-concentration oxygen by nonrebreather mask."

CRITICAL DECISION MAKING:
How or Whether to Assist with Medications

Your decisions on how to assist patients with their medications—or whether to assist them at all—are a critical part of your practice as an EMT. The following questions will test your knowledge and decision making in this vital area.

1. You are treating a patient who has chest pain. He tells you his wife has nitroglycerin. He asks if he should take her pills. What should you tell him?
2. You are treating a patient who is diabetic. She appears very sleepy and only responds to loud verbal stimulus by briefly opening her eyes. The patient's sister says, "Give her some sugar!" Should you? Why or why not?
3. Your COPD patient is breathing 48 times per minute shallowly. His wife believes his "lung problems" have been acting up. Would the patient's inhaler help him?

CHAPTER REVIEW

SUMMARY

Activated charcoal, oral glucose, and oxygen are medications carried on the ambulance that the EMT may administer to a patient under specific conditions. Prescribed inhalers, nitroglycerin, and epinephrine in auto-injectors are medications that, if prescribed for the patient, the EMT may assist the patient in taking. You may need to have permission from medical direction to administer or assist the patient with a medication. Follow local protocols.

There is a wide variety of medications that a patient may be taking. You will try to find out what medications a patient is taking when you take the SAMPLE history. These drugs may be identified by a variety of generic and trade names. Your main purpose in finding out what medications the patient is taking is to report this information to your Medical Director or hospital personnel.

KEY TERMS

activated charcoal a powder, usually premixed with water, that will adsorb some poisons and help prevent them from being absorbed by the body.

contraindications (KON-truh-in-duh-KAY-shunz) specific signs or circumstances under which it is not appropriate and may be harmful to administer a drug to a patient.

epinephrine (ep-uh-NEF-rin) a drug that helps to constrict the blood vessels and relax passages of the airway. It may be used to counter a severe allergic reaction.

indications specific signs or circumstances under which it is appropriate to administer a drug to a patient.

inhaler a spray device with a mouthpiece that contains an aerosol form of a medication that a patient can spray into his airway.

nitroglycerin (NYE-tro-GLIS-uh-rin) a drug that helps to dilate the coronary vessels that supply the heart muscle with blood.

oral glucose (GLU-kos) a form of glucose (a kind of sugar) given by mouth to treat an awake patient (who is able to swallow) with an altered mental status and a history of diabetes.

oxygen a gas commonly found in the atmosphere. Pure oxygen is used as a drug to treat any patient whose medical or traumatic condition may cause him to be hypoxic, or low in oxygen.

pharmacology (FARM-uh-KOL-uh-je) the study of drugs, their sources, characteristics, and effects.

side effect any action of a drug other than the desired action.

REVIEW QUESTIONS

1. Name the drugs that are carried on the ambulance and may be administered by the EMT under certain circumstances. (pp. 355–366)
2. Name the drugs that the EMT may assist the patient in taking if they have been prescribed for him and with approval by medical direction. (pp. 357–359)
3. Medications may take the form of tablets. Name several other forms that medications may have. (p. 360)
4. Name the four "rights" you must check before administering a medication. (p. 360)
5. Name several routes by which medications may be administered. (pp. 360, 363)

CRITICAL THINKING

- A patient is complaining of chest pain. "Here's some nitroglycerin," says a family member. "Give him that." What do you do?

MEDIA RESOURCES 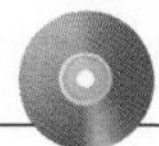

See the Student CD at the back of this book for quizzes, a case study, and other features related to this chapter. Also, visit the Companion Website for *Emergency Care* at **www.prenhall.com/limmer**, where you will find additional reinforcement and links to other resources.

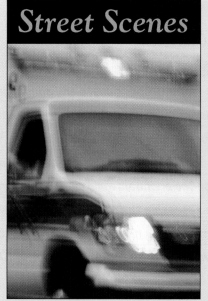

Street Scenes

It is winter and cold, so you are not too surprised when the dispatcher tells you to respond to the mall for a 62-year-old male patient with chest pain. During winter, many cardiac patients walk for exercise in the mall, and this is not the first cardiac call you have had there. When you arrive, you find the patient sitting in a chair. You introduce yourself and your partner, ask the patient his name, and then say, "Well, Mr. Edwards, why was EMS called?"

"I was doing my usual morning walk," he explains, "when I started to get chest pain. I thought it might go away but it didn't. I got concerned and asked the security guard to call 911."

As your partner administers oxygen by nonrebreather mask and takes a set of vital signs, you ask the patient: "On a scale of 1 to 10, with 10 being the worst pain you've ever had, how would you rate the chest pain you're having now?" He tells you that it is a 7. You ask him to describe the pain and to point to where it is located. He says that it feels like a dull pain and points to the center of his chest. He also says the pain does not radiate. The patient seems pale, and his skin is dry. After a bit more questioning, he tells you the last time this happened he took nitro for relief.

Street Scene Questions

1. What additional patient history should you obtain?
2. Should you let the patient take nitroglycerin? Why, or why not?
3. Are vital signs important if nitroglycerin is going to be taken by the patient?

You ask Mr. Edwards if he has nitroglycerin with him now. He says his wife has it, but she went to a store in another part of the mall and should be back shortly. You then ask about other medications, and the patient tells you he is on propranolol and a diuretic. Next, you ask if he has ever had a heart attack. The patient tells you that he had one about a year and a half ago with an angioplasty. Vital signs are: pulse 90, blood pressure 120/90, and respirations of 24 and labored. When his wife shows up, she attempts to administer a pill, but you ask her to wait.

Street Scene Questions

4. What information do you want to know about the nitroglycerin?
5. How should the nitroglycerin be administered?
6. When should vital signs be taken again?

At your request, the patient's wife gives you the nitroglycerin bottle so you can check the expiration date. At the same time, you check to make sure that it is the patient's specific prescription. It all checks. According to standing orders in your system, with these signs and symptoms including a systolic blood pressure over 100, a nitro may be given without radio contact with medical direction. You tell the patient that you are going to put the pill under his tongue and he should let it dissolve. You specifically tell Mr. Edwards not to swallow.

About a minute after the patient is given the pill, he complains of a slight headache. You tell him this is a possible side effect of taking nitro and not to be concerned. After another minute goes by, you ask the patient to rate the chest pain on a scale of 1 to 10 again. About a 2 he replies. "In fact, the pain is almost gone," he tells you. Your partner takes another set of vital signs because blood pressure can drop with nitro, but there is no change. You package the patient for transport and move to the ambulance, making sure you keep the AED close by. You give Mrs. Edwards a short update and explain to her that you will take the nitroglycerin bottle with the patient. The transport to the hospital is uneventful with another set of vital signs taken en route.

Street Scenes Sample Documentation

PATIENT NAME: Francis Edwards **PATIENT AGE:** 62

CHIEF COMPLAINT

"Chest pain"

PAST MEDICAL HISTORY

- [ ] None
- [ ] Allergy to ______
- [ ] Hypertension
- [ ] Stroke
- [ ] Seizures
- [ ] Diabetes
- [ ] COPD
- [ ] Cardiac
- [ ] Other (List)
- [ ] Asthma

Previous MI, angioplasty

Current Medications (List)

nitroglycerin, propranolol, lasix

VITAL SIGNS

TIME	RESP	PULSE	B.P.	MENTAL STATUS	R PUPILS L	SKIN
1000	Rate: 24 [ ] Regular [ ] Shallow [x] Labored	Rate: 90 [x] Regular [ ] Irregular	120/90	[x] Alert [ ] Voice [ ] Pain [ ] Unresp.	[x] Normal [x] [ ] Dilated [ ] [ ] Constricted [ ] [ ] Sluggish [ ] [ ] No-Reaction [ ]	[ ] Unremarkable [ ] Cool [x] Pale [x] Warm [ ] Cyanotic [ ] Moist [ ] Flushed [x] Dry [ ] Jaundiced
1015	Rate: 20 [x] Regular [ ] Shallow [ ] Labored	Rate: 90 [x] Regular [ ] Irregular	120/90	[x] Alert [ ] Voice [ ] Pain [ ] Unresp.	[x] Normal [x] [ ] Dilated [ ] [ ] Constricted [ ] [ ] Sluggish [ ] [ ] No-Reaction [ ]	[ ] Unremarkable [ ] Cool [x] Pale [x] Warm [ ] Cyanotic [ ] Moist [ ] Flushed [x] Dry [ ] Jaundiced
1030	Rate: 18 [x] Regular [ ] Shallow [ ] Labored	Rate: 80 [x] Regular [ ] Irregular	110/palpation	[x] Alert [ ] Voice [ ] Pain [ ] Unresp.	[x] Normal [x] [ ] Dilated [ ] [ ] Constricted [ ] [ ] Sluggish [ ] [ ] No-Reaction [ ]	[ ] Unremarkable [ ] Cool [x] Pale [x] Warm [ ] Cyanotic [ ] Moist [ ] Flushed [x] Dry [ ] Jaundiced

NARRATIVE On arrival we were met by a conscious, alert, somewhat anxious 62-year-old male with a chief complaint of a sudden onset of substernal chest pain while walking. He is sitting upright in a chair, somewhat ashen. Upon questioning, patient states that the pain is similar to previous cardiac-related chest discomfort and is 7 on the 10 scale. He denies any radiation down his arm or toward his jaw. He also denies any relief with the brief wait while sitting. Our treatment begins with O_2 at 10 LPM via nonrebreather. While we were assessing the patient, his wife arrived with his nitroglycerin prescription. Administered one of patient's 0.4 mg nitro sublingually per BLS protocol at 10:20. Patient states significant relief with the nitro and O_2 prior to transport (2 out of 10). Repeat vital signs obtained.

CHAPTER

16

Respiratory Emergencies

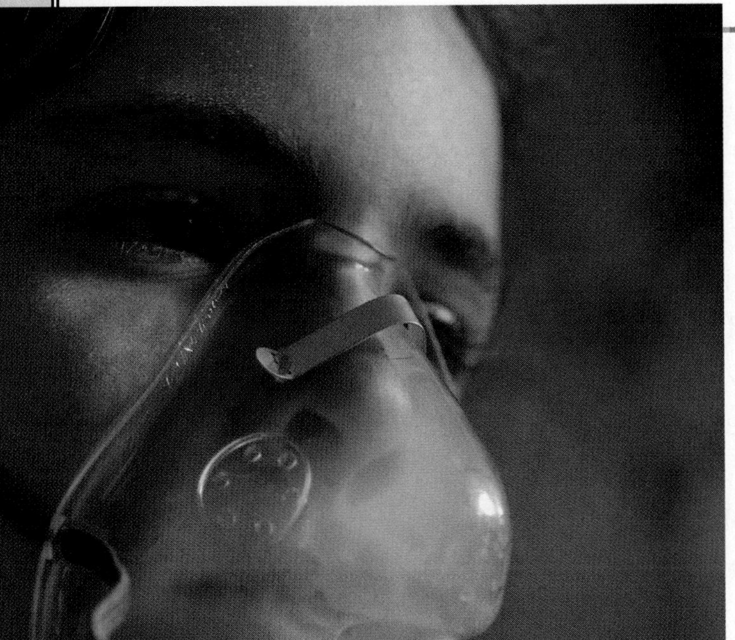

CORE CONCEPTS

The following are core concepts that will be addressed in this chapter:

- The difference between adequate and inadequate air exchange
- How to identify and treat a patient with breathing difficulty
- Use of a prescribed inhaler and how to assist a patient with one
- How to document findings and care of a patient with breathing difficulty

KEY TERMS

bronchoconstriction, p. 380
exhalation, p. 369
expiration, p. 369
inhalation, p. 369
inspiration, p. 369

DOT OBJECTIVES

*KNOWLEDGE AND ATTITUDE

4-2.1 List the structure and function of the respiratory system. (pp. 368–369)

4-2.2 State the signs and symptoms of a patient with breathing difficulty. (pp. 370–372, 374–376)

4-2.3 Describe the emergency medical care of the patient with breathing difficulty. (pp. 371–372, 376)

4-2.4 Recognize the need for medical direction to assist in the emergency medical care of the patient with breathing difficulty. (pp. 376, 381)

4-2.5 Describe the emergency medical care of the patient with breathing distress. (pp. 371–372, 376)

4-2.6 Establish the relationship between airway management and the patient with breathing difficulty. (pp. 371, 373, 374)

4-2.7 List signs of adequate air exchange. (pp. 369–370, 372)

4-2.8 State the generic name, medication forms, dose, administration, action, indications, and contraindications for the prescribed inhaler. (p. 380) (Scan 16-1, p. 382; Scan 16-2, p. 383)

4-2.9 Distinguish between the emergency medical care of the infant, child, and adult patient with breathing difficulty. (pp. 371, 373)

4-2.10 Differentiate between upper airway obstruction and lower airway disease in the infant and child patient. (p. 373)

4-2.11 Defend EMT treatment regimens for various respiratory emergencies. (pp. 371–372, 376)

4-2.12 Explain the rationale for administering an inhaler. (p. 380)

*SKILLS

4-2.13 Demonstrate the emergency medical care for breathing difficulty.

4-2.14 Perform the steps in facilitating the use of an inhaler.

As an EMT, you will encounter some patients who are having breathing difficulty but who nevertheless are breathing adequately. You will provide oxygen by nonrebreather mask to these patients and complete an on-scene assessment before transporting them to the hospital. At other times, you will encounter patients whose respiratory problems are more severe. They may be having such extreme difficulty moving air in and out of their lungs that their breathing is no longer adequate to support life. These patients will require much more rapid care, which will probably include assisted ventilations.

The difference between adequate and inadequate breathing is one of the most important concepts in this chapter.

RESPIRATION

Respiratory Anatomy and Physiology

You learned about the respiratory system in Chapter 4, "The Human Body," and in Chapter 6, "Airway Management." In preparation for this chapter, you should review in those chapters the following structures of the respiratory system: nose, mouth, oropharynx, nasopharynx, epiglottis, trachea, cricoid cartilage, larynx, bronchi, lungs, alveoli, and diaphragm.

The diaphragm is a muscular structure that divides the chest cavity from the abdominal cavity. During a normal respiratory cycle, the diaphragm and other parts of the body work together to allow the body to inhale (breathe in) and exhale (breathe out) air. The respiratory cycle progresses as follows (Figure 16-1):

- *Inspiration.* The active process that uses the contraction of several muscles to increase the size of the chest cavity is called **inspiration.** The intercostal (rib) muscles and the diaphragm contract. The diaphragm lowers and the ribs move upward and outward. The expanding size of the chest cavity causes air to flow into the lungs. Another term for inspiration is **inhalation.**
- *Expiration.* A passive process, **expiration** involves the relaxation of the rib muscles and diaphragm. The ribs move downward and inward, while the diaphragm rises. This movement causes the chest cavity to decrease in size and causes air to flow out of the lungs. Another term for expiration is **exhalation.**

inspiration
(IN-spuh-RAY-shun)
an active process in which the intercostal (rib) muscles and the diaphragm contract, expanding the size of the chest cavity and causing air to flow into the lungs.

inhalation
(IN-huh-LAY-shun)
another term for inspiration.

expiration
(EK-spuh-RAY-shun)
a passive process in which the intercostal (rib) muscles and the diaphragm relax, causing the chest cavity to decrease in size and forcing air from the lungs.

exhalation
(EX-huh-LAY-shun)
another term for expiration.

Review in Chapter 4 how oxygen and carbon dioxide are exchanged through the alveoli and capillaries of the lungs, and through the capillaries and cells throughout the body. The exchange of oxygen and carbon dioxide, both in the lungs and in the body's cells, is critical to support life. There are many things that can go wrong within the body that will alter this vital exchange. Primarily, these problems are with the respiratory system or the circulatory system. This chapter will discuss the respiratory system, problems with breathing, and their effects on the body. Problems with the circulatory system will be discussed in Chapter 17, "Cardiac Emergencies."

Adequate Breathing

It is easy to take breathing for granted. Fortunately, we do not consciously have to tell ourselves to inhale and exhale. The brain does that automatically.

As you learned in Chapter 6, "Airway Management," breathing may be classified as adequate or inadequate. Simply stated, adequate breathing is breathing that is sufficient to support life. Inadequate breathing is not. Your assessment of the adequacy of a patient's breathing may be vital to his survival.

Adequate breathing falls within certain ranges that are considered "normal." The patient will not appear to be in distress. He will be able to speak full sentences without having to catch his breath. His color, mental status, and orientation will be normal. Normal breathing may be determined by observing for rate, rhythm, and quality:

- *Rate.* Rates of breathing that are considered normal vary by age. For an adult, a normal rate is 12–20 breaths per minute. For a child, it is 15–30 breaths per minute. For an infant, it is 25–50 breaths per minute.

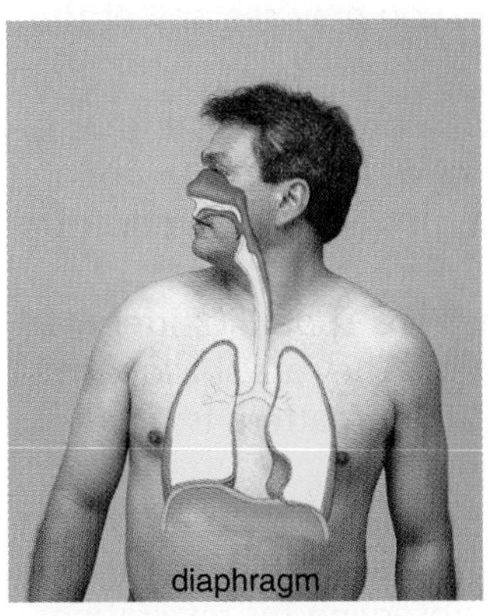

RELAXED

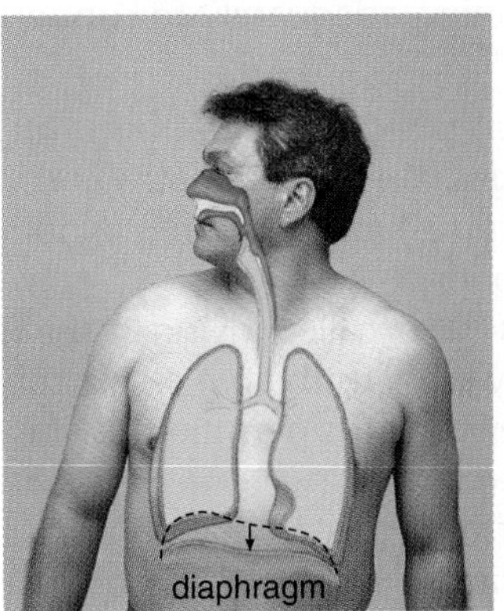

CONTRACTION
Inspiration begins

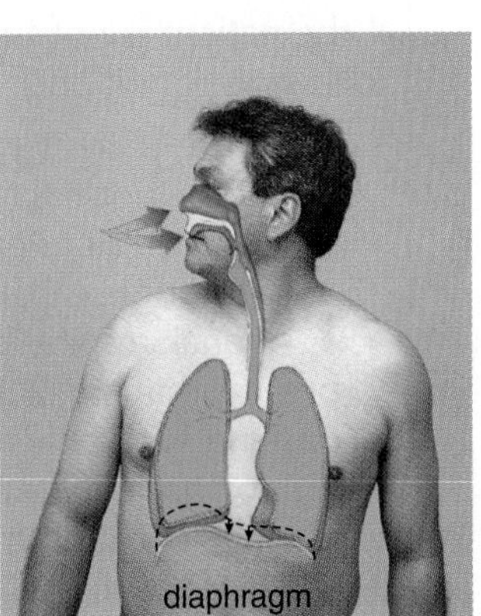

INSPIRATION

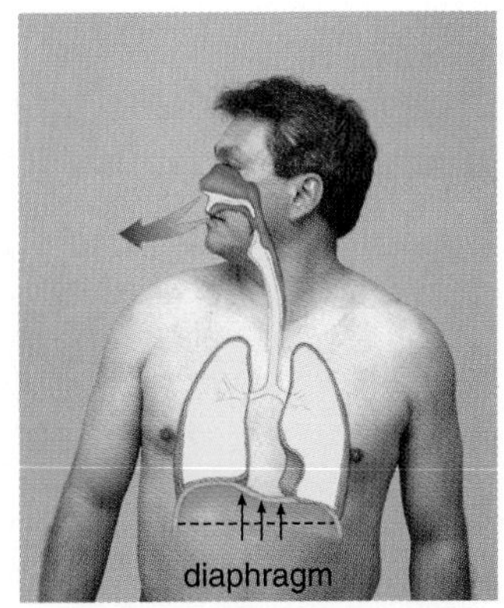

RELAXED
Passive expiration begins

Figure 16-1 • The process of respiration.

TABLE 16-1 • Adequate and Inadequate Breathing

	ADEQUATE BREATHING	INADEQUATE BREATHING
Rate	Adult: 12–20/minute Child: 15–30/minute Infant: 25–50/minute	Above or below normal rates for the patient's age group
Rhythm	Regular	May be irregular
Quality Breath Sounds Chest Expansion Effort of Breathing	Present and equal Adequate and equal Unlabored, normal respiratory effort	Diminished, unequal, or absent Inadequate or unequal Labored: increased respiratory effort; use of accessory muscles (may be pronounced in infants and children and involve nasal flaring, seesaw breathing, grunting, and retractions between the ribs and above the clavicles and sternum)
Depth	Adequate	Too shallow

- *Rhythm.* Normal breathing rhythm will usually be regular. Breaths will be taken at regular intervals and will last for about the same length of time. Remember that talking and other factors can make normal breathing slightly irregular.
- *Quality.* Breath sounds, when auscultated with a stethoscope, will normally be present and equal when the lungs are compared to each other. When observing the chest cavity, both sides should move equally and adequately to indicate a proper air exchange. The depth of the respirations must be adequate.

Inadequate Breathing

Inadequate breathing is breathing that is not sufficient to support life. If left untreated, this condition will surely lead to death. One of your most important tasks as an EMT is to identify and treat patients with inadequate breathing. Begin assessment and treatment early in the call and continue them throughout your time with the patient. Patients who are breathing adequately at first may deteriorate into inadequate breathing later on (Table 16-1).

PATIENT ASSESSMENT

INADEQUATE BREATHING

If the patient is not breathing adequately to support life, you may see any of the following conditions:

- *Rate.* The patient with inadequate breathing will have a breathing rate that is out of the normal ranges. Very slow breaths and very rapid breaths may not allow enough air to enter the lungs, resulting in not enough oxygen being distributed throughout the body.

  Agonal respirations (also called dying respirations) are sporadic, irregular breaths that are usually seen just before respiratory arrest. They are shallow and gasping with only a few breaths per minute. This breathing pattern is clearly a sign of inadequate breathing.
- *Rhythm.* The rhythm of inadequate breathing may be irregular. However, rhythm is not an absolute indicator of adequate or inadequate breathing. Remember that someone who is talking or is aware that you are observing his respirations may have slight irregularities, even though his breathing is adequate. However, a patient may have a regular rhythm, even when his breathing is inadequate.

continued

PATIENT ASSESSMENT *(continued)*

- *Quality.* When breathing is inadequate, breath sounds may be diminished or absent. The depth of respirations (tidal volume) will be inadequate or shallow. Chest expansion may be inadequate or unequal and respiratory effort increased. You may note the use of accessory muscles (e.g., muscles of the neck and abdomen) in breathing. Since oxygenation of the body's tissues is reduced, the skin may be pale or cyanotic (blue) and feel cool and clammy to the touch.

  In patients with diminished responsiveness, sounds such as snoring and gurgling also indicate a serious airway problem that requires immediate intervention. ■

PEDIATRIC NOTE

Respiratory problems can be very serious in infants and children. Since children rarely have heart attacks or other problems of adulthood, respiratory conditions are a leading killer of infants and children. With this in mind, you must begin respiratory treatment of infants and children with a thorough and accurate assessment and prompt, proper care.

The structure of infants' and children's airways differs somewhat from that of adults:

- *Airway.* All airway structures are smaller in an infant or child than in an adult and therefore are more easily obstructed.
- *Tongue.* Infants' and children's tongues are proportionately larger and therefore take up more space in the mouth than an adult's tongue.
- *Trachea.* The trachea is smaller, softer, and more flexible in infants and children, which may lead to obstruction from swelling or trauma more easily than in adults. The cricoid cartilage is less developed and less rigid.
- *Diaphragm.* Infants and children depend more heavily on the diaphragm for respiration since the chest wall is softer. This is why infants and small children in respiratory distress exhibit "seesaw breathing" in which the movement of the diaphragm causes the chest and abdomen to move in opposite directions.

Be aware that some signs of inadequate breathing are unique to or more prominent in infants and children. Therefore, be on the lookout for these signs:

- Nasal flaring (widening of the nostrils)
- Grunting
- Seesaw breathing
- Retractions (pulling in of the muscles) between the ribs (intercostal), above the clavicles (supraclavicular), and above the sternum (suprasternal)

PATIENT CARE

INADEQUATE BREATHING

There is a wide range of function between adequate respirations and complete stoppage of breathing (respiratory arrest). You must pay careful attention to the patient's breathing throughout the call. It is not enough to simply make sure he is breathing. The patient must be breathing adequately! If at any time you find that he is not breathing adequately, the treatment of this condition is your first patient-care priority (Table 16-2).

When you determine, by the signs that were discussed under the previous Patient Assessment feature, that a patient's breathing is inadequate, you will provide assisted ventilation with supplemental oxygen. In order of preference, the means of providing assisted ventilation are:

1. Pocket face mask with supplemental oxygen
2. Two-rescuer bag-valve mask with supplemental oxygen
3. Flow-restricted, oxygen-powered ventilation device
4. One-rescuer bag-valve mask with supplemental oxygen

continued

The means of providing artificial ventilation were discussed in Chapter 6, "Airway Management." Make sure that you are properly trained with the device that you are using for ventilation. If supplemental oxygen is not immediately available, begin artificial ventilation without supplemental oxygen and attach the oxygen supply to the mask as soon as it is available.

If you are uncertain about whether a patient's breathing is inadequate and requires artificial ventilation, provide artificial ventilation. In the rare circumstance when a patient with inadequate breathing is conscious enough to fight artificial ventilation, transport immediately and consult medical direction. ■

TABLE 16-2 • Respiratory Conditions with Appropriate Interventions

CONDITION	SIGNS	EMT INTERVENTION	
ADEQUATE BREATHING Patient is breathing adequately but needs supplemental oxygen due to a medical or traumatic condition	• Rate and depth of breathing are adequate • No abnormal breath sounds • Air moves freely in and out of the chest • Skin color normal	Oxygen by non-rebreather mask or nasal cannula	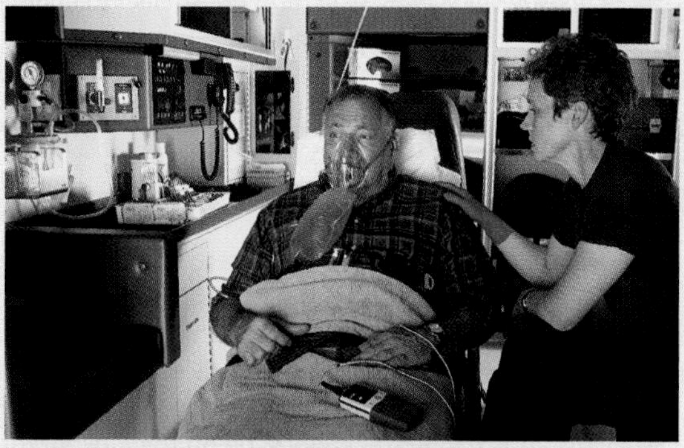
INADEQUATE BREATHING Patient is moving some air in and out but it is slow or shallow and not enough to live.	• Patient has some breathing but not enough to live • Rate and/or depth outside of normal limits • Shallow ventilations • Diminished or absent breath sounds • Noises such as crowing, stridor, snoring, gurgling, or gasping • Blue (cyanosis) or gray skin color • Decreased minute volume	Assisted ventilations (air put into the lungs under pressure) with a pocket face mask, bag-valve-mask, or FROPVD. See chapter text about adjusting rates for rapid or slow breathing. *Note: A nonrebreather mask requires adequate breathing to pull oxygen into the lungs. It DOES NOT provide ventilation to a patient who is not breathing or who is breathing inadequately.*	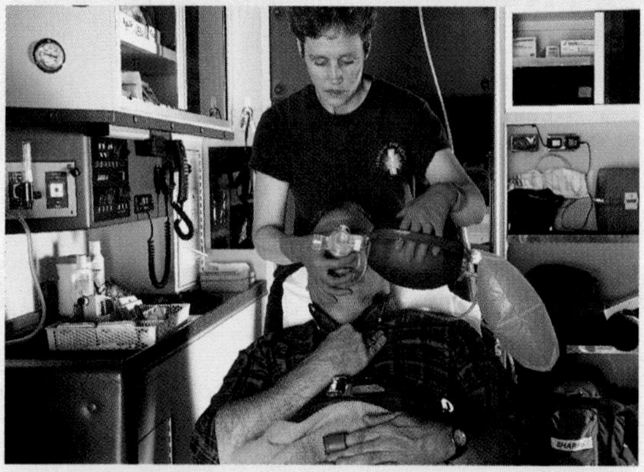
PATIENT IS NOT BREATHING AT ALL	• No chest rise • No evidence of air being moved from the mouth or nose • No breath sounds	Assisted ventilations with a pocket face mask, bag-valve mask, or FROPVD at 12/minute for an adult and 20/minute for an infant or child. *Note: DO NOT use oxygen-powered ventilation devices on infants or children.*	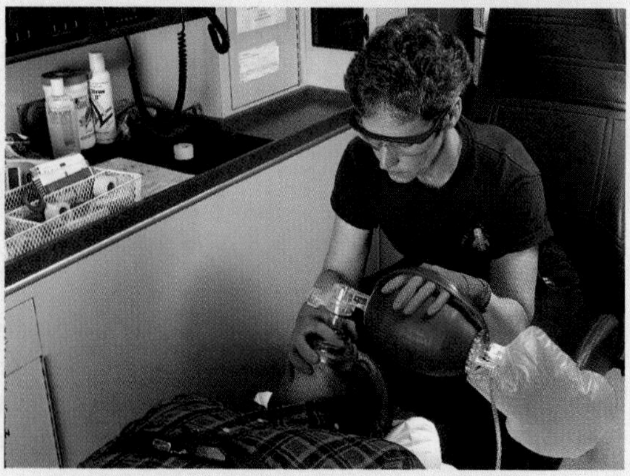

Adequate and Inadequate Artificial Ventilation

Like breathing, artificial ventilation can be adequate or inadequate. When you are performing artificial ventilation adequately, the chest will rise and fall with each artificial ventilation. The adequate rate for artificial ventilation is 12 breaths per minute for adults, and 20 per minute for infants and children.

When you provide artificial ventilation without chest compressions (patient has a pulse), monitor the pulse carefully. With adequate artificial ventilation, the rate should return to normal or near normal. Since the pulse in adults will usually rise from a lack of oxygen, a pulse that remains the same or increases may indicate inadequate artificial ventilation. Naturally, if the pulse disappears this indicates that the patient is in cardiac arrest and needs chest compressions (CPR).

PEDIATRIC NOTE

Pediatric patients differ from adults in many ways. There are few differences that are more important in emergency care than those within the respiratory system. When adult patients experience a decrease in oxygen in the bloodstream (hypoxia), their pulse increases.

In infants and children with respiratory difficulties, you may observe a slight increase in pulse early, but soon the pulse will drop significantly. A low (or bradycardic) pulse in infants and small children in the setting of a respiratory emergency usually means trouble! This is a sharp contrast from adults where it is a good sign when their pulse lowers to a more normal level.

If you observe a pulse below the expected rates for infants and children, evaluate your ventilations or oxygen therapy thoroughly. In ventilations, make sure that you have an open airway and that the chest rises with each breath. Nothing is more important for infants and children than adequate airway care! In any situation make sure that the oxygen tank has not run out and that the tubing has not kinked or slipped off the delivery device or oxygen cylinder.

For any patient—adult, child, or infant—if the chest does not rise and fall with each artificial ventilation, or the pulse does not return to normal, increase the force of ventilations. If the chest still does not rise, check that you are maintaining an open airway by the head-tilt, chin-lift maneuver (if there is no suspected spine injury) or by the jaw-thrust maneuver (if spine injury is possible). Insert an oropharyngeal or nasopharyngeal airway as needed to prevent the tongue from blocking the airway. Suction fluids and foreign matter from the airway as necessary, or perform abdominal thrusts and finger sweeps as needed to clear large airway obstructions. (Deliver alternating series of back blows and chest thrusts to clear airway obstructions in infants. Do not perform blind finger sweeps—remove only visible objects—in infants and children.) If you are using supplemental oxygen, check that all connections are secure and that the tubing has not kinked.

Review the techniques of airway maintenance and artificial ventilation in Chapter 6, "Airway Management," and in Appendix B, "Basic Cardiac Life Support Review," in the back of this book.

In infants and children, it is especially important to distinguish between an upper airway obstruction and a lower airway disease if there appears to be a blockage of the airway. If the airway is blocked by the tongue, blood, secretions, or debris, consider suctioning, performing finger sweeps, or inserting an oropharyngeal or nasopharyngeal adjunct to help maintain an open airway.

Infants and children are also subject to respiratory infections (e.g., epiglottitis) that may result in swelling of the airway passages. In such cases, probing or placing anything in the patient's mouth or pharynx may set off spasms along the airway.

Refrain from placing anything in the patient's mouth, administer oxygen, and transport as quickly as possible if you see any signs of a serious respiratory problem such as:

- Wheezing, stridor, or grunting
- Increased breathing effort
- Flared nostrils or retracted muscles of breathing
- Rapid breathing
- Pale or bluish lips or mouth

For more information about assessing and treating respiratory conditions in infants and children, see Chapter 31, "Infants and Children."

BREATHING DIFFICULTY

Breathing difficulty is a frequent chief complaint, representing a patient's feeling of labored, or difficult, breathing. Although there are objective signs associated with breathing difficulty (as the following text will show), the "difficulty" the patient reports to you is a subjective perception of the patient. The amount of distress the patient feels may or may not reflect the actual severity of his condition. His breathing may be more adequate or less adequate than he feels it is. You should not rely entirely on the patient's report to decide how serious the condition really is. Perform an assessment to help you make that determination.

It is important to remember that a patient with breathing difficulty may have either adequate or inadequate breathing. You may encounter two patients, at different times, who tell you that they are having difficulty breathing ("I can't catch my breath" or a similar complaint). One patient may be having minor difficulty due to a pre-existing respiratory condition but still have adequate breathing. His condition is not life threatening. The other patient, who has offered exactly the same complaint, may be having a problem such as an allergic reaction and severe difficulty breathing. Your examination of this patient may reveal inadequate breathing that requires immediate artificial ventilation.

Difficulty in breathing may have many causes ranging from ongoing medical conditions to illnesses such as pneumonia and other infections, to cardiac problems that cause disturbances in the respiratory system.

PATIENT ASSESSMENT

BREATHING DIFFICULTY

Symptoms of breathing difficulty include a feeling of shortness of breath or tightness in the chest and restlessness or anxiety. Signs of breathing difficulty are as follows (see also Figure 16-2):

- Increased pulse rate
- Decreased pulse rate (especially in infants and children)
- Changes in the breathing rate (above or below normal levels)
- Changes in breathing rhythm
- Pale, cyanotic, or flushed skin
- Noisy breathing which may be described as:
  - Audible wheezing (heard without stethoscope)
  - Gurgling
  - Snoring
  - Crowing
  - Stridor (harsh, high-pitched sound during breathing, usually due to upper airway obstruction)
- Inability to speak full sentences (or at all) due to breathing difficulty
- Use of accessory muscles to breathe
- Retractions
- Altered mental status
- Coughing
- Flared nostrils, pursed lips
- Patient positioning:
  - Tripod position (patient leaning forward with hands on knees or another surface)

continued

- Sitting with feet dangling, leaning forward
- Unusual anatomy (barrel chest)
- Oxygen saturation, or SpO_2, reading of less than 95 percent on the pulse oximeter

Chapter 9, "Vital Signs and SAMPLE History," discussed use of the pulse oximeter to determine the oxygen saturation of the patient's blood and identify hypoxic patients (patients with less than adequate oxygenation). While the other signs and symptoms listed previously are certainly enough to identify hypoxia, the pulse oximeter will allow you to obtain a precise numerical reading.

If you have a pulse oximeter immediately available, place the sensor on the patient's finger before applying oxygen. This will give you a "room air" reading and give you the patient's saturation before you apply oxygen. When you apply oxygen to the patient, the reading should improve. Document both readings on the report. *Never delay administration of oxygen to obtain a reading. If the pulse oximeter is not immediately available, apply oxygen immediately and apply the pulse oximeter when it becomes available.*

The oximeter reading in a normal, healthy person is typically 96 to 100 percent. An oximeter reading of 91 to 95 percent indicates hypoxia, 86 to 90 percent indicates significant hypoxia, and 85 percent or less indicates severe hypoxia. *Oxygen should be administered to all patients with respiratory distress regardless of their oxygen saturation readings. Even a patient with a saturation reading of 100 percent should receive oxygen if he has any signs of respiratory distress.*

The focused history and physical exam for patients with respiratory emergencies involves an appropriate interview and an examination of the chest and respiratory structures. Use the letters OPQRST to remember which questions to ask about the respiratory difficulty:

O—Onset. When did it begin?
P—Provocation. What were you doing when this came on?
Q—Quality. Can you describe the feeling you have?
R—Radiation. Does the feeling seem to spread to any other part of your body? Do you have pain or discomfort anywhere else in your body?
S—Severity. On a scale of 1 to 10, how bad is your breathing trouble? (10 is worst, 1 best)
T—Time. How long have you had this feeling?

Ask if the patient has taken any prescribed medications or done anything else to help relieve his condition. This may affect the treatment provided by you and the treatment provided later at the hospital. ■

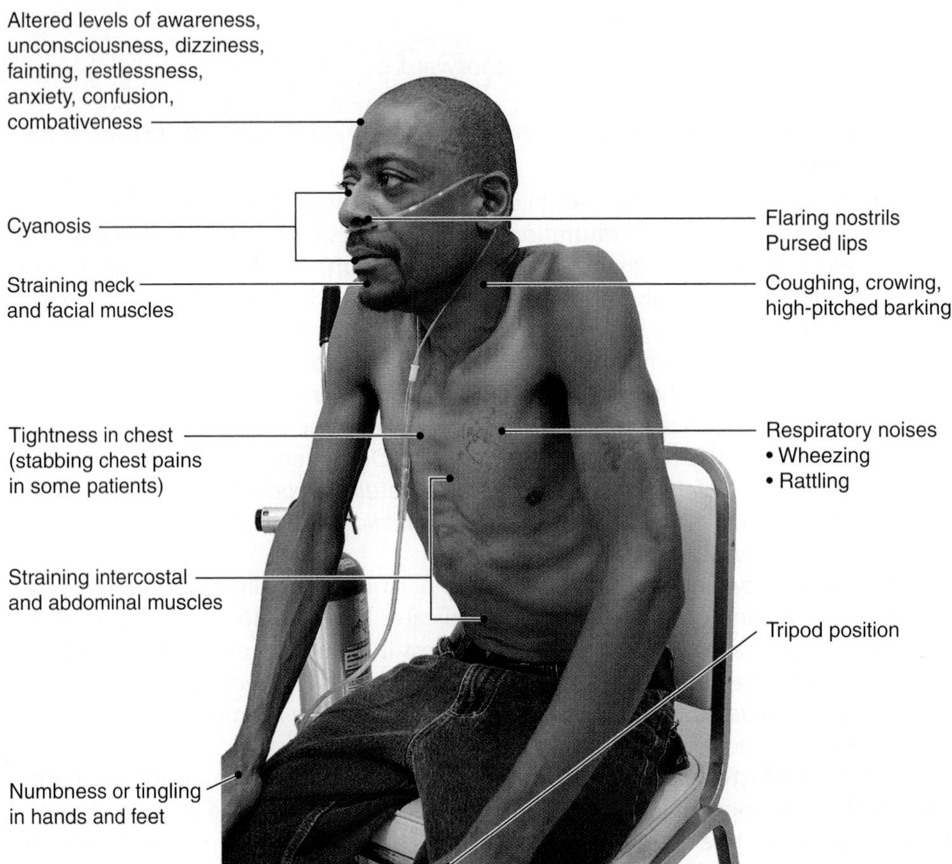

Figure 16-2 • Signs and symptoms of breathing difficulty. *(© Ray Kemp/911 Imaging)*

PATIENT CARE

BREATHING DIFFICULTY

When a patient is suffering from breathing difficulty, provide the following care:

- *Assessment.* Assess the airway during the initial assessment and then frequently throughout the call. Assist respiration with artificial ventilations and supplemental oxygen whenever the patient has or develops inadequate breathing.
- *Oxygen.* Oxygen is the main treatment for any patient in respiratory difficulty. If the patient is breathing adequately, use a nonrebreather mask at 15 liters per minute to provide oxygen. Use a nasal cannula only in cases where the patient will not tolerate a mask. If the patient has inadequate breathing, provide supplemental oxygen while performing artificial ventilation.
- *Positioning.* If the patient is experiencing breathing difficulty but is breathing adequately, place him in a position of comfort. Most patients with breathing difficulty feel they can breathe better sitting up. This is not possible if the patient has inadequate breathing, since the patient would need to be supine to receive assisted ventilations.
- *Prescribed inhaler.* If the patient has a prescribed inhaler, you may be able to assist the patient in taking this medication. This would be done after consultation with medical direction, often during transportation to the hospital. (More information will be provided on prescribed inhalers later in this chapter.) ■

ASSESSING LUNG SOUNDS

The most important sounds that you can hear through your stethoscope are the sounds of air moving in and out through the lungs. In the event you do not hear these sounds, your patient has a serious condition such as inadequate breathing, respiratory arrest, or possibly a collapsed lung (which can be caused by a pneumothorax, described in Chapter 27, "Soft Tissue Injuries").

There are other sounds you may hear. These include wheezing, rhonchi, and crackles. While an EMT is not required to know these additional sounds, it may help when communicating with medical direction to request permission to assist a patient with his medication. Listen for these lung sounds on both sides over the patient's chest (upper and lower), at the mid-axillary line, and over the patient's back (upper and lower). Figure 16-3 shows locations on the patient's body where you should listen for lung sounds.

- **Wheezes** are high-pitched sounds that will seem almost musical in nature. The sound is created by air moving through narrowed air passages in the lungs. It can be heard in a variety of diseases but is common in asthma and sometimes in chronic obstructive lung diseases such as emphysema and chronic bronchitis. Wheezing is most commonly heard during expiration.
- **Crackles** are (as the name indicates) a fine crackling or bubbling sound heard upon inspiration. The sound is caused by fluid in the alveoli or by the opening of closed alveoli.
- **Rhonchi** are lower-pitched sounds that resemble snoring or rattling. They are caused by secretions in larger airways as might be seen with pneumonia or bronchitis or when materials are aspirated (breathed) into the lungs.
- **Stridor** is a high-pitched sound that is heard on inspiration. It is an upper-airway sound indicating partial obstruction of the trachea or larynx.

When listening to the lungs, you should listen in several areas, since some sounds may be present in the lower lobes (e.g., crackles from early congestive heart failure) while others may be present throughout the lungs (e.g., wheezes from an asthma attack). You may also observe changes over time when listening to lung sounds. An asthmatic patient who has used his inhaler may feel that he is breathing easier and the wheezes have diminished. Be careful, however. Sometimes the wheezes will also disappear when a patient worsens and his breathing becomes inadequate. This is because the patient is not moving enough air in and out of the lungs any more to create the wheezing.

Remember that your patient's overall status is more important than his lung sounds.

F•Y•I

RESPIRATORY ASSESSMENT AND CONDITIONS

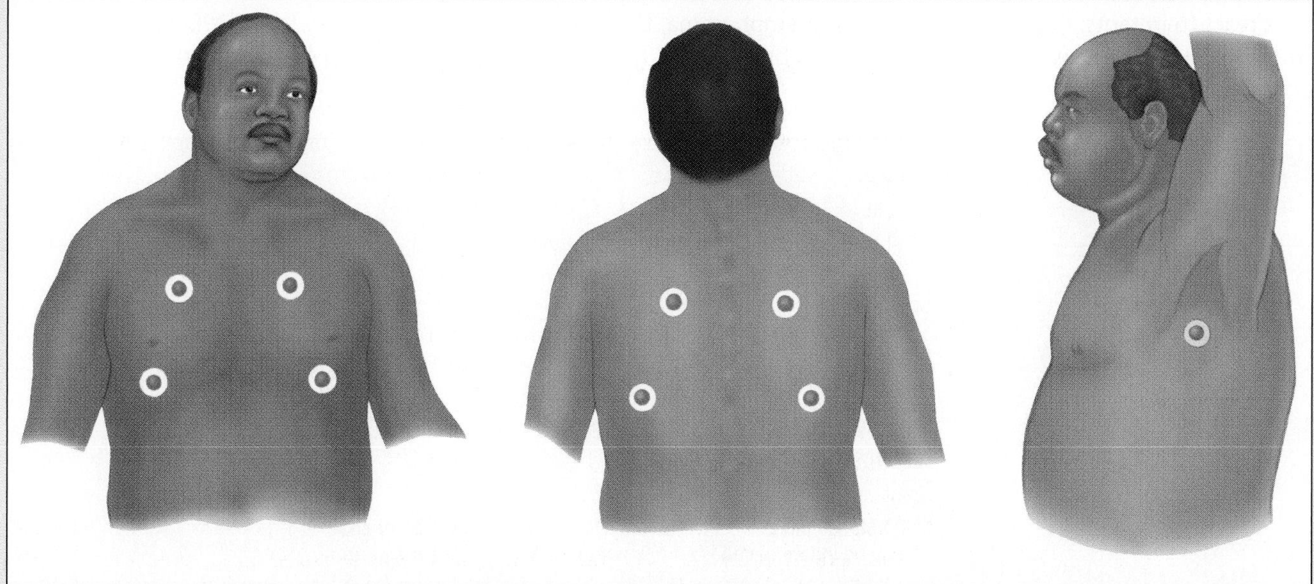

Figure 16-3 • Auscultate for breath sounds on the upper and lower chest, the upper and lower back, and at the mid-axillary line.

continued

F•Y•I

Continued

RESPIRATORY CONDITIONS

It is not necessary to diagnose a patient's condition to provide effective treatment as an EMT. In fact, the care for all respiratory conditions is essentially the same, as described earlier in this chapter. The information that follows on chronic obstructive pulmonary disease (Figure 16-4) and asthma is provided to enrich your knowledge of respiratory diseases.

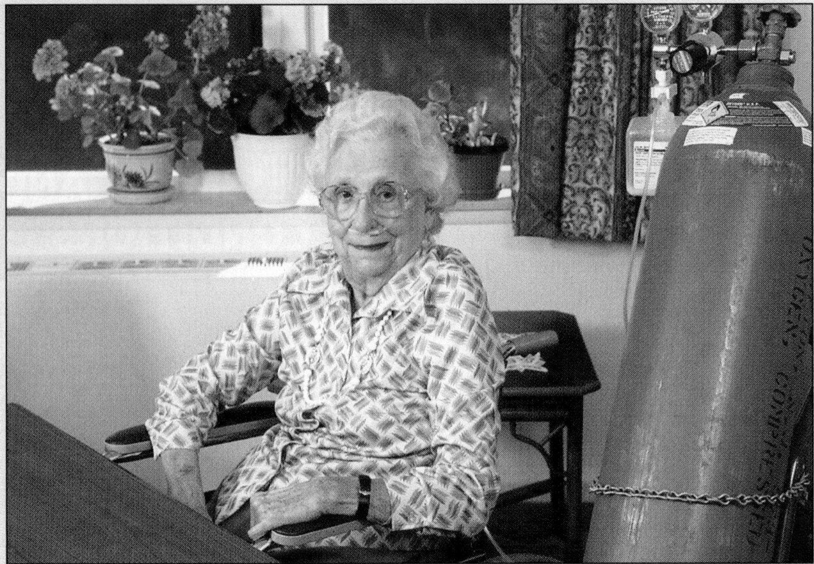

Figure 16-4 • A patient with chronic obstructive pulmonary disease (COPD).

Chronic Obstructive Pulmonary Disease (COPD)

Emphysema—as well as chronic bronchitis, black lung, and many undetermined respiratory illnesses that cause the patient problems like those seen in emphysema—are all classified as chronic obstructive pulmonary disease (COPD).

COPD is mainly a problem of middle-age or older patients. This is because these disorders take time to develop as tissues in the respiratory tract react to irritants. Cigarette smoking causes the overwhelming majority of cases of COPD. Occasionally other irritants such as chemicals, air pollutants, or repeated infections cause this condition.

Chronic bronchitis and emphysema are compared in Figure 16-5. In chronic bronchitis, the bronchiole lining is inflamed. Excess mucus is formed. The cells in the bronchioles that normally clear away accumulations of mucus are not able to do so. The sweeping apparatus on these cells, the cilia, have been damaged or destroyed.

In emphysema, the walls of the alveoli break down, greatly reducing the surface area for respiratory exchange. The lungs begin to lose elasticity. These factors combine to allow stale air laden with carbon dioxide to be trapped in the lungs, reducing the effectiveness of normal breathing efforts.

Many COPD patients will exhibit characteristics of both emphysema and chronic bronchitis. Usually the reason a COPD patient calls the ambulance is that a recent upper respiratory infection has caused an acute worsening of their chronic disease.

A very few COPD patients develop a hypoxic drive to trigger

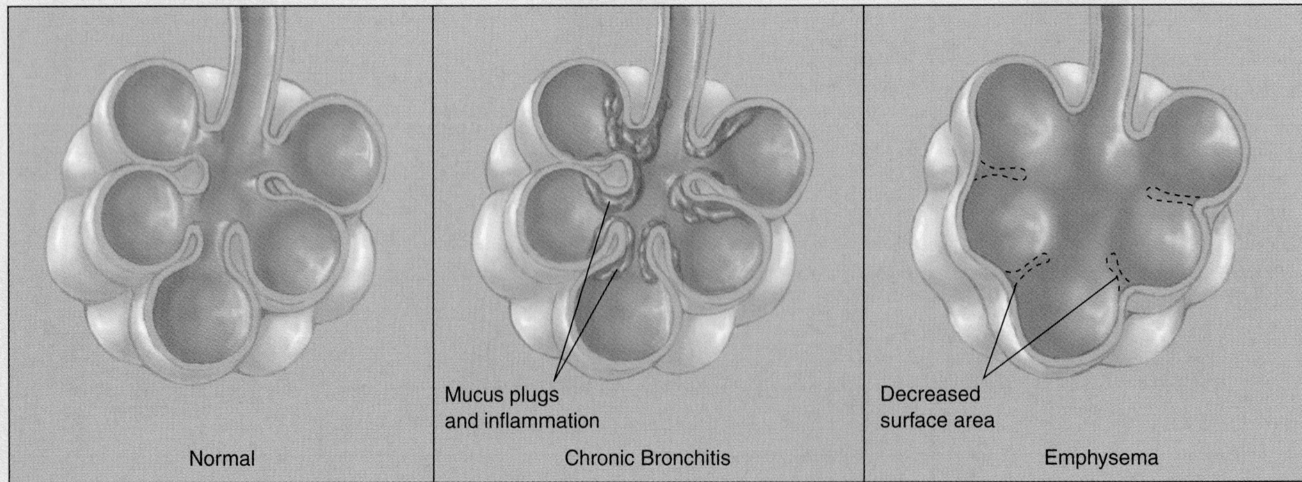

Figure 16-5 • Chronic bronchitis and emphysema are chronic obstructive pulmonary diseases.

respirations. In patients without COPD, the brain determines when to breathe based on increased levels of carbon dioxide in the blood. Since COPD patients develop a tolerance to their body's high levels of carbon dioxide, the brain learns to rely, instead, on low oxygen levels as the trigger to breathe. The higher oxygen levels that result from oxygen administration may, in rare cases, signal the COPD patient to reduce breathing or even to stop breathing (develop respiratory arrest).

In most cases, however, the hypoxic drive will not be a problem in the prehospital setting. The patient's need for oxygen will outweigh the risk involved with administration. If the patient has a possible heart attack or stroke, is developing shock, or has respiratory distress, a higher concentration of oxygen will be required in spite of the potential problems. If oxygen is required by the COPD patient, do not withhold it.

Constantly monitor the patient. If the patient's breathing becomes inadequate or stops, be prepared to assist respirations through artificial ventilation, and contact medical direction.

Asthma

Seen in young and old patients alike, asthma is a chronic disease that has episodic exacerbations or flares (a disease that only seems to affect the patient only at irregular intervals). This is far different from chronic bronchitis and emphysema, both of which continually afflict the patient. Asthma also differs from chronic bronchitis and emphysema in that it does not produce a hypoxic drive. An asthma attack or flare can be life threatening. Between episodes, the asthmatic patient can lead a normal life. Many use steroid inhalers for their chronic condition with albuterol administered only for a "rescue" during a flare.

An asthma attack may be triggered by an allergic reaction to something inhaled, swallowed, or injected into the body. Attacks can be precipitated by insect stings, air pollutants, infection, strenuous exercise, or emotional stress. When an asthma attack occurs, the small bronchioles that lead to the air sacs of the lungs become narrowed because of contractions of the muscles that make up the airway. To complicate matters, there is an overproduction of thick mucus. The combined effects of the contractions and the mucus cause the small passages to practically close down, severely restricting air flow.

The air flow is mainly restricted in one direction. When the patient inhales, the expanding lungs exert an outward pull, increasing the diameter of the airway and allowing air to flow into the lungs. During exhalation, however, the opposite occurs and the stale air becomes trapped in the lungs. This requires the patient to exhale the air forcefully, producing the characteristic wheezing sounds associated with asthma. ■

POINT OF VIEW

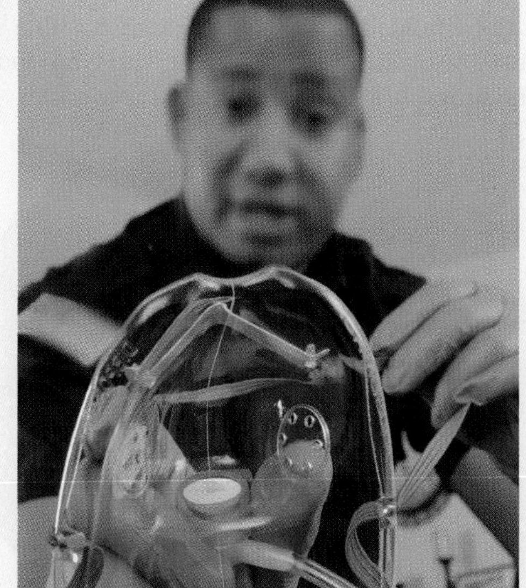

"I couldn't breathe. I mean I really couldn't breathe. I felt like I couldn't get air in and out and I was pretty sure I was going to die.

"I tell you this because I feel bad about how I yelled at the EMT. I can't remember everything, but I seem to remember being downright nasty. You see, I have asthma but have never had an attack like that before.

"My husband called the EMTs and they came to the house pretty quickly. But my breathing was getting worse and worse and, well, like I said, I wasn't sure I'd live through this one. It makes you crazy.

"When the EMT tried to put that mask on my face, I felt like I was being smothered. Even though I know it's supposed to help, I couldn't stop myself from lashing out at the EMT. I pushed his hand away and yelled. I can't imagine what it must've looked like . . . or what was going through his mind while I was yelling at him.

"He finally got me to put the mask on. He was very patient and calm. The oxygen did help me, but it wasn't easy. By the time we got to the hospital I felt a little better. And I apologized to him. He told me not to worry about it. But I do.

"I really hope this never happens again."

THE PRESCRIBED INHALER

A patient with a respiratory problem may have an inhaler prescribed by a physician. You will need to get permission from medical direction to help the patient use the inhaler. This may be accomplished by phone/radio or by standing order, depending on your local protocols. Keep in mind that a patient may overuse the inhaler prior to your arrival, so it is important to determine exactly when and how many times the inhaler has been used. Be sure to give this information to medical direction.

The metered-dose inhaler gets its name from the fact that each activation of the inhaler provides a metered, or exactly measured, dose of medication. Most patients simply refer to the device as their "inhaler" or "puffer." The inhaler is prescribed for patients with respiratory problems that cause **bronchoconstriction** (constriction, or blockage, of the bronchi that lead from the trachea to the lungs) or other types of lung obstructions. The inhalers contain a drug that dilates, or enlarges, the air passages, making breathing easier. These drugs are in the form of a fine powder. The timing of the activation of the inhaler in relation to a deep breath is very important to prevent the fine powder from coming to rest on the moist inner surface of the mouth. The medication will work only if it comes in contact with lung tissue directly. Studies have shown that inhalers can be very beneficial—but only when used properly.

bronchoconstriction constriction, or blockage, of the bronchi that lead from the trachea to the lungs.

NOTE

There are many types of drugs used in prescribed inhalers. The so-called "rescue inhalers" act immediately in an emergency to reverse airway constriction. Fast-acting emergency inhalers include albuterol inhalers (Ventolin, Proventil) and combination inhalers (Combivent). Other inhalers are not for use in emergencies; rather they are used daily to help reduce inflammation and prevent attacks. These medications (e.g., beclomethasone, Advair, Flovent) should not be used to reverse an acute attack or in the event of breathing difficulty. Additionally, you may find many different types of inhaler devices. An example is shown in Figure 16-7.

Spacer devices (Figure 16-6) make the exact timing necessary to use an inhaler less critical. The inhaler is activated into the spacer device (sometimes called an Aerochamber™). The medication stays airborne inside the chamber and can then be inhaled directly into the lungs.

When patients use an inhaler, they often are excited or nervous because they are short of breath. Many do not use their inhaler properly. Some people have never had proper instruction in use of their inhaler. Make sure to calm the patient the best you can and coach him to use the inhaler properly, as follows:

1. As with any medication, ensure that you have the right patient, the right medication, the right dose, and the right route. Check the expiration date. Make sure the inhaler is at room temperature or warmer. Shake the inhaler vigorously several times.
2. Make sure that the patient is alert enough to use the inhaler properly. Use a spacer device if the patient has one available.
3. Make sure the patient first exhales deeply.
4. Have the patient put his lips around the opening and press the inhaler to activate the spray as he inhales deeply.
5. After the patient inhales, make sure he holds his breath as long as possible so the medication can be absorbed. This may be difficult with a patient who is anxious, but unless the medication is held in the lungs, it will have minimal or no value.

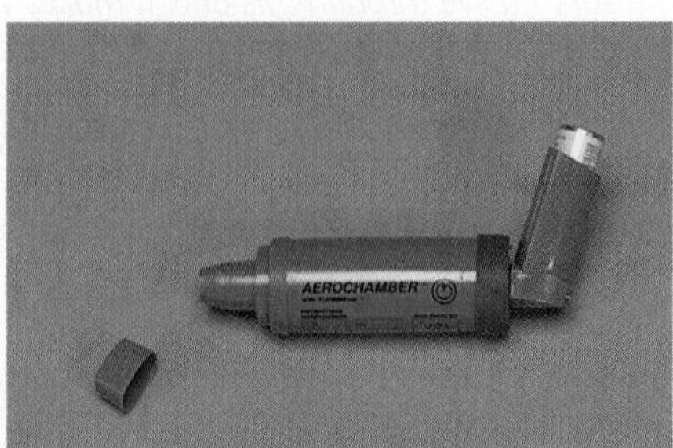

Figure 16-6 • A spacer between the inhaler and patient makes the timing during inhaler use less critical.

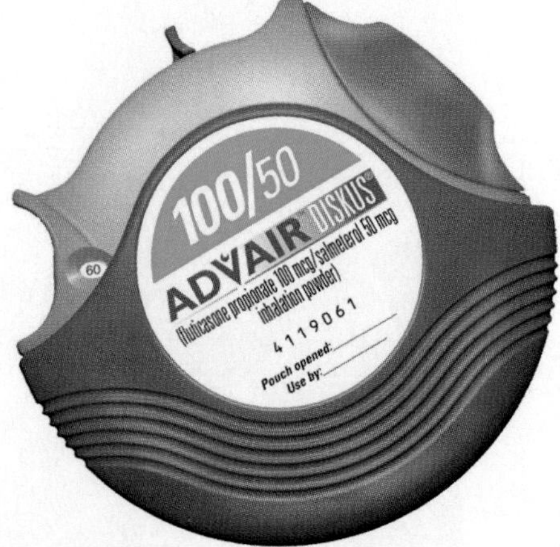

Figure 16-7 • The Advair inhaler. *(© GlaxoSmithKline)*

Your role will involve more coaching than actually administering the medication. The proper sequence for administration of a prescribed inhaler is shown in Scan 16-1. Inhalers are described in detail in Scan 16-2. Follow local protocols and consult medical direction, if required, before assisting a patient with an inhaler.

CRITICAL DECISION MAKING
Assisting with a Prescribed Inhaler

As an EMT you may be allowed to assist a patient in using his prescribed inhaler. Certain inhalers deliver a medication that relaxes narrowed airways and provides tremendous benefit to the patient when they are used properly.

For each of the situations that follows, decide whether you should or should not assist the patient with the inhaler.

1. You are called to a 14-year-old patient who complains of difficulty, breathing. He tells you he has a history of asthma. The patient's pulse is 104 strong and regular, respirations 28 with audible wheezes, blood pressure 130/84, skin warm and dry. The patient's parents are present. The inhaler is prescribed to the patient.
2. You are called to a 67-year-old patient who complains of difficulty breathing. The patient tells you she has a history of breathing problems but doesn't know specifically which ones. Her vital signs are pulse 122 strong and regular, respirations 28 with audible wheezes, blood pressure l04/64, skin cool and dry. The patient's daughter presents an inhaler, saying, "This is mine, but it's what I use when I'm wheezing."
3. You are called to a 24-year-old female who was exercising when she developed difficulty breathing. She has a history of asthma. You find her looking tired and weak. Her vital signs are pulse 142, respirations 42 and shallow, blood pressure 96/56, skin cool and moist. You do not hear any wheezes. A friend ran and got the patient's inhaler from her car.

Cultural Considerations

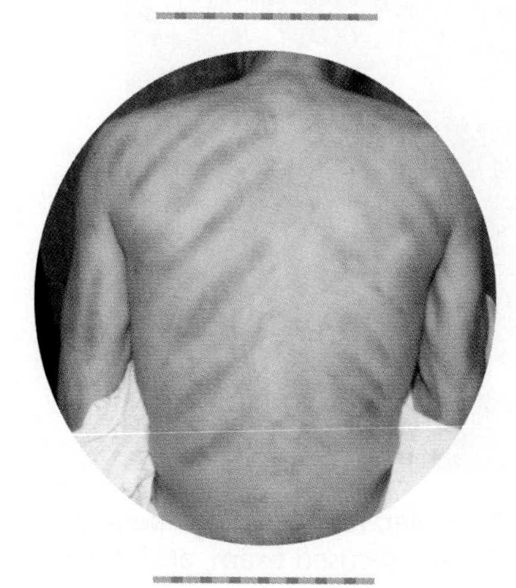

In emergency medical services, you will come to realize the wide variety of ways that people approach and respond to illness. One area that can greatly surprise the EMT is the nontraditional medical practices of certain ethnic groups. It is wrong to assume that "alternative" or "complementary" medicine is limited to chiropractic manipulation, herbal remedies, or acupuncture. Depending on the person's background, folk medicine practices can include such diverse practices as Voodoo, "cupping" (the application of heated glasses to the body to cure illness), and "coining" (the repeated rubbing of special hot or cold coins across areas of the body to cure illness).

Pictured here is a man with a lung infection who was "coined" by his family before seeking emergency care. He and his family come from an area in Vietnam where coining is a traditional part of medical practice. As you can imagine, the red marks might be startling and confusing to the EMT examining a patient. The EMT might well wonder how a complaint of respiratory distress could possibly result in red stripe marks all over the patient's back.

There have been cases where parents have been inappropriately accused of child abuse when health care workers not sensitive to cultural differences noticed the classic coining marks on a child and assumed they were the result of whippings or beatings, rather than the family's attempt to help the child.

SCAN 16-1 • Prescribed Inhaler—Patient Assessment and Management

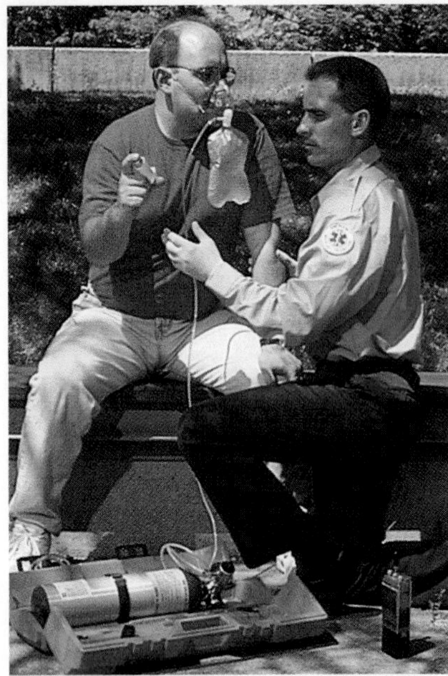

1. The patient has the indications for use of an inhaler: signs and symptoms of breathing difficulty and an inhaler prescribed by a physician.

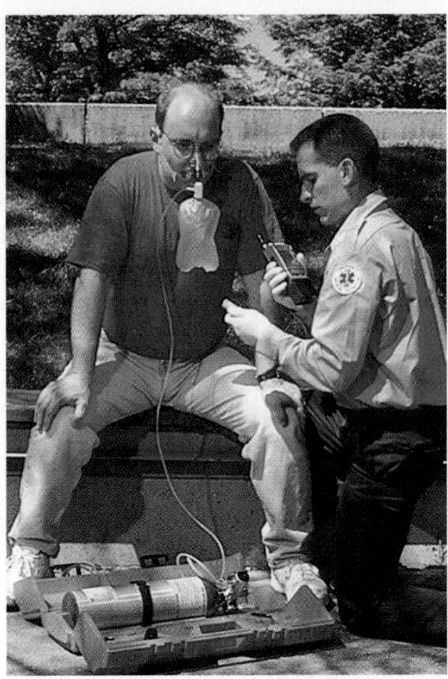

2. Contact medical direction and obtain an order to assist the patient with the prescribed inhaler.
3. Ensure the four "rights":
   - Right patient
   - Right medication
   - Right dose
   - Right route

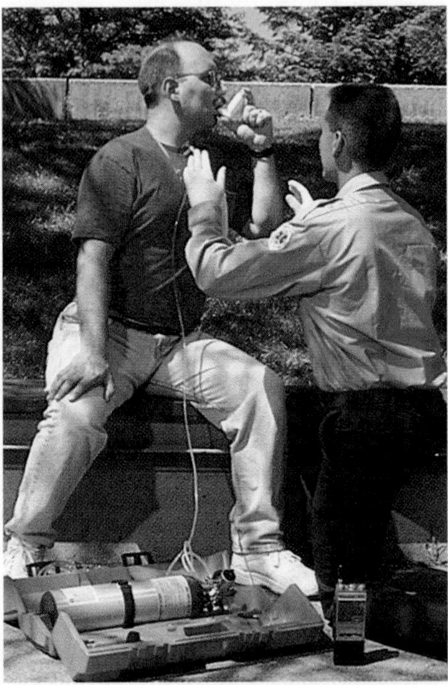

4. Coach the patient in the use of an inhaler. Tell him he should exhale deeply, press the inhaler to activate the spray, inhale, and hold his breath in so medication can be absorbed.

   Check the expiration date, shake the inhaler, make sure the inhaler is room temperature or warmer, and make sure the patient is alert.

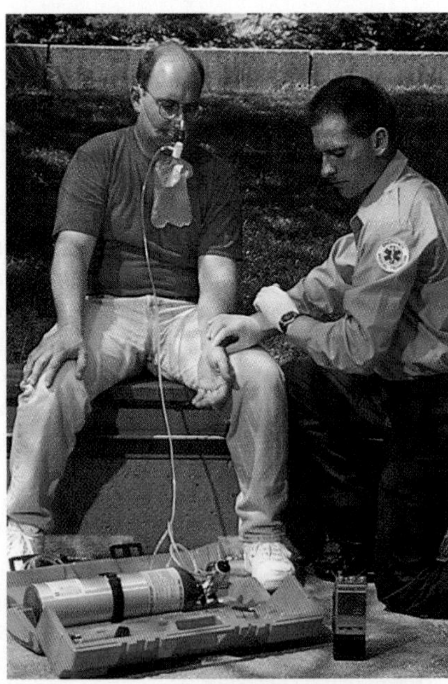

5. After use of the inhaler, reassess the patient: take vital signs, perform a focused exam, and determine if breathing is adequate.

SCAN 16-2 • Prescribed Inhaler

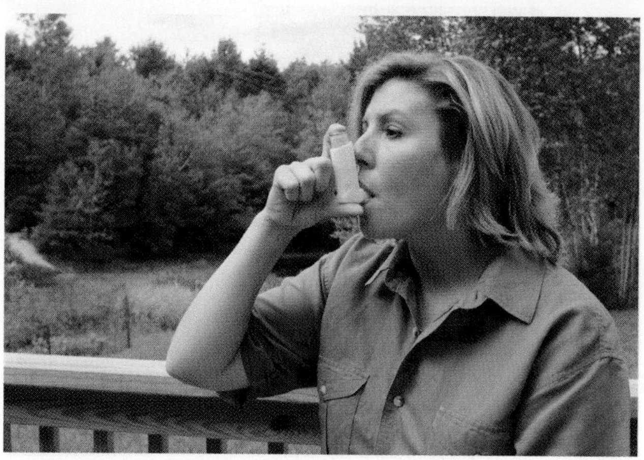

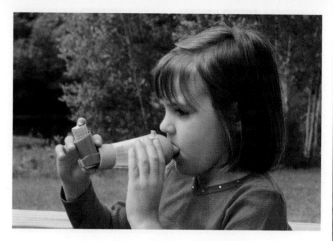

MEDICATION NAME

1. Generic: albuterol, isoetharine, metaproterenol
2. Trade: Proventil, Ventolin, Bronkosol, Bronkometer, Alupent, Metaprel

INDICATIONS

Meets all the following criteria:

1. Patient exhibits signs and symptoms of respiratory emergency.
2. Patient has physician-prescribed handheld inhaler.
3. Medical direction gives specific authorization to use.

CONTRAINDICATIONS

1. Patient is unable to use device (e.g., not alert).
2. Inhaler is not prescribed for patient.
3. No permission has been given by medical direction.
4. Patient has already taken maximum prescribed dose prior to EMT's arrival.

MEDICATION FORM

Handheld metered-dose inhaler.

DOSAGE

Number of inhalations based on medical direction's order or physician's order.

ADMINISTRATION

1. Obtain order from medical direction, either on-line or off-line.
2. Ensure right patient, right medication, right dose, right route, and patient alert enough to use inhaler.
3. Check expiration date of inhaler.
4. Check if patient has already taken any doses.
5. Ensure inhaler is at room temperature or warmer.
6. Shake inhaler vigorously several times.
7. Have patient exhale deeply.
8. Have patient put her lips around the opening of the inhaler.
9. Have patient depress the handheld inhaler as she begins to inhale deeply.
10. Instruct patient to hold her breath for as long as she comfortably can so medication can be absorbed.
11. Put oxygen back on patient.
12. Allow patient to breathe a few times and repeat second dose if so ordered by medical direction.
13. If patient has a spacer device for use with her inhaler (device for attachment between inhaler and patient to allow for more effective use of medication), it should be used.

ACTIONS

Beta agonist bronchodilator dilates bronchioles, reducing airway reistance.

SIDE EFFECTS

1. Increased pulse rate
2. Tremors
3. Nervousness

REASSESSMENT STRATEGIES

1. Gather vital signs.
2. Perform focused reassessment of chest and respiratory function.
3. Observe for deterioration of patient; if breathing becomes inadequate, provide artificial respirations.

SCAN 16-3 • Small-Volume Nebulizer (SVN)—Patient Assessment and Management

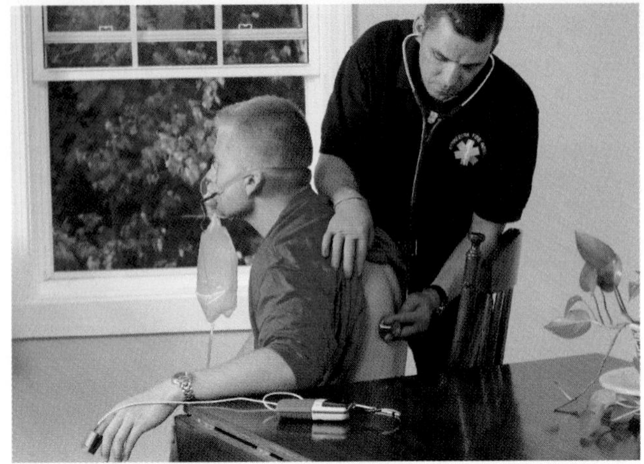

1. Identify patient as a candidate for nebulized medication per protocol (e.g., history of asthma with respiratory distress). Administer oxygen and assess vital signs. Be sure the patient is not allergic to the medication.

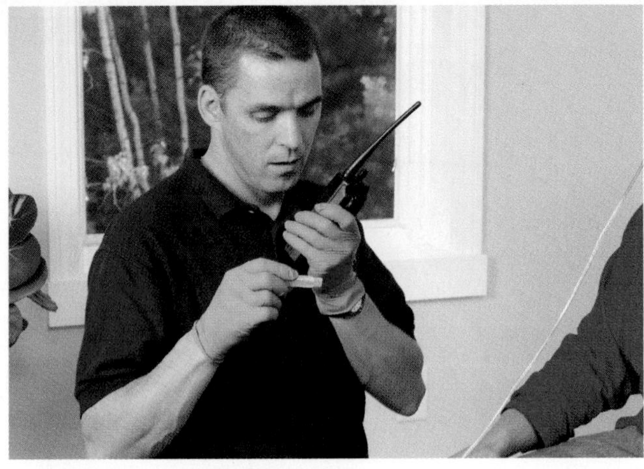

2. Obtain permission from medical direction to administer or assist with the medication.

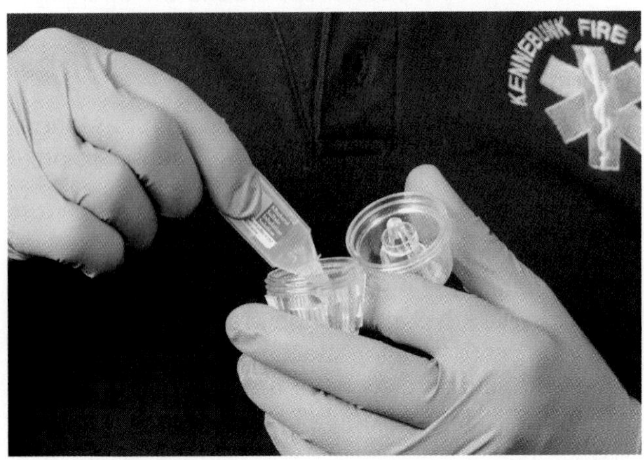

3. Ensure the four rights (right patient, right medication, right dose, right route). Prepare the nebulizer. Put the liquid medication in the chamber. Attach the oxygen tubing and set oxygen flow for 6 to 8 liters per minute (or according to manufacturer's recommendations).

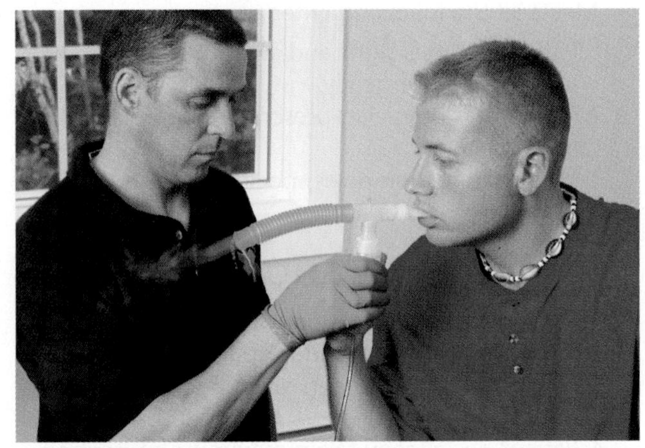

4. Have the patient seal his lips around the mouthpiece and breathe deeply. Instruct the patient to hold his breath for 2 to 3 seconds if possible. Continue until medication is gone from the chamber.

SCAN 16-3 • (Continued)

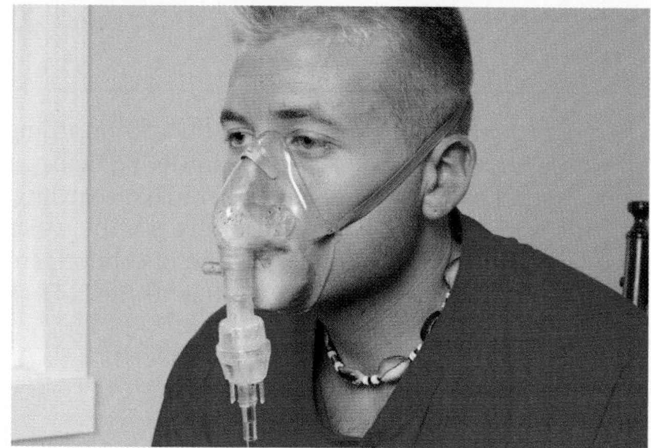

5. Alternative device—a mask delivers the medication.

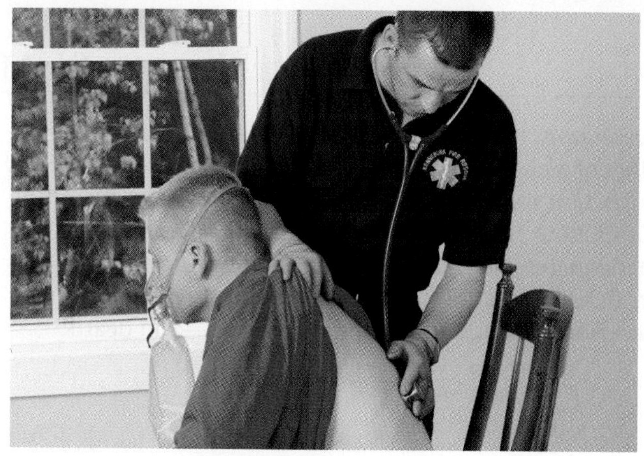

6. Reassess the patient's level of distress and vital signs. Additional doses may be authorized by medical control if the patient continues to be in distress and the patient is not having adverse effects from the medication.

F•Y•I

SMALL-VOLUME NEBULIZER

The medications used in metered-dose inhalers can also be administered by a small-volume nebulizer (SVN). Nebulizing a medication involves taking a liquid medication and running oxygen or air through it. The patient breathes the vapors created. Small-volume nebulizers are used in hospitals and ambulances as well as being prescribed to patients. Patients with chronic respiratory conditions such as asthma, emphysema, or chronic bronchitis may have these devices in their home.

Unlike the inhaler, which is only used in one breath, a nebulizer produces a continuous flow of aerosolized medication that can be taken in during multiple breaths over several minutes, giving the patient a greater exposure to the medication.

A few states have begun to allow EMTs to carry and administer nebulized medications such as albuterol, while other states may allow EMTs to assist with a home nebulizer when allowed by medical direction. Scan 16-3 demonstrates the use of an oxygen-powered nebulizer similar to ones carried on ambulances. Follow your local protocols regarding the use of nebulized medications.

The side effects and precautions with nebulized medications are the same as noted in Scan 16-2 for prescribed inhalers. Patients may experience an increased pulse rate, tremors, nervousness, or a "jittery" feeling. Patients who are not breathing adequately will not benefit from a nebulizer, since they are not breathing deeply enough to get the medication into their lungs. ■

CHAPTER REVIEW

SUMMARY

Respiratory emergencies are common calls that require diligent assessment, care, and emotional support. It is very important to evaluate your patient for adequate breathing throughout the call. If at any time you find breathing inadequate, you must assist ventilations. Providing artificial ventilation to a patient promptly may prevent him from slipping into respiratory arrest—and death!

For a patient who is experiencing difficulty breathing but whose breathing is adequate, administering high-concentration oxygen by nonrebreather mask; coaching the patient in the use of a prescribed inhaler if the patient has one; placing the patient in a position of comfort; and providing reassurance are the key treatments the EMT can provide.

KEY TERMS

bronchoconstriction constriction, or blockage, of the bronchi that lead from the trachea to the lungs.

exhalation (EX-huh-LAY-shun) another term for expiration.

expiration (EK-spuh-RAY-shun) a passive process in which the intercostal (rib) muscles and the diaphragm relax, causing the chest cavity to decrease in size and force air from the lungs.

inhalation (IN-huh-LAY-shun) another term for inspiration.

inspiration (IN-spuh-RAY-shun) an active process in which the intercostal (rib) muscles and the diaphragm contract, expanding the size of the chest cavity and causing air to flow into the lungs.

REVIEW QUESTIONS

1. List the normal rates of breathing for adults, children, and infants. List the other signs of adequate breathing. (p. 370)
2. List the signs of inadequate breathing. (pp. 370–371, 372)
3. Explain the treatment you will give, as an EMT, when a patient's breathing is inadequate. (pp. 371–372)
4. List the signs and symptoms of breathing difficulty. (pp. 374–375)
5. Explain the treatments you may give, as an EMT, for breathing difficulty when breathing is adequate. (pp. 368, 376)
6. Explain the steps to follow before, during, and after helping a patient to use a prescribed inhaler. (pp. 380–383)
7. List some differences between adult and infant/child respiratory systems. (p. 371)
8. List some special considerations in the assessment and treatment of infants and children with respiratory problems. (p. 373)

CRITICAL THINKING

For each of the following patients, state whether the patient's breathing seems adequate or inadequate—and explain your reasoning:

- A 45-year-old male patient experiencing severe difficulty in breathing. His respirations are 36/minute and very shallow. He has minimal chest expansion and can barely speak.
- A 65-year-old female who tells you that she has trouble breathing. Her respirations are 20/minute and slightly labored. Her respirations are regular and there appears to be good chest expansion.
- A 3-year-old patient who has had a respiratory infection recently. Her parents called because she is having difficulty breathing. You observe retractions of

the muscles between the ribs and above the collarbones as well as nasal flaring. The child seems drowsy. Respirations are 40/minute.

Thinking and Linking

Refer to Chapter 5, "Lifting and Moving Patients," and Chapter 6, "Airway Management," and link information from those chapters with information from this chapter as you consider the following:

- Assuming that each of the previous patients is in a second-floor bedroom in the back of the house (without an elevator), describe what patient-carrying devices you would use to get the patient to the ambulance. Your wheeled stretcher will only go as far as the front door of the house. Consider both the patient's complaint and the patient's condition as well as the patient's location within the house in choosing your transportation device.
- Once you choose the transportation device or method, explain how you will also safely transport a "D" cylinder of oxygen down the stairs with the patient.

MEDIA RESOURCES

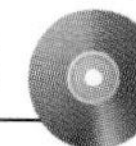

See the Student CD at the back of this book for quizzes, a case study activity, and other features related to this chapter. In particular, take a look at the Virtual Tour of the Airway, the 3D animation of the respiratory system, and the animation of an asthma attack. Also, visit the Companion Website for *Emergency Care* at **www.prenhall.com/limmer**, where you will find additional reinforcement and links to other resources.

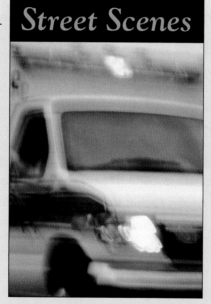

Street Scenes

Carmela Bartolone has been diagnosed with emphysema. She spends many days housebound on a home oxygen unit. But on this particular spring day, she felt that she should work in her flower garden. As she starts to pull weeds, she doesn't realize how much her rate of breathing is picking up. She soon finds that she is unable to catch her breath and unable to get back to the house. A neighbor sees Carmela having a problem breathing and asks if she needs anything. Carmela's response is, "Get help!"

Your pager is activated, and the only information the dispatcher provides is: "a female patient with difficulty breathing." The dispatcher also advises you that the ALS response unit is unavailable. Upon arrival, you find Mrs. Bartolone in a lawn chair with her husband and neighbor standing next to her, trying to get her to slow her breathing. You ask some quick medical questions and realize that the neighbor saw what happened, the husband has the medical history, and the patient can't talk in full sentences because of severe dyspnea.

Street Scene Questions

1. What is the first thing you should do for this patient?
2. What questions should you ask the husband? The neighbor?

After you perform an initial assessment, you decide to get patient information from the husband. He states that Mrs. Bartolone has emphysema from many years of smoking two packs of cigarettes a day. He says this same type of attack happened once before about 6 months ago. At that time, she was taken to the hospital and needed to be intubated and placed on a ventilator. She is on a number of medications, which he needs to get from inside the house. He reports no known allergies or other medical history.

Street Scene Questions

3. What is the significance of the medical history provided by the husband?
4. How much oxygen should the patient receive?

The fact that Mrs. Bartolone had to be put on a ventilator makes you realize that this patient is at risk of deteriorating very quickly. As you evaluate her breathing again, you note her respiration rate is still rapid. Your partner counts it at 36. You notice the patient's lips are bluish, her nostrils are flaring, and she is pushing herself up in the chair to make it easier to breathe. Your partner informs you that the patient is using the muscles of the chest and stomach to help her breathe. Mrs. Bartolone is becoming less restless because she is getting drowsy, a sign that action is needed. Your partner recommends that you assist ventilations with a bag-valve mask and you concur. As you start to hook up the oxygen reservoir, the husband returns with the patient's inhalers and tells you the patient only gets 2 liters per minute on her home unit. He also tells you that the doctor stressed she should not get more than that.

Street Scene Questions

5. Is the patient a good candidate for use of an inhaler?
6. Should this patient be considered a high priority with red light and siren for transport to the hospital?

You and your partner agree that this patient needs ventilations assisted with high-concentration oxygen and transport without delay. Her normal 2 liters per minute of oxygen are not enough to oxygenate her in this condition. You transport while assisting ventilations. You would like to help her use her inhaler but your protocol requires the patient to be alert (she is drowsy) and you know you are doing the patient a lot of good by ventilating her with high-concentration oxygen.

While en route, your partner notifies the hospital by radio of the patient's condition, treatment being provided, and an ETA of 10 minutes. You are able to ventilate the patient well by yourself, but that also means you are unable to get repeat vital signs. Keeping your priorities in mind, you continue ventilating and estimate her pulse rate by checking it quickly and frequently between ventilations. The patient seems more alert as you arrive at the emergency department. There you provide a prehospital care report to the waiting physician, which includes the patient history you obtained from the husband. As you start to leave the patient area, the doctor thanks you for being aggressive in assisting ventilations.

Street Scenes Sample Documentation

PATIENT NAME: *Carmela Bartolone* PATIENT AGE: *74*

CHIEF COMPLAINT
Dyspnea

PAST MEDICAL HISTORY
- [ ] None
- [ ] Allergy to
- [ ] Hypertension
- [ ] Stroke
- [ ] Seizures
- [ ] Diabetes
- [ ] COPD
- [ ] Cardiac
- [x] Other (List)
- [ ] Asthma

Emphysema

Current Medications (List)
2 LPM O_2 by NC, ipratropium & albuterol inhalers

VITAL SIGNS

TIME	RESP	PULSE	B.P.	MENTAL STATUS	R PUPILS L	SKIN
1028	Rate: *36*; ☐ Regular ☐ Shallow ☒ Labored	Rate: *110*; ☒ Regular ☐ Irregular	*160/90*	☑ Alert ☐ Voice ☐ Pain ☐ Unresp.	☐ Normal ☐ Dilated ☐ Constricted ☐ Sluggish ☐ No-Reaction	☐ Unremarkable ☑ Cool ☐ Pale ☐ Warm ☑ Cyanotic ☐ Moist ☐ Flushed ☑ Dry ☐ Jaundiced
1040	Rate: *12 Assisted*; ☐ Regular ☐ Shallow ☐ Labored	Rate: *Approx. 100*; ☐ Regular ☒ Irregular	/	☐ Alert ☑ Voice ☐ Pain ☐ Unresp.	☐ Normal ☐ Dilated ☐ Constricted ☐ Sluggish ☐ No-Reaction	☐ Unremarkable ☑ Cool ☐ Pale ☐ Warm ☑ Cyanotic ☐ Moist ☐ Flushed ☑ Dry ☐ Jaundiced
1055	Rate: *12 Assisted*; ☐ Regular ☐ Shallow ☐ Labored	Rate: *Approx. 110*; ☒ Regular ☐ Irregular	/	☐ Alert ☑ Voice ☐ Pain ☐ Unresp.	☐ Normal ☐ Dilated ☐ Constricted ☐ Sluggish ☐ No-Reaction	☐ Unremarkable ☑ Cool ☑ Pale ☐ Warm ☐ Cyanotic ☐ Moist ☐ Flushed ☑ Dry ☐ Jaundiced

NARRATIVE *74-year-old female patient found in her yard complaining of severe difficulty in breathing which began while working in the garden. Patient was unable to speak in full sentences. She was using accessory muscles to breathe, displayed nasal flaring, and had cyanosis about the lips. Shortly after our arrival the patient became drowsy. We provided assisted ventilations via BVM with supplemental oxygen.*

Patient has a history of smoking and emphysema. An episode similar to this about 6 months ago resulted in the patient being intubated and placed on a ventilator. Patient did not experience relief from rest. She denies chest pain or other complaints. She is on oxygen via cannula at home. Patient transported to the hospital. BVM assisted ventilations continued enroute. Patient's condition improved slightly with assisted ventilations (increased level of consciounsness). Unable to obtain second set of vital signs due to insufficient personnel and assisting ventilations.

CHAPTER 17

Cardiac Emergencies

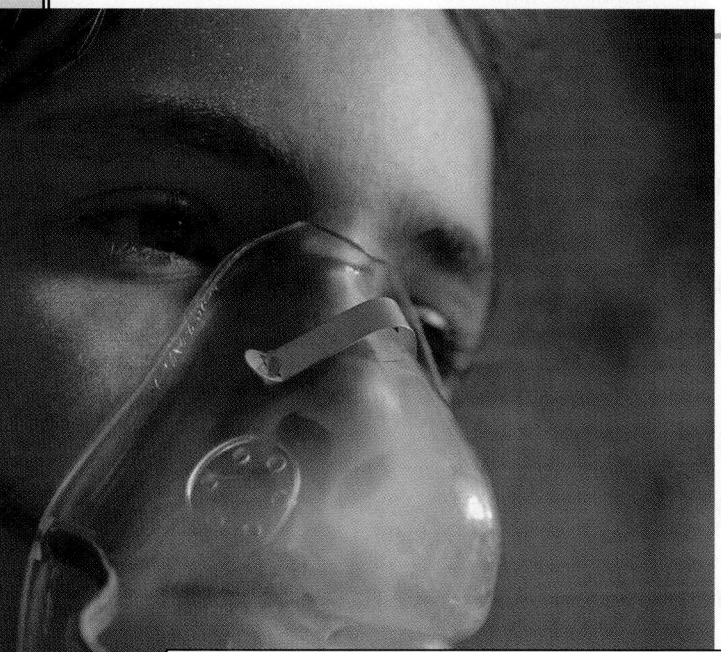

CORE CONCEPTS

The following are core concepts that will be addressed in this chapter:

- How to identify a patient with chest discomfort/pain
- How to treat a patient with chest discomfort/pain
- Your role in the administration of prescribed nitroglycerin
- How to use an AED on a patient in cardiac arrest
- How to document findings and care of patients with cardiac emergencies

KEY TERMS

acute coronary syndrome (ACS), p. 392
acute myocardial infarction (AMI), p. 406
aneurysm, p. 405
angina pectoris, p. 405
apnea, p. 414
asystole, p. 410
bradycardia, p. 393
cardiac compromise, p. 392
cardiovascular system, p. 391
congestive heart failure (CHF), p. 406
coronary artery disease (CAD), p. 405
dyspnea, p. 392
dysrhythmia, p. 405
edema, p. 406
embolism, p. 405
nitroglycerin (NTG), p. 406
occlusion, p. 405
pedal edema, p. 406
pulmonary edema, p. 406
pulseless electrical activity (PEA), p. 410
sudden death, p. 406
tachycardia, p. 393
thrombus, p. 405
ventricular fibrillation (VF), p. 409
ventricular tachycardia (V-Tach), p. 409

DOT OBJECTIVES

*KNOWLEDGE AND ATTITUDE

4-3.1 Describe the structure and function of the cardiovascular system. (pp. 391–392)

4-3.2 Describe the emergency medical care of the patient experiencing chest pain or discomfort. (pp. 393–397) (Scan 17-1, pp. 394–395)

4-3.3 List the indications for automated external defibrillation (AED). (pp. 406, 411–415, 417–418)

4-3.4 List the contraindications for automated external defibrillation. (pp. 419–420)

4-3.5 Define the role of EMT in the emergency cardiac care system. (pp. 393–397, 404–408, 417–418)

4-3.6 Explain the impact of age and weight on defibrillation. (p. 415)

4-3.7 Discuss the position of comfort for patients with various cardiac emergencies. (p. 396)

4-3.8 Establish the relationship between airway management and the patient with cardiovascular compromise. (pp. 396, 397, 399, 407, 414, 417, 418, 419, 426)

4-3.9 Predict the relationship between the patient experiencing cardiovascular compromise and basic life support. (pp. 405–406, 411, 412–414, 417)

4-3.10 Discuss the fundamentals of early defibrillation. (p. 406)

4-3.11 Explain the rationale for early defibrillation. (pp. 405, 406)

4-3.12 Explain that not all chest pain patients result in cardiac arrest and do not need to be attached to an automated external defibrillator. (pp. 392–397)

4-3.13 Explain the importance of prehospital ACLS intervention if it is available. (pp. 406, 407, 417–418)

4-3.14 Explain the importance of urgent transport to a facility with advanced cardiac life support if it is not available in the prehospital setting. (pp. 406–407)

4-3.15 Discuss the various types of automated external defibrillators. (pp. 408–409)

4-3.16 Differentiate between the fully automated and the semiautomated defibrillator. (pp. 409–410, 422)

4-3.17 Discuss the procedures that must be taken into consideration for standard operations of the various types of automated external defibrillators. (pp. 410–425)

4-3.18 State the reasons for assuring that the patient is pulseless and apneic when using the automated external defibrillator. (p. 409)

4-3.19 Discuss the circumstances which may result in inappropriate shocks. (p. 409)

4-3.20 Explain the considerations for interruption of CPR when using the automated external defibrillator. (p. 410)

4-3.21 Discuss the advantages and disadvantages of automated external defibrillators. (p. 422)

4-3.22 Summarize the speed of operation of automated external defibrillation. (pp. 422–424)

4-3.23 Discuss the use of remote defibrillation through adhesive pads. (p. 422)

4-3.24 Discuss the special considerations for rhythm monitoring. (pp. 409–410, 422)

4-3.25 List the steps in the operation of the automated external defibrillator. (pp. 415–416) (Scan 17-4, pp. 412–415)

4-3.26 Discuss the standard of care that should be used to provide care to a patient with persistent ventricular fibrillation and no available ACLS. (pp. 409, 411–420)

4-3.27 Discuss the standard of care that should be used to provide care to a patient with recurrent ventricular fibrillation and no available ACLS. (pp. 418–419)

4-3.28 Differentiate between single rescuer and multi-rescuer care with an automated external defibrillator. (p. 418)

4-3.29 Explain the reason for pulses not being checked between shocks with an automated external defibrillator. (p. 416)

4-3.30 Discuss the importance of coordinating ACLS trained providers with personnel using automated external defibrillators. (pp. 417–418)

4-3.31 Discuss the importance of post-resuscitation care. (p. 418)

4-3.32 List the components of post-resuscitation care. (p. 418)

4-3.33 Explain the importance of frequent practice with the automated external defibrillator. (pp. 409, 425)

4-3.34 Discuss the need to complete the Automated Defibrillator: Operator's Shift Checklist. (pp. 424–425)

4-3.35 Discuss the role of the American Heart Association (AHA) in the use of automated external defibrillation. (pp. 405–407)

4-3.36 Explain the role medical direction plays in the use of automated external defibrillation. (p. 425)

4-3.37 State the reasons why a case review should be completed following the use of the automated external defibrillator. (p. 425)

4-3.38 Discuss the components that should be included in a case review. (p. 425)

4-3.39 Discuss the goal of quality improvement in automated external defibrillation. (p. 425)

4-3.40 Recognize the need for medical direction of protocols to assist in the emergency medical care of the patient with chest pain. (pp. 394, 397)

4-3.41 List the indications for the use of nitroglycerin. (p. 397) (Scan 17-2, p. 398)

4-3.42 State the contraindications and side effects for the use of nitroglycerin. (p. 398)

4-3.43 Define the function of all controls on an automated external defibrillator, and describe event documentation and battery defibrillator maintenance. (pp. 412–415, 424–425)

4-3.44 Defend the reasons for obtaining initial training in automated external defibrillation and the importance of continuing education. (p. 422)

4-3.45 Defend the reason for maintenance of automated external defibrillators. (pp. 424–425)

4-3.46 Explain the rationale for administering nitroglycerin to a patient with chest pain or discomfort. (p. 397)

***SKILLS**

4-3.47 Demonstrate the assessment and emergency medical care of a patient experiencing chest pain or discomfort.

4-3.48 Demonstrate the application and operation of the automated external defibrillator.

4-3.49 Demonstrate the maintenance of an automated external defibrillator.

4-3.50 Demonstrate the assessment and documentation of patient response to the automated external defibrillator.

4-3.51 Demonstrate the skills necessary to complete the Automated Defibrillator: Operator's Shift Checklist.

4-3.52 Perform the steps in facilitating the use of nitroglycerin for chest pain or discomfort.

4-3.53 Demonstrate the assessment and documentation of patient response to nitroglycerin.

4-3.54 Practice completing a prehospital care report for patients with cardiac emergencies.

EMTs may often encounter patients who complain of chest discomfort. Sometimes this discomfort will be the result of a cardiac (heart) problem—possibly a heart attack, possibly some other cardiac disorder. As an EMT, you will be able to provide these patients with oxygen, which is the most important drug in the treatment of heart problems. You may also be able to assist patients with taking nitroglycerin. Most patients with chest pain will not be having heart attacks. In fact, they may not have a heart problem at all. Keep in mind that oxygen will not harm patients who are not having heart problems and may be of great benefit to those who are.

Occasionally, you will encounter a patient who is in cardiac arrest—whose normal heartbeat and circulation of blood have completely stopped. CPR can help postpone death for a short time, but defibrillation must be performed as quickly as possible. Defibrillation, which will be covered in the second part of this chapter, is the application of an electrical shock to the chest in order to restart the heart's normal action. Cardiac arrest is one of the few situations in which you may actually be able to save someone's life by acting quickly and efficiently.

CARDIAC ANATOMY AND PHYSIOLOGY

You learned about the **cardiovascular system** (made up of the heart and the blood vessels) and circulation of the blood in Chapter 4, "The Human Body." Before continuing through this chapter on cardiac emergencies, you should review that material. In particular, you should review:

- Flow of blood through the chambers of the heart (the atria and ventricles), and the cardiac conductive system (the electrical impulses and specialized muscles that cause the heart to contract)
- Composition of the blood (red and white blood cells, platelets, and plasma)

cardiovascular system the heart and the blood vessels.

- Flow of blood through the arteries, veins, arterioles, venules, and capillaries, and the names and positions of major blood vessels
- Circulation of blood between the heart and the lungs and between the heart and the rest of the body
- How heart function and the circulation of blood relate to pulse (review the peripheral and central pulses) and blood pressure (review systolic and diastolic pressure; also review Chapter 9, "Vital Signs and SAMPLE History")
- Shock (hypoperfusion)

You may also wish to review the diagrams of the heart, the cardiovascular system, the cardiac conductive system, and the circulatory system in Chapter 4, "The Human Body," and the diagram of the cardiovascular system in the "Anatomy and Physiology Plates" at the end of this book.

CARDIAC COMPROMISE

cardiac compromise a blanket term that refers to a heart problem with a rapid onset.

acute coronary syndrome (ACS) a blanket term used to represent any symptoms related to lack of oxygen (ischemia) in the heart muscle.

Cardiac compromise, sometimes called **acute coronary syndrome (ACS),** is a blanket term that refers to any kind of problem with the heart. There are many different ways in which patients' hearts show that they are in trouble. One reason for this is that there are many different kinds of problems the heart can experience. A coronary artery may become narrowed or blocked, a one-way valve may stop working properly, or the specialized tissue that carries electrical impulses may function abnormally.

Just as there are many different problems the heart can experience, there is a very wide variety of signs and symptoms associated with these problems. Most of these signs and symptoms can also result from problems that have nothing to do with the heart. Many patients with heart trouble will complain of pain in the center of the chest. Others may have only mild chest discomfort or no pain at all. Some may experience difficulty breathing, while still others have only the sudden onset of sweating, nausea, and vomiting.

Since the signs and symptoms of a heart problem can vary so greatly, it is much safer for the EMT to treat all patients with certain signs and symptoms as though they are having a heart problem—cardiac compromise—instead of trying to decide whether or not the patient has a heart problem or what kind of heart problem it might be. (Some common cardiovascular disorders will be discussed later in this chapter as background information, but you do not need this information to recognize and treat the symptoms associated with such disorders. Definitive diagnosis and care will be provided at the hospital.)

The best known symptom of a heart problem is chest pain. Typically, a patient describes this pain as crushing, dull, heavy, or squeezing. Sometimes the patient will vehemently deny having pain but may admit to some pressure. Some patients will describe this sensation as just a discomfort. This is a good example of why you should have a patient describe in his own words how he is feeling. If you ask some of these patients whether they are having chest pain, they will tell you they are not, because to them it is not pain. When a patient is having difficulty describing the sensation, try suggesting several choices, as you learned in Chapter 11, "Assessment of the Medical Patient".

The pain, pressure, or discomfort associated with cardiac compromise commonly radiates along the arms, down to the upper abdomen, or up to the jaw. Patients complain of radiation to the left arm more than the right, but either (or both) is possible.

dyspnea (DISP-ne-ah) shortness of breath; labored or difficult breathing.

Another frequent complaint (and sometimes the only complaint in a patient with cardiac compromise) is difficulty breathing, called **dyspnea.** If the patient does not complain of difficulty breathing, specifically ask him about it. Sometimes the pain is so

Cultural Considerations

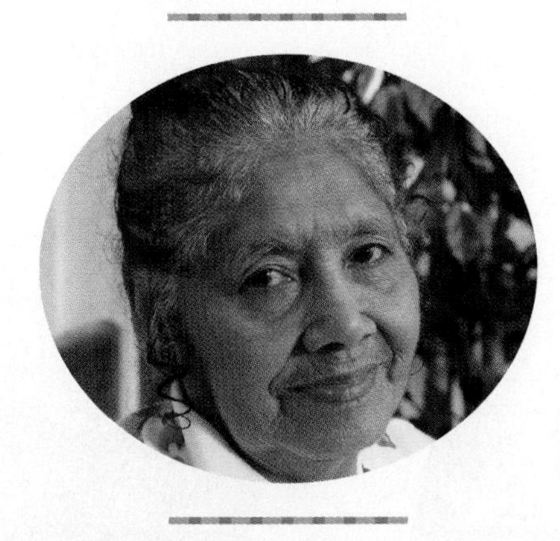

When you enter a patient's home, be sensitive to cultural cues. In most cultures, there is a designated family caretaker—possibly a mother, aunt, or grandmother. Seek her cooperation and support for any interventions. The patient is more likely to feel confidence in your care if the designated caregiver approves.

In Mexican-American families, family is a strong support. Extended family, including godparents (compadres), may want to be with the patient while you are conducting assessment and care, and more than one family member may want to accompany the patient to the hospital.

Instead of asking everyone to clear the room while you conduct assessment and care, as you might in some circumstances, be as accommodating as you can if you feel that this is a situation where family support is important to the patient. Keep in mind that, although the father in a Latino family may act as the spokesperson, mothers and other females in the family are influential in decisions about health care. Be as inclusive as possible of all the people in the family who want explanations about what is wrong with the patient and the care you are providing.

intense that patients focus their attention on that and do not mention other important symptoms.

A patient with cardiac compromise is often anxious. In some patients, this takes the form of a feeling of impending doom, which the patient may express to you or others. Occasionally, you will see a patient whose anxiety displays itself through irritability and a short temper.

Other common symptoms in patients with cardiac compromise are nausea and pain or discomfort in the upper abdomen (epigastric pain). Some of these patients also vomit. A less common finding is loss of consciousness. This may result from the heart beating too fast or too slow to adequately supply the brain with oxygenated blood. Usually, the patient regains consciousness quickly.

There are also several signs you will see in some of these patients, including the sudden onset of sweating and an abnormal pulse or blood pressure. Many patients who have sudden onset of sweating think they are coming down with the flu, but this may result from the denial that is common in these patients. They refuse to acknowledge, at least consciously, that they may be having heart problems. The pulse may be abnormally slow (slower than 60 beats per minute, called **bradycardia**) or abnormally fast (faster than 100 beats per minute, called **tachycardia**) and will frequently be irregular. Some patients complain of palpitations, which are irregular or rapid heartbeats they feel as a fluttering sensation in the chest. A few patients are hypotensive (systolic blood pressure less than 90), while others are hypertensive (systolic greater than 150 or diastolic greater than 90).

bradycardia
(bray-di-KAR-de-ah)
when the heart rate is slow, usually below 60 beats per minute.

tachycardia
(tak-e-KAR-de-ah)
when the heart rate is fast, above 100 beats per minute.

Patients with cardiac compromise can have many different presentations. Some complain of pressure or pain in the chest with difficulty breathing and a history of heart problems. Others may have just mild discomfort that they ignore for several hours or that goes away and returns. Between 10 and 20 percent of patients who are having heart attacks have no chest discomfort at all. Because of these many possibilities and because of the potentially severe complications of heart problems, it is important to have a high index of suspicion and treat patients with any of these signs and symptoms for cardiac compromise. The treatment will not hurt them and may help them.

Management of Cardiac Compromise

The management of a patient with cardiac compromise is detailed in the following text and in Scan 17-1.

SCAN 17-1 • Managing Chest Pain

First take Standard Precautions.

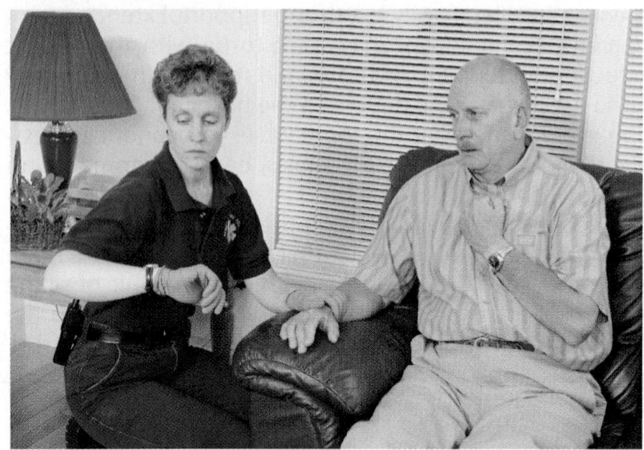

1. Perform the initial assessment.

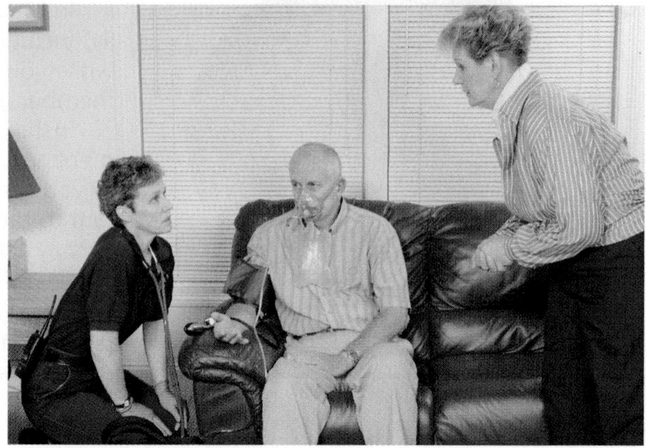

2. Provide high-concentration oxygen by nonrebreather mask. Perform the focused history and physical exam for a medical patient. Document findings.

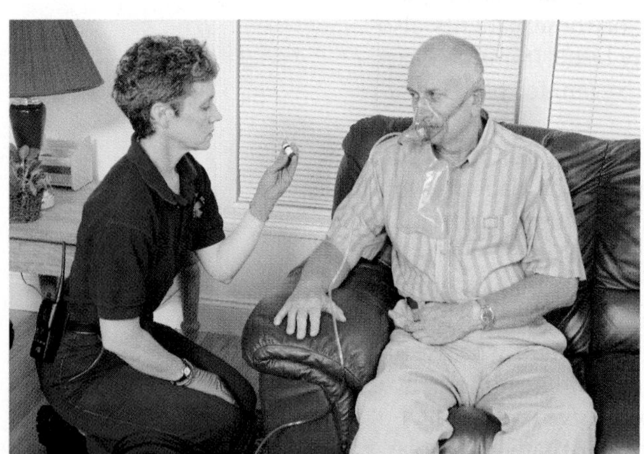

3. If the patient meets nitroglycerin criteria and has prescribed nitroglycerin, ask him about the last dose taken.

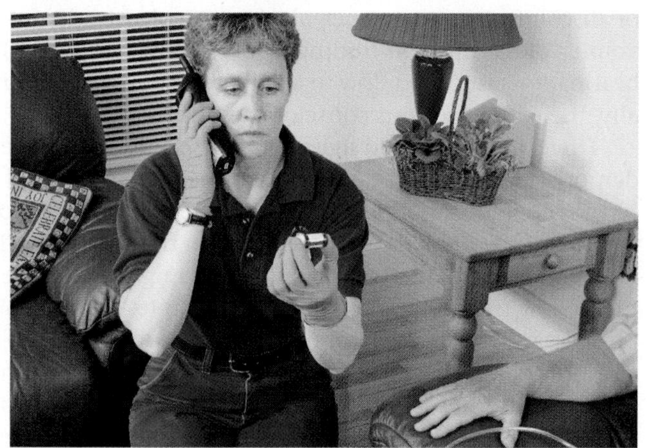

4. Check the four rights: right patient, right drug, right dose, right route. Check the expiration date. Consult medical direction before assisting the patient with taking medication.

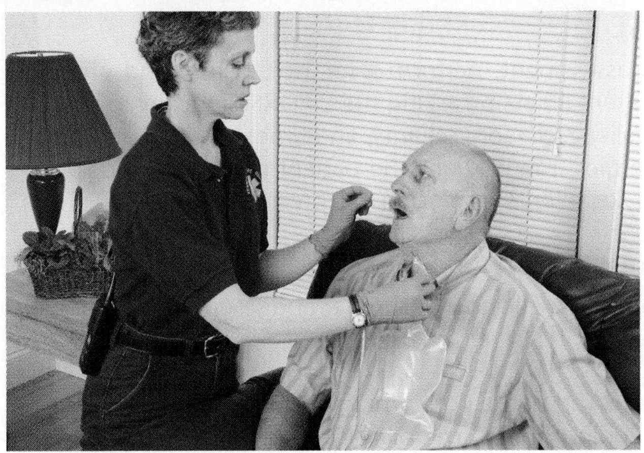

5. Remove the oxygen mask. Ask the patient to open his mouth and lift his tongue.

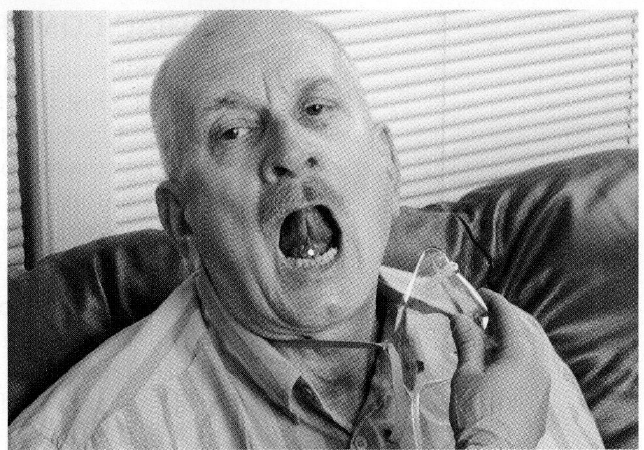

6A. Place the nitroglycerin tablet under the tongue, or . . .

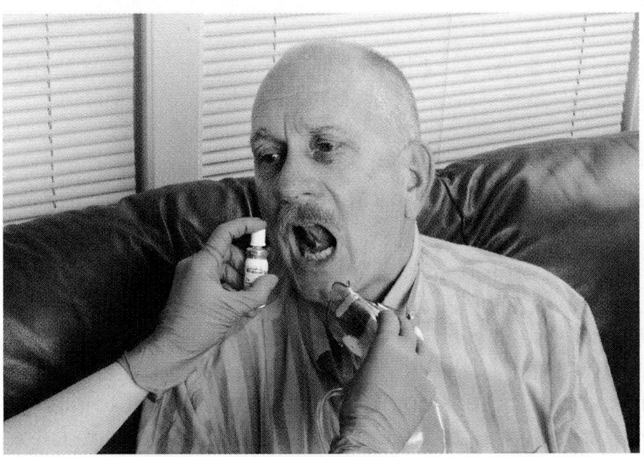

6B. If the nitroglycerin is in spray form, spray the medication under the tongue according to label directions.

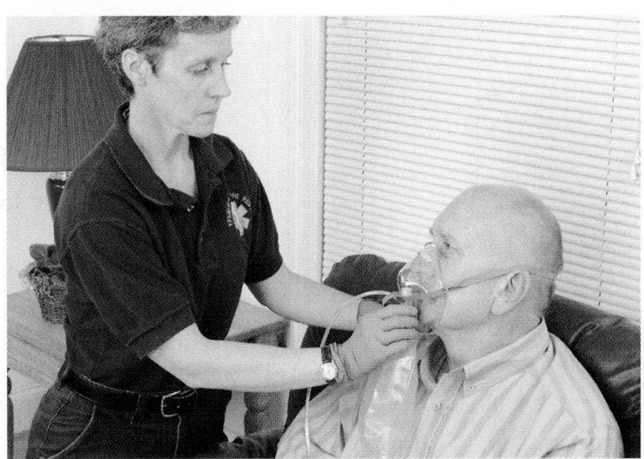

7. Have the patient close his mouth and hold the nitroglycerin under his tongue, where the medication will be quickly absorbed. Replace the oxygen mask.

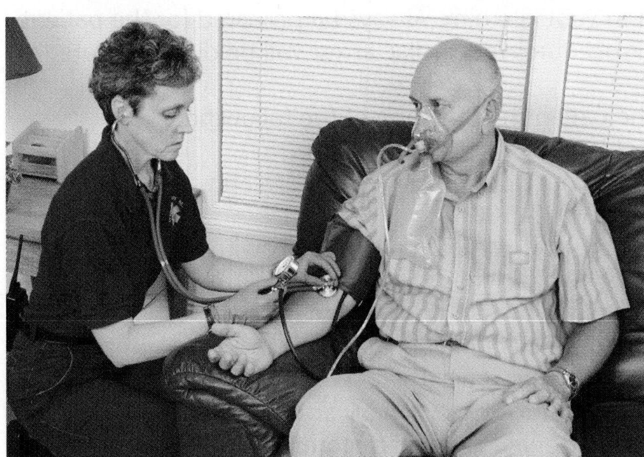

8. Reassess the patient, and document findings.

PATIENT ASSESSMENT

CARDIAC COMPROMISE

After performing your initial assessment, perform a focused history and physical exam. Get a history of the present illness by asking the OPQRST questions (inquire about onset, provocation, quality, radiation, severity, and time). Also get a SAMPLE history (signs/symptoms, allergies, medications the patient may be taking, pertinent past history, last oral intake, events leading to the present emergency). Then take baseline vital signs.

The following signs and symptoms are often associated with cardiac compromise:

- Pain, pressure, or discomfort in the chest or upper abdomen (epigastrium)
- Difficulty breathing
- Palpitations
- Sudden onset of sweating and nausea or vomiting
- Anxiety (feeling of impending doom, irritability)
- Abnormal pulse
- Abnormal blood pressure ■

PATIENT CARE

CARDIAC COMPROMISE

Follow these steps for the emergency care of a patient with suspected cardiac compromise:

1. Place the patient in a position of comfort, typically sitting up. This is especially true of patients with difficulty breathing. Patients who are hypotensive (systolic blood pressure less than 90) will usually feel better lying down. This position allows more blood to flow to the brain. Occasionally, you will see a patient who has both difficulty breathing and hypotension. It may be very difficult to find a good position in this case. The best way to determine the proper position is to ask the patient what position will relieve his breathing difficulty without making him weak or lightheaded.
2. Apply high-concentration oxygen through a nonrebreather mask if not already done. If the patient has or develops an altered mental status, you will need to open and maintain the patient's airway. If the patient is not breathing adequately, you will also need to ventilate him. Always be prepared for the patient to go into cardiac arrest. (Procedures for cardiac arrest will be discussed later in this chapter.)
3. Transport immediately if the patient has any one of the following:
   - No history of cardiac problems
   - History of cardiac problems, but does not have nitroglycerin
   - Systolic blood pressure below 90–100
4. Determine where you will transport the patient. In areas with more than one hospital, there may be one or two facilities with special treatment available for cardiac patients. Almost all hospitals can administer an intravenous drug to dissolve the clot that is causing insufficient oxygenation of the heart. Another way to unclog the coronary artery is to insert a catheter with a balloon at the tip into the arterial system and thread it into the coronary arteries. When the balloon reaches the narrow section of artery, it is inflated, compressing the obstructive material against the side of the blood vessel and opening up circulation to the

continued

heart muscle again. This method is often better than the "clotbuster drug" approach when it is done early (within a few hours of onset of symptoms). Only hospitals with special facilities and available staff can do this, however. If your EMS system has the ability to transport patients to a hospital with this capability, there will be a local protocol that you should follow describing when, where, and how you should transport patients with certain signs and symptoms.

5. Give the patient (or help the patient take) nitroglycerin (Scan 17-2) if all of the following conditions are met:
   - Patient complains of chest pain
   - Patient has a history of cardiac problems
   - Patient's physician has prescribed nitroglycerin (NTG)
   - Patient has the nitroglycerin with him
   - Patient has a pulse rate greater than 50 and below 100 beats per minute (follow local protocols)
   - Systolic blood pressure meets your protocol criteria (usually greater than 90 to 100 systolic)
   - Patient has not taken Viagra or a similar drug for erectile dysfunction within 48 to 72 hours
   - Medical direction authorizes administration of the medication
6. After giving one dose of the nitroglycerin, give a repeat dose in 5 minutes if all of the following conditions are met:
   - Patient experiences no relief or only partial relief
   - Systolic blood pressure remains greater than 90 to 100 systolic
   - Medical direction authorizes another dose of the medication

   Administer a maximum of three doses of nitroglycerin, reassessing vital signs and chest pain after each dose. If the blood pressure falls below 90 to 100 systolic, treat the patient for shock (hypoperfusion). Transport promptly.
7. If your EMS system and local protocols allow it, give the patient (or help the patient take) aspirin if *all* of the following conditions are met:
   - Patient complains of chest pain
   - Patient is not allergic to aspirin
   - Patient has no history of asthma
   - Patient is not already taking any medications to prevent clotting
   - Patient has no other contraindications to aspirin (Scan 17-3)
   - Patient is able to swallow without endangering the airway
   - Medical direction authorizes administration of the medication ■

PEDIATRIC NOTE

Children usually have very healthy hearts, so it is rare for an EMT to see a pediatric patient with a cardiac problem. Most such problems are congenital; that is, the child is born with them, so they are discovered before the newborn leaves the nursery. You may see a child who has had cardiac surgery or has learned to live with his problem through changes in lifestyle or medication. In cases like these, parents are frequently very well informed and can be of great assistance.

NOTE

Transportation of a patient with a heart condition must be carried out in a thoughtful, calm, and careful fashion. A rough ride with sudden starts, stops, and turns and siren wailing is likely to increase the patient's fear and apprehension, placing additional stress on the heart. Speed is important; the patient must reach the hospital quickly. However, the judicious use of siren or horn must be balanced against the possibility of worsening the patient's condition.

SCAN 17-2 • Nitroglycerin

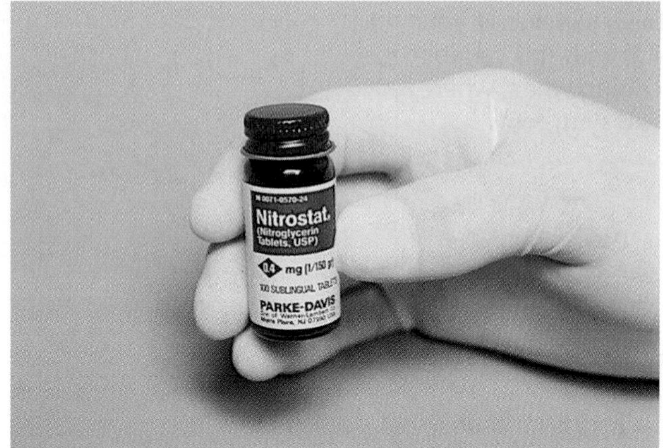

MEDICATION NAME

1. Generic: nitroglycerin
2. Trade: Nitrostat™, Nitrolingual®

INDICATIONS

All the following conditions must be met:

1. Patient complains of chest pain.
2. Patient has a history of cardiac problems.
3. Patient's physician has prescribed nitroglycerin (NTG).
4. Systolic blood pressure is greater than 90 to 100 systolic.
5. Medical direction authorizes administration of the medication.

CONTRAINDICATIONS

1. Patient has hypotension, or a systolic blood pressure below 90 to 100.
2. Patient has a pulse rate below 50 or above 100. Follow local protocols.
3. Patient has a head injury.
4. Patient is an infant or child.
5. Patient has already taken the maximum prescribed dose.
6. Patient has recently taken Viagra, Cialis, or another drug for erectile dysfunction.

MEDICATION FORM

Tablet, sublingual (under-the-tongue) spray

DOSAGE

One dose. Repeat in 5 minutes, if less than complete relief, if systolic blood pressure remains above 90 to 100, and if authorized by medical direction, up to a maximum of three doses.

ADMINISTRATION

1. Perform focused assessment for cardiac patient.

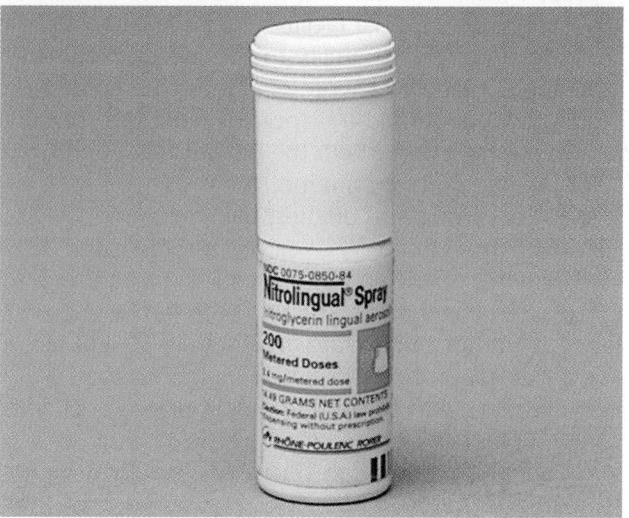

2. Take blood pressure. (Systolic pressure must be above 90 to 100.)
3. Contact medical direction, if no standing orders.
4. Ensure right medication, right patient, right dose, right route. Check expiration date.
5. Ensure patient is alert.
6. Question patient on last dose taken and effects. Ensure understanding of route of administration.
7. Ask patient to lift tongue, and place tablet or spray dose under tongue (while wearing gloves) or have patient place tablet or spray under tongue.
8. Have patient keep mouth closed with tablet under tongue (without swallowing) until dissolved and absorbed.
9. Recheck blood pressure within 2 minutes.
10. Record administration, route, and time.
11. Perform reassessment.

ACTIONS

1. Relaxes blood vessels
2. Decreases workload of heart

SIDE EFFECTS

1. Hypotension (lowers blood pressure)
2. Headache
3. Pulse rate changes

REASSESSMENT STRATEGIES

1. Monitor blood pressure.
2. Ask patient about effect on pain relief.
3. Seek medical direction before readministering.
4. Record assessments.

SCAN 17-3 • Aspirin

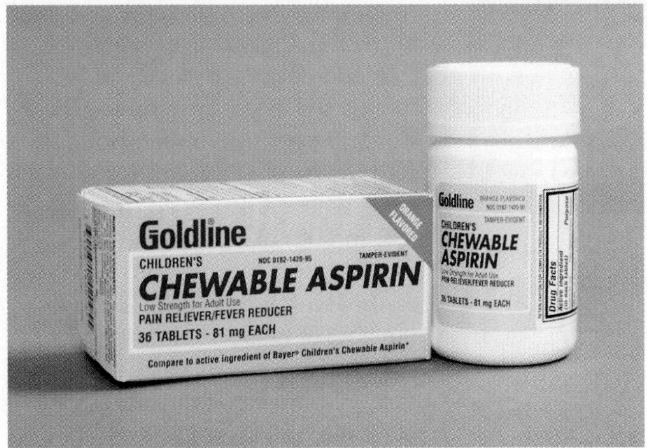

MEDICATION NAME

1. Generic: aspirin
2. Trade: many available

INDICATIONS

All the following conditions must be met:

1. Patient complains of chest pain.
2. Patient is not allergic to aspirin.
3. Patient has no history of asthma.
4. Patient is not already taking any medications to prevent clotting.
5. Patient has no other contraindications to aspirin.
6. Patient is able to swallow without endangering the airway.
7. Medical direction authorizes administration of the medication.

CONTRAINDICATIONS

1. Patient is unable to swallow without endangering the airway.
2. Patient is allergic or sensitive to aspirin.
3. Patient has a history of asthma (many people with asthma are allergic to aspirin).
4. Patient has gastrointestinal ulcer or recent bleeding.
5. Patient has a known bleeding disorder.
6. Medical direction may decide if the benefit of giving aspirin to a patient who has one of the following conditions outweighs the risk:
   a. Is already taking medication to prevent clotting (including aspirin)
   b. Pregnancy
   c. Recent surgery

MEDICATION FORM

Tablet; many EMS systems use baby aspirin, usually supplied as 81 mg chewable tablets.

DOSAGE

162 to 324 mg (two to four 81 mg tablets of chewable baby aspirin). Aspirin does not usually need to be administered more than once in the early treatment of cardiac problems.

ADMINISTRATION

1. Perform focused assessment for cardiac patient.
2. Contact medical direction, if no standing orders.
3. Ensure right medication, right patient, right dose, right route. Check expiration date.
4. Ensure patient is alert.
5. Ask patient to chew (if directed by protocol) and swallow tablets.
6. Record administration, route, and time.
7. Perform reassessment.

ACTIONS

1. Prevents blood from clotting as quickly, leading to increased survival after myocardial infarction.
2. When administered to cardiac patients, aspirin is not being used to relieve pain.

SIDE EFFECTS

1. Nausea
2. Vomiting
3. Heartburn
4. If patient is allergic, bronchospasm and wheezing
5. Bleeding

REASSESSMENT STRATEGIES

1. Perform ongoing assesssment.
2. Evaluate patient for new onset of difficulty breathing from bronchospasm.
3. Any bleeding resulting from the aspirin is very unlikely to occur before the patient arrives at a hospital.
4. Record assessments.

Cardiac compromise and its associated signs and symptoms can be caused by a number of disorders that affect the condition and function of the blood vessels and the heart. (Keep in mind that, as an EMT, you do not need to know that your patient's signs and symptoms are caused by a cardiovascular problem, much less be able to diagnose the specific disorder. The information about cardiovascular disorders given here is intended to serve only as general background.)

The majority of cardiovascular emergencies are caused, directly or indirectly, by changes in the inner walls of arteries. These arteries can be part of the systemic (total body), pulmonary (lung), or coronary (heart) circulatory systems. Problems with the heart's electrical and mechanical functions also cause cardiovascular emergencies.

CORONARY ARTERY DISEASE

The heart is a muscle—a very active muscle. Like all other muscles, it needs oxygen to contract. The blood that is pumped through the chambers of the heart does not provide oxygen to the heart itself. Instead, the heart muscle is supplied with oxygenated blood by special blood vessels: the coronary arteries.

When the coronary arteries are narrowed or blocked, blood flow is reduced, thereby reducing the amount of oxygen delivered to the heart. This might not be noticed when the body is at rest or at a low activity level. However, when the body is subject to stress or exertion, the heart rate (beats per minute) increases. With the increased heart rate comes an increased need for oxygen. Arteries that are narrowed or blocked cannot supply enough blood to meet the heart's demands.

F•Y•I

CAUSES OF CARDIAC COMPROMISE

Conditions that narrow or block the arteries of the heart are commonly called **coronary artery disease (CAD).** Coronary artery disease is a serious health problem that results in hundreds of thousands of deaths yearly in the United States.

CAD commonly involves either of two conditions, atherosclerosis and arteriosclerosis. *Atherosclerosis* is a build-up of fatty deposits on the inner walls of arteries (Figure 17-1). This build-up causes a narrowing of the inner vessel diameter, restricting the flow of blood. Fats and other particles combine to form this deposit, known as plaque. As time passes, calcium can be deposited at the site of the plaque, causing the area to harden.

Arteriosclerosis is a stiffening or hardening of the artery wall resulting from calcium deposits. Often called "hardening of the arteries," this condition causes the vessel to lose its elasticity, changing blood flow and increasing blood pressure.

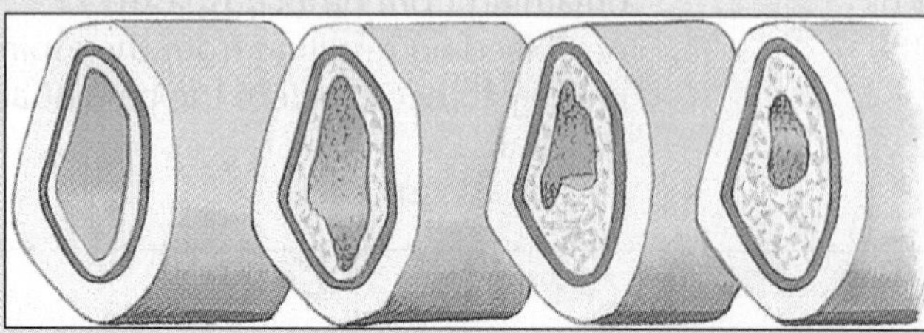

Figure 17-1 • Atherosclerosis, the process of plaque formation on the interior wall of an artery.

In CAD, the amount of blood passing through the artery is restricted. The rough surface formed inside the artery can facilitate formation of blood clots, which narrow the artery even more. The clot and debris from the plaque form a **thrombus.** A thrombus can reach a size where it causes an **occlusion** (cutting off) of blood flow, or it may break loose to become an **embolism** and move to occlude the flow of blood somewhere downstream in a smaller artery. In cases of partial or complete blockage, the tissues beyond the point of blockage will be starved of oxygen and may die. If this blockage involves a large area of the heart (as in a heart attack) or the brain (causing one kind of stroke), the results may be quickly fatal.

Some factors that put a person at risk of developing CAD, such as heredity (a close relative who has CAD) and age, cannot be changed. However, there are also many risk factors that can be modified to reduce the risk of coronary artery disease. These include hypertension (high blood pressure), obesity, lack of exercise, elevated blood levels of cholesterol and triglycerides, and cigarette smoking.

Many patients have more than one of these risk factors. Fortunately, the damage caused by the second group of risk factors may be reversed or slowed by changing behavior. Smokers can return to the risk level of a nonsmoker soon after quitting. Medication and weight loss can lower high blood pressure. Improved diet and exercise can help the other controllable factors.

In the majority of cardiac-related medical emergencies, the reduced blood supply to the myocardium (heart muscle) causes the emergency. The most common symptom of this reduced blood supply is chest pain. Patients may have symptoms that range anywhere from mild chest pain to cardiac arrest. Angina pectoris (chest pain), acute myocardial infarction (heart attack), and congestive heart failure—all conditions that can be related to CAD—are discussed later in this chapter.

ANEURYSM

Another cause of cardiovascular system disorder stems from weakened sections in the arterial walls. Each weak spot that begins to dilate (balloon) is known as an **aneurysm.** This weakening can be related to other arterial diseases, or it can exist independently. When a weakened section of an artery bursts, there can be rapid, life-threatening internal bleeding (Figure 17-2). Tissues beyond the rupture can be damaged because the oxygenated blood they need is escaping and not reaching them. If a major artery ruptures, death from shock can occur very quickly. The two most common sites of aneurysms that you will encounter in emergency situations are the aorta (see Chapter 18, "Acute Abdominal Emergencies") and the brain (see Chapter 19, "Diabetic Emergencies and Altered Mental Status"). When an artery in the brain ruptures, a severe form of stroke occurs. The severity is dependent on the site of the stroke and the amount of blood loss.

ELECTRICAL MALFUNCTIONS OF THE HEART

Electrical impulses generated within the heart are responsible for the heart's rhythmic beating that pumps blood throughout the body. A malfunction of the heart's electrical system will generally result in a **dysrhythmia,** an irregular, or absent, heart rhythm. Dysrhythmias include bradycardia (abnormally slow, less than 60 beats per minute), tachycardia (abnormally fast, greater than 100 beats per minute), and rhythms that may be present when there is no pulse (in cardiac arrest) including ventricular fibrillation, ventricular tachycardia, pulseless electrical activity, and asystole (described later in this chapter).

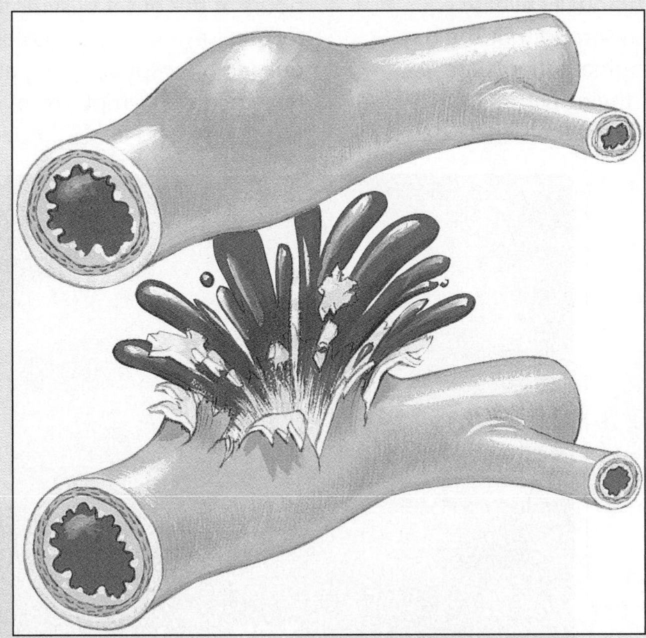

Figure 17-2 • A weakened area in the wall of an artery will tend to balloon out, forming a sac-like aneurysm, which may eventually burst.

MECHANICAL MALFUNCTIONS OF THE HEART

Another complication sometimes seen with a myocardial infarction, or heart attack, is mechanical pump failure. In this situation, a lack of oxygen causes the death of a portion of the myocardium. The dead area can no longer contract and pump. If a large enough area of the heart dies, the pumping action of the whole heart will be affected. This can lead to cardiac arrest, shock, pulmonary edema (fluids "backing up" in the lungs), or congestive heart failure (discussed later in this chapter). A few heart attack patients suffer cardiac rupture as the dead tissue area of the heart muscle bursts open. This occurs days after a heart attack.

Deterioration or malfunction of the heart valves is also a common component of cardiovascular disorders such as congestive heart failure.

ANGINA PECTORIS

Angina pectoris means, literally, a pain in the chest. Coronary artery disease has narrowed the arteries that supply the heart. During times of exertion or stress, the heart works harder. The portion of the myocardium supplied by the narrowed artery becomes starved for oxygen. When the myocardium is deprived of oxygen, chest pain—angina pectoris—is the most frequent result (Figure 17-3). This pain is sometimes called an angina attack.

Since the pain of angina pectoris comes on after stress or exertion, the pain will frequently diminish when the patient stops the exertion. As the oxygen demand of the heart returns to normal, the pain subsides. Seldom does this painful attack last longer than 3 to 5 minutes.

continued

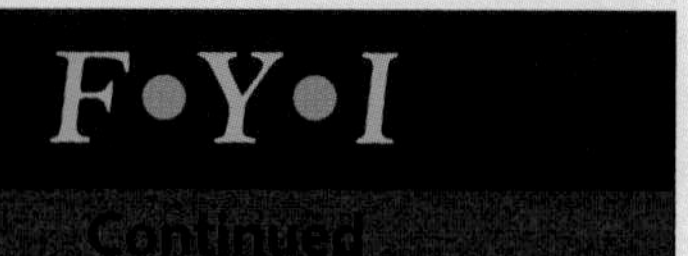

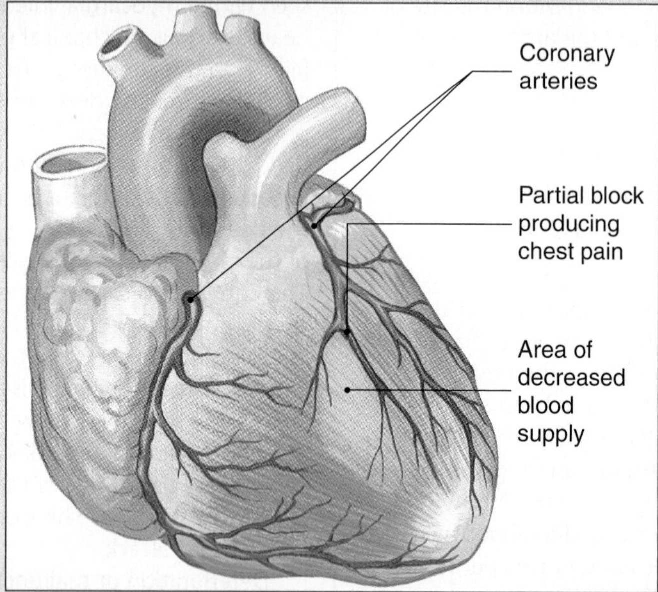

Figure 17-3 • Angina pectoris, or chest pain, results when a coronary artery is blocked, depriving an area of the myocardium of oxygen.

Possession of **nitroglycerin** is another indication that the patient has a history of this condition. Nitroglycerin is a medication that dilates the blood vessels. This results in more blood staying in the veins of the body, so there is less blood coming back to the heart. With less blood to pump out, the heart does not have to work as hard.

Nitroglycerin is available in tablets that are placed under the patient's tongue to dissolve, as well as sprays and patches. The patches have adhesive that keeps them on the skin. They gradually release nitroglycerin throughout the day.

Most angina patients are advised by their doctors to take nitroglycerin for their chest pain. Patients are usually told to rest and are allowed to take three nitroglycerin doses over a 10-minute period. If there is no relief of symptoms after that time, they are instructed to call for help.

ACUTE MYOCARDIAL INFARCTION

The condition in which a portion of the myocardium (heart muscle) dies as a result of oxygen starvation is known as **acute myocardial infarction (AMI)** (Figure 17-4). Often called a heart attack by laypersons, AMI is brought on by the narrowing or occlusion of the coronary artery that supplies the region with blood. Rarely, the interruption of blood flow to the myocardium may be due to the rupturing of a coronary artery (aneurysm).

The American Heart Association reports over a million cases of AMI in the United States each year. Cardiovascular disease causes hundreds of thousands of deaths annually. A major portion of these deaths are cases of **sudden death,** a cardiac arrest that occurs within 2 hours of the onset of symptoms. In most cases, sudden death occurs outside of hospitals. The patient may have no prior symptoms of coronary artery disease. Nearly 25 percent of

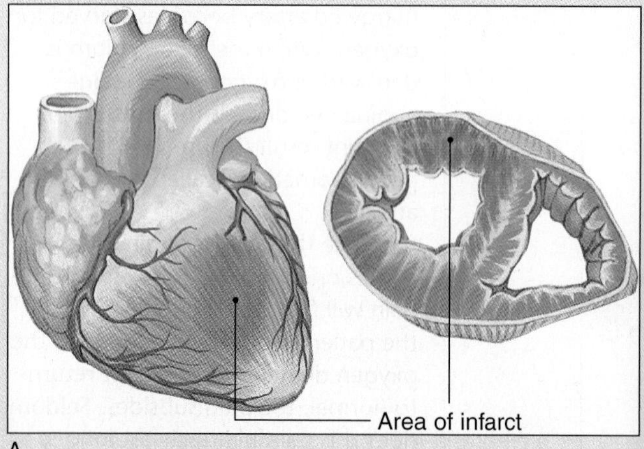

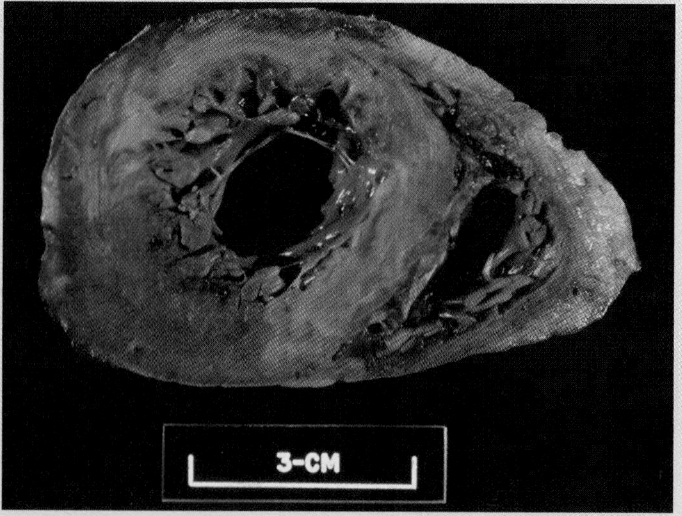

Figure 17-4 • (A) Cross-section of a myocardial infarction and (B) a heart with normal and infarcted tissue.

these individuals have no previous history of cardiac problems.

A variety of factors can cause an AMI. Coronary artery disease is usually the underlying reason for the incident. However, for some patients, factors often regarded as harmless may trigger an AMI. These factors include chronic respiratory problems, unusual exertion, or severe emotional stress.

The treatment of AMI has changed radically over recent years. Previously, patients were admitted to coronary care units where they were observed and, when emergencies occurred, treated with varying degrees of success. Now, some patients receive treatment with medications called *fibrinolytics* to dissolve the clot that is blocking the coronary artery. To be most effective, these medications must be administered early. With each hour that passes before they are administered, they become less and less likely to dissolve the clot. As noted earlier, another way to unclog the coronary artery is to insert a catheter with a balloon that can be inflated to reopen circulation to the heart, a procedure known as *balloon angioplasty* or *balloon catheterization*. Many patients with myocardial infarctions are not candidates for these treatments, but those who are must reach the hospital quickly.

A patient who leaves the hospital after an AMI will usually be told to take aspirin every day to prevent another episode. He will also probably be told to take a medication known as a "beta blocker." This group of medications slows the heart and makes it beat less strongly. This would not usually be considered a good thing, but in these patients it results in a decrease in the work the heart has to do. This actually benefits the heart and leads to longer and better lives for these patients.

CONGESTIVE HEART FAILURE

Congestive heart failure (CHF) is a condition of excessive fluid build-up in the lungs and/or other organs and body parts because of the inadequate pumping of the heart. The fluid build-up causes **edema,** or swelling. The disorder is traditionally termed *congestive* because the fluids congest, or clog, the organs. It is termed *heart failure* because the congestion both results from and also aggravates failure of the heart to function properly. The congestion may also result from and aggravate failure of the lungs to function properly.

Congestive heart failure may be brought on by diseased heart valves, hypertension, or some form of obstructive pulmonary disease such as emphysema. CHF is often a complication of AMI. Congestive heart failure often progresses as follows:

1. A patient sustains an AMI. Myocardium in the area of the left ventricle dies. (Recall the function of the heart: The left is the side of the heart that receives oxygenated blood from the lungs and pulmonary circulation and pumps it to the rest of the body.)
2. Because of the damage to the left ventricle, blood backs up into the pulmonary circulation and then the lungs. Fluid accumulation in the lungs is called **pulmonary edema.** This edema causes a poor exchange of oxygen between the lungs and the bloodstream, and the patient experiences shortness of breath, or dyspnea. Listening to this patient's lungs with a stethoscope may reveal crackling or bubbly lung sounds called crackles (rales). Some patients cough up blood-tinged sputum from their lungs.
3. Left heart failure, if untreated, commonly causes right heart failure. The right side of the heart (which receives blood from the body and pumps it to the lungs) becomes congested because the clogged lungs cannot receive more blood. In turn, fluids may accumulate in the dependent (lower) extremities, the liver, and the abdomen. Accumulation of fluid in the feet or ankles is known as **pedal edema.** The abdomen may become noticeably distended. In a bedridden patient, fluid collects in the sacral area of the spine.

The signs and symptoms of CHF may include:

- Tachycardia (rapid pulse, 100 beats per minute or more)
- Dyspnea (shortness of breath)
- Normal or elevated blood pressure
- Cyanosis
- Diaphoresis (profuse sweating), or cool and clammy skin
- Pulmonary edema, sometimes coughing up of frothy white or pink sputum
- Anxiety or confusion due to hypoxia (inadequate supply of oxygen to the brain and other tissues) caused by poor oxygen/carbon dioxide exchange
- Pedal edema
- Engorged, pulsating neck veins (late sign)
- Enlarged liver and spleen, with abdominal distention (late sign)

The CHF patient is probably on several medications for this condition. Often patients will tell you that they take a water pill for fluid build-up. This refers to a diuretic, a medication that helps remove fluid from the circulatory system. Other medications may decrease the workload of the heart, leading to improvement in the patient's condition. ■

POINT OF VIEW

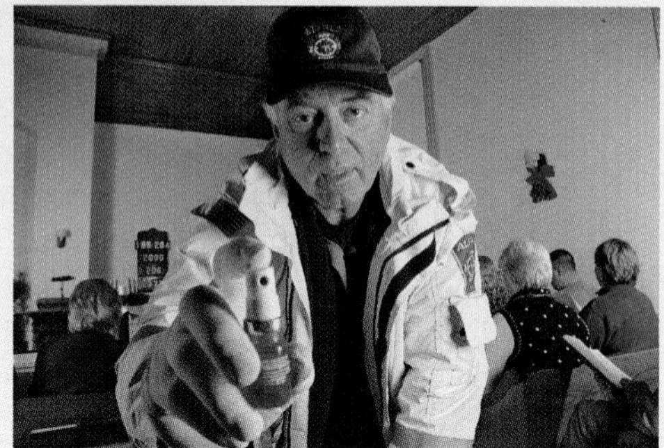

"I couldn't believe I was having chest pain. How cruel was it that I'd prayed I wouldn't have another heart attack—and where do I get chest pain again? Church. Not only did my chest hurt, but I was so embarrassed.

"I was so embarrassed and worried that I forgot I had the nitro spray with me. The EMTs came and checked me over and asked me if I'd ever had pain like this before. That was when I remembered. I never had to use it before. They put a spray under my tongue before they wheeled me out of church, because it was quite a ways to get down and to the ambulance. It actually helped.

"When we got to the ambulance I told them that my pain felt better. When they found out that I still had some pain they checked me again and then gave me another spray. I have to say I relaxed a bit when the pain went away.

"When you have chest pain, you think you are going to die. It is a great feeling suddenly realizing that the pain is gone. You really think you have a chance of living. Wow."

CRITICAL DECISION MAKING: Meeting Sublingual Nitroglycerin Criteria

You are treating a patient with chest pain. For each scenario provided, decide whether this patient meets the general criteria for sublingual nitroglycerin administration. Each of the patients has nitroglycerin prescribed by his cardiologist.

1. You are treating a patient with chest pain. He is 84 years old. His wife tells you that he began having a sensation in his chest he thought was indigestion about 2 hours ago. The patient is very pale and sweaty and appears sleepy. His pulse is 104 slightly irregular, respirations 28 and adequate, blood pressure 94/66.
2. You are treating a 68-year-old male patient who has a history of angina pectoris. He tells you that he began having chest discomfort just after eating dinner. The discomfort is in the center of his chest and is described as a heavy feeling. It feels like the last time he had a heart problem. His vital signs are pulse 92 strong and regular, respirations 20 and adequate, blood pressure 138/92, skin warm and moist.
3. You are treating a 49-year old male patient complaining of pain in his "stomach." He states the pain is below his diaphragm and radiates to the left side. He has taken one nitroglycerin spray without relief. The patient states this pain is not like his one heart attack. His vital signs are pulse 68 strong and regular, respirations 18 and adequate, blood pressure 112/68, skin warm and dry.

CARDIAC ARREST

In a typical ambulance service, only 1 to 2 percent of emergency calls are cardiac arrests. Most patients with heart problems do not go into cardiac arrest while they are under your care. Nonetheless, EMS systems exert a great deal of time and energy on attempts to resuscitate these patients. The odds of bringing a cardiac-arrest patient back to life have increased considerably over the last 15 or 20 years. As the problem of cardiac arrest has received more attention, EMS researchers, physicians, administrators, and providers have learned more about what is effective and what is not.

Chain of Survival

The American Heart Association has summarized the most important factors that affect survival of cardiac arrest patients in its chain of survival concept. The chain (Figure 17-5) has four elements: (1) early access, (2) early CPR, (3) early defibrillation, and (4) early advanced care. An EMS system where each of these links is strong is much more likely to bring back a patient from cardiac arrest than a system with weaknesses anywhere along the chain. This has been shown in systems that tried to strengthen just one link (early defibrillation) without strengthening the other links.

Early Access

Early access means that the person who sees someone collapse or finds someone unresponsive calls a dispatcher who quickly gets EMS responding to the emergency. Unfortunately, this is easier said than done. The lay public, unlike EMS providers, are not used to recognizing emergencies. It takes longer for them to realize that an emergency exists and that they should call for help right away. Even when a layperson does decide to make the call for help, there may still be obstacles.

Many areas still do not have 911. This means that emergency services have seven-digit telephone numbers that laypeople cannot be expected to remember. Even though many phone companies list emergency numbers on the inside cover of their directories, this adds an extra step to the process and delays even further the call for help. Many EMS agencies in this position have public information programs that include the distribution of telephone stickers with emergency numbers on them. Since Americans change residence frequently (and buy new telephones more often than that), emergency services must make these stickers available frequently and easily.

Early CPR

Early CPR can increase survival significantly. About the only time it does not help is when defibrillation reaches the patient within approximately 2 minutes or less. Since this rarely happens in real life, EMS agencies need to address this factor. There are at least three ways in which CPR can be delivered earlier: get CPR-trained professionals to the patient faster, train laypeople in CPR, and train dispatchers to instruct callers in how to perform CPR.

coronary artery disease (CAD) diseases that affect the arteries of the heart.

thrombus (THROM-bus) a clot formed of blood and plaque attached to the inner wall of an artery or vein.

occlusion (uh-KLU-zhun) blockage, as of an artery by fatty deposits.

embolism (EM-bo-lizm) blockage of a vessel by a clot or foreign material brought to the site by the blood current.

aneurysm (AN-u-rizm) the dilation, or ballooning, of a weakened section of the wall of an artery.

dysrhythmia (dis-RITH-me-ah) a disturbance in heart rate and rhythm.

angina pectoris (AN-ji-nah [or an-JI-nah] PEK-to-ris) pain in the chest, occurring when blood supply to the heart is reduced and a portion of the heart muscle is not receiving enough oxygen.

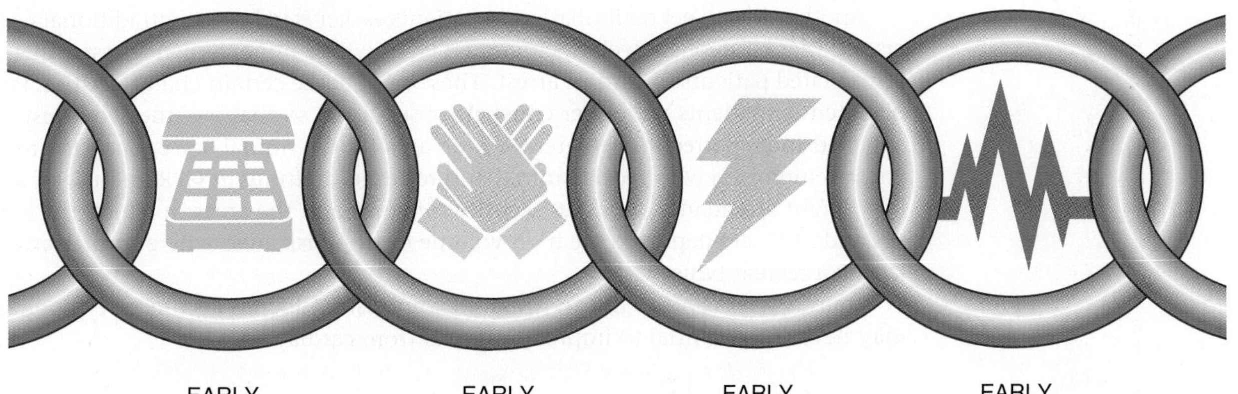

Figure 17-5 • The chain of survival. *(American Heart Association)*

nitroglycerin (NTG) a medication that dilates the blood vessels.

acute myocardial infarction (AMI) (ah-KUTE MY-o-KARD-e-ul in-FARK-shun) the condition in which a portion of the myocardium dies as a result of oxygen starvation; often called a heart attack by laypersons.

sudden death a cardiac arrest that occurs within 2 hours of the onset of symptoms. The patient may have no prior symptoms of coronary artery disease.

congestive heart failure (CHF) the failure of the heart to pump efficiently, leading to excessive blood or fluids in the lungs, the body, or both.

edema (eh-DEEM-uh) swelling resulting from a build-up of fluid in the tissues.

pulmonary edema accumulation of fluid in the lungs.

pedal edema accumulation of fluid in the feet or ankles.

An efficient way to get CPR to patients faster in many areas is to send CPR-trained professionals to the scene. This may mean police, firefighters, security officers, or lifeguards. These professionals need to receive notification of the possible need for CPR as soon as possible. They also need to be in the right place so they can respond quickly to where they are needed.

Some EMS agencies have CPR courses for the lay public as part of their public information and education programs, but too many do not. It is especially important to train the right laypeople. Teaching CPR to elementary and high school students is good, especially in the long run, but these students are not usually present when someone goes into cardiac arrest. The typical cardiac arrest patient is a male in his 60s, so it is not surprising to learn that the typical witness of a cardiac arrest is a woman in her 60s. Middle-age and older people need CPR courses at least as much as children and adolescents.

A surprisingly effective way to get a layperson to perform CPR is for a dispatcher to instruct the caller over the phone. This has been done in a number of areas and has produced significant increases in the survival rate from cardiac arrest. The quality of CPR done by untrained laypeople instructed by dispatchers is comparable to CPR done by laypeople who were trained in CPR previously. This appears to be true even when laypeople perform chest compressions without ventilating the patient. Emergency Medical Dispatchers (EMDs) are trained to give such instructions. Prearrival dispatch instructions to guide other dispatchers in this step are available.

Early Defibrillation

Early defibrillation has received a great deal of attention because it is the single most important factor in determining survival from cardiac arrest.

Although a lot of emphasis has been put on defibrillation, there is often not enough attention paid to early defibrillation. With a few thousand dollars or less, an agency can purchase an automated defibrillator. The hard part is getting this equipment to the patient in cardiac arrest early enough to be effective. If the response time of the defibrillator (time from call received to arrival of the defibrillator) is longer than 8 minutes, virtually no patients survive cardiac arrest. This is often true even if early CPR is performed. Although 8 minutes is really the maximum response time for effective defibrillation, the sooner the defibrillator arrives, the more likely it is that a patient will survive cardiac arrest. In this case, it is literally true that every minute counts.

One way to get around long ambulance response times is to provide defibrillators to other emergency services providers. Some EMS systems have used innovative ways to make sure that a defibrillator arrives in time. In urban and suburban areas, police officers and firefighters have sometimes been equipped with the machines since they may arrive on scene before the ambulance. In rural areas, some EMTs and First Responders carry defibrillators in their personal vehicles so that the patient who needs a defibrillator gets it in time.

Another way to get defibrillation to patients earlier is to have nontraditional responders use them. There are well-documented cases where nonemergency responders have resuscitated patients in cardiac arrest. These cases share certain characteristics: Patients or potential patients are under constant observation so that a witnessed arrest can be detected and reported immediately (e.g., in an airport terminal or a casino), the responders are employees who receive initial and refresher training in CPR and use of an AED (e.g., flight attendants or casino security officers), and the areas in which the employees and AEDs are deployed are high volume or high risk areas where cardiac arrests occur on a regular basis.

Training laypeople to use an AED and administer CPR has become very popular and may have the potential to improve survival from cardiac arrest.

Early Advanced Care

Early advanced care is second only to defibrillation in the drama and excitement it stirs in laypeople. Putting a breathing tube into someone's throat (endotracheal intubation),

Just as researchers continue to evaluate new interventions to improve cardiac resuscitation, they are evaluating treatments to improve cerebral or brain resuscitation. Most patients who regain a spontaneous pulse after a short period of ventricular fibrillation wake up with little or no brain damage. Some patients, however, especially those who had prolonged down times, have significant brain damage that

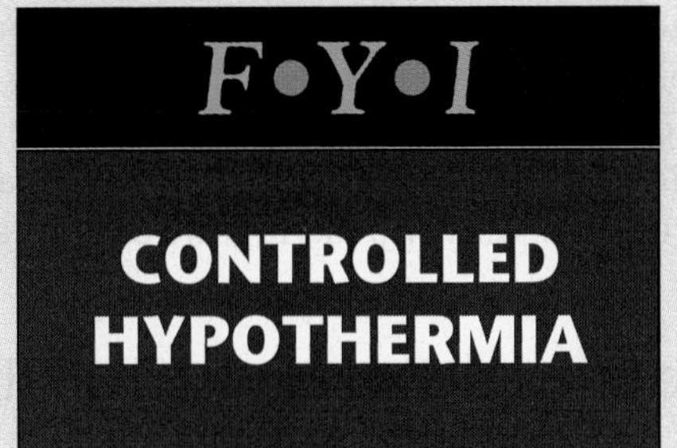

prevents them from returning to normal activities or even regaining consciousness.

One intervention that appears to reduce brain damage in some resuscitated patients is controlled hypothermia. Cooling a patient's body to around 90°F and maintaining it for up to 24 hours has led to more survivors and less brain damage than in patients who did not receive the treatment.

Deliberately putting patients into hypothermia is currently only an experimental prehospital treatment, but you may hear of treatments like this being used in hospitals. ■

putting a needle into someone's arm (starting an intravenous line), and administering medications into an IV line are all activities that laypeople may not understand, but they are actions that the public has come to expect. They may also lead to a higher survival rate.

The most common way for patients to get advanced cardiac life support (ACLS) is through EMT-Paramedics who either respond to the scene or rendezvous with a basic life support unit en route to the hospital. In some areas, there are EMTs who have more training than basic-level EMTs but less than paramedics. Their level of practice is frequently called EMT-Cardiac, EMT-Critical Care, or EMT-Intermediate. They may be able to perform interventions that can improve survival of these patients. Another method that is not quite as fast is for EMTs to transport patients not to a hospital, but to a clinic or other medical facility that is closer. Any such arrangements need to be made before they are actually needed and should be in writing in the form of protocols. These protocols should be approved by your Medical Director.

EMS systems that have early access, early CPR, early defibrillation, and early advanced care have survival rates from cardiac arrest that are higher than systems with one or more weak links in the chain of survival.

Management of Cardiac Arrest

As an EMT, you can provide two links in the chain of survival: early CPR and early defibrillation. You studied CPR in your basic life support course, which was required as a prerequisite to your EMT course. You can review CPR in Appendix B, "Basic Cardiac Life Support Review," at the end of this book.

The rest of this chapter will emphasize the role of defibrillation in treating cardiac arrest patients. Managing a patient in cardiac arrest means you need to be able to:

- Perform one- and two-rescuer CPR (Ordinarily, you will do two-rescuer CPR when you are on duty, but you must be able to perform one-rescuer CPR while your partner is preparing equipment or while you are en route to a medical facility.)
- Use an automated external defibrillator
- Request advanced life support (when available) to continue the chain of survival
- Use a bag-valve-mask device with oxygen
- Use a flow-restricted, oxygen-powered ventilation device
- Lift and move patients
- Suction a patient's airway
- Use airway adjuncts (oropharyngeal and nasopharyngeal airways)
- Take Standard Precautions to protect yourself (and patients)
- Interview bystanders and family members to obtain facts related to the arrest

Although most of the patients you see with chest pain or difficulty breathing will remain alert and in good condition while you are assessing or treating them, a few will go into cardiac arrest before you arrive at the hospital. For this reason, you must be prepared for cardiac arrest whenever you have a patient with chest discomfort or difficulty breathing. This means bringing the defibrillator to the scene when you are dispatched to one of these calls and having the defibrillator nearby while you are transporting.

Automated External Defibrillator (AED)

Types of AEDs

There are two ways someone can defibrillate. The older method (manual defibrillation) is for the operator to look at the patient's heart rhythm on a screen, decide the rhythm is shockable, lubricate and charge two paddles, and deliver a shock to the patient's chest. An automated defibrillator, in contrast, contains a computer that analyzes the patient's heart rhythm after the operator applies two monitoring–defibrillation pads to the patient's chest (Figure 17-6).

There are two types of automated external defibrillators: semiautomatic and fully automatic. Semiautomatic defibrillators, the more common type, advise the EMT to press a button that will cause the machine to deliver a shock through the pads. Semiautomatic defibrillators are sometimes called "shock advisory defibrillators." Fully automated defibrillators do not advise the EMT to take any action. They deliver the shock automatically once enough energy has been accumulated. All the EMT has to do to use

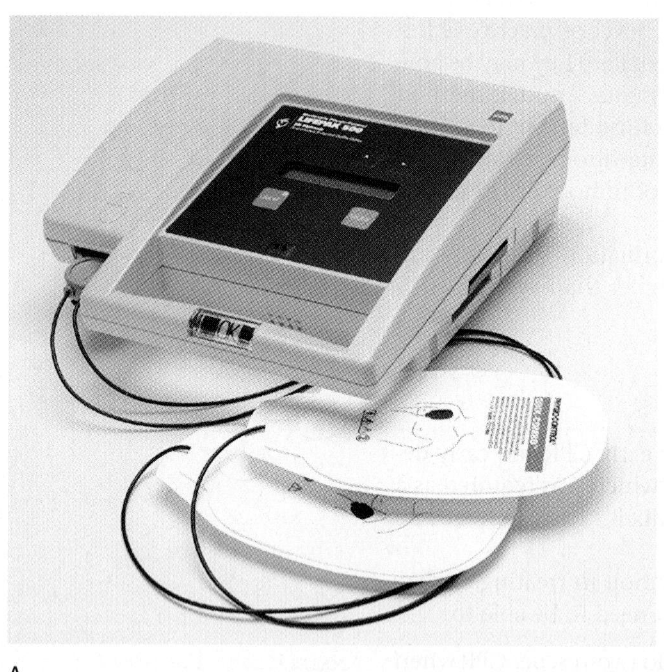

A

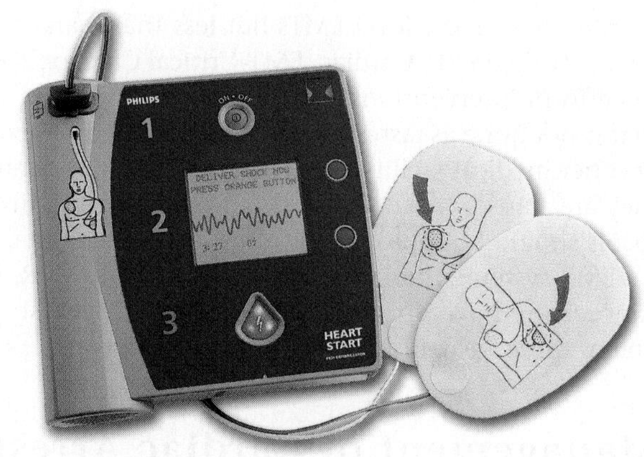

B

C

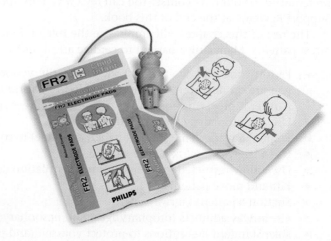

Figure 17-6 • Automated external defibrillators (AEDs) are available from various manufacturers in a variety of models. (A) Biphasic or monophasic Lifepak 500. *(© Medtronic Physiocontrol)* (B) SMART Biphasic Automated External Defibrillator, Model FR2+. *(© Philips Medical Systems)* (C) Pediatric pads for the pediatric version of the Model FR2+. *(© Philips Medical Systems)*

a fully automatic defibrillator is assess the patient, turn on the power, and put the pads on the patient's chest. The following information about how to operate an AED applies principally to a semiautomatic AED.

Another way in which AEDs can be classified is by the type of shock they deliver. The traditional monophasic defibrillator sends a single shock (this is what monophasic means) from the negative pad or paddle to the positive pad or paddle. A biphasic defibrillator sends the shock in one direction and then the other. This kind of machine also typically measures the impedance or resistance between the two pads and adjusts the energy accordingly, delivering more energy when the impedance is higher and less when it is lower. These features allow biphasic AEDs to use less energy and perhaps cause less damage to the heart. Use of biphasic AEDs does not result in higher survival rates, but they are at least as good as monophasic machines and have other advantages. Because the battery doesn't need to deliver as much energy, they are smaller and lighter than monophasic AEDs, a significant factor when an EMT has to carry several heavy pieces of equipment at once.

How AEDs Work

Like all muscles, the heart produces electrical impulses. By putting two monitoring electrodes on the chest, it is possible to "see" the heart's electrical activity. An AED can analyze this cardiac rhythm and determine whether or not it is a rhythm for which a shock is indicated. The microprocessors and the computer programs used to do this have been tested extensively and have been very accurate, both in the laboratory and in the field. Today's AEDs are very reliable in distinguishing between rhythms that need shocks and rhythms that do not need shocks.

When AEDs deliver shocks inappropriately, it is almost always the result of human error. This occurs because the operator did not assess the patient properly (AEDs are designed only for use on patients in cardiac arrest), did not use the AED properly, or did not maintain the machine. The chance of mechanical error is always present, but it is small. Maintaining the AED in good operating order; attaching an AED only to unresponsive, pulseless, nonbreathing patients; practicing frequently; and following your local protocols are the best ways to avoid making an error that could affect a patient.

Often, a cardiac event such as a spasm or blockage of a coronary artery (myocardial infarction or heart attack) is associated with a disturbance of the heart's electrical, or conduction, system, which must function normally if the heart is to continue to beat with a regular rhythm. The most common conditions that result in cardiac arrest are shockable rhythms:

- Ventricular fibrillation
- Ventricular tachycardia

The primary electrical disturbance resulting in cardiac arrest is **ventricular fibrillation (VF).** Up to 50 percent of all cardiac arrest victims will be in VF if EMS personnel arrive in the first 8 minutes or so. The heart in VF may have plenty of electrical energy, but it is totally disorganized. Chaotic electrical activity originating from many sites in the heart prevents the heart muscle from contracting normally and pumping blood. If you could see a heart in VF, it would appear to be quivering like a bag of worms. VF is considered a "shockable rhythm"; that is, VF is a rhythm for which defibrillation is effective.

Automated external defibrillators are also designed to shock a rhythm known as **ventricular tachycardia (V-tach),** if it is very fast. In ventricular tachycardia (a very unusual cardiac arrest rhythm observed in less than 10 percent of all out-of-hospital cases), the heart rhythm is organized, but it is usually quite rapid. The faster the heart rate, the more likely it is that ventricular tachycardia will not allow the heart's chambers to fill with enough blood between beats to produce blood flow sufficient to meet the body's needs, especially that of the brain. Pulseless V-tach is considered a shockable rhythm.

ventricular fibrillation (VF) (ven-TRIK-u-ler fib-ri-LAY-shun)
a condition in which the heart's electrical impulses are disorganized, preventing the heart muscle from contracting normally.

ventricular tachycardia (V-Tach) (ven-TRIK-u-ler tak-i-KAR-de-uh)
a condition in which the heartbeat is quite rapid; if rapid enough, ventricular tachycardia will not allow the heart's chambers to fill with enough blood between beats to produce blood flow sufficient to meet the body's needs.

Some patients with ventricular tachycardia are awake, even with very fast heart rates. If an AED is attached to one of these patients, it will charge up and advise a shock. Since the patient has a pulse and is awake, this action would be inappropriate. This is one of the reasons the AED should be attached only to patients in cardiac arrest.

Nonshockable rhythms include:

- Pulseless electrical activity (PEA)
- Asystole

pulseless electrical activity (PEA) a condition in which the heart's electrical rhythm remains relatively normal, yet the mechanical pumping activity fails to follow the electrical activity, causing cardiac arrest.

asystole (ay-SIS-to-le) a condition in which the heart has ceased generating electrical impulses.

In 15 to 20 percent of cardiac arrest victims, the rhythm is called **pulseless electrical activity (PEA);** that is, the heart muscle itself fails even though the electrical rhythm remains relatively normal. This condition of relatively normal electrical activity but no pumping action means that the heart muscle is severely and almost always terminally sick. Or it may mean that the patient has lost too much blood. The heart could pump if it had something to pump, but there is no fluid in the system. Defibrillation cannot help these people because their heart's electrical rhythm is already organized and slow (unlike ventricular tachycardia, where the rhythm is organized but very fast). PEA is not considered a shockable rhythm.

In the remaining 20 to 50 percent of cardiac arrest victims, the heart has ceased generating electrical impulses altogether. This condition is called **asystole.** When this happens, there is no electrical stimulus to cause the heart muscle to contract, and so it does not. As a result, there is no blood flow, and the patient has no pulse or respirations and is unconscious. (This condition is commonly called "flatline," because the wavy line displayed on an ECG when there is electrical activity goes flat with asystole.) This condition can be the result of untreated ventricular fibrillation, a sick heart, a terminal illness, or severe blood loss. Asystole is not considered a shockable rhythm.

By adding up the numbers, you can see that automated defibrillators will shock at most only about 6 or 7 of every 10 cardiac arrest patients to whom they are attached: those suffering from the disturbed rhythms of ventricular fibrillation and ventricular tachycardia. For patients suffering from pulseless electrical activity (heart muscle failure) or asystole (complete lack of electrical activity), defibrillation will not be effective.

NOTE

As an EMT, you cannot diagnose heart ailments or causes of cardiac arrest. You must initiate CPR and defibrillation as rapidly as possible and, if defibrillation is not successful in restoring heart function, continue CPR to prevent biological death until the patient's care can be taken over at a medical facility or by those with advanced skills.

Coordinating CPR and AED for a Patient in Cardiac Arrest

During your course in cardiopulmonary resuscitation, you learned to interrupt CPR only when absolutely necessary and for as short a period as possible. Since you will be using a defibrillator on patients in cardiac arrest, you need to understand some additional circumstances when you should interrupt CPR.

If you are touching the patient when the AED is analyzing the rhythm, there can be interference from the electrical impulses of your heart and from movement of the patient's muscles. This can fool the AED's computer into believing there is a shockable rhythm when there really isn't one or vice versa. It is also true that if a shock is delivered when you are touching the patient, the shock can be transmitted to you. Although this shock is not likely to cause you serious harm, you could be injured.

For these reasons, no one should ventilate, do chest compressions, or in any way touch the patient when the rhythm is being analyzed or a shock is being delivered.

Defibrillation is more effective than CPR in restoring a patient's pulse, so briefly stopping CPR to allow for rhythm analysis and defibrillation is actually better for the patient. Resume CPR immediately after delivering a shock (Figure 17-7 and Scan 17-4).

NOTE

SHOCK FIRST OR COMPRESSIONS?

Research has shown that when the response time interval is greater than 4 to 5 minutes it is more appropriate to do 2 minutes of CPR (about 5 cycles) prior to analyzing and administering the first shock. It is appropriate to "re-prime the pump" by doing CPR for 2 minutes. If you come on the scene and a citizen or other provider is already doing high-quality compressions, you can count that effort toward the first 2 minutes and proceed with applying the AED.

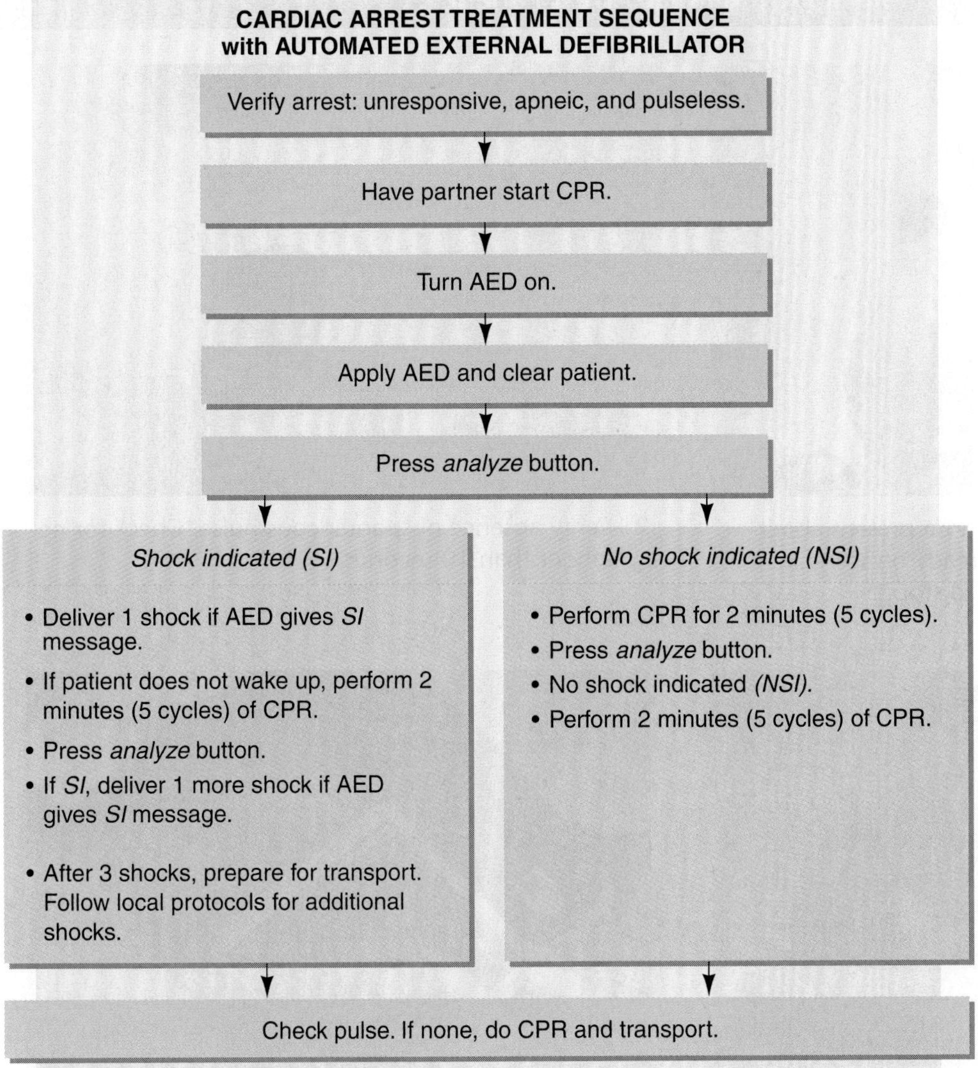

CARDIAC ARREST TREATMENT SEQUENCE with AUTOMATED EXTERNAL DEFIBRILLATOR

Verify arrest: unresponsive, apneic, and pulseless.

↓

Have partner start CPR.

↓

Turn AED on.

↓

Apply AED and clear patient.

↓

Press *analyze* button.

↓

Shock indicated (SI)

- Deliver 1 shock if AED gives *SI* message.
- If patient does not wake up, perform 2 minutes (5 cycles) of CPR.
- Press *analyze* button.
- If *SI*, deliver 1 more shock if AED gives *SI* message.
- After 3 shocks, prepare for transport. Follow local protocols for additional shocks.

No shock indicated (NSI)

- Perform CPR for 2 minutes (5 cycles).
- Press *analyze* button.
- No shock indicated *(NSI).*
- Perform 2 minutes (5 cycles) of CPR.

↓

Check pulse. If none, do CPR and transport.

Notes:

Whenever a *no shock indicated (NSI)* message appears, begin 2 minutes (5 cycles) of CPR.

If the patient regains a pulse, check breathing. Ventilate with high-concentration oxygen, or give oxygen by nonrebreather mask as needed.

If you initially shock the patient and then receive an *NSI* message before giving six shocks, follow the steps in the above right-hand column.

If you initially receive an *NSI* message and then on a subsequent analysis receive a *shock indicated (SI)* message, follow the steps in the above left-hand column.

Occasionally you may need to shift back and forth between the two columns. If this happens, follow the steps until one of the indications for transport (described below) occurs.

Transport as soon as one of the following occurs:

- You have administered three shocks.
- You have received three consecutive *NSI* messages (separated by 2 minutes of CPR).
- The patient regains a pulse.

If you shock the patient out of cardiac arrest and he arrests again, start the sequence of shocks from the beginning.

You should do no more than three cycles of analyze, shock/no shock advised, and CPR before beginning transport. Your local protocols may recommend initiating transport earlier in the sequence.

Figure 17-7 • AED cardiac arrest treatment sequence.

NOTE

APPROPRIATE DOSE OF ELECTRICITY

The proper dose of electricity for the shock depends on the type of unit you are using. For monophasic units the dose should be 360 joules (J). The ideal dose using a biphasic defibrillator is the dose at which the device has been shown to be effective in terminating VF. Biphasic defibrillators use energy levels between 120 to 200 J, depending on the device.

SCAN 17-4 • Assessing and Managing a Cardiac Arrest Patient

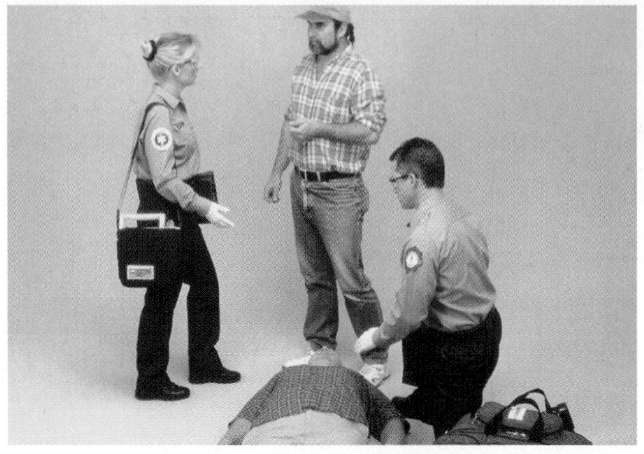

1. On arrival, briefly question those present about arrest events. (If a rescuer already on scene is performing CPR, direct him to stop.)

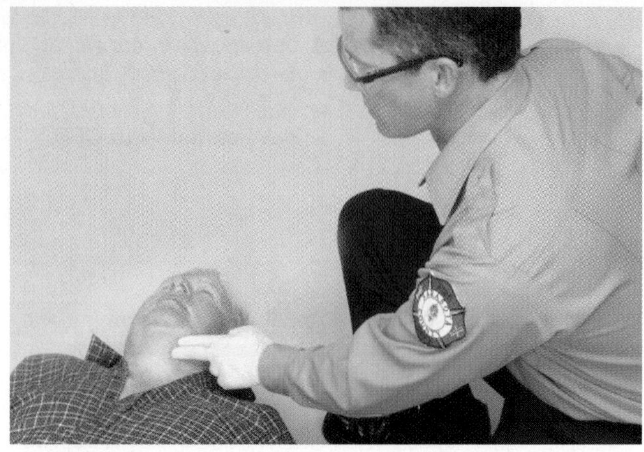

2. Verify absence of spontaneous pulse. Check for no longer than 10 seconds.

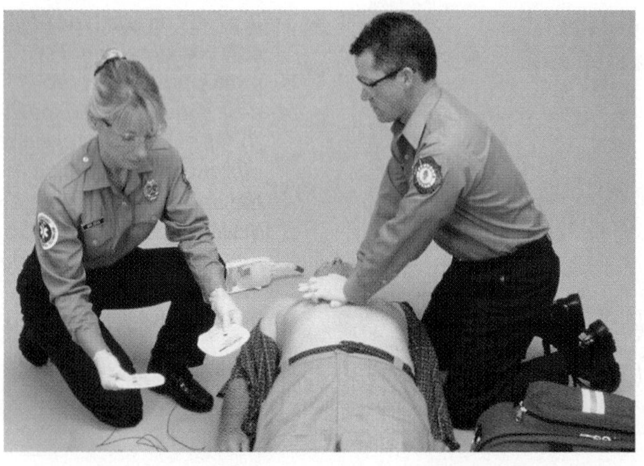

3. One EMT provides CPR; the other sets up the AED. Unless the arrest was witnessed, the patient should receive 2 minutes (5 cycles) of CPR.

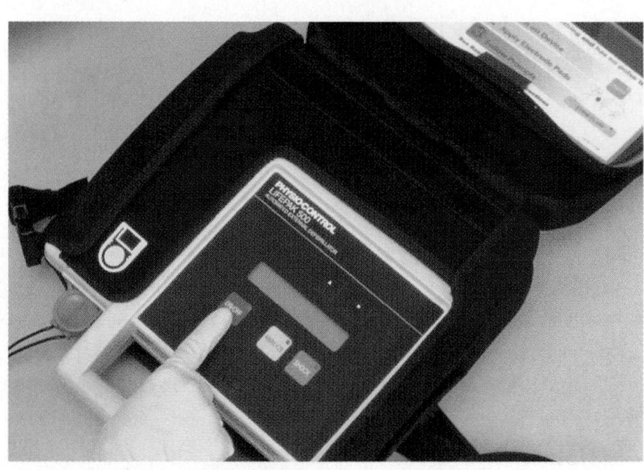

4. Turn on the AED power.

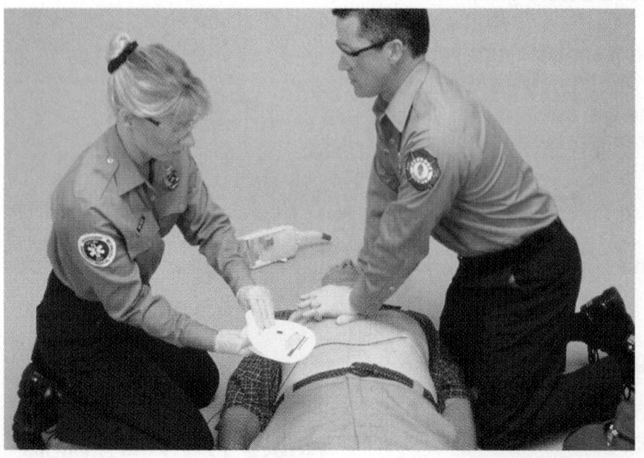

NOTE *At earliest opportunity, call for ALS intercept.*

5. Connect two defibrillator pads to cables, following the color code. Remove backing. Place one pad on the upper right chest, one on the lower left ribs.

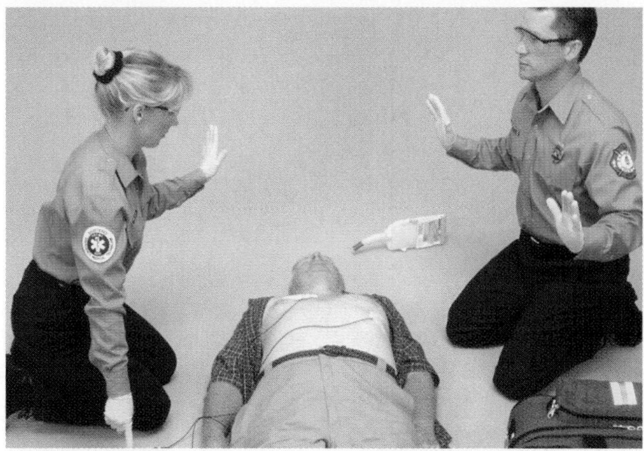

6. Say "Clear!" Ensure that all individuals are clear of patient.

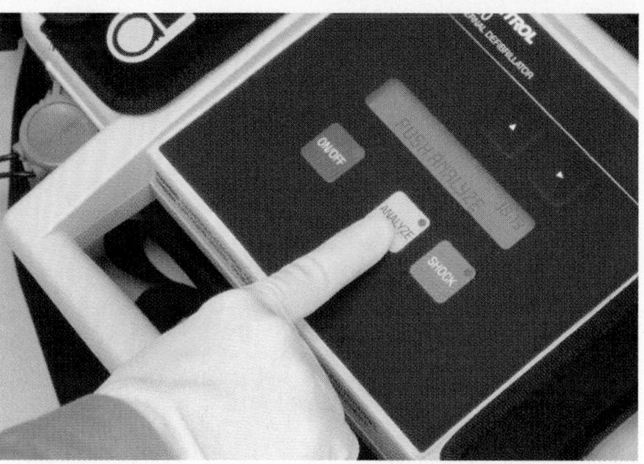

7. After everyone is clear, press the "analyze" button and wait for the AED to analyze the rhythm.

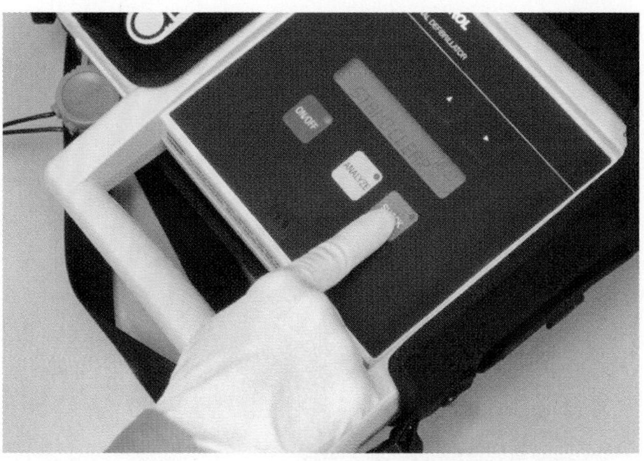

8. If advised by the AED, press the button to deliver a shock. Immediately perform compressions.

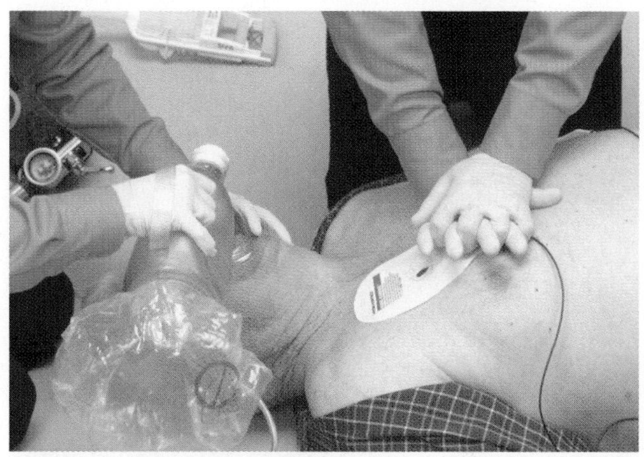

9. Perform CPR for 2 minutes (5 cycles), unless the patient wakes up.

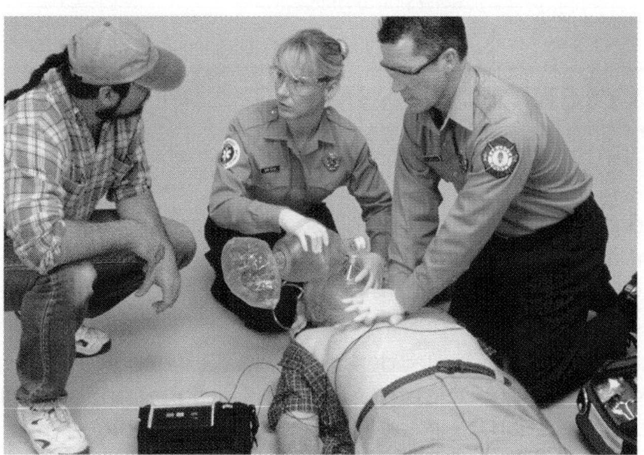

10. Gather additional information on arrest events.

continued

SCAN 17-4 • (Continued)

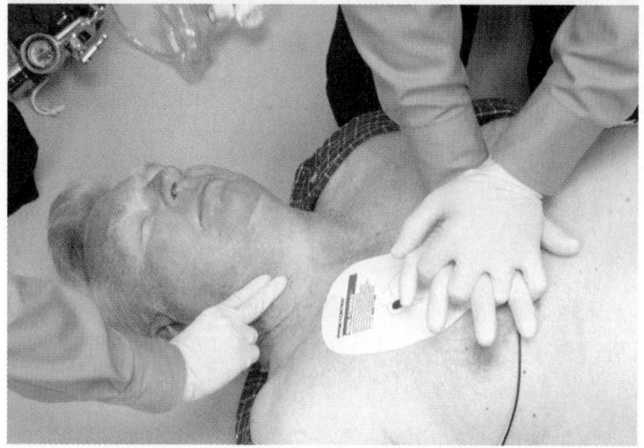

11. Check the patient's pulse during CPR to confirm effectiveness of compressions.

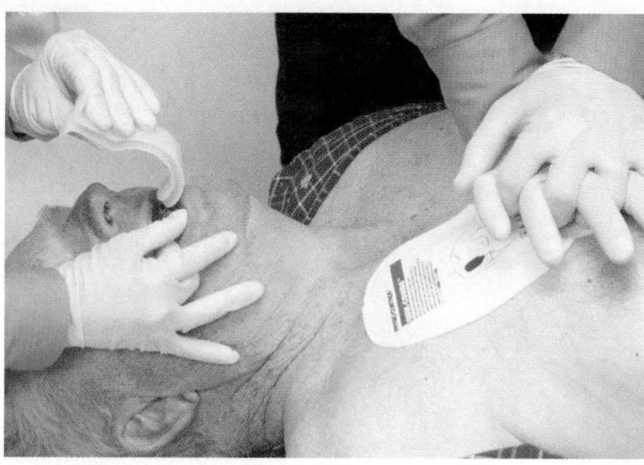

12. Direct insertion of airway adjunct.

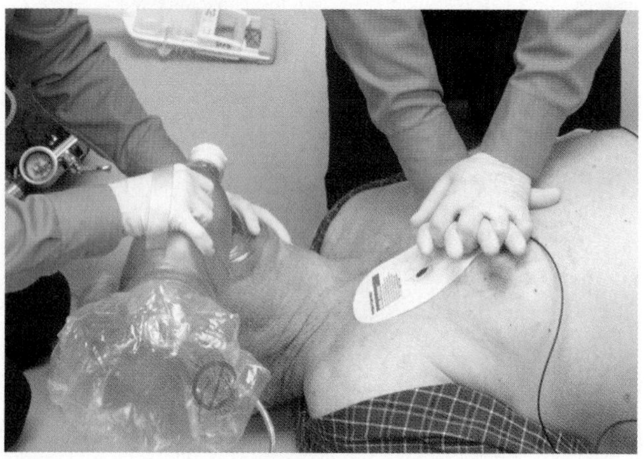

13. Direct ventilation of patient with high-concentration oxygen.

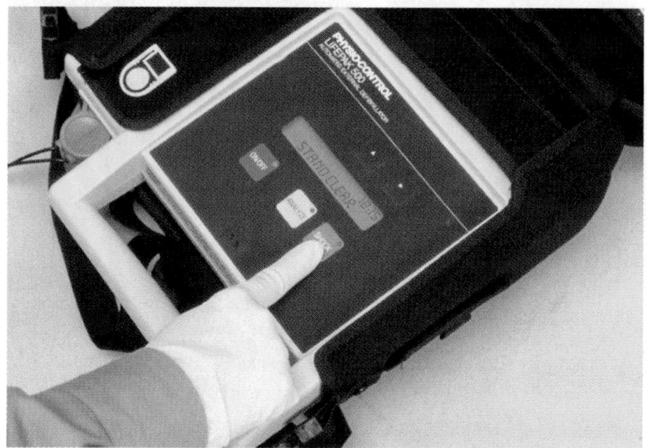

14. After 2 minutes of CPR, have all individuals stand clear and reanalyze with the AED.

PATIENT ASSESSMENT

CARDIAC ARREST

As with all calls, you should protect yourself from infectious diseases by using personal protective equipment and taking Standard Precautions. This is especially important in the case of a cardiac arrest where blood and other body fluids are commonly found. Patient assessment includes the following:

apnea (AP-ne-ah) no breathing.

- Perform the initial assessment. If a bystander is doing CPR when you arrive, have the bystander stop. Verify pulselessness (no carotid pulse) and **apnea** (no breathing) for no longer than 10 seconds. Look for external blood loss.
- Resume CPR immediately and perform a focused history and physical exam. Inquire about onset, trauma, and signs and symptoms that were present before the patient collapsed. Get a SAMPLE history if you can. However, do not let history gathering interfere with or slow down defibrillation. ■

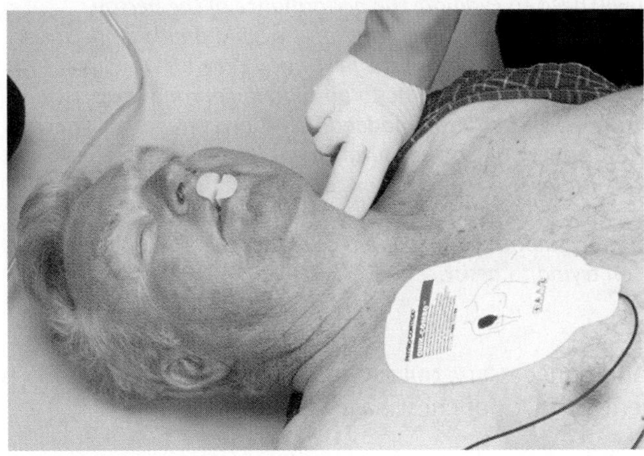

15. Check the patient's carotid pulse (maximum 10 seconds).

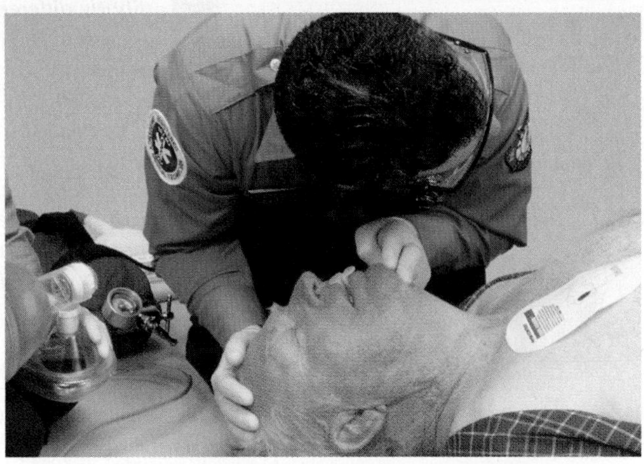

16. If there is a spontaneous pulse, check the patient's breathing. Note that in many cases, even when a pulse has returned, the patient will require ventilatory assistance.

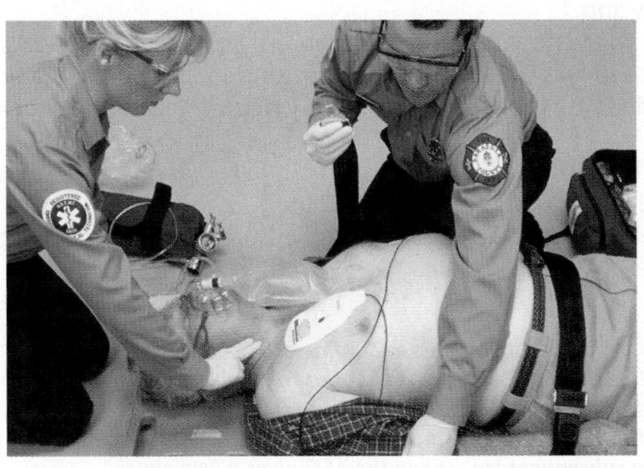

17. If breathing is adequate, provide high-concentration oxygen by nonrebreather mask. If breathing is inadequate, ventilate patient with high-concentration oxygen. Transport without delay.

PATIENT CARE

CARDIAC ARREST

Refer to Scan 17-4 as you read the steps that follow:

1. Begin or resume high-quality CPR.
2. Determine whether or not the patient is a candidate for the AED:
   - If the patient is an adult (defined by the American Heart Association as reaching puberty or older)—after 2 minutes of CPR analyze and defib if shock is indicated.
   - If the patient is a child (defined as from 1 year to puberty)—after 2 minutes of CPR analyze and defib using an AED designed to provide shocks to children.
   - If the patient is an infant (defined as the first year of life)—proceed with CPR, as this patient is not a candidate for an AED.

continued

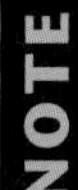

If the patient already has an AED attached when you arrive, your actions will be slightly different. You will need to evaluate the performance of the person operating the machine. If the person is analyzing or shocking and is doing it properly, allow the person to continue until the next good time for a switch occurs, usually the next time it is appropriate to do CPR. Encourage the person as needed. If the operator is not performing adequately, however, you will need to intervene, either with corrections and encouragement if the problems are easily corrected or by taking over if the operator cannot, or does not wish to, perform the steps correctly. Patient care is your highest priority, keeping in mind that roughly interrupting a smoothly functioning operation does not benefit the patient or the layperson trying to assist.

3. Bare the patient's chest and, if necessary, quickly shave the area where the pads will be placed if the patient has a lot of chest hair.
4. Turn on the AED.
5. Attach the monitoring/defibrillation electrode pads to the cables and then to the patient according to the instructions on the pads (upper right chest and lower left ribs). Many of these pads come already attached to the cables. It is helpful to remember "white to right and red to ribs."
6. Once the electrode pads are properly attached to the patient, advise all rescuers, "Stop CPR; we are analyzing."
   - The AED will search for ventricular fibrillation and, if found, automatically charge the unit. Once fully charged (the default setting for a biphasic unit is 200 joules), it will advise the EMT to clear the patient and deliver the shock to the patient.
   - If the AED does not find a shockable ECG rhythm, it will advise the EMT that no shock is indicated and to resume CPR immediately.
7. If the AED advises to deliver a shock, the EMT should ensure no one is touching the patient and then deliver a single shock.

NOTE

As stated earlier, about half of all patients in cardiac arrest have nonshockable heart rhythms. If this is the case, when you press the "analyze" button, the AED will give a "No shock" message. In other cases, the AED may provide a "Deliver shock" message and then, after one or more shocks are delivered, give a "No shock" message on a subsequent try. (When the AED gives a "No shock" message, it may be very bad news—the patient has a nonshockable heart rhythm and cannot be helped by the defibrillator. Or it may be very good news—the electrical rhythm of the patient's heart has responded successfully to earlier shocks. In the latter case, even though the heart's electrical activity has recovered, another stint of CPR may be required to get enough oxygen into the muscle cells of the heart to start it beating again.)

8. Immediately begin CPR after delivering the shock. Sometimes a defibrillation will be immediately successful in generating the return of spontaneous circulation (ROSC), and the patient may wake right up. In most cases of a successful defibrillation, the patient may no longer be in VF but is still in cardiac arrest (most likely a period of nonperfusing rhythm) and needs CPR compressions to "keep the pump primed and circulation flowing."
9. Reassess the patient—after providing 2 minutes or 5 cycles of CPR, reassess the patient (if the patient is waking up, check the pulse; if not waking up, repeat steps 6 to 8).

continued

If the patient wakes or begins to move, get a set of baseline vital signs, ensure high-concentration oxygen administration, and prepare to transport the patient to the most appropriate ED. If an ALS unit will be arriving shortly, wait for them or otherwise try to arrange for an "intercept" somewhere between the scene and the ED. Research has shown that CPR performed while moving and/or transporting a patient is not of the best quality.

Whenever providing CPR, it is essential to remember: (1) compressions must not be interrupted for any longer than 10 seconds (e.g., reassessment, pulse checks, or placement of advanced airways), (2) compressions should be 1.5 to 2 inches deep for an adult and one-third the depth of the chest for infants and children with full chest recoil, (3) the rate should be 100 per minute, and (4) ensure there is rotation of the compressors to prevent rescuer fatigue.

If the patient does not have return of spontaneous circulation after three shocks or two consecutive analyses without a shock, prepare to transport the patient to the most appropriate ED. ■

NOTE

If at any time you get a "No shock" message from the AED and determine that the patient has a pulse, check the patient's breathing. If breathing is adequate, provide high-concentration oxygen by nonrebreather mask and transport. If breathing is inadequate, provide artificial ventilations with high-concentration oxygen and transport.

Special Considerations for AED Use

General Principles

- One EMT operates the defibrillator, while another does CPR. This prevents the EMT who is operating the defibrillator from being distracted.
- Remember that CPR must include high-quality compressions.
- Defibrillation comes first. Do not hook up oxygen or do anything that delays analysis of the rhythm or defibrillation.
- You must be familiar with the particular model of AED used in your area.
- All contact with the patient must be avoided during analysis of the rhythm.
- State "Clear!" and be sure everyone is clear of the patient before delivering every shock.
- No defibrillator is capable of working without properly functioning batteries. Check the batteries at the beginning of your shift and carry a spare.
- If you have delivered three shocks (a rare occurrence) and you have no ALS backup, prepare the patient for transport. You may deliver additional shocks at the scene or en route if local medical direction approves.
- An AED cannot analyze a rhythm accurately in a moving emergency vehicle. You must completely stop the vehicle in order to analyze the rhythm if more shocks are ordered.
- It is not safe to defibrillate in a moving ambulance.
- Pulse checks should not occur during rhythm analysis.

Coordination with ALS Personnel

You do not need to have an advanced life support (ALS) team at the scene in order to use an AED, but the sooner the patient receives advanced cardiac life support (ACLS), the greater the patient's chance of survival. If you have an ALS team available, notify them of the arrest as soon as possible (preferably before you even arrive on scene). Whether you postpone transport and wait for the ALS team at the scene or start transport and rendezvous with them should be stated in local protocols approved by your

Medical Director. Your actions may depend on the location of the arrest and the estimated time of arrival of the ALS team.

If the ALS team arrives before you have finished the first shock, they should allow you to complete the shock. They should then institute the advanced care that they can give. The ALS team may allow you to defibrillate later, but that will be their decision. Since they are the most highly trained providers at the scene, the ALS team is responsible for the patient's overall care.

NOTE

The ALS personnel will initially focus on obtaining IV access to administer emergency medications and passing an advanced airway (e.g., ET tube, LMA, or Combitube®). Once an advanced airway has been inserted, you will be asked to switch the compressions and ventilations from cycles of 30:2 to an asynchronous procedure. When providing the compressions and ventilations in this manner, the compressor will push hard and fast with full chest recoil at a constant (i.e., with no interruptions) rate of 100 per minute while the ventilator provides a ventilation of 1-second duration to achieve visible chest rise at a rate of 8 to 10 per minute or every 8 seconds.

Coordination with Others Who Defibrillate Before You Arrive

First Responders, police officers, security officers, and others may defibrillate the patient before you arrive. If this happens, you should let the operator of the AED complete the shock before you take over care of the patient. After the shock is delivered, or a "No shock" message is received, work with the operator to bring about an orderly transfer of care.

In some areas, you may need to take the first AED to the hospital with the patient so that data can be retrieved from the machine. Your protocols should address this. They also should tell you whether or not to switch from the first AED to your own.

Post-Resuscitation Care

After you have run through the AED protocol, the patient will be in one of three conditions: (1) The patient has a pulse. In this case, you will need to keep a close eye on his airway and be aggressive in keeping it open. Keep the defibrillator on the patient during transportation in case the patient goes back into arrest. En route, perform a focused assessment based on what the patient tells you is bothering him, and perform an ongoing assessment every 5 minutes. (2) If the patient has no pulse, the AED will have given you a "No shock indicated" message, or (3) the AED may be prompting you to analyze the rhythm because it "thinks" there is a shockable rhythm. In either case, you will need to resume CPR. (You will not perform further defibrillation once you have completed the initial shocks of the AED protocol unless the patient has recovered a pulse and then, later, goes back into cardiac arrest.)

For all of these patients, you will need to use the techniques of lifting and moving that you learned in Chapter 5, "Lifting and Moving Patients." You will also need to consider how and where to meet ALS personnel (if available).

Patients Who Go Back into Cardiac Arrest

A patient who has been resuscitated from cardiac arrest is at high risk of going back into arrest. This change may be difficult to detect since most patients who have just been resuscitated are unconscious and many of them will need assisted ventilation. Since you are breathing for the patient, you may not notice that he no longer has a pulse. This is why, on unconscious patients who have recovered a pulse, you should check the pulse frequently (approximately every 30 seconds). The AED may alert you that it "thinks" the patient has a shockable rhythm. If you get such a prompt from the defibrillator, check for a pulse immediately. If you find that there is no pulse, then:

1. If you are en route, stop the vehicle.
2. Have someone else start CPR, if the AED is not immediately ready.
3. Analyze the rhythm.
4. Deliver a shock if indicated.

5. Continue with two shocks separated by 2 minutes (5 cycles) of CPR or as your local protocol directs.

Witnessed Arrests in the Ambulance

Occasionally, you will be transporting a conscious patient with chest pain who becomes unconscious, pulseless, and apneic (not breathing). Although there are no guarantees, you have a very good chance of getting this patient back because you can defibrillate very shortly after the patient goes into a shockable rhythm. If this happens, stop the vehicle and treat him like any other patient in cardiac arrest.

Single Rescuer with an AED

Some EMTs will be alone or have no one else nearby who can do CPR when they reach the patient. If this happens, the sequence of steps to take changes slightly. If the patient was a witnessed arrest, defibrillate immediately. If the downtime was prolonged, perform 2 minutes (5 cycles) of CPR. In this situation, you should:

1. Perform the initial assessment.
2. Ensure pulselessness and apnea. Attempt ventilation, preferably with a pocket face mask. Perform CPR for 2 minutes (5 cycles) if downtime is prolonged. Defibrillate immediately if arrest is witnessed.
3. Turn on the AED.
4. Attach the device in the usual way.
5. Initiate analysis of the rhythm.
6. Deliver a shock as advised by the AED.
7. Call for additional help, start CPR, and follow your protocol. Call for additional EMS help only after you get a "No shock" message, the patient regains a pulse, or you have delivered three shocks.

Contraindications

The only contraindications to using a defibrillator are for patients 1 year of age or less (see the following pediatric note). Any other patient in cardiac arrest will receive defibrillation. There are patients for whom defibrillation will not be the best or only remedy. An example is trauma. If a patient has a serious traumatic injury and is in cardiac arrest (unless the arrest preceded the trauma), this is most likely caused by severe blood loss or damage to one or more vital organs. Even if the patient were defibrillated, chances of success are unlikely. Also you should spend as little time as possible at the scene of a serious traumatic injury because the patient requires immediate transport to a facility where surgery can be performed.

Another case where defibrillation may not always be effective is hypothermia (very low body temperature). Patients who are severely hypothermic are usually warmed in a controlled setting before defibrillation is performed. Some systems recommend shocks in the event of cardiac arrest. If this does not work, the patient should be transported immediately.

PEDIATRIC NOTE

Unlike adults, infants have healthy hearts and go into shockable rhythms less often. Cardiac arrest in infants is more often caused by respiratory problems like foreign body airway obstruction or drowning. For this reason, aggressive airway management and artificial ventilation with chest compressions are the best way to resuscitate these patients. Applying a defibrillator to an infant would not help the patient and would result in delays to definitive in-hospital care.

AEDs are now on the market that can be adapted to pediatric use in children over 1 year of age through reducing the energy delivered and attaching smaller pads designed for children's chests (smaller pads and smaller shocks). If your service has such an AED, you should follow the protocol for its use.

For a child over 1 year of age, if an AED is available and the pads fit on the patient's chest, the potential benefits of defibrillation outweigh the potential risks. The best defibrillator in this circumstance is one that is designed for use on children. However, if an adult-sized AED is the only one available and the pads fit on the patient's chest without touching each other, it is better to use the adult AED on the child than to continue CPR without using it.

NOTE

When you defibrillate a patient, you are delivering electrical current through the patient's chest. That current can be carried or conducted to you under certain conditions. Although it is unlikely to put you into cardiac arrest, this electricity can harm you. You can prevent this and other potentially harmful effects from occurring by following a few basic principles (Figure 17-8).

Do not defibrillate a soaking-wet patient. Water is a very good conductor of electricity, so either dry the patient's chest or move him out of the wet environment (bring him inside, away from the rain, for example).

Do not defibrillate the patient if he is touching anything metallic that other people are touching. Metal is also a very good conductor of electricity. This means that you must be careful if the patient is on a metal floor or deck, and you must make sure no one is touching the stretcher when you deliver a shock. It is also a good idea to make sure no one is touching anything, including a bag-valve mask, that is in contact with the patient.

If you see a nitroglycerin patch on the patient's chest, remove it carefully before defibrillating. The plastic in the patch (not the nitroglycerin) may explode from the rapid melting that a defibrillatory shock can cause. This problem has been reported only when the patch is on the chest. Be sure to wear gloves when you remove the patch, as it is designed to release nitroglycerin through the skin, and it will not discriminate between the patient's skin and yours. One thing you don't need at a cardiac arrest is a headache from nitroglycerin.

Be absolutely sure that before every shock you say "Clear!" and look from the patient's head to his toes to ensure no one is touching the patient or any conductive material that the patient is touching.

Ask your instructor or refer to your local protocols for guidelines for defibrillating patients who have experienced trauma or are severely hypothermic. In addition, national standards established for the use of AEDs are sometimes revised as new technology and information becomes available. Your EMS system will keep you advised of these updates and may alter future protocols for AED use.

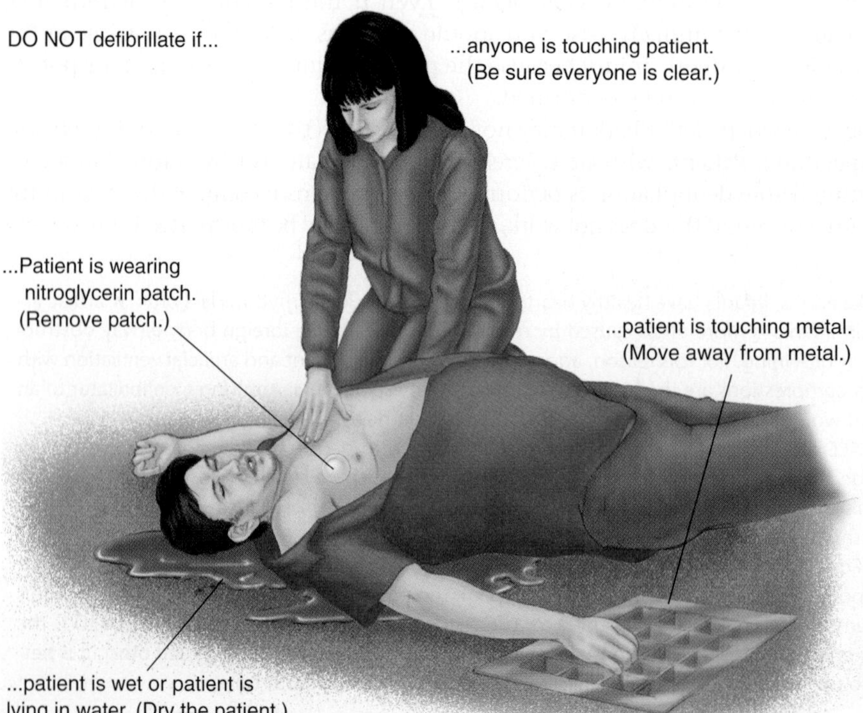
DO NOT defibrillate if...
...anyone is touching patient. (Be sure everyone is clear.)
...Patient is wearing nitroglycerin patch. (Remove patch.)
...patient is touching metal. (Move away from metal.)
...patient is wet or patient is lying in water. (Dry the patient.)

Figure 17-8 • Be alert to safety hazards when using an AED. Do not defibrillate a patient who is wet or in contact with metal. Before defibrillation, remove a nitroglycerin patch if it is on the patient's chest. Do not defibrillate until everyone is clear of the patient.

With the rapidly expanding medical technology available, the EMT may be presented with patients who have undergone surgeries or had special electronic devices implanted in the body. The ABCs, including CPR and appropriate oxygen delivery, will not change because of prior surgery or conditions. Defibrillation can be performed on such a patient, although the positioning of defibrillation pads on the patient's chest may need to be adjusted to avoid contact with an implanted device.

Some of the devices and surgeries you may observe in the field include the following:

F•Y•I

IMPLANTS AND SURGERIES

- **Cardiac pacemaker** (Figure 17-9). When the heart's natural pacemaker does not function properly, an artificial pacemaker can be surgically implanted to perform the same function. This pacemaker helps the heart beat in a normal, coordinated fashion. It is often placed below one of the clavicles, is visible as a small lump, and can be palpated. If you notice a lump under a clavicle, do not put a defibrillation pad over it. Try to put the pad at least several inches away while staying in the general area where you want the pad.

  Occasionally pacemakers malfunction. Although this situation is rare, it is possible. A malfunctioning pacemaker usually results in a slow or irregular pulse. The patient may have signs of shock due to the fact the heart is not beating properly. Pacemaker failure can be life threatening. Remember that care for patients with implanted pacemakers and signs of a cardiac emergency are the same as for those without a pacemaker. You should arrange for an ALS intercept and transport the patient immediately.
- **Implanted defibrillator.** Cardiologists are sometimes able to identify patients who are at high risk of going into ventricular fibrillation. They sometimes receive a miniature defibrillator surgically implanted in the chest or abdomen. When the patient develops a lethal cardiac rhythm, the implanted defibrillator detects it and shocks the patient. Often an implanted defibrillator is actually a defibrillator and pacemaker. The number of patients

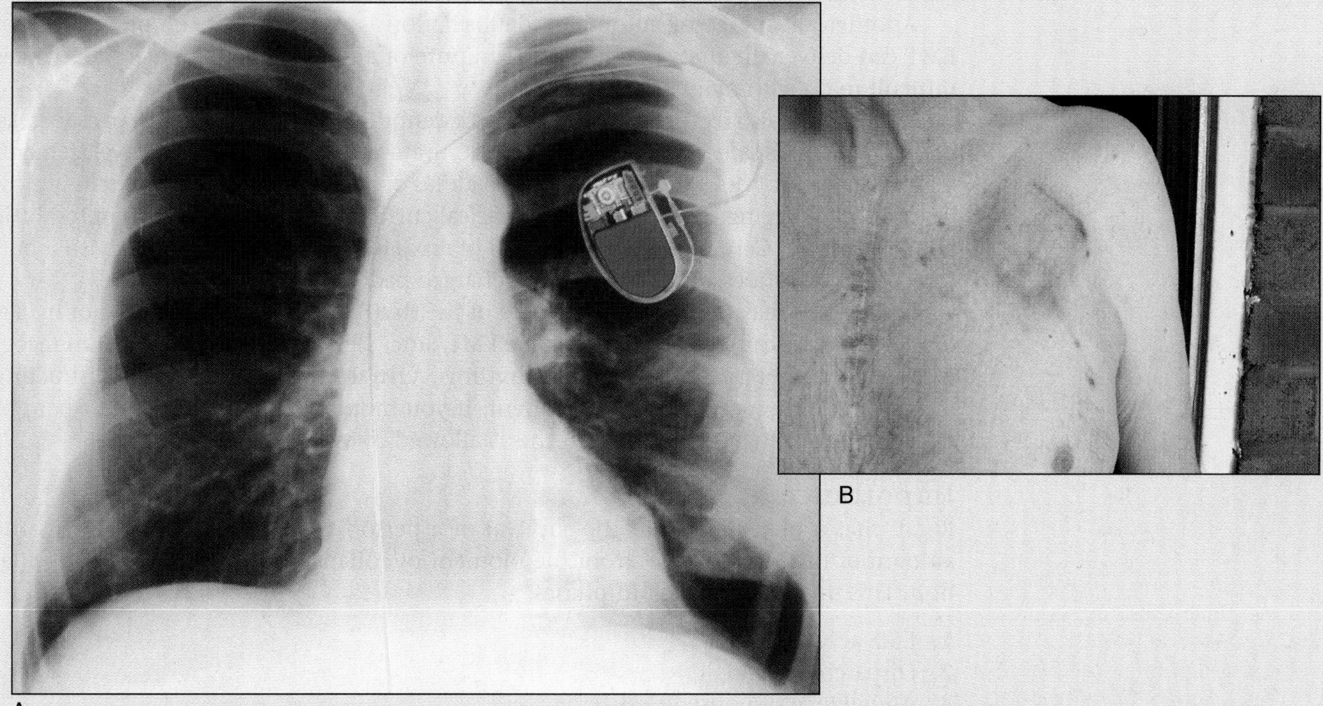

Figure 17-9 • (A) An implanted pacemaker is visible in this patient's left chest. *(© Dept. of Clinical Radiology, Salisbury District Hospital/Science Photo Library/Photo Researchers, Inc.)* (B) A combination implanted cardioverter defibrillator/pacemaker is noticeable in this patient's left chest. *(© Michael F. O'Keefe)*

continued

F•Y•I

Continued

receiving these devices will probably increase as it becomes easier to determine who is at risk of going into ventricular fibrillation. Since the implanted defibrillator is directly attached to the heart, low energy levels are needed for each shock. The presence of the implanted defibrillator should not pose a threat to the EMT. Emergency care, CPR, and defibrillation for this patient are the same as for other cardiac patients.

- **Cardiac bypass surgery.** The coronary artery bypass has become a relatively common procedure in cardiac surgery. A blood vessel from another part of the body is surgically implanted to bypass an occluded coronary artery. This helps restore blood flow to a section of the myocardium. Should a patient with a suspected myocardial infarction tell you that he has had bypass surgery, or if you observe a midline surgical scar on the chest of an unconscious patient, provide the same emergency care, including CPR and defibrillation, as for any other patient. ■

Advantages of Automated External Defibrillation

Until 25 years ago, it was unthinkable for EMTs to defibrillate patients in cardiac arrest. Now, EMTs are expected to be trained and equipped to perform this potentially life-saving intervention. The biggest reason this situation has changed is the improvement in technology that allows defibrillators to quickly and accurately determine whether a patient's rhythm is shockable.

This means that initial training and continuing education are much easier and simpler than that required for manual defibrillation in which the operator has to be able to read and analyze the heart rhythms that the AED does automatically. This is especially true in areas where EMTs see few cardiac arrests, such as in rural areas. Automated defibrillation is actually easier to learn and remember than CPR. However, this does not mean that EMTs are "well programmed robots." You still must carefully perform an initial assessment to ensure that the patient is in cardiac arrest, you must memorize the treatment sequence, and you must always act with the safety of the patient and others in mind.

Another advantage of automated defibrillation is the speed of the procedure. An EMT can deliver the first shock within 1 minute of arrival at the patient's side. This is difficult to do with manual defibrillation.

Automation also requires that the operator defibrillate through adhesive pads instead of paddles. This is safer and allows for more accurate and consistent electrode placement. Since the operator does not have to hold paddles on the patient's chest, there is almost no chance of "arcing," the passage of electrical current outside the chest from too little paddle pressure. Certainly, the EMT's level of anxiety is lower when he can push a button to deliver a shock instead of holding charged paddles on a patient's chest.

Some AEDs may allow for monitoring of the rhythm of patients who are not in cardiac arrest. This can be confusing for the EMT, since he is not trained in rhythm recognition and cannot treat nonshockable rhythms. A rhythm screen can be very distracting and take attention away from the patient. If you monitor patients with chest pain or difficulty breathing, make sure that this is allowed by your Medical Director.

Importance of Speed

Recall that a major factor in the survival of a person who is in cardiac arrest is the amount of time that elapses from the moment of collapse until the start of defibrillation. This time period has four phases:

1. EMS access interval
2. Dispatch interval
3. Ambulance response interval
4. Assessment and shock interval

For EMS to be effective, each of these time segments must be as short as possible (Table 17-1).

TABLE 17-1 • Minimizing the Time from Collapse to Defibrillation

TIME COMPONENT	OBJECTIVE	GOAL	METHOD
EMS access interval	To minimize the time from collapse until someone places a call for help	1.0 min.	An increased community awareness of the need for calling for an ambulance quickly; more public CPR programs
Dispatch interval	To minimize the time it takes for an EMS dispatcher to elicit information from a caller and get a defibrillator-equipped unit on the road	0.5 min.	Better dispatcher training; improved call-handling procedures
Response interval	To minimize the time it takes to get a trained defibrillator team to the patient	3.0 min.	Strategic placement of AEDs with first-response personnel
Shock interval	To minimize the time it takes to deliver the first shock	1.5 min.	Use AEDs; continually practice to maintain peak efficiency

EMS ACCESS INTERVAL This is the time that passes between when a person collapses in cardiac arrest until someone notifies the EMS system. A person who collapses in front of another person (a witnessed arrest) should have a far greater chance of survival than a person who collapses in an isolated place away from other people; the person seeing the collapse can call for an ambulance. Someone seeing a person collapse in cardiac arrest is no guarantee that an ambulance will be called immediately, however. In fact, most witnesses to a collapse delay calling for an ambulance for 2 minutes or more, and many delay calling for 4 to 6 minutes and longer.

Obviously, members of the public should be trained in CPR. But the public should also be trained to call for an ambulance immediately upon seeing someone collapse, even though they know CPR. Any delay in activating the community EMS system results in delayed defibrillation.

DISPATCH INTERVAL The second phase of a defibrillation effort begins with receipt of the call for help by a dispatcher and ends with the alert of an ambulance crew. This time segment should be kept as short as possible. The dispatcher rapidly determines whether the call is for a cardiac problem (by asking the caller about difficult breathing, unconsciousness, and the like). Then the dispatcher immediately sends out an EMS unit with a defibrillator. Once this is done, the dispatcher acquires additional information from the caller.

AMBULANCE RESPONSE INTERVAL The third phase of the collapse-to-defibrillation period is the time from dispatch until the ambulance arrives at the location of the stricken person. Ambulance response time varies considerably from community to community, as well as from one area to another within large communities. Response times are often long in large cities where congested streets are a problem and in small communities where volunteers must respond to the ambulance garage from homes and places of business. The fastest ambulance response times are generally in towns and small cities that are large enough to have an ambulance service staffed around the clock by in-station crews but small enough so traffic and response distances are not problems.

One way to shorten the time from dispatch to the arrival of a defibrillator in communities that do not have in-station crews is to station and equip a trained EMT in the community with an AED 24 hours a day. Thus, when a call for a potential cardiac problem is received, that trained individual can respond directly to the scene with the defibrillator while other EMTs respond to the station to get the ambulance. This approach works. In one group of small communities, the time it took to get a defibrillator on the road was reduced from 7.5 minutes to 2.5 minutes. Placing with First Responders in large cities has proved equally effective in reducing the response time of a trained individual with a defibrillator.

ASSESSMENT AND SHOCK INTERVAL The final phase of a defibrillation period is the time that elapses from the moment a rescuer arrives at the side of the stricken person to the moment the first shock is delivered. As with each of the other phases of the collapse-to-defibrillation period, this time segment must be kept as short as possible if life-saving efforts are to be effective: ideally 1 minute or less.

The shorter the collapse-to-defibrillation time, the greater the chance for survival. A person who can be shocked in 4 to 6 minutes or less after collapse has a good chance of surviving. In contrast, a person who cannot be shocked within 8 minutes of the moment of collapse has only a slim chance of surviving.

Because the ambulance response time alone approaches 8 minutes in many communities, the importance of implementing creative approaches to shortening the interval from collapse to shock cannot be overemphasized. The goals listed in Table 17-1, if achieved, should result in a witnessed VF survival rate of 25 percent or higher.

Defibrillator Maintenance

After the U.S. Food and Drug Administration received a number of reports of AED failures some years ago, the agency convened a panel of experts to review reports of these malfunctions. The experts drafted a checklist of actions that the defibrillator operator should complete on each shift. One of the most common problems with AEDs has been battery failure. It is especially important that you make sure the battery is charged and that you have a spare with the defibrillator (Figure 17-10). A defibrillator with a dead battery helps no one.

You should use the checklist at the beginning of every shift in order to be sure that you have all the supplies you will need and that the AED is functioning properly. The

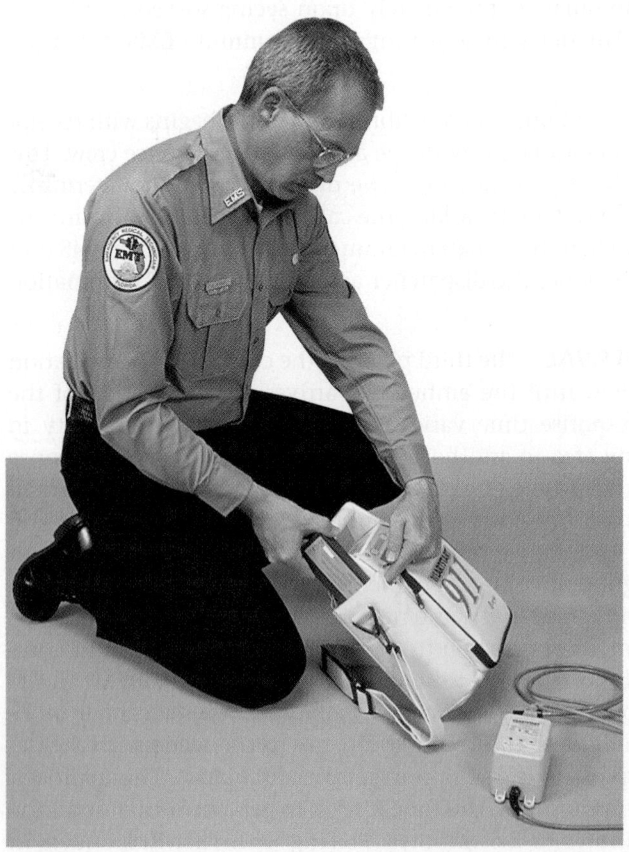

Figure 17-10 • Make sure the AED battery is charged and that you have a spare battery.

time to discover a problem is before you need the defibrillator, not when you are at the scene of a cardiac arrest.

Quality Improvement

There are many ways you can evaluate and improve your ability to resuscitate patients in cardiac arrest. These methods should be part of your service's quality improvement (QI) program. The defibrillation part of your QI program involves a number of things, including medical direction, initial training, maintenance of skills, case review, trend analysis, and strengthening the links in the chain of survival. Every participant in the EMS system has a role to play in QI, whether it is the patient who comes back to thank you, the physician who praises you for a job well done, the nurse who follows up on the patient's in-hospital course, or the EMT who uses the defibrillator and then documents the call.

Medical direction is an essential component of any defibrillation program. The Medical Director needs to be involved with all aspects of the program. This includes equipment selection (such as whether or not to get an AED with a voice recorder), initial training and evaluation, case review, continuing education, and skill maintenance. The EMT defibrillates under the Medical Director's license to practice medicine, so the Medical Director has a strong motivation to be involved.

An EMT who completes AED training in an EMT course is allowed to defibrillate only under certain conditions. He must meet the requirements of state laws and regulations and the Medical Director.

One of the best ways to improve your performance is by looking at how you performed when you actually managed an arrest. Every time an EMT uses an AED, the Medical Director or his designated representative should review the case. This can be done through several means, including the written report, voice ECG tape recorders in certain models of AED, and solid-state memory modules and magnetic tape recordings stored in the machine. The report should evaluate the timeliness of the EMT's actions, the accuracy of the machine, and any other factors that affect survival. The EMT should receive a copy of the Medical Director's report or other feedback each time he uses an AED.

Most EMTs will not use an AED very often. It becomes very easy, then, for them to forget what they learned about defibrillation. This is one of the reasons continuing education and skill maintenance are so important. These sessions should occur at least every 90 days and should include review of past cases, descriptions of changes in the program, and demonstration of cardiac-arrest management and defibrillation. The American Heart Association publishes a variety of guidelines and additional information on automated external defibrillation.

An important part of a QI program is looking at patient outcomes. Since cardiac arrests are uncommon events, few services will have enough arrest cases over a reasonable period of time to be able to conclude how well they are doing. Data collection over large regions, or even states, will give a better idea of how well things are going and where improvements need to occur. All of this depends on EMS agencies collecting and submitting the right data to the right place. This means that the information EMTs collect and document has far-reaching consequences.

Mechanical CPR Devices

Some EMS agencies have chosen to utilize mechanical CPR compressor devices to assist the EMTs with providing high-quality compressions. Realizing how important high-quality compressions are to the success of a cardiac arrest resuscitation and that the mechanical devices can provide excellent compressions, it is important that a system be in place to apply the device early in the arrest with only a minimum (maximum of 10 seconds) of interruption in the CPR. Two devices are the Thumper® and the Auto-Pulse™ (Figure 17-11). The following text shows how the devices would be worked into a typical cardiac arrest situation.

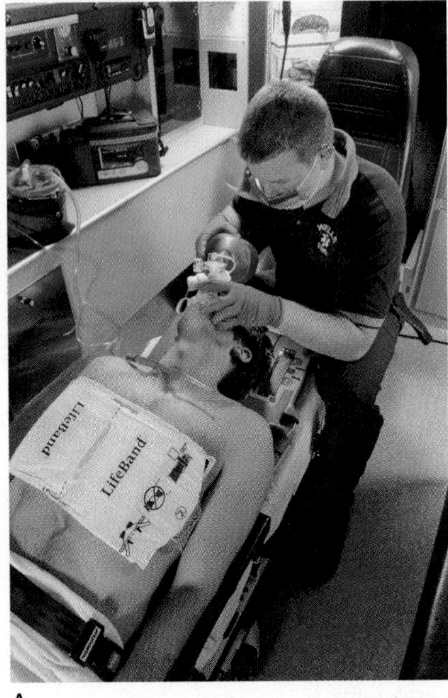

A

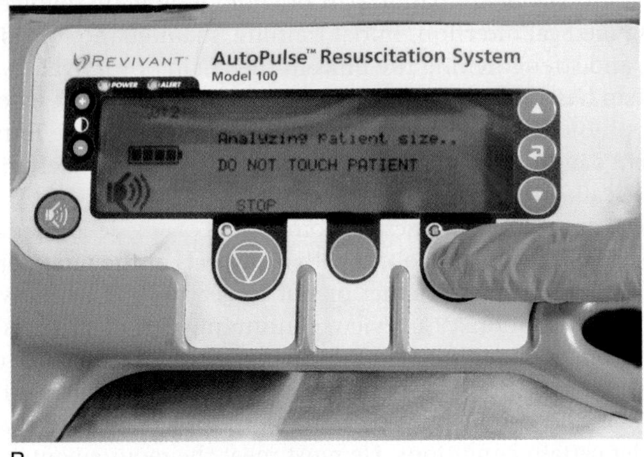

B

Figure 17-11 • The AutoPulse™ Model 100: (A) applied to a patient; (B) close-up view.

Using the Thumper®

- Take Standard Precautions.
- Ensure CPR is in progress and effective.
- Attach Thumper® base plate to long backboard.
- Stop CPR to slide long backboard under patient.*
- Restart CPR and attach shoulder straps to patient.
- Slide Thumper® piston plate into position on base plate (away from chest).
- Stop CPR and quickly pivot piston arm into place, measuring anterior/posterior and middle sternum placement.*
- Slowly adjust depth of compression to appropriate diagram.
- Adjust ventilations.
- Turn off compressions temporarily for pulse checks and defibrillation.*
- Upon termination of arrest or return of spontaneous circulation, power down unit.**

NOTE

**Always limit interruptions in chest compressions to 10 seconds or less.*

***Always store with compression depth turned down to minimum setting.*

Using the Auto-Pulse™

- Take Standard Precautions.
- Ensure CPR is in progress and effective.
- Align the patient on the Auto-Pulse™ platform.*
- Close the Lifeband chest band over the patient's chest.
- Press start (Auto-Pulse™ is designed to do the compressions automatically).
- Provide bag-mask ventilation at a rate of 2 ventilations for every 30 compressions. Each ventilation should be given over 1 second to provide visible chest rise.
- If an advanced airway is in place (ETT, LMA, or Combitube®), there are no longer cycles of compressions to ventilations. The compression rate is a continuous 100/min., and the ventilation rate is 8 to 10/min.
- After 2 minutes of CPR, reassess for pulse and/or shockable rhythm.*

NOTE

**Always limit interruptions in chest compressions to 10 seconds or less.*

CHAPTER REVIEW

SUMMARY

Patients with cardiac compromise can have many different presentations. Some complain of pressure or pain in the chest with difficulty breathing and a history of heart problems. Others may have just mild discomfort that they ignore for several hours or that goes away and returns. Between 10 and 20 percent of patients having heart attacks have no chest discomfort at all. Because of these many possibilities and because of the potentially severe complications of heart problems, it is important to have a high index of suspicion and treat patients with these symptoms for cardiac compromise. The treatment will not hurt them and may help them. These patients need high-concentration oxygen and prompt, safe transportation to definitive care. You may be able to assist patients who have their own nitroglycerin in taking it, thereby relieving pain and anxiety.

EMS agencies must strengthen the chain of survival. Early access, early CPR, early defibrillation, and early advanced care must be integrated with a quality improvement system that provides superb initial training, strong medical direction, individual case review, and encouragement to provide excellent care.

KEY TERMS

acute coronary syndrome (ACS) a blanket term used to represent any symptoms related to lack of oxygen (ischemia) in the heart muscle.

acute myocardial infarction (AMI) (ah-KUTE MY-o-KARD-e-ul in-FARK-shun) the condition in which a portion of the myocardium dies as a result of oxygen starvation; often called a heart attack by laypersons.

aneurysm (AN-u-rizm) the dilation, or ballooning, of a weakened section of the wall of an artery.

angina pectoris (AN-ji-nah [or an-JI-nah] PEK-to-ris) pain in the chest, occurring when the blood supply to the heart is reduced and a portion of the heart muscle is not receiving enough oxygen.

apnea (AP-ne-ah) no breathing.

asystole (ay-SIS-to-le) a condition in which the heart has ceased generating electrical impulses.

bradycardia (bray-di-KAR-de-ah) when the heart rate is slow, usually below 60 beats per minute.

cardiac compromise a blanket term that refers to a heart problem with a rapid onset.

cardiovascular system the heart and the blood vessels.

congestive heart failure (CHF) the failure of the heart to pump efficiently, leading to excessive blood or fluids in the lungs, the body, or both.

coronary artery disease (CAD) diseases that affect the arteries of the heart.

dyspnea (DISP-ne-ah) shortness of breath; labored or difficult breathing.

dysrhythmia (dis-RITH-me-ah) a disturbance in heart rate and rhythm.

edema (eh-DEEM-uh) swelling resulting from a build-up of fluid in the tissues.

embolism (EM-bo-lizm) blockage of a vessel by a clot or foreign material brought to the site by the blood current.

nitroglycerin (NTG) a medication that dilates the blood vessels.

occlusion (uh-KLU-zhun) blockage, as of an artery by fatty deposits.

pedal edema accumulation of fluid in the feet or ankles.

pulmonary edema accumulation of fluid in the lungs.

pulseless electrical activity (PEA) a condition in which the heart's electrical rhythm remains relatively normal, yet the mechanical pumping activity fails to follow the electrical activity, causing cardiac arrest.

sudden death a cardiac arrest that occurs within 2 hours of the onset of symptoms. The patient may have no prior symptoms of coronary artery disease.

tachycardia (tak-e-KAR-de-ah) when the heart rate is fast, above 100 beats per minute.

thrombus (THROM-bus) a clot formed of blood and plaque attached to the inner wall of an artery or vein.

ventricular fibrillation (VF) (ven-TRIK-u-ler fib-ri-LAY-shun) a condition in which the heart's electrical impulses are disorganized, preventing the heart muscle from contracting normally.

ventricular tachycardia (V-Tach) (ven-TRIK-u-ler tak-i-KAR-de-uh) a condition in which the heartbeat is quite rapid; if rapid enough, ventricular tachycardia will not allow the heart's chambers to fill with enough blood between beats to produce blood flow sufficient to meet the body's needs.

REVIEW QUESTIONS

1. What position is best for a patient with (p. 396):
   a. Difficulty breathing and a blood pressure of 100/70?
   b. Chest pain and a blood pressure of 180/90?
2. What is the best way to transfer a patient with difficulty breathing, chest pressure, and a blood pressure of 160/100 down a flight of stairs? (Chapter 5)
3. Describe how to "clear" a patient before administering a shock. (pp. 413, 414, 417, 420)
4. List three safety measures to keep in mind when using an AED. (pp. 417, 420)
5. List the steps in the application of an AED. (pp. 411–417)

CRITICAL THINKING

- Evaluate the system you work or live in with respect to the chain of survival. Which links are strong and which need work? How successful is your system in resuscitating patients from cardiac arrest?

Thinking and Linking

Think back to Chapter 3, "Medical/Legal and Ethical Issues," and link information from that chapter with information from this chapter, "Cardiac Emergencies," as you consider the following situation:

- Your patient complains of crushing pain to the center of the chest, radiating to the left shoulder. His vital signs are within normal limits. He is alert. You tell him that he needs to go to the hospital, and he says he doesn't want to go. You explain that he has signs and symptoms of a heart attack and that if he doesn't go to the hospital he could die. He says: "I understand that, but I'm not going to the hospital. Period." What should you do now?

MEDIA RESOURCES

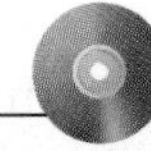

See the Student CD at the back of this book for quizzes, a case study activity, and other features related to this chapter. In particular, take a look at the 3D animation of the heart and major vessels, the animations of the cardiac cycle, blood flow to the atria, atrial and ventricular contractions, angina pectoris, and chronic heart conditions. Also, visit the Companion Website for *Emergency Care* at **www.prenhall.com/limmer,** where you will find additional reinforcement and links to other resources.

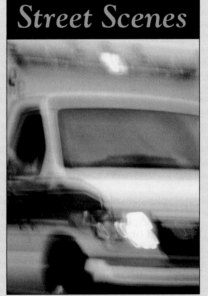

Street Scenes

Mary Anderson is an active 70-year-old who lives by herself in an apartment. She just returned home from shopping and is sitting down eating lunch when she feels some chest discomfort that she believes is indigestion. She thinks it will go away, but it doesn't. She stops eating and goes into the living room to sit on the couch, which makes her feel out of breath. She thinks about calling her doctor but doesn't want to be a bother. Unfortunately, the discomfort is now turning into pain and she feels numbness in her left arm. So, she finally calls her doctor and asks what to do. After hearing the symptoms, her doctor calls 911 to have an ambulance take her to the hospital. Almost 2 hours have passed since Mary started having signs and symptoms.

You are having a late lunch, which you have only half finished, when a tone comes over your radio. "Ambulance 32, respond to a 70-year-old cardiac at the Maple Tree Apartments, #2-D, a third-party call from a physician's office."

When you arrive on scene, your partner says he knows a stair chair will be needed to get the patient from the second floor. He gets the stair chair, and you get the first-in bag.

Street Scene Question

1. What type of emergency equipment needs to be taken to the side of every potential cardiac patient?

You proceed to the patient's apartment. As you enter, you notice the patient sitting on the couch looking pale and anxious. You ask her why EMS was called. She responds by telling you about her discomfort and her trouble breathing. She also mentions that the pain has become worse. You ask the patient on a scale of 1 to 10 (with 10 being the worst pain she ever had) what the pain was initially and what is it now. She answers, "3 in the beginning, but now it is 8." Your partner comes through the door with the AED and you give him a quick overview. You both agree that the ALS unit needs to be requested. You radio the dispatcher, who gives you an ETA of 5 minutes.

Street Scene Questions

2. What are the treatment priorities for this patient?
3. What assessment information do you need to obtain next?

Your partner gets a set of vital signs, and you place the patient on a nonrebreather mask at 15 liters per minute. You do a SAMPLE history, with the most significant additional information being high blood pressure, for which she takes medication and has been compliant. Your partner has just finished taking vital signs when the patient gasps and appears to go unconscious.

Street Scene Question

4. What should you do next?

The patient is found to be unresponsive and not breathing. As your partner ventilates the patient, you attach the AED and hit the "analyze" button. The AED indicates the need to shock. You and your partner stand clear. The AED discharges. After 2 minutes of CPR, you check the pulse and find it to be slow. You check respirations and continue assisting ventilations. As you start to check the blood pressure, the EMT-Paramedic arrives.

The paramedic starts an intravenous line and administers medication. The patient starts to breathe on her own. You prepare for transport and 20 minutes later you arrive in the emergency department with a conscious patient. A few weeks later you learn from your agency's quality improvement coordinator that Mrs. Anderson has recovered fully and is expected to return to an active lifestyle.

Street Scenes Sample Documentation

PATIENT NAME: *Mary Anderson* **PATIENT AGE:** *70*

CHIEF COMPLAINT

Chest pain, witnessed cardiac arrest

PAST MEDICAL HISTORY

☐ None
☐ Allergy to ______
☒ Hypertension ☐ Stroke
☐ Seizures ☐ Diabetes
☐ COPD ☐ Cardiac
☐ Other (List) ☐ Asthma

Current Medications (List)
Unknown antihypertensive

VITAL SIGNS

TIME	RESP	PULSE	B.P.	MENTAL STATUS	R PUPILS L	SKIN
1215	Rate: 32 ☐ Regular ☒ Shallow ☐ Labored	Rate: 120 ☒ Regular ☐ Irregular	140/84	☑ Alert ☐ Voice ☐ Pain ☐ Unresp.	☑ Normal ☑ ☐ Dilated ☐ ☐ Constricted ☐ ☐ Sluggish ☐ ☐ No-Reaction ☐	☐ Unremarkable ☑ Cool ☑ Pale ☐ Warm ☐ Cyanotic ☑ Moist ☐ Flushed ☐ Dry ☐ Jaundiced
1222	Rate: 0 ☐ Regular ☐ Shallow ☐ Labored	Rate: 0 ☐ Regular ☐ Irregular	0/0	☐ Alert ☐ Voice ☐ Pain ☑ Unresp.	☑ Normal ☑ ☐ Dilated ☐ ☐ Constricted ☐ ☐ Sluggish ☐ ☐ No-Reaction ☐	☐ Unremarkable ☑ Cool ☑ Pale ☐ Warm ☐ Cyanotic ☑ Moist ☐ Flushed ☐ Dry ☐ Jaundiced
1240	Rate: 28 ☐ Regular ☒ Shallow ☐ Labored	Rate: 110 ☒ Regular ☐ Irregular	130/80	☐ Alert ☑ Voice ☐ Pain ☐ Unresp.	☑ Normal ☑ ☐ Dilated ☐ ☐ Constricted ☐ ☐ Sluggish ☐ ☐ No-Reaction ☐	☐ Unremarkable ☐ Cool ☐ Pale ☑ Warm ☐ Cyanotic ☐ Moist ☐ Flushed ☑ Dry ☐ Jaundiced

NARRATIVE *On arrival, we met a conscious, alert, 70-year-old female who states a sudden onset of indigestion-like chest discomfort, which worsened with rest and began to radiate down her left arm. She appears somewhat anxious. She states the onset occurred after shopping and while eating her lunch. The chest discomfort quickly resulted in shortness of breath and 8 on 10 chest pain. She has been suffering from worsening pain for about 2 hours. We placed the patient on 100% O_2 via nonrebreather mask. During the assessment, she suddenly became unresponsive and was noted to be pulseless and apneic. AED was applied, and one shock was administered. Pulse returned but respirations were initially absent. Patient ventilated via two-rescuer BVM. Paramedics arrived on scene and provided ALS care. Patient began breathing adequately en route to hospital. O_2 was continued at 10 LPM via NRB. She was verbally responsive by arrival at hospital.*

Some of the material in this chapter on defibrillation and the AED has been adapted from material written by Kenneth R. Stults, M.S., former Director of the University of Iowa Hospitals and Clinics, Emergency Medical Services Learning Resources Center.

CHAPTER

18

Acute Abdominal Emergencies

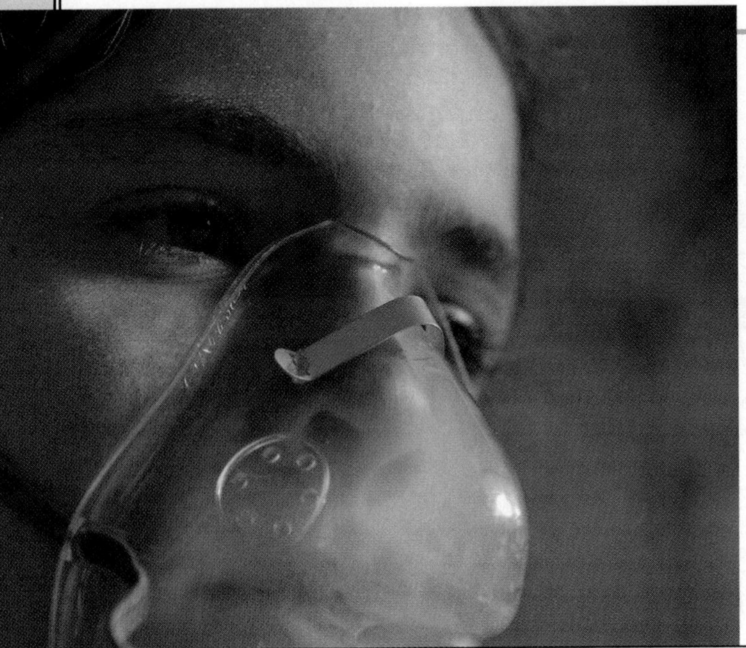

CORE CONCEPTS

The following are core concepts that will be addressed in this chapter:

- Techniques for assessing the patient with abdominal complaints
- Knowing that diagnosis of the condition is not necessary for appropriate treatment
- How to identify potential and actual shock in patients with abdominal emergencies
- How to care for patients with abdominal complaints

KEY TERMS

parietal pain, p. 433
peritoneum, p. 432
referred pain, p. 433
tearing pain, p. 433
visceral pain, p. 433

Abdominal emergencies are challenging for EMTs because the cause of the pain is not visible. Compounding the challenge is the fact that there are many organs within the abdomen that will cause pain if affected. This can cause confusion in determining the priority and stability of the patient with abdominal pain.

Fortunately these challenges can be overcome. The patient assessment process will help you determine the patient's priority. Although there are various potential causes for abdominal pain, the treatment for most conditions is the same and will not require diagnosis. This chapter will detail information about assessing and treating abdominal emergencies.

NOTE *There are no objectives in the National Standard Curriculum that pertain to the material in this chapter.*

ABDOMINAL ANATOMY AND PHYSIOLOGY

The abdomen—the area below the diaphragm and above the pelvis—contains a variety of organs that perform digestive, reproductive, endocrine, and regulatory functions. While we may think the abdomen only handles the digestion of food, in reality organs and structures within the abdomen do much more, including secreting insulin to regulate blood sugar (the islets of Langerhans of the pancreas), filtering blood and assisting with immune response (the spleen), and removing toxins from the body (the liver). Figure 18-1 shows the structures and organs of the abdomen. Table 18.1 lists the structures and organs of the abdomen with their functions.

The abdomen can be divided into quadrants. Imaginary lines drawn both vertically and horizontally through the umbilicus (the navel) create the four quadrants: right upper quadrant (RUQ), left upper quadrant (LUQ), right lower quadrant (RLQ), and left lower quadrant (LLQ). These quadrants are used to identify and describe areas of pain,

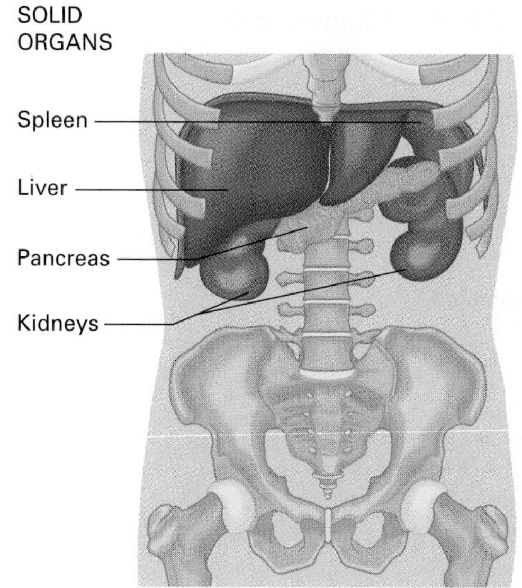

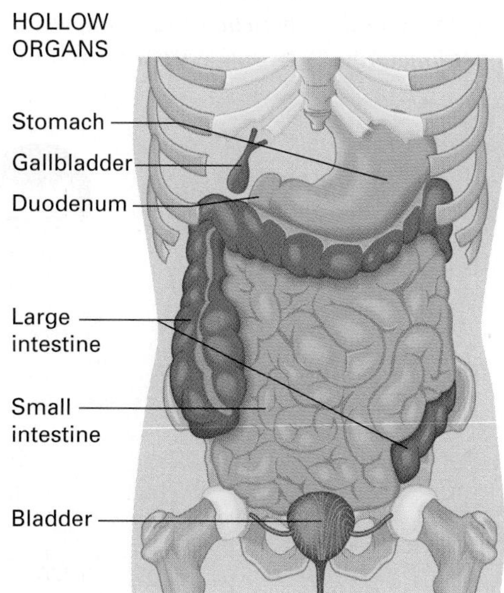

Figure 18-1 • The structures and organs of the abdomen.

TABLE 18-1 • Structures and Organs of the Abdomen

STRUCTURE OR ORGAN	TYPE OF STRUCTURE OR ORGAN	PURPOSE
Esophagus	Hollow Digestive	Carries food from the mouth and pharynx to the stomach.
Stomach	Hollow Digestive	An expandable organ located below the diaphragm and connected to the esophagus and small intestine. Begins breakdown of foods.
Small intestine	Hollow Digestive	Consisting of the duodenum, jejunum, and ileum, the small intestine takes stomach contents, removing nutrients as it passes contents to the large intestine.
Large intestine (colon)	Hollow Digestive	Absorbs fluid from contents, creating fecal waste for excretion through the rectum and anus.
Appendix	Hollow Lymphatic	A dead-ended sac of bowel rich in lymphatic tissue with no function in digestion. May become infected (appendicitis), causing pain and requiring surgery.
Liver	Solid Digestive Other functions with regulation of the blood and detoxification	Involved in regulating levels of carbohydrate and other substances in the blood. Involved in bile secretion for digestion of fats. Many other functions including detoxification of the blood.
Gallbladder	Hollow Digestive	Stores bile before release into the intestine.
Spleen	Solid Lymphatic tissue	Removes abnormal blood cells and is involved in the immune response.
Pancreas	Solid Digestive	Releases enzymes that assist in breaking down food in the small intestine into absorbable molecules. Also secretes hormones into the blood that regulate blood sugar levels.
Kidneys	Solid Urinary	Filter and excrete waste. Regulate water, blood, and electrolyte levels. Assist liver with detoxification.
Bladder	Hollow Urinary	Collects urine from kidneys prior to excretion (urination).

peritoneum the membrane that lines the abdominal cavity (the *parietal peritoneum*) and covers the organs within it (the *visceral peritoneum*).

tenderness, discomfort, injury, or other abnormalities. The abdominal quadrants are shown in Figure 18-2.

Most of the organs of the abdomen are enclosed within the **peritoneum.** There are two layers of the peritoneum: the *visceral peritoneum*, which covers the organs, and the *parietal peritoneum*, which is attached to the abdominal wall. A slight space between the two layers contains a lubricant fluid.

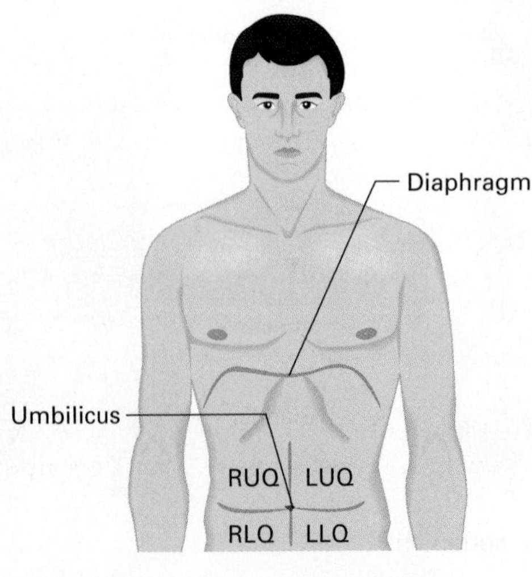

Figure 18-2 • The abdominal quadrants.

Some structures and organs are in the *retroperitoneal space*. This is the area outside of the peritoneum, between the abdomen and the back. The organs in the retroperitoneal area, which is technically not part of the abdomen, include the kidneys, the pancreas, and the aorta. This information will be important when types of pain are discussed later in the chapter.

The female reproductive organs and structures also lie within the abdomen and pelvis. These include the ovaries, fallopian tubes, and uterus, which may be sources of abdominal pain. The anatomy of the female reproductive system and the assessment and care for related emergencies are discussed in detail in Chapter 24, "Obstetrics and Gynecological Emergencies."

ABDOMINAL PAIN AND DISTRESS

The potential exists for both medical and traumatic emergencies to the abdomen. The traumatic emergencies are covered in Chapter 27, "Soft Tissue Injuries." This chapter covers the most common acute (sudden or emergent) medical abdominal emergencies.

As noted earlier in this chapter, there are many organs within the peritoneal and retroperitoneal cavities. These organs can be sources of a wide range of problems or complaints in patients of all ages. Some classic patterns and types of pain involving the abdomen include the following:

- **Visceral pain** originates from the organs (the *viscera*) within the abdomen. The organs themselves do not have a large number of nerve endings to detect pain. Therefore, visceral pain is often described as dull, achy, or intermittent and may be diffuse, or difficult to locate. (The patient may say he has abdominal pain but cannot point to a specific location.) Pain that may be described as *intermittent, crampy*, or *colicky* often comes from hollow organs of the abdomen. Pain that is *dull* and *persistent* often originates from solid organs.

visceral pain
a poorly localized, dull or diffuse pain that arises from the abdominal organs, or viscera.

- **Parietal pain,** as the name implies, arises from the parietal peritoneum, the lining of the abdominal cavity—thus it is often referred to as *peritoneal tenderness*. Because of its more widespread and efficient nerve endings, pain originating from the parietal peritoneum can be more easily located and described than pain from the visceral organs.

  Parietal pain is the direct result of local irritation of the peritoneum. Such irritation may be caused by internal bleeding (as from blood leaking into the peritoneum from an injured spleen) or infection/inflammation (such as pain in the RLQ from an infected appendix). Parietal pain may be sharp or constant and localized to a particular area. When obtaining your SAMPLE history, you may find the patient will describe this type of pain as worsening when he moves and getting better when he remains still or lies with the knees drawn up.

parietal pain
a localized, intense pain that arises from the parietal peritoneum, the lining of the abdominal cavity.

- **Tearing pain** is not the most common type of abdominal pain. Most abdominal structures or organs do not have the ability to detect tearing sensations. The exception is the aorta. In cases of abdominal aortic aneurysm (AAA), the inner layer of the aorta is damaged and blood leaks from the inner portions of the vessel to the outer layers. This causes a tearing of the vessel lining and pockets of blood resting in a weak area of the vessel. Much like a balloon, the area of collected blood creates an expanding pouch in the blood vessel wall. This is often sensed as a "tearing" pain in the back. (Remember that parts of the aorta are in the retroperitoneal space. This is why the pain is felt in the back.)

tearing pain
sharp pain that feels as if body tissues are being torn apart.

- **Referred pain** is pain felt in a place other than where the pain originates. For example, when a gallbladder is diseased, pain is often felt not in the area of the gallbladder but, instead, in the area of the right shoulder blade. This is because nerve pathways from the gallbladder return to the spinal cord by way of shared pathways with nerves that sense pain in the shoulder area.

referred pain
pain that is felt in a location other than where the pain originates.

NOTE *Pain from a heart attack (myocardial infarction) may be felt as abdominal discomfort. This pain, often described as indigestion or disgestive discomfort, is commonly felt in the epigastric region (the area below the xiphoid, in the upper center of the abdomen). If the patient complains of this type of pain, consider the possibility of cardiac involvement, as described in Chapter 17, "Cardiac Emergencies."*

Assessment and Care of Abdominal Distress

There are so many potential causes of abdominal pain that the EMT should not be concerned with diagnosing a particular cause. Diagnosing can be difficult even in a hospital, where advanced diagnostic tests are available. The focus of your assessment process (Scan 18-1) will be to accurately perform a physical examination and SAMPLE history to describe the condition and identify potentially serious conditions such as shock.

For each of the steps in the assessment process, you may observe specific concerns and points of interest in the abdominal pain patient.

Scene Size-Up

As you approach and take the important scene size-up steps, be prepared to protect your face and clothes in case vomiting occurs. Odors can be clinically important. For example, blood in vomit or feces creates a distinctly strong odor. Identifying this early will help you identify potential shock. Your search for a mechanism of injury may help you determine if this is a traumatic versus a medical condition.

Initial Assessment

NOTE *Abdominal pain or discomfort should always be considered an emergency—even if signs of shock are not present.*

The general impression you obtain as you approach the patient will be valuable in determining the seriousness of the patient's condition and the urgency of your care. First, the level of consciousness will help you determine the airway care that is required. If the patient is conscious, you will be able to begin talking to him to gain information, and if the patient is talking, you will know he has an open airway. Unconscious patients require airway care and any history will be obtained from family or bystanders.

At this stage of assessment, you will be able to notice the early signs of shock. An altered mental status; anxiety; pale, cool, or moist skin; and rapid pulse and respirations will alert you to shock—long before you would take a blood pressure or see trends in the blood pressure.

The position of the patient also provides important clues. Does the patient appear to be in pain? Is he guarding the abdomen (Figure 18-3)? Is he in the fetal position?

Apply oxygen to all patients with abdominal pain or distress at 15 lpm via nonrebreather mask.

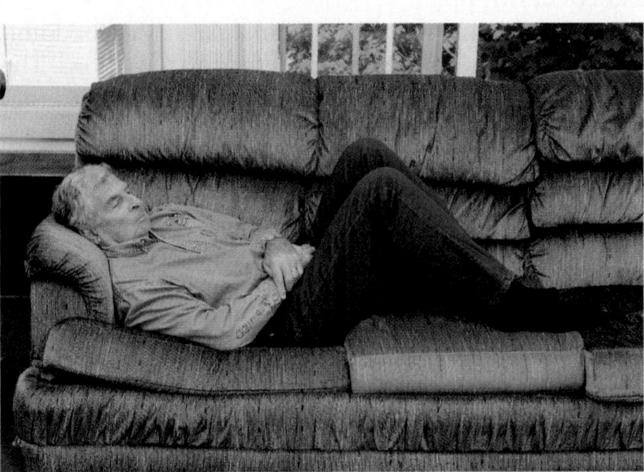

Figure 18-3 • The patient with abdominal pain will often be found in a position of guarding (knees drawn up, arms across the abdomen).

SCAN 18-1 • Assessment of the Patient with Abdominal Distress

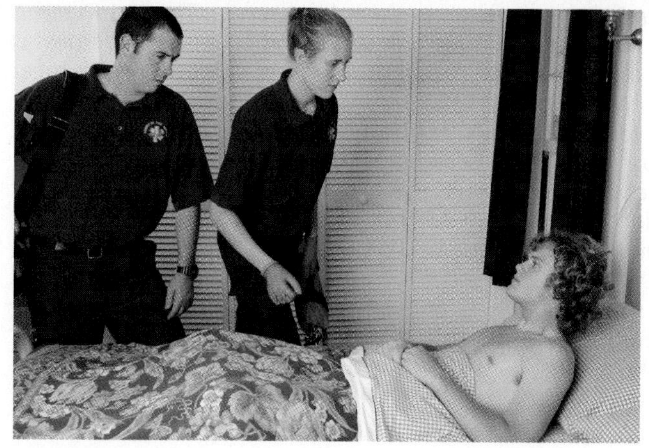
1. Perform a scene size-up.

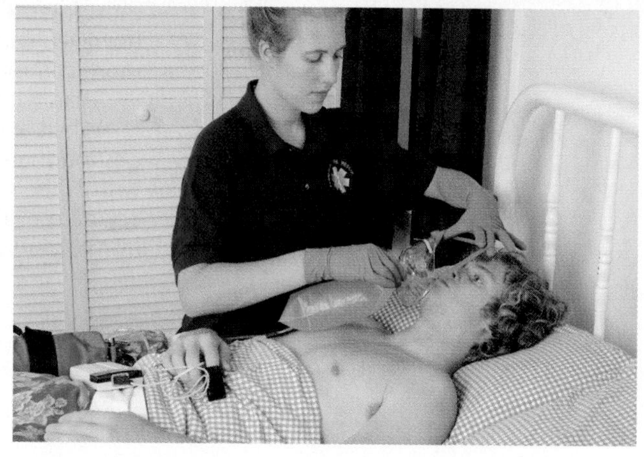
2. Perform an initial assessment and apply oxygen.

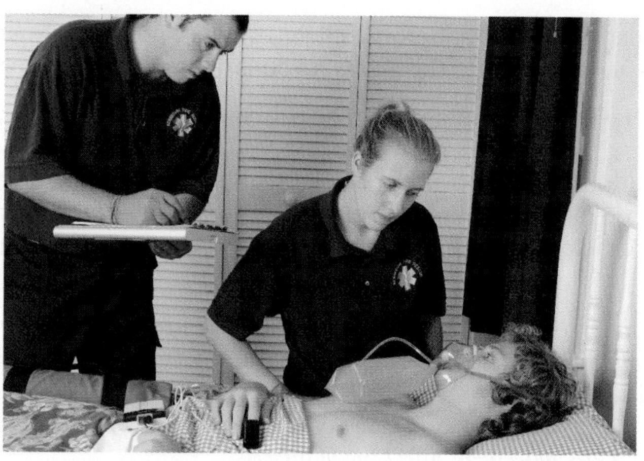
3. Take a patient history.

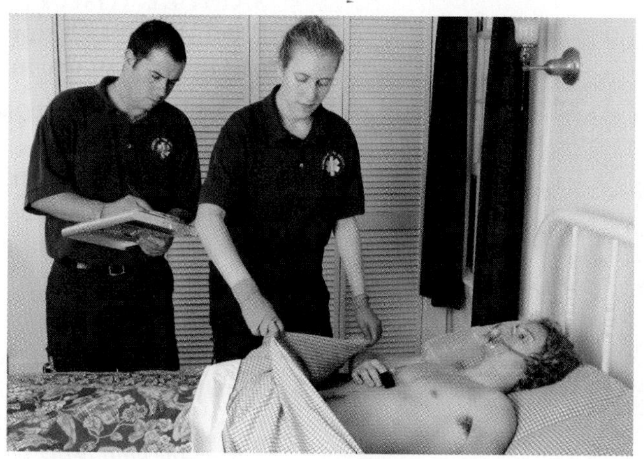
4. Expose the site.

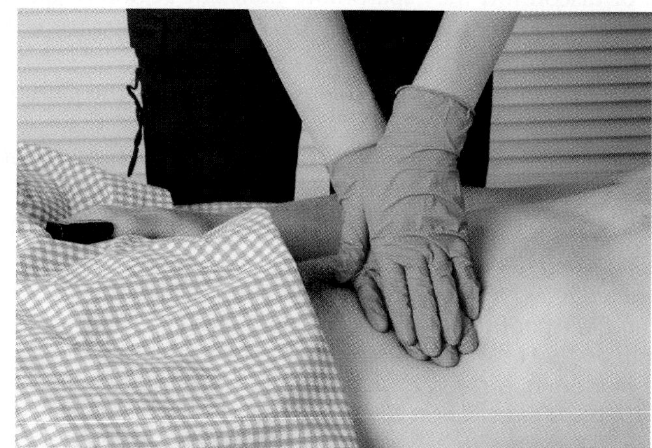
5. Palpate the abdominal quadrants.

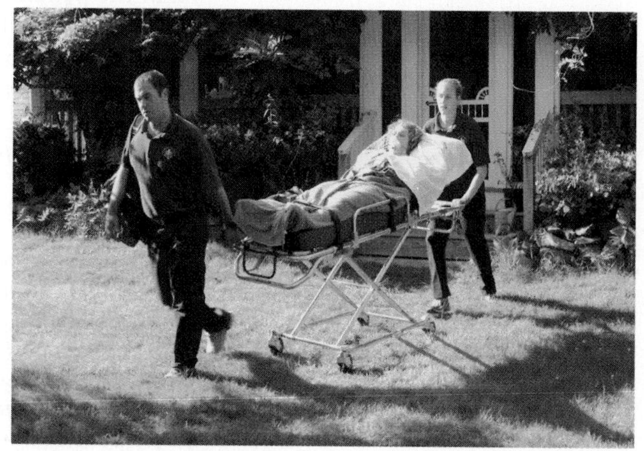
6. Transport the patient.

Cultural Considerations

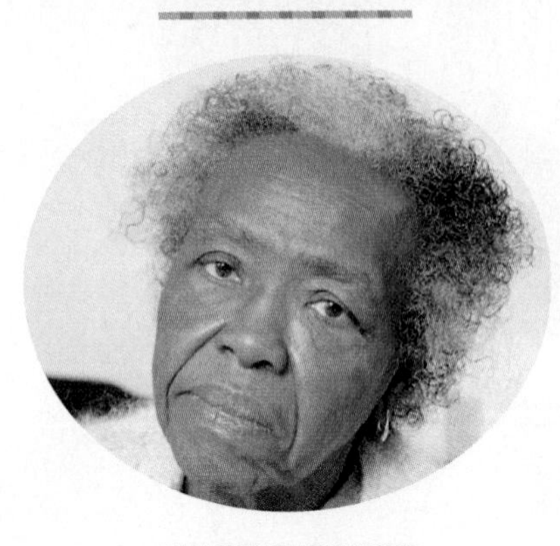

Although your patients may come from a variety of cultures, you will find considerable agreement on the meaning of terms that describe pain. *Pain* is most intense, *hurt* is less severe, and *ache* is least severe. The term *tender*, however, can be confusing. In some languages and cultures, tenderness is more commonly associated with caring or romance . . . or even with meat . . . than with soreness or pain.

When asking your patient to describe a degree of abdominal pain, suggesting that he use the 1-to-10 scale of pain intensity to describe his pain, with 10 being the worst pain he has ever felt, may help you to form a fairly accurate evaluation of what he is feeling, even if you and the patient are from different cultural or language backgrounds.

SAMPLE History

Use the SAMPLE history format (signs and symptoms, allergies, medications, pertinent past history, last oral intake, events leading to the illness) to obtain the patient's history.

SIGNS AND SYMPTOMS Have the patient describe the pain in his own words, using open-ended questions.

While gathering information about the patient's signs and symptoms, use the OPQRST mnemonic (onset, provocation/palliation, quality, region/radiation, severity, time) as a mental checklist to help you elicit information from the patient about his pain or discomfort.

- *Onset. When did the pain or discomfort begin? Did it begin while at rest or during activity? How did the pain begin?* (e.g., Did it begin as steady and severe or did it gradually build to this point?)
- *Provocation/Palliation. What makes the pain better or worse? Does any position make the pain better or worse? Does movement affect the pain?*
- *Quality. Describe the sensation in your abdomen to me.*
- *Region/Radiation. Point to or show me where the pain or discomfort is.* (Remember that the patient's pain or discomfort may span more than one region or quadrant or may be difficult for the patient to localize.) *Do you have pain anywhere else? Does the pain radiate or shoot to other parts of your abdomen, back, or body?*
- *Severity. How severe is the pain or discomfort?* Ask the patient to report the pain on a 1 to 10 scale.
- *Time. How long have you had the pain or discomfort? Has it changed over time? Better or worse?*

NOTE

Using only the word* pain *in talking to the patient about his symptoms may cause your SAMPLE history to be inaccurate. If you ask the patient if he has "pain" in his abdomen, he may reply "no." The patient may have discomfort, pressure, bloating, cramping, or another sensation that he would not call "pain." This response will reduce the effectiveness of your exam, care for the patient, and subsequent reporting. The initial use of open-ended questions will help you to get accurate information in the patient's own words.

ALLERGIES After eliciting information about the patient's signs and symptoms (the OPQRST questions), continue with the SAMPLE questions by inquiring if the patient has any allergies.

MEDICATIONS Ask if the patient takes any medications. This includes over-the-counter, herbal, and illegal medications or drugs. For example, aspirin used to prevent heart attack and stroke can cause bleeding in the stomach. Some illegal substances can cause abdominal distress in use and withdrawal. Diabetics can experience abdominal pain as a symptom of blood sugar abnormalities for which they may be taking prescribed medications.

PERTINENT PAST HISTORY The patient's medical history may provide information about past problems that may be related to the current problem. If the patient has a history of past abdominal problems, ask what these conditions are, if the pain resembles past experiences with the condition, and what happened last time. (Was it serious? Was the patient in shock? Was surgery necessary?) A patient's cardiac history with epigastric discomfort may lead you to be concerned for heart attack.

LAST ORAL INTAKE This is very important in patients with abdominal complaints. Determine the patient's last oral intake (liquids, meals, snacks). Additionally determine if this intake and the intake over the past hours-to-days has been normal for this patient.

EVENTS LEADING TO THE EMERGENCY The events leading up to the call for EMS (similar to the onset question in the OPQRST questions) can help you determine a timeline and progression of signs and symptoms. Ask again specifically about activity (even over the past few days) which seems related to the problem. Vomiting, nausea, diarrhea, and/or constipation are also important history items. Ask specifically if any dark red, bright red, or coffee-ground-like substances were noted in the vomit or feces, indicating internal bleeding.

HISTORY SPECIFIC TO FEMALE PATIENTS When female patients, especially those within childbearing years, have abdominal pain you must ask additional questions as part of the SAMPLE history.

Emergencies such as ectopic pregnancy (a pregnancy developing outside of the uterus) can be life threatening and must be considered in the history. Other conditions, such as ruptured ovarian cysts, pelvic inflammatory disease, and menstrual irregularities, can also cause significant pain.

The questions you will need to ask of a female in childbearing years who is suffering abdominal pain are highly personal but important to include in the history. Ask the questions directly, with the terminology taught in class. If the patient senses you are not at ease asking the questions, she will be uneasy answering them. Assuring privacy for the patient may help communication while you ask these questions. Remember, this is important assessment information.

Important questions to ask include the following:

Where are you in your menstrual cycle?
Is your period late?
Do you have bleeding from the vagina now that is not menstrual bleeding?
If you are menstruating, is the flow normal?
Have you had this pain before?
If so, when did it happen and what was it like?

If the patient is within childbearing years, ask if she believes she is pregnant or could be pregnant. Asking questions such as, "Is it possible you are pregnant?" leaves the answer to the patient's judgment.

Some patients may not even be fully aware of how one becomes pregnant. Some may not realize that, even if they have used birth control devices or techniques, they could be pregnant.

If the answer is yes to any of these questions, suspect ectopic pregnancy. (Even if the answers are "no," pregnancy—with ectopic pregnancy being the potential cause of the patient's pain—is still a possibility.) An ectopic pregnancy is a serious emergency, requiring *immediate* transport to the hospital.

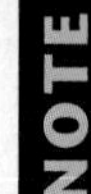

Remember that ectopic pregnancy occurs at the beginning of pregnancy. A patient with an ectopic pregnancy will not "look pregnant"—that is, will not have an abdomen that appears outwardly pregnant.

Detailed information on emergencies related to the female reproductive system can be found in Chapter 24, "Obstetrics and Gynecological Emergencies."

GERIATRIC NOTE

Geriatric patients may present some dilemmas when assessing abdominal pain. Older people may have decreased ability to perceive pain. This will, of course, make obtaining a history and description of the pain or discomfort more difficult. It is also important to remember that older patients are likely to have a more serious cause of their abdominal pain than younger patients. Research has demonstrated that elderly patients with abdominal pain are up to nine times more likely to die than younger patients with the same cause of the abdominal pain.

Many geriatric patients also take medications (e.g., beta blockers such as atenolol or metoprolol) for high blood pressure or heart conditions, which will reduce the heart rate. These medications may prevent the patient's pulse from rising during shock. An EMT could find a pulse of 72 and think that shock isn't present when in fact it is.

Physical Examination of the Abdomen

Assessment of the abdomen involves two procedures for EMS personnel: inspection and palpation. You may see some health care providers in the hospital auscultating (listening to) bowel sounds. This can be a long process (listening 3 minutes per quadrant) which will not change prehospital care and is not recommended as part of prehospital assessment.

Before you physically assess the abdomen, you will have asked the patient where it hurts. The patient may have pointed to a spot or may have moved his hand around an area indicating diffuse pain or discomfort. This will be important for your physical exam.

First, inspect the abdomen. Look for distention, bloating, discoloration, abnormal protrusions, or other signs that appear abnormal or unusual. You may have to ask the patient or family members if the current appearance of the abdomen is normal or changed, since body types and shapes vary widely.

Then palpate the abdominal quadrants. Always palpate the area that has pain or discomfort *last*. If this area is palpated first and causes additional pain, it will mask or alter the patient's response to palpation of the other quadrants.

To palpate the abdomen, use the fingertips of several fingers and gently press into the abdomen in each quadrant. While palpating, feel for rigidity or hardening and ask or observe whether this causes pain for the patient. If the initial gentle palpation does not cause pain or discomfort, you may palpate a bit deeper. Once you have found pain, discomfort, or abnormality there is no need to palpate further in that area.

You may observe that the patient is guarding the abdomen. The term *guarding* is used to describe two possible presentations: the patient drawing his arms down across

POINT OF VIEW

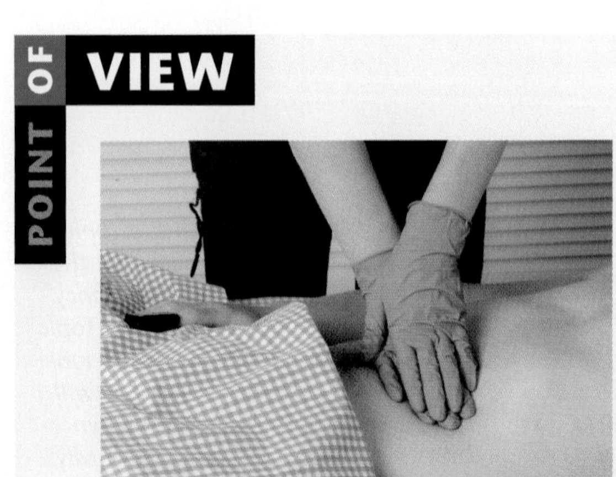

"I went to bed feeling like I had a stomachache. But I woke up with some really bad pain. It was so bad I could barely roll over and call 911 for the ambulance.

"The EMTs came and started to take care of me. They asked me questions and took my blood pressure. Then they pressed on my belly. Whoa! Did that hurt like a. . . . Well, I won't use those words here. Trust me. It hurt a lot. I yelled and almost startled the EMT. I know he had to do it to check me out.

"I found out the reason I was in so much pain. It was my appendix. They said if I hadn't gotten to surgery when I did it may have burst. I'm thankful for what the EMTs did—even if it did almost send me through the roof."

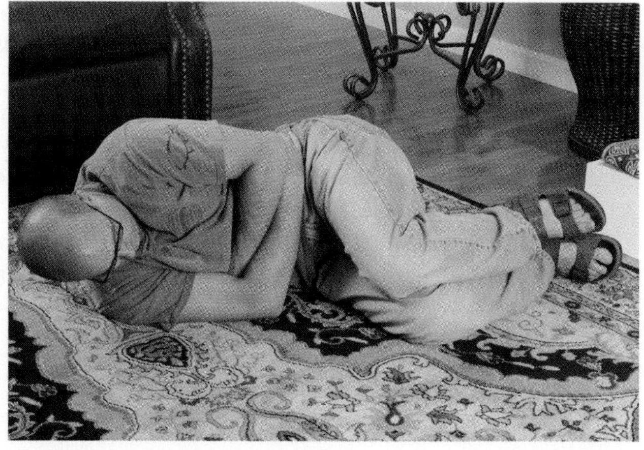

Figure 18-4 • Guarding is a common response to abdominal pain.

the abdomen (review Figure 18-4) or the patient tensing the muscles before you touch the abdomen. Guarding is a voluntary or involuntary attempt to protect the abdomen and prevent further pain.

In cases of abdominal aortic aneurysm, you may palpate a pulsating mass (abnormal bulge or lump). It may be found in conjunction with tearing or sharp pain in the back. This indicates an advanced aneurysm. If you gently palpate this mass, do not palpate it again. Report this to the receiving hospital. Some patients may have knowledge of an aneurysm which, when first found, was not serious and has worsened, or it was inoperable. This history is important.

Remember that the aorta normally creates a slight sensation of pulsing on deeper palpation of the abdomen, especially in very thin patients. The presence of the pulsating *mass* indicates an aneurysm. In larger patients, you will not be able to palpate a mass, even though an aneurysm is present. In this case, the patient's report of tearing pain may be the only indication of a possible aortic aneurysm.

NOTE

This section has talked in great detail about assessment of the abdomen, searching for abnormal findings. Keep in mind, however, that the absence of abnormal findings does not mean the patient's condition is not serious. Patients with abdominal pain should always be considered at least potentially unstable and transported promptly.

NOTE

A common assessment error is not assessing the lower quadrants properly. The lower quadrants extend from the umbilicus downward to the pelvis. In most people this extends well below the belt- or waistline and requires loosening of clothing to actually assess the lower quadrants (Figure 18-5).

Vital Signs

Vital signs should be taken initially and then every 5 minutes for a patient complaining of abdominal pain. These include pulse, respiration, blood pressure, and skin color, temperature, and condition. Mental status is also important to observe. Remember that

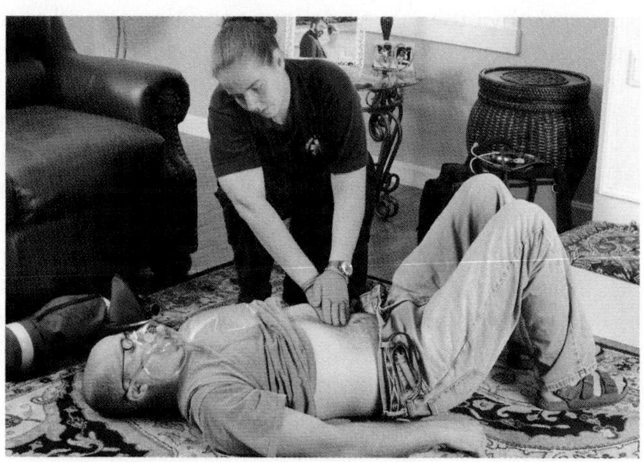

Figure 18-5 • Adequate examination of the lower abdominal quadrants, well below the beltline or waistline, requires loosening of clothing.

shock will appear initially with increased pulse and respirations; pale, moist skin; and anxiety. Falling blood pressure will be a late sign. Shock will be discussed in detail in Chapter 26, "Bleeding and Shock."

Since patients with abdominal pain may have an increased pulse simply as a result of the pain, serial vitals taken over time will help identify potentially dangerous trends. Calming, placing the patient in a position of comfort, and administering oxygen may actually reduce the pulse, which is a good sign.

Respirations may also be affected by abdominal pain. If breathing worsens the abdominal pain, the patient may be breathing shallowly and sometimes more rapidly.

PATIENT ASSESSMENT

ABDOMINAL DISTRESS

To assess a patient suffering from abdominal pain or distress:

1. Perform a scene size-up, looking for clues to a possible mechanism of injury while taking Standard Precautions as well as safety precautions.

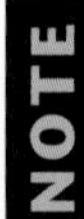

Vomiting and diarrhea will require both strict attention to Standard Precautions during patient care and careful cleaning and disinfection of the equipment and ambulance after the call.

2. Perform an initial assessment including the general impression of the patient's level of distress, mental status, airway, breathing, and circulation. Apply oxygen. Make a transport/priority decision. Vomiting may cause airway compromise, so be prepared to suction.
3. Assist the patient to a position of comfort. Calm and reassure the patient. This will help the patient and also help your next assessment steps by relaxing the patient.
4. Perform a SAMPLE history, focused physical examination, and vital signs.
5. Perform an ongoing assessment every 5 minutes en route. ■

PATIENT CARE

ABDOMINAL DISTRESS

While there are many types of abdominal emergencies, the care you will provide for all abdominal conditions is the same. You may find patients who appear unstable and obviously have a serious condition as well as those who are in pain, yet appear stable. In every case, despite the differences in patient presentation, take the following steps when treating a patient with an abdominal emergency:

1. While performing the initial assessment, maintain the airway. If the patient has an altered level of responsiveness, this will compromise the airway. Keep in mind that patients with abdominal emergencies may vomit. Suction whenever necessary.
2. Administer 15 lpm oxygen to the patient by nonrebreather mask.
3. Place the patient in a position of comfort (Figure 18-6). However, if shock and/or airway problems are present, position the patient to treat these conditions. The left laterally recumbent position will help maintain the airway. Raise the legs of a patient who is showing signs of shock.
4. Transport the patient promptly to an appropriate facility. ■

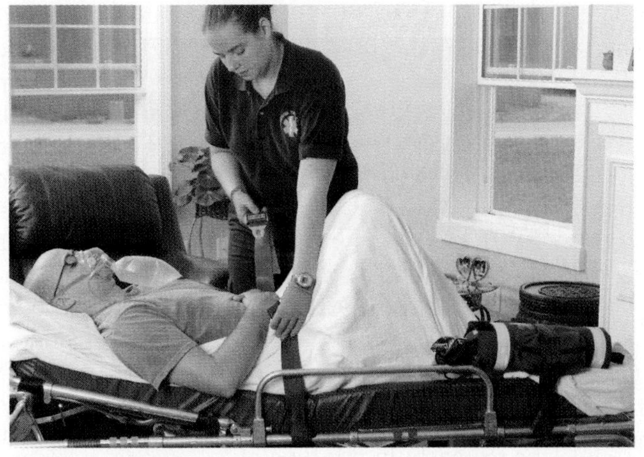

Figure 18-6 • Place the responsive patient without airway problems or signs of shock in a position of comfort and transport to an appropriate facility.

You should always work to calm the patient and reduce his anxiety. Patients who are in pain will require calming and reassurance.

Never give a patient with a complaint of abdominal pain or discomfort anything by mouth.

General Abdominal Distress

You may be called to patients who have complaints that appear nonspecific but involve the digestive system. Nausea, vomiting, and diarrhea are examples. Some of these complaints will result from digestive system disorders while others could be cardiac, diabetic, food poisoning, or the flu.

CRITICAL DECISION MAKING
Assessing a Patient with Abdominal Pain

Each patient with abdominal pain will receive a history and physical examination. In the patient presentations below determine what part or parts of the history or physical examination are missing.

1. A 26-year-old female patient complains of pain in her lower left abdominal quadrant. The pain radiates from the left to the right lower quadrant. She denies allergies or medications. The pain came on while she was sitting at her desk earlier in the day. Her vital signs are pulse 104 and slightly irregular, respirations 22, blood pressure 128/90, skin warm and dry.
2. A 14-year-old boy complains of abdominal pain. It began slowly over a day or two and has gradually become more severe. His parents are present. The patient denies medical history, allergies, or meds. He hasn't eaten since yesterday because of the pain. His vital signs are pulse 96 strong and regular, respirations 20 and adequate, blood pressure 104/72, skin warm and dry.
3. A 56-year-old man complains of severe pain in both lower quadrants of his abdomen which developed suddenly and without apparent provocation. The pain is intermittent and comes in waves. He has a history of high blood pressure and high cholesterol and takes medications for both. His pulse is 88 strong and regular, respirations 18 and adequate, blood pressure 158/104, skin cool and moist.

Many types of abdominal complaints and conditions cause abdominal complaints. The following descriptions of some of the more common conditions are presented for your information. Remember that it is not necessary or important for you to diagnose specific conditions.

F•Y•I

ABDOMINAL CONDITIONS

APPENDICITIS

Appendicitis, an infection of the appendix, is the most common cause of a person needing surgery. About 1 in 15 people will develop appendicitis at some time in their lives. Signs and symptoms include nausea and sometimes vomiting, pain in the area of the umbilicus (initially), followed by persistent pain in the RLQ.

CHOLECYSTITIS/ GALLSTONES

Cholecystitis is an inflammation of the gallbladder, often caused by gallstones. The patient will experience severe and sometimes sudden epigastric (upper central abdomen just below the xiphoid process) and/or RUQ pain, which may radiate to the shoulder or back. The pain may be caused or worsened by ingestion of foods high in fat.

PANCREATITIS

Pancreatitis, an inflammation of the pancreas, is common in patients with chronic alcohol problems. The pain from pancreatitis is found in the epigastric area. Because of the retroperitoneal location of the pancreas, behind the stomach, the pain may radiate to the back and/or shoulders. This is a serious condition which, in advanced cases, can present with signs of shock.

ULCER/INTERNAL BLEEDING

Abdominal bleeding takes two general forms. The first is bleeding from within the digestive tract, as in the case of a bleeding ulcer in the stomach. In this type of bleeding, which can arise at any location from the esophagus to the rectum, blood passes out of the GI tract either in vomit (with a bright red or coffee-ground appearance) or from the rectum (as red, maroon, or black, tarry-colored blood or stool). This type of bleeding may or may not be associated with abdominal pain.

The second form of abdominal bleeding is bleeding into the peritoneal cavity, as from a spleen that has been injured in trauma. This type of bleeding results in irritation of the peritoneum and is associated with abdominal pain and tenderness.

ABDOMINAL AORTIC ANEURYSM (AAA)

Discussed earlier in the chapter, AAA is a ballooning or weakening in the wall of the aorta as it passes through the abdomen. The weakening results in tearing of the internal layer of the blood vessel, which allows blood to escape into the weaker, outer layers. The affected area can gradually grow and rupture. Ruptured aneurysms are associated with an extremely high rate of death.

You may encounter a patient who is aware he has an aneurysm. These are sometimes found when a test for another condition, such as an abdominal ultrasound or CT scan, reveals the presence of a small aneurysm. Not all are surgically repaired immediately. If you have a patient who tells you that he has an aneurysm and he has abdominal pain, it is a serious emergency requiring prompt transportation to an appropriate hospital.

Patients with a slowly leaking AAA usually present with gradually developing abdominal pain, which can be described as sharp pain or tearing and may radiate to the back. A sudden rupture of the aorta typically causes sudden onset of excruciating abdominal and back pain. Signs of shock may be present. Depending on the location of the AAA, there may be inequality between the femoral or pedal pulses.

HERNIA

A hernia is a protrusion of intestine through the abdominal wall. This can be caused by heavy lifting or straining which causes the intestine to push through a weakened area in the abdominal wall. A hernia will cause a sudden onset of pain, usually after lifting. A hernia may be palpated as a mass or lump on the abdominal wall or in the creases of the groin. It may be very painful, but it is life threatening only if the hernia causes an obstruction or twisting of the intestine.

Because pain at the site of a hernia may indicate obstruction or strangulation of the intestine, all patients with a painful hernia should be transported for further evaluation at the hospital.

RENAL COLIC

Under certain conditions the kidneys may form small hard stones. If one of these stones begins to descend down the ureter on the way to the bladder, it can cause severe flank pain that often radiates to the groin area anteriorly. The visceral pain from such a "kidney stone" is often severe and may be associated with nausea and vomiting.

Your assessment and care for these patients, like any others discussed in this chapter, will involve providing a proper scene size-up and initial assessment with appropriate airway care. Your SAMPLE history, physical exam, and vital signs assessments will be critical for determining priority and patient condition (stable vs. unstable).

The assessment techniques discussed earlier in the chapter will apply in the same manner to these patients. Determining if there is pain, tenderness, discomfort, or any associated complaints; the time of onset (sudden vs. over a period of time); fever and malaise; and abdominal inspection and palpation are all appropriate.

Patient care will involve monitoring for airway problems if the patient is vomiting. Place the responsive patient in a position of comfort. Place the unresponsive patient or the patient who is having difficulty maintaining an airway in a left lateral recumbent position for drainage from the mouth.

CHAPTER REVIEW

SUMMARY

All complaints of abdominal pain or distress must be treated as serious emergencies requiring transport. However, as an EMT-Basic, it is not your responsibility to diagnose the cause of the complaint. Instead, you must perform a thorough assessment—including a SAMPLE history, physical exam, and vital signs—to report to the hospital staff. Emergency care will consist of protecting the patient's airway; administering high-concentration oxygen by nonrebreather mask; placing the responsive patient in a position of comfort; placing the unresponsive patient or patient with difficulty maintaining an airway in the left lateral recumbent position; and transporting to the hospital.

Take all appropriate Standard Precautions and carefully clean and disinfect equipment and the ambulance, especially if the patient has vomited or had diarrhea.

KEY TERMS

parietal pain a localized, intense pain that arises from the parietal peritoneum, the lining of the abdominal cavity.

peritoneum the membrane that lines the abdominal cavity (the *parietal peritoneum*) and covers the organs within it (the *visceral peritoneum*).

referred pain pain that is felt in a location other than where the pain originates.

tearing pain sharp pain that feels as if body tissues are being torn apart.

visceral pain a poorly localized, dull or diffuse pain that arises from the abdominal organs, or viscera.

REVIEW QUESTIONS

1. List five signs and symptoms of abdominal distress. (pp. 433–434, 436, 438–439)
2. Describe the difference between visceral and parietal pain and describe a condition that may be responsible for each. (p. 433)
3. Describe the emergency care for a patient experiencing abdominal pain or distress. (pp. 435, 440–441)
4. Name the four abdominal quadrants and explain how the quadrants are determined. (pp. 431–433)

CRITICAL THINKING

- You are called to a patient with abdominal pain. You arrive to find him sitting on the couch, doubled over with pain. He describes the pain as severe and says it began as "on and off" over the past several days. It became severe within the hour. What additional SAMPLE questions would you ask the patient? What position would he likely be most comfortable in?

MEDIA RESOURCES

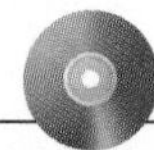

See the Student CD at the back of this book for quizzes, a case study activity, and other features related to this chapter. In particular, take a look at the 3D animations of the abdomen and pelvis, the digestive system, and the trunk and abdominal regions. Also, visit the Companion Website for *Emergency Care* at **www.prenhall.com/limmer**, where you will find additional reinforcement and links to other resources.

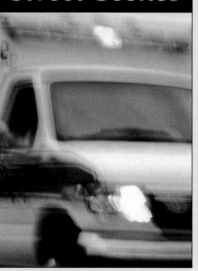

Street Scenes

You are dispatched to the Shop-Till-You-Drop supermarket for a "sick woman." You arrive at a scene that appears safe and observe store workers around an approximately 75-year-old woman who appears sweaty and somewhat pale. She is sitting in a chair brought over by a store employee. The employee tells you that the woman was standing in the checkout line and told the cashier that her stomach hurt and she felt ill. She vomited into the trash can the employee provided and then began to feel a bit weak and dizzy. She was placed in the chair to await EMS.

You introduce yourself and find the woman oriented but looking tired, breathing adequately but a bit rapidly, and having a slightly increased radial pulse. You ask the clerk to bring you the trash can the patient vomited into. She thinks you are kind of weird but complies.

Street Scene Questions

1. What is your initial impression of this patient?
2. What is the significance of the patient's initial presentation?
3. Why would you want to see the trash can?

You ask your partner to administer oxygen and get a set of vitals while you get a history. The trash can contains a considerable amount of a reddish-brown substance you believe may be partially digested blood. You radio for advanced life support before you begin the history, and realize the patient must be transported promptly.

Street Scene Questions

4. Why would you request advanced life support?
5. Do you agree with the transport priority? Why or why not?

The patient reports diffuse pain across the upper abdominal quadrants that has been increasing slightly over the past few days. It is not worsened or made better by anything in particular and is slightly tender to palpation. No rigidity is noted. She has eaten and drunk normally over the past several days and has no history of abdominal problems. She has had one "mini-stroke" a few months ago. She takes an unknown blood pressure medication and an aspirin a day to prevent further strokes. Her pulse is 104, respirations 26, BP 102/68, skin pale and moist.

You move her promptly to the stretcher and into the ambulance. An ALS engine arrives and a paramedic jumps in with her equipment. You explain that you are concerned about a potentially serious condition and shock. The paramedic agrees.

Street Scene Questions

6. Do you believe this patient is in shock? Explain your reasoning.
7. What effect might her history have on her current condition?
8. What position should the patient be placed in?

Because of the patient's apparent history of high blood pressure, you think that the blood pressure of 102/68 which would usually not be considered low, may actually indicate shock for this patient. The paramedic thinks that the aspirin taken for stroke prevention may have caused bleeding in the stomach.

The paramedic begins advanced care, including an IV and electrocardiogram. As a precaution, the patient's blood sugar level is checked and is found to be within normal limits. A second set of vital signs is obtained: pulse 112, respirations 28, blood pressure 100/64, skin unchanged. The patient insists on sitting up because she feels she may vomit again.

You arrive at the hospital a short time later and make a report to the physician. The patient is, in fact, bleeding internally and will be admitted for further care.

Street Scenes Sample Documentation

PATIENT NAME: Mary Vignola **PATIENT AGE:** 75

CHIEF COMPLAINT

"I feel sick"

PAST MEDICAL HISTORY

- [ ] None
- [ ] Allergy to
- [x] Hypertension
- [x] Stroke
- [ ] Seizures
- [ ] Diabetes
- [ ] COPD
- [ ] Cardiac
- [ ] Other (List)
- [ ] Asthma

Current Medications (List)

aspirin, unknown antihypertensive med

VITAL SIGNS

TIME	RESP	PULSE	B.P.	MENTAL STATUS	R PUPILS L	SKIN
1502	Rate: 26; [x] Regular; [ ] Shallow; [ ] Labored	Rate: 104; [x] Regular; [ ] Irregular	102/68	[x] Alert; [ ] Voice; [ ] Pain; [ ] Unresp.	R [x] Normal [x] L; [ ] Dilated [ ]; [ ] Constricted [ ]; [ ] Sluggish [ ]; [ ] No-Reaction [ ]	[ ] Unremarkable; [ ] Cool; [x] Pale; [ ] Warm; [ ] Cyanotic; [x] Moist; [ ] Flushed; [ ] Dry; [ ] Jaundiced
1510	Rate: 28; [x] Regular; [ ] Shallow; [ ] Labored	Rate: 112; [x] Regular; [ ] Irregular	100/64	[x] Alert; [ ] Voice; [ ] Pain; [ ] Unresp.	R [x] Normal [x] L; [ ] Dilated [ ]; [ ] Constricted [ ]; [ ] Sluggish [ ]; [ ] No-Reaction [ ]	[ ] Unremarkable; [ ] Cool; [x] Pale; [ ] Warm; [ ] Cyanotic; [x] Moist; [ ] Flushed; [ ] Dry; [ ] Jaundiced
	Rate: ; [ ] Regular; [ ] Shallow; [ ] Labored	Rate: ; [ ] Regular; [ ] Irregular	/	[ ] Alert; [ ] Voice; [ ] Pain; [ ] Unresp.	R [ ] Normal [ ] L; [ ] Dilated [ ]; [ ] Constricted [ ]; [ ] Sluggish [ ]; [ ] No-Reaction [ ]	[ ] Unremarkable; [ ] Cool; [ ] Pale; [ ] Warm; [ ] Cyanotic; [ ] Moist; [ ] Flushed; [ ] Dry; [ ] Jaundiced

NARRATIVE EMS called to a supermarket for a 75 year old female who felt ill and vomited. We arrived to find her sweaty, pale and appearing tired. Initial assessment revealed slightly increased respirations and a rapid radial pulse. Oxygen applied. Examination of the vomitus revealed what appears to be digested blood. Patient is given a high priority for transport due to potential shock. ALS requested. Vitals noted above. Capillary refill 3 seconds. Patient complains of diffuse pain across the upper abdominal quadrants which has increased slightly over the past few days. It is mildly tender to palpation and not worsened or decreased by anything. Patient has eaten well and normally over the past few days. History includes a "mini stroke" and high blood pressure. She takes aspirin and an unknown blood pressure medication. ALS arrived on scene and rode with this unit to the hospital performing ALS care. Patient transported to Mercy Hospital and TOT RN room #5 rails up. See ALS report 24656 for treatments performed by paramedics.

CHAPTER 19

Diabetic Emergencies and Altered Mental Status

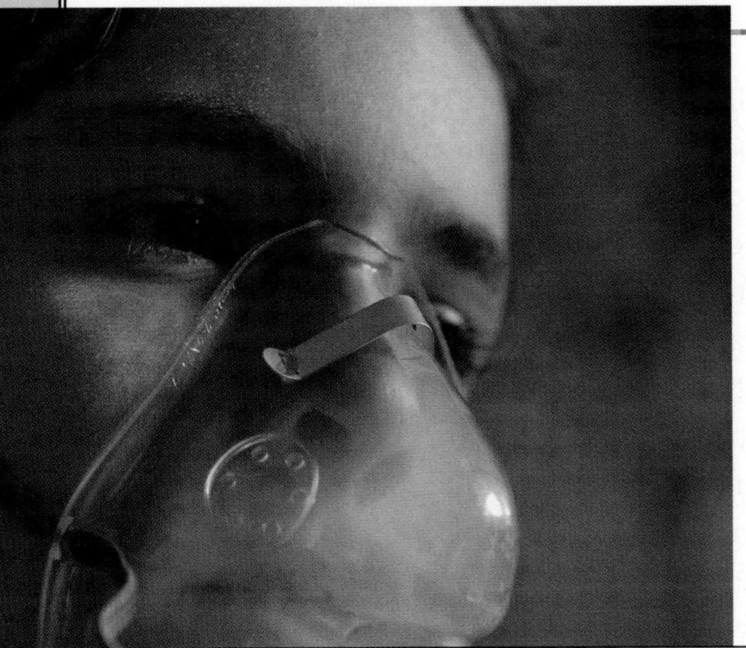

CORE CONCEPTS

The following are core concepts that will be addressed in this chapter:

- Various levels of altered mental status
- Treatment of a patient with altered mental status
- How to identify patients who should receive oral glucose and how to administer glucose
- How to document findings and care of patients with altered mental status

KEY TERMS

diabetes mellitus, p. 449
epilepsy, p. 459
glucose, p. 448
hyperglycemia, p. 449
hypoglycemia, p. 449
insulin, p. 448
seizure, p. 458
status epilepticus, p. 460
stroke, p. 462
syncope, p. 466

DOT OBJECTIVES

*KNOWLEDGE AND ATTITUDE

4-4.1 Identify the patient taking diabetic medications with altered mental status and the implications of a diabetes history. (pp. 450, 455)

4-4.2 State the steps in the emergency medical care of the patient taking diabetic medicine with an altered mental status and a history of diabetes. (p. 455) (Scan 19-1, p. 424)

4-4.3 Establish the relationship between airway management and the patient with altered mental status. (pp. 449, 455, 456, 459, 460, 465)

4-4.4 State the generic and trade names, medication forms, dose, administration, action, and contraindications for oral glucose. (p. 455) (Scan 19-3, p. 456)

4-4.5 Evaluate the need for medical direction in the emergency medical care of the diabetic patient. (pp. 453, 455, 457)

4-4.6 Explain the rationale for administering oral glucose. (pp. 449, 455, 456)

*SKILLS

4-4.7 Demonstrate the steps in the emergency medical care for the patient taking diabetic medicine with an altered mental status and a history of diabetes.

4-4.8 Demonstrate the steps in the administration of oral glucose.

4-4.9 Demonstrate the assessment and documentation of patient response to oral glucose.

4-4.10 Demonstrate how to complete a prehospital care report for patients with diabetic emergencies.

When you are called to the scene of a diabetic emergency, your task will not be to diagnose or treat diabetes but rather to recognize and treat a condition that diabetes, or the poor management of diabetes, has caused. The first indication that the patient is diabetic may be an altered mental status. There will often be other clues, such as a medical identification necklace, insulin or other diabetic medication in the refrigerator or purse, or information provided by family members, friends, or coworkers.

To do your job, you do not have to understand all the complications of diabetes, but you must be ready to administer glucose if your assessment turns up a history of diabetes, an altered mental status, and assurance that the patient can swallow. However, the following information about diabetes may provide some perspective.

DIABETES

glucose (GLU-kos) a form of sugar, the body's basic source of energy.

insulin (IN-suh-lin) a hormone produced by the pancreas or taken as a medication by many diabetics.

Glucose, a form of sugar, is the body's basic source of energy. The sugars that a person eats are converted into glucose, which is then absorbed into the bloodstream. However, this blood sugar cannot simply pass from the bloodstream into the body's cells. To enter the cells, **insulin,** a hormone produced by the pancreas, must be present. Without insulin, the cells can be surrounded by glucose but still starve for this sugar. The insulin/glucose relationship has been described as a "lock and key" mechanism. Consider insulin the key. Without the insulin "key," glucose cannot enter the locked cells (Figure 19-1).

When sugar intake and insulin production are balanced, the body can effectively use sugar as an energy source. If, for some reason, insulin production decreases, glucose cannot be used by the cells. This glucose remains in circulation, increasing in concentration as more sugars are digested by the person. The level of blood sugar climbs, eventually to be spilled over into the urine. High sugar leads to increased urine output, which in turn makes the patient abnormally thirsty.

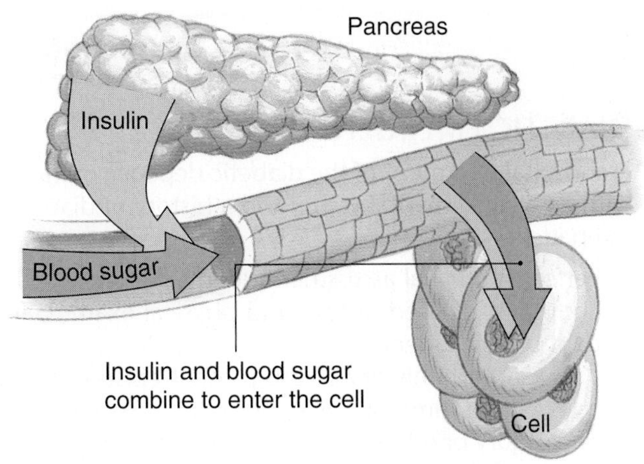

Figure 19-1 • Insulin is needed to help the cells take in glucose.

Diabetes mellitus, often called "sugar diabetes" or just "diabetes," is brought about by decreased insulin production or, more commonly in older patients, the inability of the body's cells to use insulin properly, resulting in high blood sugar. The person suffering from this condition is a diabetic.

diabetes mellitus (di-ah-BEE-tez MEL-i-tus) also called "sugar diabetes" or just "diabetes," the condition brought about by decreased insulin production or the inability of the body cells to use insulin properly. The person with this condition is a diabetic.

Diabetic Emergencies

Hypoglycemia

The most common medical emergency for the diabetic is a condition called **hypoglycemia,** or low blood sugar. (*Hypo* means "less than normal" or "deficient." *Glyc* means "sugar.") Hypoglycemia is caused when the diabetic does any one of the following:

hypoglycemia (HI-po-gli-SEE-me-ah) low blood sugar.

- Takes too much insulin (or, less commonly, oral medication used to treat diabetes), thereby putting too much sugar into the cells and leaving too little sugar in the blood
- Reduces sugar intake by not eating
- Overexercises or overexerts himself, thus using sugars faster than normal
- Vomits a meal, emptying the stomach of sugar as well as other food

When blood sugar is thus reduced, an altered mental status, possibly unconsciousness, and even permanent brain damage can occur quickly if the sugar is not replenished.

Rapid onset, abnormal behavior, and very sweaty skin are all typical of a sudden drop in blood sugar level. Quick administration of glucose, when it can be done without threatening the airway (that is, if the patient is conscious and can swallow), is critical to this patient's outcome. Glucose must be given promptly, before the patient becomes unconscious.

Hyperglycemia

Hyperglycemia is high blood sugar. (*Hyper* means "more than normal" or "excessive." *Glyc* means "sugar.") It is usually caused by a decrease in insulin, which leaves sugar in the bloodstream rather than allowing it to enter the cells. The insulin deficiency may be due to the body's inability to produce insulin or may exist because insulin injections were forgotten or not given in sufficient quantity. Infection, stress, or increasing dietary intake can also be a factor in hyperglycemia.

hyperglycemia (HI-per-gli-SEE-me-ah) high blood sugar.

Unlike hypoglycemia, hyperglycemia generally has a slower onset with the patient experiencing increased urination, thirst, and hunger. The patient may also be nauseated and have an acetone-like odor on his breath.

Remember that it is not part of the scope of practice for an EMT to diagnose an exact condition. Additional information on hyperglycemia and diabetes can be found in the FYI section titled "Additional Information on Diabetes."

PATIENT ASSESSMENT

DIABETIC EMERGENCIES

Prehospital treatment of the diabetic depends on rapid identification of the patient with an altered mental status and a history of diabetes. (See Scan 19-1.) To assess the patient:

1. Perform an initial assessment. Identify altered mental status.
2. Perform a focused history and physical exam. Gather the history from the patient or bystanders:
    - Gather a history of the present episode. Ask about how the episode occurred, time of onset, duration, associated symptoms, any mechanism of injury or other evidence of trauma, whether there have been any interruptions to the episode, seizures, or a fever.
    - During the SAMPLE history, determine if the patient has a history of diabetes. Question the patient or bystanders about such a history. Look for a medical identification bracelet, wallet card, or other identification of a diabetic condition such as a home-use blood glucose meter. Look in the refrigerator or elsewhere at the scene for medications such as insulin, a medication with a trade name for insulin (such as Humulin), or an oral medication used to treat diabetes (such as metformin, Glucotrol, Glucophage, Micronase) (Figure 19-2). Also ask about the patient's last meal, last medication dose, and any related illnesses.
    - Perform blood glucose monitoring if local protocols permit you to do so. (See the information in the next section and Scan 19-2.)
3. Determine if the patient is alert enough to be able to swallow.
4. Take baseline vital signs. (In some jurisdictions, oral glucose will be administered before the vital signs are taken.)

    The following signs and symptoms are associated with a diabetic emergency:

    - Rapid onset of altered mental status:
        - After missing a meal on a day the patient took prescribed insulin
        - After vomiting a meal on a day the patient took prescribed insulin
        - After an unusual amount of physical exercise or work
        - May occur with no identifiable predisposing factor
    - Intoxicated appearance, staggering, slurred speech, to unconsciousness
    - Cold, clammy skin
    - Elevated heart rate
    - Hunger
    - Uncharacteristic behavior
    - Anxiety
    - Combativeness
    - Seizures ■

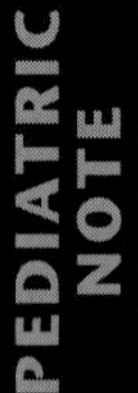

Diabetic children are more at risk for medical emergencies than diabetic adults. Children are more active and may exhaust blood sugar levels by playing hard—especially if they have taken their prescribed insulin. Children are also less likely to be disciplined about eating correctly and on time. As a consequence, children are more at risk of hypoglycemia.

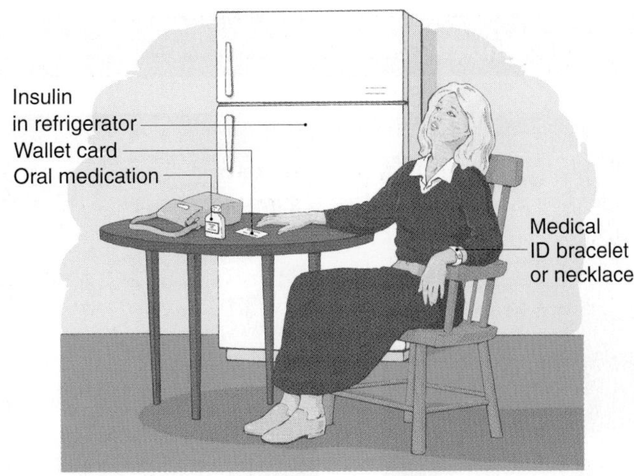

Figure 19-2 • Look for indications that the patient may have a history of diabetes.

Blood Glucose Meters

One of the many advances in managing diabetes in the last few years has been the development of portable, reliable blood glucose meters (Figure 19-3). People with diabetes now routinely test the level of glucose in their blood at least once a day, and sometimes as often as five or six times a day. By determining the amount of glucose in their blood, they can determine very precisely how much insulin they should take and how much and how often they should eat. Keeping blood glucose levels as close to normal as possible leads to significantly fewer diabetes-related complications (heart disease, blindness, and kidney failure, to name a few), so a person with diabetes has a strong motivation to keep his blood glucose level within the normal range.

A blood glucose meter is used by placing a drop of the patient's blood on a test strip. The blood is traditionally obtained from pricking a finger, although some glucose meters allow patients to obtain the blood from other areas, like the forearm. The glucose meter evaluates the change in chemical composition of the material on the strip and displays a number that correlates to the glucose concentration in the person's blood. In the United States, this number usually shows the amount of glucose in milligrams per deciliter (100 mL) of blood (expressed as mg/dl), also called milligrams percent. Outside of the United States, the meter may use a different system of measuring glucose to report results.

The portability, low cost, and accuracy of blood glucose meters has made it practical to carry them on the ambulance. They are easy to use, and since they are routinely used by patients, many EMS systems allow EMTs to use blood glucose meters that are carried on the ambulance. Your protocols will tell you whether you are allowed to carry and use a glucose meter.

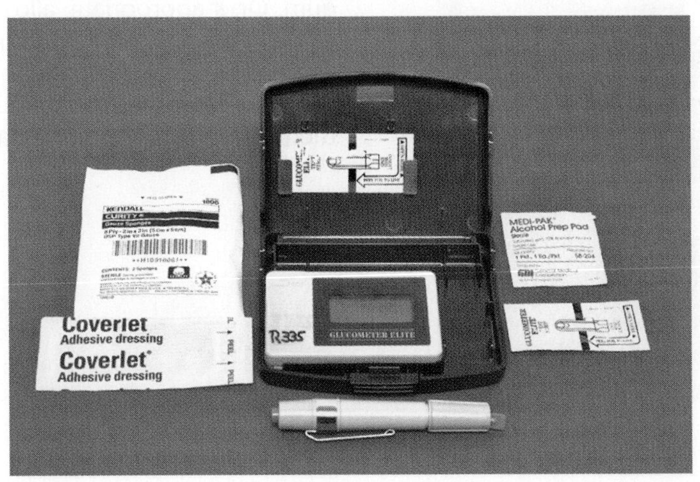

Figure 19-3 • Many diabetics use home glucometers to test their blood glucose levels.

SCAN 19-1 • Management of a Diabetic Emergency

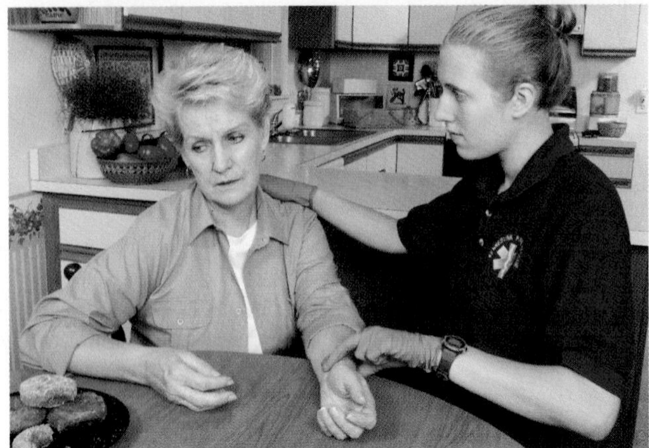

1. Perform an initial assessment. Determine if the patient's mental status is altered.

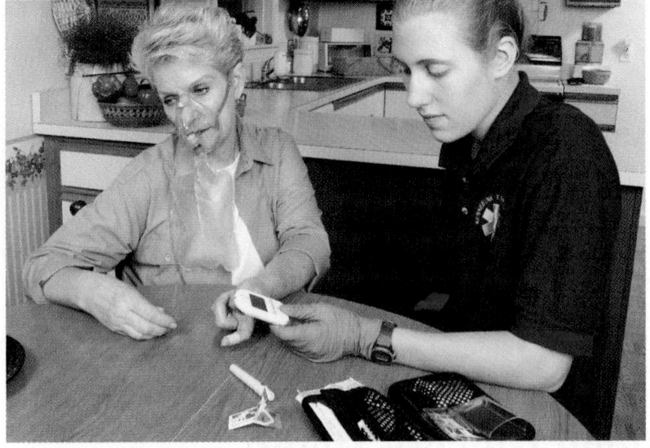

2. Perform a focused history and physical exam and take the patient's vital signs. Be sure to find out if she has a history of diabetes. Observe for a medical identification device. If your protocols allow, check the patient's blood glucose level (see Scan 19-2).

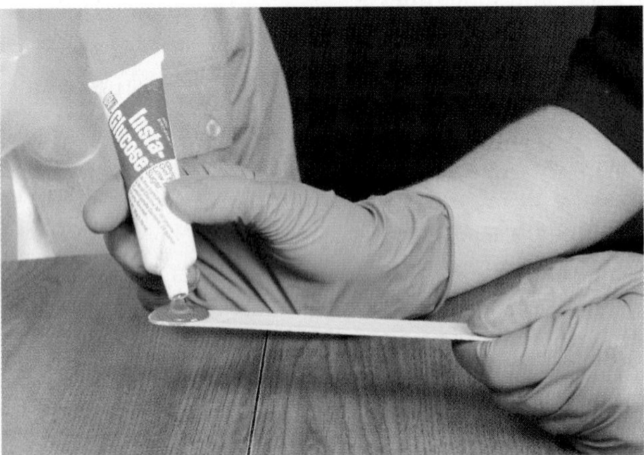

3. If the patient has a history of diabetes, has an altered mental status, and is alert enough to swallow, prepare to administer oral glucose by squeezing it onto a tongue depressor.

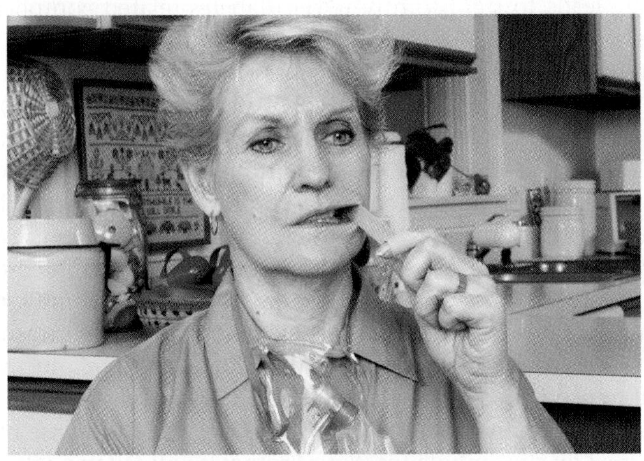

4. Then insert the tongue depressor and oral glucose into the patient's mouth between the cheek and gum. Or, if appropriate, allow the patient to do so. Leave in place until the oral glucose has been absorbed or until the patient can no longer protect her airway. The tongue depressor should then be removed from the patient's mouth.

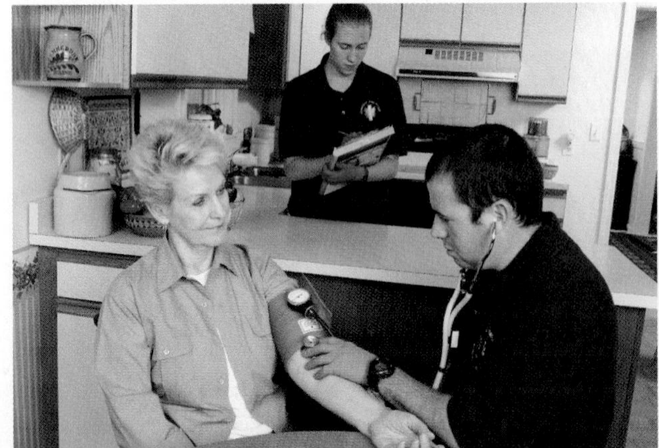

5. Reassess the patient.

SCAN 19-2 • Using a Blood Glucose Meter

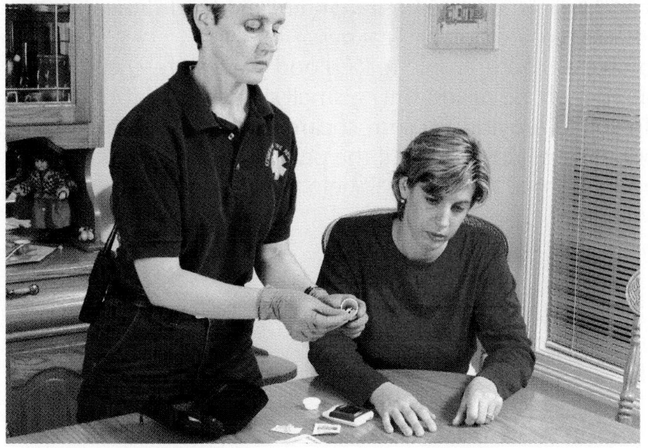

1. Prepare the blood glucose meter, including a test strip and a lancet.

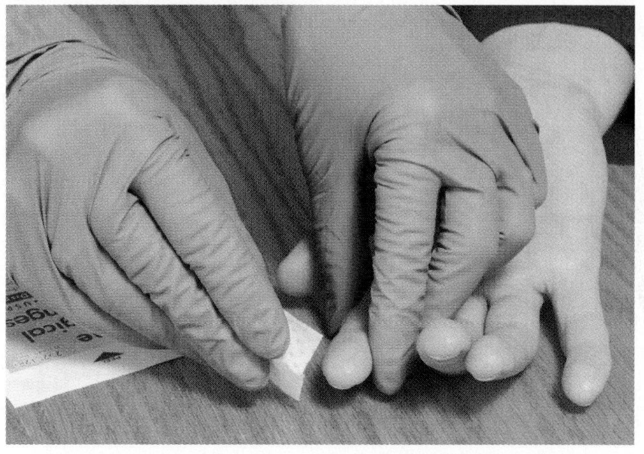

2. Cleanse the skin with an alcohol preparation. Allow the alcohol to dry before performing the finger stick.

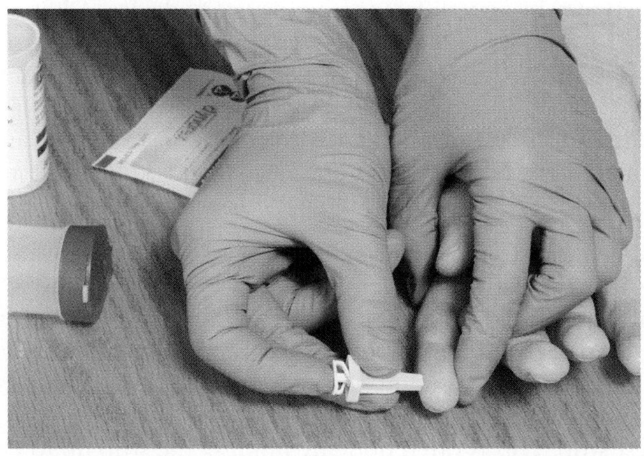

3. Use the lancet to perform a finger stick. Wipe away the first drop of blood that appears. Squeeze the finger if necessary to get a second drop of blood.

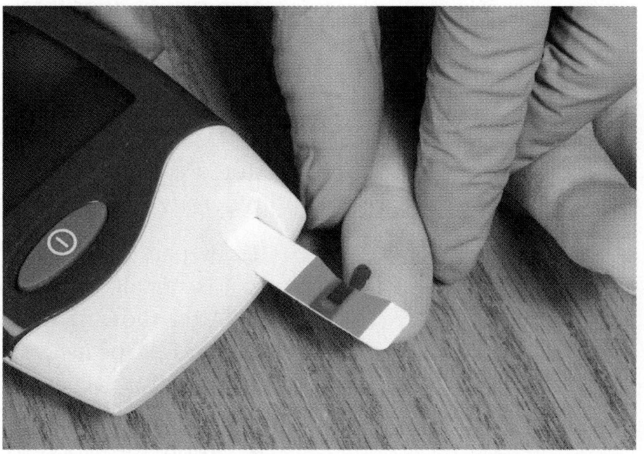

4. Apply the blood to the test strip. This may be done by holding the strip to the finger to draw the blood into the strip.

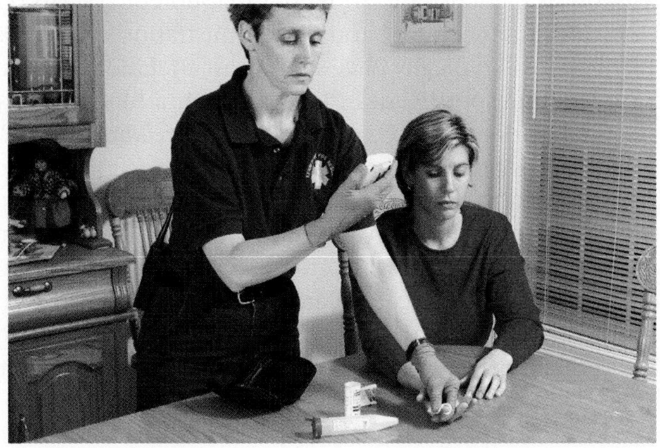

5. Read the blood glucose level displayed on the glucose meter. (It may take 15 to 60 seconds for the device to provide a reading.) Assess the puncture site and apply direct pressure or a bandage to the site if bleeding continues.

NOTE

EMTs must have permission from medical direction or by local protocol to perform blood glucose monitoring using a blood glucose meter.

Cultural Considerations

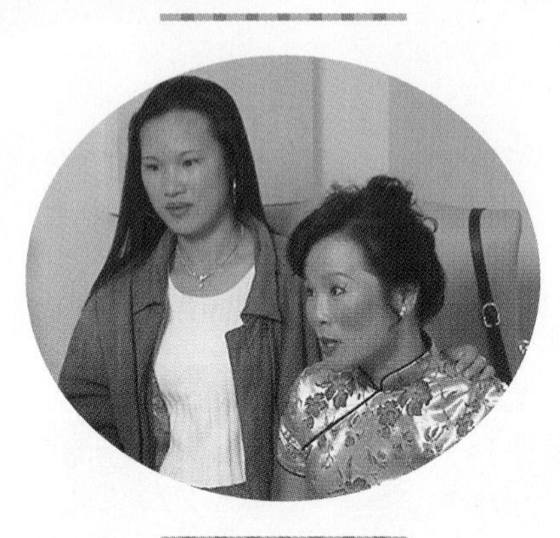

According to traditional Chinese beliefs, a person who does not feel well is lacking in *chi* (inner energy) and blood. Chinese Americans who follow traditional practices and beliefs may be hesitant to have blood drawn for fear that it will cause or exacerbate bodily weakness.

If you need to take a blood sample for a blood glucose test, emphasize to the patient that you will be taking only a small drop and that the results of the test will help you to provide the correct care. Reassure the patient that in the long run, or perhaps fairly quickly if the patient turns out to need glucose to relieve hypoglycemia, this step will help the patient to feel stronger and better, not worse.

If the patient has a glucose meter, the patient or a family member can use it to determine the patient's blood glucose level. Generally, EMTs should not use a patient's glucose meter. There are many different types of these devices on the market, each with its own instructions for use, which may be very different from device to device. Additionally, there is no way for the EMT to know whether the test strips have been stored properly or when the device was last calibrated. These facts are very important if the reading is to be accurate.

If you have blood glucose monitors on the ambulance, they must be calibrated and stored according to the manufacturer's recommendations. Take Standard Precautions. When using the glucose meter (Scan 19-2), you will follow these steps:

1. Prepare the device including a test strip and lancet.
2. Use an alcohol prep to cleanse the patient's finger.
3. After allowing the alcohol to dry, use the lancet to perform a finger stick on the patient. Wipe away the first drop of blood that appears. Squeeze the patient's finger if necessary to get a second drop of blood. Holding the patient's hand lower than the heart and warming the hand may increase blood flow.
4. Apply the blood to the test strip. This is often done by holding the strip up to the finger and then drawing the blood into the strip.
5. The blood glucose meter analyzes the sample and provides a reading—usually in less than a minute.

A value less than 60 to 80 mg/dL (milligrams per deciliter) in a symptomatic diabetic (i.e., a patient with a mild alteration in mental status or who is diaphoretic (sweaty)) is typical of hypoglycemia and indicates the need for prompt administration of glucose. Patients with values less than 50 mg/dL will typically have significant alterations in mental status that may include complete unresponsiveness. Patients with a blood glucose level that is this low will often be unable to safely receive oral glucose. A reading over 120 or 140 (depending on the manufacturer's instructions) indicates hyperglycemia, a condition that may require treatment in a health care setting more advanced than an ambulance. This will depend on the severity of the hyperglycemia and the patient's condition. Patients with glucose levels in the mid and high 100s are often without acute symptoms, although over time this level of hyperglycemia can cause damage to various body organs.

A reading inconsistent with the patient's symptoms (such as 25 mg/dL in a patient who is alert and oriented) should make the EMT question the result. There are many potential causes of inaccurate results, including insufficient blood on the test strip, a strip past its expiration date or not stored properly, or a meter that needs calibration. Although many people use blood glucose meters appropriately and accurately, it is quite common to get an inaccurate reading, especially when the device is not used properly. It is critical for any health care provider, who is using a blood glucose meter to test a patient's blood, to have the proper training in use of the device and be thoroughly familiar with its care and maintenance. Calibration and testing on a regularly scheduled basis are essential if the device is to give accurate results.

On occasion, the glucometer will display not a number but the word *HIGH*. Depending on the manufacturer, a "High" or "HI" reading indicates an extremely high glucose level, usually in excess of 500 mg/dL.

Remember that the blood glucose monitor is just one tool in your assessment of a patient with an altered mental status. Blood glucose monitoring, or any other examinations, should never be done before a thorough initial assessment has been performed. Some areas recommend that the blood glucose measurements be done while en route to the hospital.

PATIENT CARE

DIABETIC EMERGENCIES

Emergency care of a patient with a diabetic emergency includes the following (see Scans 19-1, 19-2, and 19-3):

1. Determine if all of the following criteria for administration of oral glucose are present: The patient has a history of diabetes, has an altered mental status, and is awake enough to swallow.
2. If the patient meets the criteria for administration of oral glucose, it may be given by applying it to a tongue depressor and placing it in the patient's mouth between cheek and gum. Alternatively, if he is able, let the patient squeeze the glucose from the tube directly into his mouth.
3. Reassess the patient. If the patient's condition does not improve after administration of oral glucose, consult medical direction about whether to administer more. If at any time the patient loses consciousness, remove the tongue depressor from his mouth and take steps to ensure an open airway.

If the patient is not awake enough to swallow, treat him like any other patient with an altered mental status. That is, secure the airway, provide artificial ventilations if necessary, and be prepared to perform CPR if needed. Position the patient appropriately. If the patient does not need to be ventilated, place him in the recovery position (on his side) so that he is less likely to choke on or to aspirate fluids or vomitus into his lungs. Request an ALS intercept if available. ■

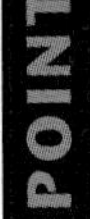

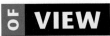

POINT OF VIEW

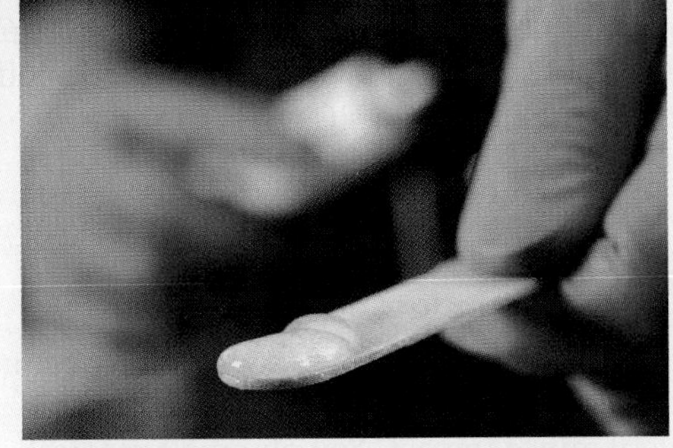

"You'd think after you've been a diabetic most of your life that the needles wouldn't bother you. Actually they've gotten better, smaller. And need less blood.

"Despite how much I try to keep my blood sugar regulated, no matter how much I see my doctor, I end up needing an ambulance a couple of times a year. It is almost embarrassing. I see the same people time after time, and they are always so nice to me.

"I remember the days before we could check my blood sugar. I'd just have to get some sugar. If it wasn't low, it would take days to get me back regulated again after all that sugar. When the EMTs came today they were right on the ball. They checked my sugar and it was the lowest I have ever seen it. They put a blob of that goop on a tongue depressor and put it in my mouth, and I was better pretty quickly.

"But I still get sick of the needles sometimes."

SCAN 19-3 • Oral Glucose

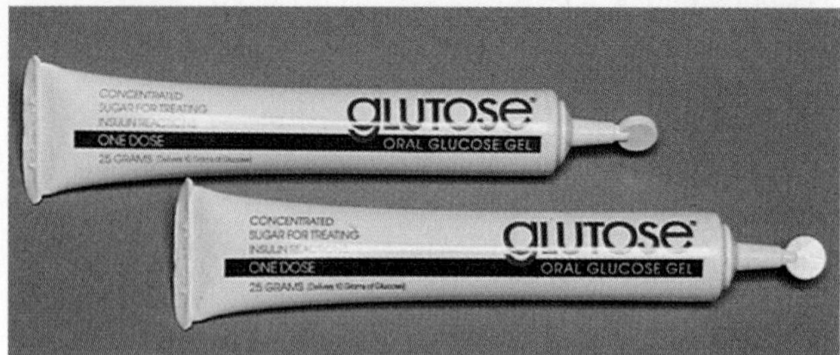

MEDICATION NAME

1. Generic: Glucose, oral
2. Trade: Glutose, Insta-glucose

INDICATIONS

Patients with altered mental status and a known history of diabetes mellitus

CONTRAINDICATIONS

1. Unconsciousness
2. Known diabetic who has not taken insulin for days
3. Unable to swallow

MEDICATION FORM

Gel, in toothpaste-type tubes

DOSAGE

One tube

ADMINISTRATION

1. Ensure signs and symptoms of altered mental status with a known history of diabetes.
2. Ensure patient is conscious.
3. Administer glucose.
   a. Place on tongue depressor between cheek and gum, or
   b. Self-administered between cheek and gum.
4. Perform ongoing assessment.

ACTIONS

Increases blood sugar

SIDE EFFECTS

None when given properly. May be aspirated by the patient without a gag reflex.

REASSESSMENT STRATEGIES

If patient loses consciousness or seizes, remove tongue depressor from mouth.

CRITICAL DECISION MAKING: The Taste of Sweet Success

For each patient below determine if the general criteria are met for you to administer glucose to the patient. Oral glucose is carried on your ambulance. For the purposes of this exercise, assume that your blood glucose monitor isn't available. (It is sometimes important to make decisions independent of devices.)

1. Your patient is confused. She doesn't know what day it is and is talking but not making any sense. Her nurse's aide tells you the patient is diabetic and has been having trouble with managing her blood sugar levels. She will occasionally take insulin but not eat and vice versa.
2. At a facility for disabled youth, a 19-year-old man recovering from a head injury was seizing prior to your arrival, but the seizure has stopped. He responds to loud verbal stimulus. He has a history of diabetes.
3. You respond to a motor vehicle collision and find one patient sitting behind the wheel of his car, rocking back and forth, muttering incoherently. The accident was low-speed with a very minor impact. You observe a medical identification bracelet that indicates the patient is diabetic.

F•Y•I

ADDITIONAL INFORMATION ON DIABETES

TYPES OF DIABETES

There are two major classifications of diabetes mellitus: Type I and Type II. Type I diabetes, which is usually insulin-dependent, occurs in individuals with little or no ability to produce insulin. It has been called "juvenile diabetes," since it tends to begin in childhood. The Type I diabetic must inject doses of supplemental insulin at least once a day.

Type II, or non-insulin-dependent, diabetes occurs in individuals who produce insulin in insufficient amounts and/or whose body cells cannot use the insulin properly. This disorder is usually associated with obesity and is seen most often in older adults. However, as childhood obesity has become more common, it is increasingly seen in children. Type II diabetes can often be controlled without supplemental insulin through supervised diets and oral medications.

The danger of undetected and untreated diabetes is severe. As the condition develops, the diabetic can become weak and lose weight even with increased sugar and fat intake. Advanced diabetes is often associated with such complications as heart disease, kidney disease, and blindness.

HYPERGLYCEMIA

Although hypoglycemia, or low blood sugar, is the most common cause of diabetic emergency, another possible problem, as discussed at the beginning of the chapter, is overly high blood sugar, or hyperglycemia. Like hypoglycemia, hyperglycemia can be life threatening.

Hyperglycemia occurs because the diabetic does not produce enough natural insulin to take sugar out of the blood and into the cells, and because of any one of the following:

- He has not taken enough insulin to make up for this deficiency.
- He has forgotten to take his insulin.
- He has overeaten.
- He has an infection that has upset his insulin/glucose balance.

With hyperglycemia, not only is there too much sugar in the blood, there is too little sugar in the cells. The body attempts to overcome the lack of sugar in the cells by using other foods for energy, particularly stored fats. However, fats are not an efficient alternative to glucose, and the waste products of fat utilization, ketones (compounds that are in the same class as those used to make fingernail polish remover), begin to concentrate in the blood, turning the blood acidic. The person will drink large quantities of water to offset the loss of fluids through excess urination, caused by the body's attempt to get rid of extra sugar. If untreated, the acidity of the blood and the loss of fluids eventually lead to a condition known as diabetic ketoacidosis, which can lead to death.

HYPOGLYCEMIA AND HYPERGLYCEMIA COMPARED

Many students find that they confuse hypoglycemia and hyperglycemia. Fortunately, it is not necessary to distinguish between the two conditions in order to give the proper treatment. There are three typical differences between hypoglycemia and hyperglycemia:

- **Onset.** Hyperglycemia usually has a slower onset, while hypoglycemia tends to come on suddenly. This is because some sugar still reaches the brain in hyperglycemic (high blood sugar) states. With hypoglycemia (low blood sugar), it is possible that no sugar is reaching the brain. Seizures may occur.
- **Skin.** Hyperglycemic patients often have warm, red, dry skin. Hypoglycemic patients have cold, pale, moist, or "clammy" skin.
- **Breath.** The hyperglycemic patient often has acetone breath (like nail polish remover), while the hypoglycemic patient does not.

Also, patients who are hyperglycemic frequently breathe very deeply and rapidly, as though they have just run a race. Dry mouth, intense thirst, abdominal pain, and vomiting are all common signs and symptoms of this condition. The proper treatment is given under close medical supervision in a hospital.

There appear to be clear-cut differences between the signs and symptoms of hyperglycemia and hypoglycemia, but distinguishing between them in the field can be difficult and is not necessary. If your system allows the use of blood glucose monitoring, it may provide the patient's actual blood glucose level. This can be used to identify someone with hypo- or hyperglycemia. Remember that this is just one tool in your assessment which, when combined with the patient's history (e.g., food intake and medications taken) and your protocols will aid in your decision-making process. Always consult medical direction if questions or concerns arise.

continued

F•Y•I

Continued

Giving glucose will help the hypoglycemic patient by getting needed sugar into the bloodstream and to the brain. Although the hyperglycemic patient already has too much sugar in his blood, the extra dose of glucose will not have time to cause damage in the short time before he reaches the hospital and can be diagnosed and treated. This is why "sugar (glucose) for everyone" is the rule of thumb for diabetic emergencies, whether the patient is hypo- or hyperglycemic, and why you do not need to distinguish between the two conditions. ■

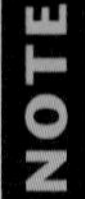

NOTE

Some hyperglycemic and hypoglycemic patients will appear to be intoxicated. Always suspect a diabetic problem in cases that seem to involve no more than intoxication. Remember that the patient intoxicated on alcohol may also be a diabetic, with the alcohol breath covering the acetone odor of diabetic ketoacidosis. The alcoholic diabetic is a good candidate for a diabetic emergency, because he tends to neglect eating and taking insulin during prolonged drinking and usually has a low blood sugar level.

OTHER CAUSES OF ALTERED MENTAL STATUS

In addition to diabetic emergencies, there are many causes of altered mental status in which the patient is confused or disoriented. Examples include alcohol use, overdose of other drugs, metabolic abnormalities, head trauma, brain tumor, infectious diseases such as meningitis, and hypoxia. In all cases, gather a careful history; calm the patient; maintain an open airway; provide high-concentration oxygen; and transport to the hospital.

The following sections provide additional information on two other causes of altered mental status: seizure disorders and stroke.

Seizure Disorders

seizure (SEE-zher) a sudden change in sensation, behavior, or movement. The most severe form of seizure produces violent muscle contractions called convulsions.

If the normal functions of the brain are upset by injury, infection, or disease, the electrical activity of the brain can become irregular. This irregularity can bring about a sudden change in sensation, behavior, or movement, called a **seizure** (also called a fit, spell, or attack by nonmedical people). Some seizures involve uncontrolled muscular movements called convulsions.

A seizure is not a disease in itself but rather a sign of some underlying defect, injury, or disease. The most common cause of seizures in adults is failure to take their prescribed anti-seizure medication. The most common cause of seizures in infants and children 6 months to 3 years of age is high fever (febrile seizures). Other categories include:

- *Toxic.* Drug or alcohol use, abuse, or withdrawal can cause seizures. (Toxic means "poisonous"—the drug or alcohol has worked as a poison.)
- *Brain tumor.* A brain tumor may occasionally cause seizures.
- *Congenital brain defects.* Seizures due to congenital defects of the brain (defects one is born with) are most often seen in infants and young children.
- *Infection.* Swelling or inflammation of the brain caused by an infection can cause seizures.
- *Metabolic.* Seizures can be caused by irregularities in the patient's body chemistry (metabolism).
- *Trauma.* Head injuries can cause seizures. So can scars formed at the site of previous brain injuries.
- *Idiopathic.* This means occuring spontaneously, with an unknown cause. This is often the case with seizures that start in childhood.

In addition, convulsive seizures may be seen with:

- Epilepsy
- Stroke
- Measles, mumps, and other childhood diseases
- Hypoglycemia
- Eclampsia (a severe complication of pregnancy)
- Hypoxia (lack of oxygen)
- Heat stroke (resulting from exposure to high temperatures)

Epilepsy is perhaps the best-known of the conditions that result in seizures. Some people are born with epilepsy, while others develop epilepsy after a head injury or surgery. Conscientious use of medications allows most epileptics to live normal lives without seizures of any type. Remember that, while a patient with seizures may be an epileptic, epilepsy is only one condition that causes seizures.

epilepsy (EP-uh-lep-see) a medical condition that causes seizures. With proper medication, many epileptic patients will no longer have seizures.

Not all seizures are alike. The type of seizure in which the person falls to the floor and has severe convulsions is the kind of seizure for which EMS will most likely be called.

PATIENT ASSESSMENT

SEIZURE DISORDERS

It is very important to be able to describe the seizure to emergency department personnel. If you have not observed the seizure (usually EMS is called after the seizure has taken place), always try to find out what it was like by asking the following questions of bystanders. Be sure to record and report your findings.

- What was the person doing before the seizure started?
- Exactly what did the person do during the seizure—movement by movement—especially at the beginning? Was there loss of bladder or bowel control?
- How long did the seizure last?
- What did the person do after the seizure? Was he asleep (and for how long)? Was he awake? Was he able to answer questions? (If you are present during the seizure, use the AVPU scale to assess mental status.) ■

PATIENT CARE

SEIZURE DISORDERS

Emergency care of a patient with a seizure disorder includes the following.

If you are present when a convulsive seizure occurs:

- Place the patient on the floor or ground. If there is no possibility of spine injury, position the patient on his side for drainage from the mouth.
- Loosen restrictive clothing.
- Remove objects that may harm the patient.
- Protect the patient from injury, but do not try to hold the patient still during convulsions (Figure 19-4).

After convulsions have ended:

- Protect the airway. A patient who has just had a generalized seizure will sometimes drool and will usually be very drowsy for a little while, so you may need to suction the airway. If there is no possibility of spine injury, position the patient on his side for drainage from the mouth.

continued

PATIENT CARE *(continued)*

- If the patient is cyanotic (blue), ensure an open airway and provide artificial ventilations with supplemental oxygen.
- Treat any injuries the patient may have sustained during the convulsions, or rule out trauma. Head injury can cause seizures, or the patient may have injured himself during the seizure. Immobilize the neck and spine if trauma is suspected.
- Transport to a medical facility, monitoring vital signs and respirations closely. ■

NOTE

Never place anything in the mouth of a seizing patient. Many objects can be broken and obstruct the patient's airway.

PEDIATRIC NOTE

Remember that seizures caused by high fevers and idiopathic seizures (with no known cause) are common in children. Seizures in children who frequently have them are rarely life threatening. However, as an EMT, you should treat any seizure in an infant or child as if it is life threatening.

The epileptic is often knowledgeable about his condition, medications, and history. Since seizures may be common for the patient, he may refuse transportation. The patient should be encouraged to accept transportation to a hospital for examination. Should the patient continue to refuse, he should not be left alone after the seizure, and he must not drive. A competent person must remain with the patient.

NOTE

Seizures usually last no more than 1 to 3 minutes. When the patient has two or more convulsive seizures lasting 5 to 10 minutes or more without regaining full consciousness, it is known as* status epilepticus. *Some systems consider all patients who are still seizing when EMS arrives on the scene to be in status epilepticus. This is a high-priority emergency requiring immediate transport to the hospital and possible ALS intercept (having an advanced life support team meet your ambulance en route). The airway must be opened and suctioned and a high concentration of oxygen should be administered at the scene and while en route.

status epilepticus (STAY-tus or STAT-us ep-i-LEP-ti-kus) a prolonged seizure or when a person suffers two or more convulsive seizures without regaining full consciousness.

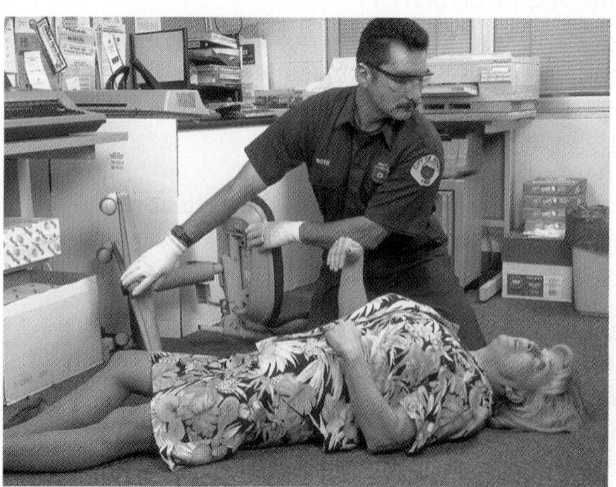

Figure 19-4 • Protect the seizure patient from injury.

Just as it is not your job to diagnose the cause of a seizure, it is not your job to identify the type of seizure. Your job as an EMT is to gather a history and provide other normal assessment and care as previously described. However, some background information about types of seizures can provide perspective.

The generalized tonic-clonic seizure (formerly called grand-mal) in which the person falls to the floor and has severe convulsions, described earlier, is only one of four common types of seizures in two classifications: partial seizures and generalized seizures.

PARTIAL SEIZURES

In a simple partial seizure (also called focal motor, focal sensory, or Jacksonian) there is tingling, stiffening, or jerking in just one part of the body. There may also be an aura, which is a sensation such as a smell, bright lights, a burst of colors, or a rising sensation in the stomach. There is no loss of consciousness. However, in some cases the jerking may spread and develop into a tonic-clonic seizure.

A complex partial seizure (also called psychomotor or temporal lobe) is often preceded by an aura. This type of seizure is characterized by abnormal behavior that varies widely from person to person. It may involve confusion, a glassy stare, aimless moving about, lip smacking or chewing, or fidgeting with clothing. The person may appear to be drunk or on drugs. He is not violent but may struggle or fight if restrained. Very rarely, such extreme behavior as screaming, running, disrobing, or showing great fear may occur. There is no loss of consciousness, but there may be confusion and no memory of the episode afterward. In some cases, the seizure may develop into a tonic-clonic seizure.

F•Y•I

TYPES OF SEIZURES

GENERALIZED SEIZURES

In a tonic-clonic seizure, there is often no aura or other warning. However, the person may cry out before falling to the floor. This type of seizure is characterized by unconsciousness and major motor activity. The patient will thrash about wildly, using his entire body. The convulsion usually lasts only a few minutes and has three distinct phases:

- **Tonic phase.** The body becomes rigid, stiffening for no more than 30 seconds. Breathing may stop, the patient may bite his tongue (rare), and bowel and bladder control could be lost.
- **Clonic phase.** The body jerks about violently, usually for no more than 1 or 2 minutes (some can last 5 minutes). The patient may foam at the mouth and drool. His face and lips often become cyanotic.
- **Postictal phase.** This begins when convulsions stop. The patient may regain consciousness immediately and enter a state of drowsiness and confusion, or he may remain unconscious for several hours. Headache is common.

An absence seizure (also called petit mal) is brief, usually only 1 to 10 seconds. There is no dramatic motor activity and the person usually does not slump or fall. Instead there is a temporary loss of concentration or awareness. An absence seizure may go unnoticed by everyone except the person and knowledgeable members of his family. A child may suffer several hundred absence seizures a day, severely interfering with his ability to pay attention and do well in school. Absence seizures often stop before adulthood but sometimes worsen and become tonic-clonic seizures.

Patient care for the generalized tonic-clonic seizure was described earlier. For a simple or complex partial seizure, do not restrain the person; simply remove objects from his path and gently guide him away from danger. For an absence seizure, if you are aware that it has occurred, simply provide the patient with any information he may have missed. ■

Stroke

stroke
a condition of altered function caused when an artery in the brain is blocked or ruptured, disrupting the supply of oxygenated blood or causing bleeding into the brain. Also formerly called a *cerebrovascular accident (CVA).*

One of the many causes of altered mental status may be a **stroke.** Formerly called a *cerebral vascular accident (CVA),* the term *stroke* refers to the death or injury of brain tissue that is deprived of oxygen. This can be caused by blockage of an artery that supplies blood to part of the brain or bleeding from a ruptured blood vessel in the brain. A stroke caused by a blockage, called an *ischemic stroke,* can occur when a clot or embolism occludes an artery or as the result of atherosclerosis. This mechanism is responsible for most strokes.

A stroke caused by bleeding into the brain, called a *hemorrhagic stroke,* frequently is the result of longstanding high blood pressure (hypertension). It also can occur when a weak area of an artery (an aneurysm) bulges out and eventually ruptures, forcing the brain into a smaller than usual space within the skull.

Different patients experiencing a stroke may have very different signs and symptoms, depending on the size and location of the arteries involved. One of the most common signs is one-sided weakness (hemiparesis). Because the left side of the brain controls movement on the right side of the body (and vice versa), someone with right-sided weakness from a stroke actually has a problem on the left side of his brain. However, the nerves that control the face muscles do not necessarily cross over in the same way, so sagging or drooping on one side of the face is not a reliable sign of injury to the opposite side.

A less common, but very important, sign of stroke is a headache caused by bleeding from a ruptured vessel. If you find in gathering a history that the patient cried out in pain, clutched his head, and collapsed, this is very important information to relay to the hospital staff. This patient may have had a particular kind of bleeding from an artery under the arachnoid layer of the meninges (the meninges are several layers of tissue that surround the brain and spinal cord). This is called a subarachnoid hemorrhage. Fortunately, most stroke patients are not hemorrhaging and do not experience headaches.

In many cases, you will find it difficult to communicate with the stroke patient. The damage to the brain sometimes causes a partial or complete loss of the ability to use words. The patient may be able to understand you but will not be able to talk or will have great difficulty with speech. Sometimes, the patient will understand you and know what he wants to say, but he will say the wrong words. This difficulty in using words is known as expressive aphasia. *Aphasia* is a general term that refers to difficulty in communication. Another form of it is receptive aphasia. In this case, the patient can speak clearly, but cannot understand what you are saying, so he will clearly say things that do not make much sense or are inappropriate for the situation.

Transient Ischemic Attack

A common occurrence is for an EMT to respond to a patient described as being confused, weak on one side, and having difficulty speaking. The EMT arrives, only to find an elderly patient who is alert, oriented, and perfectly normal. This patient may have had a transient ischemic attack (TIA), sometimes called a mini-stroke by laypeople. When this condition occurs, a patient looks as though he is having a stroke because he has the typical signs and symptoms of the condition. However, unlike stroke, a patient with a TIA has complete resolution of his symptoms without treatment within 24 hours (usually much sooner).

With TIA, small clots may be temporarily blocking circulation to part of the brain. When the clot breaks up, the patient's symptoms resolve because the affected brain tissue had only a short period of hypoxia and did not sustain permanent damage. However, this patient is at significant risk of having a full-blown stroke. If the patient refuses transport, you have a responsibility to attempt to persuade the patient to be evaluated as soon as possible so that a subsequent stroke can be prevented.

PATIENT ASSESSMENT

STROKE

A very good way to assess conscious patients for stroke is to evaluate three items that constitute the Cincinnati Prehospital Stroke Scale (Figure 19-5 and Scan 19-4):

- Ask the patient to grimace or smile. (Demonstrate to the patient what you want her to do, making sure that you show your teeth. This allows you to test control of the facial muscles.) A normal response is for the patient to move both sides of her face equally and to show you her teeth. An abnormal response is unequal movement or no movement at all.
- Ask the patient to close her eyes and extend her arms straight out in front of her for 10 seconds. A normal response is for the patient to move both arms at the same time. An abnormal response is for one arm to drift down or not move at all.

continued

Cincinnati Prehospital Stroke Scale

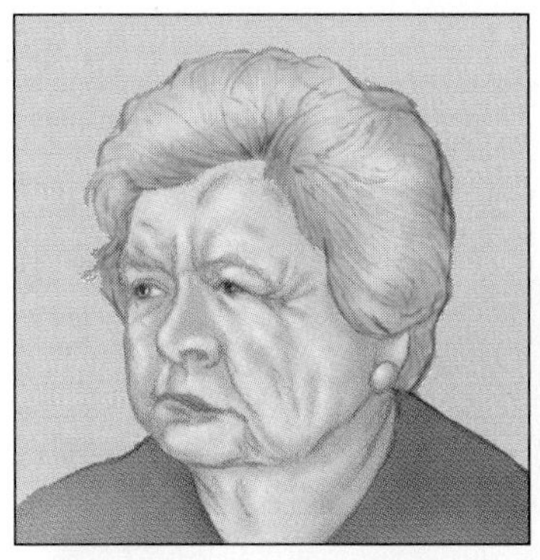

Facial Droop

Normal: Both sides of face move equally
Abnormal: One side of face does not move at all

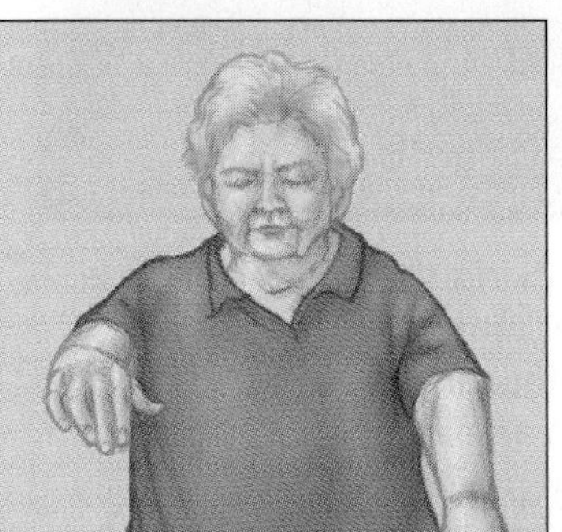

Arm Drift

Normal: Both arms move equally or not at all
Abnormal: One arm drifts compared to the other

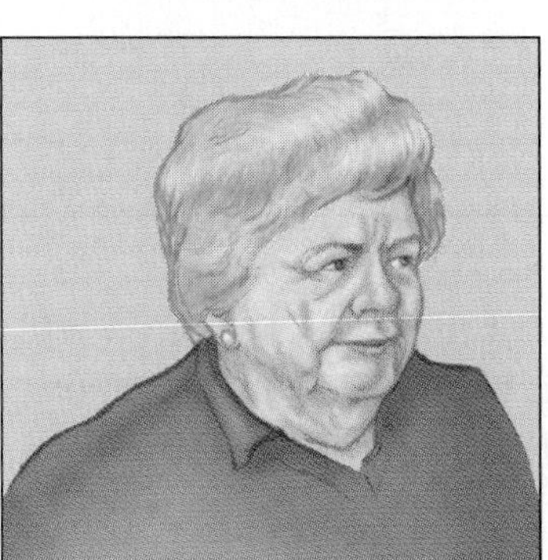

Speech

Normal: Patient uses correct words with no slurring
Abnormal: Slurred or inappropriate words or mute

Figure 19-5 • The Cincinnati Prehospital Stroke Scale.

SCAN 19-4 • Cincinnati Prehospital Stroke Scale

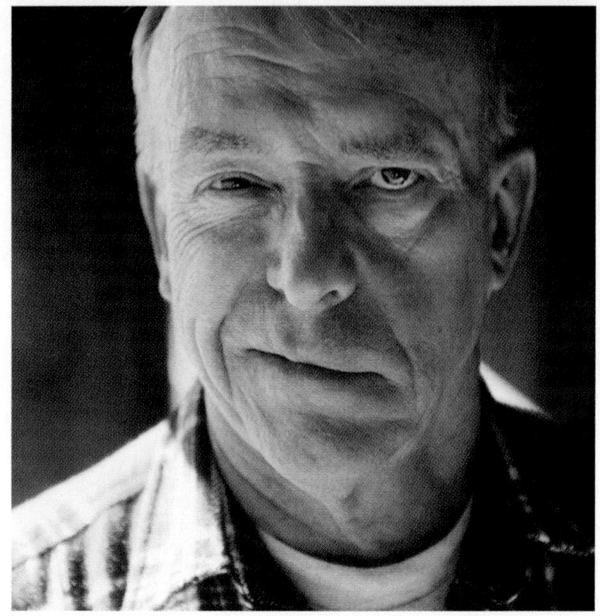

1. Assess for facial droop. The face of a stroke patient often has an abnormal drooped appearance on one side. *(© Michal Heron Photography)*

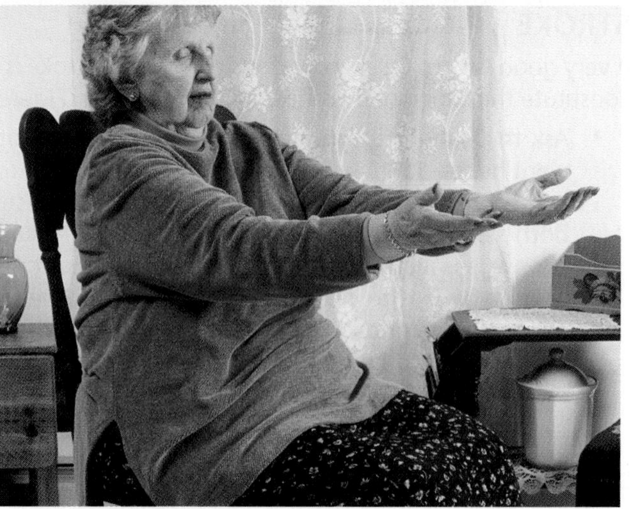

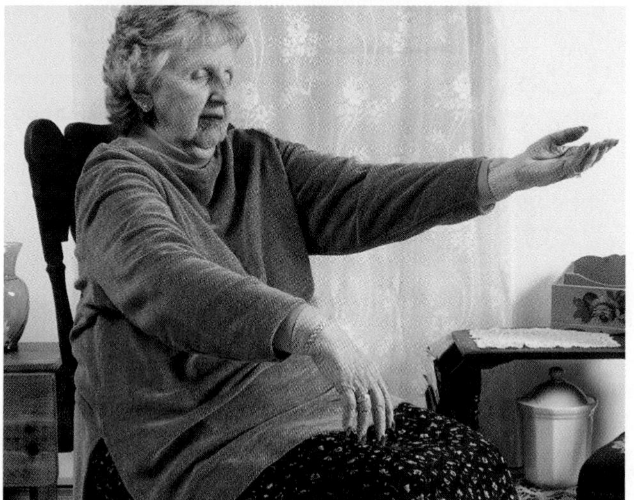

2. Assess for arm drift by asking the patient to close her eyes and extend her arms for 10 seconds. (A) A patient who has not suffered a stroke can usually hold her arms in an extended position with eyes closed. (B) A stroke patient will often display arm drift. That is, one arm will remain extended but the arm on the affected side will drift downward.

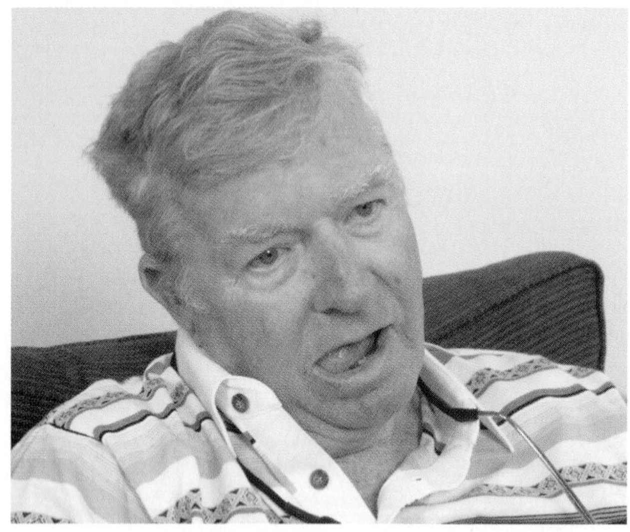

3. Assess for speech difficulties. A stroke patient will often have slurred speech, use the wrong words, or be unable to speak at all.

PATIENT ASSESSMENT *(continued)*

- Ask the patient to say something like, "The sky is blue in Cincinnati." An uninjured person's speech is usually clear. A stroke patient is more likely to show an abnormal response to the test, like slurred speech, the wrong words, or no speech at all.

continued

PATIENT ASSESSMENT *(continued)*

Other signs and symptoms of stroke, which will often fluctuate in severity while you observe the patient, include:

- Confusion
- Dizziness
- Numbness, weakness, or paralysis (usually on one side of the body)
- Loss of bowel or bladder control
- Impaired vision
- High blood pressure
- Difficult respiration or snoring
- Nausea or vomiting
- Seizures
- Unequal pupils
- Headache
- Loss of vision in one eye
- Unconsciousness (uncommon) ■

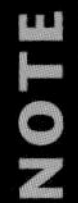

A patient who demonstrates **any one** *of the three findings of the Cincinnati Prehospital Stroke Scale has a 70 percent chance of having an acute stroke.*

PATIENT CARE

STROKE

It is not necessary to determine that a stroke has taken place, although you may suspect it. There are many problems that can mimic strokes, including tumor or infection in the brain, head injury, and hypoglycemia. Treat the patient as you would any patient with similar symptoms:

- For a conscious patient who can maintain his airway, calm and reassure him; monitor the airway; and administer high-concentration oxygen. Transport the patient in a semi-sitting position.
- For an unconscious patient, or a patient who cannot maintain his airway, maintain an open airway; provide high-concentration oxygen; and transport with the patient lying on the affected side.

Because of recent research and advances in the treatment of stroke, you may have special protocols for management and transport of patients with signs and symptoms of stroke. New treatments are being used and tried in many hospitals, but time is of the essence if any of these treatments is to be effective. There appears to be a very narrow window within which assessment must be completed and treatment must be started.

The most widespread advance in stroke care is the use of clot-busting (thrombolytic) drugs in cases of ischemic stroke. This therapy can potentially reverse the symptoms of stroke, but patients must meet very specific criteria including:

- Definite onset of stroke symptoms less than 3 hours prior to the administration of the thrombolytic drug
- An emergency CT scan of the brain confirming that there is no evidence of a hemorrhagic stroke
- Blood pressure that is not excessively hypertensive at the time the drug is administered

continued

PATIENT CARE *(continued)*

One of most important things the EMT can do to optimize the care of stroke patients who are potential candidates for thrombolytics is to determine and document the exact time of onset of symptoms. If the person who provides you with the time of onset is someone other than the patient, it is a good idea to document who that person is and how he can be contacted (e.g., cell phone number) should the physician in the emergency department have to verify any information. In cases where the exact time of onset is not known, the patient will not be able to receive thrombolytics. For example, the patient who awakens at 7 a.m. and is immediately noted by the family to have new stroke symptoms but who was last seen in a normal condition at 11:30 p.m. the night before cannot get thrombolytic therapy, because it is not known when the stroke occurred during the night. ■

NOTE

If you suspect the patient has had a stroke, it is important to transport him promptly and notify the hospital of symptoms you see and the results of the Cincinnati Prehospital Stroke Scale. If you have a choice of hospitals, your protocols may direct you to a hospital capable of providing the most recent stroke treatments.

Dizziness and Syncope

syncope (SIN-ko-pee) fainting.

Dizziness and **syncope** (SIN-ko-pee), or fainting, are common reasons EMS is called. This is especially true for the elderly population, but these problems can occur to patients of any age. Although these complaints might seem to be harmless, in fact they can be indicators of serious or even life-threatening problems. As an EMT, you can assess these patients and determine information that may be useful to the emergency department staff. Most of the time this information will not directly affect the care you give, but occasionally it will. In general, you will provide supportive treatment for these conditions.

Dizziness and syncope are separate problems that are sometimes related. It is not uncommon for someone to complain of dizziness before fainting. Because these two conditions are often caused by the same problems, we will consider them together in this chapter.

Dizziness is a common term that means different things to different people. It is important in your assessment to find out what the patient means by "dizziness." Is it weakness, a sensation of loss of strength? Is it a spinning sensation, where the surroundings are spinning around the patient (also known as *vertigo*)? Is it lightheadedness, the sensation that the patient is about to pass out (sometimes called *pre-syncope* or *near syncope*)? Is it something else?

Syncope is a brief loss of consciousness with spontaneous recovery. Typically, it is very short, from a few seconds to at most a few minutes. The patient usually regains consciousness very soon after being allowed to lie flat (Figure 19-6).

Patients will often have some warning that a syncopal episode or fainting spell is about to occur. This may include such symptoms as lightheadedness, dizziness, nausea, weakness, vision changes, sudden pallor (loss of normal skin color), or sweating. Occasionally incontinence of bladder or bowel occurs as part of the episode, but this is more common with seizures.

Patients may be able to describe specific signs or symptoms that indicate certain causes of the episode are more likely than others. This may include fluttering in the chest (palpitations), a sensation of a racing heart (tachycardia), a slow heart rate (bradycardia), or headache.

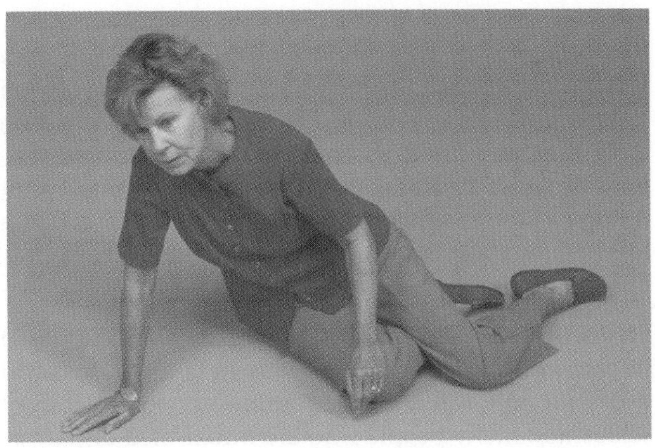

Figure 19-6 • Loss of consciousness with syncope is usually brief. The patient usually regains consciousness very soon after being allowed to lie flat.

Causes of Dizziness and Syncope

The factors that cause dizziness and syncope are generally related to something in or near the brain. Some event occurs that deprives the brain of the conditions it needs—most commonly adequate blood flow—to function properly. This may be very obvious, like a sudden severe slowing of the heart, or it may be more subtle, like slow gastrointestinal bleeding that finally reaches the point where the patient is unable to stand without losing consciousness.

There are many causes of dizziness and syncope, but some of the more common ones can be grouped into a few categories: hypovolemic, metabolic, environmental/toxicological, and cardiovascular.

HYPOVOLEMIC CAUSES Hypovolemia, or low fluid/blood volume, can cause dizziness or syncope when the patient attempts to sit up or stand. In this case, there is enough blood to perfuse the brain when the patient is lying down, but when the patient tries to get up, the body is unable to quickly divert enough blood from the legs to the brain. There are several common causes of hypovolemia, including dehydration. The most serious cause of hypovolemia is bleeding.

In a patient with dizziness or syncope, the source of the bleeding may not be obvious. A woman of childbearing age can have a ruptured ectopic pregnancy that results in significant blood loss. This is usually accompanied by lower abdominal pain. A slowly bleeding ("leaking") abdominal aortic aneurysm can also lead to life-threatening blood loss. Such an aneurysm often causes the patient to experience abdominal pain radiating to the back. Gastrointestinal bleeding is fairly common, especially among the older population, where patients often take medications that irritate the stomach or duodenum and also take medications that slow or prevent clotting (aspirin can do both), but this kind of bleed may or may not cause pain.

There are other ways to become hypovolemic besides bleeding. Dehydration results from losing more fluid than the patient takes in. This is very common in hot weather, when the patient sweats a great deal but does not drink enough liquid to keep up with this fluid loss (heat exhaustion). It can also happen when someone becomes ill with diarrhea. Because eating or drinking anything is followed by a painful, watery bowel movement, the patient is reluctant to drink any fluids at all and becomes dehydrated. Sometimes, with severe diarrhea, this happens despite the patient's efforts to drink liquids.

METABOLIC AND STRUCTURAL CAUSES When the cause of dizziness or syncope is metabolic, something is wrong with the brain or the structures near it. Because a properly functioning brain is necessary to maintain consciousness, alterations in the brain chemistry or structure can lead to a diminished level of consciousness. Similarly, because the inner and middle ear must be properly functioning for a person to maintain a sense of balance, a problem in this region can lead to dizziness. Inflammation of this area is a very common cause of dizziness. A patient who has been diagnosed with such a problem may be taking the drug meclizine.

Hypoglycemia deprives the brain of glucose, which it needs all the time to function properly. An interruption in this supply can lead to both dizziness and syncope. If the patient remains unconscious more than a few minutes, however, it is not considered syncope, or fainting. There is likely to be a more serious cause of the episode. Occasionally, a stroke will present with either dizziness or syncope. In this case, there may be other neurological signs and symptoms present, like one-sided weakness, drooping of one side of the face, or slurred speech. A seizure can cause a temporary loss of consciousness, too. You learned about managing a patient having a seizure earlier in this chapter.

ENVIRONMENTAL/TOXICOLOGICAL CAUSES Environmental and toxicological imbalances can lead to alterations in consciousness. Alcohol is the most commonly used drug and, when a patient drinks too much, it can lead to an altered level of consciousness. Many people who are intoxicated display a fluctuating level of consciousness that can appear to be syncope. Other drugs that are central nervous system depressants can cause similar effects. Syncope and near-syncope also commonly occur with carbon monoxide poisoning.

Panic attacks and anxiety attacks can lead a patient to become so anxious that the patient hyperventilates by breathing faster and deeper. When a patient breathes this hard, it can change the blood chemistry in a way that constricts the blood vessels supplying the brain with oxygen. Fortunately, when the patient loses consciousness, the hyperventilation ceases and things return at least partly to normal.

CARDIOVASCULAR CAUSES Cardiovascular causes of dizziness and syncope also deserve mention. A dysrhythmia that results in the heart beating extremely fast (a *tachycardia*) can lead to either dizziness or syncope. This is often the result of a problem with the electrical system in the heart. Ordinarily, increases in the heart rate result in increased blood being pumped out of the heart (greater cardiac output). But when the heart beats extremely fast, the ventricles do not have time to fill before they pump blood out again. So, even though the heart is beating much faster than normal, it is actually pumping out less blood than usual. A very slow heart rate (a *bradycardia*) may also lead to dizziness or syncope through reduced cardiac output, in this case because the heart is not beating fast enough to pump out sufficient blood. This may not be noticeable to the patient when he is lying flat. When the patient tries to sit or stand, though, dizziness and syncope can occur when blood goes to the legs and the brain does not get sufficient blood.

A cardiovascular cause of syncope that is not the result of a problem with the heart's electrical system is stimulation of the carotid sinus. This area is located in the carotid artery under the mandible. When stimulated, it sends signals to the heart to slow down. Some people have a very sensitive carotid sinus. All that may be needed to stimulate it in some sensitive individuals is turning the head while wearing a shirt with a tight collar.

One of the most common types of syncope is *vasovagal syncope* or simple fainting. This is thought to be the result of stimulation of the vagus nerve, which in turn signals the heart to slow down. When someone is suddenly frightened or put under significant emotional stress, this nerve can be stimulated, leading to reduced cardiac output, which in the upright individual can quickly result in syncope. When the patient reaches a horizontal position, the brain regains perfusion and the patient regains consciousness.

OTHER CAUSES The causes previously discussed are just a few of the causes of dizziness and syncope. There are many others. In some cases, you will gather information that suggests one of them is the culprit. In many cases, you will not. Determining the cause can be extremely difficult. In half of the cases of dizziness or syncope, no cause is ever found despite thorough evaluation by emergency physicians and other specialists.

PATIENT ASSESSMENT

DIZZINESS AND SYNCOPE

Dizziness or syncope is usually easily recognized by the patient's complaint of a brief loss of consciousness. The focused history and physical exam for a patient with dizziness or syncope includes an appropriate history and vital signs. Questions to ask include:

- *What do you mean by "dizziness"? weakness? a spinning sensation? lightheadedness?*
- *Did you have any warning? If so, what was it like?*
- *When did it start?*
- *How long did it last?*
- *What position were you in when the episode occurred?*
- *Have you had any similar episodes in the past? If so, what cause was found?*
- *Are you on medication for this kind of problem?*
- *Did you have any other signs or symptoms? nausea? vomiting (is there blood or material resembling coffee grounds)? black tarry stools (digested blood)?*
- *Did you witness any unpleasant sight or experience a strong emotion?*
- *Did you hurt yourself?*
- *Did anyone witness involuntary movements of the extremities (like seizures)?* ■

PATIENT CARE

DIZZINESS AND SYNCOPE

When a patient has experienced dizziness or syncope, provide the following care after attending to any threats to life:

1. Administer high-concentration oxygen.
2. Loosen any tight clothing around the neck.
3. Get the patient flat and elevate the legs if there is no reason not to do so.
4. Call ALS if it is available in your area.
5. Treat any associated injuries the patient may have incurred from the fall.
6. Transport in the position of comfort. ■

CHAPTER REVIEW

SUMMARY

Diabetic emergencies are usually caused by poor management of the patient's diabetes. Often this involves a condition brought about by hypoglycemia, or low blood sugar. The chief sign of this condition is altered mental status. Whenever a patient has an altered mental status and a history of diabetes and can swallow, administer oral glucose.

Seizures may have a number of causes. Assess and treat for possible spinal injury, protect the patient's airway, and provide oxygen as needed. Gather information about the seizure to give to hospital personnel.

A stroke is caused when an artery in the brain is blocked or ruptures. Signs and symptoms commonly include an altered mental status, numbness or paralysis on one side, and difficulty with speech, among others. Ensure an open airway and provide supplemental oxygen. Determine the exact time of onset of symptoms and transport promptly.

Dizziness and syncope (fainting) may have a variety of causes. Administer oxygen, loosen clothing around the neck, and place the patient flat with raised legs if there is no reason not to. Treat any injuries and transport.

KEY TERMS

diabetes mellitus (di-ah-BEE-tez MEL-i-tus) also called "sugar diabetes" or just "diabetes," the condition brought about by decreased insulin production or the inability of the body cells to use insulin properly. The person with this condition is a diabetic.

epilepsy (EP-uh-lep-see) a medical condition that causes seizures. With proper medication, many epileptic patients will no longer have seizures.

glucose (GLU-kos) a form of sugar, the body's basic source of energy.

hyperglycemia (HI-per-gli-SEE-me-ah) high blood sugar.

hypoglycemia (HI-po-gli-SEE-me-ah) low blood sugar.

insulin (IN-suh-lin) a hormone produced by the pancreas or taken as a medication by many diabetics.

seizure (SEE-zher) a sudden change in sensation, behavior, or movement. The most severe form of seizure produces violent muscle contractions called convulsions.

status epilepticus (STAY-tus or STAT-us ep-i-LEP-ti-kus) a prolonged seizure or when a person suffers two or more convulsive seizures without regaining full consciousness.

stroke a condition of altered function caused when an artery in the brain is blocked or ruptured, disrupting the supply of oxygenated blood or causing bleeding into the brain.

syncope (SIN-ko-pee) fainting.

REVIEW QUESTIONS

1. List the chief signs and symptoms of a diabetic emergency. (p. 450)
2. Explain how you can determine a medical history of diabetes. (p. 450)
3. Explain what treatment may be given by an EMT for a diabetic emergency and the criteria for giving it. (p. 455)
4. Tell whether treatment for a diabetic emergency should be given before or after baseline vital signs are taken. (Answer according to your local protocol.) (p. 450)
5. Explain the care that should be given to a patient who has had a seizure. (pp. 459–460)
6. Explain the care that should be given to a conscious and to an unconscious patient with suspected stroke. (pp. 465–466)
7. Explain the care that should be given to a patient who has experienced dizziness or syncope. (p. 469)

CRITICAL THINKING

- You are dispatched to a "man behaving oddly" at a train station. When you arrive, you find that the man is unconscious. "He's drunk," a bystander tells you. "He was staggering and slurring his words." As you assess the patient, you find a medical identification bracelet that tells you he is a diabetic. Do you administer oral glucose? How do you proceed?

Thinking and Linking

Think back to Chapter 9, "Vital Signs and SAMPLE History," and link information from that chapter with information from this chapter as you consider the following question:

- What parts of the patient's SAMPLE history will provide clues to the cause of a patient's altered mental status?

Think back to Chapter 3, "Medical/Legal and Ethical Issues," as well as to Chapter 14, "Documentation," as you consider the following situation:

- You have given a diabetic patient glucose. The patient is now oriented and does not want to be transported to the hospital. After you have made diligent efforts to persuade the patient to go, the patient still refuses transportation. What do you tell the patient? What do you document in relation to the refusal and your interaction with the patient?

MEDIA RESOURCES

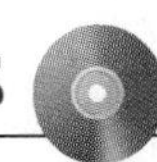

See the Student CD at the back of this book for quizzes, a case study activity, and other features related to this chapter. In particular, take a look at the animation on diabetes (hypoglycemia). Also, visit the Companion Website for *Emergency Care* at **www.prenhall.com/limmer**, where you will find additional reinforcement and links to other resources.

Street Scenes

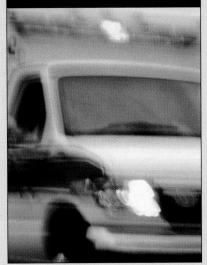

While on your day off, you receive a telephone call about working a shift at the county fair. It sounds like fun, so you agree. That Friday night, you and your partner are on stand-by with an ambulance at the first-aid tent. It is 10 p.m. and the evening has been quiet. Just when you think that it will also be uneventful, you receive a call on the radio that security has an intoxicated person they want you to examine on the midway. Upon arrival, you find a male patient in his 20s, sitting and talking in slurred speech to a deputy sheriff. A security guard tells you that the patient was wandering down the midway and talking incoherently. "I'm sure he's drunk," he tells you, "but the rules say you have to take a look before we transport to the security office."

Street Scene Questions

1. Does this patient need a thorough assessment?
2. What is the first concern when starting to assess this patient?
3. What types of underlying medical problems might make a patient appear to be drunk?

As your partner approaches the patient, he is met with what appears to be an angry patient, who says, "That's all I need—another cop." The patient then pushes the deputy sheriff away, and he turns to you. "This guy is just another drunk," your partner says, "and we are out of here." You almost buy into your partner's hasty evaluation, but you notice a bracelet on the patient's wrist. You approach, introduce yourself, and ask the patient if you can check him out. He reluctantly agrees, and as you take a pulse, which is rapid, you see that his bracelet indicates he has diabetes.

Street Scene Questions

4. Does your assessment plan change at this point?
5. How will you get a SAMPLE history if the patient is alone?
6. What is the priority level of this patient? Is there a need to call for ALS assistance?

After initial and focused assessments, you find the patient's airway is open with no mucus or other secretions noted, his breathing is at 24 breaths per minute, and his pulse rate is 110.

Just as you finish taking vital signs, a person approaches who says he is a friend of the patient. He confirms that your patient is a diabetic and that he took his insulin before they left for the fair. "He expected to eat here," the friend tells you, "but he was trying to win at the midway games and must have forgotten." You and your partner agree that he could tolerate oral glucose. You explain to your patient what you are doing and apply some to the inside of his cheek. In a few minutes he starts to become more alert, and soon he says he feels fine.

The ALS unit is now on the scene and has checked his sugar level. It is in a normal range. The patient does not want to be transported and, after you talk to medical direction, he is allowed to leave with his friend who promises to take him directly to a diner for something starchy to eat.

You call back in service and, as you walk to the ambulance, you remind your partner that you can never assume anything. Every patient needs an assessment.

Street Scenes Sample Documentation

PATIENT NAME: *John Poitier* **PATIENT AGE:** *26*

CHIEF COMPLAINT

Altered mental status

PAST MEDICAL HISTORY

- ☐ None
- ☐ Allergy to ____
- ☐ Hypertension
- ☐ Stroke
- ☐ Seizures
- ☒ Diabetes
- ☐ COPD
- ☐ Cardiac
- ☐ Other (List)
- ☐ Asthma

Current Medications (List): *Insulin*

VITAL SIGNS

TIME	RESP	PULSE	B.P.	MENTAL STATUS	R PUPILS L	SKIN
2005	Rate: *24* ☒ Regular ☐ Shallow ☐ Labored	Rate: *110* ☒ Regular ☐ Irregular	*130/80*	☐ Alert ☑ Voice ☐ Pain ☐ Unresp.	☑ Normal ☑ ☐ Dilated ☐ ☐ Constricted ☐ ☐ Sluggish ☐ ☐ No-Reaction ☐	☐ Unremarkable ☐ Cool ☐ Pale ☐ Warm ☐ Cyanotic ☑ Moist ☐ Flushed ☐ Dry ☐ Jaundiced
2012	Rate: *28* ☒ Regular ☐ Shallow ☐ Labored	Rate: *120* ☒ Regular ☐ Irregular	*120/78*	☐ Alert ☑ Voice ☐ Pain ☐ Unresp.	☑ Normal ☑ ☐ Dilated ☐ ☐ Constricted ☐ ☐ Sluggish ☐ ☐ No-Reaction ☐	☐ Unremarkable ☐ Cool ☐ Pale ☑ Warm ☐ Cyanotic ☑ Moist ☐ Flushed ☐ Dry ☐ Jaundiced
2020	Rate: *24* ☒ Regular ☐ Shallow ☐ Labored	Rate: *100* ☒ Regular ☐ Irregular	*126/84*	☑ Alert ☐ Voice ☐ Pain ☐ Unresp.	☑ Normal ☑ ☐ Dilated ☐ ☐ Constricted ☐ ☐ Sluggish ☐ ☐ No-Reaction ☐	☐ Unremarkable ☐ Cool ☐ Pale ☑ Warm ☐ Cyanotic ☐ Moist ☐ Flushed ☑ Dry ☐ Jaundiced

NARRATIVE *EMS called to the scene of what appears to be an intoxicated male patient. According to a deputy sheriff and a security guard, patient was found wandering down the midway of a fair, talking incoherently. Patient initially presents as agitated and mildly combative but eventually consents to medical evaluation. Patient is noted to be a diabetic via his medical identification bracelet. This is confirmed by a companion on scene. The patient took insulin but did not eat. The patient is verbally responsive, able to follow instructions, and able to protect his airway. We administered one tube of oral glucose on standing order. A tongue blade with the glucose was placed into patient's mouth along cheek. After administration of glucose, patient became fully alert. He refused transportation to hospital. We contacted Dr. Stiglmeier at medical direction, who agreed with the refusal as long as patient agreed to eat a starchy meal and stay with a friend. Patient was advised of the potential dangers in refusal of care and signed a release witnessed by the deputy sheriff. Patient and his companion were advised of signs of diabetic problems and advised to call again if he had problems.*

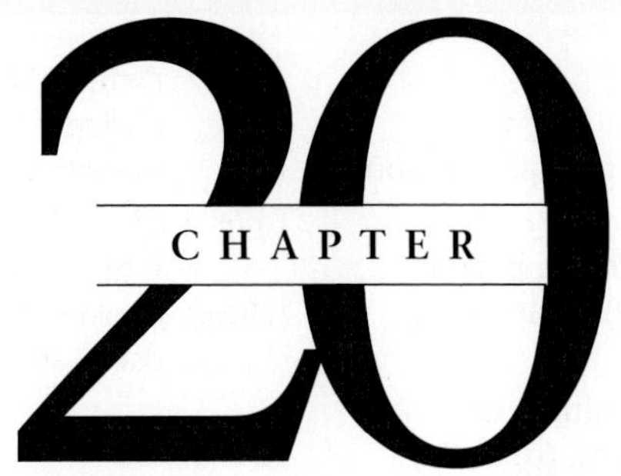

Allergic Reactions

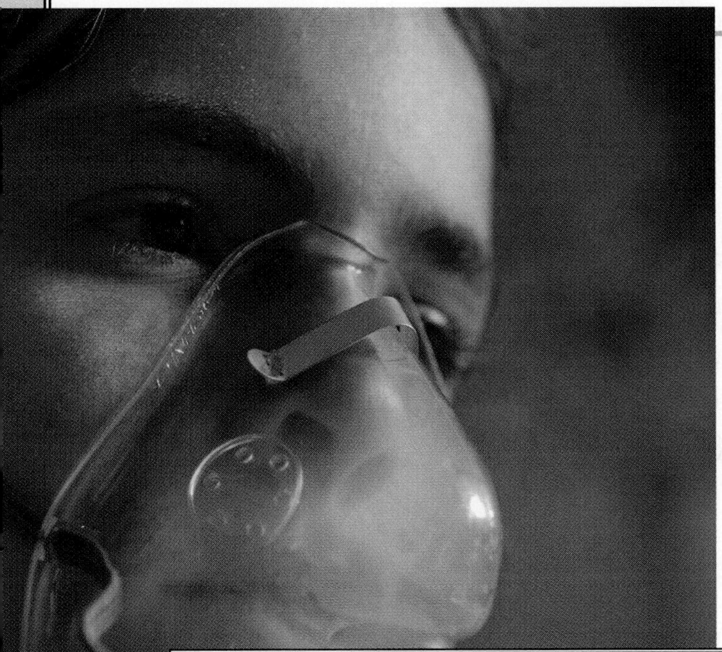

CORE CONCEPTS

The following are core concepts that will be addressed in this chapter:

- How to identify a patient experiencing an allergic reaction
- Differences between a mild allergic reaction and anaphylaxis
- How to treat a patient experiencing an allergic reaction
- Who should be assisted with an epinephrine auto-injector
- How to document findings and care of patients with allergic reactions

KEY TERMS

allergen, p. 474
allergic reaction, p. 474
anaphylaxis, p. 474
auto-injector, p. 478
epinephrine, p. 482
hives, p. 477

DOT OBJECTIVES

*KNOWLEDGE AND ATTITUDE

4-5.1 Recognize the patient experiencing an allergic reaction. (p. 477)

4-5.2 Describe the emergency medical care of the patient with an allergic reaction. (pp. 478–479) (Scan 20-1, pp. 480–482)

4-5.3 Establish the relationship between the patient with an allergic reaction and airway management. (pp. 474, 477, 478, 482, 483, 484)

4-5.4 Describe the mechanisms of allergic response and the implications for airway management. (pp. 474, 477, 478, 482, 483, 484)

4-5.5 State the generic and trade names, medication forms, dose, administration, action, and contraindications for the epinephrine auto-injector. (pp. 482–485) (Scan 20-2, p. 483)

4-5.6 Evaluate the need for medical direction in the emergency medical care of the patient with an allergic reaction. (pp. 477, 478, 479, 480, 481, 482, 483, 484)

4-5.7 Differentiate between the general category of those patients having an allergic reaction and those patients having an allergic reaction and requiring immediate medical care, including immediate use of epinephrine auto-injector. (pp. 474, 478–479)

4-5.8 Explain the rationale for administering epinephrine using an auto-injector. (pp. 482–485)

*SKILLS

4-5.9 Demonstrate the emergency medical care of the patient experiencing an allergic reaction.

4-5.10 Demonstrate the use of epinephrine auto-injector.

4-5.11 Demonstrate the assessment and documentation of patient response to an epinephrine injection.

4-5.12 Demonstrate proper disposal of equipment.

4-5.13 Demonstrate completing a prehospital care report for patients with allergic emergencies.

Allergic reactions can be mild or extremely severe. A mild allergic reaction can develop into a severe reaction rapidly. A severe allergic reaction can quickly become life threatening. For these reasons, prompt recognition and appropriate assessment and treatment of allergic reactions can be critical.

ALLERGIC REACTIONS

allergic reaction an exaggerated immune response.

allergen something that causes an allergic reaction.

anaphylaxis (an-ah-fi-LAK-sis) a severe or life-threatening allergic reaction in which the blood vessels dilate, causing a drop in blood pressure, and the tissues lining the respiratory system swell, interfering with the airway. Also called *anaphylactic shock.*

A natural response of the human body's immune system is to react to any foreign substance—to defend the body by neutralizing or getting rid of the foreign material. Sometimes the immune response is exaggerated; this exaggerated reaction is called an **allergic reaction.** Almost any of a wide variety of substances can be an **allergen,** something that causes an allergic reaction. For example, cat dander can be an allergen. A person who is allergic to cat dander will itch and sneeze whenever a cat is nearby. The reaction is unpleasant but harmless.

In some people, however, contact with certain foreign substances triggers an immune response that gets out of hand. Consider bee stings. Most people have no reaction to a bee sting other than pain and some swelling at the sting site. However, a few people have very severe, life-threatening reactions to bee stings. This kind of severe allergic reaction is called **anaphylaxis,** or *anaphylactic shock.* In anaphylaxis, exposure to the allergen will cause blood vessels to dilate rapidly and cause a drop in blood pressure (hypotension). Many tissues may swell, including those that line the respiratory system. This swelling can obstruct the airway, leading to respiratory failure.

Something that all allergic reactions share is that people do not have them the first time they are exposed to an allergen. This is because the body's immune system has not "learned" to recognize the allergen yet. The first time someone is exposed to an allergen, the immune system forms antibodies in response. These antibodies are an attempt by the body to "attack" the foreign substances. A particular antibody will combine with only the allergen it was formed in response to (or another allergen very similar to the original one). The second time the person is exposed to the allergen, the antibodies already exist in the person's body. This time, the antibody combines with the allergen, leading to the release of certain chemicals into the bloodstream. These chemicals cause dilation of the blood vessels, swelling, and difficulty breathing.

Causes of allergic reactions (in some individuals) include (Figure 20-1):

- *Insects.* The stings of bees, yellow jackets, wasps, and hornets can cause rapid and severe reactions.
- *Foods.* Foods such as nuts, eggs, milk, and shellfish can cause reactions. In most cases, the effect is slower than that seen with insect stings. An exception is peanuts. Peanut allergies are frequently very severe and very rapid in onset. Many people with allergies to one food will have allergies to related foods (for example, someone who is allergic to almonds is more likely to be allergic to walnuts). Again, peanuts are an exception. People who are allergic to peanuts do not necessarily have any other allergies, including nuts (in part because peanuts are legumes, not nuts).
- *Plants.* Contact with certain plants such as poison ivy, poison sumac, and poison oak can cause a rash that is sometimes severe (Figure 20-2). The rash associated with poison ivy is actually an allergic reaction. Approximately two-thirds of the population is allergic to the oil on poison ivy leaves. Plant pollen also causes allergic reactions in many people, but rarely anaphylaxis.
- *Medications.* Antitoxins and drugs, especially antibiotics such as penicillin, may cause severe reactions. Just as with foods, people who are allergic to one kind of antibiotic can be allergic to related antibiotics. In the course of evaluating patients, you will hear many of them say they are allergic to penicillin or other antibiotics.

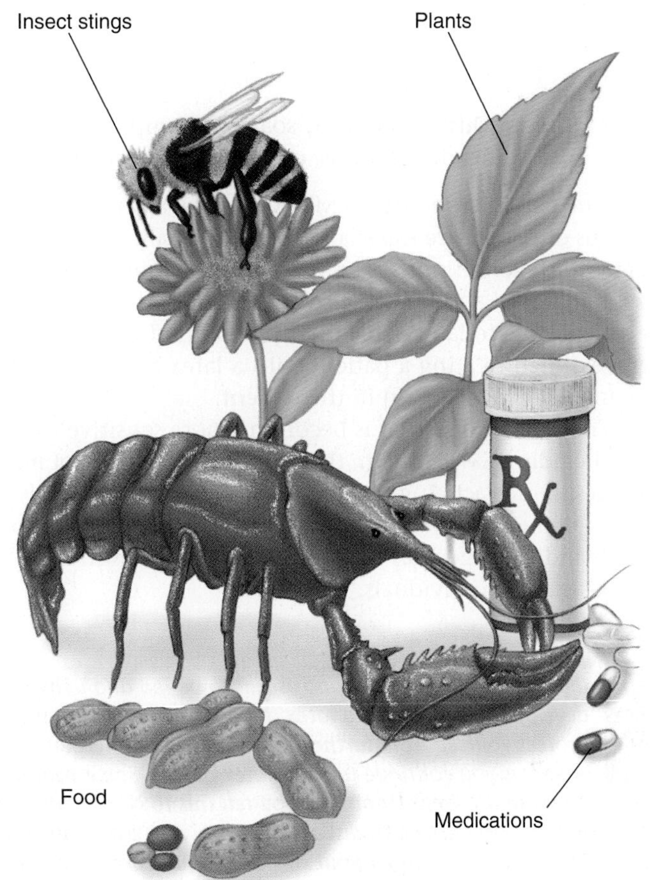

Figure 20-1 • Substances that may cause allergic reactions.

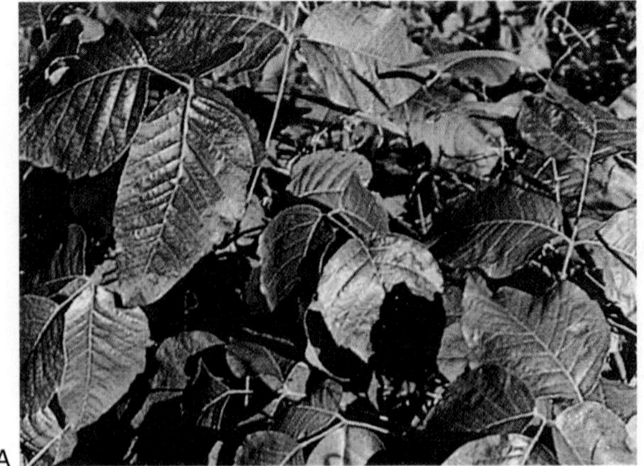

A

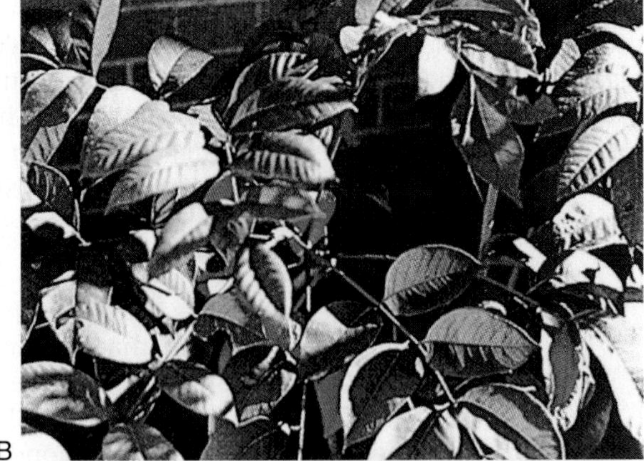

B

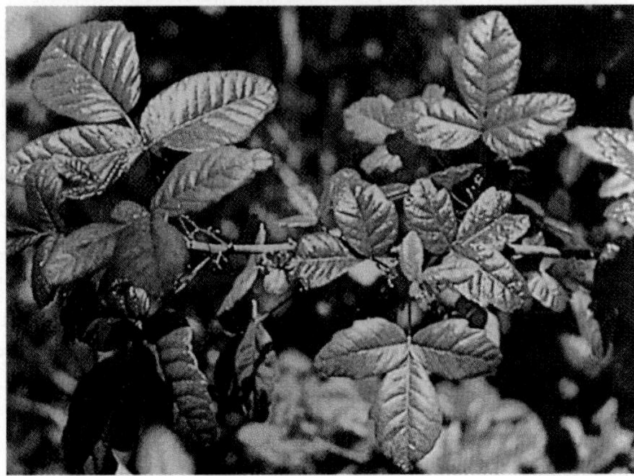

C

Figure 20-2 • (A) Poison ivy, (B) poison sumac, and (C) poison oak.

- *Others*. Dust, chemicals, soaps, makeup, and a variety of other substances can cause allergic reactions, occasionally severe, in some people.

One particular product EMTs should be aware of as a possible allergen is latex. Two groups of people are especially likely to be allergic to latex. One of these groups is patients with conditions that require multiple surgeries. The repeated exposure to the latex in doctors' and nurses' gloves is probably the reason many such patients develop a severe allergy to latex. This is very important to understand, because if you wear latex gloves when treating a patient with a latex allergy, you may actually cause an allergic or anaphylactic reaction in the patient.

The other group that is becoming more sensitive to latex is health care professionals, including EMTs. Again, this is probably because of more frequent exposure to latex as a result of practicing Standard Precautions. Fortunately, it is now possible to find virtually all medical equipment and supplies in forms that do not contain latex. Many hospitals and EMS agencies maintain latex-free environments to avoid causing reactions in latex-sensitive individuals.

NOTE

If you notice that your hands seem to be red and itchy after a call, you may be developing an allergy to latex. If you are allergic to latex, it is very important that you protect yourself from further exposure to this allergen. If you do not, the signs will get worse as you continue to wear latex gloves. Some people become extremely sensitive to latex, so it is important that you tell this to any health care provider who is caring for you as a patient. Also discuss this with your own physician so that you become as informed as possible about this topic and learn how to protect yourself.

There is no way to predict the exact course of an allergic reaction. Severe reactions most often take place immediately, but they are occasionally delayed 30 minutes or more. A mild allergic reaction may turn into more serious anaphylactic shock in a matter of minutes. When you have a patient with an exposure to a known allergen but who is displaying only minor signs and symptoms, you must closely monitor the patient for signs of the condition becoming more serious. This patient's airway may swell and close off in just a few minutes. Be prepared to manage the airway and to administer epinephrine if so advised by medical direction.

The signs and symptoms of allergic reaction or anaphylactic shock can include:

Skin:

- Itching
- **Hives** (red, itchy, possibly raised blotches on the skin—Figure 20-3), especially around an insect sting
- Flushing (red skin)
- Swelling of face (especially the eyes and lips), neck, hands, feet, or tongue
- Warm, tingling feeling in the face, mouth, chest, feet, and hands

hives
red, itchy, possibly raised blotches on the skin that often result from allergic reactions.

Respiratory:

- Patient may report a feeling of tightness in the throat or chest
- Cough
- Rapid breathing
- Labored, noisy breathing
- Hoarseness, muffled voice, or loss of voice entirely
- Stridor (harsh, high-pitched sound during inspiration)
- Wheezing (audible without a stethoscope)

Cardiac:

- Increased heart rate
- Decreased blood pressure

Generalized findings:

- Itchy, watery eyes
- Headache
- Runny nose
- Patient expresses a sense of impending doom

Signs and symptoms of shock:

- Altered mental status
- Flushed, dry skin or pale, cool, clammy skin
- Nausea or vomiting
- Changes in vital signs: increased pulse, increased respirations, decreased blood pressure

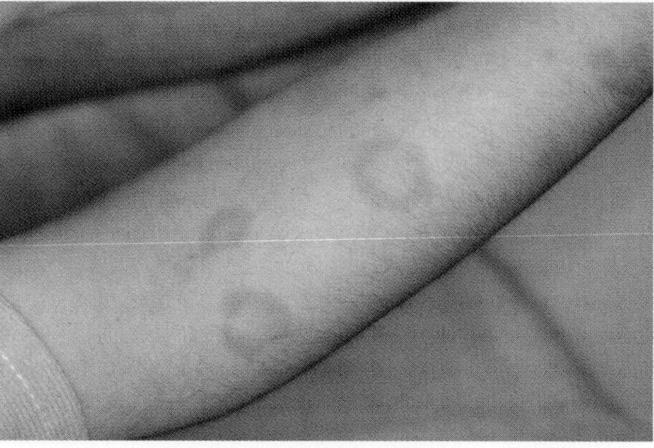

Figure 20-3 • Hives are red, itchy blotches, sometimes raised, that often accompany an allergic reaction. *(© Charles Stewart, MD and Associates)*

NOTE *When the signs and symptoms of allergic reaction include either respiratory distress or signs and symptoms of shock (hypoperfusion), assume that it is a severe allergic reaction (anaphylaxis).*

Distinguishing Anaphylaxis from Mild Allergic Reaction

Any of the signs and symptoms discussed previously can be associated with an allergic reaction. To be considered a severe allergic reaction, or anaphylaxis, the patient must have either respiratory distress or signs and symptoms of shock.

PATIENT ASSESSMENT

ALLERGIC REACTION OR ANAPHYLAXIS

Conduct the usual assessment sequence, as follows:

1. Perform the initial assessment and care for any immediately life-threatening problems with the airway, breathing, or circulation.
2. Perform a focused history and physical exam. Inquire about:
    - History of allergies
    - What patient was exposed to
    - How patient was exposed (contact, ingestion, etc.)
    - What signs and symptoms the patient is having
    - Progression (What happened first, next? How rapidly?)
    - Interventions (Has any care been provided? Has the patient taken any medication?)
3. Assess baseline vital signs and get the remainder of the SAMPLE history.

Suspect an allergic reaction whenever the patient has come in contact with a substance that has caused an allergic reaction in the past, and whenever the patient complains of itching, hives, or difficulty breathing (respiratory distress), or shows signs or symptoms of shock (hypoperfusion). ■

PATIENT CARE

ALLERGIC REACTION OR ANAPHYLAXIS

1. Manage the patient's airway and breathing. Apply high-concentration oxygen through a nonrebreather mask, if you have not already done so during the initial assessment. If the patient has or develops an altered mental status, open and maintain the patient's airway. If the patient is not breathing adequately, provide artificial ventilations.
2. You may be able to assist the patient in administering an epinephrine **auto-injector.** To find out if it is appropriate, consider each of the following:
    - IF the patient has come in contact with a substance that caused an allergic reaction in the past, AND IF the patient has respiratory distress or exhibits signs and symptoms of shock, AND IF the patient has a prescribed epinephrine auto-injector, OR IF your protocols allow you to carry and use epinephrine auto-injectors, then contact medical direction and, if so ordered, assist the patient with his prescribed auto-injector or administer epinephrine from an auto-injector you carry on the ambulance (Scan 20-1). Record the administration of the epinephrine auto-injector. Transport. Reassess 2 minutes after epinephrine administration and record reassessment findings.
    - IF the patient has come in contact with a substance that caused an allergic reaction in the past, AND IF the patient complains of respiratory distress or exhibits signs and symptoms of shock, AND IF the patient *does not* have a pre-

auto-injector a syringe preloaded with medication that has a spring-loaded device which pushes the needle through the skin when the tip of the device is pressed firmly against the body.

continued

PATIENT CARE *(continued)*

scribed epinephrine auto-injector available or has never had one prescribed, and your protocols *do not* allow you to carry and use epinephrine auto-injectors, then care for shock and transport immediately.

- IF assessment findings show that the patient has come in contact with a substance that caused an allergic reaction in the past, BUT the patient is NOT wheezing or showing signs of respiratory distress or shock (hypoperfusion), then continue with the focused assessment. Consult medical direction; if the patient has an epinephrine auto-injector and if medical direction so orders, administer epinephrine.

If the patient meets these criteria but does not have an epinephrine auto-injector and your protocols do not allow you to carry and use one, consider requesting an ALS intercept. Paramedics carry and can administer epinephrine. ■

You probably will not see many patients with allergic reactions, but most of those you see will be able to give you a history of allergies. Once in a while, you will see a patient who has no history and is having his first allergic reaction. In this case, the patient will not be carrying an epinephrine auto-injector because his physician has not prescribed one. Treat the patient for shock and transport immediately. Consider requesting ALS intercept.

CRITICAL DECISION MAKING: Is Your Patient Overreacting?

Anaphylactic reactions are truly life threatening. Fortunately, many patients carry their own epinephrine auto-injectors. Many ambulances also carry these life-saving devices. Yet not all patients who have allergic reactions have anaphylaxis. The purpose of this exercise will be to determine the difference between an allergic reaction and anaphylaxis and to determine whether epinephrine should be administered.

1. Your 24-year-old patient ate a metal that he believes contained shellfish. He is allergic to shrimp. While the kitchen staff rushes to determine if shrimp was used in or near the preparation of the patient's meal, you perform an examination. The patient is sweating and nervous. He appears to be breathing adequately. You do not note any wheezing or stridor. His face is slightly red. His pulse is 88 strong and regular, respirations 24, blood pressure 108/74, and skin warm and moist.
2. You are called to a 50-year-old woman who received a narcotic pain reliever after minor dental surgery. She believes she is allergic to some pain medication but can't remember which one. She has vomited twice. One time she believes she saw blood in her vomit. Her vital signs are pulse 92 strong and regular, respirations 22 and adequate without wheezes or stridor, blood pressure 148/86, skin warm and dry, pupils equal and reactive to light.
3. Your patient is a parent who came into his daughter's kindergarten class as a helper. After eating a cookie, he developed a funny feeling in his tongue that progressed to swelling. He is anxious and sweaty when you see him. His pulse is 126 and regular, respirations 32 and slightly labored, blood pressure 96/58, skin cool and moist, pupils equal and reactive to light.

SCAN 20-1 • Assessing and Managing an Allergic Reaction

First take Standard Precautions.

Patient suffers severe allergic reaction.

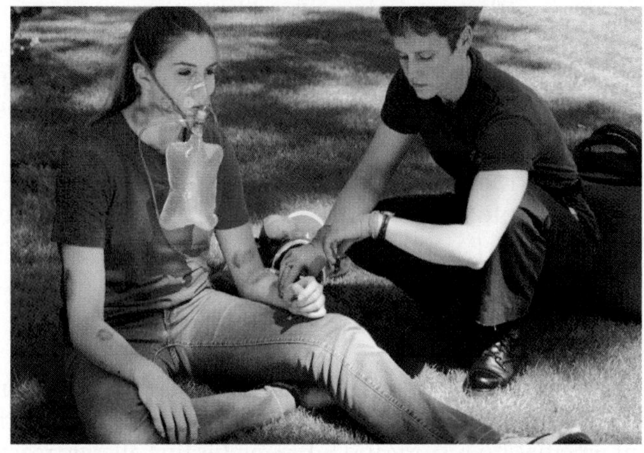

1. Perform an initial assessment. Provide high-concentration oxygen by nonrebreather mask.

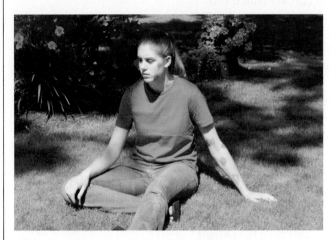

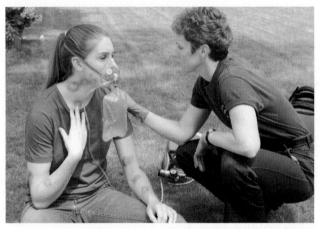

2. Perform a focused history and physical exam. Obtain a SAMPLE history.

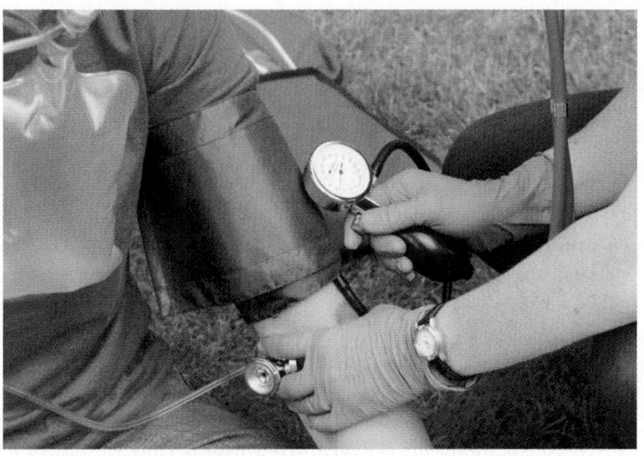

3. Take the patient's vital signs.

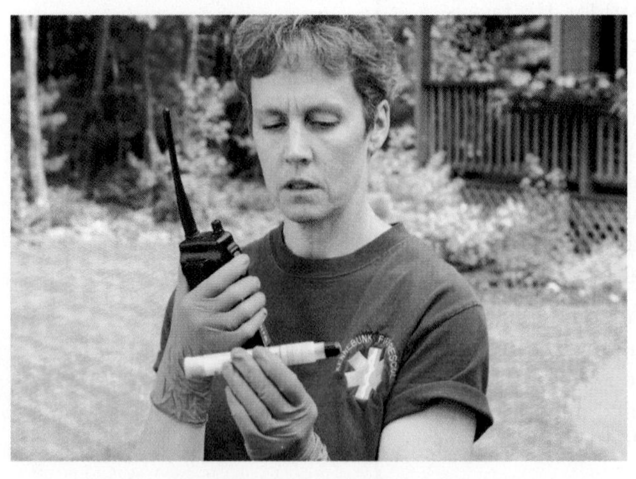

4. Find out if the patient has a prescribed epinephrine auto-injector and if it is prescribed for this patient or ensure that your protocols allow administering an epinephrine auto-injector you carry on the ambulance. Then check the expiration date and check for cloudiness or discoloration if liquid is visible. Contact medical direction.

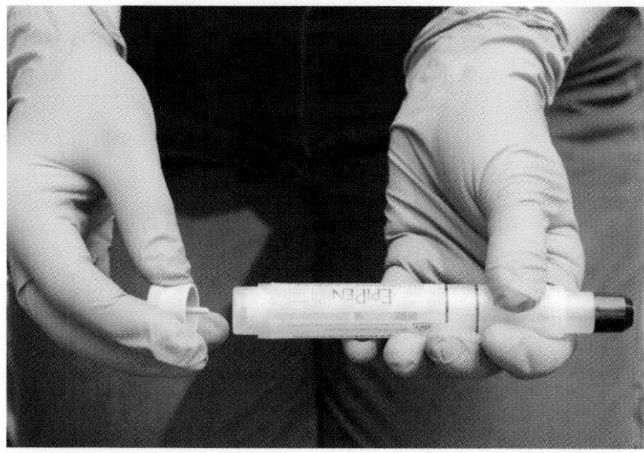

5. If medical direction orders use of the epinephrine auto-injector, prepare it for use by removing the safety cap. (Photo shows the EpiPen®.)

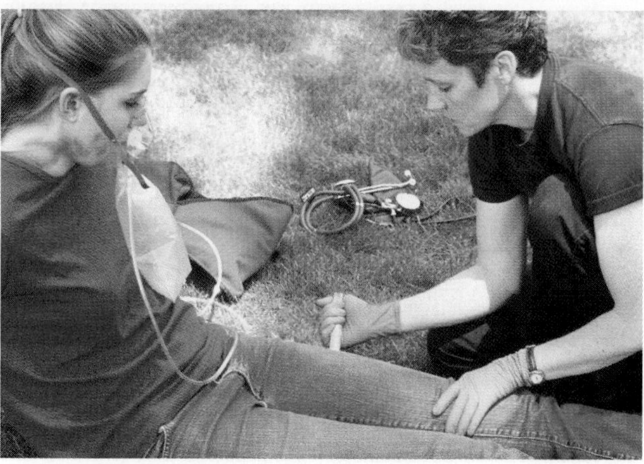

6. Press the injector against the patient's thigh to trigger release of the spring-loaded needle and inject the dose of epinephrine into the patient.

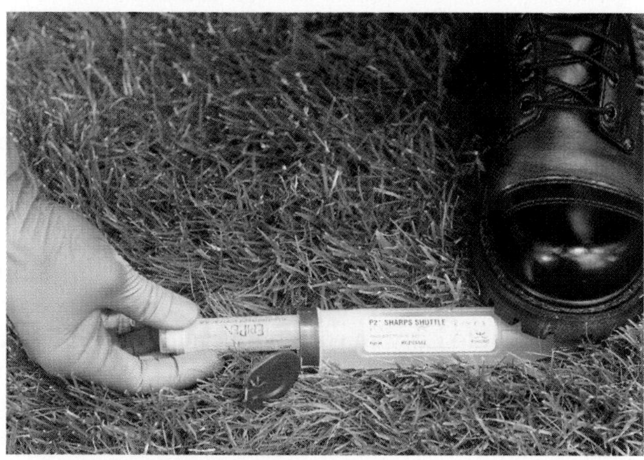

7. Dispose of the used single-dose injector in a portable biohazard container.

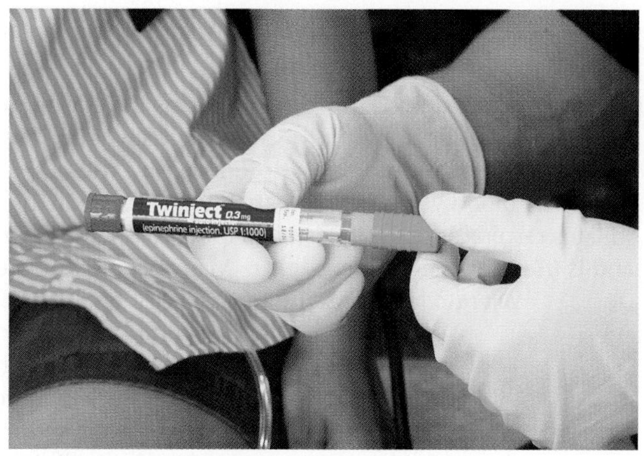

8. If using the Twinject®, follow the manufacturer's directions to remove color-coded caps and administer the first dose. Save the device and transport it with the patient in case the second dose it contains is later needed. (If needed, again follow the manufacturer's directions to remove the color-coded cap and tab to administer the second dose.)

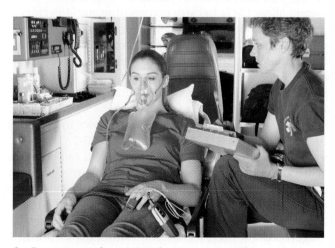

9. Document the patient's response to the medication.

continued

SCAN 20-1 • (Continued)

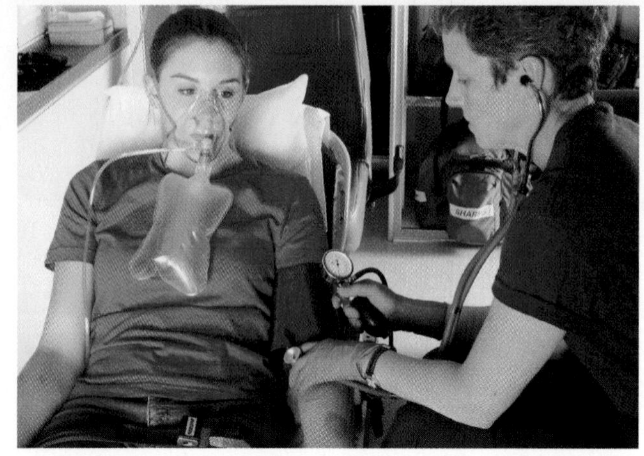

10. Perform an ongoing assessment, paying special attention to the patient's ABCs and vital signs en route to the hospital.

SELF-ADMINISTERED EPINEPHRINE

epinephrine (EP-uh-NEF-rin) a hormone produced by the body. As a medication, it constricts blood vessels and dilates respiratory passages and is used to relieve severe allergic reactions.

Physicians have long prescribed **epinephrine** in bee sting kits, AnaKits, or EpiPens® for patients who are susceptible to severe allergic reactions. Epinephrine is a hormone produced by the body. Administered as a medication, it will constrict blood vessels (helping to raise the blood pressure and improve perfusion) and dilate the bronchioles (helping to open the airway and improve respiration).

Many people who are subject to severe allergic reactions are prescribed an epinephrine auto-injector by their physician to carry with them and use when such a reaction occurs. The reason it is important for such a patient to carry an epinephrine auto-injector is that an allergic reaction can become life threatening so quickly that there is not enough time to transport the patient to a hospital to receive the medication. An auto-injector is a spring-loaded needle and syringe with a single dose of epinephrine that will automatically release and inject the medication.

When authorized by medical direction, you may administer or help the patient administer a dose of epinephrine from an auto-injector that has been prescribed for the patient by a physician. Some states allow EMTs to carry epinephrine auto-injectors on the ambulance to administer with approval from medical direction. After you make sure that the liquid is clear (if you can see it), remove the cap and press the injector firmly against the patient's thigh. Hold it there until the entire dose is injected. (Injection on the outside of the thigh midway between waist and knee is recommended.) On reassessment 2 minutes after the epinephrine is administered, in addition to some relief of symptoms, expect the patient's pulse to have increased.

The procedure for administering an epinephrine auto-injector is shown in Scan 20-1. Information about epinephrine auto-injectors is summarized in Scan 20-2.

Epinephrine is a very powerful medication. It not only saves lives, it can also occasionally take lives. One of the good things epinephrine does for patients is make the heart beat more strongly. This is beneficial when the patient is hypoperfusing (that is, when the patient is in shock), because one reason for the hypoperfusion is that the patient's blood vessels are dilated and blood is not returning to the heart as quickly. Unfortunately, once you give a drug, you cannot take it back. If the dose of epinephrine in the auto-injector is more than the patient needs, the patient's heart will be working harder than it needs to. This can be dangerous in a patient with a heart condition or who is hypertensive (has high blood pressure).

SCAN 20-2 • Epinephrine Auto-Injector

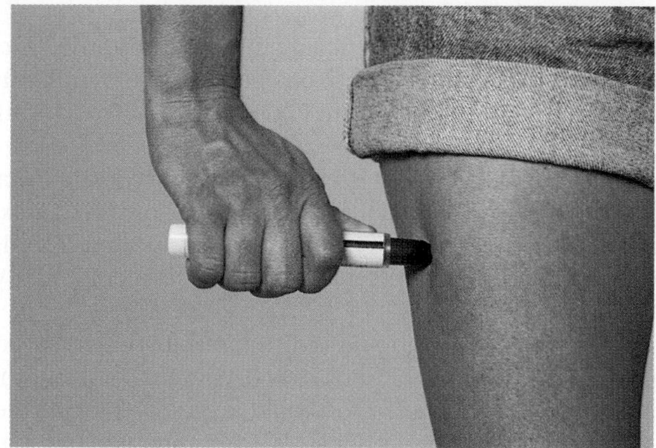

MEDICATION NAME

1. Generic: epinephrine
2. Trade: Adrenalin™
3. Delivery system: EpiPen® or EpiPen Jr.® or Twinject® (adult or child size)

INDICATIONS

Must meet the following three criteria:

1. Patient exhibits signs of a severe allergic reaction, including either respiratory distress or shock (hypoperfusion).
2. Medication is prescribed for this patient by a physician or is carried on the ambulance.
3. Medical direction authorizes use for this patient.

CONTRAINDICATIONS

No contraindications when used in a life-threatening situation.

MEDICATION FORM

Liquid administered by an auto-injector—an automatically injectable needle-and-syringe system.

DOSAGE

Adult: one adult auto-injector (0.3 mg)
Infant and child: one infant/child auto-injector (0.15 mg)

ADMINISTRATION

1. Obtain patient's prescribed auto-injector. Ensure:
   a. Prescription is written for the patient who is experiencing the severe allergic reaction or your protocols permit carrying the auto-injector on the ambulance.
   b. Medication is not discolored (if visible).
2. Obtain order from medical direction, either on-line or off-line.
3. Remove safety cap(s) from auto-injector.
4. Place tip of auto-injector against patient's thigh.
   a. Lateral portion of the thigh
   b. Midway between waist and knee
5. Push the injector firmly against the thigh until the injector activates.
6. Hold the injector in place until the medication is injected (at least 10 seconds).
7. Record activity and time.
8. Dispose of a single-dose injector, such as the EpiPen®, in a biohazard container; save a two-dose injector, such as the Twinject®, and transport it with the patient in case the second dose is later required.

ACTIONS

1. Dilates the bronchioles
2. Constricts blood vessels

SIDE EFFECTS

1. Increased heart rate
2. Pallor
3. Dizziness
4. Chest pain
5. Headache
6. Nausea
7. Vomiting
8. Excitability, anxiety

REASSESSMENT STRATEGIES

1. Transport.
2. Continue focused assessment of airway, breathing, and circulatory status.
   If patient's condition continues to worsen (decreasing mental status, increasing breathing difficulty, decreasing blood pressure):
   a. Obtain medical direction for an additional dose of epinephrine
   b. Treat for shock (hypoperfusion)
   c. Prepare to initiate basic life support procedures (CPR, AED)
   If patient's condition improves, provide supportive care:
   a. Continue oxygen
   b. Treat for shock (hypoperfusion)

This is one of the reasons why EMTs are taught to *give epinephrine only to patients who have been prescribed auto-injectors by their physicians*. They have been evaluated by physicians who have considered the patient's history and physical condition, were satisfied that a patient is a good candidate for epinephrine, and wrote a prescription.

Some patients receive instruction from their physicians in how to use the auto-injector, but others will be uncomfortable or afraid to use one because of unfamiliarity with the device and will prefer to have you help them with it. Ordinarily, when a health care provider gives an injection, the clothing over the injection site is rolled up or down and the area is cleansed with an alcohol pad. These steps are not necessary with an epinephrine auto-injector. The risk of giving a patient an infection because you did not take those steps is so small, in fact, that the manufacturer's instructions for auto-injectors do not advise patients to take those steps. Your protocols may direct you to act differently. Follow your local protocols.

One of the most difficult things you may have to do is distinguish between the patient with a (localized) allergic reaction, who should not receive epinephrine, and the patient with a (generalized) anaphylactic reaction, who should be given epinephrine. Patients can and do present in many different ways. One patient in anaphylaxis may have severe difficulty breathing with no hives or decreased blood pressure, while another patient may have a rapid heartbeat and decreased blood pressure with no difficulty breathing. The important thing to recognize in any patient is the presence of EITHER RESPIRATORY DISTRESS OR SIGNS AND SYMPTOMS OF SHOCK (HYPOPERFUSION). One of these needs to be present for the patient to be in anaphylaxis.

NOTE

A patient with an allergic reaction may have a compromised airway or respiratory function, or these conditions may develop as the allergic reaction progresses. Carefully monitor the patient's airway and breathing throughout care and transport.

In your ongoing assessment, you will frequently find that the patient's condition improves, but sometimes it will deteriorate. You may need to give additional doses of epinephrine in this case. You will be able to do this only if the patient has one or more extra auto-injectors AND you have remembered to ask the patient to bring them in the ambulance AND you obtain permission for the second dose from medical direction. Don't forget: If a patient has an extra epinephrine auto-injector, bring it along.

Most auto-injectors on the market today, such as the EpiPen® and EpiPen Jr®, can give only one dose of epinephrine (Figure 20-4a). Recently, an auto-injector became available that can provide two doses of epinephrine, the Twinject®, which also comes in adult and child sizes (Figure 20-4b). Because administering the second dose from the Twinject® requires you to disassemble part of the apparatus, you should become familiar with the auto-injector before you need to use it.

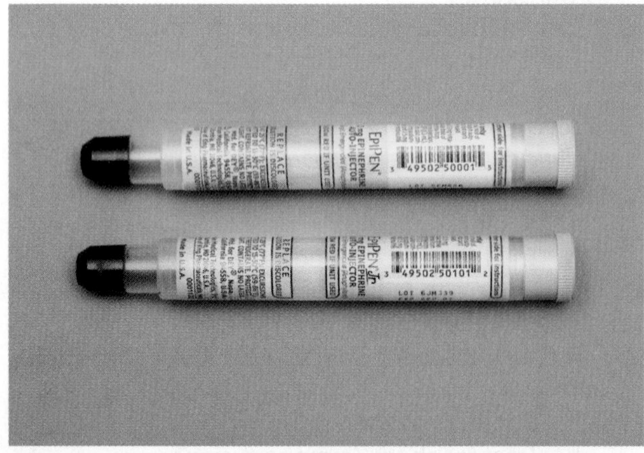

A

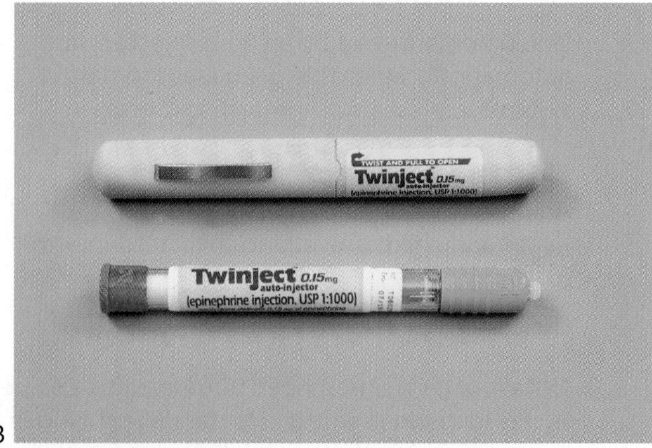

B

Figure 20-4 • Epinephrine auto-injectors: (A) EpiPen® and EpiPen Jr®; (B) the Twinject®, which also comes in child and adult sizes.

PEDIATRIC NOTE

Epinephrine auto-injectors come in two different sizes. The adult size contains an adult dose of 0.3 mg. The child size (for a child weighing less than 66 pounds) has 0.15 mg. Infants rarely experience anaphylactic reactions because their immune systems have not matured enough to develop the kinds of antibodies that cause anaphylactic reactions. Allergic reactions are common in older children, though. Fortunately, many children "grow out" of their allergies as they mature. Parents frequently will have a great deal of useful information about the child's medical history.

POINT OF VIEW

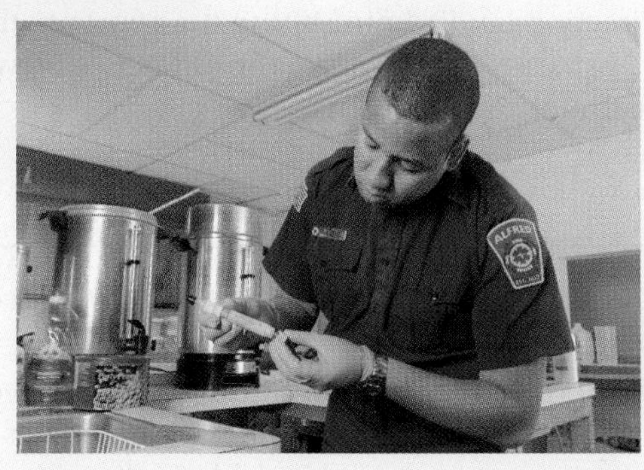

"I was at the lodge the other day. We were preparing for the holiday festival. Our biggest fundraiser of the year. It is held during tourist season. We have a dinner and bake sale. I've worked it for the past 20 years. Since I was a kid.

"Most people there know I have an allergy to nuts. It seems like all I have to do is look at them sometimes and I blow up and can't breathe. Someone brought some in, and the next thing I know it started. It seemed like seconds and I was wheezing and swelling up.

"My friends knew right away something was wrong. Mikey called 911 while Drew went out to my car to get my EpiPen®. The ambulance must have been right around the corner. They walked in with Drew. They took one look at me and I could see the concern in their eyes. I've seen it before.

"Fortunately they didn't waste time. They were putting me on oxygen and getting the stretcher while the EMT in charge got the EpiPen®. It saved my life before. It did today. They actually had to use my second EpiPen in the ambulance because it was such a bad reaction.

"The guys joked with me when I got out of the hospital. They were going to name the lodge after me if I died. They like to joke. But I'm not sure they know just how close it was."

CHAPTER REVIEW

SUMMARY

Allergic reactions are common. Anaphylaxis, a true life-threatening allergic reaction, is rare. The most common symptom in all of these cases is itching. Patients with anaphylaxis, though, will also display life-threatening difficulty breathing and/or signs and symptoms of shock (hypoperfusion). These patients will also be extremely anxious. Their bodies are in trouble and are letting the patients know it.

Fortunately, most of these patients know about their condition and manage to avoid exposure to the allergens they are sensitive to. Their physicians have often prescribed epinephrine auto-injectors for them for the times when they are exposed.

By quickly recognizing the condition, consulting medical direction, and administering the appropriate treatment, you can literally make the difference between life and death for these patients.

KEY TERMS

allergen something that causes an allergic reaction.

allergic reaction an exaggerated immune response.

anaphylaxis (an-ah-fi-LAK-sis) a severe or life-threatening allergic reaction in which the blood vessels dilate, causing a drop in blood pressure, and the tissues lining the respiratory system swell, interfering with the airway. Also called *anaphylactic shock.*

auto-injector a syringe preloaded with medication that has a spring-loaded device which pushes the needle through the skin when the tip of the device is pressed firmly against the body.

epinephrine (EP-uh-NEF-rin) a hormone produced by the body. As a medication, it constricts blood vessels and dilates respiratory passages and is used to relieve severe allergic reactions.

hives red, itchy, possibly raised blotches on the skin that often result from allergic reactions.

REVIEW QUESTIONS

1. What are the indications for administration of an epinephrine auto-injector? (p. 483)
2. List some of the more common causes of allergic reactions. (pp. 475–476)
3. List signs or symptoms of an anaphylactic reaction associated with each of the following: (p. 477)
   - Skin
   - Respiratory system
   - Cardiovascular system

CRITICAL THINKING

Thinking and Linking

Think back to Chapter 17, "Cardiac Emergencies," and link information from that chapter with information from this chapter, "Allergic Reactions," as you consider the following situation:

- Your patient is a 60-year-old who used his friend's EpiPen® and is now complaining of chest pain. He thought he might have been stung and, although he wasn't sure, his friend had said: "Here, I can help you with that," handed him the EpiPen®, and helped him inject himself with epinephrine. You know that one action of epinephrine is making the heart beat more strongly. Could this be causing the patient's chest pain? How? And how should you now proceed to assess and care for this patient?

MEDIA RESOURCES 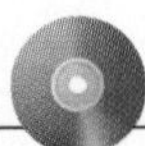

See the Student CD at the back of this book for quizzes, a case study activity, animations and other features related to this chapter. In particular, take a look at the animation on anaphylaxis. Also, visit the Companion Website for *Emergency Care* at **www.prenhall.com/limmer**, where you will find additional reinforcement and links to other resources.

Street Scenes

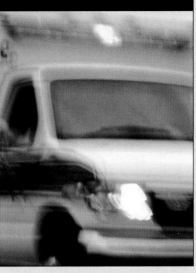

As you are responding to a remote neighborhood in your district for an unknown problem, your dispatcher gives you further information about the call. She states that an elderly male has been stung several times by hornets but has not developed difficulty breathing. The dispatcher also tells you there is an ALS unit responding from the other side of town.

As you arrive on scene, you see an older woman coming out to greet you. She appears upset as she tells you that her 68-year-old husband was doing some work in their storage shed. "I was working in the kitchen when I heard him yelling my name. As I ran outside, I could see him waving his arms around, trying to scare away the hornets."

You find Mr. Meeker sitting forward on a lawn chair at the rear of the house. You notice immediately he is using accessory muscles to breathe and that his face and neck appear flushed. He attempts to explain what has happened but is unable to speak in complete sentences.

Street Scene Questions

1. What is your impression of Mr. Meeker's condition?
2. What do you think might be happening to him?

As you apply a nonrebreather mask to the patient, Mrs. Meeker tells you that he has an allergy to hornet stings and the last time he was stung was shortly after he returned from the war in southeast Asia in the 1960s. You ask, "Does your husband carry an EpiPen®?" She tells you no. He has no other allergies, takes an aspirin daily, and had a heart attack 9 years ago.

You suspect the patient might be experiencing an allergic reaction to the insect stings and that this could be a life-threatening reaction.

As you place Mr. Meeker in the ambulance, your partner reassures the patient's wife and advises her to be careful as she follows the ambulance to the hospital. En route, you assess vital signs and find that the patient's pulse is 136 and thready, his respirations are 28 and shallow, oxygen saturation (his SpO_2) is 93 percent on 15 liters per minute O_2, and he has a blood pressure of 92/60. You notice the patient's respiratory count is falling and that he has become extremely fatigued by breathing.

Street Scene Questions

3. What do you suspect is beginning to happen to your patient?
4. What further treatment should you render?

When you reassess the patient's breathing more closely, you notice his respiratory rate has dropped significantly to about 12. Although that number is in the normal range for an adult, you realize that the depth of the patient's respirations is so shallow that he is not breathing adequately. You connect the bag-valve mask (BVM) to the oxygen tank and ventilate Mr. Meeker about 12 times a minute, making sure you ventilate him deeply enough to make his chest rise. After a few breaths, you are able to match your ventilations to the patient's so that he is not fighting against the BVM.

As you arrive at the hospital, you advise the emergency department staff that you have a 68-year-old male who has been stung by several hornets and you suspect a severe allergic reaction. The staff relieves you of patient care and thanks you for the report.

Street Scenes Sample Documentation

PATIENT NAME: Joshua Meeker **PATIENT AGE:** 68

CHIEF COMPLAINT

Hornet sting. Possible allergic reaction.

PAST MEDICAL HISTORY

- [ ] None
- [x] Allergy to Hornet stings. NKMA
- [ ] Hypertension
- [ ] Stroke
- [ ] Seizures
- [ ] Diabetes
- [ ] COPD
- [ ] Cardiac
- [ ] Other (List)
- [ ] Asthma

Heart attack 9 yrs ago

Current Medications (List)

Aspirin

VITAL SIGNS

TIME	RESP	PULSE	B.P.	MENTAL STATUS	R PUPILS L	SKIN
1147	Rate: 28 [ ] Regular [x] Shallow [ ] Labored	Rate: 136 [ ] Regular [ ] Irregular	92/60	[x] Alert [ ] Voice [ ] Pain [ ] Unresp.	[x] Normal [x] [ ] Dilated [ ] [ ] Constricted [ ] [ ] Sluggish [ ] [ ] No-Reaction [ ]	[ ] Unremarkable [ ] Cool [ ] Pale [x] Warm [ ] Cyanotic [ ] Moist [x] Flushed [x] Dry [ ] Jaundiced
	Rate: [ ] Regular [ ] Shallow [ ] Labored	Rate: [ ] Regular [ ] Irregular	/	[ ] Alert [ ] Voice [ ] Pain [ ] Unresp.	[ ] Normal [ ] [ ] Dilated [ ] [ ] Constricted [ ] [ ] Sluggish [ ] [ ] No-Reaction [ ]	[ ] Unremarkable [ ] Cool [ ] Pale [ ] Warm [ ] Cyanotic [ ] Moist [ ] Flushed [ ] Dry [ ] Jaundiced
	Rate: [ ] Regular [ ] Shallow [ ] Labored	Rate: [ ] Regular [ ] Irregular	/	[ ] Alert [ ] Voice [ ] Pain [ ] Unresp.	[ ] Normal [ ] [ ] Dilated [ ] [ ] Constricted [ ] [ ] Sluggish [ ] [ ] No-Reaction [ ]	[ ] Unremarkable [ ] Cool [ ] Pale [ ] Warm [ ] Cyanotic [ ] Moist [ ] Flushed [ ] Dry [ ] Jaundiced

NARRATIVE Dispatched for possible allergic reaction. Upon arrival, found 68 y/o male sitting upright leaning forward outside on lawn chair. Per patient and wife, patient stung several times (unknown exact number) by hornets while working in storage shed. Patient unable to ambulate back to house and alert his wife. Initial assessment showed patient oriented x 3. Patient in obvious respiratory distress; using accessory muscles to breathe. Flushed and blotchy skin noted to patient's neck and face. Immediately administered 15 LPM O_2 via NRB and placed patient into unit and transported. En route, patient became too exhausted to breathe and BVM used to assist respirations. Vitals en route are stated above. Only one set of vitals obtained due to continuous airway management. ALS intercept requested but no paramedic units available. Upon arrival to Med-Valley General, updated that staff on patient's condition and transferred patient and care. No changes at the time.

CHAPTER

21 Poisoning and Overdose Emergencies

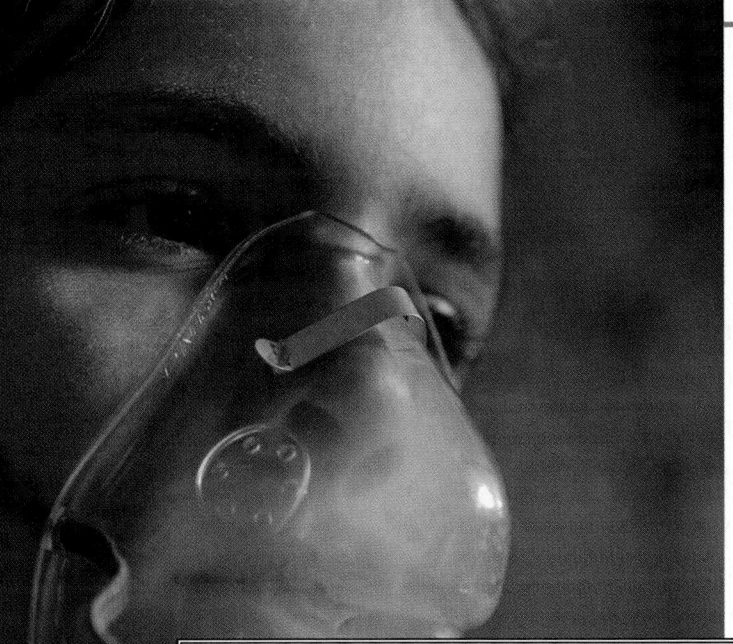

CORE CONCEPTS

The following are core concepts that will be addressed in this chapter:

- Different types of poisons and how they enter the body
- How to identify patients who have overdosed or who have had contact with poisons
- Which overdose/poisoning patients should receive activated charcoal
- Role of medical control in poisoning and overdose cases
- How to document findings and care of patients with a poisoning/overdose emergency

KEY TERMS

absorbed poisons, p. 492
activated charcoal, p. 494
antidote, p. 498
delirium tremens (DTs), p. 506
dilution, p. 497
downers, p. 508
hallucinogens, p. 508
ingested poisons, p. 491
inhaled poisons, p. 491
injected poisons, p. 492
narcotics, p. 508
poison, p. 490
toxin, p. 490
uppers, p. 508
volatile chemicals, p. 508
withdrawal, p. 506

DOT OBJECTIVES

*KNOWLEDGE AND ATTITUDE

4-6.1 List various ways that poisons enter the body. (pp. 491-492)

4-6.2 List signs and symptoms associated with poisoning. (pp. 491, 493, 498–499, 501, 502, 506, 509–510)

4-6.3 Discuss the emergency medical care for the patient with possible overdose. (pp. 511–512)

4-6.4 Describe the steps in the emergency medical care for the patient with suspected poisoning. (pp. 497–498, 499, 502, 507, 509–510) (Scan 21-1, p. 495; Scan 21-3, p. 496; Scan 21-4, p. 500)

4-6.5 Establish the relationship between the patient suffering from poisoning or overdose and airway management. (pp. 490, 493, 498, 499, 500, 501, 507, 511, 512)

4-6.6 State the generic and trade names, indications, contraindications, medication form, dose, administration, actions, side effects, and reassessment strategies for activated charcoal. (pp. 494–497) (Scan 21-2, p. 496)

4-6.7 Recognize the need for medical direction in caring for patient with poisoning or overdose. (pp. 490, 493, 494, 495, 496, 497, 498, 500, 504, 505, 511, 512)

4-6.8 Explain the rationale for administering activated charcoal. (pp. 494–497)

4-6.9 Explain the rationale for contacting medical direction early in the prehospital management of the poisoning or overdose patient. (pp. 490, 493, 494, 495, 496, 497, 498, 500, 504, 505, 511, 512)

*SKILLS

4-6.10 Demonstrate the steps in the emergency medical care for the patient with possible overdose.

4-6.11 Demonstrate the steps in the emergency medical care for the patient with suspected poisoning.

4-6.12 Perform the necessary steps required to provide a patient with activated charcoal.

4-6.13 Demonstrate the assessment and documentation of patient response.

4-6.14 Demonstrate proper disposal of equipment for the administration of activated charcoal.

4-6.15 Demonstrate completing a prehospital care report for patients with a poisoning or overdose emergency.

How can you, as an EMT, know that the patient you encounter at the scene of an emergency call has been poisoned? Family members or bystanders may, of course, report this fact when they call for help. There may be clues at the scene, such as empty pill bottles or containers of toxic substances, and the patient's signs and symptoms may indicate poisoning or overdose. After you identify and treat immediately life-threatening problems, such as airway or breathing difficulties, your main assessment task will be to gather information for medical direction, who will guide your care and management of the poisoning or overdose patient.

POISONING

poison
any substance that can harm the body by altering cell structure or functions.

toxin
a poisonous substance secreted by bacteria, plants, or animals.

A **poison** is any substance that can harm the body, sometimes seriously enough to create a medical emergency. In the United States, there are more than a million cases of poisoning annually. Although some of these result from murder or suicide attempts, most are accidental and involve young children. These accidents usually involve common substances such as medications, petroleum products, cosmetics, and pesticides. In fact, a surprisingly large percentage of chemicals in everyday use contain substances that are poisonous if misused.

We usually think of a poison as some kind of liquid or solid chemical that has been ingested by the poisoning victim. Although this is often the case, many living organisms are capable of producing a **toxin,** a substance that is poisonous to humans. For example, some mushrooms and other common plants can be poisonous if eaten. These include some varieties of house plants, including the rubber plant and certain parts of holiday plants such as mistletoe and holly berries. Bacterial contaminants in food may produce toxins, some of which can cause deadly diseases (such as botulism).

A great number of substances can be considered poisonous, with different people reacting differently to various poisons (Table 21-1). As odd as it may seem, what may be a dangerous poison for one person may have little effect on another person. For most poisonous substances, the reaction is far more serious in the ill and the elderly.

Once they are on or in the body, poisons can do damage in a variety of ways. A poison may act as a corrosive or irritant, destroying skin and other body tissues. A poisonous gas can act as a suffocating agent, displacing oxygen in the air. Some poisons are systemic poisons, causing harm to the entire body or to an entire body system. These poisons can critically depress or overstimulate the central nervous system, cause vomiting and diarrhea, prevent red blood cells from carrying oxygen, or interfere with the normal biochemical processes in the body. The actual effect and extent of damage is dependent on the nature of the poison, on its concentration, and sometimes on how it enters the body. These factors vary in importance depending on the patient's age, weight, and general health.

Poisons can be classified into four types, according to how they enter the body: ingested, inhaled, absorbed, and injected (Figure 21-1):

- **Ingested poisons** (poisons that are swallowed) can include many common household and industrial chemicals, medications, improperly prepared foods, plant materials, petroleum products, and agricultural products made specifically to control rodents, weeds, insects, and crop diseases.
- **Inhaled poisons** (poisons that are breathed in) take the form of gases, vapors, and sprays. Again, many of these substances are in common use in the home, industry, and agriculture. Such poisons include carbon monoxide (from car exhaust, wood-burning stoves, and furnaces), ammonia, chlorine, insect sprays, and the gases produced from volatile liquid chemicals (volatile means "able to change very easily from a liquid into a gas"; many industrial solvents are volatile).

ingested poisons
poisons that are swallowed.

inhaled poisons
poisons that are breathed in.

TABLE 21-1 • Common Ingested Poisons

SUBSTANCE	SIGNS AND SYMPTOMS
Acetaminophen	Nausea and vomiting. Jaundice is a delayed sign. There may be no signs or symptoms.
Acids and alkalis	Burns on or around the lips. Burning in mouth, throat, and abdomen. Vomiting.
Antihistamines and cough or cold preparations	Hyperactivity or drowsiness. Rapid pulse, flushed skin, dilated pupils.
Aspirin	Delayed signs and symptoms, including ringing in the ears, deep and rapid breathing, bruising.
Food poisoning	Different types of food poisoning have different signs and symptoms of varying onset. Most include abdominal pain, nausea, vomiting, and diarrhea, sometimes with fever.
Insecticides	Slow pulse, excessive salivation and sweating, nausea, vomiting, diarrhea, difficulty breathing, constricted pupils.
Petroleum products	Characteristic odor of breath, clothing, vomitus. If aspiration has occurred, coughing and difficulty breathing.
Plants	Wide range of signs and symptoms, ranging from none to nausea and vomiting to cardiac arrest.

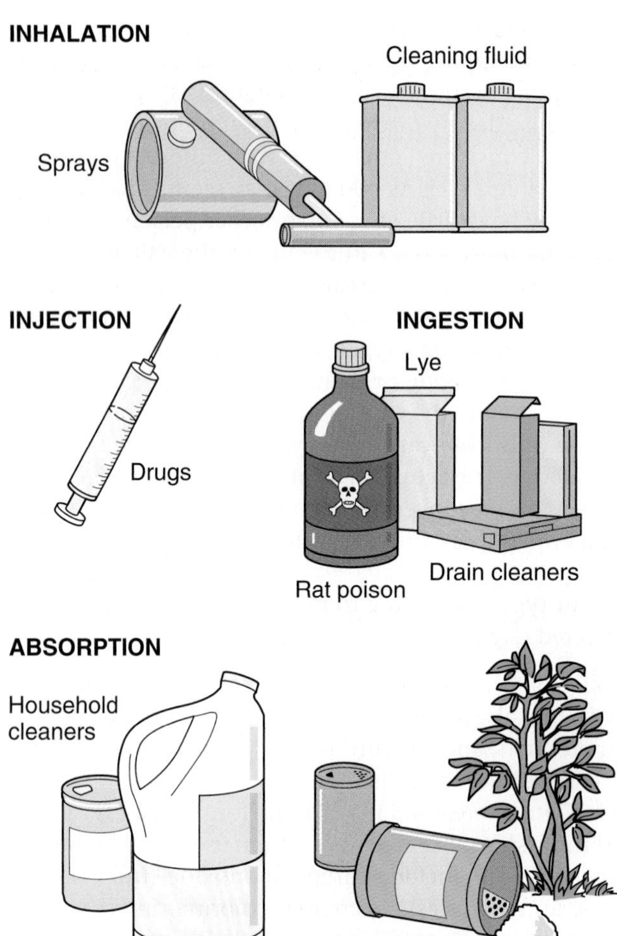

Figure 21-1 • Poisons enter the body by way of ingestion, inhalation, absorption, and injection.

absorbed poisons poisons that are taken into the body through unbroken skin.

- **Absorbed poisons** (poisons taken into the body through unbroken skin) may or may not damage the skin. Many are corrosives or irritants that will injure the skin and then be slowly absorbed into body tissues and the bloodstream, possibly causing widespread damage. Others are absorbed into the bloodstream without injuring the skin. Examples of these poisons include insecticides and agricultural chemicals. Contact with a variety of plant materials and certain forms of marine life can lead to skin damage and possible absorption into tissues under the skin.

injected poisons poisons that are inserted through the skin, for example by needle, snake fangs, or insect stinger.

- **Injected poisons** (poisons inserted through the skin). The most common injected poisons include illicit drugs injected with a needle and venoms injected by snake fangs or insect stingers. These will be discussed under "Substance Abuse," later in this chapter, and in Chapter 22, "Environmental Emergencies."

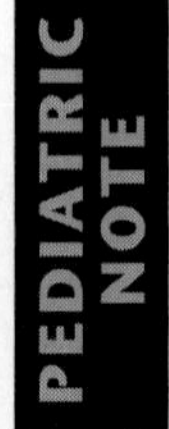

Preventing poisoning is, of course, preferable to having to treat it. The EMT's own home and the squad building should be "childproofed" against poisoning by keeping medications and other dangerous substances out of children's reach. The EMT can also share poisoning prevention information with members of the public during school visits and community outreach activities.

Ingested Poisons

Ingested poisons are those poisons that have been swallowed. An ingested poison is often a toxic substance that a curious child has eaten or drunk. In adults, an ingested poison is often a medication on which the patient has accidentally or deliberately overdosed.

PATIENT ASSESSMENT

INGESTED POISON

You must gather information quickly in cases of possible ingested poisoning. In order to determine if activated charcoal is appropriate, on-line medical direction will need certain information:

- *What substance was involved?* Many products have similar names. It is important to get the exact spelling of the substance. If it is possible and safe, bring the container to the hospital with the patient.
- *When did the exposure occur?* Some poisons act very quickly and will require immediate treatment. Others may take longer to affect the body, which may allow for other treatments to be used. It is important for emergency department personnel to know as closely as possible the time of ingestion so that appropriate testing and treatment can be done.

  It is sometimes difficult to determine the time of the exposure from family members or witnesses. If you cannot get an exact time, determine the earliest and latest possible times of exposure.
- *How much was ingested?* This may be as easy as counting the number of tablets left in a brand new prescription or as difficult as estimating the amount of gasoline spilled on a garage floor. When the amount cannot be estimated reliably, determine the maximum amount that might have been ingested.
- *Over how long a period did the ingestion occur?* Someone who takes certain medication chronically and then overdoses on it may require very different hospital treatment from the patient who has the same overdose but has never taken that medication before.
- *What interventions has the patient, family, or well-meaning bystanders taken?* Many traditional home remedies for medical problems are harmful, particularly when someone has been exposed to enough of a substance to suffer ill effects. Product labels have been improved over the last few years, but some still contain inaccurate or even dangerous instructions for management of potentially toxic exposures.
- *What is the patient's estimated weight?* This, in combination with the amount of substance ingested, may be critical in determining the appropriate treatment.
- *What effects is the patient experiencing from the ingestion?* Nausea and vomiting are two of the most common results of poison ingestion, but you may also find altered mental status, abdominal pain, diarrhea, chemical burns around the mouth, and unusual breath odors. ■

NOTE

Sometimes patients who have ingested poisons will require assisted ventilations. Direct mouth-to-mouth ventilation in such a case is dangerous, not only because of the danger of contracting an infectious disease but also because of possible contact with poisonous substances remaining on the patient's lips, in the airway, or in his vomitus. Use a pocket face mask with a one-way valve, a bag-valve-mask unit with supplemental oxygen, or positive-pressure ventilation when providing ventilations to a patient who is suspected of ingesting a poison.

If you suspect intentional poisoning or attempted suicide, approach the scene with caution and have police backup if indicated.

POINT OF VIEW

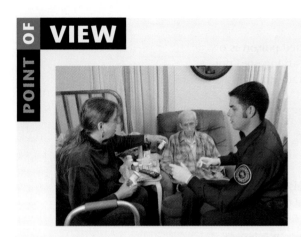

"We were sent to a call for an older patient with an altered mental status. We have a considerable older population in our community and a lot of assisted living places.

"You read in the news that people are getting older and living longer. Medicine has helped people do this. I was on a call the other day. I looked at this nice older man. You wouldn't believe how many medications he had. It was crazy.

"I'm not saying he didn't need them. That's not my place. But with just a little confusion or disorganization he could double up on powerful cardiac meds or change his blood sugar or blood pressure or thyroid levels. His daughter thought that is what happened.

"I guess, on the good side, the medications helped us figure out his medical history. We rarely get the full story from the patient and family.

"I know in this case it took 5 minutes just to get his history list of meds. It actually is an issue we see a lot."

F•Y•I

FOOD POISONING

Another way someone can be poisoned is through food that has been handled or cooked improperly. Food poisoning can be caused by several different bacteria that grow when exposed to the right conditions. This frequently happens when raw meat, poultry, or fish is left at room temperature before being cooked or the food does not reach a high enough temperature to kill the bacteria. Signs and symptoms vary somewhat, depending on the bacteria involved, but frequently include nausea, vomiting, abdominal cramps, diarrhea, and fever.

You can prevent food poisoning at home and at the station by washing hands, utensils, cutting boards, and any surface the food touches before and especially after any contact with raw meat, fish, or poultry (the bacteria can easily be spread to other foods from hands or surfaces); by storing and cooking foods at appropriate temperatures; and by not leaving raw or cooked foods at room temperature for long periods of time. ■

Activated Charcoal

To provide the proper emergency care for ingested poisons (Scan 21-1), follow the instructions given to you by medical direction or your regional poison control center. In some cases of ingested poisoning, medical direction will order administration of **activated charcoal** (Scan 21-2).

activated charcoal a substance that adsorbs many poisons and prevents them from being absorbed by the body.

Activated charcoal works through adsorption, the process of one substance becoming attached to the surface of another. Ordinary charcoal adsorbs some substances, but activated charcoal is different because it has been manufactured to have many cracks and crevices. As a result, activated charcoal has an increased amount of surface available for poisons to bind to (similar to corrugated cardboard which, if you cut it open, has many more surfaces than you would expect by looking at the smooth outer surface). Activated charcoal is not an antidote, but through the adsorption or binding process, in many cases it will prevent or reduce the amount of poison available for the body to absorb.

Many poisons are adsorbed by activated charcoal, but not all. Since there are millions of potential poisons available and the number is always increasing, it makes little sense to memorize lists of poisons where activated charcoal should not be used. Instead, medical direction (possibly in consultation with a poison control center) will determine whether the use of activated charcoal is appropriate.

SCAN 21-1 • Ingested Poisons

First take Standard Precautions.

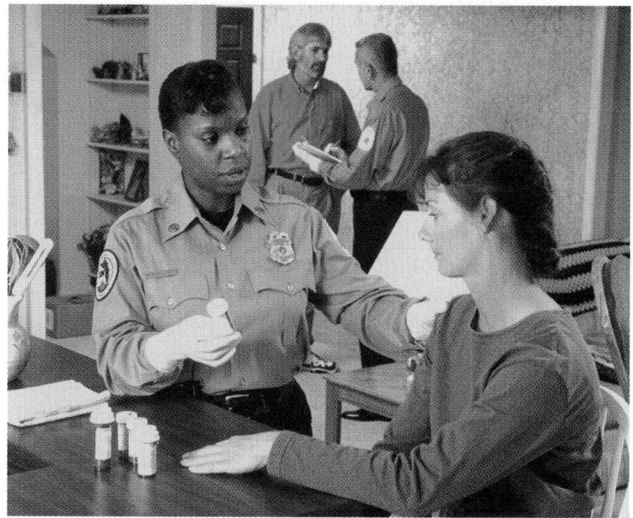

1. Quickly gather information.

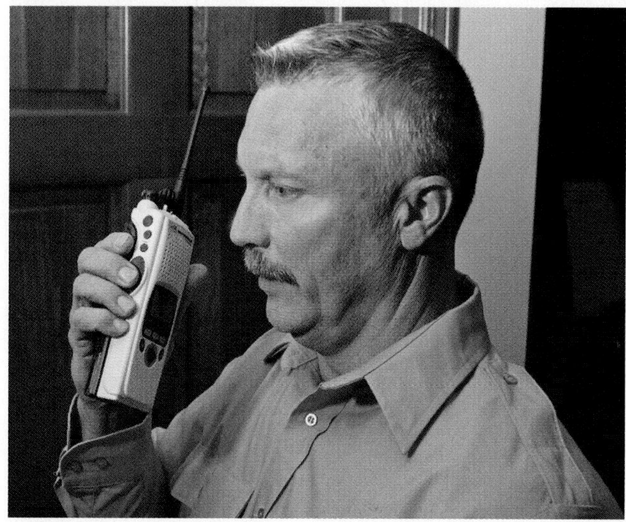

2. Call medical direction on the scene or en route to the hospital. *(© Ray Kemp/911 Imaging)*

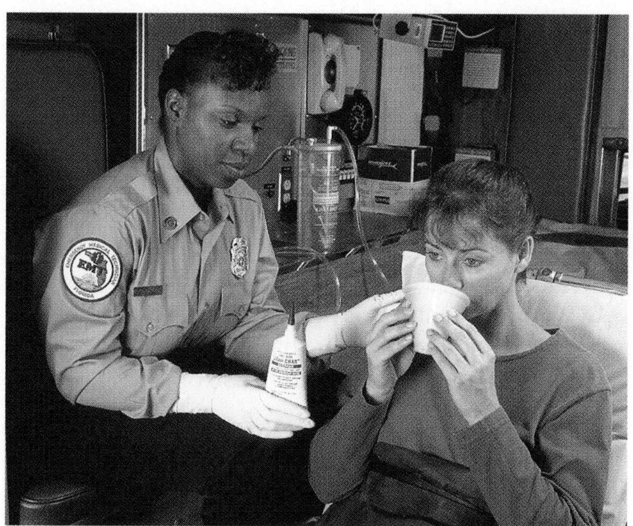

3. If directed, administer activated charcoal. You may wish to administer the medication in an opaque cup that has a lid with a hole for a straw.

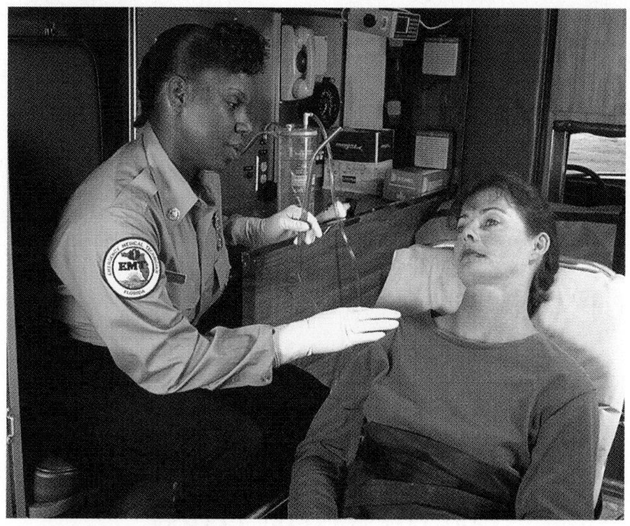

4. Position patient for vomiting and save all vomitus. Have suction equipment ready.

NOTE

When a patient has ingested a poison, it provides another reason to avoid mouth-to-mouth contact. Provide ventilations through a pocket face mask or other barrier device.

SCAN 21-2 • Activated Charcoal

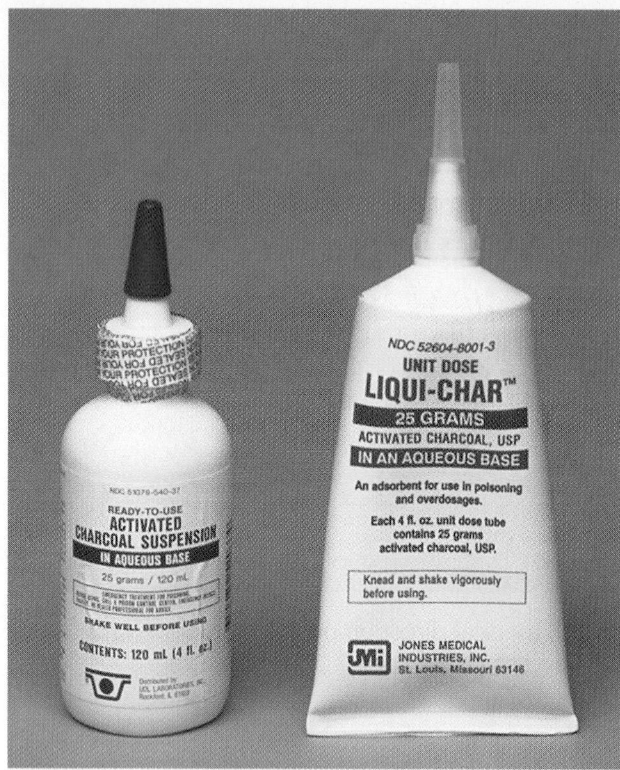

MEDICATION NAME

1. Generic: activated charcoal
2. Trade: SuperChar, InstaChar, Actidose, Liqui-Char, and others

INDICATIONS

Poisoning by mouth

CONTRAINDICATIONS

1. Altered mental status
2. Ingestion of acids or alkalis
3. Inability to swallow

MEDICATION FORM

1. Premixed in water, frequently available in plastic bottle containing 12.5 grams of activated charcoal
2. Powder—should be avoided in the field

DOSAGE

1. Adults and children: 1 gram activated charcoal/kg of body weight
2. Usual adult dose: 25 to 50 grams
3. Usual pediatric dose: 12.5 to 25 grams

ADMINISTRATION

1. Consult medical direction.
2. Shake container thoroughly.
3. Since medication looks like mud, patient may need to be persuaded to drink it. Providing a covered container and a straw will prevent the patient from seeing the medication and so may improve patient compliance.
4. If the patient does not drink the medication right away, the charcoal will settle. Shake or stir it again before administering.
5. Record the name, dose, route, and time of administration of the medication.

ACTIONS

1. Activated charcoal adsorbs (binds) certain poisons and prevents them from being absorbed into the body.
2. Not all brands of activated charcoal are the same: some adsorb much more than others, so consult medical direction about the brand to use.

SIDE EFFECTS

1. Black stools.
2. Some patients may vomit, particularly those who have ingested poisons that cause nausea. If patient vomits, repeat the dose once.

REASSESSMENT STRATEGIES

1. Be prepared for the patient to vomit or further deteriorate.

There are, however, a few instances you should know about where the use of activated charcoal is contraindicated:

- Patient who cannot swallow obviously cannot swallow activated charcoal.
- Patient with altered mental status might choke on activated charcoal and aspirate it into the lungs.

- Patient who has ingested acids or alkalis should not take activated charcoal because the caustic material may have severely damaged the mouth, throat, and esophagus. Activated charcoal cannot help the damage that has already been done, and swallowing it may cause further damage. Examples of such caustic substances are oven cleaners, drain cleaners, toilet bowl cleaners, and lye.
- Patient who has accidentally swallowed while siphoning gasoline should not be given activated charcoal. This patient will be coughing violently and possibly aspirating the gasoline. This patient will be unable to swallow activated charcoal.

Many brands of activated charcoal are on the market, but some have greater surface area than others. Medical direction can guide you in the selection of an appropriate brand.

Some patients, especially those who have taken an intentional overdose, may refuse to take activated charcoal. Never attempt to force a patient to swallow activated charcoal. If the patient refuses, notify medical direction and continue ongoing assessment and care.

ACTIVATED CHARCOAL VS. SYRUP OF IPECAC A traditional treatment for poisoning used to be syrup of ipecac. This orally administered drug causes vomiting in most people with just one dose. During recent years, however, it has been used less and less as the use of activated charcoal has increased. Ipecac stimulates both the stomach and the vomiting center in the brain, but it typically takes 15 to 20 minutes to work. If the first dose did not cause vomiting within 20 to 30 minutes, a second dose was typically given (almost everyone vomited after two doses of ipecac). When vomiting does occur, it results, on the average, in removal of less than a third of the stomach contents. Because ipecac is slow, is relatively ineffective, and has the potential to make a patient aspirate vomitus, it is rarely used today.

Although poison control centers sometimes instruct parents of young children in the proper use of syrup of ipecac, activated charcoal is the medication of first choice for health care providers in most poisoning and overdose cases. This is why the national standard EMT curriculum includes the use of activated charcoal and not syrup of ipecac.

Dilution

Occasionally, medical direction will give an order for **dilution** of a poisonous substance. This means an adult patient should drink one to two glasses of water or milk, whichever is ordered. A child should typically be given half to one glass. Dilution with water may slow absorption slightly. Milk may soothe stomach upset. This treatment is frequently advised for patients who, as determined by medical direction or poison control, do not need transport to a hospital.

dilution (di-LU-shun) thinning down or weakening by mixing with something else. Ingested poisons are sometimes diluted by drinking water or milk.

PATIENT CARE

INGESTED POISON

Emergency care of a patient who has ingested poison includes the following:

1. Detect and treat immediately life-threatening problems in the initial assessment. Evaluate the need for prompt transport for critical patients.
2. Perform a focused history and physical exam, including SAMPLE history. Use gloved hands to carefully remove any pills, tablets, or fragments from the patient's mouth.
3. Assess baseline vital signs.
4. Consult medical direction. As directed, administer activated charcoal to adsorb the poison, or water or milk to dilute it. This can usually be done en route.
5. Transport the patient with all containers, bottles, and labels from the substance.
6. Perform ongoing assessment en route. ■

Many laypeople think that every poison has an **antidote,** a substance that will neutralize the poison or its effects. This is not true. There are only a few genuine antidotes, and they can be used only with a very small number of poisons. Modern treatment of poisonings and overdoses consists primarily of prevention of absorption when possible (such as by administration of activated charcoal) and good supportive treatment (such as airway maintenance, administration of oxygen, treatment for shock). In a small number of poisonings, advanced treatments are administered in a hospital (administration of antidotes and kidney dialysis). ■

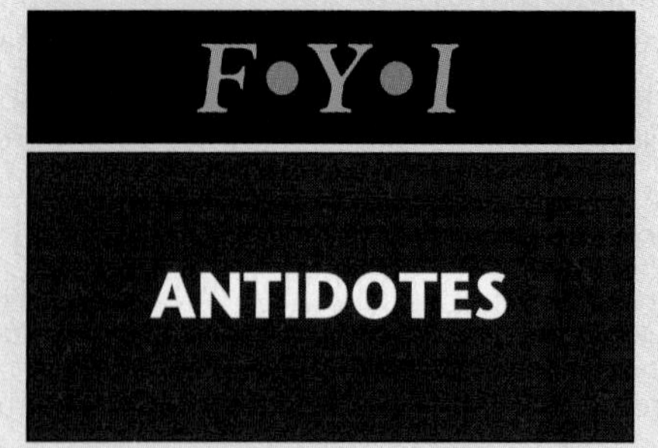

antidote
a substance that will neutralize the poison or its effects.

PEDIATRIC NOTE

It is the nature of infants and children to explore their world—and to get into and often taste whatever they find. Children will swallow substances adults cannot imagine swallowing, including horrible-tasting poisonous substances like bleach or lye. The natural curiosity of children makes them the most frequent victims of accidental poisoning.

It is important to find out an infant's or child's weight, which—in combination with the estimated amount of the poisonous substance that was ingested—will help medical direction determine appropriate treatment.

As an EMT, always assume that the infant or child has ingested a lethal amount of the poison. Because it is usually extremely difficult or impossible to be sure exactly how much the child has taken in, always treat for the worst. Call medical direction, administer the recommended treatments, and transport the child to the hospital.

Inhaled Poisons

Inhaled poisons are those that are present in the atmosphere and that you, as well as the patient, are at risk of breathing in. Carbon monoxide poisoning is a common problem. Other possible inhaled poisons include chlorine gas (often from swimming pool chemicals), ammonia (often released from household cleaners), sprayed agricultural chemicals and pesticides, and carbon dioxide (from industrial sources).

NOTE

If you suspect that a patient has inhaled a poison, approach the scene with care. Some EMS systems provide training in the use of protective clothing and self-contained breathing apparatus to be used in a hostile environment (such as chlorine gas, ammonia, or smoke). Remember that many inhaled poisons can also be absorbed through the skin. Go only where your protective equipment and clothing will allow you to go safely to perform your mission, and only after you have been trained in the use of this equipment. Do only what you have been trained to do and go only where your protective equipment will allow you to go safely. If you do not have the necessary equipment or training, get someone there who is properly equipped and trained.

PATIENT ASSESSMENT

INHALED POISON

Gather the following information as quickly as possible:

- *What substance was involved?* Get its exact name.
- *When did the exposure occur?* Estimate as well as you can when the patient was exposed to the poisonous gas by finding out the earliest and latest possible times of exposure.

continued

PATIENT ASSESSMENT *(continued)*

- *Over how long a period did the exposure occur?* The longer someone is exposed to a poisonous gas, the more poison that will probably be absorbed.
- *What interventions has anyone taken?* Did someone remove the patient or ventilate the area right away? When did this happen?
- *What effects is the patient experiencing from the exposure?* Nausea and vomiting are very common in poisoning of all types. With inhaled poisons, find out if the patient is having difficulty breathing, chest pain, coughing, hoarseness, dizziness, headache, confusion, seizures, or altered mental status. ■

PATIENT CARE

INHALED POISON

The principal prehospital treatment of inhaled poisoning consists of maintaining the airway and supporting respiration (Scan 21-3). In the case of inhaled poisoning, oxygen is a very important drug. Some inhaled poisons prevent the blood from transporting oxygen in the normal manner. Some prevent oxygen from getting into the bloodstream in the first place. In either case, your ability to keep the airway open; ventilate as needed; and give high-concentration oxygen may make the difference in the survival and quality of life of the patient who has inhaled a poison.

Emergency care steps include the following:

1. If the patient is in an unsafe environment, have trained rescuers remove the patient to a safe area. Detect and treat immediately life-threatening problems in the initial assessment. Evaluate the need to promptly transport critical patients.
2. Perform a focused history and physical exam, including SAMPLE history and vital signs.
3. Administer high-concentration oxygen. This is the single most important treatment for inhaled poisoning after the patient's airway is opened.
4. Transport the patient with all containers, bottles, and labels from the substance.
5. Perform ongoing assessment en route. ■

Carbon Monoxide

Carbon monoxide is one of the most common inhaled poisons, usually associated with motor-vehicle exhaust and fire suppression. The number of cases has increased recently because of the carbon monoxide that can accumulate from the use of improperly vented wood-burning stoves and the use of charcoal for heating and indoor cooking in areas without adequate ventilation. Malfunctioning oil-, gas-, and coal-burning furnaces and stoves can also be sources of carbon monoxide.

Since carbon monoxide is an odorless, colorless, and tasteless gas, you will not be able to directly detect its presence without special equipment (Figure 21-2). Look for indications of possible carbon monoxide poisoning like wood-burning stoves, doors that lead to a garage, bedrooms above a garage where motor repair work is in progress, and evidence that suggests the patient has spent a long period of time sitting in an idling motor vehicle. When inhaled, carbon monoxide prevents the normal carrying of oxygen by the red blood cells. Long exposure, even to low levels of the gas, can cause dramatic effects. Death may occur as hypoxia becomes more severe.

SCAN 21-3 • Inhaled Poisons

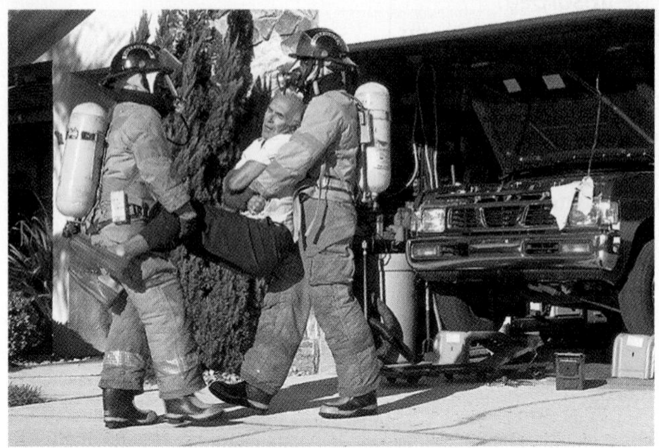

1. Remove patient from source of the poison.

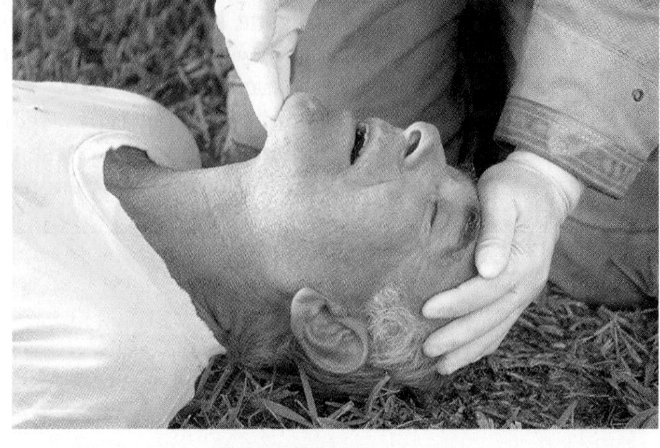

2. Establish an open airway.

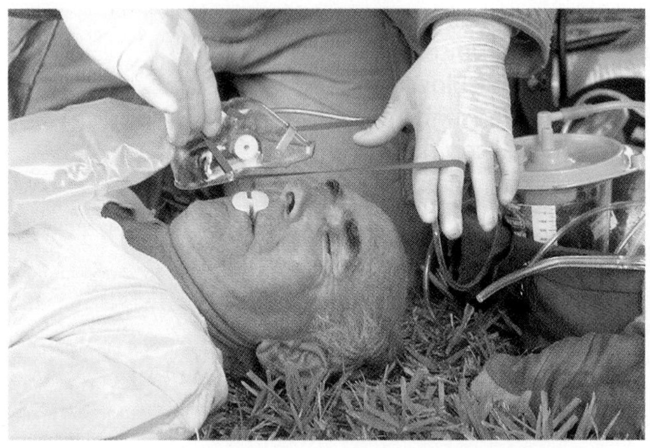

3. Insert an oropharyngeal airway and administer high-concentration oxygen by nonrebreather mask.

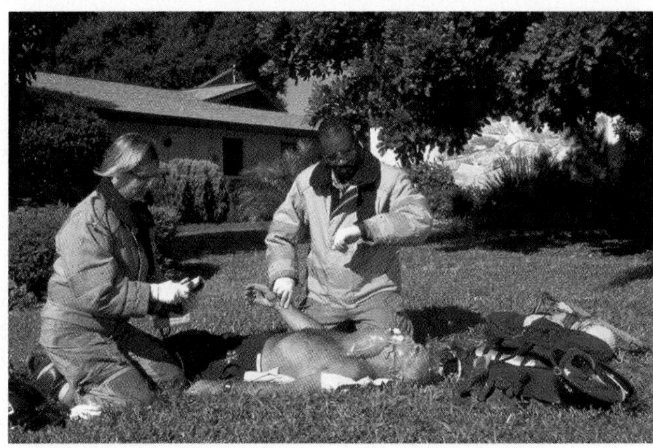

4. Gather the patient's history, take baseline vital signs, and expose the chest for auscultation.

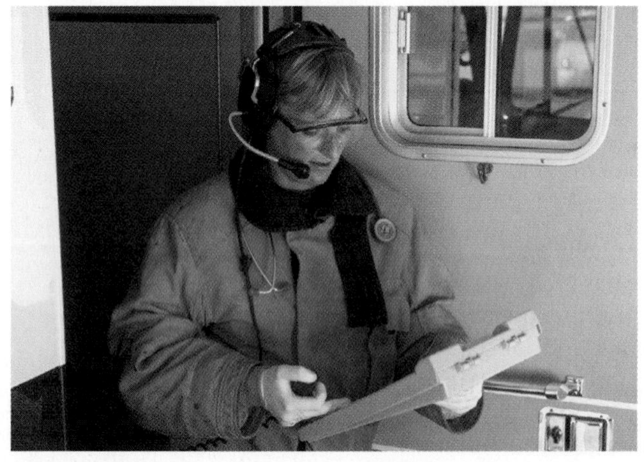

5. Contact medical direction.

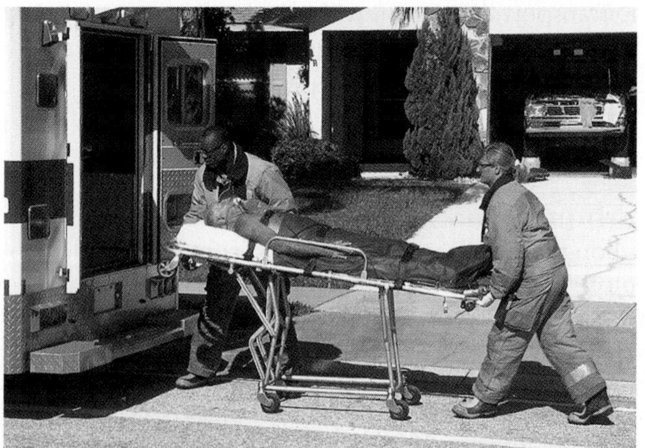

6. Transport the patient.

NOTE

In the presence of hazardous fumes or gases, wear protective clothing and self-contained breathing apparatus or wait for those who are properly trained and equipped to enter the scene and bring the patient out.

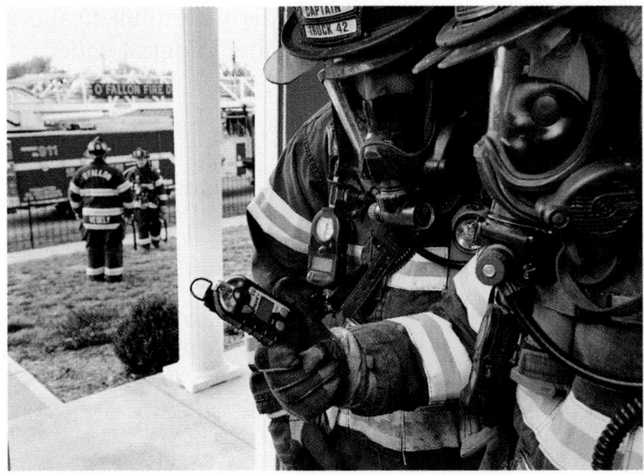

Figure 21-2 • Special monitors are needed to detect the presence of carbon monoxide in the environment. *(© Ray Kemp/911 Imaging)*

The signs and symptoms of carbon monoxide poisoning are deceptive, because they can resemble those of the flu. Specifically, you may see:

- Headache, especially "a band around the head"
- Dizziness
- Breathing difficulty
- Nausea
- Cyanosis
- Altered mental status; in severe cases, unconsciousness may result

You should suspect carbon monoxide poisoning whenever you are treating a patient with vague, flu-like symptoms who has been in an enclosed area. This is especially true when a group of people in the same area have similar symptoms. A patient with carbon monoxide poisoning may begin to feel better shortly after being removed from the dangerous environment. It is still very important to continue to administer oxygen and to transport these patients to a hospital. Oxygen is an antidote for carbon monoxide poisoning, but it takes time to "wash out" the carbon monoxide from the

NOTE

There is a commonly accepted idea that a patient exposed to carbon monoxide will have cherry red lips. In fact, cherry red skin is NOT typically seen in patients with carbon monoxide poisoning.

F•Y•I

SMOKE INHALATION

Smoke inhalation is a serious problem associated with the scenes of thermal and chemical burns. The smoke from any fire source contains many poisonous substances. Modern building materials and furnishings often contain plastics and other synthetics that release toxic fumes when they burn or are overheated. It is possible for the substances found in smoke to burn the skin, irritate the eyes, injure the airway, cause respiratory arrest, and, in some cases, cause cardiac arrest.

As an EMT, you will most likely find irritated (reddened, watering) eyes and, of far greater concern, injury to the airway associated with smoke.

Signs of an airway injured by smoke inhalation include:

- Difficulty breathing
- Coughing
- Breath that has a "smoky" smell or the odor of chemicals involved at the scene
- Black (carbon) residue in the patient's mouth and nose
- Black residue in any sputum coughed up by the patient
- Nose hairs singed from superheated air

Move the patient to a safe area and provide the same care you would provide for any inhaled poison: Assess the patient; administer high-concentration oxygen; and transport. ■

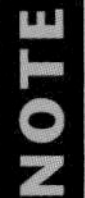

The body's reaction to toxic gases and foreign matter in the airway can often be delayed. Convince all smoke inhalation patients that they must be seen by a physician, even if they are not yet feeling serious effects.

patient's bloodstream. These patients need medical evaluation because they can have serious consequences, including neurological deficits, from their exposure.

Absorbed Poisons

Absorbed poisons frequently irritate or damage the skin. Some poisons can be absorbed with little or no damage to the skin.

NOTE

Just as poisonous substances can be absorbed by patients, they can also be absorbed by EMTs. It is critical that the EMT take protective measures to prevent exposure to these substances. It may be necessary for firefighters to decontaminate a patient before the EMT touches him.

PATIENT ASSESSMENT

ABSORBED POISON

Gather the following information as quickly as possible:

- *What substance was involved?* Get its exact name.
- *When did the exposure occur?*
- *How much of the substance was the patient exposed to?* How large an area of skin was the substance on?
- *Over how long a period did the exposure occur?* The longer someone's skin is exposed to a poison, the more likely it is to be well absorbed.
- *What interventions has anyone taken?* Did someone attempt to wash the substance off the patient? If so, with what? Did anyone attempt to use a chemical to "neutralize" the substance?
- *What effects is the patient experiencing from the exposure?* Common signs and symptoms include a liquid or powder on the patient's skin, burns, itching, irritation, and redness. ■

PATIENT CARE

ABSORBED POISON

Emergency care of a patient with absorbed poisons includes the following:

1. Detect and treat immediately life-threatening problems in the initial assessment. Evaluate the need for prompt transport of critical patients.
2. Perform a focused history and physical exam, including sample history and vital signs. This includes removing contaminated clothing while protecting oneself from contamination.
3. Remove the poison by doing one of the following:
   - *Powders.* Brush powder off the patient, then continue as for other absorbed poisons.
   - *Liquids.* Irrigate with clean water for at least 20 minutes and continue en route if possible.
   - *Eyes.* Irrigate with clean water for at least 20 minutes and continue en route if possible.
4. Transport the patient with all containers, bottles, and labels from the substance.
5. Perform ongoing assessment en route. ■

The most important part of the treatment of a patient with an absorbed poison is to get the poison off the skin or out of the eye (Scan 21-4). The best way to do this is by irrigating the skin or the eye with large amounts of clean water. A garden hose or fire hose can be used to irrigate the patient's skin, but care must be taken not to injure the skin further with high pressure.

"Neutralizing" acids or alkalis with solutions such as dilute vinegar or baking soda in water should NOT be done. When incidents like these occur, such substances are almost never readily available. Even if they were, they would not be appropriate. They have never been shown to help, and there is good reason to believe they would make matters worse. When an acid is mixed with an alkali, it is true that the two may be neutralized. It is also true, though, that this reaction produces heat. Skin that has been injured already by an acid or alkali may be further damaged by attempts to neutralize the chemical.

Injected Poisons

As mentioned earlier, the most common injected poisons are illicit drugs injected with a needle (which will be discussed later in this chapter) and the venom of snakes and insects (which will be covered in Chapter 22, "Environmental Emergencies").

ALCOHOL AND SUBSTANCE ABUSE

As an EMT, you will see many patients whose conditions are caused either directly or indirectly by alcohol or substance abuse. Although these are often thought of as urban problems, the abuse of alcohol and other drugs crosses all geographic and economic boundaries.

Alcohol Abuse

Many persons consume alcohol without having any problems. Others occasionally or chronically abuse alcohol. Although alcohol is legal (for adults), it must not be forgotten that alcohol is a drug and has a potent effect on the central nervous system. Emergencies arising from the use of alcohol may be due to the effect of alcohol that has just been consumed, or it may be the result of the cumulative effects of years of alcohol abuse.

EMTs often do not take alcohol abuse patients seriously. This may be partially due to the belligerent or unusual behavior they often exhibit. In addition, frequent calls for

CRITICAL DECISION MAKING: FIND THE CLUES

Poisoning and overdose emergencies are challenging in that you will need to figure out what toxin caused the patient's current signs and symptoms. Your ability to examine the scene and report accurate findings to Poison Control are vital to the patient's well-being. In each of the following scenarios decide what information you will need to gather—and where to obtain it—to ensure proper treatment for the patient.

1. Your patient states he has taken an overdose of prescription medications.
2. Your patient is found in a closed garage with the car running.
3. Your patient is found in the garden, confused and drooling.

SCAN 21-4 • Absorbed Poisons

First take Standard Precautions.

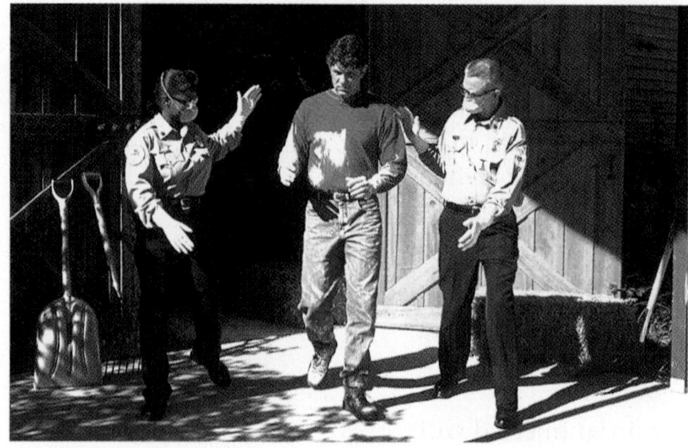

1. Remove the patient from the source or the source from the patient. Avoid contaminating yourself with the poison.

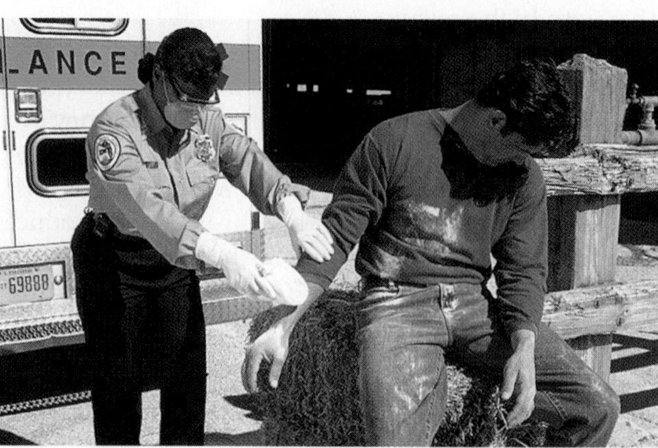

2. Brush powders from the patient. Be careful not to abrade the patient's skin.

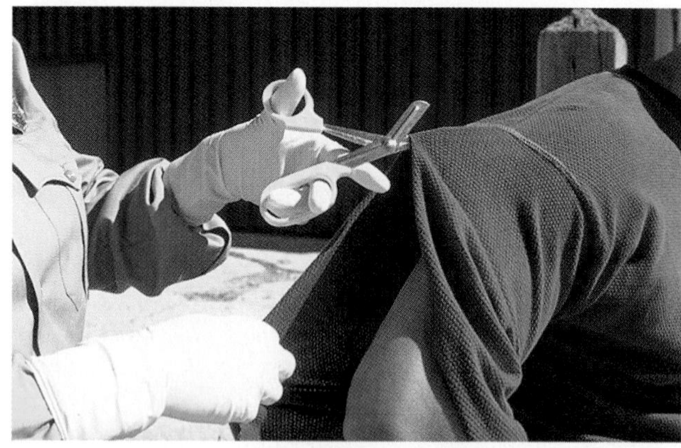

3. Remove contaminated clothing and other articles.

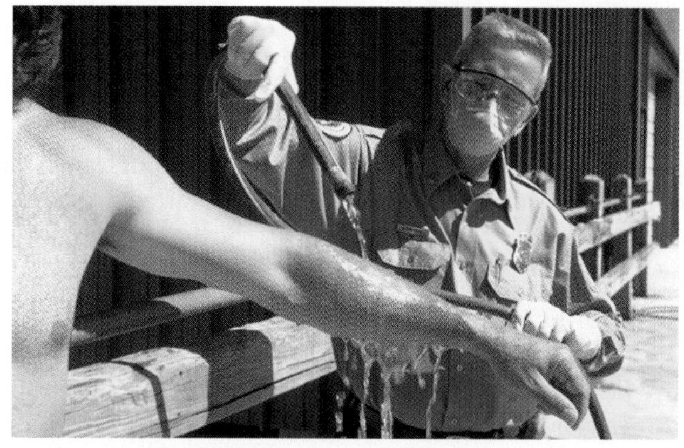

4. Irrigate with clear water for at least 20 minutes. Catch contaminated runoff and dispose of it safely.

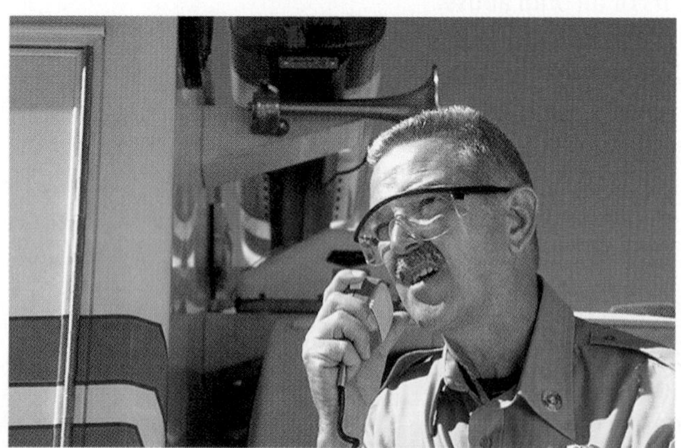

5. Contact medical direction.

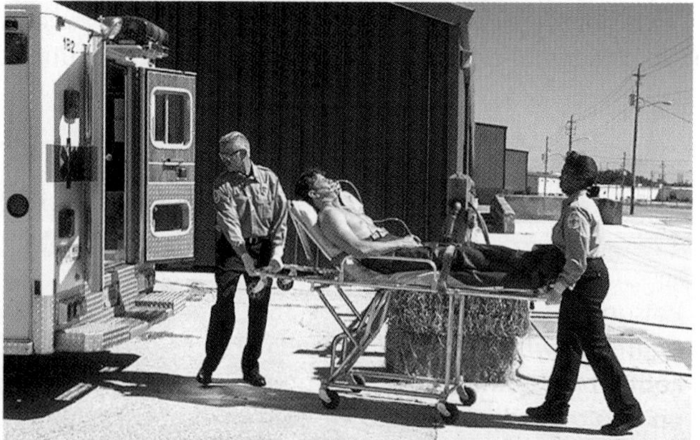

6. Transport the patient.

NOTE

Take care to protect your skin from contact with poisonous substances. Wear protective clothing. If necessary, have firefighters or others who are properly protected hose off the patient before you touch him.

Emergency care in poisoning cases presents special problems for the EMT. Signs and symptoms can vary greatly. Some poisons produce a characteristic set of signs and symptoms very quickly, while others are subtle and slow to appear. Poisons that act almost immediately usually produce obvious signs, and the particular poison or its container is often still nearby. Slow-acting poisons can produce effects that mimic an infectious disease or some other medical emergency.

There will be times when you will not know the substance that caused the poisoning. In some of these cases, an expert may be able to tell, based on the combination of signs and symptoms. Even when you know the source of the poison, correct emergency care procedures may still be in question. Ideas about proper care keep changing as more research is done on poisoning. This constant change makes it impossible to print guides and charts for poison control and care that will be up to date when you use them. Although manufacturers have improved the instructions on many container labels, some still have inaccurate or even dangerous advice.

Fortunately, a network of poison control centers exists to provide information and advice to both laypeople and health care providers.

F•Y•I

POISON CONTROL CENTERS

Throughout the United States, it is possible to reach a poison control center 24 hours a day. Dialing 1-800-222-1222 connects an EMT with the poison center covering the area the call is coming from. Your EMS agency may also have a local number for your regional poison center. Either number will work.

An EMT should consult a poison control center only when directed by local protocol. In most cases, EMTs get medical direction from physicians or nurses who are in hospital emergency departments. Unless special arrangements have been made, the poison control center staff does not have the authority to provide on-line medical direction. If the poison control center staff does have the authority to do so, they can tell you what should be done for most cases of poisoning.

If you are permitted to communicate directly with the poison control center in your area, do so by telephone. Even if you have radio contact with your local poison control center, the telephone is the preferred way to communicate. The staff member may need to talk to you for several minutes, far too long a period to monopolize the air waves. The telephone will also allow you to maintain patient confidentiality. Make certain you have memorized the number and/or carry the poison control center number with you into the residence—perhaps pasted inside your kit—so that you do not have to return to the rig to get it.

To help the poison control center staff, gather all of the information you need before you call.

Many people have the impression that the poison control center should be called only for cases of ingested poisonings. However, the center's staff can provide valuable care information for all types of poisoning.

Your community may have special poisoning problems. Not every community is exposed to rattlesnakes, jellyfish, or powerful agricultural chemicals. Many EMS systems have compiled lists of poisoning problems specific for their areas. Check to see if this has been done for the area in which you will be an EMT. ■

intoxicated persons may cause the EMT to become callous toward them. Also, the hygiene of many of these patients on the street leaves much to be desired. Nevertheless, provide care for the patient suffering from alcohol abuse the same as you would for any other patient. Patients who appear intoxicated must be treated with the same respect and dignity as those who are "sober."

Above all, you must not neglect your duty to provide medical care. Not only do alcohol-abuse patients often have injuries from accidents and falls but they are also candidates for many medical emergencies. Chronic drinkers often have derangements in blood sugar levels, poor nutrition, the potential for considerable gastrointestinal bleeding, and other problems. A person can be both intoxicated and having a heart attack or hypoglycemia. If the patient has ingested alcohol and other drugs, this can produce a serious medical emergency. When alcohol is combined with other depressants such as antihistamines and tranquilizers, the effects of alcohol can be more pronounced and, in some cases, lethal.

Since EMT safety is a critical part of all calls, do not hesitate to ask for police assistance with any patient who appears intoxicated or irrational or exhibits potentially dangerous behavior. The nature of intoxication is such that a passive person may suddenly become aggressive. Always be prepared for this event. (See Chapter 23, "Behavioral Emergencies.")

withdrawal referring to alcohol or drug withdrawal in which the patient's body reacts severely when deprived of the abused substance.

delirium tremens (duh-LEER-e-um TREM-uns) **(DTs)** a severe reaction that can be part of alcohol withdrawal, characterized by sweating, trembling, anxiety, and hallucinations. Severe alcohol withdrawal with the DTs can lead to death if untreated.

PATIENT ASSESSMENT

ALCOHOL ABUSE

Keep in mind that, while alcohol may be the patient's only problem, there may be another problem present. Conduct a complete assessment to identify any medical emergencies. Remember that diabetes, epilepsy, head injuries, high fevers, hypoxia, and other medical problems may make the patient appear to be intoxicated when he is not. Also look for injuries. Do not allow the presence of alcohol or the signs and symptoms of alcohol abuse to override your suspicions of other medical problems or injuries.

Since getting a SAMPLE history from any patient who appears intoxicated will be difficult and perhaps unreliable, your powers of observation and resourcefulness will be tested. Family members and bystanders may provide important information.

The signs and symptoms of alcohol abuse include:

- Odor of alcohol on the patient's breath or clothing. By itself, however, this is not enough to conclude alcohol abuse. Be certain that the odor is not "acetone breath," as with some diabetic emergencies.
- Swaying and unsteadiness of movement
- Slurred speech, rambling thought patterns, incoherent words or phrases
- A flushed appearance to the face, often with the patient sweating and complaining of being warm
- Nausea or vomiting
- Poor coordination
- Slowed reaction time
- Blurred vision
- Confusion
- Hallucinations, visual or auditory ("seeing things" or "hearing things")
- Lack of memory (blackout)
- Altered mental status

The alcoholic patient may not be under the influence of alcohol but, instead, may be suffering from alcohol **withdrawal.** This can be a severe reaction occurring when the patient cannot obtain alcohol, is too sick to drink alcohol, or has decided to quit drinking suddenly. The alcohol-withdrawal patient may experience seizures or **delirium tremens (DTs),** a condition characterized by sweating, trembling, anxiety, and hallucinations. In some cases, alcohol withdrawal can be fatal.

Signs of alcohol withdrawal include the following:

- Confusion and restlessness
- Unusual behavior, to the point of demonstrating "insane" behavior
- Hallucinations
- Gross tremor (obvious shaking) of the hands
- Profuse sweating
- Seizures (common and often very serious)

NOTE THAT ALL PATIENTS WITH SEIZURES OR DTs MUST BE TRANSPORTED TO A MEDICAL FACILITY AS SOON AS POSSIBLE. ■

NOTE

Be on the alert for signs—such as depressed vital signs—that the patient has mixed alcohol and drugs. Also, when interviewing the intoxicated patient or the patient suffering from alcohol withdrawal, do not begin by asking the patient if he is taking drugs. He may react to this question as if you are gathering evidence of a crime. Ask if any medications have been taken while drinking. If necessary, when you are certain that the patient knows you are concerned about his well-being, you can repeat the question using the word drugs.

PATIENT CARE

ALCOHOL ABUSE

Since alcohol abuse patients often vomit, take Standard Precautions, including gloves, mask, and protective eyewear as necessary. To provide basic care for the intoxicated patient and the patient suffering alcohol withdrawal, follow these steps:

1. Stay alert for airway and respiratory problems. Be prepared to perform airway maintenance, suctioning, and positioning of the patient should the patient lose consciousness, seize, or vomit. Help the patient during vomiting so that vomitus will not be aspirated. Have a rigid-tip suction device ready. Provide oxygen and assist respirations as needed.
2. Be alert for changes in mental status as alcohol is absorbed into the bloodstream. Talk to the patient in an effort to keep him as alert as possible.
3. Monitor vital signs.
4. Treat for shock.
5. Protect the patient from self-injury. Use restraint as authorized by your EMS system. Request assistance from law enforcement if needed. Protect yourself and your crew.
6. Stay alert for seizures.
7. Transport the patient to a medical facility if indicated. ■

NOTE

In some systems, patients under the influence of alcohol who are not suffering from a medical emergency or apparent injury are not transported. They are given over to the police. This may not be wise since some patients having an alcohol-related emergency may die if they don't receive additional care. In addition, EMS personnel may have missed a medical problem or injury. Remember that the patient's condition may worsen as the alcohol continues to be absorbed by his system. Be especially careful of patients with even minor head injuries, since subdural hematoma (see Chapter 29, "Injuries to the Head and Spine") is common in alcoholics.

Also note that A PATIENT UNDER THE INFLUENCE OF ALCOHOL CANNOT MAKE AN INFORMED REFUSAL OF TREATMENT OR TRANSPORT. If the patient refuses treatment or transport, you should nevertheless treat and arrange for transport of the patient as necessary on the basis of implied consent. Document this in your prehospital care report.

Substance Abuse

Substance abuse is a term that indicates a chemical substance is being taken for other than therapeutic (medical) reasons. Many substances have legitimate purposes when used properly. When these same substances are abused, the results can be devastating.

Individuals who abuse drugs and other chemical substances should be considered to have an illness. They have the right to the same professional emergency care as any other patient.

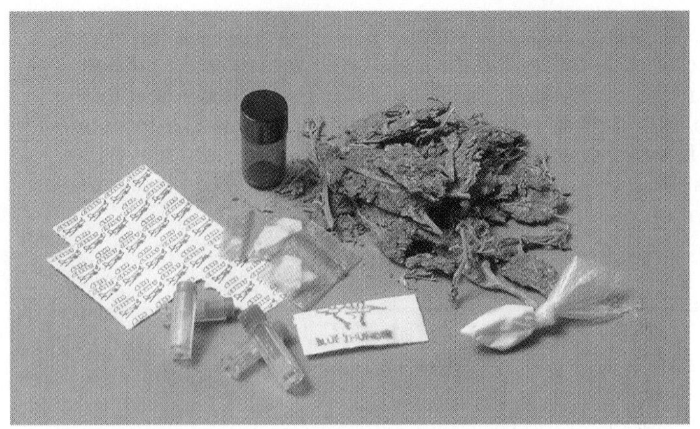

Figure 21-3 • Substances often abused.

The most common drugs and chemical substances that are abused and can lead to problems requiring an EMS response (Figure 21-3) can be classified as uppers, downers, narcotics, hallucinogens, and volatile chemicals.

uppers
stimulants such as amphetamines that affect the central nervous system to excite the user.

downers
depressants, such as barbiturates, that depress the central nervous system, often used to bring on a more relaxed state of mind.

narcotics
a class of drugs that affect the nervous system and change many normal body activities. Their legal use is for the relief of pain. Illicit use is to produce an intense state of relaxation.

hallucinogens (huh-LOO-sin-uh-jens)
mind-affecting or mind-altering drugs that act on the central nervous system to produce excitement and distortion of perceptions.

volatile chemicals
vaporizing compounds, such as cleaning fluid, that are breathed in by the abuser to produce a "high."

- **Uppers** are stimulants that affect the nervous system and excite the user. Many abusers use these drugs in an attempt to relieve fatigue or to create feelings of well-being. Examples are caffeine, amphetamines, and cocaine. Cocaine may be "snorted," smoked, or injected. Other stimulants are frequently in pill form.
- **Downers** have a depressant effect on the central nervous system. This type of drug may be used as a relaxing agent, sleeping pill, or tranquilizer. Barbiturates are an example, usually in pill or capsule form. One example of a downer that you may encounter on an EMS call is Rohypnol (flunitrazepam), also known as "Roofies." Because it is colorless, odorless, and tasteless and has been put into unsuspecting people's drinks, it has become known as a "date rape" drug. Another downer you may see is GHB (gammahydroxybutyrate), also known as Georgia Home Boy or goop. In addition to depressing the central nervous system, it produces a sense of euphoria and sometimes hallucinations. It has caused respiratory depression so severe that patients have required assisted ventilations even though some of them were still breathing.
- **Narcotics** are drugs capable of producing stupor or sleep. They are often used to relieve pain and to quiet coughing. Many drugs legitimately used for these purposes (such as codeine) are also abused, affecting the nervous system and changing many of the normal activities of the body, often producing an intense state of relaxation or feeling of well-being. A relatively new narcotic, OxyContin (oxycodone), has become a common drug of abuse. This is unfortunate, because it has done an excellent job of controlling chronic pain in patients with certain conditions. Illegal narcotics such as heroin are also commonly abused. Heroin is often injected into a vein. Other narcotics are typically in pill form. Narcotic overdoses are typically characterized by three signs: coma (or depressed level of consciousness), pinpoint pupils, and respiratory depression (slow, shallow respirations). Together, these are sometimes referred to as the opiate triad.
- **Hallucinogens** such as LSD, PCP, and certain types of mushrooms are mind-affecting drugs that act on the nervous system to produce an intense state of excitement or a distortion of the user's perceptions. This class of drugs has few legal uses. They are often eaten or dissolved in the mouth and absorbed through the mucous membranes. A newer hallucinogen is ecstasy, also known as XTC, X, or MDMA (because it is methylenedioxymethamphetamine). Often taken at "rave" parties with other drugs, this hallucinogen also has the stimulant properties of uppers.
- **Volatile chemicals** produce vapors that can be inhaled (Figure 21-4). They can give an initial "rush" and then act as a depressant on the central nervous system. Cleaning fluid, glue, model cement, and solutions used to correct typing mistakes are commonly abused volatile chemicals.

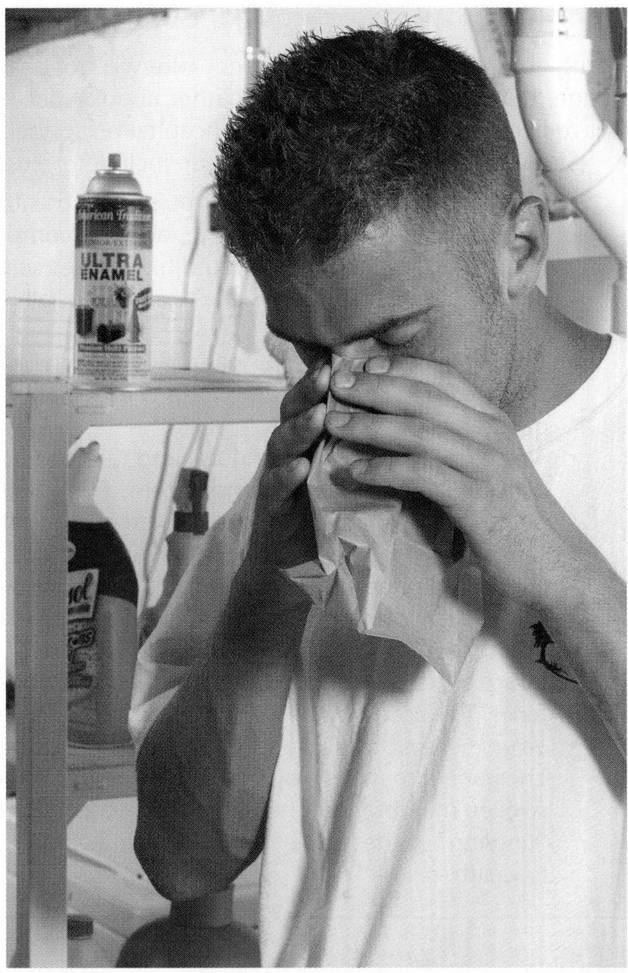

Figure 21-4 • Volatile chemicals produce vapors that can be inhaled, a practice known as "huffing."

PATIENT ASSESSMENT

SUBSTANCE ABUSE

As an EMT, you will not need to know the names of the very many abused drugs or their specific reactions. It is far more important for you to be able to detect possible drug abuse at the overdose level and to relate certain signs to certain types of drugs and drug withdrawal. Table 21-2 provides some of the names of commonly abused drugs. Do not worry about memorizing this list. Read it through so that you can place some of the more familiar drugs into categories in terms of drug type.

The signs and symptoms of substance abuse, dependency, and overdose can vary from patient to patient, even for the same drug or chemical. The problem is made more complex by the fact that many substance abusers take more than one drug or chemical at a time. Often, you will have to carefully combine the information gained from the signs and symptoms, the scene, the bystanders, and the patient in order to determine that you may be dealing with substance abuse. In many cases, you will not be able to identify the substance involved.

When questioning the patient and bystanders, you will get better results if you begin by asking if the patient has been taking any medications. Then, if necessary, ask if the patient has been taking drugs.

Some significant signs and symptoms related to specific types of drugs include those listed in the following text. These are offered to help you recognize possible

continued

drug abuse in general. Your patient care will not change as a result of this knowledge, but information you can gather about what kind of drug the patient may have been taking will be useful to hospital personnel.

Signs and symptoms of drug abuse include:

- *Uppers.* Excitement, increased pulse and breathing rates, rapid speech, dry mouth, dilated pupils, sweating, and the complaint of having gone without sleep for long periods. Repeated high doses can produce a "speed run." The patient will be restless, hyperactive, and usually very apprehensive and uncooperative.
- *Downers.* Sluggish, sleepy patient lacking typical coordination of body and speech. Pulse and breathing rates are low, often to the point of a true emergency.
- *Narcotics.* Reduced rate of pulse and rate and depth of breathing, often seen with a lowering of skin temperature. The pupils are constricted, often pinpoint in size. The muscles are relaxed and sweating is profuse. The patient is very sleepy and does not wish to do anything. In overdoses, coma is common. Respiratory arrest or cardiac arrest may develop rapidly.
- *Hallucinogens.* Fast pulse rate, dilated pupils, and a flushed face. The patient often "sees" or "hears" things, has little concept of real time, and may not be aware of the true environment. Often what he says makes no sense to the listener. The user may become aggressive or be very timid.
- *Volatile chemicals.* Dazed or showing temporary loss of contact with reality. The patient may develop coma. The linings of the nose and mouth may show swollen membranes. The patient may complain of a "funny numb feeling" or "tingling" inside the head. Changes in heart rhythm can occur. This can lead to death. ■

NOTE

When reading the just-listed signs and symptoms of drug abuse, you will have noticed that many of the indications are similar to those for quite a few other medical emergencies. As an EMT, you must never assume drug abuse is occurring by itself. You must be on the alert for medical emergencies, injuries, and combinations of drug abuse problems and other emergencies.

In addition to the effects of long-term drug use and overdose, you may encounter cases of severe drug withdrawal. Withdrawal occurs when the long-term user of certain drugs such as narcotics suddenly stops taking the drug. As in reactions to the use of various drugs, withdrawal varies from patient to patient and from drug to drug.

In most cases of drug withdrawal, you may see:

- ***Shaking***
- ***Anxiety***
- ***Nausea***
- ***Confusion and irritability***
- ***Hallucinations (both visual and auditory—"seeing things" or "hearing things")***
- ***Profuse sweating***
- ***Increased pulse and breathing rates***

TABLE 21-2 • Commonly Abused Drugs

UPPERS	DOWNERS	NARCOTICS	MIND-ALTERING DRUGS	VOLATILE CHEMICALS
AMPHETAMINE (Benzedrine, bennies, pep pills, ups, uppers, cartwheels) BIPHETAMINE (bam) COCAINE (coke, snow, crack) DESOXYN (black beauties) DEXTROAMPHETAMINE (dexies, Dexedrine) METHAMPHETAMINE (speed, crank, meth, crystal, diet pills, Methedrine) METHYLPHENIDATE (Ritalin) PRELUDIN	AMOBARBITAL (blue devils, downers barbs, Amytal) BARBITURATES (downers, dolls, barbs, rainbows) CHLORAL HYDRATE (knockout drops, Noctec) METHAQUALONE (Quaalude, ludes, Sopor, sopors) NONBARBITURATE SEDATIVES (various tranquilizers and sleeping pills: Valium or diazepam, Miltown, Equanil, meprobamate, Thorazine, Compazine, Librium or chlordiazepoxide, reserpine, Tranxene or chlorazepate and other benzodiazepines) PARALDEHYDE PENTOBARBITAL (yellow jackets, barbs, Nembutal) PHENOBARBITAL (goofballs, phennies, barbs) SECOBARBITAL (red devils, barbs, Seconal)	CODEINE (often in cough syrup) DEMEROL DILAUDID FENTANYL (Sublimaze) HEROIN ("H," horse, junk, smack, stuff) METHADONE (dolly) MORPHINE OPIUM (op, poppy) MEPERIDINE (Demerol) PAREGORIC (contains opium) TYLENOL WITH CODEINE (1, 2, 3, 4)	*Hallucinogenic:* DMT LSD (acid, sunshine) MESCALINE (peyote, mesc) MORNING GLORY SEEDS PCP (angel dust, hog, peace pills) PSILOCYBIN (magic mushrooms) STP (serenity, tranquility, peace) *Nonhallucinogenic:* HASH MARIJUANA (grass, pot, tea, wood, dope) THC	AMYL NITRATE (snappers, poppers) BUTYL NITRATE (Locker Room, Rush) CLEANING FLUID (carbon tetrachloride) FURNITURE POLISH GASOLINE GLUE HAIR SPRAY NAIL POLISH REMOVER PAINT THINNER TYPEWRITING CORRECTION FLUIDS

PATIENT CARE

SUBSTANCE ABUSE

Your care for the drug-abuse patient will be basically the same for all drugs and will not change unless you are so ordered by medical direction. When providing care for substance-abuse patients, make certain that you are safe and identify yourself as an EMT to the patient and bystanders. Since these patients often vomit, take Standard Precautions, including gloves, mask, and protective eyewear as necessary.

Emergency care includes the following:

1. Perform an initial assessment. Provide basic life support measures if required.
2. Be alert for airway problems and inadequate respirations or respiratory arrest. Provide oxygen and assist ventilations if needed.
3. Treat for shock. (Treatment for shock will be discussed in Chapter 26, "Bleeding and Shock".)
4. Talk to the patient to gain his confidence and to help maintain his level of responsiveness. Use his name often, maintain eye contact, and speak directly to the patient.

continued

PATIENT CARE *(continued)*

5. Perform a rapid trauma exam or detailed physical exam to assess for signs of injury to all parts of the body. Assess carefully for signs of head injury.
6. Look for gross soft-tissue damage on the extremities resulting from the injection of drugs ("tracks"). Tracks usually appear as darkened or red areas of scar tissue or scabs over veins.
7. Protect the patient from self-injury and attempting to hurt others. Use restraint as authorized by your EMS system. Request assistance from law enforcement if needed.
8. Transport the patient as soon as possible.
9. Contact medical direction according to local protocols.
10. Perform ongoing assessment with monitoring of vital signs. Stay alert for seizures, and be on guard for vomiting that could obstruct the airway.
11. Continue to reassure the patient throughout all phases of care. ■

NOTE

Many drug abusers may appear calm at first and then become violent as time passes. Always be on the alert and ready to protect yourself. If the patient creates an unsafe scene and you are not a trained law enforcement officer, GET OUT and find a safe place until the police arrive.

When dealing with drug abuse, you must also protect yourself from the substance itself. Many hallucinogens can be absorbed through the skin and mucous membranes. Intravenous drug users may possess hypodermic syringes, which pose a hazard of infectious disease transmission through accidental punctures. Take Standard Precautions and follow all infection exposure control procedures. Never touch or taste any suspected illicit substance.

CHAPTER REVIEW

SUMMARY

Poisonings and overdoses are frequent causes of medical emergencies. When responding to a poisoning or possible poisoning:

1. Perform initial assessment and immediately treat life-threatening problems. Ensure an open airway. Administer high-concentration oxygen if the poison was inhaled or injected.
2. Perform a focused history and physical exam, including baseline vital signs. Find out if the poison was ingested, inhaled, absorbed, or injected; what substance was involved; how much poison was taken in; when and over how long a period exposure took place; what interventions others have already done; and what effects the patient experienced.
3. Consult medical direction. As directed, administer activated charcoal or water or milk for ingested poisons. Remove the patient who has inhaled a poison from the environment and administer high-concentration oxygen; remove poisons from the skin by brushing off or diluting.
4. Transport the patient with all containers, bottles, and labels from the substance.
5. Perform ongoing assessment en route.
6. Carefully document all information about the poisoning, interventions, and the patient's responses.

KEY TERMS

absorbed poisons poisons that are taken into the body through unbroken skin.

activated charcoal a substance that adsorbs many poisons and prevents them from being absorbed by the body.

antidote a substance that will neutralize the poison or its effects.

delirium tremens (duh-LEER-e-um TREM-uns) **(DTs)** a severe reaction that can be part of alcohol withdrawal, characterized by sweating, trembling, anxiety, and hallucinations. Severe alcohol withdrawal with the DTs can lead to death if untreated.

dilution (di-LU-shun) thinning down or weakening by mixing with something else. Ingested poisons are sometimes diluted by drinking water or milk.

downers depressants, such as barbiturates, that depress the central nervous system, often used to bring on a more relaxed state of mind.

hallucinogens (huh-LOO-sin-uh-jens) mind-affecting or mind-altering drugs that act on the central nervous system to produce excitement and distortion of perceptions.

ingested poisons poisons that are swallowed.

inhaled poisons poisons that are breathed in.

injected poisons poisons that are inserted through the skin, for example by needle, snake fangs, or insect stinger.

narcotics a class of drugs that affect the nervous system and change many normal body activities. Their legal use is for the relief of pain. Illicit use is to produce an intense state of relaxation.

poison any substance that can harm the body by altering cell structure or functions.

toxin a poisonous substance secreted by bacteria, plants, or animals.

uppers stimulants such as amphetamines that affect the central nervous system to excite the user.

volatile chemicals vaporizing compounds, such as cleaning fluid, that are breathed in by the abuser to produce a "high."

withdrawal referring to alcohol or drug withdrawal in which the patient's body reacts severely when deprived of the abused substance.

REVIEW QUESTIONS

1. What are four ways in which a poison can be taken into the body? (pp. 491–492)
2. What is the sequence of assessment steps in cases of poisoning? (pp. 491, 493, 498–499, 501, 502, 506, 509–510)
3. What information must you gather in a case of poisoning before contacting medical direction? (pp. 493, 498–499, 502)
4. What are the emergency care steps for ingested poisoning? (pp. 495, 497–498)
5. What are the emergency care steps for inhaled poisoning? For absorbed poisoning? (pp. 499, 500, 502, 504)

CRITICAL THINKING

- A local farmer calls 911, concerned because one of his farm hands has tried to clean up some spilled pesticide powder with his hands. On arrival, you find that the patient insists he has brushed all the powder off, feels fine, and doesn't need to go to the hospital. As he talks, he continues to make brushing motions at his jeans on which you can see the marks of a powdery residue. How do you manage the situation?

MEDIA RESOURCES

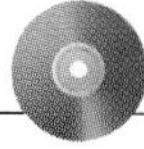

See the Student CD at the back of this book for quizzes, a case study activity, and other features related to this chapter. In particular, take a look at the animation on the use of activated charcoal in treating poisoning emergencies. Also, visit the Companion Website for *Emergency Care* at **www.prenhall.com/limmer**, where you will find additional reinforcement and links to other resources.

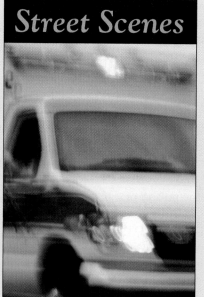

Street Scenes

You and your partner are assigned to the night shift when you are dispatched out for a "possible poisoning." You arrive on scene within 4 minutes to find a 20-year-old female sitting on the couch with a small child in her arms. The female, Anna Prince, states that she is the child's mother and she believes the child has ingested some lamp oil. The child's name is Maria, and she is 8 months old. Anna states, "I was doing the dishes when I turned around and saw Maria with the oil candle in her hands. I don't know how much she drank or how much she spilled." Maria is crying and coughing excessively, but she is alert and responds to her mother. Her skin is warm, dry, and pink. You also notice that there is some lamp oil on the front of Maria's shirt.

Street Scene Questions

1. What questions would you ask the patient's mother next?
2. What signs or symptoms should you inquire about?

You continue to gather information about the situation and discover that the time of exposure occurred approximately 3 to 4 minutes before 911 was activated. Anna also reports that she neither has the original container that the lamp oil was purchased in, nor does she remember how much oil was left in the candle. You estimate the total container size to be 100 cc and determine that half of the oil is missing. Anna also reports that she gave Maria some water, but Maria vomited after drinking a small amount.

As you continue with your assessment, you find that Maria has a clear upper airway. Her mucous membranes are pink and moist, and her pupils are equal and reactive to light. Anna states that Maria has been sick lately and that she weighed 20 pounds at her last doctor's visit. Maria is currently taking Children's Tylenol for fever reduction and has no known medical allergies. The only medical history that her mother reports is a recent fever and mild cough. Maria's current vital signs include a strong pulse of 140 and regular; respirations are 36 with crying and coughing; and an oxygen saturation of 97 percent.

Street Scene Questions

3. What treatments would you initiate?
4. Should you contact someone for advice? If yes, then who?

You provide the patient with blow-by oxygen, setting the flow rate at 10 liters per minute. You place the child in a car seat that is securely anchored to the ambulance stretcher for transport. The mother also is secured in a seat inside the ambulance. You take the lamp oil candle with you.

You contact poison control, and they advise you that the main concern for Maria is related to aspiration of the oil into the lungs. They advise you that the oil may be a petroleum product with a hydrocarbon base and that activated charcoal and syrup of ipecac are contraindicated. You also contact medical direction; they agree with the recommendations from poison control and order only supportive care.

During transport, you continually monitor your patient's airway and ventilatory status. When you repeat vital signs, respirations are 32 and slightly labored and pulse is 128, regular, and strong. As you arrive at the emergency department, Maria has stopped crying but continues to cough. No other changes occur during the transport.

Street Scenes Sample Documentation

PATIENT NAME: *Maria Prince* **PATIENT AGE:** *8 months*

CHIEF COMPLAINT

Coughing, possible ingested poisoning

PAST MEDICAL HISTORY

- ☒ None
- ☐ Allergy to
- ☐ Hypertension ☐ Stroke
- ☐ Seizures ☐ Diabetes
- ☐ COPD ☐ Cardiac
- ☐ Other (List) ☐ Asthma

Recent fever with mild cough

Current Medications (List)

Children's Tylenol

VITAL SIGNS

TIME	RESP	PULSE	B.P.	MENTAL STATUS	R PUPILS L	SKIN
2051	Rate: 36 ☐ Regular ☐ Shallow ☒ Labored	Rate: 140 ☒ Regular ☐ Irregular		☑ Alert ☐ Voice ☐ Pain ☐ Unresp.	☑ Normal ☑ ☐ Dilated ☐ ☐ Constricted ☐ ☐ Sluggish ☐ ☐ No-Reaction ☐	☐ Unremarkable ☐ Cool ☐ Pale ☑ Warm ☐ Cyanotic ☐ Moist ☐ Flushed ☑ Dry ☐ Jaundiced
2056	Rate: 32 ☐ Regular ☐ Shallow ☒ Labored	Rate: 128 ☒ Regular ☐ Irregular		☑ Alert ☐ Voice ☐ Pain ☐ Unresp.	☑ Normal ☑ ☐ Dilated ☐ ☐ Constricted ☐ ☐ Sluggish ☐ ☐ No-Reaction ☐	☐ Unremarkable ☐ Cool ☐ Pale ☑ Warm ☐ Cyanotic ☐ Moist ☐ Flushed ☑ Dry ☐ Jaundiced
	Rate: ☐ Regular ☐ Shallow ☐ Labored	Rate: ☐ Regular ☐ Irregular		☐ Alert ☐ Voice ☐ Pain ☐ Unresp.	☐ Normal ☐ ☐ Dilated ☐ ☐ Constricted ☐ ☐ Sluggish ☐ ☐ No-Reaction ☐	☐ Unremarkable ☐ Cool ☐ Pale ☐ Warm ☐ Cyanotic ☐ Moist ☐ Flushed ☐ Dry ☐ Jaundiced

NARRATIVE *Responded to a possible poisoning. Upon arrival, we found an 8-month-old female in the arms of her mother. Mother stated that she "was doing the dishes when I turned around and saw Maria with an oil candle in her hands. I do not know how much she drank or how much she spilled." Mother reports child's weight as 20 pounds. Time of exposure was approximately 3-4 minutes before 9-1-1 activation. Patient received some water, which she vomited back up, prior to our arrival. Approximate amount of lamp oil ingested may have been as much as 50 cc.*

Assessment revealed a crying and coughing infant, who appeared alert and responding to her mother. Upper airway was clear. Skin was warm and dry. Mucous membranes were moist and pink. Pupils were equal and reactive to light. Vitals above.

Treatment consisted of blow-by O_2 at 10 liters per minute. During transport, patient was kept with her mother to reduce anxiety. Lamp oil also transported for identification purposes. Poison control and medical direction contacted; both recommended only airway support and continued assessment. Upon arrival at ED, patient ceased her crying, but her cough was still present. No other changes during transport.

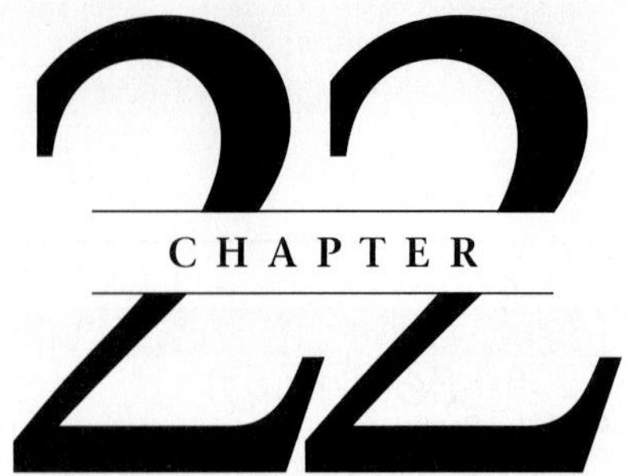

CHAPTER 22

Environmental Emergencies

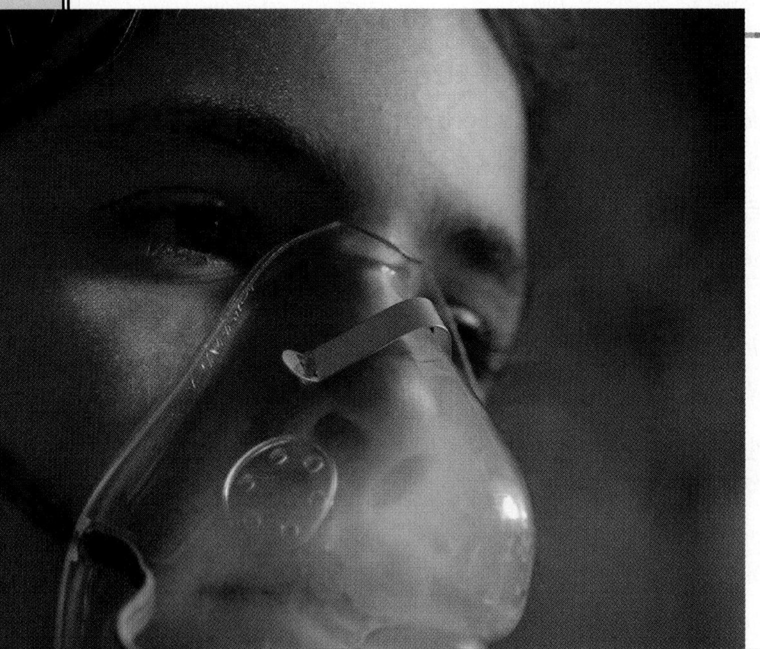

CORE CONCEPTS

The following are core concepts that will be addressed in this chapter:

- Effects of heat and cold on the body
- Treatment of conditions caused by heat and cold
- Personal safety concerns in water emergencies
- Signs, symptoms, and treatment of drowning patients
- Signs, symptoms, and treatment of patients who have experienced bites or stings
- How to document findings and care of patients with environmental emergencies

KEY TERMS

active rewarming, p. 520
air embolism, p. 534
central rewarming, p. 521
conduction, p. 517
convection, p. 518
decompression sickness, p. 534
drowning, p. 530
evaporation, p. 518
hyperthermia, p. 526
hypothermia, p. 518
local cooling, p. 523
passive rewarming, p. 520
radiation, p. 518
respiration, p. 518
toxins, p. 538
venom, p. 538
water chill, p. 518
wind chill, p. 518

DOT OBJECTIVES

*KNOWLEDGE AND ATTITUDE

4-7.1 Describe the various ways that the body loses heat. (pp. 517–518)

4-7.2 List the signs and symptoms of exposure to cold. (pp. 518–524)

4-7.3 Explain the steps in providing emergency medical care to a patient exposed to cold. (pp. 519–526)

4-7.4 List the signs and symptoms of exposure to heat. (pp. 526–528)

4-7.5 Explain the steps in providing emergency care to a patient exposed to heat. (pp. 526–528)

4-7.6 Recognize the signs and symptoms of water-related emergencies. (pp. 529–530)

4-7.7 Describe the complications of drowning. (pp. 530–534) (Scan 22-1, pp. 532–533)

4-7.8 Discuss the emergency medical care of bites and stings. (pp. 538–543)

*SKILLS

4-7.9 Demonstrate the assessment and emergency medical care of a patient with exposure to cold.

4-7.10 Demonstrate the assessment and emergency medical care of a patient with exposure to heat.

4-7.11 Demonstrate the assessment and emergency medical care of a near-drowning patient.

4-7.12 Demonstrate completing a prehospital care report for patients with environmental emergencies.

Environmental emergencies can occur in any setting—wilderness, rural, suburban, and urban areas. They include exposure to both heat and cold, drownings and other water-related injuries, and bites and stings from insects, spiders, snakes, and marine life. The keys to effective management are recognizing the patient's signs and symptoms and providing prompt and proper emergency care. However, as an EMT, you also must recognize that exposure may not be the only danger to the patient. Environmental emergencies can involve pre-existing, or cause additional, medical problems and injury.

EXPOSURE TO COLD

How the Body Loses Heat

If the environment is too cold, body heat can be lost faster than it can be generated. The body attempts to adjust by reducing perspiration and circulation to the skin—shutting down avenues by which the body usually gets rid of excess heat. Muscular activity in the form of shivering and the rate at which fuel (food) is burned within the body both increase to produce more heat. At a certain point, however, not enough heat is generated to be available to all parts of the body. This may result in damage to exposed tissues and a general reduction or cessation of body functions.

To be able to prevent or compensate for heat loss, the EMT must be aware of the ways in which a body loses heat:

- *Conduction.* The transfer of heat from one material to another through direct contact is called **conduction.** Heat will flow from a warmer material to a cooler one. Body heat transferred directly into cool air is a problem, but when the body

conduction
the transfer of heat from one material to another through direct contact.

water chill
chilling caused by conduction of heat from the body when the body or clothing is wet.

convection
carrying away of heat by currents of air or water or other gases or liquids.

wind chill
chilling caused by convection of heat from the body in the presence of air currents.

radiation
sending out energy, such as heat, in waves into space.

evaporation
the change from liquid to gas. When the body perspires or gets wet, evaporation of the perspiration or other liquid into the air has a cooling effect on the body.

respiration
breathing. During respiration, body heat is lost as warm air is exhaled from the body.

hypothermia
(HI-po-THURM-e-ah) generalized cooling that reduces body temperature below normal, life-threatening in its extreme.

NOTE *Be aware that hypothermia can develop in temperatures well above freezing.*

or clothing gets wet, **water chill** is an even greater problem because water conducts heat away from the body 25 times faster than still air. Heat loss through conduction can be a major problem when a person is lying on a cold floor or another cold surface. A person who is standing or walking around in cold weather will lose less heat than a person who is lying on the cold ground.

- *Convection.* When currents of air or water pass over the body, carrying away heat, **convection** occurs. The effects of a cold environment are worsened when moving water or air surround the body. **Wind chill** is a frequent problem. The more wind, the greater the heat loss. For example, if it is 10°F with no wind, the body will lose heat, but if there is a 20 mph wind, the amount of heat lost by the body is much greater—the same as if it were −25°F.
- *Radiation.* In conduction and convection, heat is "picked up" by the surrounding (still or moving) air or water. In **radiation,** the body's atoms and molecules send out rays of heat as they move and change. If you were in the vacuum of outer space with no air or water around to pick up heat, you would still lose heat by radiating it out into space. Most radiant heat loss occurs from a person's head and neck.
- *Evaporation.* **Evaporation** occurs when the body perspires or gets wet. As perspiration or water on the skin or clothing vaporizes, the body experiences a generalized cooling effect.
- *Respiration.* **Respiration** causes loss of body heat as a result of exhaled warm air. The amount of heat loss depends on the outside air temperature as well as the rate and depth of respirations.

Generalized Hypothermia

When cooling affects the entire body, a problem known as **hypothermia,** or generalized cooling, develops. Exposure to cold reduces body heat. With time, the body is unable to maintain its proper core (internal) temperature. If allowed to continue, hypothermia leads to death. (The stages of hypothermia are described in Table 22-1.)

Predisposing Factors

Patients with injuries, chronic illness, or certain other conditions will show the effects of cold much sooner than healthy persons. These conditions include shock (hypoperfusion), burns, head and spinal-cord injuries, generalized infection, and diabetes with hypoglycemia. Those under the influence of alcohol or other drugs also tend to be affected more rapidly and more severely than others. The unconscious patient lying on the cold ground or other cold surface is especially prone to rapid heat loss through conduction and will tend to have greater cold-related problems than one who is conscious and able to walk around.

GERIATRIC NOTE

Hypothermia is often an especially serious problem for the aged. The effects of cold temperatures on the elderly are more immediate. During the winter months, many older citizens on small fixed incomes live in unheated rooms or rooms that are kept too cool. Failing body systems, chronic illnesses, poor diets, certain medications, and a lack of exercise may combine with the cold environment to bring about hypothermia.

PEDIATRIC NOTE

Since infants and young children are small with large skin surface areas in relation to their total body mass and little body fat, they are especially prone to hypothermia. Because of their small muscle mass, infants and children do not shiver very much or at all—another reason the very young are susceptible to the cold.

TABLE 22-1 • Stages of Hypothermia

CORE BODY TEMPERATURE		SYMPTOMS
99°F–96°F	37.0°C–35.5°C	Shivering.
95°F–91°F	35.5°C–32.7°C	Intense shivering, difficulty speaking.
90°F–86°F	32.0°C–30.0°C	Shivering decreases and is replaced by strong muscular rigidity. Muscle coordination is affected and erratic or jerky movements are produced. Thinking is less clear, general comprehension is dulled, possible total amnesia. Patient generally is able to maintain the appearance of psychological contact with surroundings.
85°F–81°F	29.4°C–27.2°C	Patient becomes irrational, loses contact with environment, and drifts into stuporous state. Muscular rigidity continues. Pulse and respirations are slow and cardiac dysrhythmias may develop.
80°F–78°F	26.6°C–20.5°C	Patient loses consciousness and does not respond to spoken words. Most reflexes cease to function. Heartbeat slows further before cardiac arrest occurs.

Obvious and Subtle Exposure

At times, it is obvious that a patient has been exposed to cold and is probably suffering from hypothermia. With other patients, however, exposure is subtle—that is, not so obvious, not the first thing you may think of. Consider, for example, the elderly patient who has fallen during the night and is not discovered until morning. A broken hip or other injuries may claim your attention, but if your patient has been on the cold floor all night, he is probably also suffering from hypothermia. The patient trapped in a wrecked auto is probably suffering a variety of injuries, but if the weather is cool and extrication from the vehicle takes a while, the patient can easily develop hypothermia as well.

Consider the possibility of hypothermia in the following situations when another condition or injury may be more obvious:

- *Ethanol (alcohol) ingestion.* Has the intoxicated patient passed out on a cold floor or been wandering around outdoors in cool or cold weather?
- *Underlying illness.* Does the patient have a circulatory disorder or other condition that makes him especially susceptible to cold?
- *Overdose or poisoning.* Has the patient been lying in a cold garage or on a cold floor? Is he sweating heavily in a cool environment with evaporation causing excessive heat loss?
- *Major trauma.* Has the patient been lying on the ground or trapped in wreckage during cold weather? Is shock (hypoperfusion, or inadequate circulation of the blood) preventing parts of the body from being warmed by circulating blood?
- *Outdoor resuscitation.* Is your patient getting too cold? If your patient is a drowning victim who has been in the water, has exposure to cool water caused hypothermia?
- *Decreased ambient temperature* (for example, room temperature). Is your patient living in a home or apartment that is too cold?

GERIATRIC NOTE

Remember that older patients require an ambient temperature that would feel too warm to a younger person. If that patient's environment is slightly cool, even a temperature that might feel quite comfortable to you, consider hypothermia.

Remember that the injured patient is more susceptible to the effects of cold. Protect the patient who is entrapped or for any other reason must remain in a cool or cold environment for a period of time. The major course of action is to prevent additional body heat loss. It may be neither practical nor possible to replace wet clothing, but you can at least create a barrier to the cold with blankets, a salvage cover, an aluminized blanket, a survival blanket, or even articles of clothing. A plastic trash bag can serve as protection from wind and water. Keep in mind that the greatest area of heat loss may be the head, so provide some sort of head covering for the patient.

When the patient's injuries allow, place a blanket between his body and the cold ground. Rotate warm blankets from the heated ambulance to the patient. If the patient will remain trapped for a period of time, plug holes in the wreckage with blankets.

PATIENT ASSESSMENT

HYPOTHERMIA

Consider the impact of the following factors: air temperature, wind chill and/or water chill, the patient's age, the patient's clothing, the patient's health including underlying illness and existing injuries, how active the patient was during exposure, and possible alcohol or drug use.

The signs and symptoms of hypothermia include the following. Note that decreasing mental status and decreasing motor function both correlate with the degree of hypothermia:

- Shivering in early stages when the core body temperature is above 90°F. In severe cases shivering decreases or is absent.
- Numbness, or reduced-to-lost sense of touch.
- Stiff or rigid posture in prolonged cases.
- Drowsiness and/or unwillingness or inability to do even the simplest activities. In prolonged cases, the patient may become irrational, drift into a stuporous state, or actually remove clothing.
- Rapid breathing and rapid pulse in early stages. Slow to absent breathing and pulse in prolonged cases. Blood pressure may be low to absent.
- Loss of motor coordination, such as staggering or inability to hold things.
- Joint/muscle stiffness, or muscular rigidity.
- Decreased level of consciousness, or unconsciousness. In extreme cases, the patient has a "glassy stare."
- Cool abdominal skin temperature. (Place your hand inside the clothing with the back of your hand against the patient's abdomen.)
- Skin may appear red in early stages. In prolonged cases, skin is pale to cyanotic. In most extreme cases, some body parts are stiff and hard (frozen).

During initial assessment, be sure to check an awake patient's orientation to person, place, and time. (Can he tell you his name? Where he is? What day it is?) Perform a focused history and physical exam to help you estimate the extent of hypothermia. Assume severe hypothermia if shivering is absent. ■

passive rewarming covering a hypothermic patient and taking other steps to prevent further heat loss and help the body rewarm itself.

active rewarming application of an external heat source to rewarm the body of a hypothermic patient.

Passive and Active Rewarming

Passive rewarming allows the body to rewarm itself. It involves simply covering the patient and taking other steps, including removal of wet clothing, to prevent further heat loss. This allows the body to rewarm itself. **Active rewarming** includes application of an external heat source to the body. All EMS systems permit passive rewarming.

Although some allow the active rewarming of a hypothermic patient who is alert and responding appropriately, many do not. Follow local protocols.

Active rewarming can prove to be a dangerous process if the patient's condition is more serious than believed. If you are allowed to rewarm a patient with hypothermia who is alert and responding appropriately, do not delay transport. Rewarm the patient while en route. *The emergency care steps that follow assume a protocol that permits active rewarming of a patient who is alert and responding appropriately. Follow your local protocols.*

PATIENT CARE

HYPOTHERMIC PATIENT ALERT AND RESPONDING APPROPRIATELY

For the hypothermic patient who is alert and responding appropriately, proceed with active rewarming:

1. Remove all of the patient's wet clothing. Keep the patient dry, dress the patient in dry clothing, or wrap in dry, warm blankets. Keep the patient still and handle very gently. Do not allow the patient to walk or exert himself. Do not massage extremities.
2. During transport, actively rewarm the patient. Gently apply heat to the patient's body in the form of heat packs, hot water bottles, electric heating pads, warm air, radiated heat, and even your own body heat. *Do not warm the patient too quickly.* Rapid warming will circulate peripherally stagnated cold blood and rapidly cool the vital central areas of the body, possibly causing cardiac arrest. If transport is delayed, move the patient to a warm environment if at all possible.
3. Provide care for shock. Provide oxygen, warmed and humidified if possible.
4. Give the alert patient warm liquids slowly. When warm fluids are given too quickly, circulation patterns change, sending blood away from the core to the skin and extremities. Do not allow the patient to eat or drink stimulants.
5. Except in the mildest of cases (shivering), transport the patient. Continue to provide high-concentration oxygen and monitor vital signs. *Never allow a patient to remain in, or return to, a cold environment.*

   Take the following precautions when actively rewarming a patient:

   - Rewarm the patient slowly. Handle the patient with great care, just as if there were unstabilized cervical-spine injuries.
   - Use **central rewarming.** Heat should be applied to the lateral chest, neck, armpits, and groin. You must avoid rewarming the limbs. If they are warmed first, blood will collect in the extremities due to vasodilation (dilation of blood vessels), possibly causing a fatal form of shock (see Chapter 26, "Bleeding and Shock"). If you rewarm the trunk and leave the lower extremities exposed, you can control the rewarming process and help prevent most of the problems associated with the procedure.
   - If transport must be delayed, a warm bath is very helpful, but keep the patient alert enough so that he does not drown. Do not warm the patient too quickly.
   - Keep the patient at rest. Do not allow the patient to walk, and avoid rough handling. Such activity may set off severe heart problems, including ventricular fibrillation. Since the blood is coldest in the extremities, exercise or unnecessary movement could quickly circulate the cold blood and lower the core body temperature. ■

central rewarming application of heat to the lateral chest, neck, armpits, and groin of a hypothermic patient.

POINT OF VIEW

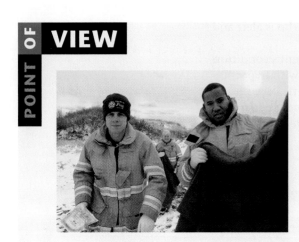

"I was riding my horse on the beach. It is a wonderful feeling. Well, it was until I got thrown. Now, I've been thrown before and you get back up. This time I broke bones.

"To make it worse, it was winter. No one was around.

"I shivered for a while. I yelled and yelled. I tried to move but no luck. Then I stopped shivering and started to get tired. It is funny looking back on that day. I kind of relaxed there at the end. Now I know that means I was on the final glide path. I was heading out.

"Someone finally saw the horse just standing there and came over to figure out why. By that time I was like an ice cube.

"I remember the EMTs coming along and warming me up. Blanket after blanket and the heat in the ambulance was blasting. Those guys must've been boiling. I'm very thankful for them—and for the person that finally called for help. Without them I wouldn't be telling this story."

PATIENT CARE

HYPOTHERMIC PATIENT UNRESPONSIVE OR NOT RESPONDING APPROPRIATELY

A patient who is unresponsive or not responding appropriately has severe hypothermia. For this patient, provide passive rewarming. Do not try to actively rewarm the patient with severe hypothermia. Remove the patient from the environment and protect him from further heat loss. Active rewarming may cause the patient to develop ventricular fibrillation.

For the patient with severe hypothermia, you should:

1. Ensure an open airway.
2. Provide high-concentration oxygen that has been passed through a warm-water humidifier. If necessary, the oxygen that has been kept warm in the ambulance passenger compartment can be used. If there is no other choice, oxygen from a cold cylinder may be used.
3. Wrap the patient in blankets. If available, use insulating blankets. Handle the patient as gently as possible. Rough handling may cause ventricular fibrillation. Do not allow the patient to eat or drink stimulants. Do not massage extremities.
4. Transport immediately. ■

Extreme Hypothermia

In cases of extreme hypothermia, you will find the patient unconscious with no discernible vital signs. The heart rate can slow to less than 10 beats per minute, and the patient will feel very cold to your touch (core body temperature may be below 80°F). Even so, it is possible that the patient is still alive! Provide emergency care as follows:

- Assess the carotid pulse for 30 to 45 seconds. If there is no pulse, start CPR immediately and prepare to apply the AED.
- If there is a pulse, follow the care steps for a patient who is unresponsive or not responding appropriately as previously listed.

Because the hypothermic patient may not reach biological death for over 30 minutes, the hospital staff will not pronounce a patient dead until after he is rewarmed and resuscitative measures have been applied. This means you cannot assume that a severe hypothermia patient is dead on the basis of body temperature and lack of vital signs. As medical personnel point out, "You're not dead until you're warm and dead!"

Localized Cold Injuries

Cold-related emergencies also can result from **local cooling.** Local cooling injuries are those affecting particular (local) parts of the body. Localized cold injuries are classified as early or superficial, and late or deep.

local cooling
cooling or freezing of particular (local) parts of the body.

Local cooling most commonly affects the ears, nose, face, hands, and the feet and toes. When a part of the body is exposed to intense cold, blood flow to that part is limited by the constriction of blood vessels. When this happens, tissues freeze. Ice crystals can form in the skin, and in the most severe cases, gangrene (localized tissue death) can set in and ultimately lead to the loss of the body part.

As you read the following pages, notice how the signs and symptoms of early or superficial cold injuries are progressive. First, the exposed skin reddens in light-skinned individuals. In dark-skinned individuals the skin color lightens and approaches a blanched (reduced-color or whitened) condition. As exposure continues, the skin takes on a gray or white blotchy appearance. Exposed skin becomes numb because of reduced circulation. If the freezing process continues, all sensation is lost and the skin becomes dead white.

PATIENT ASSESSMENT

EARLY OR SUPERFICIAL LOCAL COLD INJURY

Early or superficial local cold injuries (sometimes called *frostnip*) are brought about by direct contact with a cold object or exposure to cold air. Wind chill and water chill also can be major factors. Tissue damage is minor and response to care is good. The tip of the nose, tips of the ears, upper cheeks, and fingers (all areas that are usually exposed) are most susceptible to early or superficial local cold injuries. The injury, as its name suggests, is localized with clear demarcation of its limits. Patients are often unaware of the onset of an early local cold injury until someone indicates that there is something unusual about the person's skin color. Signs and symptoms include:

- Affected area in patients with light skin reddens; dark skin lightens. Both then blanch (whiten). Once blanching begins, the color change can take place very quickly.
- Affected area feels numb to the patient. ■

PATIENT CARE

EARLY OR SUPERFICIAL LOCAL COLD INJURY

Emergency care for early local cold injury is as follows:

1. Get the patient out of the cold environment.
2. Warm the affected area.
3. If the injury is to an extremity, splint and cover it. Do not rub or massage, and do not re-expose to the cold.

Usually, the patient can apply warmth from his own bare hands, blow warm air on the site, or, if the fingers are involved, hold them in the armpits. During recovery from an early local cold injury, the patient may complain about tingling or burning sensations, which is normal. If the condition does not respond to this simple care, begin to treat for a late or deep local cold injury. ■

PATIENT ASSESSMENT

LATE OR DEEP LOCAL COLD INJURY

Late or deep local cold injury (also known as *frostbite*) develops if an early or superficial local cold injury goes untreated. In late or deep local cold injury, the skin and subcutaneous layers of the body part are affected. Muscles, bones, deep blood vessels, and organ membranes can become frozen. Signs and symptoms include:

- Affected skin appears white and waxy. When the condition progresses to actual freezing, the skin turns mottled or blotchy, and the color turns from white to grayish yellow and finally to grayish blue. Swelling and blistering may occur (Figure 22-1).
- Affected area feels frozen, but only on the surface. The tissue below the surface is still soft and has its normal resilience, or "bounce." With freezing, the tissues are not resilient and feel frozen to the touch. (*Note:* Do not squeeze or poke the tissue. The condition of the deeper tissues can be determined by feeling gently. Do the assessment as if the affected area had a fractured bone.) ■

PATIENT CARE

LATE OR DEEP LOCAL COLD INJURY

Initial emergency care for late or deep local cold injury—frostbite and freezing—is as follows:

1. Administer high-concentration oxygen.
2. Transport to a medical facility without delay, protecting the frostbitten or frozen area by covering it and handling it as gently as possible.
3. If transport must be delayed, get the patient indoors and keep him warm. Do not allow the patient to drink alcohol or smoke, because constriction of blood vessels and decreased circulation to the injured tissues may result. Rewarm the frozen part as per local protocol, or request instructions from medical direction. ■

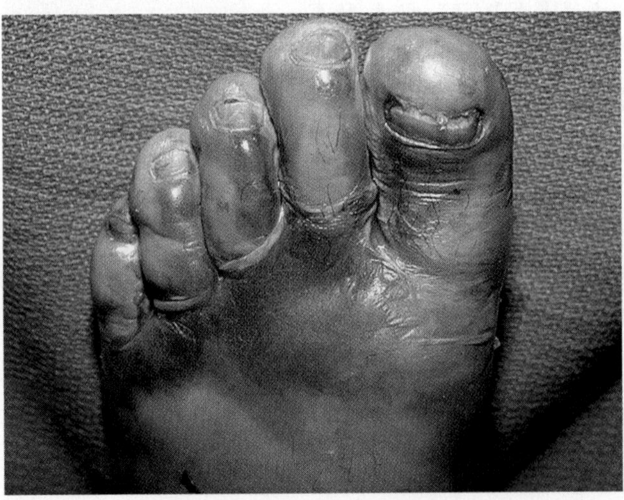

Figure 22-1 • Local cold injuries. *(© Charles Stewart, M.D. and Associates)*

NOTE

Never listen to myths and folktales about the care of frostbite. Never rub a frostbitten or frozen area. Never rub snow on a frostbitten or frozen area. There are ice crystals at the capillary level; rubbing the injury site may cause them to seriously damage the already injured tissues. Do not break blisters or massage the injured area. Do not allow the patient to walk on an affected extremity. Do not thaw a frozen limb if there is any chance it will be refrozen.

Active Rapid Rewarming of Frozen Parts

Active rewarming of frozen parts is seldom recommended. The chance of permanently injuring frozen tissues with active rewarming is too great. Consider it only if local protocols recommend it, if you are instructed to do so by medical direction, or if transport will be severely delayed and you cannot reach medical direction for instructions. If you are in a situation where you must attempt rewarming without instructions from a physician, follow the procedure described here.

You will need warm water and a container in which you can immerse the entire site of injury without the limb touching the sides or bottom of the container. If you cannot find a suitable container, fashion one from a plastic bag supported by a cardboard box or wooden crate (Figure 22-2). Proceed as follows:

1. Heat water to between 100°F and 105°F. You should be able to put your finger into the water without experiencing discomfort.
2. Fill the container with the heated water and prepare the injured part by removing clothing, jewelry, bands, or straps. Thawed areas often swell, so you need to remove potentially constricting items beforehand.
3. Fully immerse the injured part. Do not allow the injured area to touch the sides or bottom of the container. Do not place any pressure on the affected part. Continuously stir the water. When the water cools below 100°F, remove the affected part and add more warm water. The patient may complain of moderate pain as the affected area rewarms or he may experience intense pain. Pain is usually a good indicator of successful rewarming.
4. If you complete rewarming of the part (it no longer feels frozen and is turning red or blue), gently dry the affected area and apply a dry sterile dressing. Place dry sterile dressings between fingers and toes before dressing hands and feet. Next, cover the site

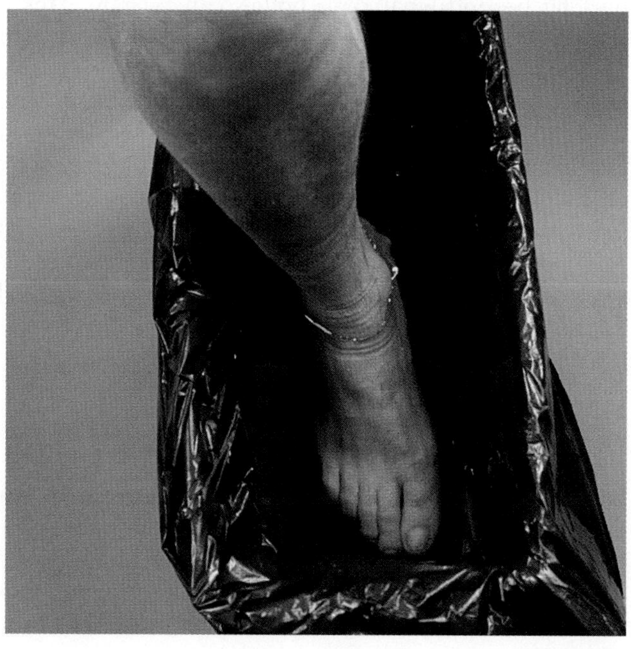

Figure 22-2 • Rewarming the frozen part.

with blankets or whatever is available to keep the area warm. Do not allow these coverings to come in direct contact with the injured area or to put pressure on the site. First try to build some sort of framework on which the coverings can be placed.

5. Keep the patient at rest. Do not allow the patient to walk if a lower extremity has been frostbitten or frozen.
6. Make certain that you keep the entire patient as warm as possible without overheating. Cover the patient's head with a towel or small blanket to reduce heat loss. Leave the patient's face exposed.
7. Continue to monitor the patient.
8. Assist circulation according to local protocol (some systems recommend rhythmically and carefully raising and lowering the affected limb).
9. Do not allow the limb to refreeze.
10. Transport as soon as possible with the affected limb slightly elevated.

EXPOSURE TO HEAT

Effects of Heat on the Body

The body generates heat as a result of its constant internal chemical processes. A certain amount of this heat is required to maintain normal body temperature. Any heat that is not needed for temperature maintenance must be lost from the body. If it is not, **hyperthermia,** an abnormally high body temperature, will be the result. Left unchecked, it will lead to death. Heat and humidity are often associated with hyperthermia.

hyperthermia (HI-per-THURM-e-ah) an increase in body temperature above normal, life-threatening in its extreme.

As you learned earlier, heat is lost through the lungs or the skin. Mechanisms of heat loss include conduction, convection, radiation, evaporation, and respiration. Consider what can happen to the body in a hot environment. Air being inhaled is warm, possibly warmer than the air being exhaled. The skin may absorb more heat than it loses. When high humidity is added, the evaporation of perspiration slows. To make things even more difficult, consider all this in an environment that lacks circulating air or a breeze, which would increase convection and evaporative heat loss.

Since evaporative heat loss is reduced in a humid environment, moist heat can produce dramatic body changes in a short time. Moist heat usually tires people quickly, frequently stopping them from harming themselves through overexertion. Dry heat, in contrast, often deceives people. They continue to work or remain exposed to excess heat far beyond what their bodies can tolerate. This is why you may see problems caused by dry heat exposure more often than those seen in moist heat exposure.

The same rules of care apply to heat emergencies as to any other emergency. You will need to perform the appropriate steps of assessment, remaining alert for problems other than those related to heat. Collapse due to heat exposure, for example, may result in a fall that can fracture bones. Pre-existing conditions such as dehydration, diabetes, fever, fatigue, high blood pressure, heart disease, lung problems, or obesity may hasten or intensify the effects of heat exposure, as will ingestion of alcohol and other drugs.

Age, diseases, and existing injuries all must be considered. The elderly may be affected by poor thermoregulation, prescription medications, and lack of mobility. Newborns and infants also may have poor thermoregulation. Always consider the problem to be greater if the patient is a child or elderly person who is injured or living with a chronic disease.

Patient with Moist, Pale, Normal-to-Cool Skin

Prolonged exposure to excessive heat can create an emergency in which the patient presents with moist pale skin that may feel normal or cool to the touch. The individual perspires heavily, often drinking large quantities of water. As sweating continues, salts are lost, bringing on painful muscle cramps (sometimes called *heat cramps*). A person who is actively exercising can lose more than a liter of perspiration per hour.

Healthy individuals who have been exposed to excessive heat while working or exercising may experience a form of shock brought about by fluid and salt loss. This condition, sometimes known as *heat exhaustion,* is often seen among firefighters, construction workers, dock workers, and those employed in poorly ventilated warehouses. It is a particular problem during prolonged heat waves.

PATIENT ASSESSMENT

HEAT EMERGENCY PATIENT WITH MOIST, PALE, NORMAL-TO-COOL SKIN

Signs and symptoms of a heat emergency patient with moist, pale, and normal-to-cool skin include:

- Muscular cramps, usually in the legs and abdomen
- Weakness or exhaustion, sometimes dizziness or periods of faintness
- Rapid, shallow breathing
- Weak pulse
- Heavy perspiration
- Loss of consciousness is possible, but is usually brief if it occurs. ■

PATIENT CARE

HEAT EMERGENCY PATIENT WITH MOIST, PALE, NORMAL-TO-COOL SKIN

Emergency care of a heat emergency patient with moist, pale, and normal-to-cool skin includes the following:

1. Remove the patient from the hot environment and place in a cool environment (such as in shade or an air-conditioned ambulance).
2. Administer oxygen by nonrebreather mask at 15 liters per minute.
3. Loosen or remove clothing to cool the patient by fanning without chilling him. Watch for shivering.
4. Put patient in a supine position with legs elevated. Keep him at rest.
5. If the patient is responsive and not nauseated, have him drink small sips of water. If this causes nausea or vomiting, do not give any more water. Be alert for vomiting and airway problems. If the patient is unresponsive or vomiting, do not give water. Transport to the hospital with the patient on his left side.
6. If the patient experiences muscular cramps, apply moist towels over cramped muscles.
7. Transport. ■

Patient with Hot and Dry or Moist Skin

When a person's temperature-regulating mechanisms fail and the body cannot rid itself of excessive heat, you will see a patient with hot, dry, or possibly moist skin. When the skin is hot—whether dry or moist—this is a true emergency. This condition is sometimes known as *heat stroke.* The problem is compounded when, in response to loss of fluid and salt, the patient stops sweating, which prevents heat loss through evaporation. Athletes, laborers, and others who exercise or work in hot environments commonly develop this condition. So do the elderly who live in poorly ventilated apartments without air conditioning, and children left in cars with the windows rolled up. More cases of patients with hot, dry skin are reported on hot, humid days. However, many cases occur from exposure to dry heat.

PATIENT ASSESSMENT

HEAT EMERGENCY PATIENT WITH HOT AND DRY OR MOIST SKIN

Signs and symptoms of a heat emergency patient with hot and dry or hot and moist skin include:

- Rapid, shallow breathing
- Full and rapid pulse
- Generalized weakness
- Little or no perspiration
- Loss of consciousness or altered mental status
- Dilated pupils
- Seizures may be seen; no muscle cramps ■

PATIENT CARE

HEAT EMERGENCY PATIENT WITH HOT AND DRY OR MOIST SKIN

Emergency care of a heat emergency patient with hot and dry or hot and moist skin is as follows (Figure 22-3):

1. Remove the patient from the hot environment and place him in a cool environment (in the ambulance with air conditioner running on high).
2. Remove clothing. Apply cool packs to neck, groin, and armpits. Keep the skin wet by applying water by sponge or wet towels. Fan aggressively.
3. Administer oxygen by nonrebreather mask at 15 liters per minute.
4. Transport immediately. Should transport be delayed, find a tub or container, immerse the patient up to the neck in cooled water, and monitor vital signs throughout the process. ■

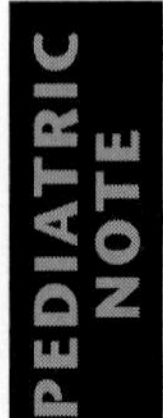

For infants or young children, cooling is started using tepid (lukewarm) water. This water can then be replaced with cooler water at the recommendation of medical direction.

Beware of what you are told by some patients. They may not believe heat emergencies are serious. Many simply want to return to work. Nevertheless, conduct a thorough initial assessment plus a focused history and physical exam. If you have any doubts, tell the patient why he should be transported and seek his permission to do so. You may have to spend a little time with some patients to gain their confidence.

WATER-RELATED EMERGENCIES

Water-Related Accidents

Drowning is the first thing people think of in connection with water-related accidents. However, there are many types of injuries resulting from many types of accidents that can occur on or in the water. Boating, water-skiing, wind surfing, jet-skiing, diving, and scuba-diving accidents can produce fractured bones, bleeding, soft-tissue injuries, and

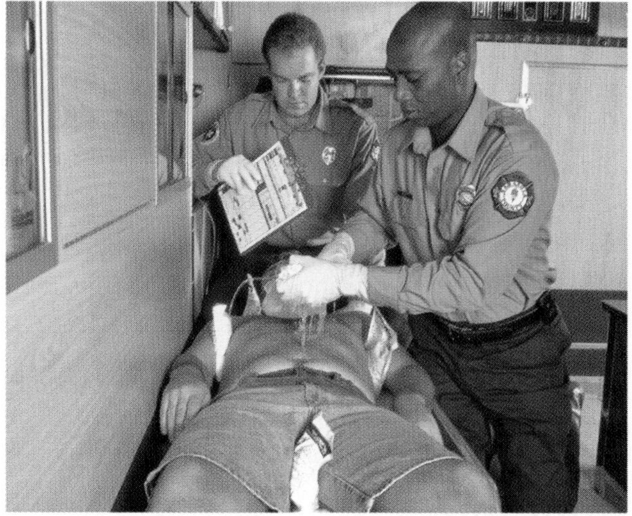

Figure 22-3 • In heat-emergency cases where the patient's skin is hot (and either dry or moist), cool aggressively.

airway obstruction. Even auto collisions can send vehicles or passengers into the water, resulting in any of the injuries usually associated with motor vehicle collisions as well as the complications caused by the presence of water.

Medical problems such as heart attacks can also cause or be caused by water accidents or can simply take place in, on, or near the water. Remember, too, that some water accidents happen far away from pools, lakes, or beaches. Bathtub drownings do occur. Adults, as well as children, can drown in only a few inches of water.

NOTE

Do not attempt a rescue in which you must enter deep water or swim, unless you have been trained to do so and are a very good swimmer. Except for shallow pools and open shallow waters with uniform bottoms, the problems faced in water rescue are too great and too dangerous for the poor swimmer or untrained person. If this bothers you—having to stand by, not being able to help—then take a course in water safety and rescue. (Both the American Red Cross and the YMCA offer water safety and rescue courses.) Otherwise, if you attempt a deep water or swimming rescue, you will probably become a victim yourself.

PATIENT ASSESSMENT

WATER-RELATED ACCIDENTS

Learn to look for the following problems in water-related-accident patients:

- *Airway obstruction.* This may be from water in the lungs, foreign matter in the airway, or swollen airway tissues (common if the neck is injured in a dive). Spasms along the airway may be present in some cases of drowning.
- *Cardiac arrest.* This is often related to respiratory arrest or occurs before drowning.
- *Signs of heart attack.* Some untrained rescuers too quickly conclude that chest pains are due to muscle cramps as a result of swimming.
- *Injuries to the head and neck.* These are expected to be found in boating, water-skiing, and diving accidents, but they are also very common in swimming accidents.
- *Internal injuries.* While doing the focused physical exam, stay on the alert for musculoskeletal injuries, soft-tissue injuries, and internal bleeding.
- *Generalized cooling, or hypothermia.* The water does not have to be very cold and the length of stay in the water does not have to be very long for hypothermia to occur.

continued

PATIENT ASSESSMENT *(continued)*

- *Substance abuse.* Alcohol and drug use are closely associated with adolescent and adult drownings. Elevated blood alcohol levels have been found in over 30 percent of drowning victims. The screening for drug use has not been as extensive as that done for alcohol, but research indicates that other drugs are a contributory factor in many water-related accidents.
- *Drowning.* The patient may be discovered under or face down in the water. He may be unconscious and without discernible vital signs or may be conscious, breathing, and coughing up water. ■

Provide assessment and care for any of the previously noted problems as you have learned in relevant chapters of this text. Drowning is discussed in detail next.

Drowning

drowning
the process of experiencing respiratory impairment from submersion/immersion in liquid, which may result in death, morbidity (illness or other adverse effects), or no morbidity.

In 2002, the World Health Organization (WHO) adopted a definition of **drowning** that is different from the traditional one. According to the WHO, "Drowning is the process of experiencing respiratory impairment from submersion/immersion in liquid. Drowning outcomes are classified as death, morbidity, and no morbidity." Morbidity means the patient experiences illness or other adverse effects, like unconsciousness or pneumonia. The WHO definition does not describe near drowning. The American Heart Association has also adopted this definition of drowning. Hence, the term *near drowning* is no longer used.

The process of drowning often begins as a person struggles to keep afloat in the water. He gulps in large breaths of air as he thrashes about. When he can no longer keep afloat and starts to submerge, he tries to take and hold one more deep breath. As he does, water may enter the airway. There is a series of coughing and swallowing actions, and the victim involuntarily inhales and swallows more water. As water flows past the epiglottis, it triggers a reflex spasm of the larynx. This spasm seals the airway so effectively that no more than a small amount of water reaches the lungs. Unconsciousness soon results from hypoxia (oxygen starvation).

About 10 percent of the people who die from drowning die just from the lack of air. In the remaining victims, the person typically attempts a final respiratory effort and draws water into the lungs, or the spasms subside with the onset of unconsciousness and water freely enters the lungs.

Some patients in cold water can be resuscitated after 30 minutes or more in cardiac arrest. Once the water temperature falls below 70°F, biological death may be delayed. The colder the water, the better the patient's chances for survival, unless generalized hypothermia produces lethal complications.

Rescue Breathing in or out of the Water

Transport for the drowning patient should not be delayed. You may initiate care when the patient is out of the water (already out when you arrive or in the water when you arrive but rescued by others before you initiate care). At other times you may need to be able to initiate care while the patient is still in the water—especially rescue breathing and immobilization for possible spine injuries. Chest compressions will be effective only after the patient is out of the water.

If needed, rescue breathing should begin without delay. If you can reach the nonbreathing patient in the water, provide ventilations as you support him in a semi-supine position. Continue providing ventilations while the patient is being immobilized and removed from the water. If the patient is already out of the water, begin rescue breathing or CPR on the land.

You may find resistance as you ventilate the drowning patient. You will probably have to ventilate more forcefully than you would other patients. Remember, you must provide air to the patient's lungs as soon as possible.

A patient with water in the lungs usually has water in the stomach, which will add resistance to your efforts to provide rescue breathing or CPR ventilations. Since the patient may have spasms along the airway, or swollen tissues in the larynx or trachea, you may find that some of the air you provide will go into the patient's stomach. Remember, the same problem will occur if you do not properly open the airway or if your ventilations are too forceful.

If gastric distention interferes with artificial ventilation, place the patient on his left side. With suction immediately available, the EMT should place his hand over the epigastric area of the abdomen and apply firm pressure to relieve the distention. This procedure should be done only if the gastric distention interferes with the EMT's efforts to artificially ventilate the patient effectively.

Care for Possible Spinal Injuries in the Water

Injuries to the cervical spine are seen with many water-related accidents. Most often, these injuries are received during a dive or when the patient is struck by a boat, skier or ski, surfer or surfboard. Even though cervical-spine injuries are the most common of the spine injuries seen in water-related accidents, there can be injury anywhere along the spine.

In water-related accidents, assume that the unconscious patient has neck and spinal injuries. Should the patient have head injuries, also assume that there are neck and spinal injuries. Keep in mind that a patient found in respiratory or cardiac arrest will need resuscitation started before you can immobilize the neck and spine. Also, realize that you may not be able to carry out a complete assessment for spinal injuries while the patient is in the water. Take care to avoid aggravating spinal injuries, but do not delay basic life support. Do not delay removing the patient from the water if the scene presents an immediate danger. When possible, keep the patient's neck rigid and in a straight line with the body's midline (Scan 22-1). Use the jaw-thrust maneuver to open the airway.

If the patient with possible spinal injuries is still in the water, you are a good swimmer with proper training, and you are able to aid in the rescue, secure the patient to a long spine board before removing him from the water. This will help prevent permanent neurological damage or paralysis. This type of rescue requires special training in the use of the spine board while in the water. This rigid device can "pop up" very easily from below the water surface. Make certain that you know how to control the board and how to work in the water.

PATIENT CARE

WATER-RELATED INCIDENTS

In all cases of water-related incidents, assume that the unconscious patient has neck and spinal injuries. If the patient is rescued by others while you wait on shore, or if the patient is out of the water when you arrive, you should:

1. Do an initial assessment, protecting the spine as much as possible.
2. Provide rescue breathing. If there is no pulse, begin CPR and prepare to apply the AED. Protect yourself by using a pocket face mask with a one-way valve or bag-valve-mask unit.
3. Look for and control profuse bleeding. Since the patient's heart rate may have slowed down, take a pulse for 60 seconds in all cold-water rescue situations before concluding that the patient is in cardiac arrest.
4. Provide care for shock (as described in Chapter 26, "Bleeding and Shock"); administer high-concentration oxygen; and transport the patient as soon as possible.
5. Continue resuscitative measures throughout transport. Initial and periodic suctioning may be needed. ■

SCAN 22-1 • Water Rescue with Possible Spinal Injury

HEAD-CHIN SUPPORT

Two Rescuers in Shallow Water

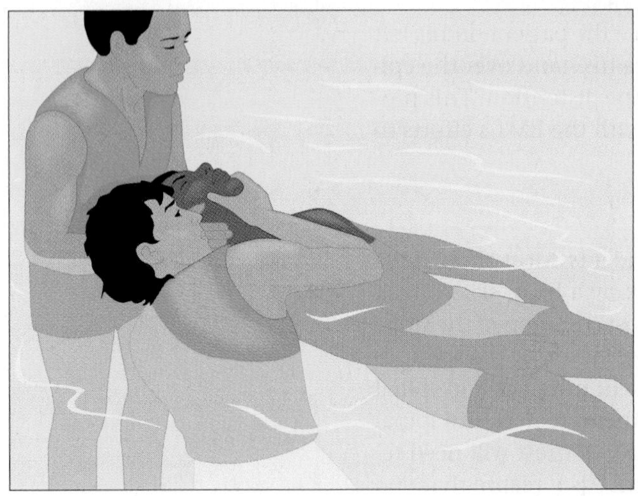

When there are two rescuers present, perform the head-chin support technique to provide in-line stabilization of a patient in shallow water.

HEAD-SPLINT SUPPORT

One Rescuer in Shallow Water

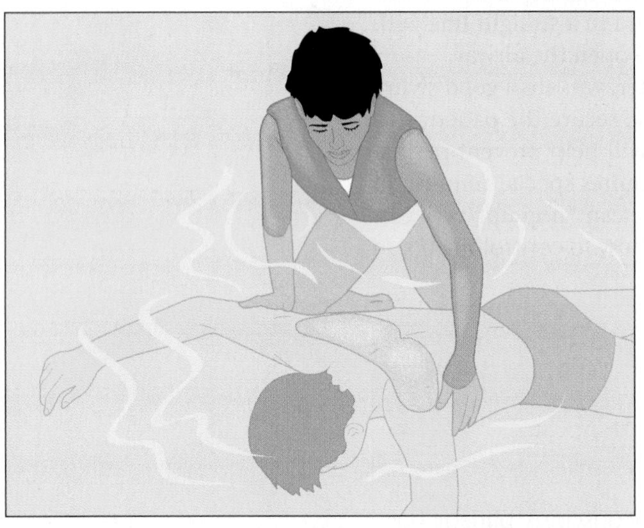

1. When you find a patient face down in shallow water, position yourself alongside the patient.

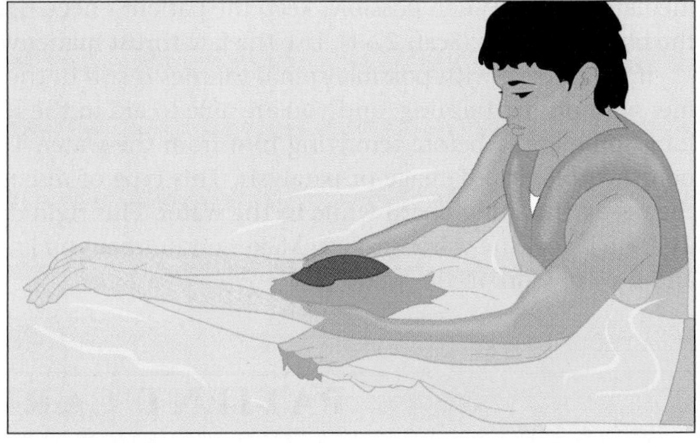

2. Extend the patient's arms straight up alongside his head to create a splint.

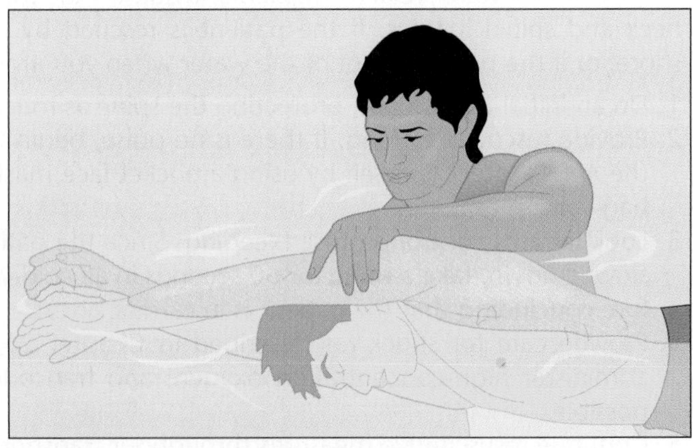

3. Begin to rotate the torso toward you.

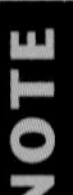

NOTE *Unless you are a very good swimmer and trained in water rescue, do not go into the water to save someone.*

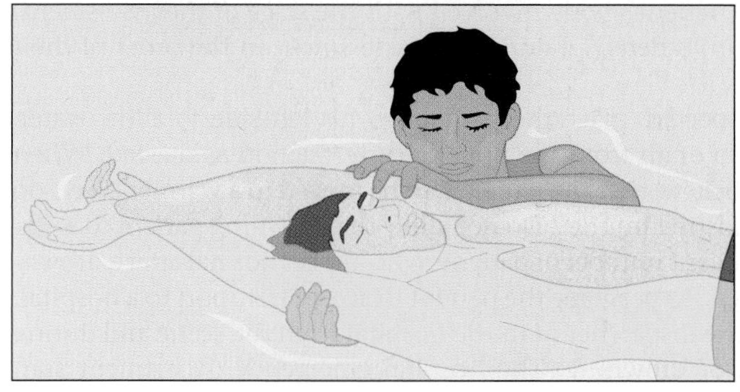

4. As you rotate the patient, lower yourself into the water.

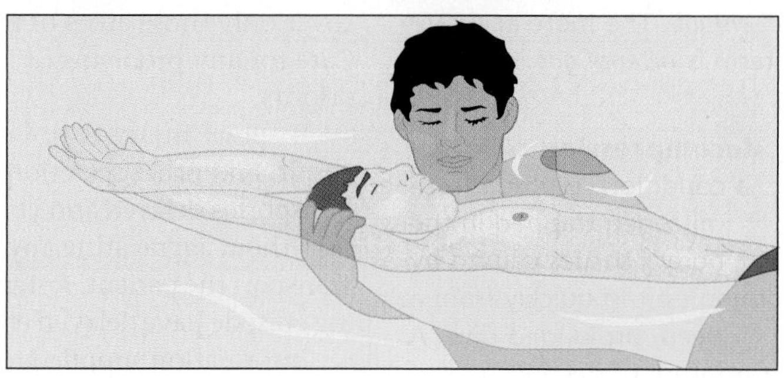

5. Maintain manual stabilization by holding the patient's head between his arms.

HEAD-CHIN SUPPORT

One Rescuer in Deep Water

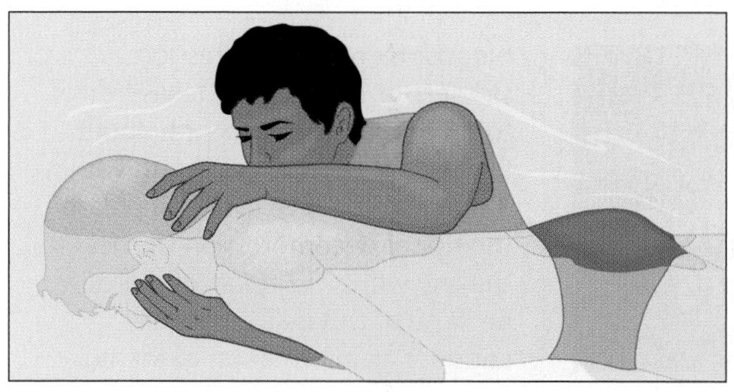

1. When you find a patient face down in deep water, position yourself beside him. Support his head with one hand and the mandible with the other.

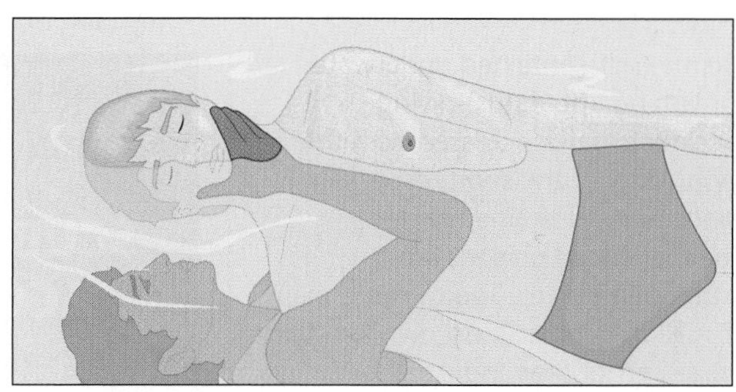

2. Then rotate the patient by ducking under him.

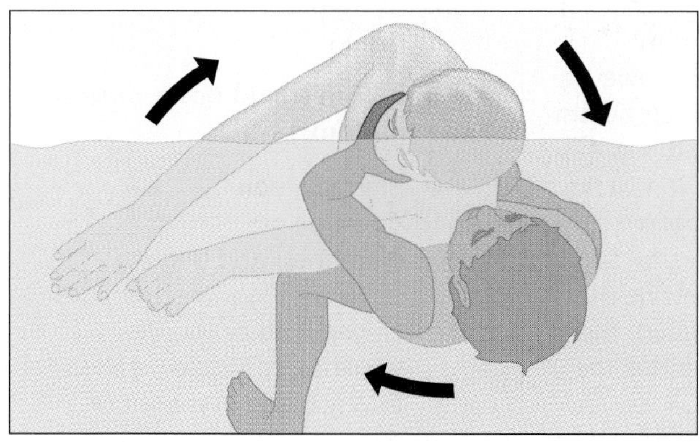

3. Continue to rotate until the patient is face up.

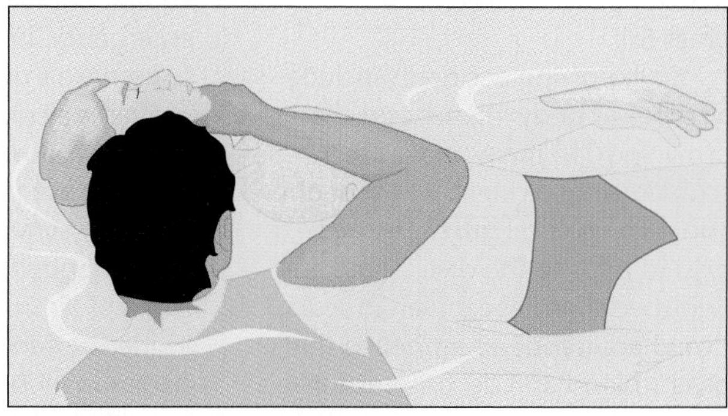

4. Maintain in-line stabilization until a backboard is used to immobilize the patient's spine.

air embolism gas bubble in the bloodstream. The plural is *air emboli.* The more accurate term is *arterial gas embolism (AGE).*

decompression sickness a condition resulting from nitrogen trapped in the body's tissues caused by coming up too quickly from a deep, prolonged dive. A symptom of decompression sickness is "the bends," or deep pain in the muscles and joints.

The drowning patient receiving rescue breathing or CPR should be transported as soon as possible. If resuscitation and immediate transport are not required, cover the patient to conserve his body heat and complete a focused history and physical exam. Uncover only those areas of the patient's body involved with the stage of the assessment. Care for any problems or injuries detected during the assessment in the order of their priority.

If spinal injury is not suspected, place the patient on his left side to allow water, vomit, and other secretions to drain from the upper airway. Suction as needed. When transport is delayed and you believe that the patient can be moved to a warmer place, do so without aggravating any existing injuries. Do not allow the drowning patient to walk. Transport the patient. A significant number of patients who appear normal after a drowning episode have delayed effects, so persuade the patient to accept transport to a hospital.

Information supplied to the dispatcher or to the hospital from the scene and during transport is critical in cases of drowning. The hospital emergency department staff needs to know if this is a fresh- or saltwater drowning, if it took place in cold or warm water, and if it is related to a diving accident. You may be asked to transport the patient to a special facility or to a center having a hyperbaric chamber when decompression therapy is needed.

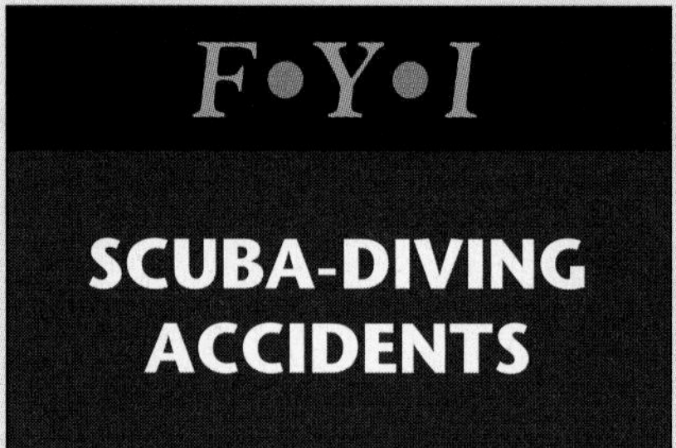

Scuba (self-contained underwater breathing apparatus)-diving accidents have increased with the popularity of the sport, especially since many untrained and inexperienced persons are attempting dives. Today, more than 2 million people scuba dive for sport or as part of their industrial or military job. Added to this are a large number who decide to "try it one time," without the benefits of lessons or supervision. Well-trained divers seldom have problems. However, those with inadequate training place themselves at great risk.

Scuba-diving accidents include all types of body injuries and drownings. In many cases, the scuba-diving accident was brought about by medical problems that existed prior to the dive. There are two special problems seen in scuba-diving accidents: air emboli in the diver's blood and decompression sickness.

An **air embolism**—more accurately called *arterial gas embolism (AGE)*—is the result of gases leaving a damaged lung and entering the bloodstream. Severe damage may lead to a collapsed lung. Air emboli (gas bubbles in the blood) are most often associated with divers who hold their breath because of inadequate training, equipment failure, underwater emergency, or when trying to conserve air during a dive. However, a diver may develop an air embolism in very shallow water (as little as 4 feet). An automobile-collision victim also may suffer an air embolism if, when trapped below water, he takes gulps of air from air pockets held inside the vehicle. When freed, the patient may develop air emboli the same as a scuba-diver.

Decompression sickness is usually caused when a diver comes up too quickly from a deep, prolonged dive. The quick ascent causes nitrogen gas to be trapped in the body tissues and then in the bloodstream. Decompression sickness in scuba divers takes from 1 to 48 hours to appear, with about 90 percent of cases occurring within 3 hours of the dive. Divers increase the risk of decompression sickness if they fly within 12 hours of a dive. Because of this delay, carefully consider all information gathered from the patient interview and reports from the patient's family and friends. This information may provide the only clues relating the patient's problems to a scuba dive.

The signs and symptoms of scuba-diving problems may include the following:

Air Embolism (rapid onset of signs and symptoms)

- Blurred vision
- Chest pains
- Numbness and tingling sensations in the extremities
- Generalized or specific weakness, possible paralysis
- Frothy blood in mouth or nose
- Convulsions
- Rapid lapse into unconsciousness
- Respiratory arrest and cardiac arrest

Diving Accidents

Water-related accidents often involve injuries that occur when individuals attempt dives or enter the water from diving boards. In the majority of these accidents, the patient is a teenager. Basically the same types of injuries are seen in dives taken from diving boards, poolsides, docks, boats, and the shore. The injury may be due to the diver striking the board or some object on or under the water. From great heights, injury may result from impact with the water.

Most diving accidents involve the head and neck, but you will also find injuries to the spine, hands, feet, and ribs in many cases. Any part of the body can be injured depending on the position that the diver is in when he strikes the water or an object. This means that you must perform an initial assessment. You must also perform a focused history and physical exam on all diving accident patients. Do not overlook the fact that a medical emergency may have led to the diving accident.

Emergency care for diving accident patients is the same as for any accident patient if they are out of the water. Care provided in the water and during removal from the water is the same as for any patient who may have neck and spine injuries. Remember, assume that any unconscious or unresponsive patient has neck and spinal injuries.

Decompression Sickness

- Personality changes
- Fatigue
- Deep pain to the muscles and joints (the "bends")
- Itchy blotches or mottling of the skin
- Numbness or paralysis
- Choking
- Coughing
- Labored breathing
- Behavior similar to intoxication (such as staggering)
- Chest pains
- Collapse leading to unconsciousness
- Skin rashes that keep changing in appearance (in some cases)

For a patient with signs and symptoms of either air embolism or decompression sickness, follow the same emergency care steps:

1. Maintain an open airway.
2. Administer the highest possible flow and concentration of oxygen by nonrebreather mask.
3. Rapidly transport all patients with possible air emboli or decompression sickness.
4. Contact medical direction for specific instructions concerning where to take the patient. You may be sent directly to a hyperbaric trauma care center.
5. Keep the patient warm.
6. Position the patient either supine or on either side (Figure 22-4). Continue to monitor the patient. You may have to reposition the patient to ensure an open airway.

The Diver Alert Network (DAN) was formed to assist rescuers with the care of underwater diving accident patients. The staff, which is available on a 24-hour basis, can be reached by phoning (919) 684-8111. Collect calls will be accepted for actual emergencies. DAN can give you or your dispatcher information on assessment and care and how to transfer the patient to a hyperbaric trauma care center. (A hyperbaric trauma care center is one that has a special pressure chamber for treatment of such conditions.) For non-emergencies, call (919) 684-2948.

Note: The well-trained scuba diver makes use of a preplanned dive chart. The dive chart, if it is available, may provide you with useful information concerning the nature and duration of the dive. This chart must be transported with the patient. ■

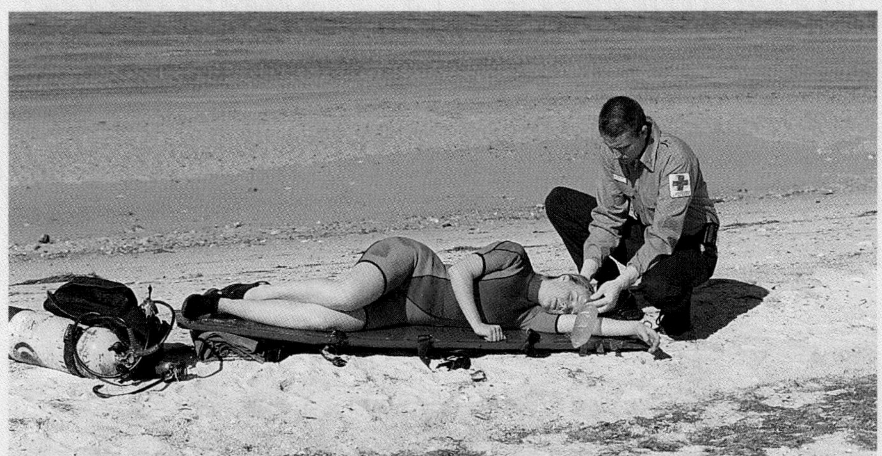

Figure 22-4 • Proper positioning of a scuba-diving accident patient.

The following is the order of procedures for a water rescue (Figure 22-5), most of which can be performed short of going into the water: *reach, throw and tow, row, go.*

- **Reach.** When the patient is responsive and close to shore or poolside, try to reach him by holding out an object for him to grab. Then pull him from the water. Make sure your position is secure. Line (rope) is considered the best choice. If no line is available, use a branch, fishing rod, oar, stick, or other such object, even a towel, blanket, or article of clothing. If no object is available or you have only one opportunity to grab the person (e.g., in strong currents), position yourself flat on your stomach and extend your hand or leg to the patient (This is not recommended for the nonswimmer). Again, make certain that you are working from a secure position.
- **Throw and tow.** Should the person be conscious and alert but too far away for you to reach and pull from the water, throw an object that will float (Figure 22-6). A personal flotation device (PFD or lifejacket) or ring buoy (life preserver) works best. Other buoyant objects include foam cushions, logs, plastic picnic containers, surf boards, flat boards, large beach balls, and plastic toys. Two empty, capped, plastic milk jugs can keep an adult afloat for hours. Inflatable splints can be used if there is nothing at the scene that will float.

  Once the conscious patient has a flotation device, try to find a way to tow him to shore. From a safe position, throw the patient a line or another flotation device attached to a line. If you are a good swimmer and you know how to judge the water, wade out no deeper than waist high, wear a personal flotation device, and have a safety line that is secured on shore.
- **Row.** When the patient is too far from shore to allow for throwing and towing, or is unresponsive, you may be able to row a boat to the patient. Do not attempt to row to the patient if you cannot swim. Even if you are a good swimmer, wearing a personal flotation device while in the boat is required.

  If the patient is conscious, tell him to grab an oar or the stern (rear end) of the boat. You must exercise great care when helping the patient into the boat. This is even trickier when you are in a canoe. Should the canoe tip over, stay with it and hold onto its bottom and side. Most canoes will stay afloat.
- **Go.** As a last resort, when all other means have failed, you can go into the water and swim to the patient. You must be a good swimmer, trained in water rescue and

F•Y•I

WATER RESCUES

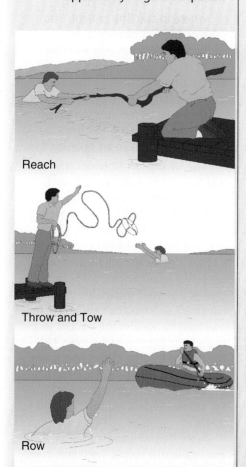

Figure 22-5 • First try to *reach* and pull the patient from the water. If that fails, *throw* him anything that will float and *tow* him from the water. If that fails, *row* to the patient.

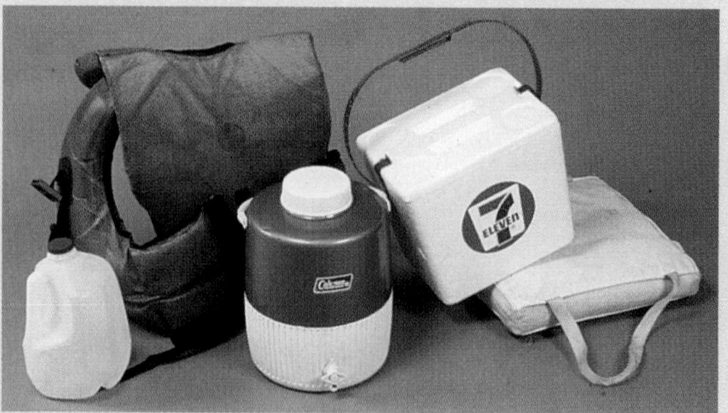

Figure 22-6 • Throw the patient any object that will float.

lifesaving. Untrained rescuers can become victims themselves.

ICE RESCUES

Every winter people fall through ice while skating or attempting to cross an ice-covered body of water. Often, the scene becomes a multiple-rescue problem as individuals try to reach the victim and also fall through the ice. The number-one rule in ice rescue is to protect yourself. Formal ice rescue training is available. A cold-water submersion suit and personal flotation device should be worn during any ice rescue attempt (Figure 22-7).

There are several ways in which you can reach a patient who has fallen through ice:

- Flotation devices can be thrown to the patient.
- A rope in which a loop has been formed can be tossed to the patient. He can put the loop around his body so that he can be pulled onto the ice and away from the danger area.
- A small, flat-bottomed aluminum boat is probably the best device for an ice rescue. It can be pushed stern (rear end) first by other rescuers and pulled to safety by a rope secured to the bow (front end). The primary rescuer will remain dry and safe should the ice break. The patient can be pulled from the water or allowed to grasp the side of the boat, although he may be unable to grasp or to hold on for long.
- A ladder is an effective tool often used in ice rescue. It can be laid flat and pushed to the patient, then pulled back by an attached rope. The ladder also can serve as a surface on which a rescuer can spread out his weight if he must go onto the ice to reach the patient. The ladder should have a line that can be secured by a rescuer in a safe position. Any rescuer on the ladder should have a safety line.

Remember that the patient may not be able to do much to help in the rescue process. Hypothermia may interfere with his mental and physical capabilities in a matter of minutes.

Whenever possible, do not work alone when trying to perform an ice rescue. If you must work alone, do not walk out onto the ice. Never go onto ice that is rapidly breaking. Never enter the water through a hole in the ice in order to find the victim. Your best course of action will be to work with others, from a safe ice surface or the shore. When there is no other choice, you and your fellow rescuers can elect to form a human chain to reach the patient. However, this is not the safest method to employ, even when all the rescuers are wearing personal flotation devices and using safety lines.

Expect to find injuries to most patients who have fallen through the ice. Treat for hypothermia according to local protocols and treat for any injuries. Transport all patients who have fallen through ice. ■

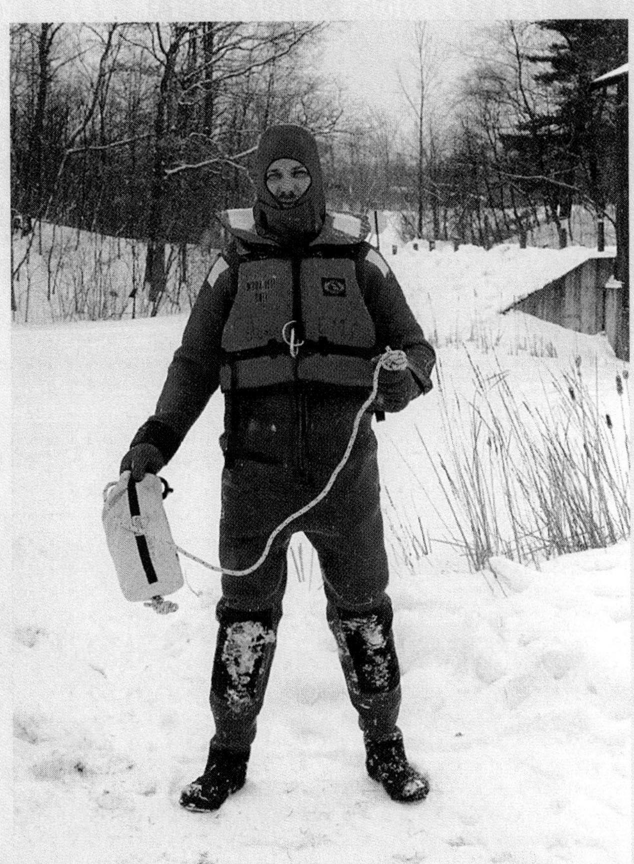

Figure 22-7 • Safe ice rescues require proper equipment.

BITES AND STINGS

Insect Bites and Stings

toxins
substances produced by animals or plants that are poisonous to humans.

venom
a toxin (poison) produced by certain animals such as snakes, spiders, and some marine life forms.

Insect stings, spider bites, and scorpion stings are typical sources of injected poisons, or **toxins**—substances produced by animals or plants that are poisonous to humans. (**Venom** is a term for a toxin produced by some animals such as snakes, spiders, and certain marine life forms.) Commonly seen insect stings are those of wasps, hornets, bees, and ants. Insect stings and bites are rarely dangerous. However, 5 percent of the U.S. population will have an allergic reaction, which may result in shock. Those who are hypersensitive develop severe anaphylactic shock that is quickly life threatening (see Chapter 20, "Allergic Reactions").

All spiders are poisonous, but most species cannot get their fangs through human skin. The black widow spider and the brown recluse, or fiddleback, spider (Figure 22-8) are two that can, and their bites can produce medical emergencies. Almost all brown recluse bites are painless, and patients seldom recall being bitten. The characteristic lesion appears in only 10 percent of cases, and then only after up to 12 hours (Figure 22-9). EMTs are seldom called to respond to a brown recluse bite. Black widow bites cause a more immediate reaction.

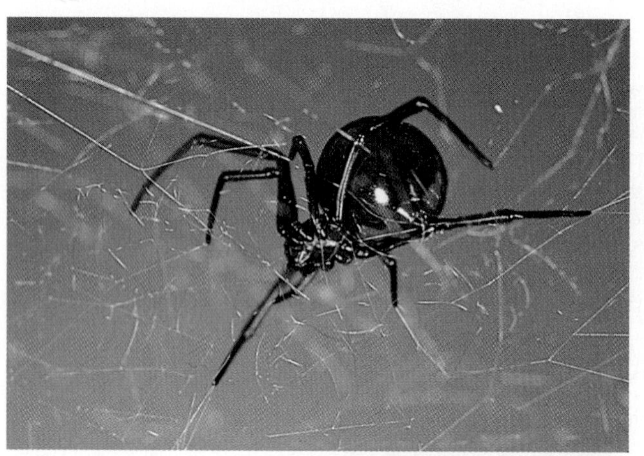

A

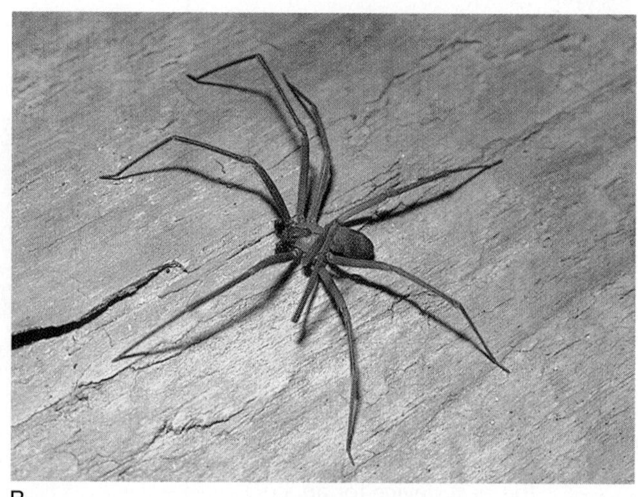

B

Figure 22-8 • (A) Black widow spider. *(© Joseph T. Collins/Photo Researchers, Inc.)* (B) Brown recluse spider. *(© Breck P. Kent)*

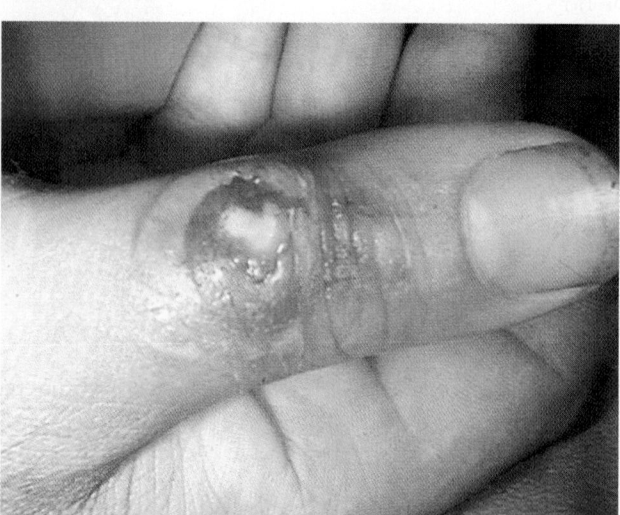

Figure 22-9 • Brown recluse spider bite.

Scorpion stings are common in the Southwest United States. They do not ordinarily cause deaths, but one rare species (*centroroides exilcauda*) is dangerous to humans and can cause serious medical problems in children, including respiratory failure.

Note: Bites and stings belong in the class of injected poisons discussed in Chapter 21, "Poisoning and Overdose Emergencies."

PATIENT ASSESSMENT

INSECT BITES AND STINGS

Gather information from the patient, bystanders, and the scene. Find out whatever you can about the insect or other possible source of the poisoning. The signs and symptoms of injected poisoning can include:

- Altered states of awareness
- Noticeable stings or bites on the skin
- Puncture marks (especially note the fingers, forearms, toes, and legs)
- Blotchy skin (mottled skin)
- Localized pain or itching
- Numbness in a limb or body part
- Burning sensations at the site followed by pain spreading throughout the limb
- Redness
- Swelling or blistering at the site
- Weakness or collapse
- Difficult breathing and abnormal pulse rate
- Headache and dizziness
- Chills
- Fever
- Nausea and vomiting
- Muscle cramps, chest tightening, joint pains
- Excessive saliva formation, profuse sweating
- Anaphylaxis ■

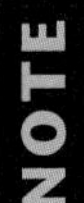

Look for medical identification devices that identify persons sensitive to certain stings or bites. Some patients sensitive to stings or bites carry medication to help prevent anaphylactic shock. This situation is described in Chapter 20, "Allergic Reactions."

PATIENT CARE

INSECT BITES AND STINGS

As an EMT, you are not expected to be able to identify insects and spiders. Proper identification of these organisms is best left to experts. If the problem has been caused by a creature that is known locally and is not normally dangerous (such as a bee, wasp, or puss caterpillar), the major concern will be anaphylactic shock. If anaphylactic shock does not develop, care is usually simple.

If the cause of the bite or sting is unknown, or the organism is unknown, the patient should be seen by a physician. Call medical direction or take the patient to a medical facility and let experts decide on the proper treatment for the patient. If

continued

PATIENT CARE *(continued)*

possible, transport the stinging object or organism in a sealed container, taking care not to handle it without proper protection, even if it is dead. If you can accomplish this safely, you may save precious minutes needed to identify the toxin.

To provide emergency care for injected toxins:

1. Treat for shock, even if the patient does not present any of the signs of shock.
2. Call medical direction. Skip this only if the organism is known and your EMS system has a specific protocol for care.
3. To remove the stinger or venom sac, the traditional advice is to scrape the site with a blade or a card and to avoid pulling with tweezers which, it was thought, might squeeze more venom into the wound. However, recent research indicates that how you remove the stinger or venom sac is far less important than doing so quickly.
4. Remove jewelry from affected limbs in case the limb swells, which would make removal more difficult later.
5. If local protocol permits and if the wound is on an extremity (not a joint), place constricting bands above and below the sting or bite site. This is done to slow the spread of venom in the lymphatic vessels and superficial veins. The band should be made of ¾-inch- to 1½-inch-wide soft rubber or other wide soft material. It should be placed about 2 inches from the wound. The band must be loose enough to slide a finger under it. It should not cut off circulation.
6. Keep the limb immobilized and the patient still to prevent distribution of the poison to other parts of the body. (*Note*: Some EMS systems recommend placing a cold compress on the wound. Most EMS systems do not use cold for any injected toxin. Follow local protocol.) ■

Snakebites

Snakebites require special care but are usually not life threatening. Nearly 50,000 people in the United States are bitten by snakes each year. Over 8,000 of these cases involve poisonous snakes, but on the average fewer than 10 deaths are reported annually. (In the United States, more people die each year from bee and wasp stings than from snakebites.) The signs and symptoms of snakebite poisoning may take several hours to appear. If death does result, it is usually not a rapidly occurring event unless anaphylactic shock develops. Most victims who die survive at least 1 to 2 days.

In the United States there are two types of native poisonous snakes—pit vipers (including rattlesnakes, copperheads, and water moccasins) and coral snakes (Figure 22-10). Up to 25 percent of pit viper bites and 50 percent of coral bites are "dry bites" without venom injection, but the venomous bite from a diamondback rattler or coral snake is considered very serious. Since each person reacts differently to snakebite, you should consider the bite from any known poisonous snake or any unidentified snake to be a serious emergency. Staying calm and keeping the patient calm and at rest is critical. Since reaction time is slow, there is time to transport the patient without haste.

NOTE

Native snakes are not the only kind of poisonous animals you may encounter. A number of people have decided to keep poisonous reptiles even though it is illegal to do so in most areas. So, even if you live in an area where there are no poisonous snakes, you may encounter a patient who has sustained a bite from one.

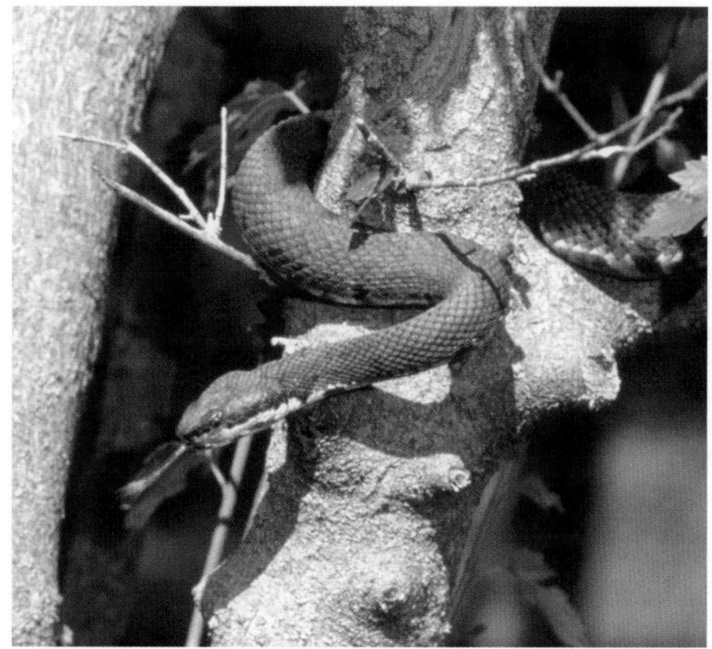

A

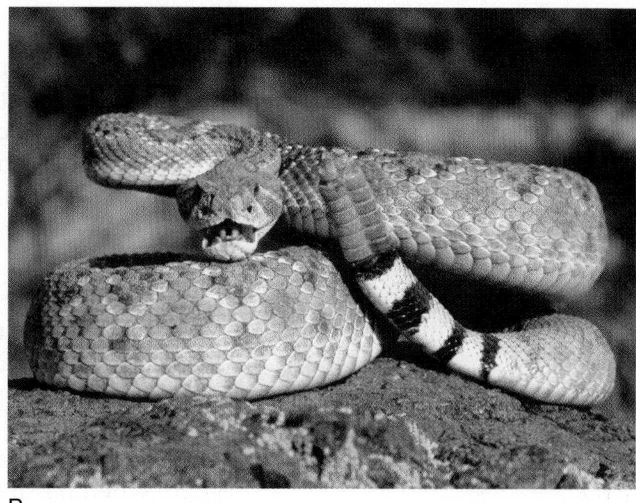

B

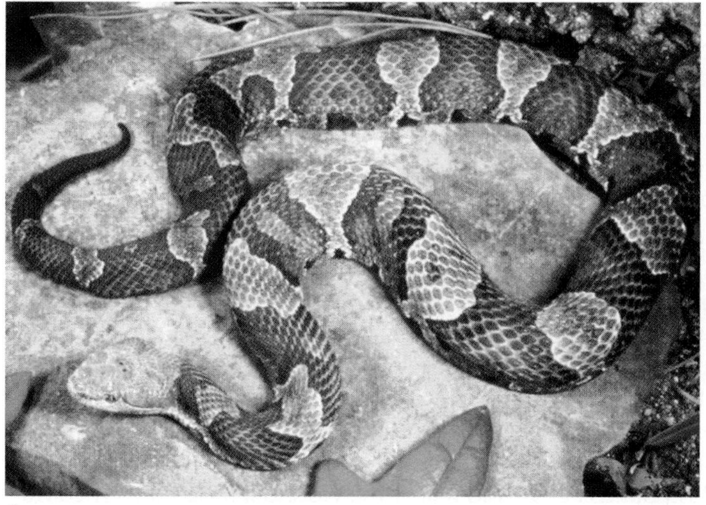

C

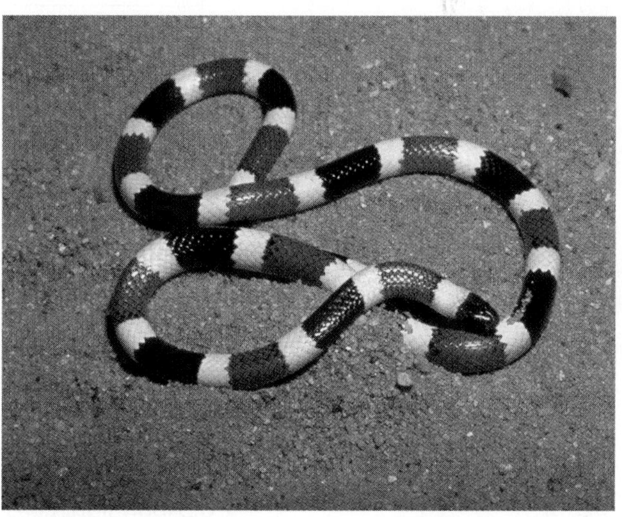

D

Figure 22-10 • The pit vipers include (A) water moccasin *(© Alan and Sandy Carey/Photo Researchers, Inc.),* (B) rattlesnake *(© CK Lorenz/Photo Researchers, Inc.),* and (C) copperhead. *(© Phil A. Dotson/Photo Researchers, Inc.)* The coral snake (D) is also poisonous. *(© J. Collins/Photo Researchers, Inc.)*

PATIENT ASSESSMENT

SNAKEBITE

Unless you are dealing with a known species of snake that is not considered poisonous, consider all snakebites to be from poisonous snakes. The patient or bystanders may say that the snake was not poisonous, but they could be mistaken. The signs and symptoms of snakebite may include the following:

- Noticeable bite on the skin. This may appear as nothing more than a discoloration.

continued

PATIENT ASSESSMENT *(continued)*

- Pain and swelling in the area of the bite. This may be slow to develop, taking from 30 minutes to several hours.
- Rapid pulse and labored breathing
- Progressive general weakness
- Vision problems (dim or blurred)
- Nausea and vomiting
- Seizures
- Drowsiness or unconsciousness

If the dead or captured snake is at the scene, your role as an EMT is not to identify the snake but to transport it in a sealed container along with the patient. Arrange for separate transport of a live specimen. Do not transport a live snake in the ambulance.

Should you see the live, uncaptured snake, take great care or you may be its next victim. When possible, note its size and coloration. Getting close enough to look for details of the eyes or for a pit between the eye and mouth is foolish. How you classify a snake, whether it is dead or alive, will probably have little to do with subsequent care. The medical facility staff will arrange to have an expert classify a captured or dead specimen, and they have protocols to determine care if the snake has not been captured. Unless you are an expert in capturing snakes, do not try to catch the snake. Never delay care and transport in order to capture the snake. ■

PATIENT CARE

SNAKEBITE

Emergency care of a patient with snakebite includes:

1. Call medical direction.
2. Treat for shock and conserve body heat. Keep the patient calm.
3. Locate the fang marks and clean the site with soap and water. There may be only one fang mark.
4. Remove any rings, bracelets, or other constricting items on the bitten extremity.
5. Keep any bitten extremities immobilized—the application of a splint will help. Try to keep the bite at the level of the heart or, when this is not possible, below the level of the heart.
6. Apply light constricting bands above and below the wound if ordered by medical direction. (See more information on constricting bands in the following text.)
7. Transport the patient, carefully monitoring vital signs. ■

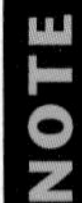

Do not place an ice bag or cold pack on the bite unless you are directed to do so by a physician or local protocol. Do not cut into the bite and suction or squeeze unless you are directed to do so by a physician. Never suck the venom from the wound using your mouth. Instead, use a suction cup. Suctioning is seldom done.

Apply constricting bands above and below the fang marks. Each band should be about 2 inches from the wound, but never place the bands on both sides of a joint, such as above and below the knee. Since the typical coral snakebite is to a finger or a toe, due to its small mouth, just a single band may be placed above a coral snakebite. If the bite is to a finger, the band can be applied to the wrist.

The purpose of the constricting bands is to restrict the flow of lymph, not of blood. The bonds should be made of $^{3}/_{4}$-inch- to $^{1}/_{2}$-inch-wide soft rubber (or non-latex equivalent). If only one band is available, place it above the wound (between the wound and the heart). If no bands are available, use a handkerchief or other wide soft material. The bands should be snug but not tight enough to cut off circulation. Monitor for a pulse at the wrist or ankle. Check to be certain that tissue swelling does not cause the constricting bands to become too tight.

Poisoning from Marine Life

Poisoning from marine life forms can occur in a variety of ways—from eating improperly prepared seafood or poisonous organisms to stings and punctures. Patients who have ingested spoiled, contaminated, or infested seafood may develop a condition that resembles anaphylactic shock. They should receive the same care as any patient in anaphylactic shock. During care, you must be prepared for vomiting. Most patients will show the signs of food poisoning. The care for seafood poisoning is the same as for all other food poisonings.

It is extremely rare for someone in the United States to eat a poisonous variety of marine life. Creatures such as puffer fish and paralytic shellfish are not readily available. For all cases of suspected poisoning due to ingestion, call your on-line medical direction or the poison control center as local protocol directs you. Be prepared for vomiting, convulsions, and respiratory arrest.

Venomous marine life forms producing sting injuries include the jellyfish, the sea nettle, the Portuguese man-of-war, coral, the sea anemone, and the hydra. For most victims, the sting produces pain with few complications. Some patients may show allergic reactions and possibly develop anaphylactic shock. These cases require the same care as rendered for any case of anaphylactic shock. Stings to the face, especially those near or on the lip or eye, require a physician's attention. Rinsing the affected area with vinegar or rubbing alcohol will reduce the pain of the sting. Be careful not to let vinegar or, especially, rubbing alcohol get into the patient's mouth or eyes.

Puncture wounds occur when someone steps on or grabs a stingray, sea urchin, spiny catfish, or other form of spiny marine animal. Although it is true that soaking the wound in non-scalding hot water for 30 minutes will break down the venom, you should not delay transport. Puncture wounds must be treated by a physician and the patient may need a tetanus inoculation. Remember, the patient could react to the venom by developing anaphylactic shock.

CRITICAL DECISION MAKING: Safety First

Environmental emergencies provide a variety of situations in which an EMT must act. Some patients need to be cooled, others warmed. But before you even get to treat the patient there are safety decisions to be made. Consider the following situations and identify the safety hazards.

1. You are talking a walk while on vacation. You hear a sound from the water and see that several hundred feet out in the water a person is struggling to stay afloat.
2. You are ice skating with the family and hear screaming. Someone has fallen through the ice. A group of people have gathered around the hole, peering downward.
3. You are on a hiking path and hear screaming. A hiker has been bitten by a snake. He is in pain and holding his leg. He is sitting by an outcropping of rocks.

CHAPTER REVIEW

SUMMARY

Patients suffering from exposure to heat or cold must be removed from the harmful environment as quickly and as safely as possible. Rewarming or cooling procedures approved by local protocol should be performed as needed. Immediate resuscitation of the water-related emergency patient may require quick and persistent intervention. For injection or ingestion of the poisons of insects, spiders, snakes, and marine life, call medical direction and follow local protocol.

KEY TERMS

active rewarming application of an external heat source to rewarm the body of a hypothermic patient.

air embolism gas bubble in the bloodstream. The plural is *air emboli*. The more accurate term is *arterial gas embolism (AGE)*.

central rewarming application of heat to the lateral chest, neck, armpits, and groin of a hypothermic patient.

conduction the transfer of heat from one material to another through direct contact.

convection carrying away of heat by currents of air or water or other gases or liquids.

decompression sickness a condition resulting from nitrogen trapped in the body's tissues caused by coming up too quickly from a deep, prolonged dive. A symptom of decompression sickness is "the bends," or deep pain in the muscles and joints.

drowning the process of experiencing respiratory impairment from submersion/immersion in liquid, which may result in death, morbidity (illness or other adverse effects), or no morbidity.

evaporation the change from liquid to gas. When the body perspires or gets wet, evaporation of the perspiration or other liquid into the air has a cooling effect on the body.

hyperthermia (HI-per-THURM-e-ah) an increase in body temperature above normal, life-threatening in its extreme.

hypothermia (HI-po-THURM-e-ah) generalized cooling that reduces body temperature below normal, life-threatening in its extreme.

local cooling cooling or freezing of particular (local) parts of the body.

passive rewarming covering a hypothermic patient and taking other steps to prevent further heat loss and help the body rewarm itself.

radiation sending out energy, such as heat, in waves into space.

respiration breathing. During respiration, body heat is lost as warm air is exhaled from the body.

toxins substances produced by animals or plants that are poisonous to humans.

venom a toxin (poison) produced by certain animals such as snakes, spiders, and some marine life forms.

water chill chilling caused by conduction of heat from the body when the body or clothing is wet.

wind chill chilling caused by convection of heat from the body in the presence of air currents.

REVIEW QUESTIONS

1. Describe when it is appropriate to treat a cold emergency with active rewarming and when you should perform passive rewarming. (pp. 520–521, 525–526)
2. List five situations in which a patient may be suffering from hypothermia along with another, more obvious medical condition or injury. (pp. 519–520)
3. Name the signs and symptoms of a late or deep localized cold injury. (p. 524)
4. Describe the management of a patient suffering from heat emergency who has moist, pale, and cool skin. (p. 527)
5. Describe the management of a patient suffering from a heat emergency who has hot, dry skin. (p. 528)
6. Describe the proper care for a patient suffering from snakebite. (pp. 542–543)

CRITICAL THINKING

Thinking and Linking

Think back to Chapter 1, "Introduction to Emergency Medical Care," Chapter 2,"The Well-Being of the EMT-Basic," and Chapter 13, "Communications." Link information from those chapters to information from this chapter as you consider the following situation:

- You respond to a snakebite. There, you find a patient and witnesses who describe a snake to you in great detail. Where would you find information on what type of snake this was, if it was poisonous, and how to treat the patient? What would you do if the snake was still present?

Think back to Chapter 1,"Introduction to Emergency Medical Care," Chapter 2, "The Well-Being of the EMT-Basic," and Chapter 5, "Lifting and Moving Patients." Link information from those chapters to information from this chapter as you consider the following situation:

- You have a patient who is experiencing hypothermia, is half a mile into the woods, and is not accessible by ambulance. Do you have clothing available that would protect you and your crew/team from hypothermia during the trip in and out? If you will be an EMT in a warm climate, change the situation. It is hot and humid. A hiker has experienced a heat emergency. Can you and your crew/team get the patient out without experiencing a heat emergency yourselves? In either case, what transport device(s) and resources would you use to remove the patient from the woods?

MEDIA RESOURCES 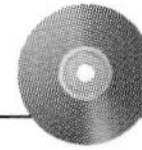

See the Student CD at the back of this book for quizzes, a case study activity, and other features related to this chapter. Also, visit the Companion Website for *Emergency Care* at **www.prenhall.com/limmer**, where you will find additional reinforcement and links to other resources.

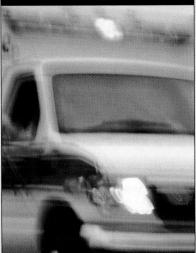

Street Scenes

It's very cold out and it's been snowing for hours. Shortly after sundown, you get dispatched to a downtown area where homeless people often sleep outdoors for an "unknown man down" call. As you pull up to the scene, you are met by a police officer who tells you that the man sitting by the heater grate in the sidewalk was going to be taken to the shelter "but something didn't seem right." You get the first-in bag and approach the patient. You ask his name and he says, "Frank." You ask for a last name but he doesn't respond.

"Well, Frank, what's going on?" He just stares. "Do you have any pain?" Again no response. He just sits with his arms folded over his chest and appears to be shivering. "Frank, we think you need to go to the hospital to get checked out."

"What?" he whispers. You ask the patient if he can stand up but his response is unintelligible. You get the cot and load for transport. The police officer asks you what's wrong and you tell him that you think the patient might be hypothermic.

Street Scene Questions

1. What concerns might you have for this patient?
2. What assessment needs to be performed?
3. Should you rewarm this patient? If so, when should you start?

When you get into the ambulance, you repeat your initial assessment, checking breathing closely and looking for any external bleeding. Again, you ask the patient if he knows where he is but he responds only with groans. You notice that his clothing is wet, so you turn up the heat in the patient compartment, take off his wet jacket and shirt, and wrap him in more blankets. He is still shivering. You take a set of vital signs and determine the BP is 90/60, pulse is 120, respiration rate is 28 and shallow, and the skin is flushed. When you feel the abdomen with the back of your hand, it feels cool. You do not smell any alcohol on the patient and when you check distal pulses, motor function, and sensation, you find that he can move all extremities but it is difficult and almost seems painful. His pupils respond to light but appear sluggish. You decide to administer oxygen by nonrebreather. You also decide not to actively rewarm the patient but keep him wrapped in blankets, covering his head and keeping the heater turned up.

Street Scene Questions

4. How often should you take vital signs?
5. When moving the patient out of the ambulance and onto the hospital stretcher, what precautions should be taken?

You decide to take another set of vital signs after 5 minutes because you think that this patient could be at risk for respiratory arrest or sudden cardiac death. You make sure the AED and the respiratory equipment are close at hand. Vital signs are about the same. You call the hospital, give your report, and advise an ETA of about 5 minutes.

When you get there, you remind your partner that this patient needs to be handled gently. You get another blanket from the emergency department before you make the move. The patient seems to be warming up and you don't want to put him at any additional risk. When you get into the emergency department, you smoothly move the patient to the stretcher and give the prehospital care report. As you are leaving, Frank looks at you and says: "Thanks, you're nice."

Street Scenes Sample Documentation

PATIENT NAME: *Frank* **PATIENT AGE:** *Unknown*

CHIEF COMPLAINT
Altered mental status

PAST MEDICAL HISTORY
- ☐ None
- ☐ Allergy to ____
- ☐ Hypertension ☐ Stroke
- ☐ Seizures ☐ Diabetes
- ☐ COPD ☐ Cardiac
- ☐ Other (List) ☐ Asthma

Unknown

Current Medications (List)
Unknown

VITAL SIGNS

TIME	RESP	PULSE	B.P.	MENTAL STATUS	R PUPILS L	SKIN
2130	Rate: *28* ☐ Regular ☒ Shallow ☐ Labored	Rate: *120* ☒ Regular ☐ Irregular	*90/60*	☐ Alert ☑ Voice ☐ Pain ☐ Unresp.	Normal ☐☐ Dilated ☐☐ Constricted ☐☐ Sluggish ☑☑ No-Reaction ☐☐	☐ Unremarkable ☑ Cool ☐ Pale ☐ Warm ☐ Cyanotic ☐ Moist ☑ Flushed ☐ Dry ☐ Jaundiced
2135	Rate: *28* ☐ Regular ☒ Shallow ☐ Labored	Rate: *120* ☒ Regular ☐ Irregular	*90/60*	☐ Alert ☑ Voice ☐ Pain ☐ Unresp.	Normal ☐☐ Dilated ☐☐ Constricted ☐☐ Sluggish ☑☑ No-Reaction ☐☐	☐ Unremarkable ☑ Cool ☐ Pale ☐ Warm ☐ Cyanotic ☐ Moist ☑ Flushed ☐ Dry ☐ Jaundiced
	Rate: ☐ Regular ☐ Shallow ☐ Labored	Rate: ☐ Regular ☐ Irregular	/	☐ Alert ☐ Voice ☐ Pain ☐ Unresp.	Normal ☐☐ Dilated ☐☐ Constricted ☐☐ Sluggish ☐☐ No-Reaction ☐☐	☐ Unremarkable ☐ Cool ☐ Pale ☐ Warm ☐ Cyanotic ☐ Moist ☐ Flushed ☐ Dry ☐ Jaundiced

NARRATIVE *EMS requested to the scene by local police, who state they found the patient sitting on a heater grate alongside the sidewalk in soaking wet clothing. They state that the patient did not appear alert, so EMS was requested. On our arrival, patient responds to loud verbal stimuli with occasional inappropriate responses. Patient is obviously shivering and initially appears to be hypothermic. Once patient is loaded in the ambulance via the cot, the heat is turned up. We removed patient's wet clothing and gently dried him prior to wrapping him in warm, dry blankets. Oxygen therapy is initiated prior to transporting the patient with as gentle a ride as possible. The patient is turned over to the hospital slightly more alert and oriented.*

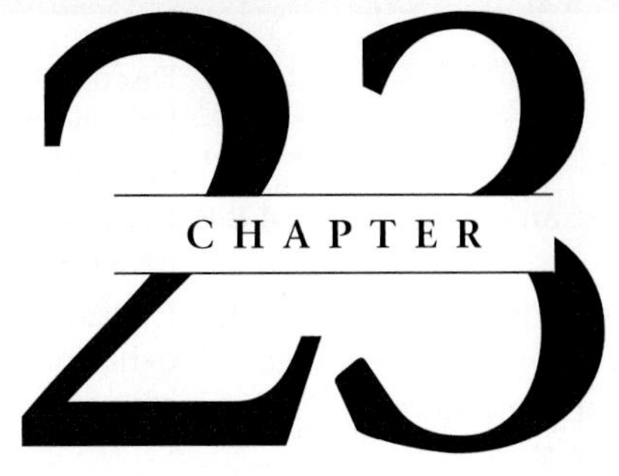

CHAPTER 23

Behavioral Emergencies

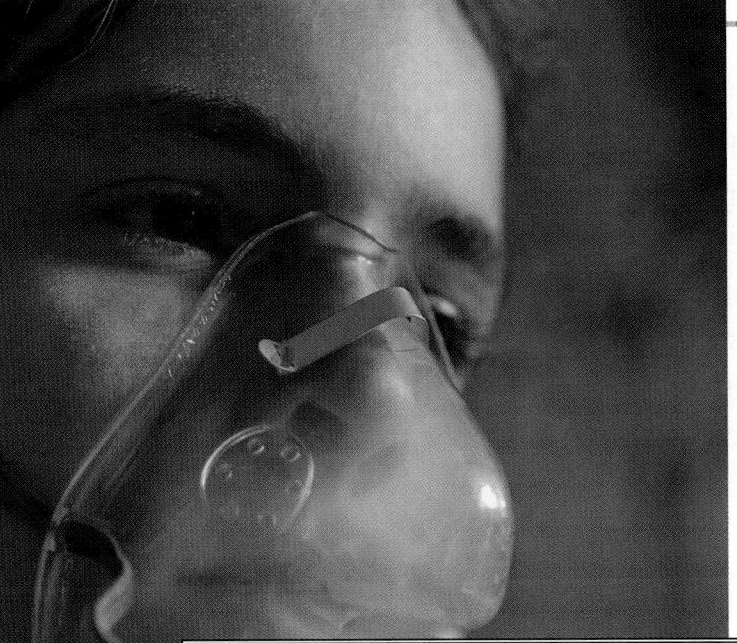

CORE CONCEPTS

The following are core concepts that will be addressed in this chapter:

- How to identify patients who are experiencing a behavioral emergency
- How to recognize potentially dangerous patients and act with safety in mind
- Methods of calming and interacting with patients experiencing behavioral emergencies
- How to restrain a patient safely and effectively
- How to document findings and care of patients with behavioral emergencies

KEY TERMS

behavior, p. 548
behavioral emergency, p. 548
positional asphyxia, p. 556

DOT OBJECTIVES

*KNOWLEDGE AND ATTITUDE

4-8.1 Define behavioral emergencies. (p. 548)

4-8.2 Discuss the general factors that may cause an alteration in a patient's behavior. (pp. 548–550)

4-8.3 State the various reasons for psychological crises. (pp. 548–550, 552–553)

4-8.4 Discuss the characteristics of an individual's behavior which suggest that the patient is at risk for suicide. (pp. 552–553)

4-8.5 Discuss special medical/legal considerations for managing behavioral emergencies. (pp. 555–556, 558) (Scan 23-1, p. 557)

4-8.6 Discuss the special considerations for assessing a patient with behavioral problems. (pp. 551, 552–553, 554)

4-8.7 Discuss the general principles of an individual's behavior which suggest that he is at risk for violence. (p. 554)

4-8.8 Discuss methods to calm behavioral emergency patients. (pp. 550, 552, 553, 555)

4-8.9 Explain the rationale for learning how to modify your behavior toward the patient with a behavioral emergency. (pp. 550, 553)

*SKILLS

4-8.10 Demonstrate the assessment and emergency medical care of the patient experiencing a behavioral emergency.

4-8.11 Demonstrate various techniques to safely restrain a patient with a behavioral problem.

As an EMT, you will respond to many emergencies in which the patient is behaving in unexpected and sometimes dangerous ways. The unusual behavior may be the result of stress, physical trauma or illness, drug or alcohol abuse, or mental illness. Whatever the apparent cause, do not hesitate to request police assistance whenever you feel it is necessary. Local protocol may even require it. Once the scene is secure, you will be able to provide appropriate emergency care.

BEHAVIORAL EMERGENCIES

What Is a Behavioral Emergency?

behavior
the manner in which a person acts.

behavioral emergency
when a patient's behavior is not typical for the situation; when the patient's behavior is unacceptable or intolerable to the patient, his family, or the community, or when the patient may harm himself or others.

We all exhibit behavior. **Behavior** is defined as the manner in which a person acts or performs. Behavior involves any or all activities of a person, including physical and mental activity. Of course, behavior differs from person to person and from situation to situation.

A **behavioral emergency** exists when a person exhibits abnormal behavior—that is, behavior within a given situation that is unacceptable or intolerable to the patient, the family, or the community.

A key part of that definition is "within a given situation." You may have observed, in your own life or in that of friends or family, that behavior varies, depending on the situation at hand. For example, if a person is notified unexpectedly of the death of a loved one, a common reaction is screaming, crying, throwing things, or other emotional outbursts. In the context of the situation, this behavior would not be unusual. If the same behaviors were exhibited for no apparent reason in the middle of a shopping center, they might indicate a behavioral emergency.

Remember that you will be exposed to persons from other cultures and with different lifestyles. Some behaviors may seem unusual to you but might be quite normal to the person performing them. Behavioral conditions require patient assessment, just like any other emergency. Remain objective. Do not judge patients hastily or solely on the way they look or act.

Physical Causes of Altered Behavior

Many medical and traumatic conditions are likely to alter a patient's behavior. These problems may include:

- *Low blood sugar*, which may be the cause of rapid onset of erratic or hostile behavior (similar to alcohol intoxication), dizziness and headache, fainting, seizures, sometimes coma, profuse perspiration, hunger, drooling, and rapid pulse but normal blood pressure. (See Chapter 19, "Diabetic Emergencies and Altered Mental Status.")
- *Lack of oxygen*, which may cause restlessness and confusion, cyanosis (blue or gray skin), and altered mental status.
- *Inadequate blood to the brain or stroke*, which may cause confusion or dizziness, impaired speech, headache, loss of function or paralysis of extremities on one side of body, nausea and vomiting, and rapid full pulse.
- *Head trauma*, which can cause personality changes ranging from irritability to irrational behavior, altered mental status, amnesia or confusion, irregular respirations, elevated blood pressure, and decreasing pulse.
- *Mind-altering substances*, which can cause highly variable signs and symptoms depending on the substance ingested. (See Chapter 21, "Poisoning and Overdose Emergencies.")
- *Excessive cold*, which may cause shivering, feelings of numbness, altered mental status, drowsiness, staggering walk, slow breathing, and slow pulse.
- *Excessive heat*, which may cause decreased or complete loss of consciousness. (See Chapter 22, "Environmental Emergencies.")

When dealing with someone who appears to be having a behavioral emergency, always consider the possibility that his unusual behavior is caused by something other than a psychological problem (Figure 23-1).

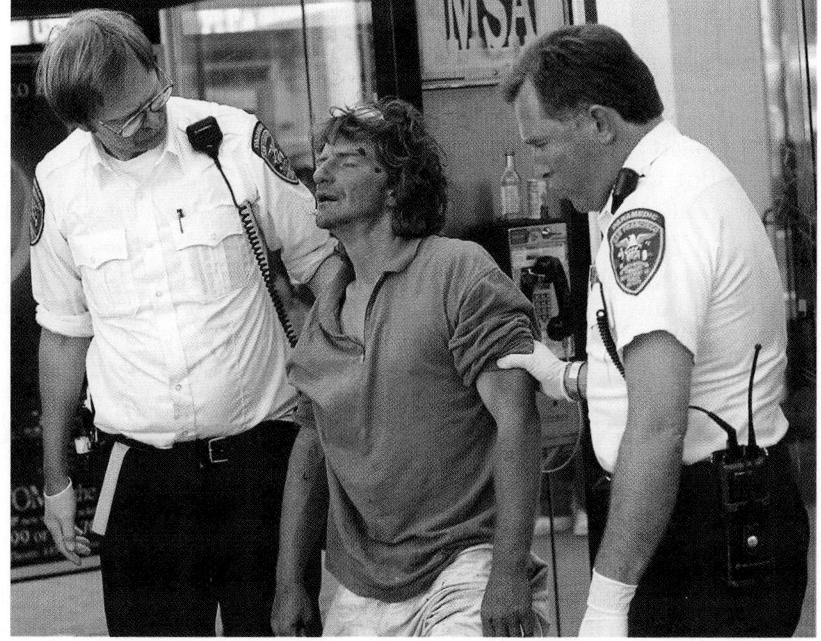

Figure 23-1 • There are many reasons why a patient may experience an altered mental status. *(© Craig Jackson/In the Dark Photography)*

CRITICAL DECISION MAKING: PSYCH CONDITION . . . OR HIDDEN MEDICAL CONDITION?

You will respond to many behavioral emergencies during your EMS experience. Sometimes patients with medical problems appear to be psychiatric patients but aren't. Other times, patients with a psychiatric history have medical problems that aren't related to their psychiatric condition. For each of these patients describe how your assessment would determine if the patient was suffering from a medical problem or a psychiatric problem.

1. Your patient is a 56-year-old man who was found to be "talking to God" and generally mumbling at the grocery store.
2. Your patient is a 21-year-old student who was found on the outskirts of his campus, acting strangely, with a slight smell of alcohol on his breath.
3. Your patient is an 84-year-old woman who is in a nursing home. She has a history of depression and cardiac problems. This morning she became agitated and angry with the staff.

Situational Stress Reactions

When faced with severe, unexpected stress, most patients will display emotions such as fear, grief, and anger. These are typical stress reactions at the accident scene and common reactions to serious illness and death. In the vast majority of cases, as you begin to take control of the situation and treat the patient as an individual, personal interaction will inspire confidence in your ability to help. The patient will begin to calm down and may even begin to feel able to cope with the emergency.

Be as unhurried as you can. If you rush your patient assessment and interview, the patient may feel as if the situation is out of control. The patient also may believe that you are concerned about the problem but not about him. Let the patient know that you are there to help.

Whenever you care for a patient who is displaying typical stress reactions, act in a calm manner, giving the patient time to gain control of his emotions. Quietly and carefully evaluate the situation, keeping your own emotions under control. Let the patient know that you are listening to what he is saying, and explain things to the patient honestly. Stay alert for sudden changes in behavior.

By acting in this manner, you are applying crisis management techniques to help the patient deal with stress. If the patient does not begin to interact with you or calm down, and if there are no apparent physical causes for the behavior, you must assume that there is a problem of a more serious nature, such as a psychiatric problem. Proceed according to the recommendations in the following segments of this chapter.

EMERGENCY CARE FOR BEHAVIORAL EMERGENCIES

Psychiatric Emergencies

There is a wide range of psychiatric problems. One patient with a psychiatric condition may be withdrawn and not wish to communicate while another may be agitated, talkative, or exhibiting bizarre or threatening behavior. Some patients may act as if they wish to harm themselves or others.

Follow these general rules to deal with a patient who is experiencing a behavioral or psychiatric emergency:

- Identify yourself and your role.
- Speak slowly and clearly. Use a calm and reassuring tone.
- Listen to the patient. You can show you are listening by repeating part of what the patient says back to him.
- Do not be judgmental. Show compassion, not pity.
- Use positive body language. Avoid crossing your arms or looking uninterested.
- Acknowledge the patient's feelings.
- Do not enter the patient's personal space. Stay at least 3 feet from the patient. Making the patient feel closed in can cause an emotional outburst.
- Be alert for changes in the patient's emotional status. Watch for increasingly aggressive behavior and take appropriate safety precautions.

PATIENT ASSESSMENT

BEHAVIORAL OR PSYCHIATRIC EMERGENCY

To assess a patient who appears to be suffering a behavioral or psychiatric emergency:

- Perform a careful scene size-up. If there are indications at the time of dispatch that the call may involve a potentially violent or agitated patient, then police should be requested to respond to the scene, arriving ahead of EMS units to assure the scene is safe ("secure") for EMS to enter.
- Identify yourself and your role. It may not be obvious to the patient who you are and what you intend to do.
- Complete an initial assessment, including assessment of the patient's mental status (level of responsiveness; orientation to person, place, and time).
- Perform as much of the focused and detailed examinations as possible. Be alert for medical and traumatic conditions that could be causing the patient's behavior.
- Gather a thorough patient history. This will alert you to past psychiatric problems, or psychiatric medications the patient may be taking (or not taking—causing the outburst). This may also alert you to conditions such as diabetes that can closely mimic a psychiatric condition.

Common presentations, or signs and symptoms, of patients experiencing psychiatric emergencies include:

- Panic or anxiety
- Unusual appearance, disordered clothing, poor hygiene
- Agitated or unusual activity, such as repetitive motions, threatening movements, or withdrawn stance
- Unusual speech patterns, such as too rapid or pressured-sounding speech (as if being forced out), or inability to carry on a coherent conversation
- Bizarre behavior or thought patterns
- Suicidal or self-destructive behavior
- Violent or aggressive behavior with threats or intent to harm others ■

PATIENT CARE

BEHAVIORAL OR PSYCHIATRIC EMERGENCY

Emergency care of a patient having a behavioral or psychiatric emergency includes:

- Be alert for personal or scene safety problems throughout the call.
- Treat any life-threatening problems during the initial assessment.
- Be alert for medical or traumatic conditions that could mimic a behavioral emergency. Treat conditions you identify (e.g., low blood sugar level).
- Be prepared to spend time talking to the patient. Use the skills listed earlier in dealing with the patient. Remember to talk in a calm, reassuring voice. Use positive body language and good eye contact. Avoid unnecessary physical contact and quick movements.
- Encourage the patient to discuss what is troubling him.
- Never play along with any visual or auditory hallucinations that a patient may be experiencing. Do not lie to the patient.
- If it appears it will help, involve family members or friends in the conversation. Evaluate the response of the patient to the presence of others. If it agitates the patient, ask the others to leave. ■

Suicide

Each year in this country, thousands of people commit suicide. Suicide is the eighth leading cause of death, but the third leading cause of death in the 15- to 24-year-old age group. Depression and suicide have also reached alarming levels in the senior citizen population. Many more suffer both physical and emotional injuries in suicide attempts. Anyone may become suicidal if emotional distress is severe, regardless of gender, age, or ethnic, social, or economic background.

People attempt suicide for many reasons, including depression caused by chemical imbalance, the death of a loved one, financial problems, the end to a love affair, poor health, loss of esteem, divorce, fear of failure, and alcohol and drug abuse. People attempt to end their lives by any one of a variety of methods. You may observe suicides or attempted suicides by drug overdose, hanging, jumping from high places, ingesting poisons, inhaling gas, wrist-cutting, self-mutilation, stabbing, or shooting.

PATIENT ASSESSMENT

POTENTIAL OR ATTEMPTED SUICIDE

Factors often associated with a risk for suicide appear in the following list. Although some or even all of them may be present in a patient, it is not possible to use these characteristics to predict who will or who will not commit suicide:

- *Depression.* Take seriously a patient's feelings and expressions of despair or suicidal thoughts.
- *High current or recent stress levels.* If so, take the threat of suicide seriously.
- *Recent emotional trauma.* This could be job loss, loss of a significant relationship, serious illness, arrest, or imprisonment.
- *Age.* High suicide rates occur at ages 15 to 25 and over age 40. The elderly are a population where suicide rates are increasing.
- *Alcohol and drug abuse.*
- *Threats of suicide.* The patient may have told others that he is considering suicide. Take all threats of suicide seriously.

continued

PATIENT ASSESSMENT *(continued)*

- *Suicide plan.* A patient who has a detailed suicide plan is more likely to commit suicide. Look for a plan that includes a method to carry out the suicide, notes, giving away personal possessions, or getting affairs in order.
- *Previous attempts or suicide threats.* These could include a history of self-destructive behavior. Often patients who have attempted suicide on a previous occasion are considered to be "looking for attention" and are not taken seriously on subsequent attempts. However, statistics reveal that a person who has attempted suicide in the past is more likely to commit suicide than one who has not.
- *Sudden improvement from depression.* A patient who has made the decision to commit suicide may actually appear to be coming out of a depression. The fact that the decision has been made and an end is in sight can cause this apparent "improvement." You may find family members and friends of suicidal patients who will report that the patient had seemed "better" in the past few days. ■

NOTE

Whenever you are called to care for a patient who has attempted or may be about to attempt suicide, your first concern must be your own safety. Not all patients will wish to harm you, but the mechanism used to attempt suicide will be capable of causing death. It could intentionally or accidentally be turned on you.

PATIENT CARE

POTENTIAL OR ATTEMPTED SUICIDE

Patients who are in an emotional, psychiatric, or attempted-suicide emergency are cared for in similar ways. In all cases, your personal interaction with the patient is key. Try to establish visual and verbal contact as soon as possible. Avoid arguing. Make no threats, and show no indication of using force.

Remember that you are the first professional to begin both the physical and mental health care of the patient. The more reassurance you can provide for the patient, the easier it will be for the hospital emergency department staff to continue care.

Emergency care includes the following:

1. Treatment must begin with scene size-up. Make sure it is safe to approach the patient. If the scene is not safe, request assistance from the police and wait until they have secured the scene. Do not leave the patient alone unless you are at risk of physical harm. Try to talk with the patient from a safe distance until the police arrive. Take Standard Precautions.
2. When the scene is secure, look for and treat life-threatening problems to the extent that the patient will permit it. Seek police assistance in restraining the patient if necessary for care of life-threatening problems.
3. As possible, perform a focused history and physical exam and provide emergency care.
4. Perform a detailed physical exam only if it is safe and you suspect the patient may have an injury.
5. Perform ongoing assessment. Watch for sudden changes in the patient's behavior and physical condition.
6. Contact the receiving hospital and report on current mental status and other essential information.

Note that a physical exam may be difficult with the emotional or psychiatric patient. You may not be able to proceed beyond the initial assessment. ■

Throughout your interaction with the patient, speak slowly and patiently await answers to your questions. As you gain the patient's confidence, explain what questions must be answered and what must be done as part of the physical exam and taking vital signs. Let the patient know that you think it would be best if he goes to the hospital and that you need his cooperation and help. Back off if necessary. If the patient's fear or aggression increases, do not push the issues of the examination or transport. Instead, try to reestablish the conversation and give the patient more time before you again say that going to the hospital is a good idea.

Transport all suicidal patients. Seek police assistance if necessary. Report any attempted suicide or expression of suicidal thoughts to the medical facility, police, or government agency designated by your state law and local protocols.

Aggressive or Hostile Patients

Aggressive or disruptive behavior may be caused by trauma to the brain and nervous system, metabolic disorders, stress, alcohol, other drugs, or psychological disorders. Sometimes you will know that your patient is aggressive from the information you receive from dispatch. Other times the scene may provide quick clues (such as drugs, yelling, unclean conditions, broken furniture). Neighbors, family members, or bystanders may tell you that the patient is dangerous or angry or has a history of aggression or combativeness. The patient's stance (tense muscles, fists clenched, or quick irregular movements, for example) or his position in the room may give you an early warning of possible violence. On rare occasions, you may start with an apparently calm patient who suddenly turns aggressive.

NOTE

When a patient acts as if he may hurt himself or others, your first concern must be your own safety. Take the following precautions:

- ***Do not isolate yourself from your partner or other sources of help. Make certain that you have an escape route. Do not let the patient come between you and the door. Should a patient become violent, retreat and wait for police assistance.***
- ***Do not take any action that may be considered threatening by the patient. To do so may bring about hostile behavior directed against you or others.***
- ***Always be on the watch for weapons. Stay out of kitchens, as they are filled with dangerous weapons. Stay in a safe area until the police can control the scene.***
- ***Be alert for sudden changes in the patient's behavior.***

PATIENT ASSESSMENT

AGGRESSIVE OR HOSTILE PATIENT

Your assessment of the aggressive or hostile patient may never go beyond the initial assessment phase. Most of your time may be spent trying to calm the patient and ensuring everyone's safety. An aggressive or hostile patient:

- Responds to people inappropriately
- Tries to hurt himself or others
- May have a rapid pulse and breathing
- Usually displays rapid speech and rapid physical movements
- May appear anxious, nervous, "panicky" ■

PATIENT CARE

AGGRESSIVE OR HOSTILE PATIENT

Follow these steps for the emergency care of an aggressive or hostile patient:

1. Treatment begins with scene size-up. Make sure it is safe to approach the patient. Request assistance from law enforcement before approaching if necessary. Practice Standard Precautions.
2. Seek advice from medical direction if the patient's behavior prevents normal assessment and care procedures.
3. As part of ongoing assessment, watch for sudden changes in the patient's behavior.
4. Seek assistance from law enforcement, as well as from medical direction, if restraint seems necessary. ■

Reasonable Force and Restraint

Reasonable force is the force necessary to keep a patient from injuring himself or others. Reasonableness is determined by looking at all circumstances involved, including the patient's strength and size, type of abnormal behavior, mental status, and available methods of restraint. Understand that you may protect yourself from attack, but otherwise you must avoid actions that can cause injury to the patient.

In addition, in most localities an EMT cannot legally restrain a behavioral emergency patient, move such a patient against his will, or force such a patient to accept emergency care—even at the family's request. The restraint and forcible moving of patients is usually within the jurisdiction of law enforcement. The police (and in some areas a physician) can order you to restrain and transport a patient to the appropriate medical facility. However, the physician is not empowered to order you to take action that could place you in danger. If police order restraint and transport, they must assist with these procedures as necessary. Remember to follow local protocol.

At times, a patient with a medical or traumatic emergency may display violent behavior to the extent that restraint is necessary before the patient can receive the medical treatment he needs. For example, a diabetic patient with hypoglycemia may be acting abnormally and even aggressively. If the patient's behavior interferes with or prevents treatment and the EMT can safely restrain the patient, he should do so in order to initiate treatment. Similarly, a patient with a head injury may be hypoxic and acting abnormally. Again, if it can be done safely, the EMT should institute the needed treatment which, in this case, includes restraint so the patient can be safely transported to a facility where his head injury can be treated.

Determining whether a particular patient has a medical or traumatic emergency that is causing his abnormal behavior can be difficult. Consider whether the patient is capable of giving or refusing informed consent, consult medical direction, and administer the care that is in the patient's best interest without endangering yourself.

Never try to assist in restraining a patient unless there are sufficient personnel to do the job. You must be able to ensure your safety as well as the safety of the patient. If you help the police or a physician to restrain a patient, make certain that the restraints are humane. Handcuffs and plastic "throwaway" criminal restraints should not be used because of the soft-tissue damage they can inflict. Initially, the police may have to use such restraints. However, in some states they can be replaced with soft restraints such as leather cuffs and belts. If authorized in your state and by local protocol, an ambulance should carry leather cuffs, a waist-size belt, and at least three short belts. Restraints for the wrists and ankles can be made from gauze roller bandages.

Do not remove police restraints until you and the police are certain that soft restraints will hold the patient. To ensure everyone's safety once they are on, do not remove soft restraints, even if the patient appears to be acting rationally.

Follow these guidelines when a patient must be restrained (Scan 23-1):

- Be sure to have adequate help.
- Plan your activities.
- Estimate the range of motion of the patient's arms and legs and stay beyond range until ready.
- Once the decision to restrain the patient has been reached, act quickly.
- Have one EMT talk to and reassure the patient throughout the restraining procedure.
- Approach with a minimum of four persons, one assigned to each limb, all to act at the same time. (Five rescuers would allow an extra person to control the head. The rescuer at the head should use caution to prevent being bitten.)
- Secure all four limbs with restraints approved by medical direction.
- Position the patient face up. The position will be dictated by what the restraining process itself permits, the patient's condition (e.g., injuries, breathing problems), and local protocols. Monitor the patient's airway. Never "hog tie" the patient or restrain the patient in any manner that will impair breathing. Patients who have been improperly restrained have died as a result of a condition called **positional asphyxia.** Monitor all restrained patients carefully.
- Use multiple straps or other restraints to ensure that the patient is adequately secured. Anticipate that the patient's behavior may turn more violent and be sure that restraint is adequate for this possibility.
- If the patient is spitting on rescuers, place a surgical mask on the patient if he has no breathing difficulty or likelihood of vomiting and if local protocols permit, or have rescuers wear protective masks, eye wear, and clothing.
- Reassess the patient's distal circulation frequently and adjust restraints as safe and necessary if distal circulation is diminished.
- Use sufficient force, but avoid unnecessary force.
- Document the reasons why the patient was restrained and the technique of restraint.

positional asphyxia
Death of a person due to a body position that restricts breathing for a prolonged time.

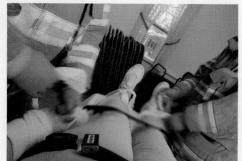

POINT OF VIEW

"I was at a group therapy session when I started noticing people were watching me. They did that for awhile. When I would talk they would whisper and giggle and point. I heard voices. They whispered, too. I couldn't see the people, but I heard the voices very clearly. They were talking about me.

"I stood up and yelled. "'Don't say those things. Oh yes, you. Stop it right now!'" They kept going. The voices got louder. I started pushing people and throwing chairs. They had no right to do this to me. The voices just laughed. People pointed and whispered. I knew what they were thinking.

"The ambulance came. The police came. I got tied down and taken to the hospital.

"Some of what I tell you is based on what my counselor told me. I don't remember it all. You see, I am schizophrenic. I guess you could say reality isn't my strong point sometimes. I can joke about it now. What I experienced are called paranoid delusions. I get them a lot. I can usually control them. But sometimes when I can't afford my pills or I get fed up with the fact that I feel groggy all the time or when I can't have sex I stop taking them.

"That's when I hear voices and get restrained and taken to the hospital. Man, there has got to be a better way."

SCAN 23-1 • Restraining a Patient

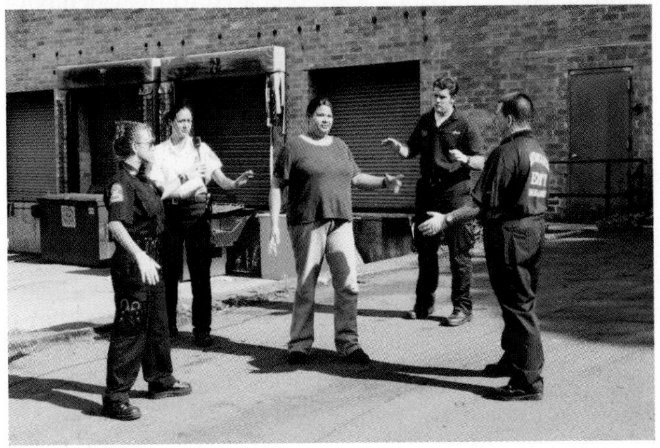

1. Plan your approach to the patient in advance and remain outside the range of arms and legs until you are ready to act.

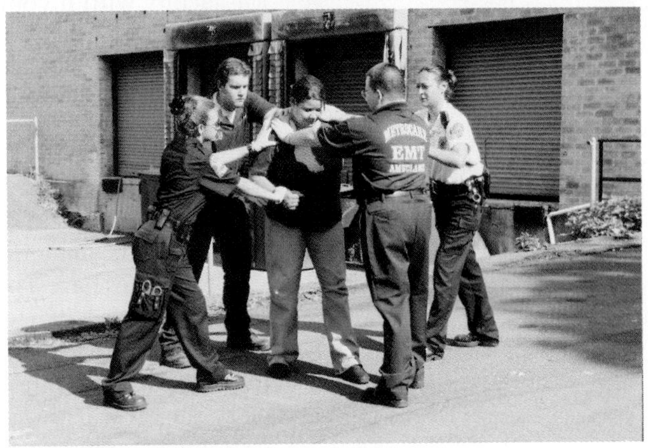

2. Assign one EMT to each limb, and approach the patient at the same time.

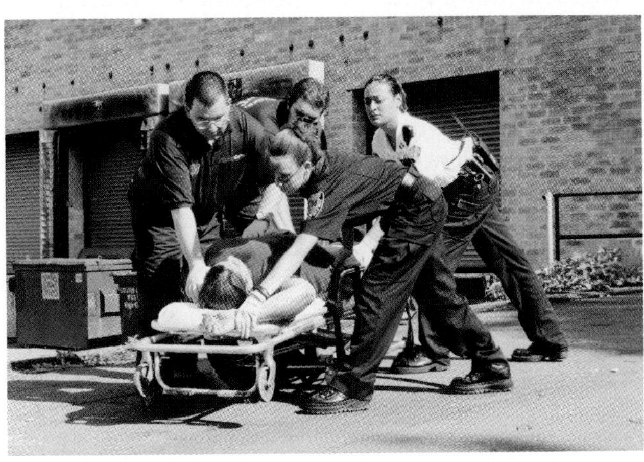

3. Place the patient on the stretcher as his/her condition and local protocols indicate. Do not let go until the patient is properly secured.

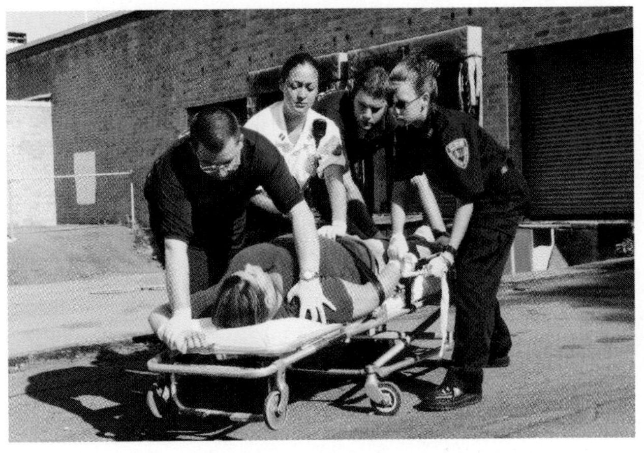

4. Use multiple straps or other soft restraints to secure the patient to the stretcher.

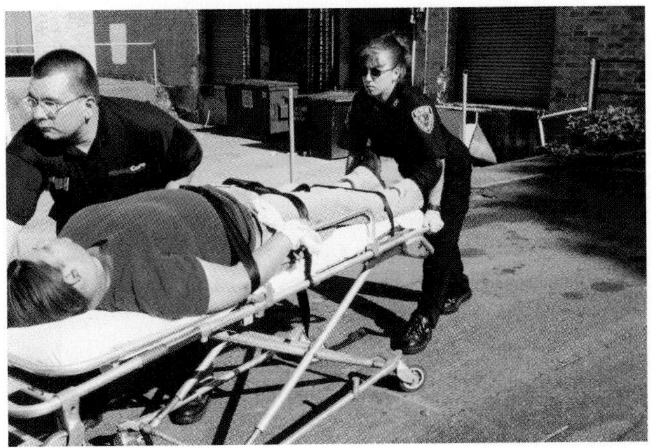

5. When the patient is secure, assess distal circulation and monitor airway and breathing continually. *(Photos 1–5 © Craig Jackson/In the Dark Photography)*

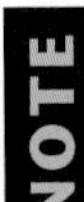

NOTE

A fifth rescuer, if available, can control the patient's head—taking special care, however, not to be bitten.

Transport to an Appropriate Facility

Your medical protocols or procedures should direct you to the most appropriate medical facility within your service area. Not all hospitals are prepared to treat behavioral emergencies.

Medical/Legal Considerations

A patient who refuses emergency care or transport is a significant medical/legal risk for EMS agencies and EMTs. What should you do when a behavioral emergency patient refuses or resists your efforts to provide care?

Most states have a provision in law that will allow a patient to be transported against his will if he is a danger to himself or others. This is an exception to the rule that patients must provide consent for their care and transportation. Know your state laws on treating patients without consent. Many states give this authority to law enforcement personnel. It will always be beneficial to have the police present if the patient must be restrained as a matter of safety.

You may also be required to contact medical direction about the psychiatric patient who refuses care. Many communities have mental health teams that will respond to the scene to help with the care of a patient with behavioral problems. This team will also help evaluate the need for transporting the patient against his will.

Emotionally disturbed patients sometimes accuse EMS personnel of sexual misconduct. If possible, EMTs of the same sex as the patient should attend to emergency care of disturbed patients. For the aggressive or violent patient, make sure law enforcement officers accompany you to the hospital to protect you and the patient. In the event of a legal problem, they can serve as third-party witnesses.

For more information on this topic, review Chapter 3, "Medical/Legal and Ethical Issues."

CHAPTER REVIEW

SUMMARY

As an EMT, you will respond to many behavioral emergencies. Because the treatment for these patients usually requires long-term management, little medical intervention can be done in the acute situation. However, how you interact with the patient during the emergency can make a difference—to the patient and to the medical professionals who take over. On these calls remember that you must ensure your own safety, consider the legal ramifications of your actions, document the circumstances, and transport the patient in a safe and effective manner to an appropriate facility. Know your local protocols.

KEY TERMS

behavior the manner in which a person acts.

behavioral emergency when a patient's behavior is not typical for the situation; when the patient's behavior is unacceptable or intolerable to the patient, his family, or the community; or when the patient may harm himself or others.

positional asphyxia death of a person due to a body position that restricts breathing for a prolonged time.

REVIEW QUESTIONS

1. Name several conditions that can alter a person's mental status and behavior. (pp. 549–550)
2. List several methods that can help calm the patient suffering a behavioral or psychiatric emergency. (pp. 552, 553, 554, 555)
3. Describe the signs and symptoms of a behavioral or psychiatric emergency. (pp. 551, 552–553, 554)
4. Describe what you can do when scene size-up reveals that it is too dangerous to approach the patient. (p. 554)
5. List several factors that can help you assess the patient's risk for suicide. (pp. 552–553)
6. Research your state law. Then describe the circumstances that must exist for you to treat and transport a behavioral emergency patient without consent. (p. 558)

CRITICAL THINKING

- You are called to respond to an intoxicated minor who is physically aggressive, threatens suicide, and whose parents permit you to treat but not transport. How would you manage this patient?

Thinking and Linking

Think back to Chapter 19, "Diabetic Emergencies and Altered Mental Status," as well as to Chapter 21, "Poisoning and Overdose Emergencies," and link information from those chapters with information from this chapter as you consider the following situation:

- You are called to a patient who is acting bizarrely. List some indications (clues at the scene, signs and symptoms) that might indicate the abnormal behavior was actually due to a diabetic condition or overdose emergency.

Think back to Chapter 5, "Lifting and Moving Patients," and link information from that chapter with information from this chapter as you consider the following situation:

- The police have subdued a violent psychiatric patient. They ask you to transport the patient to the hospital. What would you use to restrain the patient's extremities? What transport device would you use? How would you secure the patient's extremities to that device?

MEDIA RESOURCES 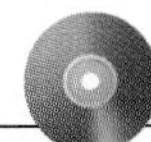

See the Student CD at the back of this book for quizzes, a case study activity, animations, and other features related to this chapter. Also, visit the Companion Website for *Emergency Care* at **www.prenhall.com/limmer**, where you will find additional reinforcement and links to other resources.

It's a sunny and relatively quiet summer afternoon when you are dispatched to a small manufacturing company for an individual "acting in a bizarre manner." The dispatcher is trying to get additional information, but it is difficult. Your response time is 5 minutes, and you are met outside by the manager. He tells you that about 15 minutes ago a worker kicked a table and disrupted some of the equipment. When he was approached by coworkers, he said, "Stay away, or I will hurt myself." The manager says the patient has a knife, but no one has seen it.

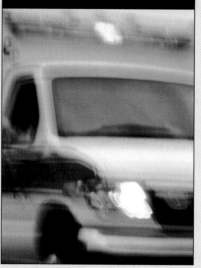

Street Scene Questions

1. What is your first and most important concern?
2. How should you handle the matter of scene safety?
3. When should you approach the patient?

You contact the dispatcher who informs you that two police officers are responding and should be on scene in 3 minutes. You make sure that your crew and bystanders are in a safe position in the event the patient exits the building. When the officers pull up, you tell them what you know. The police tell you to wait outside. They enter the building and find the patient still very agitated. While you wait outside, a coworker of the patient approaches and says that she might have some information that could help. Supposedly, the patient is on antidepressant drugs and his wife recently left him. She believes that he could hurt himself but she doubts he will hurt anyone else. At this point, one of the police officers tells you that the patient is calm and they have frisked him.

Street Scene Questions

4. How should the patient be approached?
5. What are the safety concerns when working with an agitated patient?
6. Does this patient need a medical assessment?

You decide that only you should approach the patient so as not to overwhelm him. There is already a police officer standing next to him. As you approach, you introduce yourself and tell the patient that you need to ask some questions and get some medical information. You listen to him and, during the medical history, you ask if he has taken more medication than he should. He says that he took his morning dose but that is all. You take a set of vital signs and continue to listen. After a few minutes, the patient agrees to go to the hospital with you.

You ask your partner to move the ambulance to a back door so the patient doesn't have to pass coworkers on the way out. You have discussed the situation with the police officers and you feel confident that there is no longer a safety issue and that they won't be needed for the transport. The police searched the patient for weapons and found none. The patient is placed on the stretcher with all safety straps applied. You listen to the patient all the way to the hospital, being compassionate and acknowledging the patient's feelings as well as you can. Your partner calls the hospital on the radio and gives an ETA of 5 minutes.

Later, as you walk away from the patient in the emergency department, he smiles and thanks you for listening.

Street Scenes Sample Documentation

PATIENT NAME: *Robert Lanctot* PATIENT AGE: *38*

CHIEF COMPLAINT

Threatening to injure self

PAST MEDICAL HISTORY

- ☐ None
- ☐ Allergy to ____
- ☐ Hypertension
- ☐ Stroke
- ☐ Seizures
- ☐ Diabetes
- ☐ COPD
- ☐ Cardiac
- ☒ Other (List)
- ☐ Asthma

Depression, marital problems

Current Medications (List)

Unknown antidepressant

VITAL SIGNS

TIME	RESP	PULSE	B.P.	MENTAL STATUS	R PUPILS L	SKIN
1015	Rate: 20; ☒ Regular; ☐ Shallow; ☐ Labored	Rate: 90; ☒ Regular; ☐ Irregular	120/80	☑ Alert; ☐ Voice; ☐ Pain; ☐ Unresp.	☑ Normal ☑; ☐ Dilated ☐; ☐ Constricted ☐; ☐ Sluggish ☐; ☐ No-Reaction ☐	☑ Unremarkable; ☐ Cool ☐ Pale; ☐ Warm ☐ Cyanotic; ☐ Moist ☐ Flushed; ☐ Dry ☐ Jaundiced
	Rate: ; ☐ Regular; ☐ Shallow; ☐ Labored	Rate: ; ☐ Regular; ☐ Irregular	/	☐ Alert; ☐ Voice; ☐ Pain; ☐ Unresp.	☐ Normal ☐; ☐ Dilated ☐; ☐ Constricted ☐; ☐ Sluggish ☐; ☐ No-Reaction ☐	☐ Unremarkable; ☐ Cool ☐ Pale; ☐ Warm ☐ Cyanotic; ☐ Moist ☐ Flushed; ☐ Dry ☐ Jaundiced
	Rate: ; ☐ Regular; ☐ Shallow; ☐ Labored	Rate: ; ☐ Regular; ☐ Irregular	/	☐ Alert; ☐ Voice; ☐ Pain; ☐ Unresp.	☐ Normal ☐; ☐ Dilated ☐; ☐ Constricted ☐; ☐ Sluggish ☐; ☐ No-Reaction ☐	☐ Unremarkable; ☐ Cool ☐ Pale; ☐ Warm ☐ Cyanotic; ☐ Moist ☐ Flushed; ☐ Dry ☐ Jaundiced

NARRATIVE *EMS requested to the scene by manager, who states the patient had a very sudden onset of disruptive behavior and threatened to injure himself with a knife. The patient appears very agitated when approached by police officers. According to a coworker, patient is on an unknown antidepressant and had a recent break up with his wife. After being calmed by police, patient consents to transportation for evaluation. Patient is cooperative and denies taking an overdose of his medication or any other injury.*

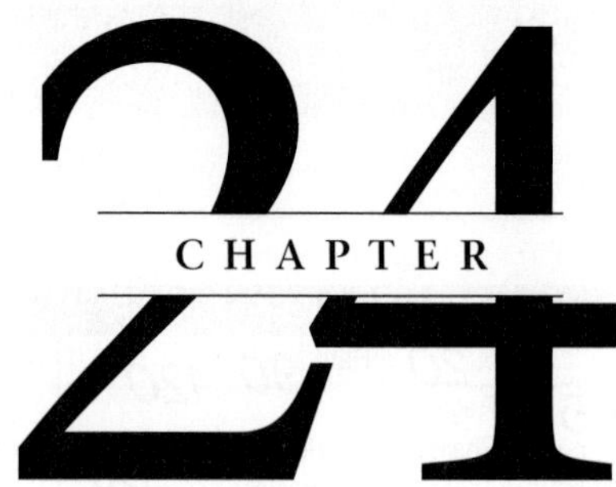

CHAPTER 24

Obstetrics and Gynecological Emergencies

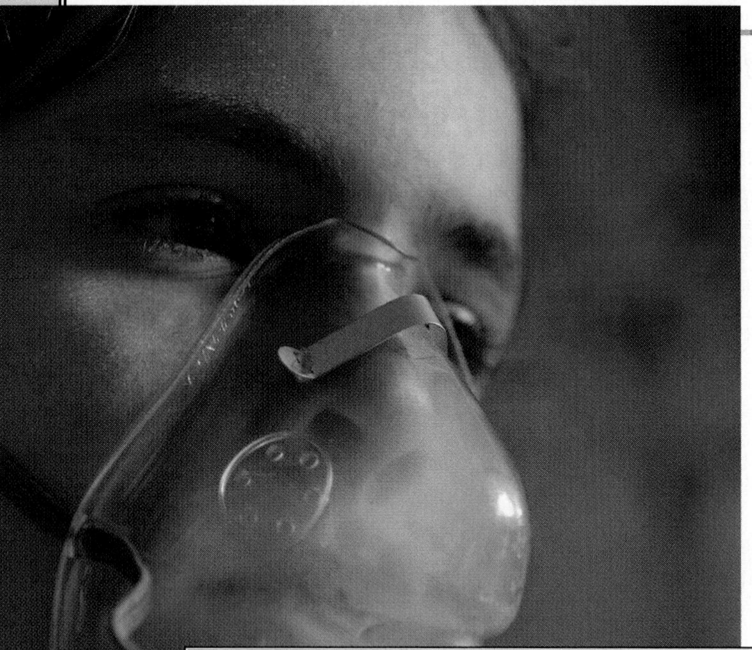

CORE CONCEPTS

The following are core concepts that will be addressed in this chapter:

- How to identify a patient at risk of immediate childbirth
- Care of the mother before, during, and after delivery
- Care of the baby during and after delivery (including potential complications)
- Neonatal resuscitation procedures
- How to document findings and care of patients with obstetric and gynecological emergencies

KEY TERMS

abortion, p. 590
abruptio placentae, p. 588
afterbirth, p. 565
amniotic sac, p. 565
breech presentation, p. 565
cephalic presentation, p. 565
crowning, p. 565
eclampsia, p. 589
ectopic pregnancy, p. 588
fetus, p. 564
labor, p. 565
limb presentation, p. 584
meconium staining, p. 566
multiple birth, p. 584
perineum, p. 581
placenta, p. 564
placenta previa, p. 588
preeclampsia, p. 589
premature infant, p. 586
prolapsed umbilical cord, p. 583
stillborn, p. 592
supine hypotensive syndrome, p. 570
umbilical cord, p. 565
uterus, p. 564

DOT OBJECTIVES

*KNOWLEDGE AND ATTITUDE

4-9.1 Identify the following structures: uterus, vagina, fetus, placenta, umbilical cord, amniotic sac, perineum. (pp. 564, 565, 581)

4-9.2 Identify and explain the use of the contents of an obstetrics kit. (pp. 567–568)

4-9.3 Identify predelivery emergencies. (pp. 570–571, 588–593)

4-9.4 State indications of an imminent delivery. (pp. 567, 568–569)

4-9.5 Differentiate the emergency medical care provided to a patient with predelivery emergencies from a normal delivery. (pp. 588–593)

4-9.6 State the steps in the predelivery preparation of the mother. (p. 571)

4-9.7 Establish the relationship between body substance isolation (Standard Precautions) and childbirth. (p. 571)

4-9.8 State the steps to assist in the delivery. (pp. 571–572, 574) (Scan 24-1, p. 573)

4-9.9 Describe care of the baby as the head appears. (pp. 572–574)

4-9.10 Describe how and when to cut the umbilical cord. (pp. 577–578)

4-9.11 Discuss the steps in the delivery of the placenta. (pp. 579–580)

4-9.12 List the steps in the emergency medical care of the mother postdelivery. (pp. 579–581)

4-9.13 Summarize neonatal resuscitation procedures. (pp. 576–577)

4-9.14 Describe the procedures for the following abnormal deliveries: breech birth, prolapsed cord, limb presentation. (pp. 582–584)

4-9.15 Differentiate the special considerations for multiple births. (pp. 584–585)

4-9.16 Describe special considerations of meconium. (p. 587)

4-9.17 Describe the special considerations of a premature baby. (p. 586)

4-9.18 Discuss the emergency medical care of a patient with a gynecological emergency. (pp. 593–595)

4-9.19 Explain the rationale for understanding the implications of treating two patients (mother and baby). (p. 579)

*SKILLS

4-9.20 Demonstrate the steps to assist in the normal cephalic delivery.

4-9.21 Demonstrate necessary care procedures of the fetus as the head appears.

4-9.22 Demonstrate infant neonatal procedures.

4-9.23 Demonstrate postdelivery care of the infant.

4-9.24 Attend to the steps in the delivery of the placenta.

4-9.25 Demonstrate the procedures for the following abnormal deliveries: vaginal bleeding, breech birth, prolapsed cord, limb presentation.

4-9.26 Demonstrate the steps in the emergency medical care of the mother with excessive bleeding.

4-9.27 Demonstrate completing a prehospital care report for patients with obstetrical/gynecological emergencies.

Childbirth is a natural process that existed long before there were EMTs. During your career as an EMT, you may be called upon to assist with an out-of-hospital delivery. One of your main responsibilities in this situation will be to help calm the patient and family members through your unruffled professional manner. However, because childbirth is not a common occurrence in the prehospital setting, it might be easy to get flustered and seem uncertain about the procedures you are performing. So it is important that you learn about childbirth and practice the procedures required to assist with delivery. If you are ever called upon to assist in a delivery, your skills will contribute to decreased stress and better care of the mother and baby.

fetus (FE-tus) the baby as he develops in the womb.

uterus (U-ter-us) the muscular abdominal organ where the fetus develops; the womb.

cervix (SUR-viks) the neck of the uterus at the entrance to the birth canal.

vagina (vah-JI-nah) the birth canal.

placenta (plah-SEN-tah) the organ of pregnancy where exchange of oxygen, nutrients, and wastes occurs between a mother and fetus.

ANATOMY AND PHYSIOLOGY OF CHILDBIRTH

Pregnancy and Delivery

The developing baby is called a **fetus** (Figure 24-1). During pregnancy, the fetus grows in the mother's **uterus,** a muscular organ also called the *womb* (Figure 24-2). When the mother is in labor, the muscles of the uterus contract at ever-shortening intervals and push the baby through the neck of the uterus, known as the **cervix.** The cervix must dilate some 4 inches (10 cm) during labor to allow the baby's head to pass into the **vagina,** or birth canal, so that delivery can take place.

More than just the fetus develops within the uterus during pregnancy. A special organ called the **placenta** is attached to the wall of the uterus. Composed of both ma-

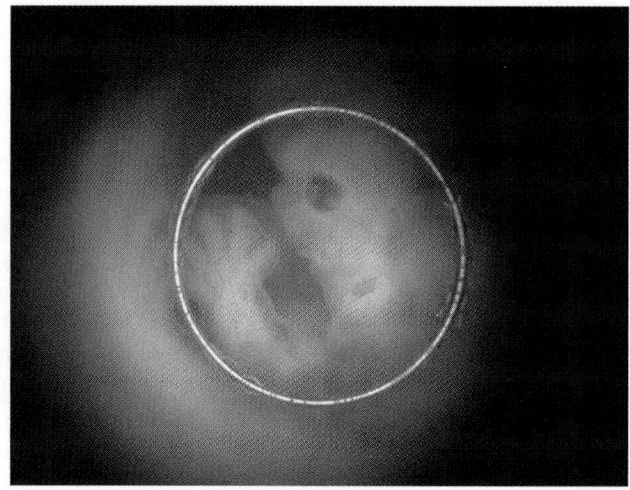

Figure 24-1 • Endoscopic photograph of a 5-week-old live fetus in the uterus. A hand and eye are clearly visible. *(© Alexander Tsiaras/Science Source/Photo Researchers, Inc.)*

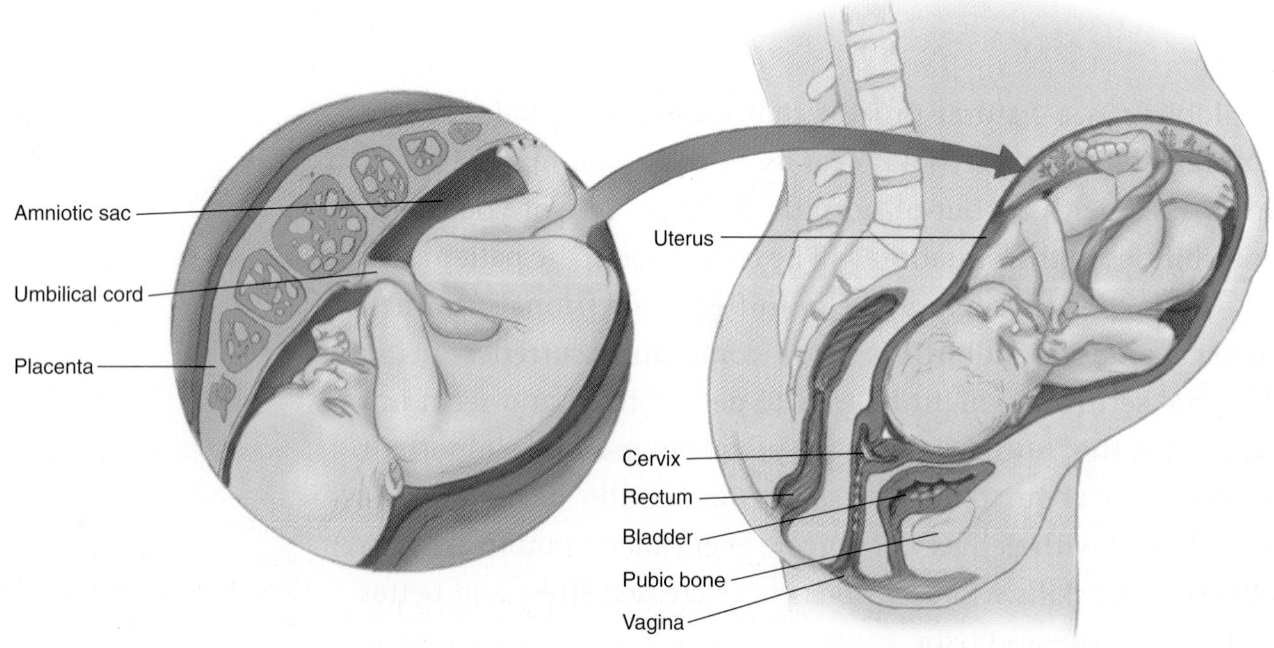

Figure 24-2 • Structures of pregnancy.

ternal and fetal tissues, the placenta serves as an exchange area between mother and fetus. Oxygen and nutrients (and drugs, nicotine, and alcohol) from the mother's bloodstream are carried across the placenta to the fetus. Carbon dioxide and certain other wastes cross from fetal circulation to maternal circulation. Since the placenta is an organ of pregnancy, it is expelled after the baby is born.

The mother's blood does not flow through the body of the fetus. The fetus has its own circulatory system. Blood from the fetus is sent through blood vessels in the **umbilical cord** to the placenta where the blood picks up nourishment from the mother, then returns through the umbilical cord to the fetus's body. The umbilical cord, about 1 inch wide and 22 inches long at birth, is fully expelled with the birth of the baby and the delivery of the placenta.

umbilical (um-BIL-i-kal) **cord**
the fetal structure containing the blood vessels that carry blood to and from the placenta.

While developing in the uterus, the fetus is enclosed and protected within a thin, membranous "bag of waters" known as the **amniotic sac.** This sac contains almost 1 quart of liquid, called amniotic fluid. It allows the fetus to float during development, acts as a cushion between the fetus and minor injury, and helps maintain a constant fetal body temperature. In the vast majority of cases, the amniotic sac breaks during labor and the fluid gushes from the birth canal. This is a normal condition of childbirth that also provides a natural lubrication to ease the infant's progress through the birth canal.

amniotic (am-ne-OT-ik) **sac**
the "bag of waters" that surrounds the developing fetus.

The 9 months of pregnancy are divided into three 3-month periods, or *trimesters.* During the first trimester, the fetus is being formed. As the fetus remains quite small, there is little uterine growth during this period. After the third month, the uterus grows rapidly, reaching the umbilicus (navel) by the fifth month and the epigastrium (upper abdomen) by the seventh month. Other changes in a woman's body during this time include increased blood volume, increased cardiac output, and increased heart rate. The blood pressure is usually decreased slightly, and there is slowed digestion. One very important change is a massive increase in vascularity (presence of blood and blood vessels) of the uterus and related structures.

Crowning occurs when the *presenting part* of the baby first bulges from the vaginal opening. The presenting part is defined as the part of the infant that is first to appear at the vaginal opening during labor. Usually, the presenting part of the baby is the head. The normal head-first birth is called a **cephalic presentation.** If the buttocks or both feet of the baby deliver first, the birth is called a **breech presentation** or breech birth.

crowning
when part of the baby is visible through the vaginal opening.

cephalic (se-FAL-ik) **presentation**
when the baby appears head first during birth. This is the normal presentation.

breech presentation
when the baby's buttocks or both legs appear first during birth.

Labor

Labor is the entire process of delivery. There are three stages of labor (Figure 24-3):

- *First stage* starts with regular contractions and the thinning and gradual dilation of the cervix and ends when the cervix is fully dilated.
- *Second stage* is the time from when the baby enters the birth canal until he is born.
- *Third stage* begins after the baby is born and lasts until the **afterbirth** (placenta, umbilical cord, and some tissues from the amniotic sac and the lining of the uterus) is delivered.

labor
the three stages of the delivery of a baby that begin with the contractions of the uterus and end with the expulsion of the placenta.

afterbirth
the placenta, membranes of the amniotic sac, part of the umbilical cord, and some tissues from the lining of the uterus that are delivered after the birth of the baby.

The first stage of labor is also called the *dilation period.* Picture the uterus as a long-neck bottle. In order to expel the contents, the neck of the bottle must be stretched to the size of a wide-mouth jar. Before the cervix can fully dilate, the long neck of the cervix must be shortened and thinned (this process is called *effacement*) to the wide-mouth-jar shape.

Sometimes several days before the onset of actual labor, uterine muscles begin mild contractions and slight dilation occurs as the cervix begins to thin. When actual labor begins, the contractions of the uterus that occur during the first stage continue the thinning and dilation process, and the infant's head begins to move downward. The cervix gradually shortens and thins enough (wide-mouth-jar shape) to become flush with the vagina or fully open to the birth canal.

The cycle of contractions starts far apart and becomes shorter as birth approaches. Typically, these contractions range from every 30 minutes at the start down to 3 minutes apart, or less. Labor pains accompany the contractions.

First stage:
beginning of contractions to full cervical dilation

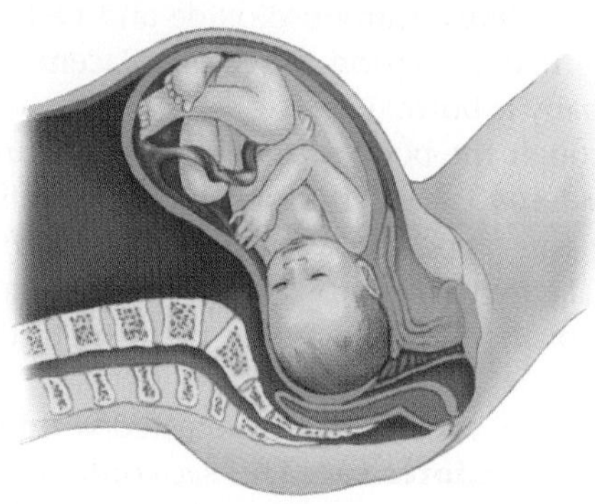

Second stage:
baby enters birth canal and is born

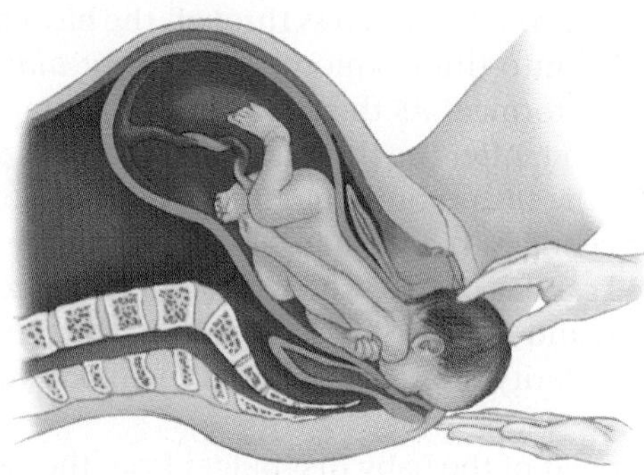

Third stage:
delivery of the placenta

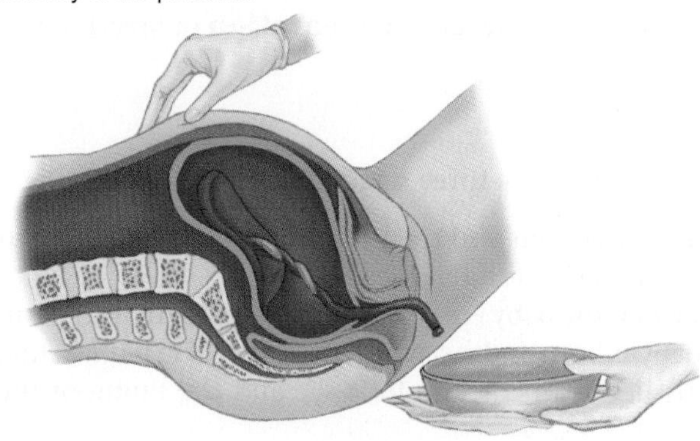

Figure 24-3 • Three stages of labor.

meconium staining amniotic fluid that is greenish or brownish-yellow rather than clear as a result of fetal defecation; an indication of possible maternal or fetal distress during labor.

As the fetus moves downward and the cervix dilates, the amniotic sac usually breaks. Normally, the amniotic fluid is clear. Fluid that is greenish or brownish-yellow in color may be an indication of maternal or fetal distress during labor and is called **meconium staining.** The full dilation of the cervix signals the end of the first stage of labor. Women giving birth for the first time will remain in this first stage for an average of 16 hours. However, some women may remain in this stage for no more than 4 hours, especially if this is not their first child.

There may be a watery, bloody discharge of mucus (not bleeding) associated with the first stage of labor. Part of this initial discharge will be from a mucus plug that was in the cervix. This is usually mixed with blood and is called the *bloody show*. It is not necessary to wipe it away. Watery, bloody fluids discharging from the vagina are typical for all three stages of labor.

The second stage of labor begins after the full dilation of the cervix. During this time, contractions become increasingly frequent, and labor pains will become more severe. In the second stage of labor, the cramping and abdominal pains associated with the first stage of labor still may be present, but most women report a major new discomfort, that of feeling they have to move their bowels. This is caused as the baby's body moves and places pressure on the rectum. The moment of birth is nearing, and the EMT will have to decide whether to transport or to keep the mother where she is and prepare to assist with delivery.

The third stage of labor begins shortly after the baby is born. Contractions will resume and continue until the placenta is delivered. The contractions and labor pains may be as painful and severe as they were in the second stage. The third stage usually lasts 10 to 20 minutes.

Labor Pains

The contractions of the uterus produce normal labor pains. Most women report the start of labor pains as an ache in the lower back. As labor progresses, the pain becomes most noticeable in the lower abdomen, with the intensity of pain increasing. The pains come at regular intervals, lasting from 30 seconds to 1 minute and occur at 2- to 3-minute intervals. When the uterus starts to contract, the pain begins. As the muscles relax, there is relief from the pain. Labor pains may start, stop for a while, then start up again.

As an EMT, you should time the following characteristics of labor pains:

- *Contraction time, or duration.* The time from the beginning of contraction to when the uterus relaxes (from start to end).
- *Contraction interval, or frequency.* The time from the start of one contraction to the beginning of the next (from start to start).

When contractions last 30 seconds to 1 minute and are 2 to 3 minutes apart, delivery of the baby may be imminent.

NORMAL CHILDBIRTH

Role of the EMT

Your primary role will be to determine whether the delivery will occur on scene and, if so, to assist the mother as she delivers her child.

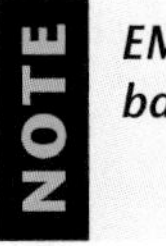

EMTs do not deliver babies; mothers do!

Assisting the mother and providing care is much easier if a few basic items are kept as part of the ambulance supplies. You will need a sterile obstetric kit that contains the items required for preparation of the mother, delivery, and initial care of the newborn (Figure 24-4). This kit should include:

- Several pairs of sterile surgical gloves to protect you from infection
- Towels or sheets for draping the mother
- 1 dozen 2 × 2 (or 4 × 4) gauze pads (sponges) for wiping and drying the baby
- 1 rubber bulb syringe (3 oz.) to suction the baby's mouth and nostrils
- Cord clamps or hemostats to clamp the umbilical cord (plus extra clamps in case of a multiple birth)
- Umbilical cord tape to tie the cord
- 1 pair of surgical scissors to cut the cord
- 1 baby blanket to wrap the baby and keep him warm
- Several individually wrapped sanitary napkins to absorb blood and other fluids
- Plastic bag

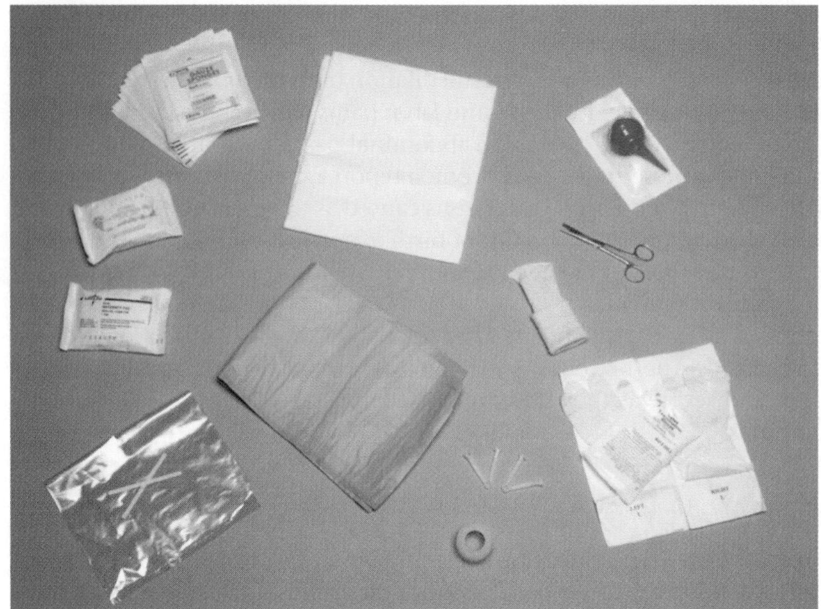

Figure 24-4 • Contents of an OB (obstetric) kit.

Occasionally, in an off-duty situation, you may need to assist in the delivery of a baby without using a sterile delivery pack. A few simple supplies can be used to assist the mother:

- Clean sheets and towels to drape the mother and wrap the newborn
- Heavy flat twine or new shoelaces to tie the cord (do not use thread, wire, or light string since these may cut through the cord)
- A towel or plastic bag to wrap the placenta after its delivery
- Clean, unused rubber gloves and eyewear. The lack of gloves and eyewear will mean possible exposure to infectious diseases.

Normal Delivery

Evaluating the Mother

NOTE *It is best to transport an expecting mother unless, based on your evaluation, you expect delivery within a few minutes.*

A simple series of questions, an examination for crowning, and determination of vital signs will allow you to make the decision for transport. However, do not let the "urgency" of this decision upset the mother. Your patient needs emotional support at this time. Your calm, professional actions will help her feel more at ease and assure her that the required care will be provided for both her and the unborn child.

To begin to evaluate the mother:

1. Ask her name, age, and expected due date.
2. Ask if this is her first pregnancy. The average time of labor for a woman having her first baby is about 16 to 17 hours. The time in labor is typically shorter for subsequent births, unless the mother has given birth to more than four or five babies already. In some women with numerous deliveries, the uterus will continue to act like a well-toned muscle; in others, it will be less effective and delivery will take longer.
3. Ask her how long she has been having labor pains, how often she is having pains, and if her "bag of waters" has broken. Ask "Have you had any bleeding or bloody show?" At this point, with a woman having her first delivery, you may think that you can make a decision about transport. However, you should continue with the evaluation procedure. Also, begin to time the frequency and length of the contractions.
4. Ask her if she is straining or if she feels as though she needs to move her bowels. If she says yes, this usually means that the baby has moved into the birth canal and is pressing the vaginal wall against the rectum. Do not allow the mother to go to the

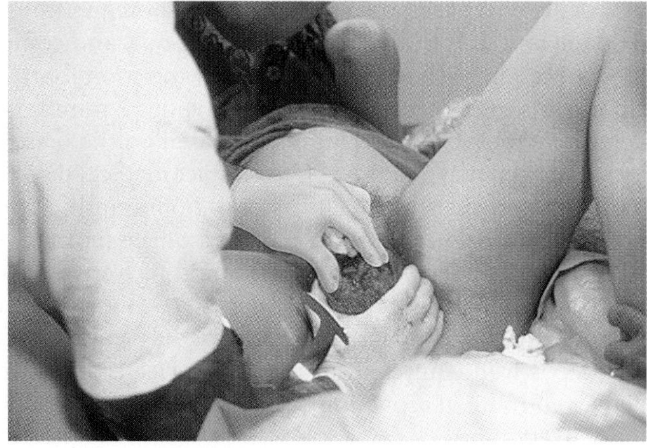

Figure 24-5 • Crowning of the infant's head.

bathroom as she may deliver the infant into the toilet. Birth will probably occur very soon. The mother may tell you that she can feel the baby trying to move out through her vaginal opening. In such cases, birth is probably very near.

5. Examine the mother for crowning (Figure 24-5). This is a visual inspection to see if there is bulging at the vaginal opening or if the presenting part of the baby is visible. If part of the baby's head or presenting part is visible with each contraction, then birth is imminent.
6. Feel for uterine contractions. You may have to delay this procedure until the patient tells you she is having labor pains. Tell her what you are going to do, then place the palm of your gloved hand on her abdomen, above the navel. This can be done over the top of the patient's clothing. You should be able to feel her uterus and its contraction. All contractions should be timed. Keep track of the duration and frequency of the contractions. The uterus and the tissues between this organ and the skin will feel more rigid as the delivery of the baby nears.
7. Take vital signs at this time if you do not have a partner to do it. Alert the medical facility staff if the mother's vital signs are abnormal.

NOTE

Do not allow the mother to go to the bathroom, even though she says that she has to move her bowels. Birth is probably only a few minutes away. Do not allow the mother to hold her legs together or use any other method to attempt to delay the delivery.

Examining for crowning may be embarrassing to the mother, the father, and any required bystanders. For this reason, it is important that you fully explain what you are doing and why. Be certain that you protect the mother from the stares of bystanders. In a polite but firm manner, ask everyone who does not belong at the scene to leave. Carefully help the patient remove enough clothing to allow you an unobstructed view of the vaginal opening.

If this is the woman's first delivery, she is not straining, and there is no crowning, there is little reason why she cannot be transported to a medical facility for delivery. (A

POINT OF VIEW

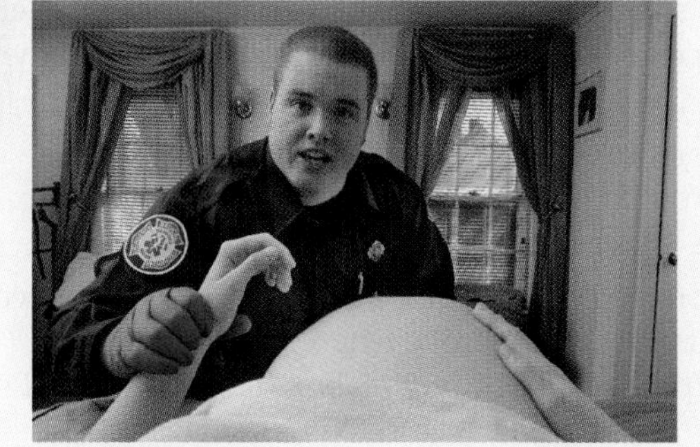

"I had planned to have a very controlled delivery. It was my first baby. And, yes, maybe I was trying to micromanage a natural process . . . when all my plans went to hell. My contractions started, my water broke, and I felt like I was going to have the baby right there.

"My husband and I freaked. All the plans to call people and have a meaningful time together before the hospital went out the window. The only call we made was to 911.

"The EMTs arrived and were great. They calmed us down. Lord knows we needed that. After they asked a few questions and timed the contractions they thought there would be time to get to the hospital before the baby was born.

"They were right. We did have time. About 8 hours. Did I mention that we totally freaked out? If we ever do this again it will be different. Honest!"

first delivery typically takes longer than subsequent ones.) However, if this is not her first delivery, and she is straining, crying out, and complaining about having to go to the bathroom, birth will probably occur too soon for transport. If the mother is having labor pains from contractions that are about 2 minutes apart, birth is very near. If you determine that delivery is imminent based on the presence of crowning or other signs, local protocol may require you to contact medical direction for the decision to commit to delivery on the site. If delivery does not occur in 10 minutes, contact medical direction for permission to initiate transport of the mother.

You may find a patient who is afraid of transport because she believes that birth will occur along the way. Assure her that you believe there is enough time before delivery. Let her know that you are trained to assist with the delivery and that the ambulance is well equipped to handle her needs and care for the newborn should she deliver en route. If crowning occurs during transport, stop the ambulance and prepare for delivery.

If your evaluation of the patient leads you to believe that birth is too near at hand for transport, you and your partner should prepare to assist the mother with delivery. Remember, as part of the preparation, the patient will need emotional support.

Supine Hypotensive Syndrome

In the third trimester, near the time of birth, the weight of the uterus, coupled with the infant's weight, placenta, and amniotic fluid, approximates 20 to 24 pounds. When the mother is in a supine position, this heavy mass will tend to compress the inferior vena cava, a major blood vessel, reducing return of blood to the heart, thereby reducing cardiac output. The resulting dizziness and drop in blood pressure constitute a set of signs and symptoms known as **supine hypotensive syndrome.** This syndrome is also referred to as *vena cava compression syndrome*. The body begins to compensate, when it senses the drop in blood pressure, by contracting the uterine arteries and redirecting blood to the major organs. This can severely affect the fetus.

supine hypotensive syndrome
Dizziness and a drop in blood pressure caused when the mother is in a supine position and the weight of the uterus, infant, placenta, and amniotic fluid compress the inferior vena cava, reducing return of blood to the heart and cardiac output.

The drop in blood pressure signals shock, but the method of treating for shock (hypoperfusion) by elevating the legs is not effective in this instance because it does not

CRITICAL DECISION MAKING: My Baby Won't Wait!

Childbirth in the field is a rare but very exciting call. For every baby you deliver you may have dozens of maternity calls in which the mother is transported to the hospital before the baby is delivered. Being able to determine whether the birth is imminent is an important skill for an EMT. For each of the scenarios presented, determine if you should stay and prepare for delivery or should transport the patient to the hospital.

1. Your patient states contractions are severe, about 30 seconds apart. She feels the need to push and suspects she has accidentally moved her bowels. There is significant bulging, and you can see the baby's head crowning. This is her fourth child.
2. Your patient reports contractions are about 5–10 minutes apart but feel strong. This is her first child. You do not observe any crowning or bulging. She is not sure if her water has broken.
3. Your patient reports contractions that are about 2 minutes apart. They have been this way for about 8 hours. Her water broke when the contractions started. She doesn't feel she is progressing through labor and is concerned for her baby.

relieve pressure on the vena cava. To counteract or avoid the possible drop in blood pressure, all third-trimester patients should be transported on their left side. A pillow or rolled blanket should be placed behind the back to maintain proper positioning.

Preparing the Mother for Delivery

When your evaluation leads you to believe birth is imminent, you must immediately prepare the mother for delivery. To do so, you should:

1. Control the scene so that the mother will have privacy. (Her birthing coach may remain.) If you are not in a private room and transfer to the ambulance is not practical (crowning is present), ask bystanders to leave.
2. In addition to surgical gloves, you and your partner should put on gowns, caps, face masks, and eye protection since there is a high probability of splashing blood and other body fluids during delivery.
3. Place the mother on a bed, floor, or the ambulance stretcher. Elevate the buttocks with blankets or a pillow. Have the mother lie with knees drawn up and spread apart. You will need about 2 feet of work space below the woman's buttocks to place and initially care for the newborn. Having the patient positioned on the stretcher may speed transport if complications arise.
4. Remove any of the patient's clothing or underclothing that obstructs your view of the vaginal opening. Use sterile sheets or sterile towels to cover the mother as shown in Figure 24-6. Clean sheets, clean cloths, towels, or materials such as tablecloths can be used if you do not have an obstetric kit.
5. Position your assistant—your partner, the father, or someone the mother agrees to have assist you—at the mother's head. This person should stay alert to help turn the mother's head should she vomit. As well, this person should provide emotional support to the mother, soothing and encouraging her.
6. Position the obstetric kit near the patient. All items must be within easy reach.

NOTE

If delivery is to take place in an automobile, position the mother flat on the seat. Arrange her legs so that she has one foot resting on the seat and the other foot resting on the floor.

Delivering the Baby

Position yourself in such a way that you have a constant view of the vaginal opening. Be prepared for the baby to come at any moment.

Be prepared for the patient to experience discomfort. Delivering a child is a natural process, but it will be accompanied by pain. Your patient may also have intense feelings of nausea. If this is her first child, she may be very frightened. All these factors may

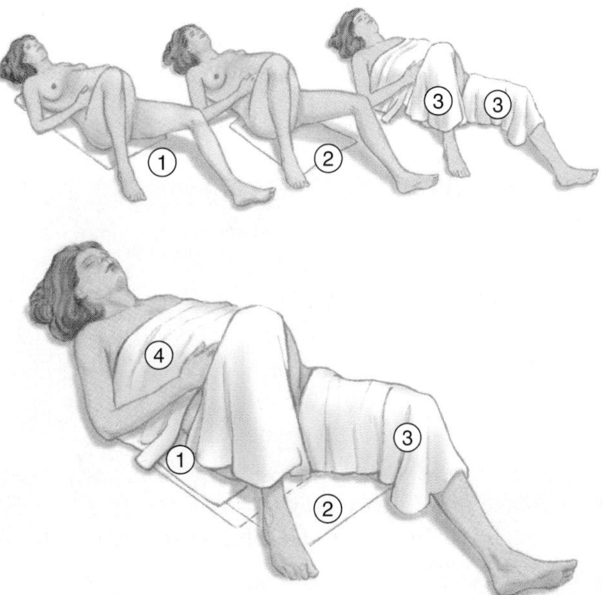

Figure 24-6 • Preparing the mother for delivery.

cause your patient to be uncooperative at times. You must remember that the patient is in pain and she may feel ill. She will need emotional support.

During delivery, talk to the mother. Encourage her to relax between contractions. Continue to time her contractions from the beginning of one contraction to the beginning of the next. Encourage her not to strain unless she feels she must. Remind her that her feeling of a pending bowel movement is usually just pressure caused by the baby moving into her birth canal. Encourage her to breathe deeply through her mouth. She may feel better if she pants, although she should be discouraged from breathing rapidly and deeply enough to bring on hyperventilation. If her "bag of waters" breaks, remind her that this is normal.

To assist the mother with a normal delivery:

NOTE *Unless there are signs of complications, consider the delivery to be normal if there is a cephalic presentation. Observe any unusual color in the amniotic fluid.*

NOTE *Some deliveries are explosive. Do not squeeze the baby, but do provide adequate support. You can prevent an explosive delivery by using one hand to maintain slight pressure on the baby's head, avoiding direct pressure to the infant's soft spots on the skull.*

1. Continue to keep someone at the mother's head to provide support, monitor vital signs, and be alert for vomiting. If no one is on hand to help, be alert for vomiting and check vital signs between contractions.
2. Position your gloved hands at the mother's vaginal opening when the baby's head starts to appear. Do not touch the area around the vagina except to assist with the delivery. For legal reasons, it is always preferable for both your protection and the patient's to have your partner present at all times when you are touching a woman's vaginal area.
3. Place one hand below the baby's head as it delivers (Figure 24-7 and Scan 24-1). Spread your fingers evenly, remembering that the baby's skull contains "soft spots," or *fontanelles*. Support the baby's head, but avoid pressure to these soft areas at the top and sides of the skull. A slight, well-distributed pressure may help prevent an explosive delivery. Keeping one hand on the baby's head and using the other hand to hold a sterile towel to support the tissue between the mother's vagina and anus can help prevent tearing of this tissue during delivery of the head. DO NOT PULL ON THE BABY!
4. If the amniotic sac has not broken by the time the baby's head is delivered, use your finger to puncture the membrane. Pull the membranes away from the baby's mouth and nose. The amniotic fluid should be clear. Examine the amniotic fluid for meconium staining, which will appear to be a dark green-black color. Meconium-stained amniotic fluid is caused by fetal feces (wastes) released during labor, usually because of maternal or fetal stress. If meconium is present, prepare to suction the infant immediately. If the meconium is aspirated (breathed in) by the fetus, the baby can develop pneumonia or other infections.
5. Once the head delivers, check to see if the umbilical cord is wrapped around the baby's neck. Tell the mother not to push while you check. If she can "pant," or take short quick breaths for just a moment, it may help relieve the urge to push while you check. Then gently loosen the cord if necessary. Even though the

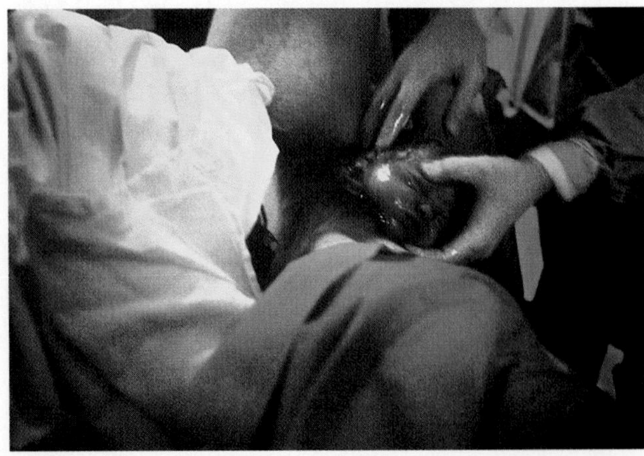

Figure 24-7 • Delivering the infant's head.

SCAN 24-1 • Assisting in a Normal Delivery

First take Standard Precautions.

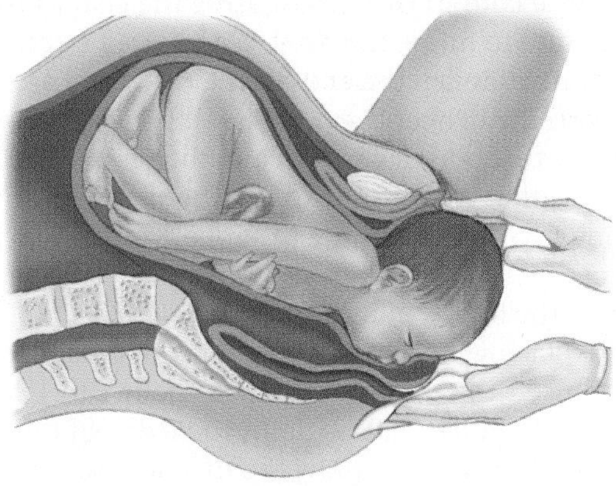

1. Support the infant's head.

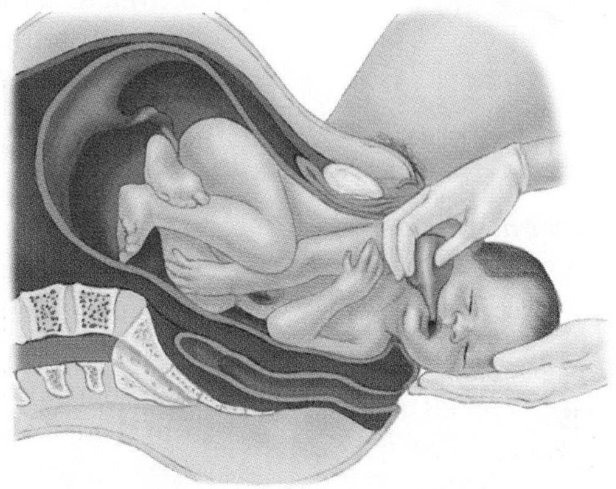

2. Suction the infant's mouth and nose.

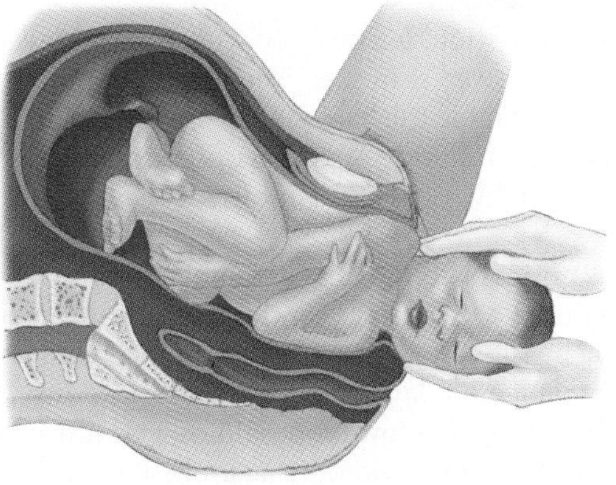

3. Aid in the birth of the upper shoulder.

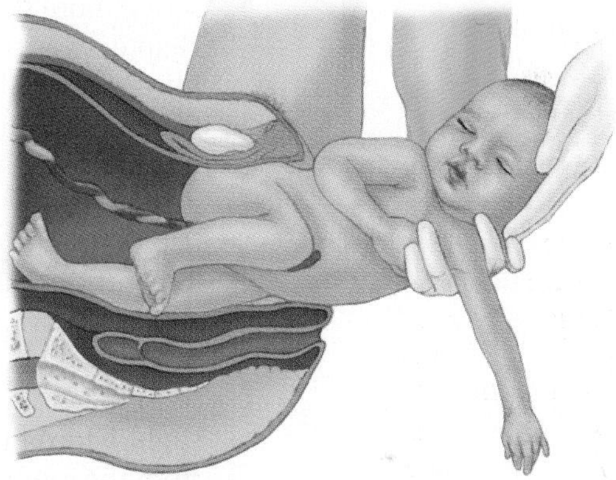

4. Support the trunk.

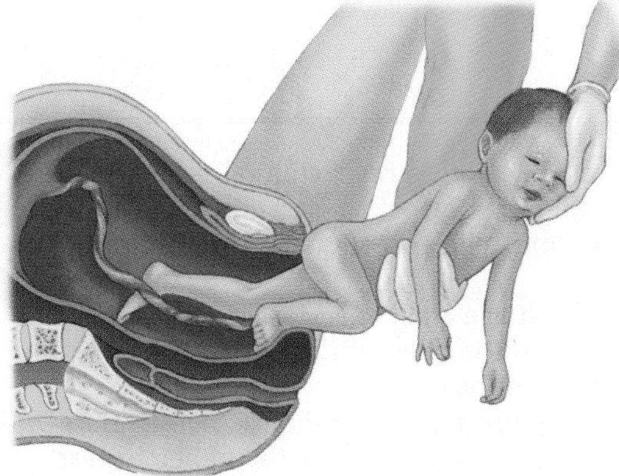

5. Support the pelvis and lower extremities.

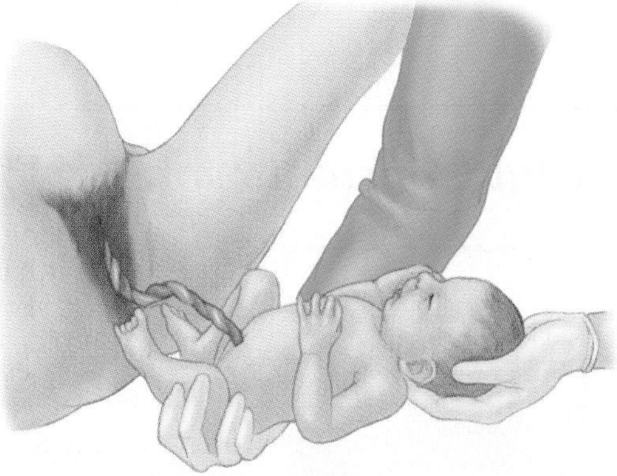

6. Keep the infant level with the vagina until the umbilical cord stops pulsating.

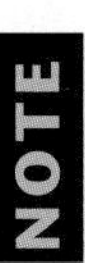

Assist the mother by supporting the baby throughout the birth process.

umbilical cord is very tough, rough handling may cause it to tear. If the cord is wrapped around the baby's neck, try to place two fingers under the cord at the back of the baby's neck. Bring the cord forward, over the baby's upper shoulder and head.

If you cannot loosen or slip the cord over the baby's head, the baby cannot be delivered. So immediately clamp the cord in two places using the clamps provided in the obstetric kit. Be very careful not to injure the baby. With extreme care, cut the cord between the two clamps. Gently unwrap the ends of the cord from around the baby's neck, and then proceed with the delivery.

6. Check the baby's airway. Most babies are born face down and then rotate to the right or left. Support the baby's head so that it does not touch the mother's anal area. When the entire head of the baby is visible, continue to support the head with one hand. With the other hand, wipe the mouth and nose with sterile gauze pads. Use the rubber bulb syringe to suction the baby's mouth, then the nose.

   Compress the syringe BEFORE placing it in the baby's mouth. Suction the mouth first, then the nostrils. Carefully insert the tip of the syringe about 1 to $1^1/_2$ inches into the baby's mouth and release the bulb to allow fluids to be drawn into the syringe. Control the release with your fingers. Withdraw the tip and discharge the syringe's contents onto a towel. Repeat this procedure two or three times in the baby's mouth and once or twice in each nostril. The tip of the syringe should not be inserted more than 1/2 inch into the baby's nostril.

NOTE

When the nostrils are suctioned, the baby may gasp or begin breathing and aspirate any meconium, blood, fluids, or mucus from his mouth into his lungs. That is why it is imperative to suction the mouth before the nostrils.

7. Help deliver the shoulders. The upper shoulder (usually with some delay) will deliver next, followed quickly by the lower shoulder. You must support the baby throughout this entire process. Gently guide the baby's head downward, to assist the mother in delivering the baby's upper shoulder. After the upper shoulder has delivered, if the lower shoulder is slow to deliver, assist the mother by gently guiding the baby's head upward.
8. Support the baby throughout the entire birth process. Remember that newborns are very slippery. As the lower extremities are born, grasp them to ensure a good hold on the baby. Never pick up a baby by the feet as they are very slippery and you could drop the child. Once the feet are delivered, lay the baby on his side with his head slightly lower than his body. This is done to allow blood, fluids, and mucus to drain from the mouth and nose. Suction the mouth and nose again with the bulb syringe. Keep the baby at the same level as the mother's vagina until the umbilical cord stops pulsating. Wrap the infant in a warm, dry blanket.
9. Note the exact time of birth.

Cultural Considerations

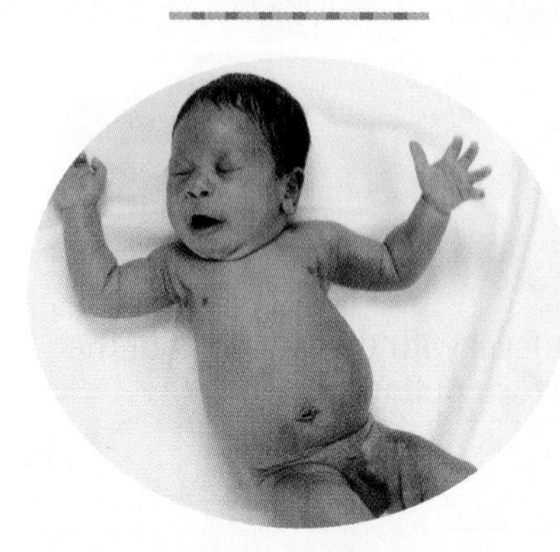

Be sensitive to the customs of various ethnic, cultural, and religious groups in your community regarding the birth of a child. If possible and the health of the mother and baby permit, allow time for the family to respond to the birth in their own way.

For example, after the birth of a child to a Muslim family, the father may call praise to Allah *(adhan)* into the newborn's right ear. The Muslim father may also want to clean the newborn.

Since it is best to leave the protective coating the baby is born with until it reaches the hospital, you might encourage the father, instead, to help dry and wrap the baby.

The Newly Born Child

Assessing the Newly Born

The vigor of an infant should be assessed as soon as he is born. If you arrive after the birth, it is still your responsibility to make the assessments based on your first observations. Remember, however, that care for the infant and the mother should not be delayed. *The assessment is meant to take place while these other activities are being performed.*

Your EMS system may call for a general or a specific evaluation protocol. A general evaluation usually calls for noting ease of breathing, the heart rate, crying, movement, and skin color. A normal newborn should have a pulse greater than 100/min, be breathing easily, be crying (vigorous crying is a good sign), be moving his extremities (the more active, the better), and show blue coloration at the hands and feet only. Five minutes later, these signs should still be apparent, with breathing becoming more relaxed. The blue coloration may or may not disappear, but it should not spread to other parts of the body.

A specific evaluation protocol that some EMS systems call for is an Apgar score. It is a way to assign a number to a newborn's condition that came about before the ABCs received the strong emphasis they do today. An Apgar score does not guide resuscitation efforts, and efforts to determine the Apgar score must never interfere with resuscitation efforts. Table 24-1 shows how an EMT assigns values to different aspects of a newly born's condition. The Apgar score is the total of the five values, and ranges from 0 to 10. It is traditionally determined 1 minute after birth and then again 5 minutes after birth. It is presented here for the sake of EMTs whose EMS systems require its use.

NOTE

A number of terms are often used interchangeably. For clarity and uniformity, it is appropriate to use the following definitions: fetus—a baby as it develops in the womb; newly born—the baby at the time of birth; newborn or neonate—the baby during its initial hospitalization; infant—a baby in its first year of life.

Caring for the Newly Born

Even with a normal delivery, each step in the care of the baby is essential for his survival. To care for the newborn, you should first place the baby on a sterile sheet on the bed or padded table surface, keeping the baby close to the level of the mother's vagina so that the infant's blood does not transfuse back into the placenta. Do not place the infant on the mother's abdomen at this time (not until after the cord is clamped and cut—see later in this chapter).

During the birth process, the newly born is passive. Once the baby is born, he very quickly becomes active. Exposure to the air is usually enough to stimulate the infant to breathe. As you suction, dry, and warm the baby, he is stimulated even more. If the newly born does not breathe on his own after suctioning, drying, and warming for 30 seconds, begin resuscitation measures.

TABLE 24-1 • The Apgar Score

	APGAR SCORE		
	0	1	2
Appearance	Blue (or pale) all over	Extremities blue, trunk pink	Pink all over
Pulse	0	<100	>100
Grimace (Reaction to suctioning or flicking of the feet)	No reaction	Facial grimace	Sneeze, cough, or cry
Activity	No movement	Only slight activity (flexing extremities)	Moving around normally
Respiratory effort	None	Slow or irregular breathing, weak cry	Good breathing, strong cry

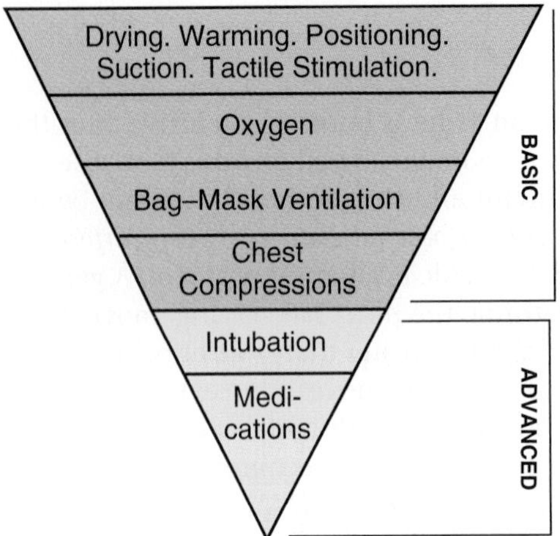

Figure 24-8 • Inverted pyramid of neonatal resuscitation.

Resuscitation of the Newly Born

Neonatal resuscitation follows an inverted pyramid (Figure 24-8). Most newly borns with abnormal assessment findings respond to relatively simple maneuvers. Few require CPR or advanced life support measures.

Follow these steps for initial care of the newly born:

1. Provide warmth and clear the baby's airway. Use a bulb syringe, suctioning the mouth first and then the nostrils. Squeeze the bulb before inserting the syringe into the baby's mouth. Release the bulb to create suction. It may be necessary to use a sterile gauze pad to clear mucus and blood from around the baby's nose and mouth.
2. Keep the baby on his side and again suction the mouth, then the nose, with a rubber bulb syringe (Figure 24-9). If necessary, you can cradle the baby in your arms. However, it is best to keep the baby on the cot or table surface.
3. Establish that the baby is breathing. Evaluate respirations, heart rate, and color. Usually the baby will be breathing on his own by the time you clear the airway. A newborn should begin breathing within 30 seconds. If he does not, then you must "encourage" the baby to breathe (Figure 24-10). Usually, a gentle but vigorous rubbing of the baby's back will promote spontaneous respiration. Should this method fail, snap one of your index fingers against the sole of the baby's foot. Do not hold the baby up by his feet and slap his bottom! Do not become alarmed if the hands and feet of a breathing newborn appear slightly blue. It is not uncommon for this blue color to remain for the first few minutes.

   If assessment of the infant's breathing reveals shallow, slow, or absent respirations, provide artificial ventilations at a rate of 40 to 60 per minute.

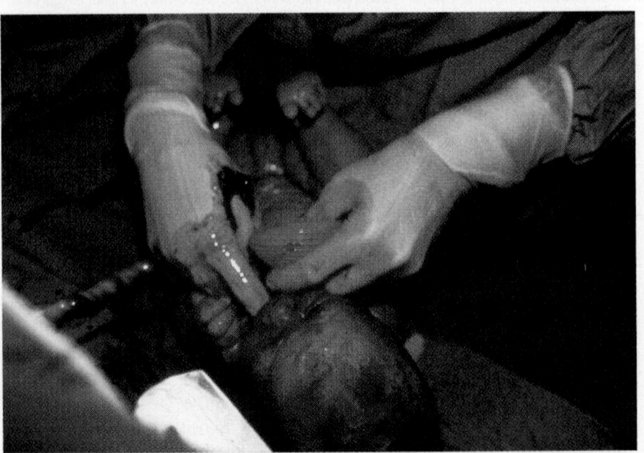

Figure 24-9 • Suction the mouth and then the nose of the newborn.

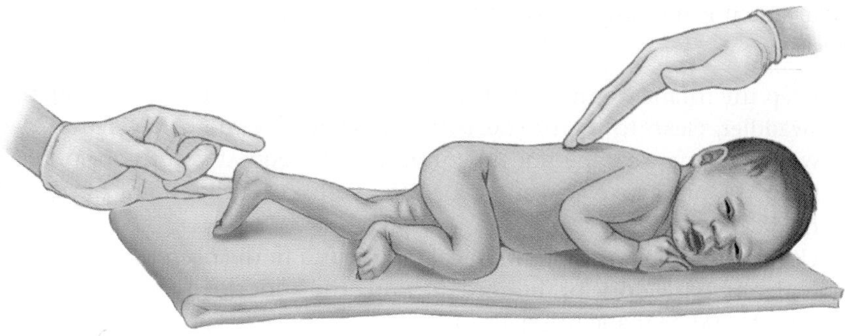

Figure 24-10 • It may be necessary to stimulate the newborn to breathe.

Remember: Provide only small puffs of air if using mouth to mask, and small squeezes on the bag if using an infant-size bag-valve-mask device. Reassess the infant's respiratory efforts after 30 seconds. If there is no change in the effort of breathing, continue with ventilations and reassessment.

4. Assess the infant's heart rate. If the heart rate is less than 100 beats per minute, then provide artificial ventilations at a rate of 40 to 60 per minute. If the heart rate is less than 60 beats per minute, initiate chest compressions, too, as shown in Figure 24-11. Chest compressions in the newly born should be delivered at a rate of 120 compressions per minute, midsternum with two thumbs, fingers supporting the back. Depth of compression is one-third to one-half the depth of the chest. Working at a 3:1 ratio of compressions to breaths in the newly born, the EMT should actually be delivering 120 "events" per minute (e.g., 90 compressions and 30 ventilations).
5. If the child has adequate respirations and a pulse rate greater than 100 per minute, but exhibits cyanosis of the face and/or torso, provide supplemental oxygen. Oxygen is best delivered at 15 liters per minute using oxygen tubing placed close to, but not directly into, the infant's face.

Cutting the Umbilical Cord

In a normal birth, the infant must be breathing on his own before you clamp and cut the cord. Before clamping and cutting the cord, palpate the cord with your fingers to

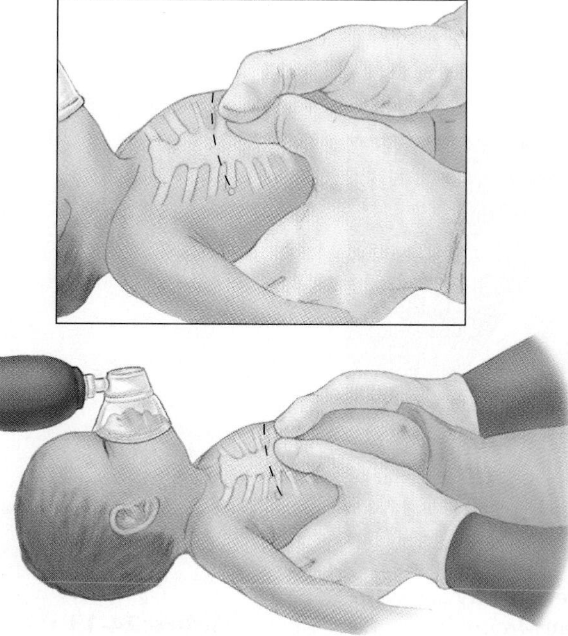

Figure 24-11 • Deliver chest compressions midsternum with two thumbs, at a depth of one-third to one-half depth of the chest. For a very small infant (inset), the thumbs may be overlapped.

NOTE *Do not tie, clamp, or cut the cord of a baby who is not breathing on his own unless you have to do so to remove the cord from around the baby's neck during birth, or unless you have to perform CPR on the infant. Do not cut or clamp a cord that is still pulsating.*

make sure it is no longer pulsating. The general procedure for umbilical cord care is as follows:

1. Keep the infant warm. Dry off the baby and wrap him in a baby blanket or infant swaddler, clean towel, or sheet prior to clamping the cord (Figure 24-12). Do not wash the infant. Sometimes the mother may request you to do so, but it is best to leave the protective coating (called the vernix) on the infant until he reaches the medical facility.
2. Use the sterile clamps or umbilical tape found in the obstetric kit. Use extreme care with any tying done to the cord, forming the knot slowly to avoid cutting the cord. Ties should be made using a square knot (right over left, then left over right).
3. Apply one clamp or tie to the cord about 10 inches from the baby. This leaves enough cord for intravenous lines to be used by paramedics or the staff at the hospital if they are needed.
4. Place a second clamp or tie about 7 inches from the baby. The proximal clamp should be about the width of 4 fingers from the distal clamp.
5. Cut the cord between the clamps or knots using sterile surgical scissors (Figure 24-13). Use caution and protect your eyes when cutting the cord as a spurt of blood is very common. Never untie or unclamp a cord once it is cut. The placental end of the cord should be placed on the drape over the mother's legs to avoid contact with expelled blood, feces, and fluids. Examine the fetal end of the cord for bleeding. Do not attempt to adjust the clamp or retie the knot. Should bleeding continue, apply another tie or clamp as close to the original as possible.
6. Be careful when moving the baby so that no trauma is brought to the clamped cord. If the cord does not remain closed off completely, the baby may bleed to death from seemingly little blood loss. In most cases, the cord vessels will collapse and seal themselves.

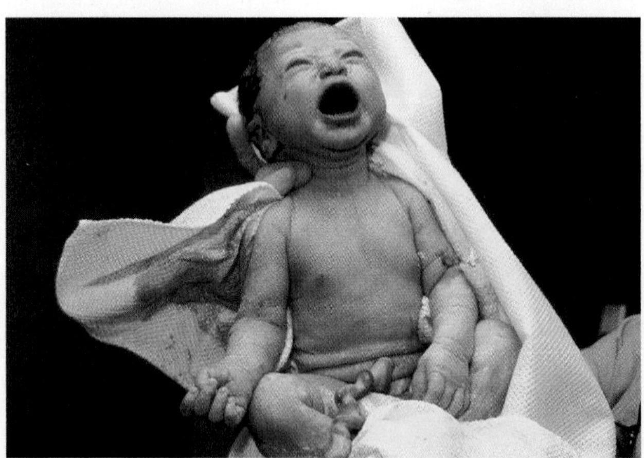

Figure 24-12 • Before clamping the cord, dry and wrap the infant to keep him warm. *(© Custom Medical Stock, Inc.)*

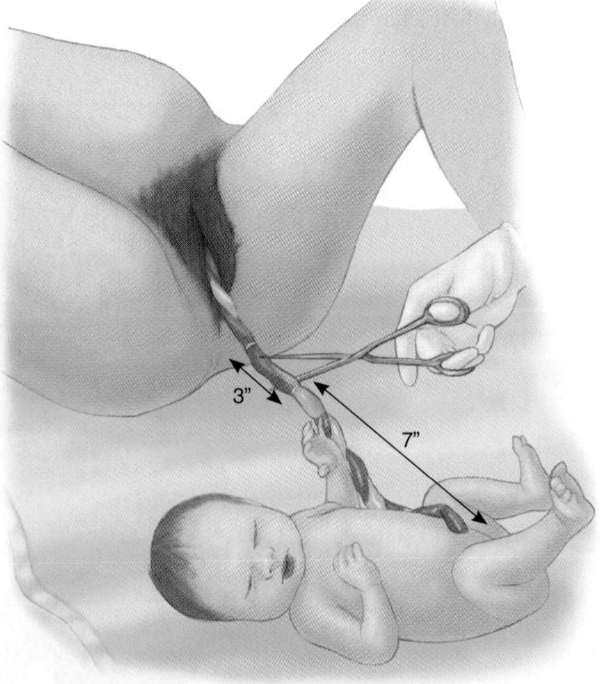

Figure 24-13 • Cutting the umbilical cord.

Keeping the Baby Warm

It is critical that the baby be kept warm. Hypothermia of babies born outside the hospital is a common and potentially serious condition that can be avoided by simple interventions. First, ensure that the baby has been properly dried. Discard towels initially used to dry the baby, as the moisture contained in them cools quickly. Wrap the newborn in an infant swaddler and a warmed blanket or towel and let the mother hold the infant on her abdomen (Figure 24-14). Bubble wrap can also be used. It provides padded protection, warmth (pre-warm it), and allows visual monitoring of the infant. Be sure to cover the infant's head (but not the face). During the delivery of the placenta, have your partner hold the baby unless the mother insists otherwise. Keep the ambulance warm.

Assisting at a Birth When Off Duty

If you are assisting at a birth when off duty, you will probably be able to find all the items you need to tie and cut the cord. If no clamps or tying devices are on hand, use clean shoelaces or similar soft, clean ties. You may delay clamping and tying the cord if the infant will receive this care within 30 minutes. If you tie the cord, if you believe it will be some time before transport and transfer, and if you do not have sterile scissors, soak scissors in alcohol for several minutes and use them to cut the cord. If the baby is still attached to the placenta when the organ is delivered, wrap the placenta in a towel and transport the infant and placenta as a unit. The placenta should be placed at the same level as the baby, or slightly higher. Careful monitoring of the baby must be maintained.

Caring for the Mother

Remember that you have two patients to care for: the infant and the mother. Care for the mother includes helping her deliver the placenta, controlling her vaginal bleeding, and making her as comfortable as possible.

Delivering the Placenta

The third stage of labor is the delivery of the placenta with its umbilical cord section, membranes of the amniotic sac, and some of the tissues lining the uterus (Figure 24-15). (All of these together are known as the afterbirth.) Placental delivery begins with a brief return of the labor pains that stopped when the baby was born. You will notice a lengthening of the cord, which indicates the placenta has separated from the uterus. In most cases, the placenta will be expelled within a few minutes after the baby is born.

Although the process may take 30 minutes or longer, avoid the urge to put pressure on the abdomen over the uterus to hasten delivery of the placenta. If mother and baby are doing well, and there are no respiratory problems or significant uncontrolled bleeding, transportation to the hospital can be delayed up to 20 minutes while awaiting delivery of the placenta.

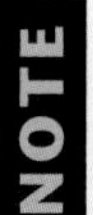

Some EMS systems recommend transport without waiting for delivery of the placenta. There may be a condition in which the placenta does not separate from the uterine wall, and it is important for mother and baby to get to the hospital. You can always stop the ambulance to deliver the placenta if it crowns en route.

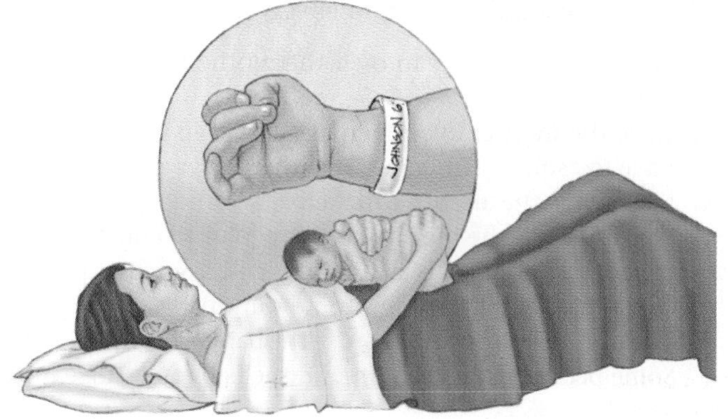

Figure 24-14 • Place the baby on the mother's abdomen. Write the mother's last name and time of delivery on a tape, fold it so the adhesive does not touch the baby's skin, and place it around the baby's wrist.

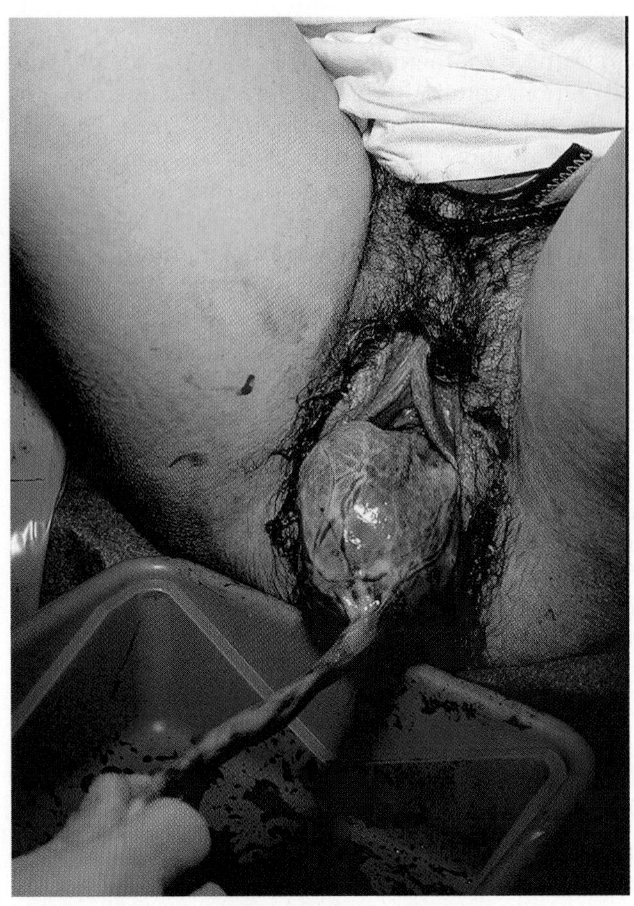

Figure 24-15 • Delivery of the placenta. *(© Fred McConnaughey/Photo Researchers, Inc.)*

Save all afterbirth tissues. The attending physician will want to examine the placenta and other tissues for completeness since any afterbirth tissues remaining in the uterus pose a serious threat of infection and prolonged bleeding to the mother. Try to catch the afterbirth in a container. Place the container in a plastic bag, or wrap it in a towel, paper, or plastic. If no container is available, catch the afterbirth in a towel, paper, or a plastic bag. Label this material "placenta" and include the name of the mother and the time the tissues were expelled.

Remember: If the placenta does not deliver within 20 minutes of the baby's birth, transport the mother and baby to a medical facility without delay.

Controlling Vaginal Bleeding After Birth

Delivery of the baby and placenta is ALWAYS accompanied by some bleeding from the vagina. Although the blood loss is usually no more than 500 cc, it may be profuse. To control vaginal bleeding after delivery of the baby and placenta, you should:

1. Place a sanitary napkin over the mother's vaginal opening. Do not place anything in the vagina.
2. Have the mother lower her legs and keep them together. Tell her that she does not have to "squeeze" her legs together. Elevate her feet.
3. Massaging the uterus will help it contract (Figure 24-16). This will help control bleeding. Feel the mother's abdomen until you note a "grapefruit-sized" object. This is her uterus. Rub this area lightly with a circular motion. It should contract and become firm, and bleeding should diminish.
4. The mother may want to nurse the baby. This will aid in the contraction of the uterus. Some pediatricians recommend the baby not nurse until a doctor has examined it.

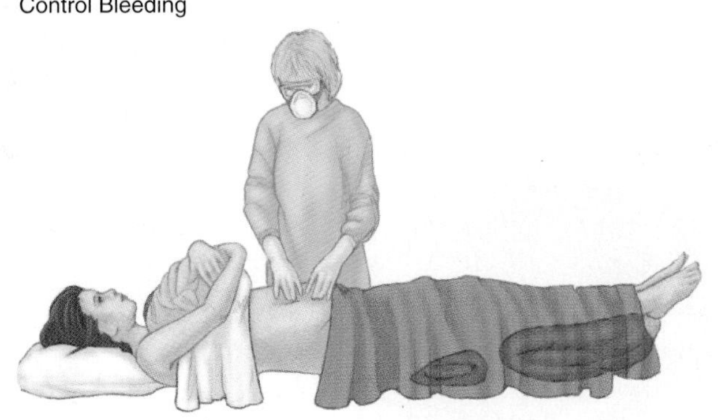

Figure 24-16 • After delivery of the placenta, massage the uterus to help control vaginal bleeding.

The skin between the vagina and the anus is known as the **perineum.** A tearing of tissue can occur in the perineum at the vaginal opening during the birth process. The mother may feel the discomfort from this torn tissue. Let her know that this is normal and that the problem will be quickly cared for at the medical facility. Treat the torn perineum as a wound. Dress by applying a sanitary napkin and applying some pressure.

perineum (per-i-NE-um) the surface area between the vagina and anus.

Providing Comfort to the Mother

Keep contact with the mother throughout the entire birth process and after she has delivered. Your care for the mother does not end when you have completed your duties with the placenta and vaginal bleeding. Take her vital signs frequently. Be aware that she has just undergone a tremendous emotional experience and small acts of kindness will be appreciated and remembered. Childbirth is a rigorous task, and a woman is physically exhausted at the conclusion of delivery. Wiping her face and hands with a damp washcloth and then drying them with a towel will do wonders to refresh her and prepare her for the trip to the hospital. Replace blood-soaked sheets and blankets. Make sure that both she and the baby are warm.

When delivery occurs at home, ask a member of the family or a trusted neighbor to help you clean up. You should clean up whatever disorder EMS care has caused in the house; however, you should not delay transport in order to complete these activities. In some areas, local protocol may have you return to the house after transport in order to complete the clean-up process. If you do, you will have to be accompanied by a member of the family. Be sure to properly dispose of items that have been in contact with blood and other body fluids in a biohazard container.

NOTE

Keep in mind that birth is an exciting and joyous event. Talking to the mother and paying attention to her new baby are part of total patient care. A good rule to follow is to treat your patient as you would wish a member of your family to be treated.

CHILDBIRTH COMPLICATIONS

Complications of Delivery

Although most babies are born without difficulty, complications may occur during and after delivery. We have already considered three such complications: the cord around the neck, an unbroken amniotic sac, and infants who need encouragement to breathe. These problems can be handled by simple procedures. However, there are other complications that can threaten the life of both mother and newborn and for which definitive treatment is beyond the EMT's level of training. For emergencies such as breech presentation, prolapsed umbilical cord, and limb presentation, you will provide high-concentration oxygen and rapid transport to the hospital.

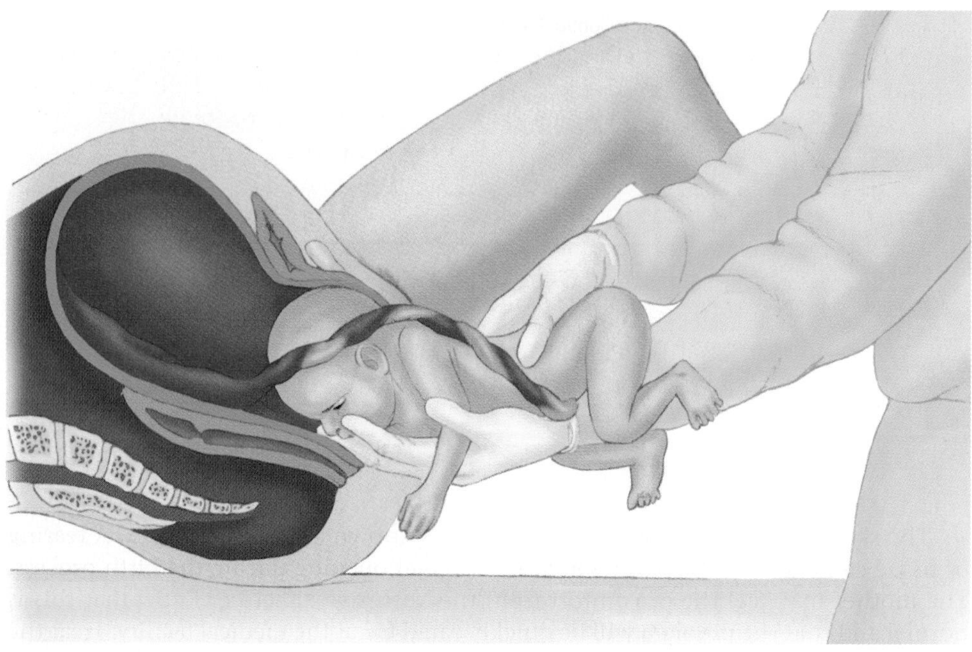

Figure 24-17 • Breech delivery.

Breech Presentation

Breech presentation, the most common abnormal delivery, involves a buttocks-first or both-legs-first delivery (Figure 24-17). The risk of birth trauma to the baby is high in breech deliveries. In addition, there is an increased risk of prolapsed cord (see the next section). Meconium staining often occurs with breech presentations.

PATIENT ASSESSMENT

BREECH PRESENTATION

If you evaluate a woman in labor and find the baby's buttocks or both legs presenting, rather than the head, this is a breech presentation. Breech presentations can spontaneously deliver successfully, but the complication rate is high. ■

PATIENT CARE

BREECH PRESENTATION

Emergency care of a patient with a breech presentation includes the following:

1. Initiate rapid transport upon recognition of a breech presentation.
2. Never attempt to deliver the baby by pulling on his legs.
3. Provide high-concentration oxygen.
4. Place the mother in a head-down position with the pelvis elevated.
5. If the body delivers, support it and prevent an explosive delivery of the head. Insert gloved index and middle fingers into the vagina to form a "V" on either side of the baby's nose to lift it away from the vaginal wall in case the baby begins to breathe spontaneously.
6. Care for baby, cord, mother, and placenta as in after cephalic delivery. ■

Prolapsed Umbilical Cord

Sometimes during delivery, the umbilical cord presents first (this is most common in breech births) and the cord is squeezed between the vaginal wall and the head of the baby. The cord is pinched, and oxygen supply to the baby may be totally interrupted. This occurrence is known as a **prolapsed umbilical cord.**

prolapsed umbilical cord when the umbilical cord presents first and is squeezed between the vaginal wall and the baby's head.

PATIENT ASSESSMENT

PROLAPSED UMBILICAL CORD

If, upon viewing the vaginal area, you see the umbilical cord presenting, the cord is prolapsed. ■

PATIENT CARE

PROLAPSED UMBILICAL CORD

Follow these steps when the umbilical cord is prolapsed (Figure 24-18):

1. Position the mother with her head down and buttocks raised with a blanket or pillow, using gravity to lessen pressure on the birth canal.
2. Provide the mother with high-concentration oxygen by way of a nonrebreather mask to increase the concentration carried over to the infant.
3. Check the cord for pulses and wrap the exposed cord, using a sterile towel from the obstetric kit. The cord must be kept warm.
4. Insert several fingers of your gloved hand into the mother's vagina so that you can gently push up on the baby's head or buttocks to keep pressure off of the cord. You will be pushing up through the cervix. This may be the only chance that the baby has for survival, so continue to push up on the baby until a physician relieves you. You may feel the cord pulsating when pressure is released.
5. Keeping mother, child, and EMT as a unit, transport immediately to a medical facility. Be prepared to stay in this position until you reach the hospital.
6. All patients with prolapsed cords require rapid transport. Have your partner obtain vital signs while en route to the hospital if possible. ■

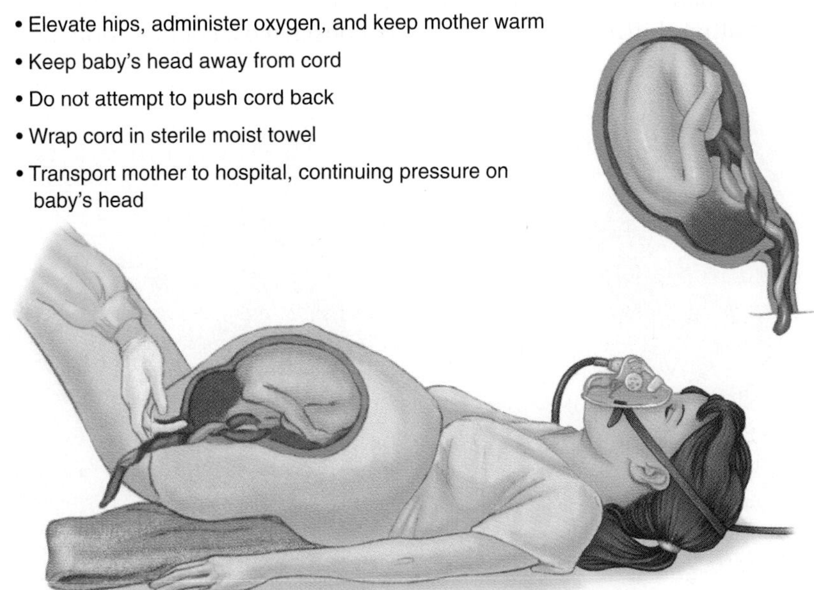

• Elevate hips, administer oxygen, and keep mother warm
• Keep baby's head away from cord
• Do not attempt to push cord back
• Wrap cord in sterile moist towel
• Transport mother to hospital, continuing pressure on baby's head

Figure 24-18 • Prolapsed umbilical cord.

Limb Presentation

limb presentation when an infant's limb protrudes from the vagina before the appearance of any other body part.

A **limb presentation** occurs when a limb of an infant protrudes from the vagina. The presenting limb is commonly a foot when the baby is in the breech position. Limb presentations cannot be delivered in the prehospital setting. Rapid transport is essential to the baby's survival.

PATIENT ASSESSMENT

LIMB PRESENTATION

When checking for crowning, you may see an arm, a single leg, an arm and leg together, or a shoulder and an arm (Figure 24-19). If one or more limbs present, there is often a prolapsed umbilical cord as well. ■

PATIENT CARE

LIMB PRESENTATION

When you discover a limb presentation, take these emergency care steps:

1. If there is a prolapsed cord, follow the same procedures as you would for any delivery involving a prolapsed cord. Remember, you have to keep pushing up on the baby until relieved by a physician. The baby must be kept off of the cord if he is to survive.
2. Transport the mother immediately to a medical facility.
3. Place the mother in a head-down position with the pelvis elevated.
4. Administer high-concentration oxygen with a nonrebreather mask. ■

NOTE *For a limb presentation, do not try to pull on the limb or replace the limb into the vagina. Do not place your gloved hand into the vagina unless there is a prolapsed cord.*

Multiple Birth

multiple birth when more than one baby is born during a single delivery.

When more than one baby is born during a single delivery, it is called a **multiple birth.** A multiple birth, usually twins, is not considered a complication, provided that

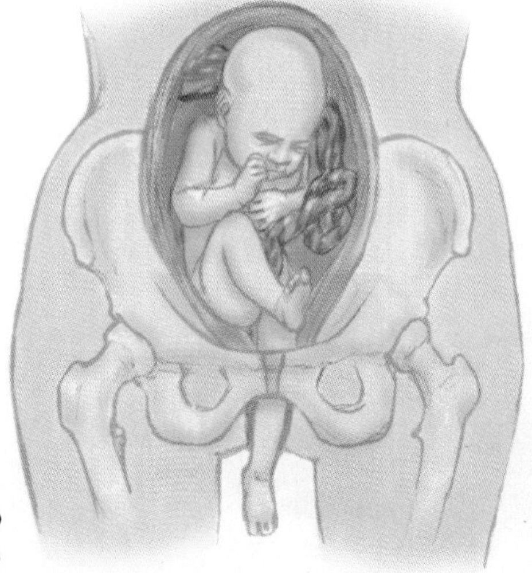

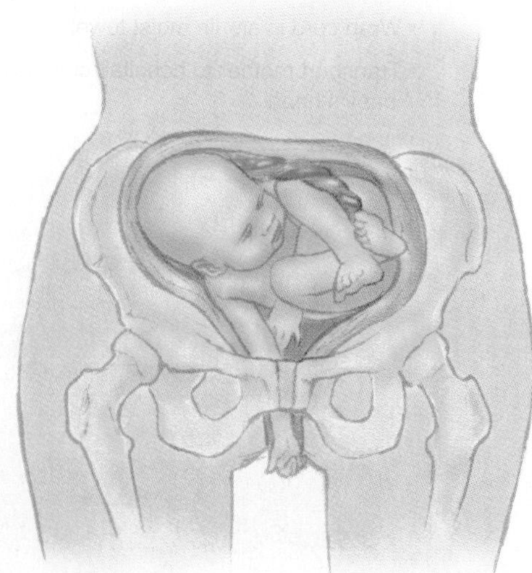

Figure 24-19 • Limb presentation.

the deliveries are normal. Twins are generally delivered in the same manner as a single delivery, one birth following the other. However, if a multiple birth is encountered, you should have enough personnel and equipment to be prepared for multiple resuscitations. Call for assistance if needed.

When delivering twins, identify the infants as to order of birth (one and two, or A and B).

PATIENT ASSESSMENT

MULTIPLE BIRTH

If the mother is under a physician's care, she will probably be aware that she is carrying twins. Without this information, you should consider a multiple birth to be a possibility if the mother's abdomen appears unusually large before delivery, or it remains very large after delivery of one baby. If the birth is multiple, labor contractions will continue and the second baby will be delivered shortly after the first. The second baby may present in a breech position, usually within minutes of the first birth. The placenta(s) are delivered normally (Figure 24-20). ■

PATIENT CARE

MULTIPLE BIRTH

When assisting in the delivery of twins, follow these steps:

1. Clamp or tie the cord of the first baby before the second baby is born.
2. The second baby may be born either before or after the placenta is delivered. Assist the mother with the delivery of the second baby.
3. Provide care for the babies, umbilical cords, placenta(s), and the mother as you would in a single-baby delivery.
4. The babies will probably be smaller than in a single birth, so special care should be taken to keep them warm during transport. ■

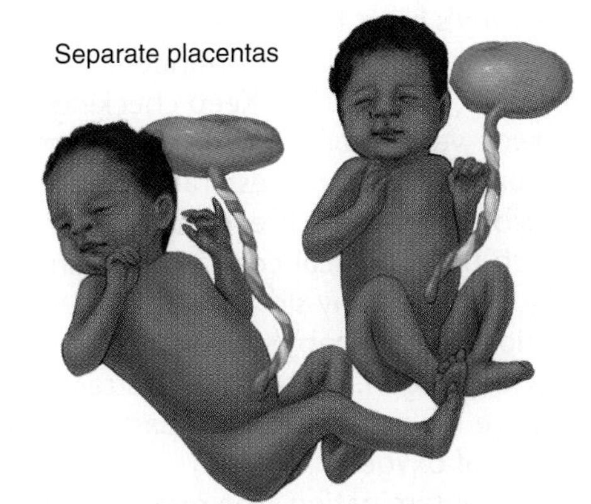

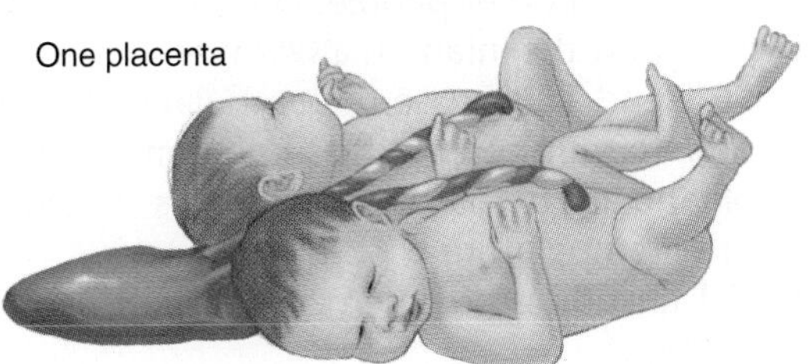

Figure 24-20 • Multiple births.

Premature Birth

premature infant any newborn weighing less than $5^1/_2$ pounds or born before the 37th week of pregnancy.

By definition, a **premature infant** is one who weighs less than $5^1/_2$ pounds ($2^1/_2$ kilograms) at birth, or one who is born before the 37th week of pregnancy.

PATIENT ASSESSMENT

PREMATURE BIRTH

Since you probably will not be able to weigh the baby, make a determination as to whether the baby is full-term or premature based on the mother's information and the baby's appearance. By comparison with a normal full-term baby, the head of a premature infant is much larger in proportion to the small, thin, red body (Figure 24-21). ■

PATIENT CARE

PREMATURE BIRTH

Premature babies need special care from the moment of birth. The smaller the baby, the more important is the initial care. You should take the following steps when providing care for the premature infant:

1. Keep the baby warm. Premature infants are at great risk of developing hypothermia. Once breathing, the baby should be dried and wrapped snugly in a warm blanket. Additional protection can be provided by an outer wrap of plastic bubble wrap (keep away from the face) or a small reflective blanket. Premature babies lack fat deposits that would normally keep them warm. Some EMS systems in cold regions use plastic, bubble wrap, or a bag for the infant, covered by a blanket. This helps maintain warmth and allows for easier visual inspection of the clamped cord to check for bleeding. A stockinet cap should be placed on the baby's head to help reduce heat loss.
2. Keep the airway clear. Continue to suction fluids from the nose and mouth using a rubber bulb syringe. Keep checking to see if additional suctioning is required.
3. Provide ventilations and/or chest compressions as outlined earlier based upon the baby's pulse and respiratory effort. In some cases, resuscitation may not be possible if the baby is extremely premature.
4. Watch the umbilical cord for bleeding. Examine the cut end of the cord carefully. If there is any sign of bleeding, even the slightest, apply another clamp or tie closer to the baby's body.
5. Provide oxygen. Do not blow a stream of oxygen directly on the baby's face, but arrange for oxygen to flow past the baby's face. If available, use a humidified source of oxygen.
6. Avoid contamination. The premature infant is susceptible to infection. Keep him away from other people. Do not breathe on his face.
7. Transport the infant in a warm ambulance. The desired temperature is between 90°F and 100°F. Use the ambulance heater to warm the patient compartment prior to transport. In the summer months, the air conditioning should be turned off and all compartment windows should be closed or adjusted to keep the desired temperature.
8. Call ahead to the emergency department. ■

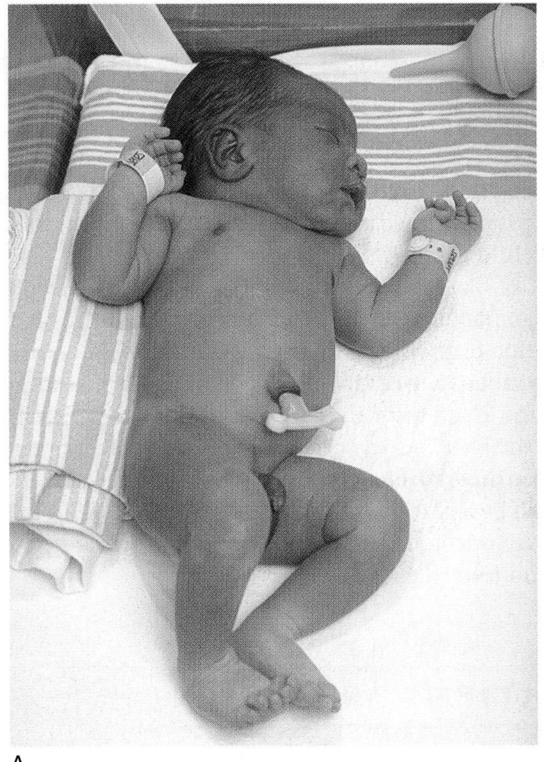

A

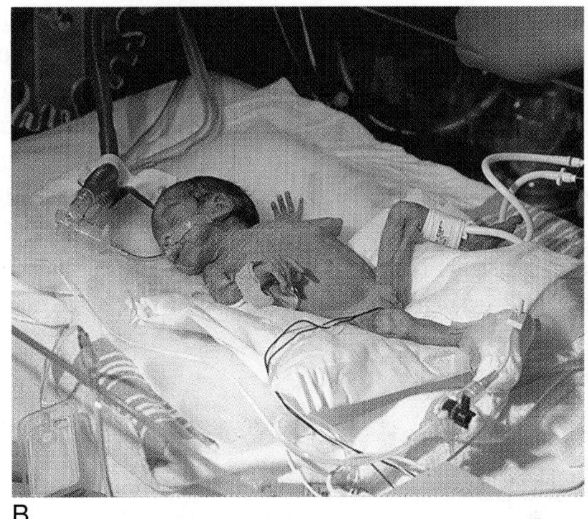

B

Figure 24-21 • (A) Full-term newborn *(© Will and Deni McIntyre/Photo Researchers, Inc.)* and (B) a premature newborn after 24 weeks of gestation. *(© Susan Leavines/Photo Researchers, Inc.)*

Meconium

As noted earlier, meconium is a result of the fetus defecating (putting out wastes). It is a sign of fetal or maternal distress.

PATIENT ASSESSMENT

MECONIUM

Meconium stains amniotic fluid greenish or brownish-yellow in color. Infants born with meconium are at increased risk for respiratory problems, especially if aspiration of the meconium occurs at birth. ■

PATIENT CARE

MECONIUM

If you see meconium staining in the amniotic fluid, follow these steps:

1. To reduce the risk of aspiration, do not stimulate the infant before suctioning the oropharynx.
2. Suction the mouth and then the nose.
3. Maintain an open airway.
4. Provide artificial ventilations and/or chest compression as indicated by effort of breathing and heart rate.
5. Transport as soon as possible. ■

Emergencies in Pregnancy

There are a number of predelivery emergencies that can arise in the pregnant patient prior to labor or childbirth.

Excessive Prebirth Bleeding

A number of conditions can cause excessive prebirth bleeding late in pregnancy. Whether the vaginal bleeding is associated with abdominal pain or not, the risk to both the mother and the unborn child is great.

A pregnant woman does not have to be in labor to have excessive bleeding from the vagina. Bleeding in early pregnancy may be due to a miscarriage. If the bleeding occurs late in pregnancy, it may be due to problems involving the placenta.

placenta previa (plah-SEN-tah PRE-vi-ah) a condition in which the placenta is formed in an abnormal location (low in the uterus and close to or over the cervical opening) that will not allow for a normal delivery of the fetus; a cause of excessive prebirth bleeding.

abruptio placentae (ab-RUPT-si-o plah-SENT-ta) a condition in which the placenta separates from the uterine wall; a cause of prebirth bleeding.

In one such condition, **placenta previa,** the placenta is formed in an abnormal location (low in the uterus and close to or over the cervical opening) that will not allow for a normal delivery of the fetus. As the cervix dilates, the placenta tears. Another such condition is **abruptio placentae,** a condition in which the placenta separates from the uterine wall. This can be a partial or a complete abruption. Either placenta previa or abruptio placentae may occur in the third trimester. Both are potentially life threatening to the mother and fetus.

PATIENT ASSESSMENT

EXCESSIVE PREBIRTH BLEEDING

Signs and symptoms of excessive prebirth bleeding include the following:

- Main sign is usually profuse bleeding from the vagina.
- Mother may or may not experience associated abdominal pain.
- During initial assessment, look for signs of shock.
- Obtain baseline vital signs. A rapid heartbeat may indicate significant blood loss. ■

PATIENT CARE

EXCESSIVE PREBIRTH BLEEDING

- If signs of shock exist, treat with high-concentration oxygen and rapid transportation.
- Place a sanitary napkin over the vaginal opening. Note the time of napkin placement. DO NOT PLACE ANYTHING IN THE VAGINA. Replace pads as they become soaked, but save all pads for use in evaluating blood loss.
- Save all tissue that is passed. ■

oviduct fallopian tube; tube that carries eggs from an ovary to the uterus.

ectopic (ek-TOP-ik) **pregnancy** when implantation of the fertilized egg is not in the body of the uterus, occurring instead in the oviduct (fallopian tube), cervix, or abdominopelvic cavity.

Ectopic Pregnancy

In normal pregnancy, the fertilized egg will begin to divide in the **oviduct** (fallopian tube) and eventually implant in the wall of the uterus. In an **ectopic pregnancy,** the egg may implant outside the uterus—for example, in the cervix or pelvic cavity. Ectopic pregnancies usually occur in the tubular oviduct, which ruptures as the fetus grows, resulting in internal bleeding.

PATIENT ASSESSMENT

ECTOPIC PREGNANCY

The problems related to this condition are seen early in pregnancy. Indeed, some women with an ectopic pregnancy may be unaware that they are even pregnant at the time of onset of signs and symptoms. Women may have signs and symptoms including those indicating shock due to internal bleeding. This condition can be life threatening and, as the saying goes, "Any woman of childbearing age with abdominal pain has an ectopic pregnancy until proven otherwise by the physician in the emergency department."

Be alert to recognize the following signs and symptoms as they develop:

- Acute abdominal pain, often beginning on one side or the other
- Vaginal bleeding (often accompanies pain)
- Rapid and weak pulse (a later sign)
- Low blood pressure (a very late sign) ■

PATIENT CARE

ECTOPIC PREGNANCY

Emergency care includes the following:

1. Consider the need for immediate transport.
2. Position the patient for shock.
3. Care for shock.
4. Provide high-concentration oxygen by nonrebreather mask.
5. Do not give the patient anything by mouth. ■

Seizures in Pregnancy

Seizures in pregnancy, sometimes caused by a condition called **eclampsia,** tend to occur late in pregnancy. The seizures are usually associated with high blood pressure and **preeclampsia,** or swelling of the extremities. Seizures in pregnancy pose a serious threat to both the mother and unborn baby.

eclampsia (e-KLAMP-se-ah) a severe complication of pregnancy that produces seizures and coma.

preeclampsia (pre-e-KLAMP-se-ah) a complication of pregnancy where the woman retains large amounts of fluid and has hypertension. She may also experience seizures and/or coma during birth, which is very dangerous to the infant.

PATIENT ASSESSMENT

SEIZURES IN PREGNANCY

A seizure may be associated with any of the following:

- Elevated blood pressure, which increases the risk of abruptio placentae
- Excessive weight gain
- Extreme swelling of face, hands, ankles, and feet
- Headache ■

PATIENT CARE

SEIZURES IN PREGNANCY

Emergency care of a pregnant patient with seizures includes the following:

1. Ensure and maintain an open airway.
2. Administer high-concentration oxygen by nonrebreather mask.
3. Transport the patient positioned on her left side.
4. Handle her gently at all times. Rough handling may induce more seizures.
5. Keep her warm, but do not overheat.
6. Have suction ready.
7. Have a delivery kit ready. ■

Miscarriage and Abortion

For a number of reasons, the fetus and placenta may deliver before the 28th week of pregnancy—generally before the baby can live on his own. This occurrence is an **abortion.** When it happens on its own, it is called a **spontaneous abortion,** more commonly known as a **miscarriage.** An **induced abortion** is an abortion that results from deliberate actions taken to stop the pregnancy.

abortion spontaneous (miscarriage) or induced termination of pregnancy.

spontaneous abortion when the fetus and placenta deliver before the 28th week of pregnancy; commonly called a miscarriage.

miscarriage *see* spontaneous abortion.

induced abortion expulsion of a fetus as a result of deliberate actions taken to stop the pregnancy.

PATIENT ASSESSMENT

MISCARRIAGE AND ABORTION

Women having a miscarriage that requires them to seek emergency care generally have the following signs and symptoms:

- Cramping abdominal pains not unlike those associated with the first stage of labor
- Bleeding ranging from moderate to severe
- A noticeable discharge of tissue and blood from the vagina

Ask the patient about the starting date of her last menstrual period. If it has been more than 24 weeks, be prepared with a delivery pack. Premature infants may survive if they receive rapid neonatal intensive care. ■

PATIENT CARE

MISCARRIAGE AND ABORTION

1. Obtain baseline vital signs.
2. If signs of shock are present, provide high-concentration oxygen by a nonrebreather mask. Treatment should be based on signs and symptoms.
3. Help absorb vaginal bleeding by placing a sanitary napkin over the vaginal opening. Do not pack the vagina.
4. Transport as soon as possible.
5. Replace and save all blood-soaked pads.
6. Save all tissues that are expelled. Do not attempt to replace or pull out any tissues that are being expelled through the vagina.

continued

PATIENT CARE *(continued)*

7. Provide emotional support to the mother. Emotional support is very important. When speaking to the patient, her family, or where bystanders may hear you, ALWAYS use the term *miscarriage* instead of spontaneous abortion. Most people associate the word *abortion* with an induced abortion, not a miscarriage. It is essential to talk with the patient to gain her confidence and to allow you to provide emotional support. ■

Trauma in Pregnancy

Obviously the pregnant patient, like any other patient, can sustain injury. However, especially during the last two trimesters, the uterus and fetus are also subject to injuries when the mother is injured. Injuries to the uterus may be blunt or penetrating. In both cases, the greatest danger to the mother and baby is hemorrhage (bleeding) and shock.

The most common cause of blunt trauma is automobile collisions, but falls or beatings also account for many injuries. The uterus is well designed to protect the baby. The fetus is inside the uterus, a muscular chamber filled with fluid. The uterus acts as an efficient shock absorber. Thus most minor trauma to the abdomen, such as a blow or fall, does not harm the fetus.

Automobile collisions are a different story. The magnitude of forces is great. Because of its size and location, the uterus is frequently injured. Sudden blunt trauma to the abdomen during the later months of pregnancy may cause uterine rupture or premature separation of the placenta (abruptio placentae). Other blunt trauma injuries, such as a ruptured spleen or liver, may also occur. Rupture of the diaphragm may occur with blunt trauma during later pregnancy. Multiple trauma with fractures of the pelvis can cause laceration or tearing of the vessels in the pelvis with massive hemorrhage. The common problem with most blunt injuries to the pregnant abdomen or pelvis is massive bleeding and shock.

If a pregnant woman is injured in an incident such as a motor-vehicle collision or a fall, perform a patient assessment and treat her injuries as you would those of any other trauma patient.

PATIENT ASSESSMENT

TRAUMA IN PREGNANCY

Follow these patient assessment steps:

- During initial assessment and assessment of vital signs, remember the following about the physiology of pregnant women:
  - The pregnant patient has a pulse that is 10 to 15 beats per minute faster than the nonpregnant female. Vital signs may be interpreted as being suggestive of shock when they are normal for the pregnant female.
  - A woman in later pregnancy may have a blood volume that is up to 48 percent higher than her nonpregnant state. With hemorrhage, 30 to 35 percent blood loss may occur before otherwise healthy pregnant females exhibit signs or symptoms.
  - Although shock is more difficult to assess in the pregnant patient, it is the most likely cause of prehospital death from injury to the uterus.
- Question the conscious patient to determine if she has received any blows to the abdomen, pelvis, or back.
- Ask the patient if she has had bleeding or rupture of the bag of waters. When in doubt, examine the vaginal area for bleeding, being certain to provide privacy.
- Examine the unconscious patient for abdominal injuries, remembering to consider the mechanism of injury. ■

PATIENT CARE

TRAUMA IN PREGNANCY

Remember that maintenance of respiration and circulation and the control of bleeding are vital not only to the mother but also to the fetus. A developing fetus is critically dependent on the uninterrupted oxygenated blood supply that enters the placenta. What is good for the mother is good for the baby. Since the mother-to-be may have undetected internal bleeding or the fetus may be injured, provide the following care to the injured mother:

1. Provide resuscitation if necessary.
2. Provide high-concentration oxygen by using a nonrebreather mask. (Oxygen requirements of the woman in later pregnancy are 10 to 20 percent greater than normal. If in doubt, give oxygen.)
3. Because of slowed digestion and delayed gastric emptying, there is a greater risk the patient will vomit and aspirate. Be ready with suction.
4. Transport as soon as possible. All pregnant women should be transported in the left lateral recumbent position, supported with pillows or blankets, unless a spinal injury is suspected. If so, first secure the mother to a spine board, then tip the board and patient as a unit to the left, relieving pressure on the abdominal organs and vena cava. Be sure to monitor and record vital signs.
5. Provide emotional support. A pregnant woman who is a trauma victim will naturally worry about her unborn child. Remind her that the developing baby is well protected in the uterus. Let her know that she is being transported to a medical facility that can take care of her needs and the needs of the unborn child. ■

Stillbirths

stillborn born dead.

Some babies die in the womb several hours, days, or even weeks before birth. Such a baby is called **stillborn.**

Nothing is quite so sad as a baby born dead or one who dies shortly after birth. It is a tragic moment for the parents and other family members. Your thoughtfulness may provide the distraught parents with comfort. In addition, do not lie to the mother. Many death-and-dying experts believe that she should be allowed to view her baby if she so desires. Do not stop her from seeing the dead baby if she wants to.

All resuscitative efforts should be continued until transfer to the hospital. Also, keep accurate records of the time of stillbirth and the care rendered for completion of the fetal death certificate.

PATIENT ASSESSMENT

STILLBIRTH

When a baby has died some time before birth, death is obvious by the presence of blisters, foul odor, skin or tissue deterioration and discoloration, and a softened head. At other times, a baby may be born in pulmonary or cardiac arrest but in otherwise good condition and with the possibility of being resuscitated. ■

PATIENT CARE

STILLBIRTH

Emergency care for a stillborn baby is as follows:

1. Stillborn babies who have obviously been dead for some time before birth are not to receive resuscitation.
2. Any other babies who are born in pulmonary or cardiac arrest are to receive basic life support measures.
3. When the baby is alive but respiratory or cardiac arrest appears to be imminent, prepare to provide life support. ■

Accidental Death of a Pregnant Woman

If a woman in advanced pregnancy dies from trauma and you begin CPR on her immediately, there is a chance of saving the life of the infant. CPR must be continued until an emergency cesarean section can be performed. Reposition your hands for compressions 1 to 2 inches higher on the sternum to make up for shifting of the heart due to the large fetus. If CPR is delayed 5 to 10 minutes, chances of saving the baby are fair, while a 25-minute delay reduces the chances to almost zero. Continue CPR on the mother until you are relieved in the emergency department.

GYNECOLOGICAL EMERGENCIES

Several emergencies are unique to the reproductive systems of women who are not, or are not necessarily, pregnant.

Vaginal Bleeding

Vaginal bleeding that is not a result of direct trauma or a woman's normal menstrual cycle may indicate a serious gynecological emergency.

PATIENT ASSESSMENT

VAGINAL BLEEDING

Since it will be impossible for the EMT to determine a specific cause of the bleeding, it is important that all women who have vaginal bleeding be treated as though they have a potentially life-threatening condition. This is especially true if the bleeding is associated with abdominal pain. The most serious complication of vaginal bleeding is hypovolemic shock due to blood loss. ■

PATIENT CARE

VAGINAL BLEEDING

1. Take Standard Precautions. Wear gloves, gown, protective eyewear, and mask as indicated.
2. Ensure an adequate airway.
3. Assess for signs of shock.
4. Administer high-concentration oxygen by nonrebreather mask.
5. Transport. ■

Trauma to the External Genitalia

Trauma to a woman's external genitalia can be difficult to care for because of the patient's modesty and the severe pain often involved with such injuries.

PATIENT ASSESSMENT

TRAUMA TO THE EXTERNAL GENITALIA

Injuries in this area tend to bleed profusely because of the rich blood supply to the area. Injuries to the female external genitalia are frequently the result of straddle-type injuries:

- In sizing up the scene, observe for mechanisms of injury.
- During initial assessment, look for signs of severe blood loss and shock. ■

PATIENT CARE

TRAUMA TO THE EXTERNAL GENITALIA

1. Control bleeding with direct pressure over a bulky dressing or sanitary pad. (If the patient is alert, she will probably prefer to do this herself.) Do not remove undergarments unless necessary. Do not pack the vagina.
2. If signs of shock are present, treat with high-concentration oxygen.
3. Maintain a professional attitude.
4. Respect the patient's privacy. Remove unneeded bystanders and expose the patient's body only to the extent necessary to provide appropriate care. ■

Sexual Assault

Situations where a sexual assault has occurred are always a challenge to the EMT. Care of the patient must include both medical and psychological considerations. In addition, law enforcement agencies are also frequently involved.

There is no question that the victim of sexual assault is under tremendous stress. You must be prepared to deal with a wide range of emotions that the patient may exhibit. The best approach is to be nonjudgmental and to maintain a professional but compassionate attitude. It is generally preferable that an EMT of the same sex as the patient establish rapport and be the primary provider of emergency care.

PATIENT ASSESSMENT

SEXUAL ASSAULT

- Since you may be entering a potential crime scene, ensure that the scene is safe prior to entering. It may be necessary to "stage" your unit near the scene until it is rendered safe by police.
- During assessment, identify and treat both the medical and the psychological needs of the patient. ■

PATIENT CARE

SEXUAL ASSAULT

1. Provide an open airway.
2. Be careful not to disturb potential criminal evidence unless it is absolutely necessary for patient care.
3. Examine the genitals only if severe bleeding is present.
4. Discourage the patient from bathing, voiding, or cleansing any wounds as this may result in loss of important evidence.
5. Fulfill any reporting requirements that are locally mandated. ■

CHAPTER REVIEW

SUMMARY

Birth is a natural process that usually takes place without complications. The EMT's role at a birth is generally to provide reassurance and to assist the mother in the delivery of her baby. During the normal delivery, the EMT will evaluate the mother to determine if there should be immediate transport to a medical facility or if birth is imminent and will take place at the scene. If birth is to take place at the scene, the EMT prepares the mother for delivery, assists in the delivery, assesses the newborn, and cares for the newborn and the mother.

Occasionally there will be some complications to delivery, including breech presentation, prolapsed umbilical cord, limb presentation, multiple birth, premature birth, or meconium staining of the amniotic fluid. There may also be predelivery emergencies, or emergencies associated with pregnancy (such as excessive bleeding, ectopic pregnancy, seizures, abortion, or trauma to the pregnant mother) that the EMT must be prepared to treat. Stillbirth and death of the mother are difficult emergencies the EMT is occasionally called upon to manage, as are gynecological emergencies (such as vaginal bleeding, trauma, or sexual assault).

KEY TERMS

abortion spontaneous (miscarriage) or induced termination of pregnancy.

abruptio placentae (ab-RUPT-si-o plah-SENT-ta) a condition in which the placenta separates from the uterine wall; a cause of prebirth bleeding.

afterbirth the placenta, membranes of the amniotic sac, part of the umbilical cord, and some tissues from the lining of the uterus that are delivered after the birth of the baby.

amniotic (am-ne-OT-ik) **sac** the "bag of waters" that surrounds the developing fetus.

breech presentation when the baby's buttocks or both legs appear first during birth.

cephalic (se-FAL-ik) **presentation** when the baby appears head first during birth. This is the normal presentation.

cervix (SUR-viks) the neck of the uterus at the entrance to the birth canal.

crowning when part of the baby is visible through the vaginal opening.

eclampsia (e-KLAMP-se-ah) a severe complication of pregnancy that produces seizures and coma.

ectopic (ek-TOP-ik) **pregnancy** when implantation of the fertilized egg is not in the body of the uterus, occurring instead in the oviduct (fallopian tube), cervix, or abdominopelvic cavity.

fetus (FE-tus) the baby as he develops in the womb.

induced abortion expulsion of a fetus as a result of deliberate actions taken to stop the pregnancy.

labor the three stages of the delivery of a baby that begin with the contractions of the uterus and end with the expulsion of the placenta.

limb presentation when an infant's limb protrudes from the vagina before the appearance of any other body part.

meconium staining amniotic fluid that is greenish or brownish-yellow rather than clear as a result of fetal defecation; an indication of possible maternal or fetal distress during labor.

miscarriage *see* spontaneous abortion.

multiple birth when more than one baby is born during a single delivery.

oviduct fallopian tube; tube that carries eggs from an ovary to the uterus.

perineum (per-i-NE-um) the surface area between the vagina and anus.

placenta (plah-SEN-tah) the organ of pregnancy where exchange of oxygen, foods, and wastes occurs between a mother and fetus.

placenta previa (plah-SEN-tah PRE-vi-ah) a condition in which the placenta is formed in an abnormal location (low in the uterus and close to or over the cervical opening) that will not allow for a normal delivery of the fetus; a cause of excessive prebirth bleeding.

preeclampsia (pre-e-KLAMP-se-ah) a complication of pregnancy where the woman retains large amounts of fluid and has hypertension. She may also experience seizures and/or coma during birth, which is very dangerous to the infant.

premature infant any newborn weighing less than $5^1/_2$ pounds or born before the 37th week of pregnancy.

prolapsed umbilical cord when the umbilical cord presents first and is squeezed between the vaginal wall and the baby's head.

spontaneous abortion when the fetus and placenta deliver before the 28th week of pregnancy; commonly called a miscarriage.

stillborn born dead.

supine hypotensive syndrome dizziness and a drop in blood pressure caused when the mother is in a supine position and the weight of the uterus, infant, placenta, and amniotic fluid compress the inferior vena cava, reducing return of blood to the heart and cardiac output.

umbilical (um-BIL-i-kal) **cord** the fetal structure containing the blood vessels that carry blood to and from the placenta.

uterus (U-ter-us) the muscular abdominal organ where the fetus develops; the womb.

vagina (vah-JI-nah) the birth canal.

REVIEW QUESTIONS

1. Name and describe the anatomical structures of a woman's body that are associated with pregnancy. (pp. 564–565)
2. Describe the three stages of labor. (pp. 565–567)
3. Explain how to evaluate and to prepare the mother for delivery. (pp. 568–571)
4. Name, in the order of the inverted pyramid, the steps that may be taken to resuscitate a newly born infant. (pp. 576–577)
5. Name and describe several possible complications of delivery. (pp. 581–588)
6. Name and describe several possible predelivery emergencies. (pp. 570–571, 588–593)

CRITICAL THINKING

- You are called to respond to a pregnant woman who is in labor. During your evaluation, you find that this is the woman's first pregnancy, the baby's head is not yet crowning, and contractions are 10 minutes apart. You ask the mother if she feels she needs to move her bowels, and she says she does not. Do you prepare for delivery at the scene? Or do you transport the mother to the hospital? Explain your reasoning.

Thinking and Linking

Think back to Chapter 2, "The Well-Being of the EMT-Basic," and link information from that chapter with information from this chapter, "Obstetrics and Gynecological Emergencies," as you consider the following situation:

- While assisting with an emergency out-of-hospital childbirth, you are sprayed with amniotic fluid. Afterwards, you find out that the mother is HIV positive. Who should you go to with this information? What should you do?

MEDIA RESOURCES

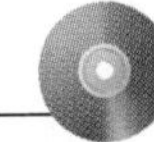

See the Student CD at the back of this book for quizzes, a case study activity, animations, videos, and other features related to this chapter. In particular, take a look at the 3D animation of the female reproductive system as well as the videos on stages of delivery, birth, delivery of the placenta, and care of the infant. Also, visit the Companion Website for *Emergency Care* at **www.prenhall.com/limmer**, where you will find additional reinforcement and links to other resources.

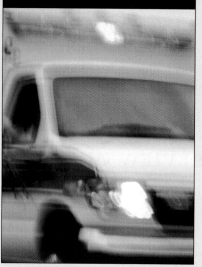

Street Scenes

Your sleep is interrupted by the tones of the radio and the dispatcher saying, "Bravo 3, stand-by for a call." You swing your feet onto the floor and grab the radio. "Go ahead, dispatch," you say.

"Bravo 3, respond to 77 Cherry Tree Lane for a pregnant patient in labor. The other dispatcher is still on the phone with the husband. Additional information to follow."

You and your partner head to the ambulance and start toward the scene. About 3 minutes from the patient's house, the dispatcher tells you that the baby appears to be crowning and the husband is still on the phone getting instructions. You and your partner decide you need a plan. You agree that both the adult and pediatric equipment need to be brought in, as well as the OB kit. You also agree that you will focus on the baby after delivery and your partner will provide care to the mother.

Street Scene Questions

1. What should be the first priority when entering the scene?
2. Should ALS assistance be requested?
3. What questions should you ask the mother or the father?

As you move toward the house, you ask the dispatcher if ALS has responded. You are told they are already en route. When you walk into the room, you see the mother on the bed and the father with the telephone cradled on his shoulder talking to the dispatcher. The father immediately stands aside, and you and your partner see crowning and realize that the delivery will take place any minute. You put on gloves and set up the OB kit while getting assessment information from the mother. It is her second delivery but it is 2 weeks early. Labor started about an hour ago, and the pains have been more frequent and very intense. The water broke just before they called 911. While your partner is obtaining a set of vital signs, the baby starts to deliver. The head comes out and you notice that the umbilical cord is around the baby's neck. You are able to slip it over the baby's head, and the baby continues to deliver. The shoulders and the rest of the baby's body follow quickly.

Street Scene Questions

4. What immediate care should be provided to the newborn?
5. What care should your partner be giving to the mother?

You immediately start down the inverted pyramid for neonate resuscitation. You suction the mouth and then the nose. The baby starts to cry immediately. You dry the baby off and wrap the swaddling blanket around her, making sure that the top of the baby's head is covered. The baby is pink and actively moving. You check the pulse, and it is at least 150 beats per minute. Your partner clamps the cord and makes the cut. You call the dispatcher to log in the time of the delivery and announce that it is a girl. At that time, dispatch reports that ALS has been diverted to a cardiac arrest. After 20 minutes, the placenta still has not delivered and you transport to the hospital without any further delay.

When you arrive back at the station, there is still time to get a couple of hours sleep but you are too excited so you turn on the television.

Street Scenes Sample Documentation

PATIENT NAME: *Doris Garfinkel* PATIENT AGE: *32*

CHIEF COMPLAINT: *Imminent childbirth*

PAST MEDICAL HISTORY

- [ ] None
- [ ] Allergy to
- [ ] Hypertension
- [ ] Stroke
- [ ] Seizures
- [ ] Diabetes
- [ ] COPD
- [ ] Cardiac
- [x] Other (List) *Second child*
- [ ] Asthma

Current Medications (List) *None*

VITAL SIGNS

TIME	RESP	PULSE	B.P.	MENTAL STATUS	R PUPILS L	SKIN
0145	Rate: 28; Shallow	Rate: 100; Regular	130/84	Alert	Normal (R, L)	Moist
0157	Rate: 28; Shallow	Rate: 100; Regular	138/82	Alert	Normal (R, L)	Moist
0210	Rate: 28; Regular	Rate: 88; Regular	120/78	Alert	Normal (R, L)	Moist

NARRATIVE: *On arrival, crew met the patient and her husband. They state that the baby is about two weeks early and labor began an hour ago. Labor progressed very quickly and the pains and contractions are very intense and frequent. At the time of the 911 call, the patient's water broke. Delivery is imminent. A second unit with ALS requested in the event that there are complications, but they were diverted. We assisted with a normal cephalic delivery. The umbilical cord is loosened around the baby's neck and a normal delivery is observed. The baby is suctioned, stimulated, dried, and warmed. The cord is clamped and cut. The baby is placed on the mother's abdomen for transport and warmth. Transport is initiated prior to delivery of the placenta. See Form #107 for PCR on baby.*

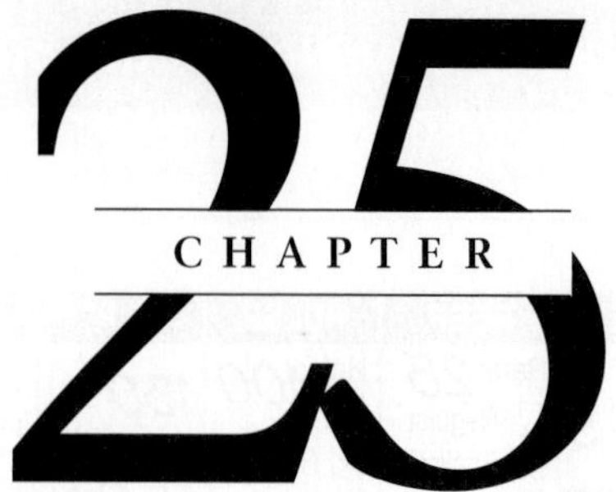

CHAPTER 25

Putting It All Together for the Medical Patient

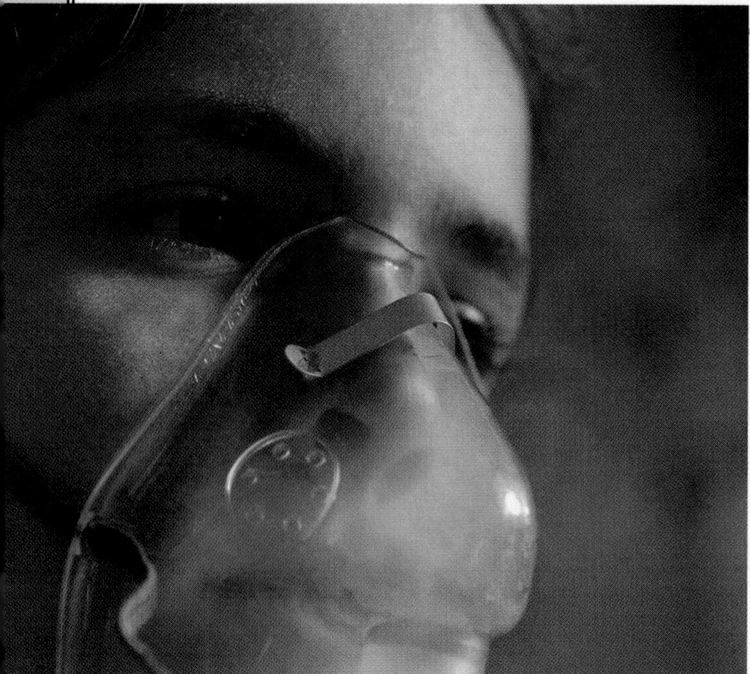

CORE CONCEPTS

The following are core concepts that will be addressed in this chapter:

- Management of patients with more than one medical complaint
- Management of patient conditions not covered in a basic EMT course

In previous chapters in this module, you learned how to look for, recognize, and manage a number of medical complaints patients may have. However, each of those chapters assumed the patient had only the problem described in that chapter. What should an EMT do when a patient has two or more presenting problems? How should the EMT handle situations in which the patient has a chief complaint that is not covered in a basic EMT course? This chapter will help answer these and other questions about applying knowledge and skills from a basic EMT course to the real world.

NOTE

There are no objectives in the National Standard Curriculum that pertain to the material in this chapter.

MULTIPLE MEDICAL COMPLAINTS

Many EMTs feel more comfortable dealing with injuries than illnesses. This may be because it is relatively easy to look at a mechanism of injury, look at the injured patient, and get a good idea of what the patient's problem might be. After all, a deformed leg can only be caused by one of a very few things, such as a fracture or dislocation.

However, medical conditions present a very different picture. A medical patient's chest pain might be the result of any number of conditions, including myocardial infarction (heart attack), angina, a collapsed lung, a pulmonary embolus (a clot in one of the pulmonary arteries), pneumonia, or plain old heartburn to name just a few. This presents a confusing picture to the EMT.

Fortunately, since there are a limited number of interventions an EMT can administer, there are also a limited number of decisions that the EMT must make. For the medical patient, these decisions are:

- *Airway.* Does the airway need to be cleared with suction? Should the EMT position the patient on his side or insert an oral or nasal airway to maintain a patent airway?
- *Breathing.* Should the patient receive high-concentration oxygen by nonrebreather mask? Should the EMT ventilate the patient with oxygen?
- *Circulation.* Is there bleeding that needs to be controlled? Should the patient receive chest compressions? Should the EMT apply an AED?
- *Priority determination.* How promptly and rapidly does this patient need transport?
- *Interventions.* Does the EMT have any interventions that might help the patient? Specifically, does the patient meet local criteria for assistance with an inhaler, nitroglycerin, or an epinephrine auto-injector; administration of oral glucose or activated charcoal; cooling or warming; talking down or restraining; or assisting in childbirth?

MANAGING THE PATIENT WITH MULTIPLE MEDICAL COMPLAINTS

It can be very challenging for the EMT to manage a patient who presents with more than one condition or a familiar condition but under unusual circumstances. When faced with this kind of situation, you should assess the patient as usual. Then determine whether the patient meets the criteria for one or more of your interventions. If there is

POINT OF VIEW

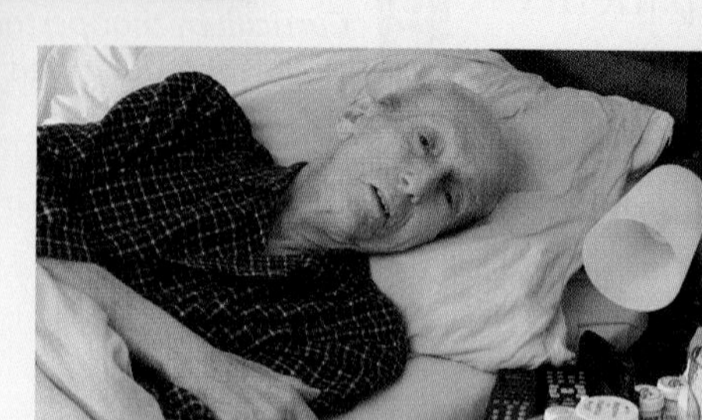

"We got the call for a 'sick person.' This kind of call never gives us a lot of information. It certainly offers no idea where to start.

"At this call we got there and found an older man lying in bed. He could talk to us and answer questions, but he said he was weak and just couldn't seem to get out of bed. I remember EMT class. We learned a lot about a lot of conditions but never what to do when you didn't even know what the problem was. So we did what we were taught in class—follow the assessment process. We put some oxygen on after we made sure he was breathing adequately and began a history. And wow, what a history. He had a little bit of everything. Some he told us, some his family told us, and some we pieced together from his medications. He was taking one medication for a condition his family outright denied he had!

"We took vitals, did a stroke scale, checked his blood sugar. There was nothing that jumped out as his problem, that's for sure. He did have a bit of a cough and a slight fever. Sometimes that is enough for our geriatric patients to knock them for a loop. We didn't find anything else.

"We took good care of him, monitored him throughout the call, and brought him to the hospital. Sometimes that is all you can do . . . just treat people well and take care of them."

any reason to believe the patient is at greater risk of harm from the intervention, or that unusual circumstances make the situation difficult to assess, consult medical direction, even if it is not required by your protocols. By consulting on-line medical direction, you will be able to find out which intervention, if any, you should employ.

Typical Calls

The cases that follow—all in EMS systems where advanced life support is not available—demonstrate these principles in action.

Case #1: Overdose in a Patient with Diabetes

You receive a call for a female who has taken an overdose of pills. As you approach the scene, you note that the house is dirty and unkempt but appears to be safe. Your general impression is of a teenage female who looks sleepy. She is awake and answers questions slowly, although she continues to appear drowsy. Her airway is

Cultural Considerations

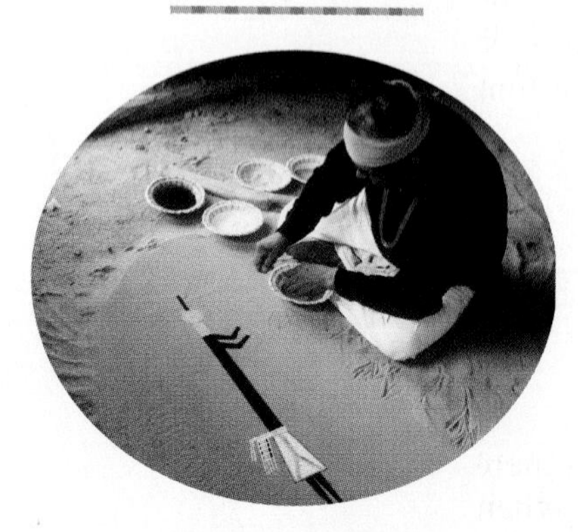

Members of some cultures may not believe in the germ theory of disease causation. They may consider illness to be a punishment for some type of behavior, as a curse placed by an enemy, or as the action of an evil spirit.

Native Americans have a very strong tradition of respect for the natural world. Some may view illness as being caused by the patient or the group having lived or acted in disharmony with nature. They may take the medicines a doctor prescribes. They may also, or instead, perform traditional rites or use traditional cures such as herbs to treat the illness.

open, and her breathing appears adequate in rate and depth. There is no blood or bleeding visible, and her radial pulse feels rapid and full.

You decide that her condition is serious and requires transport soon, but you have a few minutes to gather more information, which the emergency department will need to institute the proper treatment. From the patient's mother, you learn that the patient is a 16-year-old who had a fight with her boyfriend and then decided to swallow all the pills she could find in the house. To wash the pills down, she had a "couple" of beers. All of this occurred about 10 to 15 minutes ago. The medications include propranolol 80 mg (up to 6 tablets missing), amitriptyline 50 mg (up to 15 tablets missing), and extra-strength acetaminophen 500 mg (up to 50 tablets missing).

Through slurred speech, the patient tells you she feels nauseated but has not vomited. Her last meal was lunch 3 hours ago. The only medication she is supposed to take is insulin for her diabetes. She refuses to say when she last took her insulin or how much she took. She has no other medical history and has no known medication allergies.

Vital signs are pulse 96 and full, BP 100/70, respirations 14 and adequate, skin warm and dry. Your partner places a nonrebreather mask with 15 liters per minute of oxygen on the patient.

Your standing orders allow you to give one tube of oral glucose to a diabetic with an altered mental status who can swallow without threatening her airway. Your protocols also direct you to call medical direction for conscious overdose patients so that activated charcoal can be considered. Activated charcoal prevents many drugs from being absorbed by the body. You wonder whether you should give the oral glucose now and then call medical direction about the activated charcoal. You decide against doing that, because this case is so unusual and because you are not sure whether oral glucose will work if the patient also receives activated charcoal. You think to yourself that you are glad you will be speaking to a physician in a few minutes anyway.

You contact on-line medical direction. You describe the patient's condition, her history of insulin-dependent diabetes, and the names and amounts of the medications involved in the present emergency. When you ask the doctor whether you should give oral glucose or not, he asks if there is any way to find out what her blood sugar is. Your partner tells you he just checked it with your blood glucose meter and reports it is 105 mg/dL. The doctor is satisfied with this and directs you to withhold oral glucose and to administer 25 grams of activated charcoal orally, if you can get her to swallow without aspirating it. He also advises you to be prepared for the possibility of vomiting and ventricular fibrillation because of the medications involved. You attempt to give the patient the activated charcoal, but she refuses. Otherwise, transport is uneventful.

After you turn over patient care to the emergency department staff, you get a chance to think about the case. Although this patient's condition technically fulfilled the criteria in your standing orders for administration of oral glucose, you wonder if the authors of the protocol ever pictured a situation where the patient had also taken an overdose. You had to consider the possibility that the patient might need activated charcoal. You also did not know whether activated charcoal might prevent the glucose from working or whether the glucose might prevent the activated charcoal from working. For these reasons, it was prudent to consult on-line medical direction before giving the patient something that might end up harming her.

Later, the on-line physician catches you on your way out of the hospital emergency department and tells you he is glad you called in. She is being evaluated now and will be admitted to the hospital. He appreciated your report on the patient and was not doubting you when he asked for a blood glucose reading. He just wanted to confirm what he thought was the case: that the patient's depressed mental status was a result of the medications, not hypoglycemia.

Case #2: A Surprising Change in a Patient with Chest Pain

You receive a call for a male with chest pain (Figure 25-1). The scene is safe, so you proceed to introduce yourself to the patient and perform an initial assessment. Your general impression is of an older man who appears anxious and uncomfortable. His mental status is alert. His airway is patent, and his breathing appears adequate, although it is a little rapid and shallow. There is no blood or bleeding visible, and his radial pulse feels weak. You decide to assess the patient quickly and get underway to the hospital.

The patient, who is 68, tells you he has had dull substernal pain without radiation for about 15 minutes. It came on at rest. He denies shortness of breath but admits to some nausea. He has a prescription for nitroglycerin, but cannot find the bottle. His medications include ibuprofen, nitroglycerin, and diltiazem. He has a history of arthritis, angina, and high blood pressure. He has no known allergies to medications.

Vital signs are pulse 84 and weak, BP 118/90, respirations 22, skin pale and sweaty. Breath sounds are equal on both sides of his chest. His oxygen saturation is 98 percent on room air.

As your partner puts a nonrebreather mask on the patient, the wife finds the nitroglycerin. Your protocol calls for you to contact on-line medical direction before assisting a patient with his nitro, so you call and speak to a doctor in the emergency department. She advises one sublingual nitro now and another in 5 minutes if he still has chest pain and his systolic blood pressure is greater than 100. You help the patient take his nitroglycerin and transport him sitting up. Four minutes later, just after you take his blood pressure, the patient vomits a mixture of material that looks like coffee grounds and bright red blood. You are 15 minutes from the hospital. The patient received some relief after the nitroglycerin and oxygen, but he still has a little bit of pain in his chest. His pulse is 92, weak and regular, BP 102/80, respirations 22, skin pale and sweaty.

The patient fulfills the conditions described by your protocol and the physician you spoke to, but you do not think this is what she expected. You contact her again, inform her of the vomiting and the patient's most recent vital signs, and she directs you to withhold any more nitro for the moment and to

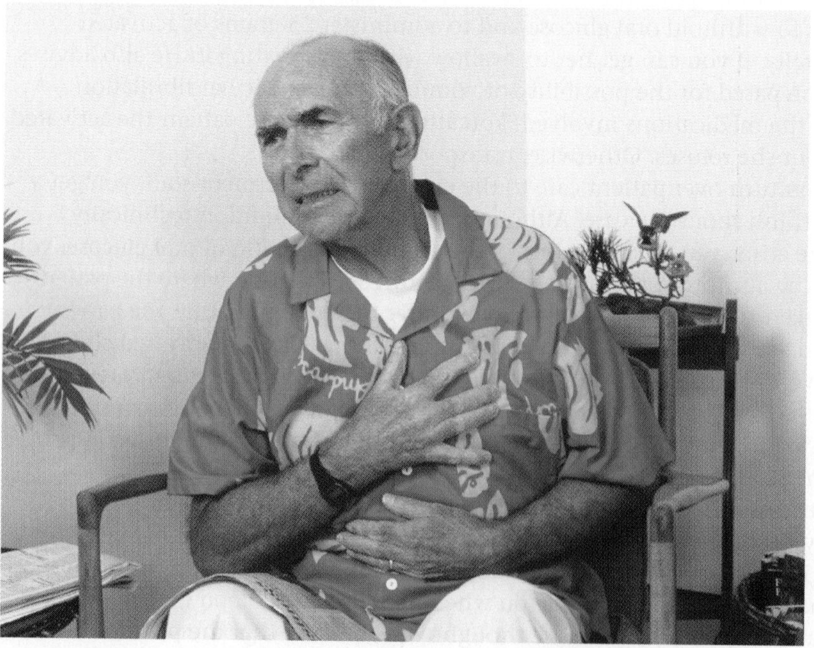

Figure 25-1 • Male patient in his 60s with chest pain.

inform her of any further changes. The patient's condition and vital signs remain essentially the same for the remainder of the trip, and you turn the patient over to the emergency department staff.

This case began as a very straightforward presentation of chest pain in a patient with a prescription for nitroglycerin. Then it took a sudden unexpected turn when the patient vomited blood (blood that has been in the stomach for a while frequently looks like coffee grounds when it is vomited). Since you are not familiar with this condition, you ask the emergency physician what happened to this patient.

She explains that the ibuprofen the patient was taking for his arthritis is irritating to the stomach and sometimes causes gastrointestinal bleeding. A patient with angina is sensitive to a decrease in the amount of oxygen getting to his heart. If enough blood is lost, there are not enough red blood cells to carry sufficient oxygen to the heart. In a patient with angina, this can lead to chest pain. You are grateful for the explanation and relieved, because you had feared the nitro you gave the patient might have caused the bleeding.

She praises you for giving the patient high-concentration oxygen despite the normal oxygen saturation reading. This patient had lost a significant number of red blood cells, so saturating the red blood cells and the plasma they are dissolved in gave the patient's hypoxic heart as much oxygen as could be given short of a transfusion.

The doctor also commends you on not going ahead with her original instructions but instead using good judgment and advising her of the vomited blood. Most of the patient's pain had been relieved by the nitro and oxygen, so she weighed the risks and benefits of another nitro and decided to wait until the patient arrived at the hospital.

Case #3: A Not-So-Simple Allergic Reaction

You receive a call for a pregnant woman stung by a bee. The scene is safe, so you proceed to introduce yourself to the patient and perform an initial assessment. Your general impression is of a woman in her mid-20s who looks a little anxious and who has some hives on her neck and arms. Her mental status is alert. Her airway is patent, and her breathing appears adequate. There is no blood or bleeding visible, and her radial pulse feels weak. You decide that her condition is potentially serious, but that you need more information to determine how urgently you need to transport her.

The patient is a 26-year-old female who is 5 months pregnant with her first child. She was stung 5 minutes ago on her hand by a bee. She is complaining of slight difficulty breathing and itching on her neck and arms.

The patient has a history of allergic reactions to bee stings and has an epinephrine auto-injector, but she does not like needles and was afraid to use it.

As you examine her, you notice that you do not hear any wheezes. She has hives on her neck and arms, but no swelling of the tongue, mouth, face, or neck. There is no stinger visible at the sting site. Vital signs are pulse 88, BP 110/80, respirations 20, skin warm and dry. You have her on high-concentration oxygen by nonrebreather.

Since your protocol requires you to contact on-line medical direction in cases like this one, you contact a physician in the emergency department and advise him of the patient's condition and the availability of an epinephrine auto-injector. He wants you to hold off on the epinephrine auto-injector for the moment, but he also wants you to watch her closely, monitor her vital signs every 5 minutes, and report back with any changes in the patient's condition immediately.

About 5 minutes later, you can hear wheezes without a stethoscope. Her difficulty breathing has increased, and the hives have spread over most of her upper body. Vital signs are pulse 104, BP 96/80, respirations 24 and labored, skin warm and dry. When you advise the physician of these changes, he orders use of the epinephrine auto-injector. Five minutes after the epinephrine, the patient's hives have cleared up, her wheezes are no longer audible, and the patient is no longer short of breath. You arrive at the emergency department a few minutes later with the patient looking and feeling much better.

The emergency department is not too busy today, so you get a chance to speak briefly with the physician. He explains he asked you to hold off on using the epinephrine auto-injector because the patient is pregnant and her condition was not initially serious enough to warrant the injection. Epinephrine causes many blood vessels to constrict, including those in the uterus of this pregnant patient. He felt the risk of reducing circulating oxygen to the fetus outweighed the benefit of the epinephrine as long as she had only minor symptoms. Once you advised him of her turn for the worse, the benefit to both mother and baby outweighed the risks. He thanks you for monitoring the patient closely and relaying that important information.

Analysis of the Calls

In each of these cases, the EMT was confronted with situations that called for judgment. Most patients you will see will have straightforward complaints, but occasionally you will run into a situation where the usual rules may not be applicable. In these cases, it is essential that you treat any immediate life-threats and then consider the risk to the patient your usual treatment might pose. If the risk appears greater or it is unknown, your best plan of action is to consult on-line medical direction. (See the flowchart in Figure 25-2.)

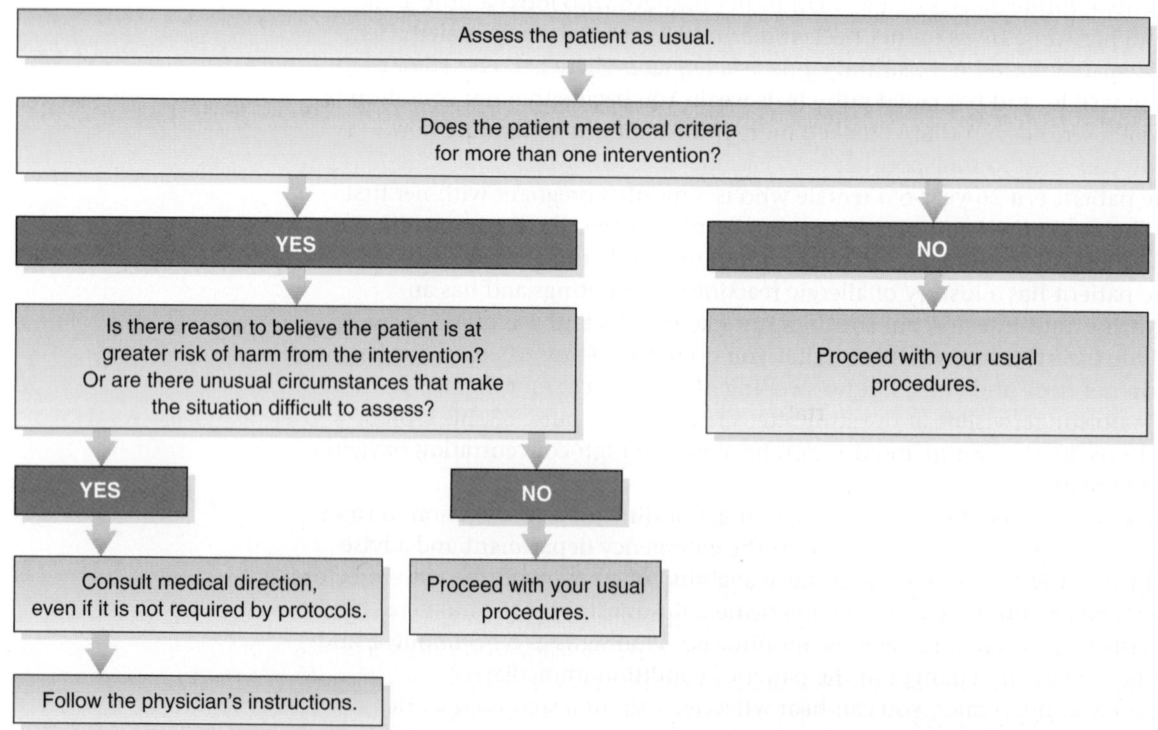

Approach to the Patient with Multiple Complaints
Assess the patient as usual.
Does the patient meet local criteria for more than one intervention?
YES
NO
Is there reason to believe the patient is at greater risk of harm from the intervention? Or are there unusual circumstances that make the situation difficult to assess?
Proceed with your usual procedures.
YES
NO
Consult medical direction, even if it is not required by protocols.
Proceed with your usual procedures.
Follow the physician's instructions.

Figure 25-2 • Approach to the patient with multiple complaints.

PATIENT CONDITIONS NOT COVERED IN THE BASIC EMT COURSE

One of the most important purposes of a basic EMT course is to help you learn when to employ the interventions you have available to you. In the second module of this book, you learned how to detect and treat immediate threats to the airway. Chapters in this module have described the appropriate use of specific interventions for specific medical problems:

- Assisting a patient in using his own inhaler (respiratory difficulty)
- Assisting a patient in taking his own nitroglycerin (cardiac compromise)
- Application of an automated defibrillator (cardiac arrest)
- Administration of oral glucose (diabetics with altered mental status)
- Assisting a patient in using his own epinephrine auto-injector (allergic reaction)
- Administration of activated charcoal (overdose or poisoning)
- Cooling or warming (environmental emergencies)
- Talking down and restraining (behavioral emergencies)
- Assisting in delivery of an infant (patient in labor)

For a number of reasons, common chief complaints for which EMTs have no specific treatment are not covered in the typical basic EMT course. In each of these conditions, the appropriate course of action for the EMT is to assess the patient and provide the appropriate supportive treatment, such as airway management and treatment for shock (hypoperfusion). For example, there is no intervention an EMT has available that should be administered specifically for abdominal pain, as you learned in Chapter 18, "Acute Abdominal Emergencies." If the patient with abdominal pain has signs and symptoms of shock (hypoperfusion), the patient should be treated for shock. If the patient has a compromised airway, the EMT should clear the patient's airway. In neither of these cases did the treatment for the patient depend on the cause of the abdominal pain. There also are no specific EMT interventions for patients with postsurgical complications, headache, or sickle-cell crisis. In each case, the EMT should assess the patient and treat the problems found (control bleeding in a surgical incision that has opened, for instance).

Confronting common problems for which an EMT has no treatment can leave the EMT feeling lost or inadequate. There are a number of important principles to keep in mind:

- Assess the patient as you learned to do in your basic EMT class.
- Look for and treat the problems for which you have treatments.
- If you work in a system where more advanced providers are available, follow your protocols and procedures for calling for assistance.
- Keep in mind that patients generally do not realize you are providing basic-EMT-level care, but they do know if you are polite, respectful, and empathetic when you are with them. An air of confidence and warmth will do wonders to make an anxious patient more comfortable.

An even more alarming situation for an EMT, especially a new one, is assessing a patient who tells you his problem is caused by some disease he names and it is one you have never heard of nor can even pronounce. In this case, being honest with the patient is usually the best approach. A simple statement like, "I have to admit I'm not familiar with that disease. Could you tell me a little bit about it?" is likely to result in the patient happily informing you about his condition. Most patients will respond very well to this approach. They know you are not a physician, and they do not expect you to be as knowledgeable as one. Often, though not always, the patient is extremely knowledgeable about the condition and the treatment for it. If it is a rare condition, the patient will in all likelihood be very accustomed to explaining it to others (including doctors and nurses).

A very similar situation can arise when the patient is using medical equipment at home that the EMT is not familiar with. In this case, the patient or a family member is usually very knowledgeable about the device and its use. You will learn more about high technology treatments at home in Chapter 31, "Infants and Children."

CRITICAL DECISION MAKING:
PROBLEMS, PROBLEMS

It is not unusual to have a patient who has more than one problem—or more than one potential cause for a single problem. Each brief patient presentation below details a patient with dual problems—or two potential causes for the same problem. You will be asked how to differentiate one from the other. (Note: Solutions for these questions are drawn from material throughout the Medical Emergencies module.)

1. You are treating a patient who is experiencing difficulty breathing. The patient has a history of COPD and congestive heart failure. He has a prescribed inhaler and wants to know if he should use it.
2. You are called by a wife who reports her husband suddenly became confused. He has a history of diabetes and recently had a stroke. He is alert enough to receive sugar, but how can you tell the difference between this possible diabetic condition and stroke?
3. A patient who has a history of heart problems calls because he has had a feeling of indigestion for several hours. He also has a history of acid reflux—which he thought this was—but his medication wasn't working. He wants to know if you think he should go to the hospital.

CHAPTER REVIEW

SUMMARY

Most patients you encounter will have straightforward presentations of common problems. When a patient presents with more than one complaint, evaluate the situation, determine any unusual or increased risks from your interventions, and consult on-line medical direction. Similar principles apply to the situation where the patient has a complaint for which you have no specific intervention or a complaint related to a disease you are not familiar with. Assess the patient as you usually do, provide supportive care, and consult on-line medical direction as needed.

REVIEW QUESTIONS

1. What are the decisions an EMT must make for a medical patient with regard to interventions? (p. 601)
2. What steps should the EMT follow when a patient seems to require two interventions? (pp. 602–603)
3. What are the advantages to consulting on-line medical direction in a difficult medical case? (p. 602)
4. How can an EMT learn more about a patient's complaint that is not covered in the EMT curriculum? (p. 607)
5. What is an appropriate response on the part of an EMT when a patient tells him she has Crohn's disease? (p. 607)

CRITICAL THINKING

- You are treating a 65-year-old male for carbon monoxide poisoning. He is responsive only to pain, and he is tolerating a nasal airway well. He is breathing adequately, so you apply high-concentration oxygen by nonrebreather mask. His wife tells you that he is not supposed to get any more than 2 liters per minute of oxygen because he has emphysema. What should you do? Explain your answer.

MEDIA RESOURCES 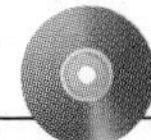

See the Student CD at the back of this book for quizzes, a case study activity, and other features related to this chapter. Also, visit the Companion Website for *Emergency Care* at **www.prenhall.com/limmer,** where you will find additional reinforcement and links to other resources.

Street Scenes

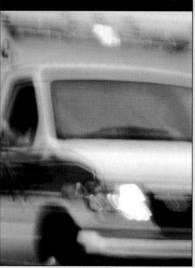

At 3:00 in the morning, your rescue squad is toned-out for a "sick person." Arriving at the residence 6 minutes later, you are met by a woman identifying herself as Mrs. Jones. She tells you that she called 911 because her husband has been sick and running a fever. She says he is in the bedroom.

In the bedroom you observe a man lying in bed with a wash cloth on his head. In response to your query, he identifies himself as Wilson Jones, 56 years old. He is alert and verbally responsive. He proceeds to tell you that he has been running a fever for the past 48 hours and that it was his wife, not he, who called 911. Your assessment reveals a clear airway, respirations of adequate rate and depth, and skin that appears pink, warm, and dry.

Street Scene Questions

1. What pertinent signs or symptoms should you inquire about?
2. What further patient assessment should you perform?

Mr. Jones informs you that he believes he has the "flu." He says he has not been nauseated and he has not vomited. He states he has been eating and drinking normal amounts of fluid. His vital signs include pulse 80 and regular; blood pressure 150/70, respirations 20 and regular. You determine that Wilson is taking no medications other than an over-the-counter one for his fever. He has no allergies and no significant past medical history. He states he does not want to go to the hospital. The patient denies shortness of breath, chest pain, dizziness, headache, or other complaints.

Contacting medical direction, you are advised that Mr. Jones does not need to go to the emergency department but instead should contact his personal physician in the morning if symptoms persist. Mr. Jones states he understands and will contact his physician in the morning. You and your partner then leave the residence.

Two hours later, you are once again dispatched to the Jones's residence. Mrs. Jones again meets you at the door, and states that she once again called 911. She says that her husband was now shaking and it "scared her." Once in the bedroom, you find Mr. Jones still in bed. Though his eyes are open, he is not alert, and he responds to verbal commands by groaning. His airway is open and respirations are regular. He is not shaking, but instead repeatedly rolls from his back onto his left side, and then onto his back.

Street Scene Question

3. What treatment should you provide to Mr. Jones at this time?

You administer high-concentration oxygen by way of a nonrebreather mask. Mr. Jones's vitals include pulse 110 and regular; BP 160/76; respirations 28; skin, hot and dry; pupils, normal. You and your partner place Mr. Jones on your cot, and load him into the ambulance. As you reassess this patient, you find he is now becoming more responsive and wants to know, "What happened?" You arrive at the hospital emergency department with no further medical problems.

Street Scenes Sample Documentation

PATIENT NAME: *Wilson Jones* PATIENT AGE: *56*

CHIEF COMPLAINT		TIME	RESP	PULSE	B.P.	MENTAL STATUS	R PUPILS L	SKIN
Altered mental status	V I T A L	*0507*	Rate: *28* ☒ Regular ☐ Shallow ☐ Labored	Rate: *110* ☒ Regular ☐ Irregular	*160/76*	☐ Alert ☑ Voice ☐ Pain ☐ Unresp.	☑ Normal ☑ ☐ Dilated ☐ ☐ Constricted ☐ ☐ Sluggish ☐ ☐ No-Reaction ☐	☐ Unremarkable ☐ Cool ☐ Pale ☑ Warm ☐ Cyanotic ☐ Moist ☐ Flushed ☑ Dry ☐ Jaundiced
PAST MEDICAL HISTORY ☐ None ☐ Allergy to ____ ☐ Hypertension ☐ Stroke ☐ Seizures ☐ Diabetes ☐ COPD ☐ Cardiac ☒ Other (List) ☐ Asthma *Previous EMS call (Run 5428)*	S I		Rate: ☐ Regular ☐ Shallow ☐ Labored	Rate: ☐ Regular ☐ Irregular	/	☐ Alert ☐ Voice ☐ Pain ☐ Unresp.	☐ Normal ☐ ☐ Dilated ☐ ☐ Constricted ☐ ☐ Sluggish ☐ ☐ No-Reaction ☐	☐ Unremarkable ☐ Cool ☐ Pale ☐ Warm ☐ Cyanotic ☐ Moist ☐ Flushed ☐ Dry ☐ Jaundiced
Current Medications (List) *Tylenol*	G N S		Rate: ☐ Regular ☐ Shallow ☐ Labored	Rate: ☐ Regular ☐ Irregular	/	☐ Alert ☐ Voice ☐ Pain ☐ Unresp.	☐ Normal ☐ ☐ Dilated ☐ ☐ Constricted ☐ ☐ Sluggish ☐ ☐ No-Reaction ☐	☐ Unremarkable ☐ Cool ☐ Pale ☐ Warm ☐ Cyanotic ☐ Moist ☐ Flushed ☐ Dry ☐ Jaundiced

NARRATIVE *We initially responded to patient's house earlier this morning (see patient run #5428). Past medical history of "flu-like" symptoms for past 48 hours, per patient on previous EMS incident. No other pertinent medical history. Upon arrival, patient's wife stated she initiated EMS because husband was "shaking." We observed a 56-year-old male responsive to verbal stimuli by groaning. Patient has no purposeful movement, although he moves from a supine to left lateral recumbent position and then back to supine repeatedly. Airway clear; breathing rapid and unlabored; pupils equal and reactive to light; no vomiting noted; patient unable to ambulate; patient placed on cot by EMS personnel and high-concentration oxygen initiated. Due to short transport time, no other treatment/reassessment initiated.*

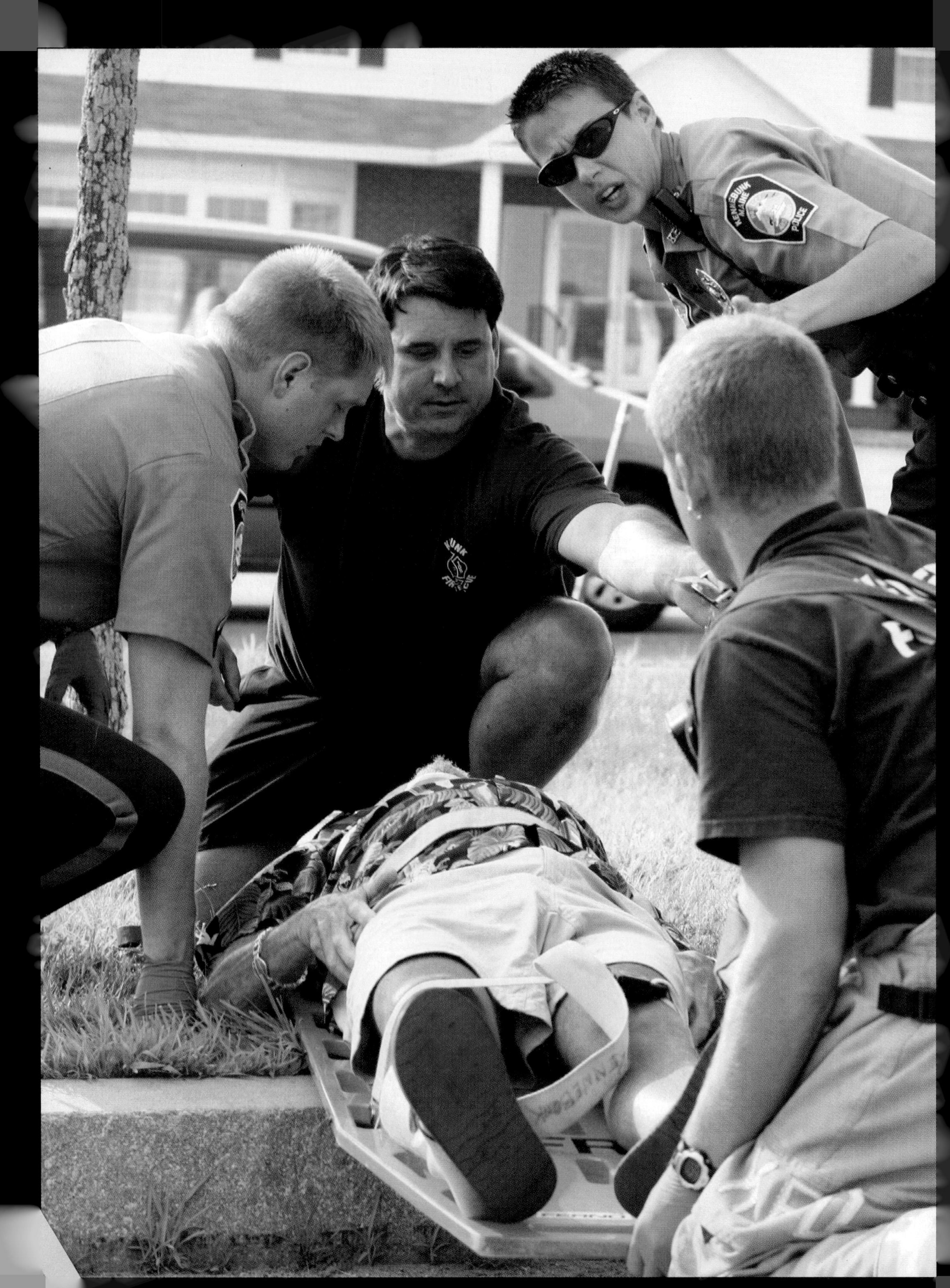
POLICE

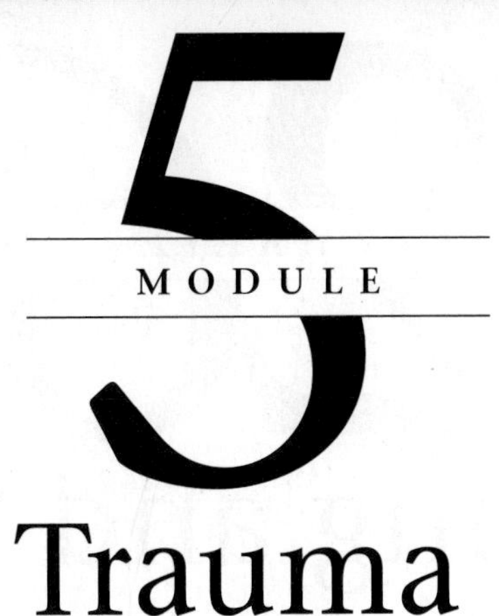

MODULE

Trauma

Trauma is another word for "injury." Falls, vehicle collisions, and violence are just a few causes of trauma. The loss of blood, either externally or internally, can cause serious complications, the most critical of which is hypoperfusion, also known as shock. Both severe blood loss and shock (Chapter 26, "Bleeding and Shock") are life-threatening conditions.

Soft-tissue injuries, which include a wide range of trauma to the skin, underlying tissues, and internal organs, as well as burns, are the topic of Chapter 27, "Soft-Tissue Injuries." Injuries to the bones, joints, and muscles, while seldom life-threatening, are a frequent cause of severe pain and emergency calls. They will be covered in Chapter 28, "Musculoskeletal Injuries." Head and spinal trauma can cause serious physical injury, paralysis, and even death. They are the topic of Chapter 29, "Injuries to the Head and Spine." A final discussion of trauma with an emphasis on multiple trauma is found in Chapter 30, "Putting It All Together for the Trauma Patient."

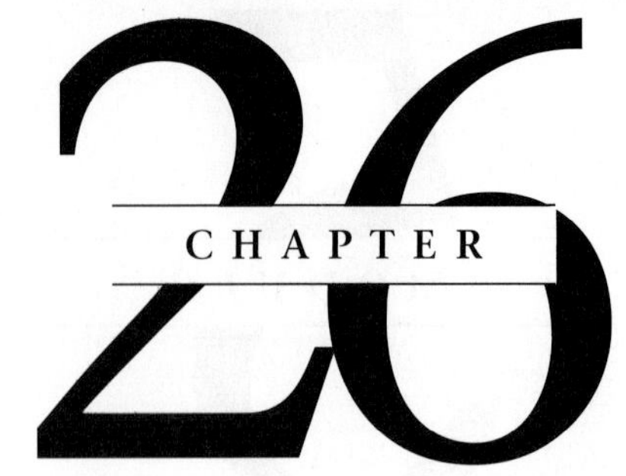

CHAPTER 26

Bleeding and Shock

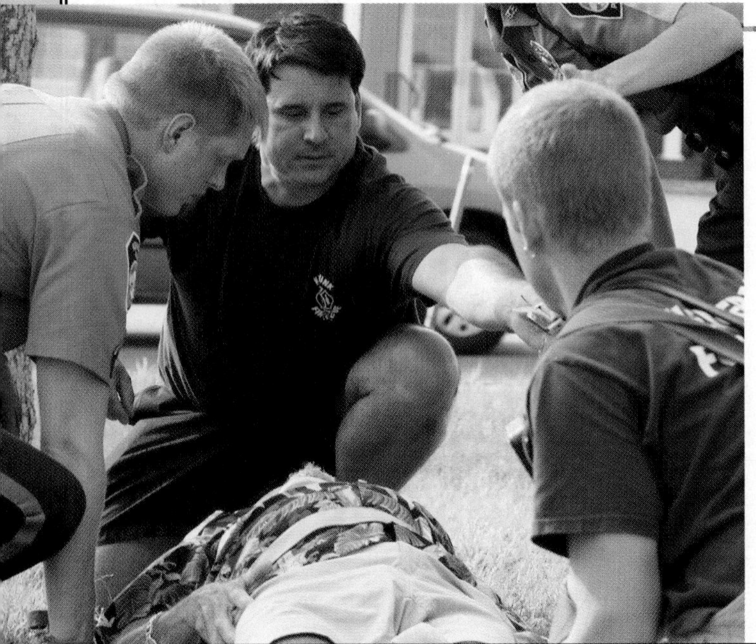

CORE CONCEPTS

The following are core concepts that will be addressed in this chapter:

- How to recognize arterial, venous, and capillary bleeding
- When to use Standard Precautions with a bleeding patient
- Steps for controlling bleeding
- Signs, symptoms, and care of a patient with internal bleeding
- Signs, symptoms, and care of a patient with shock
- How to use the mechanism of injury to identify potential internal injuries

KEY TERMS

arterial bleeding, p. 618
brachial artery, p. 627
capillary bleeding, p. 619
cardiogenic shock, p. 632
compensated shock, p. 631
decompensated shock, p. 633
femoral artery, p. 627
hemorrhage, p. 617
hemorrhagic shock, p. 632
hypoperfusion, p. 617
hypovolemic shock, p. 632
irreversible shock, p. 633
neurogenic shock, p. 632
perfusion, p. 617
pressure dressing, p. 623
pressure point, p. 626
shock, p. 617
tourniquet, p. 623
venous bleeding, p. 619

This chapter includes updated information on bleeding control/shock management.

DOT OBJECTIVES

*KNOWLEDGE AND ATTITUDE

5-1.1 List the structure and function of the circulatory system. (pp. 615–617)[†]

5-1.2 Differentiate between arterial, venous, and capillary bleeding. (pp. 618–619)[†]

5-1.3 State methods of emergency medical care of external bleeding. (pp. 621, 623–628) (Scan 26-1, p. 622)[†]

5-1.4 Establish the relationship between Standard Precautions (body substance isolation) and bleeding. (pp. 618, 621, 636)[†]

5-1.5 Establish the relationship between airway management and the trauma patient. (pp. 621, 626, 628, 630, 633, 636)[†]

5-1.6 Establish the relationship between mechanism of injury and internal bleeding. (pp. 629–630)[†]

5-1.7 List the signs of internal bleeding. (pp. 629–630)[†]

5-1.8 List the steps in the emergency medical care of the patient with signs and symptoms of internal bleeding. (p. 630)[†]

5-1.9 List signs and symptoms of shock (hypoperfusion). (p. 633)[†]

5-1.10 State the steps in the emergency medical care of the patient with signs and symptoms of shock (hypoperfusion). (pp. 633–636) (Scan 26-2, p. 637; Scan 26-3, p. 638)[†]

5-1.11 Explain the sense of urgency to transport patients that are bleeding and show signs of shock (hypoperfusion). (pp. 633–634, 636)[†]

*SKILLS

5-1.12 Demonstrate direct pressure as a method of emergency medical care of external bleeding.[†]

5-1.13 Demonstrate the use of diffuse pressure as a method of emergency medical care of external bleeding.[†]

5-1.14 Demonstrate the use of pressure points and tourniquets as a method of emergency medical care of external bleeding.[†]

5-1.15 Demonstrate the care of the patient exhibiting signs and symptoms of internal bleeding.

5-1.16 Demonstrate the care of the patient exhibiting signs and symptoms of shock (hypoperfusion).

5-1.17 Demonstrate completing a prehospital care report for patient with bleeding and/or shock (hypoperfusion).

[†] Taken from the 1994 Department of Transportation EMT-B Curriculum. This objective no longer reflects current bleeding control practices.

The leading cause of death in the United States for persons between the ages of 1 and 44 is trauma. As an EMT, you will be called upon to provide emergency care to victims of traumatic injuries varying in severity from minor to life-threatening. It is vital that you learn to recognize the signs and symptoms of serious trauma and shock. Early identification, appropriate care, and expeditious transport contribute greatly to the patient's chance of survival. Understanding the signs, symptoms, and management of bleeding and shock is a vital part of good prehospital care.

CIRCULATORY SYSTEM

Main Components

The circulatory (or cardiovascular) system is responsible for the distribution of blood to all parts of the body. This system has three main components: the heart, blood vessels, and the blood that flows through them. All components must function properly for the system to remain intact. (You may wish to review the information about the heart and the circulatory system in Chapter 4, "The Human Body.")

The heart is a muscular organ that lies within the chest, behind the sternum. Its job is to pump blood, which supplies oxygen and nutrients to the body's cells. To provide a sufficient supply of oxygen and nutrients to all parts of the body, the heart must pump

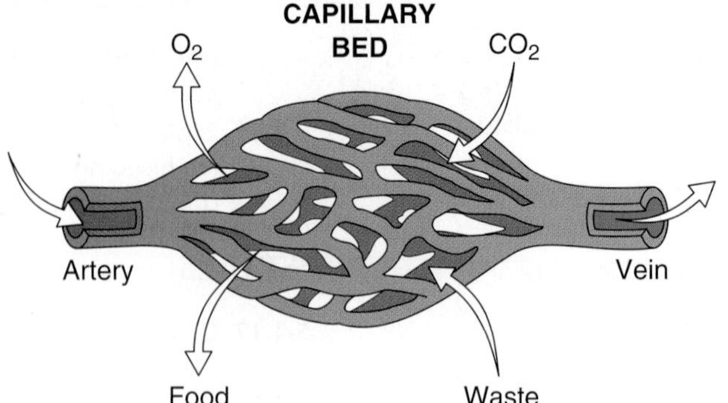

Figure 26-1 • Blood vessels.

at an adequate rate and rhythm. The blood is circulated throughout the body through three major types of blood vessels (Figure 26-1):

- *Arteries.* The arteries carry oxygen-rich blood away from the heart. They are under a great deal of pressure during the heart's contractions. (Taking the patient's blood pressure is a means of measuring arterial pressure.) An artery has a thick, muscular wall that enables it to dilate or constrict, depending on the need for oxygen and nutrients of the cells or organs it feeds (Figure 26-2).
- *Capillaries.* Oxygen-rich blood is emptied from the arteries into microscopically small capillaries, which supply every cell of the body. Where capillaries and body

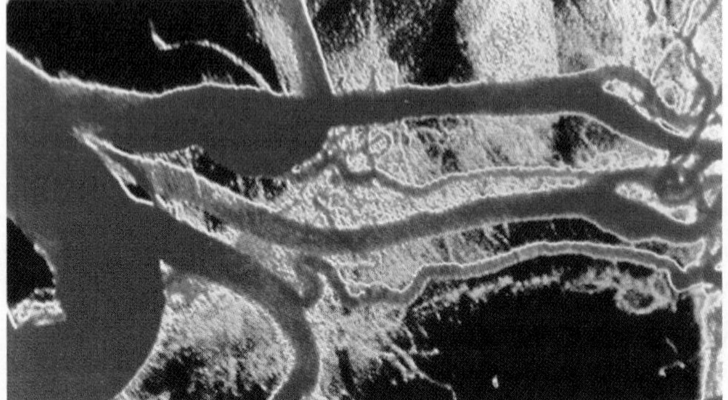

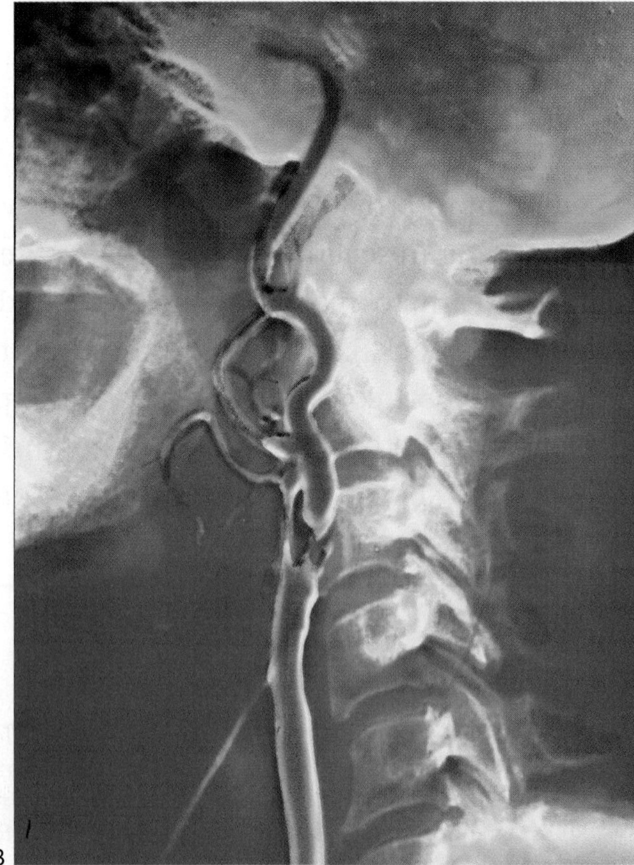

Figure 26-2 • An arteriogram of (A) a normal, healthy artery and (B) an artery that has been damaged. *(Both: © CNRI/Science Photo Library/Photo Researchers, Inc.)*

F•Y•I

FUNCTIONS OF THE BLOOD

The blood has several functions. These include:

- **Transportation of gases.** Blood carries inhaled oxygen from the lungs to the body's cells, and it carries carbon dioxide from the body cells back to the lungs where it is then exhaled.
- **Nutrition.** Blood circulates nutrients from the intestines or storage tissues (such as fatty tissue, the liver, and muscle cells) to the other body cells.
- **Excretion.** Blood carries waste products from the cells to organs, such as the kidneys, that excrete (eliminate) them from the body.
- **Protection.** Blood carries antibodies and white blood cells, which help fight disease and infection.
- **Regulation.** Blood carries substances that control the functions of the body, such as hormones, water, salt, enzymes, and chemicals. Blood also helps regulate body temperature by carrying body heat to the lungs and skin surface where it is dissipated.

cells are in contact, a vital "exchange" takes place. Oxygen and nutrients are given up by the blood and pass through the extremely thin capillary walls into the cells. At the same time, carbon dioxide and other waste products given up by the cells pass through the capillary walls and are taken up by the blood.

- *Veins.* Blood that has been depleted of oxygen and loaded with carbon dioxide and other wastes in the capillaries empties into the veins, which carry it back to the heart. Veins have one-way valves that prevent the blood from flowing in the wrong direction. Blood in a vein is under much less pressure than blood in an artery.

The adequate circulation of blood throughout the body, which fills the capillaries and supplies the cells and tissues with oxygen and nutrients, is called **perfusion.** If, for some reason, blood is not adequately circulated, some of the cells and organs of the body do not receive adequate supplies of oxygen, and dangerous waste products build up. Inadequate perfusion of the body's tissues and organs is called **hypoperfusion,** which is also known as **shock.** (*Hypo-* means "low," so *hypoperfusion* means "low perfusion.")

Recall that the heart, blood vessels, and blood are the three main components of the circulatory system. These components may be likened to a pump, pipes, and fluid in the pipes. For the circulatory system to function properly, all three components must function properly. If any component fails, or "leaks," the body will try in various ways to compensate and maintain adequate perfusion. However, if the problem is not corrected and the condition is quickly reversed, adequate perfusion cannot be maintained and shock (hypoperfusion) will result.

perfusion
the supply of oxygen to and removal of wastes from the cells and tissues of the body as a result of the flow of blood through the capillaries.

hypoperfusion
(HI-po-per-FEW-zhun) inability of the body to adequately circulate blood to the body's cells to supply them with oxygen and nutrients. *See also* shock.

shock
also known as *hypoperfusion.* The inability of the body to adequately circulate blood to the body's cells to supply them with oxygen and nutrients. A life-threatening condition.

hemorrhage (HEM-o-rej)
bleeding, especially severe bleeding.

BLEEDING

Severe bleeding, or **hemorrhage,** is the major cause of shock (hypoperfusion). The body contains a certain amount of blood to circulate through the blood vessels. If enough blood volume is lost, perfusion of all cells will not occur. Inadequate perfusion of the body's cells will eventually lead to the death of tissues and organs. The cells and tissues of the brain, the spinal cord, and the kidneys are the most sensitive to inadequate perfusion.

Bleeding, or hemorrhage, is classified as either external or internal, as explained in the next sections.

NOTE

A growing number of patients that you will encounter are on prescription medications that are designed to impair the body's natural ability to form blood clots. Often referred to as **blood thinners**, *these medications are commonly prescribed to patients with a history of stroke, an irregular heartbeat (atrial fibrillation), artificial heart valves, or a history of a heart attack. These medications, which include warfarin (Coumadin) and clopidogrel (Plavix), act to prevent strokes or heart attacks, but in the setting of external or internal bleeding can result in life-threatening bleeding in injuries that might be relatively minor for a patient who is not on one of these medications. When treating patients with external or internal bleeding, it is important to determine whether or not they are on blood thinners as part of your SAMPLE history.*

External Bleeding

Whenever bleeding is anticipated or discovered, the use of Standard Precautions is essential to avoid exposure of the skin and mucous membranes. Blood and open wounds pose a high risk of infection to the EMT. Protective gloves must be worn when caring for any bleeding patient. A mask and protective eyewear should also be worn if there is a chance of splattered blood. With profuse or spurting (arterial) bleeding, or if the patient is spitting or coughing blood, masks should be worn. Gowns should be considered if clothing may become contaminated.

While Standard Precautions decrease the possibility of exposure to blood and body fluids, you should ALWAYS cleanse your hands with either an alcohol-based hand rub or soap and water immediately after each call. Gloves may develop tears or small holes without your knowledge. Always remove the gloves carefully, turning them inside out as you take them off. This reduces the possibility of blood or fluid on the gloves coming in contact with your hands.

External bleeding may be classified according to which of the three types of blood vessels is injured and losing blood (Figure 26-3):

- Arterial bleeding
- Venous bleeding
- Capillary bleeding

arterial bleeding bleeding from an artery, which is characterized by bright red blood and as rapid, profuse, and difficult to control.

Arterial bleeding is usually bright red in color, because it is still rich in oxygen. It is often rapid and profuse, spurting with each heartbeat, though as the patient's systolic blood pressure drops, the strength of the spurting may decrease. As explained earlier, blood in an artery is under high pressure, and arteries have thick, muscular walls that maintain the pressure. For this reason, arterial bleeding is the most difficult bleeding to control. Control measures may need to continue throughout transport to the hospital.

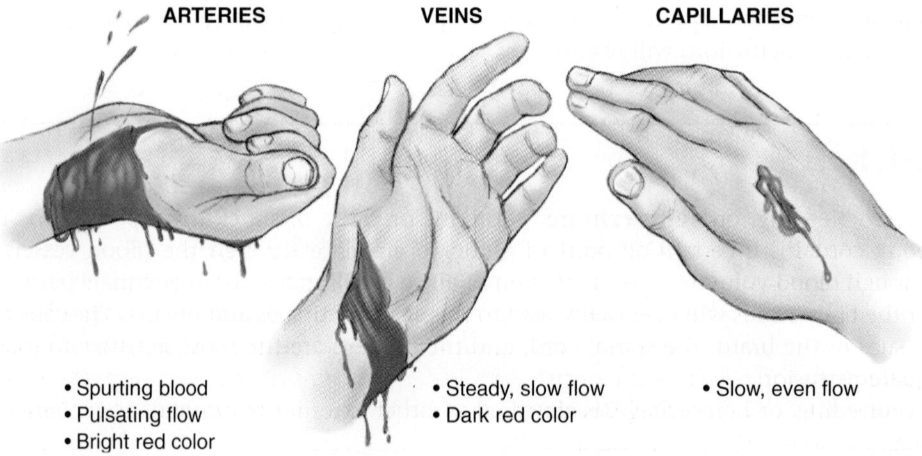

Figure 26-3 • Three types of external bleeding.

Venous bleeding is usually dark red or maroon in color, because it has already passed its oxygen to the cells and picked up carbon dioxide and wastes. Bleeding from the veins has a steady flow. It is usually easy to control (although it can be profuse), because veins return blood to the heart under low pressure. Because venous pressure may be lower than atmospheric pressure, large veins may actually suck in debris or air bubbles. Bleeding from the large veins in the neck is an especially serious problem. An air bubble, or embolism, may be carried directly to the heart, interfering with the regular heart rhythm, or even stopping it completely. An air embolism also can cause damage to the brain or lungs if lodged there.

venous bleeding bleeding from a vein, which is characterized by dark red or maroon blood and as a steady flow, easy to control.

Capillary bleeding is usually slow and "oozing" due to the capillaries small size and low pressure. Most capillary bleeding is considered minor and is easily controlled. It often clots spontaneously, or with minimal treatment. As you would expect, the color of capillary blood is usually somewhere between the bright red of arterial blood and the darker red of venous blood. Capillary bleeding usually results from a minor injury such as a scrape. However, these wounds can easily become contaminated, leading to infection. You may also see capillary bleeding from the edges of more serious wounds.

capillary bleeding bleeding from capillaries, which is characterized by a slow, oozing flow of blood.

Severity of External Bleeding

An important skill for the EMT to develop is determining the severity of blood loss. The severity of the bleeding is somewhat dependent on the amount of blood lost in relation to the physical size of the patient. While a sudden loss of 1 liter (1,000 cc) of blood is considered serious in the average adult, half that amount (500 cc) is considered serious in a child. In a 1-year-old infant, with a total blood volume of only about 800 cc, a loss of even 150 cc is considered serious.

Severity is dependent on the patient's condition, as well as on the relative amount of blood lost. If, at any time, the patient begins to exhibit signs and symptoms of shock (hypoperfusion), the bleeding is immediately considered serious.

The body's natural response to bleeding is constriction of the injured blood vessel and clotting. However, a serious injury may prevent effective clotting, allowing continued bleeding. Wounds that are large or deep may not clot well. Uncontrolled bleeding or significant blood loss can eventually lead to death.

PATIENT ASSESSMENT

EXTERNAL BLEEDING

It is important for you to learn to estimate the amount of external blood loss in order to predict potential shock (hypoperfusion), triage (prioritize) patients properly, and identify bleeding that must be treated during the initial assessment.

It is sometimes difficult to estimate blood loss when the blood has flowed onto the floor or when carpeting or clothing has absorbed it. An exercise that may help you better estimate external blood loss is pouring a pint of liquid on the floor to note its appearance, and soaking an article of clothing in a pint of fluid to note how wet it feels and looks. Since estimating external blood loss is difficult, it is important for you to watch for signs and symptoms of shock (hypoperfusion), which are listed in Table 26-1.

No matter how small blood loss appears to be, if the patient shows any signs or symptoms of shock (hypoperfusion), the bleeding is considered serious. However, do not wait for signs and symptoms to appear before beginning treatment. Any patient with a significant amount of blood loss should be treated to prevent the development of shock. Many of the signs and symptoms of shock appear late in the process. By the time they develop, it may be too late for the patient to recover. ■

TABLE 26-1 • Signs of Shock

SIGNS (IN ORDER OF APPEARANCE)	DESCRIPTION
Altered mental status	Altered mental status occurs because the brain is not receiving enough oxygen. The brain is very sensitive to oxygen deficiencies. When it is deprived of oxygen, even slightly, behavioral changes may be noted. These changes may begin as anxiety and progress to restlessness and sometimes combativeness.
Pale, cool, clammy skin	When the body senses low blood volume, natural mechanisms take over in an attempt to correct the problem. One of these mechanisms is to divert blood from nonvital areas to vital organs. Blood is quickly directed away from the skin to such organs as the brain and heart. This results in the loss of color and temperature in the skin. Infants and children may exhibit capillary refill times of greater than 2 seconds. Note: In neurogenic shock (rare) the skin is typically warm, flushed, and dry because the circulatory system has lost the ability to constrict blood vessels in the skin.
Nausea and vomiting	In the body's continuing effort to keep blood perfusing vital organs, blood is diverted from the digestive system. This causes feelings of nausea and occasionally vomiting.
Vital sign changes	The first vital signs to change are the pulse and respirations: • The pulse will increase in an attempt to pump more blood. As the pulse gradually increases, it becomes weak and thready. • Respirations also increase in an attempt to increase the amount of oxygen in the blood. The respirations will become more shallow and labored as shock progresses. • Blood pressure is one of the last signs to change. When blood pressure drops, the patient is clearly in a state of serious, life-threatening shock. • A narrowing of the pulse pressure may also occur. This means that the difference between the systolic and diastolic pressures will decrease (become closer together).
	Other signs of shock that you may encounter include thirst, dilated pupils, and in some cases cyanosis around the lips and nail beds.

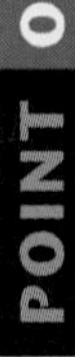

VIEW

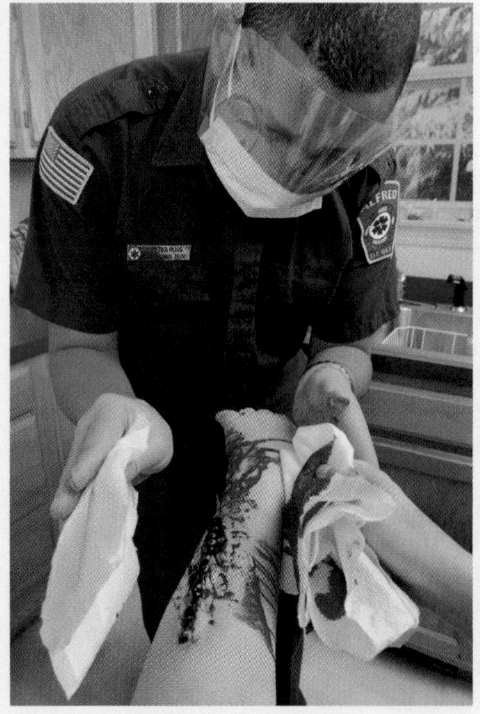

"I remember waiting to see if it would hurt.

"It wasn't the blood. That didn't bother me. I just sat there and waited for the pain. Things were in slow motion. The knife had gone into my forearm. Everyone stopped what they were doing and stared. I grabbed my arm and felt the warm blood drip down over my fingers. But it still didn't seem real.

"I heard someone scream. Someone else called 911. It took me a minute to get my head around what happened. It seemed like only a few seconds had gone by when the EMS people showed up. They put a bandage on my arm and made sure the bleeding had stopped.

"As I look back on it now, I am amazed at how detached I was from the whole thing. I guess some would call that shock.

"And for the record, once I got composed again, it hurt. Oh yes, trust me. It hurt."

Controlling External Bleeding

The control of external bleeding is one of the most important elements in the prevention and management of shock (hypoperfusion). If bleeding is not controlled, shock will continue to develop and worsen, leading to the patient's death.

PATIENT CARE

EXTERNAL BLEEDING

Patient assessment and care always begin with the ABCs. After taking Standard Precautions, maintain an open airway, monitor respirations, and ventilate if necessary. Assess circulation by taking a radial pulse; assessing skin color, temperature, and condition; and controlling external bleeding. Severe external bleeding must be identified and controlled during the initial assessment. The major methods of controlling external bleeding are (Scan 26-1):

- Direct pressure and elevation
- Hemostatic dressings
- Tourniquet

The techniques presented in this section are dramatically different from what EMT students have been taught in previous years. The medical experience gained in the battlefield during recent wars has given us greater insight into how bleeding may be safely and most effectively controlled. The methods presented in this section may also be different from what was taught to EMS providers who have recently graduated from EMT class and are now providing care in the field.

Since these techniques are recent changes, you may find that there are differences in the ways your EMS system protocols instruct you to control bleeding in the field. This does not mean that one way is right and another is wrong. Rather, the medical directors in various states, regions and systems review science and medical literature to determine what they believe is best for the patients in your care.

While we have listed the primary and preferred methods of bleeding control above, there are other methods which have been traditionally used in the past. We will review them in the section that follows in the event your system uses any of these techniques. These include pressure points, splinting, cold application, and use of the pneumatic anti-shock garment (PASG).

In addition to controlling external bleeding, an important treatment for any trauma patient is administration of oxygen. Blood loss decreases perfusion. This means that less oxygen is delivered to the tissues. The administration of supplemental oxygen will increase the oxygen saturation of the blood that is still in the patient's circulatory system, improving oxygenation of the tissues. ■

Standard Precautions and infection control are mandatory when attempting to control external bleeding. Always wear disposable gloves when caring for the patient and cleaning up after the call. Follow your local infection exposure control plan regarding cleaning and disposal of contaminated bandages, sheets, and other materials and supplies.

DIRECT PRESSURE The most common and effective way to control external bleeding is by applying direct pressure to the wound. This can be done with your gloved hand, a dressing and your gloved hand, or by a pressure dressing and bandage.

1. Apply pressure to the wound until bleeding is controlled. If the bleeding is mild, use a sterile dressing. If the bleeding is severe or spurting, immediately place your gloved hand directly on the wound. Do not waste time trying to find a dressing (Figure 26-4).

SCAN 26-1 • Controlling Bleeding

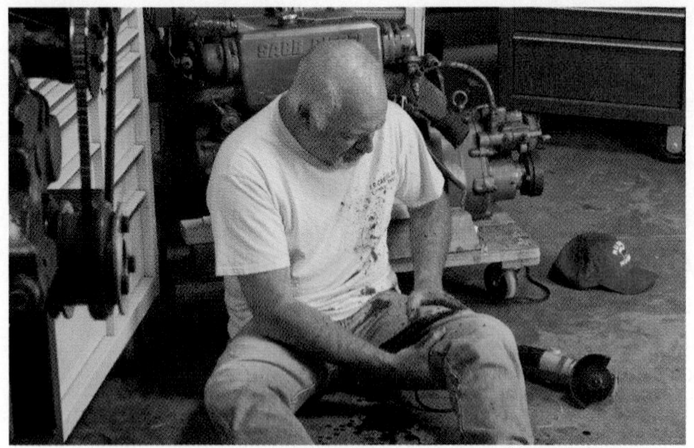

1. Perform a scene size-up look for hazards and determine the necessary Standard Precautions.

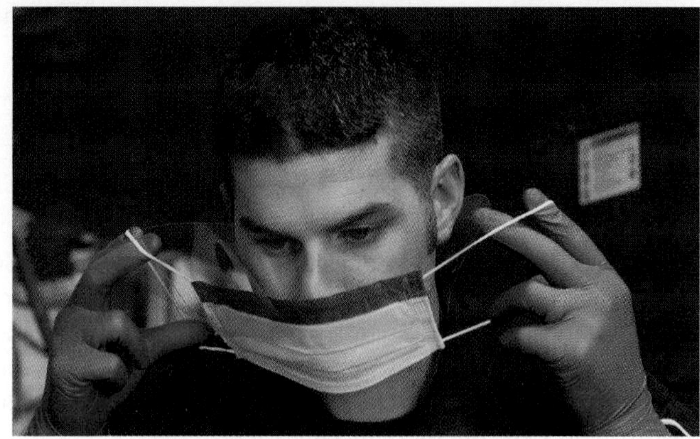

2. Take Standard Precautions.

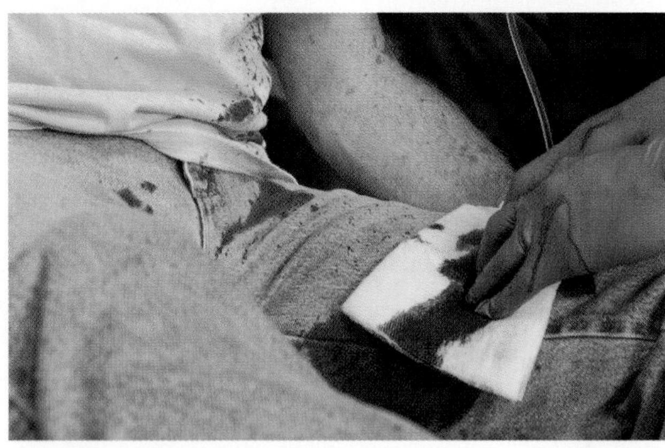

3. Apply direct pressure. If another EMT is available, administer oxygen.

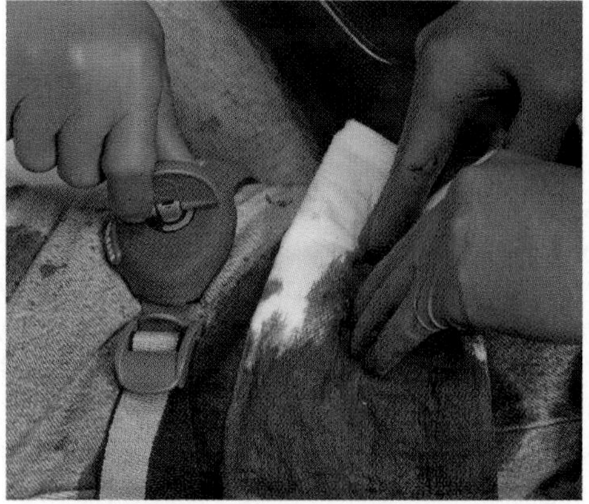

4. If pressure does not stop the bleeding apply and tighten a tourniquet until the bleeding stops.

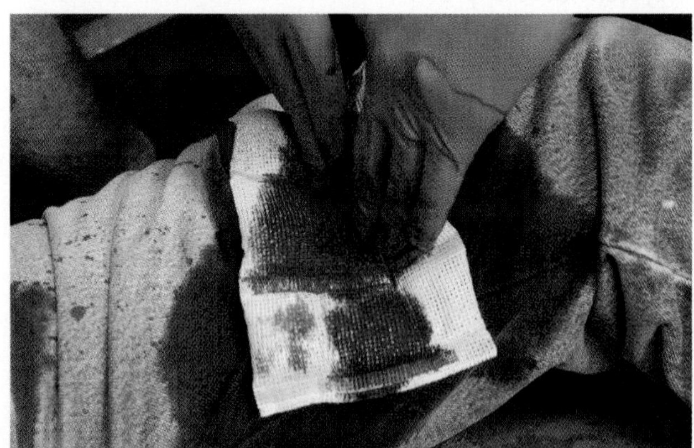

5. Hemostatic dressings may be used to stop bleeding if pressure alone doesn't work. Use your gloved hand to push the dressing into the wound.

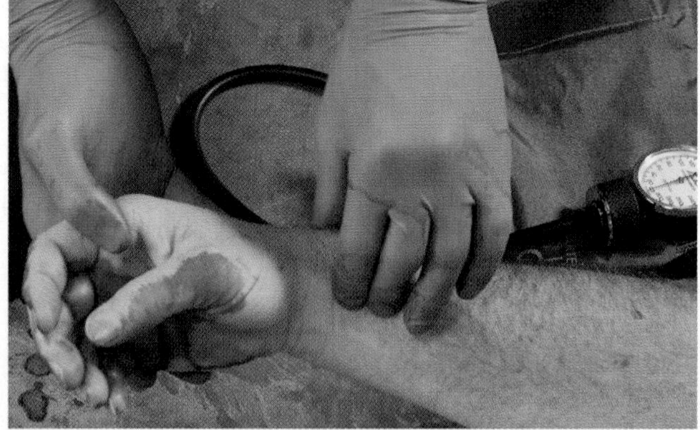

6. Assess and treat the patient for shock.

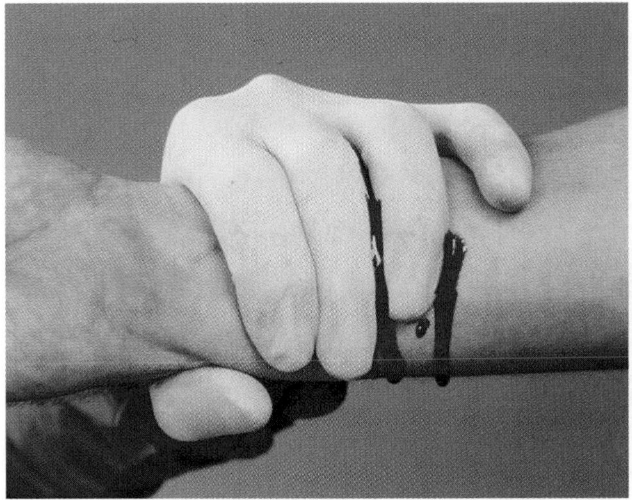

Figure 26-4 • In cases of profuse bleeding, do not waste time finding a dressing. Instead, use your gloved hand to apply direct pressure.

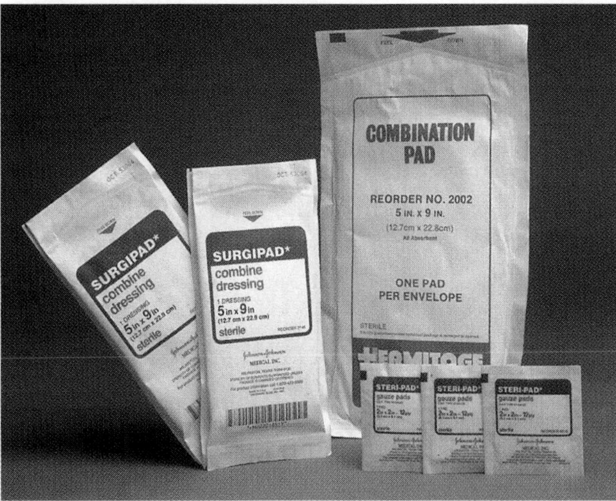

Figure 26-5 • Various types of dressings.

2. If the bleeding is from an extremity and you do not suspect musculoskeletal injury (e.g., broken bones), elevate the extremity above the level of the heart.
3. Maintain firm pressure over the wound. In deeper wounds you may place fingertip pressure deeper into the wound to more effectively stop bleeding.
4. Evaluate your efforts to determine if bleeding has stopped. If not, move to the next step. If bleeding has been controlled (many cases of bleeding can be controlled by direct pressure alone) never remove a dressing once it has been placed on the wound. Removal of a dressing may destroy clots or cause further injury to the site. If a dressing becomes blood soaked, apply additional dressings on top of it and hold them firmly in place. You may need to continue holding direct pressure on the wound until arrival at the hospital.

NOTE

After controlling bleeding from an extremity using a pressure dressing, always check for a distal pulse to make sure that the dressing has not been applied too tightly. If you do not feel a pulse, adjust the pressure applied by the dressing to reestablish circulation. Check distal pulses frequently while the patient is in your care.

Application of a **pressure dressing** will assist in the control of most external bleeding and will help keep pressure in place when your attention has been diverted elsewhere during patient care. Place several gauze pads on the wound. Hold the dressings in place with a self-adhering roller bandage wrapped tightly over the dressings, and above and below the wound site. The pressure bandage will hold the dressing in place and maintain some pressure on the wound. The pressure dressing is not a tourniquet and should not be applied so tightly that it occludes blood flow.

pressure dressing
a bulky dressing held in position with a tightly wrapped bandage to apply pressure to help control bleeding.

Use the pressure dressing after bleeding has been controlled. If bleeding is not controlled, move to the next steps instead. Several types of dressings may be used to control external bleeding (Figure 26-5).

You may be unable to apply an effective pressure dressing to some areas of the body. For example, bleeding from the armpit may require you to hold continuous direct pressure with your gloved hand and a dressing. Remember that direct pressure is usually the quickest and most effective method of controlling external bleeding.

ELEVATION Elevation of an injured extremity may be used at the same time as direct pressure. When you elevate an injury above the level of the heart, gravity helps reduce the blood pressure in the extremity, slowing bleeding. However, do not use this method if you suspect possible musculoskeletal injuries, impaled objects in the extremity, or spine injury.

To use elevation in controlling external bleeding, apply direct pressure to the injury site. Elevate the injured extremity, keeping the injury site above the level of the heart.

TOURNIQUET A **tourniquet** (Figure 26-6) is a device that closes off blood flow to and from an extremity. Previously believed to be an extreme last resort, tourniquets have moved into mainstream care for patients with severe bleeding that can't be controlled

tourniquet (TURN-i-ket)
a device used for bleeding control that constricts all blood flow to and from an extremity.

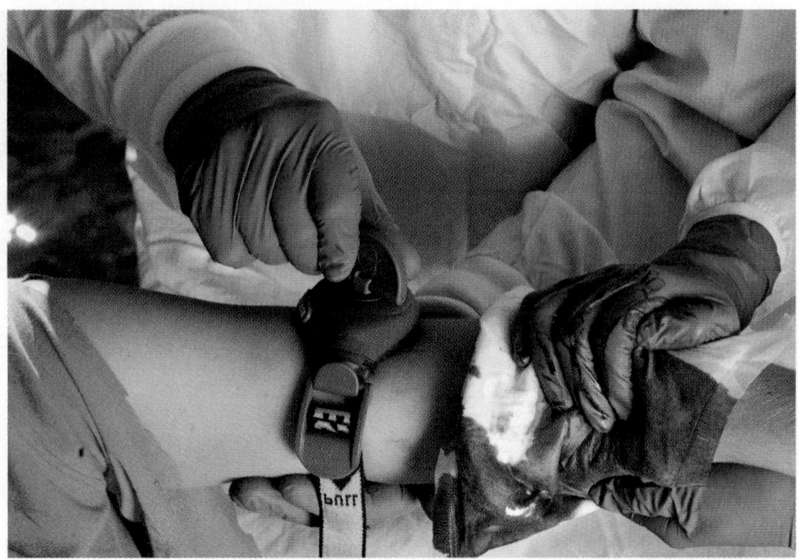

Figure 26-6 • The Mechanical Advantage Tourniquet (MAT)

by direct pressure. At one point it was believed that the use of a tourniquet was a "life or limb" decision, that is, use of a tourniquet will stop blood flow and likely result in amputation of the limb.

Testing in battle has shown that the risks, while present, are believed to be justified in the presence of bleeding that can't otherwise be controlled. In civilian use, with the exception of wilderness applications or prolonged entrapment, it is extremely rare for transport time to take longer than an hour. In these cases it appears that the risk of permanent damage to an extremity is considerably less than the risk of death from uncontrolled bleeding.

Remember that patients who have severe bleeding may also have other injuries or conditions such as airway compromise, inadequate breathing or chest injury which will also require your urgent attention. In these cases the use of a tourniquet offers the additional benefit of allowing you to treat these conditions.

The decision to use a tourniquet is an important one. You must recognize a situation where you have been unable to stop bleeding with direct and fingertip pressure. When the bleeding remains severe you will then apply and tighten a tourniquet. (NOTE: some systems may also authorize the use of hemostatic agents in this situation as an alternative.)

Tourniquets are used only on extremity injuries. Do not apply the tourniquet over a joint (elbow or knee). Place the tourniquet approximately two inches above the bleeding wound. There are several brands of commercial tourniquets available (Figure 26-6). These devices fasten around the extremity and are tightened by a turning or twisting mechanism.

Tourniquets can also be made from ambulance equipment such as a cravat. Improvised tourniquets should be at least 2–4 inches wide and several layers thick. Never use narrow material such as rope or wire that may cut into the skin. A blood-pressure cuff may be used as a tourniquet (Figure 26-7). Monitor the cuff pressure to be sure the cuff does not gradually deflate.

Once a tourniquet has been applied, do not remove or loosen it unless ordered by medical direction. Loosening a tourniquet may dislodge clots that have formed, resulting in further bleeding. If you must use a tourniquet, keep it in place.

While you are applying a tourniquet, have another rescuer (if available) continue to apply direct pressure. This may slow the bleeding until the tourniquet is applied. To properly apply a tourniquet, follow these steps:

1. Select a site no farther than 2 inches from the wound. If the wound is on a joint, or just distal to the joint, apply the tourniquet above the joint. The tourniquet should be between the wound and the heart.
2. If using a commercial tourniquet, place the strap around the limb, pull the free end through the buckle or catch, and tighten this end over the pad. Tighten to the point where bleeding is controlled. Do not tighten beyond that point.

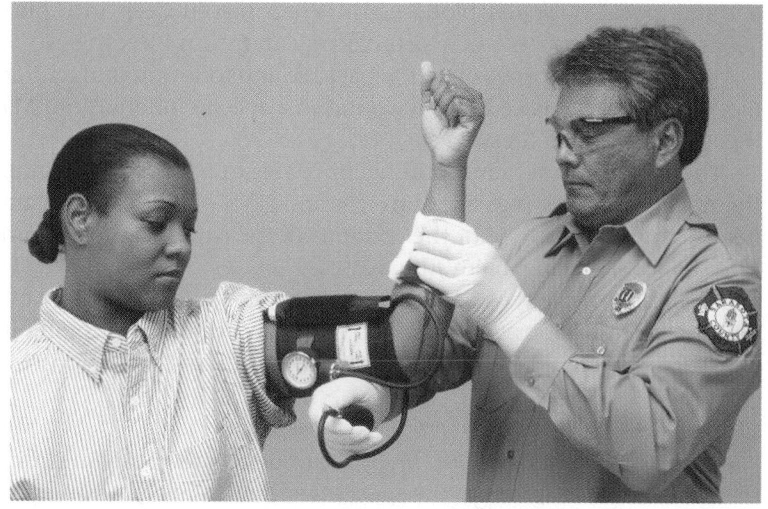

Figure 26-7 • A blood pressure cuff used as a tourniquet.

If you are using cravats, or triangular bandages, wrap the material around the injured limb and tie a knot over the pad. Slip a pen, stick, or similar device into the knot and rotate to tighten the tourniquet. Tighten to the point that bleeding is controlled; no more. Secure the device in place with tape or by tying with the ends of the cravat.

3. Attach a notation to the patient to alert other rescuers and hospital staff that a tourniquet has been applied, and the time of the application. Note this on your prehospital care report also. Do not cover the extremity. You must visually monitor the wound site and the effectiveness of the tourniquet. Leave the tourniquet in open view. Advise hospital staff of the application of a tourniquet during your radio report and in person on your arrival at the emergency department.

You may arrive at a scene to find that well-meaning bystanders have already applied a tourniquet to an injury. It may or may not have been necessary. If the EMT determines that the bleeding is not severe, and other means would control it, medical direction may be contacted about removing the tourniquet. If the bleeding is severe, remove it immediately and follow the steps for controlling bleeding. A tourniquet applied by a well-meaning layperson may very well have been applied improperly. If the tourniquet restricts venous flow but not arterial flow, it may actually lead to worse bleeding than if no "tourniquet" had been applied at all. Always follow your local protocols for this situation. If you are directed to remove the tourniquet, have another rescuer apply direct pressure to the wound while the tourniquet is released.

HEMOSTATIC AGENTS Hemostatic agents are relatively new to civilian EMS. They have been used extensively in the military and are frequently carried on ambulances and may also be purchased at pharmacies and sporting goods stores.

Most of the hemostatic agents seen in the field today are hemostatic dressings (Figure 26-8). These dressings, placed directly into wounds, contain a substance that is

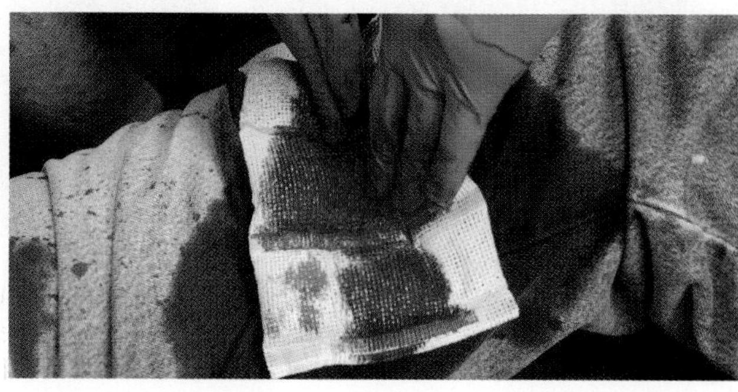

Figure 26-8 • Hemostatic dressing.

absorbent and traps red blood cells. When placed deep into bleeding wounds it is believed that this speeds or assists clotting and stops bleeding.

To use these dressings open the package and follow manufacturer's directions. Some dressings must be placed into a wound in a specific orientation. Maintain pressure on the wound over the dressing.

The other type of hemostatic agent comes in a powder or granular form. Although the hemostatic dressings are more common, you may see the granular version in the field. To use this form, pour the contents of the package into a wound and then pack it into the wound using a gloved hand.

Regardless of the type of agent, continue manual pressure and monitor the patient's bleeding. Hemostatic agents are frequently successful in stopping bleeding. If they do not work you should use a tourniquet. Always follow local protocols.

Other Methods of Bleeding Control

While the methods of bleeding control listed previously in the chapter are the ones that most experts agree are the most effective, there are a variety of other techniques which may have a benefit in limited or specific applications or may still be part of the protocols in some areas. These methods include:

pressure point
a site where a main artery lies near the surface of the body and directly over a bone. Pressure on such a point can stop distal bleeding.

PRESSURE POINTS If direct pressure, or direct pressure with elevation, fails to control the external bleeding, your next method is the use of a **pressure point.** A pressure point is a site where a large artery lies close to the surface of the body and directly over a bone. Simply put, any site where a pulse can be felt is a pressure point. In emergency medical care, there are four sites (two on each side) used as pressure points to control profuse bleeding in extremities: the brachial arteries for bleeding from the upper extremities, and the femoral arteries for bleeding from the lower extremities (Figure 26-9A and B).

The pressure-point method of controlling external bleeding should be used only after direct pressure and elevation have failed. To properly use pressure points, you need to know exactly where the points are located and how much pressure to apply. Note that use of the pressure point may not be effective if the wound is at the distal end of the limb. Blood is being sent to this area of the arm from many other smaller arteries.

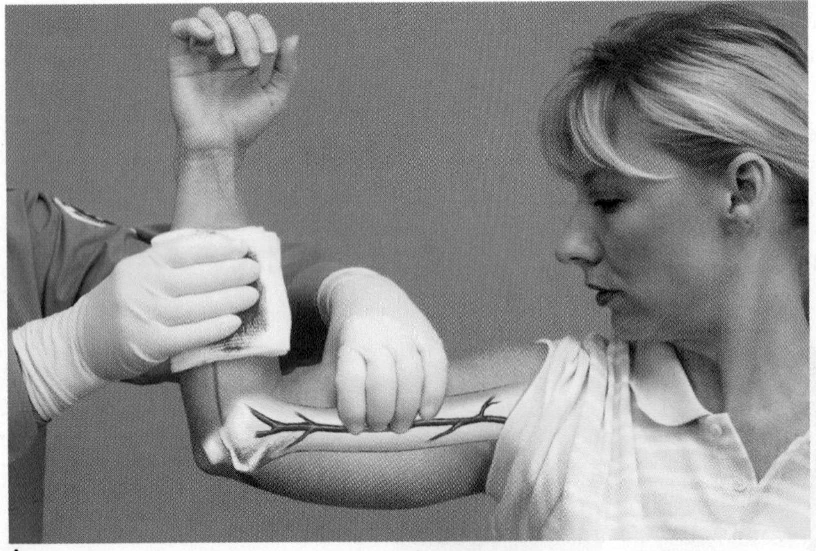

A

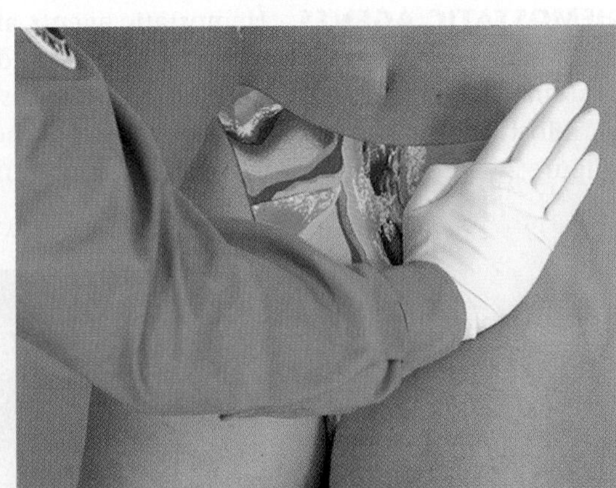

B

Figure 26-9 • (A) Brachial pressure point. (B) Femoral pressure point.

For bleeding from an upper extremity, apply pressure to a point over the **brachial artery**. To find the artery:

brachial (BRAY-ke-al) **artery** the major artery of the upper arm.

1. Hold the patient's arm out at a right angle to his body with the palm of the hand facing up. Do not use force to raise the arm, if the movement causes pain or may aggravate an injury. If it is not possible to raise the arm this far, do the best you can, leaving the arm in the position in which it was found.
2. Locate the groove between the biceps muscle and the upper arm bone (humerus) about midway between the elbow and armpit. Cradle the upper arm in the palm of your hand and position your fingers in this medial groove.
3. Compress the artery against the underlying bone by pressing your finger into the groove. If pressure is properly applied, no radial pulse should be felt.

For bleeding from a lower extremity, apply pressure to a point over the **femoral artery**. Locate the femoral artery on the medial side of the anterior thigh where it joins the lower trunk of the body. You should be able to feel a pulse at a point just below the groin. Place the heel of your hand over the site and apply pressure toward the bone until the bleeding is controlled.

femoral (FEM-or-al) **artery** the major artery supplying the thigh.

Due to the amount of muscle and tissue in the thigh, you will need to apply more pressure than you apply to the brachial artery pressure point. Even more force will be needed if the patient is very muscular or obese. As with the brachial artery pressure point, if pressure is properly applied, a distal pulse will not be felt. As noted for upper extremity injuries, this method may not control the bleeding of distal wounds.

SPLINTING Bleeding associated with a musculoskeletal injury may be controlled by proper splinting of the injury. Since the sharp ends of broken bones may cause tissue and vessel injury, stabilizing them and preventing further movement of the bone ends prevents additional damage. There are several types of splints used for stabilizing injured extremities. (Splinting musculoskeletal injuries will be discussed in detail in Chapter 28, "Musculoskeletal Injuries.")

Inflatable splints, also called air splints, may be used to control internal and external bleeding from an extremity. This type of splint may be used to control bleeding even if there is no suspected bone injury. The splint produces a form of direct pressure. Air splints are useful if there are several wounds to the extremity or one that extends over the length of the extremity. Air splints are most effective for venous and capillary bleeding. They are not usually effective for the high-pressure bleeding caused by an injured artery—at least not until the arterial pressure has decreased below that of the splint. However, you may use an air splint to maintain pressure on a bleeding wound after other manual methods, such as a pressure dressing, have already controlled the bleeding.

NOTE *Never apply ice or cold packs directly to the skin. This can cause frostbite and further damage to the tissue. Always wrap ice or a cold pack in a cloth or towel before applying it to the skin. Do not leave it in place for longer than 20 minutes at a time.*

COLD APPLICATION A centuries-old method of controlling bleeding is the application of ice or a cold pack to the injury. The cold minimizes swelling and reduces the bleeding by constricting the blood vessels. Application of cold should not be used alone but in conjunction with other manual techniques. Application of cold will also reduce pain at the injury site.

PNEUMATIC ANTI-SHOCK GARMENT (PASG) Although the use of the PASG is controversial, many experts agree that it is useful in controlling bleeding from the areas the garment covers. The PASG controls external bleeding from the lower extremities by direct pressure, similarly to the air splint. It is also useful in providing indirect pressure to help control internal bleeding in the pelvic and abdominal cavities. NEVER inflate only the abdominal section of the PASG. Use of the PASG when there is shock present with a chest wound is generally not advised. Follow your local protocols regarding the use of the PASG or contact medical direction for advice.

If your local protocols call for PASG use, remove the patient's lower outer garments to improve application of the garment and to allow for easier insertion of a urinary catheter later. If clothing cannot be removed, remove the patient's belt and any sharp objects from the pockets. Since transport will be required, place the PASG on the spine board before placing the patient on the PASG. An inflated anti-shock garment should be removed only when a physician is present and under the direction of the physician. Removal should only take place when vital signs have just been monitored and indicate that the patient is stable, and when an operating room is immediately available.

Use of the PASG in the treatment of shock (hypoperfusion) will be discussed later in this chapter.

BLOOD PRESSURE CUFF A blood pressure cuff may be used, temporarily, as a tourniquet to control life-threatening arterial bleeding from an extremity while a pressure dressing is applied. Place the cuff above the wound and inflate to approximately 150 mmHg. When the bleeding is controlled, a pressure dressing and bandage are applied. You may then slowly release the pressure in the cuff. Keep the cuff inflated only as long as necessary to secure the pressure dressing and bandage.

HEMOSTATIC AGENTS For many years bleeding control has been performed using the same steps, as just described (direct pressure, elevation, and so on). In addition, hemostatic agents are approved as a new bleeding control method in the protocols of many EMS systems. Hemostatic agents, available as both powders and dressings, are applied to wounds to stop bleeding. Hemostatic dressings were studied and used in the military during Operation Iraqi Freedom and Operation Enduring Freedom.

Hemostatic agents are applied directly to open, bleeding wounds. There are several brands on the market. Follow your local protocols and manufacturers' recommendations on use of these products.

Special Situations Involving Bleeding

Bleeding most often occurs from a wound caused by direct trauma (striking or being struck or cut by something, such as in a collision, a fall, a stabbing, or a shooting). However, you may also find external bleeding from other causes, such as bleeding from the ears caused indirectly by a head injury or a nosebleed caused by high blood pressure.

HEAD INJURY Traumatic injuries resulting in a fractured skull may cause bleeding or loss of cerebrospinal fluid (CSF) from the ears or nose. This fluid loss is not due to direct trauma to the ears or nose. Instead, the head injury results in increased pressure within the skull, which forces fluid out of the cranial cavity. You should not attempt to stop this bleeding or fluid loss, as doing so may increase the pressure in the skull. Do not apply pressure to the ears or nose. Allow the drainage to flow freely, using a gauze pad to collect it.

NOSEBLEED Nosebleeds, also called *epistaxis*, may be caused by direct trauma to the nose. However, bleeding from the nose may also be caused by medical problems such as high blood pressure (hypertension). Tiny capillaries in the nose may burst because of increased blood pressure, sinus infection, or digital trauma (nose picking). Controlling bleeding from the nose is sometimes more difficult if the patient is taking certain medications, such as an anticoagulant like Coumadin. To stop a nosebleed, follow these steps:

1. Have the patient sit down and lean forward.
2. Apply or instruct the patient to apply direct pressure to the fleshy portion around the nostrils.
3. Keep the patient calm and quiet.
4. Do not let the patient lean back. This can allow blood to flow down the esophagus to the stomach, resulting in nausea and vomiting.
5. If the patient becomes unconscious or is unable to control his own airway, place the patient in the recovery position (on his side) and be prepared to provide suction and aggressive airway management.

Internal Bleeding

Internal bleeding is bleeding that occurs inside the body. The bleeding itself is not visible, but many of the signs and symptoms are very apparent. There are several reasons why internal bleeding can be very serious:

- Damage to the internal organs and large blood vessels can result in loss of a large quantity of blood in a short period of time.
- Blood loss cannot be seen. While external bleeding is easy to identify, internal bleeding is hidden. Patients may die of blood loss without having any external bleeding.
- Severe internal blood loss may even occur from injuries to the extremities. Sharp bone ends of a fractured femur can cause enough tissue and blood vessel damage to cause shock (hypoperfusion).

PATIENT ASSESSMENT

INTERNAL BLEEDING

Since internal bleeding is not visible, and may not be obvious, you must identify patients who may have internal bleeding by performing a thorough history and physical exam. Suspicion of internal bleeding and estimates of its severity should be based on the mechanism of injury as well as clinical signs and symptoms. If a patient has a mechanism of injury that suggests the possibility of internal bleeding, treat as though the patient has internal bleeding.

Blunt trauma is the leading cause of internal injuries and bleeding. Mechanisms of blunt trauma that may cause internal bleeding include:

- Falls
- Motor-vehicle or motorcycle crashes
- Auto-pedestrian collisions
- Blast injuries

Penetrating trauma is also a common cause of internal injuries and bleeding. It is often difficult to judge the severity of the wound even when the size and length of the penetrating object are known. Always assess your patient for exit wounds. Mechanisms of penetrating trauma include:

- Gunshot wounds
- Stab wounds from a knife, ice pick, screwdriver, or similar object
- Impaled objects

SIGNS OF INTERNAL BLEEDING

Many of the signs of internal bleeding that you will see are also signs of shock (hypoperfusion). These signs have developed as a result of uncontrolled internal bleeding. They are late signs, indicating that a life-threatening condition has already developed. If you wait for signs of internal bleeding or shock to develop before beginning treatment, you have waited too long. Signs of internal bleeding are:

- Injuries to the surface of the body, which could indicate underlying injuries.
- Bruising (Figure 26-10), swelling, or pain over vital organs (especially in the chest and abdomen). Basic knowledge of anatomy is important for this reason.
- Painful, swollen, or deformed extremities.
- Bleeding from the mouth, rectum, vagina, or other body orifice.
- A tender, rigid, or distended abdomen.
- Vomiting a coffee-ground-like substance or bright red vomitus, indicating the presence of blood. (Red blood is usually "new." Dark blood is usually "old.")

continued

PATIENT ASSESSMENT *(continued)*

- Dark, tarry stools or bright red blood in the stool.
- Signs and symptoms of shock. Remember that the signs listed in Table 26-1 are late signs. They will appear only after internal bleeding has already resulted in significant blood loss.

Remember, your best clue to the possibility of internal bleeding may be the presence of a mechanism of injury that could have caused internal bleeding. ■

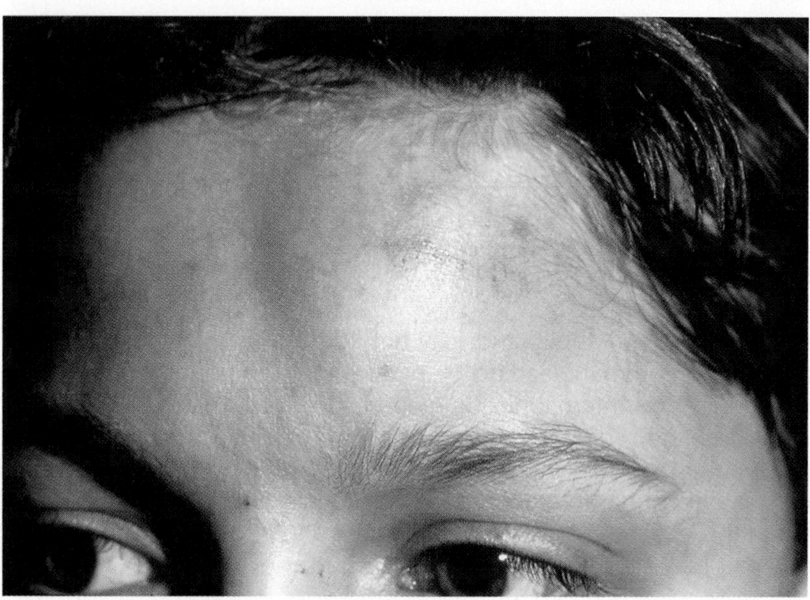

Figure 26-10 • Bruising is one sign of internal bleeding. *(© Dr. P. Marazzi/Photo Researchers, Inc.)*

PATIENT CARE

INTERNAL BLEEDING

Care for the patient with internal bleeding centers on the prevention and treatment of shock (hypoperfusion). Definitive treatment for internal bleeding can only take place in the hospital. Patients with suspected internal bleeding must be considered serious and warrant immediate transport to the hospital.

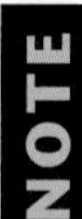

NOTE

Treatment for internal injuries will cause no harm if it is not needed. But death may be the result of not treating a patient who needs it.

As with all patients, your first priority is the standard ABCs; that is, ensure an open airway, adequate breathing, and circulation. Patients with internal bleeding may deteriorate quickly. Monitor the ABCs and vital signs often. Be prepared to maintain the patient's airway, to provide or assist ventilations, or to administer CPR as needed.

1. Maintain the ABCs and provide support as needed.
2. Administer high-concentration oxygen by nonrebreather mask, if oxygen administration has not already begun.
3. Control any external bleeding. If you suspect internal bleeding in an injured extremity, apply an appropriate splint.
4. Provide prompt transport to an appropriate medical facility. Internal bleeding must often be controlled in the operating room. ■

SHOCK (HYPOPERFUSION)

Shock, also known as hypoperfusion, is inadequate tissue perfusion. (Perfusion and hypoperfusion were defined at the beginning of this chapter.) It is the inability of the circulatory system to supply cells with oxygen and nutrients. Hypoperfusion also causes the inadequate removal of waste products from the cells. The result of untreated shock is death.

Causes of Shock

As discussed previously, the circulatory system consists of three components: the heart, blood vessels, and blood. Failure of any of these components—the pumping of the heart, the supply of blood, the integrity of the blood vessels, or the ability of the vessels to dilate and constrict—means that perfusion of the brain, lungs, and other body organs will not be adequate.

Blood vessels can play an important role in the development of shock (if they are *not* functioning properly) or in the body's ability to compensate for shock (if they are functioning properly). Blood vessels can change their diameter, either by dilating or constricting. These changes in size are governed by the need for blood in various areas of the body. In an area of the body that is doing more work, blood vessels dilate to allow more blood to flow to that area. At the same time, in another area of the body that is not working as hard, vessels will constrict. For example, if you are running, blood flow to the muscles in the legs increases through dilated arteries. At the same time, blood flow to the digestive system lessens because vessels supplying these organs have been constricted to compensate for the dilation of the arteries in the legs.

Since the amount of blood in the body does not change, this balance between dilation of some vessels and constriction of others is necessary to keep the system full. The same amount of blood is in the body, but it is distributed differently. If all the blood vessels in the body dilated at one time, there would not be enough blood to fill the entire circulatory system. Circulation would fail, and tissues would not be adequately perfused. The result would be the development of shock.

As shock develops, the failure of one component of the system may cause adverse effects on another. If blood is being lost through external bleeding, the heart rate will increase in an effort to circulate the remaining blood to all the tissues. However, the increased heart rate causes increased bleeding. As more blood is lost, the heart tries to compensate by increasing its rate even more. Left untreated, the process continues until the patient dies.

In early shock, the body attempts to compensate for blood loss. Most of the signs and symptoms of shock are caused by the body's compensating mechanisms attempting to adequately perfuse the tissues. Shock may develop if (1) the heart fails as a pump, (2) blood volume is lost, or (3) blood vessels dilate, creating a vascular container capacity that is too great to be filled by the available blood.

Severity of Shock

Shock (hypoperfusion) is the body's reaction to decreased blood circulation to the organ systems. It is the result of the inadequate perfusion of tissues with oxygen and nutrients and the inadequate removal of metabolic waste products. If untreated, shock will cause cell and organ malfunction and, finally, it will result in death. Prompt recognition and aggressive treatment are vital to patient survival.

Shock is classified into three categories of severity. These are compensated shock, decompensated shock, and irreversible shock:

- **Compensated shock.** The body senses the decrease in perfusion and attempts to compensate for it. For a time, the body's compensating mechanisms work, and

compensated shock when the patient is developing shock but the body is still able to maintain perfusion. *See* shock.

F•Y•I

TYPES OF SHOCK

Regardless of the cause, shock is the failure of the circulatory system to provide sufficient blood and oxygen to all the vital tissues of the body. The three major types of shock are hypovolemic shock, cardiogenic shock, and neurogenic shock:

- **Hypovolemic shock.** This is the type of shock most commonly seen by EMTs. When it is caused by uncontrolled bleeding, or hemorrhage, it can be called **hemorrhagic shock.** The bleeding can be internal, external, or a combination of both. Hypovolemic shock may also be caused by burns or crush injuries, where plasma is lost.
- **Cardiogenic shock.** Patients suffering a myocardial infarction, or heart attack, may develop shock from the inadequate pumping of blood by the heart. The strength of the heart's contractions may be decreased because of the damage to the heart muscle. Or the heart's electrical system may be malfunctioning, causing a heartbeat that is too slow, too fast, or irregular. Other cardiac problems, such as congestive heart failure, may also cause shock. Watch for low blood pressure, edema in the feet and ankles, and other signs of heart failure. (Review Chapter 17, "Cardiac Emergencies.")
- **Neurogenic shock.** Shock may result from the uncontrolled dilation of blood vessels due to nerve paralysis caused by spinal cord injuries. While there is no actual blood loss, the dilation of the blood vessels increases the circulatory system's capacity to the point where the available blood can no longer adequately fill it. With sepsis (massive infection) or anaphylactic (severe allergic) reaction, vasodilation may also cause shock. Neurogenic shock is rarely seen in the field.

Keep in mind that, as an EMT, you do not need to diagnose the type of shock. Instead, you must recognize and treat for shock whenever there is a mechanism of injury or signs that indicate the possibility of shock.

blood pressure is maintained. Some early signs of shock are actually caused by the body's compensating mechanisms at work. You will note an increased heart rate (to increase blood flow) and increased respirations (to increase oxygenation of the blood). Constriction of the peripheral circulation (to redirect blood to the vital core organs) results in pale, cool skin and, in infants and children, increased capillary refill time.

- **Decompensated shock.** At the point when the body can no longer compensate for the low blood volume or lack of perfusion, decompensated shock begins. Late signs of shock, such as falling blood pressure, develop.
- **Irreversible shock.** Irreversible shock exists when the body has lost the battle to maintain perfusion to the organ systems. Cell damage occurs, especially in the liver and kidneys. Even if adequate vital signs can be restored, the patient may die days later due to the failure of irreparably damaged organs.

hypovolemic (HI-po-vo-LE-mik) **shock** shock resulting from blood or fluid loss.

hemorrhagic (HEM-or-AJ-ik) **shock** shock resulting from blood loss.

cardiogenic shock shock, or lack of perfusion, brought on not by blood loss, but by inadequate pumping action of the heart. It is often the result of a heart attack or congestive heart failure.

neurogenic shock hypoperfusion due to nerve paralysis (sometimes caused by spinal cord injuries) resulting in the dilation of blood vessels that increases the volume of the circulatory system beyond the point where it can be filled.

PEDIATRIC NOTE

Infants and children present a special problem when assessing for shock. They have such efficient compensating mechanisms that they can maintain a normal blood pressure until over half of their blood volume is gone. By the time their blood pressure drops, they are already near death. Shock must be considered and cared for early. Do not wait for signs of shock to appear.

PATIENT ASSESSMENT

SHOCK (HYPOPERFUSION)

Many of the signs and symptoms of shock are the same no matter what the cause (hypovolemic, cardiogenic, or neurogenic). The symptoms follow a logical progression as shock develops and worsens. The signs and symptoms, in the order they appear, are as follows (Figure 26-11 and Table 26-1):

- *Altered mental status.* The brain is very sensitive to any decrease in oxygen supply. When the brain is deprived of oxygen, even slightly, mental and behavioral changes may be seen. These may include anxiety, restlessness, and combativeness.
- *Pale, cool, clammy skin.* When the body senses inadequate tissue perfusion, it attempts to correct the problem by diverting, or shunting, blood from nonvital areas to the vital organs. Blood is quickly directed away from the skin and sent to organs such as the heart and brain. This results in loss of skin color and temperature. Infants and young children may have a capillary refill time of greater than 2 seconds. (Delayed capillary refill time is considered an unreliable sign of shock in patients over the age of 5 when capillary refill time can more readily be influenced by other factors.) Note that in neurogenic shock (rare) the skin is typically warm, flushed, and dry because the circulatory system has lost the ability to constrict blood vessels in the skin.
- *Nausea and vomiting.* In the body's efforts to direct blood to the vital organs, blood is diverted from the digestive system, resulting in nausea and sometimes vomiting.
- *Vital sign changes.* The first vital signs to change are the respiratory and pulse rates:
  - The pulse will increase in an attempt to pump more blood. As it continues to increase and blood loss worsens, the pulse becomes weak and thready.
  - Respirations increase in an attempt to raise the oxygen saturation of the blood left in the system. As shock progresses, respirations become more rapid, labored, shallow, and sometimes irregular.
  - Blood pressure drops because the body's compensating mechanisms can no longer keep up with the decrease in perfusion or blood loss. Decreased blood pressure is a LATE sign of shock. By the time the blood pressure drops, the patient is in a truly life-threatening condition.
  - Pulse oximetry might not be accurate in patients with shock. Oximeters rely on adequate perfusion to get an accurate reading. Patients with shock may not be adequately perfusing their extremities.
- *Other signs.* Other signs of shock include thirst, dilated pupils, and sometimes cyanosis around the lips and nail beds. ■

decompensated shock occurs when the body can no longer compensate for low blood volume or lack of perfusion. Late signs such as decreasing blood pressure become evident. *See* shock.

irreversible shock when the body has lost the battle to maintain perfusion to vital organs. Even if adequate vital signs return, the patient may die days later due to organ failure.

Emergency Care for Shock

Emergency care for the patient in shock includes airway maintenance and the administration of high-concentration oxygen. Increasing the blood's oxygen saturation will improve oxygen supply to the tissues. You must also attempt to stop what is causing the shock, such as external bleeding, and attempt to maintain perfusion.

Remember that TRANSPORTATION IS AN INTERVENTION. Your most significant treatment for the shock patient may be early recognition of the problem and prompt transportation to a hospital where the patient will receive definitive care.

The term *golden hour* has been used to describe the optimal time from the infliction of a traumatic injury until the patient receives definitive treatment in a hospital—usually

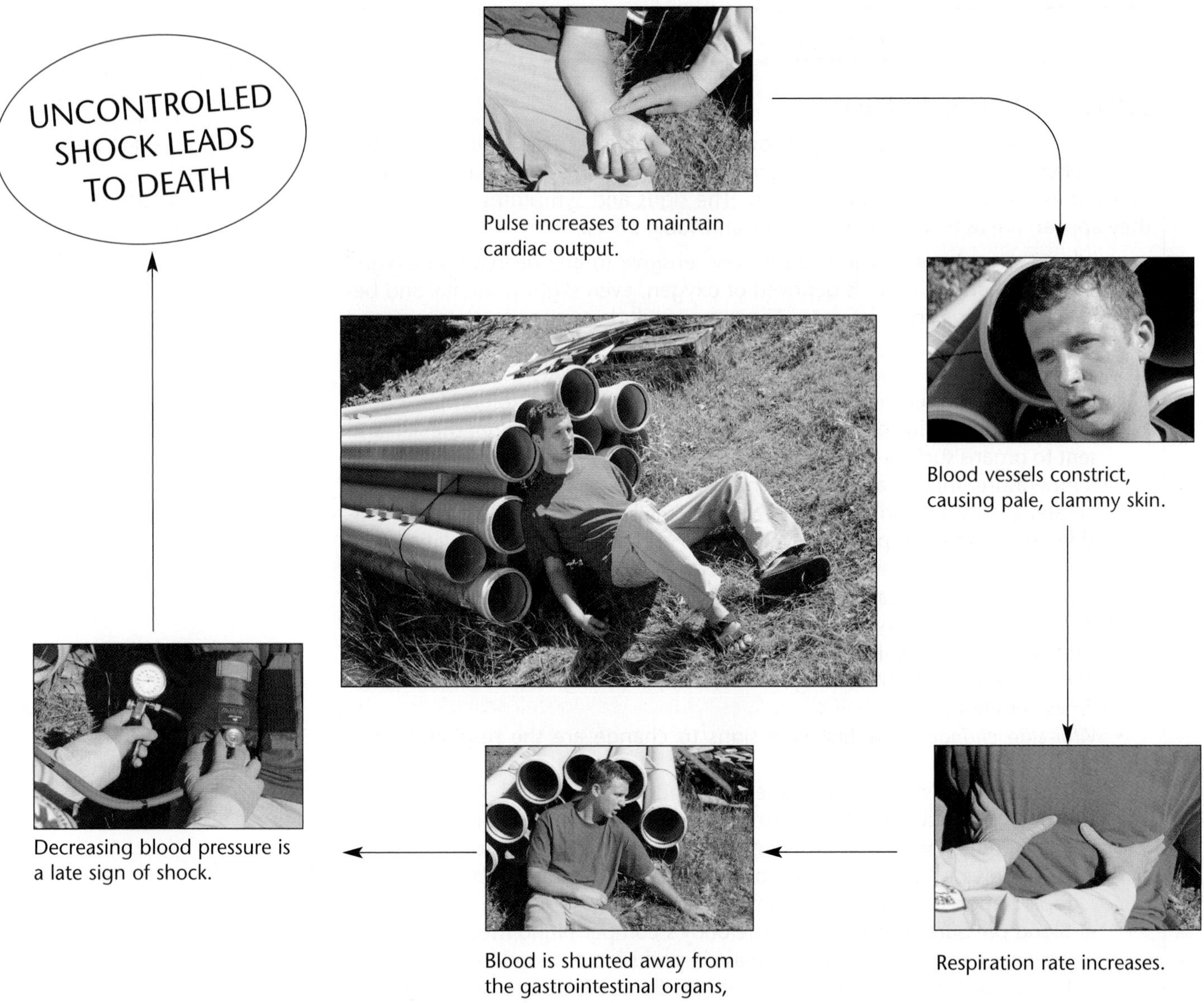

UNCONTROLLED SHOCK LEADS TO DEATH
Pulse increases to maintain cardiac output.
Blood vessels constrict, causing pale, clammy skin.
Respiration rate increases.
Blood is shunted away from the gastrointestinal organs, causing nausea.
Decreasing blood pressure is a late sign of shock.

Figure 26-11 • Signs of shock will be detectable during the patient assessment.

surgery. Many experts believe that survival rates from traumatic injuries are best if needed surgery takes place within this first hour after the injury. Survival rates decrease rapidly thereafter.

Recently, trauma programs have ceased using the term *golden hour* because there is no research that clearly identifies the optimal time between injury and definitive care. Furthermore, EMTs should never consider an hour the ideal time if less time can be taken. Perhaps a better statement is that *every minute between the time of injury and the patient getting to an operating suite is, in fact, like gold to the patient—and to his chances of survival.*

Note that the clock begins running at the time of injury, not the time of your arrival on scene. If the patient is not quickly found, or you have a long response time to the scene, much of this critical time, formerly called the golden hour, may have already ticked away. Therefore, your goal in caring for trauma and shock patients is to limit on-scene time and provide immediate transportation to the hospital. Be sure to alert the receiving hospital as soon as possible, as they may need to call in a surgeon. The clock does not stop with the patient's arrival at the hospital. It stops in the operating room.

Cultural Considerations

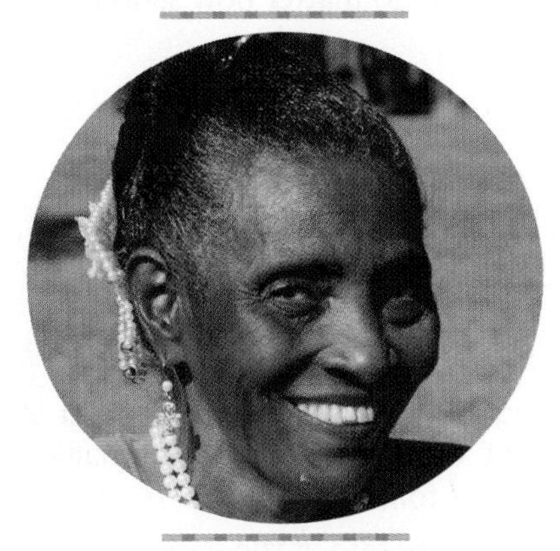

Your patients will, of course, have a wide variety of skin tones. If your patient is dark-skinned, how do you check for pallor or cyanosis—critical signs of the development of shock?

In all patients, skin color is best evaluated where the epidermis (the outer layer of the skin) is thinnest. This includes the fingernails and lips. Open the patient's mouth, or ask him to open it, so that you can examine the color of the mucous membranes inside the mouth. Pull down the patient's lower eyelids and note the color of the conjunctiva (the mucous membrane that lines the eyelids). These are places where pallor or cyanosis will be evident, and these examinations are the same for patients of any skin color.

In dark-skinned patients, you can also check the palms of the hands and soles of the feet, where the skin is lighter, to observe for other colorations such as the yellowish color of jaundice or the small round purplish spots called petechiae that are the result of capillary bleeding. You can also ask the patient or his family if the patient's skin color looks normal, since they may be aware of changes such as an "ashy" look to the skin that would not be obvious to you.

For the reasons just discussed, limiting the time spent at the scene is vital. The goal for on-scene time when caring for a trauma or shock patient has been stated as a maximum of 10 minutes (unless lengthy extrication is required). This time limit is often called the *platinum 10 minutes*. Like the golden hour, there is no research that proves 10 minutes is the ideal on-scene time. The best rule is simply to take as little time as possible at the scene.

In order to stay within optimal time spans, procedures done at the scene must be kept to a minimum. In patients showing signs of shock, or a mechanism of injury that suggests that possibility, some elements of patient assessment, such as detailed exams

CRITICAL DECISION MAKING:
No Pressure, No Problem

Falling blood pressure is a late sign of shock. In the following patients, use material you learned in this chapter to determine if your early decision making would lead you to expedite the call because you suspected shock or if, instead, you believe the patient will likely be stable. You will not be provided a blood pressure—but in each patient you will find enough information to make a proper early decision without a blood pressure reading.

1. Your patient was working on scaffolding that collapsed causing him to fall one story (about 10 feet). He is conscious, is alert but anxious, and complains of pain to the right side of his chest. His pulse is 102 and regular, respirations 26, skin cool and moist, pupils equal and reactive to light.
2. Your patient is found sitting in a bathroom stall at an upscale restaurant. He is pale, sweaty, and leaning against the wall. He tells you he has had a problem with bleeding hemorrhoids recently. There is bright red blood in the toilet bowl. When you stand the patient up to move him to the stretcher, he feels like he is going to pass out.
3. You are called to an assault. A 26-year-old man was struck in the head by his girlfriend. She used a telephone to strike him once in the nose and again in the forehead. The police called you to evaluate a nosebleed. The patient's shirt has blood streaked down it. His nose is oozing blood now. He is alert and oriented. His pulse is 78 strong and regular, respirations 14, skin warm and dry.

and treatments, are best done in the ambulance en route to the hospital. On-scene assessment and care should consist of the ABCs with spinal precautions, a rapid trauma exam, immobilization, and moving the patient to the ambulance.

Always drive safely and responsibly to the hospital no matter how serious your patient's condition may be.

PATIENT CARE

SHOCK (HYPOPERFUSION)

Care for shock is similar to the care for bleeding described earlier. Remember Standard Precautions when caring for any patient who is bleeding externally. The emergency care steps for shock (Scan 26-2) are as follows:

1. Maintain an open airway and assess the respiratory rate. If the patient is breathing adequately, apply high-concentration oxygen by nonrebreather mask. Assist ventilations or perform CPR if necessary.
2. Control any external bleeding.
3. Apply and inflate the PASG if approved or ordered by your local medical direction (Scan 26-3). The PASG is usually indicated for bleeding in areas covered by the garment, pelvic injury, and some abdominal trauma. Always follow your local protocols for use of the PASG. Alternative treatments for pelvic injuries, which also help treat for shock, are discussed in Chapter 28, "Musculoskeletal Injuries."

   Use of the PASG is usually contraindicated in cardiogenic shock, or if there are abnormal lung sounds. Special consideration should be taken if your patient has bleeding in areas not covered by the garment.

   Use of the PASG when there is shock in the presence of a chest wound is generally not advised. If your female patient is pregnant, inflate only the leg sections. If your patient is a child, it is recommended that only the leg sections be inflated. This is because the top of the abdominal section of the pediatric-size garment often covers the lower portion of a child's chest, which can interfere with the child's respirations.
4. If there is no possibility of spine injury, elevate the legs 8 to 12 inches. This position will assist the body in maintaining perfusion to the vital organs. Elevation is not necessary if you have applied and inflated the PASG.
5. Splint any suspected bone injuries or joint injuries. If your patient is in shock, do not use your valuable on-scene time for this. Splints should be applied en route to the hospital. Do not take time to individually splint multiple injuries. Splint the entire body by securing the patient to a long spine board. This will adequately stabilize the injuries until further care can be given.
6. Prevent loss of body heat by covering the patient with a blanket.
7. Transport the patient immediately. Detailed exams and care procedures should be done en route to the hospital. Notify the receiving hospital as soon as possible. Give them information on the patient's injuries and condition. Contact medical direction if necessary. If your on-scene time is extended due to extrication, or your transport time to the hospital is lengthy, request an ALS intercept if available. This may be a ground ambulance or a helicopter service. If you have the patient loaded in your ambulance, begin transport and ask that the ALS unit intercept your unit en route. Time is of the essence.
8. If the patient is conscious, speak calmly and reassuringly throughout assessment, care, and transport. Fear increases the body's work and worsens developing shock. ■

SCAN 26-2 • Managing Shock

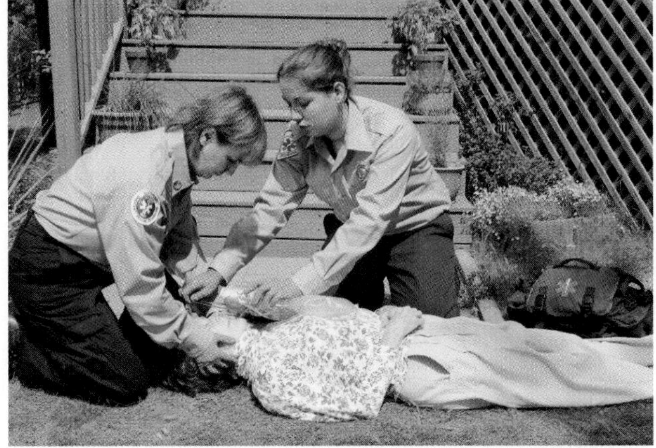

1. Maintain an open airway, and give high-concentration oxygen by nonrebreather mask. Control external bleeding. Assist ventilations and perform CPR, if needed.

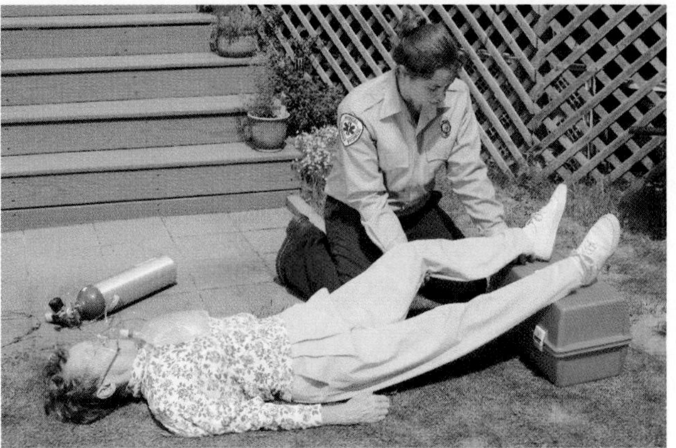

2. If there is no serious injury, elevate the patient's legs 8 to 12 inches, or . . .

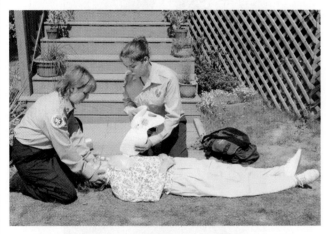

. . . If there is any possibility of spine injury, position the patient with NO elevation of the extremities.

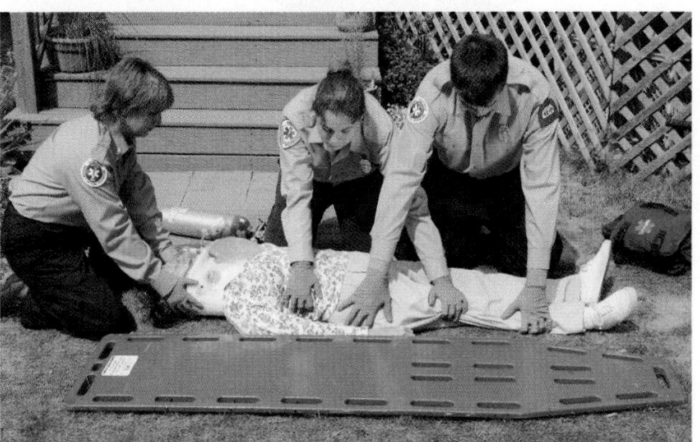

3. Place the patient on a spine board to splint the entire body. Splinting of individual bone and joint injuries should be done en route.

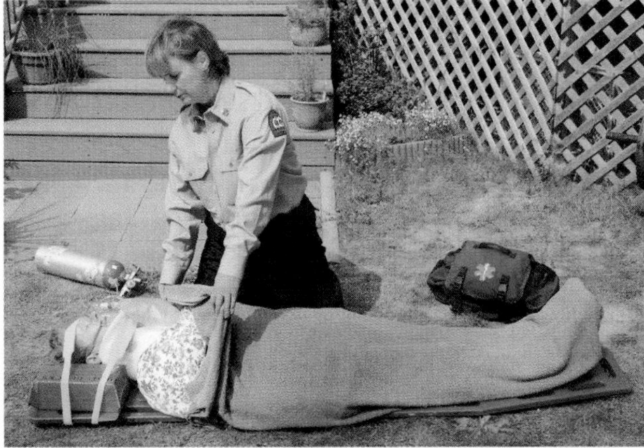

4. Protect the patient from heat loss.

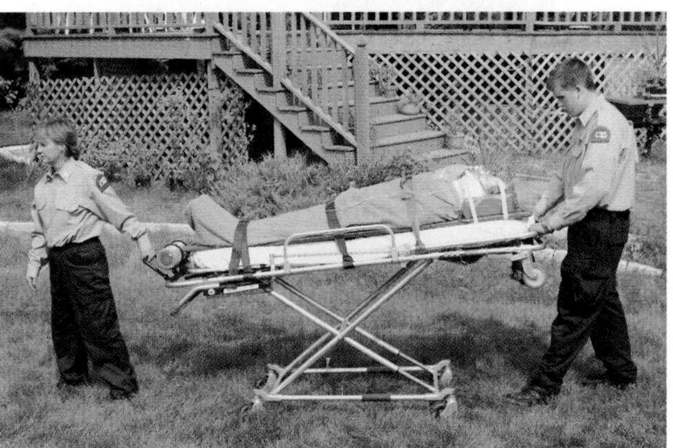

5. Transport immediately.

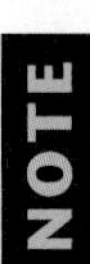

NOTE

FIRST take Standard Precautions.

SCAN 26-3 • Applying the Anti-Shock Garment

FOLLOW LOCAL PROTOCOLS REGARDING APPLICATION AND INFLATION.

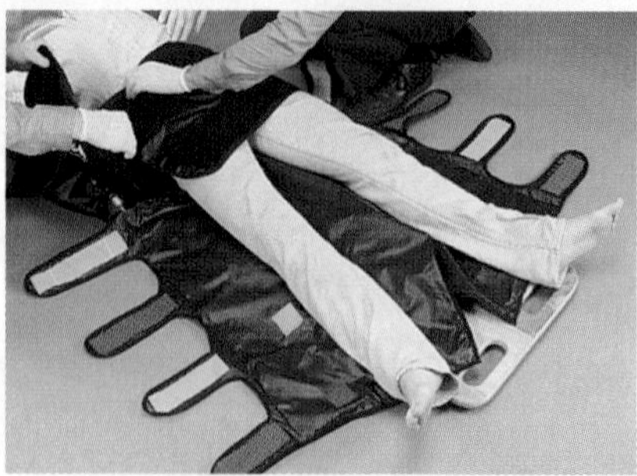

1. Log roll the patient onto the garment, so the upper edge is below the patient's bottom rib.

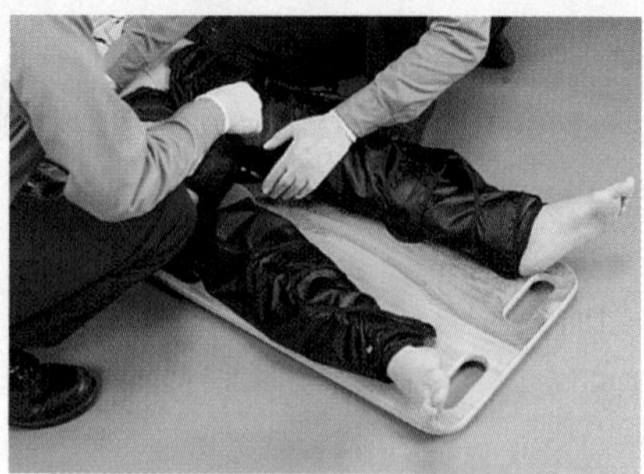

2. Enclose the legs, one at a time, securing the Velcro straps.

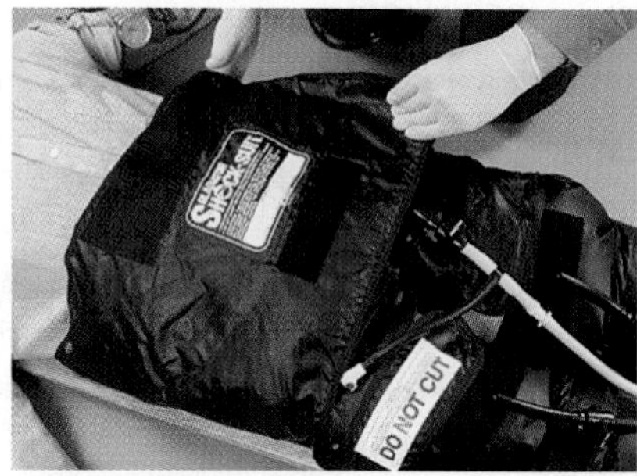

3. Enclose the abdomen and pelvis, securing the Velcro straps.

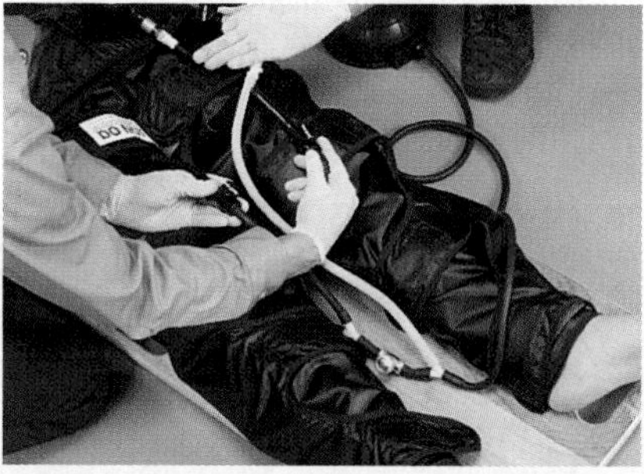

4. Check the tubes. Open the stopcocks to the legs; close the abdominal compartment stopcock.

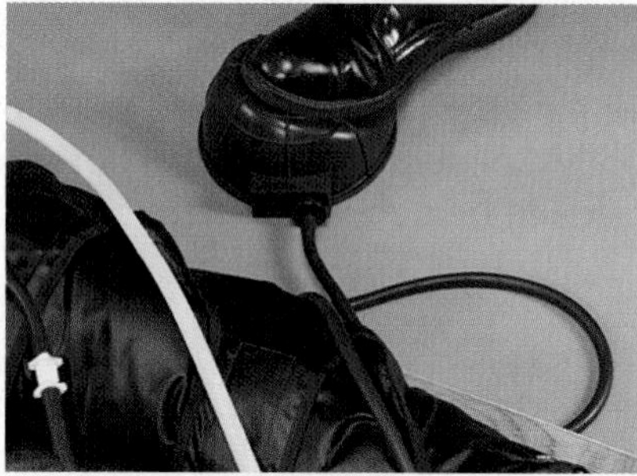

5. Inflate the lower compartments until the Velcro crackles. Close the stopcocks.

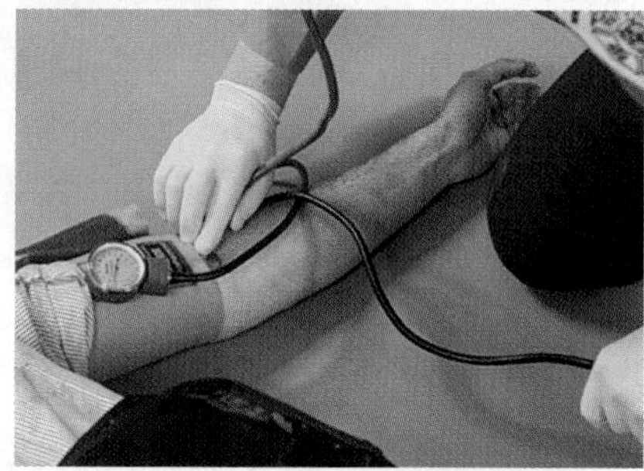

6. If systolic blood pressure is below 90, open the stopcock, inflate the abdominal compartment, and close the stopcock.

Monitor and record vital signs every 5 minutes. If the garment loses pressure, add air as needed. Some protocols call for the inflation of all three compartments of the garment simultaneously. Always follow local protocols. Some systems require direct medical direction.

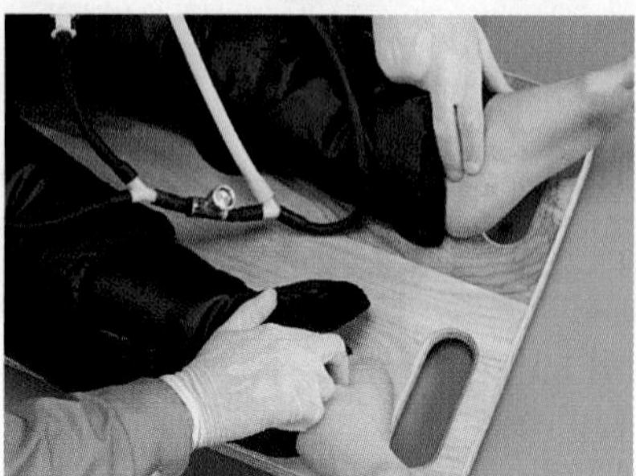

7. Check both extremities for a distal pulse.

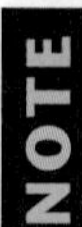

The patient's clothing remains on for demonstration purposes. In actual use, clothing should be removed.

CHAPTER REVIEW

SUMMARY

Blood loss can be external or internal. External bleeding can be controlled by direct pressure, elevation, and the use of a tourniquet. Emergency care for internal bleeding is based on the prevention and treatment of shock.

Shock is usually first seen in a patient as restlessness or anxiety. Skin becomes pale, and the pulse and respirations increase. If shock remains uncontrolled, the patient's blood pressure begins to fall. A decrease in blood pressure is a late sign of shock. Signs and symptoms of shock may not be evident early in the call, so treatment based on the mechanism of injury may be life-saving.

Treat shock by airway maintenance; administration of high-concentration oxygen; controlling bleeding; and keeping the patient warm. One of the most important treatments is early recognition of shock and immediate transport to a hospital.

KEY TERMS

arterial bleeding bleeding from an artery, which is characterized by bright red blood and as rapid, profuse, and difficult to control.

brachial (BRAY-ke-al) **artery** the major artery of the upper arm.

capillary bleeding bleeding from capillaries, which is characterized by a slow, oozing flow of blood.

cardiogenic shock shock, or lack of perfusion, brought on not by blood loss, but by inadequate pumping action of the heart. It is often the result of a heart attack or congestive heart failure.

compensated shock when the patient is developing shock but the body is still able to maintain perfusion. *See* shock.

decompensated shock occurs when the body can no longer compensate for low blood volume or lack of perfusion. Late signs such as decreasing blood pressure become evident. *See* shock.

femoral (FEM-or-al) **artery** the major artery supplying the thigh.

hemorrhage (HEM-o-rej) bleeding, especially severe bleeding.

hemorrhagic (HEM-or-AJ-ik) **shock** shock resulting from blood loss.

hypoperfusion (HI-po-per-FEW-zhun) inability of the body to adequately circulate blood to the body's cells to supply them with oxygen and nutrients. *See also* shock.

hypovolemic (HI-po-vo-LE-mik) **shock** shock resulting from blood or fluid loss.

irreversible shock when the body has lost the battle to maintain perfusion to vital organs. Even if adequate vital signs return, the patient may die days later due to organ failure.

neurogenic shock hypoperfusion due to nerve paralysis (sometimes caused by spinal cord injuries) resulting in the dilation of blood vessels that increases the volume of the circulatory system beyond the point where it can be filled.

perfusion the supply of oxygen to and removal of wastes from the cells and tissues of the body as a result of the flow of blood through the capillaries.

pressure dressing a bulky dressing held in position with a tightly wrapped bandage to apply pressure to help control bleeding.

pressure point a site where a main artery lies near the surface of the body and directly over a bone. Pressure on such a point can stop distal bleeding.

shock also known as *hypoperfusion.* The inability of the body to adequately circulate blood to the body's cells to supply them with oxygen and nutrients. A life-threatening condition.

tourniquet (TURN-i-ket) a device used for bleeding control that constricts all blood flow to and from an extremity.

venous bleeding bleeding from a vein, which is characterized by dark red or maroon blood and as a steady flow, easy to control.

REVIEW QUESTIONS

1. Name the three main types of blood vessels, and describe the type of bleeding you would expect to see from each one. (pp. 616–617, 618–619)
2. List the patient care steps for external bleeding control. (p. 621)

3. Define perfusion and hypoperfusion. (p. 617)
4. List the signs and symptoms of shock. Which would you expect to see early? Which are late signs? Explain what causes each of them. (pp. 620, 633, 634)
5. List the three major types of shock and what causes each one. (p. 632)
6. List the emergency care steps for treating a patient in shock. (pp. 633–637)
7. In gauging the optimal time between injury and definitive care, when does the clock start running and when does the clock stop running? (pp. 633–635)

CRITICAL THINKING

- A patient has been involved in a motor-vehicle collision. There is considerable damage to his vehicle. The steering column and wheel are badly deformed. The patient complains of a "sore chest." You note no external bleeding. The patient's vital signs are pulse 116, respirations 20, blood pressure 106/70. How would you proceed to assess and care for this patient?

Thinking and Linking

Think back to Chapters 7–12 on scene size-up and patient assessment as well as Chapters 16–25 on medical emergencies. Link information from those chapters with information from this chapter as you consider the following questions:

- You respond to a shopping center parking lot for a motor-vehicle collision. You find an older male patient unresponsive in his vehicle. What facts could you gather at the scene that would help you determine whether the patient's unresponsiveness was caused by trauma and shock or a medical condition?
- What medical conditions can cause shock or present with signs and symptoms similar to shock?

MEDIA RESOURCES

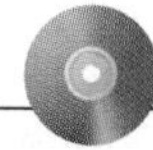

See the Student CD at the back of this book for quizzes, animations, a case study activity, and other features related to this chapter. In particular, take a look at the animation on shock. Also, visit the Companion Website for *Emergency Care* at **www.prenhall.com/limmer**, where you will find additional reinforcement and links to other resources.

Street Scenes

Arnold Johnson likes to do odd jobs around the house. Today's project is to fix a loose shelf in the kitchen. He gets out his ladder and tools and starts to work. As he reaches to hammer his first nail, he loses his footing and falls a few feet, hitting his left side on the corner of the kitchen table. It hurts but he goes back to finish the shelf. After a few minutes, he realizes he is in considerable discomfort. As the pain increases and Arnold starts to feel worse, he knows something is wrong and calls 911. Your ambulance is dispatched with a First Response unit from the fire department, Squad 31, to a 46-year-old male with injuries from a fall. Squad 31 is on scene first, gathering a history and taking a set of vital signs. You arrive about 3 minutes later. Mr. Johnson is sitting in a chair and looks anxious.

Street Scene Questions

1. What is the priority for this patient? Does an initial assessment still need to be done?
2. What assessment information do you want to receive from Squad 31?
3. Is the mechanism of injury important information for this patient?

You approach the patient as your partner gets the First Responder information. You notice that Mr. Johnson is pale and seems to have an increased respiratory rate. Your partner gives you the patient history from Squad 31, including their impression that the patient may have broken some ribs. The First Responders report the following vital signs: a thready pulse of 110, respiratory rate of 24 and labored, and a blood pressure of 130/85. As you move on to the focused assessment, your partner prepares the stretcher.

You are becoming more concerned. You ask the wife if this is his normal color and she tells you he is very pale. At that point, the patient tells you he feels nauseated and thinks he might throw up.

Street Scene Questions

4. What is the treatment priority for this patient?
5. How often should you get a new set of vital signs?

You load the patient on the stretcher, ask him how he feels, and notice he is not as alert as when you arrived on the scene about 10 minutes ago. You administer oxygen by way of nonrebreather mask and move toward the ambulance, concerned that this patient may be bleeding internally. Once en route to the hospital, you get another set of vital signs and realize the pulse is weak and has increased by 10 beats per minute. The respiratory rate is now 28 and seems more labored. The blood pressure is 124/80. You do a detailed assessment of the abdomen, and the patient reacts with tenderness in the left upper quadrant. The closest hospital is a trauma center, and you tell your partner this is a high priority. You continue patient care with 15 liters per minute of oxygen by nonrebreather mask and keep the patient warm. Another set of vital signs is taken, followed by a radio report to the hospital. You end the transmission by advising ETA in 7 minutes.

A short time after you give your prehospital care report to ED personnel, you overhear a surgeon turn to a nurse and quietly say, "Get an operating room set up. This patient likely has a severe spleen injury."

Street Scenes Sample Documentation

PATIENT NAME: *Arnold Johnson* PATIENT AGE: *46*

CHIEF COMPLAINT: *Tenderness LUQ*

PAST MEDICAL HISTORY

- [x] None
- [ ] Allergy to
- [ ] Hypertension
- [ ] Stroke
- [ ] Seizures
- [ ] Diabetes
- [ ] COPD
- [ ] Cardiac
- [ ] Other (List)
- [ ] Asthma

Current Medications (List): *None*

VITAL SIGNS

TIME	RESP	PULSE	B.P.	MENTAL STATUS	R PUPILS L	SKIN
0922	Rate: *24* [ ] Regular [ ] Shallow [x] Labored	Rate: *110* [x] Regular [ ] Irregular	*130/85*	[x] Alert [ ] Voice [ ] Pain [ ] Unresp.	[x] Normal [x] [ ] Dilated [ ] [ ] Constricted [ ] [ ] Sluggish [ ] [ ] No-Reaction [ ]	[ ] Unremarkable [ ] Cool [x] Pale [ ] Warm [ ] Cyanotic [x] Moist [ ] Flushed [ ] Dry [ ] Jaundiced
0928	Rate: *28* [ ] Regular [ ] Shallow [x] Labored	Rate: *120* [x] Regular [ ] Irregular	*124/80*	[ ] Alert [x] Voice [ ] Pain [ ] Unresp.	[x] Normal [x] [ ] Dilated [ ] [ ] Constricted [ ] [ ] Sluggish [ ] [ ] No-Reaction [ ]	[ ] Unremarkable [x] Cool [x] Pale [ ] Warm [ ] Cyanotic [x] Moist [ ] Flushed [ ] Dry [ ] Jaundiced
0935	Rate: *28* [ ] Regular [ ] Shallow [x] Labored	Rate: *120* [x] Regular [ ] Irregular	*118/78*	[ ] Alert [x] Voice [ ] Pain [ ] Unresp.	[x] Normal [x] [ ] Dilated [ ] [ ] Constricted [ ] [ ] Sluggish [ ] [ ] No-Reaction [ ]	[ ] Unremarkable [x] Cool [x] Pale [ ] Warm [ ] Cyanotic [x] Moist [ ] Flushed [ ] Dry [ ] Jaundiced

NARRATIVE *Our patient states that he fell several feet while standing on a ladder. While falling, he struck his left side on the edge of a protruding kitchen table. Patient denies striking his head, neck, or back. He denies any loss of consciousness. 0922 vital signs were reported by First Responders. Patient is now ashen, respiration has become more rapid and labored, and pulse has become weak and more rapid. Patient has a decreasing level of responsiveness, and is becoming nauseated. Our physical exam reveals a very tender LUQ. Patient placed on 15 LPM via nonrebreather. Monitored and managed patient's body temperature en route to trauma center.*

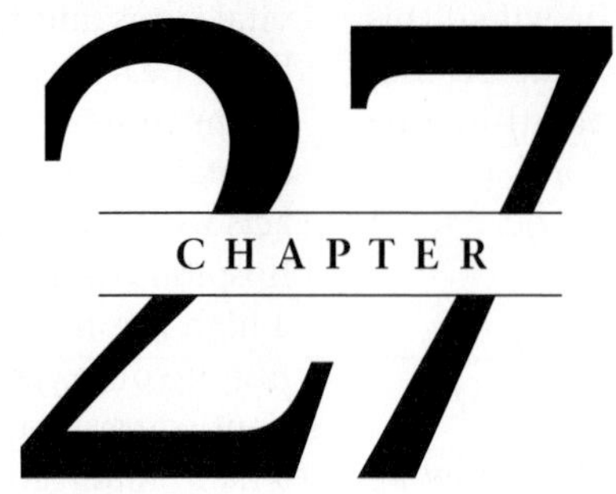

CHAPTER 27

Soft-Tissue Injuries

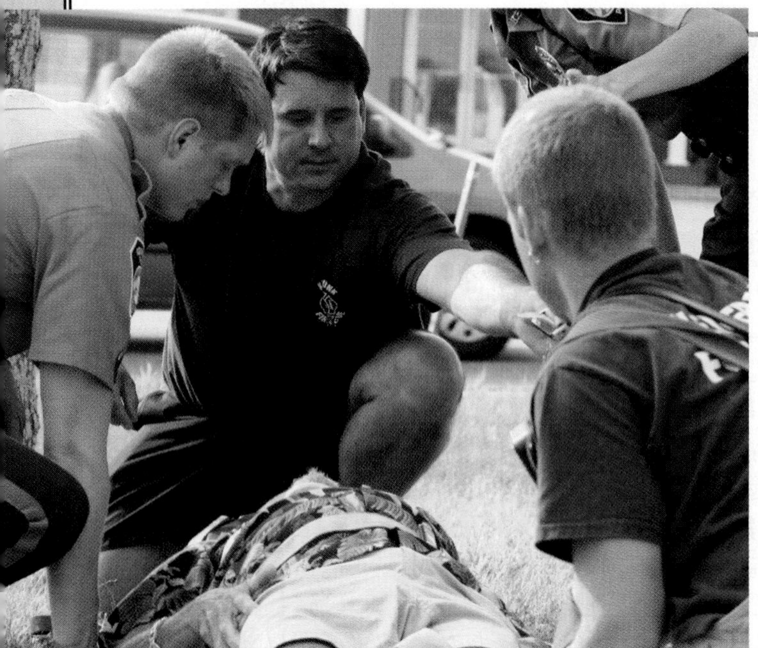

CORE CONCEPTS

The following are core concepts that will be addressed in this chapter:

- Emergency care for burns, amputations, chest and abdominal wounds, impaled objects, and both open and closed soft-tissue injuries
- How to recognize and treat the different types of burns and electrical injuries
- How to dress and bandage wounds

KEY TERMS

abrasion, p. 648
air embolus, p. 658
amputation, p. 651
avulsion, p. 650
closed wound, p. 645
contusion, p. 646
crush injury, p. 647
dermis, p. 645
epidermis, p. 645
evisceration, p. 668
flail chest, p. 660
full thickness burn, p. 673
hematoma, p. 647
laceration, p. 648
open wound, p. 648
paradoxical motion, p. 661
partial thickness burn, p. 672
pneumothorax, p. 663
puncture wound, p. 649
rule of nines, p. 674
rule of palm, p. 674
subcutaneous layers, p. 645
sucking chest wound, p. 663
superficial burn, p. 671
tension pneumothorax, p. 663

DOT OBJECTIVES

*KNOWLEDGE AND ATTITUDE

5-2.1 State the major functions of the skin. (p. 644)

5-2.2 List the layers of the skin. (p. 645)

5-2.3 Establish the relationship between Standard Precautions (body substance isolation) and soft-tissue injuries. (pp. 648, 652, 653, 686)

5-2.4 List the types of closed soft-tissue injuries. (pp. 646–647)

5-2.5 Describe the emergency medical care of the patient with a closed soft-tissue injury. (p. 648)

5-2.6 State the types of open soft-tissue injuries. (pp. 648–652)

5-2.7 Describe the emergency medical care of the patient with an open soft-tissue injury. (p. 653)

5-2.8 Discuss the emergency medical care considerations for a patient with a penetrating chest injury. (pp. 659, 662–664)

5-2.9 State the emergency medical care considerations for a patient with an open wound to the abdomen. (pp. 668–669) (Scan 27-2, p. 670)

5-2.10 Differentiate the care of an open wound to the chest from an open wound to the abdomen. (pp. 662–670)

5-2.11 List the classifications of burns. (pp. 671–677)

5-2.12 Define superficial burn. (p. 671)

5-2.13 List the characteristics of a superficial burn. (pp. 671–672)

5-2.14 Define partial thickness burn. (p. 672)

5-2.15 List the characteristics of a partial thickness burn. (p. 672)

5-2.16 Define full thickness burn. (p. 673)

5-2.17 List the characteristics of a full thickness burn. (p. 673)

5-2.18 Describe the emergency medical care of the patient with a superficial burn. (p. 678)

5-2.19 Describe the emergency medical care of the patient with a partial thickness burn. (p. 678)

5-2.20 Describe the emergency medical care of the patient with a full thickness burn. (p. 678)

5-2.21 List the functions of dressing and bandaging. (pp. 683, 685) (Scan 27-3, p. 684)

5-2.22 Describe the purpose of a bandage. (p. 683)

5-2.23 Describe the steps in applying a pressure dressing. (p. 685)

5-2.24 Establish the relationship between airway management and the patient with chest injury, burns, and blunt and penetrating injuries. (pp. 648, 652, 654, 656, 657, 659, 663, 668, 669, 671, 675, 676, 678, 681, 683)

5-2.25 Describe the effects of improperly applied dressings, splints, and tourniquets. (pp. 685–686). (Air splints and tourniquets were discussed in Chapter 26, "Bleeding and Shock." Splints will be discussed in Chapter 28, "Musculoskeletal Injuries.")

5-2.26 Describe the emergency medical care of a patient with an impaled object. (pp. 654–657)

5-2.27 Describe the emergency medical care of a patient with an amputation. (p. 658)

5-2.28 Describe the emergency care for a chemical burn. (pp. 679–680)

5-2.29 Describe the emergency care for an electrical burn. (pp. 681–683)

*SKILLS

5-2.30 Demonstrate the steps in emergency medical care of closed and open soft-tissue injuries.

5-2.31 Demonstrate the steps in emergency medical care of a patient with an open chest wound.

5-2.32 Demonstrate the steps in emergency medical care of a patient with open abdominal wounds.

5-2.33 Demonstrate the steps in emergency medical care of a patient with an impaled object.

5-2.34 Demonstrate the steps in emergency medical care of a patient with an amputation.

5-2.35 Demonstrate the steps in emergency medical care of an amputated part.

5-2.36 Demonstrate the steps in emergency medical care of a patient with superficial burns.

5-2.37 Demonstrate the steps in emergency medical care of a patient with partial thickness burns.

5-2.38 Demonstrate the steps in emergency medical care of a patient with full thickness burns.

5-2.39 Demonstrate the steps in emergency medical care of a patient with a chemical burn.

5-2.40 Demonstrate completing a prehospital care report for patients with soft-tissue injuries.

EMTs are frequently called to deal with injuries to the soft tissues of the body. These injuries may range from minor scrapes and bruises to life-threatening injuries to the chest and abdomen. It is the EMT's responsibility to identify and treat each of these injuries skillfully and professionally. Many soft-tissue injuries are open wounds, which can be very upsetting to the patient. Your emotional care and demeanor will mean a great deal. Overall, the assessment and care of the patient with a soft-tissue injury will be a challenging part of your responsibilities as an EMT.

SOFT TISSUES

The soft tissues of the body include the skin, fatty tissues, muscles, blood vessels, fibrous tissues, membranes (tissues that line or cover organs), glands, and nerves (Figure 27-1). Teeth, bones, and cartilage are considered hard tissues.

The most obvious soft-tissue injuries involve the skin (Figure 27-2). Most people do not think of the skin as a body organ, but it is. In fact, it is the largest organ of the human body. The skin's total surface area is over 20 square feet. The major functions of the skin include:

- *Protection.* The skin is a barrier that keeps out microorganisms (germs), debris, and unwanted chemicals. Underlying tissues and organs are protected from environmental contact.
- *Water balance.* The skin helps prevent water loss and stops environmental water from entering the body. This helps preserve the chemical balance of body fluids and tissues.
- *Temperature regulation.* Blood vessels in the skin can dilate (increase in diameter) to carry more blood to the skin, allowing heat to radiate away from the body. When the body needs to conserve heat, these vessels constrict (decrease in diameter) to prevent heat loss. The sweat glands found in the skin produce perspiration, which will evaporate and help cool the body. The fat that is part of the skin serves as a thermal insulator.
- *Excretion.* Salts, carbon dioxide, and excess water can be released through the skin.
- *Shock (impact) absorption.* The skin and its layers of fat help protect the underlying organs from minor impacts and pressures.

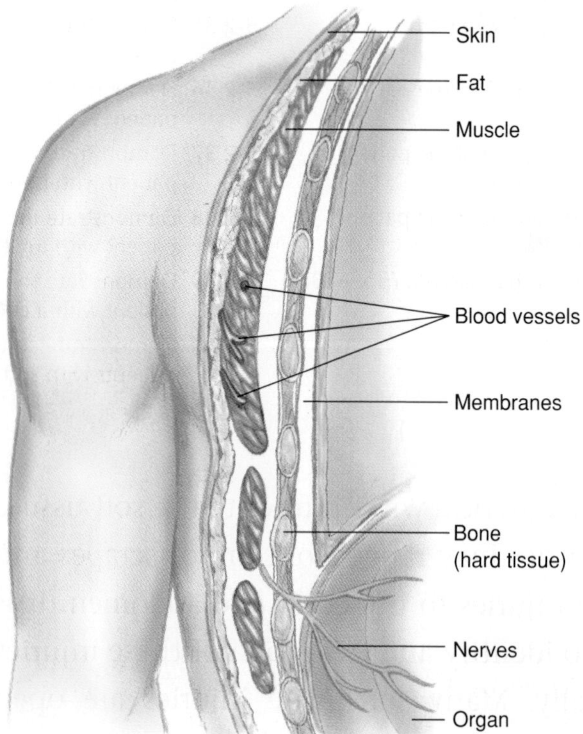

Figure 27-1 • Soft tissues.

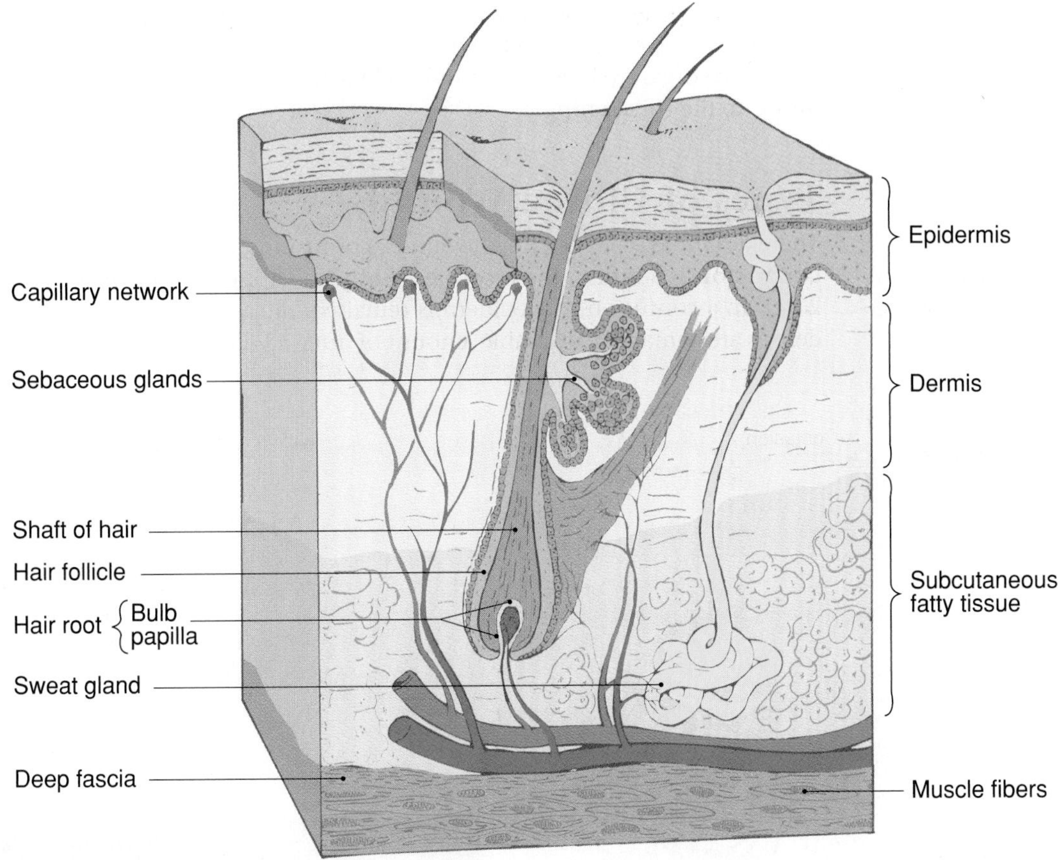

Figure 27-2 • The skin.

The skin has three major layers: the epidermis, the dermis, and the subcutaneous layer. The outer layer of the skin is the **epidermis.** The outermost epidermis is composed of dead cells, which are rubbed off or sloughed off and are replaced. The pigment granules of the skin and living cells are found deeper in the epidermis. The cells of the innermost portion are actively dividing, replacing the dead cells of the outer layers. The epidermis contains no blood vessels or nerves. Except for certain types of burns and injuries due to cold, injuries of the epidermis present few problems in EMT-level care.

epidermis (ep-i-DER-mis) the outer layer of the skin.

The layer of skin below the epidermis is the **dermis.** This layer is rich with blood vessels, nerves, and specialized structures such as sweat glands, sebaceous (oil) glands, and hair follicles. Specialized nerve endings in the dermis are involved with the senses of touch, cold, heat, and pain. Once the dermis is opened to the outside world, contamination and infection become major problems. Such wounds can be serious, accompanied by profuse bleeding and intense pain.

dermis (DER-mis) the inner (second) layer of the skin found beneath the epidermis. It is rich in blood vessels and nerves.

The layers of fat and soft tissue below the dermis are called the **subcutaneous layers.** Shock absorption and insulation are major functions of this layer. Again, when these layers are injured there are problems of tissue and bloodstream contamination, bleeding, and pain.

Soft-tissue injuries are generally classified as closed wounds or open wounds.

subcutaneous (SUB-ku-TAY-ne-us) **layers** the layers of fat and soft tissues found below the dermis.

CLOSED WOUNDS

closed wound an internal injury with no open pathway from the outside.

A **closed wound** is an internal injury; that is, there is no open pathway from the outside to the injured site. These wounds usually result from the impact of a blunt object. Although the skin itself may not be broken, there may be extensively crushed tissues beneath it. Closed wounds can be simple bruises, internal lacerations (cuts), and internal punctures caused by fractured bones, crushing forces, or the rupture (bursting open) of internal organs (Figure 27-3). Internal bleeding from a closed wound can range from minor to life threatening.

Types of Closed Wounds

contusion (kun-TU-zhun) a bruise.

There are three types of closed wounds: contusions, hematomas, and crush injuries. A **contusion** is a bruise, the most frequently encountered type of closed wound (Figure 27-4). In a contusion, the epidermis remains intact, but cells and blood vessels in the dermis are damaged. A variable amount of internal bleeding occurs at the time of injury

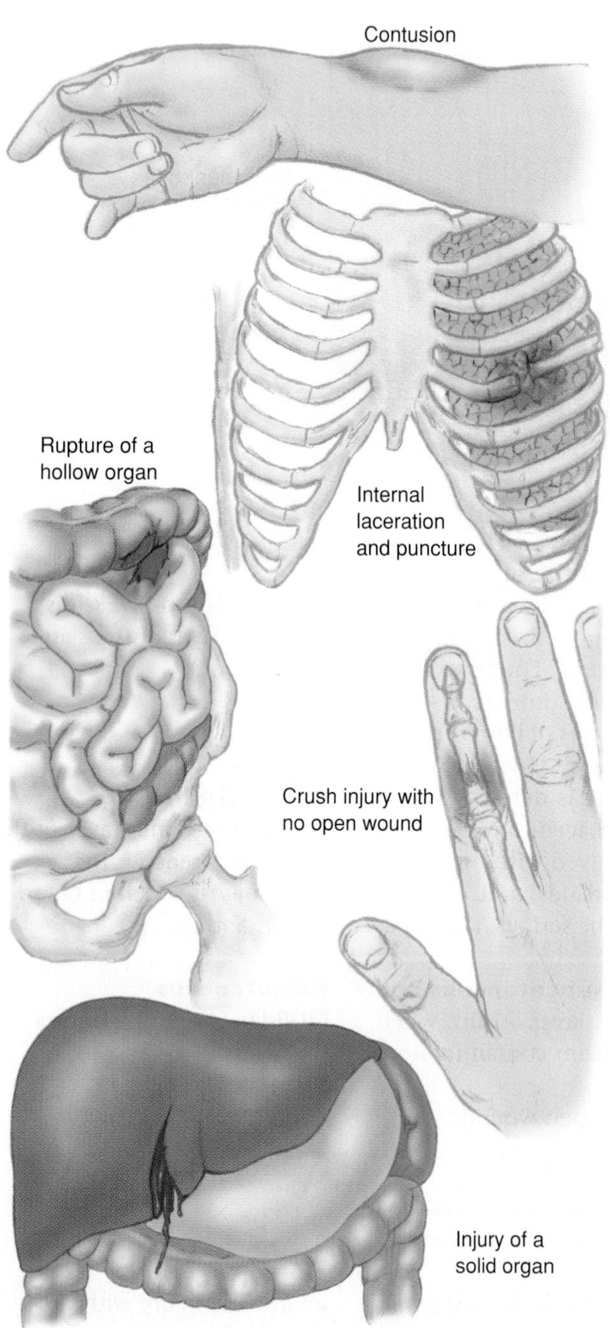

Figure 27-3 • Closed wounds.

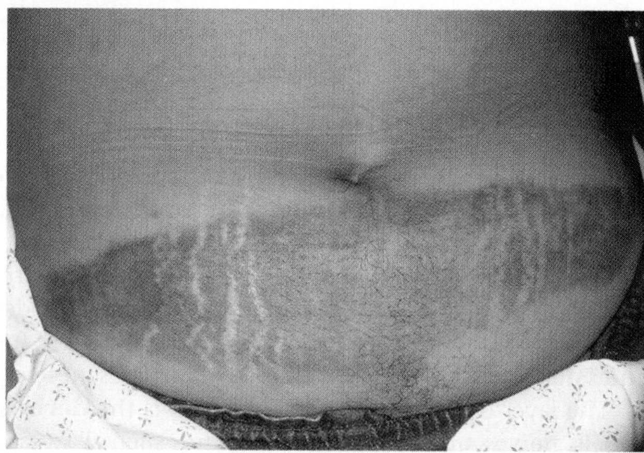

Figure 27-4 • Contusions are the most common type of closed wound. *(© Charles Stewart, M.D. and Associates)*

and may continue for a few hours. There is pain, swelling, and discoloration at the wound site. Swelling and discoloration may occur immediately or may be delayed as much as 24 to 48 hours. The swelling is caused by a collection of blood under the skin or within the damaged tissues. Other organs such as the kidneys or brain may also be contused.

Blood almost always collects at the injury site. This results in a **hematoma.** A hematoma differs from a contusion in that hematomas involve a larger amount of tissue damage, including damage to larger blood vessels with greater internal blood loss. As much as a liter of blood may be lost in a hematoma.

hematoma
(hem-ah-TO-mah)
a swelling caused by the collection of blood under the skin or in damaged tissues as a result of an injured or broken blood vessel.

Force can be transmitted from the body's exterior to its internal structures, even when the skin remains intact and even when the only indication of injury is a simple bruise. This force can cause the internal organs to be crushed or ruptured, causing internal bleeding. This is called a **crush injury.** Solid organs such as the liver and spleen normally contain considerable amounts of blood. When crushed, they bleed severely and cause shock. Contents of hollow organs, such as digested food or urine, can leak into the body cavities, causing severe inflammation and tissue damage.

crush injury
an injury caused when force is transmitted from the body's exterior to its internal structures. Bones can be broken; muscles, nerves, and tissues damaged; and internal organs ruptured, causing internal bleeding.

PATIENT ASSESSMENT

CLOSED WOUNDS

Bruising may be an indication of internal injuries and related internal bleeding (Table 27-1). In addition, consider the possibility of closed soft-tissue injuries whenever there is swelling, pain, or deformity, and a mechanism of blunt trauma. Always consider the mechanism of injury (MOI) when you examine a patient with a closed wound. Crush injuries may be difficult or impossible to identify during assessment, so you must rely on the MOI. Patients with a significant MOI should be considered to have internal bleeding and shock until they are ruled out in the emergency department. ■

TABLE 27-1 • Contusions (Bruises) as Signs of Soft-Tissue Injury

SIGN	INDICATES
Large bruise or bruised areas directly over body	Possible injury to underlying organs such as the spleen, liver, or kidneys.
Swelling or deformity at site of bruise	Possible underlying fracture.
Bruise on the head or neck	Possible injury to the cervical spine or brain. Search for blood in the mouth, nose, and ears.
Bruise on the trunk or signs of damage to the ribs or sternum	Possible chest injury. Determine if the patient is coughing up frothy red blood, which may indicate a punctured lung, and assess for difficult breathing. Use your stethoscope to listen for equal air entry and any unusual breath sounds.
Bruise on the abdomen	Possible injury to the abdominal organs. Look to see if the patient has vomited. If so, is there any substance in the vomitus that looks like coffee grounds (partially digested blood)? Palpate to detect if patient's abdomen is rigid or tender.

Note: Treatment for internal bleeding is discussed in Chapter 26, "Bleeding and Shock"; treatment of head injury in Chapter 29, "Injuries to the Head and Spine"; treatment of chest and abdominal injuries in this chapter.

PATIENT CARE

CLOSED WOUNDS

Take the appropriate Standard Precautions and follow these steps for emergency care of a patient with closed wounds:

1. Manage the patient's airway, breathing, and circulation. Apply high-concentration oxygen by nonrebreather mask.
2. MANAGE AS IF THERE IS INTERNAL BLEEDING and PROVIDE CARE FOR SHOCK, if you believe that there is any possibility of internal injuries.
3. Splint extremities that are painful, swollen, or deformed.
4. Stay alert for the patient to vomit.
5. Continue to monitor the patient for the development of shock and transport as soon as possible. ■

OPEN WOUNDS

open wound an injury in which the skin is interrupted, exposing the tissue beneath.

An **open wound** is an injury in which the skin is interrupted, or broken, exposing the tissues underneath. The interruption can come from the outside, as a laceration, or from the inside when a fractured bone end tears outward through the skin.

Types of Open Wounds

Abrasions

abrasion (ab-RAY-zhun) a scratch or scrape.

The classification of **abrasion** includes simple scrapes and scratches in which the outer layer of the skin is damaged but not all the layers are penetrated (Figure 27-5). Skinned elbows and knees, *road rash*, *mat burns*, *rug burns*, and *brush burns* are examples of abrasions. With abrasions, there may be no detectable bleeding or only the minor ooze of blood from capillary beds. The patient may be experiencing great pain, even if the injury is minor. Because of dirt or other substances ground into the skin, the opportunity for infection is great.

Lacerations

laceration (las-er-AY-shun) a cut.

A **laceration** is a cut. It may be smooth or jagged (Figure 27-6). This type of wound is often caused by an object with a sharp edge, such as a razor blade, broken glass, or a

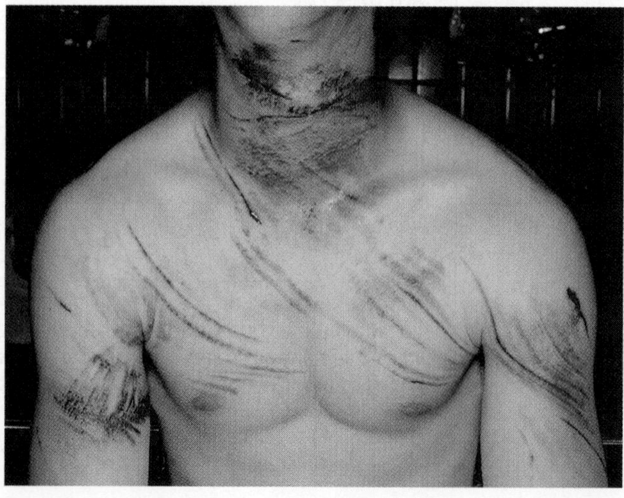

Figure 27-5 • Abrasions are usually the least serious type of open wound. *(© Charles Stewart, M.D. and Associates)*

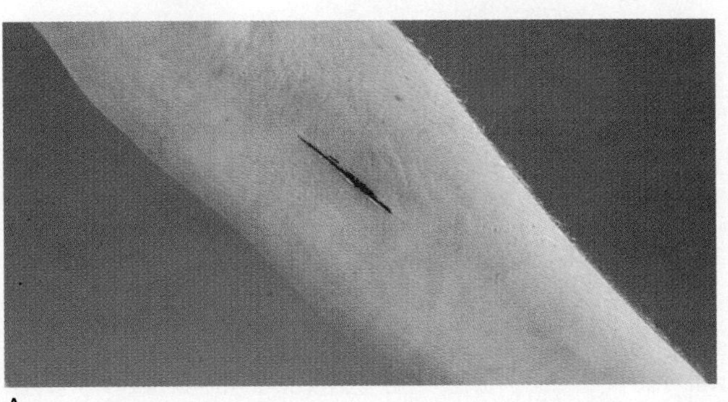

A

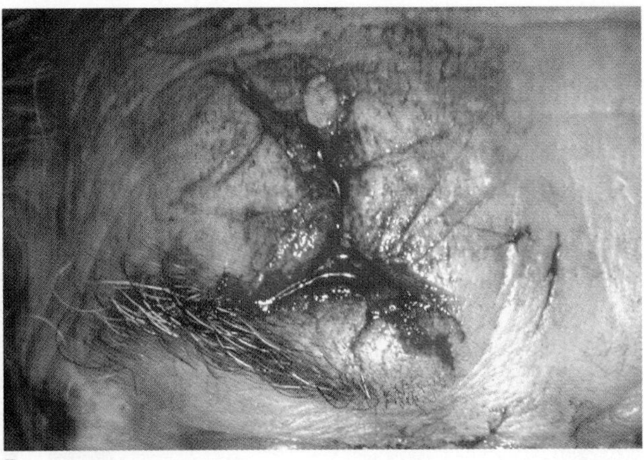

B

Figure 27-6 • (A) Some lacerations have smooth edges, and (B) some have jagged edges. *(Photo B: © Dr. Paula Moynahan, Moynahan Medical Center)*

jagged piece of metal. However, a laceration can also result from a severe blow or impact with a blunt object. If the laceration has rough edges, it may tend to fall together and obstruct the view as you try to determine the wound depth. It is usually impossible to look at the outside of a laceration and determine the extent of the damage to underlying tissues. If significant blood vessels have been torn, bleeding will be considerable. Sometimes the bleeding is partially controlled when blood vessels are stretched and torn. This is due to the natural retraction and constriction of the cut ends that aid in rapid clot formation.

puncture wound
an open wound that tears through the skin and destroys underlying tissues. A *penetrating puncture wound* can be shallow or deep. A *perforating puncture wound* has both an entrance and an exit wound.

Punctures

When a sharp, pointed object passes through the skin or other tissue, a **puncture wound** has occurred. Typically, puncture wounds are caused by objects such as nails, ice picks, splinters, or knives (Figure 27-7). Often, there is no severe external bleeding,

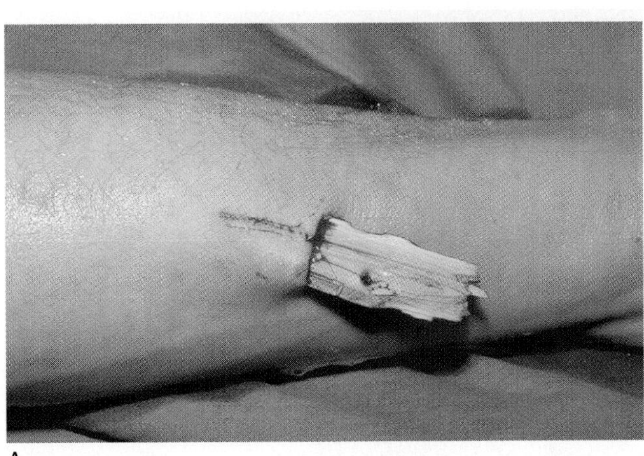

A

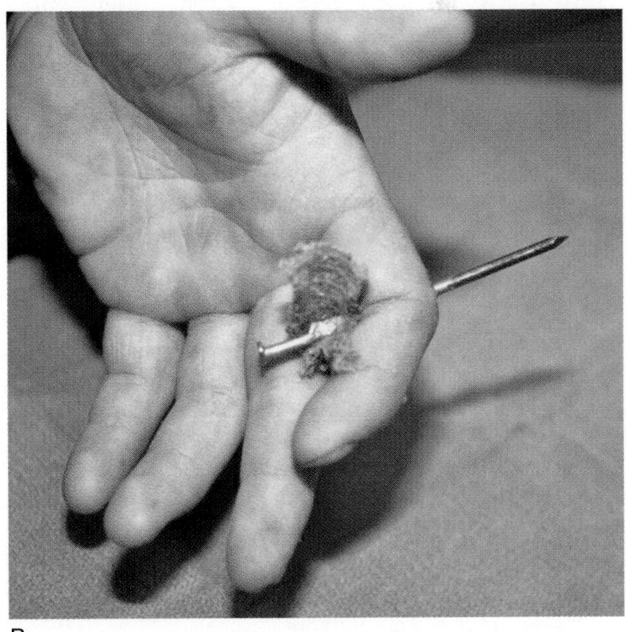

B

Figure 27-7 • (A) A penetrating puncture wound *(© Charles Stewart, M.D. and Associates)* and (B) a perforating puncture wound. *(© Edward T. Dickinson, M.D.)*

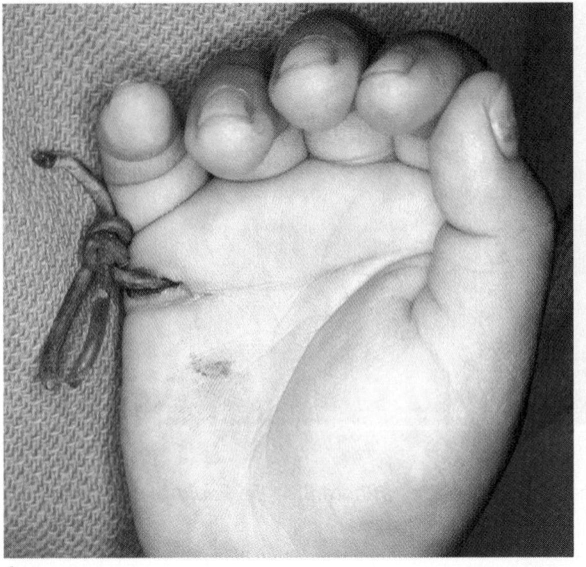

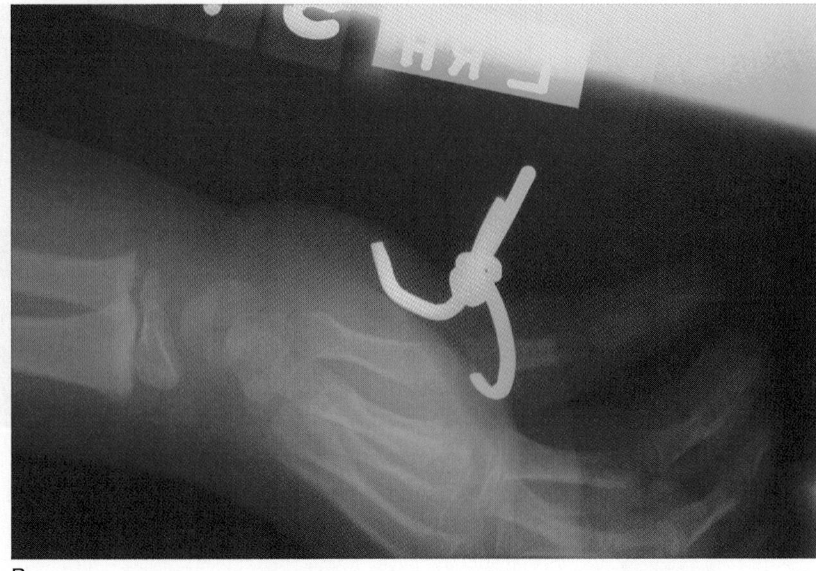

A B

Figure 27-8 • (A) A penetrating puncture wound, external view, and (B) an X-ray of the same wound. *(Both: © Charles Stewart, M.D. and Associates)*

but internal bleeding may be profuse. The threat of contamination must always be seriously considered.

There are two types of puncture wounds. A *penetrating puncture wound* can be shallow or deep (Figures 27-7 and 27-8). In either case, tissues and blood vessels are injured. A *perforating puncture wound* has both an entrance wound and an exit wound (Figure 27-9). The object causing the injury passes through the body and out again. In many cases, the exit wound is more serious than the entrance wound. A "through-and-through" gunshot wound is an example of a perforating puncture wound.

avulsion (ah-VUL-shun) the tearing away or tearing off of a piece or flap of skin or other soft tissue. This term also may be used for an eye pulled from its socket or a tooth dislodged from its socket.

Avulsions

In an **avulsion,** flaps of skin and tissues are torn loose or pulled off completely (Figure 27-10). When the tip of the nose is cut or torn off, this is an avulsion. The same applies to the external ear. A degloving avulsion occurs when the hand is caught in a roller. In this type of incident, the skin is stripped off like a glove. An eye pulled from its socket

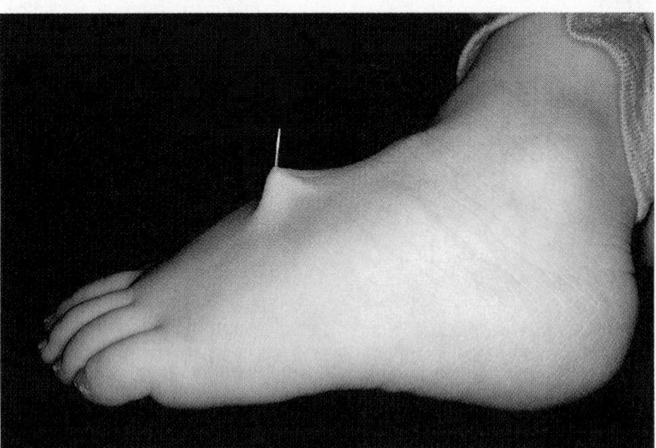

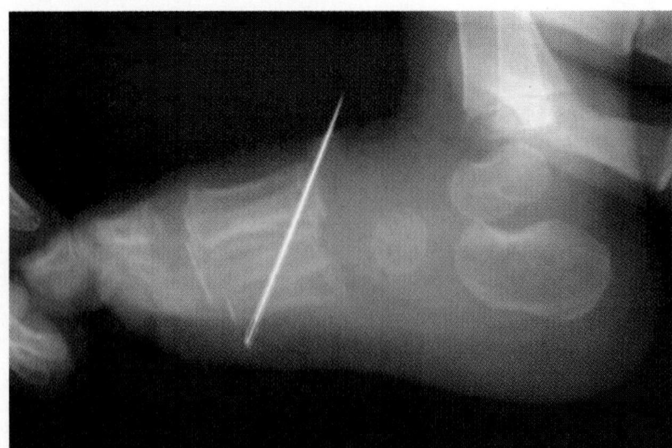

Figure 27-9 • This perforating puncture wound has both an entry wound (at the bottom of the foot) and an exit wound (at the top of the foot). *(Both: © Charles Stewart, M.D. and Associates)*

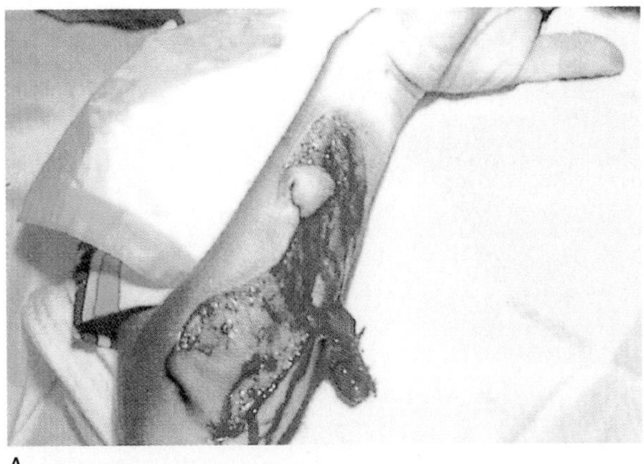
A

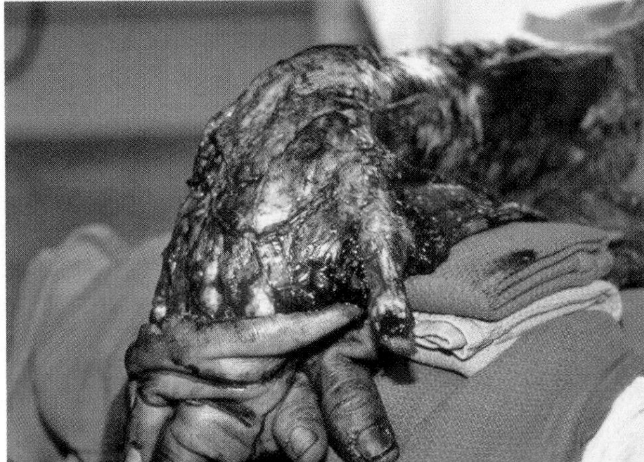
B

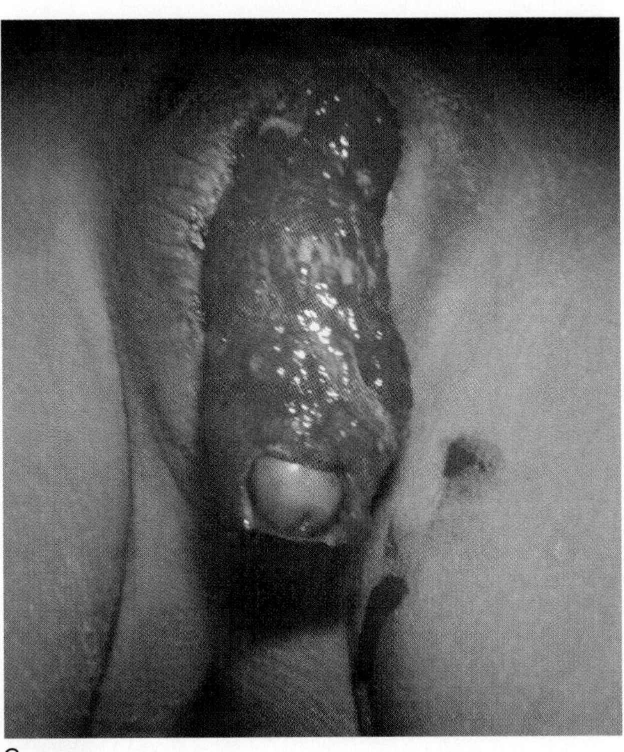
C

Figure 27-10 • (A) An avulsion, (B) an avulsion injury that caused a degloving *(© Edward T. Dickinson, M.D.),* and (C) an avulsion of male genitalia. *(© Dr. Paula Moynahan, Moynahan Medical Center)*

(extruded) is also a form of avulsion. The term *avulsed* is used in reporting the wound, as in "an avulsed eye" or "an avulsed ear." When tissue is avulsed, it is cut off from its oxygen supply and will soon die.

Amputations

The extremities are sometimes subject to **amputation.** Amputated fingers, toes, hands, feet, or limbs are completely cut through or torn off (Figure 27-11). Jagged skin and bone edges can sometimes be observed. There may be massive bleeding; or the force that amputates a limb may close off torn blood vessels, limiting the amount of bleeding. Often, blood vessels collapse, or they retract and constrict, which limits bleeding from the wound site.

amputation
(am-pyu-TAY-shun)
the surgical removal or traumatic severing of a body part, usually an extremity.

Crush Injuries

Crush injuries were discussed earlier in this chapter as closed wounds, but crush injuries also can be open wounds. An open crush injury can result when an extremity is caught between heavy items, such as pieces of machinery. Blood vessels, nerves, and muscles are involved, and swelling may be a major problem with resulting loss of blood supply distally. Bones are fractured and may protrude through the wound site. Soft tissues and

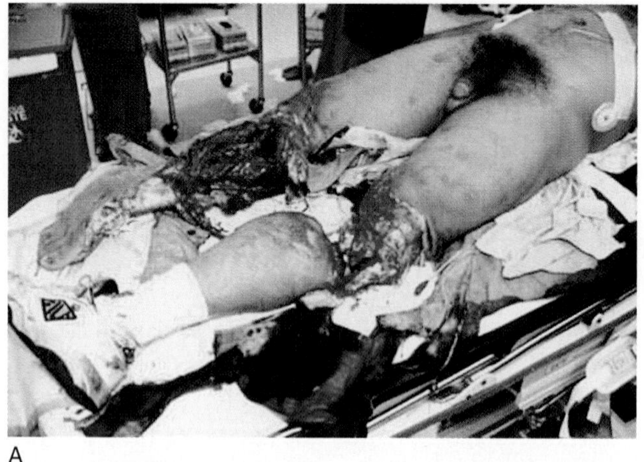

A

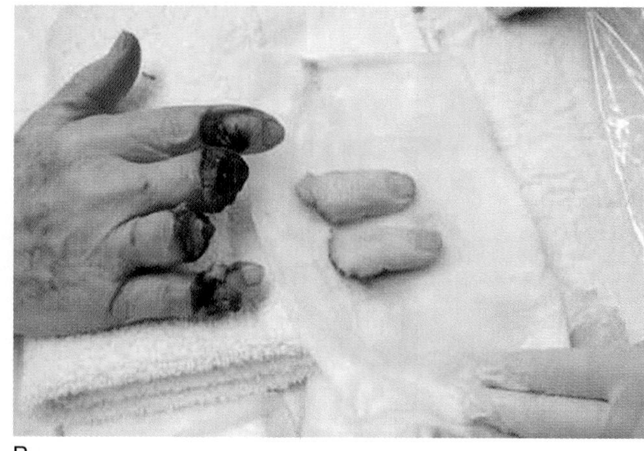

B

Figure 27-11 • (A) Amputated leg. (B) Amputated fingers. *(Both: © Edward T. Dickinson, M.D.)*

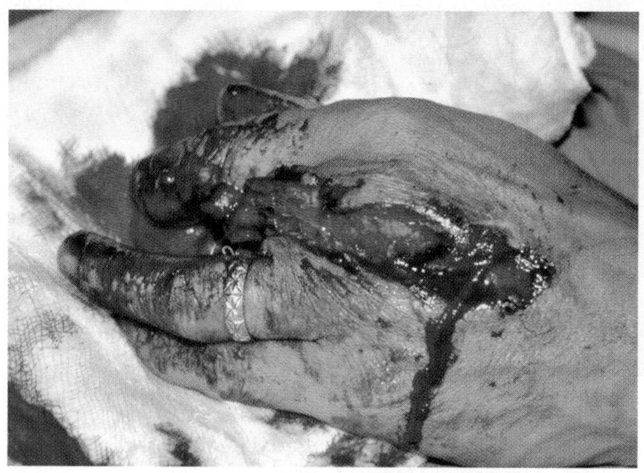

Figure 27-12 • An open crush injury. Consider early removal of the ring, as swelling may occur. *(© John Callan/Shout Picture Library)*

internal organs can be crushed to produce profuse bleeding, both externally and internally (Figure 27-12).

Emergency Care for Open Wounds

Open wounds require strict attention to Standard Precautions. In addition to wearing gloves, a gown and protective eyewear may also be required. Remember to properly dispose of all soiled materials and wash your hands after each call.

PATIENT ASSESSMENT

OPEN WOUNDS

Airway, breathing, circulation, and severe bleeding are identified and treated in the initial assessment. Once the initial assessment and the appropriate physical examination have been completed, care for the individual wounds begins. ■

PATIENT CARE

OPEN WOUNDS

The following steps are general guidelines for emergency care of open wounds. Steps for specific kinds of open wounds appear on the following pages. Take appropriate Standard Precautions and:

1. Expose the wound. Clothing that covers a soft-tissue injury must be lifted, cut, or split away. For some articles of clothing, this is best done with scissors or a seam cutter. Do not attempt to remove clothing in the usual manner, which can aggravate existing injuries and cause additional damage and pain.
2. Clean the wound surface. Do not try to pick embedded particles and debris from the wound. Simply remove large pieces of foreign matter from the surface. When possible, use a piece of sterile dressing to brush away large debris while protecting the wound from contact with your soiled gloves. Do not spend much time cleaning the wound. Control of bleeding is the priority.
3. Control bleeding. Start with direct pressure, or direct pressure and elevation. If bleeding does not stop use a tourniquet or hemostatic dressings as directed in your local protocols (see Chapter 26, "Bleeding and Shock").
4. For all serious wounds, provide care for shock, including administration of high-flow, high-concentration oxygen (see Chapter 26, "Bleeding and Shock").
5. Prevent further contamination. Use a sterile dressing. When none is available, use the cleanest cloth material at the scene.
6. Bandage the dressing in place after bleeding has been controlled. If an extremity is involved, check for a distal pulse to make certain that circulation has not been interrupted by the application of a tight bandage. With the exception of a pressure dressing, bleeding must be controlled before bandaging is started. Periodically recheck the bandage to make certain that bleeding has not restarted.
7. Keep the patient lying still. Any movement will increase circulation and could restart bleeding.
8. Reassure the patient. This will help ease the patient's emotional response and perhaps lower his pulse rate and blood pressure. In some cases this may help to reduce the bleeding rate. Also, a patient who feels reassured will usually be more willing to lie still, reducing the chances of restarting bleeding. ■

TREATING SPECIFIC TYPES OF OPEN WOUNDS

Treating Abrasions and Lacerations

In treating abrasions, take care to reduce wound contamination. Bleeding from a long, deep laceration may be difficult to control, but direct pressure over a dressing usually works well. The air-inflated splint can be useful in the management of this type of wound when it is applied over a dressing. Do not pull apart the edges of a laceration in an effort to see into the wound.

Most lacerations can be cared for by bandaging a dressing in place. Some EMS systems recommend using a butterfly bandage for minor lacerations. (A butterfly bandage is made up of thin strips of adhesive bandaging and is designed to bring the sides of a laceration together.) Bandage a gauze dressing over the butterfly strip.

NOTE

Do not underestimate the effects of a laceration. When evaluating a laceration, check the pulse, as well as motor and sensory function, distal to the injury. The patient may need stitches, plastic surgery, or a tetanus shot at the hospital, so do not put on butterfly bandages and leave the patient at the scene. Serious infection or scarring could result.

Treating Puncture Wounds

Use caution when caring for puncture wounds. An object that appears to be embedded only in the skin may actually go all the way to the bone. In such cases, it is possible that the patient may not have any serious pain. Even an apparently moderate puncture wound may cause extensive internal injury with serious internal bleeding. What appears at first to be a simple, shallow puncture wound may be only part of the problem. There also could be a severe exit wound that requires immediate care, so be sure to search for one.

Gunshot wounds are puncture wounds that can fracture bones and cause extensive soft-tissue and organ injury. The seriousness of the wound cannot be determined by the caliber of the bullet or the point of entry and exit. The bullet may have tumbled through tissues, been deflected off a bone, fragmented, or exploded inside the body (Figure 27-13). All bullet wounds are considered serious. If the bullet has penetrated the body, you must assume that there is considerable internal injury. Close-range shootings often have burns around the entry wound. Remember that any gunshot wound to the face, no matter how minor, can create airway problems. Air guns fired at close range can cause serious damage by injecting air into the tissues.

All stab wounds should be considered serious, especially when they involve the head, neck, chest, abdomen, or groin.

Care for a patient with a moderate or serious puncture wound includes these steps:

1. Reassure the alert patient. Such wounds can be frightening.
2. Search for an exit wound, especially when there is a gunshot wound. Control bleeding and provide adequate wound treatment to both the entry and exit wounds.
3. Assess the need for basic life support whenever there is a gunshot wound. Care for shock, administering high-concentration oxygen.
4. Immobilize the spine when the patient's head, neck, or torso is involved.
5. Transport the patient. If the object that caused the puncture wound is available, take it to the emergency department for examination also.

Treating Impaled Objects

A puncture wound may contain an impaled object. The object may be a knife, a fence post or guard rail, a shard of glass, or even a wooden stick, piercing any part of the body. Even though it is rare, you may be confronted with an impaled object that is long

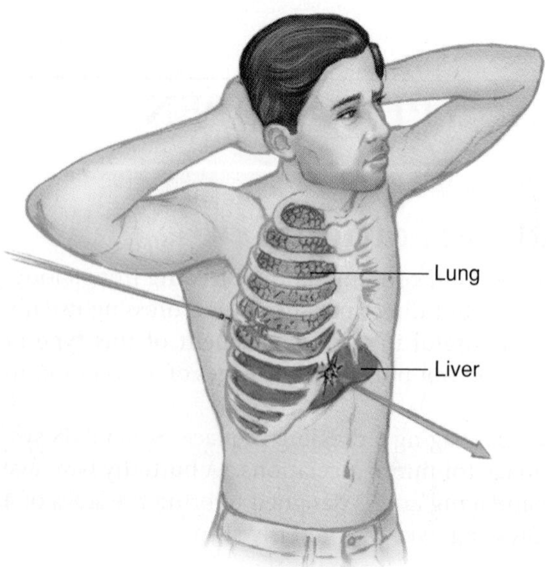

Figure 27-13 • Bullets travel an unpredictable path once inside the body and can cause damage to multiple organs and bones.

enough to make transport impossible unless the object is shortened. In such cases, contact the emergency department physician for specific directions. Usually, someone must hold the object, keeping it very stable, while you gently saw through it at the desired length. A fine-toothed saw with rigid blade support (e.g., a hack saw or reciprocating saw) should be used. In some cases, you may need to leave the object in place as found. The challenge in these cases is stabilization of the object.

In general, when caring for a patient with a puncture wound involving an impaled object, DO NOT REMOVE THE IMPALED OBJECT. The object may be plugging bleeding from a major artery while it is in place. Removing may cause severe bleeding when the pressure is released. Removal of the object also may cause further injury to nerves, muscles, and other soft tissues. Any movement of the impaled object at the skin's surface will be magnified several times in the inner tissues. Proceed as follows:

1. Expose the wound area. Cut away clothing, taking great care not to disturb the object. Do not attempt to lift clothing over the object; you may accidentally move it. Long impaled objects may have to be stabilized by hand during exposure, bleeding control, and dressing.
2. Control profuse bleeding by direct pressure if possible. Be careful to position your gloved hands on either side of the object and exert pressure downward. *Do not put pressure on the object.* Apply pressure with great care if the object has a cutting edge, such as a knife or a shard of glass; otherwise, you may cause additional injury to the patient. Be careful not to injure your hands or damage your gloves.
3. While you continue to stabilize the object and control bleeding, have another trained rescuer place several layers of bulky dressing around the injury site so that the dressings surround the object on all sides (Figure 27-14). Manual stabilization must continue until the stabilizing dressings are secured in place.

   Have the other rescuer begin by placing folded universal pads, sanitary napkins, or some other bulky dressing material on opposite sides of the object. For long or large objects, folded towels, blankets, or pillows may have to be used in place of dressing pads. Remove your hands from under the pads. Place them on top and apply pressure as each layer is placed in position. The next layer of pads should be placed on opposite sides of the object, perpendicular to the first layer. Continue this process until as much of the object as possible has been stabilized.

   Once bandaged in place, the dressings will stabilize the object and exert downward pressure on bleeding vessels. Keep in mind that there is a limited amount of time that can be given to stabilizing an impaled object. Stay in contact with the Medical Director for directions and recommendations.
4. Secure the dressings in place. Although adhesive strips may hold the dressings in place, blood around the wound site, sweat, and body movements may not allow you to use tape. Triangular bandages folded into strips (cravats) can be applied by tying one above and one below the impaled object. The cravats should be wide (no less than 4 inches

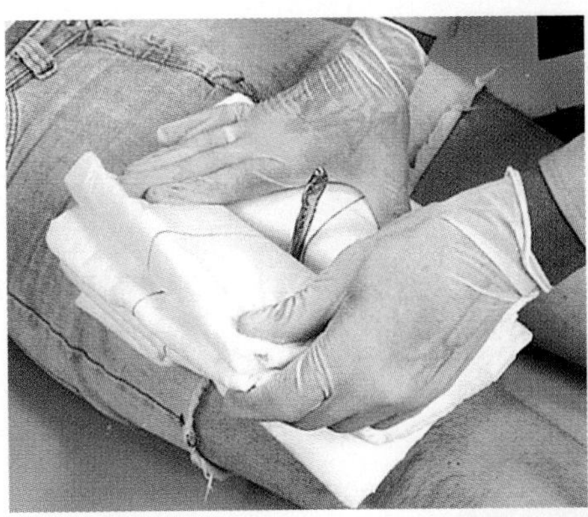

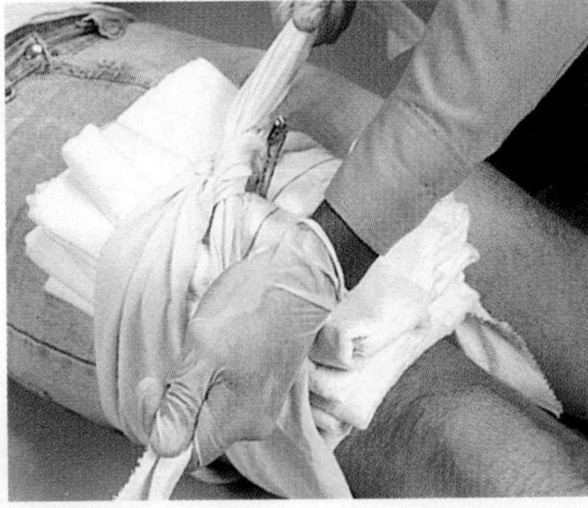

Figure 27-14 • Stabilize an impaled object with a bulky dressing.

in width once folded). A thin rigid splint can be used to push the cravats under the patient's back when they are needed to care for objects impaled in the trunk of the body.

5. Care for shock. Provide oxygen at the highest possible flow and concentration. When appropriate, oxygen administration and heat conservation measures should be accomplished as soon as possible. When working by yourself, these may have to be delayed while you attempt to control bleeding.
6. Keep the patient at rest. Position the patient for minimum stress. If possible, immobilize the affected area, for example with a splint or a spine board. Provide emotional support.
7. Transport the patient carefully and as soon as possible. Avoid any movement that may jar, loosen, or dislodge the object. If the object was removed by bystanders before you arrived, bring it to the hospital for examination.
8. Reassure the patient throughout all aspects of care. An alert patient with an impaled object is usually very frightened.

Object Impaled in the Cheek

A dangerous situation exists when the cheek has been penetrated by a foreign object. First, the object may go into the oral cavity and create an airway obstruction, or it may stay impaled in the cheek wall but work its way free and enter the oral cavity later. Second, when the cheek wall is perforated, bleeding into the mouth and throat can be profuse and interfere with breathing, or it may make the patient nauseated and induce vomiting. External wound care will not stop the flow of blood into the mouth.

If you find a patient with an object impaled in the cheek, you should (Figure 27-15):

1. Examine the wound site. Gently inspect both the external cheek and the inside of the mouth. Use your penlight and look into the patient's mouth. If need be, carefully use your gloved fingers to probe the inside cheek to determine if the object has passed through the cheek wall. This is best done with a dressing pad used to protect your fingers and any wound you touch.
2. Remove the object, IF you find perforation and you can SEE BOTH ENDS of the object. Pull it out in the direction that it entered the cheek. If this cannot be done easily, leave the object in place. Do not twist the object. OR IF you find perforation but the tip of the object is also IMPALED INTO A DEEPER STRUCTURE (e.g., the palate), STABILIZE THE OBJECT. Do not try to remove it.
3. Position the patient. Make certain that you allow for drainage (the possibility of spine injuries may require you to immobilize the head, neck, and spine first, then tilt the patient and the spine board as a unit).
4. Monitor the patient's airway, once the object is removed or stabilized. *Be prepared to suction as necessary.* Keep in mind that an object penetrating the cheek wall also may have caused teeth or dentures to break, creating potential airway obstruction. Pay

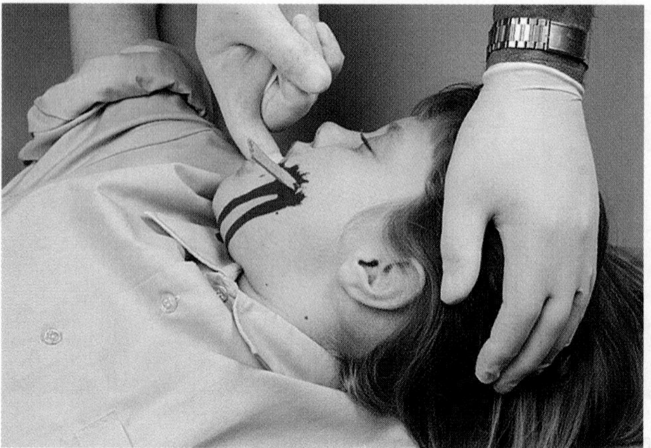

Figure 27-15 • Removing an impaled object from the cheek.

close attention, especially if the patient is not alert. Blood in the patient's mouth can compromise the airway.

5. Dress the outside of the wound using a pressure dressing and bandage or apply a sterile dressing and use direct hand pressure to control the bleeding. You may be able to place gauze on the inside of the cheek to help control bleeding into the mouth, but only if the patient is alert and cooperative. Monitor the patient's mental status closely, and make sure the dressing does not work its way into the airway.
6. Provide oxygen and care for shock. You may have to use a nasal cannula if constant suctioning is required. If any dressing materials are placed in the patient's mouth, use of standard face masks can be dangerous unless you leave 3 to 4 inches of the dressing outside of the patient's mouth.

Puncture Wound or Object Impaled in the Eye

Use loose dressings for a puncture wound to the eye with no impaled object. If you find an object impaled in the eye, you should (Figure 27-16):

1. Stabilize the object. Place a roll of 3-inch gauze bandage or folded 4 × 4s on either side of the object, along the vertical axis of the head in a manner that will stabilize the object.
2. Apply rigid protection. Fit a disposable paper drinking cup or paper cone over the impaled object and allow it to come to rest on the dressing rolls. Do not allow it to touch the object. Do not use a Styrofoam cup, which can flake.
3. Have another rescuer stabilize the dressings and cup while you secure them in place with a self-adherent roller bandage or with a wrapping of gauze. Do not secure the bandage on top of the cup.
4. Dress and bandage the uninjured eye. This will help to reduce sympathetic eye movements.
5. Provide oxygen and care for shock.
6. Reassure the patient and provide emotional support.

This method can also be used as a pressure dressing to control bleeding in the area of the eye.

An alternative to the previous method calls for the rescuer to make a thick dressing with several layers of sterile gauze pads or universal dressings. A hole is cut in the center of this pad, approximately the size of the impaled object. The rescuer then carefully passes this dressing over the impaled object and positions the pad so that the impaled object is centered in the opening. The rest of the procedure remains the same as previously described. If your EMS system has you use this technique, remember that you must take great care not to touch the object as the dressing is set in place.

NOTE

In some EMS systems, step 3 is not part of the recommended treatment for an injured eye. Covering both eyes often makes a patient anxious. Covering the uninjured eye seems to make little, if any, difference in patient outcome. Follow your local protocols.

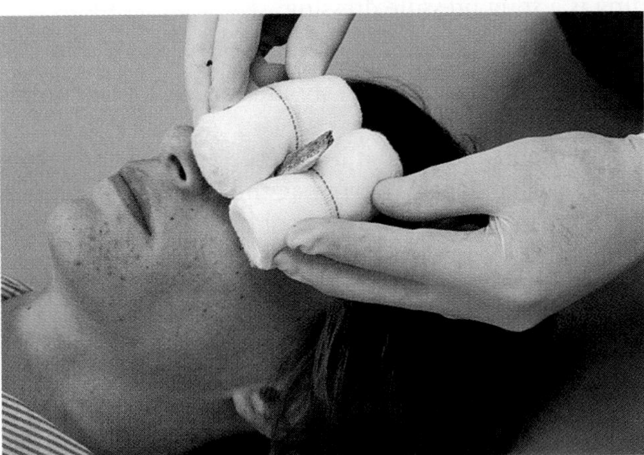

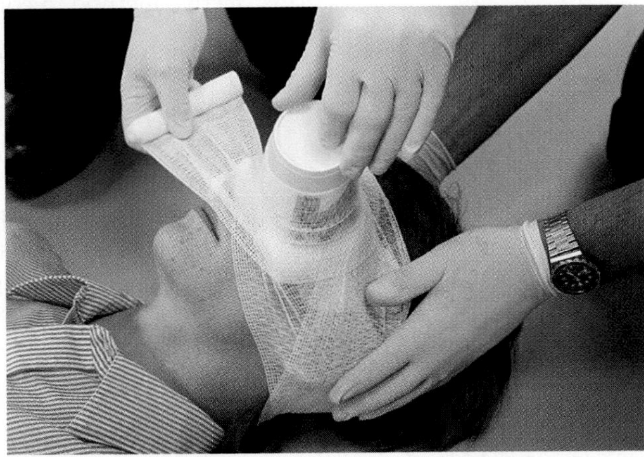

Figure 27-16 • Managing a patient with an object impaled in the eye.

Treating Avulsions

Emergency care for avulsions requires the application of large, bulky pressure dressings. In addition, you should make every effort to preserve any avulsed parts and transport them to the medical facility along with the patient. It may be possible to surgically restore the part or to use it for skin grafts.

In cases in which flaps of skin have been torn loose but not off, follow these steps:

1. Clean the wound surface.
2. Fold the skin back to its normal position as gently as possible.
3. Control bleeding and dress the wound using bulky pressure dressings.

Should skin or another body part be torn from the body, control bleeding and dress the wound using a bulky pressure dressing. Save the avulsed part by wrapping it in a dry sterile gauze dressing secured in place by self-adherent roller bandage. Then place it in a plastic bag, plastic wrap, or aluminum foil, in accordance with local protocol. If none of these items is available at the scene, wrap the avulsed part in a lint-free, dry sterile dressing. (Some research suggests that the sterile wrap should be soaked in sterile saline to make a moist dressing. Follow local protocols.)

Make certain that you label the avulsed part with what it is, the patient's name and date, and the time the part was wrapped and bagged. Your records should show the approximate time of the avulsion. Be sure to keep the part as cool as possible, without freezing it, by placing it in a cooler or any other available container so that it is on top of a cold pack or a SEALED bag of ice. Do not use dry ice. Do not immerse the avulsed part in ice, cooled water, or saline. Label the container the same as the label used for the saved part.

NOTE

The care of avulsed tissues is directed by local protocols, which are often written to match the reimplantation procedures of the hospitals in your EMS system. Some EMS systems prefer that the dressing used to wrap the avulsed part be moistened with sterile normal saline (sterile distilled water is not recommended). This saline must be from a fresh sterile source. Keep in mind that once a sterile source of saline has been opened, it is no longer considered sterile. Take great care if you use this method, since the saline may carry microorganisms from your gloved hand through the dressing to the avulsed part. During your care, remember that avulsions appear grotesque and will be frightening to your patient. Provide reassurance to your patient throughout the call.

Treating Amputations

Never complete an amputation. As in other external bleeding situations, the most effective method to control bleeding is a snug pressure dressing:

1. Apply the pressure dressing. Place it over the stump.
2. Use pressure points to control bleeding. A tourniquet should not be applied unless other methods used to control bleeding have failed.
3. Care for the amputated part. When possible, wrap it in a sterile dressing and secure the dressing with self-adhesive gauze bandage. Wrap or bag the amputated part in a plastic bag and place the bag in a pan with water kept cool by cold packs. Do not immerse the amputated part directly in water or saline. Do not let the part come in direct contact with ice or it may freeze.

Wounds to the Neck

air embolus (EM-bo-lus) a bubble of air in the bloodstream.

Because large arteries and veins lie close to the surface of the neck, the potential for serious bleeding from an open wound is great. Since the pressure in a large vein is likely to be lower than atmospheric pressure, the possibility of an **air embolus** (air bubble) being sucked in through a vein is also great. An air embolus can be carried to the heart and interfere with the heart's ability to circulate blood or actually cause cardiac arrest. The treatment of neck veins is aimed at stopping bleeding and preventing an embolus from entering the circulation.

PATIENT ASSESSMENT

OPEN NECK WOUND

An injury that has severed a major artery or vein of the neck will produce severe bleeding. Arterial bleeding will be profuse, with bright red blood spurting from the wound. Venous bleeding will be profuse with dark red to maroon-colored blood flowing steadily from the wound. ■

PATIENT CARE

OPEN NECK WOUND

Follow these steps for providing emergency care to a patient with an open neck wound (Scan 27-1):

1. Ensure an open airway.
2. Place your gloved hand over the wound.
3. Apply an occlusive dressing to the wound. The dressing should be a thick material that will not be sucked into the wound and must extend 2 inches past the sides of the wound.
4. Place a dressing over the occlusive dressing.
5. Apply pressure as needed to stop the bleeding. Be careful not to compress both carotid arteries at once.
6. Once bleeding has stopped, bandage the dressing in place. Take care not to restrict the airway or the arteries and veins of the neck.
7. If the mechanism of injury could have caused cervical injury, immobilize the spine. ■

Chest Injuries

The chest can be injured in a number of ways, including by blunt trauma, penetrating objects, and compression:

- *Blunt trauma.* A blow to the chest can fracture the ribs, the sternum, and the costal (rib) cartilages. Whole sections of the chest can collapse. With severe blunt trauma, the lungs and airway can be damaged and the great vessels (aorta and venae cavae) and the heart may be seriously injured.
- *Penetrating objects.* Bullets, knives, pieces of metal or glass, steel rods, pipes, and various other objects can penetrate the chest wall, damaging internal organs and impairing respiration.
- *Compression.* This results from severe blunt trauma in which the chest is rapidly compressed, as when a driver in a motor-vehicle collision strikes his chest on the steering column. The heart can be severely squeezed, the lungs can be ruptured, and the sternum and ribs can be fractured.

SCAN 27-1 • Dressing an Open Neck Wound

First take Standard Precautions.

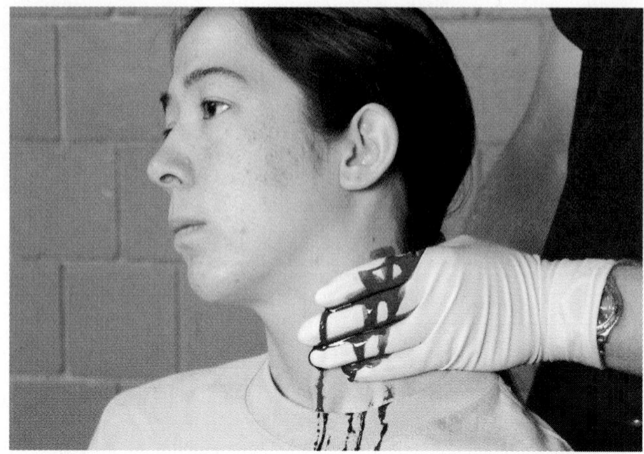

1. Do not delay! Place your gloved palm over the wound.

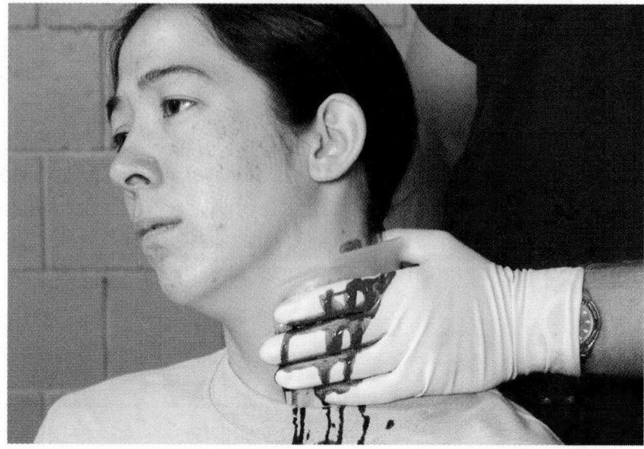

2. Place an occlusive dressing over the wound. It must be heavy plastic, sized to be 2 inches larger in diameter than the wound site.

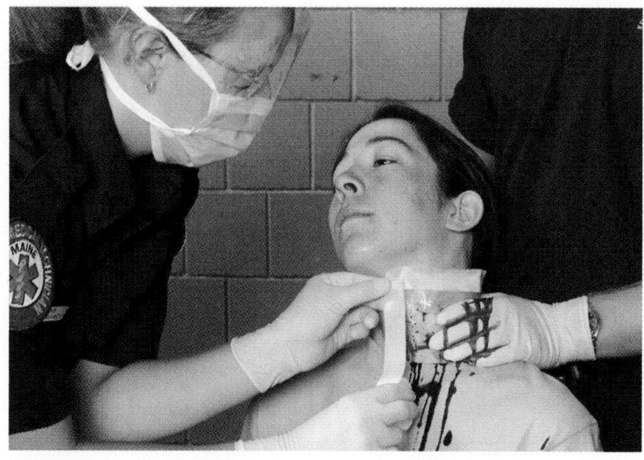

3. Seal the dressing with tape on all four sides.

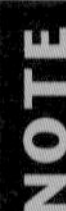

For demonstration purposes, the patient is upright.

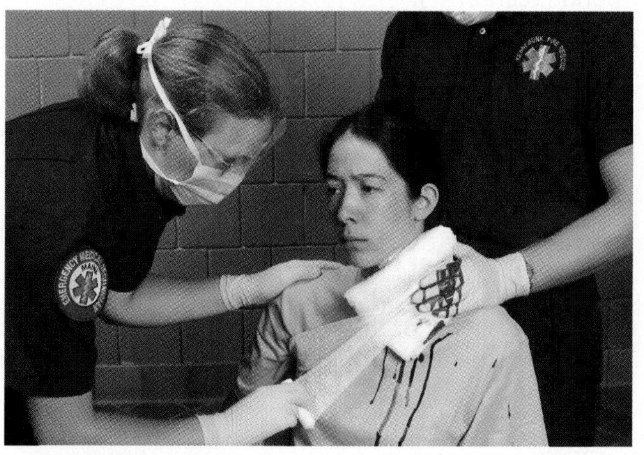

4. Cover the occlusive dressing with a large gauze dressing. Bring a bandage over the dressing and wrap it in a figure-eight configuration, winding the bandage under the arm opposite the wound. Never wind the bandage around the neck.

Closed Chest Injuries

flail chest
fracture of two or more adjacent ribs in two or more places that allows for free movement of the fractured segment.

Chest injuries are classified as closed or open. In a closed chest injury, the skin is not broken, leading many people to think that the damage done is not serious. However, such injuries, sustained through blunt trauma and compression injuries, can cause contusions and lacerations of the heart, lungs, and great vessels.

Closed chest injuries may cause a condition known as **flail chest** (Figure 27-17). This condition is defined as a fracture of two or more consecutive ribs in two or more

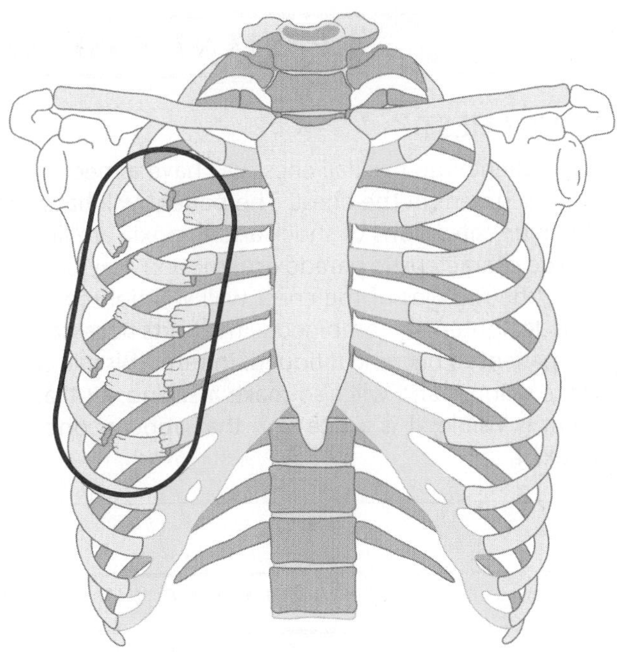

Figure 27-17 • Flail chest occurs when blunt trauma creates a fracture of two or more ribs in two or more places.

places. (Some sources say three or more ribs in two or more places.) The most important factor to remember—even more than the number of broken ribs—is that flail chest leaves a portion of the chest wall unstable, which affects breathing and reduces lung expansion. This can lead to inadequate breathing and hypoventilation.

Because the flail segment is not attached, it is free to move independently. When the patient's chest expands to inhale, negative pressure draws air into the lungs, and this negative pressure also draws the flail segment inward. When the patient's chest moves inward, positive pressure is created that pushes air out of the lungs, and this positive pressure also pushes the flail segment outward. Thus the movement of the flail segment is opposite to the movement of the remainder of the chest cavity. This is called **paradoxical motion** (Figure 27-18).

paradoxical motion movement of ribs in a flail segment that is opposite to the direction of movement of the rest of the chest cavity.

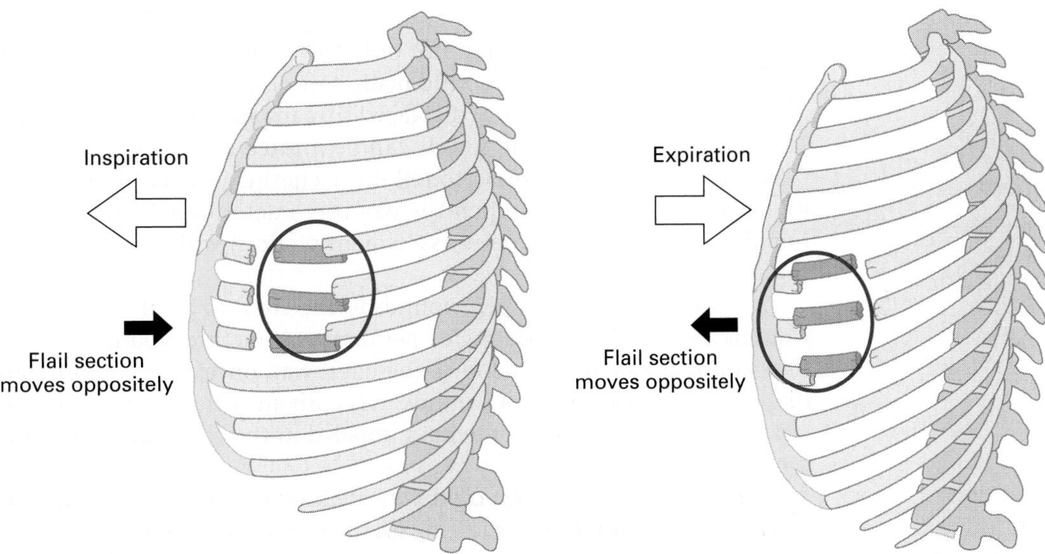

Figure 27-18 • Paradoxical motion.

PATIENT ASSESSMENT

FLAIL CHEST

The patient who has flail chest will have a mechanism of injury capable of causing a flail segment in the chest. The patient will have difficulty breathing with pain at the injury site. Signs of shock and hypoxia are likely.

The characteristic paradoxical motion may be difficult to observe in early stages since the muscles of the chest wall will tighten and naturally splint the area. This muscle tightening combined with efforts necessary to breathe will eventually cause the patient to become fatigued. In turn, this will cause the flail segment to become more visible—and will also make assisting ventilations necessary. When a flail segment is visible, it is a late sign that appears once the patient becomes tired and weak. ■

PATIENT CARE

FLAIL CHEST

1. Perform an initial assessment. Flail segments should be identified as early in the assessment as possible since they pose a threat to life.
2. Administer oxygen. If the patient is breathing inadequately, assist ventilations.
3. Use a bulky dressing to stabilize the flail segment. Tape the dressing into place. The tape or bandage used should not encircle the chest or interfere with chest expansion.
4. Monitor the patient carefully. Watch the patient's respiratory rate and depth. If respirations become too shallow, assist ventilations. ■

Open Chest Injuries

When the skin is broken, the patient has an open wound. However, the term *open chest wound* usually means that not only the skin but the chest wall is penetrated, as for example by a bullet or a knife blade. An object can pass through the wall from the outside, or a fractured and displaced rib can penetrate the chest wall from within. The heart, lungs, and great vessels can be injured at the same time the chest wall is penetrated. It may be difficult to tell if the chest cavity has been penetrated by looking at the wound. Do not open the wound to determine its depth. Specific signs (as noted in the following Patient Assessment section) will indicate possible open chest injury.

You must consider all open wounds to the chest to be life-threatening. Open chest wounds are usually penetrating or perforating puncture wounds. A penetrating puncture wound is one that penetrates the chest wall once; a perforating puncture wound (for example, many gunshot wounds) has both an entrance and an exit wound. An object producing a wound may remain impaled in the chest, or the wound may be completely open.

When air enters the chest cavity, the delicate pressure balance within the chest cavity is destroyed. This causes the lung on the injured side to collapse. (Injuries associated with air in the chest cavity are discussed in more detail under "Injuries within the Chest Cavity.")

PATIENT ASSESSMENT

OPEN CHEST WOUND

The term **sucking chest wound** is used when the chest cavity is open to the atmosphere. Each time the patient breathes, air can be sucked into the opening. This patient will develop severe difficulty breathing. Signs include:

- The patient has a wound to the chest.
- There may or may not be the characteristic sucking sound associated with an open chest wound.
- The patient may be gasping for air.

Keep in mind that the object penetrating the chest wall may have seriously damaged a lung, major blood vessel, or the heart itself. ■

sucking chest wound an open chest wound in which air is "sucked" into the chest cavity.

PATIENT CARE

OPEN CHEST WOUND

An open chest wound is a TRUE EMERGENCY that requires rapid initial care and immediate transport to a medical facility. Follow these steps:

1. Maintain an open airway. Provide basic life support if necessary.
2. Seal the open chest wound as quickly as possible. If need be, use your gloved hand. Do not delay sealing the wound to find an occlusive dressing.
3. Apply an occlusive dressing to seal the wound. When possible, the dressing should be at least 2 inches wider than the wound. If there is an exit wound in the chest, apply an occlusive dressing over this wound, too. Create a flutter-valve dressing with one corner or side unsealed. These dressings will be discussed in detail later under "Occlusive and Flutter-Valve Dressings."
4. Administer high-concentration oxygen.
5. Care for shock.
6. Transport as soon as possible. Unless other injuries prevent you from doing so, keep the patient positioned on the injured side. This allows the uninjured lung to expand without restriction.
7. Consider advanced life support intercept if it will not delay the patient's arrival at the hospital. ■

Occlusive and Flutter-Valve Dressings

Care for an open chest wound involves application of a dressing that will allow air to escape the chest cavity while preventing air from entering. These dressings—called occlusive, one-way, or flutter-valve dressings—involve taping the dressing in place, leaving a side or corner of the dressing unsealed (Figures 27-19 and 27-20). As the patient inhales, the dressing will seal the wound. As the patient exhales, the free corner or edge will act as a flutter valve to release air that is trapped in the chest cavity.

The danger of a **pneumothorax** developing into a **tension pneumothorax** (see the description of pneumothorax and tension pneumothorax in the section "Injuries within the Chest Cavity") is the reason why medical authorities recommend the flutter-valve (three-sided) occlusive dressing instead of an occlusive dressing sealed on all four sides. If you find that blood or tissue begins to accumulate under the dressing and prevents air escape, you may need to briefly remove the dressing, wipe away the accumulated material, and reseal the dressing on three sides.

pneumothorax air in the chest cavity.

tension pneumothorax a type of pneumothorax in which air that enters the chest cavity is prevented from escaping.

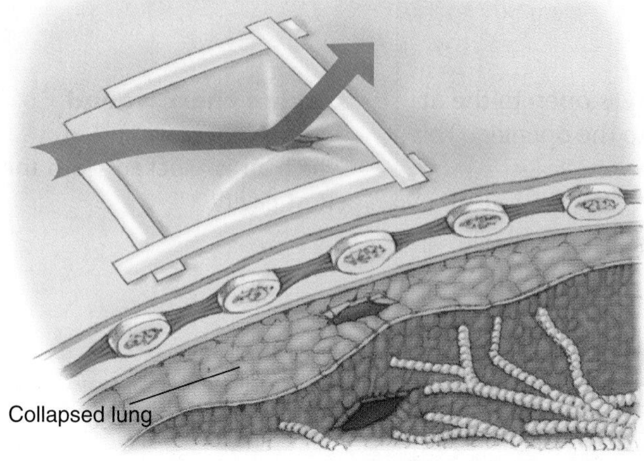
On inspiration, dressing seals wound, preventing air entry
Collapsed lung

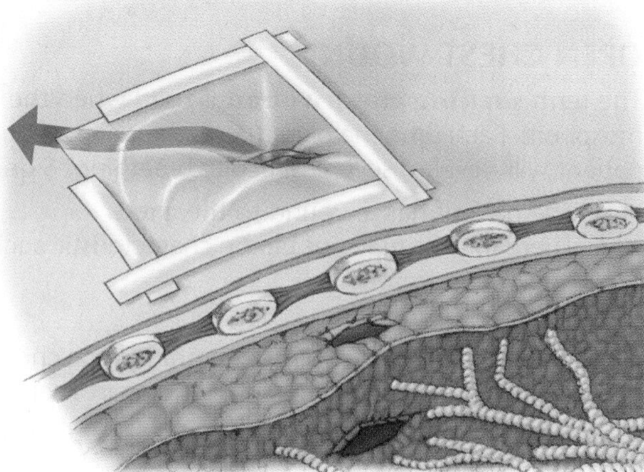
Expiration allows trapped air to escape through untaped section of dressing

Figure 27-19 • Creating a flutter valve to allow air to escape from the chest cavity.

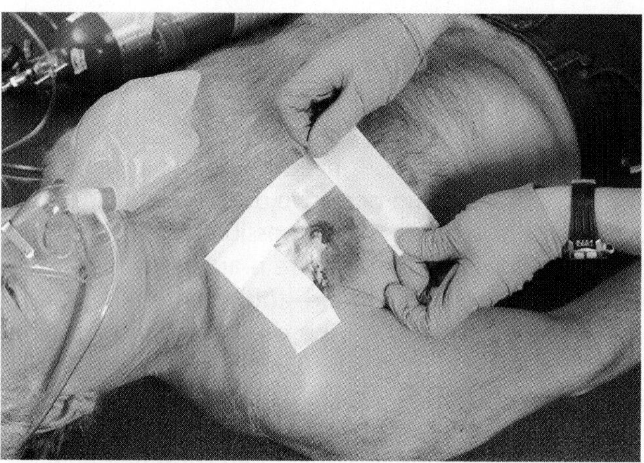

Figure 27-20 • Seal three edges of an occlusive dressing for an open chest wound.

You may have to maintain hand pressure over the occlusive dressing en route to the hospital. The tape also may not stick well to bloody skin or to skin that is sweaty from shock.

Note that if a commercial occlusive dressing is not available, you may have to improvise. Most ambulances carry sterile disposable items that are wrapped in plastic. The inside surface of the plastic is sterile. If you do not have an occlusive dressing, use one of these wrappers or an IV bag. Keep in mind that household plastic wrap is not thick enough to make an effective occlusive dressing for an open chest wound. If nothing else is available, household wrap can be used, but it must be folded several times to be of the proper thickness. Even then, it may fail. If there is no other choice, aluminum foil may be used to make the seal. Be careful, however, as foil edges may lacerate skin and may tear when lifted to release pressure.

NOTE

Once a chest wound is sealed, you must continue to monitor the patient and stay alert for complications. Even if you use a flutter valve, you still must monitor the patient for a buildup of pressure. The free corner or edge of the dressing may stick to the chest, blood may accumulate under the dressing, or the dressing may be drawn into the wound, causing the valve to fail.

Injuries Within the Chest Cavity

Because each of the organs inside the chest cavity is vital to life, any chest injury has the potential to be serious. The blood vessels that run through the chest are the largest in the body, and injury to these vessels is often fatal. In fact, the chest can hold over 3 liters of blood. It is possible to bleed to death within the chest cavity and never spill a drop outside the body.

Since chest injuries have the potential to be serious—even fatal—it is important to describe some of the specific injuries that may occur within the chest cavity. It isn't necessary to diagnose or differentiate between the injuries, just to be familiar with them and to assess and care for them effectively as described at the end of this section.

- *Pneumothorax and tension pneumothorax.* Pneumothorax occurs when air enters the chest cavity, possibly causing collapse of a lung. The air can enter through an external wound (Figure 27-21), the air may enter the cavity through a punctured lung, or both may occur. Especially critical is tension pneumothorax, which is most often found with a closed chest injury or after a sealed occlusive dressing has been applied to an open chest wound. The lung may be punctured by a broken rib or other cause. If there is no opening to the outside of the chest, air that leaks from the lung has no avenue of escape. It builds up in the chest cavity and puts pressure on the heart, great blood vessels, and the unaffected lung, reducing cardiac output and the ability of the lungs to oxygenate the blood.

  Patients with pneumothorax will have diminished or absent lung sounds on the affected side. As the pneumothorax progresses to a tension pneumothorax the jugular veins in the neck may become distended (unless blood volume is low). Signs of shock will also be present. The trachea may shift to the opposite side but this is a very late sign and one which is difficult to detect.
- *Hemothorax and hemopneumothorax* (Figure 27-22). Hemothorax is a condition in which the chest cavity fills with blood. With hemopneumothorax, the chest cavity fills with both blood and air. It is easy to compare these two complications with pneumothorax if you remember that *pneumo* means "air" and *hemo* means "blood." In pneumothorax, there is a buildup of air in the thorax. In hemothorax and hemopneumothorax, blood creates or adds to the pressure.

  Hemothorax can be caused when lacerations within the chest cavity are produced by penetrating objects or fractured ribs. Blood will flow into the space around the lung, the lung may collapse, and the patient will experience a loss of blood leading to shock. Hemopneumothorax is a combination of blood and air, usually producing the same results: a collapsed lung and loss of blood leading to shock.

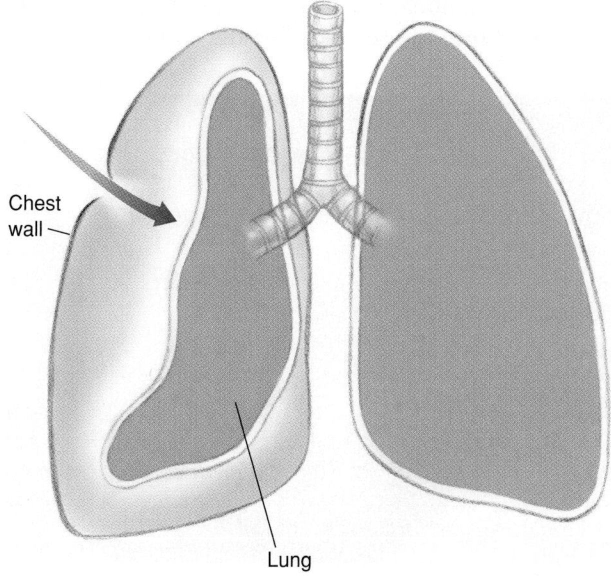

Figure 27-21 • Air can enter the chest cavity through a puncture in the chest wall. This can cause a collapse of a lung and impaired breathing.

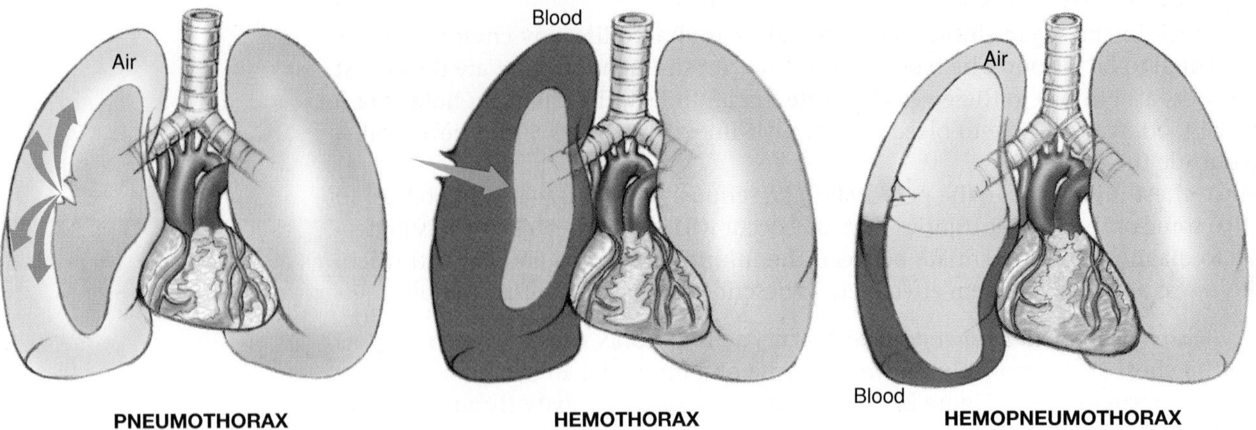

Figure 27-22 • Pneumothorax, hemothorax, hemopneumothorax.

Patients with hemothorax usually present with signs of shock.

- *Traumatic asphyxia.* Traumatic asphyxia is associated with sudden compression of the chest. When this occurs, the sternum and the ribs exert severe pressure on the heart and lungs, forcing blood out of the right atrium and up into the jugular veins in the neck. The pressure of the blood being forced into the head and neck will usually result in blood vessels rupturing, causing extensive bruising of the face and neck (Figure 27-23).

  Patients with traumatic asphyxia present with a mechanism of injury that can cause compression of the chest. The patient's neck and face will be a darker color than the rest of the body (red, purple, or blue). Depending on the amount of pressure and how long the pressure was exerted on the torso, the patient may also have bulging eyes, distended neck veins, and broken blood vessels in the face.
- *Cardiac tamponade.* When an injury to the heart causes blood to flow into the surrounding pericardial sac, the condition produced is cardiac tamponade. The heart's unyielding sac fills with blood and compresses the chambers of the heart to a point where they will no longer fill adequately, backing up blood into the veins.

  Patients who experience cardiac tamponade will usually have distended neck veins. The patient will exhibit signs of shock and a narrowed pulse pressure.
- *Aortic injury and dissection.* Trauma can also cause injury to the aorta, the largest artery in the body. Damage to this large, high-pressure vessel causes massive, often fatal bleeding. Penetrating trauma can cause direct damage to the aorta. Blunt trauma, such as deceleration from a severe motor-vehicle collision (e.g., head-on), can sever or tear the aorta.

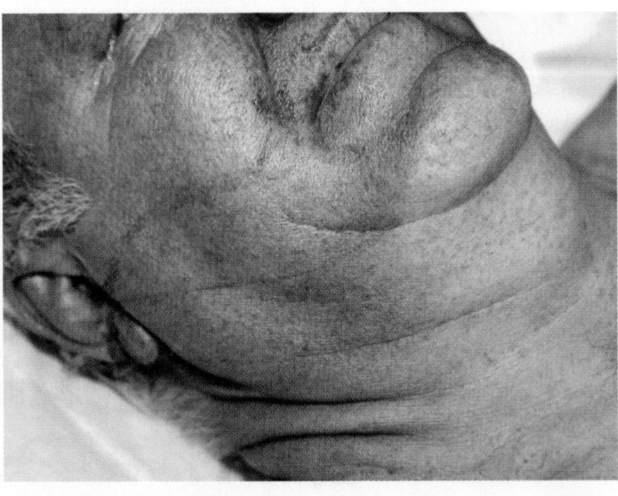

Figure 27-23 • A patient suffering traumatic asphyxia. *(© Edward T. Dickinson, M.D.)*

The aorta can also be damaged without trauma. Degeneration of the aorta, often worsened by high blood pressure or other diseases, causes weakening of this large vessel. Aortic dissection is a condition where the inner layer of the wall of the aorta begins to tear. Blood from the interior of the vessel leaks into the outer layers and eventually causes a balloon-like protrusion (aneurysm). As pressure builds in the aneurysm, risk of rupture and death is great. The aorta runs from the left ventricle through the chest and abdomen, and these injuries can occur anywhere along its path.

The patient with an aortic injury may complain of pain in the chest, abdomen or back—depending on where the injury is. The patient will often exhibit signs of shock. The patient may have differences in pulse or blood pressure between the right and left arms (in proximal aortic injury) or differences in pulses between the arms and the legs or the legs themselves (in abdominal aortic injury). In thin patients or those with a large aneurysm in the abdomen, the aneurysm may occasionally be palpated. Other than routine abdominal palpation, however, it is not recommended to probe the abdomen specifically for aneurysms to avoid causing injury to the patient, such as rupture of the aorta.

PATIENT ASSESSMENT

INJURIES WITHIN THE CHEST CAVITY

Signs of pneumothorax or tension pneumothorax include:

- Increasing respiratory difficulty
- Indications of developing shock, including rapid, weak pulse; cyanosis; narrowing pulse pressure; and low blood pressure due to decreased cardiac output
- Distended neck veins
- Tracheal deviation to the uninjured side (a late sign and difficult to observe)
- Uneven chest wall movement
- Reduction of breath sounds heard in the affected side of the chest (listen with stethoscope)

Signs of hemothorax or hemopneumothorax include:

- Signs of pneumothorax plus coughed-up frothy red blood

Signs of traumatic asphyxia include:

- Distended neck veins
- Head, neck, and shoulders appearing dark blue or purple
- Eyes may be bloodshot and bulging
- Tongue and lips may appear swollen and blue
- Chest deformity may be present

Signs of cardiac tamponade include:

- Distended neck veins
- Very weak pulse
- Low blood pressure
- Steadily decreasing pulse pressure (Pulse pressure is the difference between systolic and diastolic readings.)

Signs of aortic injury or dissection include:

- Tearing chest pain radiating to the back
- Differences in pulse or blood pressure between right and left extremities or between arms and legs
- Palpable pulsating mass
- Cardiac arrest ■

PATIENT CARE

INJURIES WITHIN THE CHEST CAVITY

The treatment for any type of injury within the chest cavity just described is the same:

1. Maintain an open airway. Be prepared to apply suction.
2. Administer high-concentration oxygen.
3. Follow local protocols as to the preferred type of dressing for any open wound.
4. Care for shock.
5. Transport as soon as possible.
6. Consider ALS intercept if it will not delay the patient's arrival at the hospital. ALS personnel can perform procedures such as chest decompression that can greatly benefit a patient suffering chest injury complications. ■

Abdominal Injuries

Abdominal injuries can be open or closed, with a closed injury usually due to blunt trauma. Internal bleeding can be severe if organs and major blood vessels are lacerated or ruptured. Very serious and painful reactions can occur when the hollow organs are ruptured and their contents leak into the abdominal cavity. Penetrating wounds to the abdomen can be caused by objects such as knives, ice picks, arrows, and the broken glass and twisted metal of vehicular collisions and structural accidents. Very serious perforating wounds can be caused by bullets, even when the bullet is small caliber. Open wounds of the abdomen may be so large and deep that organs protrude through the wound opening. This is known as an **evisceration.**

evisceration (e-vis-er-AY-shun) an intestine or other internal organ protruding through a wound in the abdomen.

Information on abdominal emergencies from medical causes may be found in Chapter 18, "Acute Abdominal Emergencies."

PATIENT ASSESSMENT

ABDOMINAL INJURY

Gunshot wounds without exit wounds can cause serious abdominal damage, just as those with exit wounds do. A misconception about bullet wounds is that internal damage can be assessed easily. On the contrary, any projectile entering the body can be deflected, or it can explode and send out pieces in many directions. Do not believe that only the structures directly under the entrance wound have been injured. Also, keep in mind that the pathway of a bullet between entrance wound and exit wound is seldom a straight line.

Complicating the problem even more is the fact that penetrating abdominal wounds can be associated with wounds in adjacent areas of the body. For example, a bullet can enter the chest cavity, pierce the diaphragm, and cause widespread damage in the abdomen. A complete patient assessment is essential in determining the probable extent of injuries. Always assess for an exit wound.

Signs and symptoms of abdominal injury include:

- Pain, often starting as mild pain then rapidly becoming intolerable.
- Cramps.
- Nausea.

continued

PATIENT ASSESSMENT *(continued)*

- Weakness.
- Thirst.
- Obvious lacerations and puncture wounds to the abdomen.
- Lacerations and puncture wounds to the pelvis and middle and lower back or chest wounds near the diaphragm.
- Indications of blunt trauma, such as a large bruised area or an intense bruise on the abdomen.
- Indications of developing shock, including restlessness; pale, cool, and clammy skin; rapid shallow breathing; a rapid pulse; and low blood pressure. (Sometimes patients with abdominal injury who are in extreme pain show an initial elevated blood pressure.)
- Coughing up or vomiting blood. The vomitus may contain a substance that looks like coffee grounds (partially digested blood).
- Rigid and/or tender abdomen. The patient tries to protect the abdomen (guarded abdomen).
- Distended abdomen.
- The patient tries to lie very still, with the legs drawn up in an effort to reduce the tension on the abdominal muscles. ■

PATIENT CARE

ABDOMINAL INJURY

Some emergency care steps apply to both closed and open abdominal injuries. Some additional care steps are necessary for open abdominal injuries.

For both closed and open abdominal injuries:

1. Stay alert for vomiting and keep the airway open.
2. Place the patient on his back, legs flexed at the knees, to reduce pain by relaxing abdominal muscles.
3. Administer high-concentration oxygen.
4. Care for shock.
5. Apply anti-shock garments, if indicated and local protocols recommend.
6. Give nothing to the patient by mouth. This could induce vomiting or pass through open wounds in the esophagus, stomach, or intestine and enter the abdominal cavity.
7. Constantly monitor vital signs.
8. Transport as soon as possible.

Additional steps for open abdominal injuries:

9. Control external bleeding and dress all open wounds.
10. Do not touch or try to replace any eviscerated, or exposed, organs. Apply a sterile dressing moistened with sterile saline over the wound site before you apply an occlusive dressing. Maintain warmth by placing layers of bulky dressing or a lint-free towel over the occlusive dressing (Scan 27-2).
11. Do not remove any impaled objects. Stabilize impaled objects with bulky dressings that are bandaged in place. Leave the patient's legs in the position in which you found them to avoid muscular movement that may move the impaled object. ■

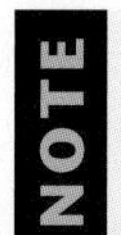

Do not use aluminum foil. Aluminum foil occlusive dressings have been known to cut eviscerated organs.

SCAN 27-2 • Dressing an Open Abdominal Wound

First take Standard Precautions.

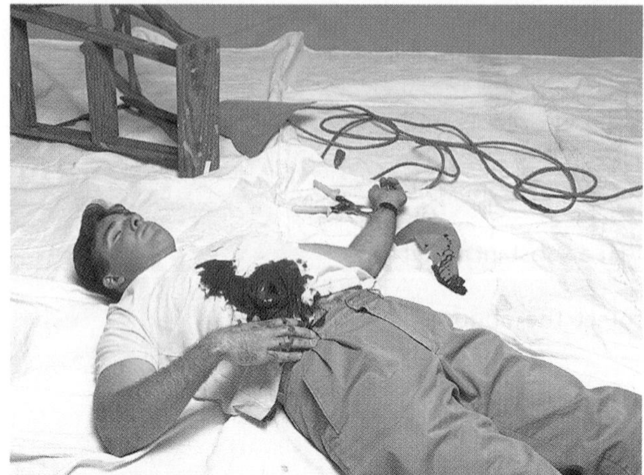

Open abdominal wound with evisceration.

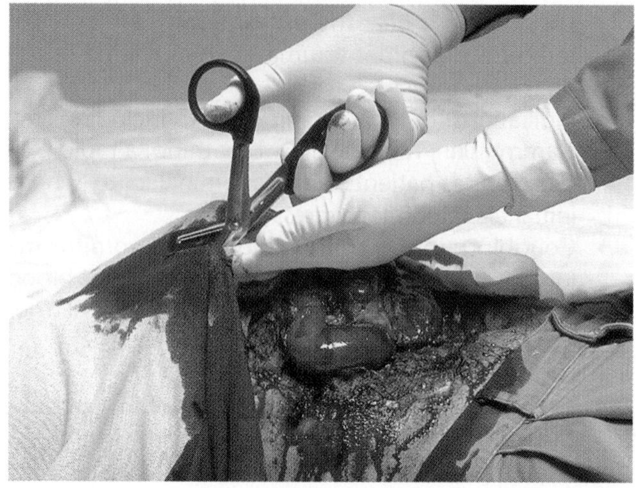

1. Cut away clothing from the wound.

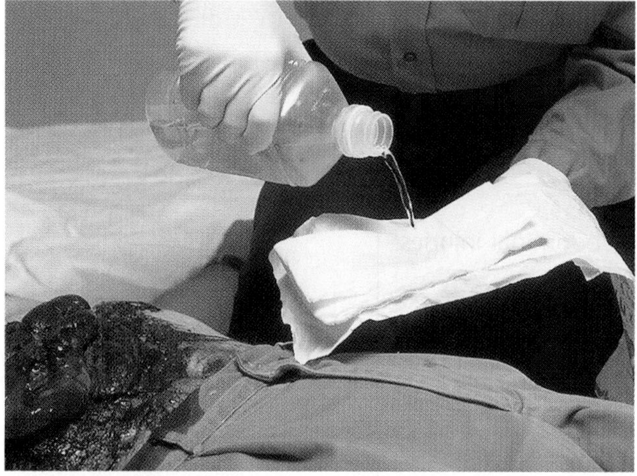

2. Soak a dressing with sterile saline.

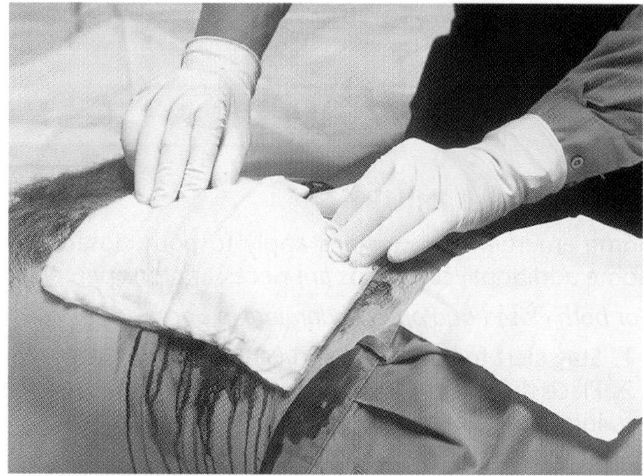

3. Place the moist dressing over the wound.

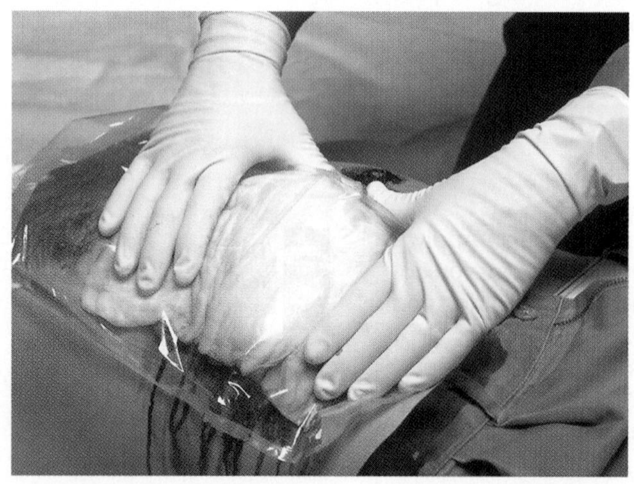

4. Apply an occlusive dressing over the moist dressing if local protocols recommend that you do so.

Cover the dressed wound to maintain warmth. Secure the covering with tape or cravats tied above and below the position of the exposed organ.

BURNS

Most people think of burns as injuries to the skin, but burns can do much more. Burn injuries often involve structures below the skin, including muscles, bones, nerves, and blood vessels. Burns can injure the eyes beyond repair. Respiratory system structures can be damaged, producing airway obstruction due to tissue swelling, and even cause respiratory failure and respiratory arrest. In addition to the physical damage caused by burns, patients often suffer emotional and psychological problems that begin at the emergency scene and may last a lifetime.

When caring for a burn patient, always think beyond the burn. For example, a medical emergency or accident may have led to the burn. The patient may have had a heart attack while smoking a cigarette, and the unattended cigarette caused a fire. During the patient assessment, the EMT should detect the heart problem even though the burn may be the most obvious injury. Conversely, a fire or burn may cause or aggravate another injury or medical condition. Someone trying to escape a fire may fall and suffer spinal damage and fractures. The EMT should not only detect the burn but detect the spinal damage and fractures as well.

PATIENT ASSESSMENT

BURNS

When your patient has been burned, patient assessment involves classifying, then evaluating, the burns. Burns can be classified and evaluated in three ways:

- By agent and source
- By depth
- By severity

All three are important in deciding the urgency and the kind of emergency care the burn requires. These classifications are discussed in detail in the following text. ■

NOTE

Patient assessment should not be neglected in order to begin immediate burn care.

Classifying Burns by Agent and Source

Burns can be classified according to the agent causing the burn (e.g., chemicals or electricity). Noting the source of the burn (e.g., dry lime or alternating current) can make the classification more specific. You should report the agent and also, when practical, the source of the agent (Table 27-2). For example, a burn can be reported as "chemical burns from contact with dry lime."

Never assume the agent or source of the burn. What may appear to be a thermal burn could in fact be caused by radiation. You may find minor thermal burns on the patient's face and forget to consider light burns to the eyes. Always gather information from your observations of the scene, bystanders' reports, and the patient interview.

Classifying Burns by Depth

Burns involving the skin are classified as superficial, partial thickness, and full thickness burns (Figure 27-24). These classifications are also sometimes called first-degree, second-degree, and third-degree burns, with first-degree burns corresponding to superficial burns, and so on, as described next (Figure 27-25):

- **Superficial burn.** This burn involves only the epidermis (the outer layer of the skin). It is characterized by reddening of the skin and perhaps some swelling. An

superficial burn
a burn that involves only the epidermis, the outer layer of the skin. It is characterized by reddening of the skin and perhaps some swelling. An example is a sunburn. Also called a first-degree burn.

TABLE 27-2 • Agents and Sources of Burns

AGENTS	SOURCES
Thermal	Flame; radiation; excessive heat from fire, steam, hot liquids, hot objects
Chemicals	Various acids, bases, caustics
Electricity	Alternating current, direct current, lightning
Light (typically involving the eyes)	Intense light sources; ultraviolet light can also be considered a source of radiation burns
Radiation	Usually from nuclear sources; ultraviolet light can also be considered a source of radiation burns

example is a sunburn. The patient will usually complain about pain (sometimes severe) at the site. The burn will heal of its own accord, without scarring. Superficial burns are also called first-degree burns.

partial thickness burn a burn in which the epidermis (first layer of skin) is burned through and the dermis (second layer) is damaged. Burns of this type cause reddening, blistering, and a mottled appearance. Also called a second-degree burn.

- **Partial thickness burn.** In this type of burn, the epidermis is burned through and the dermis (the second layer of the skin) is damaged, but the burn does not pass through to underlying tissues. There will be deep intense pain, noticeable reddening, blisters, and a mottled (spotted) appearance to the skin. Burns of this type cause swelling and blistering for 48 hours after the injury, as plasma and tissue fluids are released and rise to the top layer of skin. When treated with reasonable care, partial thickness burns will heal themselves, producing very little scarring. Partial thickness burns are also called second-degree burns.

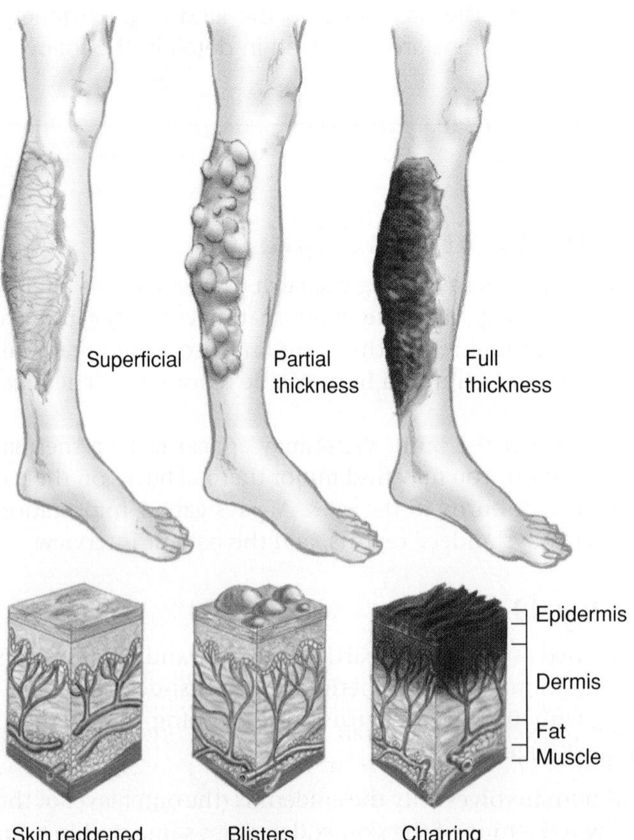

Figure 27-24 • Burns are classified by depth.

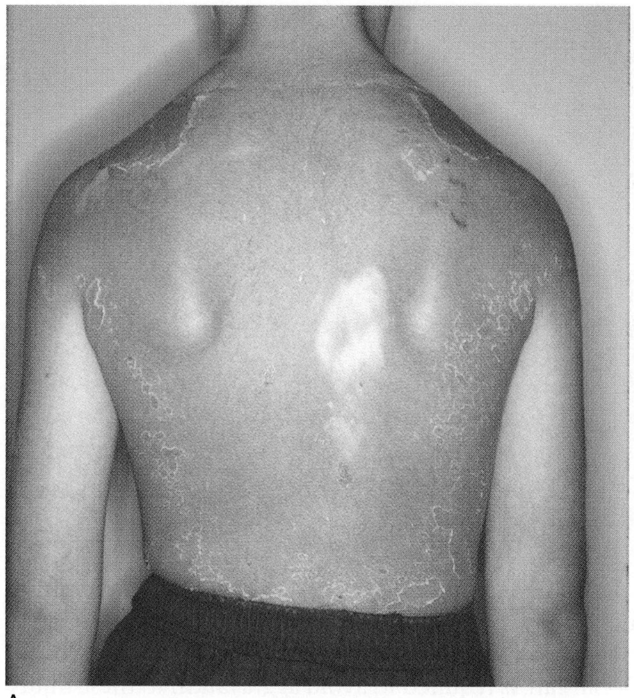

A

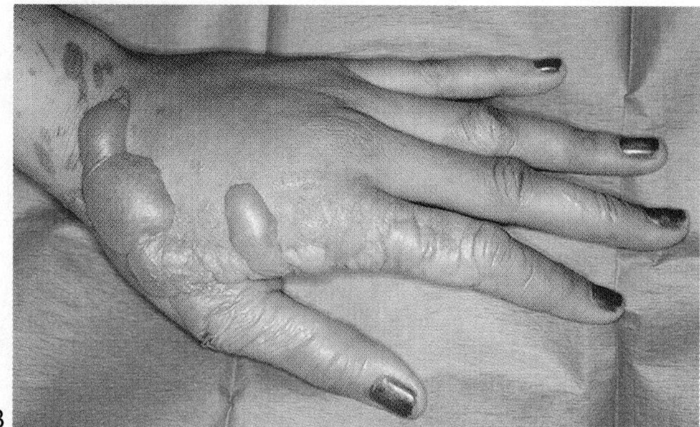

B

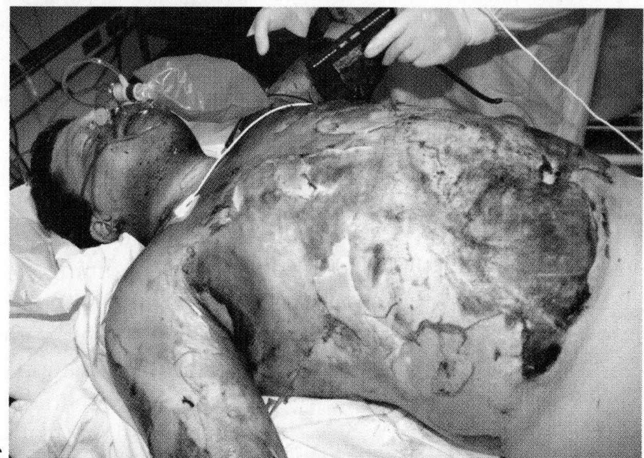

C

Figure 27-25 • (A) A superficial burn *(Charles Stewart, M.D. and Associates),* (B) a partial thickness burn *(© Charles Stewart, M.D. and Associates),* and (C) a full thickness burn. *(© Edward T. Dickinson, M.D.)*

- **Full thickness burn.** This is a burn in which all the layers of the skin are damaged. Some full thickness burns are difficult to tell from partial thickness burns; however, there are usually areas that are charred black or brown or areas that are dry and white. The patient may complain of severe pain, or if enough nerves have been damaged, he may not feel any pain at all (except at the periphery of the burn where adjoining partial thickness burns may be causing pain). This type of burn may require skin grafting. As these burns heal, dense scars form. Full thickness burns damage all layers of the skin and additionally may damage subcutaneous tissue, muscle, bone, and underlying organs. These burns are sometimes called third-degree burns.

full thickness burn
a burn in which all the layers of the skin are damaged. There are usually areas that are charred black or areas that are dry and white. Also called a third-degree burn.

Determining the Severity of Burns

When determining the severity of a burn, consider the following factors:

- Agent or source of the burn
- Body regions burned
- Depth of the burn
- Extent of the burn
- Age of the patient
- Other illnesses and injuries

The agent or source of the burn can be significant in terms of patient assessment. A burn caused by electrical current may cause only small areas of skin injury but pose a great risk of severe internal injuries. Chemical burns are of special concern since the chemical may remain on the skin and continue to burn for hours or even days, eventually entering the bloodstream. This is sometimes the case with certain alkaline chemicals.

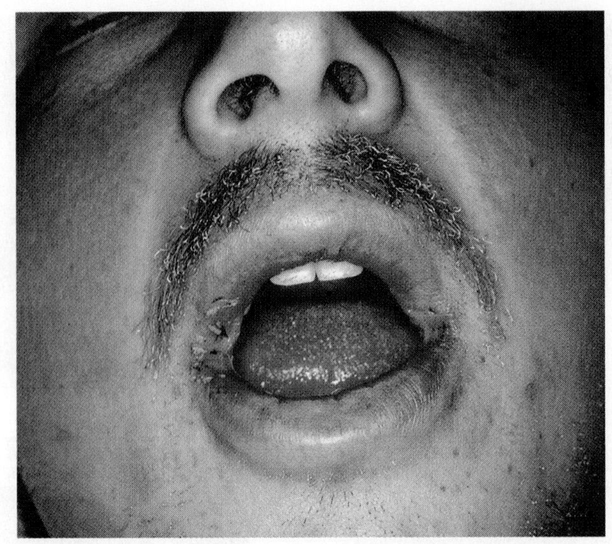

Figure 27-26 • A singed mustache and burns to the tip of the tongue signal danger of airway burns or burns to the eyes. *(© Charles Stewart, M.D. and Associates)*

When you are considering the body regions burned, keep in mind that any burn to the face is of special concern since it may involve injury to the airway or the eyes (Figure 27-26). The hands and feet also are areas of concern because scarring may cause loss of movement of fingers or toes. Special care is required to avoid aggravation to these injury sites when moving the patient and to prevent the damaged tissues from sticking to one another. When the groin, genitalia, buttocks, or medial thighs are burned, potential bacterial contamination can be far more serious than the initial damage to the tissues. Note that circumferential burns (burns that encircle the body or a body part) can be very serious because they constrict the skin. When they occur to an extremity, they can interrupt circulation to the distal tissues. In addition, the burn healing process can be very complicated. This is particularly true when circumferential burns occur to joints, the chest, and the abdomen where the encircling scarring tends to limit normal functions.

rule of nines
a method for estimating the extent of a burn. For an adult, each of the following areas represents 9 percent of the body surface: the head and neck, each upper extremity, the chest, the abdomen, the upper back, the lower back and buttocks, the front of each lower extremity, and the back of each lower extremity. The remaining 1 percent is assigned to the genital region. For an infant or child the percentages are modified so that 18 percent is assigned to the head, 14 percent to each lower extremity.

rule of palm
a method for estimating the extent of a burn. The palm of the patient's hand, which equals about 1 percent of the body's surface area, is compared with the patient's burn to estimate its size.

The depth of the burn is important to determining severity. In partial thickness and full thickness burns, the outer layer of the skin is penetrated. This can lead to contamination of exposed tissues and the invasion of the circulatory system by harmful chemicals and microorganisms.

You also will need to estimate roughly the extent of the burn area. The amount of skin surface involved can be calculated quickly by using the **rule of nines** (Figure 27-27). For an adult, each of the following areas represents 9 percent of the body surface: head and neck, each upper extremity, chest, abdomen, upper back, lower back and buttocks, the front of each lower extremity, and the back of each lower extremity. These make up 99 percent of the body's surface. The remaining 1 percent is assigned to the genital region.

In the rule of nines, the percentages are modified for infants and young children, whose heads are much larger in relationship to the rest of the body. An infant's or young child's head and neck are counted as 18 percent; each upper extremity as 9 percent; chest and abdomen as 18 percent; the entire back as 18 percent; each lower extremity as 14 percent; and the genital region as 1 percent. (This adds up to 101 percent, but it is only used to give a rough determination. Some systems count each lower limb as 13.5 percent to achieve an even 100 percent.)

An alternative way to estimate the extent of a burn is the **rule of palm,** which uses the patient's hand to approximate the surface area. The rule of palm can be applied to any patient—infant, child, or adult. Since the palm of the hand equals about 1 percent of the body's surface area, mentally compare the patient's palm with the size of the burn to estimate its extent. (For example, a burn the size of five palms = 5 percent of the body.) The rule of palm may be easier to apply to smaller or localized burns, whereas the rule of nines may be easier for larger or more widespread burns.

The age of the patient is a major factor in considering the severity of burns. Infants, children under age 5, and adults over age 55, because of their anatomy and physiology,

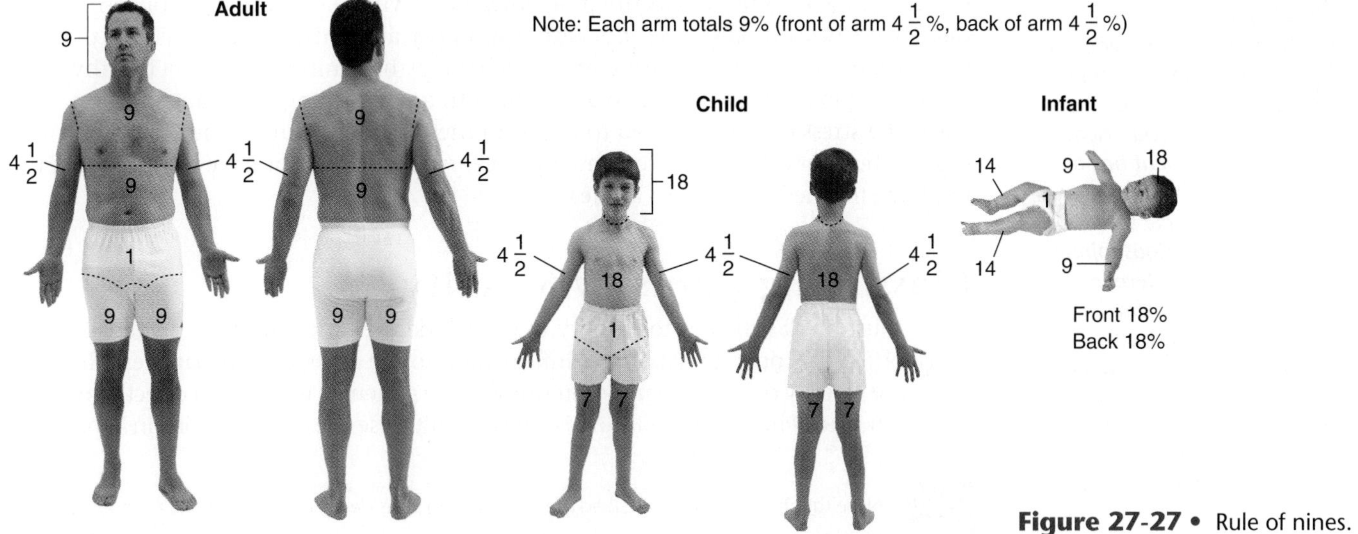

Figure 27-27 • Rule of nines.

have the most severe responses to burns and the greatest risk of death. They also have different healing patterns than other age groups.

When determining the severity of a burn, you also must consider the other illnesses and injuries a patient may have. Obviously, a patient with an existing respiratory illness will be especially vulnerable to exposure to heated air or chemical vapors. Likewise, the

GERIATRIC NOTE

Burn intensity and body-area involvement that would be minor to moderate in a young adult could be fatal for an aged person. In late adulthood, the body's ability to cope with injury is reduced by aging tissues and failing body systems. The ability of tissues to heal from any injury is lessened and the time of healing is increased.

CRITICAL DECISION MAKING:
Burns—by the Numbers

Burns are a type of soft-tissue injury. Decisions about burn care and transportation are often determined by an approximation of body surface area affected. For each of the following patients, determine the approximate body surface area burned and the degree of the burn.

1. Your patient fell asleep by the pool and was sunburned over the backs of both legs, his back, and the backs of both arms. The skin is bright red.
2. Your patient works at a fast food restaurant. She was by the fryer when someone threw in an ice cube as a joke to scare her. Hot grease splashed up and covered the anterior portion of her left forearm and her entire right hand. The skin is red and blistered.
3. Your patient fell asleep while smoking. He has circumferential burns on both legs and has burned the entire right arm. The legs are red and blistered. The patient's right arm is severely charred and peeling.

NOTE

All burns are to be treated as more serious if accompanied by other injuries or medical problems. If you discover that the patient has a decreased blood pressure, always assume that he has other serious injuries. Attempt to determine the patient's problem through standard assessment techniques.

stress of a fire or other environmental emergency will be of particular concern for patients with heart disease. Patients with respiratory ailments, heart disease, or diabetes will react more severely to burn damage. What may be a minor burn for a healthy adult could be of major significance to a patient with a pre-existing medical condition. Similarly, the stress of a burn added to other injuries sustained during the emergency may lead to shock or other life-threatening problems that would not have resulted from the nonburn injuries or the burn alone.

Classifying Burns by Severity

Burns must be classified as to severity to determine the order and type of care, order of transport, and to provide maximum information to the emergency department. In some cases, the severity of the burn may determine if the patient is to be taken directly to a hospital with special burn-care facilities. For most adults, use the classifications in Table 27-3.

GERIATRIC NOTE

Note that burns usually classified as moderate are considered critical in adults over 55 years of age.

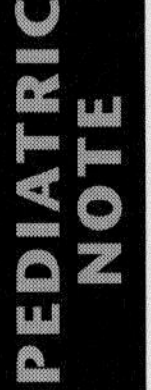

Burns pose greater risks to infants and children. This is because their body surface area is greater in relation to their total body size. This results in greater fluid and heat loss than would be found in an adult patient. Infants have a higher risk of shock, airway problems, and hypothermia from burns. Additionally, the classification of burn severity differs in patients less than 5 years of age as shown in Table 27-4. When a child has been burned, consider the possibility of child abuse.

TABLE 27-3 • Classification of Burn Severity: Adults

CLASSIFICATIONS BY THICKNESS, PERCENT OF BODY SURFACE AREA, AND COMPLICATING FACTORS

Minor Burns

- Full thickness burns of less than 2 percent, excluding face, hands, feet, genitalia, or respiratory tract
- Partial thickness burns of less than 15 percent
- Superficial burns of 50 percent or less

Moderate Burns

- Full thickness burns of 2 to 10 percent, excluding face, hands, feet, genitalia, or respiratory tract
- Partial thickness burns of 15 to 30 percent
- Superficial burns that involve more than 50 percent

Critical Burns

- All burns complicated by injuries of the respiratory tract, other soft-tissue injuries, and injuries of the bones
- Partial thickness or full thickness burns involving the face, hands, feet, genitalia, or respiratory tract
- Full thickness burns of more than 10 percent
- Partial thickness burns of more than 30 percent
- Burns complicated by musculoskeletal injuries
- Circumferential burns

Note: Burns which, by the prior classification, are moderate should be considered critical in a person less than 5 or greater than 55 years of age. See Table 27-4 for classifications for children less than 5 years of age.

POINT OF VIEW

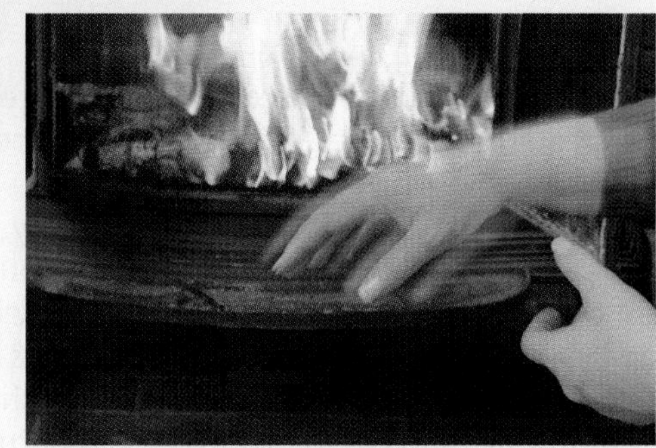

"I was tending the fire. I do it all the time. We were about to put in a movie, so I may have gotten a bit greedy and wanted to load the fireplace up so it would burn long and hot.

"The wood was nice and dry and a small fire had been going for awhile. But like I said, I decided it would be a good idea to build up the fire, and I put too much wood in. The wood shifted. I moved to catch some of the pieces, and then I heard a whoosh. *The shift must've created an airflow that fed the fire. Well that fire certainly caught. And so did my hand.*

"I didn't think my hand was in the fire for that long, but it must've been. I felt the heat first. I'm not sure why, but I noticed hairs burning on my wrist before I even noticed the pain...and redness...and blistering. It got most of my hand and up my wrist a little.

"The EMTs came and put a dressing on my hand. I knew it was bad by looking at it. They were even more concerned, because they knew a burn to the hand can be really serious. They called the doctor on the radio who said to go to a hospital different than my normal one. They took me to a hospital with a specialty in treating burns.

"I'll tell you this: I'll never try to overfeed a fire again. Burns hurt a lot—and for a long time."

TABLE 27-4 • Classification of Burn Severity: Children Less Than 5 Years of Age

CLASSIFICATIONS BY THICKNESS AND PERCENT OF BODY SURFACE AREA

Minor Burns

- Partial thickness burns of less than 10 percent of body surface

Moderate Burns

- Partial thickness burns of 10 to 20 percent of body surface

Critical Burns

- Full thickness burns of any extent or partial thickness burns of more than 20 percent of body surface

Treating Specific Types of Burns

There are special approaches to the care of thermal burns, general chemical burns, and chemical burns to the eyes (Figure 27-28).

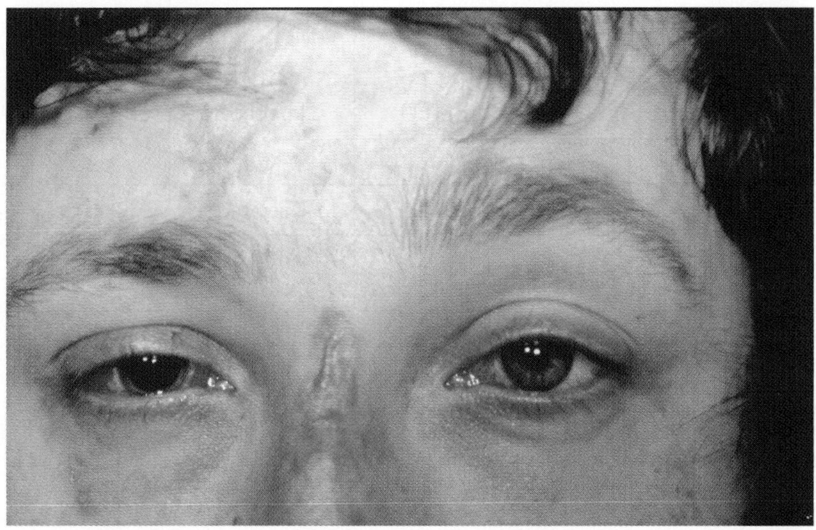

Figure 27-28 • Chemical burns to the eyes. *(© Western Ophthalmic Hospital/Science Photo Library/Photo Researchers, Inc.)*

NOTE

Do not attempt to rescue persons trapped by fire unless you are trained to do so and have the equipment and personnel required. The simple act of opening a door might cost you your life. In some fires, opening a door or window may greatly intensify the fire or even cause an explosion.

PATIENT ASSESSMENT

THERMAL BURNS

As an EMT you will have to care for thermal burns caused by scalding liquids, steam, contact with hot objects, flames, flaming liquids, and gases. Sunburn can also be severe in infants and young children, who may have other heat-related injuries.

The steps for basic care of thermal burns are given in Table 27-5. Currently, dry sterile dressings are recommended by the national EMT curriculum for all burns. The standing orders for burn care are determined by your EMS Medical Director and the regional EMS system. Some EMS systems state that all partial thickness and full thickness burns are to be wrapped with dry sterile dressing or a burn sheet, while some burn centers recommend moist dressings for partial thickness burns to less than 10 percent of the body and dry dressings for more severe cases. The latter protocol is now being adopted by most EMS systems.

Note that EMTs must manage burns correctly until the patient can be transferred to the care of the staff of a medical facility. Never apply ointments, sprays, or butter (which would trap the heat against the burn site and have to be scraped off by the hospital staff). Do not break blisters. Do not apply ice to any burn (it can cause tissue damage). Keep the burn site clean to prevent infection. Keep the patient warm, as the temperature regulation function of the skin may be affected by the burn. ■

TABLE 27-5 • Care for Thermal Burns

1. STOP THE BURNING PROCESS!
   Flame—Wet down, smother, then remove clothing.
   Semi-solid (grease, tar, wax)—Cool with water. Do not remove substance.
2. Ensure an open airway. Assess breathing.
3. Look for signs of airway injury: soot deposits, burnt nasal hair, facial burns.
4. Complete the initial assessment.
5. Treat for shock. Provide high-concentration oxygen. Treat serious injuries.
6. Evaluate burns by depth (see below), extent (rule of nines or rule of palm), and severity.

DEPTH OF BURN	OUTER SKIN LAYER IS BURNED	SECOND SKIN LAYER IS BURNED	TISSUE BELOW SKIN IS BURNED	COLOR CHANGES	PAIN	BLISTERS
Superficial	Yes	No	No	Red	Yes	No
Partial thickness	Yes	Yes	No	Deep red	Yes	Yes
Full thickness	Yes	Yes	Yes	Charred black or white	Yes/No	Yes/No

7. **Do not** clear debris. Remove clothing and jewelry.
8. Wrap with dry sterile dressing.
9. **Burns to hands or feet**—Remove rings or jewelry that may constrict with swelling. Separate fingers or toes with sterile gauze pads.
   Burns to the eyes —Do not open eyelids if burned. Be certain burn is thermal, not chemical. Apply sterile gauze pads to **both** eyes to prevent sympathetic movement. (If burn is chemical, flush eyes for 20 minutes en route to hospital.)
   FOLLOW LOCAL BURN CENTER PROTOCOLS, AND TRANSPORT ALL BURN PATIENTS AS SOON AS POSSIBLE.

PATIENT CARE

CHEMICAL BURNS

Chemical burns require immediate care. It is hoped that people at the scene will begin this care before you arrive. At many industrial sites, workers and First Responders are trained to provide initial care for incidents involving the chemicals in use. Most major industries have emergency deluge-type safety showers to wash dangerous chemicals from the body. However, this will not always be the case. Be prepared for situations in which nothing has been done and there is no running water near the scene.

Emergency care for a patient with chemical burns includes the following (Figure 27-29):

1. The primary care procedure is to WASH away the chemical with flowing water. If a dry chemical is involved, BRUSH away as much of the chemical as possible and then flush the skin. Simply wetting the burn site is not enough. Continuous flooding of the affected area is required, using a copious but gentle flow of water. Avoid hard sprays that may damage badly burned tissues. Continue to wash the area for at least 20 minutes, and continue the process en route to the hospital. Remove contaminated clothing, shoes, socks, and jewelry from the patient as you apply the wash. *Do not contaminate skin that has not been in contact with the chemical.*
2. Apply a sterile dressing or burn sheet.
3. Treat for shock.
4. Transport.

Continue to be on the alert for delayed reactions that may cause renewed pain or interfere with the patient's ability to breathe. Should the patient complain of increased burning or irritation, wash the burned areas again with flowing water for several minutes. ■

NOTE *Protect yourself during the washing process for a chemical burn. Wear protective gloves and eyewear and control the wash to avoid splashing.*

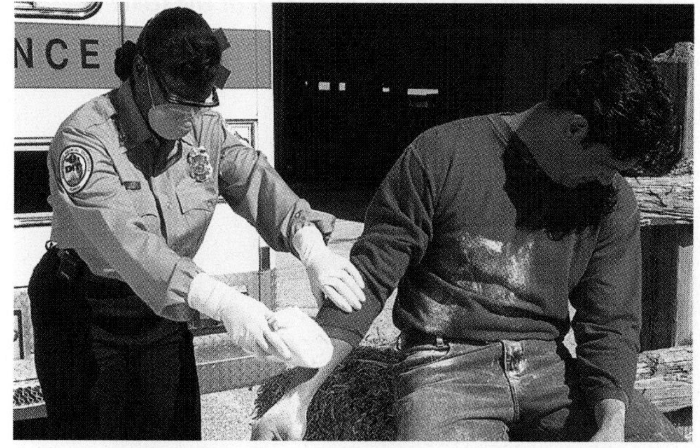

A

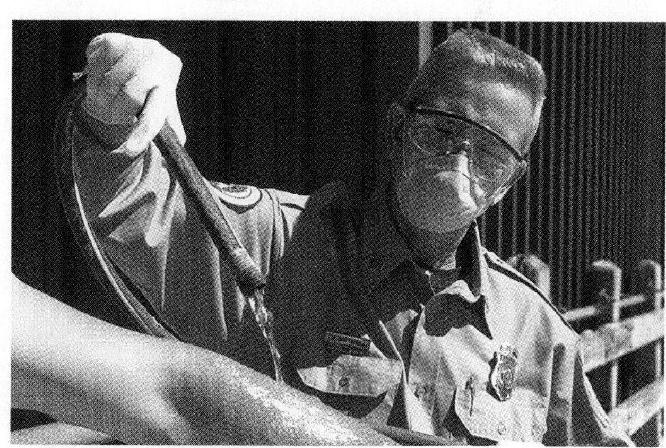

B

Figure 27-29 • For a chemical burn, (A) brush away dry powders, and then (B) flood the area with water.

PATIENT CARE

CHEMICAL BURNS TO THE EYES

A corrosive chemical can burn the globe of a person's eye before he can react and close the eyelid. Even with the lid shut, chemicals can seep through onto the globe.

To care for chemical burns to the eye, you should take the following steps:

1. IMMEDIATELY flood the eyes with water. Often the burn will involve areas of the face as well as the eye. When this is the case, flood the entire area. Avoid washing chemicals back into the eye or into an unaffected eye (Figure 27-30).
2. Keep running water from a faucet, low-pressure hose, bucket, cup, bottle, rubber bulb syringe, IV setup, or other such source flowing into the burned eye. The flow should be from the medial (nasal) corner of the eye to the lateral corner. Since the patient's natural reaction will be to keep the eyes tightly shut, you may have to hold the eyelids open.
3. Start transport and continue washing the eye for at least 20 minutes or until the patient's arrival at the medical facility.
4. After washing the eye, cover both eyes with moistened pads.
5. Wash the patient's eyes for 5 more minutes if he begins to complain about renewed burning sensations or irritation. ■

NOTE

Do not use neutralizers such as vinegar or baking soda in a patient's eyes.

NOTE

Some scenes where chemical burns have taken place can be very hazardous. Always evaluate the scene. There may be large pools of dangerous chemicals around the patient. Acids could be spurting from containers. Toxic fumes may be present. If the scene will place you in danger, do not attempt a rescue unless you have been trained for such a situation and have the needed equipment and personnel at the scene.

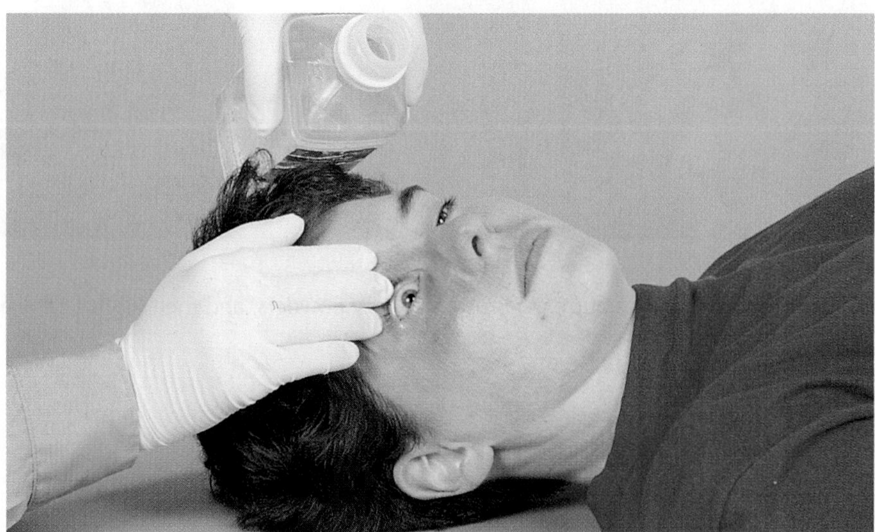

Figure 27-30 • Emergency care of chemical burns to the eye.

SPECIFIC CHEMICAL BURNS

When possible, find out the exact chemical or mixture of chemicals that were involved in the incident. Some special chemical burns require specific care procedures.

- **Mixed or strong acids or unidentified substances.** Many of the chemicals used in industrial processes are mixed acids. Their combined action can be immediate and severe. The pain produced from the initial chemical burn may mask any pain being caused by renewed burning due to small concentrations left on the skin.

  When the chemical is a strong acid (e.g., hydrochloric acid or sulfuric acid), a combination of acids, or an unknown, play it safe and continue washing even after the patient claims he is no longer experiencing pain.
- **Dry lime.** If dry lime is the burn agent, do not wash the burn site with water. To do so will create a corrosive liquid. Brush the dry lime from the patient's skin, hair, and clothing. Make certain that you do not contaminate the eyes or airway.

  Use water only after the lime has been brushed from the body, contaminated clothing and jewelry have been removed, and the process of washing can be done quickly and continuously with running water.
- **Carbolic acid (phenol).** Carbolic acid does not mix with water. When available, use alcohol for the initial wash of unbroken skin, followed by a long steady wash with water. (Follow local protocols.)
- **Sulfuric acid.** Heat is produced when water is added to concentrated sulfuric acid, but it is still preferable to wash rather than leave the contaminant on the skin.
- **Hydrofluoric acid.** This acid is used for etching glass and in many other manufacturing processes. Burns from it may be delayed, so treat all patients who may have come into contact with the chemical, even if burns are not in evidence. Flood with water. Do not delay care and transport to find neutralizing agents. (Follow local protocols.)
- **Inhaled vapors.** Whenever a patient is exposed to a caustic chemical and may have inhaled the vapors, provide a high flow and concentration of oxygen (humidified, if available) and transport as soon as possible. This is very important when the chemical is an acid that is known to vaporize at standard environmental temperatures. (Examples include hydrochloric acid and sulfuric acid.) ■

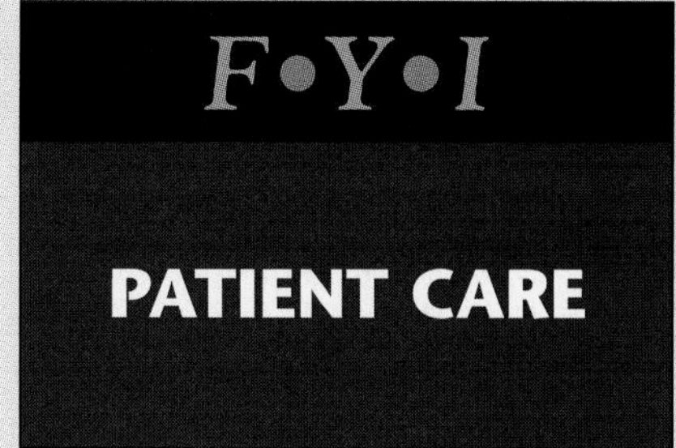

ELECTRICAL INJURIES

Electric current, including lightning, can cause severe damage to the body. The skin is burned where the energy enters the body and where it flows into a ground. Along the path of this flow, tissues are damaged due to heat. In addition, significant chemical changes take place in the nerves, heart, and muscles, and body processes are disrupted or may completely shut down.

NOTE *The scenes of injuries due to electricity are often very hazardous. Assume that the source of electricity is still active unless a qualified person tells you that the power has been turned off. Do not attempt a rescue unless you have been trained to do this kind of rescue and have the necessary equipment and personnel. For information about electrical hazards at the scene of a vehicle collision, see Chapter 7, "Scene Size-Up," and Chapter 35, "Gaining Access and Rescue Operations."*

PATIENT ASSESSMENT

ELECTRICAL INJURIES

The victim of an electrical accident may have any or all of the following signs and symptoms (Figure 27-31):

- Burns where the energy enters and exits the body
- Disrupted nerve pathways displayed as paralysis
- Muscle tenderness, with or without muscular twitching
- Respiratory difficulties or respiratory arrest
- Irregular heartbeat or cardiac arrest
- Elevated blood pressure or low blood pressure with the signs and symptoms of shock
- Restlessness or irritability if conscious, or loss of consciousness
- Visual difficulties
- Fractured bones and dislocations from severe muscle contractions or from falling (This can include the spinal column.)
- Seizures (in severe cases) ■

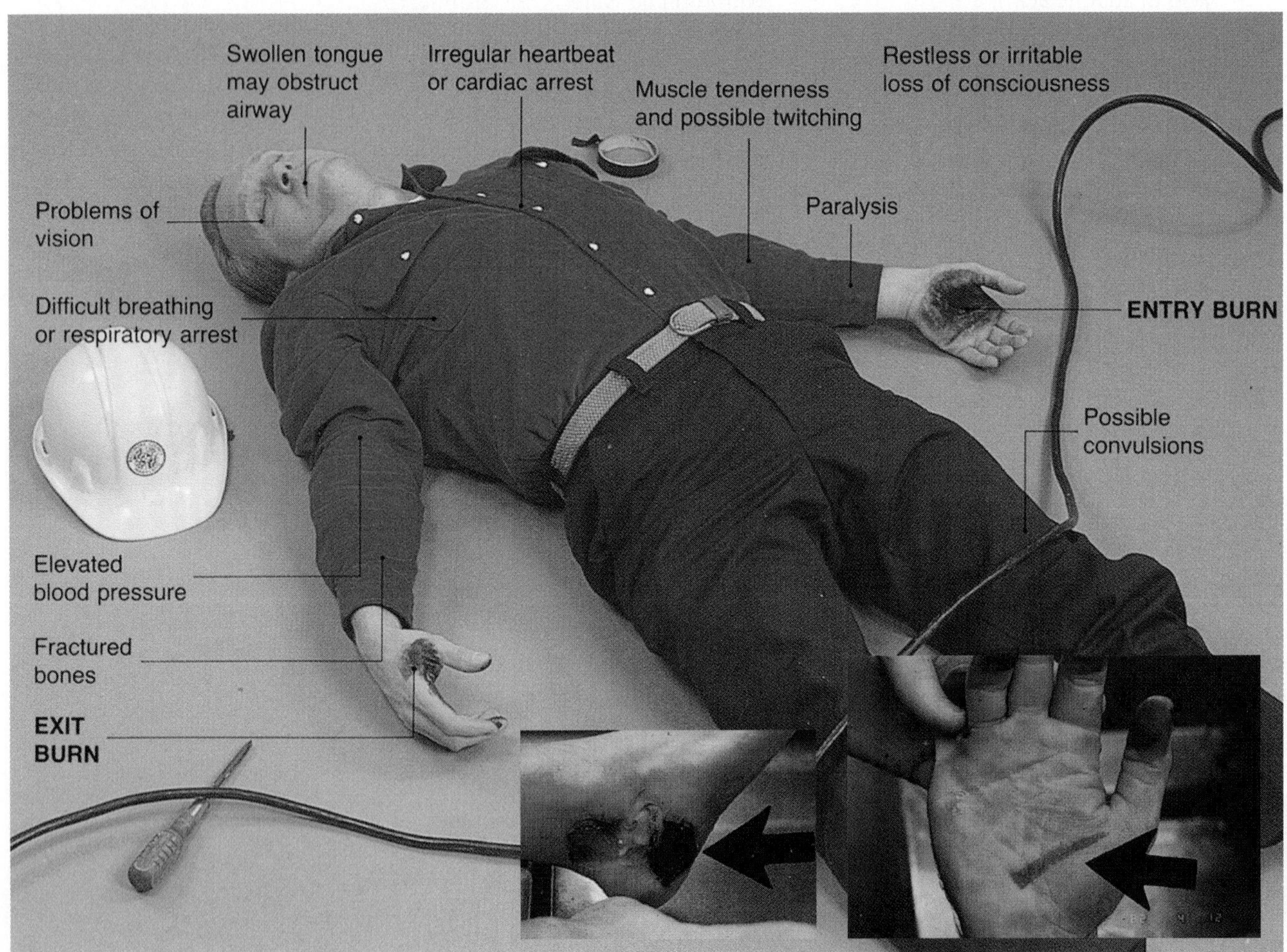

Figure 27-31 • Injuries due to electrical shock (top), and detail of entry and exit burns (bottom).

PATIENT CARE

ELECTRICAL INJURIES

Follow these steps to provide emergency care to a patient with electrical injuries:

1. Provide airway care. Electrical shock may cause severe swelling along the airway.
2. Provide basic cardiac life support as required. Since cardiac rhythm disturbances are common, be prepared to perform defibrillation if necessary.
3. Care for shock and administer high-concentration oxygen.
4. Care for spine injuries, head injuries, and severe fractures. All serious electrical shock patients should be fully immobilized because electrical current can cause severe muscular contraction. Also, the patient may have been thrown by a high-voltage current. In either case, there is the possibility of spine injury that requires immobilization.
5. Evaluate electrical burns, looking for at least two external burn sites: contact with the energy source and contact with a ground.
6. Cool the burn areas and smoldering clothing the same as you would for a flame burn.
7. Apply dry sterile dressings to the burn sites.
8. Transport as soon as possible. Some problems have a slow onset. If there are burns, there also may be more serious hidden problems. In any case of electrical shock, heart problems may develop.

Remember that the major problem caused by electrical shock is usually not the burn. Respiratory and cardiac arrest are real possibilities. Be prepared to provide basic cardiac life support measures with automated defibrillation. ■

NOTE *Make certain that you and the patient are in a SAFE ZONE (not in contact with any electrical source and outside the area where downed or broken wires or other sources of electricity can reach you).*

DRESSING AND BANDAGING

Most cases of open wound care require the application of a dressing and a bandage (Figure 27-32 and Scan 27-3). A **dressing** is any material applied to a wound in an effort to control bleeding and prevent further contamination. Dressings should be sterile. A **bandage** is any material used to hold a dressing in place. Bandages need not be sterile.

dressing
any material (preferably sterile) used to cover a wound that will help control bleeding and help prevent additional contamination.

bandage
any material used to hold a dressing in place.

NOTE *Be certain to wear disposable gloves and other barrier devices to avoid contact with the patient's blood and body fluids. Follow infection control procedures.*

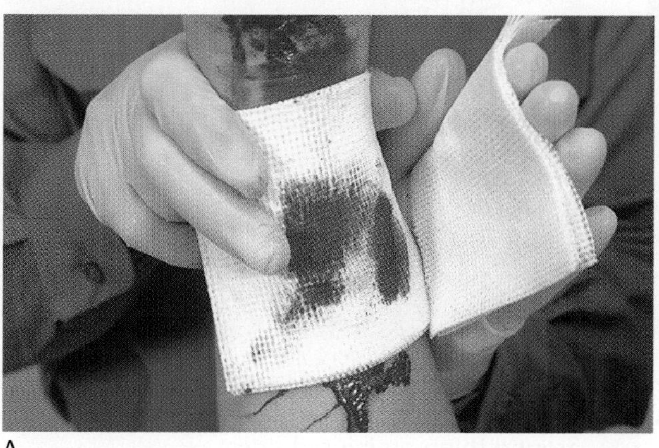
A

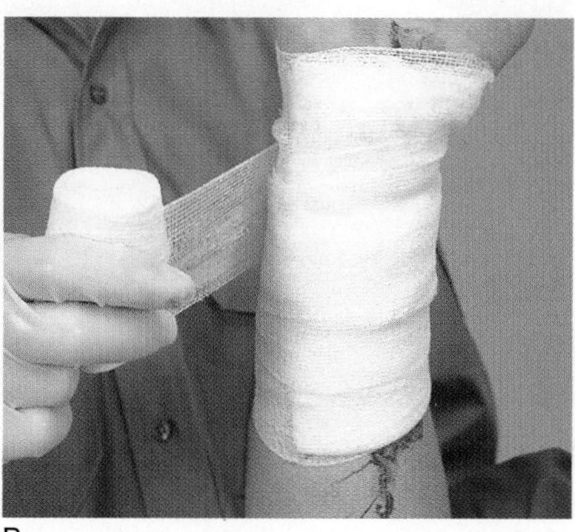
B

Figure 27-32 • (A) Dressings cover wounds and (B) bandages hold dressings in place.

SCAN 27-3 • Dressing and Bandaging

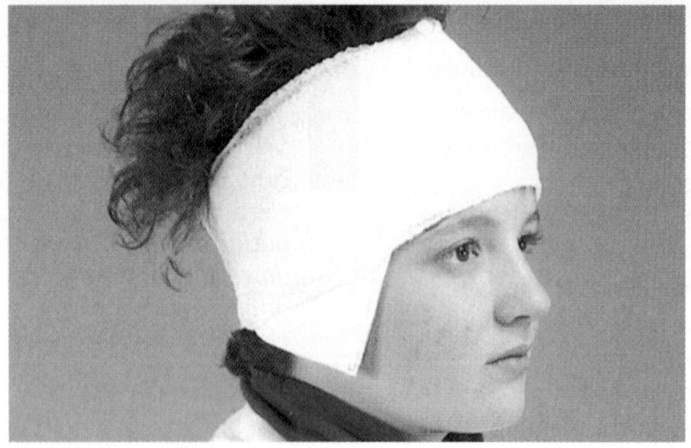

FOREHEAD OR EAR (NO SKULL INJURY). Place dressing and secure with self-adherent roller bandage.

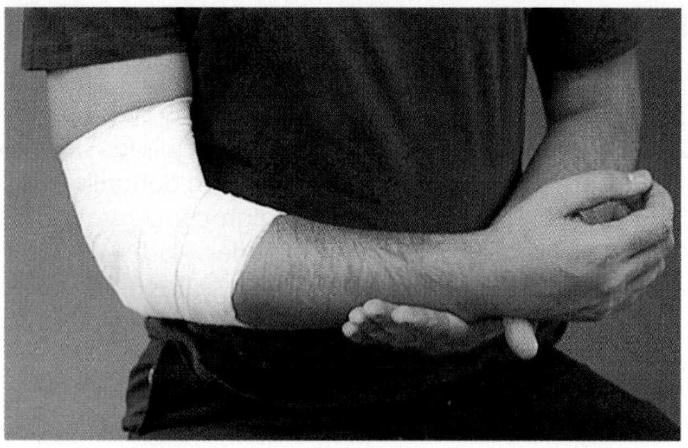

ELBOW OR KNEE. Place dressing and secure with cravat or roller bandage. Apply roller bandage in figure-eight pattern.

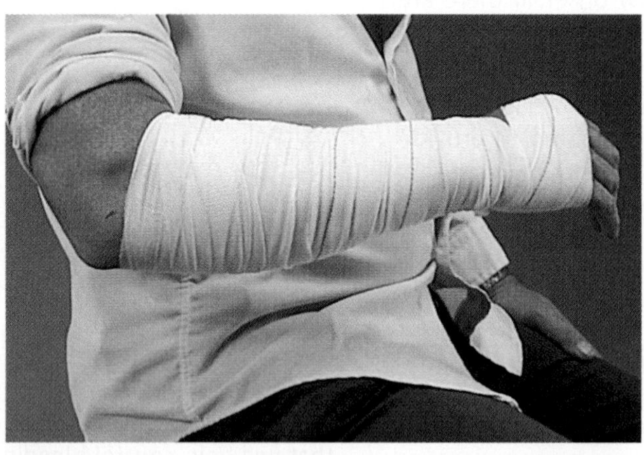

FOREARM OR LEG. Place dressing and secure with roller bandage, distal to proximal. Better protection is offered if palm or sole is wrapped.

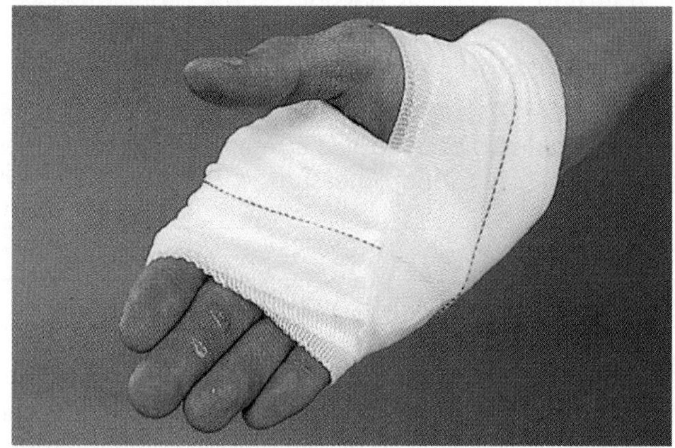

HAND. Place dressing, wrap with roller bandages, and secure at wrist. When possible, bandage in position of function.

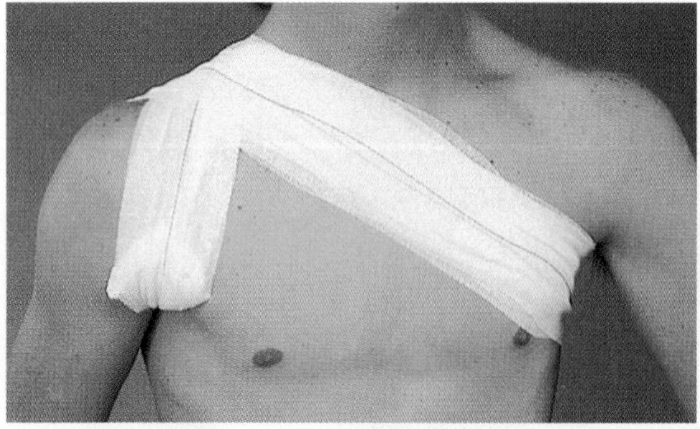

SHOULDER. Place dressing and secure with figure-eight of cravat or roller dressing. Pad under knot if cravat is used.

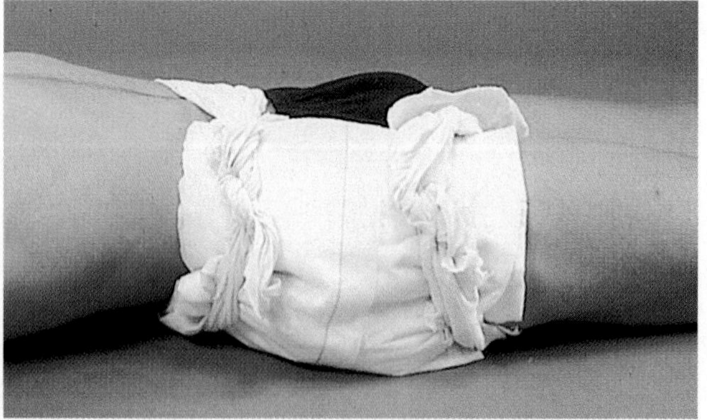

HIP. Place bandage and large dressing to cover hip. Secure with first cravat around waist and second cravat around thigh on injured side.

Various dressings are carried in emergency care kits. These dressings should be sterile, meaning that all microorganisms and spores that can grow into active organisms have been killed. Dressings also should be aseptic, meaning that all dirt and foreign debris have been removed. Many EMS systems now also carry hemostatic dressings used to stop bleeding. In emergency situations, when commercially prepared dressings are not available, clean cloth, towels, sheets, handkerchiefs, and other similar materials may be suitable alternatives.

The most popular dressings are individually wrapped sterile gauze pads, typically 4 inches square. A variety of sizes are available, referred to according to size in inches, such as 2 × 2s, 4 × 4s, 5 × 9s, and 8 × 10s.

Large bulky dressings, such as the multitrauma or **universal dressing,** are available when bulk is required for profuse bleeding or when a large wound must be covered. These dressings are especially useful for stabilizing impaled objects. Sanitary napkins can sometimes be used in place of the standard bulky dressings. Although not sterile, they are separately wrapped and have very clean surfaces. (Do not apply any adhesive surface of the napkin directly to the wound.) Of course, bulky dressings can be made by building up layers of gauze pads.

universal dressing
a bulky dressing.

A **pressure dressing** is used to control bleeding. Gauze pads are placed on the wound and a bulky dressing is placed over the pads. A self-adherent roller bandage is wrapped tightly over the dressing and above and below the wound. Distal pulse must be checked and frequently rechecked, and you may need to readjust the pressure to ensure distal circulation.

pressure dressing
a dressing applied tightly to control bleeding.

An **occlusive dressing** is used when it is necessary to form an airtight seal. This is done when caring for open wounds to the abdomen, for external bleeding from large neck veins, and for open wounds to the chest. Sterile, commercially prepared occlusive dressings are available in two different forms: plastic wrap and petroleum-gel-impregnated gauze occlusive dressings. Local protocols vary as to which form to use. Nonsterile wrap and foil also can be used in emergency situations. In emergencies, EMTs have been known to fashion occlusive dressings from plastic credit cards, plastic bags, sterile medical equipment wrappers, and defibrillator pads.

occlusive dressing
any dressing that forms an airtight seal.

NOTE

Most EMS systems recommend against the use of aluminum foil for covering an abdominal evisceration because it may injure exposed abdominal organs.

Large dressings are sometimes needed in emergency care. Sterile, disposable burn sheets are commercially available. Bed sheets can be sterilized and kept in plastic wrappers to be later used as dressings. These sheets can make effective burn dressings or may be used in some cases to cover exposed abdominal organs.

Bandages are provided in a wide variety of types. The preferred bandage is the self-adhering, form-fitting roller bandage (Figure 27-33). It eliminates the need to know many specialized bandaging techniques developed for use with ordinary gauze roller bandages.

Dressings can be secured using adhering or nonadhering gauze roller bandage, triangular bandages, strips of adhesive tape, or an air splint. In a situation where one of these is not available, you can use strips of cloth, handkerchiefs, and other such materials. Elastic bandages that are used in the general care of strains and sprains should not be used to hold dressings in place. They can become constricting bands, interfering with circulation. This is very likely to occur as the tissues around the wound site begin to swell after the elastic bandage is in place.

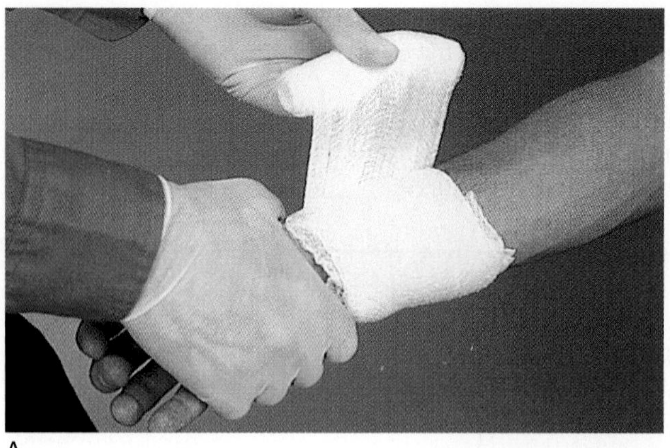
A

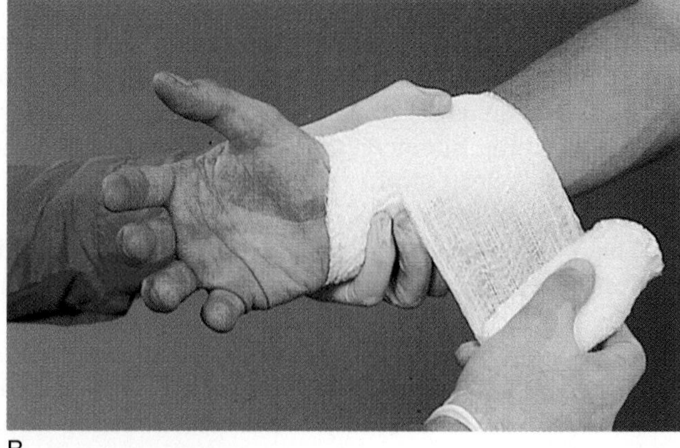
B

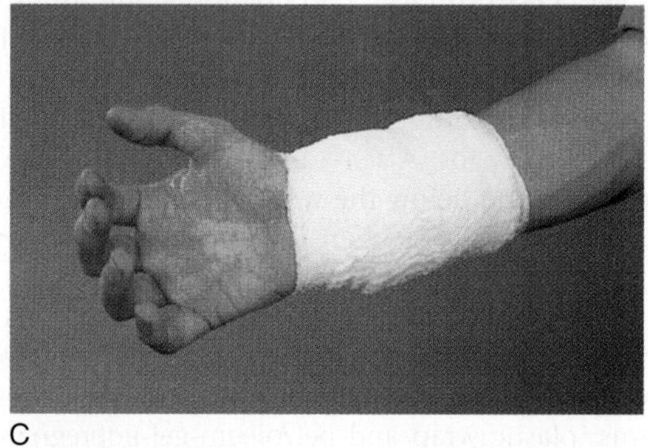
C

Figure 27-33 • To apply a self-adhering roller bandage, (A) secure it with several overlapping wraps, (B) keep it snug, and (C) cut and tape or tie it in place.

PATIENT CARE

DRESSING OPEN WOUNDS

The following rules apply to the general dressing of wounds (Figure 27-34):

1. Take Standard Precautions.
2. Expose the wound. Cut away any clothing so the entire wound is exposed.
3. Use sterile or very clean materials. Avoid touching the dressing in the area that will come into contact with the wound. Grasp the dressing by the corner, taking it directly from its protective pack, and place it on the wound.
4. Cover the entire wound. The entire surface of the wound and the immediate surrounding areas should be covered.
5. Control bleeding. With the exception of the pressure dressing, a dressing should not be bandaged into place if it has not controlled the bleeding. You should continue to apply dressings and pressure as needed for the proper control of bleeding.
6. Do not remove dressings. Once a dressing has been applied to a wound, it must remain in place. Bleeding may restart and tissues at the wound site may be injured if the dressing is removed. If the bleeding continues, put new dressings over the blood-soaked ones. ■

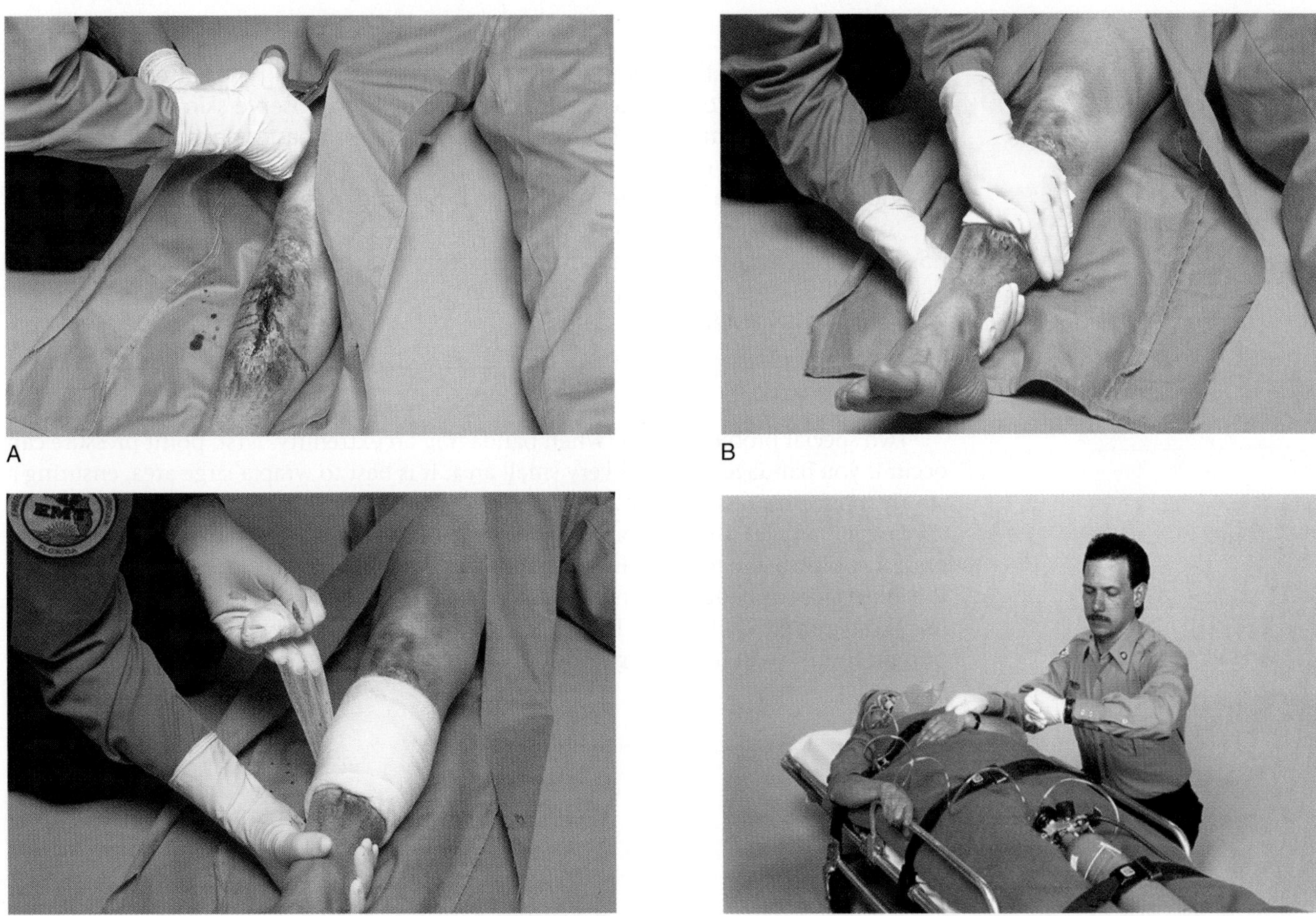

Figure 27-34 • To dress an open wound, (A) expose the wound site, (B) control bleeding, (C) dress and bandage the wound, and (D) keep the patient at rest.

There is an exception to the rule prohibiting the removal of dressings. If a bulky dressing has become blood-soaked, it may be necessary to remove the dressing so that direct pressure can be reestablished or a new bulky dressing can be added and a pressure dressing created. Protection for the wound site is better maintained if one or more gauze pads are placed over the injured tissues before placing the bulky dressing. This will allow for the removal of a bulky dressing without disturbing the wound.

PATIENT CARE

BANDAGING OPEN WOUNDS

The following rules apply to general bandaging:

1. Do not bandage too tightly. All dressings should be held snugly in place, but they must not restrict the blood supply to the affected part.
2. Do not bandage too loosely. Hold the dressing by bandaging snugly, so the dressing does not move around or slip from the wound. Loose bandaging is a common error in emergency care.
3. Do not leave loose ends. Any loose ends of gauze, tape, or cloth may get caught on objects when the patient is moved.

continued

PATIENT CARE *(continued)*

4. Do not cover the tips of fingers and toes. When bandaging the extremities, leave the fingers and toes exposed whenever possible to observe skin color changes that indicate a change in circulation and to allow for easier neurologic reassessment. Pain, pale or blue-colored skin, cold skin, numbness, and tingling are all indications that a bandage may be too tight. The exception is burned fingers or toes, which have to be covered.
5. Cover all edges of the dressing. This will help to reduce additional contamination. The flutter-valve dressing for an open chest wound is an exception (see earlier in this chapter). ■

Two special problems occur when bandaging an extremity. First, point pressure can occur if you bandage around a very small area. It is best to wrap a large area, ensuring a steady, uniform pressure. Apply the bandage from the smaller diameter of the limb to the larger diameter (distal to proximal) to help ensure proper pressure and contact. Second, the joints have to be considered. You can bandage across a joint, but do not bend the limb once the bandage is in place. To do so may restrict circulation, loosen the dressing and bandage, or do both. In some cases, it may be necessary to apply an inflatable or rigid splint, or to use a sling and swathe to prevent movement of the joint.

CHAPTER REVIEW

SUMMARY

Injuries to the soft tissues of the body are common calls for the EMT. Soft-tissue injuries may be closed (internal, with no pathway to the outside) or open (an injury in which the skin is interrupted, exposing the tissues below). An open chest or abdominal wound is considered to be one that penetrates not only the skin but the chest or abdominal wall to expose internal organs. Closed injuries include contusions (bruises), hematomas, and crush injuries. Open wounds include abrasions, lacerations, punctures, avulsions, amputations, and crush injuries. Open neck, chest, and abdominal wounds are life-threatening.

For open wounds, expose the wound, control bleeding, and prevent further contamination. For an open neck, chest, or abdominal wound apply an occlusive dressing. For both open and closed injuries, take appropriate Standard Precautions; note the mechanism of injury; protect the patient's airway and breathing; administer high-concentration oxygen by nonrebreather mask; treat for shock; and transport.

Burn severity is determined by considering the source of the burn, body regions burned, depth of burn (superficial, partial thickness, and full thickness), extent of burn (by rule of nines or rule of palm), age of patient (children under 5 and adults over 55 react most severely), and other patient illnesses or injuries. Care for burns includes stopping the burning process (water for a thermal burn, brushing away chemicals), covering a thermal burn with a dry sterile dressing, flushing a chemical burn with sterile water, protection of the airway, administration of oxygen, treatment for shock, and transport.

For treatment of electrical injuries, be sure that you and the patient are in a safe zone away from possible contact with electrical sources. Protect airway, breathing, and circulation. Be prepared to care for respiratory or cardiac arrest. Treat for shock, care for burns, and transport.

KEY TERMS

abrasion (ab-RAY-zhun) a scratch or scrape.

air embolus (EM-bo-lus) a bubble of air in the bloodstream.

amputation (am-pyu-TAY-shun) the surgical removal or traumatic severing of a body part, usually an extremity.

avulsion (ah-VUL-shun) the tearing away or tearing off of a piece or flap of skin or other soft tissue. This term also may be used for an eye pulled from its socket or a tooth dislodged from its socket.

bandage any material used to hold a dressing in place.

closed wound an internal injury with no open pathway from the outside.

contusion (kun-TU-zhun) a bruise.

crush injury an injury caused when force is transmitted from the body's exterior to its internal structures. Bones can be broken; muscles, nerves, and tissues damaged; and internal organs ruptured, causing internal bleeding.

dermis (DER-mis) the inner (second) layer of the skin found beneath the epidermis. It is rich in blood vessels and nerves.

dressing any material (preferably sterile) used to cover a wound that will help control bleeding and help prevent additional contamination.

epidermis (ep-i-DER-mis) the outer layer of the skin.

evisceration (e-vis-er-AY-shun) an intestine or other internal organ protruding through a wound in the abdomen.

flail chest fracture of two or more adjacent ribs in two or more places that allows for free movement of the fractured segment.

full thickness burn a burn in which all the layers of the skin are damaged. There are usually areas that are charred black or areas that are dry and white. Also called a third-degree burn.

hematoma (hem-ah-TO-mah) a swelling caused by the collection of blood under the skin or in damaged tissues as a result of an injured or broken blood vessel.

laceration (las-er-AY-shun) a cut.

occlusive dressing any dressing that forms an airtight seal.

open wound an injury in which the skin is interrupted, exposing the tissue beneath.

paradoxical motion movement of ribs in a flail segment that is opposite to the direction of movement of the rest of the chest cavity.

partial thickness burn a burn in which the epidermis (first layer of skin) is burned through and the dermis (second layer) is damaged. Burns of this type cause reddening, blistering, and a mottled appearance. Also called a second-degree burn.

pneumothorax air in the chest cavity.

pressure dressing a dressing applied tightly to control bleeding.

puncture wound an open wound that tears through the skin and destroys underlying tissues. A *penetrating puncture wound* can be shallow or deep. A *perforating puncture wound* has both an entrance and an exit wound.

rule of nines a method for estimating the extent of a burn. For an adult, each of the following areas represents 9 percent of the body surface: the head and neck, each upper extremity, the chest, the abdomen, the upper back, the lower back and buttocks, the front of each lower extremity, and the back of each lower extremity. The remaining 1 percent is assigned to the genital region. For an infant or child the percentages are modified so that 18 percent is assigned to the head, 14 percent to each lower extremity.

rule of palm a method for estimating the extent of a burn. The palm of the patient's hand, which equals about 1 percent of the body's surface area, is compared with the patient's burn to estimate its size.

subcutaneous (SUB-ku-TAY-ne-us) **layers** the layers of fat and soft tissues found below the dermis.

sucking chest wound an open chest wound in which air is "sucked" into the chest cavity.

superficial burn a burn that involves only the epidermis, the outer layer of the skin. It is characterized by reddening of the skin and perhaps some swelling. An example is a sunburn. Also called a first-degree burn.

tension pneumothorax a type of pneumothorax in which air that enters the chest cavity is prevented from escaping.

universal dressing a bulky dressing.

REVIEW QUESTIONS

1. List three types of closed soft-tissue injury. (pp. 646–647)
2. List four types of open soft-tissue injury. (pp. 648–652)
3. Describe the care for an open wound to the chest. (p. 663)
4. Describe the care for impaled objects in the eye. (p. 657)
5. Explain when you would remove an object impaled in the cheek and when you would, instead, stabilize an object impaled in the cheek. (pp. 656–657)
6. Describe the three classifications (depths) of burns. (pp. 671–673)
7. Differentiate between a dressing and a bandage. (p. 683)
8. List the qualities and purpose of an effective bandage. How could you tell if a bandage were improperly applied? (pp. 683–688)

CRITICAL THINKING

- You have been caring for a patient who shot himself in the chest with a nail gun. You applied an occlusive dressing around the wound. The patient is now suddenly beginning to deteriorate. He is having extreme difficulty breathing and his color has worsened. Breath sounds have become almost totally absent on the side with the impaled nail. What complication might you suspect is causing his worsening condition? How could this be corrected?

Thinking and Linking

Think back to Chapter 2, "The Well-Being of the EMT," as you consider the following question:

- What Standard Precautions are required for the following calls?
  a. An agitated person with a lip laceration and missing teeth
  b. A small cut to the left hand, oozing blood
  c. A laceration to the right forearm with bright red spurting blood

Think back to Chapter 1, "Introduction to Emergency Medical Care," and the discussion of specialized trauma and other treatment centers under "Components of the EMS System" as you consider the following question:

- Which specialty centers should the following patients be transported to (if the center is available in your region)?
  a. A patient with a collapsed lung
  b. A patient with partial thickness burns on 35 percent of his body
  c. A patient with suspected internal bleeding and trauma
  d. A patient with an amputated hand

MEDIA RESOURCES 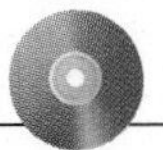

See the Student CD at the back of this book for quizzes, a case study activity and other features related to this chapter. Also, visit the Companion Website for *Emergency Care* at **www.prenhall.com/limmer**, where you will find additional reinforcement and links to other resources.

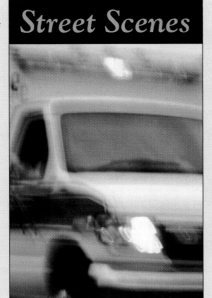

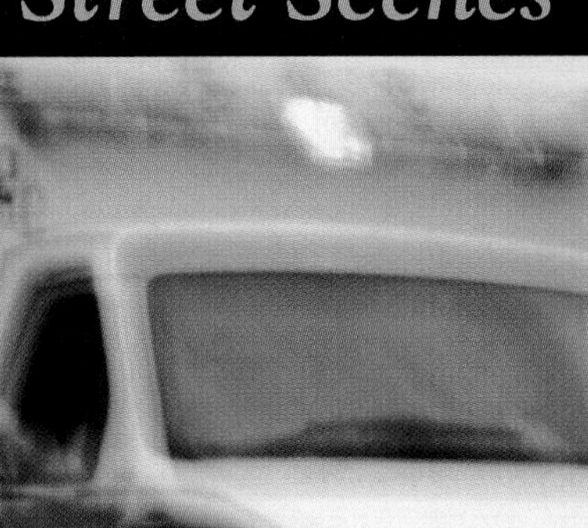

Late Sunday evening you respond to #4 Mountain View Apartments. You and your partner are met by the manager and a security guard, who lead you to Mary, a 42-year-old female sitting in a chair in the manager's office with a thick towel wrapped around her right forearm. Standard Precautions are in place. "Hi, my name's Jim Morrow," you say, "and I'm with the ambulance service. What happened?" You note the trail of blood spots on the floor leading to an outside door.

"I locked myself out of my apartment. So, I wrapped my coat around my arm and broke the glass window above my kitchen sink. I thought the coat would protect me," she tells you, "but I was wrong."

Street Scene Questions

1. What is your general impression of this patient?
2. What priority would you assign to her?
3. What interventions are appropriate at this time?

Your general impression is of an alert female patient holding a blood-soaked towel to her right forearm. Initial assessment shows her airway open and clear, respirations normal, and a regular pulse in her right wrist. You assign her a low transport priority.

You ask Norma, your partner, to go to Mary's apartment accompanied by the security guard to see if she can learn anything more about the mechanism of injury. Meanwhile, you observe that the bleeding is being controlled and begin a focused history and physical exam. You gently remove the towel and note there is no active bleeding from a smooth and deep laceration with muscle and tendons visible. You dress and bandage the wound.

There are no other injuries or medical problems present. You do, however, detect an odor of alcohol on Mary's breath. "Have you had any alcohol today?" you ask.

"Yes, I drank two beers about 3 hours ago. That's all!" she exclaims. However, you figure with the odor on her breath, she must have had more than two beers. Focusing on her right arm, you find pulses still present in that extremity. She is also able to feel your finger touch her palm. However, when asked to wiggle her fingers, the ring and little fingers remain motionless. She also tells you it hurts to move her fingers. Norma returns and tells you there is a pool of blood on Mary's patio.

Street Scene Questions

4. Would you change the priority of transport of this patient based on what you now know? Why or why not?
5. What interventions are appropriate for this patient?

While you continue with the patient history, Norma obtains baseline vital signs. You learn Mary is taking thyroid medication and a blood-thinner for a medical condition. You ask when her last tetanus shot had been. She tells you she cannot remember.

Norma informs you that Mary's pulse is equal in both extremities at a rate of 128 and regular; her blood pressure is 156/94, her respirations are 24 and unlabored; pupils are equal and reactive to light; and her skin is warm, dry, and a normal color.

You contact medical direction, concerned about the loss of movement in her affected extremity. The doctor tells you that you should stabilize Mary's arm with a sling.

You apply a sling, reassess vitals, and find no significant changes. Reassessing pulse, motor function, and sensation, you find Mary still unable to move her fourth and fifth digits on her right hand. You place her on your cot, load her into the ambulance, and transport her to the closest facility, monitoring her condition throughout the 15-minute ride. You find no other significant changes occurring.

Street Scenes Sample Documentation

PATIENT NAME: *Mary Brighton* PATIENT AGE: *42*

CHIEF COMPLAINT

"wrapped coat around arm and broke glass window"

PAST MEDICAL HISTORY

- [ ] None
- [ ] Allergy to
- [ ] Hypertension
- [ ] Stroke
- [ ] Seizures
- [ ] Diabetes
- [ ] COPD
- [ ] Cardiac
- [x] Other (List)
- [ ] Asthma

Thyroid problems

Current Medications (List)

Synthroid, Coumadin

VITAL SIGNS

TIME	RESP	PULSE	B.P.	MENTAL STATUS	R PUPILS L	SKIN
2355	Rate: 24; [x] Regular; [ ] Shallow; [ ] Labored	Rate: 128; [x] Regular; [ ] Irregular	156/94	[x] Alert; [ ] Voice; [ ] Pain; [ ] Unresp.	R [x] Normal L [x]; [ ] Dilated [ ]; [ ] Constricted [ ]; [ ] Sluggish [ ]; [ ] No-Reaction [ ]	[x] Unremarkable; [ ] Cool; [ ] Pale; [ ] Warm; [ ] Cyanotic; [ ] Moist; [ ] Flushed; [ ] Dry; [ ] Jaundiced
0005	Rate: 26; [x] Regular; [ ] Shallow; [ ] Labored	Rate: 126; [x] Regular; [ ] Irregular	152/96	[x] Alert; [ ] Voice; [ ] Pain; [ ] Unresp.	R [x] Normal L [x]; [ ] Dilated [ ]; [ ] Constricted [ ]; [ ] Sluggish [ ]; [ ] No-Reaction [ ]	[x] Unremarkable; [ ] Cool; [ ] Pale; [ ] Warm; [ ] Cyanotic; [ ] Moist; [ ] Flushed; [ ] Dry; [ ] Jaundiced
0011	Rate: 24; [x] Regular; [ ] Shallow; [ ] Labored	Rate: 128; [x] Regular; [ ] Irregular	156/94	[x] Alert; [ ] Voice; [ ] Pain; [ ] Unresp.	R [x] Normal L [x]; [ ] Dilated [ ]; [ ] Constricted [ ]; [ ] Sluggish [ ]; [ ] No-Reaction [ ]	[x] Unremarkable; [ ] Cool; [ ] Pale; [ ] Warm; [ ] Cyanotic; [ ] Moist; [ ] Flushed; [ ] Dry; [ ] Jaundiced

NARRATIVE *Upon arrival, noted patient sitting upright in a chair in the manager's office of apartment complex. Patient was alert and oriented, with a large towel wrapped around her right forearm. Blood had soaked through the towel, and spots of blood noted on floor. Further investigation revealed a pool of blood approx. 12" in diameter on patient's patio. Patient attempted to break into her own apartment by breaking glass window; suffered a laceration with muscle and tendons visible. Upon EMS arrival, bleeding arrested by direct pressure. Patient has pulse and sensation, but unable to move fourth and fifth digits on affected limb. She c/o pain when moving fingers. Patient denies any other pain/medical problems at this time other than aforementioned. Patient states she had "two beers 3 hours ago"; significant fruity odor apparent on breath. Patient's extremity dressed, bandaged, and stabilized with a sling. Medical direction established and advised EMS to transport immediately to appropriate facility. No significant change noted en route. O_2 administered via nonrebreather at 15 LPM.*

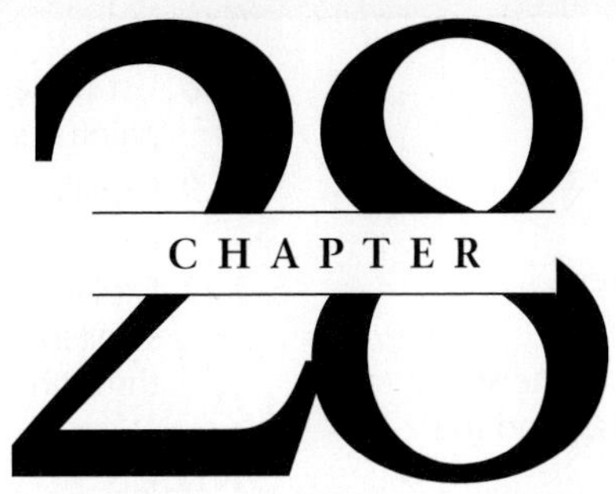

CHAPTER

Musculoskeletal Injuries

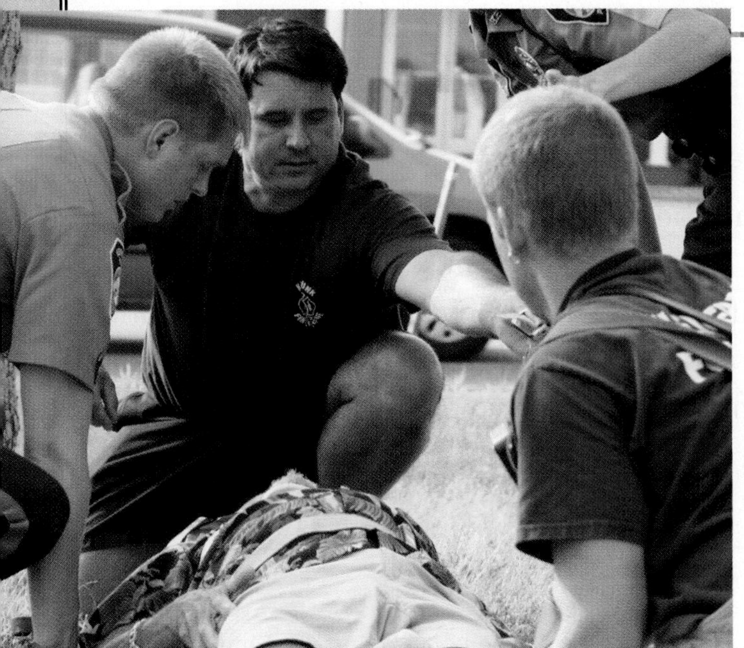

CORE CONCEPTS

The following are core concepts that will be addressed in this chapter:

- Major bones and regions of the musculoskeletal system
- How to identify open and closed extremity injuries
- Purposes and general procedures for splinting
- How to splint injured extremities

KEY TERMS

bones, p. 694
cartilage, p. 699
closed extremity injury, p. 702
crepitus, p. 704
dislocation, p. 701
extremities, p. 694
fracture, p. 701
joints, p. 694
ligaments, p. 699
manual traction, p. 706
muscles, p. 699
open extremity injury, p. 702
sprain, p. 702
strain, p. 702
tendons, p. 699
traction splint, p. 701

DOT OBJECTIVES

*KNOWLEDGE AND ATTITUDE

5-3.1 Describe the function of the muscular system. (pp. 694, 699–700)

5-3.2 Describe the function of the skeletal system. (pp. 694–699)

5-3.3 List the major bones or bone groupings of the spinal column, the thorax, the upper extremities, and the lower extremities. (pp. 695–698)

5-3.4 Differentiate between an open and a closed painful, swollen, or deformed extremity. (p. 702)

5-3.5 State the reasons for splinting. (p. 705)

5-3.6 List the general rules of splinting. (pp. 706–707) (Scans 28-1 through 28-4, pp. 708–713)

5-3.7 List the complications of splinting. (p. 707)

5-3.8 List the emergency medical care for a patient with a painful, swollen, deformed extremity. (p. 704–705)

5-3.9 Explain the rationale for splinting at the scene versus load and go. (pp. 705, 707)

5-3.10 Explain the rationale for immobilization of the painful, swollen, deformed extremity. (pp. 705–706) (Scans 28-5 through 28-17, pp. 726–743)

*SKILLS

5-3.11 Demonstrate the emergency medical care of a patient with a painful, swollen, deformed extremity.

5-3.12 Demonstrate completing a prehospital care report for patients with musculoskeletal injuries.

Musculoskeletal injuries are common. As an EMT, you will be called upon to treat injuries to muscles and bones, which range from minor to life threatening. Many musculoskeletal injuries can have a grotesque appearance. You will be called upon to fully evaluate the patient and not be distracted from life-threatening conditions by a deformed limb.

MUSCULOSKELETAL SYSTEM

The musculoskeletal system is composed of all the bones, joints, and muscles of the body, as well as cartilage, tendons, and ligaments. As an EMT, you do not need to know every structure found in the body. However, you do need to remember how complex the structures are and what kinds of damage may be done in case of injury. Examine the skeleton and its major divisions in Figures 28-1 and 28-2. Also review the musculoskeletal system in Chapter 4, "The Human Body."

extremities (ex-TREM-i-teez) the portions of the skeleton that include the clavicles, scapulae, arms, wrists, and hands (upper extremities) and the pelvis, thighs, legs, ankles, and feet (lower extremities).

In this chapter, we will pay special attention to the **extremities**—the portions of the skeleton that include the clavicles, scapulae, arms, wrists, and hands (upper extremities, Figure 28-3) and the pelvis, thighs, legs, ankles, and feet (lower extremities, Figure 28-4).

Anatomy of Bone

bones hard but flexible living structures that provide support for the body and protection to vital organs.

joints places where bones articulate, or meet.

Bones are formed of dense connective tissue. As components of the skeleton, they provide the body's framework. They are strong to provide support and protection for the internal organs, but they are also flexible to withstand stress. The bones store salts and metabolic materials and provide a site for the production of red blood cells. **Joints** are the places where bones articulate, or meet, and are a critical element in the body's ability to move.

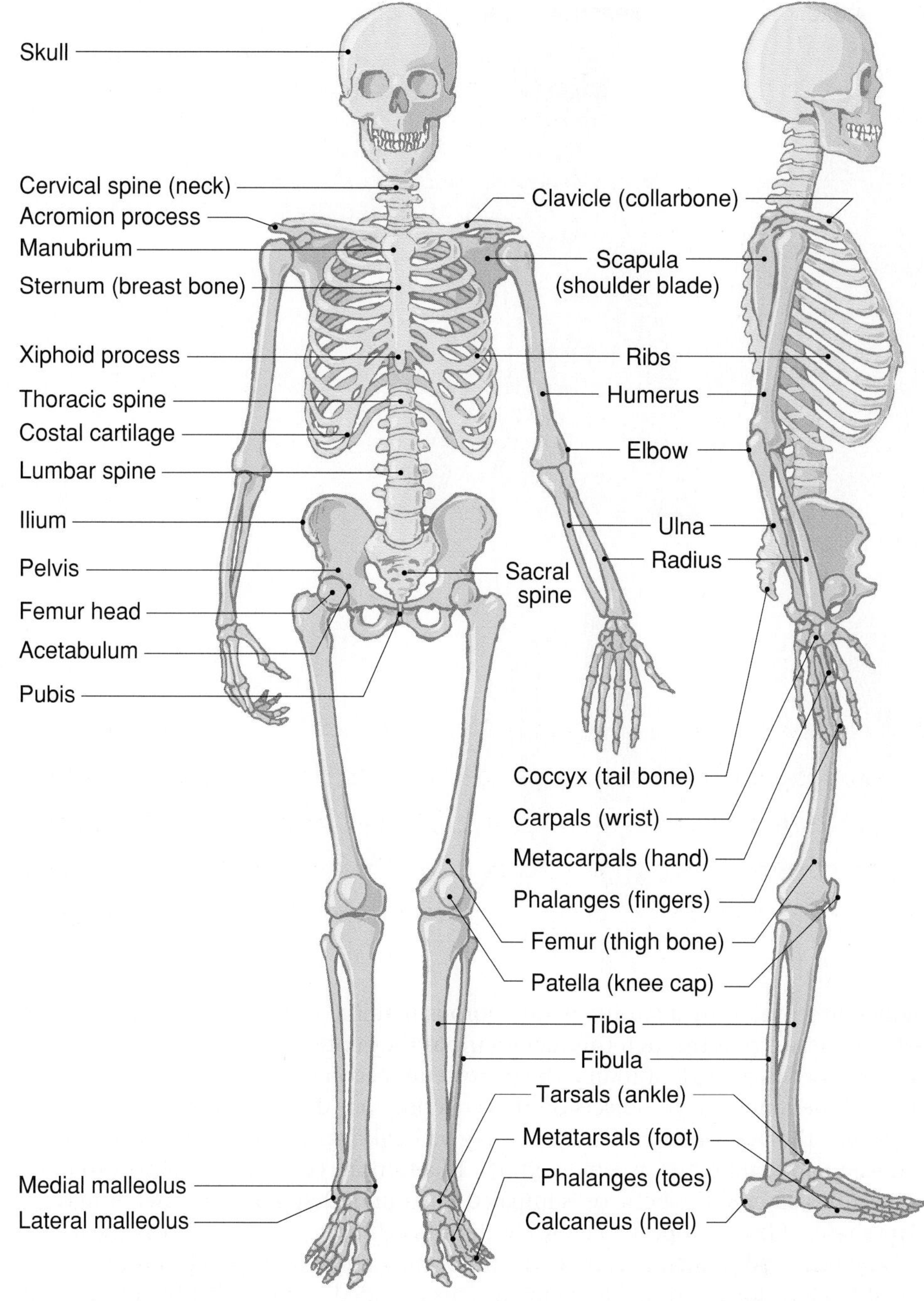

Figure 28-1 • Human skeleton.

Generally, bones are classified according to their appearance—long, short, flat, and irregular (Figure 28-5). The bones found in the arm and thigh are examples of long bones. The major short bones of the body are in the hands and feet. The flat bones include the sternum, shoulder blades, and ribs. The vertebrae of the spinal column are examples of irregular bones.

The outward appearance of a typical long bone creates the impression that it is a simple, rigid structure made of the same material throughout. Actually, it is quite complex. Most people are aware that bone contains calcium, which helps to make it very hard. Bone also contains protein fibers that make it somewhat flexible. The strength of our bones is a combination of this hardness and flexibility. As we age, less protein is formed in the bones, less calcium is stored, and as a result, bones become brittle and break more easily.

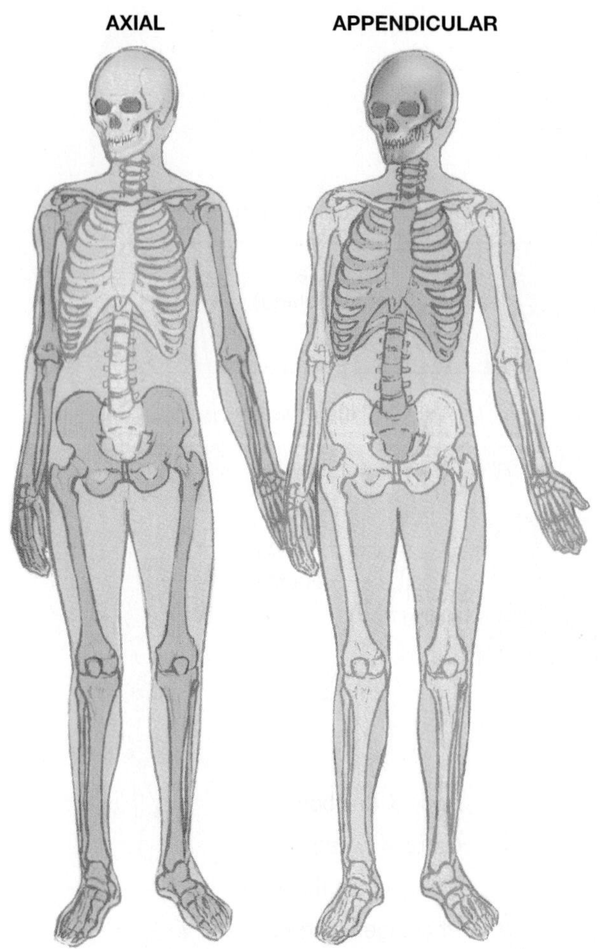

Figure 28-2 • The axial skeleton is made up of the skull, spine, ribs, and sternum. The extremities comprise the appendicular skeleton.

Bones are covered by a strong, white, fibrous material called the *periosteum*. Blood vessels and nerves pass through this membrane as they enter and leave the bone. When bone is exposed as a result of injury, the periosteum becomes visible. You may see fragments of bones and foreign objects on this covering, but do not remove them. If they have pierced the periosteum, the objects may be held firmly in place and offer a great resistance to any pulling or sweeping efforts. In addition, you will not be able to tell if the object has entered the bone or is impaled in an underlying blood vessel or nerve.

The shafts of bones appear to be straight, but each bone has its own unique curvature. When the end of a bone is involved in forming a ball-and-socket joint, it will be rounded to allow for rotational movement. This rounded end is called the head of the bone. It is connected to the shaft by the neck. Bone marrow, which is contained in the center of bones, is the site of red blood cell production.

Self-Healing Nature of Bone

The most common bone injury is a break, or fracture (Figure 28-6). The first effects of an injury to bone are swelling of soft tissue and the formation of a blood clot in the area of the fracture. Both the swelling and the clotting are due to the destruction of blood vessels in the periosteum and the bone as well as to loss of blood from adjacent damaged vessels.

Interruption of the blood supply causes death to the cells at the injury site. Cells a little farther from the fracture remain intact and, within a few hours, begin to divide rapidly. They soon grow together to form a mass of tissue that completely surrounds the fracture site. New bone is generated from this mass to eventually heal the damaged

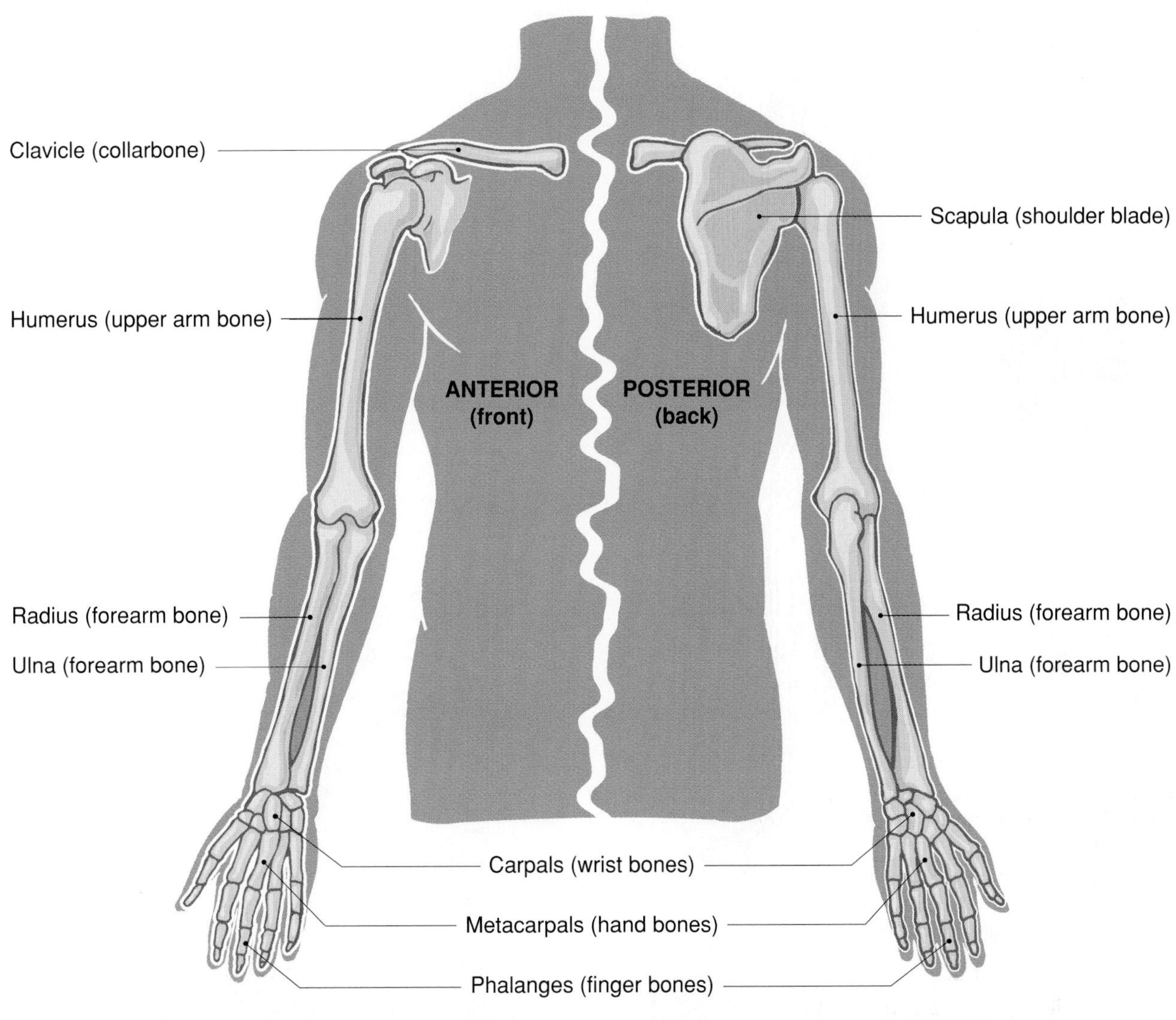

THE UPPER EXTREMITIES

COMMON NAME	*ANATOMICAL NAME*
Shoulder girdle	Pectoral girdle (PEK-tor-al): clavicle, scapula, and head of humerus
Collarbone (1/side)	Clavicle (KLAV-i-kul)
Shoulder blade (1/side)	Scapula (SKAP-u-lah)
Arm bone (1/limb, from shoulder to elbow)	Humerus (HU-mer-us)
Forearm bones (2/limb, from elbow to wrist: 1/medial, 1/lateral)	Ulna (UL-nah)–medial Radius (RAY-de-us)–lateral
Wrist bones (8/wrist)	Carpals (KAR-pals)
Hand bones (5/palm, palm bones)	Metacarpals (meta-KAR-pals)
Finger bones (14/hand)	Phalanges (fah-LAN-jez)

Figure 28-3 • Bones of the upper extremities.

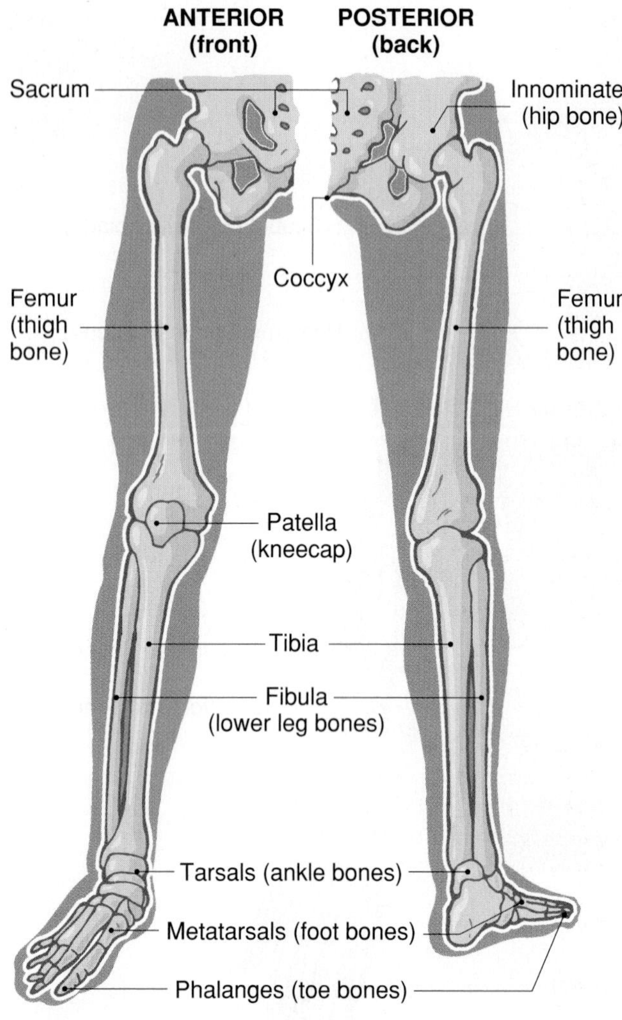

THE LOWER EXTREMITIES

COMMON NAME	*ANATOMICAL NAME*
Pelvic girdle (pelvis or hips)	Innominate on each side made up of the fused ilium, ischium, and pubis bones, as well as sacrum and coccyx posteriorly
Thigh bone (1/limb)	Femur (FE-mer)
Kneecap (1/limb)	Patella (pah-TEL-lah)
Leg bones (shin bones, 2/leg, 1 medial, 1 lateral)	Tibia (TIB-e-ah) – medial Fibula (FIB-yo-lah) – lateral
Ankle bones (7/foot)	Tarsals (TAR-sals)
Foot bones (5/foot)	Metatarsals (meta-TAR-sals)
Toe bones (14/foot. Some people have two bones in their little toe, others may have three.)	Phalanges (fah-LAN-jez)

Figure 28-4 • Bones of the lower extremities.

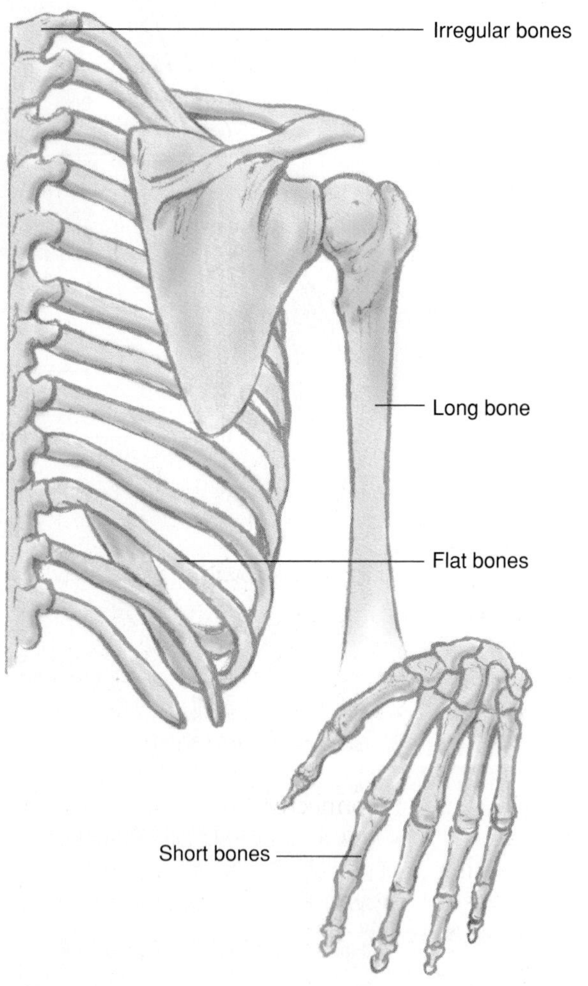

Figure 28-5 • Bones are classified by shape.

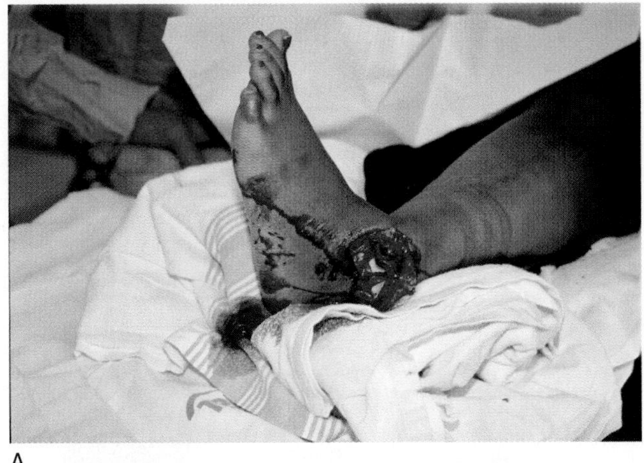

A

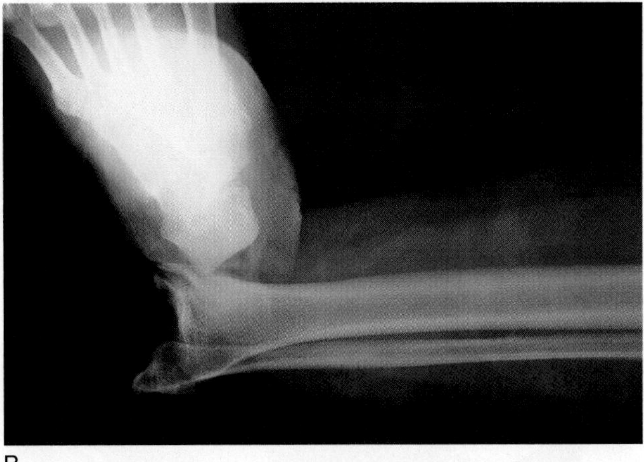

B

Figure 28-6 • (A) An open fracture to the ankle. (B) An X-ray of the same fracture. *(Both: © Edward T. Dickinson, M.D.)*

bone. The whole process can take weeks or months, depending on the bone that has been fractured, the type of fracture, and the health and age of the patient.

It is very important for a broken bone to be immobilized quickly and remain immobilized to heal properly. Should the fractured bone be mishandled early in care, more soft tissue may be damaged, which would require a longer period for the formation of a tissue mass and replacement of bone. If the bone ends are disturbed during regeneration, proper healing will not take place and a permanent disability may result. In children, the majority of growth of a long bone occurs in the area known as the growth plate, which is near the end of the shaft. If a fracture in this area is not properly handled, the child may grow up with one limb shorter than the other.

Muscles, Cartilage, Ligaments, and Tendons

In addition to bones, the elements of the musculoskeletal system are the muscles, cartilage, ligaments, and tendons. **Muscles** are the tissues or fibers that cause movement of body parts or organs. There are three kinds of muscles: skeletal (voluntary), smooth (involuntary), and cardiac (myocardial) (Figure 28-7). Smooth, or involuntary, muscles are found in the walls of organs and digestive structures. These are the muscles that move food through the digestive system. Cardiac muscle is found in the walls of the heart. The muscles that are of chief concern in trauma and musculoskeletal injury are the skeletal, or voluntary, muscles. These are the muscles that control all conscious or deliberate motions. The skeletal or voluntary muscles include all the muscles that are connected to bones as well as the muscles in the tongue, pharynx, and upper esophagus.

muscles
tissues or fibers that cause movement of body parts and organs.

Cartilage is connective tissue that covers the outside of the bone end (epiphysis) and acts as a surface for articulation, allowing for smooth movement at joints. Cartilage, which is less rigid than bone, forms or helps to form some of the more flexible structures of the body, such as the septum of the nose (the wall between the nostrils), the external ear, the trachea, and the connections between the ribs and sternum (breastbone).

cartilage
tough tissue that covers the joint ends of bones and helps to form certain body parts such as the ear.

Tendons are bands of connective tissue that bind the muscles to bones. The tendons allow for the power of movement across the joints. **Ligaments** are connective tissue that supports joints by attaching the bone ends and allowing for a stable range of motion. Two mnemonics can help you distinguish between the connective functions of tendons and ligaments: MTB = muscle-tendon-bone; BLB = bone-ligament-bone (Figure 28-8).

tendons
tissues that connect muscle to bone.

ligaments
connective tissues that connect bone to bone.

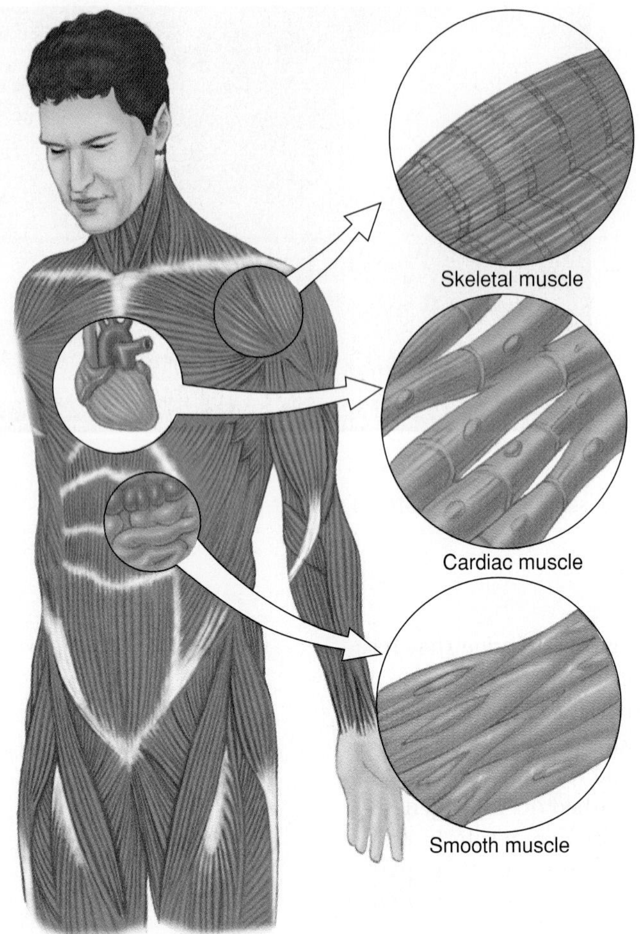

Figure 28-7 • Three types of muscles.

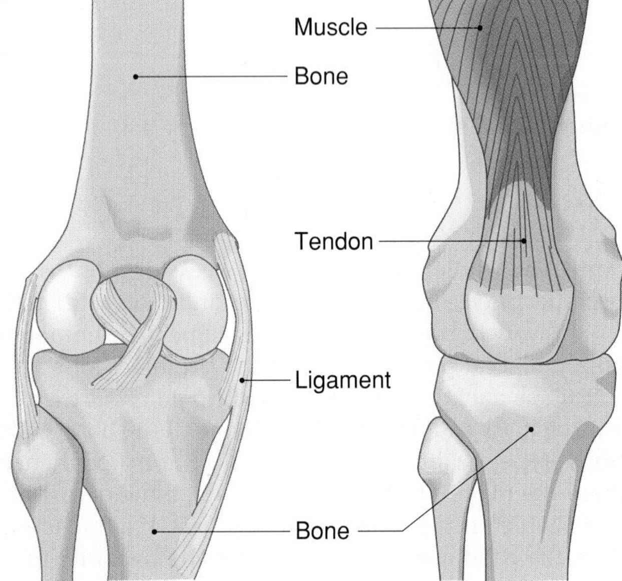

Figure 28-8 • Tendons tie muscle to bone. Ligaments tie bone to bone.

GENERAL GUIDELINES FOR EMERGENCY CARE

Mechanisms of Musculoskeletal Injury

There are basically three types of mechanisms that cause musculoskeletal injuries: direct force, indirect force, and twisting force (Figure 28-9). An example of *direct force* is a person being struck by an automobile, causing crushed tissue and fractures. *Twisting or rotational forces* can cause stretching or tearing of muscles and ligaments, as well as broken bones, such as occur when a ski digs into the snow while the skier's body rotates. Sporting activities such as football, basketball, soccer, in-line skating, skiing, snowboarding, and wrestling—in addition to motor-vehicle collisions—account for many musculoskeletal injuries.

It is easy to see how direct forces cause injuries, but an *indirect force* can be just as powerful. For example, a well-known injury pattern occurs when people fall from heights and land on their feet. The direct forces cause injuries to the feet and ankles, while indirect forces usually cause injuries to the knees, femurs, pelvis, and spinal column. In fact, most injuries to the upper extremities are caused by forces applied to an outstretched arm. In the course of a fall, the person reaches out with an arm in an effort to break the fall and, in doing so, often breaks the radius, ulna, or clavicle, or dislocates the shoulder.

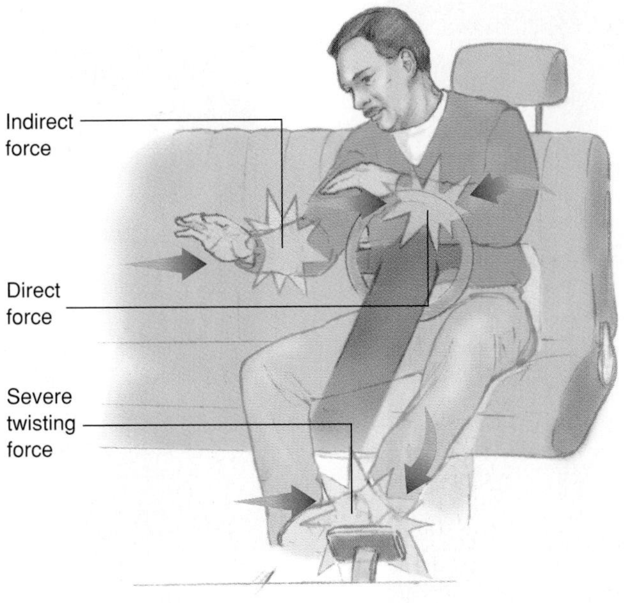

Figure 28-9 • Three basic mechanisms of musculoskeletal injury.

Painful, Swollen, or Deformed Extremity

Unless there is very obvious deformity, it is not possible or even important for you to decide if a patient's injury is a fracture, a dislocation, a sprain, or a severe bruise. Most patients simply present with pain, swelling, and—sometimes—deformity. It will take an X-ray or other imaging process to diagnose the injury precisely (Figure 28-10). So in the field the worst must be assumed, and a patient with a painful, swollen, or deformed extremity should be treated as though he has a fracture. Though most fractures are not life-threatening, remember that bones are living tissue. Even in simple uncomplicated fractures, bones bleed. For example, a simple closed tibia-fibula fracture typically causes a 1-pint (500 cc) blood loss. Fractures of the femur typically cause a 2-pint (1,000 cc) blood loss, and pelvic fractures cause a 3- to 4-pint (1,500–2,000 cc) blood loss (Figure 28-11).

In World War I, the battlefield death rate from a closed fracture of the femur was about 80 percent, because of complications such as blood loss. Two surgeons noticed that large muscle groups in the thigh go into spasms (contract, or shrink), forcing the broken femoral ends to override each other, injuring the blood vessels. To correct the problem, they invented the **traction splint,** a splint that applies constant pull along the length of the leg to help stabilize the fractured bone and reduce muscle spasms. With early application of a traction splint, the mortality rate from femur fractures dropped to under 20 percent (and much lower today).

traction splint
a splint that applies constant pull along the length of a lower extremity to help stabilize the fractured bone and to reduce muscle spasm in the limb. Traction splints are used primarily on femoral shaft fractures.

Remember that splinting a painful, swollen, or deformed extremity can prevent additional blood loss, pain, and complications from nerve and blood vessel injury. Therefore, treat for the worst (a fracture) and immobilize. Physicians in the hospital will diagnose the actual injury with an X-ray.

While it is not important for you to attempt to diagnose the underlying problem, it may be helpful for you to know the terminology health professionals use to define various musculoskeletal injuries:

- **Fracture.** A fracture is any break in a bone (Figure 28-12). Fractures can be classified as open or closed, and are also classified by the way a bone is broken, such as comminuted if broken in several places, or greenstick if the break is incomplete, or angulated if the broken bone is bent at an angle.
- **Dislocation.** The disruption or "coming apart" of a joint is called a dislocation. In order for a joint to dislocate, the soft tissue of the joint capsule and ligaments must be stretched beyond the normal range of motion and torn.

fracture (FRAK-cher)
any break in a bone.

dislocation
the disruption or "coming apart" of a joint.

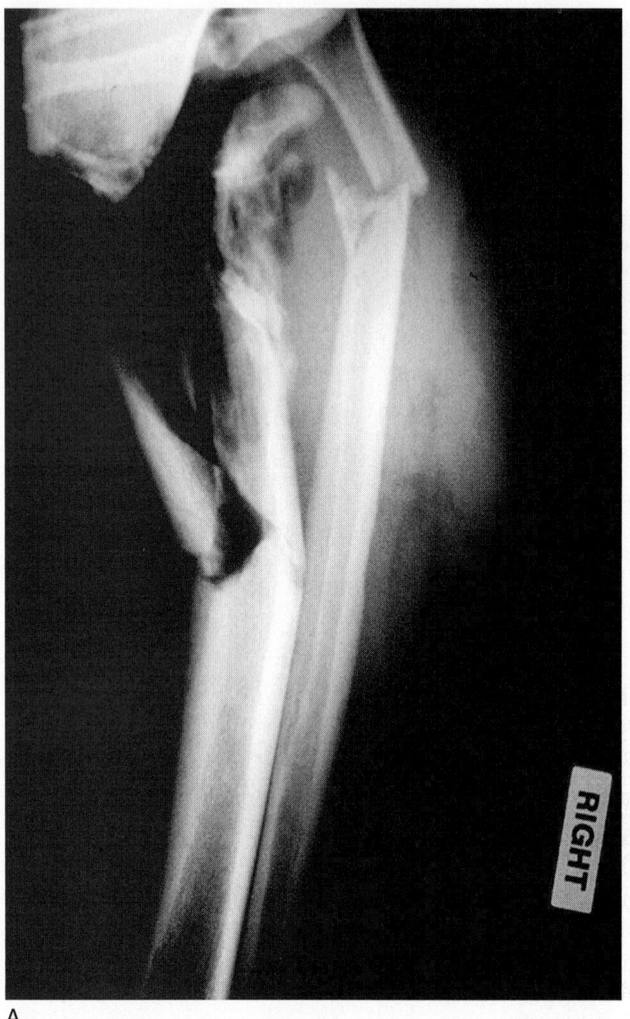

A

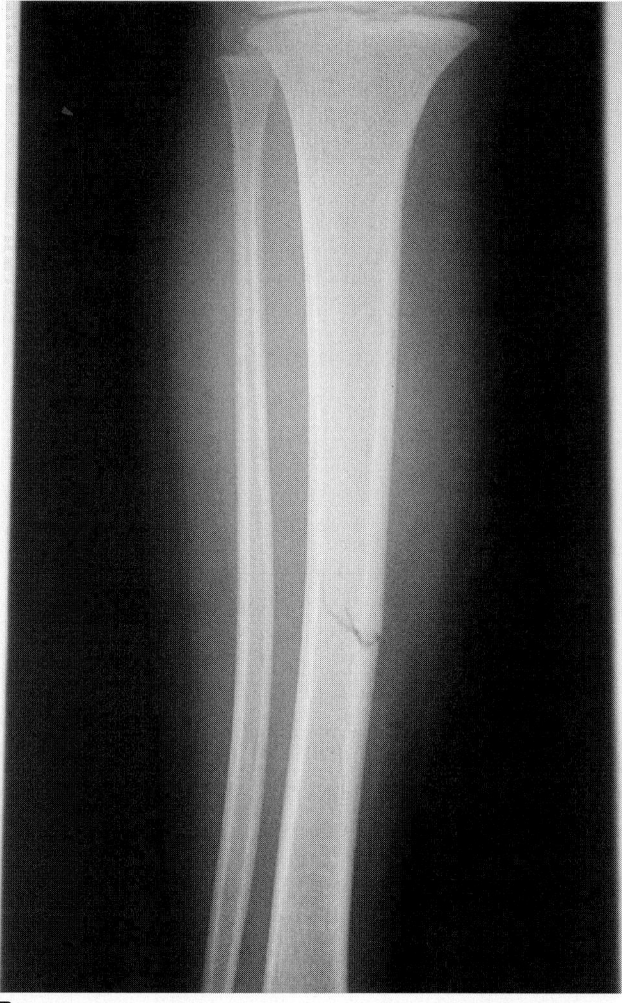

B

Figure 28-10 • (A) Some fractures are severe and obvious during external exams, while (B) others are subtle and difficult to detect without an X-ray. *(Both: © Charles Stewart, M.D. and Associates)*

sprain
the stretching and tearing of ligaments.

strain
muscle injury resulting from overstretching or overexertion of the muscle.

closed extremity injury
an extremity injury with no opening in the skin.

open extremity injury
an extremity injury in which the skin has been broken or torn through.

- **Sprain.** A sprain is caused by the stretching and tearing of ligaments. It is most commonly associated with joint injuries.
- **Strain.** A strain is a muscle injury caused by overstretching or overexertion of the muscle.

A **closed extremity injury** is one in which the skin is not broken. An **open extremity injury** is one in which the skin has been broken or torn through from the inside by the injured bone or from the outside by something that has caused a penetrating wound with associated injury to the bone. An open injury is a serious situation because of the increased likelihood of infection.

While many closed injuries can be handled simply in the hospital emergency department, all patients with open fractures require surgery. Proper splinting and prehospital care of musculoskeletal injuries help prevent closed injuries from becoming open ones.

Assessment of Musculoskeletal Injuries

Examination involves your senses and the skills of inspection (looking), palpation (feeling), and auscultation (listening). One of the basic principles of assessment is that it is difficult to do a proper examination on patients when they are fully clothed. However, it often is difficult, impractical, or inadvisable to completely disrobe or cut away a patient's

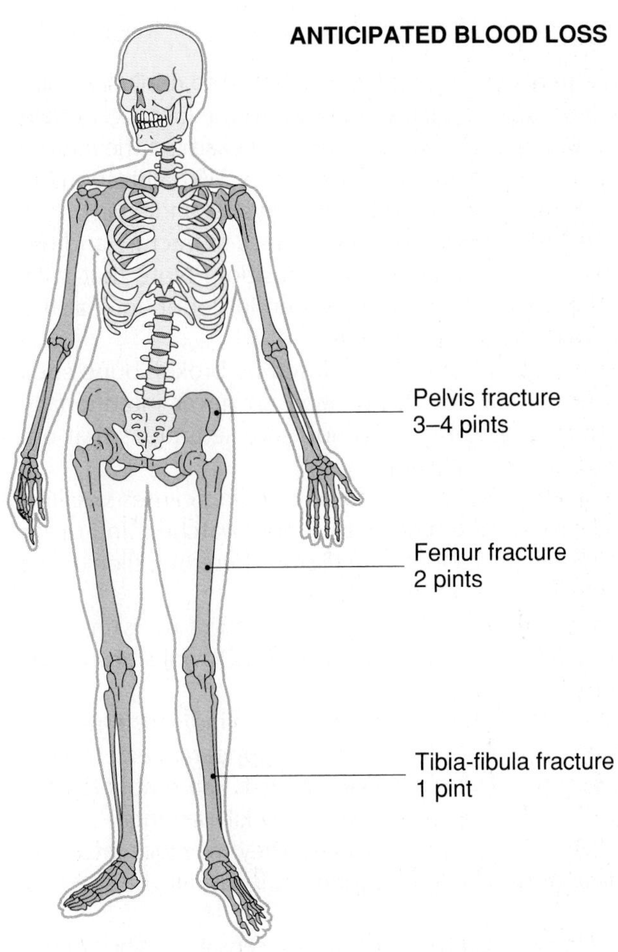

Figure 28-11 • Bones bleed. In fact, there may be considerable blood loss, even from an uncomplicated closed fracture.

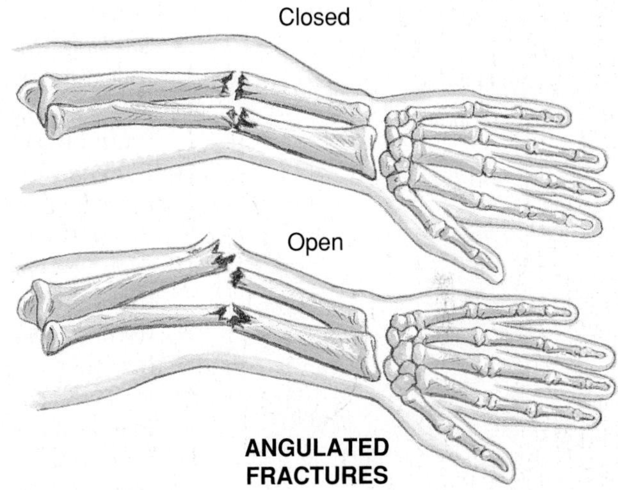

Figure 28-12 • Angulated bone injuries may be open or closed.

clothing due to weather, the patient's modesty, or patient refusal. A good rule of thumb is to cut or remove clothing according to the environment and severity of the situation.

In cases of severe extremity trauma, injuries can be very obvious. However, when treating trauma patients, *your priority must be to rapidly identify and treat life-threatening conditions first.* Do not let a grotesque but relatively minor extremity injury sidetrack you—or the patient. The pain or terrible appearance of an extremity injury may distract the patient from awareness of other injuries or symptoms. Be sure to assess the patient fully and ask appropriate questions to avoid missing another injury. After your initial assessment and focused exam rules out obvious life-threatening airway, breathing, or circulation problems and injuries to the head, spine, chest, and abdomen, focus your attention on musculoskeletal injuries to the extremities.

PATIENT ASSESSMENT

MUSCULOSKELETAL INJURIES

Signs and symptoms of musculoskeletal injuries in a patient include the following:

- *Pain and tenderness.* The patient with a painful, swollen, or deformed extremity experiences pain when the injured part is touched or moved. Generally, a

continued

patient will hold the injured part still, or guard it, in an effort to minimize pain. When examining a conscious patient, ask him to point to the location of pain if possible. Then, initially avoiding that location, carefully examine the injured part to assess if there are any other painful or injured areas. With unresponsive patients, suspicion of injury must be based on other physical findings.

- *Deformity or angulation.* The force of trauma causes bones to fracture and become deformed, or angulated, out of anatomical position. Note that with joint injuries, sometimes the deformity is subtle. When in doubt, look at the uninjured side and compare it to the injured one.
- *Grating,* or **crepitus.** This is a sound or feeling caused by broken bone ends rubbing together. It can be painful for the patient, so never intentionally cause crepitus. The patient may report grating noises or sensations that occurred prior to your arrival and examination.

crepitus (KREP-i-tus) a grating sensation or sound made when fractured bone ends rub together.

- *Swelling.* When bones break and soft tissue is torn, bleeding causes swelling that may increase the proportions of a deformity. Rings, watches, and other jewelry can easily constrict and injure underlying tissue. Therefore, slide or cut them off as soon as possible if swelling is likely to occur.
- *Bruising.* Ecchymosis, or large black-and-blue discoloration of the skin, indicates an underlying injury that may be hours or days old. Obvious bruises indicate the need for splinting.
- *Exposed bone ends.* Bone ends protruding through the skin indicate a fracture that requires splinting. Again, the more gruesome the appearance of the extremity, the greater the temptation to treat that injury first. Remember to care for life-threatening injuries first. Extremity injuries rarely kill patients.
- *Joints locked into position.* When joints are dislocated, they may lock into normal or abnormal anatomical positions. Joint injuries must usually be splinted as found.
- *Nerve and blood-vessel compromise.* Examine for pulses, sensation, and movement distal to the injury site. This must be accomplished before and after splinting. Check for nerve injury by asking the patient if he can sense your touch and can move all fingers or toes. Any problem of sensation or movement must be noted. Then feel for pulses in the wrist (radial), ankle (posterior tibial), or foot (dorsalis pedis). Obviously, to accurately examine for sensation, movement, and pulses, the patient's gloves and footwear must be removed.

Another method of assessing compromise to an extremity when a musculoskeletal injury is suspected is to learn and follow the "five p's": pain or tenderness; pallor (pale skin or poor capillary refill); paresthesia, or the sensation of "pins and needles"; pulses diminished or absent in the injured extremity; and paralysis or the inability to move. ■

PATIENT CARE

MUSCULOSKELETAL INJURIES

Emergency care of a patient with musculoskeletal injuries includes the following:

1. Take and maintain appropriate Standard Precautions.
2. Perform the initial assessment. Remember, do not get distracted from your initial assessment and from determining patient priority by a dramatic-looking or painful extremity injury. Keep in mind, however, that multiple fractures, especially to the femurs, can cause life-threatening external or internal bleeding.

continued

PATIENT CARE *(continued)*

3. During the rapid trauma exam, apply a cervical collar if spine injury is suspected.
4. After life-threatening conditions have been addressed, any patient with a painful, swollen, or deformed extremity must be splinted. For a low-priority (stable) patient, splint individual injuries before transport. For a high-priority (unstable) patient, immobilize the whole body on a long spine board, then "load and go." If time and the patient's condition permit, you may be able to splint a specific injury en route.
5. If appropriate, cover open wounds with sterile dressings, elevate the extremity, and apply a cold pack to the area to help reduce swelling. ■

NOTE

If an initial assessment reveals that your patient is unstable, managing extremity injuries becomes a low priority. An unstable patient with "load and go" problems must have the ABCs managed and the entire body splinted or immobilized on a long spine board. Do not take time to splint each injury individually. It is not in the patient's best interest to waste time treating minor injuries and delivering a perfectly packaged but unsavable patient to the hospital.

Splinting

Emergency care for all painful, swollen, or deformed extremities starts by splinting. *For any splint to be effective, it must immobilize adjacent joints and bone ends.* Effective splinting minimizes the movement of disrupted joints and broken bone ends, and it decreases the patient's pain. It helps prevent additional injury to soft tissues such as nerves, arteries, veins, and muscles. It can prevent a closed fracture from becoming an open fracture, a much more serious condition, and it can help to minimize blood loss. In the case of the spine, splinting on a backboard prevents injury to the spinal cord and helps to prevent permanent paralysis.

Realignment of the Deformed Extremity

The object of realignment (straightening) is to assist in restoring effective circulation to the extremity and to fit it to a splint. Some injuries, such as certain wrist fractures, may be completely splintable because they are only slightly deformed. In this case, the only reason to attempt realignment would be to restore circulation to the hand if it appeared to be cyanotic or lacked pulses.

The thought of realigning an angulated injury can be a frightening one. However, remember these points:

- If the extremity is not realigned, the splint may be ineffective, causing increased pain and possible further injury (including an open fracture) during transportation.
- If the extremity is not realigned, the chance of nerves, arteries, and veins being compromised increases. When distal circulation is compromised or shut down, tissues beyond the injury become starved for oxygen and die.
- Pain is increased for only a moment during realignment under traction. Pain is reduced by effective splinting.

Due to the size and weight of extremities, attempting to splint one in the deformed position is usually futile and only increases the chance of its becoming an open fracture. When angulated injuries to the tibia or fibula, femur, radius or ulna, or humerus cannot be fit into a rigid splint, realign the bone. Also realign a long bone when the distal extremity is cyanotic or lacks pulses, indicating compromised circulation.

The general guidelines for realigning an extremity are as follows (Figure 28-13):

1. One EMT grasps the distal extremity, while a partner places one hand above and one hand below the injury site.

manual traction the process of applying tension to straighten and realign a fractured limb before splinting. Also called *tension.*

2. The partner supports the site while the first EMT pulls gentle **manual traction** in the direction of the long axis of the extremity. If resistance is felt or if it appears that bone ends will come through the skin, stop realignment and splint the extremity in the position found.
3. If no resistance is felt, maintain gentle traction until the extremity is properly splinted.

Generally, injured joints should be splinted in the position found unless the distal extremity is cyanotic or lacks pulses. If so, an attempt should be made to align the joint to a neutral anatomical position using gentle traction, provided that no resistance is felt.

Strategies for Splinting

Effective splinting may require some ingenuity. Even though you carry different types of splinting devices, many situations will require you to improvise. In a pinch, you can use pillows or rolled blankets as soft splints. For rigid splints you can use a piece of lumber, cardboard, a rolled newspaper, an umbrella, a cane, a broom handle, a catcher's shin guard, or a tongue depressor for a finger. A bystander can often rummage through his car trunk and find something suitable.

Splints carried on EMS units come in three basic types: rigid splints, formable splints, and traction splints (Figure 28-14). Rigid splints require the limb to be moved to the anatomical position. They tend to provide the greatest support and are ideally used to splint long-bone injuries. Examples are cardboard, wood, pneumatic splints such as air splints and vacuum splints, and the pneumatic anti-shock garment. Formable splints are capable of being molded to different angles and generally allow for considerable movement. They are most commonly used to immobilize joint injuries in the position found. Examples are pillow and blanket splints. Traction splints are used specifically for femur fractures.

Regardless of the method of splinting, general rules that apply to all types of immobilization are as follows:

- *Expose the injury site.* Before moving the injured extremity, expose the area and control any bleeding.
- *Assess distal PMS.* Because complications of musculoskeletal injury include nerve and blood vessel injury, assess and record distal pulse, motor function, and sensation (PMS) both before and after splinting. (Review Scan 10-5 in Chapter 10, "Assessment of the Trauma Patient,"which illustrates how to assess distal function.)
- *Align long-bone injuries to anatomical position.* Do this under gentle traction, if severe deformity exists or distal circulation is compromised.
- *Do not push protruding bones back into place.* However, when you realign deformed open injuries, they may slip back into position under traction.

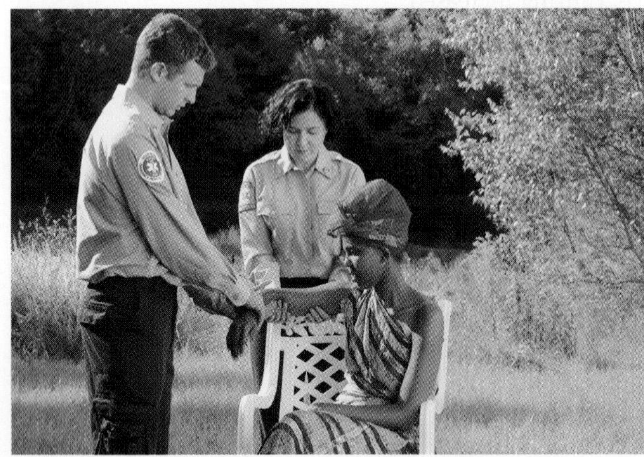

Figure 28-13 • Aligning an extremity.

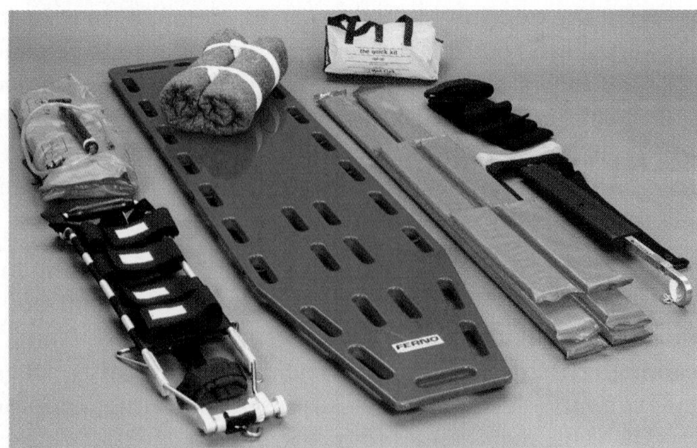

Figure 28-14 • Splints and accessories for musculoskeletal injuries.

- *Immobilize both the injury site and adjacent joints.* In order for splints to be effective, they must keep the injury site and the joints above and below still. (If the joint is injured, splint to immobilize the joint and the adjacent bones.)
- *Splint before moving the patient to a stretcher or other location, if possible.* A good rule of thumb is "least handling causes least damage." Sometimes patients must be extricated from where they are before ideal splinting techniques can occur. Attempt to immobilize the extremity as well as you can. (For example, prior to extrication, the injured extremity might be immobilized to the uninjured one.)
- *Pad the voids.* Many rigid splints do not conform to body curves and allow too much movement of the limb. Pad the voids, or spaces between the body part and the splint, to ensure proper immobilization and increase patient comfort.
- *Choose a method of splinting.* This is always dictated by the severity of the patient's condition and priority decision. If the patient is a high priority for "load and go" transport, choose a fast method of splinting. If the patient is a low priority for transport, choose a slower-but-better splinting method. The methods of splinting from slowest to fastest are: each site is individually splinted (slowest but best); the limb is secured to the torso or an uninjured leg (a bit faster, but second choice to individual splints); and the entire body is secured to a spine board (fastest, but only better than no splint at all).
- *Care for life-threatening problems first.* If the patient is unstable, do not waste time with splinting. You can align the injuries in anatomical position and immobilize the whole body to a long spine board.

Hazards of Splinting

By far the most serious hazard of splinting is "splinting someone to death"—splinting before life-threatening conditions are addressed, or spending time splinting a high-priority patient instead of immediately getting the patient into the ambulance and to the hospital. Always ensure airway, breathing, and circulation before going on to care for other injuries. Remember, the method of splinting is always dictated by the severity of the patient's condition and by the priority for transportation.

Other hazards include improper or inadequate splinting. If a splint is applied too tightly, it can compress soft tissue and injure nerves, blood vessels, and muscles. If it is applied too loosely or inappropriately, it will allow so much movement that further soft-tissue injury or an open fracture may occur. In addition, because rescue workers may be insecure about realigning a deformed injury, they may attempt to splint it in a deformed position and actually do more harm than good. Remember, it can be very difficult to splint deformed long-bone injuries well enough to prevent excessive movement.

Splinting Long-Bone and Joint Injuries

Before you start the splinting process, select a splint appropriate to the severity of the patient's condition and method of transportation. Be sure to have cravats, padding, and roller bandages immediately at hand.

The splinting of joints usually requires considerable ingenuity. In most cases formable splints are used to splint the joint in the position it is found. If the distal extremity is pulseless or cyanotic, try to align it to anatomical position using gentle traction. As with long-bone splinting, get all of your equipment ready before starting the splinting process.

To splint long-bone or joint injuries, follow these guidelines (Scans 28-1 and 28-2):

1. Take appropriate Standard Precautions and, if possible, expose the area to be splinted.
2. Manually stabilize the injury site. This can be done either by you or by a helper.
3. Assess pulses and circulation, motor function, and sensation (PMS). Check for pulses and see if the patient can feel your touch distal to the injury. Ask the patient to wiggle his fingers or toes, grasp your fingers, or push his feet against your hands.
4. Realign the injury if deformed or if the distal extremity is cyanotic or pulseless. Be sure to attempt to realign an injured joint only if the distal extremity is pulseless or cyanotic.

SCAN 28-1 • Immobilizing a Long Bone

First take Standard Precautions.

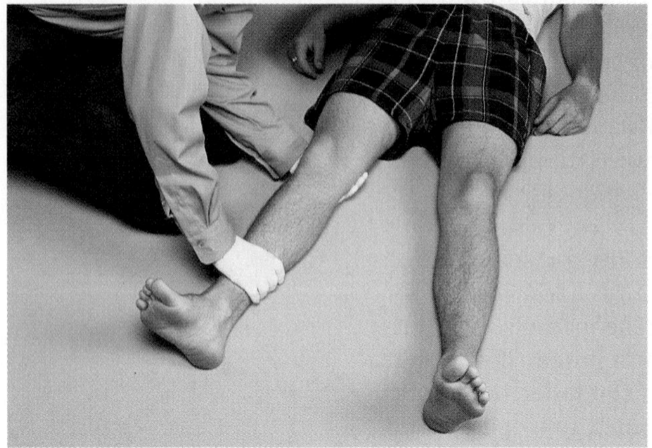

1. Manually stabilize the injured limb.

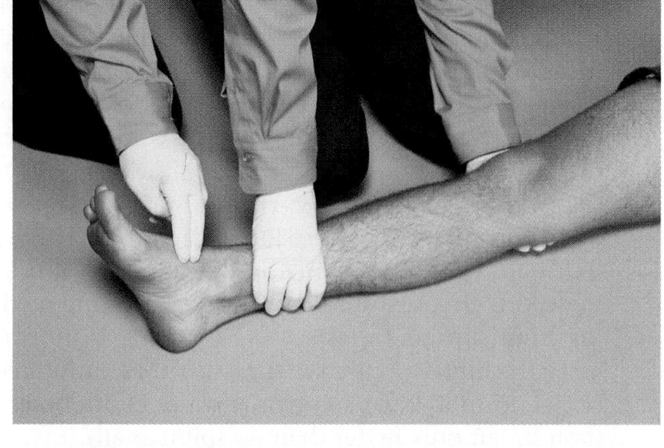

2. Assess distal pulse, motor function, and sensation (PMS).

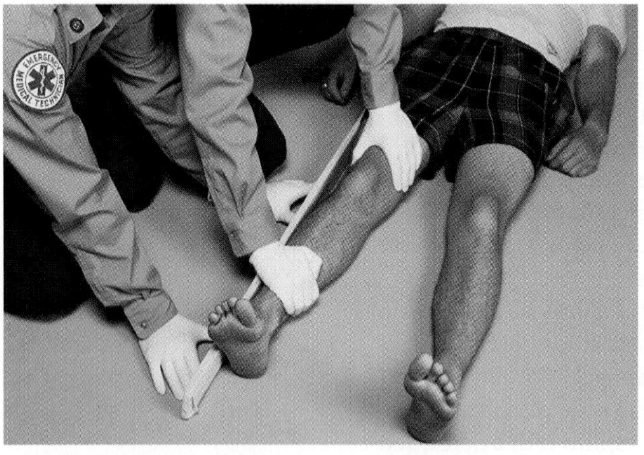

3. Measure the splint. It should extend several inches beyond the joints above and below injury.

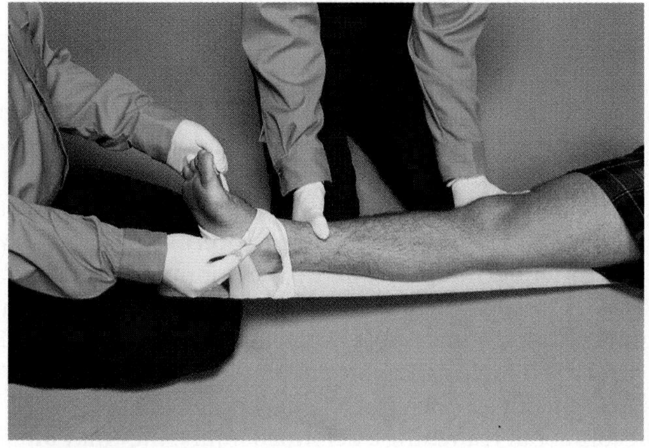

4. Apply the splint and immobilize the joints above and below the injury.

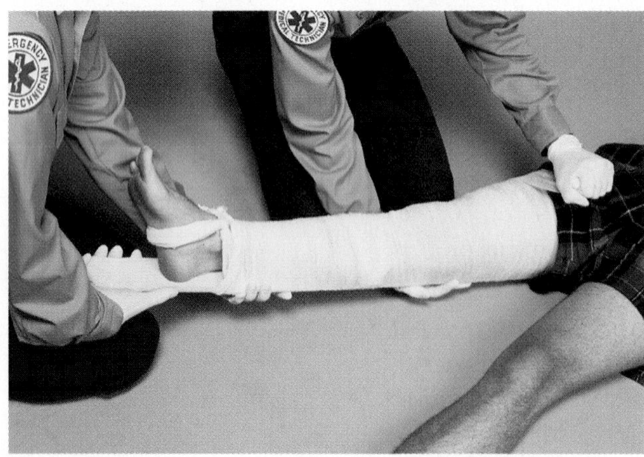

5. Secure the entire injured extremity.

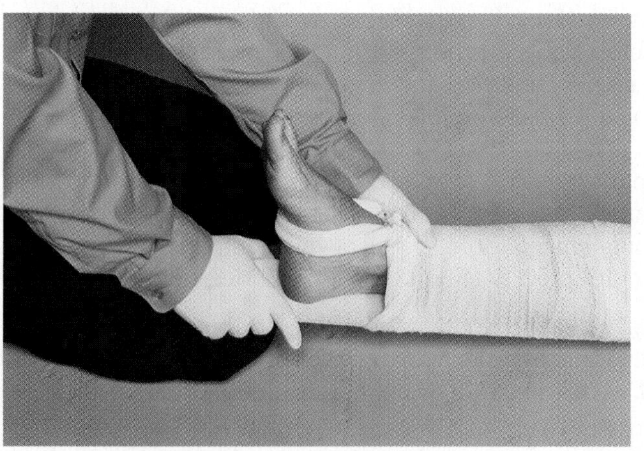

6. Secure the foot in position of function . . .

SCAN 28-1 • (Continued)

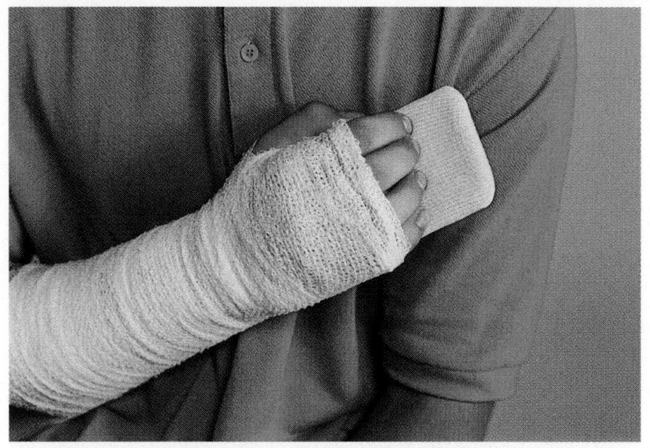

. . . Or if splinting an arm, secure the hand in the position of function. This is the position the hand would be in if the patient were holding a palm-sized ball. A roll of bandage can be placed in the patient's hand to help maintain the position of function.

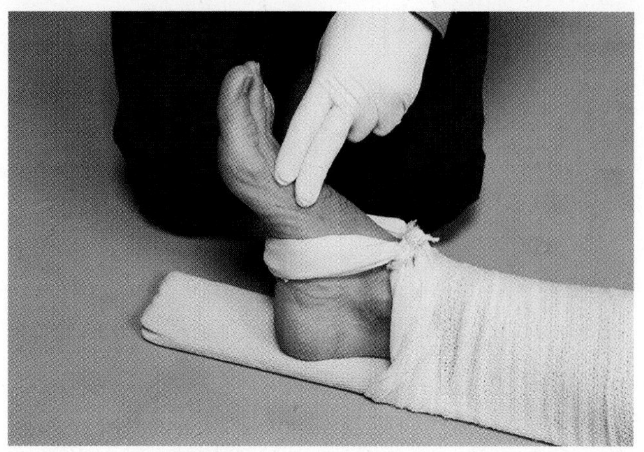

7. Reassess distal PMS function.

5. Measure or adjust the splint and move it into position under or alongside the limb. Maintain manual stabilization or traction during positioning and until the splinting procedure is complete.
6. Apply and secure the splint to immobilize adjacent joints and the injury site.
7. Reassess PMS distal to the injury.

If using a vacuum splint (Scan 28-3), use the previous steps to assess and prepare the extremity for splinting. Move the vacuum splint into position. Place the splint around the extremity, leaving the distal end (fingers or toes) exposed. Using the pump, withdraw the air from the splint until it is firm. Secure the Velcro straps. Monitor the patient.

Traction Splint

Splinting a femur injury is different from splinting other long bone or joint injuries. The major problem with femur fractures is the tendency for the large muscle groups of the thigh (quadriceps and hamstrings) to go into spasm, forcing the bone ends to override each other, causing pain and further soft-tissue injury. A traction splint counteracts the muscle spasms and greatly reduces the pain.

Traction splints come in two basic varieties: bipolar and unipolar. A bipolar splint cradles the leg between two metal rods; a unipolar splint has a single metal rod that is placed alongside the leg. Examples of the bipolar splint are the half-ring splint, Hare, and Fernotrac. Examples of the unipolar splint are the Sager and the Kendrick traction devices. (General traction splinting will be shown later in Scan 28-4. Traction splinting using Fernotrac bipolar and Sager unipolar devices will be shown later in Scans 28-10, 28-11, and 28-12.)

One of the most common EMT questions is, "How much traction should I pull?" An answer commonly given is, "Pull enough traction to give the patient some relief from the pain." This answer can be misleading. When the thigh muscles begin to spasm and the bones begin to override, the patient is in real pain. When manual or mechanical traction is applied, you are pulling against a muscle spasm, and that hurts too. Most patients do not begin to feel relief with the traction splint until it has been applied for several minutes and the muscle spasm begins to subside. With the Sager unipolar splint,

SCAN 28-2 • Immobilizing a Joint

First take Standard Precautions.

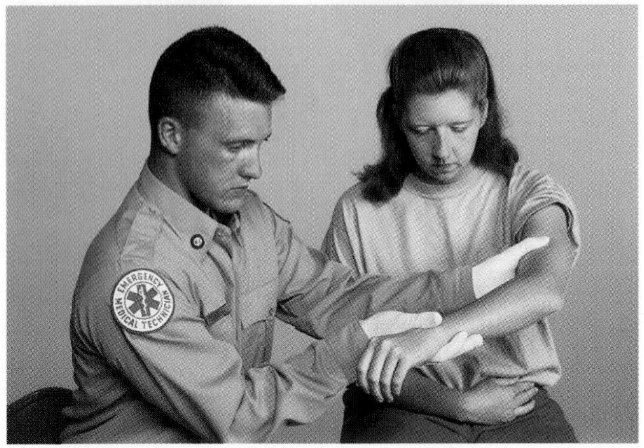

1. Manually stabilize the injured limb, in this case an injured elbow.

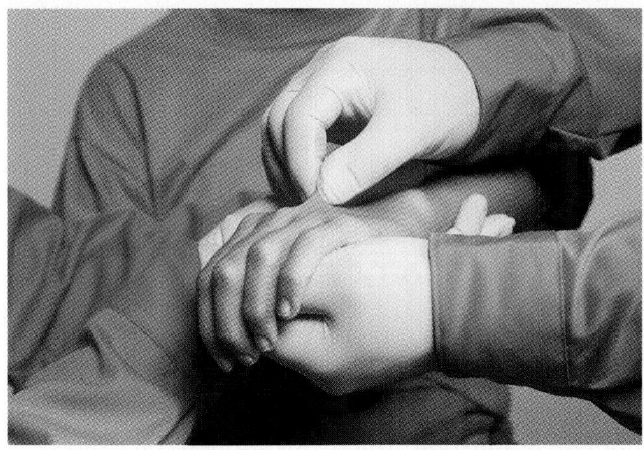

2. Assess distal pulse, motor function, and sensation (PMS).

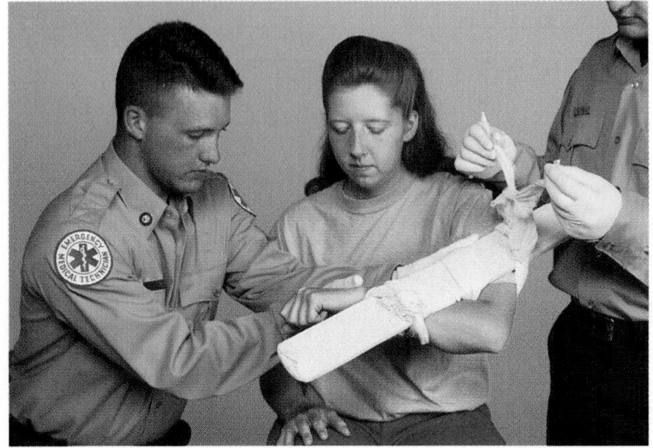

3. Select proper splint material. Immobilize site of injury and bones above and below.

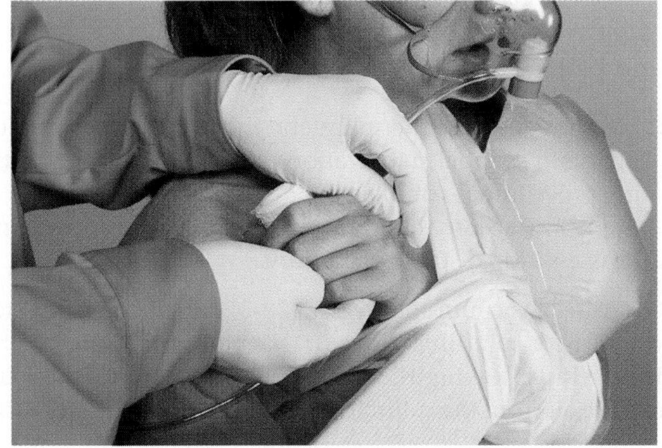

4. Reassess distal PMS function.

traction can be measured. The amount of traction applied should be roughly 10 percent of the patient's body weight and not exceed 15 pounds. With a bipolar splint, firm traction should be applied to align the limb. Exert and maintain a firm pull to prevent bones from continuing to override.

No traction splint applied in the field pulls true traction. All exert "countertraction." The splint pulls on an ankle hitch and the splint frame is anchored against the pelvis. Once anchored, a pull is felt on the leg. With bipolar splints, any movement of the pelvis off the ground causes a shifting of the splint and loss of traction. Unipolar splints, such as the Sager, are anchored against the pubis between the legs and are less apt to shift and cause a loss of traction during patient movement.

The indications for a traction splint are a painful, swollen, deformed mid-thigh with no joint or lower leg injury. A traction splint is contraindicated if there is a pelvis, hip, or knee injury; if there is an avulsion or partial amputation where traction could separate the extremity; or if there is an injury to the lower third of the leg that would interfere with the ankle hitch.

SCAN 28-3 • Applying a Vacuum Splint

First take Standard Precautions.

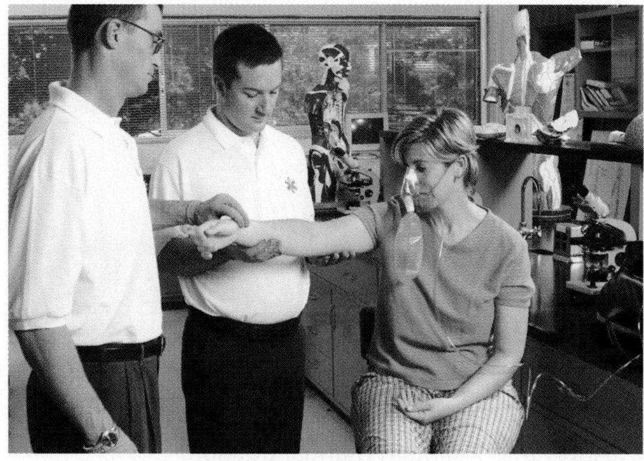

1. Stabilize the extremity and check distal pulse, motor function, and sensation (PMS).

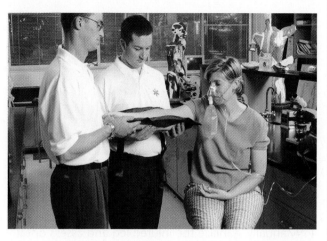

2. Apply the splint to the extremity and secure it with the straps.

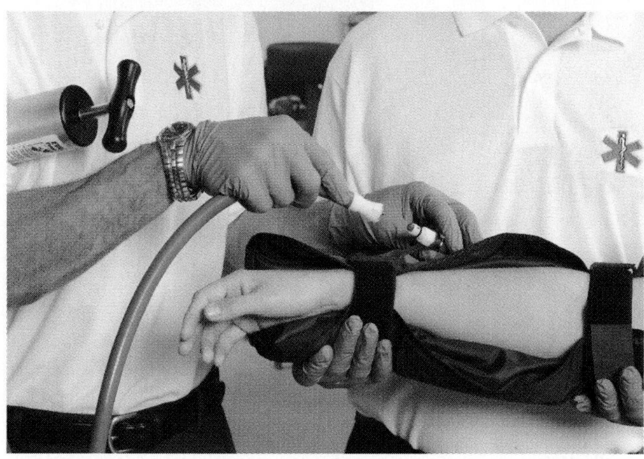

3. Remove the air from the splint with the pump provided by the manufacturer.

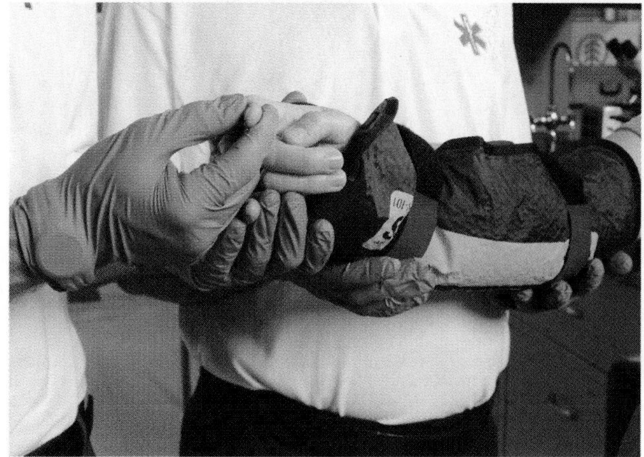

4. Reassess distal PMS function.

When possible, use three rescuers to apply a traction splint. One can support the injury site when the limb is lifted to position the traction splint.

General guidelines for the application of a traction splint are as follows (Scan 28-4):

1. Take Standard Precautions and, if possible, expose the area to be splinted.
2. Manually stabilize the leg and apply manual traction.
3. Assess PMS distal to the injury.
4. Adjust the splint to the proper length, and position it at or under the injured leg.
5. Apply the proximal securing device (ischial strap).
6. Apply the distal securing device (ankle hitch).
7. Apply mechanical traction.
8. Position and secure support straps.
9. Re-evaluate the proximal and distal securing devices, and reassess PMS distal to the injury.
10. Secure the patient's torso and the traction splint to a long spine board to immobilize the hip and to prevent movement of the splint.

SCAN 28-4 • Applying a Traction Splint

First take Standard Precautions.

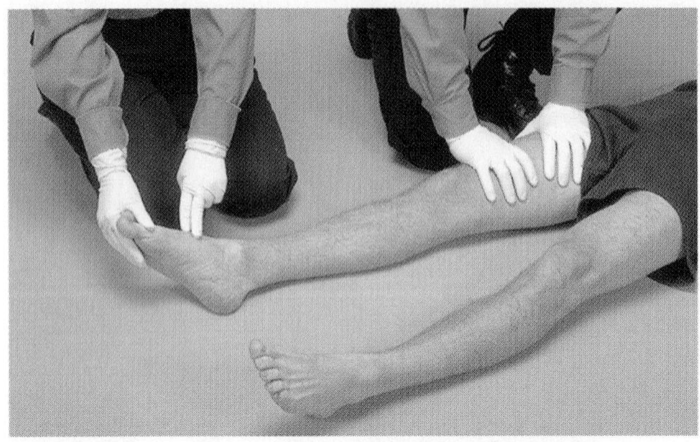

1. Manually stabilize the injured leg and assess distal pulse, motor function, and sensation (PMS).

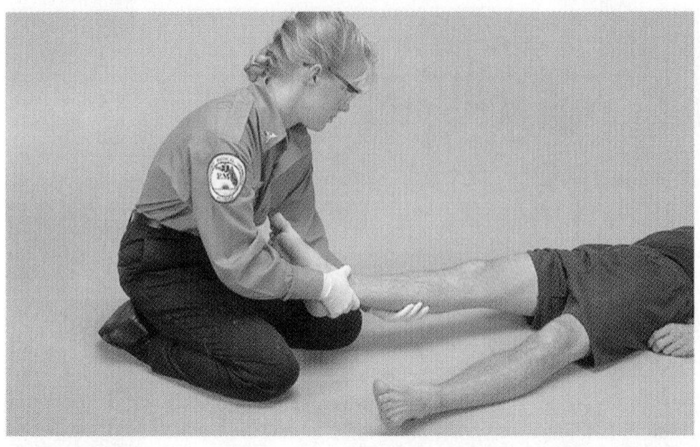

2. Apply and maintain manual traction.

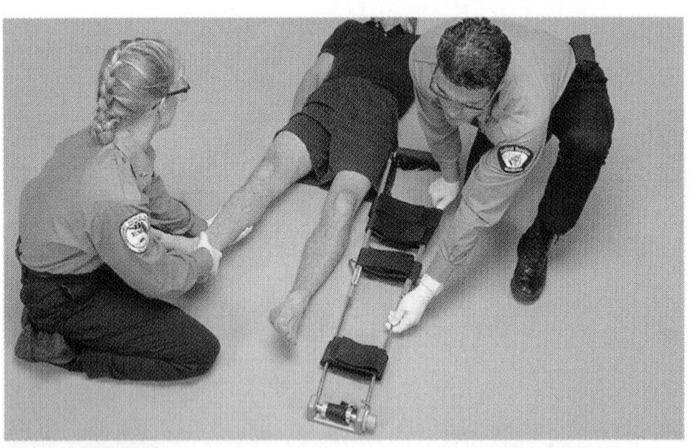

3. Measure the splint.

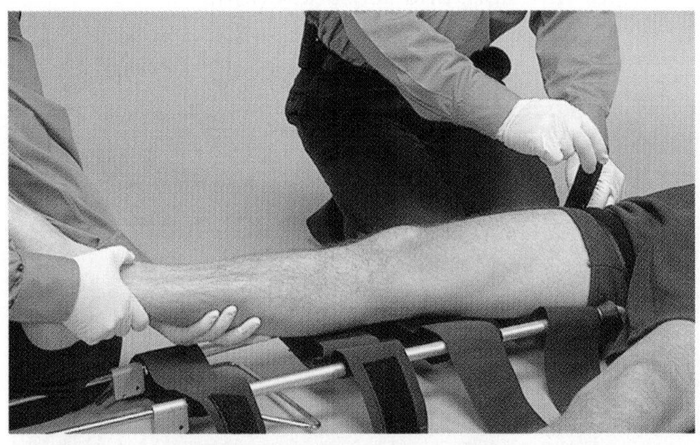

4. Apply the proximal securing device (e.g., ischial strap).

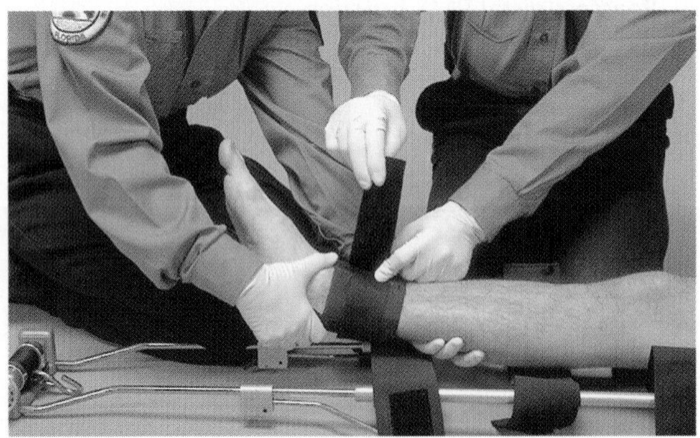

5. Apply the distal securing device (e.g., ankle hitch).

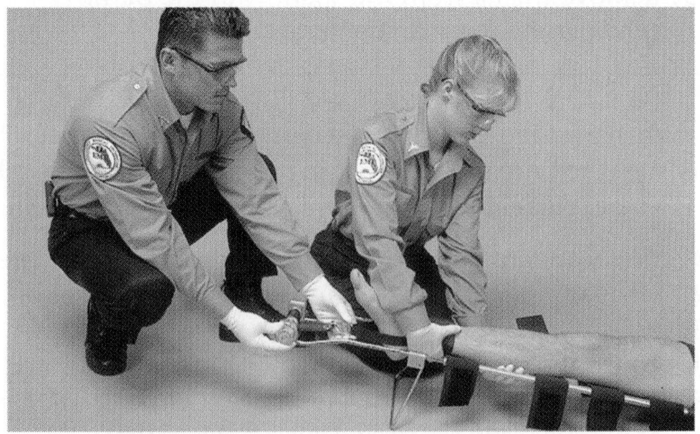

6. Apply mechanical traction.

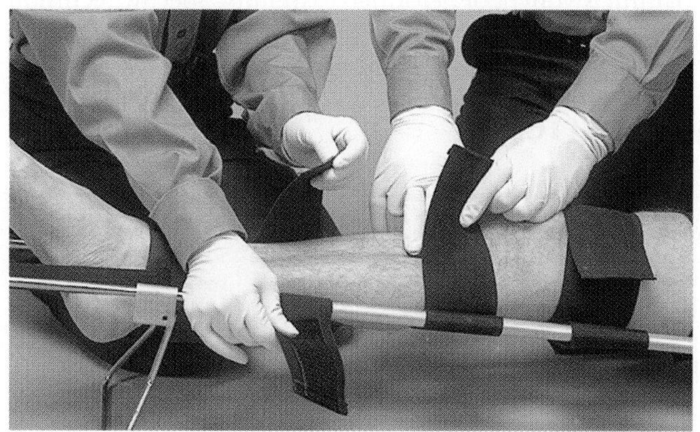

7. Position and secure the support straps.

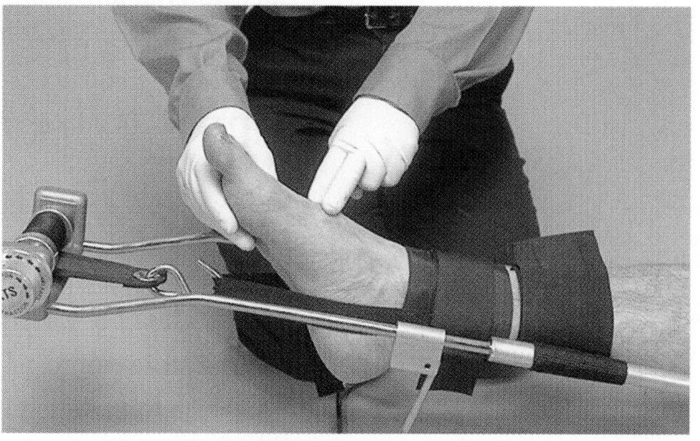

8. Reassess distal PMS function.

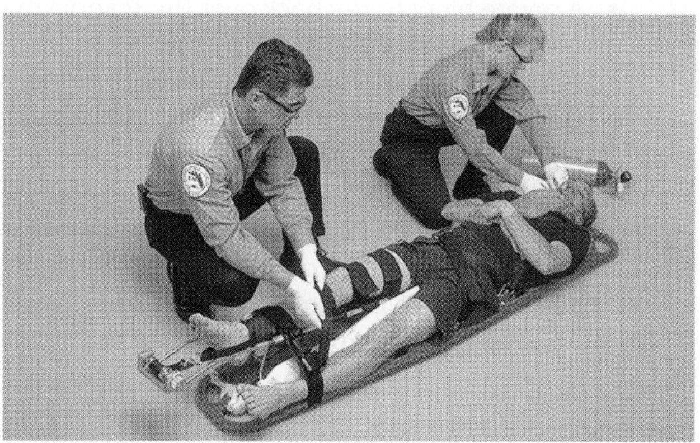

9. Secure the patient's torso and traction splint to a long board for transport.

EMERGENCY CARE OF SPECIFIC INJURIES

The specific injuries described in this section are usually identified as fractures or dislocations. Remember that you do not need to determine the exact nature of an extremity injury. You will immobilize any painful, swollen, or deformed extremity. Specific techniques are discussed on the following pages and illustrated later in Scans 28-5 through 28-17.

Upper Extremity Injuries

PATIENT ASSESSMENT

SHOULDER GIRDLE INJURIES

Signs and symptoms of an injury to the shoulder girdle include the following:

- Pain in the shoulder may indicate several types of injury. Look for specific signs.
- A dropped shoulder, with the patient holding the arm of his injured side against the chest, often indicates a fracture of the clavicle.
- A severe blow to the back over the scapula may cause a fracture of that bone. (All the bones of the shoulder girdle can be felt except the scapula. Only the superior ridge of the scapula, called its spine, can be easily palpated. Injury to the scapula is rare but must be considered if there are indications of a severe blow at the site of this bone.)

Check the entire shoulder girdle. Check for deformity where the clavicle attaches to the sternum. Feel for deformity where the clavicle joins the scapula. Feel and look along the entire clavicle for deformity. Note if the head of the humerus can be felt or moves in front of the shoulder. This is a sign of possible anterior dislocation, which may be due to a fracture. ■

PATIENT CARE

SHOULDER GIRDLE INJURIES

Emergency care of a patient with a shoulder girdle injury includes the following:

1. Assess distal PMS function. If distal PMS function is impaired, immobilize and transport as soon as possible, notifying the receiving facility.
2. It is not practical to use a rigid splint for injuries to the clavicle, scapula, or the head of the humerus. Use a sling and swathe (Scan 28-5). If there is possible cervical-spine injury, do not tie a sling around the patient's neck.
3. If there is evidence of a possible anterior dislocation of the head of the humerus (the bone head is pushed toward the front of the body), place a thin pillow between the patient's arm and chest before applying the sling and swathe.
4. Do not attempt to straighten or reduce any dislocations.
5. Reassess distal PMS function. ■

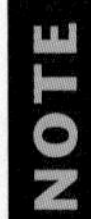

Sometimes a dislocated shoulder will reduce itself (the displaced head of the humerus "pops back into place"). When this happens, check for distal PMS function. Apply a sling and swathe and transport the patient. The patient must be seen by a physician.

Lower Extremity Injuries

PATIENT ASSESSMENT

PELVIC INJURIES

Fractures of the pelvis may occur with falls, in motor-vehicle collisions, or when a person is crushed by being squeezed between two objects. Pelvic fractures may be the result of direct or indirect force. Signs and symptoms of a pelvic injury in a patient include:

- Complaint of pain in the pelvis, hips, groin, or back. This may be the only indication, but it is significant if the mechanism of injury indicates possible fracture. Usually, obvious deformity is associated with the pain.
- Painful reaction when pressure is applied to the iliac crests (wings of the pelvis) or to the pubic bones.
- Patient complains that he cannot lift his legs when lying on his back. (Do not test for this, but do check for sensation.)
- Foot on the injured side may turn outward (lateral rotation). This also may indicate a hip fracture.
- Patient has an unexplained pressure on the urinary bladder and the feeling of having to empty the bladder. ■

NOTE *Indications of pelvic fractures mean that there may be serious damage to internal organs, blood vessels, and nerves. Internal bleeding may be profuse and lead to shock. Any force strong enough to fracture the pelvis also can cause injury to the spine.*

PATIENT CARE

PELVIC INJURIES

Emergency care includes the following:

1. Move the patient as little as possible, moving the patient as a unit when necessary. Never lift the patient with the pelvis unsupported. Warning: Use caution when using a log roll to move a patient with a suspected pelvic fracture. Roll the patient gently to the uninjured side when possible.
2. Determine PMS function distal to the injury site.
3. Straighten the patient's lower limbs into the anatomical position if there are no injuries to the hip joints and lower limbs and if it can be done without meeting resistance or causing excessive pain.
4. Prevent additional injury to the pelvis by stabilizing the lower limbs. Place a folded blanket between the patient's legs, from the groin to the feet, and bind them together with wide cravats. Thin rigid splints can be used to push the cravats under the patient. The cravats can then be adjusted for proper placement at the upper thigh, above the knee, below the knee, and above the ankle.
5. Apply a pneumatic anti-shock garment (PASG) to stabilize the pelvis in a patient with hypotension (blood pressure below 90).
6. Assume that there are spinal injuries. Immobilize the patient on a long spine board. When securing the patient, avoid placing the straps or ties over the pelvic area.

continued

PATIENT CARE *(continued)*

7. Reassess distal PMS function.
8. Care for shock, providing high-concentration oxygen.
9. Transport the patient as soon as possible.
10. Monitor vital signs.

Once the patient is in the ambulance, some EMTs are allowed to make adjustments to improve patient comfort and reduce muscle spasms of the abdomen and lower limb by gently flexing the legs and placing a pillow under the knees. If you are allowed to follow this protocol, be extremely careful not to move the spine, since the patient may have associated spinal injuries. ■

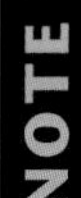

It may be very difficult to tell a fractured pelvis from a fracture of the upper femur. When there is doubt, care for the patient as if there is a pelvic fracture to protect blood vessels and nerves associated with the joint. Remember, there may be spinal injuries.

Pelvic Wrap

A new method of treating pelvic injuries is the pelvic wrap. Performed with commercially available devices (Figure 28-15) or formed from a sheet (steps described in the following text), the wrap is reported to reduce internal bleeding and pain while providing stabilization to the pelvis. It may also prevent further injury. Since many systems no longer carry the pneumatic anti-shock garment (PASG), the pelvic wrap provides an alternative treatment for suspected pelvic fracture.

The pelvic wrap should be performed on patients who have pelvic deformity or instability (movement upon palpation) whether or not signs of shock are present. Some systems may also recommend use of the pelvic wrap with a mechanism of injury that would indicate pelvic injury (e.g., motorcycle crashes, auto-pedestrian collisions) even if obvious deformity is not present. A sheet may be placed on the backboard even if the wrap is not immediately secured in the event evidence of instability or shock develops. Always follow your local protocols.

To apply a sheet as a pelvic wrap:

1. Complete a scene size-up and initial assessment.
2. Once you determine the patient is a candidate for a pelvic wrap (unstable pelvis with or without signs of shock or positive MOI), prepare a backboard with a sheet, folded flat, approximately 10 inches wide and lying across the backboard (Figure 28-16a).

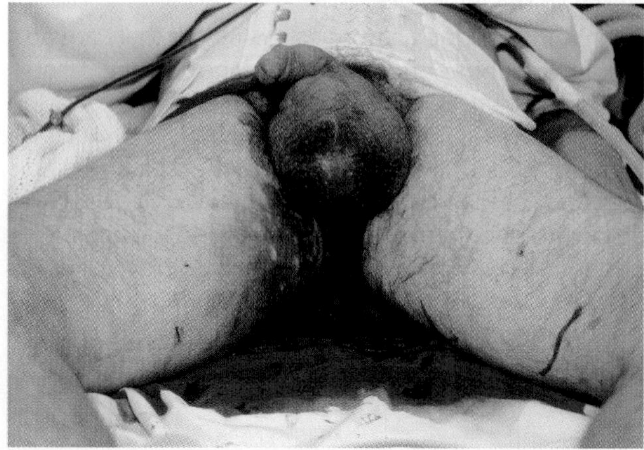

Figure 28-15 • A pelvic wrap can help to stabilize a fractured pelvis. Shown here is a commercial device ready for use on a severely injured patient. *(© Edward T. Dickinson, M.D.)*

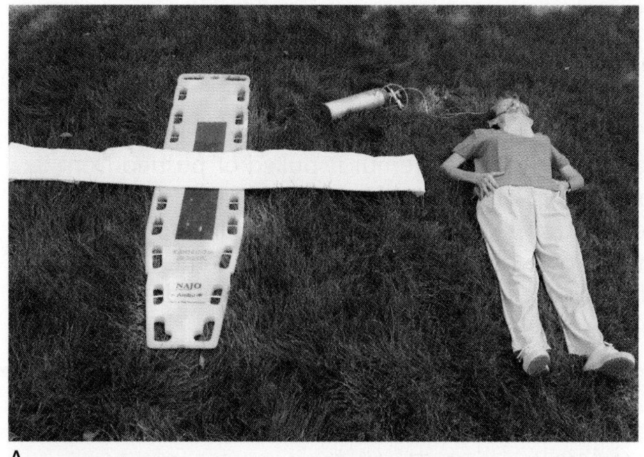
A

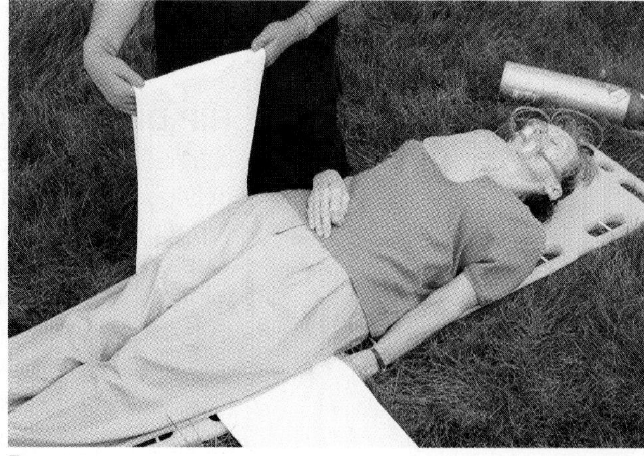
B

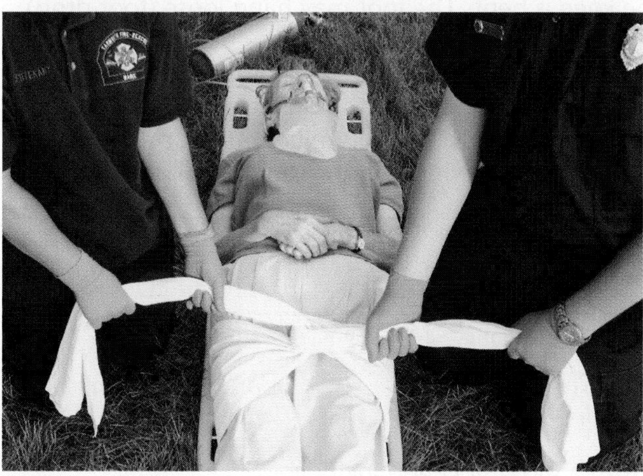
C

Figure 28-16 • (A) For a pelvic wrap, lay a sheet, folded flat, approximately 10 inches wide onto the backboard. (B) Bring the sides of the sheet together. (C) Tie the sheet firmly without overcompression to complete the pelvic wrap.

3. Carefully roll the patient to the backboard. Center the sheet at the patient's greater trochanter (the bony prominence at the proximal end of the femur). This will position the sheet lower than the iliac "wings." This is the correct position.
4. Bring the sides of the sheet around to the front of the patient (Figure 28-16b). As you bring the sides of the sheet together and tie them, you will cause compression and stabilization of the pelvis. The sheet should feel firm enough on the pelvis to keep it in normal position without overcompression (Figure 28-16c).
5. Secure the sheet using ties or clamps so that the compression is maintained.

Pneumatic Anti-Shock Garment

The pneumatic anti-shock garment (PASG, also known as a MAST garment) may be used (where available) for splinting a suspected pelvic fracture in a patient with hypotension (blood pressure below 90). Some EMS systems also use the anti-shock garment for splinting hip, femoral, and multiple leg fractures. An anti-shock garment is to be applied in accordance with local protocols. In many localities, application requires an order from a physician. (Review Chapter 26, "Bleeding and Shock," Scan 26-3, "Applying the Anti-Shock Garment.")

When pelvic fracture is a possibility, always be alert for shock and possible injuries to internal organs. Always take vital signs before applying an anti-shock garment and monitor the vital signs every 5 minutes thereafter.

PATIENT ASSESSMENT

HIP DISLOCATION

A hip dislocation occurs when the head of the femur is pulled or pushed from its pelvic socket. It is difficult to tell a hip dislocation from a fracture of the proximal (uppermost portion of the) femur. Conscious patients will complain of intense pain with both types of injury. Patients who have had a surgical replacement of the hip joint are at increased risk of hip dislocation. The hip can be dislocated either anteriorly or posteriorly.

Signs and symptoms of a hip dislocation include:

- *Anterior hip dislocation.* The patient's entire lower limb is rotated outward and the hip is usually flexed.
- *Posterior hip dislocation* (most common). The patient's leg is rotated inward, the hip is flexed, and the knee is bent. The foot may hang loose (foot drop), and the patient is unable to flex the foot or lift the toes. Often, there is a lack of sensation in the limb. These signs indicate possible damage, caused by the dislocated femoral head, to the sciatic nerve, the major nerve that extends from the lower spine to the posterior thigh. This injury often occurs when a person's knees strike the dashboard during a motor-vehicle collision. ■

PATIENT CARE

HIP DISLOCATION

Emergency care of a patient with a hip dislocation includes:

1. Assess distal PMS function.
2. Move the patient onto a long spine board. Some systems use a scoop-style stretcher. When this device is used, the limb should be immobilized.
3. Immobilize the limb with pillows or rolled blankets.
4. Secure the patient to the long spine board with straps or cravats.
5. Reassess distal PMS function. If there is a pulse, motor, or sensory problem, notify medical direction and transport immediately.
6. Care for shock, providing high-concentration oxygen.
7. Transport carefully, monitor vital signs, and continue to check for nerve and circulation impairment.

Note that if you find a painful, swollen, or deformed thigh and the leg is flexed and will not straighten, the patient may also have a fractured femur. ■

PATIENT ASSESSMENT

HIP FRACTURE

As noted earlier, a hip fracture is a fracture of the proximal femur, not the pelvis. The fracture can occur to the femoral head, the femoral neck, or at the portion of the femur just below the neck of the bone.

continued

PATIENT ASSESSMENT *(continued)*

Signs and symptoms of a hip fracture include the following:

- Pain is localized, but some patients complain of pain in the knee.
- Sometimes the patient is sensitive to pressure exerted on the lateral prominence of the hip (greater trochanter).
- Surrounding tissues are discolored. Discoloration may be delayed.
- Swelling may be evident.
- Patient is unable to move limb while on his back.
- Patient complains about being unable to stand.
- Foot on injured side usually turns outward; however, it may rotate inward (rarely).
- Injured limb may appear shorter. ■

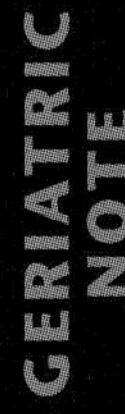

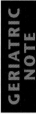

GERIATRIC NOTE

Direct force (as occurs in a motor-vehicle collision) and twisting forces (as may occur in falls) can cause a hip fracture. Elderly people are more susceptible to this type of injury because of brittle bones or bones weakened by disease.

PATIENT CARE

HIP FRACTURE

Be certain to assess distal PMS function before and after splinting and during transport. The patient should be managed for shock and receive oxygen at a high flow and concentration. It is recommended that the patient be placed on a long spine board or orthopedic stretcher after splinting.

One of the following emergency care methods can be used to stabilize a hip fracture (Figure 28-17):

- *Bind the legs together.* Place a folded blanket between the patient's legs and bind the legs together with wide straps, Velcro-equipped straps, or wide cravats. Carefully place the patient on a long spine board and use pillows to support the lower limbs. Secure the patient to the board. An orthopedic stretcher can be used in place of the long spine board.
- *Padded boards.* Use thin splints to push cravats or straps under the patient at the natural voids (such as the small of the back and back of the knees) and readjust them so that they will pass across the chest, the abdomen just below the belt, below the crotch, above and below the knee, and at the ankle. Splint with two long padded boards. Ideally, one should be long enough to extend from the patient's armpit to beyond the foot. The other should be long enough to extend from the crotch to beyond the foot. Cushion with padding in the armpit and crotch and pad all voids created at the ankle and knee. Secure the boards with the cravats or straps.
- *Apply an anti-shock garment.* Do this if local protocols indicate. ■

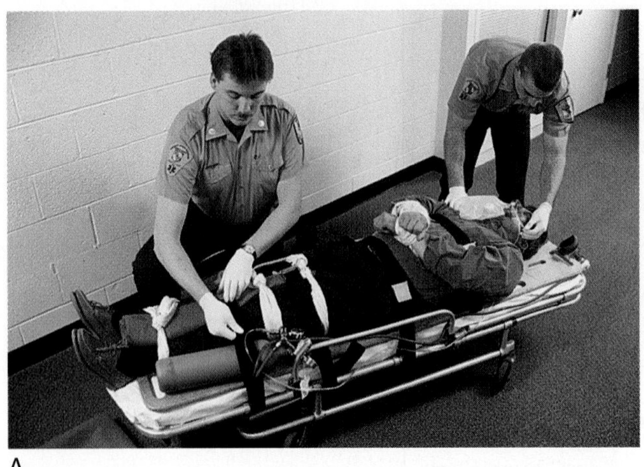

A

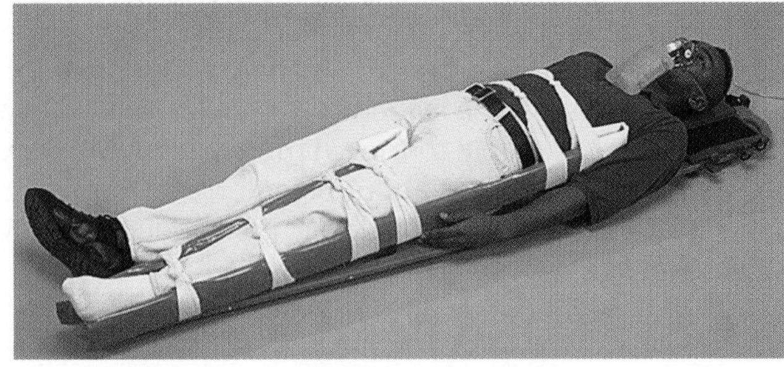

B

Figure 28-17 • For a patient with a hip or pelvic injury, (A) bind the legs together or (B) splint with a padded long board. Apply an anti-shock garment, if local protocols indicate.

PATIENT ASSESSMENT

FEMORAL SHAFT FRACTURE

Because the femur is a large, strong bone, considerable force is necessary to cause a fracture of the femoral shaft. Remember also that muscle contractions can cause bone ends to ride over each other. The bone ends may or may not protrude from an open wound. Never assume that a wound on the thigh is superficial because you do not see bone ends. Always check for signs and symptoms that this may be an open fracture.

Signs and symptoms of a femoral shaft fracture include:

- Pain, often intense.
- Often there will be an open fracture with deformity and sometimes with the end of the bone protruding through the wound. When the injury is a closed fracture, often there will be deformity with possible severe angulation.
- Injured limb may appear to be shortened because the contraction of the thigh muscles caused the bone ends to override each other. ■

POINT OF VIEW

"I was builiding this really cool indoor driving range in the loft over the barn. I put down green artifical turf. It was going to be great. I was hanging the net when the ladder gave way and I fell.

"It's funny, but on the way down I had time to get a sinking feeling. Knowing it was going to hurt when I landed. Hoping I didn't break anything. And thinking that probably no one would even hear me. I hit the floor and broke my leg. I knew, because I heard—and felt—the twist, then the break.

"I yelled for about 5 minutes before a neighbor heard me. But then the EMTs came pretty quickly, and they were good guys. They didn't sugar coat the situation. They said it might hurt when they put the splint on and when they carried me down the narrow barn stairs. I hadn't even thought of how they would get me downstairs. I'm not a small guy.

"But they did it. They did it well. They were right, it hurt some, but I appreciate them telling me the truth.

"I guess I've got about 8 weeks before I get to take the first swing in my new driving range."

PATIENT CARE

FEMORAL SHAFT FRACTURE

Emergency care of a patient with a femoral shaft fracture includes:

1. Control any bleeding by applying direct pressure (avoiding the fracture site) forcefully enough to overcome the barrier of muscle mass. If bleeding cannot be controlled use a tourniquet or hemostatic dressing per local protocols.
2. As soon as possible, manage the patient for shock (hypoperfusion) and provide high-concentration oxygen.
3. Assess distal PMS function.
4. Apply a traction splint. (See Scans 28-10, 28-11, and 28-12.) If a traction splint is not available, bind the legs together after placing them in the anatomical position.
5. Reassess distal PMS function. ■

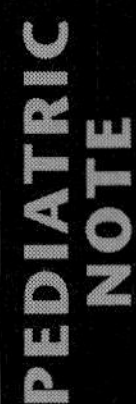

When traction-splinting thigh injuries in children, be sure to use appropriately sized splints. Warning: Studies of mechanisms of injury indicate that infants and children with fractured femurs often have injury to internal organs.

NOTE

The traction splint should not be applied if you suspect that there may be additional injuries or fractures to the area of the knee or tibia/fibula of the same limb. If local protocols permit, an anti-shock garment may be used if there are multiple leg fractures. It is not, however, a good splint for the lower leg since it does not immobilize the ankle.

PATIENT ASSESSMENT

KNEE INJURY

The knee is a joint and not a single bone. Fractures can occur to the distal femur, to the proximal tibia and fibula, and to the patella (kneecap). Signs and symptoms of a knee injury include:

- Pain and tenderness
- Swelling
- Deformity with obvious swelling ■

PATIENT CARE

KNEE INJURY

There are two general emergency care methods of immobilizing the knee—one if the knee is bent, the other if it is straight:

- *Knee is bent.* Assess distal PMS function. Immobilize in the position in which the leg is found. Tie two padded board splints to the thigh and above the ankle so that the knee is held in position. A pillow can be used to support the leg. Reassess distal PMS function. (See Scan 28-13.)

continued

PATIENT CARE *(continued)*

- *Knee is straight or returned to anatomical position.* Assess distal PMS function. Immobilize with two padded board splints or a single padded splint. When using two padded boards, one medial and one lateral offer the best support. Remember to pad the voids created at the knee and ankle. Reassess distal PMS function. (See Scans 28-14 and 28-15.) ■

Do not confuse a knee dislocation with a patella dislocation. The patella can become displaced by ligament damage when the lower leg and knee are twisted, as in a skiing or racquetball accident. A knee dislocation occurs when the tibia itself is forced either anteriorly or posteriorly in relation to the distal femur. Always check for a distal pulse, since the dislocated knee joint can compress the popliteal artery and stop the major blood supply to the lower leg. If there is no pulse, this is a true emergency. Contact medical direction for permission to gently move the lower leg anteriorly to allow for a pulse, and transport immediately.

What may appear to be a dislocation may prove to be a fracture or a combined fracture and dislocation. Even if you believe that the patient has suffered a dislocated patella and the kneecap has repositioned itself, realize that other damage may be hidden. Whether you suspect a fracture, a dislocation, a sprain, or a strain, always splint and transport.

Once splinting is done, monitor the patient. If there is a loss of distal PMS function, or if the foot becomes discolored (white, mottled, or blue) and turns cold, transport the patient without delay. Notify medical direction while en route.

PATIENT ASSESSMENT

TIBIA OR FIBULA INJURY

Signs and symptoms of a tibia or fibula injury include:

- Pain and tenderness
- Swelling
- Possible deformity (You might expect to see a deformity of the lower leg when the tibia or fibula is fractured. However, such deformity is often absent.) ■

PATIENT CARE

TIBIA OR FIBULA INJURY

Emergency care of a patient with a tibia or fibula injury includes providing care for shock and administering high-concentration oxygen. Because immobilizing the leg can help to relieve pain and control bleeding, apply a splint using one of the following methods. Remember to assess distal PMS function before and after application.

- *Air-inflated splint.* Apply an air-inflated splint (Figure 28-18). Slide the uninflated splint over your hand and gather it in place until the lower edge clears your wrist. Using your free hand, grasp the patient's foot and leg just above the injury site. While maintaining manual traction, have your partner slide the splint over your hand and onto the injured leg. Your partner must

continued

PATIENT CARE *(continued)*

make sure that the splint is relatively wrinkle free and that it covers the injury site. Continue to maintain traction while your partner inflates the splint. Test to see if you can cause a slight dent in the plastic with fingertip pressure. Remember to check periodically to see that the pressure in the splint has remained adequate and has not decreased or increased.

- *Two-splint method.* You can immobilize the fracture using two rigid board splints (Scan 28-16).
- *Single splint with ankle hitch.* A single splint with an ankle hitch can be applied (Scan 28-17). ■

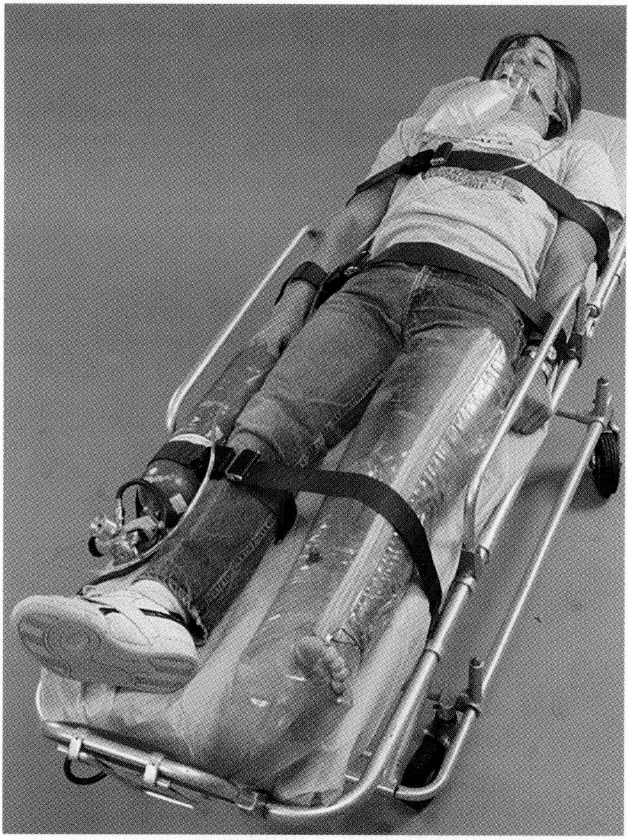

Figure 28-18 • An air splint may be used for a lower leg injury.

PATIENT ASSESSMENT

ANKLE OR FOOT INJURY

Sprains (torn ligaments) and fractures are the most common musculoskeletal injuries to the ankle and foot. It is often difficult to distinguish between them, so always treat for a fracture. Signs and symptoms of an ankle or foot injury include:

- Pain
- Swelling
- Possible deformity ■

CRITICAL DECISION MAKING: STICKS AND STONES MAY BREAK MY BONES, BUT TRAUMA CENTERS SAVE ME

Care for patients with musculoskeletal injuries depends on the overall patient condition. Patients with isolated fractures may be splinted and transported routinely, while those with multiple fractures are at an increased risk of shock and should be treated as multiple-trauma patients. For each of these patients, determine whether you would stay and splint or, as a higher priority, consider transport to a trauma center, using a backboard as the main splinting device.

1. You are called to a patient who tripped and tried to catch himself with an outstretched arm. He believes he broke his wrist and hit his head when he fell. He is alert and oriented. His vital signs are pulse 88 strong and regular, repirations 16, blood pressure 140/84, skin warm and dry, pupils equal and reactive to light.

2. You are called to an industrial complex where a large spool pinned a man by the legs. The workers are able to move the spool for you to safely access the patient. The patient is in extreme pain. Your physical examination reveals deformity in both thighs and the patient's left lower leg. The patient is agitated. His pulse is 112 and regular, respirations 24 and adequate, blood pressure 108/64, pupils equal and reactive to light.

3. Your patient was ejected from a vehicle and found about 20 feet away. He complains only of a broken arm. Your physical assessment doesn't reveal any other injuries. The patient is alert and oriented. His pulse is 130 and weak, respirations 28 and adequate, blood pressure 88/56, skin cool and moist, pupils equal and reactive to light.

PATIENT CARE

ANKLE OR FOOT INJURY

Long splints, extending from above the knee to beyond the foot, can be used. However, soft splinting is an effective, rapid method and is recommended for most patients (Figure 28-19). To soft splint, you should follow the emergency care steps described in the following list:

1. Assess distal PMS function.
2. Stabilize the limb. Remove the patient's shoe if possible, but only if it removes easily and can be done with no movement to the ankle.
3. Lift the limb, but do not apply manual traction (tension).
4. Place three cravats on the floor under the ankle. Then place a pillow lengthwise under the ankle on top of the cravats. The pillow should extend 6 inches beyond the foot.
5. Gently lower the limb onto the pillow, taking care not to change the position of the ankle. Stabilize by tying the cravats, and adjust them so they are at the top of the pillow, midway, and at the heel.
6. Tie the pillow to the ankle and foot.
7. Tie a fourth cravat loosely at the arch of the foot.
8. Elevate with a second pillow or blanket. Reassess distal PMS function.

continued

PATIENT CARE *(continued)*

9. Care for shock (hypoperfusion) if needed.
10. Apply an ice pack to the injury site to reduce bleeding and swelling, if appropriate. Do not apply the ice pack directly to the skin.

Note that a commercial splint with a foot and leg that extends above the knee may be better than a pillow since it will also immobilize the knee, the joint adjacent to the ankle. ■

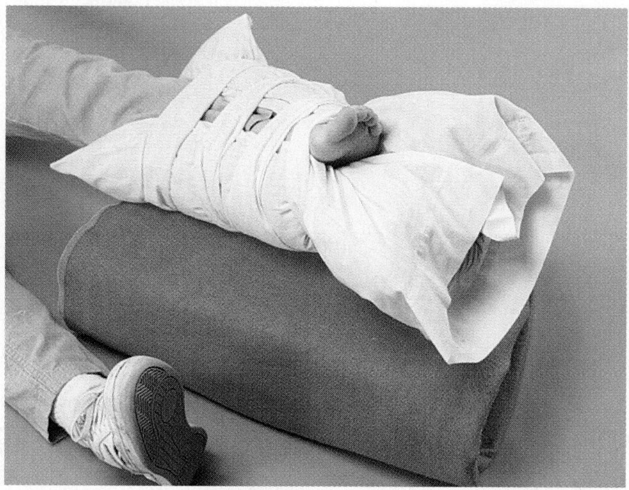

Figure 28-19 • A pillow splint may be used for an injured ankle.

SCAN 28-5 • Applying a Sling and Swathe

A sling is a triangular bandage used to support the shoulder and arm. Once the patient's arm is placed in a sling, a swathe can be used to hold the arm against the side of the chest. Commercial slings are available. Velcro straps can be used to form a swathe. Use whatever materials you have on hand, provided they will not cut into the patient. Also, remember to assess distal pulse, motor function, and sensation both before and after immobilizing or splinting an extremity.

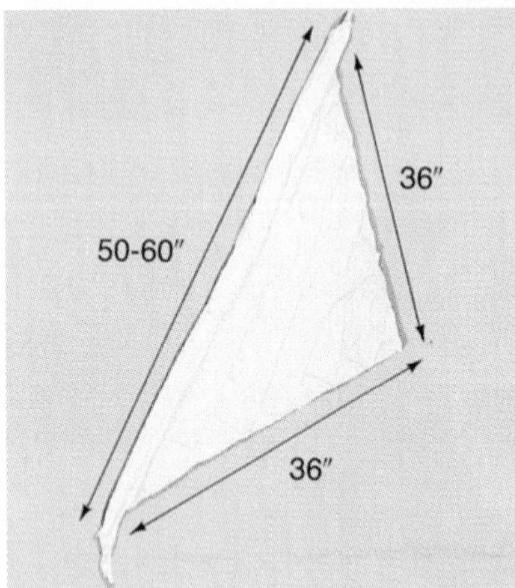

1. Prepare the sling by folding cloth into a triangle.

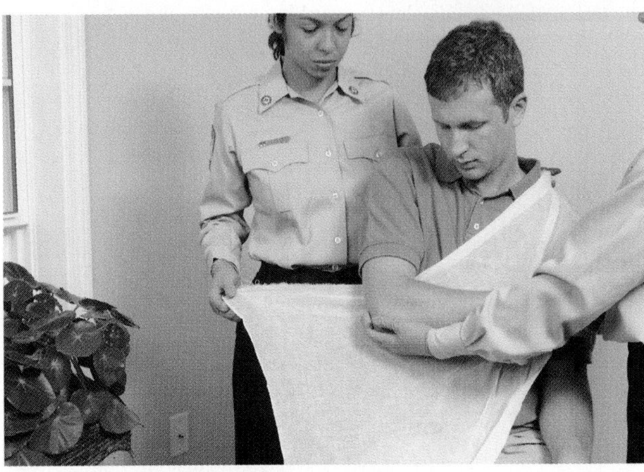

. . . If the patient cannot hold his arm, have someone assist him until you tie the sling.

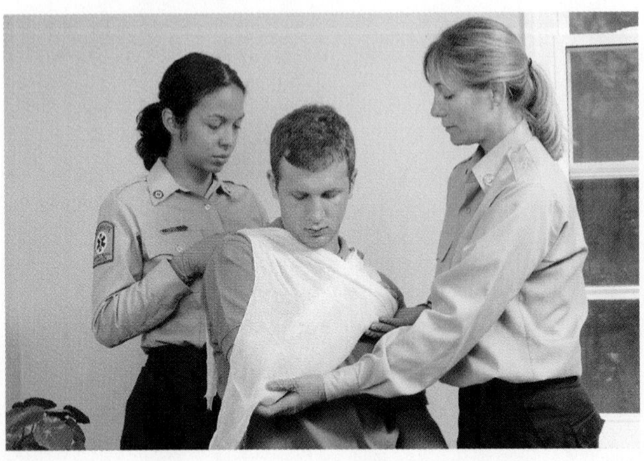

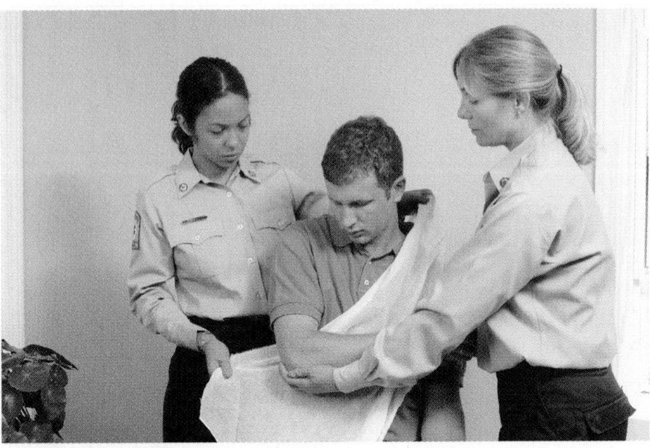

2. Position the sling over the top of the patient's chest as shown. Fold the injured arm across his chest. And . . .

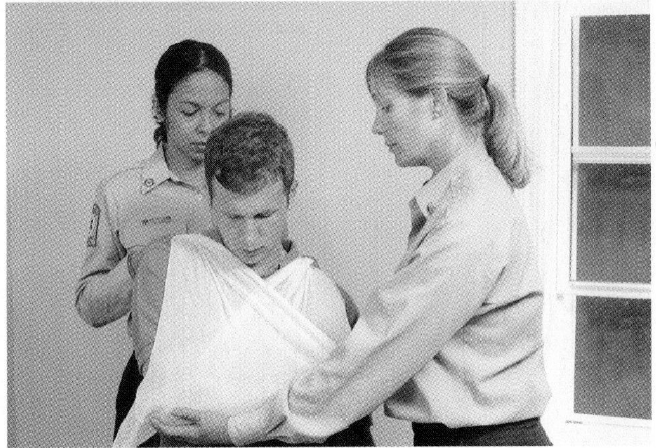

3. Extend one point of the triangle beyond the elbow on the injured side. Take the bottom point and bring it up over the patient's arm. Then take it over the top of the injured shoulder.

4. If appropriate, draw up the ends of the sling so that the patient's hand is about 4 inches above the elbow.

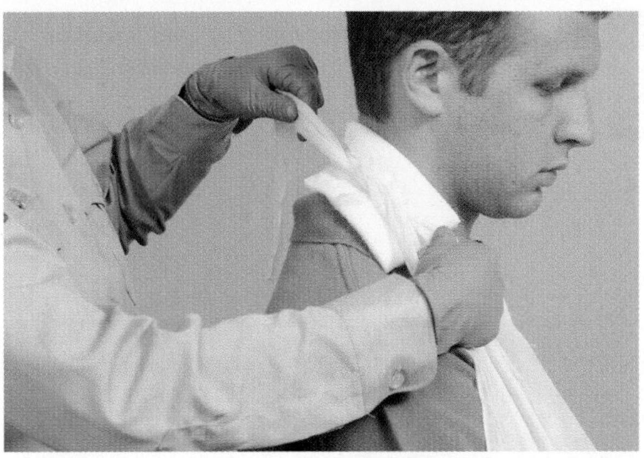

5. Tie the two ends of the sling together, making sure that the knot does not press against the back of the patient's neck. Pad with bulky dressings. (If spine injury is possible, pin ends to clothing. Do not tie around the neck.)

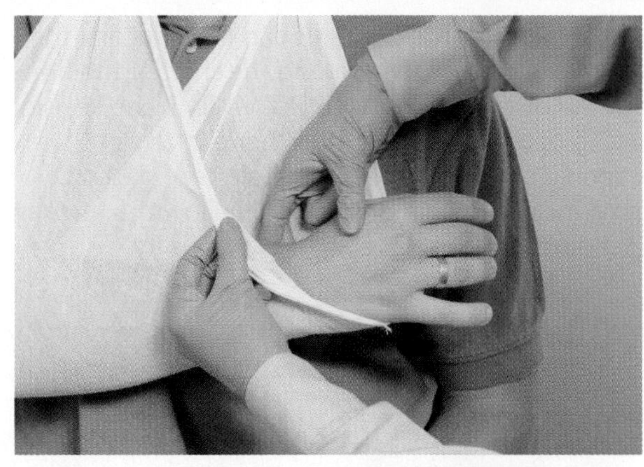

6. Check to be sure you have left the patient's fingertips exposed. Then assess distal pulse, motor function, and sensation (PMS). If the pulse has been lost, take off the sling and repeat the procedure. Then check again.

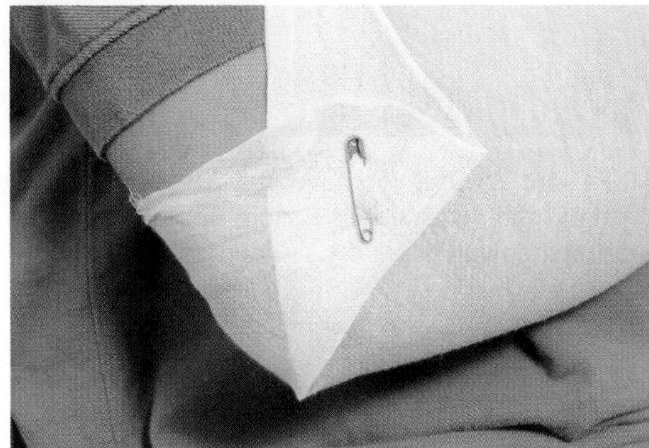

7. To form a pocket for the patient's elbow, take hold of the point of material at the elbow and fold it forward, pinning it to the front of the sling. Or . . .

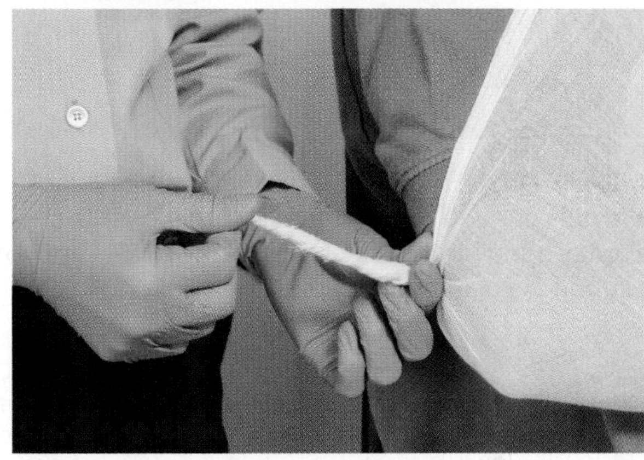

. . . If you do not have a pin, twist the excess material and tie a knot in the point.

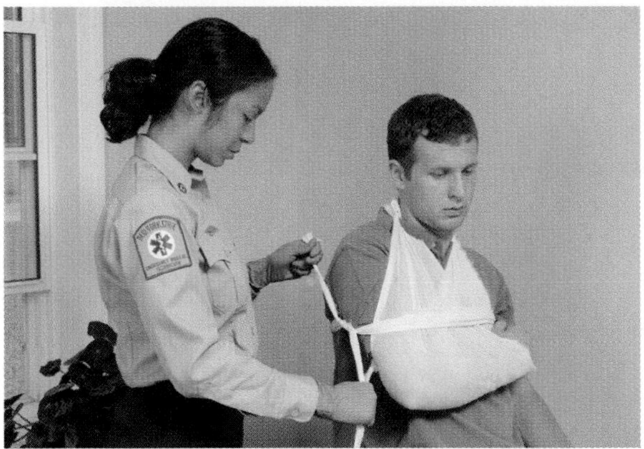

8. Form a swathe from a second piece of material. Tie it around the chest and the injured arm, over the sling. Do not place it over the patient's arm on the uninjured side.

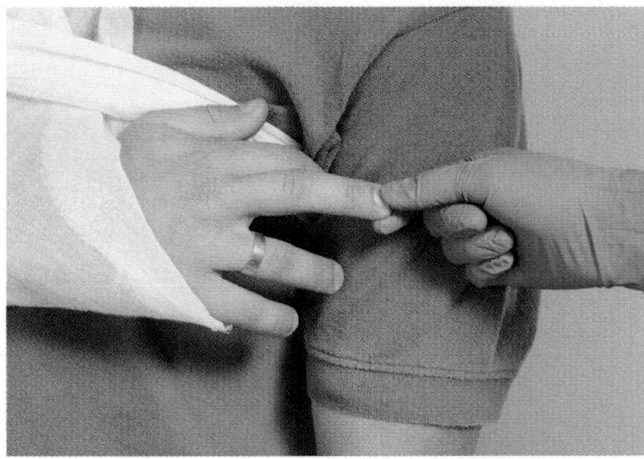

9. Reassess distal pulse, motor function, and sensation (PMS). Treat for shock, and provide high-concentration oxygen. Take vital signs. Perform detailed and ongoing assessments as appropriate.

SCAN 28-6 • Splinting an Injured Humerus

SIGNS: Injury to the humerus can take place at the proximal end (shoulder), along the shaft of the bone, or at the distal end (elbow). Deformity is the key sign used to detect fractures to this bone in any of these locations; however, assess for all signs of skeletal injury, including pain or swelling. Follow the rules and procedures for care of an injured extremity.

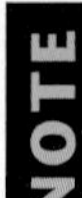

NOTE *Assess distal pulse, motor function, and sensation both before and after immobilizing or splinting an extremity.*

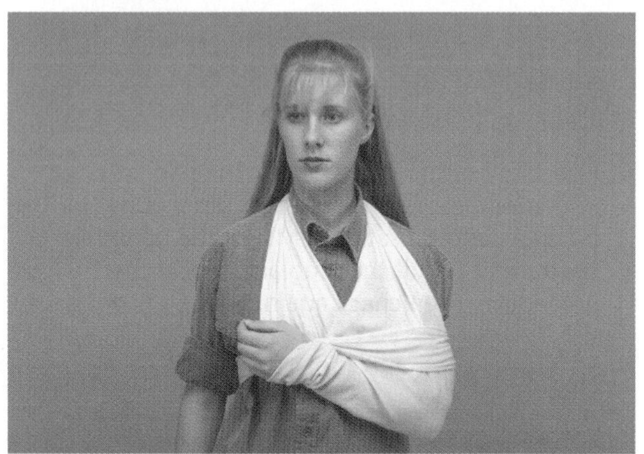

VARIATION ONE: Apply a sling and swathe. If you have only enough material for a swathe, bind the patient's upper arm to her body, taking great care not to cut off circulation to the forearm.

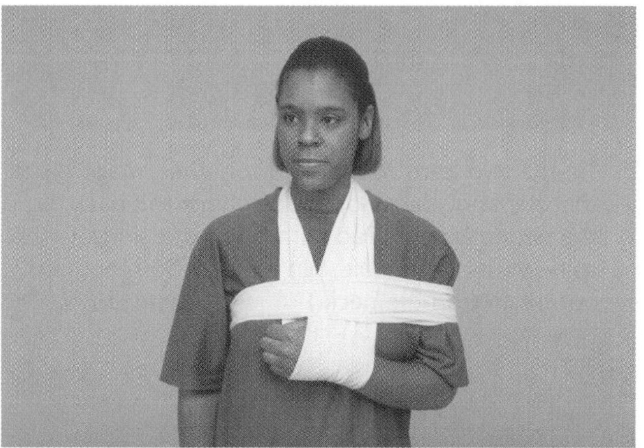

VARIATION TWO: If you have only a narrow or short length of material to use as a sling, apply it so that it supports the wrist only.

NOTE *Before applying a sling and swathe to care for injuries to the humerus, check for distal pulse, motor function, and sensation (PMS). If you do not feel a pulse, attempt to straighten any slight angulation if the patient has a closed fracture (follow local protocol). Otherwise, prepare for immediate immobilization and transport. Should straightening of the angulation fail to restore the pulse or function, splint with a medium board splint, keeping the forearm extended. If there is no sign of circulation or sensory or motor function, you will have to attempt a second splinting. If this fails to restore distal function, transport immediately. Do not try to straighten angulation of the humerus if there are any signs of fracture or dislocation of the shoulder or elbow.*

SCAN 28-7 • Splinting Arm and Elbow Injuries

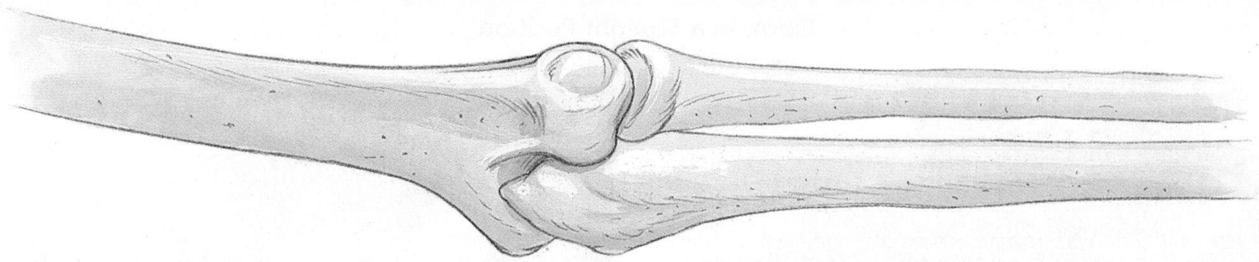

SIGNS: The elbow is a joint and not a bone. It is composed of the distal humerus and the proximal ulna and radius, forming a hinge joint. You will have to decide if the injury is truly to the elbow. The location of deformity and tenderness will direct you to the injury site.
CARE: If there is a distal pulse, the dislocated elbow should be immobilized in the position in which it is found. The joint has too many nerves and blood vessels to risk movement. When a distal pulse is absent, make one attempt to slightly reposition the limb after contacting medical direction. Do not force the limb into anatomical position.

Elbow in or Returned to Bent Position

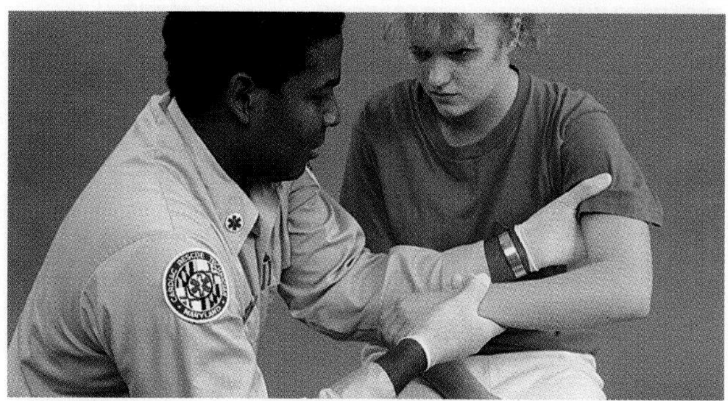

1. Move the limb only if necessary for splinting or if pulse is absent. STOP if you meet resistance or significantly increase the pain.

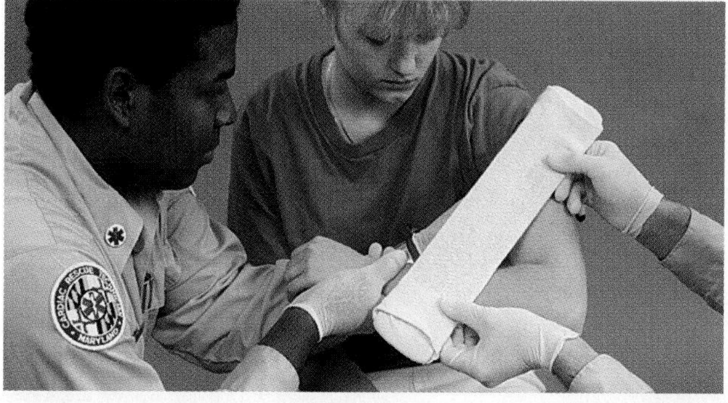

2. Use a padded board splint that will extend 2 to 6 inches beyond the arm and wrist when placed diagonally.

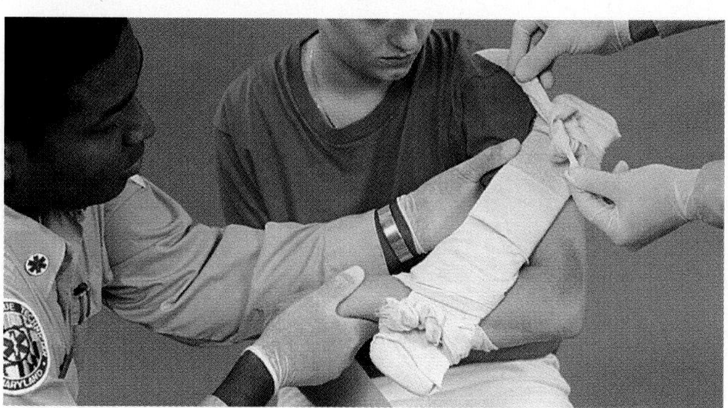

3. Place the splint so it is just proximal to the elbow and wrist. Use cravats to secure it to the forearm, then the arm.

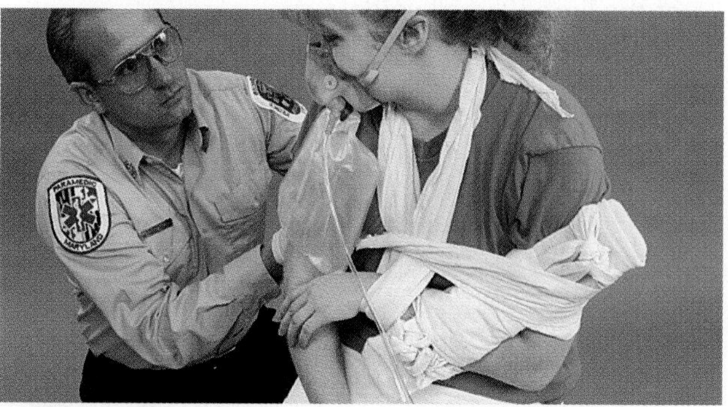

4. A wrist sling can be applied to support the limb. Keep the elbow exposed. Apply a swathe if possible.

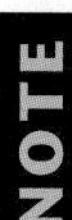

NOTE

Assess distal pulse, motor function, and sensation both before and after immobilizing or splinting an extremity.

continued

SCAN 28-7 • (Continued)

Elbow in a Straight Position

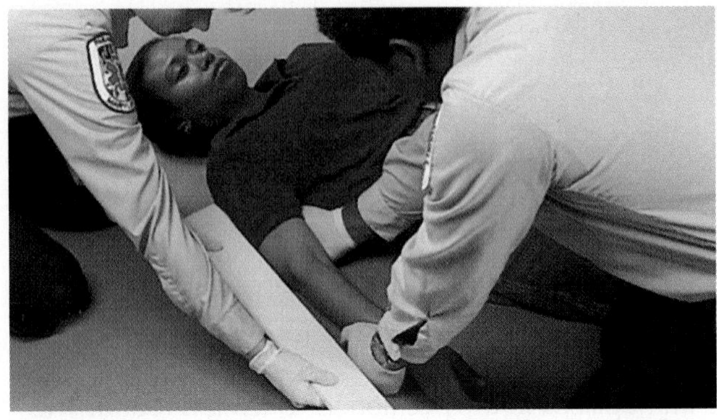

1. Assess distal pulse, motor function, and sensation (PMS).

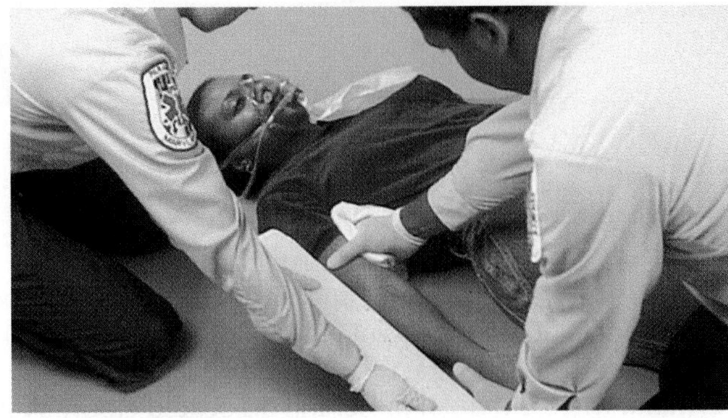

2. Use a padded board splint that extends from under the armpit to a point past the fingertips. Pad the armpit.

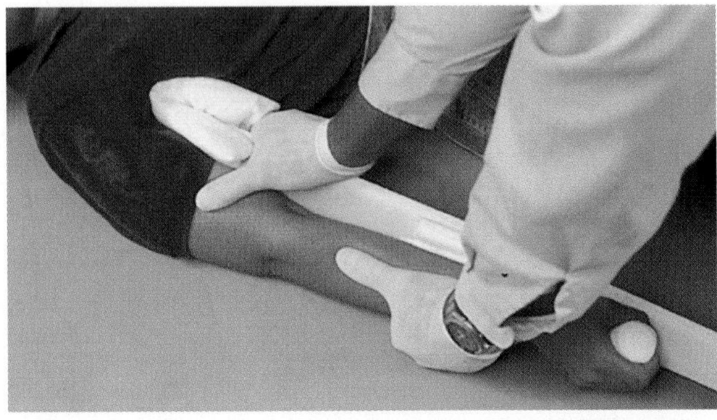

3. Place a roll of bandages in the patient's hand to help maintain position of function. Place the padded side of the board against the medial side of the limb. Pad all voids.

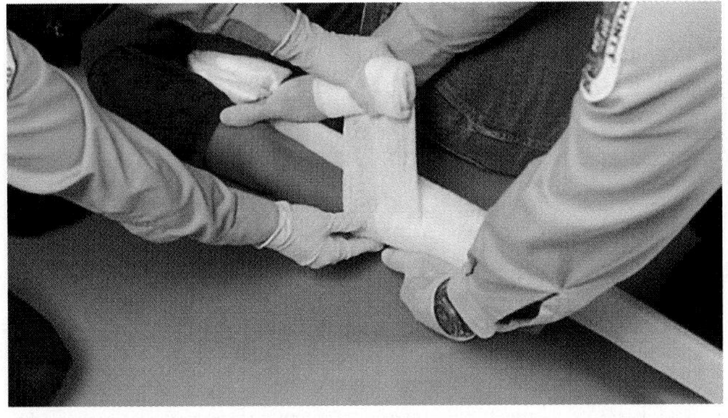

4. Secure the splint. Leave the patient's fingertips exposed.

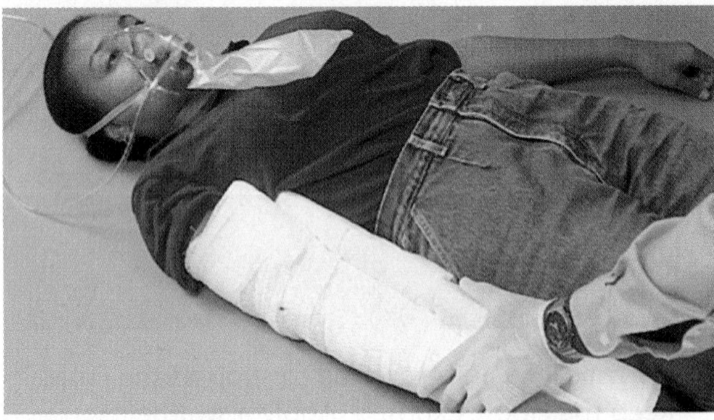

5. Place pads between the patient's side and the splint.

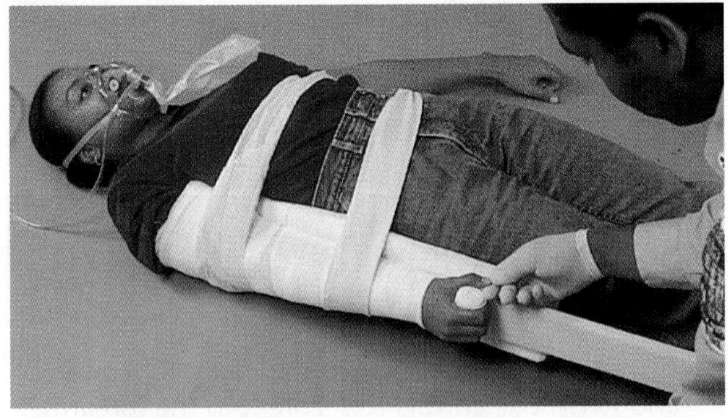

6. Secure the splinted limb to the body with two cravats. Avoid placing the cravats over the suspected injury site. Reassess distal pulse, motor function, and sensation (PMS).

SCAN 28-8 • Splinting Forearm, Wrist, and Hand

SIGNS:

- *Forearm.* Deformity and tenderness. If only one bone is broken, deformity may be minor or absent.
- *Wrist.* Deformity and tenderness.
- *Hand.* Deformity and pain. Dislocated fingers are obvious.

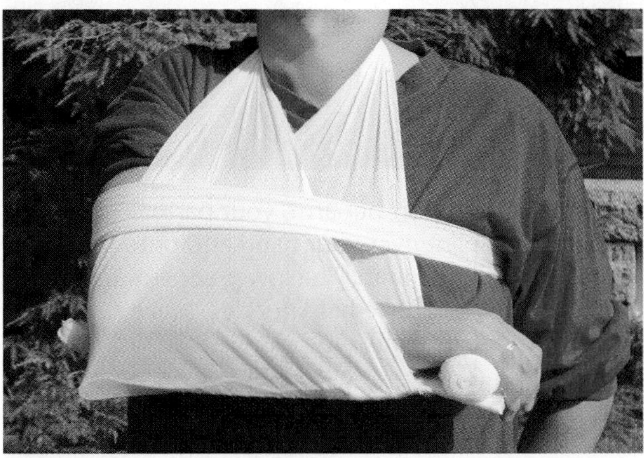

CARE: Injuries occurring to the forearm, wrist, or hand can be splinted using a padded rigid splint that extends from the elbow past the fingertips. The patient's elbow, forearm, wrist, and hand all need the support of the splint. Tension must be provided throughout the splinting. A roll of bandage should be placed in the hand to ensure the position of function. After rigid splinting, apply a sling and swathe.

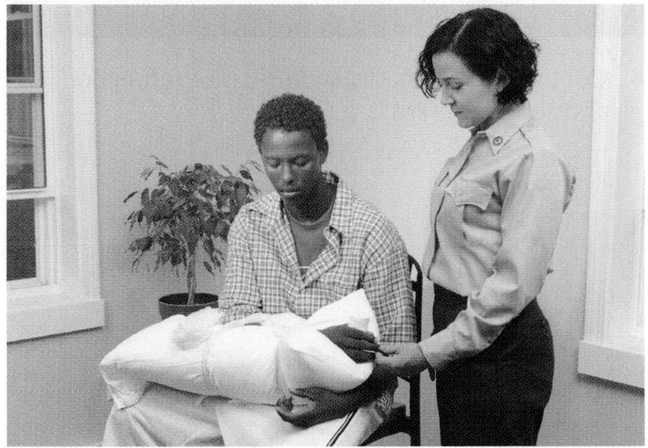

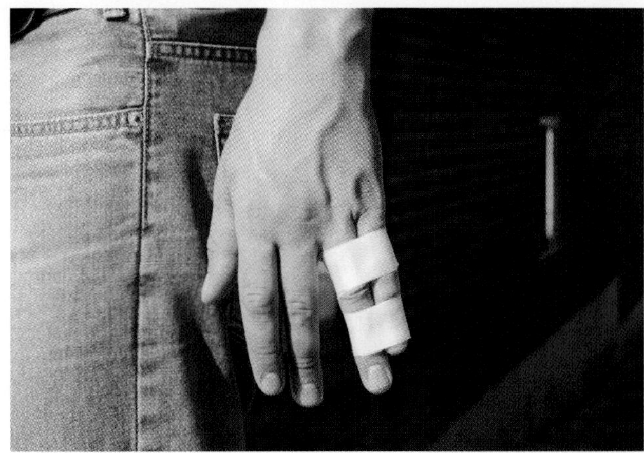

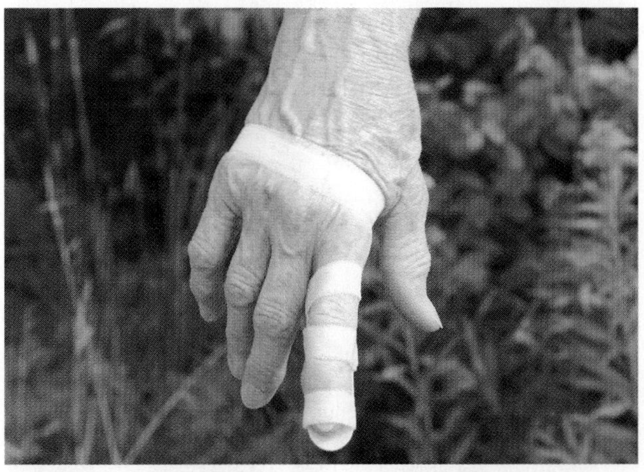

ALTERNATIVE CARE: Injuries to the hand and wrist can be cared for with soft splinting by placing a roll of bandages in the hand to maintain position of function, then tying the forearm, wrist, and hand into the fold of one pillow or between two pillows. An injured finger can be taped to an adjacent uninjured finger or splinted with a tongue depressor. Some emergency department physicians prefer that care be limited to a wrap of soft bandages. Do not try to "pop" dislocated fingers back into place.

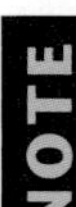

Assess distal pulse, motor function, and sensation both before and after immobilizing or splinting an extremity.

SCAN 28-9 • Applying an Air Splint

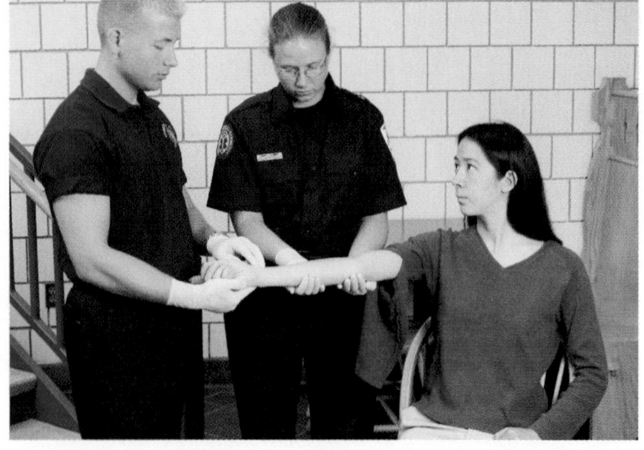

1. Check distal pulse, motor function, and sensation (PMS). Grasp the hand of the patient's injured limb as though you were going to shake hands and apply steady tension.

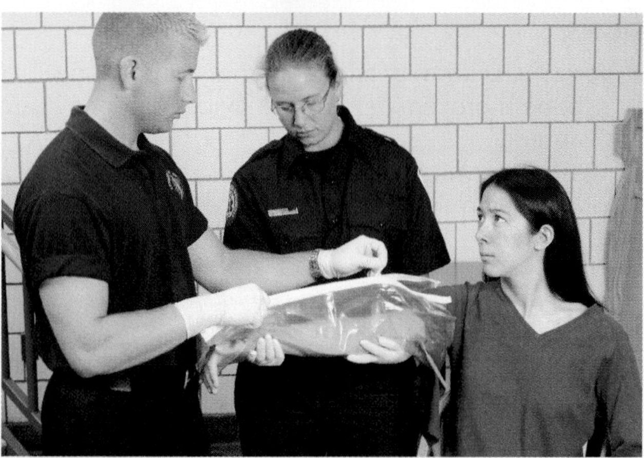

2. While you support her arm, your partner gently slides the splint over your hand and onto the patient's injured limb. The lower edge of the splint should be just above her knuckles. Make sure the splint is free of wrinkles.

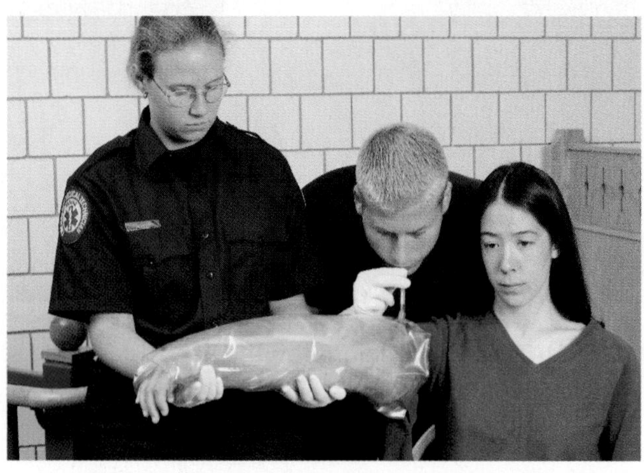

3. Continue to support the arm while your partner inflates the splint by mouth to a point where you can make a slight dent in the plastic when you press it with your thumb.

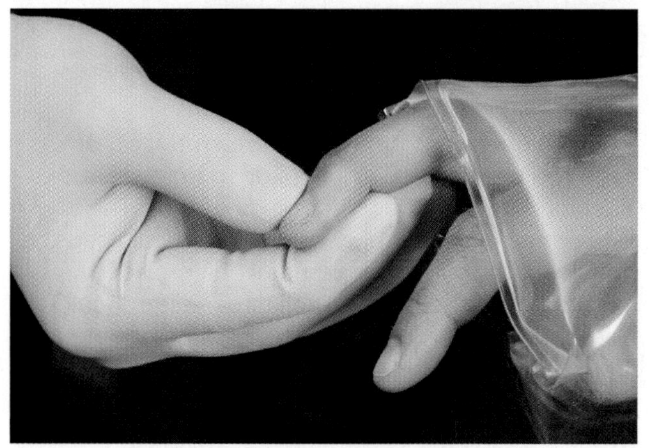

4. Continue to assess distal pulse, motor function, and sensation (PMS).

NOTE

Air-inflated splints may leak. When applied in cold weather, an inflatable splint will expand when the patient is moved to a warmer place. Variations in pressure also occur if the patient is moved to a different altitude. Frequently monitor the pressure in the splint with your fingertip. Air-inflated splints may stick to the patient's skin in hot weather.

SCAN 28-10 • Preparing the Fernotrac Traction Splint

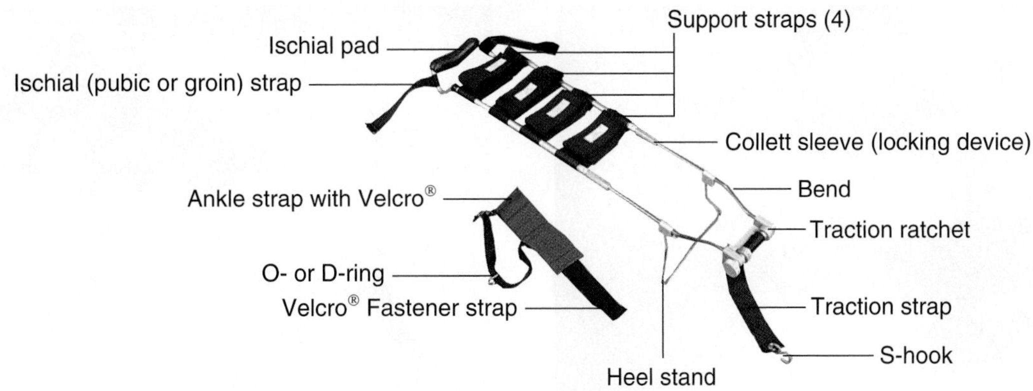

Fernotrac Traction Splint

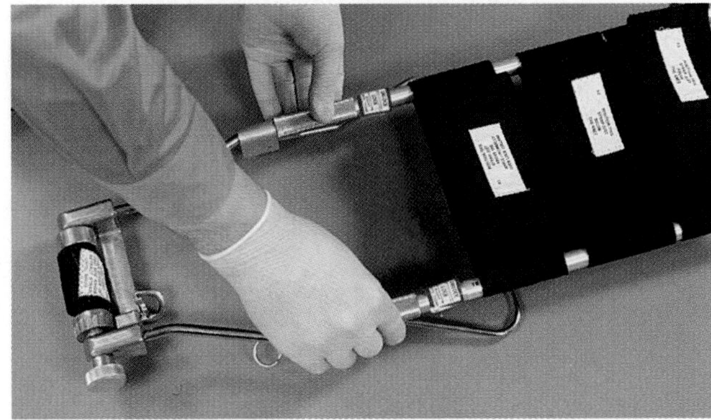

1. Loosen the sleeve locking device.

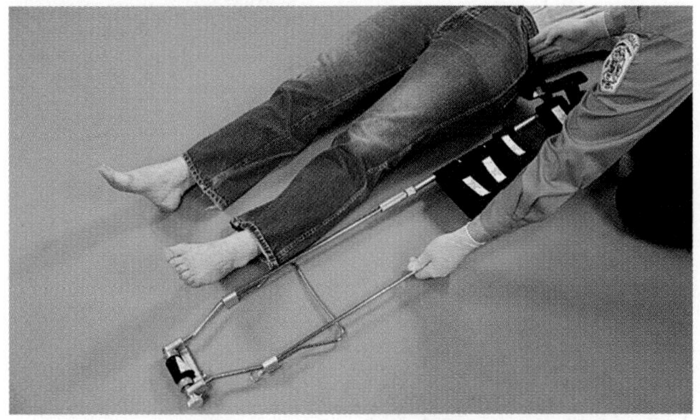

2. Place the splint next to the uninjured leg, ischial pad next to the iliac crest.

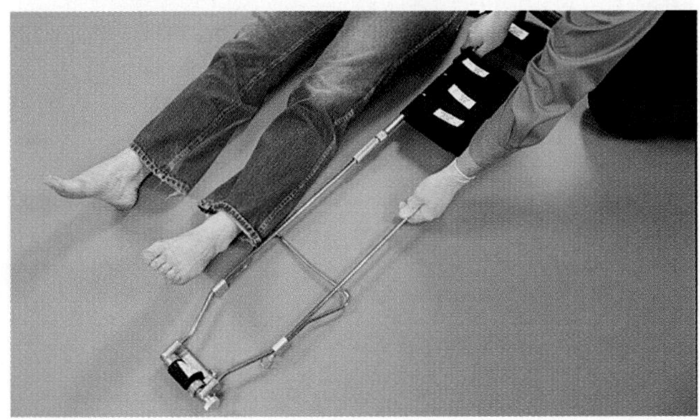

3. Hold the top and move the bottom until the bend is at the heel.

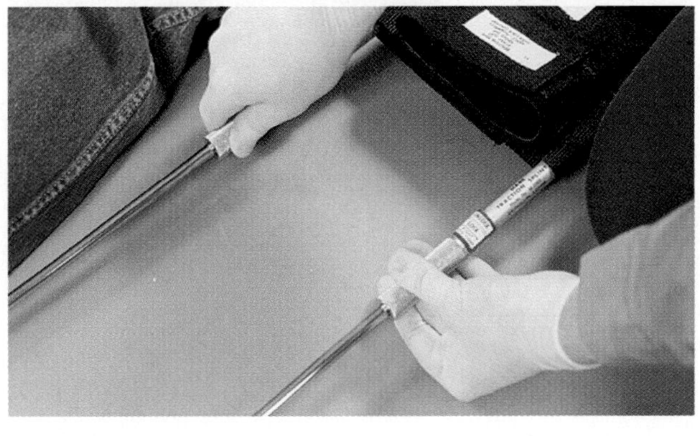

4. Lock the sleeve.

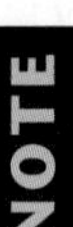

Assess distal pulse, motor function, and sensation both before and after immobilizing or splinting an extremity.

continued

SCAN 28-10 • (Continued)

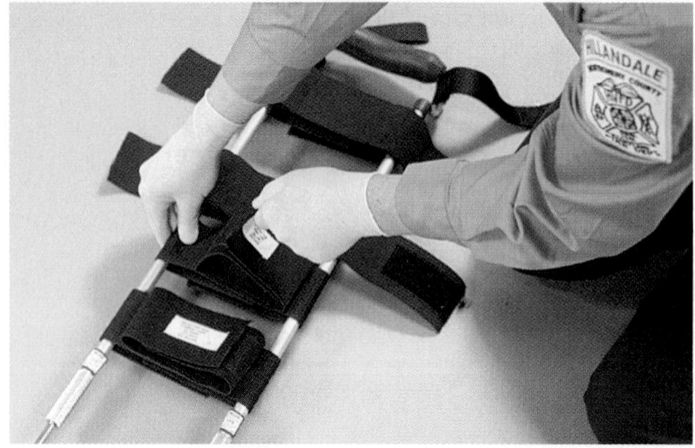

5. Open the support straps.

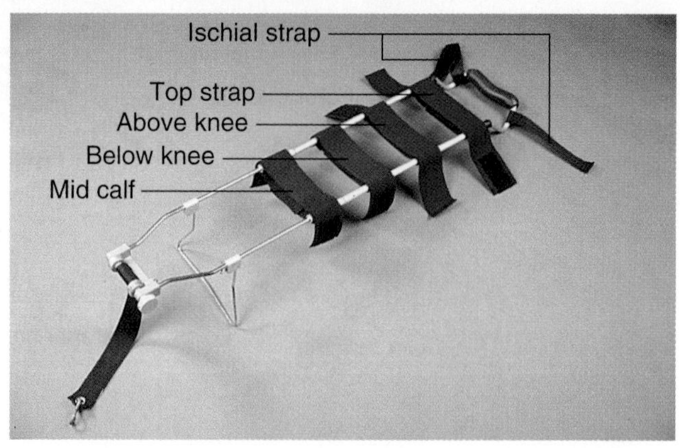

6. Place the straps under the splint.

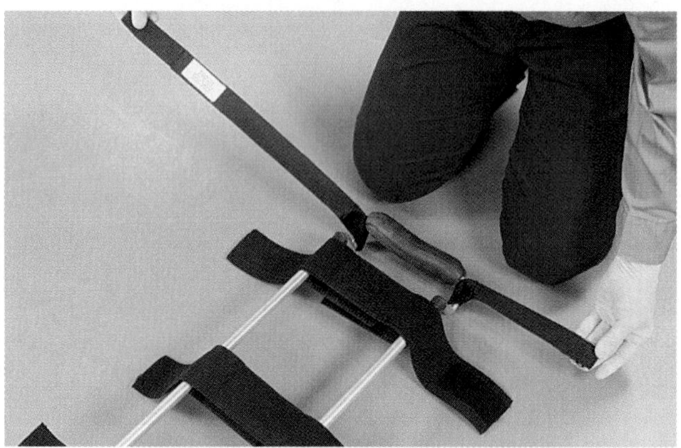

7. Release the ischial strap. Attached ends should be next to the ischial pad.

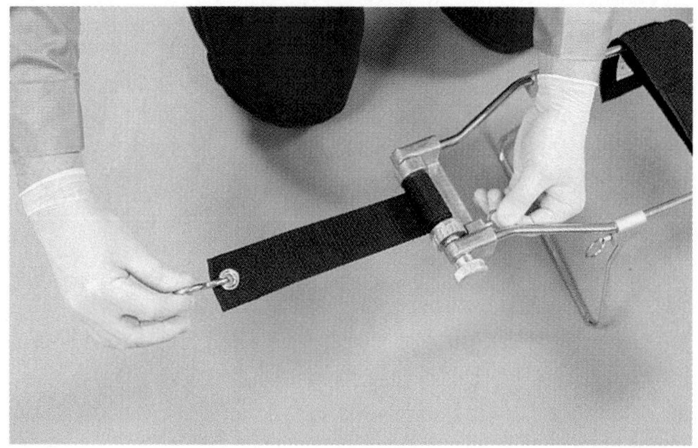

8. Pull release ring on ratchet and . . .

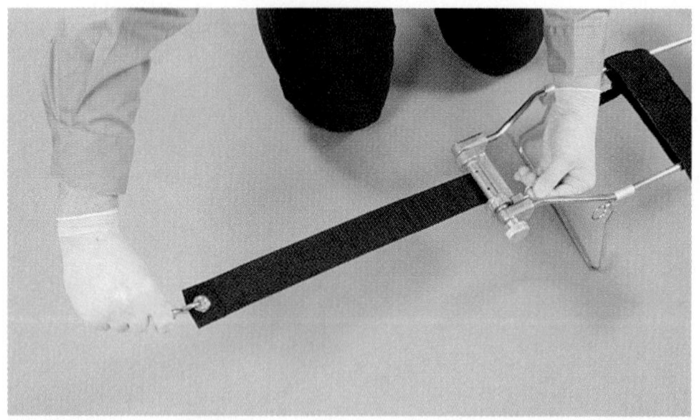

. . . Release the traction strap.

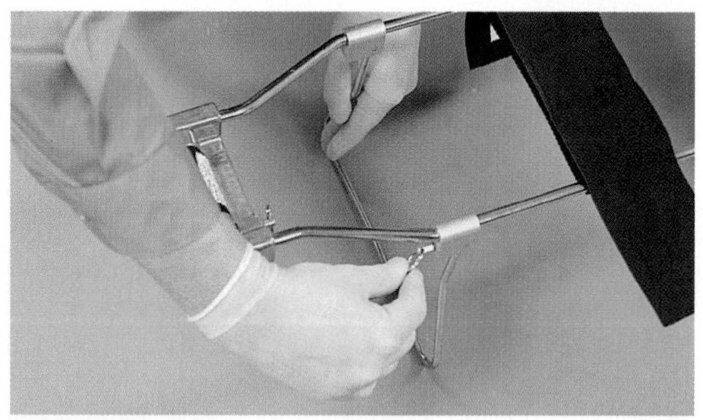

9. Extend and position the heel stand after the splint is in position under the patient.

NOTE

Traction splints vary depending on the manufacturer. Some splints in use are measured by placing the ring at the level of the bony prominence that can be felt in the middle of each buttock (ischial tuberosity) and the distal end of the splint placed 8 to 10 inches beyond the foot. Learn to use the equipment supplied in your area and keep up to date with new equipment as it is approved for use.

SCAN 28-11 • Traction Splinting

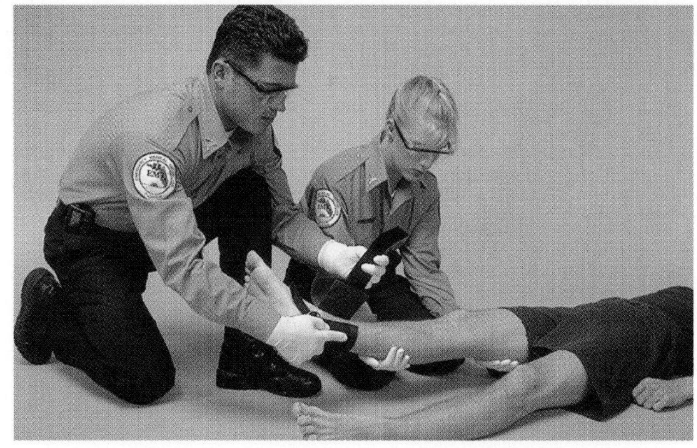

1. Some systems attach the ankle hitch prior to applying manual traction (tension). EMT #1 should apply the hitch while EMT #2 stabilizes the patient's limb.

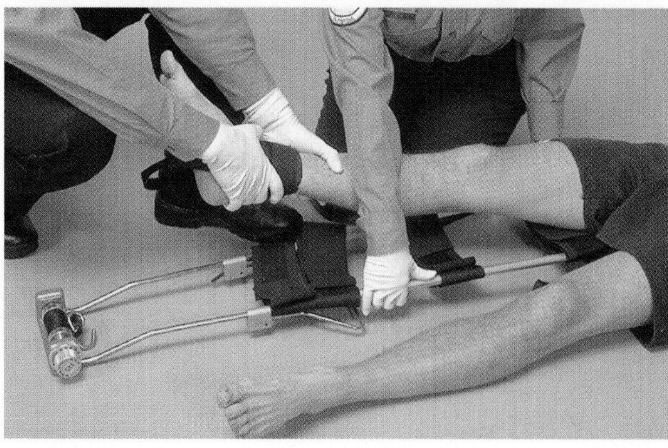

2. While EMT #1 applies manual traction (tension), EMT #2 can position the splint. Note . . .

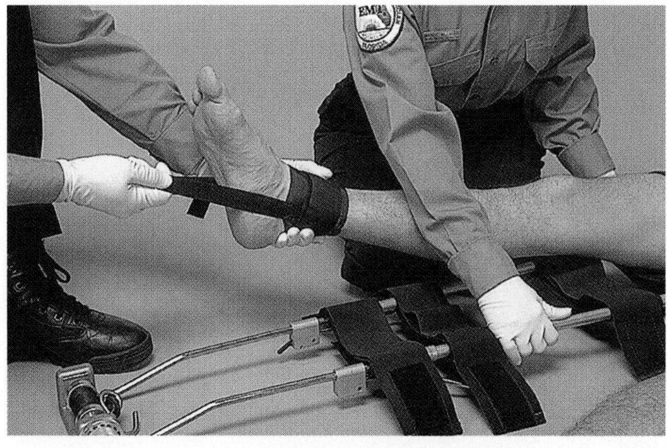

. . . Some systems allow manual traction to be applied by grasping the D-ring and ankle.

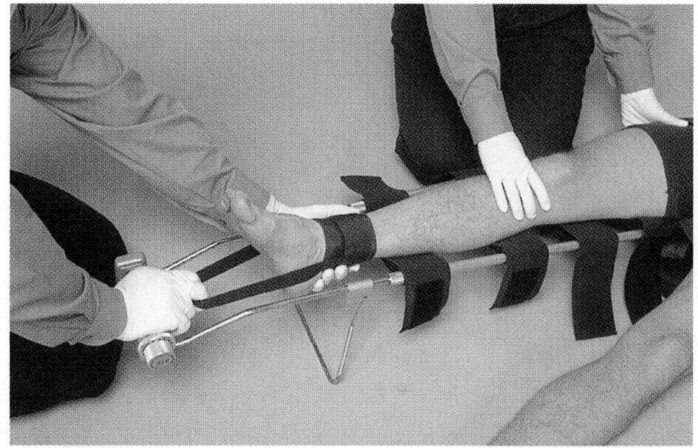

3. EMT #1 maintains manual traction (tension) and lowers the limb onto the cradles of the splint.

NOTE

Assess distal pulse, motor function, and sensation both before and after immobilizing or splinting an extremity.

continued

SCAN 28-11 • (Continued)

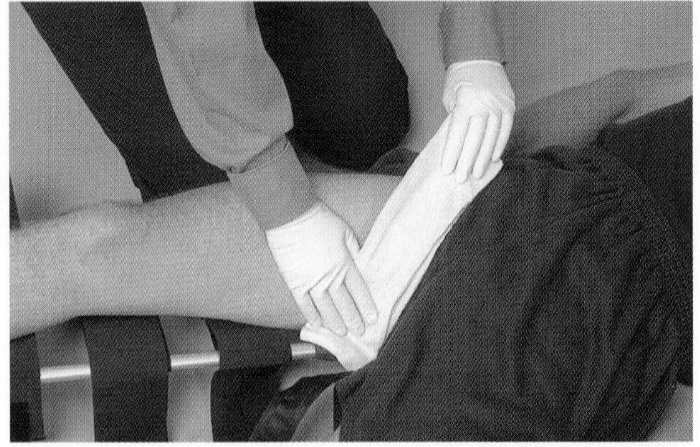

4. While EMT #1 maintains manual traction, EMT #2 applies padding to the groin area before securing the ischial strap. *Note:* Some EMS systems do not apply padding in order to reduce slippage.

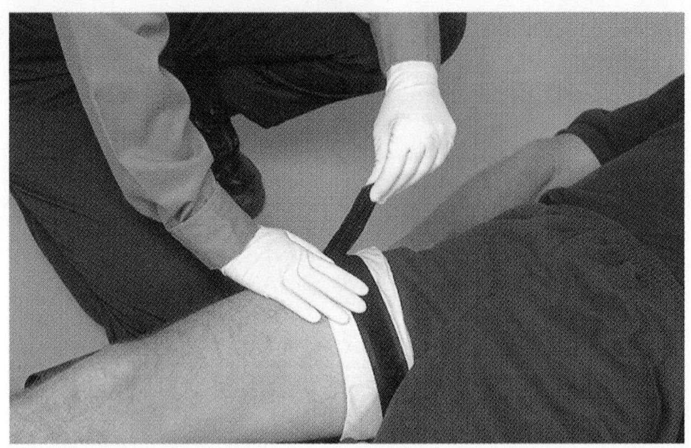

5. EMT #2 secures the ischial strap.

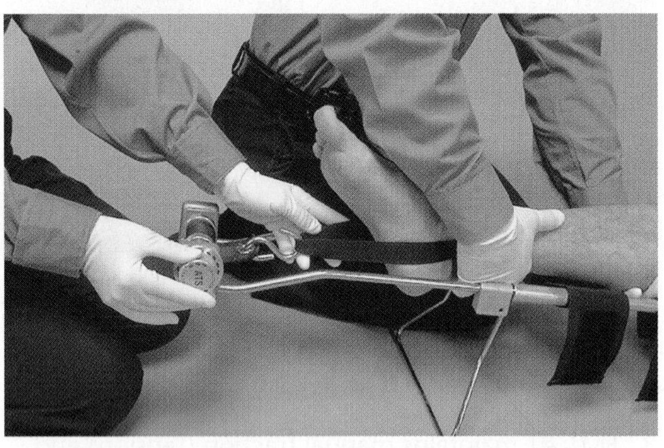

6. EMT #2 connects the ankle hitch to the windlass and tightens the ratchet to equal manual traction (tension).

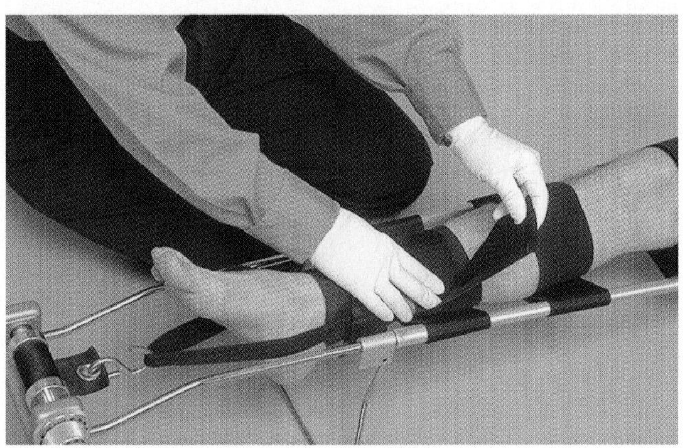

7. EMT #2 secures the cradle straps.

NOTE

Assess distal pulse, motor function, and sensation both before and after immobilizing or splinting an extremity.

SCAN 28-12 • Applying the Sager Traction Splint

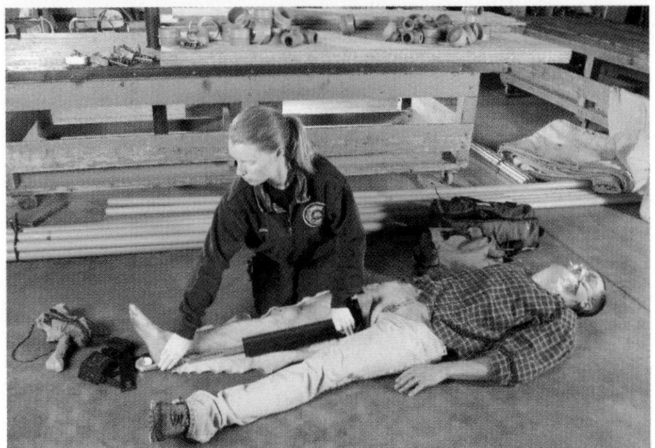

1. Place the splint medially.

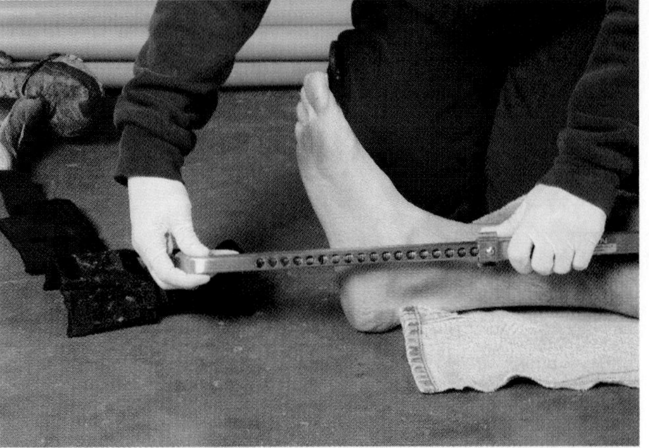

2. The length of the splint should be from groin to 4 inches below the heel. Unlock the clasp to extend the splint.

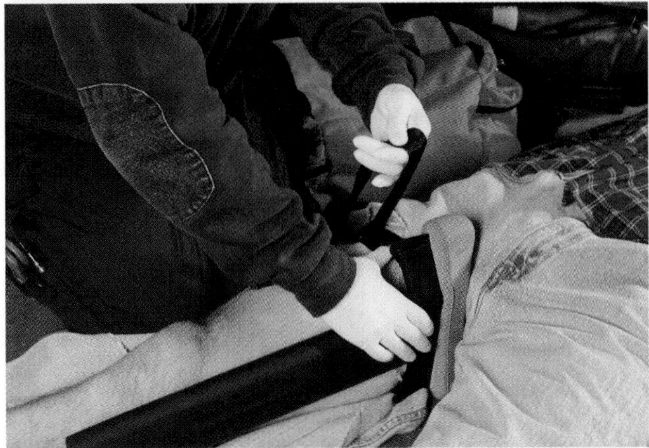

3. Secure the thigh strap.

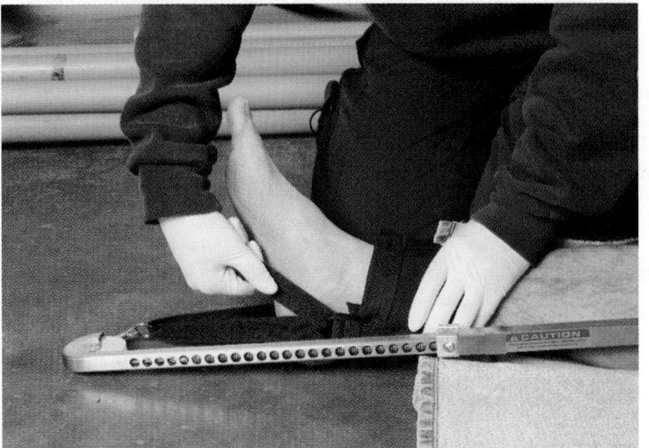

4. Wrap the ankle harness above the ankle (malleoli) and secure it under the heel.

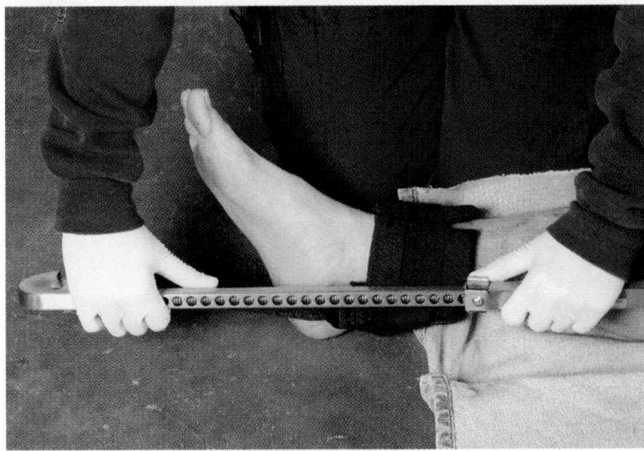

5. Release the lock and extend the splint to achieve desired traction (in pounds on pulley wheel).

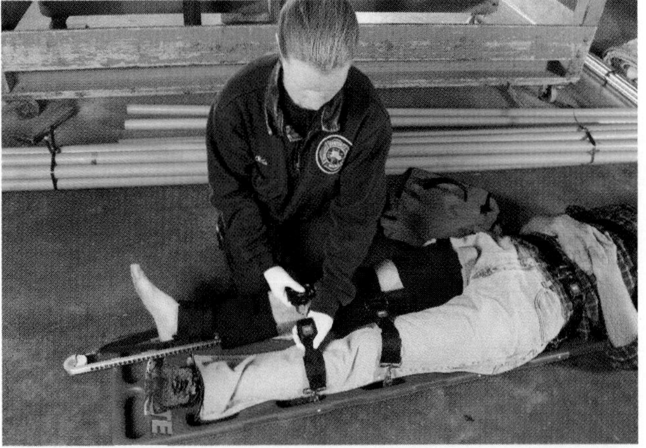

6. Secure the straps at thigh, lower thigh and knee, and lower leg. Strap the ankles and feet together. Secure the patient to the spine board.

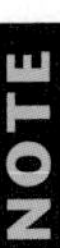
NOTE

Assess distal pulse, motor function, and sensation both before and after immobilizing or splinting an extremity.

SCAN 28-13 • Two-Splint Method—Bent Knee

If there is a distal pulse and nerve function, or the limb cannot be straightened without meeting resistance or causing severe pain, knee injuries should be splinted with the knee in the position in which it is found.

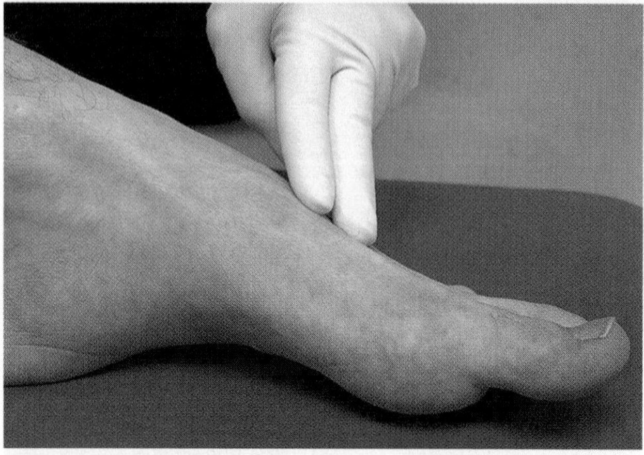

1. Assess distal PMS function.

2. Stabilize the knee above and below the injury site.

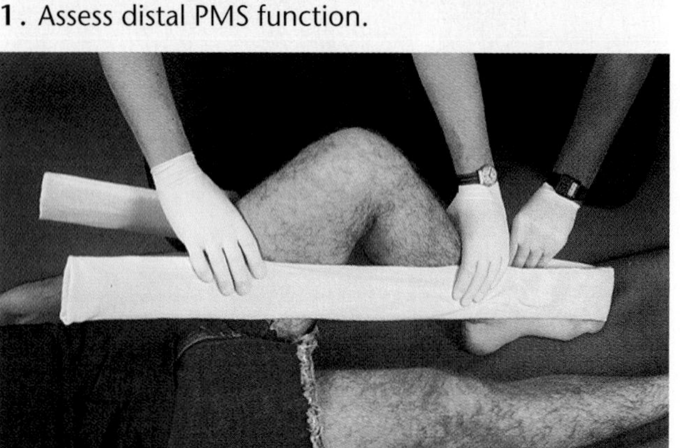

3. Place the padded side of the splints next to the injured extremity. Note that they should be equal in length and extend 6 to 12 inches beyond the mid-thigh and mid-calf.

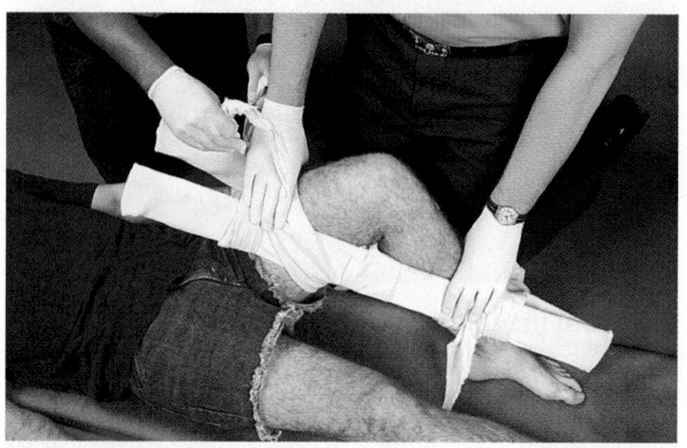

4. Place a cravat through the knee void and tie the boards together.

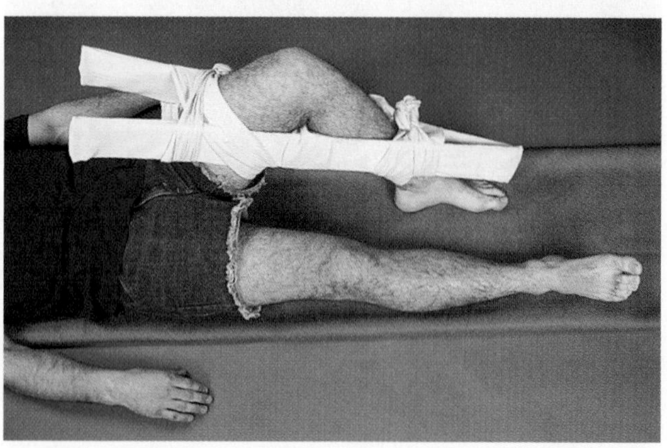

5. Using a figure-eight configuration, secure one cravat to the ankle and the boards, and the second cravat to the thigh and the boards. Reassess distal PMS function.

SCAN 28-14 • One-Splint Method—Straight Knee

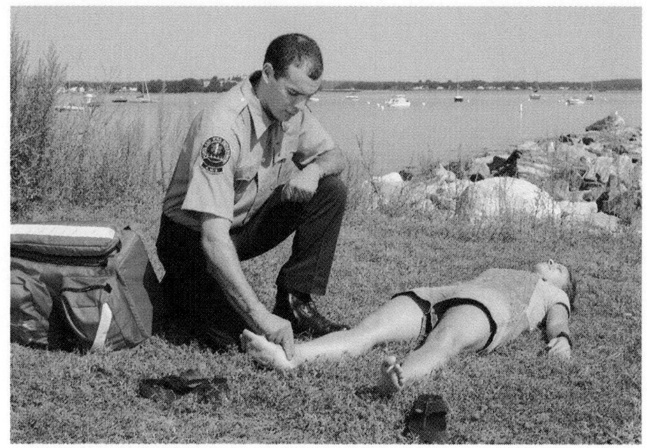

1. Assess distal PMS function.

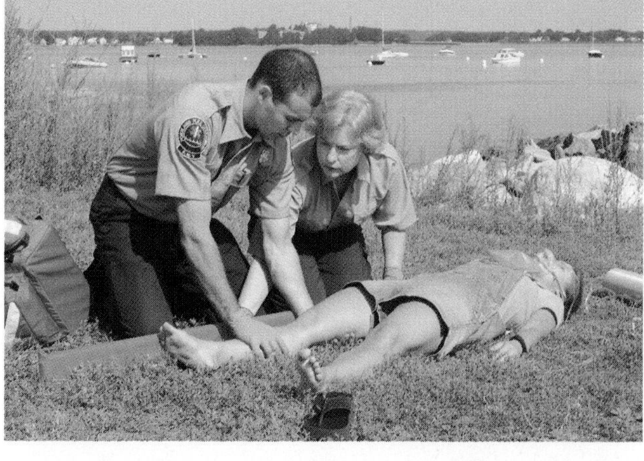

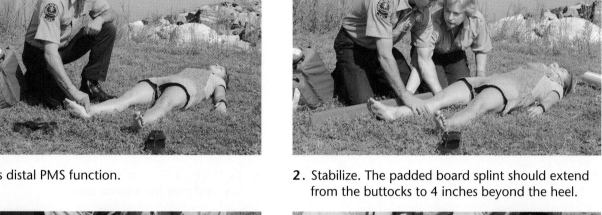

2. Stabilize. The padded board splint should extend from the buttocks to 4 inches beyond the heel.

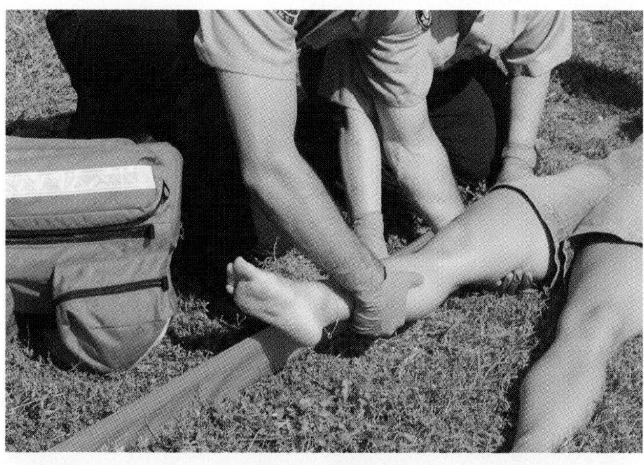

3. Maintain stabilization and lift the limb.

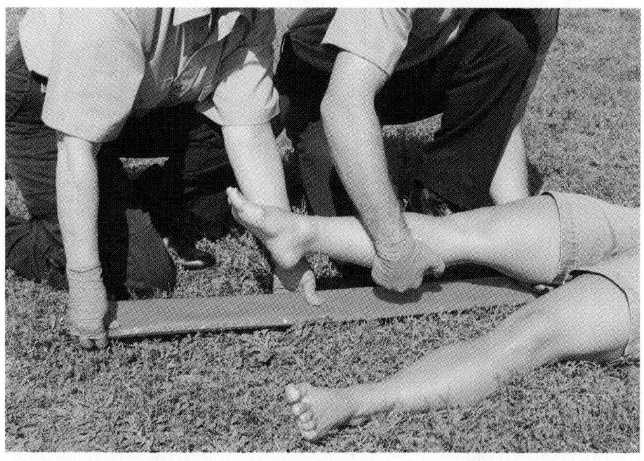

4. Place the splint along the posterior of the limb.

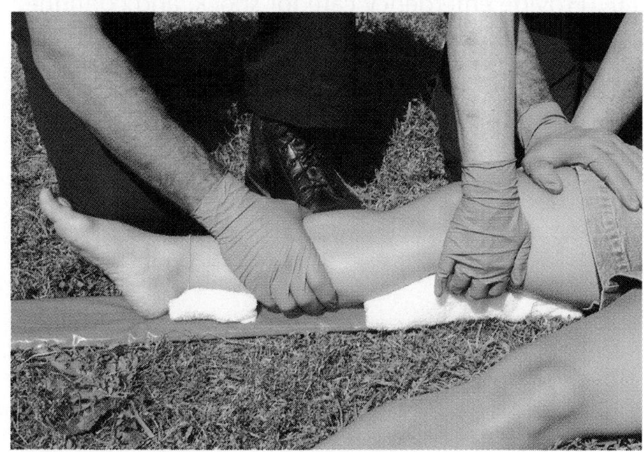

5. Pad the voids.

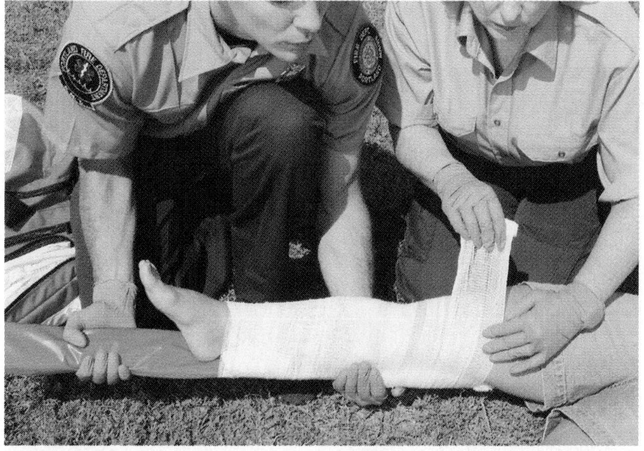

6. Use a 6-inch roller bandage or cravats to secure the injured leg to the splint.

continued

SCAN 28-14 • (Continued)

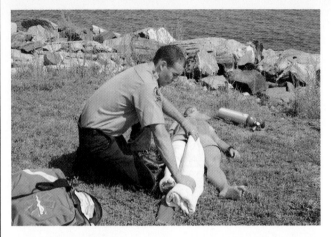

7. Place the folded blanket between legs, groin to feet.

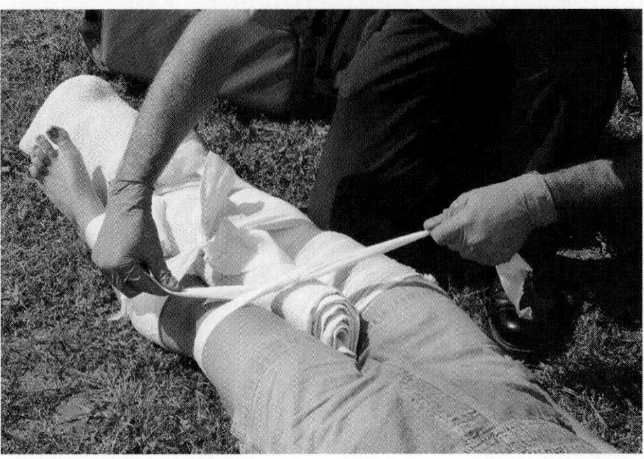

8. Tie thighs, calves, and ankles together. Do not tie the knot over the injured area.

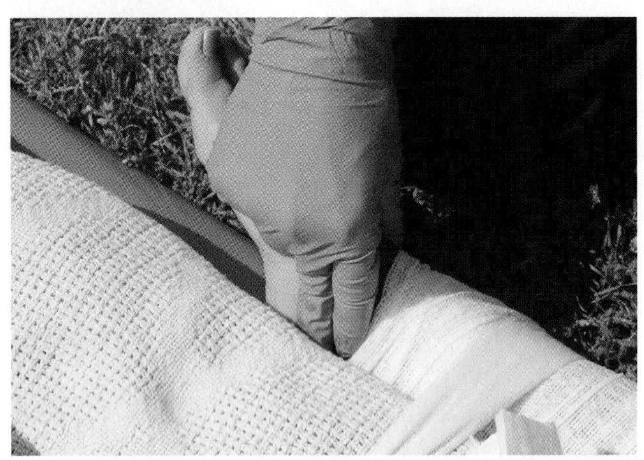

9. Reassess distal PMS function.

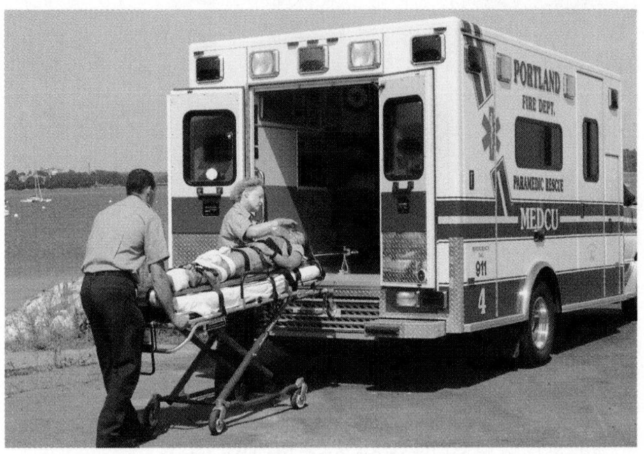

10. Provide emergency care for shock, and continue to administer high-concentration oxygen.

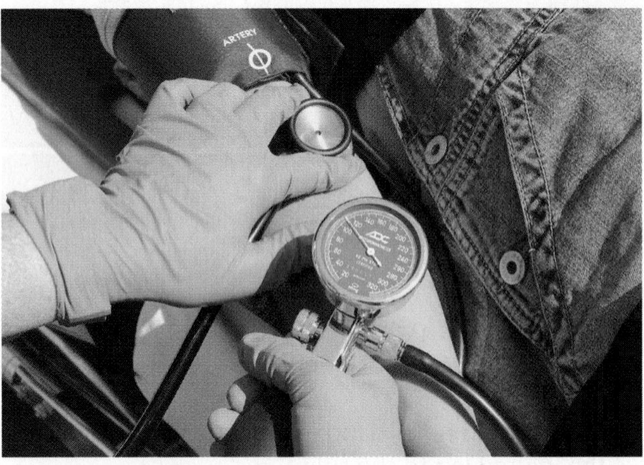

11. Monitor distal pulse and vital signs.

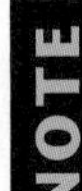

Assess distal pulse, motor function, and sensation both before and after immobilizing or splinting an extremity.

SCAN 28-15 • Two-Splint Method—Straight Knee

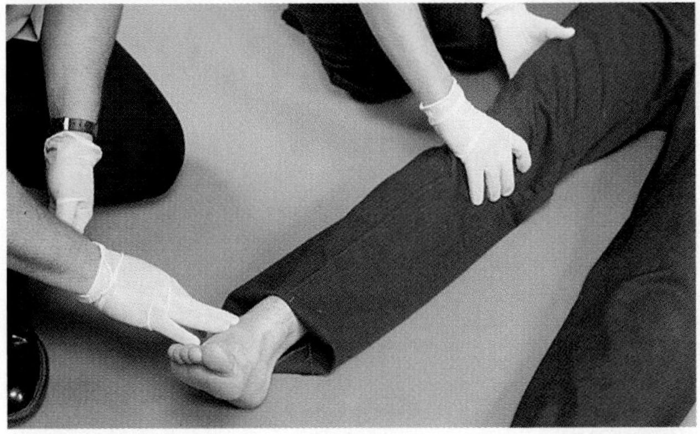

1. Stabilize the injured limb, and assess distal PMS function.

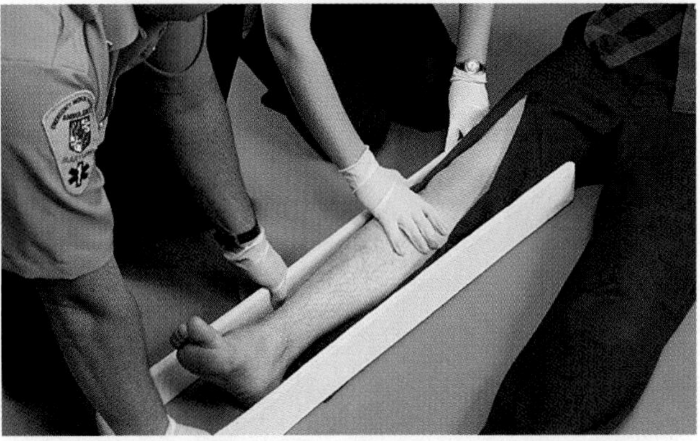

2. Measure the padded board splints, medial from groin, lateral from iliac crest, both to 4 inches beyond foot.

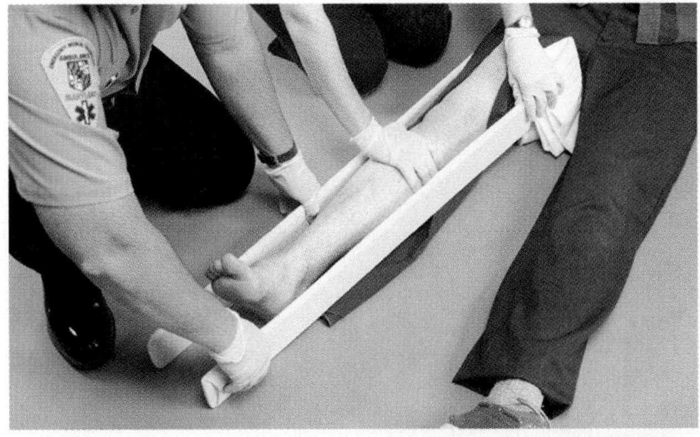

3. Position the splints.

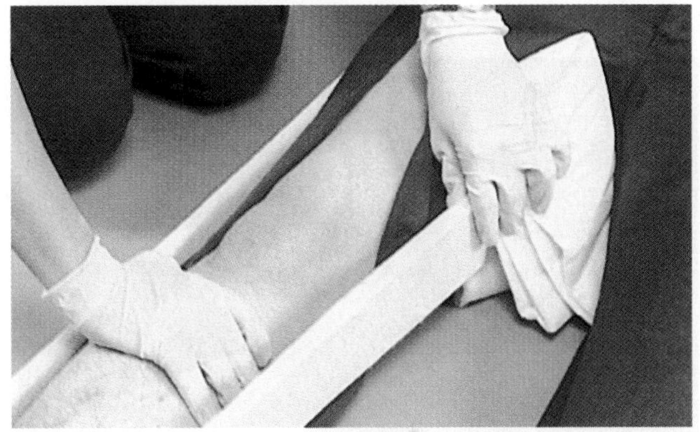

4. Pad the groin.

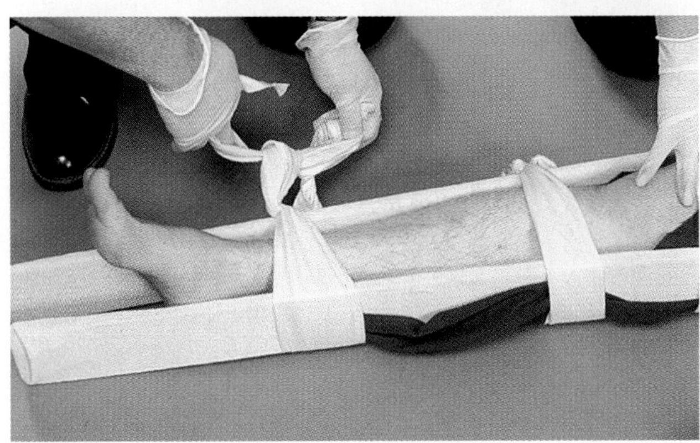

5. Secure splints at thigh, above and below knee, and at mid-calf. Pad all voids.

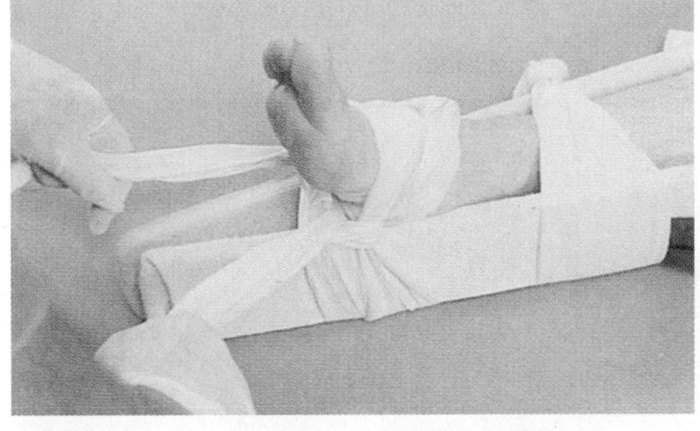

6. Cross and tie two cravats at the ankle or hitch the ankle. Reassess distal PMS function, care for shock, and provide high-concentration oxygen.

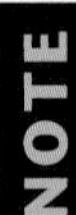

NOTE

Assess distal pulse, motor function, and sensation both before and after immobilizing or splinting an extremity.

SCAN 28-16 • Two-Splint Method—Leg Injuries

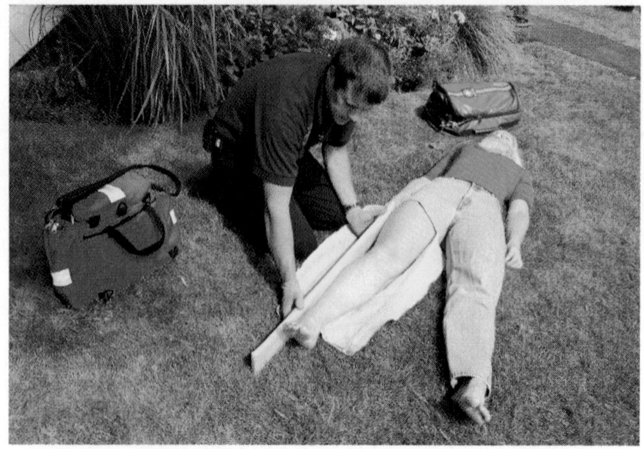

1. Assess distal PMS function. Measure the splints. They should extend above the knee and below the ankle.

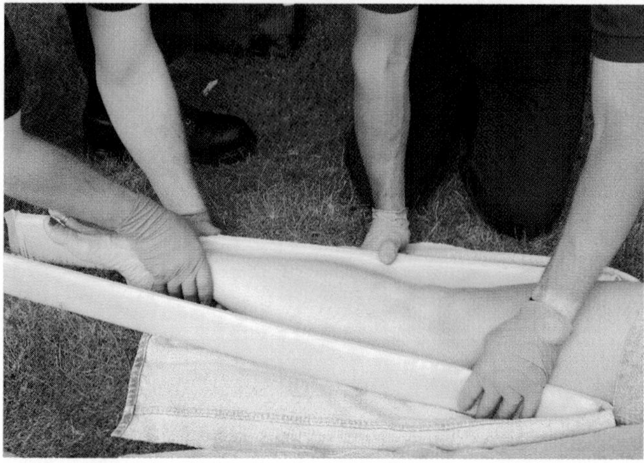

2. Apply manual traction (tension) and place one splint medially and one laterally. Padding is toward the leg.

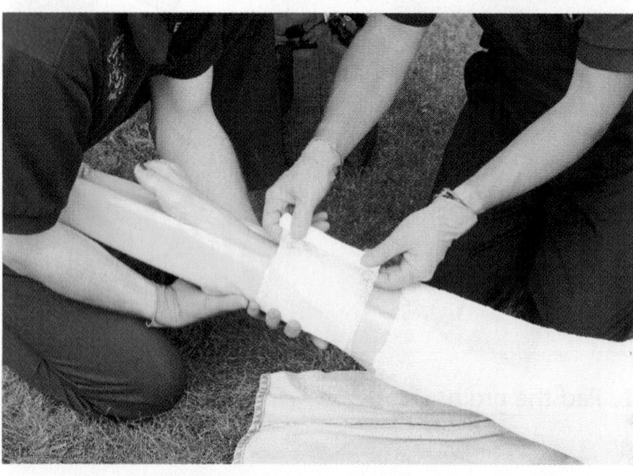

3. Secure splints, padding voids.

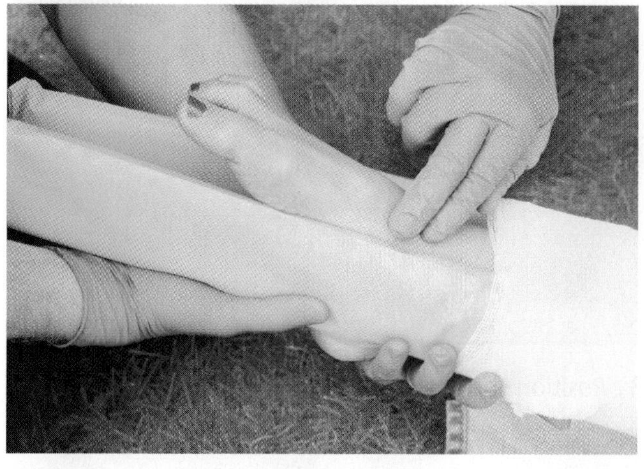

4. Reassess distal PMS function.

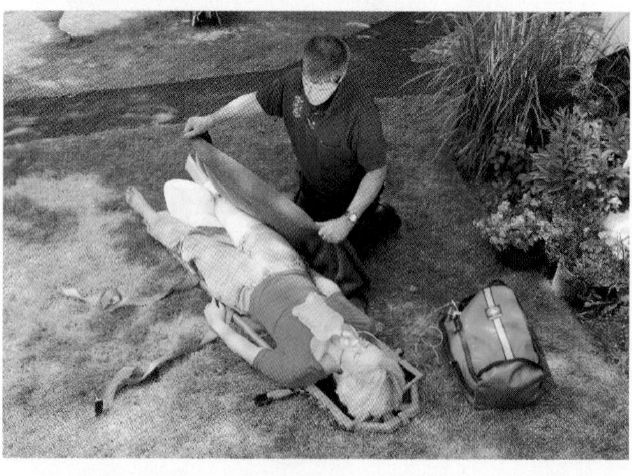

5. Provide emergency care for shock, and administer high-concentration oxygen. Transport on a long spine board.

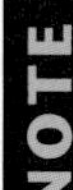

NOTE *Assess distal pulse, motor function, and sensation both before and after immobilizing or splinting an extremity.*

SCAN 28-17 • One-Splint Method—Leg Injuries

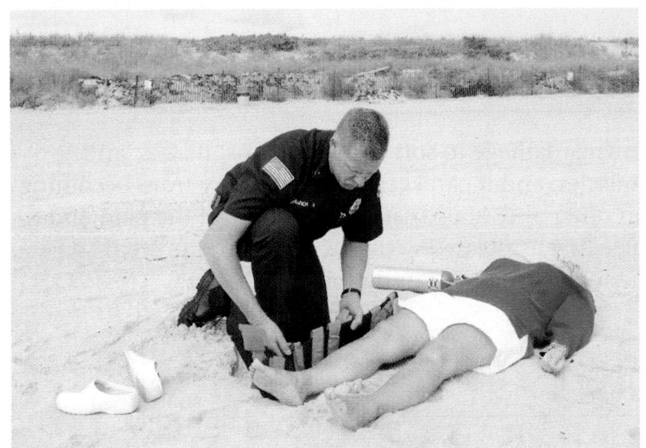

1. Assess distal PMS function. Measure the splint.

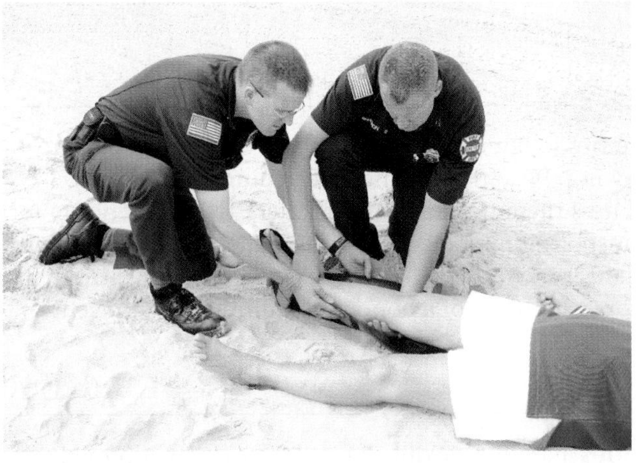

2. Lift limb off the ground.

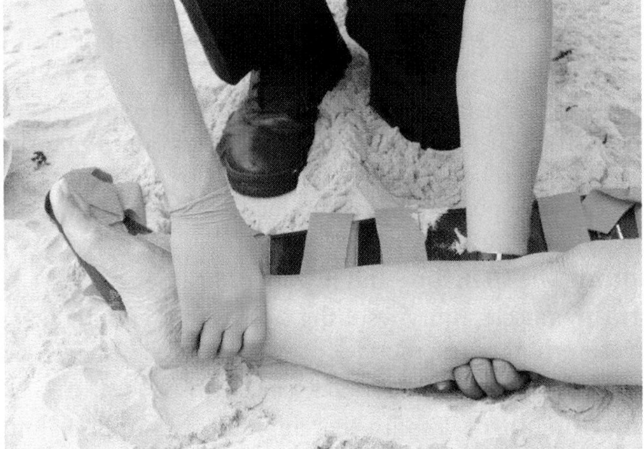

3. Apply manual traction (tension).

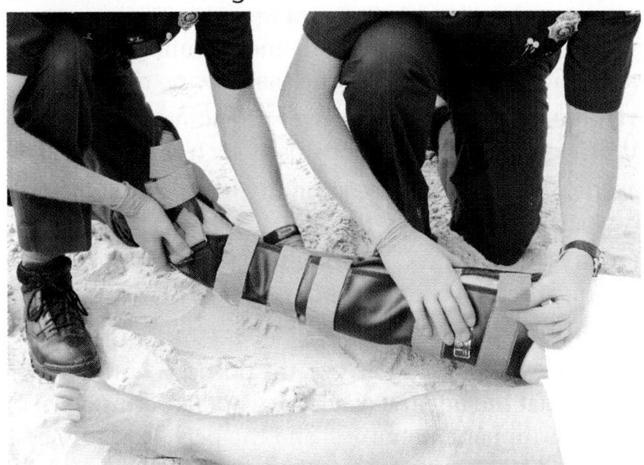

4. Secure the splint to the injured leg.

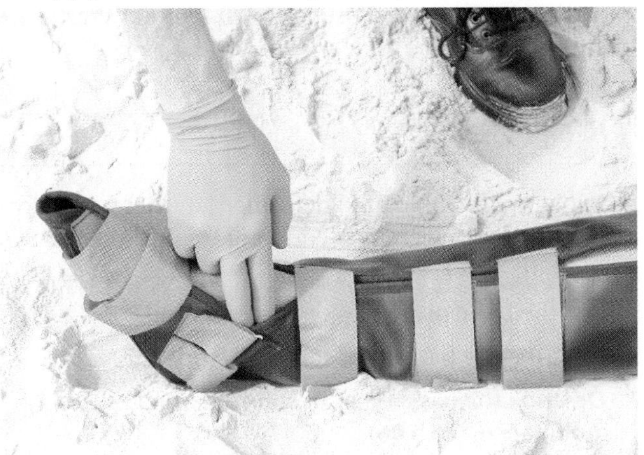

5. Reassess distal PMS function.

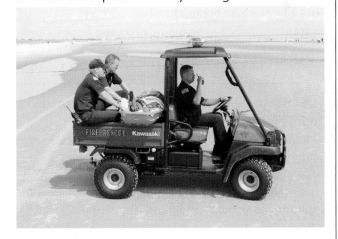

6. Care for shock, and continue to administer high-flow, high-concentration oxygen. Package the patient and prepare to transport.

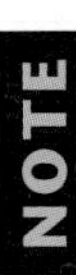

Assess distal pulse, motor function, and sensation both before and after immobilizing or splinting an extremity.

CHAPTER REVIEW

SUMMARY

Injuries to bones and joints should be splinted prior to moving the patient. If life-threatening injuries exist, address them first and, if the patient is a high priority for transport, immobilize the whole patient on a long spine board. When time and the patient's condition permit, proper splinting of a bone or joint injury can prevent further damage to soft tissues, organs, nerves, and muscles, and it can keep a closed injury from becoming an open one. It also can help to control the pain and bleeding associated with the injury, and prevent permanent damage or disability.

KEY TERMS

bones hard but flexible living structures that provide support for the body and protection to vital organs. Types of bones are long, short, flat, and irregular. The typical long bone has a cylindrical shaft and a rounded end or head, which is connected to the shaft by the neck.

cartilage tough tissue that covers the joint ends of bones and helps to form certain body parts such as the ear.

closed extremity injury an injury to an extremity with no associated opening in the skin.

crepitus (KREP-i-tus) a grating sensation or sound made when fractured bone ends rub together.

dislocation the disruption or "coming apart" of a joint.

extremities (ex-TREM-i-teez) the portions of the skeleton that include the clavicles, scapulae, arms, wrists, and hands (upper extremities) and the pelvis, thighs, legs, ankles, and feet (lower extremities).

fracture (FRAK-cher) any break in a bone.

joints places where bones articulate, or meet.

ligaments connective tissues that connect bone to bone.

manual traction the process of applying tension to straighten and realign a fractured limb before splinting. Also called *tension*.

muscles tissues or fibers that cause movement of body parts and organs.

open extremity injury an extremity injury in which the skin has been broken or torn through from the inside by an injured bone or from the outside by something that has caused a penetrating wound with associated injury to the bone.

sprain the stretching and tearing of ligaments.

strain muscle injury resulting from overstretching or overexertion of the muscle.

tendons tissues that connect muscle to bone.

traction splint a splint that applies constant pull along the length of a lower extremity to help stabilize the fractured bone and to reduce muscle spasm in the limb. Traction splints are used primarily on femoral shaft fractures.

REVIEW QUESTIONS

1. Describe the basic anatomy of bone and its purposes. (pp. 694–696)
2. Identify the signs and symptoms of musculoskeletal injury. (pp. 703–704)
3. Describe basic emergency care for painful, swollen, or deformed extremities, including general guidelines for splinting long bones and joints. (pp. 704–707)
4. Explain why angulated deformed injuries to the long bones should be realigned to anatomical position. (pp. 705–706)
5. List the basic principles of splinting. (pp. 706–707)
6. Describe the hazards of splinting. (pp. 707, 709)
7. Describe the basic types of splints carried on ambulances. (p. 706)

CRITICAL THINKING

- A hiker drives his boot under an old tree root and is tossed head over heels down the slope of a small hill. When he finally comes to rest, his left leg is bent below the knee at an unusual angle. Your initial assessment shows an alert adult male guarding a grossly deformed left leg. He hasn't lost consciousness and has no other pain. You find he has a strong radial pulse, normal skin, and no bleeding. How should you proceed?

Thinking and Linking

Think back to Chapter 26, "Bleeding and Shock," and link information from that chapter with information from this chapter as you consider the following situations:

- Blood loss can be significant with a fracture—even with a closed fracture. For each of the following, describe the signs and symptoms of shock you might see and whether you would expect the patient to compensate or eventually decompensate for the blood loss:
  - Fractured tibia and fibula
  - Both tibias and fibulas fractured
  - Femur fracture
  - Pelvic fracture

Think back to Chapter 5, "Lifting and Moving Patients," and Chapter 7, "Scene Size-Up," and link information from those chapters with information from this chapter as you consider the following situation:

- You have a patient who was thrown from an ATV deep in the woods. He complains of pain to his thigh and hip. What treatment and transportation devices would you use? What assistance would you call for in the scene size-up?

MEDIA RESOURCES

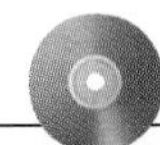

See the Student CD at the back of this book for quizzes, a case study activity, animations, and other features related to this chapter. Also, visit the Companion Website for *Emergency Care* at **www.prenhall.com/limmer**, where you will find additional reinforcement and links to other resources.

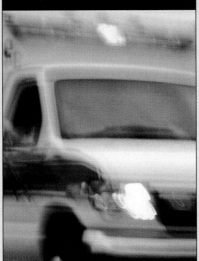

Street Scenes

You and your crew arrive for duty at the firehouse when you are called out for a "fall injury." A police unit is already on scene. They inform you that it is safe. Exiting your engine and taking Standard Precautions, you observe a tall woman in her 20s in jogging clothes leaning on the front hood of a car. She is wincing. The police officer standing next to her approaches and introduces you to your patient.

"How're you doing?" you ask. "My name's Len."

"Hi, Len, I'm Desta," she replies.

Your initial assessment reveals that Desta has a good airway and that she is breathing fine. "What happened, Desta, and why did you call EMS this morning?"

"I fell off that wall while trying to climb over it," she answers, simultaneously pointing to a 4-foot rock wall approximately 100 feet away. "When I landed, I heard something crack in my right leg. I hopped on one foot to this car, and called for help." You quickly make a mental note that the surface she landed on is asphalt.

Street Scene Questions

1. What priority would you assign to this patient? Why?
2. How would you continue your assessment?

Desta's mental status seems normal. There are no signs of bleeding anywhere on her body. You assign a low priority to her, and continue your assessment by performing a focused history and physical exam. Desta tells you that she is taking no medications. You ask if she has any allergies and she replies smiling, "Rock walls, apparently." She laughs, then suddenly grimaces in pain as she unintentionally shifts her weight onto her right leg.

Baseline vitals are obtained and you learn Desta's pulse is 88 and regular, respirations are 16 and unlabored, and blood pressure is 108/72. Her pupils are equal and reactive. She states she has no pain anywhere but in her lower right leg.

Street Scene Questions

3. What signs might you expect to find with a broken long bone?
4. What are your major concerns with possible broken bones in the extremities?

You assist Desta from her standing position onto your cot, carefully supporting her right leg. Then you expose the extremity. About 2 inches above the ankle, you observe swelling and a noticeable, unnatural curve to her leg. The skin is not broken. You are concerned that she might have nerve and muscle damage below the injury, but she is able to move her toes and feel you touch her foot. You also detect a pulse below the injury site.

Street Scene Question

5. What interventions are appropriate for this patient?

A member of your crew brings an air splint, which provides immobilization to the joint above and below the injury site. You maintain manual traction, being careful not to move the extremity unnecessarily, and apply the splint. After application, the patient states the leg feels more secure. You reassess her vitals as well as pulses, motor function, and sensation below the injury site. Everything appears to be normal. During transport, you continue to check distal pulses, motor function, and sensation on the affected extremity. Transport to the hospital is uneventful.

Street Scenes Sample Documentation

PATIENT NAME: *Modesta Salerno* **PATIENT AGE:** *24*

CHIEF COMPLAINT

Pain in lower right extremity

PAST MEDICAL HISTORY

- [X] None
- [ ] Allergy to
- [ ] Hypertension
- [ ] Stroke
- [ ] Seizures
- [ ] Diabetes
- [ ] COPD
- [ ] Cardiac
- [ ] Other (List)
- [ ] Asthma

Current Medications (List)

VITAL SIGNS

TIME	RESP	PULSE	B.P.	MENTAL STATUS	R PUPILS L	SKIN
0630	Rate: *16*; [X] Regular; [ ] Shallow; [ ] Labored	Rate: *88*; [X] Regular; [ ] Irregular	*108/72*	[✓] Alert; [ ] Voice; [ ] Pain; [ ] Unresp.	[✓] Normal [✓]; [ ] Dilated [ ]; [ ] Constricted [ ]; [ ] Sluggish [ ]; [ ] No-Reaction [ ]	[✓] Unremarkable; [ ] Cool; [ ] Pale; [ ] Warm; [ ] Cyanotic; [ ] Moist; [ ] Flushed; [ ] Dry; [ ] Jaundiced
0640	Rate: *16*; [X] Regular; [ ] Shallow; [ ] Labored	Rate: *86*; [X] Regular; [ ] Irregular	*108/72*	[✓] Alert; [ ] Voice; [ ] Pain; [ ] Unresp.	[✓] Normal [✓]; [ ] Dilated [ ]; [ ] Constricted [ ]; [ ] Sluggish [ ]; [ ] No-Reaction [ ]	[✓] Unremarkable; [ ] Cool; [ ] Pale; [ ] Warm; [ ] Cyanotic; [ ] Moist; [ ] Flushed; [ ] Dry; [ ] Jaundiced
	Rate:; [ ] Regular; [ ] Shallow; [ ] Labored	Rate:; [ ] Regular; [ ] Irregular	/	[ ] Alert; [ ] Voice; [ ] Pain; [ ] Unresp.	[ ] Normal [ ]; [ ] Dilated [ ]; [ ] Constricted [ ]; [ ] Sluggish [ ]; [ ] No-Reaction [ ]	[ ] Unremarkable; [ ] Cool; [ ] Pale; [ ] Warm; [ ] Cyanotic; [ ] Moist; [ ] Flushed; [ ] Dry; [ ] Jaundiced

NARRATIVE *Upon arrival, noted a 24-year-old female patient leaning back onto the hood of a car. States she attempted to climb over an approximately 4-foot rock wall when she fell, landing on an asphalt surface. She states she heard a "crack" as she landed. Focused physical exam reveals no bleeding. Trauma isolated to lower right tibia/fibula. Noted swelling and tenderness, as well as an unnatural curve to extremity approximately 2 inches above ankle. Good pulse, motor function, and sensation before and after application of full-leg air splint. No change noted during transport.*

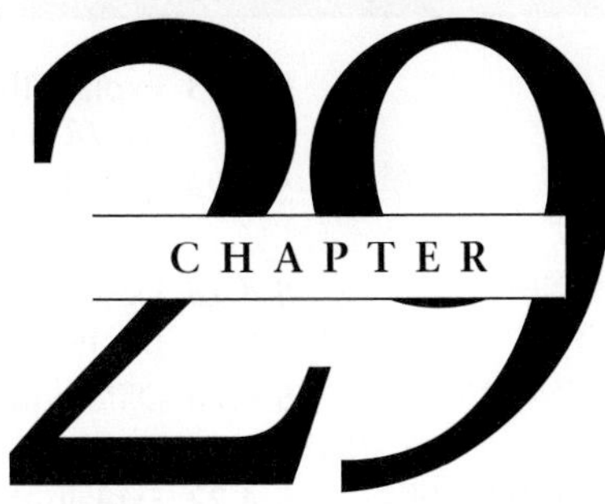

CHAPTER 29

Injuries to the Head and Spine

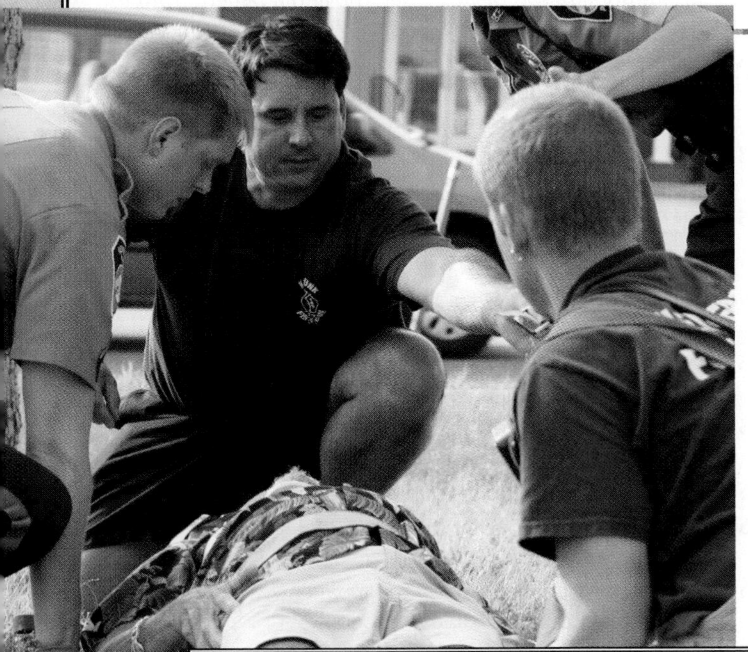

CORE CONCEPTS

The following are core concepts that will be addressed in this chapter:

- Identification of mechanisms of head and spine injury
- Stabilization of the cervical spine
- Application of a cervical spine immobilization device
- How and when to perform a rapid extrication
- Immobilization using short and long backboards
- Procedures for helmet removal

KEY TERMS

autonomic nervous system, p. 751
central nervous system, p. 749
cerebrospinal fluid (CSF), p. 752
concussion, p. 753
contusion, p. 753
cranium, p. 751
hematoma, p. 753
laceration, p. 753
malar, p. 751
mandible, p. 751
maxillae, p. 751
nasal bones, p. 751
nervous system, p. 749
orbits, p. 751
peripheral nervous system, p. 749
spinous process, p. 752
temporal bone, p. 751
temporomandibular joint, p. 751
vertebrae, p. 752

DOT OBJECTIVES

*KNOWLEDGE AND ATTITUDE

5-4.1 State the components of the nervous system. (pp. 749–751)

5-4.2 List the functions of the central nervous system. (pp. 749–751)

5-4.3 Define the structure of the skeletal system as it relates to the nervous system. (pp. 751–752)

5-4.4 Relate mechanism of injury to potential injuries of the head and spine. (pp. 752–755)

5-4.5 Describe the implications of not properly caring for potential spine injuries. (p. 760)

5-4.6 State the signs and symptoms of a potential spine injury. (pp. 762–763)

5-4.7 Describe the method of determining if a responsive patient may have a spine injury. (pp. 762–763)

5-4.8 Relate the airway emergency medical care techniques to the patient with a suspected spine injury. (p. 764)

5-4.9 Describe how to stabilize the cervical spine. (p. 764)

5-4.10 Discuss indications for sizing and using a cervical spine immobilization device. (p. 764)

5-4.11 Establish the relationship between airway management and the patient with head and spine injuries. (pp. 756–758, 764)

5-4.12 Describe a method for sizing a cervical spine immobilization device. (p. 766)

5-4.13 Describe how to log roll a patient with a suspected spine injury. (pp. 772–776) (Scan 29-3, p. 773)

5-4.14 Describe how to secure a patient to a long spine board. (pp. 772–776) (Scan 29-4, pp. 774–775; Scan 29-5, p. 778)

5-4.15 List instances when a short spine board should be used. (pp. 766, 771)

5-4.16 Describe how to immobilize a patient using a short spine board. (pp. 766, 771) (Scan 29-1, pp. 767–768)

5-4.17 Describe the indications for the use of rapid extrication. (p. 766)

5-4.18 List steps in performing rapid extrication. (pp. 766, 771) (Scan 29-2, pp. 769–770; Scan 29-8, pp. 784–786)

5-4.19 State the circumstances when a helmet should be left on the patient. (p. 777)

5-4.20 Discuss the circumstances when a helmet should be removed. (p. 781)

5-4.21 Identify different types of helmets. (p. 777)

5-4.22 Describe the unique characteristics of sports helmets. (p. 777)

5-4.23 Explain the preferred methods to remove a helmet. (p. 781) (Scan 29-6, pp. 782–783)

5-4.24 Discuss alternative methods for removal of a helmet. (p. 781) (Scan 29-6, p. 783)

5-4.25 Describe how the patient's head is stabilized to remove the helmet. (pp. 782–783)

5-4.26 Differentiate how the head is stabilized with a helmet compared to without a helmet. (pp. 782–783)

5-4.27 Explain the rationale for immobilization of the entire spine when a cervical spine injury is suspected. (pp. 757, 760–761)

5-4.28 Explain the rationale for utilizing immobilization methods apart from the straps on the cot. (pp. 772, 774–776, 781, 787–788)

5-4.29 Explain the rationale for utilizing a short spine immobilization device when moving a patient from the sitting to supine position. (pp. 766, 771–772)

5-4.30 Explain the rationale for utilizing rapid extrication approaches only when they indeed will make the difference between life and death. (pp. 766, 771–772)

5-4.31 Defend the reasons for leaving a helmet in place for transport of a patient. (p. 777)

5-4.32 Defend the reasons for removal of a helmet prior to transport of a patient. (p. 781)

*SKILLS

5-4.33 Demonstrate opening the airway in a patient with suspected spinal cord injury.

5-4.34 Demonstrate evaluating a responsive patient with a suspected spinal cord injury.

5-4.35 Demonstrate stabilization of the cervical spine.

5-4.36 Demonstrate the four person log roll for a patient with a suspected spinal cord injury.

5-4.37 Demonstrate how to log roll a patient with a suspected spinal cord injury using two people.

5-4.38 Demonstrate securing a patient to a long spine board.

5-4.39 Demonstrate using the short board immobilization technique.

5-4.40 Demonstrate the procedure for rapid extrication.

5-4.41 Demonstrate preferred methods for stabilization of a helmet.

5-4.42 Demonstrate helmet removal techniques.

5-4.43 Demonstrate alternative methods for stabilization of a helmet.

5-4.44 Demonstrate completing a prehospital care report for patients with head and spinal injuries.

You have probably noticed that throughout the earlier chapters of this book there have been many cautions for patients with possible injuries to the head and spine. This is because injuries to these areas are extremely serious and may result in severe permanent disability or death if improperly treated or missed during your assessment. Second only to proper assessment and care of the ABCs, proper assessment and care for head and spine injuries will be your most important responsibility as an EMT.

NERVOUS AND SKELETAL SYSTEMS

The following segments briefly review the anatomy of the nervous system, head, and spine. For more information, review Chapter 4, "The Human Body."

Nervous System

The major components of the **nervous system** are the brain and the spinal cord. The nervous system provides overall control of thought, sensations, and motor functions. The skeletal system provides support and protection. The skull protects the brain, while the bones of the spine protect the spinal cord (Figure 29-1). Whenever the skull or the spine is injured, suspect nervous system damage as well.

The nervous system (Figure 29-2) is divided into two subsystems: the central nervous system and the peripheral nervous system. The **central nervous system** consists of the brain and the spinal cord. The **peripheral nervous system** includes the pairs of nerves that enter and exit the spinal cord between each pair of vertebrae, the 12 pairs of cranial nerves that travel from the brain without passing through the spinal cord, and all of the body's other motor and sensory nerves (Figure 29-3).

nervous system provides overall control of thought, sensation, and the voluntary and involuntary motor functions of the body. The major components of the nervous system are the brain and the spinal cord.

central nervous system the brain and the spinal cord.

peripheral nervous system the nerves that enter and exit the spinal cord between the vertebrae and the 12 pairs of cranial nerves that travel between the brain and organs without passing through the spinal cord, and all of the body's other motor and sensory nerves.

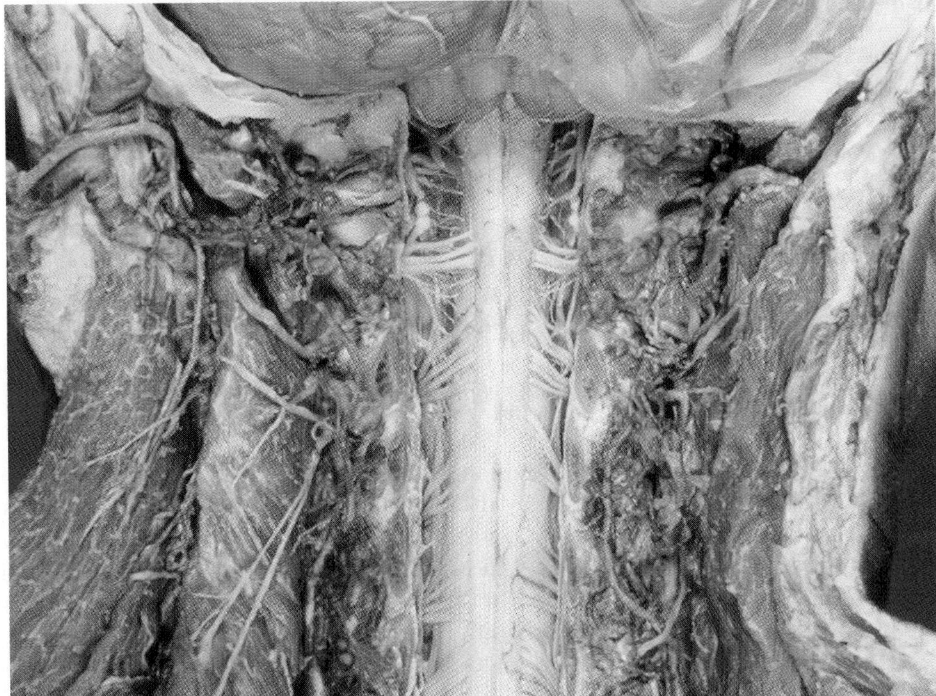

Figure 29-1 • Enhanced color spinal cord. *(© Photo Researchers, Inc.)*

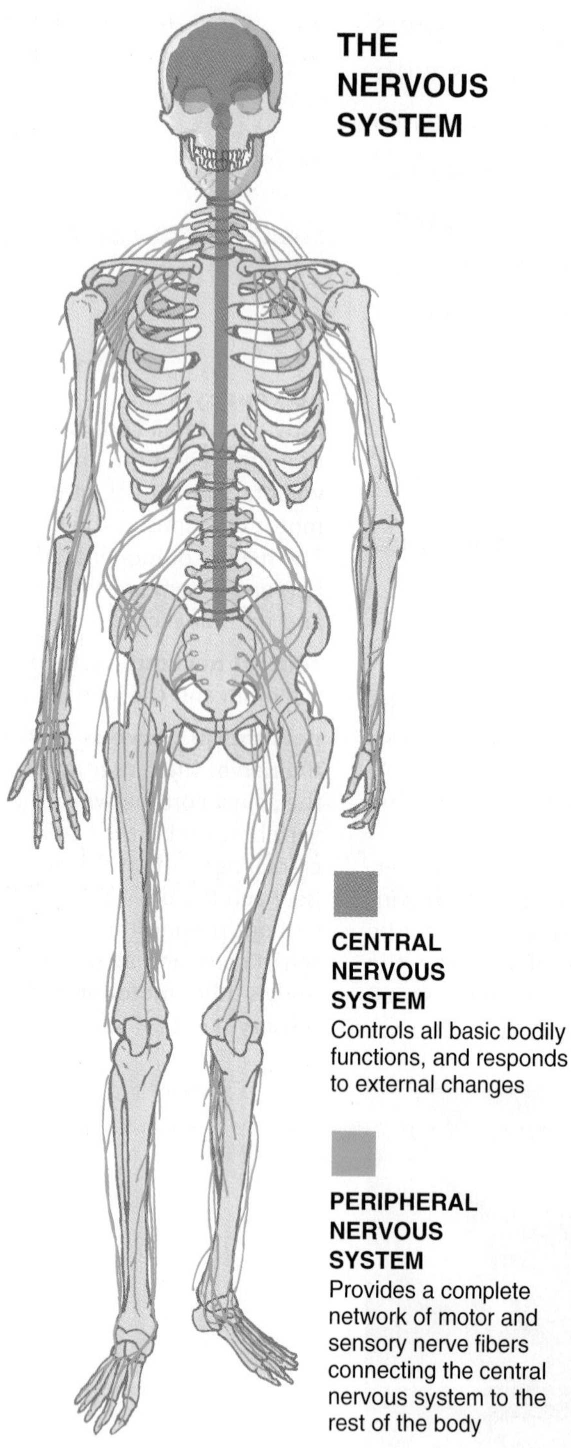

THE NERVOUS SYSTEM
CENTRAL NERVOUS SYSTEM
Controls all basic bodily functions, and responds to external changes
PERIPHERAL NERVOUS SYSTEM
Provides a complete network of motor and sensory nerve fibers connecting the central nervous system to the rest of the body

Figure 29-2 • Nervous system.

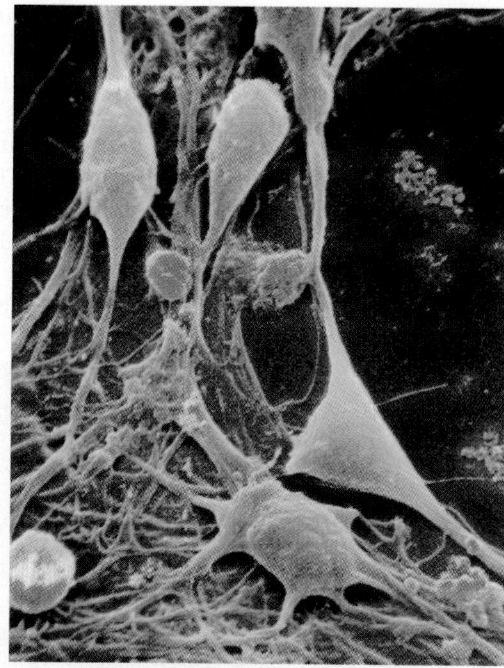

Figure 29-3 • The neuron is the specialized nerve cell that transmits the nervous system impulses throughout the body. *(© Photo Researchers, Inc.)*

Messages from the body to the brain are carried by sensory nerves. Messages from the brain to the muscles are carried by motor nerves. These nerves control voluntary movements, or those we consciously control such as running or grasping. As the nerves exit the brain, prior to traveling down the spinal cord, they cross over to the opposite side of the body. This is why an injury to the left side of the brain may produce effects such as weakness or lack of sensation on the right side of the body.

Some nerves control involuntary functions—those we do not consciously control—including heartbeat, breathing, control of the diameter of your vessels, control of the round sphincter muscles closing your bladder and bowel, and digestion. These nerves are part of the **autonomic nervous system** (autonomic means automatic).

The brain is the master organ of life. Messages from all over the body are received by the brain, which determines the body's response. The brain sends messages to the muscles so that we can move, or to a particular organ so that it will carry out a desired function. (For example, it may tell the adrenal gland to dump epinephrine into the bloodstream, which increases heart rate.) Any major head injury can damage the brain, causing vital body functions to fail.

The spinal cord is a relay between most of the body and the brain. A large number of the messages to and from the brain are sent through the spinal cord. Damage to the cord can isolate a part of the body from the brain. Function of this region can be lost, possibly forever.

The healing power of nerve tissue is limited. This is especially true in certain areas. If nerve tissue in the brain or spinal cord is damaged, to a certain extent function is lost and cannot be restored. As an EMT, your initial care will often prevent additional damage to the brain, spinal cord, and major nerves of the body.

Anatomy of the Head

The skull is made up of the **cranium** and the facial bones (Figure 29-4). The cranium, the portion of the skull that encloses the brain, is formed by the forehead, top, back, and upper sides of the skull. The cranial floor is the inferior wall of the brain case, the bony floor beneath the brain. The cranial bones are fused together to form immovable joints.

There are 14 irregularly shaped bones forming the face. The facial bones are fused into immovable joints, except for the **mandible,** which joins on each side of the cranium with a **temporal bone** to form the **temporomandibular joint.** This joint is sometimes referred to as the TM joint.

The upper jaw is made up of two fused bones called the **maxillae.** Each is known as a *maxilla.* The upper third, or bridge, of the nose contains two **nasal bones.** There is a cheek bone on each side of the skull. The cheek bone can be called the **malar** or the *zygomatic bone.* The malars and the maxillae form a portion of the **orbits** (sockets) of the eyes.

The brain is held within the skull. The spinal cord exits the base of the brain and leaves the skull through a large hole where the spinal column is attached. The brain is

autonomic nervous system controls involuntary functions.

cranium (KRAY-ne-um) the bony structure making up the forehead, top, back, and upper sides of the skull.

mandible (MAN-di-bl) the lower jaw bone.

temporal (TEM-po-ral) **bone** bone that forms part of the side of the skull and floor of the cranial cavity. There is a right and a left temporal bone.

temporomandibular (TEM-po-ro-mand-DIB-yuh-lar) **joint** the movable joint formed between the mandible and the temporal bone, also called the TMJ.

maxillae (mak-SIL-e) the two fused bones forming the upper jaw.

nasal (NAY-zul) **bones** the bones that form the upper third, or bridge, of the nose.

malar (MAY-lar) the cheek bone, also called the *zygomatic bone.*

orbits the bony structures around the eyes; the eye sockets.

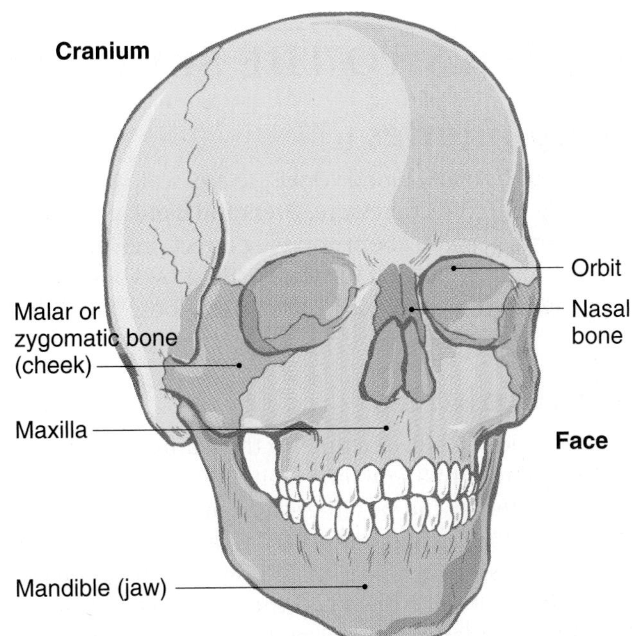

Figure 29-4 • Skull: cranium and face.

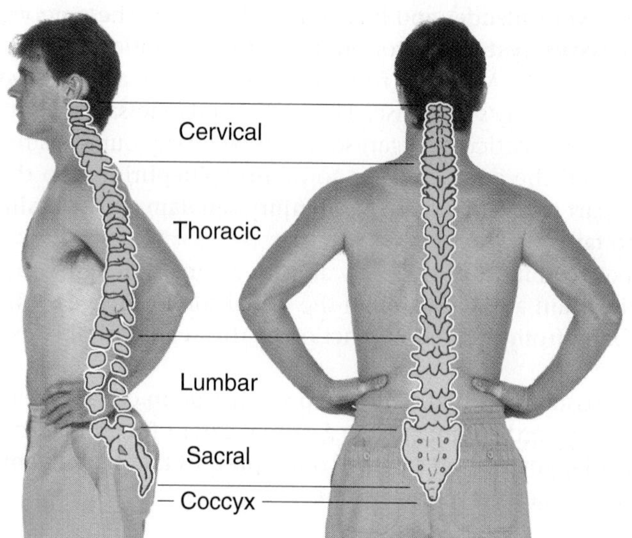

Figure 29-5 • Divisions of spinal column.

cerebrospinal (suh-RE-bro-SPI-nal) **fluid (CSF)** the fluid that surrounds the brain and spinal cord.

vertebrae (VERT-uh-bray) the bones of the spinal column (singular vertebra).

spinous (SPI-nus) **process** the bony bump on a vertebra.

bathed in a fluid called **cerebrospinal fluid (CSF).** This fluid also circulates down the spine around the spinal cord.

Anatomy of the Spine

The spine is made up of 33 irregularly shaped bones, called **vertebrae** (singular *vertebra*), which sit one on top of another to form the spinal column. Each vertebra has a **spinous process,** a bony bump you can feel along the center of a person's back. Every vertebra has a hollow space like the hole in a donut. These hollow spaces form a channel that runs the length of the spinal column and contains the spinal cord, which is cushioned by the cerebrospinal fluid.

The vertebrae are divided into five areas (shown in Figure 29-5). From top to bottom, they are: 7 cervical (in the neck), 12 thoracic (to which the ribs attach), 5 lumbar (mid-back), 5 sacral (lower back), and 4 coccygeal (in the coccyx, or tailbone). Both the sacral and coccygeal vertebrae are fused together, forming the posterior portion of the pelvis.

INJURIES TO THE SKULL AND BRAIN

Scalp Injuries

The scalp has many blood vessels, so any scalp injury may bleed profusely. Control scalp bleeding with direct pressure. Dress and bandage as you would other soft-tissue injuries. However, be careful about applying direct pressure when there is a possible skull injury. Do not apply pressure if the injury site shows bone fragments or depression of the bone or if the brain is exposed. Instead, use a loose gauze dressing.

Skull Injuries

Skull injuries include fractures to the cranium and the face. If severe enough, there can also be injuries to the brain.

NOTE *Whenever you suspect skull or brain injury, also suspect spine injury.*

Skull injuries can be either open or closed. With most injuries, the words *open* and *closed* refer to whether or not the skin and its underlying tissues have been broken. With head injuries, the words *open* and *closed* refer to the cranial bones. When the bones of the cranium are fractured, and the overlying scalp is lacerated, the patient has an *open head injury*. If the scalp is lacerated but the cranium is intact, it is considered to be a *closed head injury*. In practice, you may not be able to determine if a head injury is open or closed. It is safest to assume that there may be an open head injury beneath any contusion or laceration of the scalp.

concussion
mild closed head injury without detectable damage to the brain. Complete recovery is usually expected.

contusion
in brain injuries, a bruised brain caused when the force of a blow to the head is great enough to rupture blood vessels.

laceration (las-uh-RAY-shun)
in brain injuries, a cut to the brain.

hematoma (HE-mah-TO-mah)
in a head injury, a collection of blood within the skull or brain.

Brain Injuries

Brain injuries can be classified as direct or indirect. *Direct injuries* to the brain can occur in open head injuries, with the brain being lacerated, punctured, or bruised by the broken bones or by foreign objects. *Indirect injuries* to the brain may occur with either closed or open head injuries. In an indirect injury, the shock of impact on the skull is transferred to the brain. Indirect injuries to the brain include concussions and contusions.

NOTE

One of the first and most significant signs of head injury is altered mental status. In some patients it would be easy to assume the patient was intoxicated or on drugs when the true underlying problem is a head injury. Never assume a patient with an altered mental status is simply intoxicated or on drugs. Use your assessment (palpation) and history.

F•Y•I

TYPES OF BRAIN INJURIES

An EMT does not need to determine or diagnose the exact type of brain injury in order to assess and care for a patient with head trauma, but the following will provide some background information on brain injuries.

A **concussion** (Figure 29-6) may be so mild that the patient is unaware of the injury. When a person strikes his head in a fall, or is struck by a blunt object, a certain amount of the force is transferred through the skull to the brain. Usually there is no detectable damage to the brain and the patient may or may not become unconscious. Most patients with a concussion will feel a little "groggy" after receiving a blow to the head. Headache is common. If there is a loss of consciousness, it usually lasts only a short time and does not tend to recur. Sometimes, after a head blow, bystanders will say the patient "just sat there staring off into space for a few minutes." Some loss of memory (amnesia) of the events surrounding the incident is fairly common. A common saying is that the fighter did not see the punch that did him in. Actually, he probably did see the punch but then forgot it because of the concussion.

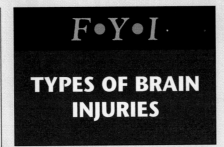

A bruised brain, or brain **contusion,** can occur with closed head injuries, when the force of the blow is great enough to rupture blood vessels on or within the brain. A contusion is often caused by a collision or blow that causes the brain to hit the inside of the skull, bounce off the opposite side, and then rebound to strike the first side of the skull again. When the bruising of the brain occurs on the side of the blow, it is called a *coup*; when it occurs on the side opposite the blow, it is called a *contrecoup*.

A **laceration,** or cut, to the brain can occur from the same forces that might cause a contusion. The inner skull has many sharp, bony ridges that can lacerate a moving brain. A laceration or a puncture wound can also be caused by an object penetrating the cranium.

A **hematoma** is a collection of blood within tissue. A hematoma inside the cranium is named according to its location. It may be located inside or outside the dura, the brain's protective outer covering (Figure 29-7), or within the brain itself. A *subdural hematoma* is a collection of blood between the brain and the dura. An *epidural hematoma* is blood between the dura and the skull. An *intracerebral hematoma* occurs when blood pools within the brain (Figure 29-8).

Head injury is made worse by several problems. There is limited room for expansion inside the hard skull. When a hematoma develops, pressure inside the skull increases, making it difficult for normal blood flow to enter the head. To meet this challenge, the blood pressure is forced to increase. As a result of decreased blood flow, the brain becomes starved for oxygen and high in waste carbon dioxide, causing even more swelling. Finally, head injury may cause decreased respiratory effort, which further worsens oxygen starvation and swelling in the brain.

continued

F•Y•I

Continued

CONCUSSION

- Mild injury, usually with no detectable brain damage
- May have brief loss of consciousness
- Headache, grogginess, and short-term memory loss common

BLUNT FORCE

CONTUSION

- Unconsciousness or decreased level of responsiveness
- Bruising of brain tissue

Figure 29-6 • Closed head injuries.

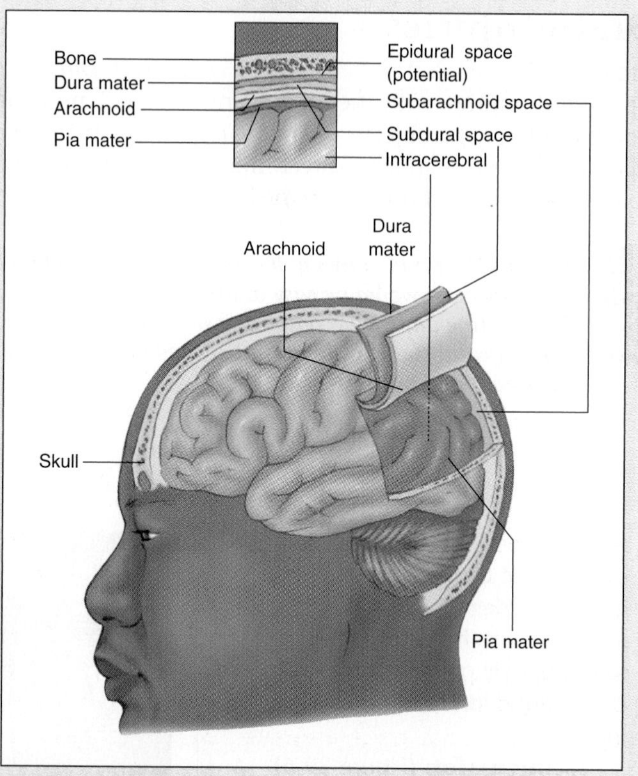

Figure 29-7 • Meninges (covering layers) of the brain.

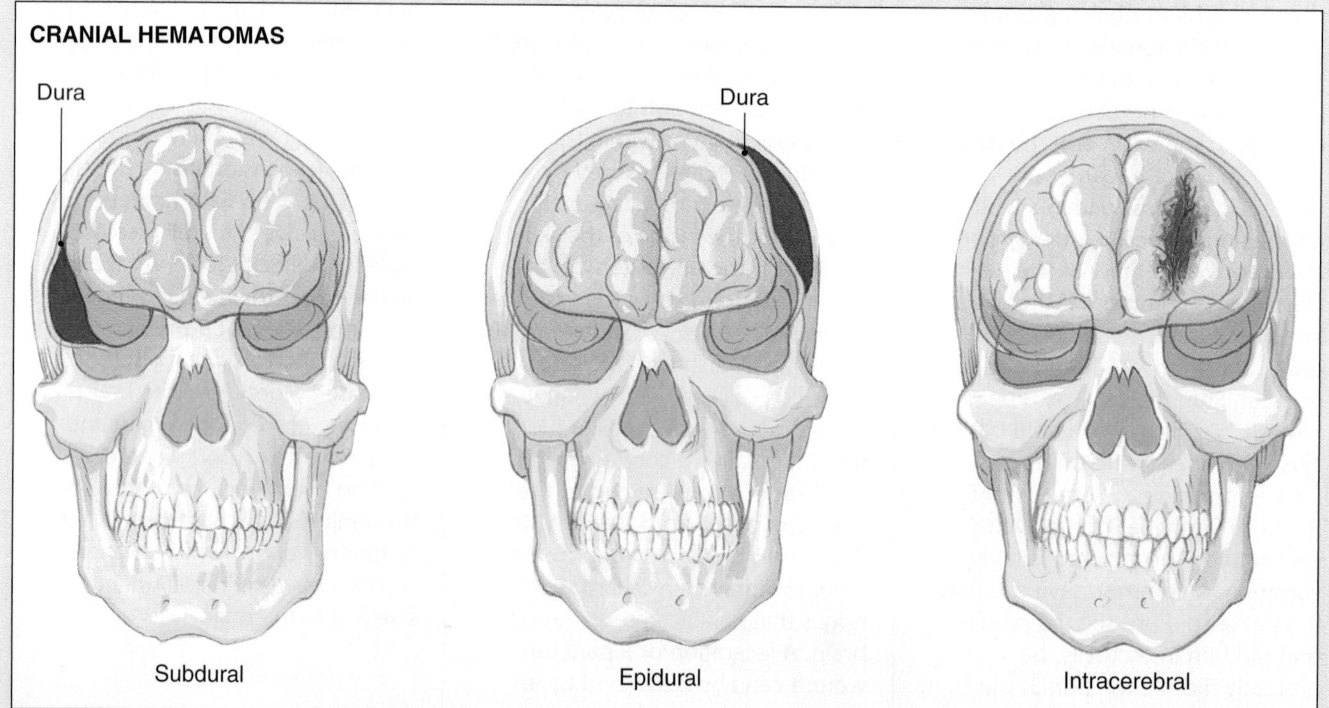

Figure 29-8 • Hematomas within the cranium.

PATIENT ASSESSMENT

SKULL FRACTURES AND BRAIN INJURIES

The signs of skull fracture and of brain injury are very similar, as noted in the following list (Figure 29-9):

- Visible bone fragments and perhaps bits of brain tissue are the most obvious signs of skull fracture, but most skull fractures do not produce these signs.
- Altered mental status. Check mental status by using the AVPU scale (alert, verbal stimulus, painful stimulus, unresponsive). If the patient is alert, check for orientation to person, place, and time. Some EMS agencies also use the Glasgow Coma Scale (described later in this chapter).
- Deep laceration or severe bruise or hematoma to the scalp or forehead. Do not probe or separate the wound opening to determine wound depth.
- Depressions or deformity of the skull, large swellings ("goose eggs"), or anything unusual about the shape of the cranium.
- Severe pain at the site of a head injury. Pain may range from a headache to severe discomfort. Do not palpate the injury site with your fingertips as you may push bone fragments into the injury.
- "Battle's sign," a bruise behind the ear (late sign).
- Pupils unequal or unreactive to light (Figure 29-10).
- "Raccoon eyes," black eyes, or discoloration of the soft tissues under both eyes (late sign).
- One eye that appears to be sunken.
- Bleeding from the ears and/or nose.
- Clear fluid flowing from ears and/or nose.
- Personality change, ranging from irritable to irrational behavior (a major sign).
- Increased blood pressure and decreased pulse rate (Cushing's triad, also called Cushing's reflex).
- Irregular breathing patterns.
- Temperature increase (late sign due to inflammation, infection, or damage to temperature-regulating centers).
- Blurred or multiple-image vision in one or both eyes.
- Impaired hearing or ringing in the ears.
- Equilibrium problems. The patient may be unable to stand still with his eyes closed or may stumble when attempting to walk. (Do not test for this.)
- Forceful or projectile vomiting.
- Posturing. The patient may exhibit neurological posturing, such as flexing arms and wrists and extending legs and feet (decorticate posture) or extending arms with the shoulders rotated inward and wrists flexed, legs extended (decerebrate posture). These postures may be assumed spontaneously or in response to a painful stimulus.
- Paralysis or disability on one side of the body.
- Seizures.
- Deteriorating vital signs.

Note that shock (hypoperfusion) from blood loss is generally not a sign of head injury, except in infants. There simply is not enough room within the adult skull to permit enough bleeding to cause shock. If there is head injury with shock, look for indications of blood loss somewhere else on the body.

With so many factors to consider, possible skull or brain injury can be very difficult to determine definitively. Therefore, assume skull or brain injury when the mechanism of injury and the location of the injury indicate a possible head injury. ■

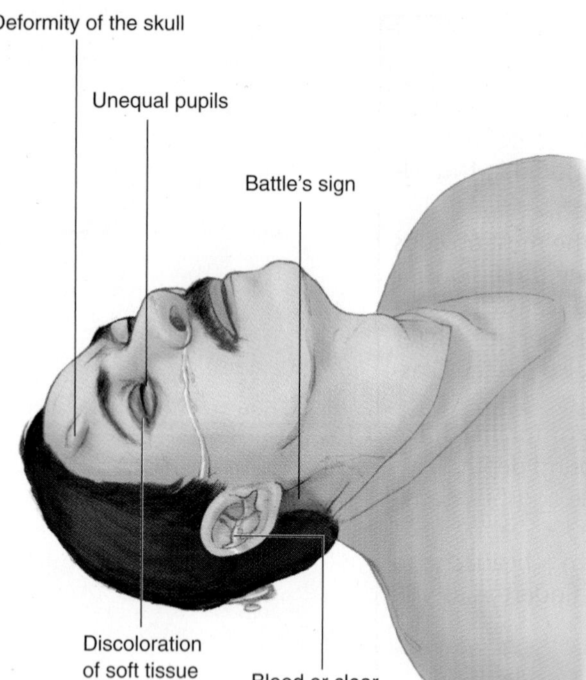

Figure 29-9 • Signs of cranial fracture or brain injury.

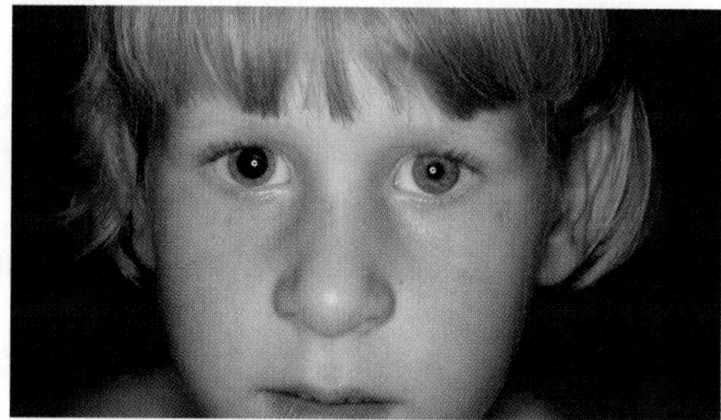

Figure 29-10 • Unequal pupils. *(© Charles Stewart, M.D. and Associates)*

PATIENT CARE

SKULL FRACTURES AND BRAIN INJURIES

Emergency care of a patient with skull fractures and brain injuries includes the following:

1. Take appropriate Standard Precautions.
2. Assume spine injury. Provide manual stabilization of the head on first patient contact, and use the jaw-thrust maneuver to open the airway. For the unconscious patient, insert an oropharyngeal airway without hyperextending the neck. Have suctioning equipment ready, since these patients are prone to vomiting.
3. Monitor the unconscious patient for changes in breathing. Provide artificial ventilations if breathing is inadequate.
4. Apply a rigid cervical collar, immobilize the neck and spine, and, if appropriate, determine the method of extrication, either normal or rapid (discussed later in this chapter).
5. Administer high-concentration oxygen by nonrebreather mask, and evaluate the need for artificial ventilations with supplemental oxygen. This is critical should there be any brain damage. In some EMS systems, if the patient shows signs of a critical brain injury (such as decreased mental status associated with increased blood pressure and decreased pulse or unequal pupils), EMTs are instructed to ventilate the patient with supplemental oxygen at the rate of approximately 20 breaths per minute. Hyperventilation will help reduce brain tissue swelling by lowering carbon dioxide levels and raising oxygen levels, but it can also decrease blood flow to the brain. It is reserved for patients with critical head injuries, where the benefit is felt to outweigh the risk.

continued

PATIENT CARE *(continued)*

Hyperventilating a breathing patient with a bag-valve mask and oral airway is extremely difficult to do and runs a serious risk of inflating the stomach and causing aspiration of stomach contents. Follow your local protocol. Hyperventilation is not a routine part of the management of patients with mild or moderate head injuries.

6. Control bleeding. Do not apply direct pressure if the injury site shows bone fragments or depression of the bone or if the brain is exposed. Do not attempt to stop the flow of blood or cerebrospinal fluid from the ears or the nose. If the skull is fractured, you may increase intracranial pressure and the risk of infection. Instead, use a loose gauze dressing.
7. Keep the patient at rest. This can be critical.
8. Talk to the conscious patient, providing emotional support. Ask the patient questions so that he will have to concentrate. This procedure also will help you to detect changes in the patient's mental status.
9. Dress and bandage open wounds. Stabilize any penetrating objects. (Do not remove any objects or fragments of bone.)
10. Manage the patient for shock even if signs of shock are not yet present. However, do not elevate the legs unless signs of shock are present and your local protocols permit. Avoid overheating.
11. Be prepared for vomiting. Have a suction unit ready for use.
12. Transport the patient promptly.
13. Monitor vital signs every 5 minutes en route to the hospital. ■

If you are not certain of the severity of the patient's injuries, or if there is evidence of cervical-spine injury, or if the patient with a head injury is unconscious, then the patient must be immobilized to a long spine board. With the entire head, neck, and body rigidly immobilized, the patient may be rotated into a lateral recumbent position so that blood and saliva can drain freely. If the patient vomits, the vomitus is less likely to cause an airway obstruction or be aspirated (breathed into the lungs). Some patients with a head injury will vomit without warning. Many vomit without first experiencing nausea. If injuries prevent such positioning, constant monitoring and frequent suctioning are required.

Cranial Injuries with Impaled Objects

If there is an object impaled in the cranium, do not remove it. Instead, stabilize the object in place with bulky dressings. (See information on stabilizing impaled objects in Chapter 27, "Soft-Tissue Injuries.") This, with care in handling, will minimize accidental movement of the object.

A lengthy impaled object can make transporting the patient impossible until the object is cut or shortened. Pad around the object with bulky dressings, then carefully (and rigidly) stabilize the object on both sides of where the cut will be made. Cutting should be done with a tool that will not cause the object to move or vibrate when it is finally severed. A hand hacksaw with a fine-tooth blade can be carefully controlled and produces only a small amount of heat. In any case in which you may have to cut an impaled object, seek advice from medical direction or the emergency department physician.

Injuries to the Face and Jaw

Facial fractures are usually caused by an impact, as when a child is struck in the face by a baseball bat or when someone is thrown against a windshield. Bone fragments may lodge in the back of the pharynx and cause airway obstruction. So may blood,

NOTE

The face is part of the skull. Brain injury may accompany a blow of sufficient force to the face. Treat this patient as you would any patient with a suspected skull or brain injury.

blood clots, dislodged teeth, or a separated palate. Signs of a facial fracture are shown in Figure 29-11.

The mandible is subject to dislocation as well as to fracture. As with any facial injury, there may be pain, discoloration, swelling, and facial distortion. In addition, when the mandible is injured or dislocated, the patient may be unable to move the lower jaw or may have difficulty speaking. There may be an improper alignment of the upper and lower teeth and bleeding around the teeth.

The primary concern with facial fractures is the patient's airway (Figure 29-12). Be prepared to suction to remove debris and blood from the airway. Because of possible spinal injury, use the jaw-thrust maneuver to open the airway. Control profuse bleeding. (See Chapter 27, "Soft-Tissue Injuries," for care of an object impaled in the cheek.) Apply a rigid collar and immobilize the patient on a spine board. If possible, position the patient for drainage from the mouth. Care for shock.

Nontraumatic Brain Injuries

Many of the signs of brain injury may be caused by an internal brain event such as a hemorrhage or blood clot. (See the information on stroke in Chapter 19, "Diabetic Emergencies and Altered Mental Status.") The signs of nontraumatic (not caused by external trauma) brain injury will be the same as those for a traumatic injury, except that there will be no evidence of trauma and no mechanism of injury.

Glasgow Coma Scale

All head-injury patients must be constantly monitored during transport. Be prepared in case the patient vomits or has a seizure. What you observe and report can have a great bearing on the initial actions that will be taken by the emergency department staff. The early signs of deterioration are subtle changes in mental status that may be overlooked if you are not watching for them.

Some EMS agencies use the Glasgow Coma Scale (GCS) (Figure 29-13), in addition to AVPU, for ongoing neurological assessment. Some systems would immediately transport a patient with a GCS score of 8 or less directly to the trauma center if they are

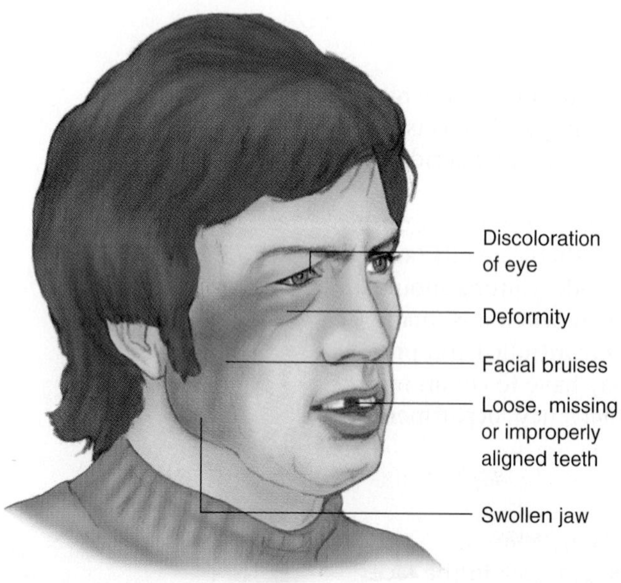

Figure 29-11 • Signs of facial fracture.

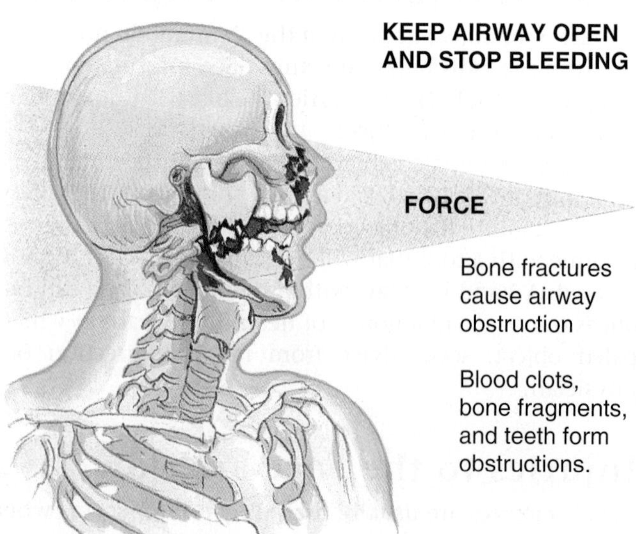

Figure 29-12 • Complications of facial fracture.

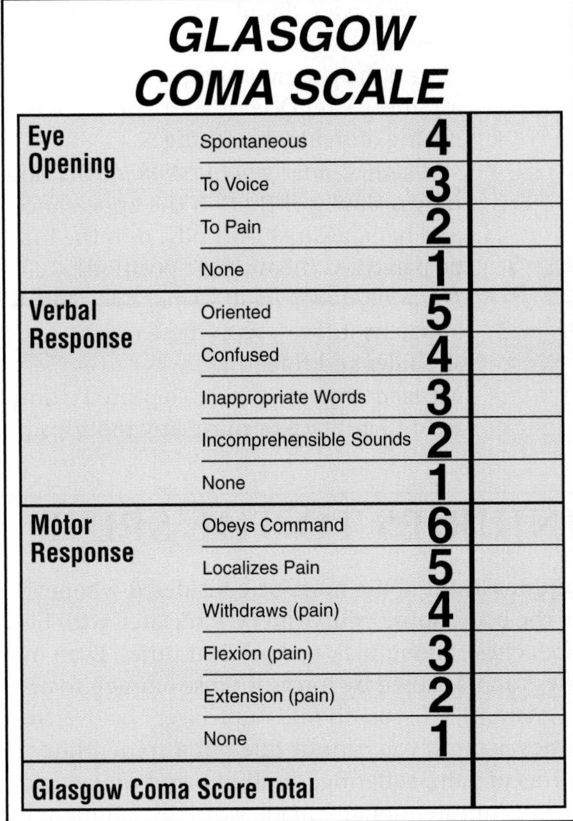

GLASGOW COMA SCALE

Eye Opening	Spontaneous	4	
	To Voice	3	
	To Pain	2	
	None	1	
Verbal Response	Oriented	5	
	Confused	4	
	Inappropriate Words	3	
	Incomprehensible Sounds	2	
	None	1	
Motor Response	Obeys Command	6	
	Localizes Pain	5	
	Withdraws (pain)	4	
	Flexion (pain)	3	
	Extension (pain)	2	
	None	1	
Glasgow Coma Score Total			

Figure 29-13 • Glasgow Coma Scale.

within 30 minutes transport time. When using this score, keep the following considerations in mind:

NOTE

Do not spend extra time at the scene calculating a GCS score. Calculate the score en route to the hospital to avoid prolonged scene times.

- *Eye opening.* Spontaneous eye opening means that the patient opens his eyes without your having to do anything. If his eyes are closed, say "Open your eyes" to see if he will obey. Try a normal level of voice. If this fails, shout the command. Should the patient's eyes remain closed, apply an accepted painful stimulus (such as pinch a toe, scratch the palm or sole, rub the sternum). Note any eye injuries or injuries to the face that prevent the patient from opening the eyes. If the injuries are more than minor ones, do not ask the patient to open his eyes.
- *Verbal response.* When evaluating the patient's verbal responses, use the following criteria:
  - *Oriented.* The patient, once aroused, can tell you who he is, where he is, and the day of the week. A person who can answer all three of these questions appropriately is said to be alert on the AVPU scale.
  - *Confused.* The patient cannot answer the previous questions, but he can speak in phrases and sentences.
  - *Inappropriate words.* The patient says or shouts a word or several words at a time. Usually this requires physical stimulation. The words do not fit the situation or a particular question. Often, the patient curses.
  - *Incomprehensible sounds.* The patient responds with mumbling, moans, or groans.
  - *No verbal response.* Repeated stimulation, verbal and physical, does not cause the patient to speak or make any sounds.
- *Motor response.* The following criteria are used to evaluate motor response:
  - *Obeys command.* The patient must be able to understand your instruction and carry out the request. For example, you may ask the patient (when appropriate) to hold up two fingers.

- *Localizes pain.* Should the patient fail to respond to your commands, apply pressure to one of the nail beds for 5 seconds or firm pressure to the sternum. Note if the patient attempts to remove your hand. Do not apply pressure over an injury site. Do not apply pressure to the sternum if the patient is experiencing difficulty breathing.
- *Withdraws, after painful stimulation.* Note if the elbow flexes, if the patient moves slowly, if there is the appearance of stiffness, if he holds his forearm and hand against the body, or if the limbs on one side of the body appear to be paralyzed (hemiplegic position).
- *Posturing, after painful stimulation.* Note if the legs and arms extend, if there is apparent stiffness with these moves, and if there is an internal rotation of the shoulder and forearm.
- *No motor response to pain.* Repeated painful stimulation does not cause the patient to grimace or make any motions.

INJURIES TO THE SPINE

Injuries to the spine must be considered whenever there is serious trauma to any part of the body. Spine injury can be associated with head, neck, and back injuries—and also with chest, abdominal, and pelvic injuries. Even injuries to the upper and lower extremities can be caused by forces intense enough to also produce spine injury.

As an EMT, you should "uptriage," or overtreat, patients with potential spine injuries because you cannot rule out a spine injury in the field and because the costs in terms of pain, suffering, disability, and dollars are very high when a spine-injured patient is unintentionally made worse by failure to immobilize the spine.

Injuries to the spinal column include fractures with and without bone displacement, dislocations, muscular strains, and disk injury including compression. The vertebral column may be injured without damage to the spinal cord or spinal nerves. For example, a fractured coccyx is below the level of the spinal cord. Muscular strains are relatively simple injuries. However, when displaced fractures or dislocations occur, the cord, disk, and spinal nerves may be severely injured.

Mechanisms of Spine Injury

A simple rule of thumb is: If the mechanism of injury exerts great force on the upper body (Figure 29-14) or if there is any soft-tissue damage to the head, face, or neck due to trauma (such as from being thrown against a dashboard), assume possible cervical-spine injury. Any blunt trauma above the clavicles may damage the cervical spine.

Some parts of the spine are more susceptible to injury than others. Because it is somewhat splinted by the attached ribs, the thoracic spine is not usually damaged except in the most violent collisions or in gunshot wounds. The pelvic-sacral spine attachment helps to protect the sacrum in the same way. However, the cervical and lumbar vertebrae are susceptible to injury because they are not supported by other bony structures.

The spine is most often injured by compression or excessive flexion, extension, or rotation from falls, diving injuries, and motor-vehicle collisions. Spine injuries in EMS workers often result from not adhering to the proper lifting techniques, causing lateral bending or disk injuries. When the spine is excessively pulled, it can cause a "distraction" injury. This mechanism of spine injury occurs in a hanging. Years ago, rescuers were taught to pull traction on the neck of an injured patient sitting in an automobile. This actually had the potential to cause injury, so today EMTs are taught to manually stabilize the head and neck, or hold it still.

Maintain a high degree of suspicion of a potential spine injury when your patient is a victim of a motor-vehicle or motorcycle collision, was struck by a vehicle, received blunt injury to the spine or above the clavicles, was involved in a diving incident, was found hanging by his neck, or was found unconscious due to trauma.

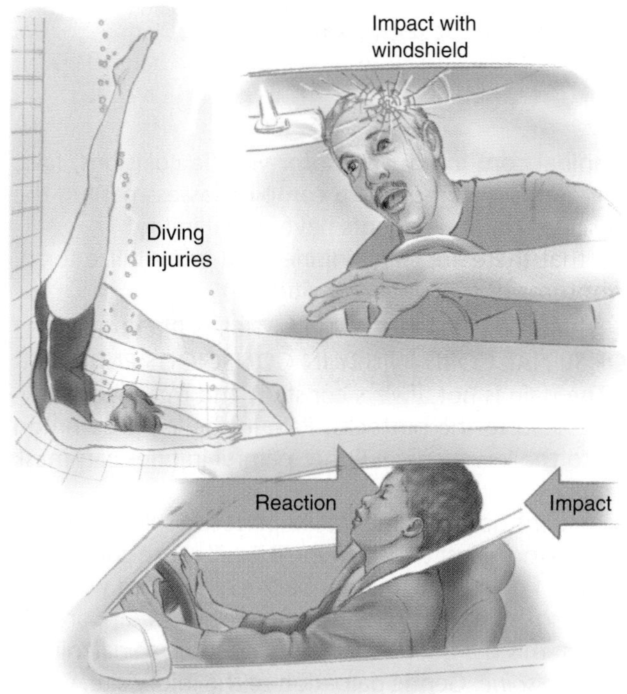

Figure 29-14 • Mechanisms of injury to the upper body.

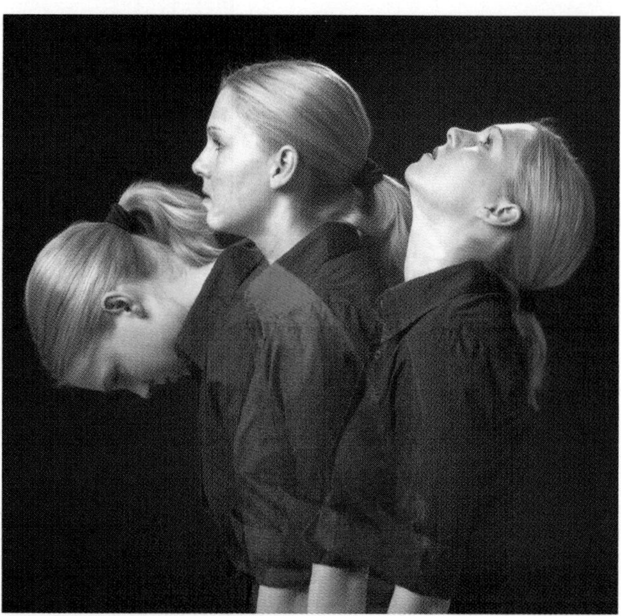

Figure 29-15 • Usually, whiplash is caused by a poorly adjusted or absent head rest during a rear-end collision.

The adult skull weighs more than 17 pounds and rests on a very small area of the cervical spine (like a pumpkin on a broom handle). Motor-vehicle collisions produce violent whiplash injuries because of the speed and sudden deceleration of the vehicle (Figure 29-15). When a vehicle strikes another vehicle or a fixed object head on, the neck can whip quickly back and forth. The vehicle decelerates abruptly, but the head continues to travel forward at the same speed that the vehicle was traveling, even though the body is held by seat restraints. This neck movement may exceed the normal range of motion. Virtually the same thing occurs when the vehicle is struck from behind.

A fall can generate enough force to fracture or dislocate vertebrae. Assume that any fall three times the patient's height or with enough force to cause open fractures to the ankles will also be accompanied by a spine injury. Needless disability has been caused when head injuries or other injuries resulting from a fall were noted and cared for but spinal injuries were overlooked.

Today more and more people are participating in sports of all kinds: in-line skating, mountain biking, surfing, rock climbing, and others too numerous to mention. Many sports mishaps can cause spine injury. Sledding or skiing can hurl a person into a tree or other fixed object, twisting or compressing the spinal column. There may be no open wound or fracture of an extremity, or signs of injury may be hidden by bulky clothing. As a result, improper care may be rendered as the patient with a possible spinal injury is placed on a stretcher without adequate examination and immobilization.

Diving incidents often produce injury to the cervical spine. When the diver strikes the diving board, the side or bottom of the pool, or an underwater object, the head can be severely forced beyond its normal limits of motion (flexion, extension, or compression). Cervical vertebrae may be fractured or dislocated, ligaments may be severely sprained, and the spinal cord may be compressed or otherwise traumatized in the cervical region and at other spots along the cord.

Football and other contact sports can generate forces severe enough to produce spinal injury. Spear tackling, using the head, has been outlawed in grade schools and high schools for a number of years due to the incidence of cervical compression fractures. Whenever a game involves player contact or falling to the ground, be on the alert for spinal injury.

PATIENT ASSESSMENT

SPINAL INJURY

The most common causes of spinal cord injury are motor-vehicle collisions, falls, diving incidents, and gunshot wounds. You must do a complete assessment of the patient. Assume that all unconscious trauma patients have spinal injury.

Whenever in doubt, assume that there are spine injuries and immobilize torso, head, and neck. Signs and symptoms of spine injury include:

- *Paralysis of the extremities.* PARALYSIS OF THE EXTREMITIES IS PROBABLY THE MOST RELIABLE SIGN OF SPINAL CORD INJURY IN CONSCIOUS PATIENTS.
- *Pain without movement.* The pain is not always constant and may occur anywhere from the top of the head to the buttocks. Pain in the leg is common for certain types of injury to the lower spine. Other painful injuries can mask this symptom of spinal injury.
- *Pain with movement.* The patient normally tries to lie perfectly still to prevent pain. Do not ask the patient to move just to determine if it will cause pain. However, if the patient complains of pain in the neck or back experienced with voluntary movements, including spinal pain with movement in apparently uninjured shoulders and legs, this is a good indicator of possible spinal injury.
- *Tenderness anywhere along the spine.* Gentle palpation of the injury site, when accessible, may reveal point tenderness.

These signs and symptoms are reliable indicators of possible spinal injury in the conscious patient. If any one of them is present, you have sufficient reason to immobilize the patient. In the field, it is not possible to rule out spinal injury even when the patient has no pain and is able to move his limbs. The mechanism of injury alone may be the deciding factor. Additional signs of spinal injury may include:

- *Impaired breathing.* Watch the patient breathe. If there is only a slight movement of the abdomen, with little or no movement of the chest, it is safe to assume that the patient is breathing with the diaphragm alone (diaphragmatic breathing). This is also true if there is a reversal of normal breathing patterns with the rib cage collapsing on inspiration and rising on expiration. Damage to the nerves that control the movement of the rib cage can cause this breathing pattern. The nerves that control the diaphragm are located high in the cervical area (the third, fourth, and fifth cervical nerves) and are often unharmed, but the intercostal (between-the-ribs) nerves that control the chest muscles are often damaged in cervical and thoracic injuries. As a result, when the diaphragm moves downward to pull in air, the ribs, instead of expanding, collapse. When the diaphragm relaxes and air is expelled, the rib cage rises—the opposite of the normal pattern.

  Impaired breathing is characteristic of spinal cord injury. Check abdominal movement from the side by placing your hand on the patient's abdomen and looking for reversed movements during respiration. Panting due to respiratory insufficiency may develop.

GERIATRIC NOTE

Keep in mind that fractured spines in the elderly are often caused by falls or spontaneous fractures of brittle bones that, in turn, cause falls.

continued

PATIENT ASSESSMENT *(continued)*

- *Deformity.* Removing clothing to check for deformity of the spine is not recommended. OBVIOUS SPINAL DEFORMITIES ARE RARE. However, if you note a gap between the spinous processes (bony extensions) of the vertebrae, or if you can feel a broken spinous process, you must consider the patient to have serious spinal injuries. It is also possible to feel tight muscles in spasm.
- *Priapism.* Persistent erection of the penis is a sign of spinal injury affecting nerves to the external genitalia.
- *Loss of bowel or bladder control.* This may indicate spinal injury.
- *Nerve impairment to the extremities.* The patient may experience loss of use, weakness, numbness, tingling, or loss of feeling in the upper and/or lower extremities—especially below the suspected level of the injury.
- *Severe spinal shock.* This kind of shock (neurogenic shock) can be caused by the failure of the nervous system to control the diameter of blood vessels. The pulse rate may be normal—or even slow in the setting of a low or falling blood pressure—because a message to "speed up" the heart may be prevented from getting to the heart due to the cord injury.
- *Soft-tissue injuries associated with trauma.* Traumatic soft-tissue injuries to the head and neck may signal injury of the cervical spine. Traumatic soft-tissue injuries to the shoulders, back, or abdomen may signal injury of the thoracic or lumbar spine. Traumatic soft-tissue injuries to the lower extremities may signal injury of the lumbar or sacral spine.

Assessment strategies for a responsive patient with suspected spinal injury include the following:

- Ascertain the mechanism of injury.
- Ask these questions (and tell the patient not to move while answering):
  - What happened?
  - Where does it hurt? Does your neck or back hurt?
  - Can you move your hands and feet?
  - Can you feel me touching (lightly) your fingers? Your toes?
  - Do you feel "pins and needles" (tingling) in your legs? Anywhere?
- Inspect for contusions, deformities, lacerations, punctures, penetrations, swelling.
- Palpate for tenderness or deformity.
- Assess equality of strength in the extremities by checking hand grip or pushing against the patient's hands and feet.

Assessment strategies for an unresponsive patient with suspected spinal injury include the following:

- Ascertain from bystanders the mechanism of injury and information about the patient's mental status prior to your arrival.
- Inspect for contusions, deformities, lacerations, punctures, penetrations, swelling.
- Palpate for area of tenderness (some unresponsive patients will withdraw from or react to pain) or deformity. ■

NOTE

The ability to walk, move the extremities, feel sensation, or experience a lack of pain in the spinal area does not rule out the possibility of spinal column or spinal cord injury.

PATIENT CARE

SPINAL INJURY

Regardless of where the apparent spinal injury is located on the cord, care is the same. Perform the initial assessment and rapid trauma exam and determine the patient's priority, since this will be important in deciding how to immobilize him (Figure 29-16).

NOTE

Do not spend much time trying to rule out spinal injury in an unresponsive patient. If there is a mechanism of injury associated with spinal injury, immobilize the patient and treat as if there is a spinal injury.

For all patients with possible spinal injury, and for all trauma victims when there is doubt as to the extent of injury, emergency care includes the following:

1. Provide manual in-line stabilization for the head and neck on first patient contact. Place the head in a neutral in-line position unless the patient complains of pain or the head is not easily moved into that position. If that is the case, steady the head in the position found. Maintain manual stabilization until the patient is properly secured to a backboard.
2. Assess airway, breathing, and circulation. If necessary, open and control the airway with the jaw-thrust maneuver, maintaining in-line stabilization of the head.
3. In your rapid trauma exam, assess the head and neck, then apply a rigid cervical collar. Make sure the collar is properly sized. A wrong-size collar may do more harm than good by hyperextending the neck if too large or allowing flexion if too small. Also make sure the collar is not applied in a way that will obstruct the airway. Maintain manual stabilization even after the collar is in place until the patient is secured to a backboard, since no collar completely restricts motion.
4. Quickly assess sensory and motor function in all four extremities if the patient is responsive.
5. Based on the patient's priority, apply the appropriate spinal immobilization device at the appropriate speed. (Scans 29-1 through 29-8 are provided in this chapter in order to demonstrate the proper procedure to use based upon the condition of the patient and the position in which the patient is found.)
6. If the patient has paralysis or weakness of the extremities, administer high-concentration oxygen via nonrebreather mask and evaluate the need for artificial ventilations with supplemental oxygen. This is critical should there be any cord damage.
7. Reassess sensory and motor function in all four extremities if the patient is responsive. ■

PEDIATRIC NOTE

For an infant or child, be sure to use a pediatric-sized collar. If you do not have the right pediatric size, use a rolled towel, maintaining manual support of the infant's or child's head.

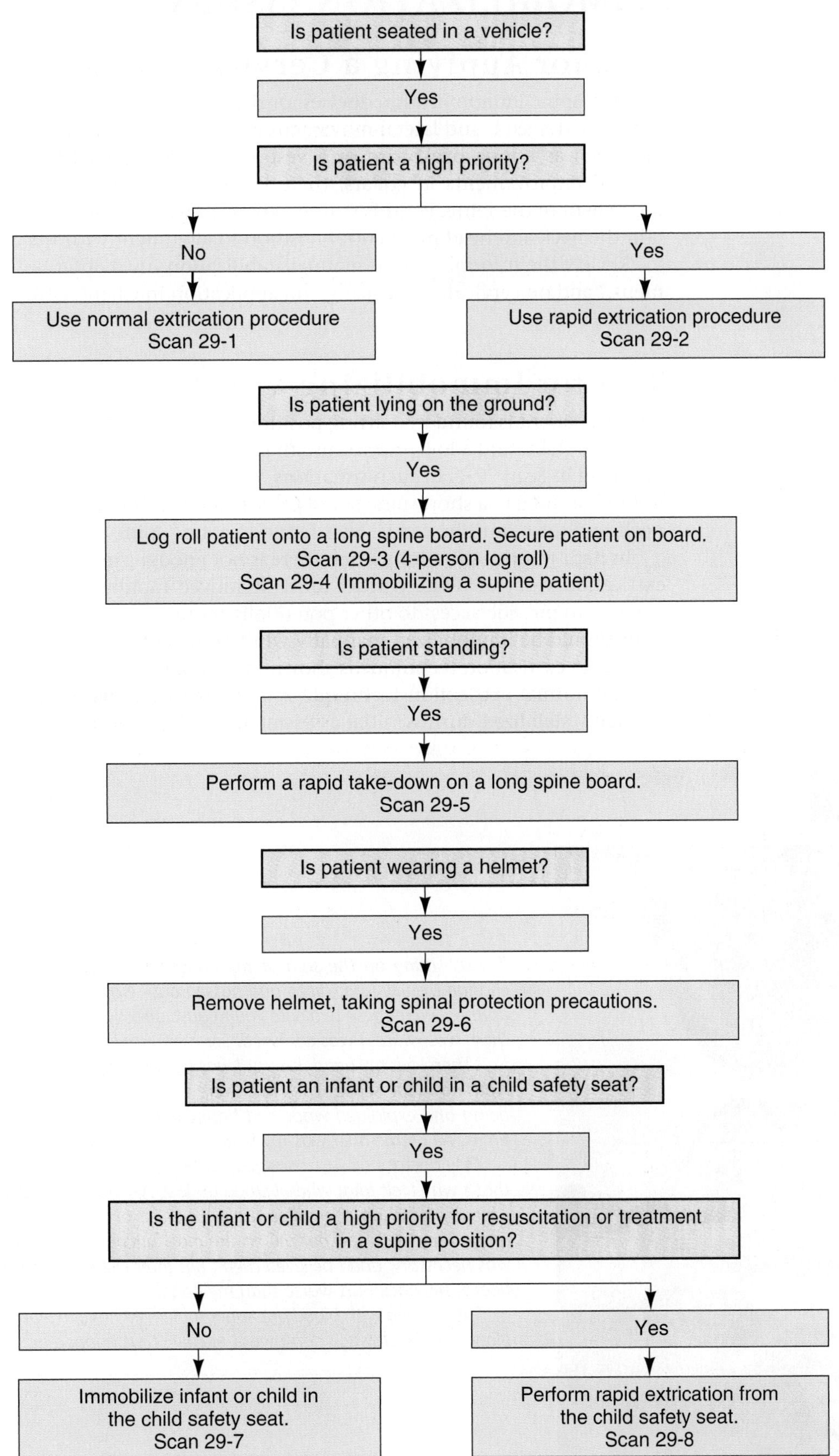

Figure 29-16 • Choose appropriate extrication and immobilization procedures.

IMMOBILIZATION ISSUES

Tips for Applying a Cervical Collar

Cervical spine immobilization devices, or rigid extrication collars, are designed to limit flexion, extension, and lateral movement when combined with an immobilization device such as a long backboard or a vest-style device. Even though there have been marked improvements in collars, there is still no collar that completely eliminates movement of the spine. For this reason, when applying a collar, always manually maintain the neck and head in a neutral position in alignment with the rest of the body.

Review the information on manual stabilization in Chapter 8, "The Initial Assessment," and on cervical-collar sizing and application in Chapter 10, "Assessment of the Trauma Patient."

Tips for Immobilizing a Seated Patient

When a patient is found in a sitting position, you will need to decide his priority. If the patient is stable and a low priority, use the normal procedure for spinal immobilization as shown in Scan 29-1. In such situations, where time is not of the essence, the patient must be secured to a short spine board or extrication vest that will immobilize the head, neck, and torso until he can be transferred to a long spine board.

In high-priority situations when there is not enough time to apply a short board or extrication vest—or if the patient must be moved rapidly because of dangers at the scene or to provide access to other potentially more seriously injured patients—the patient should be immobilized manually while moving him onto the long spine board. This rapid extrication technique is shown in Scan 29-2.

The normal extrication technique is as follows: The patient's head and neck are manually stabilized during initial assessment. After the head and neck are assessed in

POINT OF VIEW

"I was sitting on the sofa at my daughter's house, and when I got up to change the TV, I got dizzy and passed out—passed out good! When I woke up there were these two cute young guys directly over me. Everything around them was white. I was confused. For a minute I thought I was in heaven.

"Then I felt my head. It hurt. I was trying to figure out what was going on. Nothing made sense. The EMTs were so kind. They stopped what they were doing and explained what had happened. They had to explain a couple of times. All I remember was my head hurting and being confused.

"My doctor had just changed my blood pressure medication, and I guess that's why I felt faint when I stood up fast. My daughter said that when I fell I hit my head on the coffee table. Because of that, the EMTs put a collar around my neck and put me on the most uncomfortable board. They said it was necessary, and I believed them. But after the ride to the hospital on that board, my back hurt worse than my head.

"At 75, and with blood pressure problems, I have to learn to take my time. Now I get up slowly. I don't want to have that happen again!"

SCAN 29-1 • Spinal Immobilization of a Seated Patient

First take Standard Precautions.

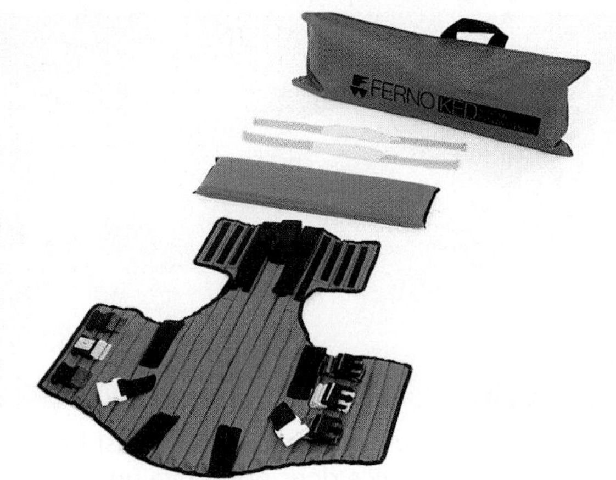

1. Select an immobilization device.

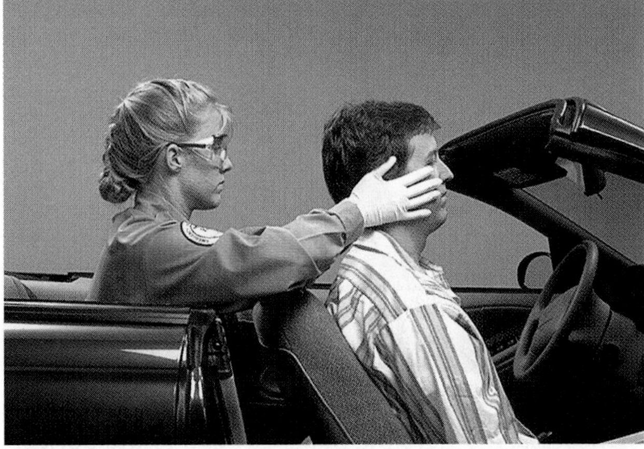

2. Manually stabilize the patient's head in neutral, in-line position.

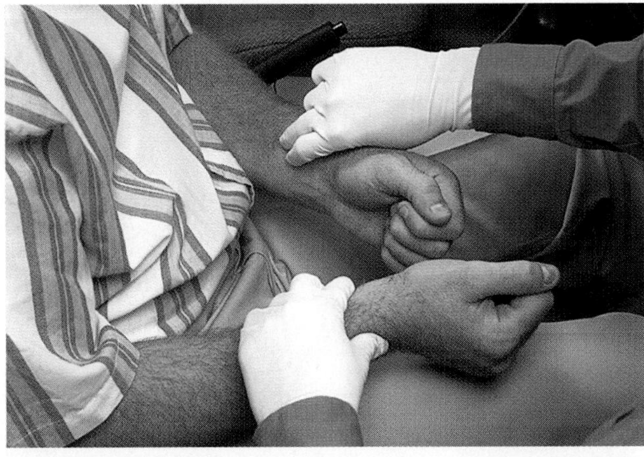

3. Assess distal pulse, motor function, and sensation (PMS).

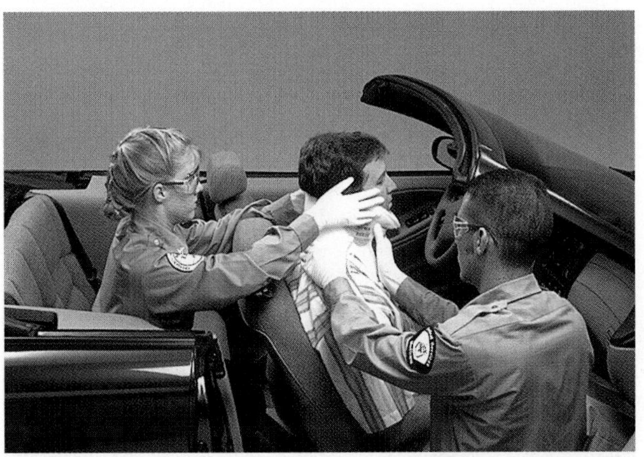

4. Apply the appropriately sized extrication collar.

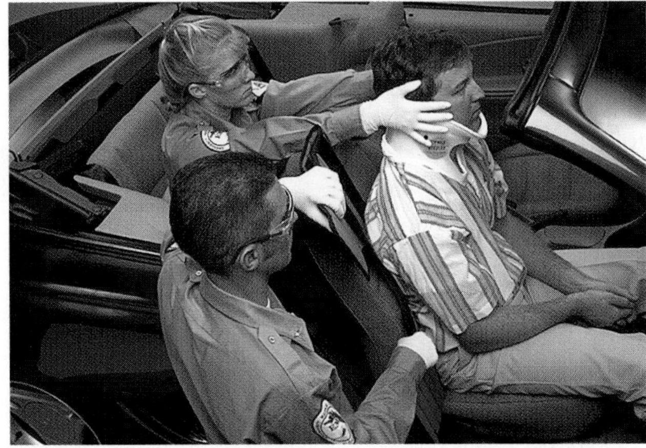

5. Position the immobilization device behind the patient.

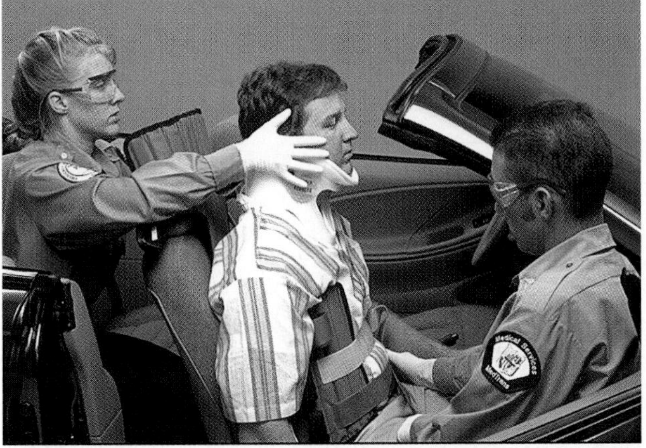

6. Secure the device to the patient's torso.

continued

SCAN 29-1 • (Continued)

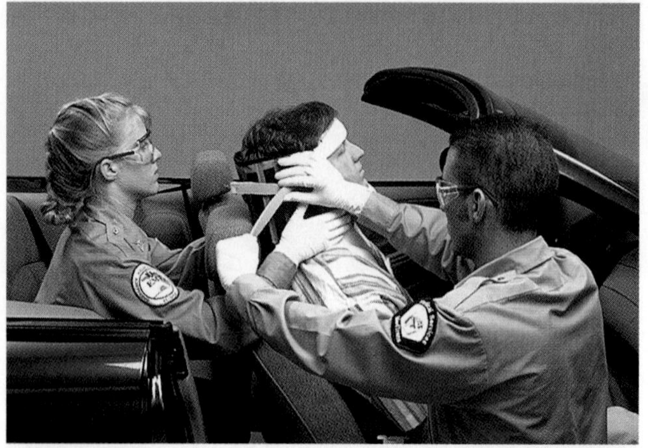

7. Evaluate and pad behind the patient's head as necessary. Secure the patient's head to the device.

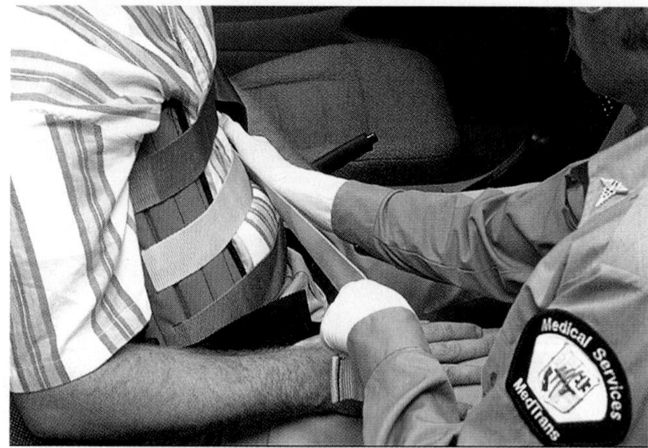

8. Evaluate and adjust the straps. They must be tight enough so the device does not move up, down, left, or right excessively, but not so tight as to restrict the patient's breathing.

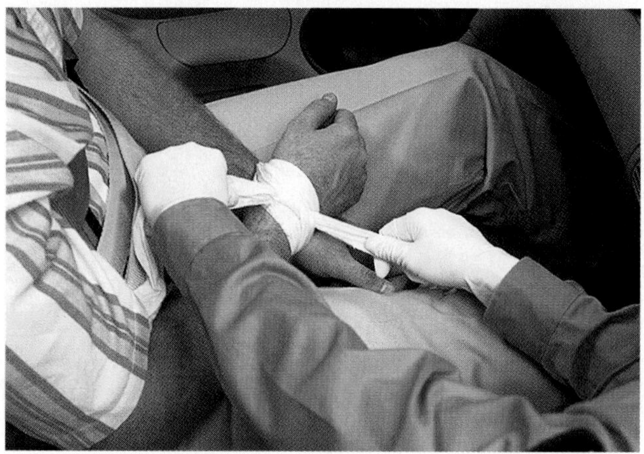

9. As needed, secure the patient's wrists and legs.

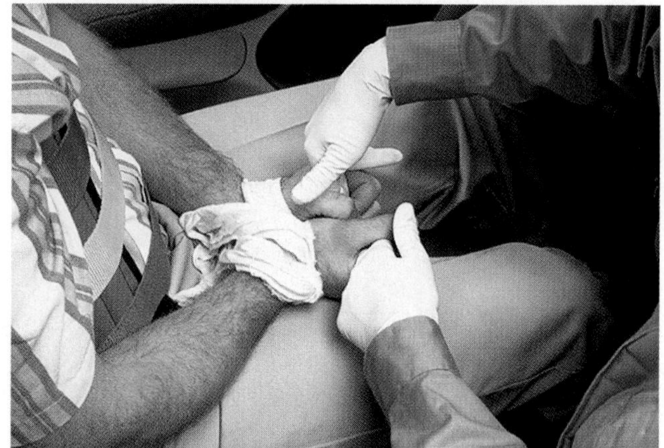

10. Reassess distal pulse, motor function, and sensation (PMS), and transfer the patient to the long board.

NOTE *In the photos, the roof of the vehicle has been removed to allow for easier illustration of the positions of the EMTs. In most cases, this procedure will be done and should be practiced with the roof intact.*

SCAN 29-2 • Rapid Extrication Procedure for High-Priority Patients Only

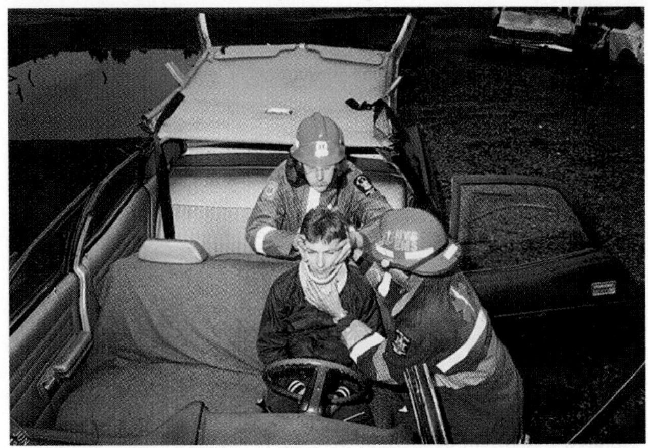

1. Manually stabilize the patient's head and neck and have a second EMT apply a cervical collar.

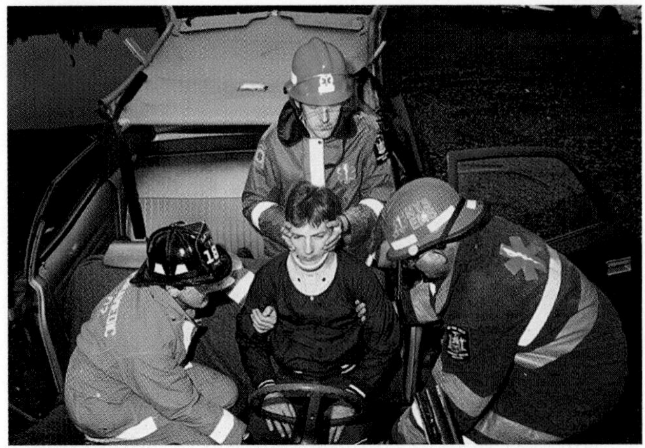

2. At the direction of the EMT stabilizing the head and neck, two EMTs each lift the patient by the armpits and buttocks/thighs just enough for a bystander or additional rescuer to slide a long spine board between the patient and the vehicle seat.

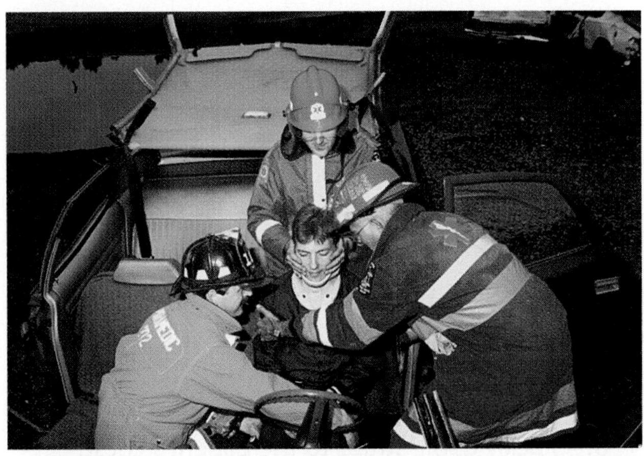

3. The EMTs reposition their hands so the EMT on the front seat inside the vehicle holds the patient's legs and pelvis, while the EMT outside the vehicle holds the upper chest and arms.

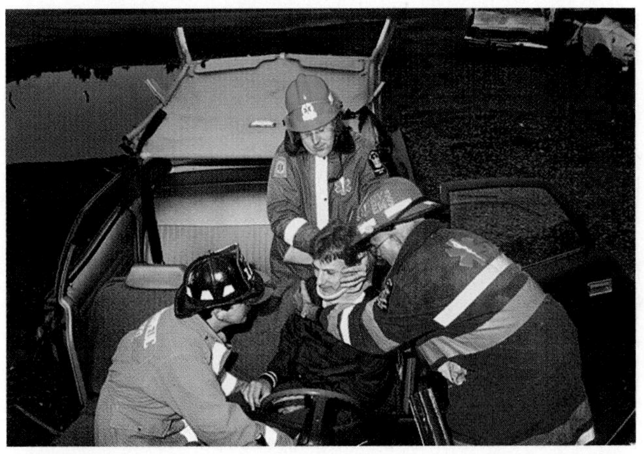

4. At the direction of the EMT holding the head and neck, carefully turn the patient a quarter turn so his back is toward the door of the vehicle.

NOTE *The rapid extrication procedure is only for critical or unstable high-priority patients who must be moved in less time than would be required to apply a short spine board or extrication vest inside the vehicle before moving the patient to the long spine board (Scan 29-1).*

continued

SCAN 29-2 • (Continued)

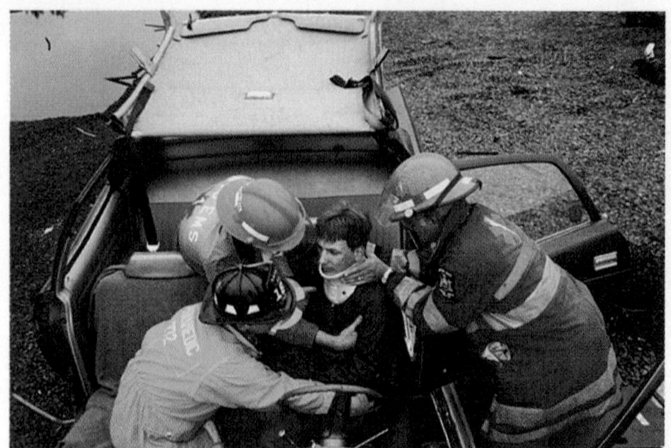

5. The EMT who was holding the pelvis temporarily holds the chest so the EMT who was holding the chest can take over head and neck stabilization. The EMT in the back seat can then reach over the seat and assist with the chest, and the EMT inside on the front seat can move his hands back to the pelvis.

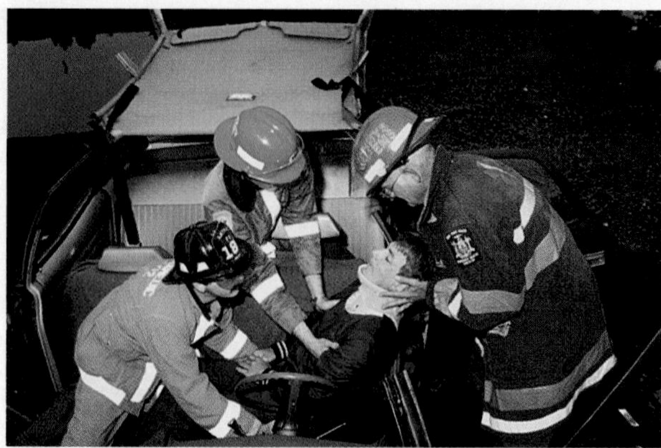

6. At the direction of the EMT at the head and neck, gently lower the patient to the spine board. *Note:* Sometimes it may be necessary to move the patient inside the vehicle a few inches so there is ample room to lay him down without touching the upper door opening.

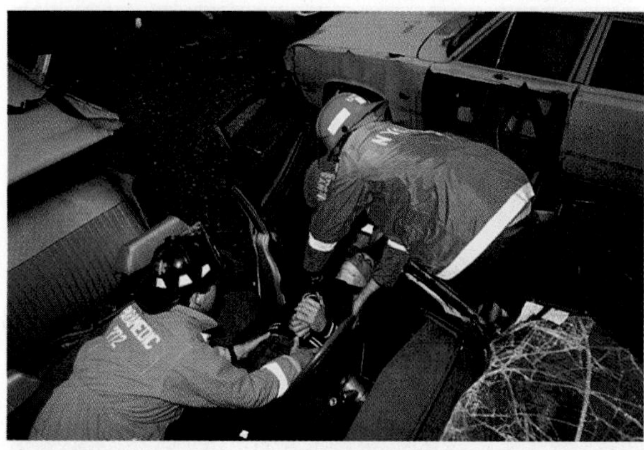

7. As a bystander or additional rescuer holds the end of the spine board, the EMTs slide the patient to the head end of the board.

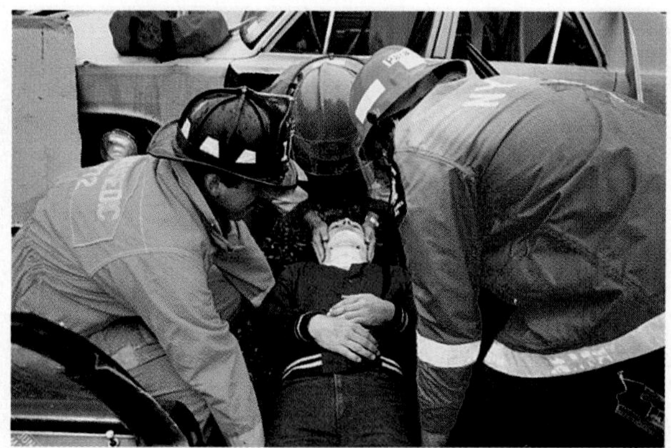

8. Quickly apply straps to the patient's chest, pelvis, and legs and remove the patient to a stretcher or the ground, under the direction of the EMT stabilizing the head and neck. *Note:* Since the patient's head is not yet fully immobilized (it is only being manually held stable by the EMT and collar), DO NOT walk more than a few steps with the patient. Once on stable ground or the stretcher, apply a head immobilizer or blanket roll and wide tape.

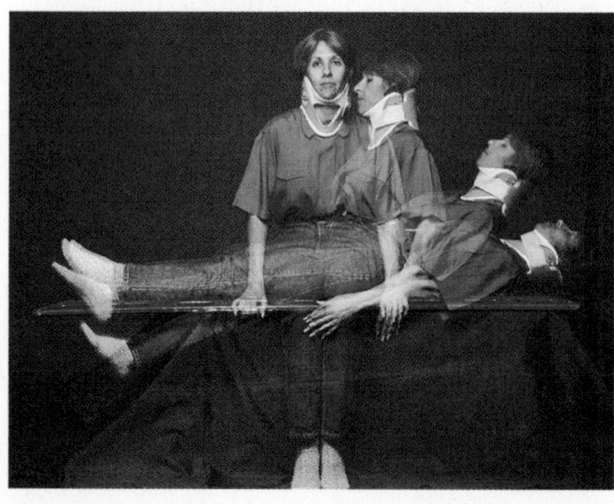

As you move the patient from a sitting to a supine position, her spine must not bend, twist, or get jolted. Handle her very gently, and make sure you have enough assistance to perform the move correctly.

the rapid trauma exam, a rigid collar is applied. Then the patient is secured to a short spine board or extrication vest.

A vest-style extrication device (such as the one shown in Figure 29-17) is a flexible piece of equipment useful for immobilizing patients with possible injury to the cervical spine. It can be used when the patient is found in a bucket seat, in a short compact car seat, in a seat with a contoured back, or in a confined space. It is also useful when the short spine board cannot be inserted into a car because of obstructions. A number of commercial vest-style extrication devices, such as the KED, Kansas Backboard, XP-1, and LSP Halfback Vest, are available. Use the devices approved by your EMS system.

A short spine board (Figure 29-18) is just a shortened version of a long spine board. It is the original extrication device and has been used for many years. It is used less frequently now, because today's contoured automobile seat backs do not accommodate a flat board. Also, the short spine board is often too wide and too high to be used effectively in a small car.

A particular sequence must be followed in all applications, whether of a flexible extrication device or a short spine board. That sequence is: secure the torso first and the head last. This ensures greater stability during the strapping process and may help prevent compression of the cervical spine. If the patient has suffered abdominal injuries or displays diaphragmatic breathing that prevents adequate securing of the torso, the torso straps will still be needed but care must be taken so as not to interfere with breathing.

There are a number of special considerations when applying a short board to the patient:

- Assessment of the back, shoulder blades, arms, or collarbones must be done before the device is placed against the patient.
- The EMT applying the board must angle it, without striking or jarring, to fit between the arms of the rescuer who is stabilizing the head from behind the patient.
- To provide full cervical support, the uppermost holes must be level with the patient's shoulders. The base of the board should not extend past the coccyx.
- Never place a chin cup or chin strap on the patient, as it can prevent him from opening his mouth if he has to vomit.
- Avoid applying the first torso strap too tightly. This could aggravate an abdominal injury or limit respirations for the diaphragmatic breathing patient.
- Some buckles have quick-release mechanisms. Be careful not to accidentally loosen these buckles when moving the patient.
- Do not pad between collar and board. This will create a pivot point that may cause the hyperextension of the cervical spine when the head is secured. Instead, pad the occipital region, but only enough to fill any void. This will help keep the head in a neutral position. Sometimes when the shoulders are rolled back to the board, the head will come back to the board far enough so padding is not needed. Never use excessive padding behind the head, because when the patient is placed in a supine position, the shoulders will fall back but the head will not be able to. This will place the patient in an undesirable position of flexion.

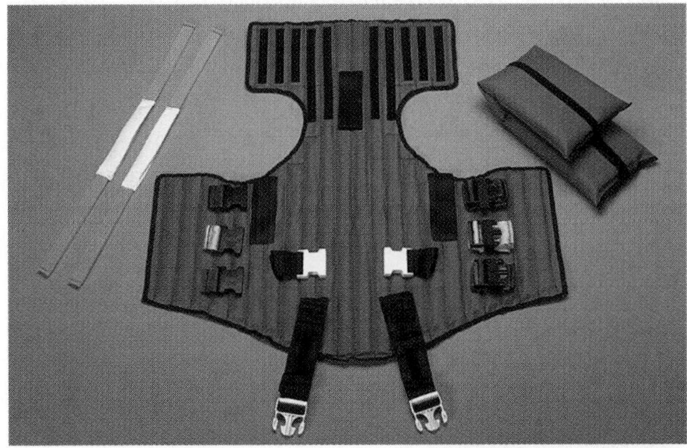

Figure 29-17 • Ferno KED (Kendrick Extrication Device).

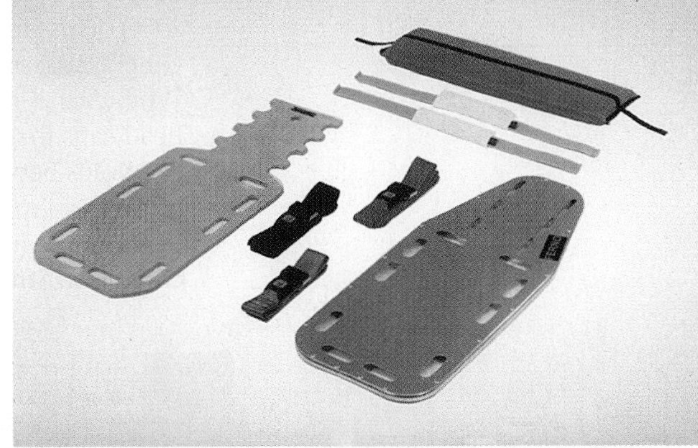

Figure 29-18 • Short spine board.

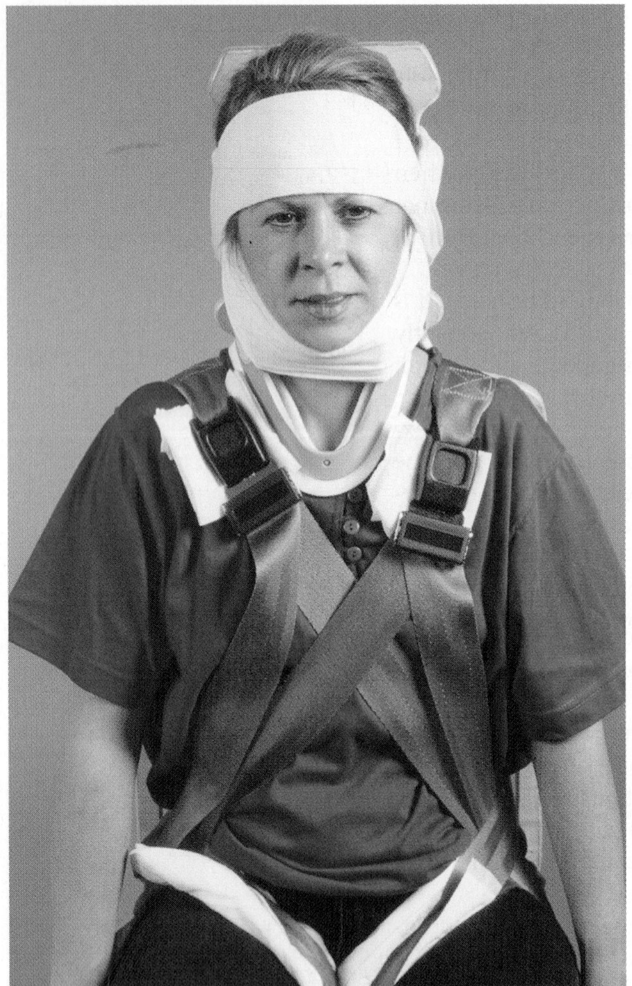

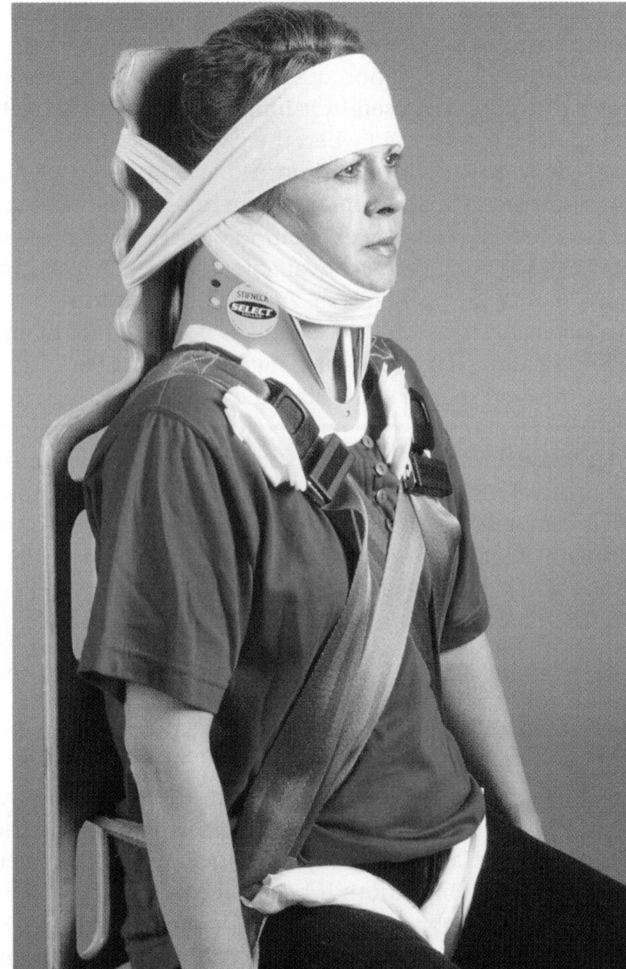

Figure 29-19 • Seated patient, "packaged."

- Follow the instructions of the manufacturer of the device you are using.
- After applying the short spine board, the packaging of the patient will be completed as shown in Figure 29-19.

Tips for Applying a Long Backboard

The following tips relate to immobilization of the supine patient:

- You will need to log roll the patient to apply the long backboard (Scans 29-3 and 29-4). This procedure must be done carefully, keeping the spine in alignment. Quickly assess the posterior body before rolling the patient back onto the board. Whenever a move is done involving neck stabilization, the EMT holding the head calls for the move ("We will turn on three: One . . . two . . . three").
- Pad voids between the patient's head and torso and the board. Be careful not to cause extra movement or to move the patient's spine out of alignment.
- When a patient is secured to a long spine board (Figure 29-20), the head is secured last. Strapping is easier with Velcro or speed-clip straps.

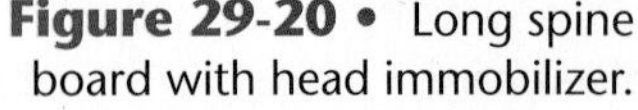

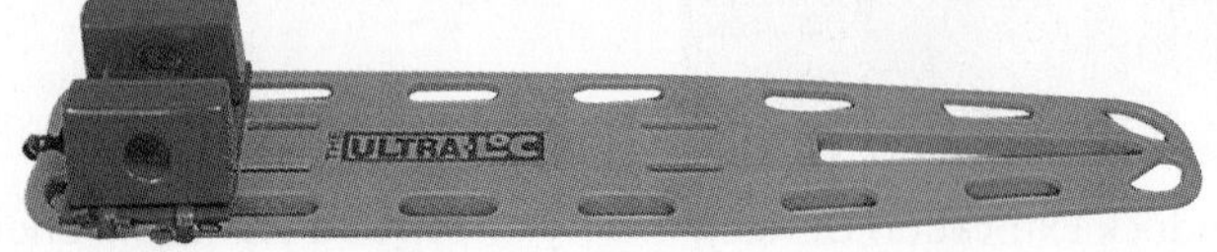

Figure 29-20 • Long spine board with head immobilizer.

SCAN 29-3 • Four-Rescuer Log Roll

First take Standard Precautions.

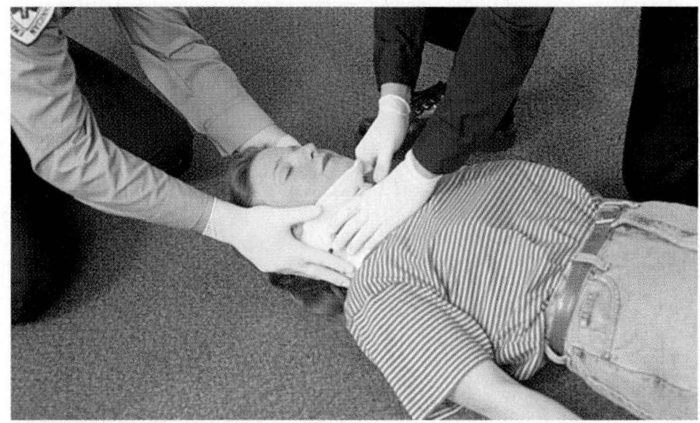

1. Stabilize the head and neck. Apply a rigid cervical collar.

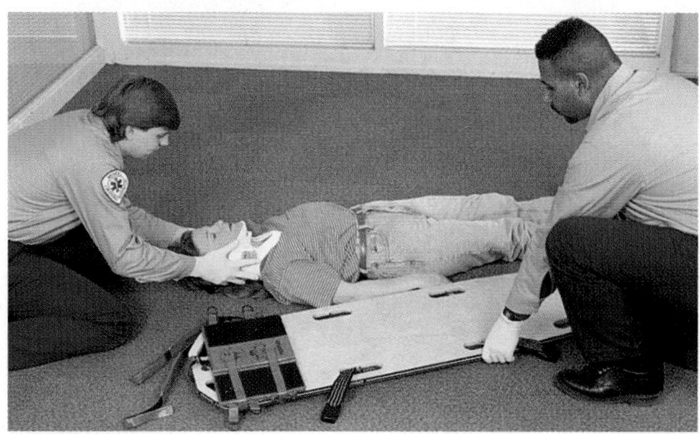

2. Place the board parallel to the patient.

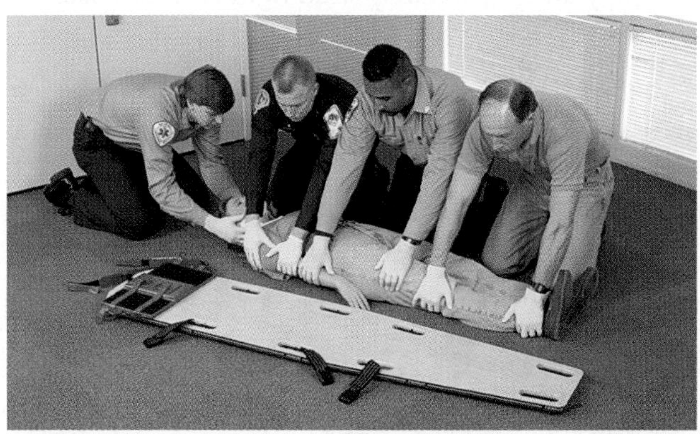

3. Have three rescuers kneel at the patient's side opposite the board, leaving room to roll the patient toward them. Place rescuers at the shoulder, waist, and knee. One EMT will continue to stabilize the head, while the others reach across the patient to position their hands properly.

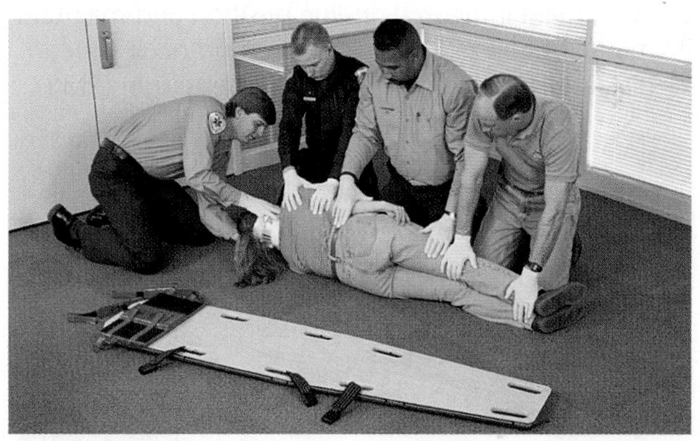

4. The EMT at the head and neck directs the others to roll the patient as a unit.

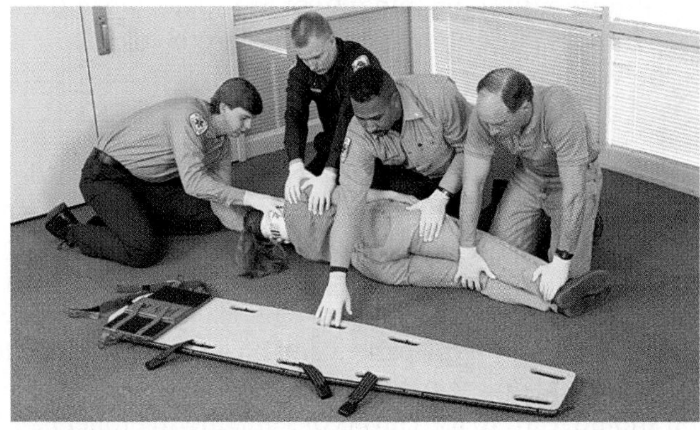

5. The EMT at the patient's waist grips the spine board and pulls it into position against the patient. (This can be done by a fifth rescuer.)

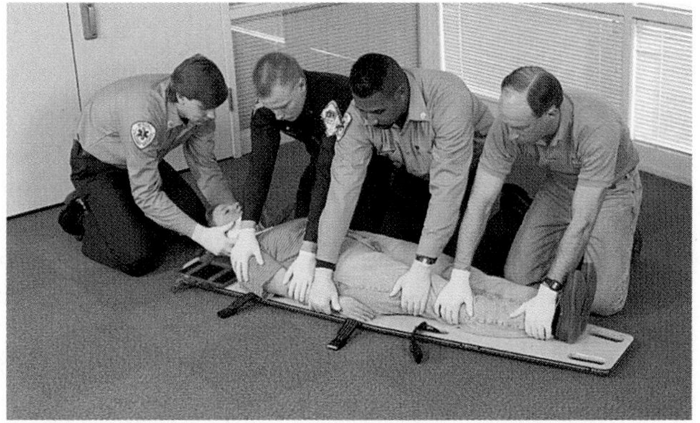

6. Roll the patient as a unit onto the board.

SCAN 29-4 • Spinal Immobilization of a Supine Patient

First take Standard Precautions.

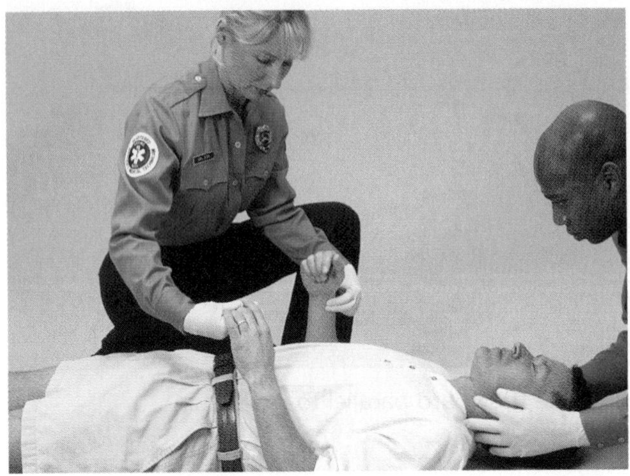

1. Place head in neutral, in-line position and maintain manual stabilization of the head and neck. Assess distal pulse, motor function, and sensation (PMS).

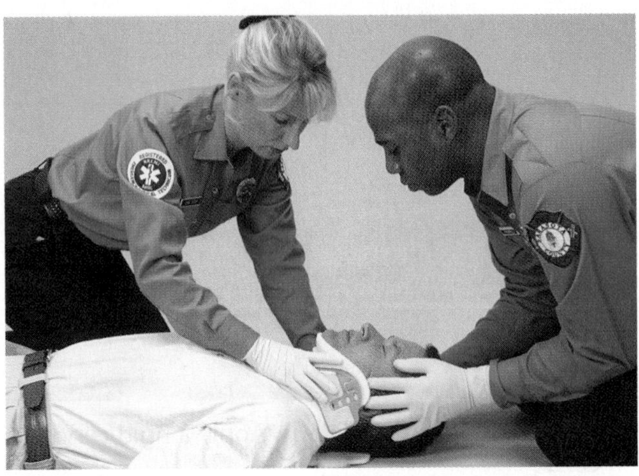

2. Apply an appropriately sized rigid cervical collar.

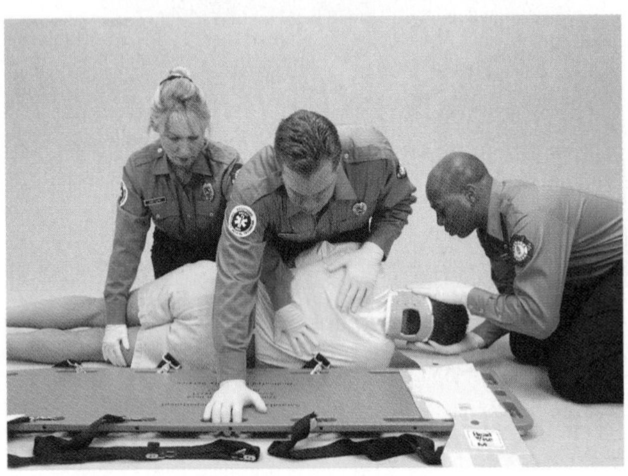

3. Position an immobilization device.

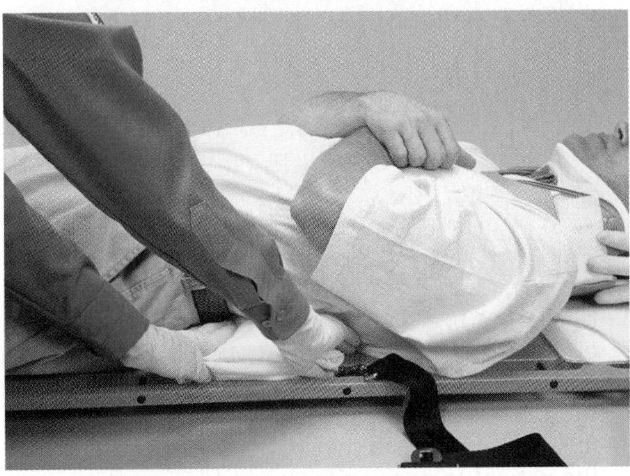

4. Move the patient onto the device without compromising the integrity of the spine. Once the patient is in position, apply padding to voids between the torso and board.

- Additional immobilization for the head and neck can be provided with light foam-filled cushions, a commercial head immobilization device (such as the Ferno Washington head immobilizer, Bashaw CID, or the Laerdal Head Bed), or a blanket roll (Figure 29-21). If used, these are applied after securing the patient's body to the long backboard. Secure the head with 3-inch hypoallergenic adhesive tape. The tape offers support, especially if the patient and board are to be tilted to allow for drainage. However, blood on the patient's skin and hair may make using tape impractical. You should learn to use cravats or self-adhering roller bandages as a backup method. Do not tape or tie the cravats across the patient's eyes.
- If the patient is a full-term pregnant woman, after immobilizing on the backboard, tilt the board to the left by propping up the right side to minimize the effect of the uterus compressing the vena cava and causing hypotension and dizziness.

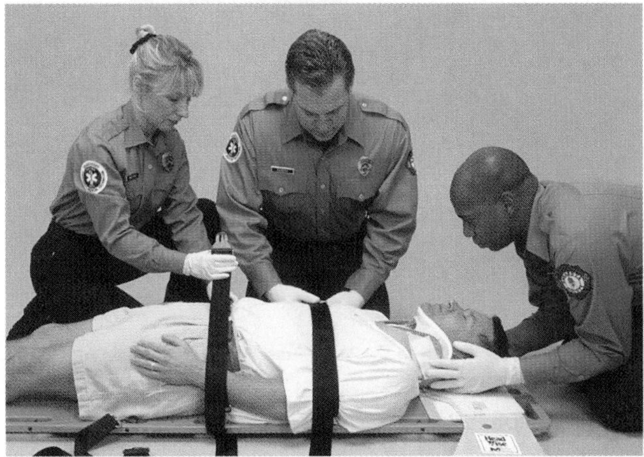

5. Secure the patient's torso to the board first.

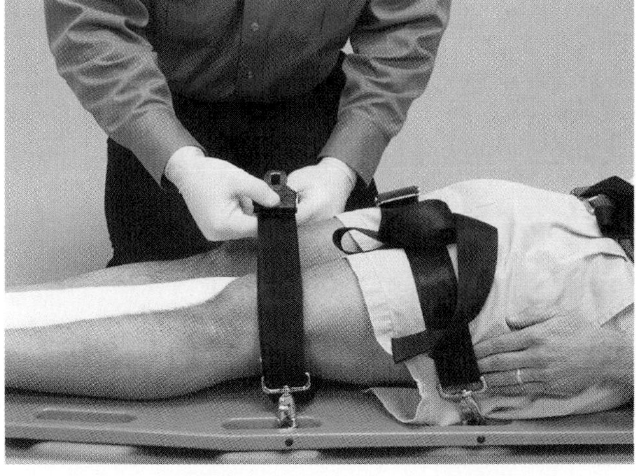

6. Then the patient's legs (above and below the knee).

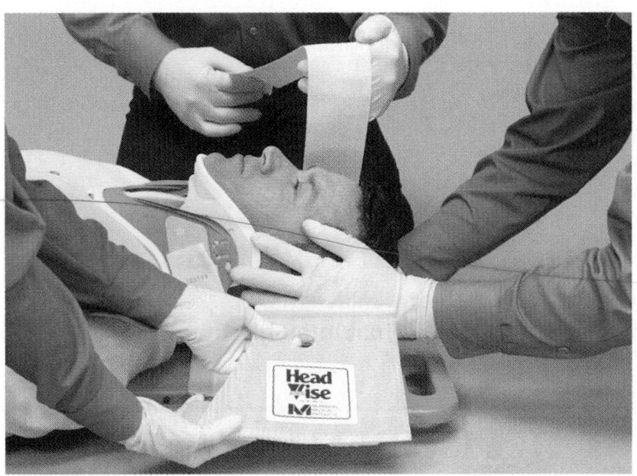

7. Pad and immobilize the patient's head last.

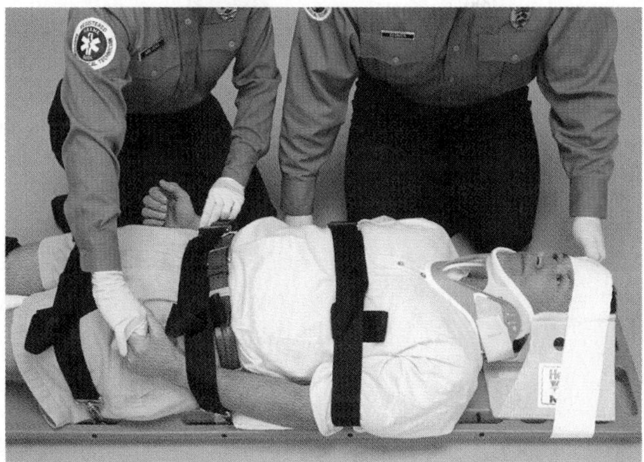

8. Reassess the patient's distal pulse, motor function, and sensation (PMS).

- Unless the spine board has straps specifically intended to criss-cross the shoulders and chest, it is best to strap across the upper chest, the pelvis, and the thighs. If you will need to stand the patient up to carry him out of a tight building, up a basement stairwell, or into a small elevator, make sure the straps are secure under the armpits and tight on the thighs.
- If your service transports to a helicopter, make sure that your backboard fits. There are some restrictions on the size or taper of the long backboard, depending on the helicopter's loading configuration, so find this out ahead of time.
- For a water rescue or diving injury there are various specialty backboards, such as the Miller board, that are designed to float up beneath the patient and use Velcro closures for ease of application.

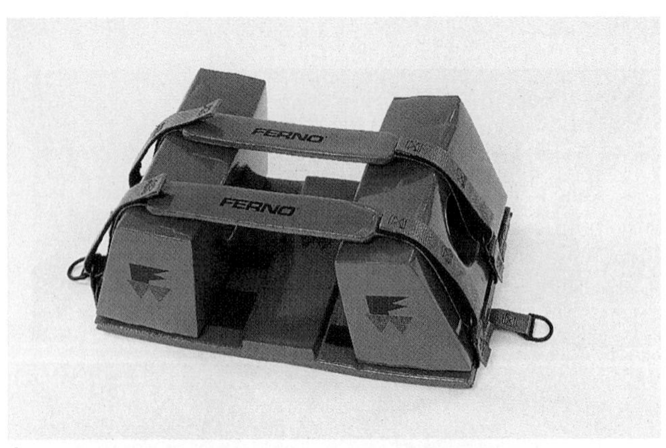

A

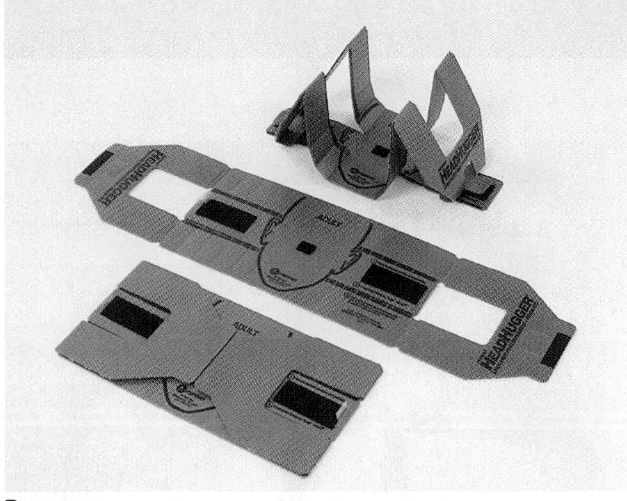

B

Figure 29-21 • (A) Ferno head immobilizer and (B) disposable head immobilizer. *(Both: © Ferno, Inc.)*

PEDIATRIC NOTE

When immobilizing a 6-year-old or younger child, provide padding beneath the shoulder blades to compensate for the large head. Pad from shoulders to toes as needed to establish a neutral position.

If you do not carry a pediatric long spine immobilization device, then practice immobilizing children using adult equipment and lots of towels or blankets to pad around the child. EMTs are usually very good at improvising. In this case, however, the first time you improvise should be in the classroom so you will work quickly in the field!

Tips for Dealing with a Standing Patient

When you approach a vehicle and see the tell-tale spider-web-cracked windshield, you know whoever sat behind that crack needs full spinal immobilization. Sometimes this

CRITICAL DECISION MAKING:
More Than a Pain in the Neck

You have learned the procedure for immobilizing patients. The decision-making process that leads up to the immobilization is equally important. Which patients do you immobilize and which do not require immobilization? (*Note:* Use the general concepts from this chapter to make your determination. Your protocols in the field may vary.)

1. Your patient was the driver of a vehicle that was struck in the rear end while stopped at a light. The patient denies pain, but you observe her rubbing her neck and looking like she may have some pain.
2. Your patient was in the back seat of a car that was hit broadside (T-bone). She doesn't complain of neck pain, but her head was knocked into the side of the car during the collision. She has a large hematoma on the right side of her head from the impact.
3. Your patient was a passenger in a car that was struck in the driver's side in a minor collision. She denies all injury and isn't sure she wants to go to the hospital.

patient is up and walking around at the collision scene. He still has the potential for a spine injury but may not yet have dislocated the fracture or ligament injury site. It would be dangerous to have him sit down or lie down on your long backboard, so instead use a backboard to carefully but rapidly take him down to the supine position without compromising his spine.

Some EMS providers advocate strapping the patient onto the long board while the patient is standing. However, this is often not practical in the field. (It works in the classroom because the simulated patients are not in shock, intoxicated, head injured, combative, or just dizzy!)

The easiest technique is the rapid takedown which, like all skills in this text, should be demonstrated by a qualified instructor and practiced in the classroom prior to use in the field. The procedure takes three EMTs, a set of collars, and a long backboard. (See Figure 29-22 and Scan 29-5.)

Patient Found Wearing a Helmet

Helmets are worn in many sporting events and by many motorcycle riders. Even ski resorts are starting to advocate the use of helmets. Sporting helmets are typically open in the front, making it easier to access the patient's airway than with a motorcycle helmet, which has a shield and often a full face section that is not removable.

Face, neck, and spine care and airway management or resuscitation may call for the removal of the helmet, especially if the helmet will prevent you from reaching the patient's mouth or nose. If the helmet is left on, shields can be lifted and face guards removed. One EMT must manually steady the patient's head and neck while the other cuts, snaps off, or unscrews the guard. Do not attempt to remove a helmet if doing so causes increased pain, or if the helmet proves difficult to remove, unless there is a possible airway obstruction or ventilatory assistance must be provided. Indications for leaving the helmet in place or for removing the helmet are summarized in the following text:

Indications for leaving the helmet in place:

- Helmet fits snugly, allowing little or no movement of the patient's head within the helmet.
- There are absolutely no impending airway or breathing problems nor any reason to resuscitate or ventilate the patient.
- Removal would cause further injury.
- Proper spinal immobilization can be done with the helmet in place.
- There is no interference with the EMT's ability to assess the airway or breathing.

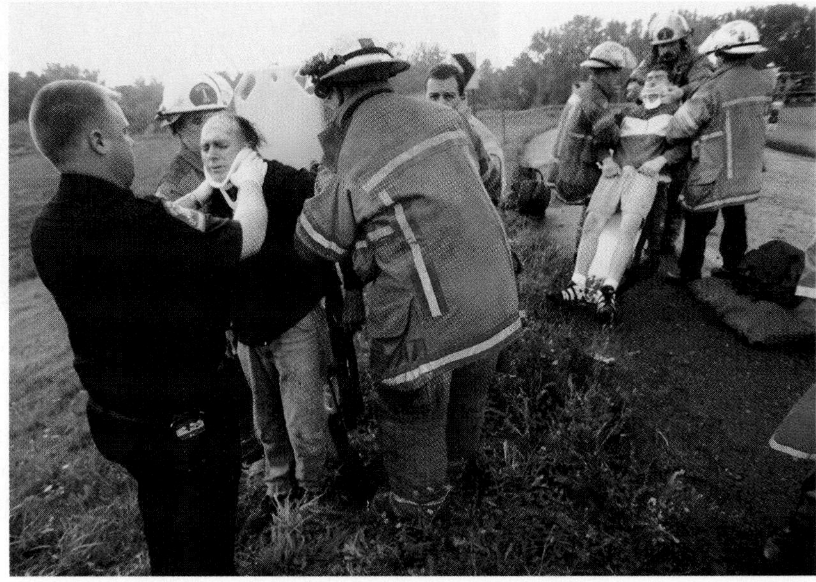

Figure 29-22 • Standing takedown at the scene of an emergency. *(© Howard Paul/Emergency! Stock)*

SCAN 29-5 • Rapid Takedown of a Standing Patient

First take Standard Precautions.

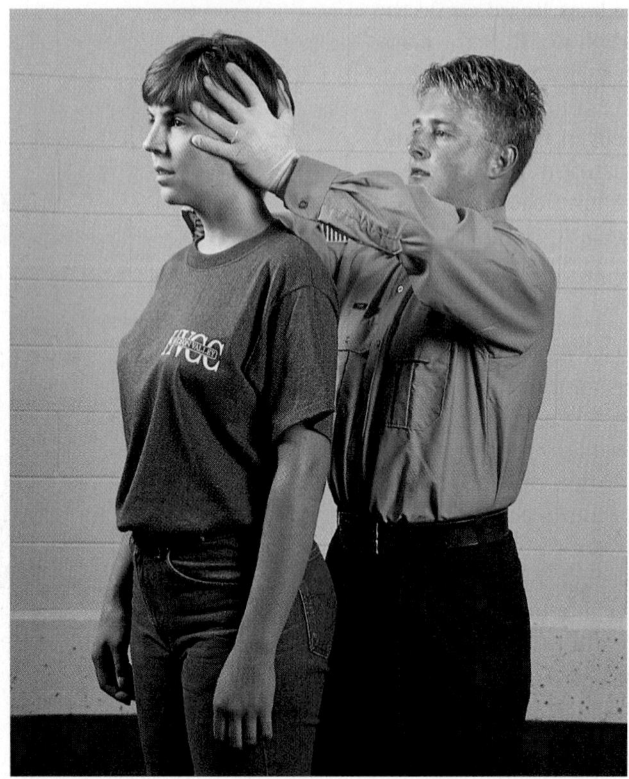

1. Position your tallest crew member (EMT #1) behind the patient and have him manually stabilize the head and neck. His hands should not leave the patient's head until the entire procedure is complete and the head is secured to the long spine board.

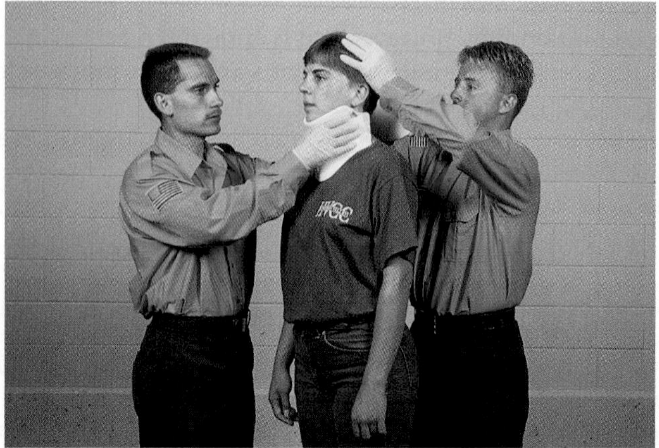

2. EMT #2 applies a properly sized cervical collar to the patient. EMT #1 continues manual stabilization (collar aids, but does not replace, manual stabilization).

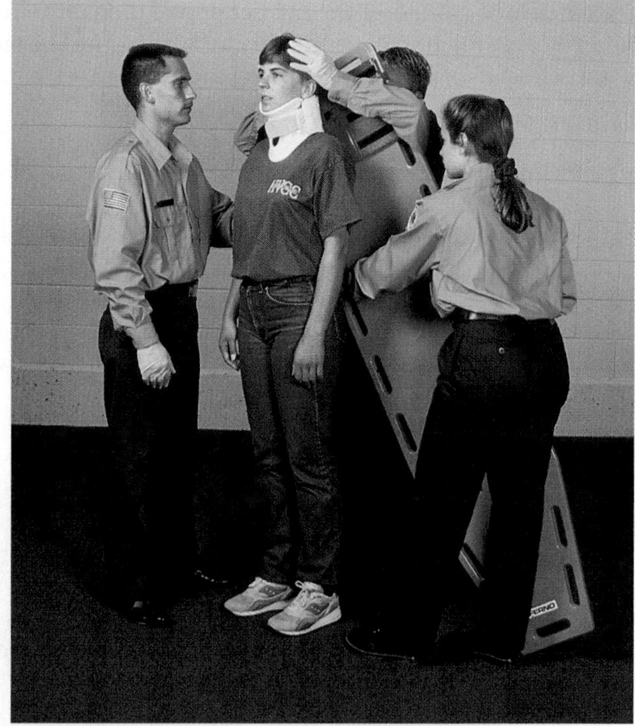

3. EMT #1 continues manual stabilization, as EMT #2 and another rescuer position a long spine board behind the patient, being careful not to disturb EMT #1's manual stabilization of the patient's head and neck. It will help if EMT #1 spreads elbows to give the other rescuers more room to maneuver the spine board.

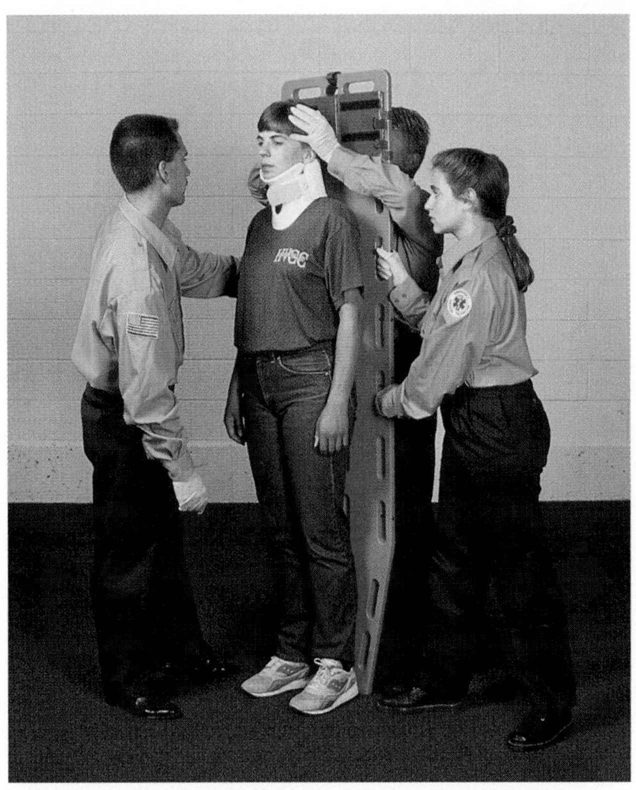

4. EMT #1 continues manual stabilization. EMT #2 looks at the spine board from the front of the patient and does any necessary repositioning to be sure it is centered behind the patient.

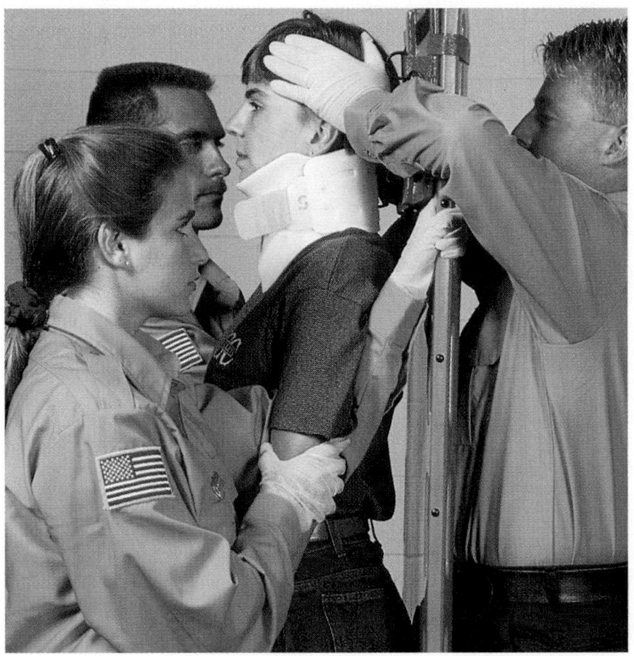

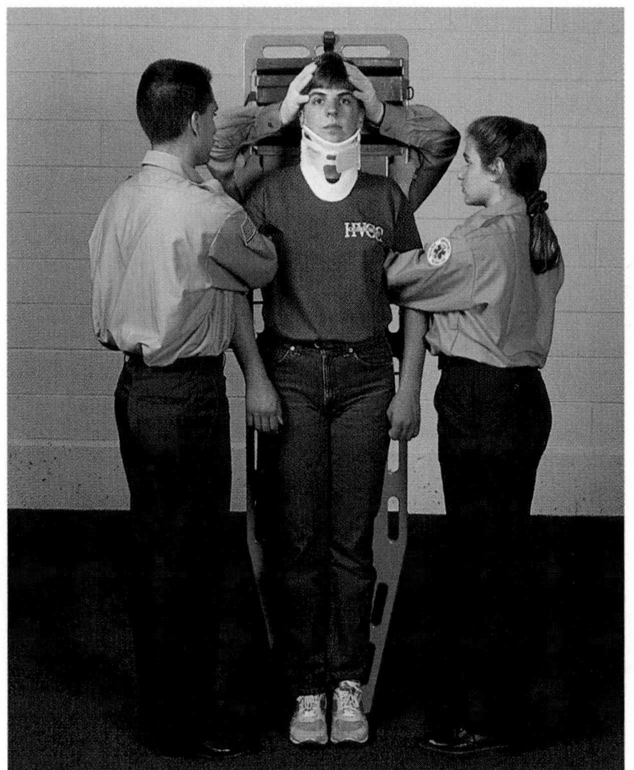

5. EMT #1 continues manual stabilization. EMT #2 and the third rescuer reach the arm that is nearest the patient under the patient's armpits and grasp the spine board. (Once the board is tilted down, the patient will actually be temporarily suspended by the armpits.) To keep the patient's arms secure, they will use the other hand to grasp the patient's arm just above the elbow and hold it against the patient's body.

6. EMT #2 and the third rescuer, when reaching under the patient's armpits, must grasp a handhold on the spine board at the patient's armpit level or higher.

continued

SCAN 29-5 • (Continued)

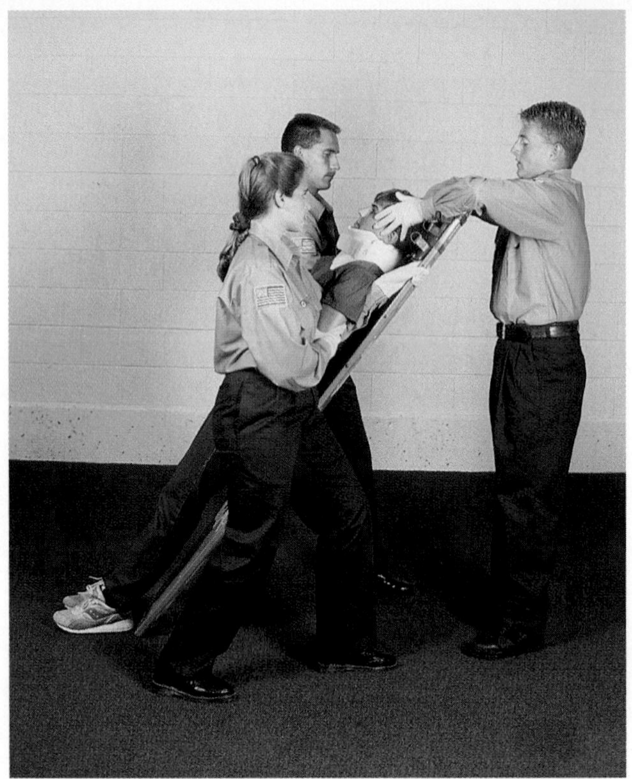

7. EMT #1 continues manual stabilization. EMT #2 and the third rescuer maintain their grasp on the spine board and patient. EMT #1 explains to the patient what is going to happen, then gives the signal to begin slowly tilting the board and patient to the ground. As the board is lowered, EMT #1 walks backward and crouches, keeping up with the board as it is lowered and allowing the patient's head to slowly move back to the neutral position against the board. EMT #1 must accomplish all this without holding back or slowing the lowering of the board. EMT #1 may need to rotate somewhat so that, once the board is almost flat, he is holding the head down on the board. Once the patient's head comes in contact with the board, it must not be allowed to leave the board, to avoid flexing the neck. The job of the two rescuers doing the lowering is to control it so that it is slow and even on both sides. They should also move into a squatting position as they lower the board to avoid injuring their backs.

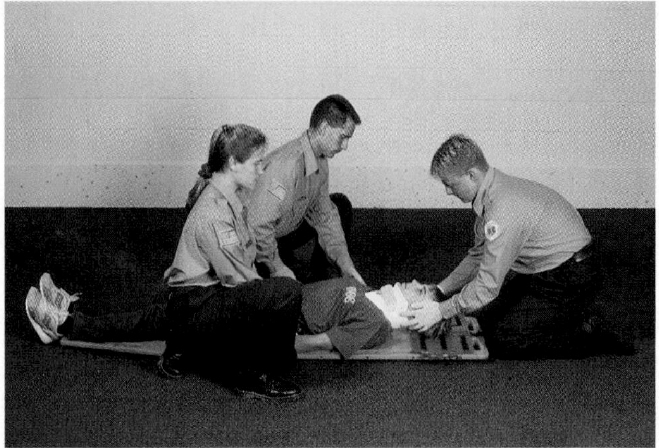

8. EMT #1 maintains manual in-line stabilization throughout the procedure.

Indications for removing the helmet:

- Helmet interferes with the ability to assess and manage airway and breathing.
- Helmet is improperly fitted, allowing excessive head movement.
- Helmet interferes with immobilization.
- Cardiac arrest.

Many experienced EMS providers put the controversy of removal versus nonremoval into the following perspective: If your child injured his neck playing football, would you want the trainer and the EMT to work together carefully to remove the helmet at the scene, or would you prefer this be left to emergency department personnel who probably will not have the help of the trainer nor the benefit of lots of practice in the helmet removal technique?

Note that if a football player is wearing shoulder pads and a helmet, you should either remove the pads and the helmet or you should leave them both on. Taking off one, but not the other, will result in hyperflexion or hyperextension because of the space the pads occupy behind the patient's shoulders.

When a helmet must be removed, it is a two-rescuer procedure, as shown in Scan 29-6.

PEDIATRIC NOTE

Occasionally, EMTs are confronted at a motor-vehicle collision with an infant or young child who was riding in a child safety seat. Placing a child in a supine position with the legs elevated, as you will need to do if you are going to tip the seat backward and move the child onto a spine board, places a great deal of pressure on the abdominal organs and diaphragm, making respiration difficult. So, provided the patient is not in need of immediate resuscitative measures, or for any other reason needs to be placed in the supine position, it makes sense to let the child remain sitting upright and use the child safety seat as an immobilization device.

The key decision on whether to immobilize the child in the seat or to rapidly remove the child from the seat onto a spine board is based upon the patient's priority and need to be in a supine position. The procedure for immobilization in the child safety seat is described in Scan 29-7 and the procedure for rapid extrication from the car seat is shown in Scan 29-8.

SCAN 29-6 • Removing a Helmet from an Injured Patient

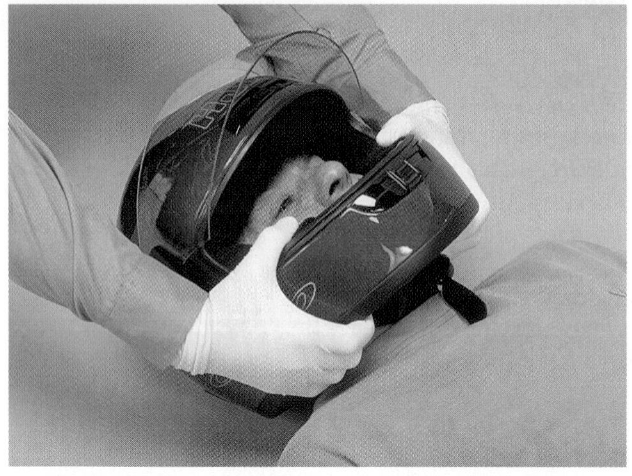

1. EMT #1 is positioned at the top of the patient's head and maintains manual stabilization. Two hands hold the helmet stable while the fingertips hold the lower jaw.

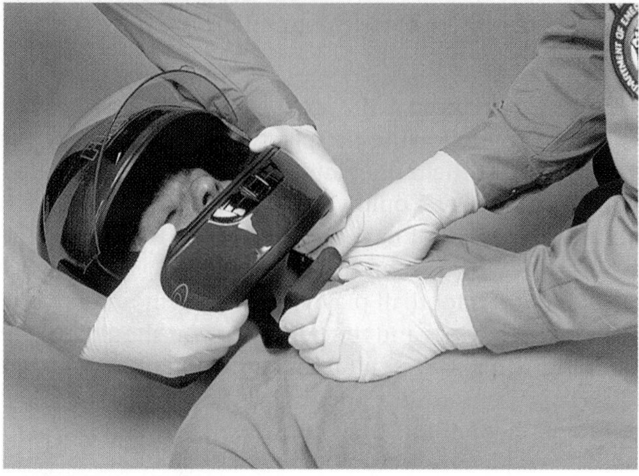

2. EMT #2 opens, cuts, or removes the chin strap.

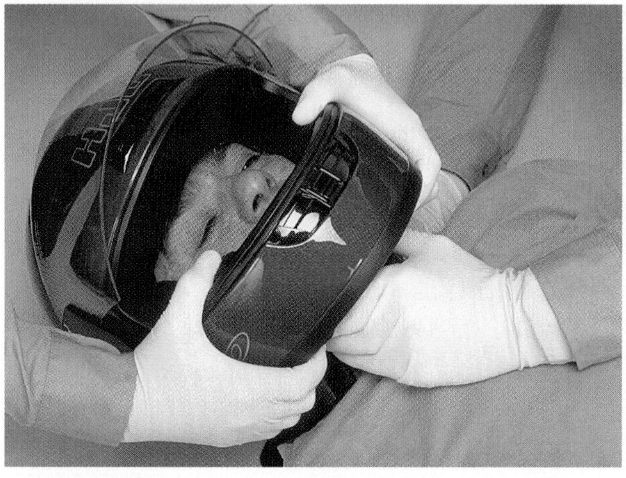

3. EMT #2 then places one hand on the patient's mandible and, using the other hand, reaches in behind the neck and stabilizes the occipital region. Using the combination of the hand in front of the chin and the hand behind the neck, EMT #2 should be able to hold the head securely. If the patient has glasses on, they should be removed now, prior to removal of the helmet.

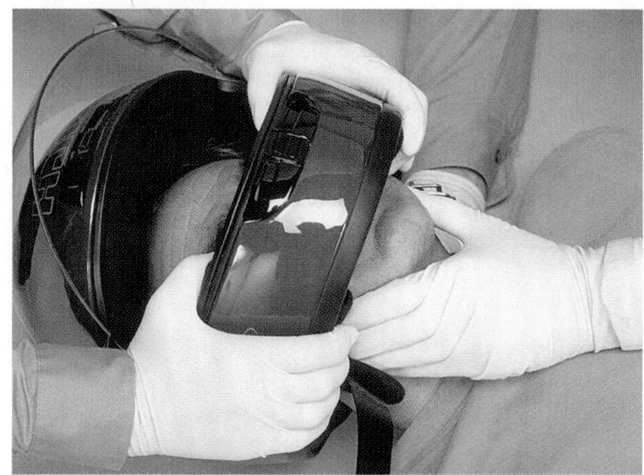

4. EMT #1 can now release manual stabilization and slowly remove the helmet. The lower sides, or ear cups, of the helmet will have to be gently pulled out to clear the ears.

NOTE *If the patient has shoulder pads and you are removing a football helmet, remember to remove the shoulder pads or pad behind the head to keep it aligned with the padded shoulders. With either helmet-removal method, manual stabilization must be maintained until the patient is secured to a long spine board with full immobilization of the head.*

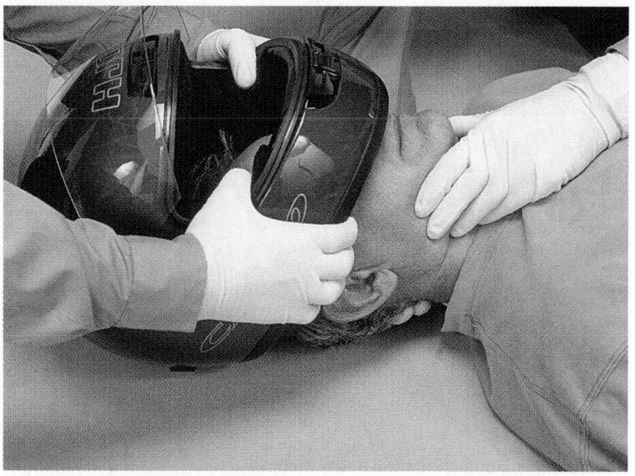

5. The helmet should come off straight with no backward tilting. A full-face helmet may need to be tilted just enough for the chin guard to clear the nose. EMT #2 must support and prevent the head from moving as the helmet is removed.

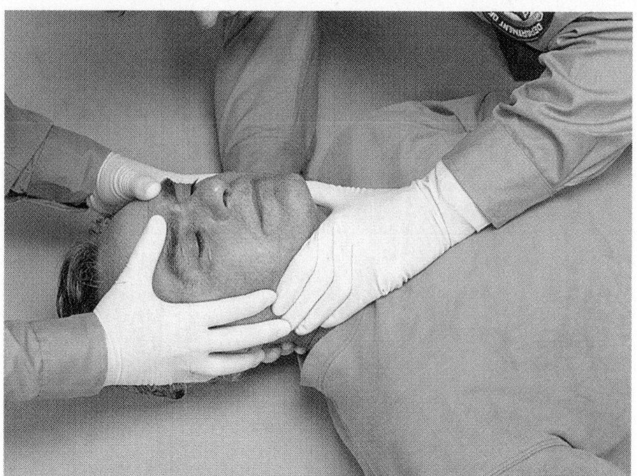

6. EMT #1, after removing the helmet, re-establishes manual stabilization and maintains an open airway by using the jaw-thrust.

HELMET REMOVAL—ALTERNATIVE METHOD

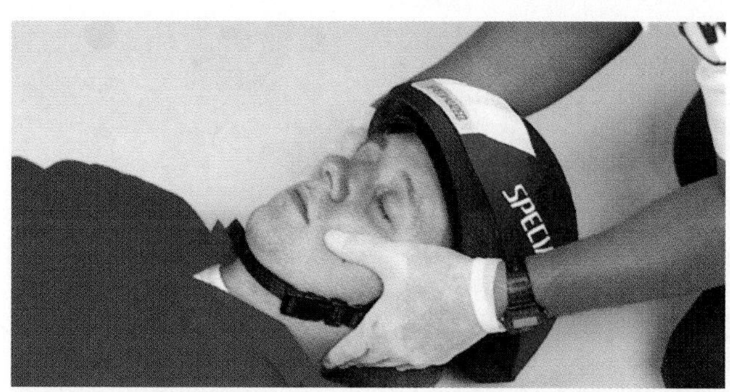

1. EMT #1 applies manual stabilization with the patient's neck in neutral position.

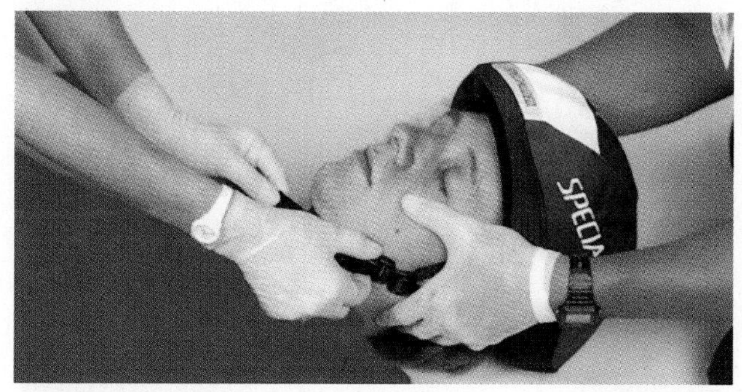

2. EMT #2 removes the chin strap.

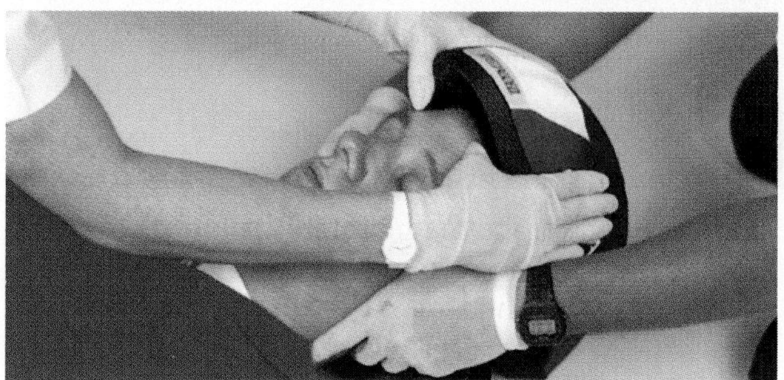

3. EMT #2 removes the helmet, pulling out on each side to clear the ears.

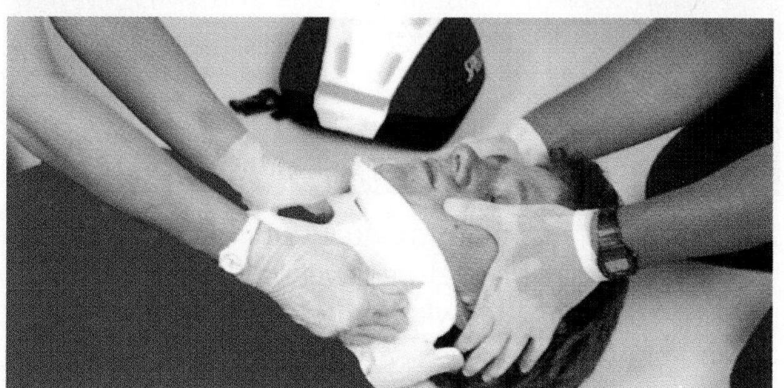

4. EMT #1 maintains manual stabilization as EMT #2 applies a cervical collar.

SCAN 29-7 • Immobilizing in a Child Safety Seat

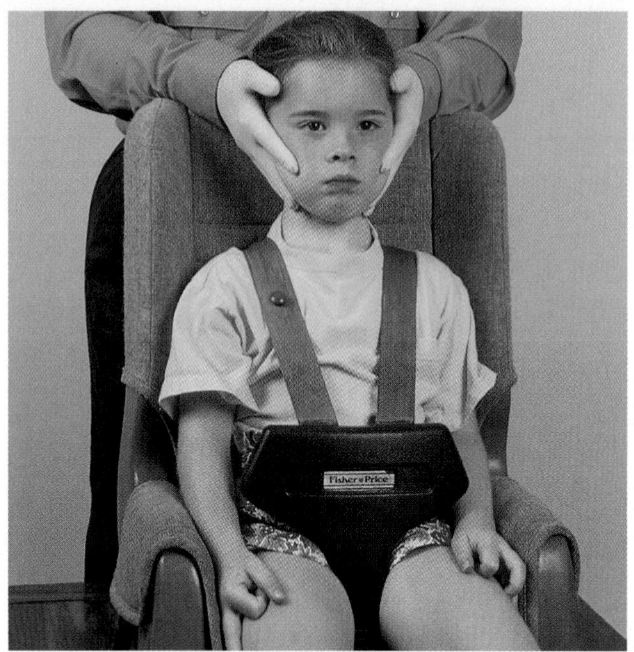

1. EMT #1 stabilizes the car seat in the upright position, applies manual stabilization to the head and neck . . .

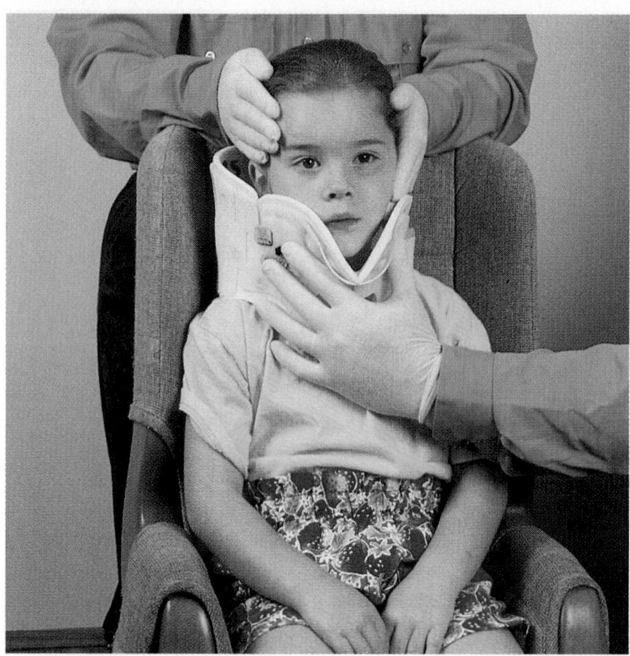

. . . as EMT #2 prepares equipment, then applies the cervical collar, or improvises with a rolled hand towel for the newborn or infant.

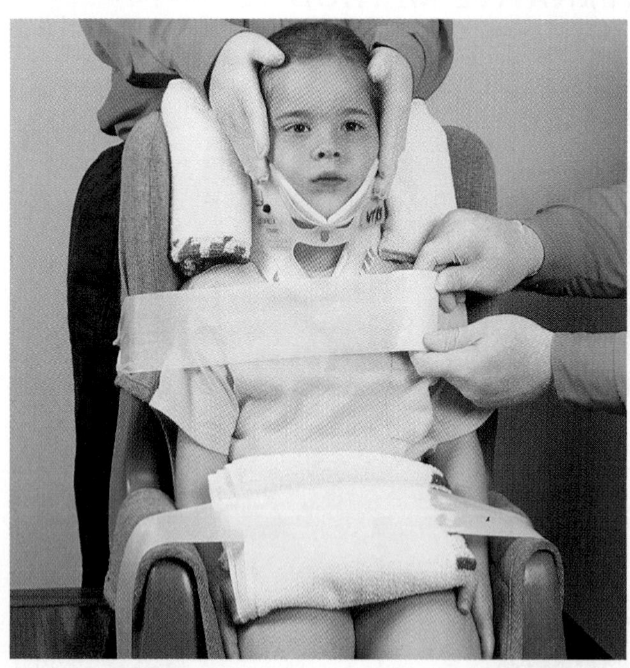

2. As EMT #1 maintains manual stabilization, EMT #2 places a small blanket or towel on the child's lap, then straps or uses wide tape to secure the pelvis and chest area to the seat.

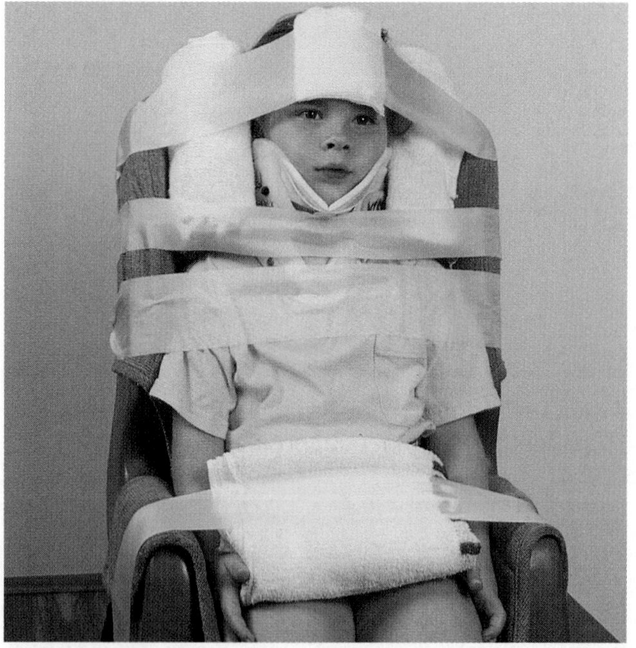

3. EMT #1 maintains manual stabilization, as the patient and seat are carried to the ambulance and strapped onto the stretcher with stretcher head raised. EMT #2 places a towel roll on both sides of the head to fill voids, tapes forehead in place, then tapes across the collar. (Avoid taping chin, which would place pressure on the child's neck.)

SCAN 29-8 • Rapid Extrication from a Child Safety Seat

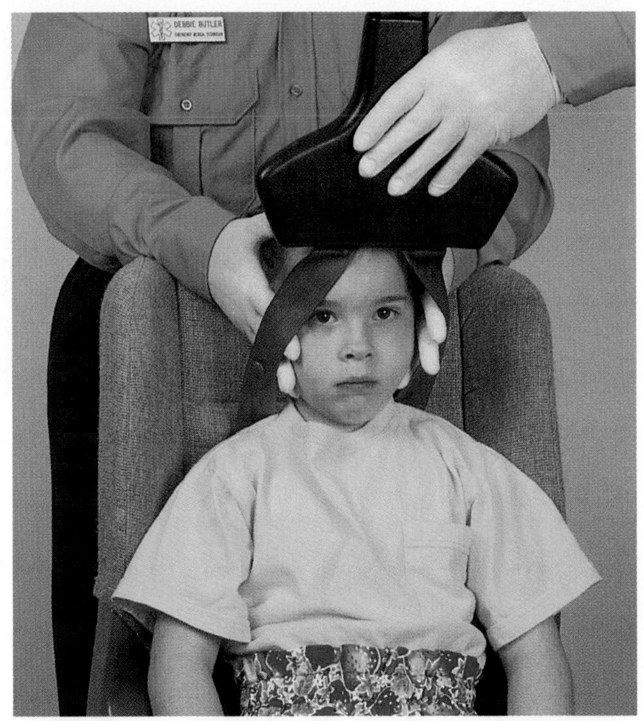

1. EMT #1 stabilizes the car seat in the upright position and applies manual stabilization of the head and neck. EMT #2 prepares equipment, and then loosens or cuts the seat straps and raises the front guard.

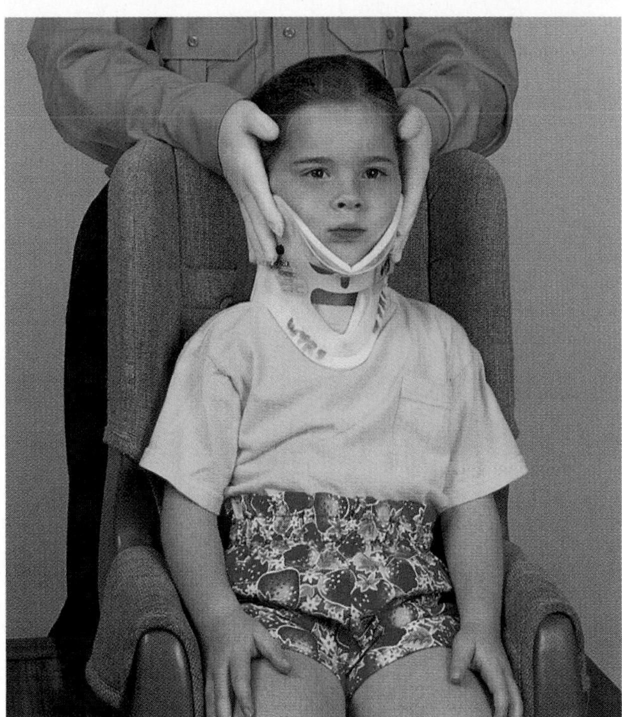

2. Cervical collar is applied to the patient as EMT #1 maintains manual stabilization of the head and neck.

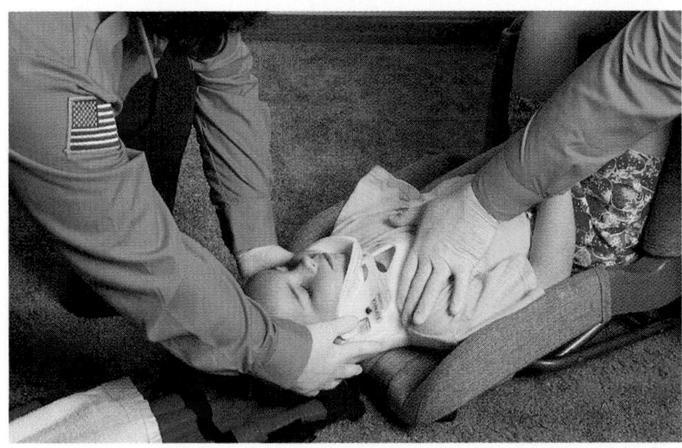

3. As EMT #1 maintains manual stabilization, EMT #2 places the child safety seat on the center of the backboard and slowly tilts it into the supine position. EMTs are careful not to let the child slide out of the chair. For the child with a large head, place a towel under the area where the shoulders will eventually be placed on the board to prevent the head from tilting forward.

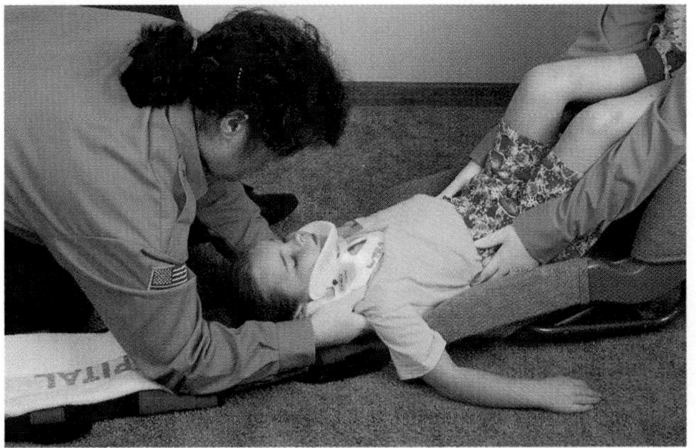

4. EMT #1 maintains manual stabilization and calls for a coordinated long axis move onto the backboard.

continued

SCAN 29-8 • (Continued)

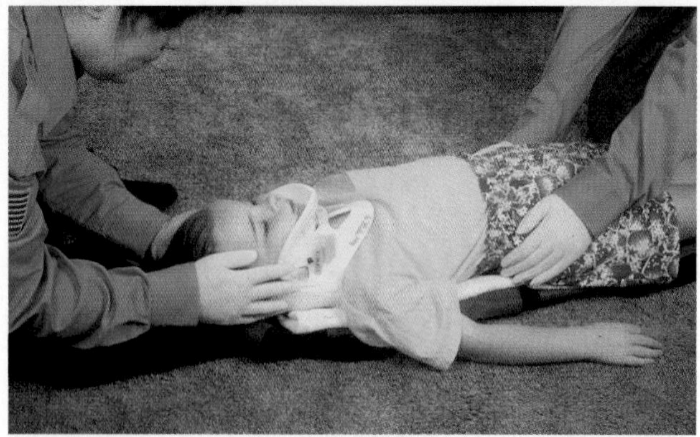

5. EMT #1 maintains manual stabilization, as the move onto the board is completed, with the child's shoulders over the folded towel.

6. EMT #1 maintains manual stabilization, as EMT #2 places rolled towels or blankets on both sides of the patient.

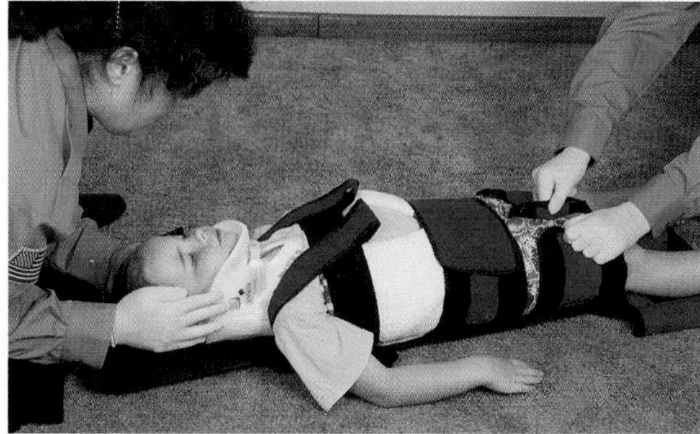

7. EMT #1 maintains manual stabilization, as EMT #2 straps or tapes the patient to the board at the level of the upper chest, pelvis, and lower legs. DO NOT STRAP ACROSS THE ABDOMEN.

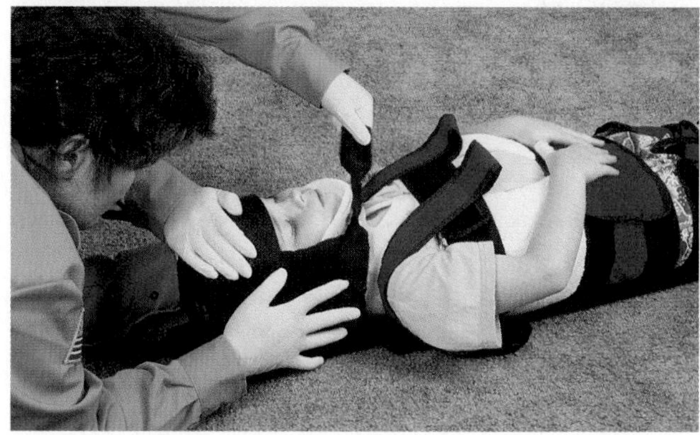

8. EMT #1 maintains manual stabilization, as EMT #2 places rolled towels on both sides of the head, then tapes the head securely in place across the forehead and cervical collar. DO NOT TAPE ACROSS THE CHIN TO AVOID PRESSURE ON THE NECK.

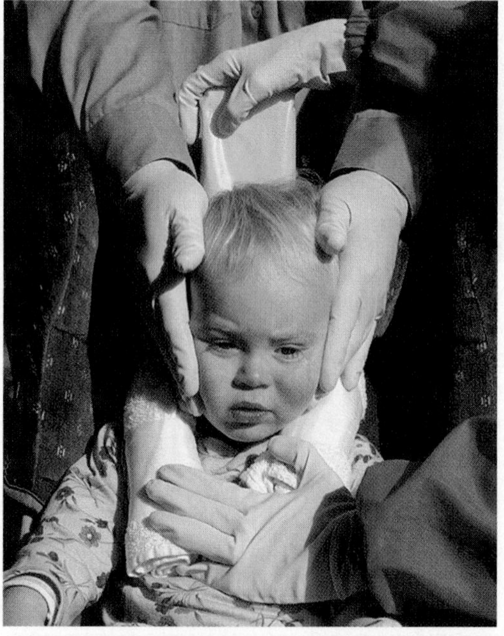

The newborn and infant procedure is exactly the same as for a child, except that an armboard is inserted behind the child in Step 2. If the infant is very small, the armboard may actually be used as the spine board.

Selective Spine Immobilization

The traditional approach to spine immobilization in EMS has been to immobilize any patient whose assessment or mechanism of injury suggests the possibility of spine injury. But what exactly does that mean? A serious MOI to one EMT may not seem serious to another EMT. In some EMS systems, providers now have specific indications for spine immobilization. Use of these indications may be limited to advanced level providers in some systems. In others, EMT level providers may be authorized to use them.

This approach is sometimes incorrectly referred to as a "spine clearance protocol." EMTs do not clear spines (i.e., determine there is no spine injury). Instead, in systems that employ this approach, each patient's condition and circumstances are evaluated and compared to a protocol to determine whether spine immobilization is indicated for that patient. In some cases, an EMT may immobilize patients he would not have immobilized before institution of such a protocol.

Typical elements of such a protocol (Table 29-1 and Figure 29-23) include evaluation of both the mechanism of injury and the patient's condition. Patient condition is further broken down into injury-related conditions such as paralysis and non-injury-related conditions such as intoxication that limit the reliability of the assessment.

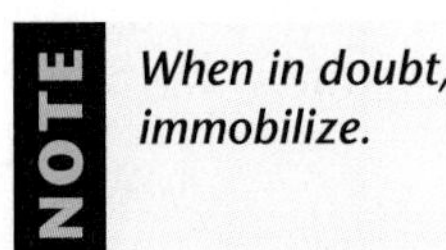

NOTE

When in doubt, immobilize.

These protocols may also differentiate patients by age. Differences in elderly and pediatric patients (as compared to adults) pose special assessment and immobilization challenges.

Most protocols also allow the EMT an "out" by encouraging the provider to immobilize a patient when clinical judgment suggests that it is appropriate, even if none of the other conditions are present.

Although spine immobilization causes pain and discomfort in some patients, that concern is insignificant when compared to the devastating lifelong consequences of failure to immobilize an injured spine. Before you use a selective spine immobilization protocol, be sure you have been trained in the specific indications and contraindications of such a protocol and that your Medical Director has approved it.

TABLE 29-1 • Typical Elements of a Selective Spine Immobilization Protocol

Immobilize the patient's spine if one or more of the following are present:

MECHANISM OF INJURY	PATIENT CHARACTERISTICS INJURY RELATED
• Violent impact to head, neck, torso, or pelvis • Moderate-to-high-speed motor-vehicle incident • Pedestrian struck by a vehicle • Explosion • Ejection from a vehicle • Shallow-water diving incident • Fall: Some protocols include all falls, while others include only falls greater than a particular height, commonly three times the patient's height (There may be differences with elderly patients.) • Axial load • Penetrating trauma in or near the spine • Sports injury to the head or neck	• Spine pain, tenderness, or deformity • Neurological deficit or complaint • Pain on movement of the neck or back
PATIENT CHARACTERISTICS NOT DIRECTLY INJURY RELATED	**EMT CHARACTERISTICS**
• Altered mental status • Intoxication from alcohol or other drugs • Inability to communicate • Distracting injury (e.g., a leg injury so painful the patient might not feel a less obvious injury to the spine) • Stress significant enough to prevent the patient from feeling pain	• The EMT suspects that the patient is not being truthful. • The EMT suspects that there is more to the incident than meets the eye or • The EMT's clinical judgment or suspicions suggest the patient should be immobilized.

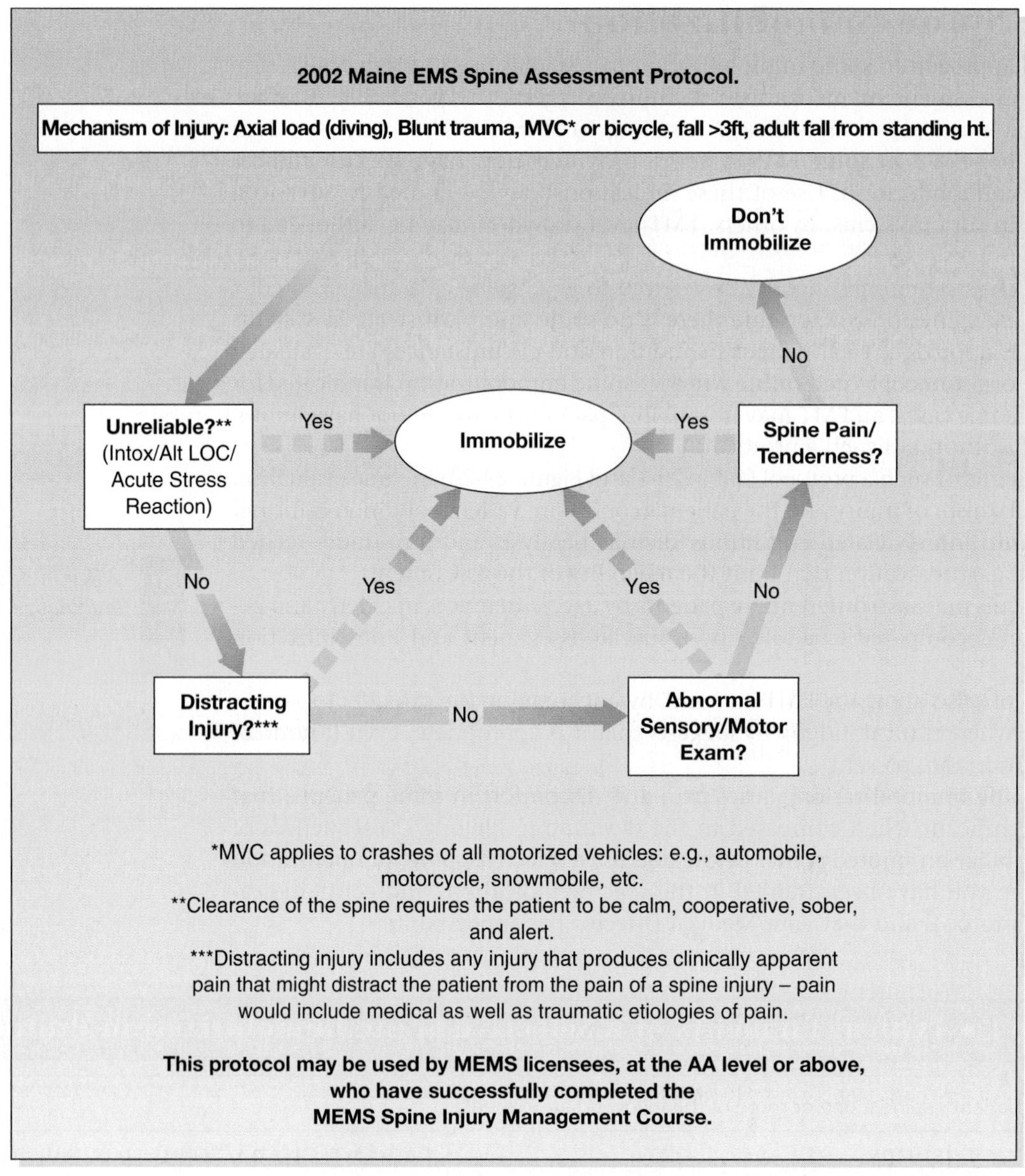

Figure 29-23 • Maine EMS spine assessment protocol. *Note*: This is an example. Local protocols will determine your ability to make the judgments necessary for selective spine immobilization.

CHAPTER REVIEW

SUMMARY

It is important to maintain a high index of suspicion for head or spine injury whenever there is a relevant mechanism of injury. When there is a head injury, assume a brain injury as well as a spine injury. Provide high-concentration oxygen, immobilize, and transport.

Assume a spine injury whenever there is a mechanism of injury of sufficient force or an injury to the head, neck, or upper body. Provide manual stabilization of the head and neck and apply a cervical collar, continuing manual stabilization until the patient is fully immobilized on a long spine board.

In the event of a suspected head or spine injury, ascertain if there has been a loss of consciousness, however brief, and carefully assess the patient's mental status, including orientation to person, place, and time. Monitor and document any changes in the patient's mental status.

KEY TERMS

autonomic nervous system controls involuntary functions.

central nervous system the brain and the spinal cord.

cerebrospinal (suh-RE-bro-SPI-nal) **fluid (CSF)** the fluid that surrounds the brain and spinal cord.

concussion mild closed head injury without detectable damage to the brain. Complete recovery is usually expected.

contusion in brain injuries, a bruised brain caused when the force of a blow to the head is great enough to rupture blood vessels.

cranium (KRAY-ne-um) the bony structure making up the forehead, top, back, and upper sides of the skull.

hematoma (HE-mah-TO-mah) in a head injury, a collection of blood within the skull or brain.

laceration (las-uh-RAY-shun) in brain injuries, a cut to the brain.

malar (MAY-lar) the cheek bone, also called the *zygomatic bone.*

mandible (MAN-di-bl) the lower jaw bone.

maxillae (mak-SIL-e) the two fused bones forming the upper jaw.

nasal (NAY-zul) **bones** the bones that form the upper third, or bridge, of the nose.

nervous system provides overall control of thought, sensation, and the voluntary and involuntary motor functions of the body. The major components of the nervous system are the brain and the spinal cord.

orbits the bony structures around the eyes; the eye sockets.

peripheral nervous system the nerves that enter and exit the spinal cord between the vertebrae and the 12 pairs of cranial nerves that travel between the brain and organs without passing through the spinal cord, and all of the body's other motor and sensory nerves.

spinous (SPI-nus) **process** the bony bump on a vertebra.

temporal (TEM-po-ral) **bone** bone that forms part of the side of the skull and floor of the cranial cavity. There is a right and a left temporal bone.

temporomandibular (TEM-po-ro-mand-DIB-yuh-lar) **joint** the movable joint formed between the mandible and the temporal bone, also called the TMJ.

vertebrae (VERT-uh-bray) the bones of the spinal column (singular vertebra).

REVIEW QUESTIONS

1. Name the two components of the nervous system and discuss their functions. (pp. 749–751)
2. List five signs of a brain injury and explain why mechanism of injury is important in determining possible brain injury. (p. 755)
3. Describe the appropriate emergency treatment of a patient with possible head or brain injury. (pp. 756–757)
4. List five mechanisms of injury that would support suspicion of a spine injury. (pp. 760–761)
5. Describe the appropriate emergency care for a patient with a possible spine injury. (p. 764)

CRITICAL THINKING

- You are called to the scene of a motor-vehicle collision. After ensuring scene safety and taking Standard Precautions, you approach the car, which has struck a bridge abutment, and note a deformed steering wheel. The driver's side door is open and, out on the middle of the bridge, you see a person you presume to be the driver wandering erratically toward the opposite side of the bridge. How should you proceed?

MEDIA RESOURCES

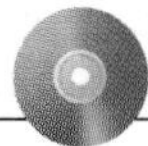

See the Student CD at the back of this book for quizzes, a case study activity, animations, and other features related to this chapter. In particular, take a look at the 3D animations for skeletal, nervous system, and circulatory system aspects of the head and spine. Also, visit the Companion Website for *Emergency Care* at **www.prenhall.com/limmer**, where you will find additional reinforcement and links to other resources.

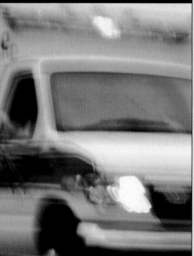

Street Scenes

You and your partner are dispatched to the city park for a patient with head injury. Arriving on scene, you determine the scene is safe and observe a group of teenage boys huddled around a person who is lying on the ground. Taking Standard Precautions, you grab your equipment and approach the patient. Your partner asks, "What happened?"

"We were jumping ramps on our bicycles when Lee tried to do a flip," states one of the boys. "He hit the ground head first. I told that fool he should be wearing a helmet!" You observe a young male lying supine on the asphalt parking lot, eyes closed, with blood oozing from the top of his head from what appears to be an abrasion.

One of the boys identifies himself as Lee's brother and tells you that Lee is 13 years old. He states he lives just around the corner. You ask if his mother is home and he says she is. You ask him to go tell his mother what happened and to come to the park immediately.

Street Scene Questions

1. What is your general impression of this patient?
2. What immediate treatment should be provided?

Your general impression is of an unconscious male with a head and possible spine injury, so your partner provides manual stabilization of the head and neck. Lee's airway is patent, he is breathing normally, and you observe no other bleeding other than the laceration on the top of his head. You decide this is a high-priority trauma patient.

"Lee," you call out. "Lee, can you hear me?"

Lee opens his eyes and asks, "What happened?" Though the patient responds to verbal stimuli, it is apparent that he does not know what happened. He is able to tell you what day it is (Saturday), but not the date.

"Lee, I am going to give you a number to remember. It's number 51. Can you say that?" you ask.

He replies, "51." About this time, Lee's mother arrives. You briefly recount what you know. She seems concerned, but not overly upset. You apply a rigid collar to further restrict the motion of the patient's neck. You learn that Lee is on no medications, has no allergies, and has no medical history. He ate lunch 2 hours before. You obtain baseline vitals and find his pulse is 80 and normal; respirations are 24 and unlabored; blood pressure is 108/74, skin is pink, warm, and dry; and pupils are equal and reactive to light.

Street Scene Question

3. How should you monitor changing levels of responsiveness in a patient with a head injury?

"Lee, tell me what day it is today. Then tell me that number I asked you to keep in mind," you say.

"Saturday. But what number?" he responds.

You place Lee on a nonrebreather mask at 15 liters per minute and also apply a loose dressing to the abrasion on his forehead. There is no other sign of injury on his body. Lee denies any neck pain and has good pulses, motor function, and sensation in all extremities.

The fire department rescue squad is now on scene, and they help you restrict motion of the patient's neck and spine by securing Lee to a rigid board. Lee continues to have good pulses, motor function, and sensation in all extremities. When asked to recall the number again, he states, "I think it was 37." You tell him it is "51" and ask him to repeat it. "51," he says.

On-line medical direction has no other orders for you, but tells you to keep an eye on his airway and mental status. You allow his mother to ride in the ambulance with you. You assess vitals once more en route, noting no significant changes. You once again ask Lee what day and what number and this time he looks at you and says, "Saturday, and I think it's 51." You tell him he's correct. He groans and states he has a headache. The rest of the transport is uneventful.

Street Scenes Sample Documentation

PATIENT NAME: *Lee Zhu* PATIENT AGE: *13*

CHIEF COMPLAINT: *Loss of consciousness*

PAST MEDICAL HISTORY

- [X] None
- [ ] Allergy to
- [ ] Hypertension
- [ ] Stroke
- [ ] Seizures
- [ ] Diabetes
- [ ] COPD
- [ ] Cardiac
- [ ] Other (List)
- [ ] Asthma

Current Medications (List)

VITAL SIGNS

TIME	RESP	PULSE	B.P.	MENTAL STATUS	R PUPILS L	SKIN
1830	Rate: *24*; ☒ Regular ☐ Shallow ☐ Labored	Rate: *80*; ☒ Regular ☐ Irregular	*108/74*	☐ Alert ☑ Voice ☐ Pain ☐ Unresp.	☑ Normal ☑; ☐ Dilated ☐; ☐ Constricted ☐; ☐ Sluggish ☐; ☐ No-Reaction ☐	☑ Unremarkable; ☐ Cool ☐ Pale; ☐ Warm ☐ Cyanotic; ☐ Moist ☐ Flushed; ☐ Dry ☐ Jaundiced
1835	Rate: *24*; ☒ Regular ☐ Shallow ☐ Labored	Rate: *83*; ☒ Regular ☐ Irregular	*110/74*	☐ Alert ☑ Voice ☐ Pain ☐ Unresp.	☑ Normal ☑; ☐ Dilated ☐; ☐ Constricted ☐; ☐ Sluggish ☐; ☐ No-Reaction ☐	☑ Unremarkable; ☐ Cool ☐ Pale; ☐ Warm ☐ Cyanotic; ☐ Moist ☐ Flushed; ☐ Dry ☐ Jaundiced
1840	Rate: *25*; ☒ Regular ☐ Shallow ☐ Labored	Rate: *85*; ☒ Regular ☐ Irregular	*108/76*	☑ Alert ☐ Voice ☐ Pain ☐ Unresp.	☑ Normal ☑; ☐ Dilated ☐; ☐ Constricted ☐; ☐ Sluggish ☐; ☐ No-Reaction ☐	☑ Unremarkable; ☐ Cool ☐ Pale; ☐ Warm ☐ Cyanotic; ☐ Moist ☐ Flushed; ☐ Dry ☐ Jaundiced

NARRATIVE *13-year-old male rode bicycle and jumped off ramp approx. 3 feet high at approx. 15 mph; landed on head; no helmet; landed on asphalt surface. Apparent loss of consciousness; responded to verbal; oriented to person, place, and day. Patient given number 51 to recall, but unable to recall that number while on scene. Airway, breathing, and circulation normal. Abrasion noted on forehead approx. 2" above bridge of the nose with minimal bleeding. Patient denies neck and back pain; good pulse/motor function/sensation in all four extremities. Mother arrived on scene approx. 10 minutes post EMS arrival; related history and other pertinent information as well as permission to treat.*

Treatment: manual stabilization of C-spine with rigid collar and full spinal motion restriction; nonrebreather at 10 LPM; vitals; dressing for abrasion; on-line medical direction established; transport uneventful.

Reassess: En route, patient able to recall number 51 for first time; c/o headache. No change.

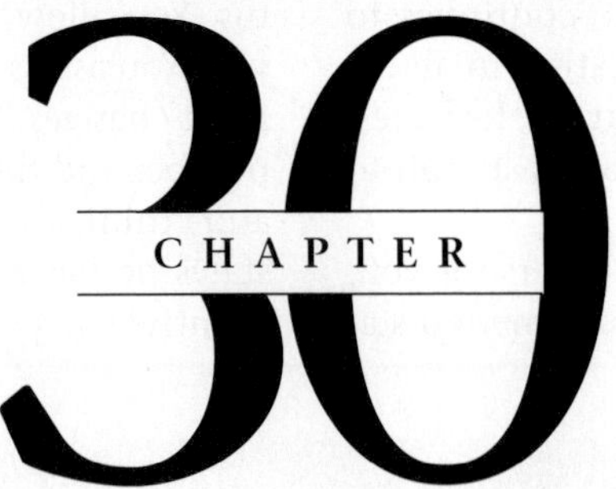

CHAPTER 30

Putting It All Together for the Trauma Patient

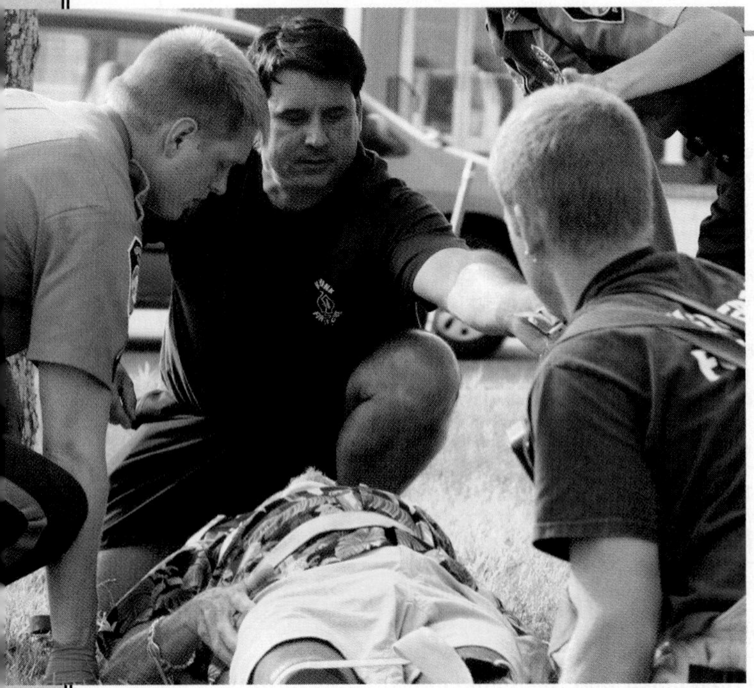

CORE CONCEPTS

The following are core concepts that will be addressed in this chapter:

- How to balance the critical trauma patient's need for prompt transport against the time needed to treat all of the patient's injuries at the scene
- How to select the critical interventions to implement at the scene of a multiple-trauma patient
- How to choose an appropriate destination for a critical trauma patient

In Chapter 7, "Scene Size-Up," you learned about mechanism of injury. Although using a mechanism of injury to predict specific injuries is not yet an exact science, you learned that you can still gain important information about the amount of force involved, the directions of those forces, and the obstacles the patient might have struck. This can give you a general indication of the nature and severity of injury to expect.

Then, in the last few chapters, you learned how to manage those injuries. In each case, there was an assumption that the patient had at most one other problem. (For example, the presence of a head injury would lead you to suspect a spine injury.) This is often the case, but not always. Although the number of deaths from vehicular trauma is decreasing, EMTs must be prepared for situations where the patient has multiple injuries, also known as "multiple trauma."

NOTE *There are no objectives in the National Standard Curriculum that pertain to the material in this chapter.*

MULTIPLE TRAUMA

The multiple-trauma patient has more than one serious injury. For example, a patient with crush injuries to the chest and a painful, swollen, deformed extremity is a multiple-trauma patient. Although multiple internal organs may be involved, a patient who has a crush injury to the chest, and no other apparent injuries, is not considered to be a multiple-trauma patient.

When the mechanism of injury suggests that your patient has more than one injury, decisions beyond what are called for on more typical EMS runs become necessary. For example, consider the patient who is reported to have an angulated forearm: Your initial assessment reveals him to be unresponsive with the airway partially occluded by his tongue. Do you spend the time applying a rigid splint to the limb? The answer in this case is no. This patient has life-threatening injuries that can only be treated in a hospital emergency department or operating room. Spending additional time at the scene to treat an injury that is not life-threatening may reduce the patient's chances of survival.

Now consider an alert patient with no signs or symptoms of shock who has pain and tenderness in the middle of his thigh as well as an angulated forearm. In this case, the patient is stable enough to allow you a few minutes to apply a splint and prevent further injury. In each of these two examples, an EMT's actions should be intended to provide the most benefit to the patient, while at the same time reducing the risk as much as possible.

These decisions are made easier when your crew works well together, each member knowing what to expect from another. This is called *teamwork*. Crew members also must be aware of the importance of moving a multiple-trauma patient to definitive care as soon as possible, since it is rarely possible for EMS providers (even EMT-Paramedics) to truly stabilize a trauma patient in the field. This is called *timing*. Finally, the appropriate destination must be chosen for the patient. This is a *transport* decision. In areas where some hospitals are designated trauma centers, it is important that protocols specify which patients need to be taken there and when it is (and is not) appropriate for EMS to bypass another hospital.

Cultural Considerations

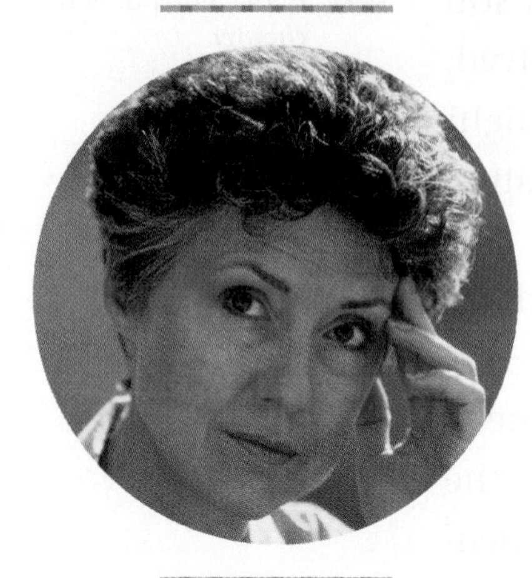

Some ethnic groups, such as Asian, Anglo-Saxon, and Irish, do not openly express pain. People of Italian and Jewish descent are more likely to use both verbal and nonverbal methods to express pain freely.

Children have individualized responses, and younger children have had less time to acquire culturally learned behaviors. If your patient is an adult, however, you might keep in mind that she may belong to one of those groups that values stoicism—in other words, she may be experiencing more pain than she is letting on.

Integrating the three "Ts"—*teamwork, timing,* and *transport*—into your management of a multiple-trauma patient will help things go smoother and more efficiently for the patient.

MANAGING THE MULTIPLE-TRAUMA PATIENT

The following scenario describes a typical multiple-trauma call. As you read, ask yourself these questions: When does the EMT recognize that the patient has multiple injuries? What is his first decision about managing those injuries, and why do you think he made it? What priorities does he set for his patient?

A Typical Call

You receive a call for a motorcyclist who was hit by a car. The scene is safe, so you approach the patient, an adult male you estimate to be about 25 years old. He appears unresponsive in a pool of blood on the road and is not wearing a helmet (Figure 30-1). Police point about 20 feet away to the motorcycle he was riding.

The patient responds purposefully to a painful stimulus; that is, he tries to push your hand away. He is making gurgling sounds with each breath, so you suction some blood out of his airway. He also is making snoring sounds, so you insert an oropharyngeal airway, which he tolerates and which eliminates the snoring sounds. His breathing is shallow and labored at a rate of about 30, so you have your partner ventilate him with a bag-valve mask and high-concentration oxygen as she simultaneously stabilizes his head with her knees.

There is a pool of blood around the patient's left thigh, which appears angulated. You quickly cut away the left leg of his pants so you can apply direct pressure with a sterile dressing and a pressure bandage to an apparent compound angulated midshaft femur fracture. The patient's radial pulse is rapid and weak. Skin is pale and sweaty.

You assign this patient a high priority for rapid treatment and transport based on mechanism of injury, altered mental status, and presence of shock (hypoperfusion). You cannot request ALS backup, because you work in a BLS system.

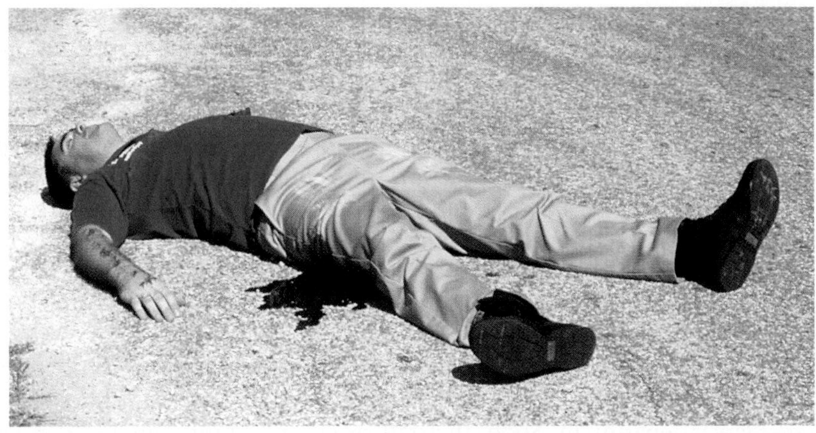

Figure 30-1 • Unresponsive adult male patient, victim of a motorcycle-passenger vehicle collision.

You perform a rapid trauma assessment. At the same time, a firefighter with whom you have worked before gets a long backboard and the other equipment necessary to immobilize the patient. By the time he returns, you have finished the rapid trauma assessment and gained the following information: a hematoma (lump) is present on the left side of the patient's head, neck veins are flat, there is no deformity of the cervical spine, breath sounds are decreased on the left side of his chest, his abdomen is soft, pelvis seems stable, there is an obvious compound angulated midshaft femur fracture on the left side, there are some nonbleeding lacerations on the left forearm and lower leg, and pulses are weak but palpable in all extremities.

With a cervical collar in place on the patient, you roll him as a unit and examine his spine and posterior trunk. You find no further injuries. You roll him down on the board, taking care to move the injured leg as little as possible once it is in the anatomical position.

As you quickly immobilize the patient on the board (using the board as a splint for the fractured femur), you make sure the firefighter is available to drive the ambulance so you and your partner can tend to the patient in back. You make sure the firefighter knows you are to go to the trauma center, not the community hospital that is 5 minutes closer. Your protocols specify that you are to go directly to the trauma center under conditions such as these because of the comprehensive care available there.

You move the patient and board onto the stretcher and into the ambulance, making sure your partner is able to continue ventilating him during the move. Once inside the patient compartment, you repeat the initial assessment. Your general impression is of a young adult male with multiple injuries. His mental status remains unchanged: he again tries to brush your hand away when you apply a painful stimulus. His tongue is prevented from obstructing his airway by an oropharyngeal airway. There is a little bit of gurgling when you listen carefully, so you suction some more blood out of his mouth. There are now no abnormal sounds as your partner ventilates him. Oxygen is flowing, and you see the patient's chest rise with each breath. The pressure dressing you applied to the open thigh wound has not bled through, and you see no other wounds that are bleeding. Radial pulse is rapid and weak. The patient is still a high priority.

With a second initial assessment completed, you call the trauma center and notify them of the patient's condition and your estimated time of arrival (10 minutes). You tell them you will give them vital signs as soon as you get them. With the hospital preparing for the patient's arrival, you turn to obtaining vital signs. Pulse is 108, weak and regular, blood pressure 100/80, respirations assisted at 12 per minute, skin pale and sweaty. You relay this information to the trauma center.

You have a few minutes before you arrive, so you check with your partner to make sure she is still able to ventilate the patient well before you perform a detailed physical exam. You find equal pupils that are slow to react, a hematoma (lump) on the left side of his head, nothing unusual in or behind the ears, deformity on both sides of his mandible (you conclude this is what is causing the bleeding into his airway), flat neck veins (you are unable to palpate the cervical spine because the cervical collar is in place), breath sounds are still decreased on the left side of his chest, his abdomen seems to be firmer than before, pelvis seems stable, there is an obvious compound midshaft femur fracture on the left side (it is no longer angulated because you straightened it out when you put the patient on the board), and there are some nonbleeding lacerations on the left forearm and lower leg. It is more difficult now to palpate peripheral pulses.

You would like to apply a traction splint but realize you do not have enough time or personnel. With just a few minutes before you arrive at the trauma center, you repeat the initial assessment one more time. The patient still responds purposefully to painful stimuli, but now he also opens his eyes briefly when you pinch him. You find no other changes. You get another set of vital signs: pulse 120, blood pressure 90 by palpation, respirations assisted at 12 per minute, skin pale and sweaty.

You arrive at the emergency department and give a report to the team as you transfer your patient to their bed. The patient's mental status continues to improve in the emergency department. Soon, the staff stops ventilating him and removes the airway. The patient becomes conscious, although confused and disoriented. The staff stabilizes his vital signs for the moment. There will be a slight delay before the patient leaves the emergency department for further tests, so the staff asks you and your partner to apply a traction splint to the patient's fractured femur. You are able to do so quickly and efficiently. The patient goes off for further tests and surgery.

Later you learn that the patient had a cerebral contusion (bruise of the brain), bilateral fracture of the mandible, left hemothorax (blood in the left side of the chest cavity), and a fractured femur.

After a lengthy stay, the patient is able to walk out of the hospital with some temporary assistance from a pair of crutches.

Analysis of the Call

The previous scenario shows an example of a patient who has critical injuries. Immediate threats to his life included shock (hypoperfusion) and bleeding into an airway that was partially obstructed by his tongue. Other serious injuries included an apparent head injury, inadequate ventilation, a presumed chest injury, a mandible injury, a compound angulated femur fracture, and a suspected spine injury (based on mechanism of injury). The EMT in the scenario gave his patient the best possible chance of survival by following the priorities determined by his assessments.

The initial assessment revealed several immediate threats to life that the EMT could do something about:

- The airway was partially obstructed by blood, which he suctioned.
- The patient's tongue was partially blocking the airway, causing snoring sounds with breathing, for which he inserted an artificial airway.
- Breathing was shallow and labored at a rate of about 30, which described inadequate ventilation, for which the EMT's partner instituted assisted ventilations with high-concentration oxygen.

The EMT then picked up on the seriousness of the patient's condition and made the decision not to treat some injuries the way he ordinarily would. That is, normally he would have applied a traction splint and dressed and bandaged the limb lacerations. Although it was tempting to do so, he realized this would delay transport for a patient who might have very little time to waste. A patient who has bleeding into his airway does not have any time to spare. Accordingly, he used a backboard as a universal splint for the femur and did not bandage the lacerations because they were not bleeding.

Some might say the EMT in the scenario was wrong and should have applied the traction splint in the field. After all, the emergency department staff later asked him to do it, right? In fact, the EMT showed good judgment. The appropriate place to apply a traction splint to this patient was in the emergency department, not in the field. When the emergency department staff asked him to apply the splint, it was because the patient was stable enough (and because the EMT was more familiar with the device than they were). If the patient's condition had not improved, they would not have asked him to put the splint on. Instead, the patient would have been whisked away for surgery or further tests.

There were two ways in which the EMT showed good judgment: he postponed taking vital signs, and he gave the hospital staff time to prepare. That is, the patient was ready to be put in the ambulance before the EMT was able to get vital signs, so he appropriately postponed taking them until they were en route. As tempting as it might be to complete an assessment all at once, the EMT realized that vital signs were not going to change anything he could do and taking them would delay transport. He also called the hospital and gave them an admittedly incomplete report so that they could prepare properly. He made sure to tell them he would get vital signs as soon as possible and then he did. This gave the hospital some additional time to notify the trauma team.

General Principles of Multiple-Trauma Management

Prepare for a call to a multiple-trauma patient by practicing for it. If you are on a regular crew, determine roles beforehand. For example, someone should be designated to manually immobilize the patient's head and, if necessary, ventilate with a bag-valve mask. Depending on the number of people available, you may have to have each person handle several roles. En route to the call, if you have reason to believe you might care for a multiple-trauma patient, review the roles each person will have.

At the scene, follow the steps of assessment as you learned them in your EMT course. Follow the priorities you discover in your initial assessment (airway, breathing, and circulation). Then balance the need for scene interventions with the time needed to perform them. As you may recall, the concept of the "golden hour" refers to the need for critical trauma patients to get to surgery within 1 hour of injury (not 1 hour from when you get to the patient). Although the time the patient has to get to surgery has not been scientifically proven to be an hour, the concept is still a useful one in avoiding delays at the scene.

For most critical patients, limit scene treatment to:

- Suctioning the airway
- Inserting an oral or nasal airway
- Restoring a patent airway by sealing a sucking chest wound
- Ventilating with a bag-valve mask
- Administering high-concentration oxygen
- Controlling bleeding
- Immobilizing the patient with a cervical collar and a long backboard

Principles of multiple-trauma management also include the following:

- *Scene safety is paramount.* Different kinds of trauma tend to have different kinds of dangers. Blunt trauma, which is more common in rural and suburban areas, can be associated with such dangers as bent power poles, leaking fuel, sharp glass and metal edges, and passing traffic. Penetrating trauma, such as stab wounds and gunshot wounds, tend to occur more commonly in urban areas. Risks you will need to consider include presence of the assailant (especially one who is upset because you are trying to save a person he tried to kill), presence of multiple weapons (on the victim, assailant, and bystanders), absent or delayed police response, and angry crowds.
- *Ensure an open airway.* If you are unable to ventilate your patient without assistance, try other approaches until you find one that works. You might get another person to assist you en route or you might have to switch places with your partner. Other alternatives include using a different device to ventilate, such as a pocket mask with supplemental oxygen, or you and your partner may have to work together to ventilate the patient.

- *Perform urgent or emergency moves as necessary.* For example, if a critical patient is sitting in a vehicle, you will need to perform a rapid extrication.
- *Adapt to the situation.* When a patient is trapped, for example, and part of the patient's body is not accessible, assess as much of him as you can. Keep in mind that when he is extricated you will need to perform a complete examination.

For a multiple-trauma patient, your overall goal is to treat immediate threats to life, which you can treat with prompt transportation to a facility that will provide definitive care (or as close to it as is available). Guard against the temptation in these cases to spend time at the scene treating all of the patient's injuries and immobilizing him perfectly. It is not good patient care to arrive at the hospital with the world's best-packaged corpse.

Trauma Scoring

In some EMS systems, hospitals ask EMTs and other providers not only to perform the usual assessment of trauma patients but also to evaluate trauma patients according to a numerical rating system. By evaluating certain patient characteristics and assigning a number to each of them, the provider can determine a score (a trauma score) that may do two things.

First, calculating the trauma score may help to determine whether a patient should go to a trauma center. A patient who needs the resources that a trauma center can provide (like 24-hour-a-day availability of trauma surgeons and nurses, operating rooms, special intensive care beds, etc.) should be transported there expeditiously. In rural areas, this typically means EMS transports to the local hospital where the patient receives enough care to quickly stabilize his condition as much as possible before he is transferred to a distant trauma center. In more densely populated areas where some local hos-

POINT OF VIEW

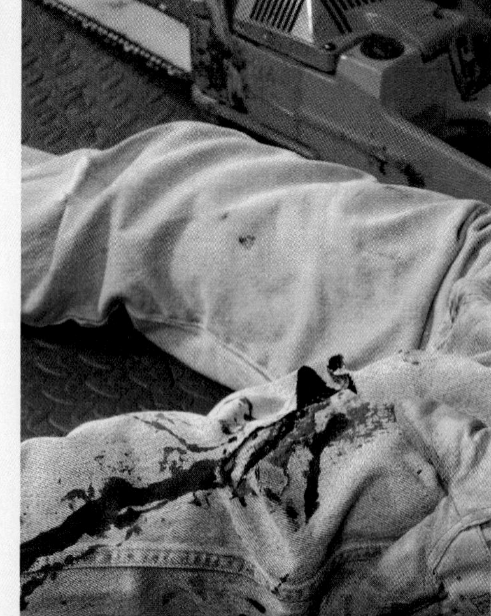

"I pulled the cord on my chainsaw. I really didn't think it would start. It had been in the garage for 2 or 3 years. Imagine my surprise when it fired up—which was nothing compared to my surprise when the saw slipped and cut into my leg.

"I don't remember much else, not even how I got to the ground. I do remember seeing blood and the room getting darker. Then I saw my wife . . . then the EMTs.

"As I came around, I figured it was just a bad cut on my leg. But the EMTs seemed pretty concerned. They were moving quickly. My wife looked worried. I heard the EMTs talking about my vital signs, and then they were moving me to the ambulance.

"On the way, I was a little more coherent. The EMTs told me that they were taking precautions because my pulse was a little high. The leg wound was pretty deep. They took me to a larger hospital close to the city—not my usual hospital. Turns out it was a good thing. I had a lot of muscle and nerve damage, and the hospital where they took me had the staff and equipment to deal with it.

"It was a tough day. My surgeon said the EMTs did a good job by realizing that my leg—and me—were in bad shape and deciding to take me to a hospital that could handle special surgery. A good decision. One I am very grateful for."

pitals are trauma centers and some are not, there will be local protocols describing when EMS should transport a patient directly to a trauma center, even if it is necessary to go past a hospital that is not a trauma center. This is where a trauma scoring system can help. By objectively describing the severity of a patient's condition, the score can direct more severely injured patients directly to trauma centers and allow less seriously injured patients to go to local hospitals.

The second major function of a trauma scoring system is to allow trauma centers to evaluate themselves in comparing the outcomes of trauma patients who have similar severity of injuries. In this way, they can improve the quality of care their trauma patients receive and conduct research on trauma care.

Several systems are in use to achieve these purposes. One of the most useful and widely utilized is the Revised Trauma Score (RTS). The RTS evaluates three characteristics of the patient's condition: Glasgow Coma Scale or GCS (which you learned about in Chapter 29, "Injuries to the Head and Spine"), systolic blood pressure, and respiratory rate. The original trauma score included other characteristics that were difficult to evaluate consistently under field conditions and turned out to be unnecessary.

Figure 30-2 shows the values assigned to the EMT's assessment findings in the Revised Trauma Score. Up to four points are assigned for each of the elements of the RTS. The lower the score, the more seriously injured the patient is and the less likely he will survive, even with excellent care.

Follow your local protocol for use of a trauma scoring system, but do not let it interfere with patient care. Manage airway problems and control other immediate threats to life before trying to use a score. In some systems, EMTs are asked to determine the score en route. In others, they may be asked simply to gather all the elements used to calculate the score, but not to assign numerical values. By reporting this information, a physician or nurse at an emergency department can calculate the score and advise you on the appropriate destination for your patient. Follow your local protocol.

REVISED TRAUMA SCORE

Characteristic	Criterion	RTS Points	
Glasgow Coma Scale	13-15	4	
	9-12	3	
	6-8	2	
	4-5	1	
	3	0	
Systolic Blood Pressure	> 89 mmHg	4	
	76-89 MmHg	3	
	50-75 MmHg	2	
	1-49 MmHg	1	
	0	0	
Respiratory Rate	10-29/min	4	
	> 29/min	3	
	6-9/min	2	
	1-5/min	1	
	0	0	
Revised Trauma Score (Total)			

Source: Champion HR, Sacco WJ, Copes WS, et al. A Revision of the Trauma Score. J Trauma 29 (5): 623-9, 1989

Figure 30-2 • Revised Trauma Score.

CRITICAL DECISION MAKING:
FALLING FOR YOUR ATTENTION

A determination of criticality (whether the patient has a serious condition or not) is one of the most important decisions you can make for the trauma patient. Just identifying when the *potential* for serious injury exists is vital. Your patient priority and transport decisions are based on these determinations. Assume you have a local hospital 15 minutes away and a trauma center 25 minutes away. Determine which patients should be transported to the trauma center and which could be transported to the local hospital—and explain why.

1. Your 30-year-old patient fell 4 feet from a ladder and got his lower leg caught in a rung. He believes he broke his lower left leg. His pulse is 96 strong and regular, respirations 18 and adequate, blood pressure 126/86, pupils equal and reactive to light, skin warm and dry. He is alert. There are distal pulses in the extremity.
2. Your patient is an 8-year-old male who fell 8–10 feet from a tree to the ground. He is holding his right wrist and says it hurts. As you talk with him and his parents, you note that he appears confused. As you move him to the ambulance, you believe his mental status is decreasing. Pulse 82 strong and regular, respirations 24, blood pressure 122/86, pupils equal and sluggishly reactive to light, mental status as noted above.
3. Your patient is a 32-year-old female who is 30 weeks pregnant and fell down a flight of stairs. She struck her head and has pain in her left shoulder. Her main concern is the brisk vaginal bleeding that began since the fall.

CHAPTER REVIEW

SUMMARY

The multiple-trauma patient has conflicting needs. He requires treatment of his injuries at the same time that he requires prompt transport to a facility that can provide definitive treatment. The EMT must balance and meet these competing needs in a way that provides the most benefit for the patient. Teamwork, timing, and transport are important elements in a plan to provide quality trauma care. Practice and planning are also essential if a critical trauma patient is to get the care he needs in the field and in the hospital.

REVIEW QUESTIONS

1. What considerations must the EMT weigh when considering whether to perform an intervention at the scene? (pp. 797–798)
2. What are the interventions that should generally be performed for a critical trauma patient at the scene? (p. 797)
3. When might it be appropriate for EMTs to bypass a closer hospital for a trauma center? (pp. 793, 798)
4. What are the three "Ts" of multiple-trauma patient management? (pp. 793–794)
5. When might it be appropriate not to apply a traction splint in the field to an obviously fractured femur? (pp. 796–797, 798)

CRITICAL THINKING

A controversy exists regarding whether patients with penetrating trauma, such as stab and gunshot wounds, should have spine immobilization before transport.

- What factors would have to be considered in this type of case?
- What do your local protocols say about this topic?

Thinking and Linking

Think back to Chapter 17, "Cardiac Emergencies," and link information from that chapter with information from this chapter, "Putting It All Together for the Trauma Patient," as you consider the following situation:

- Your patient is a 50-year-old male who has been electrocuted and knocked forcefully to the ground. He's an electrician who thought the power was off when it wasn't. You are taking his vital signs, which seem to be normal, when suddenly he goes into cardiac arrest. Should you use the AED and treat it as a medical arrest . . . or should you transport him immediately without using the AED as for a trauma arrest? Why?

MEDIA RESOURCES 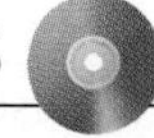

See the Student CD at the back of this book for quizzes, a case study activity and other features related to this chapter. In particular, look at the Case Study about setting priorities when treating a multiple-trauma patient. Also, visit the Companion Website for *Emergency Care* at **www.prenhall.com/limmer**, where you will find additional reinforcement and links to other resources.

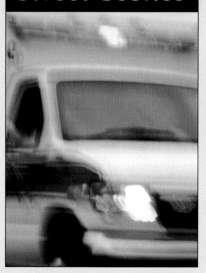

Street Scenes

At 9:15 a.m. your BLS ambulance is dispatched to a busy intersection for a motor-vehicle collision. While responding, you are advised by dispatch that she has had several 911 calls regarding this collision and that there are two vehicles involved. As you arrive on scene, you observe that a full-size pick-up truck apparently struck a smaller compact vehicle head on. Your partner strategically places the ambulance to protect the scene. You notice two occupants slumped over inside the small vehicle, which has fluid draining from under the engine.

Street Scene Questions

1. What is your initial impression of the collision?
2. What additional resources will be necessary on-scene?

The driver of the pick-up truck walks over to you and says that he bumped his head but he feels okay. Since he can walk and talk, you move toward the smaller car. As you approach, you note that both air bags have deployed and that the leaking fluid appears to be antifreeze, which does not pose a danger. You call for additional ambulances and make sure the police are en route. The male driver is wearing a full shoulder and lap restraint and appears conscious but "dazed." You notice his unrestrained passenger lying on her left side across the console motionless. Your initial assessment of the passenger reveals an approximately 25-year-old female responding to verbal stimuli, verbally abusive, and unaware of her surroundings. She is crying and complaining of pain to her right arm. Her airway appears clear as you notice she has sustained severe facial trauma. Her respirations appear slightly labored and shallow. You note a strong and rapid radial pulse and warm and dry skin.

Street Scene Questions

3. Which patient should be transported first?
4. What is your critical decision regarding the female patient?
5. What critical interventions should you perform on-scene?

You realize that the woman is the priority because of her altered mental status and labored respirations. She has a large laceration, which extends from her upper lip up through her hair line, and you observe angulation to her right humerus. Because of the mechanism of injury and the patient's current status, you decide to perform a rapid extrication. You place a cervical collar on her and spin her onto a board. When she yells, "My baby! Don't hurt my baby!" you note her large abdomen, which is consistent with pregnancy. You place padding under the right side of the backboard, which moves the patient onto her left side. This prevents the baby from compressing the vena cava, which could lower blood pressure. You move her to the ambulance with 15 liters of oxygen by nonrebreather mask in place.

Once in the ambulance, you suction blood that has begun to drain into her mouth from the facial laceration. Her initial vital signs show a pulse rate of 122, slightly labored respirations at a rate of 28, and a blood pressure of 142/94. Her pupils appear equal and reactive, and you notice no fluid exiting the ears. Her neck veins are flat and her trachea appears midline. You expose the patient, auscultate lung sounds, and find the right side sounds diminished, coinciding with tenderness to the right side of her chest. As you assess her large abdomen, she winces and again yells about her baby. You recheck her arm and notice angulation and crepitus. You align it and secure her arm alongside her torso, which acts as a splint. Her remaining extremities appear unremarkable. Your patient's level of responsiveness is not reliable enough for a medical history, but you notice she is wearing a medical identification tag, which states she is allergic to sulfa medication.

Street Scene Questions

6. What further information would you like to obtain about the female patient?
7. To what type of receiving facility should your patient be transported?

While en route to the hospital, you notice the patient's heart rate has increased to 128, her blood pressure has fallen to 122/86, and she is now guarding her abdomen with her left arm. You have contacted medical direction and have been advised to transport the patient to the nearest trauma center. Upon arrival at the trauma center, you update the staff and transfer the patient to their care.

Street Scenes Sample Documentation

PATIENT NAME: *Jan Jackson* PATIENT AGE: *Approx. 25*

CHIEF COMPLAINT

Multi-trauma

PAST MEDICAL HISTORY

- [ ] None
- [x] Allergy to *Sulfa*
- [ ] Hypertension
- [ ] Stroke
- [ ] Seizures
- [ ] Diabetes
- [ ] COPD
- [ ] Cardiac
- [ ] Other (List)
- [ ] Asthma

Unknown

Current Medications (List)

Unknown

VITAL SIGNS

TIME	RESP	PULSE	B.P.	MENTAL STATUS	R PUPILS L	SKIN
0922	Rate: *28*; [x] Shallow; [x] Labored; [ ] Regular	Rate: *122*; [x] Regular; [ ] Irregular	*142/94*	[x] Voice; [ ] Alert; [ ] Pain; [ ] Unresp.	R: [x] Normal; L: [x] Normal	[x] Warm; [x] Dry
0927	Rate: *28*; [x] Shallow; [x] Labored; [ ] Regular	Rate: *128*; [x] Regular; [ ] Irregular	*122/86*	[x] Voice; [ ] Alert; [ ] Pain; [ ] Unresp.	R: [x] Normal; L: [x] Normal	[x] Warm; [x] Dry
	Rate: ; [ ] Regular; [ ] Shallow; [ ] Labored	Rate: ; [ ] Regular; [ ] Irregular	/	[ ] Alert; [ ] Voice; [ ] Pain; [ ] Unresp.	[ ] Normal; [ ] Dilated; [ ] Constricted; [ ] Sluggish; [ ] No-Reaction	[ ] Unremarkable; [ ] Cool; [ ] Pale; [ ] Warm; [ ] Cyanotic; [ ] Moist; [ ] Flushed; [ ] Dry; [ ] Jaundiced

(Unchecked options in the first two rows: Pupils — Dilated, Constricted, Sluggish, No-Reaction; Skin — Unremarkable, Cool, Pale, Cyanotic, Moist, Flushed, Jaundiced.)

NARRATIVE *Responded to a motor-vehicle collision at Algonquin intersection. Upon arrival, found approximately 25-year-old female lying left lateral recumbent across center of vehicle. Patient appeared to be the unrestrained passenger of compact vehicle that received head-on impact from full-size pick-up truck travelling approx. 45 mph. Airbags were deployed. Initial assessment showed patient responsive to verbal stimuli but unaware of surroundings and unable to recall incident. Obvious bleeding noted to facial region with no apparent compromise to airway. Skin warm and dry. Rapidly extricated patient onto spine board and immobilized with straps, c-collar, and head blocks and initiated high-concentration O_2 and rapid transport. Change in patient position (recumbent on backboard) required constant suctioning of airway from facial laceration (full thickness from patient's upper lip to unknown point on top of head). Head, ears, eyes, nose, and throat clear except for facial laceration. Neck/trachea unremarkable. Chest—noted point tenderness to right chest wall with accompanied diminished lung sounds to that side; left side normal. Abdomen is tender to touch in all four quadrants, with pregnancy noted. Padding placed under right side of backboard to displace patient to left. Deformed right humerus splinted in place. Pulses, motor function, and sensation intact x 4. Contacted the emergency department and received orders to divert to nearest Level One trauma center. Upon arrival, updated the waiting staff and transferred patient and care. No changes at the time.*

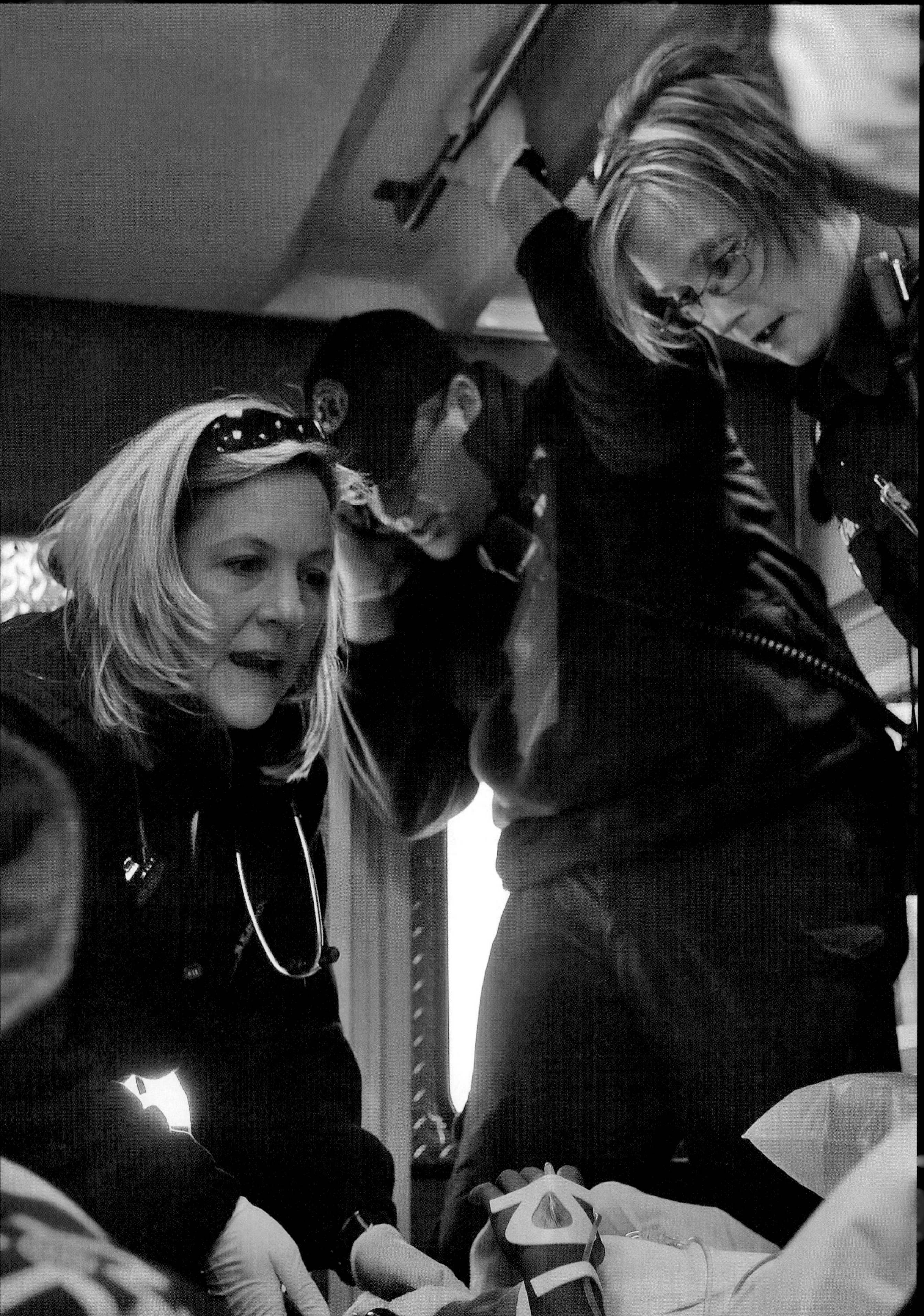

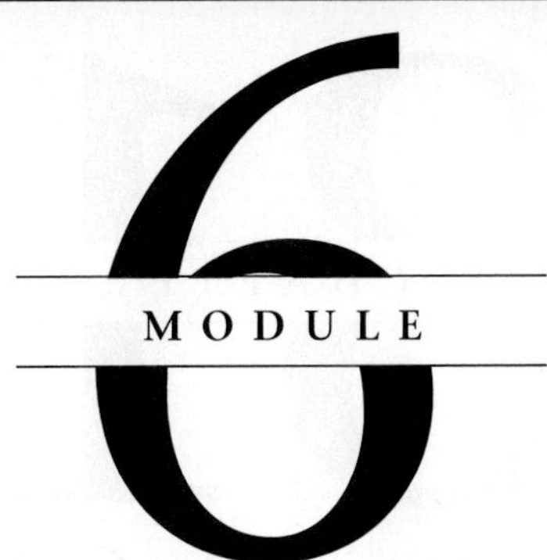

MODULE

Special Patient Populations

There are special considerations when it comes to younger and older patients, but for these patients you will find that you will be able to adapt the basics of patient assessment and care that you have already learned.

Emergencies involving infants and children (Chapter 31) are less common than those for adults. However, there is a special emotional component to treating a critically injured or ill child. Children often have the same medical and trauma problems as adults. The difference in treating them often lies in understanding the differences in their anatomy and physiology and their behavioral and emotional development.

Today the EMT is likely to encounter a number of patients with special needs (Chapter 32) who have advanced medical devices in their homes that enable them to live and function outside a hospital setting. The emergency call to such a patient may involve the underlying medical condition or may involve the medical device the patient depends on.

Elderly patients (Chapter 33) often have the same medical or trauma problems as other adults, but there are changes in human anatomy and physiology as we age, signs and symptoms may differ from those of younger adults, and there can be special communication challenges.

CHAPTER 31

Infants and Children

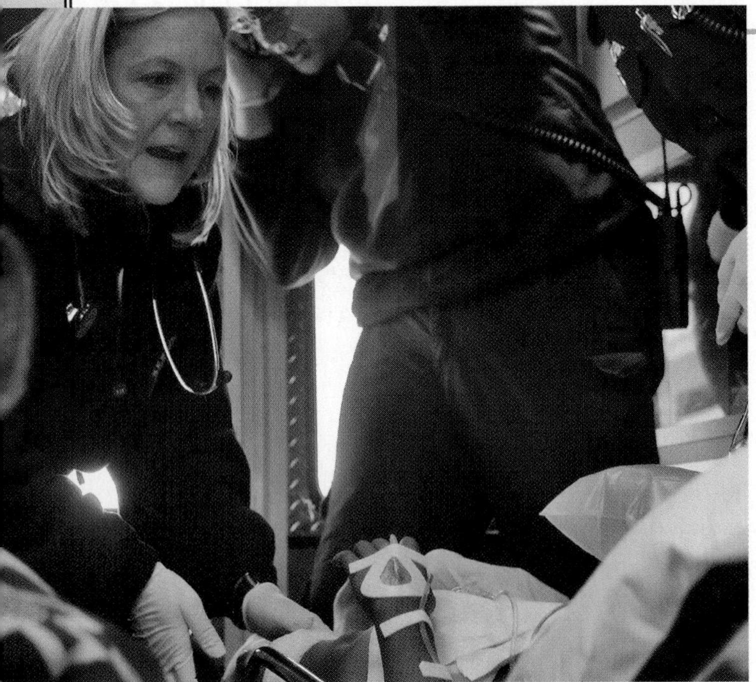

CORE CONCEPTS

The following are core concepts that will be addressed in this chapter:

- Ways of dealing with children of different ages and their parents or care providers
- Differences in anatomy between children and adults
- How to assess the pediatric patient
- How to maintain the pediatric patient's airway, oxygenation, and ventilation
- How to identify and treat respiratory conditions and other medical conditions in infants and children
- Differences between children and adults when identifying and dealing with shock and trauma
- How to deal with issues of child abuse and neglect and children with special needs

DOT OBJECTIVES

*KNOWLEDGE AND ATTITUDE

6-1.1 Identify the developmental considerations for the following age groups: (pp. 807–811)
- Infants
- Toddlers
- Preschool
- School age
- Adolescent

6-1.2 Describe differences in anatomy and physiology of the infant, child, and adult patient. (pp. 811–816)

6-1.3 Differentiate the response of the ill or injured infant or child (age specific) from that of an adult. (pp. 807–816)

6-1.4 Indicate various causes of respiratory emergencies. (pp. 837–841)

6-1.5 Differentiate between respiratory distress and respiratory failure. (pp. 837–841)

6-1.6 List the steps in the management of foreign body airway obstruction. (pp. 830–832)

6-1.7 Summarize emergency medical care strategies for respiratory distress and respiratory failure. (pp. 838–839)

6-1.8 Identify the signs and symptoms of shock (hypoperfusion) in the infant and child patient. (pp. 835–837)

6-1.9 Describe the methods of determining end organ perfusion in the infant and child. (pp. 835–837)

6-1.10 State the usual cause of cardiac arrest in infants and children versus adults. (pp. 837, 841)

6-1.11 List the common causes of seizures in the infant and child patient. (p. 844)

6-1.12 Describe the management of seizures in the infant and child patient. (p. 845)

6-1.13 Differentiate between the injury patterns in adults, infants, and children. (pp. 849–851)

6-1.14 Discuss the field management of the infant and child trauma patient. (p. 851)

6-1.15 Summarize the indicators of possible child abuse and neglect. (pp. 853–856)

6-1.16 Describe the medical/legal responsibilities in suspected child abuse. (pp. 856–857)

6-1.17 Recognize the need for EMT-Basic debriefing following a difficult infant or child transport. (p. 860)

6-1.18 Explain the rationale for having knowledge and skills appropriate for dealing with the infant and child patient. (pp. 807, 813–816)

6-1.19 Attend to the feelings of the family when dealing with an ill or injured infant or child. (p. 816)

6-1.20 Understand the provider's own response (emotional) to caring for infants or children. (p. 860)

*SKILLS

6-1.21 Demonstrate the techniques of foreign body airway obstruction removal in the infant.

6-1.22 Demonstrate the techniques of foreign body airway obstruction removal in the child.

6-1.23 Demonstrate the assessment of the infant and child.

6-1.24 Demonstrate bag-valve-mask artificial ventilations for the infant.

6-1.25 Demonstrate bag-valve-mask artificial ventilations for the child.

6-1.26 Demonstrate oxygen delivery for the infant and child.

The principles of assessing and managing the pediatric patient are similar to those for an injured or ill adult. Yet children are not just little adults. The EMT must be aware of the special characteristics of pediatric patients as well as some of the medical and trauma problems to which they are susceptible.

DEVELOPMENTAL CHARACTERISTICS OF INFANTS AND CHILDREN

Some important differences should be kept in mind when you are caring for a young patient. For example, since young children do not like to be separated from their parents, you will want to let the child sit in the parent's lap, if possible, during assessment and treatment (Figure 31-1). Children will exhibit different characteristics as they grow

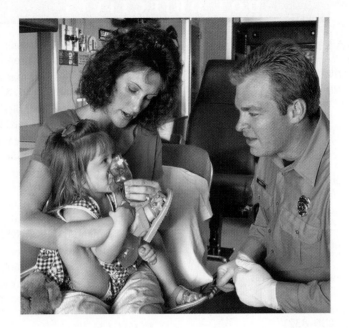

Figure 31-1 • If at all possible, let a young child sit in the parent's lap during assessment and care. (During transport, the child should be in a car seat or immobilized to a backboard.)

older, and these will require the EMT to adapt treatment strategies, depending on the patient's developmental age (Table 31-1). However, the psychological and social characteristics of infants and children cannot be specifically defined by their age. Key anatomical and physiological characteristics and their potential impact on care are summarized in Table 31-2.

Just as a 6-year-old child is different from a 35-year-old adult, so is a 4-week-old infant different from a 12-year-old child. Children are constantly growing and learning and hence changing. In an ideal world, we might be able to tell exactly how a 4-year-old will behave. In reality, we have to put children into broad categories according to how children of their age group behave on the average. No system of categorizing children is perfect, but each has advantages for particular uses. As this applies to the psychological and social characteristics, it is also true for physical development. Children grow at different rates, and size may not match social development.

After determining a child's age, if you are able to, attempt to have age-appropriate conversation with the child. If that doesn't seem to work, then observe the interaction with parent or caregiver for clues that might help you with assessment and treatment strategies.

For basic life support (rescue breathing and CPR), the American Heart Association defines an infant as ages birth to 1 year, a child as 1 year to puberty (where puberty can be identified by breast development in females and hair observed on the face, chest, or underarms of males). These age ranges defined for basic life support do not always apply to the care of children in other medical or trauma cases. In general emergency care, the following age categories are more useful to keep in mind:

- Newborns and infants: birth to 1 year
- Toddlers: 1 to 3 years
- Preschool: 3 to 6 years
- School age: 6 to 12 years
- Adolescent: 12 to 18 years

Age ranges will vary somewhat in different listings; for example, in vital sign ranges as shown in Table 31-3. There will be calls when it will not be possible to find out the patient's age and you will have to guess at the age, based on the child's physical size and emotional reactions.

TABLE 31-1 • Developmental Characteristics of Infants and Children

AGE GROUP	CHARACTERISTICS	ASSESSMENT AND CARE STRATEGIES
Newborns and Infants Birth to 1 year 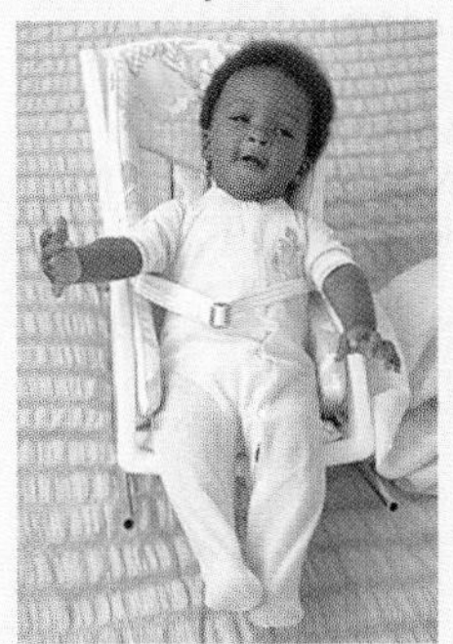	• Infants do not like to be separated from their parents. • There is minimal stranger anxiety. • Infants are used to being undressed but like to feel warm, physically and emotionally. • The younger infant follows movement with his eyes. • The older infant is more active, developing a personality. • They do not want to be "suffocated" by an oxygen mask.	• Have the parent hold the infant while you examine him. • Be sure to keep him warm—warm your hands and stethoscope before touching the infant. As infants can easily become hypothermic, keep the ambulance compartment warm and the child properly covered during cool or cold weather. • It may be best to observe breathing from a distance, noting the rise and fall of the chest, the level of activity, and skin color. • Examine the heart and lungs first and the head last. This is perceived as less threatening to the infant and therefore less likely to start him crying. • A pediatric nonrebreather mask may be held near the face to provide "blow-by" oxygen.
Toddlers 1 to 3 years 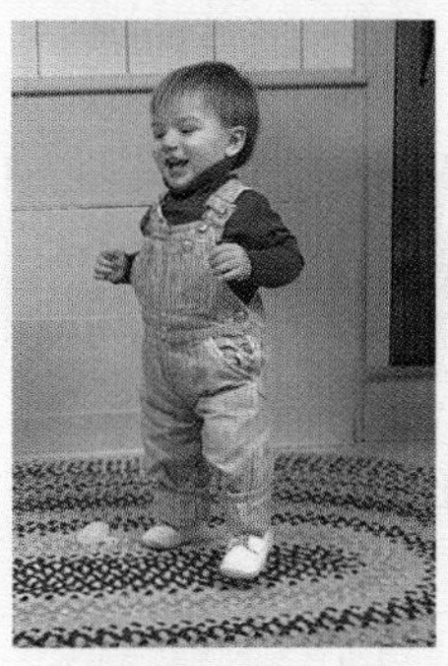	• Toddlers do not like to be touched or separated from their parents. • Toddlers may believe that their illness is a punishment for being bad. • Unlike infants, they do not like having their clothing removed. • They frighten easily, overreact, and have a fear of needles, pain. • Toddlers may understand more than they communicate. • They begin to assert their independence. • They do not want to be "suffocated" by an oxygen mask.	• Have a parent hold the child while you examine him. • Assure the child that he was not bad. • Remove an article of clothing, examine, and then replace the clothing. • Examine in a trunk-to-head approach to build confidence. (Touching the head first may be frightening.) • Explain what you are going to do in terms the toddler can understand (taking the blood pressure becomes a squeeze or a hug on the arm).
Preschool 3 to 6 years 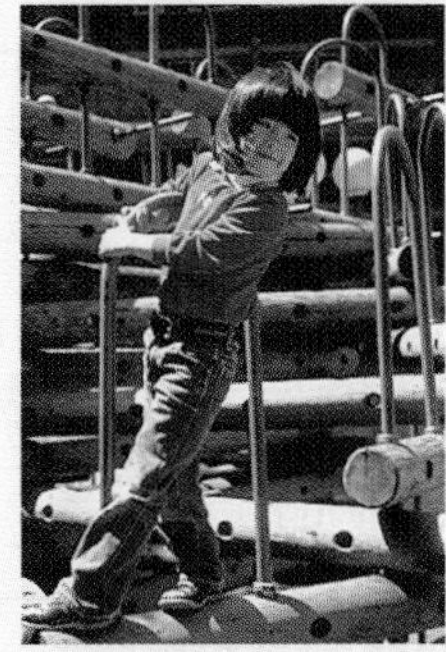	• Preschoolers do not like to be touched or separated from their parents. • They are modest and do not like their clothing removed. • Preschoolers may believe that their illness is a punishment for being bad. • Preschoolers have a fear of blood, pain, and permanent injury. • They are curious, communicative, and can be cooperative. • They do not want to be "suffocated" by an oxygen mask.	• Have a parent hold the child while you examine him. • Respect the child's modesty. Remove an article of clothing, examine, and then replace the clothing. • Have a calm, confident, reassuring, respectful manner. • Be sure to offer explanations about what you are doing. • Allow the child the responsibility of giving the history. • Explain as you examine. • A pediatric nonrebreather mask may be held near the face to provide "blow-by" oxygen.
School age 6 to 12 years 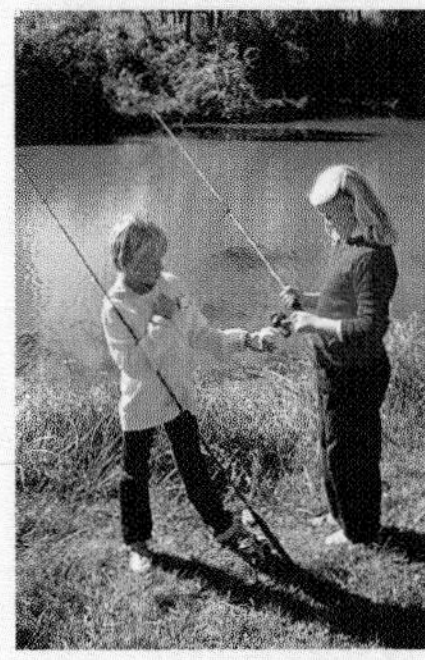	• This age group cooperates but likes their opinions heard. • They fear blood, pain, disfigurement, and permanent injury. • School-age children are modest and do not like their bodies exposed. (All photos on this page © Michal Heron.)	• Allow the child the responsibility of giving the history. • Explain as you examine. • Present a confident, calm, respectful manner. • Respect the child's modesty. *continued*

TABLE 31-1 • (Continued)

AGE GROUP	CHARACTERISTICS	ASSESSMENT AND CARE STRATEGIES
Adolescent 12 to 18 years	• Adolescents want to be treated as adults. • Adolescents generally feel that they are indestructible but may have fears of permanent injury and disfigurement. • Adolescents vary in their emotional and physical development and may not be comfortable with their changing bodies. (© Index Stock)	• Although they wish to be treated as adults, they may need as much support as children. • Present a confident, calm, respectful manner. • Be sure to explain what you are doing. • Respect modesty. You may consider assessing them away from their parents. Have the physical exam done by an EMT of the same sex as the patient if possible.

TABLE 31-2 • Anatomical and Physiological Characteristics of Infants and Children

ANATOMICAL AND PHYSIOLOGICAL DIFFERENCES COMPARED TO ADULTS	POTENTIAL IMPACT ON ASSESSMENT AND CARE
Tongue proportionally larger	More likely to block airway
Smaller airway structures	More easily blocked
Abundant secretions	Can block the airway
Deciduous (baby) teeth	Easily dislodged; can block the airway
Flat nose and face	Difficult to obtain good face mask seal
Head heavier relative to body and less-developed neck structures and muscles	Head may be propelled more forcefully than body, creating a higher incidence of head injury
Fontanelle and open sutures (soft spots) palpable on top of young infant's head	Bulging fontanelle can be a sign of intracranial pressure (but may be normal if infant is crying); sunken fontanelle may indicate dehydration
Thinner, softer brain tissue	Susceptible to serious brain trauma
Head larger in proportion to body	Head tips forward when supine, causing flexion of neck, making neutral alignment of cervical spine and airway difficult
Shorter, narrower, more elastic (flexible) trachea	Can close off trachea with hyperextension of neck
Short neck	Difficult to stabilize or immobilize
Abdominal breathers	Difficult to evaluate breathing
Faster respiratory rate	Muscles easily fatigue, causing respiratory distress
Newborns breathe primarily through the nose (obligate nose breathers)	May not automatically open mouth to breathe if nose is blocked; airway more easily blocked
Larger body surface relative to body mass	Prone to hypothermia
Softer bones	More flexible, less easily fractured; traumatic forces may be transmitted to, and injure, internal organs without fracturing ribs or other bones
More flexible ribs	Traumatic forces may be transmitted to chest cavity without fracturing ribs; lungs easily damaged with trauma
Spleen and liver more exposed	Injury likely with significant force to abdomen

Author: Andrew Stern, NREMT-P, MPA, MA.

TABLE 31-3 • Normal Vital Sign Ranges: Infants and Children		
NORMAL PULSE RATE (BEATS PER MINUTE, AT REST)		
Newborn	120 to 160	
Infant 0–5 months	90 to 140	
Infant 6–12 months	80 to 140	
Toddler 1–3 years	80 to 130	
Preschooler 3–5 years	80 to 120	
School age 6–10 years	70 to 110	
Adolescent 11–14 years	60 to 105	
NORMAL RESPIRATION RATE (BREATHS PER MINUTE, AT REST)		
Newborn	30 to 50	
Infant 0–5 months	25 to 40	
Infant 6–12 months	20 to 30	
Toddler 1–3 years	20 to 30	
Preschooler 3–5 years	20 to 30	
School age 6–10 years	15 to 30	
Adolescent 11–14 years	12 to 20	
BLOOD PRESSURE NORMAL RANGES		
	SYSTOLIC:	DIASTOLIC:
	APPROX. 80 PLUS 2 × AGE	APPROX. 2/3 SYSTOLIC
Preschooler 3–5 years	Average 99 (78 to 116)	Average 65
School age 6–10 years	Average 105 (80 to 122)	Average 69
Adolescent 11–14 years	Average 114 (88 to 140)	Average 76

Note: A high pulse in an infant or child is not as great a concern as a low pulse. A low pulse may indicate imminent cardiac arrest. Blood pressure is usually not taken in a child under 3 years. In cases of blood loss or shock, a child's blood pressure will remain within normal limits until near the end, then fall swiftly.

Psychological and Personality Characteristics

Each age group has its own general characteristics of psychology and personality that will affect the way you assess and care for the patient. These were outlined in Table 31-1.

Anatomical and Physiological Differences

Infants and children differ from adults not only in psychology but also in anatomy and physiology. (Review Table 31-2. Also review the special characteristics of infants and children in Chapter 4, "The Human Body.") Understanding some of these differences will help you do a better job of assessing and caring for young patients. Key differences have to do with the head, airway and respiratory system, chest and abdomen, body surface, and blood volume.

Head

A child's head is proportionately larger and heavier than an adult's until about the age of 4. The implication for emergency care is that you should suspect head injury whenever there is a serious mechanism of injury because a child is likely to be propelled forward head first.

Infants up to about 1 year or 18 months of age will have a "soft spot," or anterior fontanelle, which is flat and soft while the child is quiet. The fontanelle is just anterior to the center of the skull. A sunken fontanelle may indicate dehydration. A bulging fontanelle may indicate elevated intracranial pressure. The fontanelle also normally bulges when the infant is crying.

Airway and Respiratory System

The infant's and child's neck muscles are immature and the airway structures are narrower and less rigid than an adult's. There are several other special characteristics you should be aware of (Figure 31-2):

- The mouth and nose are smaller and more easily obstructed than in adults.
- The tongue takes up more space proportionately in the mouth than in adults.
- Newborns and infants are obligate nose breathers. This means they will not know to open their mouths to breathe when the nose becomes obstructed.
- The trachea (windpipe) is softer and more flexible in infants and children.
- The trachea is narrower and is easily obstructed by swelling or foreign objects.
- The chest wall is softer, and infants and children tend to depend more on their diaphragms for breathing.

These differences in respiratory anatomy pose several implications for the emergency treatment you provide to an infant or a child:

- Because infants are obligate nose breathers, be sure to suction secretions from the nose as needed to help the patient breathe.
- Hyperextension or flexion of the neck (tipping the head too far back or letting it fall forward) may result in airway obstruction. A folded towel under the shoulders of a supine infant or young child will help to keep the airway in a neutral in-line position (Figure 31-3).
- "Blind" finger sweeps are not performed when trying to clear an airway obstruction in an infant or child because your finger might force the obstruction back and wedge it in the narrow trachea. An attempt to remove a foreign body airway obstruction should be done only when the obstruction is directly observed.

Chest and Abdomen

The less developed and more elastic chest structures of an infant or child make labored or distressed breathing obvious from a distance. The muscles above the sternum and

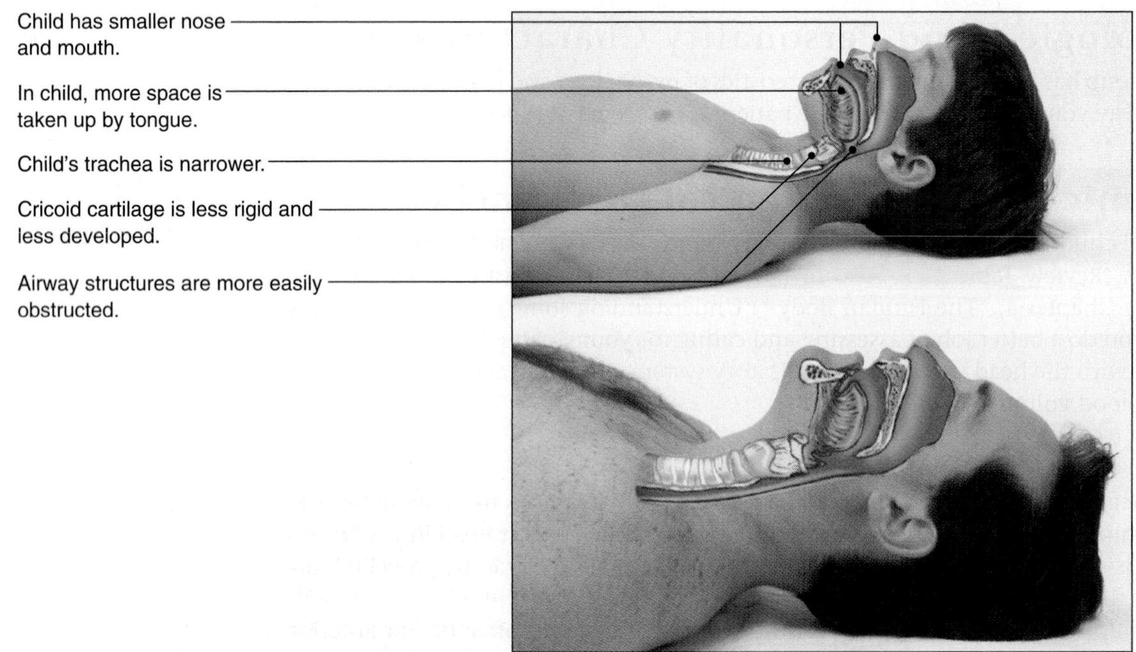
Child has smaller nose and mouth.
In child, more space is taken up by tongue.
Child's trachea is narrower.
Cricoid cartilage is less rigid and less developed.
Airway structures are more easily obstructed.

Figure 31-2 • Comparison of child and adult respiratory passages.

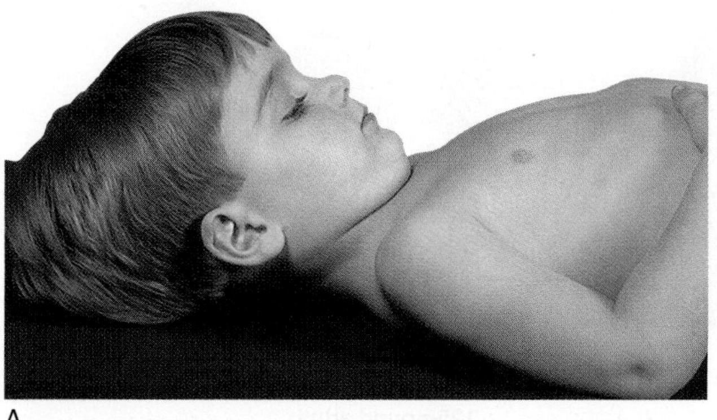

A

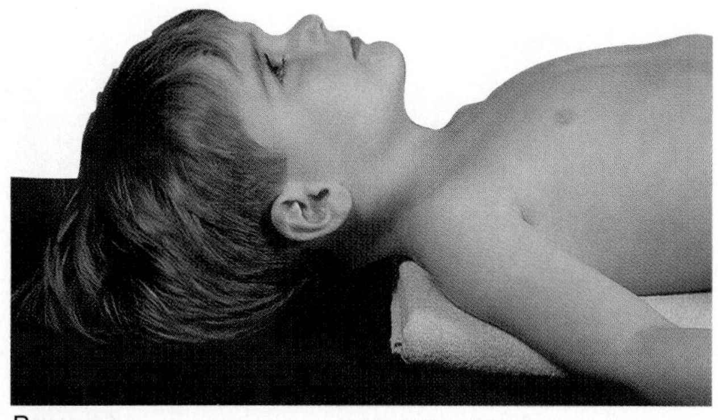

B

Figure 31-3 • (A) When an infant or young child is supine, the head will tip forward, obstructing the airway. (B) To keep the airway aligned, place a folded towel under the shoulders.

between the ribs, and the ribs themselves, will pull inward when breathing is labored. Infants and young children are abdominal breathers, using their diaphragms for breathing more than adults. Watch the abdomen as well as the chest to evaluate breathing.

In addition, the fact that musculoskeletal structures of the chest and abdomen are less well developed means that the vital organs are not as well protected from injury as are those of adults.

Body Surface

A child's body surface area is larger in proportion to the body mass, making the child more prone to heat loss through the skin. This makes infants and children more vulnerable to hypothermia, an abnormally low body temperature. (See Chapter 22, "Environmental Emergencies".) They must be kept covered and warm. Climate control in the patient compartment of the ambulance is very important.

With regard to burns, because an infant's or child's head, body, and extremities are proportioned differently from an adult's (the head being larger, for example), the extent of a burn is estimated differently for a child, using a special formula that was described in Chapter 27, "Soft-Tissue Injuries."

Blood Volume

As you would expect, the blood volume of a pediatric patient is less than the blood volume of an adult (Figure 31-4). A newborn does not have enough blood to fill a 12-ounce soda can, and an 8-year-old has only about 2 liters of blood. Therefore, a blood loss that might be considered moderate in an adult can be a life-threatening situation for a child.

Interacting with the Pediatric Patient

You will not be able to interview infants, and most toddlers are poor communicators. However, the parents or the care providers who called for help can usually provide a history of a small child's illness or injury.

Preschoolers can usually be interviewed if you take your time and keep your language simple. School-age children will be able to describe more clearly how they feel and what happened. They will talk with you honestly but may feel that the injury or illness is a punishment for something they did. They must be reassured and told it is all right to feel sick or hurt or to cry. Before telling the child something or asking him a question, take a second to think about how the child might interpret what you are about to say. This may help you to minimize the child's confusion or anxiety.

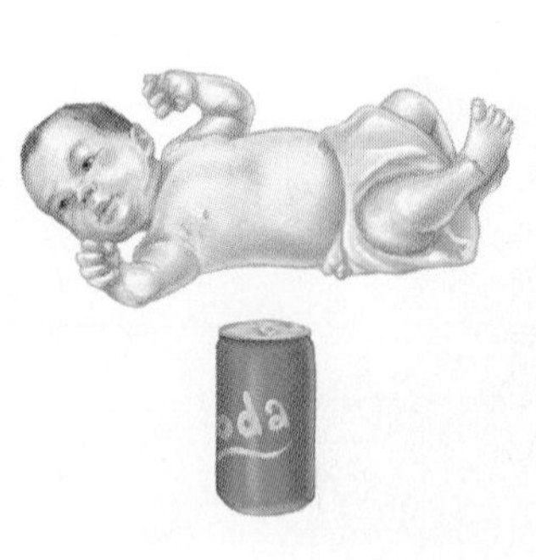

9-pound newborn:
Blood volume equals less than a 12-oz (335 ml) can of a soft drink

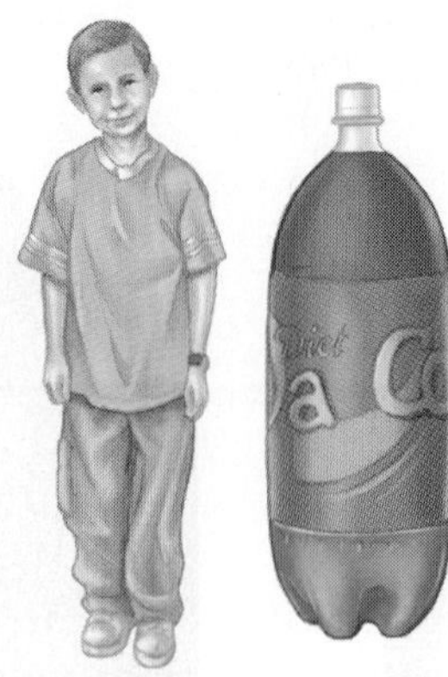

60-pound child:
Blood volume equals about a 2-liter bottle of a soft drink

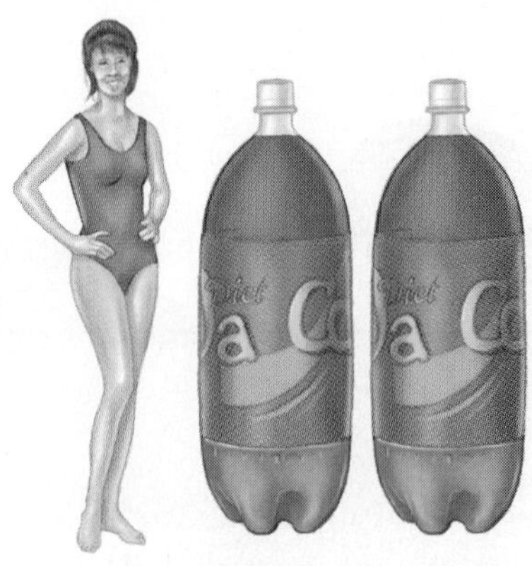

125-pound adult:
Blood volume equals about two 2-liter bottles of a soft drink

Figure 31-4 • Infant, child, and adolescent/adult blood volumes compared.

If parents, teachers, or care providers are at the scene, talk with them but do not exclude the child. Seeing that familiar adults are being included gains the child's confidence if you follow up by talking directly to the child. If the parents are injured, you may not be able to get information from them, and the child needs to know that someone is caring for his parent as well.

All patients have some degree of fear at the emergency scene. Infants and children are usually more fearful than adults because they lack experience with illness and injury. In addition to this, children are easily frightened by the unknown. Since so many details of the emergency scene are unknowns, it is easy to see why emergencies can be scary for children. The elements associated with the emergency (pain, noise, bright lights, cold) can set off a panic reaction in infants.

At an emergency, if the child does not understand you, or believes that you do not understand in return, fear will increase. If the child is to communicate, he must remain calm. Putting the child at ease is a very important part of the care you must provide. Some children, when stressed, will act like a younger child. This is called regression.

Any problems faced by the child will be intensified if the parents are not at the scene. Children find security by being with their parents when facing new problems or emergencies. Asking for mom or dad may be the child's first priority, even above that of having your help.

When dealing with pediatric patients you should:

1. Identify yourself simply by saying, "Hi, I'm Pat. What's your name?"
2. Let the child know that someone will call his parents.
3. Determine if there are life-threatening problems and treat them immediately. If there are no problems of this nature, continue at a relaxed pace. Fearful children cannot take the pressure of a rapidly paced assessment and confusing questions fired at them by a stranger.
4. Let the child have any nearby toy that he may want.
5. Kneel or sit at the child's eye level. Ensure that bright light is not directly behind you and shining into the child's eyes.
6. SMILE. This is a familiar sign from adults that reassures children.
7. Touch the child or hold his hand or foot. Very young children sometimes like to have their toes played with. A child who does not wish to be touched will let you know. Do not force the issue; smile and provide comfort through your conversation.
8. Do not use any equipment on the child without explaining what you will do with it. Many children fear the medical items that are so familiar to the EMT, thinking

they will cause pain. Always tell the child what you are going to do as you take vital signs and do a physical exam. Do not try to explain the entire procedure at once. Instead, explain each step as you do it. Use simple language and remember that children tend to take things literally. If you tell a young child, "I'm going to take your pulse," he may think you are going to take something away from him. Instead say, "I'm going to hold your wrist for a minute." If the child is older, explain why.

9. Let the child see your face, and make eye contact without staring at the child. (Staring makes children uncomfortable.) Speak directly to the child, making a special effort to speak clearly and slowly in words he can understand. Be sure the child can hear you.
10. Stop occasionally to find out if the child understands. Never assume the child understood you, but find out by asking questions if the child is old enough to respond.
11. NEVER LIE TO THE CHILD. Tell him when the examination may hurt. If the child asks if he is sick or hurt, be honest, but be sure to add that you are there to help and will not leave. Let the child know that other people also will be helping.

The Adolescent Patient

In many ways, adolescent patients are almost like adult patients. Certainly they like to be treated as adults and are very sensitive to violations of their dignity or a manner they believe is patronizing. However, when ill or injured or frightened, they often need as much emotional support as younger children (Figure 31-5).

Adolescents should be able to tell you exactly what happened and how they feel. However, in the presence of parents or peers, an adolescent patient may not be completely communicative or cooperative. When injured, scared, or anxious, an adolescent may act immaturely or "act out." He may be embarrassed, intimidated by the attention, trying to hide the fact that he was doing something wrong, or feel pressure to show bravado. Tact may be required to get information from the adolescent patient, and assessment may be more productive if this patient can be taken aside or into a private area.

Adolescents are especially sensitive to their peers and what they think. Adolescents may also be intimidated by those in authority, such as parents or teachers. Therefore, it is important to be very discrete when asking sensitive questions about drug or alcohol use and medical issues like a possible pregnancy. Such discussions should take place

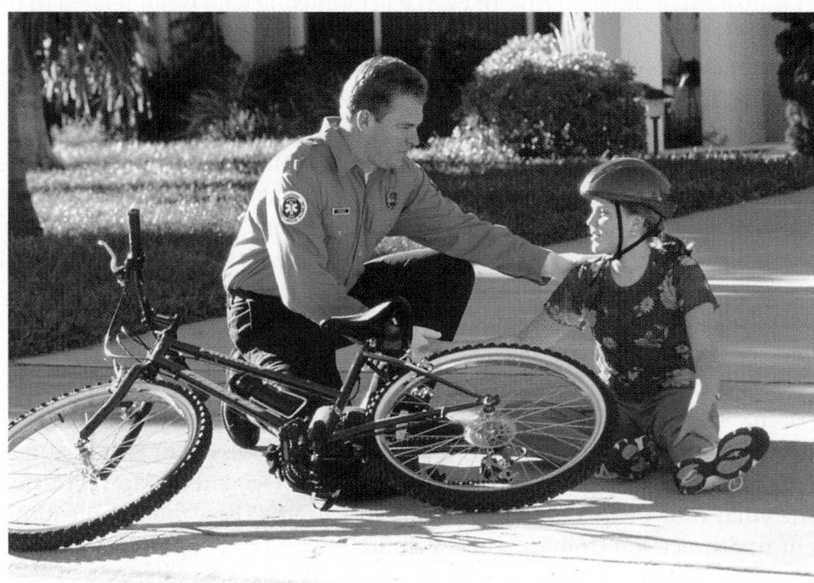

Figure 31-5 • Treat the adolescent with respect.

away from anyone who might overhear the conversation (for example, in the back of the ambulance or, if necessary, by waiting until you arrive at the hospital).

The young adolescent is often embarrassed or worried about the changes occurring to his or her body and uncertain if these changes are "normal." Handling the clothing of a teenager of the opposite sex can be awkward for the EMT as well as for the patient. In most cases, a simple preliminary description of the examination will set the patient at ease. However, you should make sure that both the adolescent and the parents understand what you are going to do and why it must be done. When possible, have the exam conducted by or in the presence of an EMT of the same sex as the patient.

However, do not delay patient evaluation and care because you or the patient may be embarrassed. As a professional, you must put such feelings aside and act in a manner that will allow the patient to relax and understand that there is no need for embarrassment.

SUPPORTING THE PARENTS OR OTHER CARE PROVIDERS

When your patient is young, you will need to make some adjustments in how you proceed with the assessment and care. This is especially true with regard to communicating with parents or other caregivers or providers. Children are very perceptive and will pick up on confidence as well as fear and anxiety in those they trust. What an EMT says, how he says it, and the calming influence he demonstrates can all make a difference in how a parent may respond and ultimately how effectively the EMT can interact with the patient.

Parents may react in one of several ways when their child suffers a sudden life-threatening injury or illness. Their first reaction may be one of denial or shock. Some parents will react by crying, screaming, or becoming angry. Another common reaction is self-blame and guilt. In all of these instances, be calm, reassuring, and supportive. Use simple language to explain what has happened and what is being done to and for their child.

In some cases, an upset parent may interfere with your care of the child. This is a natural reaction to protect the child from further harm. Usually, you can persuade the parent to assist you by asking him to hold the child's hand, give you a medical history, or comfort the child. If the parent is out of control, however, and cannot or will not cooperate, have a friend or relative of the parent remove him from the scene.

At this point, it should be noted that not all children live with two parents in a traditional nuclear family. The child may have a single parent or may be living with a grandparent or other relative or even with someone who is not related to the child. Whoever the child's full-time caretaker or guardian is, that person is likely to have the same emotional responses in an emergency as any parent. The EMT should be sensitive to the fact that the child may or may not call this person "Mommy" or "Daddy" and may be upset if asked where his mother or father is. Tact is often required to find out who is responsible for the child and what the child calls that person. Though "parent" or "mom and dad" appear in this chapter, keep in mind that the terms are being used to stand for any person or persons who act as parents, guardians, or principal caretakers to the child.

You need to gain confidence and calm the emotions of all the people around the scene in order to be able to treat the child effectively. Your interactions with the child will show everyone present your concern, and the manner in which you provide care will show your professionalism.

In general, involving the parent in the care of the child helps both the child and the parent. The most effective method may be to have the parent hold the child in a position of comfort on his lap, if appropriate, during assessment and treatment procedures. Offer as much emotional support as possible to the parent. However, never forget that the child (not the parent) is your patient. Do not allow communication with the parent to distract you from care of the child.

ASSESSING THE PEDIATRIC PATIENT

Assessment is the key to good quality patient care. A good assessment leads to the right care for the right presenting problem in the right amount of time. Assessment is an ongoing process that continues from initial patient contact until care is transferred to the emergency department. The EMT must continually be looking, asking, and reassessing vital signs. Patient conditions can change—sometimes very quickly—and if assessment is not an ongoing process, a problem can be missed.

Patient assessment is an extremely important skill for EMTs to learn, and with pediatric patients it may be even more significant for two reasons: First, the condition of sick and traumatized kids can change rapidly. Second, sometimes signs and symptoms are subtle and will be missed without close observation. Therefore, two approaches to assessment will be reviewed.

The first approach we will discuss is the *pediatric assessment triangle (PAT)*, which provides an easy and systematic format for keeping the assessment process organized and provides a way of identifying presenting problems and conditions that require immediate attention.

The second approach we will discuss will be the step-by-step assessment sequence you are already familiar with for adults, with additional information that pertains to infants and children. This second approach will follow the general format for assessment that was presented in Chapters 7 through 14.

Pediatric Assessment Triangle (PAT)

The pediatric assessment triangle (PAT) (Figure 31-6) is a method of pediatric assessment from two viewpoints. The first is the general impression formed as you approach the child, often referred to as an assessment "from the doorway." The second is the impression based on the remainder of the initial assessment that is done next to the patient. Each of the three sides of the triangle represents a different patient presentation that should be evaluated:

- Appearance
- Work of breathing
- Circulation to skin

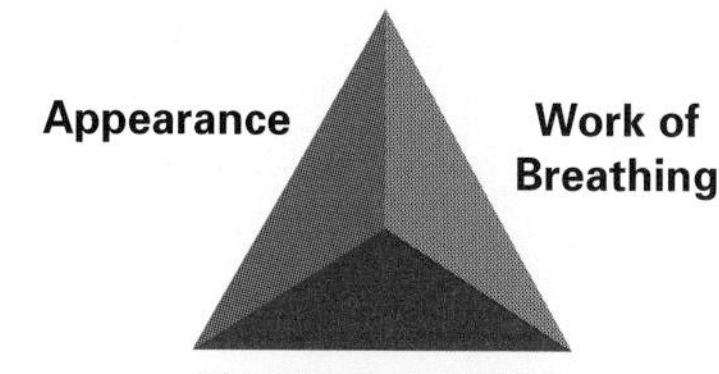

Figure 31-6 • The pediatric assessment triangle. *(Used with permission of the American Academy of Pediatrics)*

The first impressions are those formed as you enter the scene and approach the patient ("from the doorway"). These first few seconds will provide you with a great deal of information that can be important in determining the seriousness of the patient's condition. For the first side of the triangle, you look at the patient's *appearance*. Consider the child's mental status using the "AV" part of AVPU (alertness, verbal response).What are the patient's apparent muscle tone, interactiveness, consolability, look or gaze, speech or cry? For the second side of the triangle, you observe *breathing (including airway)*. Are there any abnormal airway/breathing sounds such as hoarseness, muffled speech, grunting, wheezing, stridor, or crowing? Is there any abnormal body position such as sniffing position, tripoding, or refusing to lie down? Are there retractions, nasal flaring, "see-saw" breathing, or head bobbing? For the base of the triangle, you look at those signs that might indicate a *circulation* problem, such as pallor, mottling, or cyanosis (a gray-blue coloration).

The remainder of the initial assessment is done up close and hands on. This confirms what you may already have surmised from your first, from-the-doorway impressions and may identify additional presenting problems requiring immediate interventions. During the hands-on initial assessment, the triangle again looks at appearance, breathing including airway, and circulation—but with more precision. For *appearance*, you look at mental status using the "PU" part of AVPU (response to pain or unresponsiveness). For *breathing*, you start by ensuring that the airway is open and closely observing the quality of the patient's breathing. For *circulation*, you check for pulse, subtle cyanosis, and capillary refill.

As part of the initial assessment, you will need to make continual decisions about "treat as you go" care, which means that as soon as a problem is identified, you immediately start to provide care—before moving on to the next part of the initial assessment. In other words, any needed care should be performed as each part of the assessment (each side of the assessment triangle) is completed. For example, if the patient appears to be unconscious and the mechanism of injury suggests some type of cervical-spine trauma, then in-line stabilization should be initiated before and maintained while assessing the airway and breathing. If the patient is not breathing, you must ensure an open airway and initiate ventilations as needed before checking circulation. The information from the assessment is what guides your decisions for patient care and treatment.

Remember, assessment is an ongoing process!

The overall sequence of assessment steps is the same for the pediatric patient as for the adult patient. In the following sections, special concerns for assessment of the pediatric patient are discussed.

Scene Size-Up and Safety—Pediatric

When entering an area where there is a pediatric patient, enter slowly and make some important observations. The first is to determine if the scene is safe. Even though it is a rare occurrence, sometimes there may be a risk from violence or abusive behavior, possibly directed toward the child. Look around carefully for any mechanism of injury.

Standard Precautions must be taken for the usual reasons. Additionally, be aware that ordinary childhood diseases can be devastating when contracted by an adult.

Initial Assessment—Pediatric

Forming a General Impression

A great deal of information can and should be gathered from the doorway, before you approach and possibly upset the patient. From across the room, you can gain a general impression of the child. First decide: Is the child well or sick? The child's general appearance and behavior will usually provide the answer.

A child who is alertly watching your approach, squirming and able to talk with you, or vigorously crying obviously has an open airway, is breathing, and has a pulse and blood pressure. If the child is silent, appears to be sleeping deeply, or is unresponsive, the child's airway, breathing, and circulation must be assessed immediately.

As you approach and form your general impression, make the following observations:

- *Mental status.* The well child is alert. The sick child may be drowsy, inattentive, or sleeping.
- *Effort of breathing.* The well child's breathing should be unlabored. The sick child will be making a visible effort to breathe, including flared nostrils and retractions or pulling in of the tissues between the ribs.
- *Skin color.* A sick child may be pale, cyanotic, or flushed.
- *Quality of cry or speech.* In general, a strong cry or normal speech indicates a well child with good air exchange. The child who can speak only in short sentences or grunts has significant respiratory distress.
- *Interaction with the environment or others.* The healthy child exhibits normal behavior for his age. He moves around, plays, is attentive, establishes eye contact, and interacts with his parents. The sick child may be silent, listless, or unconscious.
- *Emotional state.* The well child's emotional state is appropriate to the situation. Crying may be his normal response to pain or fear. A withdrawn child or one who is emotionally flat is probably a sick child.

- *Response to you.* A well child may be interested in you or afraid of you. A sick child will give little attention to a stranger.
- *Tone and body position.* A sick child may be limp with poor muscle tone. Pediatric patients with respiratory distress often assume characteristic positions that seem to help them breathe (e.g., leaning forward with hands on knees, referred to as tripoding).

Assessing Mental Status

Use the AVPU method of assessing mental status, taking the child's age and developmental characteristics into account. You may need to shout to elicit a response to verbal stimulus. Tap or pinch the patient to test for response to painful stimulus. Never shake an infant or child.

Assessing the Airway

Consider not only whether the airway is open but whether it is endangered. A depressed mental status, secretions, blood, vomitus, foreign bodies, face or neck trauma, and lower respiratory infections may all compromise the airway. Be careful not to hyperextend the child's neck.

Assessing Breathing

First assess if the patient is breathing or not. If the patient is not breathing or is breathing inadequately, provide artificial ventilations with supplemental oxygen. If the patient is experiencing respiratory distress, provide high-concentration oxygen by pediatric nonrebreather mask. (See Chapter 16, "Respiratory Emergencies.")

To assess breathing, observe the following:

- *Chest expansion.* There should be equal movement on both sides of the chest.
- *Effort of breathing.* Watch for nasal flaring when the patient inhales, and retractions or "pulling in" of the sternum and ribs with inhalation.
- *Sounds of breathing.* Listen for stridor, crowing, or other noisy respirations. Breath sounds should be present and equal on both sides of the chest. Note the presence of grunting at the end of expiration, which is a worrisome sign.
- *Breathing rate.* Normal respiratory rates for infants and children are 12 to 20 per minute in an adolescent, 15 to 30 per minute in a child, 25 to 50 per minute in an infant. Breathing that is either faster or slower than normal is inadequate and requires artificial ventilation as well as oxygen.
- *Color.* Cyanosis (blue or gray color) indicates that the patient is not getting enough oxygen.

Assessing Circulation

As with an adult, check for normal warm, pink, and dry skin and normal pulse as indications of adequate circulation and perfusion. For assessment, check the radial pulse in a child, the brachial pulse in an infant. For basic life support, check the carotid pulse in a child, the brachial or femoral pulse in an infant (Figure 31-7). In infants and children 5 years old or younger, also check capillary refill. When you press on the nail bed or press the top of a hand or foot, the area will turn white. If circulation is adequate, the normal pink color will return in less than 2 seconds, or in less time than it takes to say "capillary refill." Check for and control any blood loss.

Identifying Priority Patients

A patient who is a high priority for immediate transport is one who:

- Gives a poor general impression
- Is unresponsive or listless
- Does not recognize the parent or primary caregiver
- Is not comforted when held by parent but becomes calm and quiet when set down

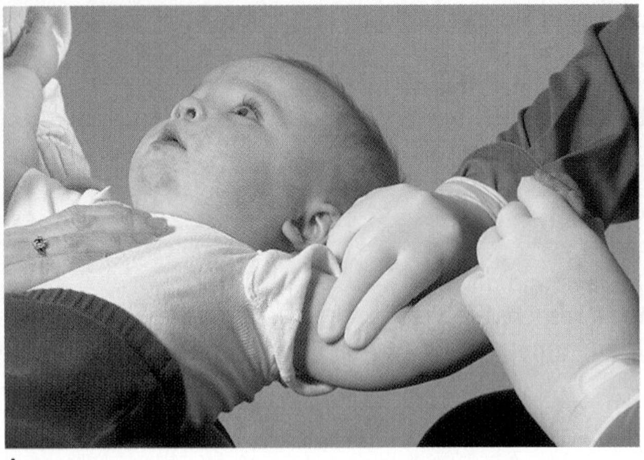
A

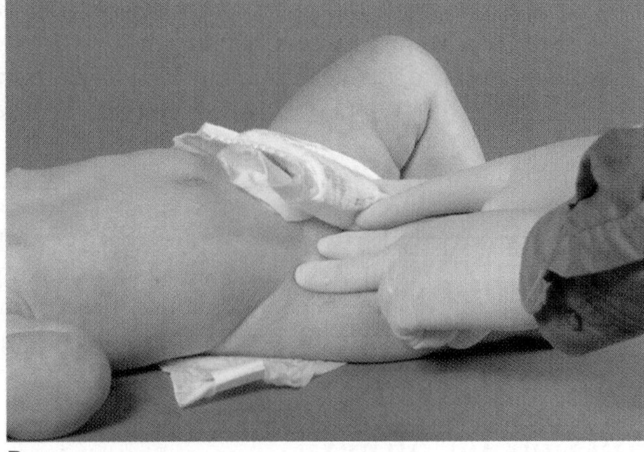
B

Figure 31-7 • For basic life support, check the (A) brachial pulse or (B) femoral pulse in an infant.

- Has a compromised airway
- Is in respiratory arrest or has inadequate breathing or respiratory distress
- Has a possibility of shock
- Has uncontrolled bleeding

Focused History and Physical Exam—Pediatric

At times, the child may be the only source of a history. He may be at school or another place where medical records are not kept or where adults who know his medical history are not present. Get as much history as you can from the child by asking simple questions that cannot be answered with a yes or no. A child who cannot tell you where it hurts can usually point to the area.

Perform a focused physical exam for a medical patient and a rapid trauma exam for a trauma patient, as you would for an adult. Explain to the awake child what you are doing, and do the exam in trunk-to-head order to avoid frightening the child.

Take and record vital signs, assessing blood pressure only in children older than 3, using an appropriately-sized cuff (Figure 31-8). See Table 31-3 for normal ranges of pediatric vital signs. It may be helpful to carry a pocket guide or reference card with pediatric vital signs when responding to pediatric calls.

Detailed Physical Exam—Pediatric

The EMT normally performs the physical examination or body assessment in head-to-toe order; however, on alert infants and small children this is reversed. Starting with the toes or trunk and working your way toward the head will let the child get used to you and your touch before you attempt to touch him around the head and face. Playing with infants' feet often puts them at ease.

Unless there are possible injuries that indicate the child should not be moved, a young child should be held on the parent's lap during the physical exam. Many EMS teams carry clean stuffed animals (like teddy bears) that can be given to a child during the physical exam. The toys can provide comfort to the child and allow you to explain the examination by using the toy as a model. Point to an area on the toy to show the child where you must touch and where you will bandage when you need to provide emergency care. This type of one-to-one communication also helps build parent and bystander confidence, letting them know that a professional, compassionate EMT is caring for the child. (If you use a toy, allow the child to keep it.)

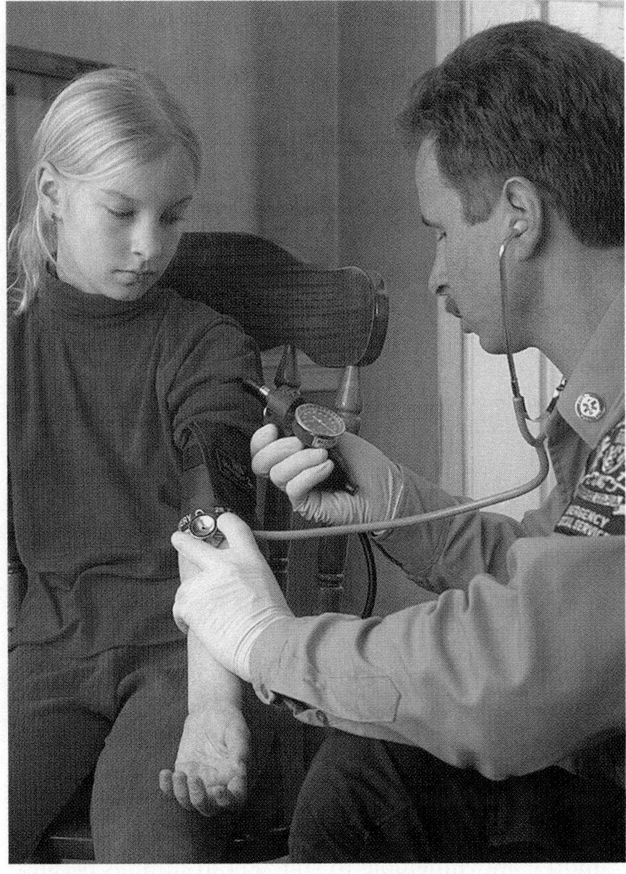

Figure 31-8 • Take blood pressure in patients older than 3 years.

Most very young children will suffer no embarrassment when clothing is removed or repositioned during the exam. Nonetheless, protect the child from the stares of onlookers. Many children around the age of 5 to 8 go through a stage of intense modesty. You may have to keep explaining why you must remove certain articles of clothing. Many parents, teachers, and day care personnel teach children that strangers should not remove their clothing or touch them. The children that you examine may not understand your intentions and may resist. Some children may become upset because they feel you are taking something away from them. Take your time and do not rush children into accepting all that is happening. Remember that children lose body heat rapidly, so if you expose them, quickly cover them with a blanket.

The assessment of an infant or child is done to look for the same signs of injury and illness as in the case of the adult patient. However, you should take special care with components of the exam as discussed in the following sections (Figure 31-9 and Scan 31-1).

Head

Do not apply pressure to the "soft spots" (fontanelles) of an infant. The skin over the anterior fontanelle is normally level with the top of the skull, or slightly sunken. It may bulge naturally when the infant cries or be abnormally sunken if the infant is dehydrated. Meningitis and head trauma cause the fontanelle to bulge due to increased intracranial pressure. Collisions involving infants and children can often produce head injuries.

Nose and Ears

Look for blood and clear fluids from the nose and ears. Suspect skull fractures if present. Children are nose breathers, so mucus or blood clot obstructions will make it hard for them to breathe.

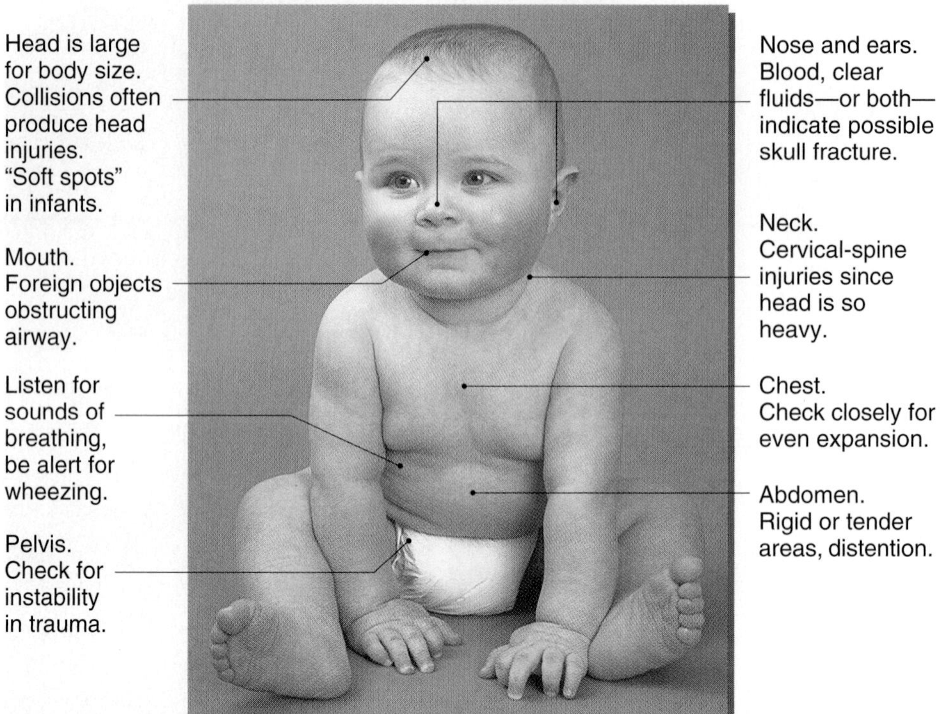
Head is large
for body size.
Collisions often
produce head
injuries.
"Soft spots"
in infants.
Mouth.
Foreign objects
obstructing
airway.
Listen for
sounds of
breathing,
be alert for
wheezing.
Pelvis.
Check for
instability
in trauma.
Nose and ears.
Blood, clear
fluids—or both—
indicate possible
skull fracture.
Neck.
Cervical-spine
injuries since
head is so
heavy.
Chest.
Check closely for
even expansion.
Abdomen.
Rigid or tender
areas, distention.

Figure 31-9 • Special areas to consider during pediatric assessment.

Neck

Children are vulnerable to spinal cord injuries because of their proportionately larger and heavier heads. The neck offers less support because muscles and bone structures are less developed. In medical emergencies, the neck may be sore, stiff, or swollen.

Airway

Keep the infant's head in the neutral position and the child's head in the neutral-plus or sniffing position (chin thrust forward to maintain an open airway). If there is no suspicion of spinal injury, place a flat, folded towel under the patient's shoulders to get the appropriate airway alignment. Children's airways are more pliable and smaller than an adult's. Hyperextension or hyperflexion may close off the airway. For medical respiratory problems, the child will probably want to sit up.

Chest

Listen closely for even air entry and the sounds of breathing on both sides of the chest. Be alert for wheezes and other noises. Check for symmetry, bruising, paradoxical movement, and retraction of the sternum or the muscles between the ribs. Remember that a child's soft ribs may not break, but there may be underlying injuries to the organs within the chest.

Abdomen

Note any rigid or tender areas and distention. Because a child's abdominal organs (especially the spleen and liver) are large in relation to the size of the abdominal cavity, and because there is little protection offered by the still-undeveloped abdominal muscles, these organs are more susceptible to trauma than an adult's. Any injury that impedes the movement of the diaphragm will compromise a young child's breathing, as most children 8 years of age or younger are abdominal breathers.

Pelvis

In trauma, check for stability of the pelvic girdle.

SCAN 31-1 • The Pediatric Physical Examination

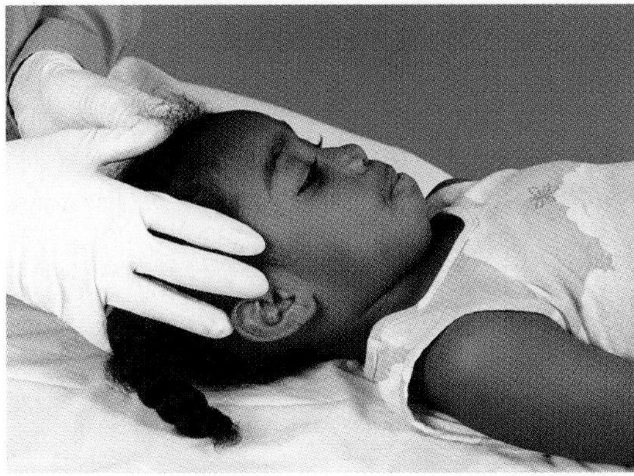

1. Examine the head. Look for bruising or blood or clear fluid draining from the nose or ears. Palpate gently for soft or spongy areas, skull irregularities, or crepitus (feeling of grinding bone fragments). Check the fontanelle in infants.

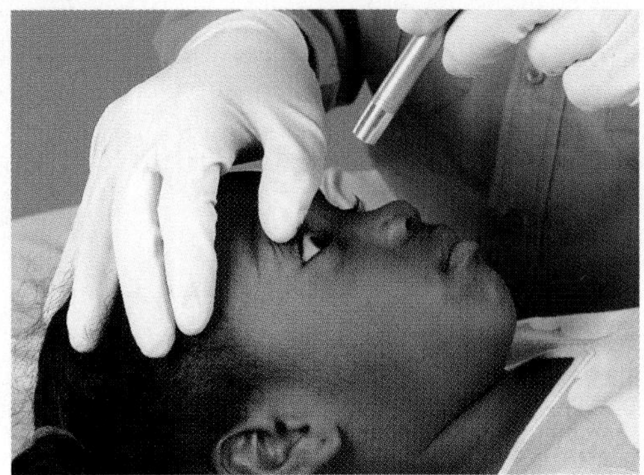

2. Check the eyes. The pupils should be equal in size and reactivity to light.

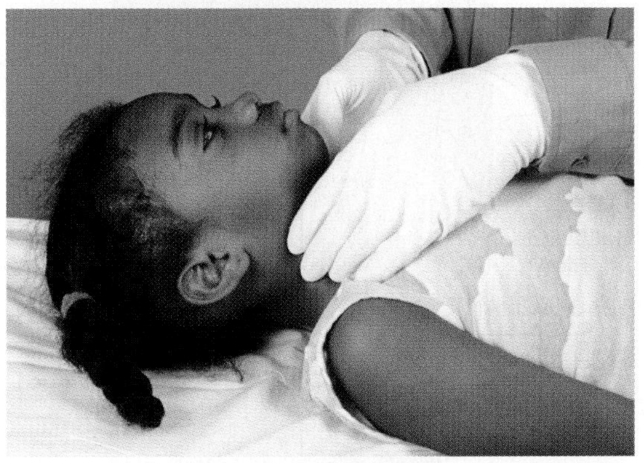

3. Examine the neck. Check for the position of the trachea, swollen neck veins, stiffness, tenderness, or crepitus.

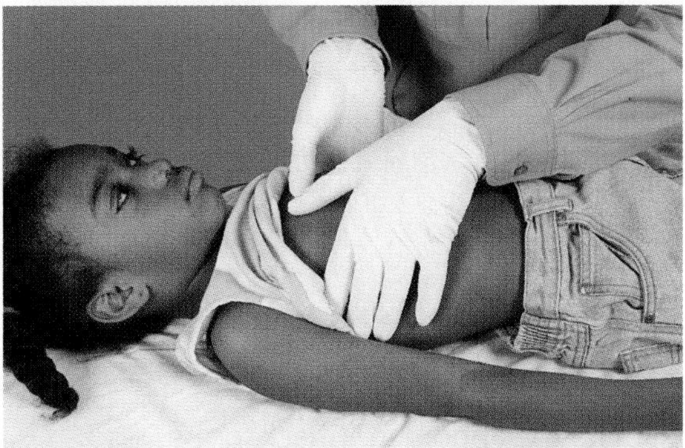

4. Examine the chest. Check for bruising, equal chest rise and fall, and crepitus. Watch for signs of breathing difficulty.

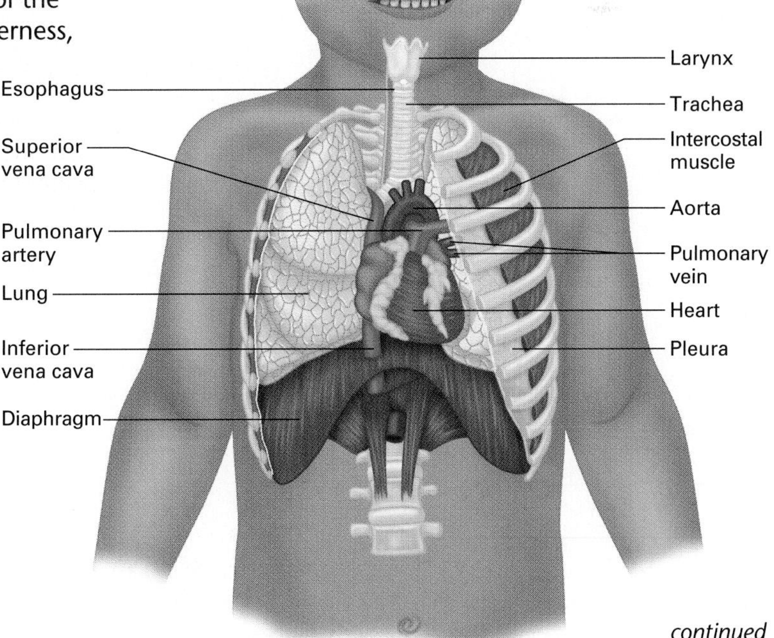

While examining the chest, be aware of the contents of the thorax.

continued

SCAN 31-1 • (Continued)

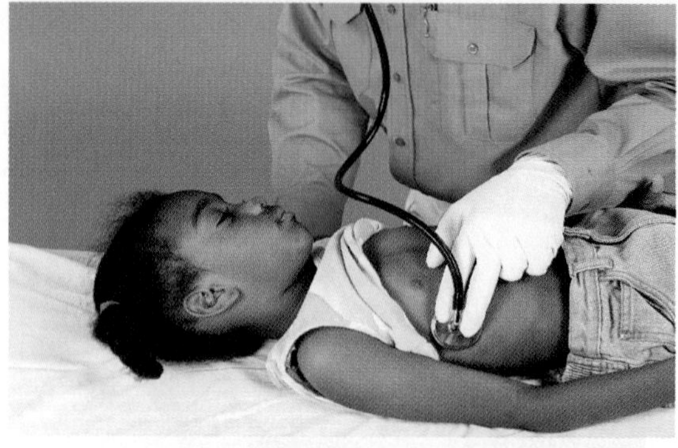

5. Auscultate for breath sounds over all lung fields.

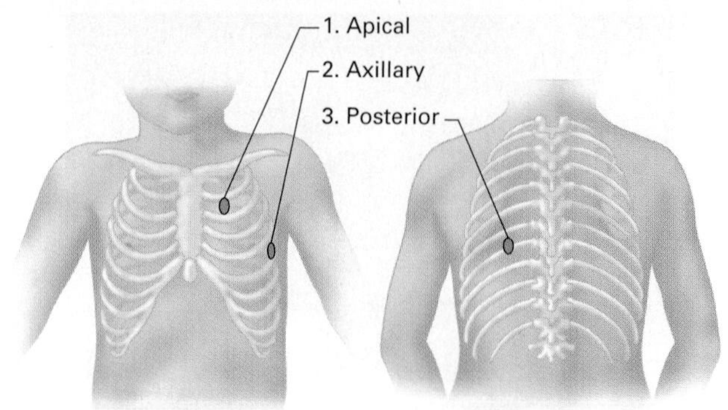

Auscultation sites.

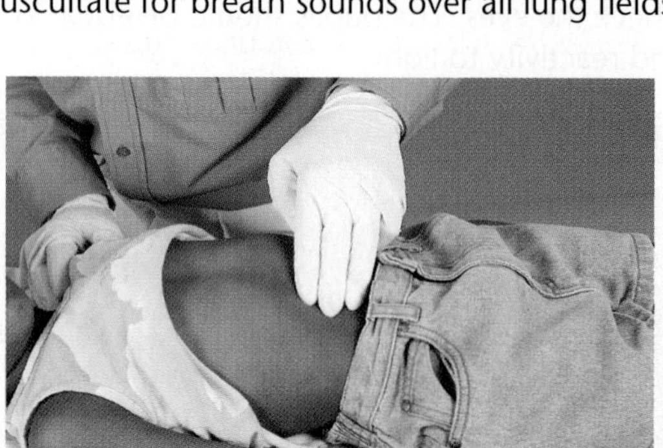

6. Examine the abdomen. Check for bruising, tenderness, or guarding. Look for swelling that may indicate swallowed air.

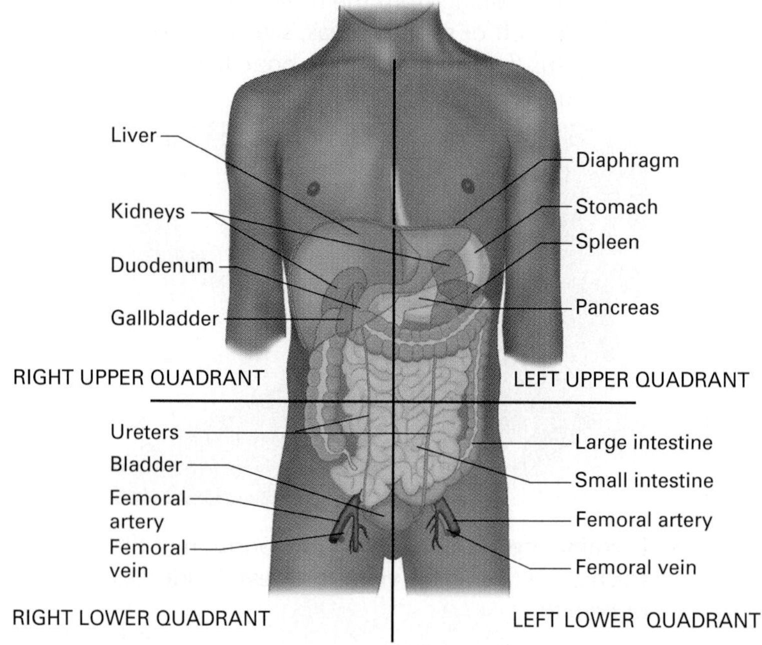

Divide the abdomen into quadrants and examine each one, while remembering which organs are located in each quadrant.

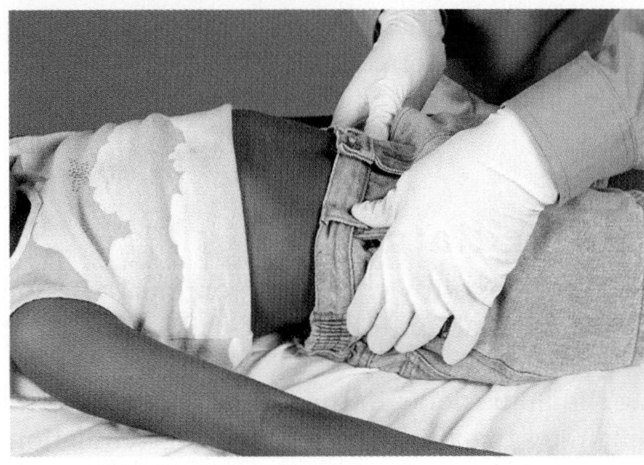

7. Examine the pelvis for tenderness, swelling, bruising, or crepitus. If the patient complains of pain, injury, or other problems in the genital area, assess for bruising, swelling, or tenderness in that area.

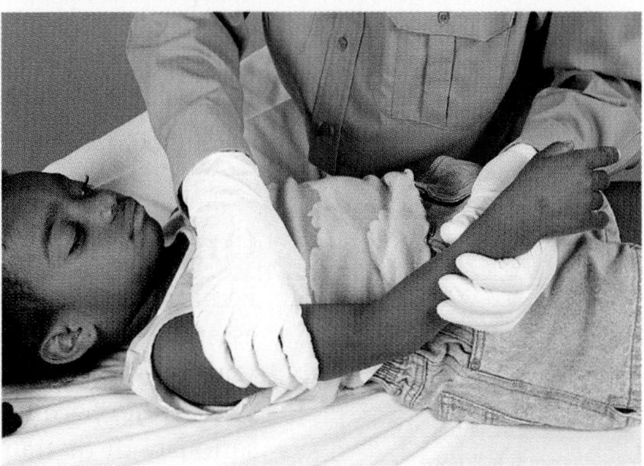

8. Examine the extremities. Evaluate pulses, sensation, and warmth. Look for unequal movement.

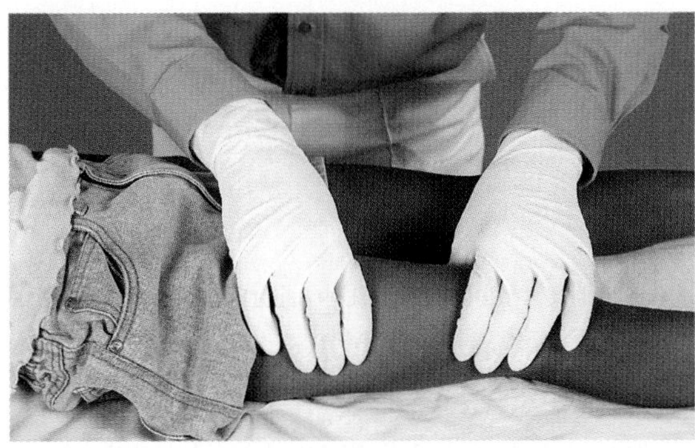

9. If you have immobilized an extremity, check capillary refill and peripheral pulses and compare with the other arm or leg.

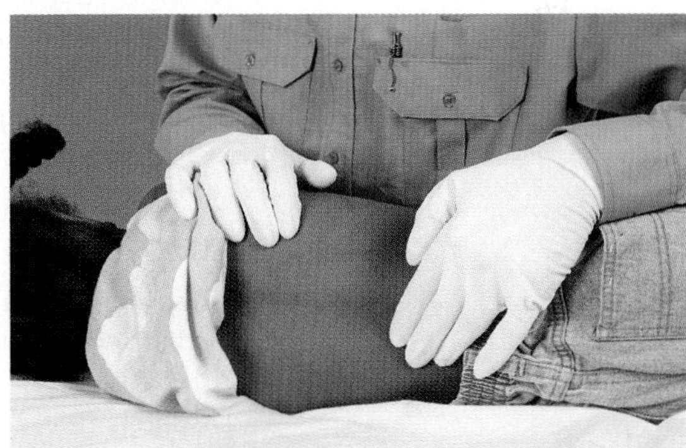

10. Examine the back. Assess for tenderness, bruising, and crepitus. If the child requires immobilization, the back can be checked while the child is being log rolled onto the spine board.

Extremities

Perform an assessment with capillary refill and distal pulse, including a neurological component for motor function with a sensation check. With an infant or young child, you do not have to press on a nail bed. You can quickly check capillary refill by squeezing a hand or foot, forearm or lower leg. Check for painful, swollen, and deformed injury sites. (The bones of an infant or child are more pliable so they bend, splinter, and buckle before they fracture.)

Ongoing Assessment—Pediatric

Pediatric patients are dynamic—that is, constantly changing. Continual assessment is essential to good patient care. A rule of thumb for infants and children is: Don't take your eyes off them for a minute!

As time permits, the following should be done. In some cases where the patient is seriously ill or traumatized, maintaining the airway and supporting ventilations will keep the EMT from performing a detailed physical exam and a complete history:

1. Reassess mental status
2. Maintain open airway
3. Monitor breathing
4. Reassess pulse
5. Monitor skin color, temperature, and moisture
6. Reassess vital signs:
   - Every 5 minutes in unstable patients
   - Every 15 minutes in stable patients
7. Ensure that all appropriate care and treatment are being given.

Comparing Assessments

The following scenario may help you see the special considerations involved in assessing pediatric patients.

Dispatch

Two ambulance crews, including you and three other EMTs, have been dispatched to care for three victims of carbon monoxide inhalation: Andrea (16 years old), Megan (10 years old), and Eddie (11 months old). You find the patients inside a neighbor's home, Megan supine on the floor, Eddie crying in Andrea's arms.

Assessment of 10-Year-Old Girl (Megan)

Initial Assessment

Your partner's general impression is of a moaning 10-year-old girl. Megan's mental status is awake and crying. Her airway is open and her breathing is adequate in both rate and depth. Your partner's assessment of circulation reveals a strong, rapid radial pulse. Skin is flushed and dry. There is no apparent external bleeding. Megan's priority is high because of the nature of the illness: carbon monoxide poisoning. Your partner calms the child as she begins administering oxygen by pediatric nonrebreather mask at 15 liters per minute and continues with her assessment.

Focused History and Physical Exam—Medical

At first, like many sick children, Megan is withdrawn and not interested in communicating with your partner, who is a stranger to her. However, by treating Megan in a calm and friendly manner, your partner is able to gain her attention and confidence. The history your partner can gather is scant, however. The firefighter says Megan was found lying on the living room floor, very drowsy, and was quickly carried out of the house. Megan confides that the whole family started feeling sick at the same time and that right now her head hurts. A rapid physical exam reveals no injuries or other abnormalities. Baseline vital signs are pulse 140, regular and strong; blood pressure 100/70; and respirations of 28 and regular.

Assessment of 11-Month-Old Infant (Eddie)

Initial Assessment

The general impression formed by the EMT from the other ambulance is of an infant who appears to be in no acute distress. Eddie's mental status is awake and calm. He is moving energetically in Andrea's arms and looking around curiously at all the activity in the room. His airway is open and his breathing is adequate in both rate and depth. The assessment of circulation reveals a strong, rapid brachial pulse. Skin is warm, pink, and dry. There is no apparent external bleeding. Although Eddie does not appear to be in distress, his priority is high because of the nature of the illness, carbon monoxide poisoning. The EMT starts to administer high-concentration oxygen. Eddie fights the mask, but he tolerates "blow-by" administration with his big sister holding the mask near his face.

Focused History and Physical Exam—Medical

Eddie's history—provided by Andrea—includes the fact that his sister had placed him upstairs in a crib when the family started feeling ill, so he was relatively far from the malfunctioning furnace. The EMT who is assessing Eddie gets him giggling happily by playing with his toes, then conducts a rapid physical exam in toe-to-head sequence. The exam reveals no injuries or other abnormalities. Baseline vital signs are pulse 128, regular and strong; respirations of 30 and regular.

Assessment of 16-Year-Old Girl (Andrea)

Initial Assessment

The general impression is of a teenage girl who appears in no acute distress. Andrea's mental status is awake and oriented, although she is quite anxious about her sister and brother. Her airway, breathing, and circulation are all normal. Although she appears to be well, her priority is high because she has been exposed to carbon monoxide. The EMT gives her high-concentration oxygen, but first thinks to enlist Andrea's help in showing the mask to Eddie, smiling, and saying, "Look what I get to put on!" so Eddie won't be frightened by the mask on his sister's face.

En Route

Focused History and Physical Exam—Medical

Andrea's history includes the fact that she had been upstairs with her baby brother and, like him, farther from the furnace than her little sister. The female EMT has gained Andrea's confidence by treating her with professionalism and respect. Andrea admits that she is afraid she has done herself some permanent injury by breathing carbon monoxide and also feels guilty that she didn't do more to help her siblings. The EMT is able to comfort and reassure her. She explains to Andrea the elements of the rapid physical exam before she conducts it. She is careful to protect Andrea's privacy during the exam, which reveals no injuries or other abnormalities. Baseline vital signs are pulse 70, regular and strong; blood pressure 94/60; respirations of 18 and regular.

Backup drivers have been sent to the scene so members of each ambulance crew can attend to their patients en route. You continue administering oxygen to Andrea. She remains alert and is complaining of a slight headache and some nausea by the time you arrive at the emergency department. Her vital signs remain in the normal range as you turn her care over to emergency department staff. Megan's head still hurts, but she is far less drowsy and is looking and feeling better. In the other ambulance, Eddie, being comforted by one EMT as the other continues to administer oxygen, seems quite well by the time they arrive at the emergency department.

At the hospital, blood tests on the patients confirm that they all were exposed to carbon monoxide. Megan had a moderate exposure, and Andrea and Eddie had only a minor exposure. All three are expected to make a good recovery.

SPECIAL CONCERNS IN PEDIATRIC CARE

Like adults, infants and children may be subject to either medical problems or trauma. Concerns that frequently apply to both medical emergencies and trauma are: airway maintenance, providing supplemental oxygen, supporting ventilations, caring for shock, and protecting the infant or child from hypothermia (Figure 31-10).

Maintaining an Open Airway

Just as with an adult, it is important to position the child's head and neck to align and open the airway. It is important not to hyperextend or to permit flexion of a child's neck. The child's head should be positioned in a more neutral position than an adult's because of the danger of closing the airway when the neck is flexed or hyperextended. Placing a folded towel under the shoulders of a young infant or child will help to keep the airway aligned. To achieve the proper position, perform a head-tilt, chin-lift if there is no trauma, or a jaw-thrust with spinal immobilization if trauma is suspected.

Be prepared to suction the airway as needed. Use suction catheters that are sized for infant and child patients. Do not touch the back of the patient's throat, as this may activate the gag reflex, causing vomiting. It is also possible to stimulate the vagus nerve in the back of the throat, which can slow the heart rate. Do not suction for more than a few seconds at a time, as cutting off the body's oxygen supply is especially dangerous to infants and children, causing cardiac arrest more quickly than in adults. You may give a few extra breaths after suctioning.

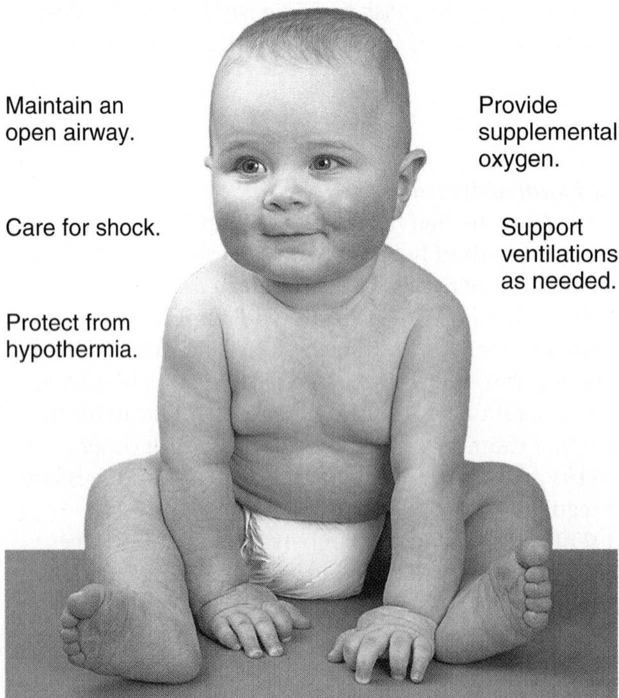

Maintain an open airway.
Provide supplemental oxygen.
Care for shock.
Support ventilations as needed.
Protect from hypothermia.

Figure 31-10 • Special considerations apply to the treatment of many pediatric medical and trauma emergencies.

SCAN 31-2 • Inserting an Oropharyngeal Airway in a Child

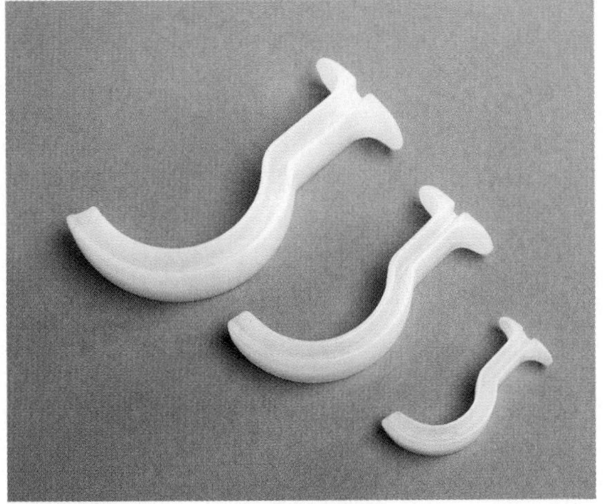

1. Oropharyngeal airways come in a variety of sizes.

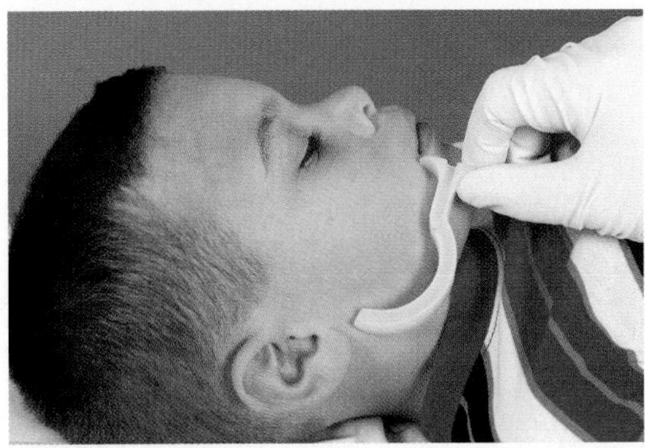

2. Size the airway by measuring from the corner of the mouth to the tip of the earlobe.

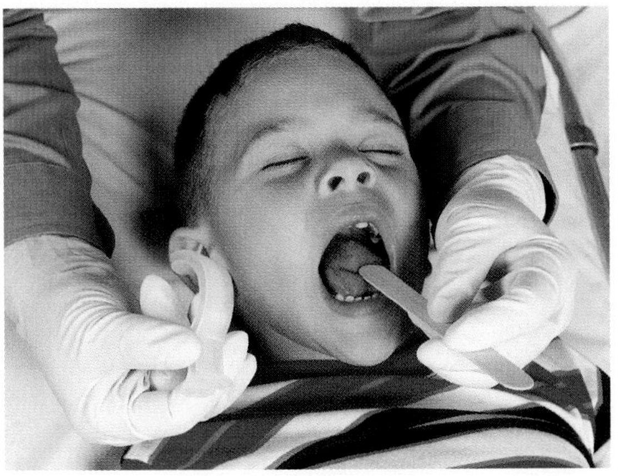

3. Use a tongue depressor to hold the tongue in position. Insert the airway with the tip pointing downward, toward the tongue and throat—the same position it will be in after insertion.

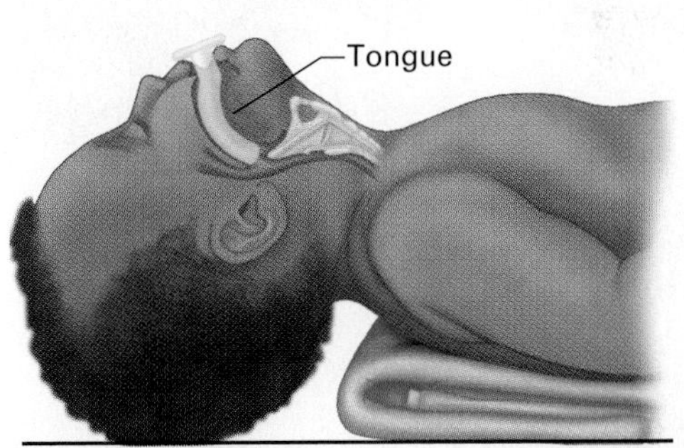

4. The oropharyngeal airway in position.

As with adults, the tongues of infants and children are likely to slide back into the pharynx and block the airway. In fact, airway blockage by the tongue is even more likely with infants and children because their tongues are proportionately larger compared to the size of the mouth and pharynx.

If the patient is unconscious and does not have a gag reflex, you may insert an oropharyngeal airway to prevent the tongue from blocking the airway. To insert an oropharyngeal airway, insert a tongue depressor to the base of the tongue. Push down against the tongue while lifting the jaw upward. Then insert the oropharyngeal airway. An important difference to note is that when an oropharyngeal airway is inserted in an adult, it is inserted with the tip pointing toward the roof of the mouth, then rotated 180 degrees into position. For an infant or child, the oropharyngeal airway is inserted with the tip of the airway pointing downward, toward the tongue and throat, in the same position it will be in after insertion (Scan 31-2).

SCAN 31-3 • Inserting a Nasopharyngeal Airway in a Child

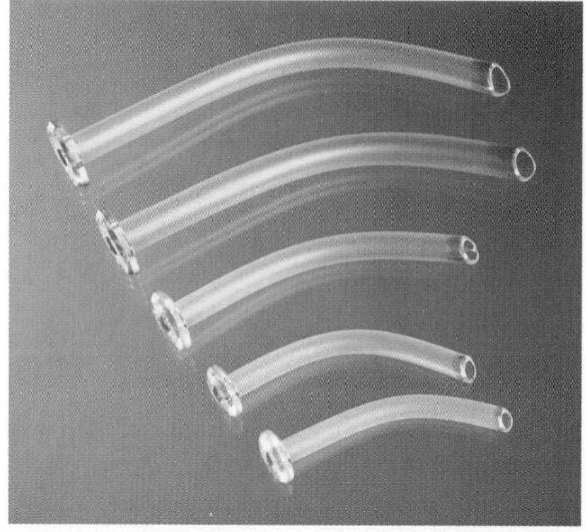

1. Nasopharyngeal airways come in a variety of sizes.

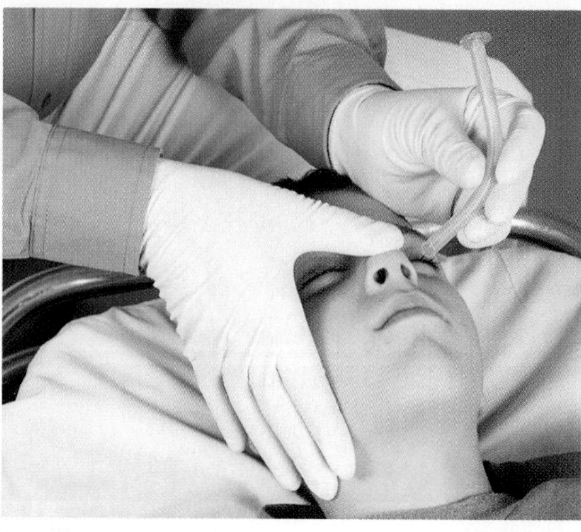

2. The airway should be about the thickness of the patient's little finger and should measure from the nostril to the tragus (cartilage at the front) of the ear.

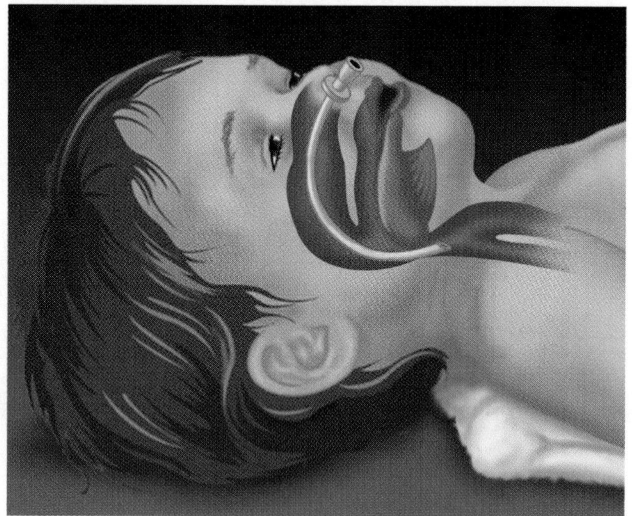

3. The nasopharyngeal airway in position.

If the patient is conscious but cannot maintain an open airway, a nasopharyngeal airway can be inserted (Scan 31-3). Note, however, that a nasopharyngeal airway should not be used if the child has facial trauma or head injuries, because the airway could penetrate a breach in the cranium.

Clearing an Airway Obstruction

Infants and children are naturally curious. They explore their environment and often put things in their mouths. They can easily choke on a foreign object as well as on a piece of food.

An airway obstruction can be mild or severe. With many mild obstructions, the child is still able to breathe and get enough oxygen. With other mild obstructions or with severe obstruction of the airway, the supply of air is cut off to a significant extent or completely. The assessment and care summaries that follow detail how to determine if an obstruction is mild or severe and how to manage an obstruction.

PATIENT ASSESSMENT

MILD AIRWAY OBSTRUCTION

Signs of a mild airway obstruction in a pediatric patient include the following:

- Noisy breathing (stridor, crowing)
- Retractions of the muscles around the ribs and sternum when inhaling
- Skin is still pink
- Peripheral perfusion is satisfactory (capillary refill under 2 seconds in a child 5 years old or less)
- Still alert, not unconscious ■

PATIENT CARE

MILD AIRWAY OBSTRUCTION

Emergency care of a pediatric patient with a mild airway obstruction is as follows:

1. Allow the child to assume a position of comfort, sitting up, not lying down. Assist an infant or younger child into a sitting position. Allow the child to sit on the parent's lap.
2. Offer high-concentration oxygen by pediatric nonrebreather mask or blow-by technique (described later in this chapter).
3. Transport.
4. Do not agitate the child. Do a limited exam. Do not assess blood pressure. ■

PATIENT ASSESSMENT

SEVERE AIRWAY OBSTRUCTION

The obstruction may be complete, or a partial obstruction may be severe enough to prevent adequate intake of oxygen. Signs include:

- Cyanosis
- Child's cough becomes ineffective; child cannot cry or speak
- Increased respiratory difficulty accompanied by stridor or respiratory arrest
- Altered mental status or child has lost or loses consciousness ■

PATIENT CARE

SEVERE AIRWAY OBSTRUCTION

Follow these steps for emergency care:

1. Perform airway clearance techniques. For infants less than 1 year old, alternate back blows and chest thrusts (Figure 31-11) and use finger sweeps to remove visible objects (no blind sweeps). For children older than 1 year, provide abdominal thrusts when conscious and chest compressions with attempted ventilation and finger sweeps to remove visible objects when unconscious. (Airway clearance sequences are summarized in Table 31-4.)
2. Attempt artificial ventilations with a pocket mask or bag-valve-mask unit in the appropriate pediatric size and supplemental oxygen (Table 31-5). ■

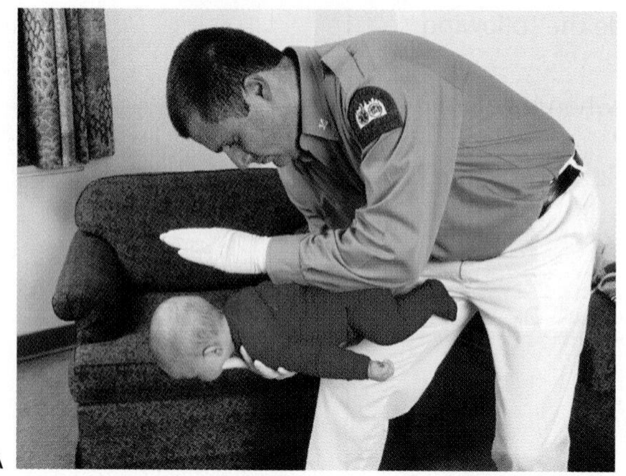

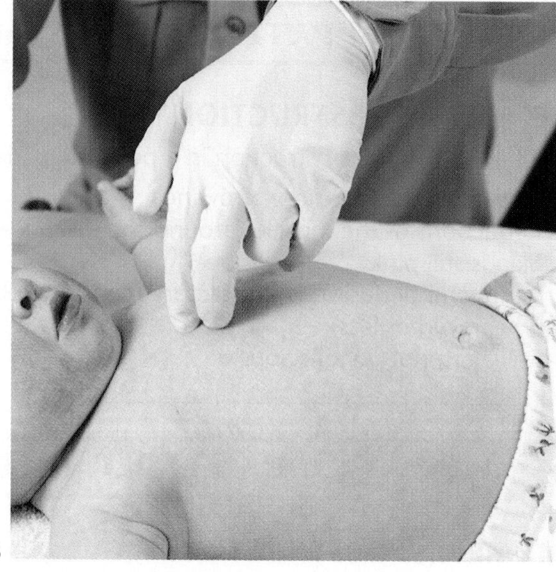

Figure 31-11 • For a complete airway obstruction in an infant, alternate (A) back blows with (B) chest thrusts.

TABLE 31-4 • Pediatric Airway Clearance Sequences

	CHILD: 1 YEAR TO PUBERTY	INFANT: BIRTH TO 1 YEAR
Conscious	Ask, "Are you choking?" Perform abdominal thrusts.	Observe signs of choking (small objects or food, wheezing, agitation, blue color, not breathing). Series of five back blows, five chest thrusts
Loses Consciousness During Procedure	Assist patient to floor. Open airway. Remove visible objects (NO blind sweeps). Attempt to ventilate. If unsuccessful, reposition head and attempt to ventilate again. If unsuccessful, perform CPR. If alone, call for help after 2 minutes.	Open airway. Remove visible objects (NO blind sweeps). Attempt to ventilate. If unsuccessful, reposition head and attempt to ventilate again. If unsuccessful, perform CPR. If alone, call for help after 2 minutes.
Unconscious When Found	Establish unresponsiveness. Open airway. Attempt to ventilate. If unsuccessful, reposition head and attempt to ventilate again. If unsuccessful, perform CPR. Remove visible objects (NO blind sweeps). If alone, call for help after 2 minutes.	Establish unresponsiveness. Open airway. Attempt to ventilate. If unsuccessful, reposition head and attempt to ventilate again. If unsuccessful, perform CPR. Remove visible objects (NO blind sweeps). If alone, call for help after 2 minutes.

Note: Perform CPR, attempting compressions to ventilations at a 30:2 ratio. Remove visible objects from airway (no blind sweeps). Continue CPR until ventilations are successful.

TABLE 31-5 • Artificial Ventilation

	PUBERTY AND OLDER	OVER AGE 1 TO PUBERTY	BIRTH TO 1 YEAR
Ventilation Duration	1 sec.	1 sec.	1 sec.
Ventilation Rate	10 to 12 breaths/min.	12 to 20 breaths/min.	12 to 20 breaths/min.

POINT OF VIEW

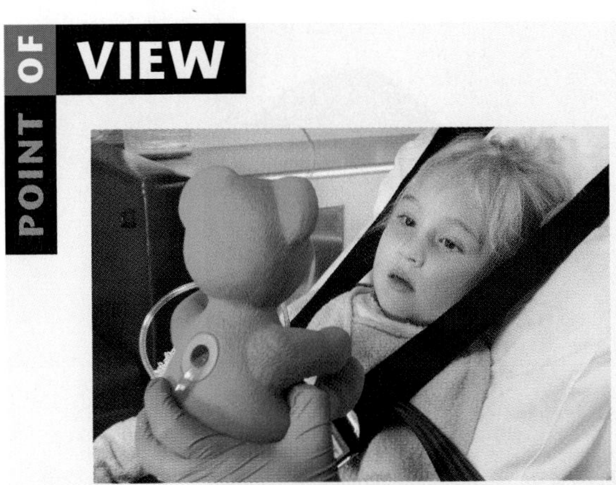

"We don't get a lot of pediatric calls. That's a good thing. When we do get them, it is a bit unnerving. I don't have kids myself so sometimes I think it's harder for me. The EMTs I volunteer with that have kids seem to be more natural.

"Well wouldn't you know I get a peds call while I am crew chief of the all-bachelor-no-kids crew. The little girl had trouble breathing and had a real barky cough. Her parents were worried. I was, too. But, you know, I did it. I got down on her level and talked with her. She was sitting with her mother and seemed alert. By the time we were headed to the ambulance I think she even liked me.

"What really clinched it was the oxygen bear. There wasn't any way I could have got a mask on her face without freaking her out. She liked the bear, and it gave her some blow-by oxygen.

"Maybe I do have some potential getting along with kids."

Infant and Child BCLS Review

For a review of infant and child basic cardiac life support, including CPR (ventilations and chest compressions) and airway clearance techniques, see Appendix B, "Basic Cardiac Life Support Review."

Providing Supplemental Oxygen and Ventilations

As for adults, high-concentration oxygen should be administered to children in respiratory distress, with inadequate respirations, or in possible shock. Hypoxia (oxygen starvation) is the underlying reason for many of the most serious medical problems with children. Inadequate oxygen will have immediate effects on the heart rate and the brain, as shown by a slowed heart rate and an altered mental status.

However, infants and young children are often afraid of an oxygen mask. For these patients, try a "blow-by" technique. That is, hold, or have a parent hold, the oxygen tubing or the pediatric nonrebreather mask 2 inches from the patient's face so the oxygen will pass over the face and be inhaled. Some departments use blow-by oxygen devices that resemble stuffed animals. These commercially made products may be less threatening to a child than traditional oxygen devices. Use the liter flow per minute recommended by the manufacturer when using these devices.

Some children respond well when oxygen tubing is pushed through the bottom of a paper cup, especially if the cup is colorful or has a picture drawn inside it (Figure 31-12). Hand the cup to the child or ask a parent to hold it. Infants and young children instinctively explore new things by bringing them up to their mouths. As the patient handles and explores the cup, he will breathe in the oxygen. *Do not use a Styrofoam cup.* Styrofoam may flake and the particles can be inhaled.

Artificial ventilations should be provided at the rate of 12 to 20 per minute (one every 3 to 5 seconds) for an infant or child up to puberty, at 10 to 12 per minute (one every 5 to 6 seconds) if the child has reached puberty. Use a pocket face mask (Figure 31-13) or a bag-valve-mask unit (Figure 31-14) in the correct infant or child size. Follow these guidelines when ventilating the infant or child patient:

- Avoid breathing too hard through the pocket face mask or using excessive bag pressure and volume. Use only enough force to make the chest rise.
- Use properly sized face masks to ensure a good mask seal (Figure 31-15).
- Flow-restricted, oxygen-powered ventilation devices are contraindicated in infants and children.

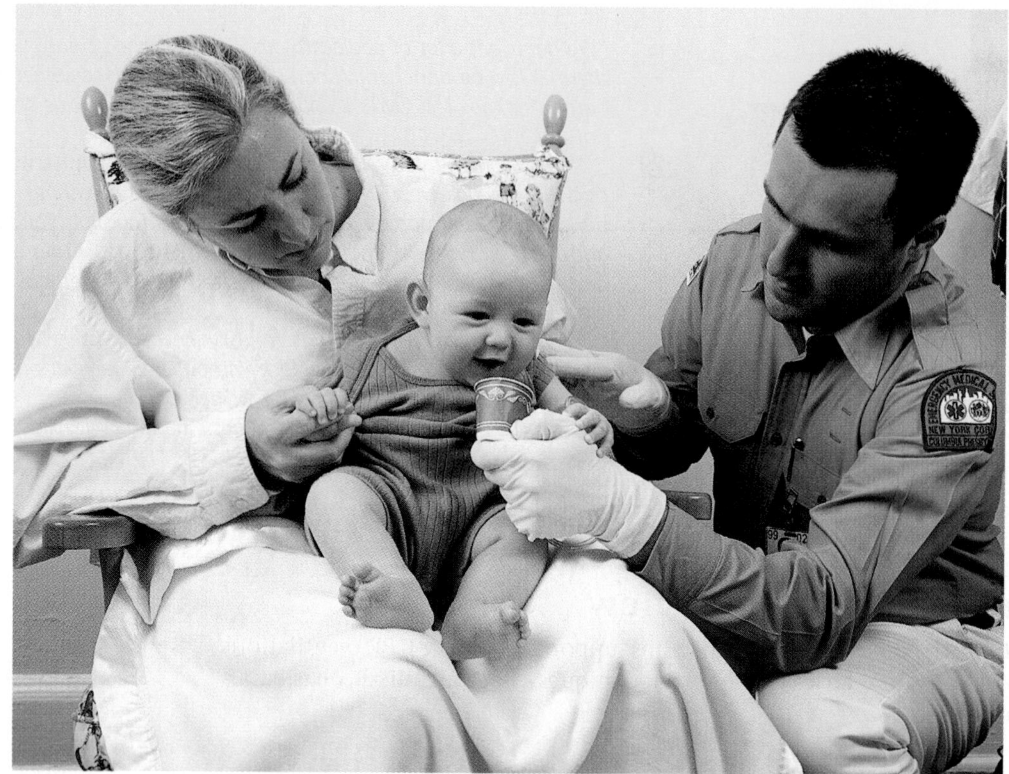

Figure 31-12 • You can deliver oxygen to an infant using the blow-by method.

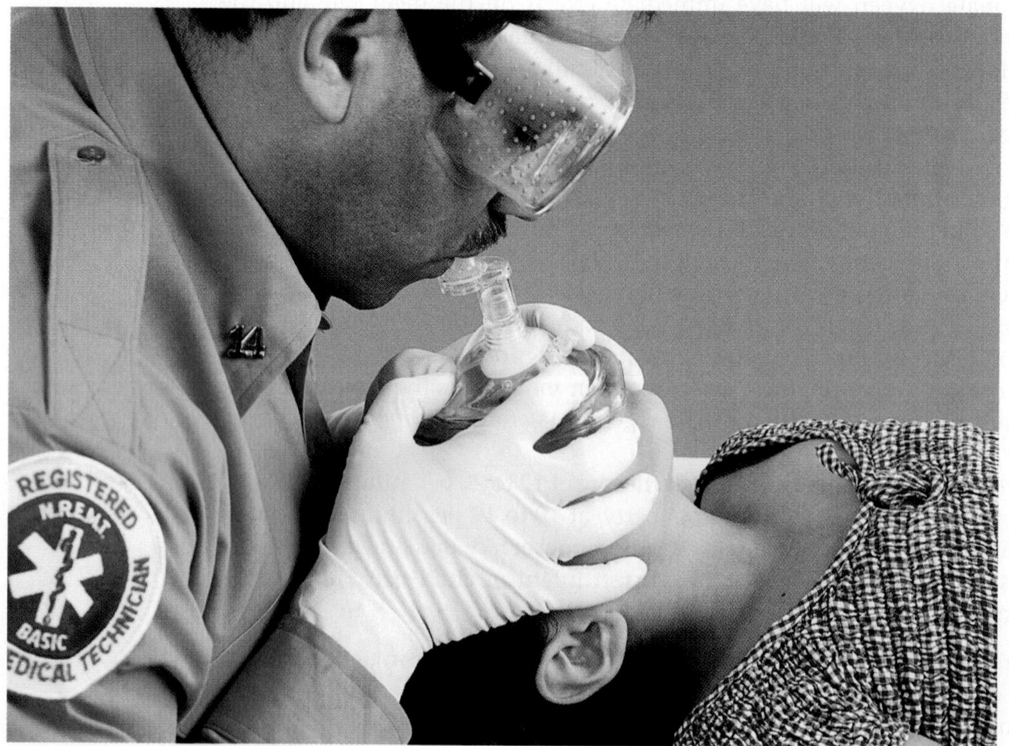

Figure 31-13 • Ventilation of a child using a pocket face mask.

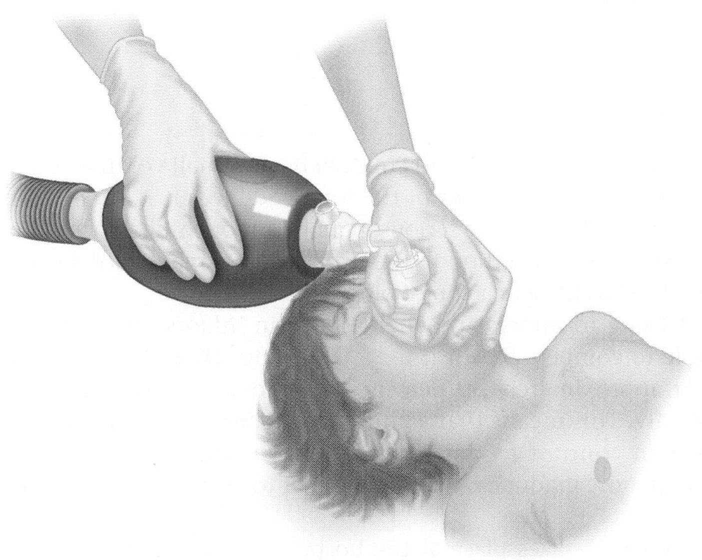

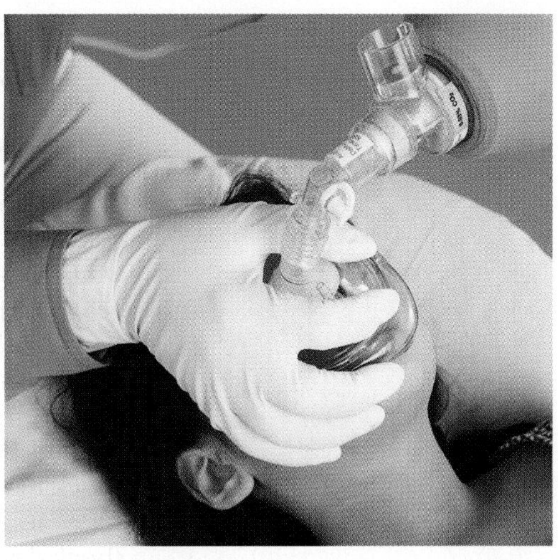

Figure 31-14 • Ventilation of a child using a bag-valve-mask device. If using one hand to squeeze the bag, achieve a good mask seal with the other hand by placing your fingers in an E-C configuration. The thumb and index finger form a C around the mask chimney while the other three fingers form an E along the child's jaw.

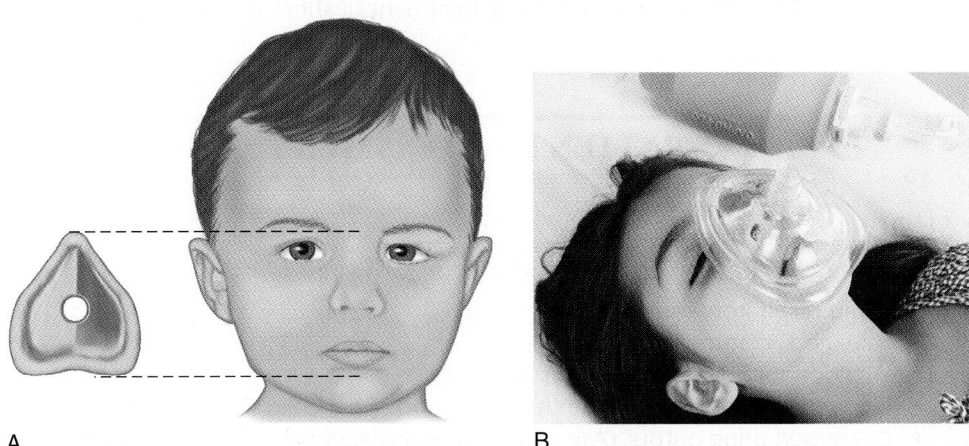

Figure 31-15 • Correct placement of a properly sized mask is necessary to ensure a good mask seal. (A) shows correct placement of the mask. (B) shows the mask placed on a child.

- If ventilation is not successful in raising the patient's chest, perform procedures for clearing an obstructed airway. Then try to ventilate again. (Review Tables 31-4 and 31-5.)

Caring for Shock (Hypoperfusion)

Shock is another term for hypoperfusion, or the inadequate circulation of blood and oxygen throughout the body. One common cause of shock in adults—a failure of heart function or of the cardiovascular system—is rare in infants and children. Common causes of shock in infants and children include:

- Diarrhea and/or vomiting with resulting dehydration
- Infection
- Trauma (especially abdominal injuries)
- Blood loss

Less common causes include:

- Allergic reactions
- Poisoning
- Cardiac events (rare)

It is important to remember that infants and children have a small volume of blood compared to adults (approximately 8 percent of the total body weight). Bleeding that would not be dangerous in an adult may be serious in an infant or child. Shock can develop in the small child who has a laceration to the scalp (with its many blood vessels) or in the 3-year-old who loses as little as a cup of blood.

The most important thing to understand about shock in infants and children is that their bodies are able to compensate for it for a long time. Then the compensating mechanisms fail, at approximately 30 percent blood loss, and decompensated shock develops very rapidly. This means that a child may appear to be fine, then "go sour" in a hurry. This is in contrast to the adult patient in whom decompensated shock develops earlier and more gradually, making it easier to assess and treat than in a child.

The definitive care for shock takes place at the hospital (usually in the operating room). Since infants and children are prone to go into decompensated shock so suddenly, IT IS IMPORTANT NOT TO WAIT FOR SIGNS OF DECOMPENSATED SHOCK TO DEVELOP. Instead, in any situation in which shock is a possibility, provide oxygen (which boosts the supply of oxygen to poorly perfused tissues and helps keep up heart function) and transport as quickly as possible.

The signs (Figure 31-16) and emergency treatment of shock are as follows.

PATIENT ASSESSMENT

SHOCK

Signs of shock in pediatric patients include the following:

- Rapid respiratory rate
- Pale, cool, clammy skin
- Weak or absent peripheral pulses
- Delayed capillary refill, more than 2 seconds (in a child 5 years or younger)
- Decreased urine output (Ask parents about diaper wetting; look at diaper.)
- Mental status changes
- Absence of tears, even when crying ■

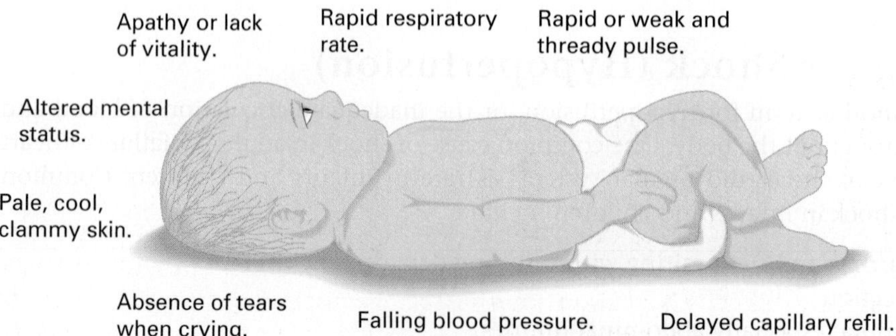
Apathy or lack of vitality.
Rapid respiratory rate.
Rapid or weak and thready pulse.
Altered mental status.
Pale, cool, clammy skin.
Absence of tears when crying.
Falling blood pressure.
Delayed capillary refill.

Figure 31-16 • Signs of shock in an infant or child.

PATIENT CARE

SHOCK

Follow these steps for emergency care:

1. Ensure an open airway.
2. Provide high-concentration oxygen. Be prepared to artificially ventilate.
3. Manage external bleeding, if present.
4. Elevate legs if there is no trauma.
5. Keep warm.
6. Transport immediately. Perform any additional assessment and treatments en route. ■

Protecting Against Hypothermia

Hypothermia, or cooling of the body, is a condition that in extreme cases is life-threatening. People lose heat more readily if their clothes are wet, if they are exposed to wind, or if they are submerged in cold water. The body attempts to compensate for a decrease in body temperature, but as these compensatory functions begin to fail, the core body temperature drops. Because children have a large surface area in proportion to their body mass, exposure to cool weather and water can result in hypothermia more easily than with adults. Therefore, hypothermia is always a concern with a pediatric patient.

Other causes of hypothermia, in children as well as in adults, include ingestion of alcohol or drugs that dilate peripheral vessels and cause loss of body heat, metabolic problems such as hypoglycemia, brain disorders that interfere with temperature regulation, severe infection or sepsis, and shock.

Hypothermia may be a concern in both medical and trauma emergencies. For example, a sick child in a cool room or in sheets or nightclothes that have become wet from perspiration or loss of bladder control may be hypothermic. When trauma occurs outdoors, caregivers attending to injuries may forget to protect the patient from a cool or damp environment, and may exacerbate the situation by exposing the patient's body during the physical exam.

Field care for children is the same as for adults. It is important to keep the patient warm. Cover the patient to avoid further loss of body heat. Special attention should be paid to covering the head, as the head is a major area of heat loss. Also, be aware of the temperature in the patient compartment of the ambulance. Consult medical direction for advice on active rewarming by application of hot water bottles or other heat sources to the body if the patient is awake and responding appropriately. Avoid rough handling and inserting anything in the mouth as these actions may cause ventricular fibrillation or cardiac arrest in the severely hypothermic child. Suction very gently if suctioning is necessary, being alert to the possibility of cardiac arrest.

PEDIATRIC MEDICAL EMERGENCIES

Respiratory Disorders

Respiratory disorders are a great concern in infants and children. For example, it is important to remember that while cardiac arrest in the adult is likely to be caused by a heart problem, the likeliest cause of cardiac arrest in a child, other than trauma, is respiratory failure. For the pediatric patient, it is important to distinguish whether the probable cause of breathing difficulty is an airway obstruction or a respiratory disease, because the care will be very different. The care that you would give for an airway obstruction can be lethal in a child with a respiratory disease. Also, because respiratory problems can have such serious consequences in infants and children, it is critical to be alert for early signs of respiratory distress.

Differentiating Airway Obstruction from Respiratory Disease

In infants and children, it is especially important to try to distinguish between an airway obstruction and an airway disease. Many of the signs of an airway obstruction are the same as the signs of airway respiratory disease, since respiratory infection or disease will also often swell and obstruct the airway passages.

With some of these diseases, it is dangerous to perform finger sweeps or to place a tongue depressor or any other instrument in the patient's mouth or pharynx because this may set off spasms along the airway. Do not attempt to clear the airway of a foreign obstruction unless it is clear that this is the problem—that is, the child has been observed ingesting a foreign object or the signs of such ingestion are clear.

In general, with suspected airway diseases you should transport as quickly as possible if you see or hear wheezing, breathing effort on exhalation, or rapid breathing.

NOTE

Airway obstruction usually occurs in the upper airway—roughly the larynx and the structures above the larynx (epiglottis, pharynx).

Airway diseases are more likely to affect the lower airway—the larynx and the structures below it (trachea, bronchi, bronchioles, alveoli).

Respiratory Distress

There are a number of respiratory diseases or disorders an infant or child may have that will cause respiratory distress, including serious ones like epiglottitis, and less serious ones like a cold. It is not easy to determine which respiratory problem the child may have. Many signs and symptoms are similar, and age ranges for occurrence overlap.

As an EMT, you do not need to decide what respiratory disorder a child is suffering from. Instead, use the following guidelines for recognizing and managing respiratory distress. It is especially important to recognize the signs of early respiratory distress and treat it before it advances to a life-threatening stage or to respiratory arrest.

PATIENT ASSESSMENT

RESPIRATORY DISTRESS

Gather information quickly from the parents and do a rapid assessment of the child. Unless there are clear indications of foreign body airway obstruction, do not put a tongue depressor in the child's mouth to examine the airway. This may cause spasms that can totally obstruct the airway. Rely on any of the following signs of early respiratory distress (Figure 31-17):

- Nasal flaring
- Retraction of the muscles above, below, and between the sternum and ribs
- Use of abdominal muscles
- Stridor (high-pitched, harsh sound)
- Audible wheezing
- Grunting
- Breathing rate greater than 60

In addition to these signs of early respiratory distress, watch for these additional signs:

- Cyanosis
- Decreased muscle tone

continued

PATIENT ASSESSMENT *(continued)*

- Poor peripheral perfusion (capillary refill greater than 2 seconds)
- Altered mental status
- Decreased heart rate (a late sign) ■

PATIENT CARE

RESPIRATORY DISTRESS

PROVIDE OXYGEN TO ALL CHILDREN WITH RESPIRATORY EMERGENCIES. For children in early respiratory distress:

- Provide oxygen by pediatric nonrebreather mask or blow-by technique.

For children in severe respiratory distress (those with respiratory distress and altered mental status, cyanosis even when oxygen is administered, poor muscle tone, or inadequate breathing):

- Provide assisted ventilations with pediatric pocket mask or bag-valve mask and supplemental oxygen.

For children in respiratory arrest:

- Ventilate with pediatric pocket mask or bag-valve mask and supplemental oxygen. ■

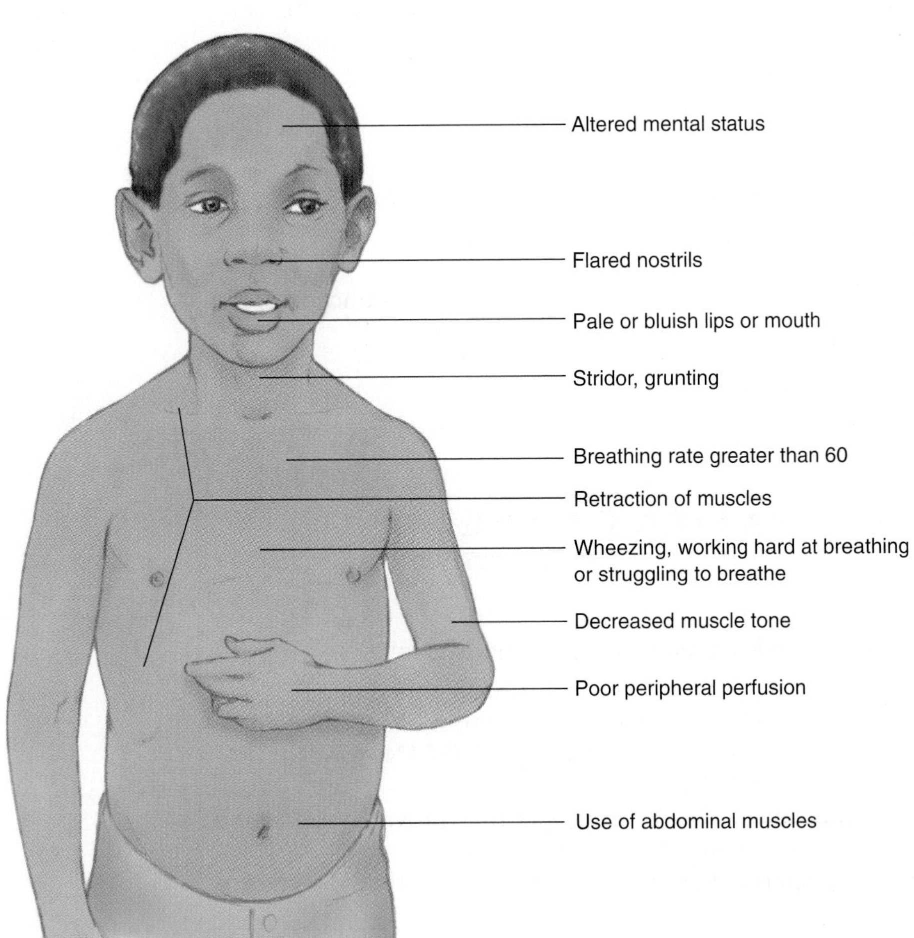

Figure 31-17 • Signs of respiratory distress.

Two illnesses that sometimes cause airway problems in children are croup and epiglottitis.

CROUP

Croup is caused by a group of viral illnesses that result in inflammation of the larynx, trachea, and bronchi. It is typically an illness of children 6 months to about 4 years of age that often occurs at night. This problem sometimes follows a cold or other respiratory infection. Tissues in the airway (particularly the upper airway) become swollen and restrict the passage of air.

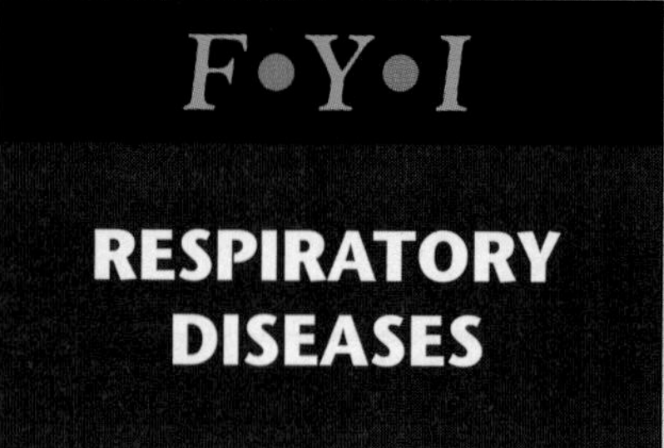

EPIGLOTTITIS

Epiglottitis is most commonly caused by a bacterial infection that produces swelling of the epiglottis and partial airway obstruction. The typical patient will be between 3 and 7 years old. Although epiglottitis has become much less common with the development of vaccines, it is a life-threatening illness that must be suspected when treating any child with stridor (a high-pitched sound caused by air moving through narrowed passageways). ■

NOTE *All cases of epiglottitis must be considered life-threatening, no matter how early the detection.*

PATIENT ASSESSMENT

CROUP

During the day, the child usually will have these signs:

- Mild fever
- Some hoarseness

At night, the child's condition will worsen and he will develop:

- A loud "seal bark" cough
- Difficulty breathing
- Signs of respiratory distress including nasal flaring, retraction of the muscles between the ribs, tugging at the throat
- Restlessness
- Paleness with cyanosis ■

PATIENT CARE

CROUP

Emergency care of a pediatric patient with croup is as follows:

1. Place the patient in a position of comfort (usually sitting up).
2. Administer high-concentration oxygen. When possible, this should be from a humidified source. (DO NOT DELAY OXYGEN ADMINISTRATION IN ORDER TO HUMIDIFY.)
3. Walk to the ambulance. The cool night air may provide relief as the cool air reduces the edema in the airway tissues.
4. Do not delay transport unless ordered to do so by medical direction. ■

PATIENT ASSESSMENT

EPIGLOTTITIS

Signs include:

- A sudden onset of high fever
- Painful swallowing (the child often will drool to avoid swallowing)
- Patient will assume a "tripod" position, sitting upright and leaning forward with the chin thrust outward (sniffing position) and the mouth wide open in an effort to maintain a wide airway opening.
- Patient will sit very still, but the muscles will work hard to breathe, and the child can tire quickly from the effort.
- Child appears more generally ill than with croup. ■

PATIENT CARE

EPIGLOTTITIS

Emergency care for the pediatric patient with epiglottitis is as follows:

1. Immediately transport the child, with the child sitting on the parent's lap.
2. Provide high-concentration oxygen from a humidified source. Do not increase the child's anxiety. If he or she resists the mask, let the parent hold it in front of the child's face. (DO NOT DELAY OXYGEN ADMINISTRATION IN ORDER TO HUMIDIFY.)
3. Constantly monitor the child for respiratory distress or arrest and be ready to resuscitate.
4. DO NOT PLACE ANYTHING INTO THE CHILD'S MOUTH, including a thermometer, tongue blade, or oral airway. To do so may set off spasms along the upper airway that will totally obstruct the airway.

The child will not want to lie down, and you should not force him to do so. The child must be handled gently, since rough handling and stress could lead to a total airway obstruction from spasms of the larynx and swelling tissues. ■

ALL RESPIRATORY DISORDERS IN CHILDREN MUST BE TAKEN SERIOUSLY. RESPIRATORY DISEASE IS THE PRIMARY CAUSE OF CARDIAC ARREST NOT DUE TO TRAUMA. If you treat the respiratory system, the heart will also respond. The EMT's primary concern when caring for infants and children with respiratory problems, whether medical or trauma related, is to establish and maintain an open airway. About one-third of all pediatric trauma deaths are related to airway mismanagement.

Fever

Above-normal body temperature is one of the most important signs of an existing or impending acute illness. Fever usually accompanies infections (ear infections are common) as well as such childhood diseases as chicken pox, mononucleosis, pneumonia, epiglottitis, and meningitis. The fever also may be due to heat exposure, any infection, or some other noninfectious disease problem.

PATIENT ASSESSMENT

FEVER

Never regard a fever as unimportant. Parents may have an opinion about what they believe may be the problem, but the EMT is not qualified to diagnose or determine what is likely to happen over the next few hours.

Use relative skin temperature as a sign. Generally oral or rectal temperatures are not taken in the prehospital setting unless permitted by local medical direction. Either a skin thermometer or information provided by the parents should be used for determining the patient's temperature. Applying the ungloved back of your hand to the patient's forehead or to the abdomen beneath the clothing is another way to determine relative skin temperature. A high relative skin temperature is always enough reason to transport and seek medical opinion. Other signs include:

- Fever with a rash is a sign of a potentially serious condition.
- A seizure or seizures may accompany a high fever. ■

PATIENT CARE

FEVER

Children can tolerate a high temperature, and only a small percent will have a seizure due to fever (febrile seizure). It is the rapid rise in temperature rather than the temperature itself that causes seizures. Cooling the child without bringing on hypothermia is an important care objective. Should you find an infant or child with a high fever, take the following steps:

1. Remove the child's clothing, but do not allow him to be exposed to conditions that may bring on hypothermia. If the child objects to having clothing removed, let the child keep on light clothing or underwear.
2. If the condition is a result of heat exposure, and if local protocols permit, cover the child with a towel soaked in tepid water. This will cool the child quickly.
3. Monitor for shivering and avoid hypothermia. This may develop quickly in children. If shivering develops, stop the cooling activities and cover the child with a light blanket.
4. If local protocols permit, give the child fluids by mouth or allow him to suck on chipped ice. This may not prevent dehydration but will increase comfort.
5. Be aware that a mild fever can quickly turn into a high fever that may indicate a serious, if not life-threatening, problem. If the infant or child feels very warm-to-hot to the touch, then prepare the patient for transport. Transport all children who have suffered a seizure as quickly as possible, protecting the patient from temperature extremes.

   There are also some "do nots" in treating an infant or child with fever:

   - Do not submerge the child in cold water, or cover with a towel soaked in ice water (which can cause hypothermia rapidly).
   - DO NOT USE RUBBING ALCOHOL TO COOL THE PATIENT. (IT CAN BE ABSORBED IN TOXIC AMOUNTS AND IS A FIRE HAZARD.) ■

Meningitis is caused by either a bacterial or a viral infection of the lining of the brain and spinal cord (the meninges). The majority of meningitis cases occur between the ages of 1 month and 5 years. ■

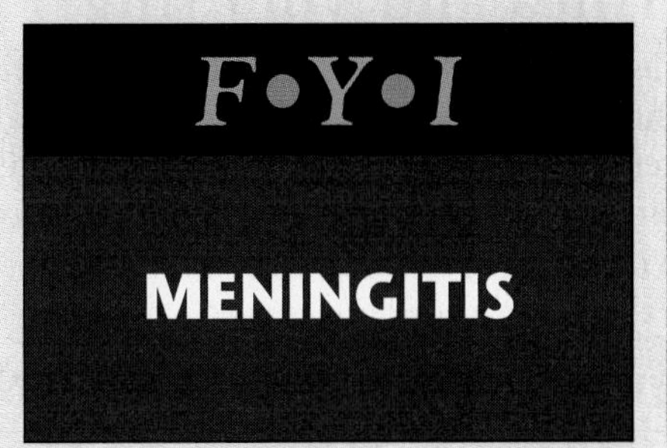

PATIENT ASSESSMENT

MENINGITIS

The following are signs and symptoms of meningitis:

- High fever
- Lethargy
- Irritability
- Headache
- Stiff neck
- Sensitivity to light
- In infants, the fontanelles may be bulging unless the child is dehydrated.
- Movement is painful and the child does not want to be touched or held.
- Seizures
- A rash may be present in the bacterial-type infection. ■

PATIENT CARE

MENINGITIS

It is most important to carefully take appropriate Standard Precautions. Wear a surgical mask, since this is an airborne disease. When meningitis is suspected, provide the following care:

1. Monitor airway, breathing, circulation, and vital signs.
2. Provide high-concentration oxygen by nonrebreather mask.
3. Ventilate with a pediatric pocket mask or bag-valve mask with supplemental oxygen if necessary.
4. Provide CPR if necessary.
5. Be alert for seizures.
6. Transport immediately. This is a TRUE EMERGENCY. Do not delay. ■

NOTE

Some forms of meningitis may be highly infectious, requiring that EMS personnel be evaluated and provided antibiotic treatment by a physician.

Diarrhea and Vomiting

Diarrhea and vomiting are common in childhood illness. Either one can cause dehydration that worsens whatever other condition the child may have and may lead to life-threatening shock. Infants are more susceptible to the effects of dehydration because, compared to adults, a greater percentage of their body is water and their fluid maintenance needs are greater.

PATIENT ASSESSMENT

DIARRHEA AND VOMITING

For any pediatric patient with diarrhea or vomiting:

1. Monitor the airway.
2. Monitor respiration.
3. Be alert for signs of shock. ■

PATIENT CARE

DIARRHEA AND VOMITING

Emergency care includes the following:

1. Maintain an open airway and be prepared to provide oral suctioning.
2. Provide oxygen if respirations are compromised.
3. If signs of shock are present, contact medical direction immediately and transport.
4. If your protocols or medical direction permits, offer the child sips of clear liquids or chipped ice if only diarrhea is present. Many physicians recommend nothing by mouth if there is nausea or vomiting.
5. Save a sample of vomitus and rectal discharge (e.g., a soiled diaper). ■

Seizures

Fever is the most common cause of seizures in infants and children. Epilepsy, infections, poisoning, hypoglycemia, trauma including head injury, or decreased levels of oxygen can also bring on seizures. Some seizures in children are idiopathic; that is, they have no known cause. They may be brief or prolonged. They are rarely life-threatening in children who have them frequently. However, THE EMT SHOULD CONSIDER SEIZURES, INCLUDING THOSE CAUSED BY FEVER, TO BE LIFE-THREATENING.

Usually, you will arrive after the convulsion has passed.

PATIENT ASSESSMENT

SEIZURES

Interview the patient as well as family members and bystanders who saw the convulsion. Ask them if the child has a history of seizures. Ask:

- Has the child had prior seizures?
- If yes, is this the child's normal seizure pattern? (How long did the seizure last? What part of the body was seizing?)

continued

PATIENT ASSESSMENT *(continued)*

- Has the child had a fever?
- Has the child taken any anti-seizure medication? other medication?

Assess the child for signs and symptoms of illness or injury, taking care to note any injuries sustained during the convulsion. All infants and children who have undergone a seizure require medical evaluation. The seizure itself may not be serious but it may be a sign of an underlying condition. Be aware that seizures may be caused by a head injury. ■

PATIENT CARE

SEIZURES

If the patient has a seizure in your presence, possibly during transport, provide the following care:

1. Maintain an open airway. Do not insert an oropharyngeal airway or bite stick.
2. Position the patient on his side if there is no possibility of spinal injury.
3. Be alert for vomiting. Suction as needed.
4. Provide oxygen. If the patient is in respiratory arrest, provide artificial ventilations with supplemental oxygen.
5. Transport.
6. Monitor for inadequate breathing and/or altered mental status, which may occur following a seizure. ■

Altered Mental Status

Altered mental status may be caused by a variety of conditions, including hypoglycemia, poisoning, infection, head injury, decreased oxygen levels, shock, or the aftermath of a seizure.

PATIENT ASSESSMENT

ALTERED MENTAL STATUS

Assessment of the patient with altered mental status focuses on life-threatening problems discovered during the initial assessment:

- Be alert for a mechanism of injury that may have caused the altered mental status, such as head injury.
- Be alert for signs of shock.
- Look for evidence of poisoning by ingested, inhaled, or absorbed substances.
- Attempt to quickly obtain a history of any seizure disorder or diabetes. ■

PATIENT CARE

ALTERED MENTAL STATUS

Emergency care of a pediatric patient with altered mental status includes the following:

1. Ensure an open airway. Be prepared to suction.
2. Protect the spine while managing the airway if a head injury or other trauma is present.
3. Administer high-concentration oxygen by pediatric nonrebreather mask or blow-by technique. Be prepared to perform artificial ventilations by pediatric pocket mask or bag-valve mask with supplemental oxygen.
4. Treat for shock.
5. Transport. ■

Poisoning

Children are often the victims of accidental poisoning, often resulting from the ingestion of household products or medications. Certain poisons can quickly depress the respiratory system, cause respiratory arrest, and cause life-threatening conditions of the circulatory and nervous systems. The airway and gastrointestinal tract can also be burned by corrosive substances upon ingestion and with subsequent vomiting.

Review Chapter 21, "Poisoning and Overdose Emergencies," for information on ingested, inhaled, absorbed, and injected poisons. This information applies to children as well as to adults.

PATIENT ASSESSMENT

POISONING

Some types of poisonings are not often associated with adult patients but are common to children. These special cases include:

- *Aspirin poisoning.* Look for hyperventilation, vomiting, and sweating. The skin may feel hot. Severe cases cause seizures, coma, or shock.
- *Acetaminophen poisoning.* Many medications have this compound, including Tylenol, Comtrex, Bancap, Excedrin PM, and Datril. Initially, the child may have no abnormal signs or symptoms. The child may be restless (early) or drowsy. Nausea, vomiting, and heavy perspiration may occur. Loss of consciousness is possible.
- *Lead poisoning.* This usually comes from ingesting chips of lead-based paint. It is often chronic (building up over a long time). Look for nausea with abdominal pain and vomiting. Muscle cramps, headache, muscle weakness, and irritability are often present.
- *Iron poisoning.* Iron compounds such as ferrous sulfate are found in some vitamin tablets and liquids. As little as 1 gram of ferrous sulfate can be lethal to a child. Within 30 minutes to several hours, the child will show nausea and bloody vomiting, often accompanied by diarrhea. Typically the child will develop shock, but this may be delayed for up to 24 hours as the child appears to be getting better.
- *Petroleum product poisoning.* The patient will usually be vomiting with coughing or choking. In most cases, you will smell the distinctive odor of a petroleum distillate (e.g., gasoline, kerosene, heating fuel). ■

PATIENT CARE

POISONING

Emergency care for a responsive patient includes:

1. Contact medical direction or the poison control center.
2. Consider the need to administer activated charcoal.
3. Provide oxygen.
4. Transport.
5. Continue to monitor the patient. The patient may become unresponsive.

Emergency care for an unresponsive patient includes:

1. Ensure an open airway.
2. Provide oxygen.
3. Be prepared to provide artificial ventilation.
4. Transport.
5. Contact medical direction or the poison control center.
6. Rule out trauma as a cause of altered mental status. ■

Drowning

As explained in Chapter 22, "Environmental Emergencies," drowning is the process of experiencing respiratory impairment from submersion/immersion in liquid, which may result in death, morbidity (illness or other adverse effects), or no morbidity. Water temperature may affect outcomes from drowning. Patients who have been submerged in *cold* water have been revived 30 minutes or more after submersion.

PATIENT ASSESSMENT

DROWNING

Assess as for any unresponsive patient:

1. Establish unresponsiveness, breathlessness, and pulselessness.
2. Perform five cycles of compressions and ventilations (30:2 ratio) at a rate of 100 compressions per minute before activating the emergency response system if this has not already been done.
3. If trauma may have been a cause or result of the submersion incident (such as injury from a dive), maintain spinal stabilization and follow trauma assessment procedures. Remember, however, that resuscitation is your first priority.
4. Consider possible ingestion of alcohol as a cause of the drowning, especially in adolescents.
5. Consider the possibility of "secondary drowning syndrome"—deterioration after normal breathing resumes, minutes to hours after the event. ■

PATIENT CARE

DROWNING

For the drowning patient, provide the following care:

1. Provide artificial ventilation or CPR as necessary. This is your first treatment priority.
2. Protect the airway. Suction if necessary.

continued

PATIENT CARE *(continued)*

3. Protect against possible hypothermia, especially if the patient has been in cool or cold water. As soon as practical, remove wet clothing, dry the skin, and cover with a blanket.
4. Treat any trauma.
5. Transport all drowning patients to the hospital, even if they seem to have recovered. ■

Sudden Infant Death Syndrome

In the United States, sudden infant death syndrome (SIDS)—the sudden unexplained death during sleep of an apparently healthy baby in its first year of life—occurs in between 2,000 and 2,500 babies each year. These babies were usually receiving proper care and frequently have passed physical examinations within days of their sudden death.

Many possible causes have been investigated but are not well understood. The problem is not caused by external methods of suffocation or by vomiting or choking. The problem may possibly be related to nerve cell development in the brain or the tissue chemistry of the respiratory system or the heart. Some relationships have been drawn to family history of SIDS and respiratory problems, but there is still no accepted reason why these babies die.

When asleep, the typical SIDS patient will show periods of cardiac slowdown and temporary cessation of breathing known as sleep apnea. Eventually, the infant will stop breathing and will not start again on its own. Unless reached in time, the episode can be fatal. The baby's condition is most commonly discovered in the early morning when the parents go to wake the baby.

It is not up to you, as an EMT, to diagnose SIDS. All you or the parents will know is that the baby is in respiratory and cardiac arrest. You will treat the baby as you would any patient in this condition:

1. Unless there is rigor mortis (stiffening of the body after death), provide resuscitation and transport to the hospital. Let the pronouncement of death come from hospital personnel, not from you. (Depending on the circumstances, some EMS systems do not transport. In these situations follow local protocol and contact medical direction as necessary.)
2. Be certain that the parents receive emotional support and that they understand that everything possible is being done for the child at the scene and during transport.

Parents who lose a child to SIDS often suffer intense guilt feelings from the moment they find the child. Whether or not the parents express such guilt, remind them that SIDS occurs to apparently healthy babies who are receiving the best of parental care. Do not speak with a suspicious tone or ask inappropriate questions. Do not be embarrassed to express your sorrow for their loss, but be sure to do so only after a physician has officially informed them of the child's death.

PEDIATRIC TRAUMA EMERGENCIES

Trauma is the number one cause of death in infants and children. Blunt trauma far exceeds penetrating trauma in this age group. Much of this trauma occurs because children are curious and learning about their environment. Exploring often leads to injury from accidental falls or things falling on them, burns, entrapment, crushing, and other mechanisms of injury.

When providing emergency care for the injured child, always tell him what you are going to do before you do it. If the child cries, let him know this is all right and you know he is trying to be brave, but everyone gets scared when hurt. Carry brightly colored adhesive bandages to hold dressings in place, and let the child know these are especially for him as a reward for bravery. You can carry along other small rewards like sheets of peel-off stickers. (Be sure the rewards are not small items that can be swallowed.)

Injury Patterns

Injury management is basically the same for children as for adults (Figure 31-18). However, their anatomic and physiological differences cause children to have different patterns of injury (Table 31-6).

During motor-vehicle collisions:

- Unrestrained child passengers (those without seat belts or restraint in a child safety seat) tend to have head and neck injuries.
- Restrained passengers may have abdominal and lower spine injuries.

Children who are struck by autos while bicycle riding often have head, spinal, and abdominal injuries. The child who has been struck by a vehicle may present with the following triad of injuries:

- Head injury
- Abdominal injury with possible internal bleeding
- Lower extremity injury (possibly a fractured femur)

Other common injuries include diving injuries with associated head and neck injury; sports injuries, which also often involve the head and neck; and injuries from child abuse.

You will need to have a good understanding of pediatric anatomic and physiologic characteristics as they relate to trauma in order to deliver expert emergency care. These include features of the head, chest, abdomen, and extremities, as described in the following paragraphs.

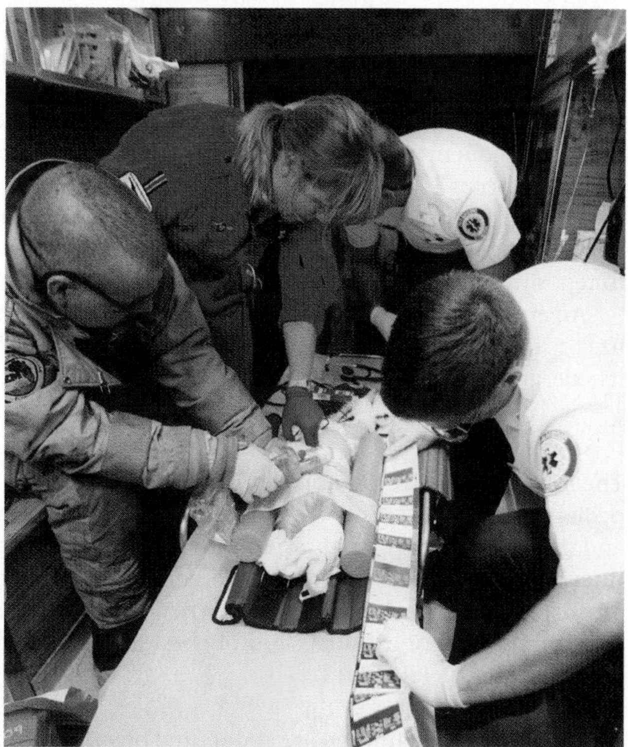

Figure 31-18 • Infant receiving emergency care. *(© Craig Jackson/In the Dark Photography)*

TABLE 31-6 • High-Risk Mechanisms of Injury and Pediatric Injury Patterns

HIGH-RISK MECHANISM	TYPE OF INJURY TO PEDIATRIC PATIENT
Motor-vehicle collision: Improperly restrained/unrestrained passenger	Serious head and neck injury, facial abrasions and lacerations. Soft-tissue injury of the neck from shoulder belt used without lap belt or shoulder belt used on a too-small child Internal abdominal injury from lap belt used without shoulder belt or lap belt improperly positioned over abdomen Fracture of lower vertebrae and spinal cord damage from violent flexion at waist when lap belt is used without shoulder belt
Pedestrian struck by car Child thrown onto hood/windshield or minimal distance on impact	Severe head injury, especially if thrown any distance, by force of high speed at impact Multiple head, chest, abdominal, and leg injuries Fracture of long bones, especially the femur Internal injury and bleeding of the liver, spleen. (Kidney, liver—blows to right upper quadrant; spleen—blows to flank and torso)
Pedestrian run over by car	Internal chest injury, often without obvious external damage Internal abdominal injury, often without obvious external damage Fractures of upper and lower extremities and the pelvis
Child struck by deployed air bag	Severe head and neck injury. Burns to the eye and face caused by the caustic powder released when air bag deploys
Falls Seriousness depends on (1) height of fall, (2) surface on which child fell, and (3) child's age. (Infants may have serious head injury from falls of 3–4 ft. from a changing table)	Head and upper neck injury and fractures to upper and lower extremities from moderate falls, 5–15 ft. Head, neck, spine injury, abdominal and chest injury, and fractures of upper and lower extremities from high falls over 15 ft.

Head

Recall that the head is proportionately larger and heavier in the small child. This leads to head injury when the head is propelled forward in a collision. This is often combined with internal injuries. Suspect internal injuries whenever a child with a head injury presents with shock, since head injury itself is seldom a cause of shock. Respiratory arrest is a common secondary effect of head injury, so be alert to this possibility. Although the most frequent sign of head injury is an altered mental status, nausea and vomiting also often occur.

The most important common cause of hypoxia in the unconscious head-injury patient is the tongue falling back and blocking the airway. Use the jaw-thrust maneuver to reposition the tongue and open the airway.

An error to avoid in caring for the child with a head injury is using sandbags to stabilize the head. Should the patient begin to vomit, the backboard will need to be turned on its side, and the weight of the heavy sandbag on the child's head may cause further injury.

Chest

The less-developed respiratory muscles of the chest and the more elastic ribs make the pediatric chest more easily deformed. The immature respiratory muscles may tire easily and cannot maintain rapid respiratory rates for long. The more elastic ribs rarely fracture; however, there is more likely to be injury to the structures beneath the ribs. You must suspect internal chest injuries when the mechanism of injury is significant, despite the absence of external signs of chest injury.

Abdomen

Infants and young children are abdominal breathers; that is, they use their diaphragms for breathing. Thus, they may not have significant movement of their chests while breathing. Watch the abdomen to evaluate breathing. In addition, abdominal muscles are immature and therefore provide less protection to internal organs than do adult abdominal muscles.

The abdomen can be a site of "hidden" injuries. You must suspect an internal abdominal injury when the patient deteriorates even without evidence of external injury. In addition, air in the stomach can distend the abdomen and interfere with artificial ventilation. This may also lead to vomiting. Be prepared to suction the patient.

Extremities

Despite the more flexible bones in the pediatric patient, their extremity injuries are managed the same way as extremity injuries in adults.

Pneumatic Anti-Shock Garments

In some EMS systems, pneumatic anti-shock garments (PASG) may be employed for the treatment of shock and bleeding in pediatric patients. Some general principles for their use in pediatric patients include the following:

- Use them only if they fit the patient. Never place the infant in one leg of an adult garment.
- Do not inflate the abdominal compartment. This may compromise breathing.
- PASG may be indicated for the treatment of the pediatric trauma patient with signs of severe hypoperfusion and pelvic instability.

Burns

Burns are a common pediatric injury. Review the "rule of nines" in Chapter 27, "Soft-Tissue Injuries," as it applies to estimating the extent of burns in children and infants. Follow these guidelines when managing patients with burns:

- Identify candidates for transportation to burn centers. Local protocols should guide your determination.
- Cover the burn with sterile dressings. Nonadherent dressings are the best, but sterile sheets may be used.

Moist dressings should be used with caution in the pediatric patient. Remember that the child's body surface area is larger proportionately to their body mass, making them more prone to heat loss. Burned patients who become hypothermic have a higher death rate. You must keep the infant or child covered to prevent a drop in body temperature.

PATIENT CARE

TRAUMA

Emergency care steps for the pediatric trauma patient should include the following:

1. Ensure an open airway. Use the jaw-thrust maneuver.
2. Suction as necessary, using a rigid suction catheter.
3. Provide high-concentration oxygen.
4. Ventilate with a pediatric pocket mask or bag-valve mask as needed.
5. Provide spinal immobilization (Figure 31-19 and Scan 31-4).
6. Transport immediately.
7. Continue to reassess en route.
8. Assess and treat other injuries en route if time permits. ■

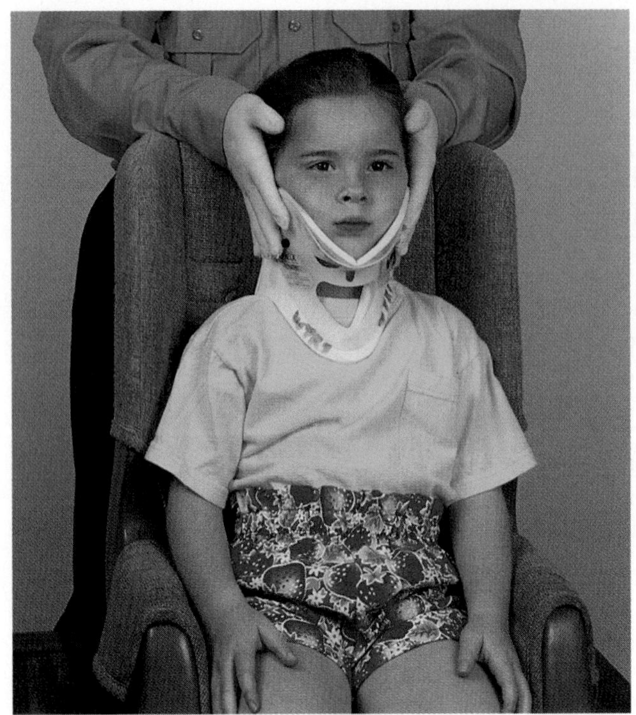

Figure 31-19 • Some protocols allow a child who is secured in an undamaged child safety seat to be immobilized and transported in the safety seat.

SCAN 31-4 • Immobilizing a Child Using a KED

Many pediatric immobilization devices are available, but an adult Kendrick Extrication Device (KED) can also be used successfully to immobilize a child if adjusted to suit the child's size and anatomy.

Manually stabilize the child's neck and spine throughout, and apply a cervical spine immobilization collar before securing the child to the KED.

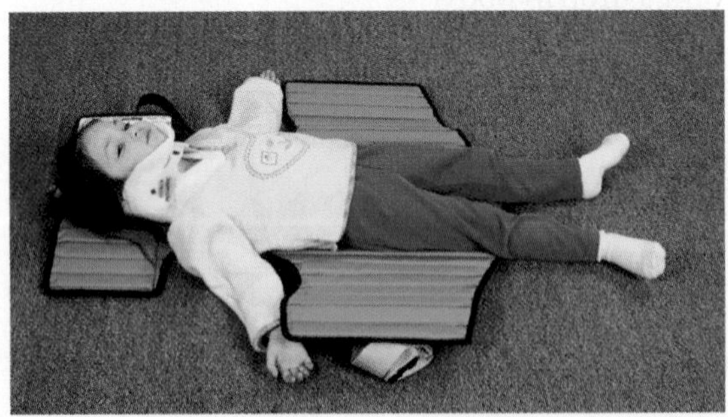

1. Open the KED and place padding on it to properly position and align the child's head and body. Log roll the child onto the KED.

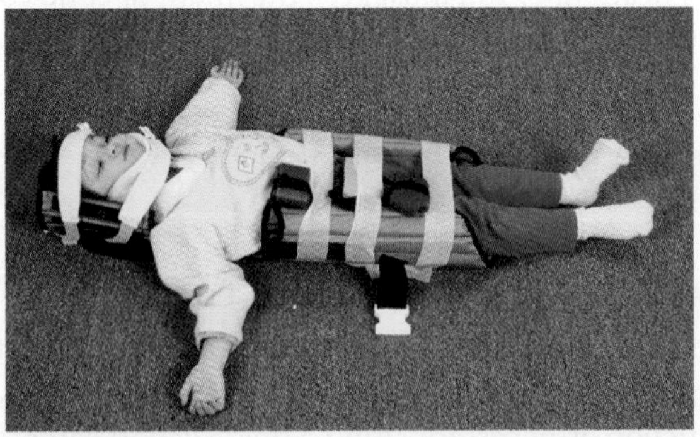

2. Fold the side pieces inward to provide side padding and support and to allow visualization of the chest and abdomen. Since the torso straps will be rolled to the inside, secure the torso with tape. Fold the head flaps securely against the child's head and tape across the head and chin.

CRITICAL DECISION MAKING:
The Little Ones Make Us Nervous

Pediatric patients cause stress because the stakes are high and we (fortunately) don't get a lot of pediatric calls. The decision making in this section will involve your "from-the-doorway" pediatric assessment. With the information provided, determine if the patient is in a serious or a less serious condition.

1. You are met at the door by an upset mother who is holding a limp 13-month-old child in her arms.
2. A 3-year-old child is reported as having a croupy cough and difficulty breathing. She is screaming and clinging to her mother as you approach.
3. A child has fallen from a high sliding board. You arrive to find the child holding his left forearm against his body while quietly clinging to his mother.

CHILD ABUSE AND NEGLECT

The number of known child abuse cases is large but the real number may be even larger than the statistics indicate. Experts believe that for every abused child seen by the emergency department or family physician, there are many more unreported cases who never receive care.

Child abusers are mothers, fathers, sisters, brothers, grandparents, stepparents, baby-sitters and other caregivers, white-collar workers, blue-collar workers, and those who are unemployed, rich, or poor. There is no distinction as to race, creed, ethnicity, or economic background.

Child abuse can take several different forms, often occurring in combination. These forms include:

- Psychological (emotional) abuse
- Neglect
- Physical abuse
- Sexual abuse

What constitutes neglect is a serious legal question. If a child goes without proper food, shelter, clothing, supervision, treatment of injuries and illnesses, a safe environment, and love, the effects surely will be seen but will seldom directly trigger an emergency call. Physical and sexual abuse are the problems likely to be seen by EMTs. If signs of neglect are observed in the course of a call, they should also be reported to the proper authorities.

Physical and Sexual Abuse

Abusers inflict almost every imaginable kind of injury and maltreatment. Physically abused children—often called "battered" children—are beaten with fists, hair brushes, straps, electric cords, pool cues, razor straps, bottles, broom handles, baseball bats, pots and pans, and almost any other object that can be used as a weapon. They are intentionally burned by hot water, steam, open flames, cigarettes, and other thermal sources. Battered children may be severely shaken, thrown into their cribs or down steps, pushed out of windows and over railings, and even pushed from moving cars. Some are shot, stabbed, electrocuted, or suffocated.

Sexual abuse ranges from adults exposing themselves to children to sexual intercourse or sexual torture. Adults exposing themselves to children are often reported to the authorities. Cases in which sexual abuse results in serious physical injury also are typically reported. The cases in between, especially those in which emotional injury or minor physical injury were done, are usually not reported, and therefore are difficult to estimate.

PATIENT ASSESSMENT

PHYSICAL ABUSE

In child physical abuse cases, you will find (Figure 31-20):

- Slap marks, bruises, abrasions, lacerations, and incisions of all sizes and with shapes matching the item used. You may see wide welts from belts, in a looped shape from cords, or in the shape of a hand from slapping. You may find swollen limbs, split lips, black eyes, and loose or broken teeth. Often the injuries are to the back, legs, and arms. The injuries may be in various stages of healing, as evidenced by different-colored bruises.
- Broken bones are common and all types of fractures are possible. Many battered children have multiple fractures, often in various stages of healing, or have fracture-associated complications.
- Head injuries are common, with concussions and skull fractures being reported. Closed head injuries occur to many infants and small children who have been severely shaken.
- Abdominal injuries include ruptured spleens, livers and lungs lacerated by broken ribs, internal bleeding from blunt trauma and punching, and lacerated and avulsed genitalia.
- Bite marks may be present showing the teeth size and pattern of the adult mouth.
- Burn marks that are small and round from cigarettes; "glove" or "stocking" burn marks from dipping in hot water; burns on buttocks and legs (creases behind the knees and at the thighs are protected when flexed); and demarcation burns in the shape of an iron, stove burner, or other hot utensil are frequently found.
- Indications of shaking an infant include a bulging fontanelle due to increased intracranial pressure from the bleeding of torn blood vessels in the brain, unconsciousness, and typical signs and symptoms of head and brain injury. Injuries to the central nervous system from "the shaken baby syndrome" are the most lethal child abuse injuries.

Sometimes you will treat an injured child and never think that he has been abused. The child relates well with the parents and there appears to be a strong bond between them. However, there can be certain indications that abuse may be occurring in or outside the home, with the family feeling they must not admit to the problem. Be on the alert for:

- Repeated responses to provide care for the same child or children in a family. Remember that in areas with many hospitals, you may see the child more frequently than any one hospital.
- Indications of past injuries. This is one reason why you must do a physical examination and why you must remove articles of clothing. Pay special attention to the back and buttocks of the child.
- Poorly healing wounds or improperly healed fractures. It is extremely rare for a child to receive a fracture, be given proper orthopedic care, and then show angulations and large "bumps" and "knots" of bone at the "healed" injury site.
- Indications of past burns or fresh bilateral burns. Children seldom put both hands on a hot object or touch the same hot object again (true, some do—this is only an indication, not proof). Some types of burns are almost always linked to child abuse, such as cigarette burns to the body and burns to the buttocks and lower extremities that result from the child being dipped in hot water.

continued

PATIENT ASSESSMENT *(continued)*

- Many different types of injuries to both sides or the front and back of the body. This gains even more importance if the adults on the scene keep insisting that the child "falls a lot."
- Fear on the part of the child to tell you how the injury occurred. The child may seem to expect no comfort from the parents and may have little or no apparent reaction to pain.
- The parent or caregiver at the scene who does not wish to leave you alone with the child, tells conflicting or changing stories, overwhelms you with explanations of the cause of the injury, or faults the child may rouse your suspicions and cause you to assess the situation more carefully.

Pay attention to the adults as you treat the child:

- Do they seem inappropriately unconcerned about the child?
- Do they have trouble controlling anger?
- Do you feel that at any moment there may be an emotional explosion?
- Do any of the adults appear to be in a deep state of depression?
- Are there indications of alcohol or drug abuse?
- Do any of the adults speak of suicide or seeking mercy for their unhappy children?

Parents or caregivers may have called for help for the child, yet be reluctant to provide a history of the injury and refuse transport. Take note of any parent who refuses to have his child sent to the nearest hospital or to a hospital where the child has been seen before. This may indicate fear of the staff remembering or seeing a record of past injuries. (You cannot transport without parental consent; however, you may be able to convince the parents the child needs to be seen by a doctor because of certain signs and symptoms that are "difficult to determine" in the field.) Be the child's advocate, but do not accuse the parent. ■

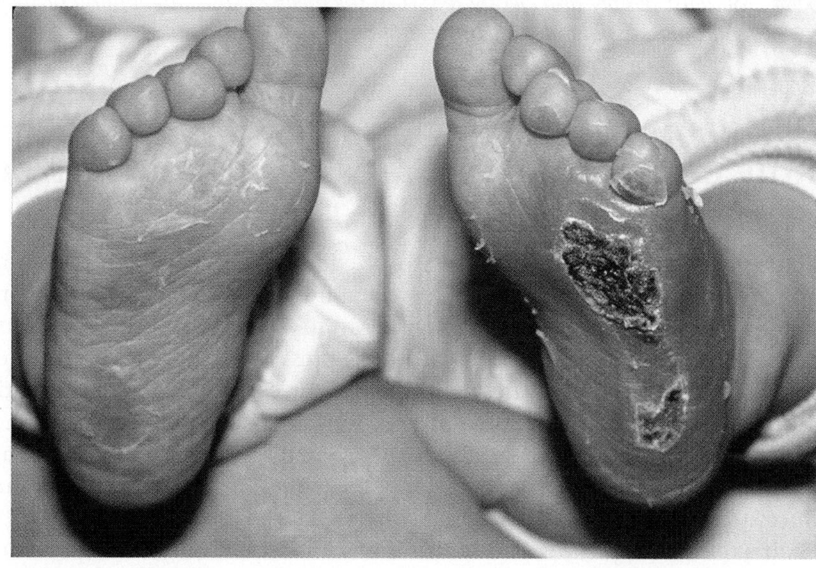

Figure 31-20 • Child abuse injuries. *(© Robert A. Felter, M.D.)*

PATIENT ASSESSMENT

SEXUAL ABUSE

Rearrange or remove clothing only as necessary to determine and treat injuries. This will help preserve evidence where possible. Examine the genitalia only if there is obvious injury or the child tells you of a recent injury. The child may be hysterical, frightened, or withdrawn and unable to give you a history of the incident. Be calm and as reassuring as possible. Signs of sexual abuse include:

- Obvious results of sexual assault, including burns or wounds to the genitalia.
- Any unexplained genital injury such as bruising, lacerations, or bloody discharge from genital orifices (openings).
- Seminal fluid on the body or clothes or other discharges associated with sexually transmitted diseases.
- In rare cases, the child may tell you that he was sexually assaulted.

Remain professional and control your emotions. Protect the child from embarrassment. Say nothing that may make the child believe that he is to blame for the sexual assault. (Many believe that they are.) ■

PATIENT CARE

PHYSICAL OR SEXUAL ABUSE

Emergency care includes the following:

1. Dress and provide other appropriate care for injuries as necessary.
2. Preserve evidence of sexual abuse if it is suspected:
   - Discourage the child from going to the bathroom (for both defecation and urination).
   - Give nothing to the patient by mouth.
   - Do not have the child wash or change clothes.
3. Transport the child. ■

NOTE *You must plainly and clearly report to the medical staff any finding or suspicion regarding possible physical or sexual abuse.*

Role of the EMT in Cases of Suspected Abuse or Neglect

Remember that you are charged with providing emergency care for an injured child. You are not a physician trained to detect abuse or neglect, a police officer, court investigator, social worker, judge, or one-person jury. Gather information from the parents or caregiver away from the child without expression of disbelief or judgment. Talk with the child separately about how an injury occurred. As you assess the patient and provide appropriate care, control your emotions and hold back accusations. Do not indicate to the parents or other adults at the scene that you suspect child abuse or neglect. Do not ask the child if he has been abused. Doing so when others are around could produce stress too great for the injured child to handle.

If you are suspicious about the mechanism of injury, transport the child even though the severity of injury may not warrant such action.

Cultural Considerations

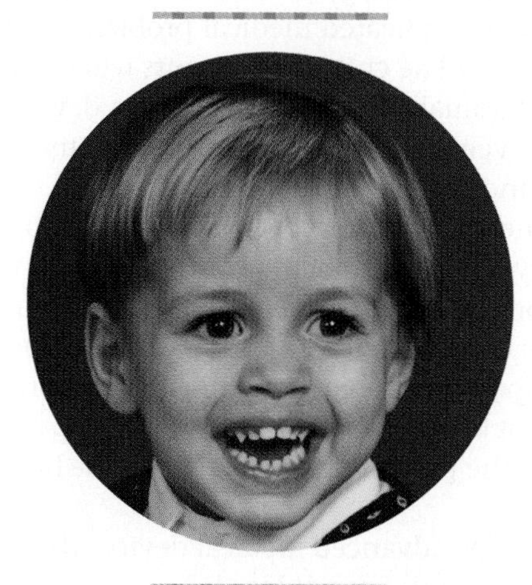

Conflicts can occur when traditional rituals and practices of a family or of a religious group the family belongs to do not conform with current medical practices. As an EMT, you need to be sensitive to the potential implications for the child's medical care. When parents refuse medical care for a child, is it just a cultural or religious difference to be respected? Or does it constitute child neglect or abuse?

As always, of course, be polite and respectful toward the family. However, do not shirk your responsibility to the child, who is your patient. Make every effort to persuade the family to permit the treatment and transport you feel the child should have, patiently explaining the medical reasons. And always report any refusal of care and any suspicions you may have regarding abuse or neglect, according to the laws of your state and the protocols of your EMS agency.

ALWAYS report your suspicions to the emergency department staff and in accordance with local policies. Every medical facility should take action to see if your fears are well founded. If you fear that the medical staff has not taken you seriously, then you must report your suspicions to the juvenile authorities of the local police department. In some states, EMTs are mandatory reporters; that is, they are required by law to report suspicions of child abuse or neglect. Be familiar with your state laws. Even if reporting possible child abuse or neglect is not a legal requirement in your state, it is a professional obligation. As an EMT you may be the only advocate an abused child has. Be conscientious.

Maintain patient and family confidentiality. You cannot name the child or the family or give any details concerning the family to anyone other than the medical staff, the police, your superior officer, or the agency that deals with child abuse. Follow department requirements and state laws in reporting the problem.

Past responses can be checked and future responses noted in case a pattern develops to indicate possible abuse. However, even when talking to your partner, the hospital staff, the police, and your superiors, use the terms *suspected* and *possible*. Do not call someone a child abuser. Keep in mind that the courts can deal harshly with those who provide patient care and then violate the confidentiality of the patient, the family, and the home. Keep in mind that rumors about abuse may, in the long run, cause mental or physical harm to your child patient.

It may be difficult, but keep in mind that the parent or caregiver needs help also. Your actions, response, and concern directed toward suspected abusers can help them recognize their problem and may encourage them to seek therapy and rehabilitation. Also bear in mind that your suspicions may be unfounded. Not every injury to a child is the result of child abuse. Suspicions should be aroused not by individual injuries but by patterns of injuries and behavior.

INFANTS AND CHILDREN WITH SPECIAL NEEDS

Over the years, medical expertise has improved significantly, allowing many children who would formerly have died to live. The group of children with special needs includes:

- Premature infants with lung disease
- Infants and children with heart disease

- Infants and children with neurological disease
- Children with chronic disease or altered function from birth

Often these children are able to live at home with their parents. This means that you may receive calls to care for children who have complicated medical problems and are dependent on various technologies (Figure 31-21). The children's parents will be familiar with the various devices and can serve as a valuable resource. Common devices include tracheostomy tubes, home artificial ventilators, central intravenous lines, gastrostomy tubes and gastric feeding tubes, and shunts.

Emergency care of children with special needs has often been complicated by the lack of information that EMTs and emergency department staff are able to quickly obtain about their medication, condition, history, precautions needed, and special management plans. In 1999, the American College of Emergency Physicians (ACEP) and the American Academy of Pediatrics (AAP) developed the Emergency Information Form for Children with Special Needs that should be kept up to date and on hand by the patient's caregivers. If a copy of this form is available at the patient's home, it should be brought along if the child is transported to the hospital.

More about patients with special needs and the advanced medical devices they may rely on will be discussed in Chapter 32, "Patients with Special Needs."

Tracheostomy Tubes

Tracheostomy tubes are tubes that have been placed into the child's trachea to create an open airway (Figure 31-22). They are often used when a child has been on a ventila-

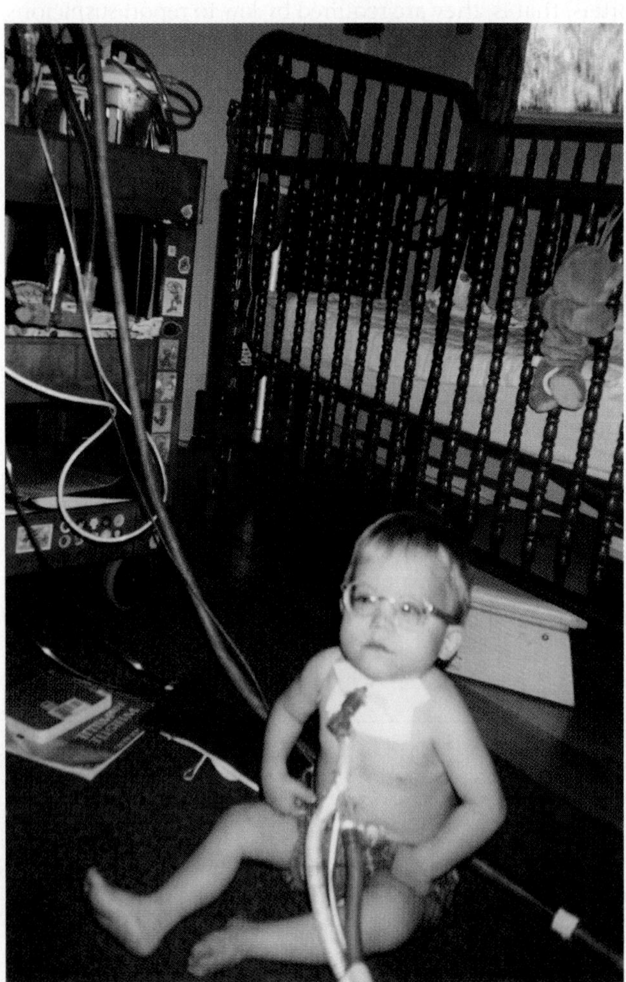

Figure 31-21 • Children who have complicated medical problems are often dependent on various technologies. *(© Family Voices)*

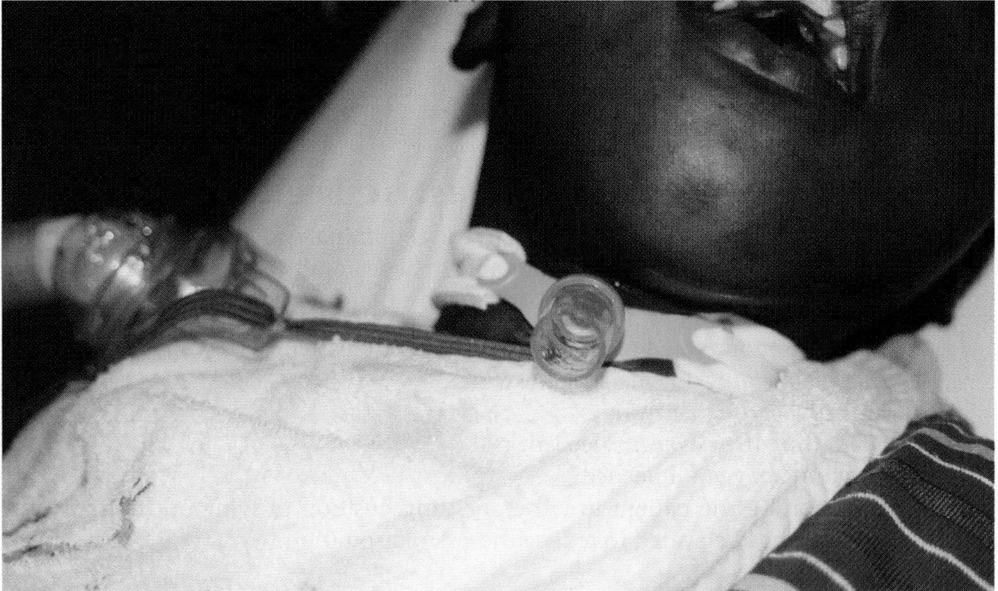

Figure 31-22 • Various emergencies may arise when a child has a tracheostomy. *(© Fran Nadel, M.D.)*

tor for a prolonged time. Although there are various types of tubes, the potential complications are identical. You may be called to help when there is:

- Obstruction
- Bleeding from the tube or around the tube
- Air leak around the tube
- Infection
- Dislodged tube

Your emergency care will consist of:

- Maintaining an open airway
- Suctioning the tube as needed
- Allowing the patient to remain in a position of comfort, perhaps on the parent's lap
- Transporting the patient to the hospital

Home Artificial Ventilators

Artificial ventilators in the home are becoming more common. The parents will be trained in the ventilator's use but will call EMS when there is trouble. Regardless of the problem, your emergency care will include:

- Maintaining an open airway
- Artificially ventilating with a pocket mask or bag-valve mask with oxygen
- Transporting the patient

Central Intravenous Lines

Central lines are intravenous lines that are placed close to the heart. Unlike most peripheral IV lines, central lines may be left in place for long-term use. Possible complications of central lines are:

- Infection
- Bleeding
- Clotting-off of the line
- Cracked line

Your emergency care will include:

- Applying pressure if there is bleeding
- Transporting the patient

Gastrostomy Tubes and Gastric Feeding

Gastrostomy tubes are tubes placed through the abdominal wall directly into the stomach. These are used when a patient is not able to be fed orally. The most dangerous potential problem involves respiratory distress. The emergency care will include:

- Being alert for altered mental status in diabetic patients. They may become hypoglycemic quickly when unable to eat.
- Ensuring an open airway.
- Suctioning the airway as needed.
- Providing oxygen if needed.
- Transporting the patient in either a sitting position or lying on the right side with the head elevated to reduce the risk of aspiration.

Shunts

A shunt is a drainage device that runs from the brain to the abdomen to relieve excess cerebrospinal fluid. There will be a reservoir on the side of the skull. Should the shunt malfunction, pressure inside the skull will rise, causing an altered mental status. An altered mental status may also be caused by an infection. These patients are prone to respiratory arrest. Your emergency care will include:

- Maintaining an open airway
- Ventilating with a pocket mask or bag-valve mask and high-concentration oxygen if needed
- Transporting the patient

THE EMT AND PEDIATRIC EMERGENCIES

Many types of pediatric illnesses and injuries have been discussed. The focus has been on the patient. Now we will look at the psychological responses of the EMT.

It is well known that pediatric calls can be among the most stressful for the EMT, even when they are uneventful. EMTs who have children often identify their patients with their own children. Other EMTs have no experience with children and feel anxiety about communicating with them and treating them—even about estimating their ages. However, the skills of communicating with and treating children can be learned and applied. Often the EMT who starts out "knowing nothing about children" turns out to have a real knack for dealing with them.

Most of the care of children consists of applying what you have learned about the care of adult patients with knowledge of the key differences in developmental characteristics, anatomy, and physiology of children.

Often the most serious stresses an EMT faces result from pediatric calls that involve a very sick, injured, or abused child, or a child who has died or who dies during or after emergency care. Such calls are, fortunately, rare, and can be prepared for with advance training.

When you have had an experience like this, talk with other EMTs. If your squad or service has a counselor, see this person for advice. You may think that you can handle the stress or sorrow by yourself, but experienced EMTs know better. Unless you resolve the impact of stressful events, the problems created may compound and could lead to "burnout."

CHAPTER REVIEW

SUMMARY

For the most part, assessment and treatment for the illnesses and injuries of infants and children are like the assessment and treatment for adults. However, children do have some special developmental characteristics, as well as special characteristics of anatomy and physiology. To assess and treat infants and children effectively, you should know something about these special characteristics of children and the illnesses and injuries to which they are prone.

REVIEW QUESTIONS

1. Name one psychological/social characteristic that you would be likely to find in a patient of each of the following ages and explain how you would tailor your actions as an EMT to accommodate this characteristic: 2-year-old, 6-year-old, and 15-year-old. (pp. 809–810)
2. Describe how each of the differences you named for question 1 will affect your assessment of the infant or child patient. (pp. 809–810)
3. Describe key differences in the anatomy and physiology of infants and children with regard to the following: (pp. 810–813)
    - Head
    - Airway and respiratory system
    - Chest
    - Abdomen
    - Body surface
    - Blood volume
4. Describe ways of calming and interacting effectively with the infant or child patient and with the parent or caregiver. (pp. 813–816)
5. Explain some of the elements of a general impression of the infant or child patient that you can obtain "from the doorway"—before you approach the patient. (pp. 817–819)
6. Explain how to differentiate between an upper airway obstruction and a lower airway disease or disorder. Explain how and why the two should be treated differently. (p. 838)
7. Explain the main steps of emergency treatment for any infant or child trauma patient. (p. 851)
8. Explain how suspicion of child abuse should or should not affect the care you provide for an infant or child patient. Explain the reporting requirements regarding child abuse and neglect in your state or locality. (pp. 853–857)

CRITICAL THINKING

- You are called to the scene of a collision between a vehicle and a 5-year-old on a bicycle. The child is lying near the curb. Based on what you know about the developmental characteristics of children as well as common injury patterns in children, explain some of the special elements you should take into consideration as you proceed to assess and care for this patient.

Thinking and Linking

Think back to Chapter 8, "The Initial Assessment," and link information from that chapter with information from this chapter, "Infants and Children," as you consider the following situation:

- You are called to respond to a "sick baby." When you arrive, you are led to a baby in its crib. The baby's eyes are closed. How do you conduct your initial assessment?

MEDIA RESOURCES 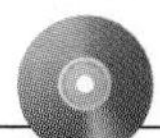

See the Student CD at the back of this book for quizzes, a case study activity, animations, and other features related to this chapter. In particular, take a look at the animations on the ear and eye. Also, visit the Companion Website for *Emergency Care* at **www.prenhall.com/limmer**, where you will find additional reinforcement and links to other resources.

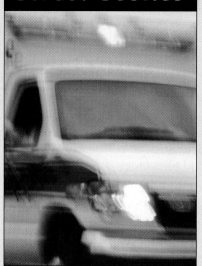

Street Scenes

Shawna Simon is an active 2-year-old who has been playing most of the afternoon since her nap. After dinner, her mother notices that her face seems flushed, her forehead is warm, and she is not her usual self. After getting Shawna ready for bed, the mother sits with her for a while. Just as she is about to leave the room, Shawna arches her back and starts to shake. The mother is frightened, and when she turns on the light, Shawna appears not to be breathing. The mother calls 911 immediately. The dispatcher has trouble calming her down, but he does hear her say, "My baby isn't breathing."

While one dispatcher continues to calm the mother, another dispatches you to 143 Pine Lane for "a child not breathing. More information to follow."

Street Scene Questions

1. What is your assessment plan for this patient?
2. What equipment should be brought into the house?
3. Should ALS be dispatched to the scene prior to your arrival?

Your response time is less than 5 minutes. Your partner radios the dispatcher and asks for an ALS response before you arrive at the scene. Dispatch has informed you that the mother is still very upset and he has no additional information. About a minute before arriving, you discuss with your partner the equipment that needs to go into the house, and you both agree to take in the pediatric bag that contains the airway equipment, including the BVM, an oxygen tank, and suction.

You volunteer to get the equipment, while your partner goes to the patient. Your partner enters the house just before you and he sees the mother holding a limp child. He takes Shawna and places her on the couch.

Your partner immediately evaluates the airway and breathing. He then performs a head-tilt, chin-lift maneuver, which brings the tongue forward. He sees mucus around the mouth, so he clears the airway by suctioning. Shawna becomes more responsive and cries. Her respirations are deep and adequate. (They would have to be for her to cry that loudly.) You and your partner realize that it is a good sound.

Street Scene Questions

4. What care should be provided next?
5. What additional assessment needs to be done?
6. What information needs to be relayed to the ALS unit?

You administer blow-by oxygen to the patient, while your partner gets a full set of vital signs. You reassure the mother that Shawna is breathing and tell her that she can help by answering some questions. You proceed to ask all the SAMPLE questions. Shawna's mother describes what led up to this event. You radio the ALS unit with this information and are informed of a 2-minute ETA, so you start to package the patient for transport to the hospital. As you are doing this, Shawna opens her eyes. She continues to cry and you ask her mother to hold her hand and talk to her. Although she is not fully alert, she is breathing well and her skin color is improving.

As you arrive at the ambulance, the ALS unit pulls up and a paramedic gets into your patient compartment. She does an assessment and is confident that a BLS transport is all that is required. She calls medical direction and provides a patient history with vital signs. Medical direction concurs that a BLS transport is appropriate. As she returns to her vehicle, the paramedic compliments you and your partner on a job well done.

Street Scenes Sample Documentation

PATIENT NAME: *Shawna Simon* **PATIENT AGE:** *2 years*

CHIEF COMPLAINT

"Isn't breathing"

PAST MEDICAL HISTORY

- [x] None
- [ ] Allergy to ______
- [ ] Hypertension
- [ ] Stroke
- [ ] Seizures
- [ ] Diabetes
- [ ] COPD
- [ ] Cardiac
- [ ] Other (List)
- [ ] Asthma

Current Medications (List)

VITAL SIGNS

TIME	RESP	PULSE	B.P.	MENTAL STATUS	R PUPILS L	SKIN
1905	Rate: 32 [ ] Regular [x] Shallow [ ] Labored	Rate: 120 [x] Regular [ ] Irregular	/	[ ] Alert [ ] Voice [ ] Pain [x] Unresp.	[x] Normal [x] [ ] Dilated [ ] [ ] Constricted [ ] [ ] Sluggish [ ] [ ] No-Reaction [ ]	[ ] Unremarkable [ ] Cool [ ] Pale [x] Warm [ ] Cyanotic [x] Moist [x] Flushed [ ] Dry [ ] Jaundiced
1915	Rate: 30 [x] Regular [ ] Shallow [ ] Labored	Rate: 110 [x] Regular [ ] Irregular	/	[ ] Alert [x] Voice [ ] Pain [ ] Unresp.	[x] Normal [x] [ ] Dilated [ ] [ ] Constricted [ ] [ ] Sluggish [ ] [ ] No-Reaction [ ]	[ ] Unremarkable [ ] Cool [ ] Pale [x] Warm [ ] Cyanotic [x] Moist [ ] Flushed [ ] Dry [ ] Jaundiced
1925	Rate: 30 [x] Regular [ ] Shallow [ ] Labored	Rate: 110 [x] Regular [ ] Irregular	/	[ ] Alert [x] Voice [ ] Pain [ ] Unresp.	[x] Normal [x] [ ] Dilated [ ] [ ] Constricted [ ] [ ] Sluggish [ ] [ ] No-Reaction [ ]	[ ] Unremarkable [ ] Cool [ ] Pale [x] Warm [ ] Cyanotic [ ] Moist [ ] Flushed [x] Dry [ ] Jaundiced

NARRATIVE *On arrival, mom was holding the child, who was limp in her arms. Mother stated the patient became flushed, lethargic, and felt warm to the touch, and suddenly began to shake and appeared not to be breathing. The patient was unresponsive initially. While assessing the patient, she was noted to be breathing with mucus around her mouth. After suctioning, oxygen was initiated at 10 LPM with a pediatric nonrebreather via blow-by technique. Patient gradually became more responsive and was crying prior to transport. ALS arrived at the scene but did not come with us to the hospital. Both the paramedics and medical direction felt the patient was stable and appropriate for BLS transport.*

CHAPTER

32 Patients with Special Needs

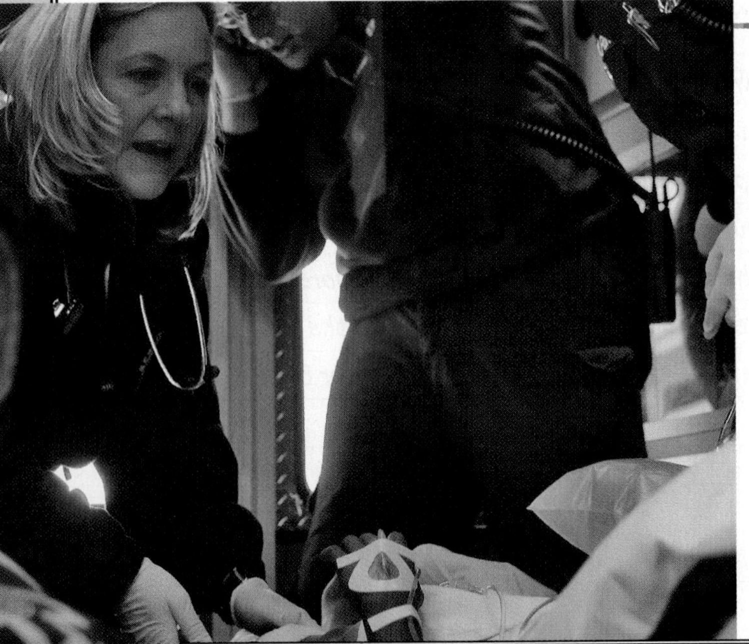

CORE CONCEPTS

The following are core concepts that will be addressed in this chapter:

- The trend toward patients surviving at home with the aid of advanced medical devices
- Congenital and acquired diseases and conditions
- Types of advanced medical devices that may be found in patients' homes
- EMT assessment and transport of patients with special needs

KEY TERMS

acquired disease/condition, p. 867
automatic implanted cardiac defibrillator (AICD), p. 871
central IV catheter, p. 875
congenital disease/condition, p. 867
continuous positive airway pressure (CPAP), p. 868
dialysis, p. 874
feeding tube, p. 873
left ventricular assist device (LVAD), p. 872
ostomy bag, p. 874
pacemaker, p. 870
stoma, p. 869
tracheostomy, p. 869
urinary catheter, p. 873
ventilator, p. 870

In today's world of medicine, EMTs are discovering that a number of people in their communities have advanced medical devices in their homes. These devices go beyond the usual assortment of medications to include machines that extend a patient's ability to function and be comfortable, even machines that keep the patient alive. The limitations these machines compensate for may be the result of medical, traumatic, emotional, behavioral, or developmental disorders.

NOTE *There are no objectives in the National Standard Curriculum that pertain to the material in this chapter.*

RESPONDING TO PATIENTS WITH SPECIAL NEEDS

In many respects, responding to and caring for a person with special needs is like any other call for service in that it may be for an emergency such as a fall, general illness, chest pain, seizures, or shortness of breath. What is different for you, the EMT, is that the patient's pre-existing condition can complicate and quickly overwhelm your ability to assess and treat the patient. To ensure proper care for such a patient, you must be able to recognize, understand, and evaluate the patient's specific special health care needs in addition to the presenting problem or chief complaint that led to the 911 call.

Advanced Medical Devices in the Home

In recent years, medical advances and insurance coverage changes have allowed more and more people to have medical devices and care at home that were formerly seen only in the hospital environment. Patients who previously may have been unable to survive at home are now afforded the opportunity and relative comfort of living and working in a normal, nonhospital environment. As a result, prehospital providers are faced with an increasing number of calls to patients with devices and conditions that were previously not encountered by EMTs (Figure 32-1). These calls may be for a problem with the device the patient relies on or it may be for a medical or traumatic problem unrelated to the device.

Variety of Health Care Settings

Patients with special care needs can be encountered in a variety of locations. With the proliferation of varied levels of health care settings, an EMT may respond to calls at private residences, nursing homes, specialty rehabilitation centers, and specialized care facilities. As an EMT, you should take the time to become familiar with any special health care settings in your community so you can be better prepared for calls of this nature.

In addition to identifying the locations of such facilities, EMTs should meet and develop plans with facility representatives in order to minimize confusion that could occur during an emergency call. Facility representatives may be able to arrange for you to see various medical devices in operation prior to any problems or medical distress.

Some communities have programs in place through their dispatch system to help identify people who may require additional help with medical devices in case of a disaster or evacuation from a building.

Knowledgeable Caregivers

One of the advantages of encounters with patients with special needs is that they will often have on site, or will be accompanied by, a person who has been trained regarding the patient's devices and conditions. This person may be medically trained, such as a

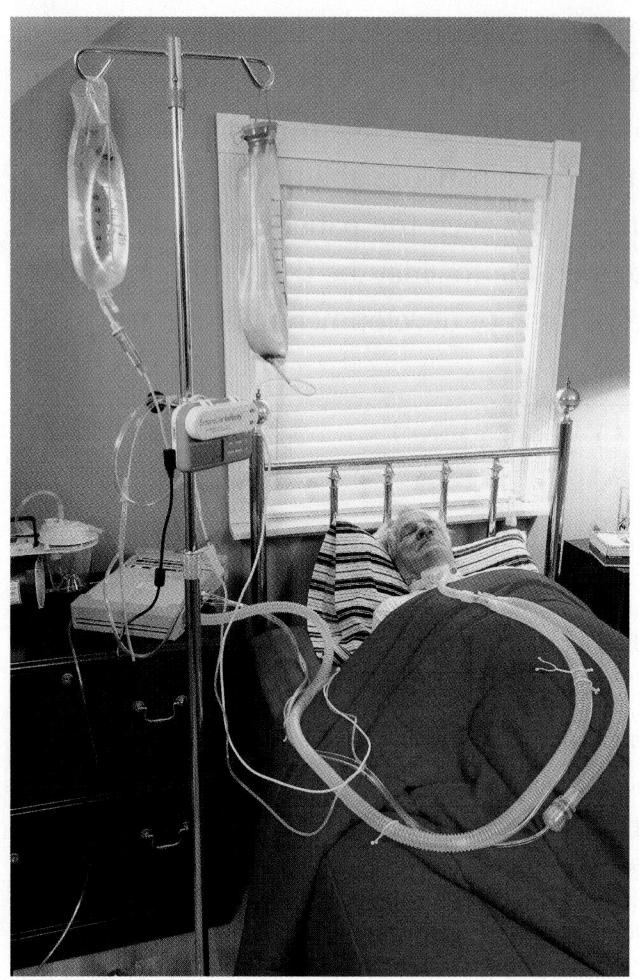

Figure 32-1 • EMTs are now frequently called to assist patients who use a variety of advanced medical devices at home. This patient has a feeding line and a home ventilator connected to a tracheostomy. *(© Ray Kemp/911 Imaging)*

Registered Nurse, a Certified Nursing Assistant, or a home health aide, but more often it will be a family member or friend.

Although family members may not have had formal medical training or certification, they are generally very familiar and comfortable with using the devices the patient relies on. The knowledge and techniques they have were taught to them by medical professionals before the discharge of their family member (the patient) from a hospital. Because they have a vested interest in being competent with the devices, family members are very thorough and deliberate with their understanding and application of the devices and their features. Therefore, it is advisable to seek their input on any problem that may be occurring with devices the patient has and to ask if they have been in a similar situation before. Some general questions should include:

Has this problem ever occurred before? If so, what fixed it?
Have you (or other family members/caregivers) been taught how to fix this problem?
Have you tried to fix the problem? If so, what happened?

Additionally, asking questions such as: "How do you normally move him?" or "Has she ever been transported by ambulance, and what worked well for the transfer?" will allow family members to be part of the solution. Family members do not necessarily expect the arriving members of EMS to know or be familiar with the patient's medical device, and they can help guide the EMTs in the device's use and function. It is a good idea to assign a member of the EMS team to work with the family member regarding the medical device while others on the team concentrate on assessment, treatment, and moving the patient to the ambulance.

Despite the family's willingness to help you, they will still be apprehensive about the problem that occasioned the EMS call and eager to ensure that the device is not damaged or allowed to malfunction. Therefore, proceed with deliberate steps and explain all of your actions to the family.

A Knowledgeable Patient

The patient may also be a great help to the EMT regarding his condition, need for the device, functioning of the device, and how the device operates. The patient has likely been using and/or watching the use of this device for some time and has most likely been trained by medical providers to use the device correctly. Ask the patient about the device and any problems he may be having with it (Figure 32-2).

This approach will depend greatly on the patient's mental status and baseline level of functioning. If the patient has an altered mental status or if medical conditions dictate otherwise, the family will be the primary source of knowledge. Regardless of the patient's mental status or condition, always explain what you are doing. One of the last senses a patient may lose is hearing, so talking and explaining your actions to the patient may help alleviate any stress the patient may be feeling yet unable to show.

Following Protocols

One note of caution is that, as an EMT, your actions fall under specific regional and state scopes of practice. Thus, you should confer with medical direction if the treatment or skill required is not something you are trained in or allowed to do under these protocols. Specific considerations should be given, such as:

Is the problem with the device life-threatening?
Do I have the knowledge to fix this problem?
Do I have the supplies needed to fix this problem?
Is this within my protocols or within medical control authorization?

DISEASES AND CONDITIONS

A disease or condition may be congenital or acquired. A **congenital disease** or condition is one that is present at birth. Some congenital diseases may be genetic, others may not. One example of a congenital disease is congenital heart disease (the most common birth defect), where the heart or large blood vessels of the heart are malformed. Other examples include cleft palates and congenital deafness.

congenital disease/condition a disease or condition that is present at birth.

An **acquired disease** or condition is one that occurs after birth and may be the result of exposure to a virus or bacteria or may be the result of another medical condition

acquired disease/condition a disease or condition that occurs after birth.

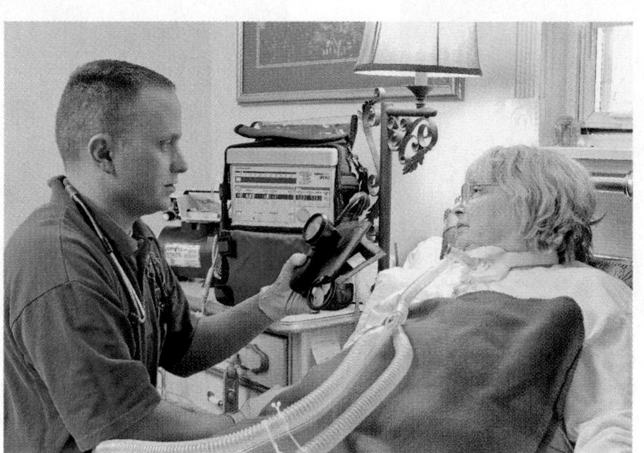

Figure 32-2 • The patient is often an expert on the device or devices she depends on. Enlist the patient's advice as you discuss her condition, special devices, and the assessments and care you plan to perform. *(© Ray Kemp/911 Imaging)*

or trauma. Examples of acquired diseases include COPD, AIDS, and traumatic spinal cord injury.

Some diseases or conditions may be either congenital or acquired, depending on how they occurred. An example of this would be deafness. A patient may be deaf from a congenital birth defect or may become deaf from a disease or from a loud explosion in a work environment.

It is important to understand that a patient with a chronic disease, whether it is congenital or acquired, may develop a sudden, acute worsening of the disease that prompts a call to 911. In addition, the patient with a chronic disease may develop an acute illness, and this acute illness may be potentially more devastating than the same disease would be for a patient who did not have a coexisting chronic disease.

ADVANCED MEDICAL DEVICES

As an EMT, you may encounter patients of any age or physical condition who have advanced medical devices. Take into consideration what the device is doing for the patient and how important the device is to the patient's survival. Some devices are intended to allow the patient to have the fullest life possible while others actually sustain life. Many patients who rely on such devices for life support have limited life expectancies. Even with proper use of the devices, their diseases or conditions may be terminal.

As already noted, you should include family caregivers, as appropriate, in care decisions and patient transportation.

Respiratory Devices

Continuous Positive Airway Pressure Devices

continuous positive airway pressure (CPAP) a device that exerts constant pressure through a tube and mask worn by a patient to keep airway passages from collapsing at the end of a breath.

A **continuous positive airway pressure (CPAP)** device is a machine that provides constant pressure, through a tube and mask, to prevent airway passages from collapsing at the end of a breath. It is often prescribed to patients who suffer sleep apnea (periods when breathing stops during sleep) to help keep airway passages open as the patient sleeps (Figure 32-3). CPAP can help such patients prevent exacerbation of other medical conditions and conquer the chronic fatigue and irritability that are likely to result from interrupted sleep caused by the apneic periods, and may be especially helpful in moderating behavioral problems that can occur in children with sleep apnea (Figure 32-4).

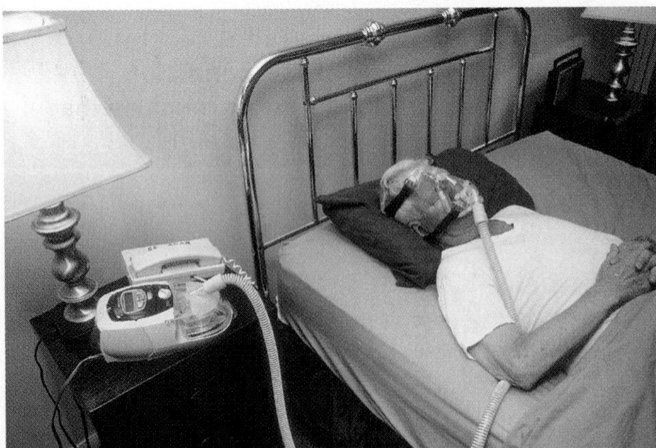

Figure 32-3 • A continuous positive airway pressure (CPAP) device provides constant pressure to keep airway passages open. It is often prescribed to patients with sleep apnea. *(© Don Garbera/Phototake USA)*

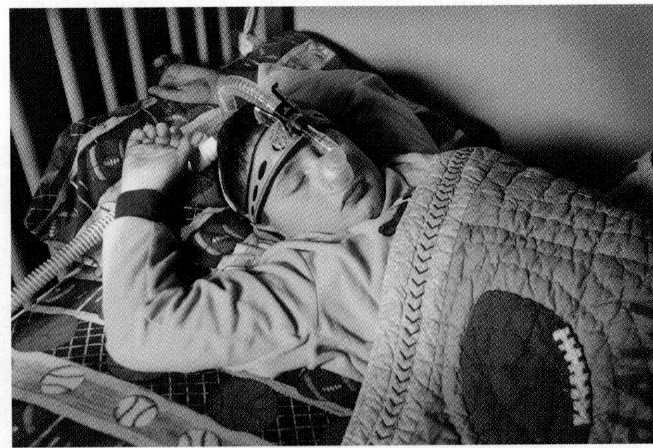

Figure 32-4 • This 9-year-old was thought to have behavior problems but then was diagnosed with sleep apnea. A nasal CPAP machine now helps him sleep through the night. *(© AP Photo/The Herald, Julie Busch)*

EMT ASSESSMENT AND TRANSPORT A patient who uses a CPAP device at night is unlikely to have a medical emergency directly related to the device and will not need the device during transport. However, the patient may wish to bring the device along to the hospital. Hospital personnel should also be alerted that the patient uses a CPAP device during sleep.

Tracheostomy Tubes

A **tracheostomy** is a surgical opening through the neck into the trachea. When the opening created is permanent, it is called a **stoma.** A tracheostomy is usually created near the second to fourth tracheal ring. A tracheostomy tube (a short breathing tube and flange) is inserted into the airway to allow the patient to breathe through the stoma instead of through the nose and mouth. It is often called a "trach" (trayk) tube.

tracheostomy
a surgical opening in the neck into the trachea.

stoma
a surgically created opening into the body, as with a tracheostomy, colostomy, or ileostomy.

Tracheostomy tubes used by older children and adults are usually double-cannula tubes. A double-cannula tube has an inner cannula (a tube within a tube) that can be locked into place and removed periodically for cleaning. Tracheostomy tubes for young children are usually single-cannula tubes that don't have the removable inner cannula. A bag-valve mask can be connected to either type of trach tube—to the inner cannula of a double-cannula tube or directly to a single-cannula tube.

Trach tubes usually come with an obturator, which is a long "plug" that is placed inside the tube to help guide it during insertion and that also prevents material from getting into and clogging the tube during insertion. The obturator is removed after the trach tube is in place.

A tracheostomy procedure may be performed for long-term reasons in patients with neuromuscular disorders, spinal cord injuries, tumors, congenital deformities, coma, and a variety of other conditions that affect the ability to breathe. A patient with a tracheostomy tube may or may not be on a home ventilator. Tracheostomy patients who are on ventilators may be on them all the time or only when sleeping.

Tracheostomy patients range from newborns to the very elderly. A patient with a tracheostomy may or may not be able to speak, depending on his condition. Some are able to speak by covering the tracheostomy tube briefly and making use of a speaker valve attached to the tube or an electronic box applied to the larynx. Do not assume that a patient with a tracheostomy either can or cannot speak.

A frequent problem with tracheostomy tubes is a buildup of mucus that forms in the tube. Because the tube bypasses the upper airway's function of warming, filtering, and humidifying inspired air, suctioning of the tube is needed regularly, often every few hours. This is especially common during times of distress, the first few weeks after tube insertion, or if the patient has an infection. Other problems with the tube can range from dislodgement to infection around the stoma to general respiratory distress.

A patient with a tracheostomy requires extensive care, and caregivers are given substantial training. Caregivers should be very familiar with the procedures used to suction the tube. Caregivers may also know how to change and replace the tracheostomy tube, since it needs to be cleaned regularly. These procedures are outside the scope of practice for most EMTs, so check with local protocols before attempting them.

EMT ASSESSMENT AND TRANSPORT Carefully assess the tracheostomy tube for any blockage, and clear it (under protocol, or by having caregivers perform this). To clear a blockage, carefully insert a whistle-tip catheter (a soft, flexible catheter used to suction tracheostomy or endotracheal tubes) into the stoma. Determine the correct depth of insertion by measuring the suction tubing against the length of the obturator, which is the same length as the trach tube itself. You will usually be able to find the obturator among the patient's tracheostomy supplies. If you can't locate the obturator for measurement, stop insertion of the suction catheter when you feel resistance. Suction as the catheter is being withdrawn, using a twisting motion as it is slowly removed. The patient may "buck" during this procedure. If the patient requires further suctioning (indicated by visible or audible mucus), insert the suction tip into a container of sterile water to remove any mucus left in the catheter, then repeat. If the patient is on a ventilator, he may need to be ventilated by a BVM between suctionings. During transport, the patient should be positioned with his head slightly elevated to allow for mucus drainage.

Home Ventilators

ventilator
a device that breathes for a patient.

A **ventilator** is a device that breathes for a patient. A home ventilator weighs anywhere from several pounds to over 20 pounds and can range from the size of a desktop computer to the size of this textbook. It is programmed to take over the functions of inhalation, exhalation, timing, and rate of breathing.

The ventilator is attached to a ribbed tube called a ventilator circuit, which may come in various lengths, that enters the trachea. The tube from the ventilator may be attached to a plastic or metal port (called a cannula) that enters through a stoma in the neck. It may also be attached to an endotracheal tube through the mouth.

Although the patient is dependent on the ventilator for breathing, he may still lead an active life. One of the best examples of this was Christopher Reeve, the actor who once played Superman, who was paralyzed from the neck down in a 1995 riding accident. With the assistance of a ventilator, he was able to lead an active professional and family life until his death in 2004.

The patient on a home ventilator may call EMS for a variety of problems with his device. As with a tracheostomy tube, mucus plugs and secretions develop that require suctioning, and the patient may develop infections or respiratory distress. Additionally, the home ventilator depends on AC power, and power failures may be cause for concern. Ventilators do have backup batteries that generally last an hour or more.

Home ventilators are tailored with settings that are the most comfortable for the patient. In the case of a mechanical failure, or during transport of the patient, a bag-valve-mask (BVM) device can take over the function of the ventilator. During this procedure, you should adjust the rate, volume, and pressure of the BVM to the patient's comfort level. This can often be accomplished with guidance from the patient or his caregivers. If the patient or caregivers are unable to provide guidance, you should observe for adequate chest rise and improving skin color.

EMT ASSESSMENT AND TRANSPORT While caring for a patient with a home ventilator, ensure that the ventilator tube does not have any mucus buildup, and suction as needed. During transport, it may be easier to use a BVM while moving the patient to the ambulance, depending on the location and situation (e.g., stairs or a heavy patient). If you use a BVM at any point, ensure that it is the appropriate size for the patient and that it is connected to oxygen. If the patient has a tracheostomy tube and the BVM does not fit the tube attachment, use the face mask from the BVM to cover the stoma and secure the mask to provide a good seal against the neck, then ventilate as normal.

If the ventilator is left attached to the patient, firmly affix it to the stretcher. Secure the ventilator to prevent movement in the ambulance during transport. Consider transport time versus battery life, and plug the ventilator into the ambulance's inverter if available. If a BVM will be used during transport, obtain extra help so you can continue to provide assessment and care.

Cardiac Devices

Implanted Pacemakers and Cardiac Defibrillators

A patient may have an implanted pacemaker or automatic implanted cardiac defibrillator. These devices are both designed to respond to potentially lethal electrical rhythm changes in the heart.

pacemaker
a device that uses electrical impulses to regulate rhythms of the heart, which is usually implanted under the skin.

In the case of a **pacemaker,** a small device is implanted under the skin and wires are implanted into the heart. The pacemaker is designed to prevent the heart rate from becoming too slow. Early pacemakers were set at a fixed rate, but modern pacemakers are "rate-responsive"; that is, they detect what the patient is doing and modify the heart rate accordingly. For example, if the patient is moving around and performing an action, a sensor will detect this and increase the rate to allow for the activity. Addition-

POINT OF VIEW

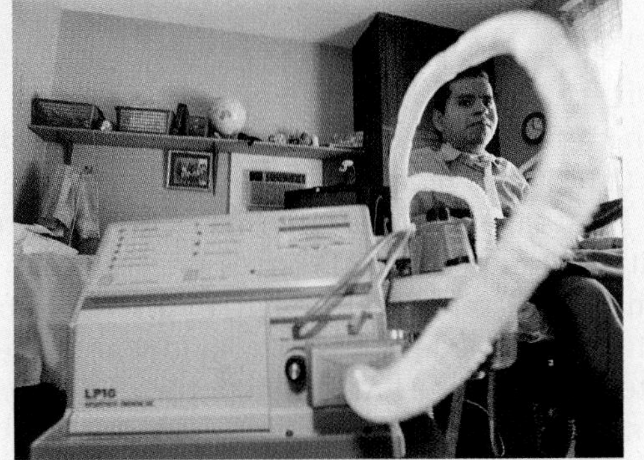
© AP Photo/Journal Times, Jim Slosiarek/AP Images

"I went to school with a guy who got into a motorcycle crash. He was hurt pretty bad. He had an injury to his spine that put him in a wheelchair and on a ventilator. I think about him from time to time. When I became an EMT and started transporting patients, it really got me thinking. What if he ever needed an ambulance?

"The logistics of either taking the ventilator, or ventilating him with a BVM, is probably more scary to him than it is to me. But it is pretty intimidating to me, too, let me tell you. I'd do it. But I'd be nervous.

"Do you think it's normal to feel that way?"

ally, if the breathing rate increases, the pacemaker will increase the heart rate as well. The pacemaker delivers a series of low-energy pulses at set intervals to stimulate the heart to beat at a faster rate. These pulses are not felt by the patient and cannot be detected on the skin or felt by providers. The pacemaker does not squeeze the heart or fix damaged muscle; rather, it helps regulate the timing of each beat.

Like a pacemaker, an **automatic implanted cardiac defibrillator (AICD)** is placed under the skin with wires inserted into the heart. The AICD varies in size from slightly larger than a 9-volt battery to the size of a wallet. It is usually implanted in the upper left chest area, although occasionally it may be implanted in the area of the left upper quadrant of the abdomen. It is generally palpable through the skin.

automatic implanted cardiac defibrillator (AICD)
a device implanted under the skin that can detect a life-threatening cardiac dysrhythmia and respond by delivering one or more shocks to correct the rhythm.

The implanted defibrillator is designed to detect life-threatening cardiac rhythms (ventricular fibrillation and ventricular tachycardia). Newer models may have a pacemaker feature built in as well. The AICD delivers a single shock when a life-threatening rhythm is detected. This shock is often very painful to the patient, generally rated as 6 on a 1-to-10 pain scale. If the single shock does not correct the rhythm, or if the rhythm returns, other shocks will be delivered, one at a time, until the dysrhythmia is resolved or the machine is turned off. The AICD can be turned off only by a special magnet and generally only in a hospital setting.

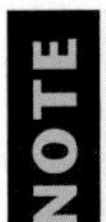

NOTE *The occurrence of an AICD shock is often very upsetting to the patient. Be prepared to provide emotional support.*

Although muscle twitches may be seen on the patient, providers and caregivers will not be shocked or harmed if the AICD shocks while they are touching the patient. The AICD is not dangerous if it shocks when the patient is wet. Patients are generally instructed to call their doctor if they feel fine after a shock. However, if they have any symptoms such as dizziness, chest pain, shortness of breath, not feeling well, or if they are shocked more than twice in any 24-hour period, they should go to the hospital or call EMS.

The functioning of pacemakers and AICDs can be affected by certain electromagnetic and radio frequency signals, so people with these devices should not stand still in the doorway of a business with an electronic anti-theft device nor stand still in a walk-through metal detector (although walking through either of these without stopping is not harmful). Stereo speakers and cellular telephones should not be held against a pacemaker or AICD device. Additionally, electric motors (as in power tools) and gas-powered tools (such as chainsaws and snow blowers) must be kept at least 6 inches away from the AICD or pacemaker when they are running.

Most patients who have one or both of these devices have had a significant cardiac medical history. They may be on multiple medications and may carry wallet cards or wear bracelets stating that they have one of these devices in use.

EMT ASSESSMENT AND TRANSPORT Depending on the nature of the call and chief complaint, the EMT may wish to have ALS transport for a patient with a pacemaker or AICD device. A patient who merely has a pacemaker as part of his medical history may not need ALS, but if the pacemaker is malfunctioning or if an AICD has discharged, this patient is a high-risk cardiac patient and should be treated as such with high-concentration oxygen and frequent reassessment. If the patient goes into cardiac arrest, CPR and an AED should be used as indicated.

Left Ventricular Assist Devices

left ventricular assist device (LVAD)
a battery-powered mechanical pump implanted in the body to assist a failing left ventricle in pumping blood to the body.

A recent advance in cardiac care is the **left ventricular assist device (LVAD).** The left ventricle is the cardiac chamber that pumps blood through the aorta to the body. When there is severe left ventricular heart failure, a heart transplant may be required. While the patient is waiting for a suitable donor, the LVAD serves as a "bridge to transplant." The LVAD moves blood from the left ventricle through an inserted tube to a pump implanted in the abdomen where the blood is pressurized and sent to the aorta for transport to the body. A tube extends from the LVAD through the abdominal wall to an external pump battery and control panel.

Problems that may be associated with LVADs are infection, air leakage, and battery failure. All require rapid transport to a hospital.

EMT ASSESSMENT AND TRANSPORT The patient with an LVAD will have an external battery pack that may be the size of a small backpack or briefcase (Figure 32-5). This should be carefully secured and prevented from tugging on the attached tubing. Failures of the battery system should first be addressed by attempting to plug the unit into an AC source in the home, inverter in an ambulance, or other power source. This will begin recharging the battery, and allow functioning of the pump. If the pump itself fails, a hand or foot pump is included with the system as a backup. The pump looks similar to the bulb on a blood pressure cuff and must be squeezed for each beat of the heart. Heart transplant centers will generally provide training to local EMS personnel if someone in the community has an LVAD. The training is specific to the model used by local patients.

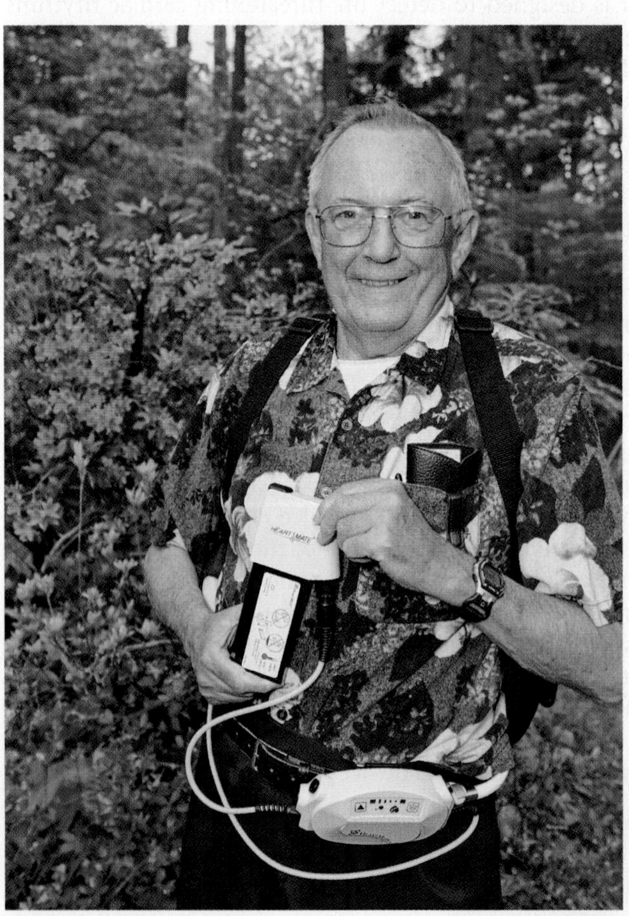

Figure 32-5 • This patient holds one of the two batteries that powers his implanted left ventricular assist device. The LVAD's controller is attached to his belt. *(© AP Photo/George Widman)*

Gastrourinary Devices

Feeding Tubes

A **feeding tube** is used in a patient who is unable to feed himself or can't swallow. It may be used short term (during recovery from surgery) or long term (for chronic conditions). A feeding tube is most commonly seen in one of two forms: a nasogastric tube or a gastric tube.

feeding tube
a tube used to provide delivery of nutrients to the stomach. A nasogastric feeding tube is inserted through the nose and into the stomach; a gastric feeding tube is surgically implanted through the abdominal wall and into the stomach.

A *nasogastric tube (NG tube)* is a long tube inserted through the nose into the stomach that can be used to deliver nutrients. Additionally, the device can be used in emergency departments and by some ALS providers to suction out the stomach's contents, for example with certain overdoses. The NG tube is generally taped to the patient's nose or cheek to prevent the tube from dislodging. A *gastric tube (G-tube)* is a feeding tube surgically implanted through the abdominal wall and into the stomach (Figure 32-6). It is used to provide longer term nutrient delivery than would be provided by an NG tube. The G-tube is held in place by a balloon inside the stomach. It can also be used by hospital personnel to drain stomach contents. Some feeding tubes are placed through the abdominal wall, directly into the small intestine. For example, a *J-tube* is placed into the jejunum section of the small intestine.

With both NG tubes and G-tubes, common problems include dislodgement, infection at the site of insertion, or a clog that prevents nutrients from being provided to the patient. All of these conditions warrant transport and evaluation in a hospital setting.

EMT ASSESSMENT AND TRANSPORT Ensure that the feeding tube is secured with tape to the patient's body before transport (Figure 32-7). If protocols allow, and nutrients are being administered during transport, keep the nutrient source higher than the level of the NG tube or G-tube and hang it like an IV bag. Although the tube is not pressurized when nutrients are not being administered, the protective end cap should be placed on the tube to prevent leakage.

Urinary Catheters

A **urinary catheter** is used for a patient who has lost the ability to urinate or has lost the ability to control when he urinates. Most commonly seen as indwelling Foley catheters, other types include the externally applied condom catheter. Most catheters are inserted into the bladder through the urethra and use a balloon to hold the tubing

urinary catheter
a tube inserted into the bladder through the urethra to drain urine from the bladder.

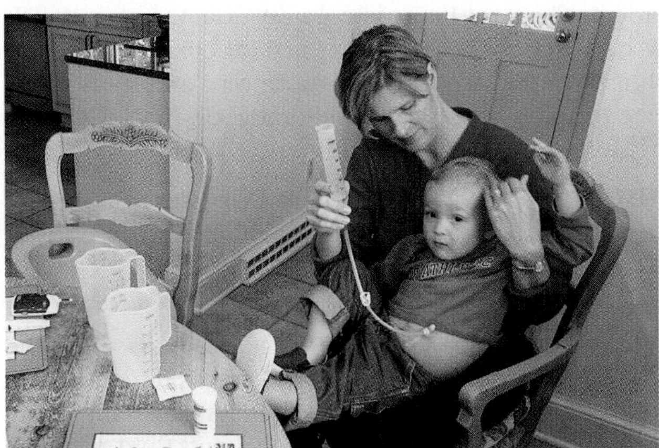

Figure 32-6 • In her home kitchen, this mother is administering a liquid cornstarch solution to her child through an implanted gastric feeding tube. The child has a rare disease that requires him to ingest cornstarch every 4 hours to avoid seizures and hospitalization. *(© AP Photo/The Charlotte Observer, David T. Foster III)*

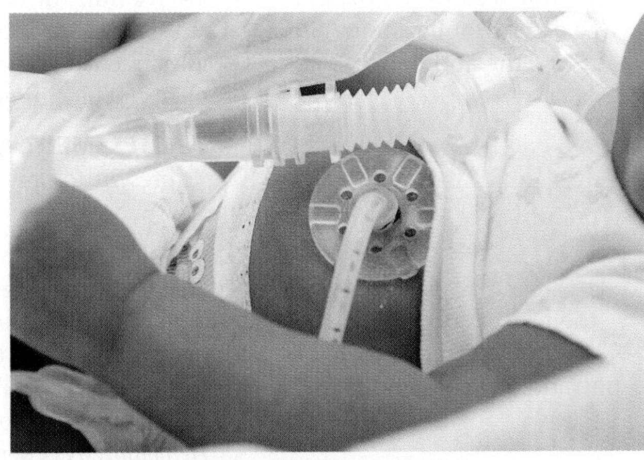

Figure 32-7 • A gastric tube (G-tube) implanted in a baby's abdomen. Use tape to secure such a feeding tube to the patient's body before transport. *(© Ray Kemp/911 Imaging)*

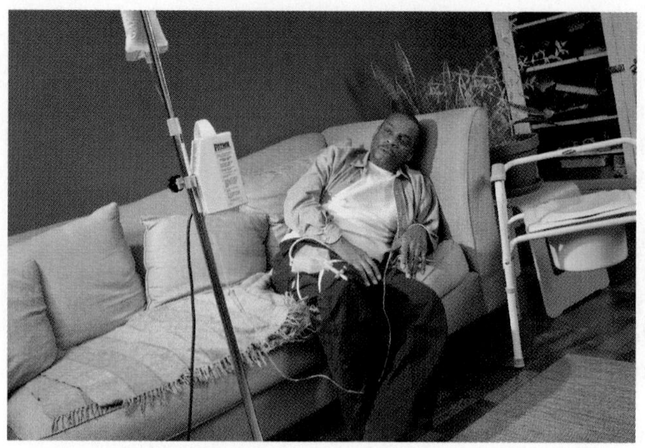

Figure 32-8 • This patient, who has a urinary catheter, wears a collection bag strapped to his leg. *(© Phototake USA/ Yoav Levy)*

in place. The external tubing is connected to a collection bag (Figure 32-8), which may be a bag strapped to a leg or a larger drainage bag, called a down drain, that hangs on the side of a patient's bed. Patients with leg bags are generally those who are more active than patients with down drains, as the leg bag may be hidden under clothing when the patient is in public. Common problems EMS providers see with urinary catheters include infection, blockages causing lack of urinary output, discoloration of urine, and dislodgement of the catheter.

EMT ASSESSMENT AND TRANSPORT During transport, keep the catheter bag lower than the level of the patient (but not on a floor), and use care not to damage the bag with a stretcher or lifting device. Document and report any discoloration of the urine or any odors from the urine itself. Drainage bags should be emptied when they are a third to half full. EMS providers may want caregivers to empty the bag before transport to prevent overfilling, which will cause backflow into the bladder. Some patients are required to keep track of their total urine output every day, so document the amount emptied.

Ostomy Bags

ostomy bag
an external pouch that collects fecal matter diverted from the colon or ileum through a surgical opening (colostomy or ileostomy) in the abdominal wall.

As an EMT, you may also encounter a patient who has an **ostomy bag,** also called an ostomy pouch. An ostomy bag is connected to the site of a colostomy or an ileostomy. A colostomy or ileostomy is the result of a surgery that brings a section of the intestine through the abdominal wall in order to divert the flow of stool away from the normal path to the rectum. An ostomy may be necessary because of a medical condition such as Crohn's disease or ulcerative colitis or cancer, especially colon cancer. An ostomy bag is usually attached to the patient's leg and often will not be visible under clothing. Common problems include infection at the stoma site, blockage or, in some cases, dislodgement.

EMT ASSESSMENT AND TRANSPORT Use care when moving a patient if an ostomy bag is present to prevent breakage or dislodgement through rough handling.

Dialysis

dialysis
the process of filtering the blood to remove toxic or unwanted wastes and fluids.

A patient who requires **dialysis** has renal failure. The kidneys are unable to remove the buildup of toxins that occurs with the metabolism of daily life. Dialysis removes these toxins and filters the blood, taking over some of the roles the kidneys play in detoxifying the blood. Dialysis serves two important roles: waste removal and fluid removal. There are two forms of dialysis: hemodialysis and peritoneal dialysis.

Hemodialysis is performed by attaching the patient to an external machine called a dialyzer. The procedure is usually performed at a dialysis center, although home units do exist. Hemodialysis works by inserting a needle that drains blood into the machine, which then filters the blood through a semipermeable membrane to remove waste products and fluid. Another inserted needle allows the filtered blood to be returned to the patient. Treatment takes place over 3 to 5 hours and is usually done three times a week. The dialysis is performed by staff at the dialysis center.

Hemodialysis requires the use of large needles and tubing to remove and return the blood. The needles are inserted into one of three locations: an arteriovenous (AV) shunt, an arteriovenous (AV) fistula, or an arteriovenous (AV) graft. In each of these, the term *arteriovenous* indicates the connection of an artery and a vein. An AV shunt connects an artery and vein via two external plastic tubes. When not in use, the AV shunt tubes are connected to each other and taped or bandaged to the skin. An AV shunt is often used for short-term dialysis or for new dialysis patients. Long-term dialysis patients will have an AV fistula, which is a surgical connection of an artery and a vein underneath the skin, which may be felt or seen as a large bump. If veins are too small for proper surgical connection, an AV graft may be placed, which is a surgically implanted tube that connects the artery and vein. A normally functioning AV graft or AV fistula will have a soft vibrating feeling (called a "thrill") when it is gently palpated. Common complications encountered with patients on hemodialysis include bleeding from the AV fistula site after dialysis and infection at the site of external dialysis catheters.

Peritoneal dialysis is performed by a solution containing minerals and glucose that is run into the abdominal cavity through a surgically implanted plastic tube. Fluid surrounds the intestines and the intestinal walls act as the semipermeable membrane. The fluid inside the abdominal cavity is drained and replaced with fresh solution four to five times a day. Although not as efficient as hemodialysis, the frequent fluid changes in peritoneal dialysis achieve similar filtration results. The procedure can often be performed at home with minimal equipment, but the daily treatment schedule it requires makes peritoneal dialysis more reliant on patient and/or caregiver compliance than does hemodialysis. Common complications encountered with patients on peritoneal dialysis include dislodging of the catheter and infection in the peritoneal cavity (peritonitis), which results in the normally clear dialysis fluid turning cloudy.

EMT ASSESSMENT AND TRANSPORT Do not take a blood pressure on any arm with an AV shunt, fistula, or graft, which could cause damage that would require surgical repair.

If a shunt, graft, or fistula ruptures, significant blood loss (up to 500 mL/min. or more) will occur very quickly. In the case of a bleeding shunt, stop the bleeding by direct pressure. In the case of a fistula or graft bleed, which may be indicated by significant swelling under the skin at the site, apply direct pressure. DO NOT release the pressure until advised by a physician to do so, because the pressure is unlikely to allow clotting that would stop the bleeding. In all cases of bleeding from a shunt, fistula, or graft, the patient should be treated for shock, transported, and carefully monitored.

Central IV Catheters

Sometimes a patient you encounter will have a **central IV catheter.** A patient who receives frequent IV therapy, such as with chemotherapy or total parenteral nutrition, may have one of a variety of such catheters. Inserted in a hospital with surgery or under radiography, central IV catheters prevent patients from having to endure multiple needlesticks in their arms. A common problem with central IV catheters is infection at the site. Central IV catheters are usually inserted via a surgical venous puncture to introduce medications or fluids into the central circulation.

central IV catheter
a catheter surgically inserted for long-term delivery of medications or fluids into the central circulation.

One form of central IV catheter is the *peripherally inserted central catheter (PICC) line,* which has an external tube slightly larger than IV tubing, which is inserted into a peripheral vein from which it is threaded into the central circulation. A PICC line is often found inserted into the patient's arm.

Another form of central IV catheter is a *central venous line*, which may be inserted through a subclavian, jugular, or femoral vein. Central venous lines carry a variety of brand names, such as a Groshong®, a Hickman®, or a Broviac® catheter. These catheters may have one, two, or three external IV tubes that are attached to the patient's chest.

Finally, a central IV catheter may be in the form of an *implanted port* that can be felt under the skin. This port has no external tubing; special needles are required to access these ports. Brand names include Port-a-Cath® and Mediport®.

EMT ASSESSMENT AND TRANSPORT In most cases, neither the EMT nor a family caregiver will use a central IV catheter to administer medications to the patient or for any other purpose. Use of a central IV catheter is usually restricted to hospital personnel. However, awareness of the presence of a central IV device is important for the EMT, who must exercise caution to avoid any tugging or contamination of the catheter site.

Physical Impairments

Patients who call EMS may have a variety of impairments that affect their hearing, sight, or speech. When one of these senses has been adversely affected or removed, you should take extra care and time to help the patient adjust. It is important to remember, however, that these impairments do NOT necessarily affect the patient's ability to think. Each limitation requires different approaches and considerations when you are assessing and treating the patient.

Hearing loss is more common in the elderly than in younger persons, but it is not restricted to the older patient. Approach each patient individually and ascertain their abilities. Not all patients with hearing loss can read lips, and in most cases yelling or slowing down your speech will only make matters worse. One of the easiest ways to communicate with a patient with hearing loss is to write your questions and explain your actions on a piece of paper. Many dispatch centers and communities also have TDD/TTY phones, and may be able to relay information through these devices.

NOTE

TDD/TTY stands for Telecommunication Device for the Deaf/TeleTYpewriter. *The system consists of a keyboard, display screen, and modem connected to an analog telephone line. The user can type in a message and receive a response that is displayed on the screen.*

Impairments to sight can be partial or complete. Determine if the patient has poor vision or no vision. Blind patients may not use lights in their home or may not notice lights that have burned out. It is good practice for the EMT always to carry a small flashlight, even during the day. The patient may know the layout of his home very well, so if anything is moved for transport of the patient, be careful to return it to its original position. If the patient has a guide dog, federal law allows for the patient to bring the dog along in an ambulance, unless the dog is a direct threat to others (for example, if barking or growling).

A patient who is unable to speak (aphasic) may need to write answers to your questions, use a TDD/TTY phone, or have a computer that speaks the words they type.

Many elderly persons contend with difficulty walking or standing, but problems with gait and balance can occur at any age. Carefully assist people who have such disabilities, and make sure to bring along any helping devices they want to have with them, such as a cane, a walker, or braces. Patients in wheelchairs may be difficult to assess completely as they may be unable to stand or turn for complete physical assessment. If a patient in a wheelchair is moved to a stretcher, ensure that the patient's wheelchair either safely accompanies them or is secured from theft or loss.

EMT ASSESSMENT AND TRANSPORT Approach and treat each patient with one or more physical impairments by providing whatever extra assistance he requires. Carefully assess to determine if an impairment is the patient's baseline or if it is a new problem (for example, a person suffering a stroke and has lost the ability to speak). Determine the patient's comfort level and any abilities or tools he uses to compensate. During care, carefully explain all of your actions and treatments. Bring any devices the patient uses, such as a walker, a hearing aid, glasses, speech computer, or other items to help communicate with hospital staff, and make his environment more comfortable. If the patient has a wheelchair, consider the use of a wheelchair van if one is available.

CRITICAL DECISION MAKING:
EMTs Need to Know

Patients with special needs pose challenges for EMS providers at all levels. For each of the following situations, explain how you would handle it and where you might turn for help or advice.

1. You are treating an unresponsive diabetic patient when you notice he has an insulin pump. You believe you should turn it off but are not sure how.
2. You are treating a patient who had just performed peritoneal dialysis at home. She complains of excruciating pain with even the least little movement.
3. You are called for a possible respiratory infection in a child. You arrive to find the patient has a trach and a ventilator. You are not sure how to transport the ventilator.

CHAPTER REVIEW

SUMMARY

As an EMT, you may occasionally respond to an emergency for a patient with special needs—a patient who relies on one or more advanced medical devices that enable him to live at home rather than in a hospital or other medical facility. Whether or not the emergency relates to the device the patient depends on, your primary job, as always, is assessment of the patient, care of the patient's medical condition, and transport of the patient to a medical facility as needed. You may not be able to fix a problem with a medical device but, if necessary, you can provide support of life functions.

As preparation for such responses, you should become as familiar as possible with advanced medical devices in use in your community. You should also be aware that the caregiver of the patient with special needs, usually a family member, is likely to be very familiar with the patient's condition and the devices he depends on. That person may be your best source of information in the emergency situation. Attend to the patient's medical condition and follow your local protocols.

KEY TERMS

acquired disease/condition a disease or condition that occurs after birth.

automatic implanted cardiac defibrillator (AICD) a device implanted under the skin that can detect a life-threatening cardiac dysrhythmia and respond by delivering one or more shocks to correct the rhythm.

central IV catheter a catheter surgically inserted for long-term delivery of medications or fluids into the central circulation.

congenital disease/condition a disease or condition that is present at birth.

continuous positive airway pressure (CPAP) a device that exerts constant pressure through a tube and mask worn by a patient to keep airway passages from collapsing at the end of a breath.

dialysis the process of filtering the blood to remove toxic or unwanted wastes and fluids.

feeding tube a tube used to provide delivery of nutrients to the stomach. A nasogastric feeding tube is inserted through the nose and into the stomach; a gastric feeding tube is surgically implanted through the abdominal wall and into the stomach.

left ventricular assist device (LVAD) a battery-powered mechanical pump implanted in the body to assist a failing left ventricle in pumping blood to the body.

ostomy bag an external pouch that collects fecal matter diverted from the colon or ileum through a surgical opening (colostomy or ileostomy) in the abdominal wall.

pacemaker a device that uses electrical impulses to regulate rhythms of the heart, which is usually implanted under the skin.

stoma a surgically created opening into the body, as with a tracheostomy, colostomy, or ileostomy.

tracheostomy a surgical opening in the neck into the trachea.

urinary catheter a tube inserted into the bladder through the urethra to drain urine from the bladder.

ventilator a device that breathes for a patient.

REVIEW QUESTIONS

1. List several advanced medical devices you might find when responding to patients with special needs at home. (pp. 868–876)
2. Differentiate congenital diseases from acquired diseases or conditions. (pp. 867–868)
3. If a tracheostomy tube is blocked and your protocols allow, describe a method of clearing the blockage. (pp. 869–870)
4. If a ventilator that a patient relies on to breathe malfunctions, what life support care should you perform? (p. 870)
5. If a patient's pacemaker or AICD malfunctions, in addition to transport to the hospital, what care should you provide? (pp. 871–872)
6. If a patient cannot hear or cannot speak, describe several methods that might facilitate communication with him. (p. 876)

CRITICAL THINKING

- You are called to respond to a patient who has an arteriovenous (AV) fistula that is used during his triweekly visits to the dialysis center. The patient presents as pale, sweaty, anxious, and almost incoherent. Could the cause of his condition be related to the AV fistula? How might you determine if this is the case? What actions should you take?

Thinking and Linking

Think back to your training in Basic Life Support. What BLS training might you draw on to help you deal with a patient with special needs whose life-sustaining equipment has malfunctioned?

MEDIA RESOURCES

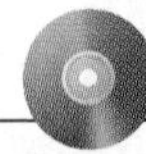

See the Student CD for quizzes, a case study activity, videos, and other features related to patient assessment. Also, visit the Companion Website for *Emergency Care* at **www.prenhall.com/limmer**, where you will find additional reinforcement and links to other resources.

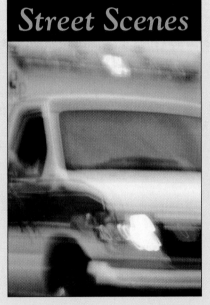

Street Scenes

Eighteen-month-old Amber's parents have left their daughter in the care of her Aunt Dorothy while they get away for a day to themselves. Dorothy is familiar with Amber's tracheostomy but has not had any experience with anything going wrong. Unfortunately, something does go wrong. Late in the afternoon, Amber experiences a fever and begins to look a little gray. Dorothy calls EMS.

Your initial impression as you enter Amber's room is that she is alert but in some respiratory distress with cyanosis around the lips. When you examine her tracheostomy, you see that there is a small amount of mucus coming from her trach tube. Her radial pulse is rapid and weak.

Street Scene Questions

1. What is this patient's priority?
2. What additional information do you need to treat the patient?

Next to Amber you see several small soft suction catheters. You remove one from the package, attach it to your suction device, measure the length to insert by comparing it to the obturator on the table next to the patient, and suction some mucus out of her trach tube. Amber's color begins to improve. Your partner tells you the patient's pulse is 128 and her respiratory rate is 44.

Street Scene Questions

3. How should you reassess the patient?
4. What equipment should you take to the hospital with Amber?

You listen to Amber's breathing through her trach tube and no longer hear the gurgling sounds that were initially audible. She is moving air well. Although her color is better than when you found her, she appears pale and still in some respiratory distress, although less than before you suctioned her. Amber's pulse oximeter reading has increased from 85 percent to 91 percent. You gather Amber's "Ready-To-Go" bag with her medical records and Emergency Information Form as you prepare her for transport. You administer high-concentration oxygen and suction her trach tube a few more times on the trip to the Emergency Department.

Later, Amber's parents call your station to thank you for what you did. Amber had a respiratory infection that is responding well to treatment. Dorothy was very impressed with your calm professionalism, and the entire family is very grateful.

Street Scenes Sample Documentation

PATIENT NAME: *Amber Brown* **PATIENT AGE:** *18 months*

CHIEF COMPLAINT

Not breathing right

PAST MEDICAL HISTORY

- ☐ None
- ☐ Allergy to
- ☐ Hypertension ☐ Stroke
- ☐ Seizures ☐ Diabetes
- ☐ COPD ☐ Cardiac
- ☒ Other (List) ☐ Asthma

Tracheostomy

Current Medications (List)

Unknown

VITAL SIGNS

TIME	RESP	PULSE	B.P.	MENTAL STATUS	R PUPILS L	SKIN
1610	Rate: 44 ☐ Regular ☐ Shallow ☐ Labored	Rate: 128 ☐ Regular ☐ Irregular	/	☑ Alert ☐ Voice ☐ Pain ☐ Unresp.	☐ Normal ☐ ☐ Dilated ☐ ☐ Constricted ☐ ☐ Sluggish ☐ ☐ No-Reaction ☐	☐ Unremarkable ☑ Cool ☐ Pale ☐ Warm ☑ Cyanotic ☐ Moist ☐ Flushed ☐ Dry ☐ Jaundiced
1623	Rate: 40 ☐ Regular ☐ Shallow ☐ Labored	Rate: 116 ☐ Regular ☐ Irregular	/	☑ Alert ☐ Voice ☐ Pain ☐ Unresp.	☐ Normal ☐ ☐ Dilated ☐ ☐ Constricted ☐ ☐ Sluggish ☐ ☐ No-Reaction ☐	☐ Unremarkable ☑ Cool ☑ Pale ☐ Warm ☐ Cyanotic ☐ Moist ☐ Flushed ☐ Dry ☐ Jaundiced
1628	Rate: 40 ☐ Regular ☐ Shallow ☐ Labored	Rate: 120 ☐ Regular ☐ Irregular	/	☑ Alert ☐ Voice ☐ Pain ☐ Unresp.	☐ Normal ☐ ☐ Dilated ☐ ☐ Constricted ☐ ☐ Sluggish ☐ ☐ No-Reaction ☐	☐ Unremarkable ☑ Cool ☑ Pale ☐ Warm ☐ Cyanotic ☐ Moist ☐ Flushed ☐ Dry ☐ Jaundiced

NARRATIVE *18-month-old female with tracheostomy had onset this afternoon of respiratory distress accompanied by fever and cyanosis around the lips. Pt. alert with small amount of mucus coming from the trach tube. Gurgling audible with each breath. Caregiver aunt unable to assist pt.*

Suctioned mucus out of trach tube with improvement in breathing sounds and skin color. Pt moving air well, but still pale and in some respiratory distress. Administered 15 lpm of oxygen by NRB.

Transported pt sitting up with Ready-To-Go bag and medical records. No change in pt. condition en route to hospital.

CHAPTER 33

Geriatric Patients

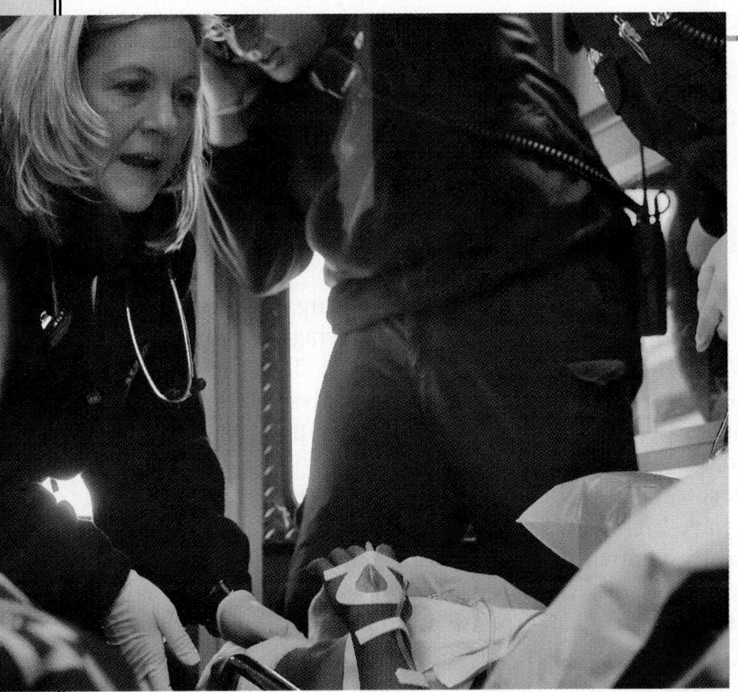

CORE CONCEPTS

The following are core concepts that will be addressed in this chapter:

- Communicating with the geriatric patient
- Assessing the geriatric patient
- Common reasons the elderly encounter EMS

NOTE

There are no objectives in the National Standard Curriculum that pertain to the material in this chapter.

You learned how to assess a patient in Chapters 8 through 12 and how to treat a patient's problems in later chapters. The principles you learned pertain to all patients. However, when your patient is at one of the extremes of age, you will need to make some adjustments in how you proceed. In Chapter 31, "Infants and Children," you learned about infants and children and how they are different. Elderly patients have some characteristics that make them different from the typical young or middle-age adult, too. No definition of elderly that specifies an age range can do justice to the many different conditions, presentations, and ages you will see in older patients, so we will not attempt to define the term. Instead, you should use your common sense, experience, and EMS knowledge to guide you in dealing with these patients. This chapter will describe many of the differences in older patients.

THE GERIATRIC PATIENT

Most people living in the United States today can remember visiting their grandparents when they were growing up. This was not always the case. The average age has increased significantly over the last two centuries. Today, one out of every eight persons in the United States is 65 years or older. By the year 2040, one of every five persons will be at least 65. Fortunately, with longer lives we are also seeing healthier lives. Those over 85 are the fastest growing age group.

Among those over 65 years, certain medical conditions are common: almost half have arthritis, about a third have high blood pressure and heart disease, more than a quarter have some kind of hearing impairment, and about one tenth have diabetes or some kind of visual impairment. Despite these medical problems, more than half of those 85 years or older live alone or with just a spouse. In the 65 to 74 age group, even more live independently. Contrary to popular opinion, only about 5 percent of the older population resides in nursing homes.

Some medical authorities believe that starting at about age 30, our organ systems lose about 1 percent of their function each year (the "1 percent rule"), which can make it difficult to distinguish between the normal effects of aging and the effects of disease. This is one reason why it is important to find out early what a patient's normal or baseline condition is. One way to do this is to ask how the patient is different compared to a week ago. This information can be very helpful in distinguishing a chronic condition from a new problem.

Just as children change as they get older, so do adults, though not always in ways that are apparent. The function of many body systems diminishes as a person ages. Table 33-1 describes some of these changes and their implications for assessment by the EMT.

Older patients make up a much higher proportion of patients transported by EMS than their numbers in society would indicate. In fact, older patients are at least twice as likely to use EMS. They also are more likely than younger patients to have a medical problem, rather than an injury.

The most common reasons for EMS to be called to an older person include cardiac and respiratory problems, neurological problems like stroke and altered mental status, injuries from a fall, and hazy complaints like dizziness, weakness, and malaise.

TABLE 33-1 • Physiological Effects of Aging and Implications for Assessment

CHANGE	RESULT	IMPLICATIONS FOR ASSESSMENT
Depositing of cholesterol on arterial walls that have become thicker	Increased risk of heart attack and stroke, hypertension	Heart attack and stroke more likely
Decreased cardiac output	Diminished activity and tolerance of physical stress	More prone to falls
Decreased elasticity of lungs and decreased activity of cilia	Decreased ability to clear foreign substances from lungs	Higher risk of pneumonia and other respiratory infections
Fewer taste buds, less saliva; less acid production and slower movement in digestive system	Difficulty chewing and swallowing; less enjoyment of eating; difficulty digesting and absorbing food; constipation; early feeling of fullness when eating	Weight loss; abdominal pain common
Diminished liver and kidney function	Increased toxicity from alcohol and medications; diminished ability of blood to clot	Need for reduced doses of medication; bleeding tendencies
Diminished function of thyroid	Decreased energy and tolerance of heat and cold	Increased risk of hypothermia and hyperthermia
Decreased muscle mass, loss of minerals from bones	Decreased strength	Falls more likely; minor falls more likely to cause fractures
Multiple medical conditions	Many different medications, sometimes prescribed by different physicians	Increased risk of medication error; potentially harmful medication interactions common
Death of friends and family	Depression; loss of social support	Increased risk of suicide
Loss of skin elasticity, shrinking of sweat glands	Thin, dry, wrinkled skin	Increased risk of injury (The EMT must handle the patient gently to avoid injuring skin and subcutaneous tissues.)

Communicating with the Geriatric Patient

Although most elderly people are healthy and able to live on their own, a sizable number of them have conditions that can hamper communication, such as hearing loss or deterioration of vision. Many also wear dentures that, if not fitted properly, can make speech difficult or even painful. Table 33-2 lists some of the physiological effects of aging that may affect communication and EMT actions that can help to offset these problems.

TABLE 33-2 • Effects of Aging with Implications for Communication

CHANGE	RESULT	EMT COMMUNICATION STRATEGIES
Clouding and thickening of lens in eye	Cataracts; poor vision, especially peripheral vision	Position yourself in front of patient where you can be seen; put hand on arm of blind patient to let patient know where you are.
Shrinkage of structures in ear	Decreased hearing, especially ability to hear high-frequency sounds; diminished sense of balance	Speak clearly; check hearing aids as necessary
Deterioration of teeth and gums	Patient needs dentures, but they may inflict pain on sensitive gums, so patient doesn't always wear them	If patient's speech is unintelligible, ask patient to put his dentures in.

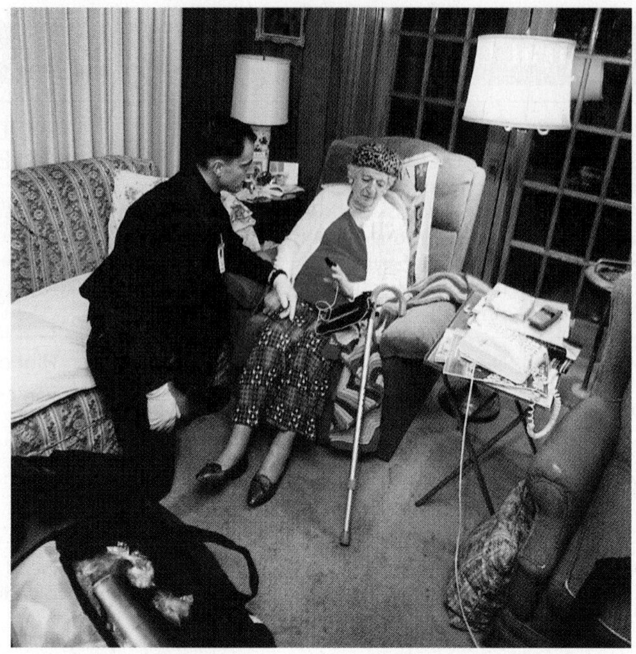

Figure 33-1 • Position yourself at the patient's level, make good eye contact, and speak slowly and clearly. *(© Craig Jackson/In the Dark Photography)*

A few of the elderly have a significant deterioration of memory and overall intellectual ability from Alzheimer's disease (a chronic organic disorder resulting in dementia) or other conditions. However, do not assume that confusion in your elderly patient is "normal," or the result of long-term mental deterioration. Unless someone who knows the patient can confirm that this is a chronic condition, suspect that an altered mental status may be the result of the present illness or injury.

When you are speaking to any patient, it is important that the patient see and hear you. This is especially true in the elderly patient who has a hearing impairment or poor peripheral vision. Keep in mind that speaking loudly to a patient does not mean speaking down to a patient. Treat the patient with respect and dignity (Figure 33-1). Begin by calling the patient by a title and her last name, for example, Mrs. Sanchez. Ask the patient how she would like to be addressed before assuming that you may use her first name. Whenever possible, speak to the patient at the same level. This may involve crouching, or even kneeling down.

Assessing the Geriatric Patient

The steps of assessment for geriatric patients are the same as those for other patients. Some particular things to be aware of and to look for include the following.

Scene Size-Up and Safety—Geriatric

When you approach an elderly person's residence, look both outside and inside for clues as to the patient's physical and mental abilities. Is the outside of the house conscientiously cared for, or is the paint on the house peeling and the garden untended? When you enter the home, besides looking for potential dangers to you and your crew, look at the general condition of the residence. Is half-eaten food sitting in the living room? Is something unrecognizable drying up in a pan on the stove? Is the house dirty? Are items left out in the open where someone can trip on them?

A very important question to ask is what is the temperature? Like infants, older people cannot regulate their body temperatures very well. They need an environment that frequently feels uncomfortably warm to younger people. Even at such temperatures, some older people still wear several layers of clothing to retain sufficient heat. This can become a problem when a heat wave occurs and the older person fails to feel the temperature rising. A life-threatening rise in body temperature can result. (See Chapter 22, "Environmental Emergencies.")

Initial Assessment—Geriatric

FORMING A GENERAL IMPRESSION Now that you have looked at the patient's surroundings, look at the patient. What is the level of his distress? Is he leaning forward with hands on knees gasping for breath? Is he lying on a hospital bed apparently unresponsive and breathing through an open mouth? Is he sitting in a chair in no acute distress?

ASSESSING MENTAL STATUS This can be very challenging, because some older people have an abnormal mental status as part of their baseline condition. If family members or caregivers are available, it is important you find out from them what normal status is for this patient.

ASSESSING THE AIRWAY Evaluating the airway of an older patient is very similar to evaluating the airway of other patients with two major exceptions. You may find it difficult to extend the head and flex the neck of an older patient because of arthritic changes in the bones of the neck. The best thing to do in this case is not to try to force the head back, but instead to thrust the jaw forward to pull the tongue out of the airway.

The other difficulty you may come across is dentures. If a patient's dentures are secure, there is usually no reason to remove them. If, however, they are loose or ill-fitting, it is best to remove them from the mouth of an unresponsive patient to prevent them from becoming an airway obstruction.

ASSESSING BREATHING Older patients are at higher risk of foreign body airway obstruction. Two major risk factors are large, poorly chewed pieces of food and dentures. If you are unable to ventilate an older patient, reposition the head and try to ventilate again. If this does not work, initiate the sequence of steps to relieve a foreign body airway obstruction.

ASSESSING CIRCULATION Finding a radial pulse in an older patient is usually no different from finding a pulse in other patients. What you may notice in these patients, though, is that the pulse is often irregularly irregular (i.e., completely without any kind of cycle or regularity). This is the result of a very common dysrhythmia (abnormal heart rhythm) in older people. The irregularity is not a reason for concern in itself.

IDENTIFYING PRIORITY PATIENTS Older patients are less likely to show severe symptoms in certain conditions, so it can be difficult to determine a patient's priority. For example, most people having a heart attack experience significant chest pain. An older person is more likely to have just the sudden onset of weakness with no chest pain. Keep a high index of suspicion for serious conditions in elderly patients, even if symptoms are seemingly mild or vague.

Focused History and Physical Exam—Geriatric

HISTORY Obtaining a history of the present illness can be challenging when the patient is elderly. He may answer questions very slowly or even inappropriately. It may be difficult to understand his speech, or he may have difficulty understanding your questions. Regardless of the particular circumstances, you must gather as much information as you can from the patient and from other sources.

When interviewing the patient, be sure to introduce yourself, speak slowly and clearly, and position yourself where the patient can easily see you. If he is answering your questions slowly and your initial assessment did not reveal any immediate threats to life, give him additional time. Be sure to ask just one question at a time. Similarly, if the patient's speech is slurred but still understandable, do not rush him. Doing so could easily fluster him, delaying responses even more, and destroy any rapport you have established. If the patient's speech is difficult to understand because his dentures are not in place, ask him to put them in if appropriate.

Cultural Considerations

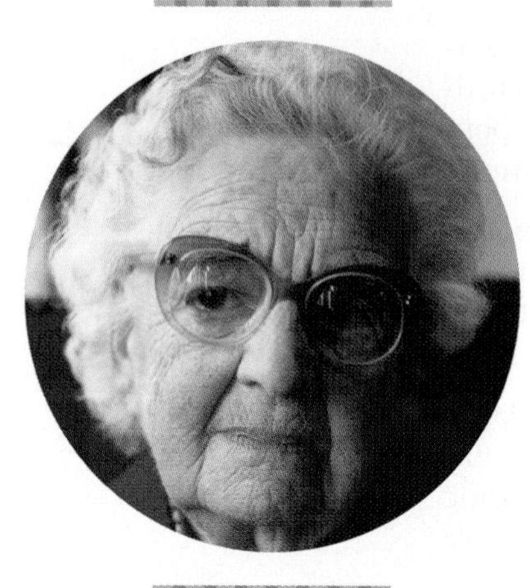

Older patients sometimes prefer to use traditional treatments instead of "what the doctor ordered." Perhaps they cannot afford to fill the prescriptions the doctor has given them or perhaps they decide to take the prescribed pill every other day to cut the cost in half. Perhaps they feel that homemade remedies like chicken soup, the old-fashioned jar of smelly chest-rub, or the herbal tea that Grandma taught them how to make will do the trick. These "cures" may remind them of the "good old days" when doctors made house calls, had an encouraging bedside manner, and carried enough pills in his bag to take care of any problem. At least that's how the patient may remember, or rationalize, it.

A careful history, patiently taken, with time allowed for the patient to tell you what his medical conditions are, what the doctor has prescribed, and whether he is doing what the doctor advised (or, perhaps, something else) will go a long way toward helping you to find out about—and document—your older patient's true situation.

Sometimes a patient will answer questions very slowly because he is clinically depressed, or so sad or blue that his eating and sleeping habits are altered, he feels fatigued, his memory or concentration is impaired, his self-confidence is low, and he may even have thoughts of suicide. About one-tenth of older people have clinical depression. However, do not be fooled into thinking that a depressed patient has no other problems. Depression can both mimic and mask other serious medical problems.

Another possibility you may find when interviewing a patient is that the family tells you he was wrong in some of his responses. This is sometimes a result of a neurological condition, but it can also be caused by medications the patient is taking, especially if there are many of them (Figure 33-2) or the dose for some is too high.

A variation of this is the patient who gives you a story of having gone out to the movies last night but who, according to family members, has not left the house in years. This is called *confabulation*. The patient is replacing lost circumstances with imaginary ones. These made-up experiences are usually quite believable and the patient is typically very pleasant to talk to. Nonetheless, the experiences are not real and may very

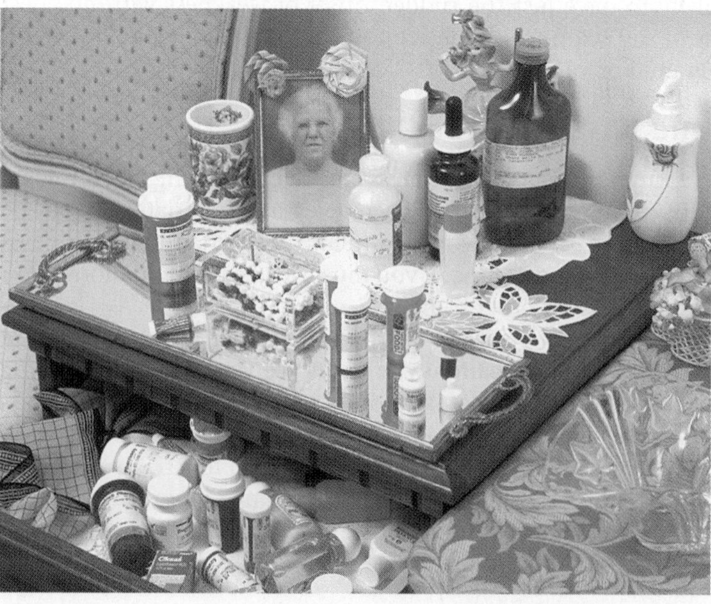

Figure 33-2 • Older patients often take multiple medications.

well change if you ask the same question a few minutes later. Confabulation can be caused by a number of neurological conditions.

This points out the importance of gathering information from family members and others who are familiar with the patient's condition. If the patient lives with a spouse or other family members, they can frequently be an excellent source of information about his medications, SAMPLE history, and even the history of the present illness. Similarly, visiting nurses can often provide or confirm a great deal of this information.

PHYSICAL EXAM When performing a physical exam on an older person, keep the patient's dignity in mind. Explain what you are going to do before you do it and replace any clothing you remove as soon as possible. Many older people have a high threshold for pain. An extremity that is obviously fractured may cause very little discomfort to some patients. On the other hand, some of these patients have a very low threshold for pain. You will need to judge this for yourself when doing the physical exam.

BASELINE VITAL SIGNS Vital signs of the elderly are similar to those of other adults with only a few exceptions. As people age, the systolic blood pressure has a tendency to increase. Many older patients you meet will be on medication for hypertension, usually defined as a diastolic pressure over about 90 mmHg. These medications can have significant side effects, including weakness and dizziness, especially on standing up quickly from a sitting or supine position.

The skin loses much of its elasticity as it ages, leading to dry skin that is thin and fragile. Applying pressure that is too heavy, even with just your fingertips, can be enough to cause the skin to tear in some patients. Be careful when pulling or lifting a patient to be as gentle as possible.

The pupils are not round and reactive to light in some older patients. Eye surgery or pre-existing conditions may have given the pupil an abnormal shape or the inability to react to light normally. Certain eye drops can also prevent normal reactions to light. When you find this condition, inquire as to whether it is normal before assuming the patient has a serious condition based on this sign.

Detailed Physical Exam—Geriatric

The detailed physical exam for older patients is the same as for other adults. You may come across some unusual findings because of the patient's age or condition, though.

HEAD AND NECK When evaluating the head, be especially attentive. Injuries to the head and face are very common in older patients who have sustained a fall or been involved in a motor-vehicle collision. In fact, falls and motor-vehicle collisions account for the overwhelming majority of injuries in patients over 65 years.

The neck may be stiff and the head may be far forward of where it normally is because of changes in the spine. This can be a challenge to deal with when you suspect a neck injury and must immobilize the patient. Use folded towels or other materials to keep the head in its normal position, prevent hyperextension, and make the patient more comfortable.

CHEST AND ABDOMEN The chest and abdomen are not commonly injured, but keep in mind the decreased sensitivity to pain that many older people have. Serious abdominal problems that would cause a younger person agony may produce only slight discomfort for older patients.

PELVIS AND EXTREMITIES The hip or proximal femur is commonly fractured in a fall, especially in women. This is partly because more women than men survive to be old, but even more so because women are more prone to loss of calcium from bone. This leads to so much weakening of the bone that a fracture is sometimes the cause of a fall rather than a result. Other areas on the extremities are also injured sometimes because of this weakening of the bone.

SPINE The back is sometimes injured in a fall, but it is very commonly injured in motor-vehicle collisions. Again, because of abnormal curvature that sometimes accompanies

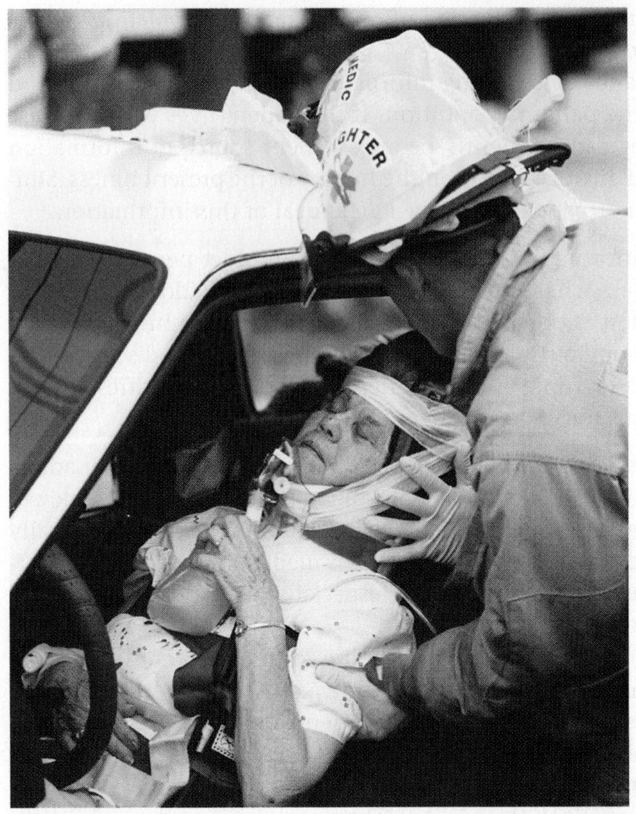

Figure 33-3 • Extrication of an elderly patient from a motor-vehicle collision. *(© Eddie Sperling Photography)*

aging, immobilizing these patients can be very challenging. Do your best to keep the vertebrae in alignment and to reduce the patient's discomfort (Figure 33-3).

Ongoing Assessment—Geriatric

Children who deteriorate are likely to exhibit sudden changes in condition. Although that can happen in elderly patients, it is more common for them to show a slow, steady decline in condition. This can be deceiving because the patient does not suddenly tell you or show sudden signs that his condition is going downhill. Instead, you may be lulled into a false sense of security because there is little or no appreciable change from one minute to the next. Guard against this by performing an ongoing assessment at regular intervals and comparing your findings to those you recorded previously. Look for trends that indicate trouble.

Keep in mind the elements of the ongoing assessment:

1. Reassess mental status
2. Maintain open airway
3. Monitor breathing
4. Reassess pulse
5. Monitor skin color, temperature, and moisture
6. Reassess vital signs
   - Every 5 minutes in unstable patients
   - Every 15 minutes in stable patients
7. Ensure that all appropriate care and treatments are being given

Reasons the Elderly Encounter EMS

Pharmacology

The elderly use far more medications than other age groups. This is true not only because of the numerous diseases and conditions they have but also because modern medicine is producing more medications to treat these conditions. A significant number of

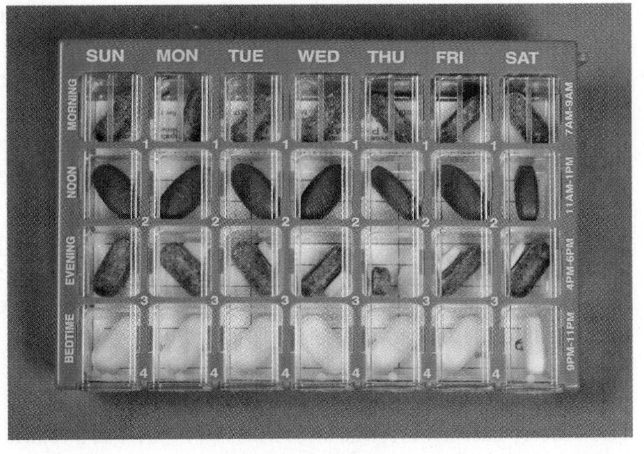

Figure 33-4 • Many elderly persons use a pill organizer to help them remember when to take medications.

the elderly take more than just one medication; some take as many as six, eight, ten, or even more. Keeping track of which pill to take and when to take it can be extremely challenging even for the best-organized person. A handy way to help prevent problems like this is the use of a pill organizer with the pills for each day (or for each time of day) in a separate compartment (Figure 33-4). Another potential problem is that pills that have very different effects may have very similar appearances. If someone with vision problems and limited manual dexterity drops several pills on the floor, it becomes very easy to mix them up.

Many of these medications are expensive. Some elderly people must unfortunately make the choice between food and medication because they cannot afford both. Obviously, this can lead to noncompliance with medication schedules. This can be even worse when a missed pill is supposed to correct some of the undesirable effects of another drug that the patient is still taking.

Even when a medication is taken as directed, it can have a number of adverse effects. For example, many elderly patients take a medication from a class known as nonsteroidal anti-inflammatory drugs (NSAIDs). These medications, such as ibuprofen and ketoprofen (both available without a prescription), relieve the pain and inflammation associated with conditions such as arthritis. Unfortunately, these and other NSAIDs are also irritating to the gastrointestinal tract and often cause internal bleeding. More than 16,000 people die every year in the United States because of gastrointestinal bleeding when these medications are taken for arthritis.

Drug-patient interactions can occur because of the older patient's inability to clear medications from the body as quickly as before. Most drugs are broken down by the liver and kidneys before excretion, but liver and kidney function decrease with age. A dose that would be fine for a 30-year-old may be incapacitating to a 75-year-old.

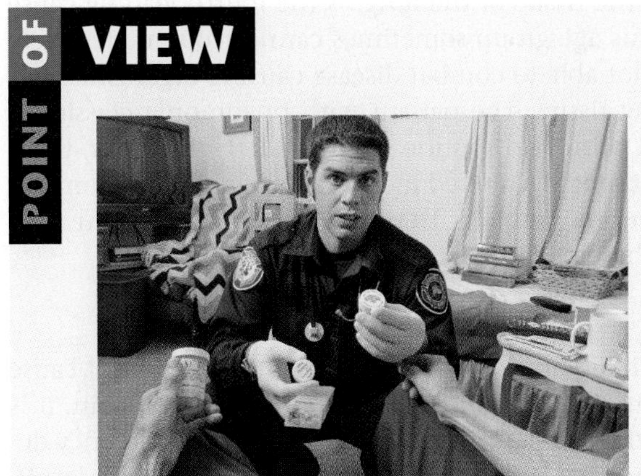

"I wasn't feeling well. It happens at my age—93. I didn't think much of it, but my daughter called the ambulance. She read that it could be a stroke or my heart or something.

"The men and women from the ambulance are always nice to me. A lot of them know my name. Some of them even know my medical problems by heart. This time the man was new. I have so many medications and medical problems it seems like it takes 20 minutes to get them all straight.

"But he listened and wrote things down. Then he listened some more and wrote more down. He was very nice. He actually looked at my medications and reminded me about a condition I forgot I had. Pretty sharp fellow, that youngster.

"It's nothing personal, but I hope I don't see the people from the ambulance again for awhile."

Drug-drug interactions are very common in this age group, especially as the number of medications goes up. When two drugs interact, there are two possibilities: one may block or reduce the effect of the other, or one may increase the effect of the other. This outcome can be so severe that it becomes life-threatening. The likelihood of a drug-drug interaction increases when a patient goes to different doctors for different problems and fills prescriptions at different pharmacies. Patients sometimes forget to tell the doctor or pharmacist about the other medications they are taking.

Drug-drug interactions are not limited to just prescription drugs. Prescription medications can have serious interactions with over-the-counter drugs, nutrient or herbal preparations, and even food (for example, grapefruit juice can increase the effects of certain cardiac medications).

Shortness of Breath

The elderly can experience shortness of breath as a result of the same diseases that cause this symptom in younger patients, such as asthma. The older population, however, is more likely to have conditions such as emphysema and heart failure (pulmonary edema) or a combination of these diseases that causes shortness of breath. Shortness of breath is also often the chief complaint of elderly patients having myocardial infarctions (heart attacks). As a patient gets older, the patient experiencing a cardiac problem is more likely to complain of shortness of breath *without* chest pain. The EMT must maintain a high index of suspicion for cardiac problems in these patients.

Chest Pain

A complaint of chest pain can arise from many conditions. Some that are more common in the elderly are angina, myocardial infarction, pneumonia, and aortic aneurysm. An aneurysm is an abnormal widening of a blood vessel, usually an artery. As the vessel walls are stretched, they become thinner and weaker, so the vessel can rupture, leading to catastrophic bleeding. The pain from a thoracic aortic aneurysm as it dissects (separates the layers of the artery) is classically described as "tearing."

Altered Mental Status

The list of conditions that can cause alteration of mental status is nearly endless. Some of the more common ones in the elderly include adverse effects from medications (many drugs have sedating effects that are more pronounced in the elderly), hypoglycemia (perhaps from taking too much diabetic medication), stroke (from chronic or untreated hypertension), generalized infection in the bloodstream (the immune system may not fend off microbes as well as it used to), and hypothermia (the elderly patient may lose heat at a temperature that is comfortable for others). Do not assume that an altered mental status is normal for an elderly patient until you check with someone who knows the patient and can describe the patient's baseline status.

Pneumonia, an inflammation in the tissue of the lung, is the fourth leading cause of death in the elderly. Patients in this age group sometimes cannot cough effectively and have immune systems that are not able to combat disease-causing organisms very well, leading to infection in the lung tissue. The patient with pneumonia classically presents with fever and a cough that brings up sputum. In the elderly, however, these signs may be very subtle or entirely absent. An altered mental status, resulting from hypoxia, may be the only outward sign of a problem. Despite aggressive treatment with antibiotics in the hospital, some of these patients will not survive.

Abdominal Pain

Conditions that would cause abdominal pain in a younger patient often do not cause pain in the older patient, so when an older person complains of abdominal pain, it is often a sign of a serious condition and will be taken very seriously in the emergency department. One of the most serious causes of abdominal pain in this population is an abdominal aortic aneurysm, which you may hear experienced providers refer to as a "triple A." If it is stable in size or growing very slowly, the patient may not even know about it. Like the aneurysm in the thoracic aorta, though, as it grows it sometimes causes pain with a tearing nature. The pain is often excruciating in intensity and will be accompanied by severe shock if the artery has ruptured. If it is leaking slowly, the problem can sometimes be surgically repaired if the patient is able to withstand the stress of surgery.

Another common cause of abdominal pain in the elderly is bowel obstruction or blockage, which can cause severe pain and may require surgery for repair. Also common in this age group is diverticulitis, a condition where a diverticulum, an outpouching of the intestine, provides a sac where food can lodge and cause inflammation (diverticulitis). Ask the patient with abdominal pain if he has had black, tarry stools, caused by the remains of red blood cells that have gone through the digestive tract, which is one indicator of internal bleeding.

Dizziness, Weakness, and Malaise

Dizziness, weakness, and malaise are vague symptoms that are easy for the EMT to take lightly. Don't! These complaints can be associated with a number of serious conditions, including some life-threatening ones. Dizziness, especially upon standing, may be the only indication that a patient is experiencing significant internal bleeding. Weakness can be the result of cardiac dysrhythmias. When an 80-year-old's heart is beating 180 times a minute, there isn't time for the heart to fill between contractions. More commonly in the elderly, the heart experiences bradycardia, a pulse rate less than 60 per minute. Fortunately, either condition can be treated with medications, a pacemaker, or both. Many other extremely serious conditions may present in an elderly patient with no more than the complaint that "I'm not feeling myself today." Be diligent in your assessment of this seemingly minor problem.

Depression and Suicide

Depression is very common in the elderly, sometimes because of medical conditions that limit activity, medications that sap the patient's energy, loss of friends or a spouse (especially widowers), or just a biochemical imbalance in the brain. For this reason, many elderly patients are on antidepressants. When evaluating a patient's illness or injury, observe the patient's mood, speech, and activity. Referral to an appropriate source of assistance may be life-saving.

The segment of the population most likely to be successful in a suicide attempt is elderly males. It is not possible to predict accurately who will attempt or complete suicide, so mention any suspicions of this nature to the emergency department staff when you turn over the patient.

Unusual Problems

A condition much more common in the older population is herpes zoster or shingles. This condition is the result of varicella, the same virus that causes chicken pox. In shingles, the virus reawakens after years of inactivity. The patient experiences pain, often quite severe, on one side of the body over a dermatome, the area associated with one of the nerves coming from the spinal cord (Figure 33-5). Within a few days, small blisters appear in that area. After a few more days, the blisters dry out and scab over. Further healing takes a few more weeks. Unfortunately for many older patients, this is not the end of the problem. In almost half of patients over 60 years, the area remains quite painful, requiring strong pain medication for relief. The pain of this condition commonly occurs somewhere on one side of the torso, but it also can occur higher up. A severe headache may be the result of shingles.

Note: Until the lesions scab over, an EMT who has not had varicella infection can contract it from the fluid. Standard Precautions and attention to hygiene should keep the uninfected EMT healthy.

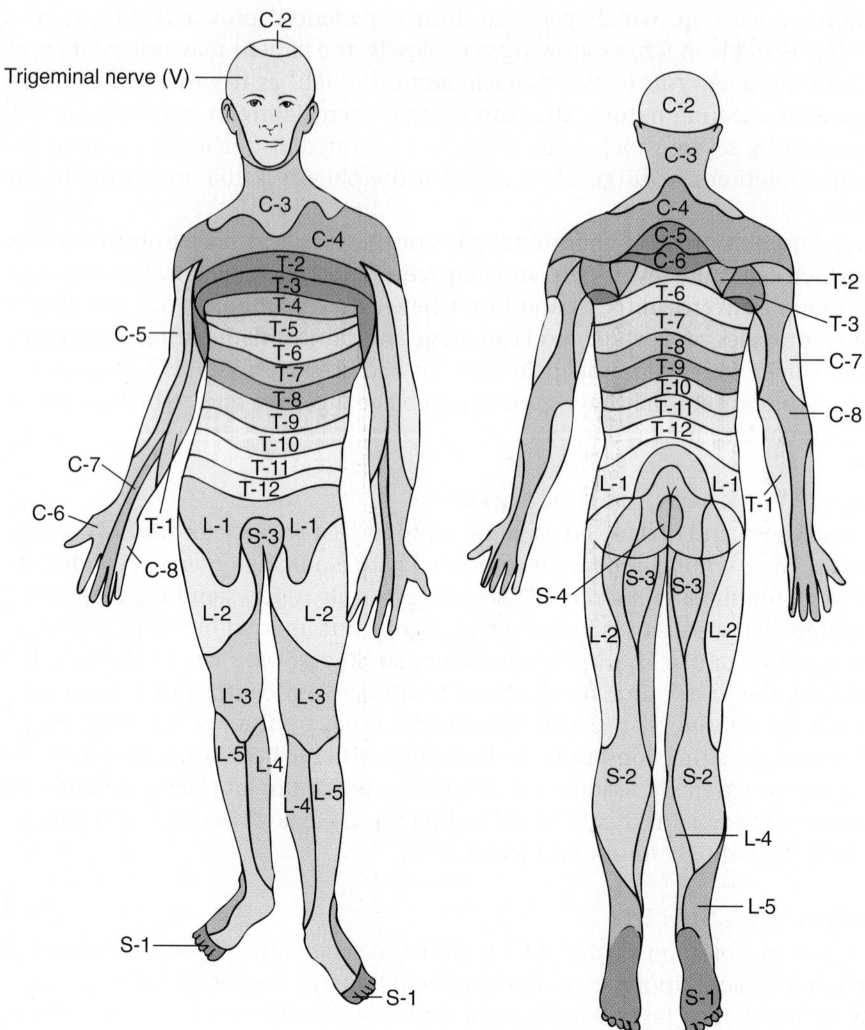

Figure 33-5 • Dermatomes are areas of the skin that are innervated by various segments of the spinal cord. Those marked "C" are innervated by levels of the cervical spine, "T" the thoracic spine, "L" the lumbar spine, and "S" the sacral spine.

Falls

The significance of a fall for an older person should not be underestimated. Of older patients seen in an emergency department for a fall, one quarter will die within a year. Death may not be a direct result of the fall, but instead may result from complications of the fall. For example, while recuperating from bruised ribs sustained in a fall, a 74-year-old woman may not breathe as deeply as normal because of the pain associated with inhalation. As a result of not being able to cough, as well as other changes in the aging lungs, if this patient comes down with pneumonia, she is more likely to die from it.

Often, a fall is just an indication of a more serious problem. A number of older people fall because of abnormal heart rhythms. Others fall because of a stroke or internal bleeding from an ulcer. Whenever possible and when time allows, assess the patient not only for injuries from the fall, but also for a cause of the fall.

EMTs can help prevent falls. When you enter an older person's home, look for potential hazards. Table 33-3 lists a number of hazards and what you or the patient's family or friends can do to correct them.

Elder Abuse and Neglect

Elder abuse and neglect have occurred for many years but have only recently received the attention they deserve. There are essentially three ways in which elders can be abused or neglected: physically, psychologically, and financially. Physical abuse in-

TABLE 33-3 • Making a Home Safer for the Elderly

HAZARD	INTERVENTION	REASON
Torn or slippery rugs	Repair or replace.	To prevent tripping and slipping
Chair without armrests	Install armrests.	To provide leverage in getting out of chair
Chair with low back	Replace with a chair with high back.	To support neck; prevent falling backward for patients who must rock to get out of chair
Chair with wheels	Replace with a chair with sturdy legs.	To prevent chair from sliding when person is getting into or out of it
Temperature too low	Maintain temperature at 72°F in winter.	To prevent hypothermia
Obstructing furniture	Move items so that clutter is minimized and pathways are clear.	To help those with poor mobility and poor peripheral vision
Slippery bathtub	Install skid-resistant strips or mat.	To provide more stable footing
Missing handrails on stairways	Install handrail.	To allow person to grab onto support

cludes pushing, shoving, hitting, or shaking of an older person. It occasionally includes sexual abuse. Physical neglect includes improper feeding, poor hygiene, or inadequate medical care. Psychological abuse and neglect include threats, insults, or ignoring an older person ("the silent treatment"). Financial abuse and neglect include exploitation or misuse of an older person's belongings or money.

Detecting elder abuse and neglect can be difficult. Don't automatically assume that an injury is the result of a simple fall, even though falls are common among the elderly. Evaluate any injury in this age group with an eye toward recognizing signs of abuse or neglect. Many states have laws that require the reporting of such suspicions. Be aware of the laws in your state and local protocols and take whatever actions you are permitted to take to help the victim of abuse.

Loss of Independence

It is hard for younger adults to understand how disruptive a serious injury or illness can be to an older person. Years of independence can vanish in an instant, leaving the patient in the care of strangers. Even worse, he goes to a hospital where many friends and perhaps a spouse have gone, never to return. The EMT can help by treating the patient with dignity. Do not minimize the patient's fears and concerns. Instead, acknowledge them and try to put them in perspective.

Ask the patient if he would like you to lock up before you leave the house. Inquire about the care of any pets and whether there is a trusted neighbor who can take care of them for awhile. If you can honestly say it, reassure the patient that most patients you have seen with this particular problem do well and return home in good condition. A friendly hand on the forearm, if you feel the patient will accept it, can be very reassuring. Talking with the patient during transport about what he has done over the course of a lifetime can be not only therapeutic for the patient, but enlightening for you as well. Above all, treat the patient in a respectful, empathetic manner.

CRITICAL DECISION MAKING:
CHANGES WITH AGE

Geriatric patients differ from those in other age groups. This exercise asks you to apply your understanding of these differences to your assessment and decision making.

1. You are treating a geriatric patient who, you suspect, has fractured her hip. The patient is pale and is breathing rapidly. You suspect shock, but her pulse is 84. She is a diabetic, has a cardiac history and hypertension, and takes several medications. If she is in shock, why isn't her pulse rate more rapid?
2. Your geriatric patient hasn't felt well for the past several days. She complains of a cough and flu-like symptoms. She has become increasingly weak. Her family suspects the flu, but she doesn't have a fever. Why?
3. You are called to an assisted living facility for a man who is "just not right." He was fine last night. The man complains of suddenly feeling very weak and is having a little difficulty breathing. The nurse wants him sent to the hospital in case he is having a heart attack. Why would she think this?

CHAPTER REVIEW

SUMMARY

People are most dependent on others for help, especially when illness or injury strikes, at the extremes of age. By taking into account an elderly patient's prior conditions and illnesses, you will be able to perform a more thorough assessment that will lead to more accurate information for you and less stress for the patient. These patients are very similar to younger adults, but they often have numerous illnesses and medications. The most striking characteristic shared by this age group is the lack of reserve. Something that causes moderate stress for a middle-age adult may inflict severe stress that can be life-threatening in an older patient.

REVIEW QUESTIONS

1. Describe how to approach an elderly patient who has vision and hearing impairments. (pp. 883–884, 885)
2. What question should you ask to determine if an elderly patient's condition is normal or a change from baseline? (p. 885)
3. Name some of the most common medical conditions that cause EMS to be called for elderly patients. (pp. 888–893)
4. Name the two most common mechanisms of injury to patients over age 65. (p. 887)

CRITICAL THINKING

- You respond to an elderly woman who has fallen and injured her hip. When you arrive, you find a 90-year-old woman lying on the kitchen floor, alert and oriented, complaining of hip pain. She is somewhat hard of hearing. Her 91-year-old husband is very upset over what happened and blaming himself for her fall. How should you approach your assessment of the patient? How should you deal with her husband?

MEDIA RESOURCES

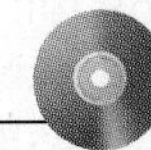

See the Student CD at the back of this book for quizzes, a case study activity, and other features related to this chapter. Also, visit the Companion Website for *Emergency Care* at **www.prenhall.com/limmer,** where you will find additional reinforcement and links to other resources.

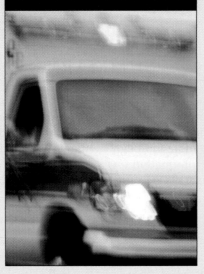

Street Scenes

"Unit 10, respond to the senior citizen housing center on Martin Luther King, Jr. Avenue for a patient having difficulty breathing." When you arrive, you stop for a moment at the doorway and notice that the apartment is messy. The patient is a 67-year-old male sitting upright in a chair with rapid respirations and wheezing. You ask why he has called EMS, and he responds in short sentences, telling you that he is having trouble catching his breath and may be having an asthma attack. Your partner tells the patient she wants to give him oxygen. While a nonrebreather mask is set up, you perform an initial assessment.

Street Scene Questions

1. What is your initial priority for providing care to this patient?
2. After the initial assessment is completed, what assessment information should be obtained next?
3. Why is the condition of the apartment significant?

The patient's airway is open and his respirations are 24 per minute with wheezing upon exhalation. Your partner continues to obtain additional vitals, and you get a SAMPLE history. When you ask the patient if he is taking any medications, he asks if you could speak up because he doesn't hear well. You reposition yourself in front of the patient and speak clearly, without shouting, at a greater volume. He responds by pointing to a shoe box full of pill bottles and two inhalers. You ask if he has been taking his medications and, appearing confused, he says he doesn't remember which ones he took today. When asked if someone knows about his medication schedule, he states that he lives alone. Your partner reports the following vital signs: respirations are 28, pulse is 110, blood pressure is 160/100, skin is moist, and pupils equal and reactive. You and your partner tell the patient that you want to take him to the hospital. He agrees, and you package and move him to the ambulance, bringing his box of medications along.

Street Scene Questions

4. Based on the assessment, would you expect this patient's condition to worsen? How should you be prepared if it does?
5. What additional assessment should be done en route to the hospital? How often should the vital signs be taken?
6. What information about the patient's living situation should you provide to the hospital staff?

You briefly discuss the patient situation with your partner and you decide that a transport with red lights and siren seems appropriate as the patient's breathing rate is increasing and you may need to assist ventilations with a bag-valve mask. You also decide, based on the patient's confused state and inability to breathe deeply, not to assist him with one of his inhalers. As you proceed to the hospital, with your partner driving, you reassess vital signs and find the patient's respiratory rate has returned to 24 and the patient is starting to talk in longer sentences. You ask some additional medical history questions about previous asthma attacks and the patient seems more lucid. You are communicating well with the patient, and he is hearing you. In fact, he provides the name of his daughter and gives you a telephone number. The patient seems less anxious and, about 5 minutes before arrival at the hospital, he has a respiratory rate of 20 with wheezing still present. You contact the hospital by radio, provide patient information, and give an ETA.

While completing your prehospital care report, you remember the condition of the apartment and that this patient lives alone. Before leaving, you share this information with the charge nurse and suggest that if this patient is sent home, he may need living assistance as well as help with his care, such as medications. The nurse thanks you and tells you that she will ask a case manager to follow up.

Street Scenes Sample Documentation

PATIENT NAME: Paul Minkler | **PATIENT AGE:** 67

CHIEF COMPLAINT
Difficulty breathing

PAST MEDICAL HISTORY

☐ None	
☐ Allergy to	
☐ Hypertension	☐ Stroke
☐ Seizures	☐ Diabetes
☐ COPD	☐ Cardiac
☐ Other (List)	☒ Asthma

Current Medications (List)
Albuterol and Flovent inhalers; multiple other meds

VITAL SIGNS

TIME	RESP	PULSE	B.P.	MENTAL STATUS	R PUPILS	L PUPILS	SKIN
1240	Rate: 28 ☐ Regular ☐ Shallow ☑ Labored	Rate: 110 ☑ Regular ☐ Irregular	160/100	☑ Alert ☐ Voice ☐ Pain ☐ Unresp.	☑ Normal ☐ Dilated ☐ Constricted ☐ Sluggish ☐ No-Reaction	☑ Normal ☐ Dilated ☐ Constricted ☐ Sluggish ☐ No-Reaction	☐ Unremarkable ☐ Cool ☐ Pale ☐ Warm ☐ Cyanotic ☑ Moist ☐ Flushed ☐ Dry ☐ Jaundiced
1250	Rate: 24 ☐ Regular ☐ Shallow ☑ Labored	Rate: 104 ☑ Regular ☐ Irregular	150/P	☑ Alert ☐ Voice ☐ Pain ☐ Unresp.	☑ Normal ☐ Dilated ☐ Constricted ☐ Sluggish ☐ No-Reaction	☑ Normal ☐ Dilated ☐ Constricted ☐ Sluggish ☐ No-Reaction	☐ Unremarkable ☐ Cool ☐ Pale ☐ Warm ☐ Cyanotic ☑ Moist ☐ Flushed ☐ Dry ☐ Jaundiced
1255	Rate: 20 ☐ Regular ☐ Shallow ☑ Labored	Rate: 108 ☑ Regular ☐ Irregular	150/P	☑ Alert ☐ Voice ☐ Pain ☐ Unresp.	☑ Normal ☐ Dilated ☐ Constricted ☐ Sluggish ☐ No-Reaction	☑ Normal ☐ Dilated ☐ Constricted ☐ Sluggish ☐ No-Reaction	☐ Unremarkable ☐ Cool ☐ Pale ☐ Warm ☐ Cyanotic ☑ Moist ☐ Flushed ☐ Dry ☐ Jaundiced

NARRATIVE Dispatched for difficulty breathing. Found confused 67 y/o male sitting upright, wheezing, speaking only a few words at a time and complaining of "trouble catching my breath." Patient appears to be in significant resp. distress. He has asthma and unknown other medical problems. Patient has two inhalers, but can't remember if he used them today. Administered 15 lpm O_2 via NRB, transferred patient to unit and transported. En route, patient became more lucid, appeared to be in less distress and began speaking in longer sentences. Further medical history not obtained because of patient's initial mental status and short transport time. Gave report to E.D. staff and transferred patient and care. No other changes in patient's condition.

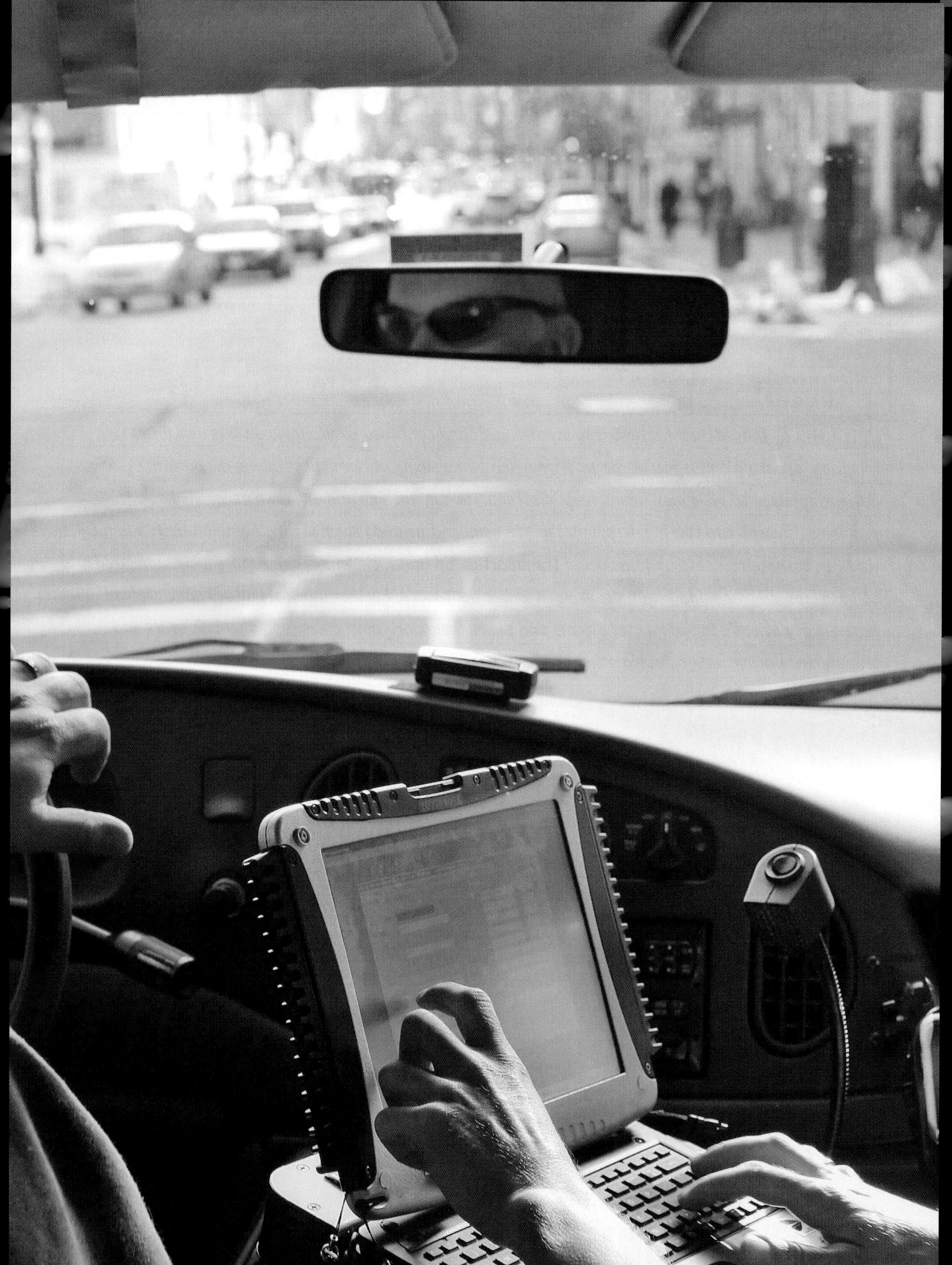

7 MODULE

Operations

This module deals with EMS operations and organization, both for the day-to-day conduct of your job as an EMT and for certain special situations.

Chapter 34 will lead you through the sequence of tasks you will perform before, during, and after an ambulance call—from the moment you report for duty at the beginning of your shift until the ambulance is back in quarters at the end of the last call of your day. In Chapter 35 you will learn about access to and rescue for entrapped patients and about your role as an EMT at the scene of a rescue.

Chapter 36 covers incidents that involve large numbers of patients and those that involve hazardous materials. Chapter 37 discusses domestic and international terrorism and the kinds of terrorist attacks that may involve an EMS response. A special section on your own self-protection is included.

CHAPTER

34 Ambulance Operations

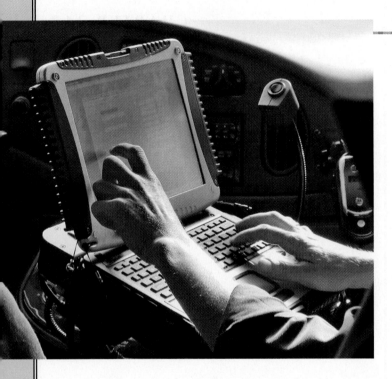

CORE CONCEPTS

The following are core concepts that will be addressed in this chapter:

- Phases of an ambulance call
- Preparation for a call
- Emergency driving laws and regulations
- Operating an emergency vehicle
- How to clean and disinfect EMS equipment

DOT OBJECTIVES

*KNOWLEDGE AND ATTITUDE

7-1.1 Discuss the medical and nonmedical equipment needed to respond to a call. (pp. 902–907)

7-1.2 List the phases of an ambulance call. (p. 901)

7-1.3 Describe the general provisions of state laws relating to the operation of the ambulance and privileges in any or all of the following categories: (pp. 911–918) (Scan 34-2, p. 917)
- Speed
- Warning lights
- Sirens
- Right-of-way
- Parking
- Turning

7-1.4 List contributing factors to unsafe driving conditions. (pp. 915–916)

7-1.5 Describe the considerations that should be given to: (pp. 914–915)
- Request for escorts
- Following an escort vehicle
- Intersections

7-1.6 Discuss "Due Regard for Safety of All Others" while operating an emergency vehicle. (pp. 912–913, 914)

7-1.7 State what information is essential in order to respond to a call. (pp. 910–911)

7-1.8 Discuss various situations that may affect response to a call. (pp. 915–916)

7-1.9 Differentiate between the various methods of moving a patient to the unit based upon injury or illness. (pp. 918–919)

7-1.10 Apply the components of the essential patient information in a written report. (p. 923)

7-1.11 Summarize the importance of preparing the unit for the next response. (pp. 923–931) (Scan 34-4, p. 926; Scan 34-5, pp. 928–929; Scan 34-6, p. 930)

7-1.12 Identify what is essential for completion of a call. (p. 923) (Scan 34-3, p. 924)

7-1.13 Distinguish among the terms *cleaning, disinfection, high-level disinfection*, and *sterilization*. (pp. 930–931) (Scan 34-6, p. 930)

7-1.14 Describe how to clean or disinfect items following patient care. (pp. 930–931) (Scan 34-5, pp. 928–929) (Scan 34-6, p. 930)

7-1.15 Explain the rationale for appropriate report of patient information. (pp. 921–923)

7-1.16 Explain the rationale for having the unit prepared to respond. (pp. 907–910) (Scan 34-1, p. 908)

Your responsibilities may differ somewhat depending on the type of EMS agency you join. However, most nonmedical operational responsibilities include the following five phases:

- Preparing for the ambulance call
- Receiving and responding to a call
- Transferring the patient to the ambulance
- Transporting the patient to the hospital
- Terminating the call

PREPARING FOR THE AMBULANCE CALL

The modern ambulance has come a long way from its primitive beginnings. Far more than just a means of transport, today's ambulance is a well-equipped and efficiently organized mobile pre-hospital emergency department and communications unit.

The U.S. Department of Transportation has issued specifications for Type I, Type II, and Type III ambulances. Because of the extra equipment now placed on ambulances for specialty rescue, advanced life support, and hazardous materials operations, the gross vehicle weight has been easily exceeded in some communities. This has necessitated introduction of a medium-duty truck chassis built for rugged durability and large storage and work areas (Figure 34-1). As needs evolve, ambulance standards will also continue to evolve.

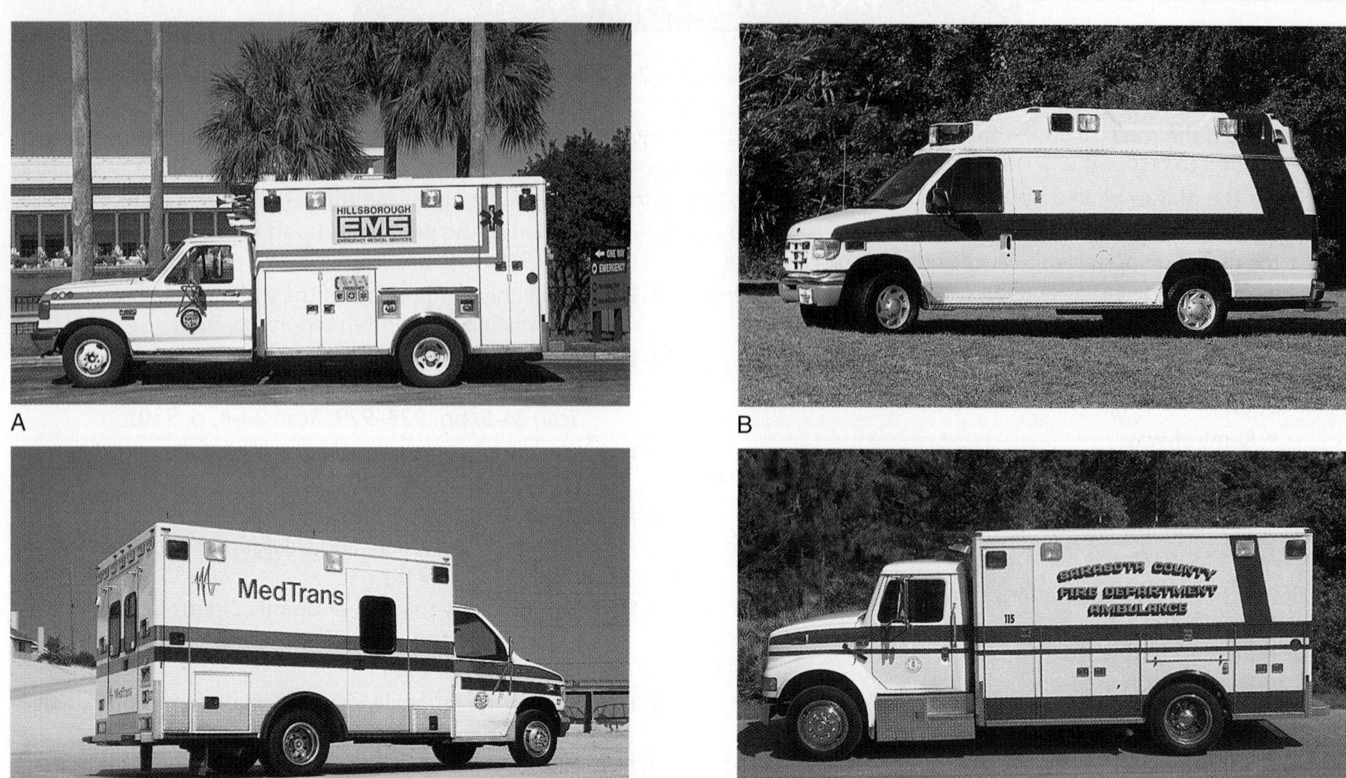

Figure 34-1 • Four types of ambulances: (A) Type I, (B) Type II, (C) Type III, and (D) medium duty.

Ambulance Supplies and Equipment

If an ambulance does not have the proper equipment for patient care and transportation, it is just another truck. Following are lists of supplies and equipment that should be carried in an ambulance. The lists are based on recommendations of the American College of Surgeons, the American College of Emergency Physicians, and various ambulance services. Your region or state may have specific requirements that differ slightly from the list included here. Refer to your state or regional office for specific details.

Patient Infection Control, Comfort, and Protection Supplies

The following supplies should be carried in the ambulance:

- Two pillows
- Four pillow cases
- Two spare sheets
- Four blankets
- Six disposable emesis (vomit) bags or basins
- Two boxes of facial tissues
- Disposable bedpan, urinal, and toilet paper
- One package of drinking cups
- One package of wet wipes
- Four liters of sterile water or saline
- Four soft restraining devices (upper and lower extremities)
- Packages of large and small red biohazard bags for waste or severed parts
- One package of large yellow bags for used linens or garbage (or otherwise color-coded or labeled according to your service's Exposure Control Plan)
- EPA-registered, intermediate-level disinfectant (which destroys mycobacterium tuberculosis)

- EPA-registered, low-level disinfectant such as Lysol
- An empty plastic spray bottle with lines at the 1:100 level, a plastic bottle of water, and a plastic bottle of bleach for cleaning up blood spills (Measure a fresh mixture of 1 part bleach to 100 parts water each day as needed.)
- Eye shields or other protective eyewear for each crew member
- Sharps container for the vehicle (BLS or ALS unit) and (for ALS unit) drug box
- Disposable vinyl or other synthetic gloves: a box of each size
- N-95 or HEPA respirator for each crew member

Initial and Focused Assessment Equipment

Portable first-in kits come in all shapes and sizes, in hard cases or soft bags. A first-in kit should include supplies for:

- *Airway.* Airways, suction, infection control, personal protective equipment; if permitted for EMT use by local protocols, equipment for adult and pediatric orotracheal intubation
- *Breathing.* Stethoscope, pocket mask with one-way valve and oxygen inlet, bag-valve mask, oxygen, oxygen delivery devices
- *Circulation.* Blood pressure cuff, bandages and dressings, occlusive dressings, AED (automated external defibrillator)
- *Neck and spine stabilization.* Set of rigid cervical collars
- *Exposure.* Scissors and blankets to expose and deal with exposure
- *Vital signs:*
    - Sphygmomanometer kit with separate cuffs for average-size and obese adults as well as child sizes
    - Adult and pediatric stethoscopes
    - Pulse oximeter if required by your service
    - Thermometer and a hypothermia thermometer that goes down to at least 82°F
    - One penlight

Many services carry a pocket guide with pediatric vitals and other information.

Equipment for Transfer of Patient

The following carrying devices should be included:

- Wheeled ambulance stretcher designed so that a sick or injured person can be transported in the Fowler's (sitting), supine, or Trendelenburg position. Also called a cot or gurney, the wheeled stretcher should have a number of features. It should be adjustable in height and have detachable supports for intravenous fluid containers. Restraining devices should be provided to prevent a patient from falling off the stretcher or sliding past the foot end or head end.
- Reeves stretcher for carrying a patient who must lie supine down stairs when a cot is too heavy or wide
- Folding stair chair for moving patients down stairs in a sitting position
- Scoop stretcher, also called an orthopedic stretcher, for picking up patients found in tight spaces with a minimum of movement
- Stokes or basket stretcher for long-distance carries, as well as high-angle or off-the-road rescues
- Child safety seat for transporting infants and small children in the ambulance

Equipment for Airway Maintenance, Ventilation, and Resuscitation

A number of devices should be carried for maintaining an open airway and assisting breathing:

- Oropharyngeal airways in sizes suitable for adults, children, and infants
- Soft rubber nasopharyngeal airways in sizes 14 through 30

- Two pocket face masks with one-way valves and filters for times when ventilation is necessary or when you are the only person ventilating a patient who does not have an endotracheal tube inserted
- Three manually operated, self-refilling bag-valve-mask units (infant, child, adult) capable of delivering 100 percent oxygen to a patient by the addition of a reservoir. Masks of various sizes should be designed to ensure a tight face seal and should have an air cushion. The masks should be clear so you can see vomitus and the clouding caused by exhalations.

Oxygen Therapy and Suction Equipment

An ambulance should have two oxygen supply systems (one fixed, one portable) so oxygen can be supplied to two patients at once:

- Fixed oxygen delivery system supplies oxygen to a patient in the ambulance. A typical installation consists of a minimum 3,000-liter reservoir, a two-stage regulator, plus yokes, reducing valve, and non-gravity-type flowmeter. Oxygen delivery tubing, transparent masks, and controls should all be located within easy reach when you are sitting at the patient's head. The system should be capable of delivering at least 15 liters of oxygen per minute and adaptable to the bag-valve-mask units carried on the ambulance.
- Two portable oxygen delivery systems that have a capacity of at least 350 liters. Each system should have a regulator capable of delivering at least 15 liters of oxygen per minute. Many ambulances are equipped with multiple function regulators that can be used for liter-flow oxygen, suctioning, and positive pressure ventilation.

In addition, an ambulance should have the following:

- Spare D, E, or jumbo D oxygen cylinders with a current hydrostat test date seal imprinted on the tank
- Six adult and four pediatric nonrebreather masks
- Six adult and four pediatric nasal cannulas
- One flow-restricted, oxygen-powered ventilation device
- One automatic transport ventilator (ATV) (optional)
- One plastic colorful or comic cup for administering blow-by oxygen to a child

The fixed suction system should be sufficient to provide an air flow of over 30 liters per minute at the end of the delivery tube. A vacuum of at least 300 mmHg should be reached within 4 seconds after the suction tube is clamped. The suction should be controllable. The installed system should have a large-diameter, non-kinking tube fitted with a rigid tip. There should be a spare nonbreakable, disposable suction bottle and a container of water for rinsing the tubing, as well as an assortment of sterile catheters. The suction system should be usable by a person seated at the head of the patient.

The portable suction unit can be one of the many models powered by battery, hand or foot action, oxygen, or compressed air. The unit should be fitted with a nonkinking tube as well as a large-bore Yankauer tip.

Equipment for Assisting with Cardiac Resuscitation

The following equipment for assisting with cardiopulmonary resuscitation and defibrillation should be carried on the ambulance:

- Short or long spine board to provide rigid support during CPR efforts
- An automated external defibrillator (AED)
- A mechanical CPR compressor (e.g., Thumper)—especially helpful for doing CPR for services with transports over 15 minutes to the hospital (optional)

Supplies and Equipment for Immobilization of Suspected Bone Injuries

The ambulance should carry a variety of devices for immobilization of injured extremities and suspected spine injuries:

- Adult and pediatric traction splints (e.g., Sager or Hare) for the immobilization of a painful, swollen, or deformed thigh
- Padded board splints for the immobilization of upper and lower extremities. Recommended are two 3″×54″ splints, two 3″×36″ splints, and two 3″×15″ splints.
- Variety of splints: air-inflatable splints, vacuum splints, cardboard splints, soft rubberized splints with aluminum stays and Velcro fasteners, padded aluminum (SAM) splints, and splints that are inflated with cryogenic (cold) gas
- Tongue depressors to immobilize broken fingers
- Triangular bandages for use with splints and for making slings and swathes
- Several rolls of self-adhering roller bandage for securing the various splints
- Six chemical cold packs for use on injured extremities
- Two long spine boards for full-body immobilization, preferably with speed clips or Velcro straps (The long spine board can also be used for patient transfer.)
- Rigid cervical collars in a variety of adult and child sizes
- One KED, XP1, Kansas Board, or LSP halfback board for seated persons with possible spinal injuries
- Six 9′ by 2″ web straps with aircraft-style buckles or D-rings for securing patients to carrying devices
- Head immobilizer device such as the Headbed, Bashaw CID, Ferno Head Immobilizer, or a rolled blanket

Supplies for Wound Care and Treatment of Shock

A variety of dressings and bandaging materials should be carried on the ambulance:

- Sterile gauze pads (2″×2″ and 4″×4″)
- 5″ × 9″ combine dressings
- Sterile universal dressings (multitrauma dressings) approximately 10″×36″
- Self-adhering roller bandages in 4″ and 6″ width × 5 yards
- Occlusive dressings (Vaseline gauze) for sealing open (sucking) chest wounds and eviscerations
- Aluminum foil (sterilized in a separate package) for various uses such as occlusive dressings and also to maintain body heat or to form an oxygen tent for a newborn infant
- Sterile burn sheets or prepackaged burn kit
- Adhesive strip bandages for minor wound care (3″×3/4″ and 3″×1/2″), individually packaged
- Hypoallergenic adhesive tape (1″ and 3″ rolls)
- Large safety pins for the securing of slings and swathes
- Bandage scissors
- Pneumatic anti-shock garments (PASG) in sizes for adults and children
- Aluminum blankets (survival blankets) for maintaining body heat

Supplies for Childbirth

A sterile childbirth kit, either provided by a local medical facility or a commercially available disposable kit, as mandated by your system, should contain:

- Several pairs of sterile surgical gloves
- Four umbilical cord clamps or umbilical tape
- One pair of sterile surgical scissors
- One rubber bulb syringe (3 oz.)

- Twelve 4″×4″ gauze pads
- Four pairs of sterile disposable gloves
- Five towels
- One baby blanket (receiving blanket)
- Infant swaddler
- Sanitary napkins
- Two large plastic bags
- Two stockinette infant caps

Also carry items that you can wear to minimize contamination of or by the mother and baby during and after childbirth:

- Two surgical gowns
- Two surgical caps
- Two surgical masks
- Two pairs of goggles or eye shields

Supplies, Equipment, and Medications for the Treatment of Acute Poisoning, Snakebite, Chemical Burns, and Diabetic Emergencies

A number of poison control kits are available from emergency care equipment suppliers. Whether purchased intact or handmade, a poison control kit should include these items:

- Drinking water to dilute poisons
- Activated charcoal
- Paper cups and other equipment for oral administration
- Equipment for irrigating a patient's eyes or skin with sterile water
- Constriction bands for snakebites
- Blood glucose meter if required by your service
- Instant glucose paste

Specialized kits for treatment of chemical agents or other specific poisons (e.g., nerve agents, cyanide). Kit availability varies by local protocol.

Special Equipment for Paramedics and Physicians

Depending on state laws and your Medical Director, some ambulances are provided with locked kits of supplies and equipment that can be used by paramedics or physicians, especially in rural areas. This equipment may include supplies for:

- Endotracheal intubation, orotracheal and endotracheal suctioning, and pediatric nasogastric intubation (In some areas EMTs will be trained to perform these procedures.)
- Chest decompression
- Drug administration
- Advanced airways such as the Combitube® airway or the laryngeal mask airway (LMA)
- Cricothyrotomy
- Cardiac monitoring and defibrillation

Safety and Miscellaneous Equipment

Ambulances should also be provided with personal protective equipment for you; equipment for warning, signaling, and lighting; hazard control devices; and tools for gaining access and disentanglements including:

- The most current edition of the *Emergency Response Guidebook*
- Binoculars
- Clipboard, prehospital care reports (PCRs), and other documentation forms
- Ring cutter

- Portable radio
- Multiple-casualty incident management logs
- Triage tags and destination logs
- Command vests
- Tarps in red, green, black, and yellow for multiple-casualty incident field treatment areas
- Disposable Tyvek jumpsuits
- Flares
- Jumper cables
- Set of turnout gear (coat, helmet, protective eyewear, gloves) for each crew member
- Large floodlight/spotlight
- Concentrated sports drink (e.g., Gatorade) and a cooler for rehabilitation sector (optional)
- Self-contained breathing apparatus (SCBA) (optional)
- Spring-loaded center punch
- Glas-Master or flathead ax
- Small sledgehammer, prybar, Biel tool, and other tools for gaining access
- Wheel chocks
- Utility rope
- Stuffed animal for child patients

Compare the items listed in this chapter with the inventory of your ambulance. Learn where each item is stored, what every item is for, and when it should be used. If the item is a mechanical device, also learn how it works and how it should be maintained.

Ensuring Ambulance Readiness for Service

The most modern, well-equipped ambulance is not worth the room it takes up in the garage unless it is ready to respond at the time of an emergency. A planned preventive maintenance program includes periodic servicing. Oil should be changed regularly, tires rotated, the vehicle lubricated, and so on.

Let us say that you and your partner have just reported for duty. As soon as it is practical, speak with the crew going off duty. Learn whether they experienced any problems with either the ambulance or its equipment during their shift. Make a thorough bumper-to-bumper inspection of the ambulance (Scan 34-1), using the checklist provided by your service.

Ambulance Inspection, Engine Off

Following are inspection steps that can be taken while the ambulance is in quarters:

1. Inspect the body of the vehicle. Look for damage that could interfere with its safe operation. A crumpled fender, for example, may prevent the front wheels from turning the maximum distance.
2. Inspect the wheels and tires. The tires take a beating in normal operation. At collision scenes they may contact shards of glass and sharp pieces of metal and other debris. Check for damage or worn wheel rims and tire sidewalls. Check the tread depth. Use a pressure gauge to ensure that all tires are properly inflated. Do not forget to inspect the inside rear tires.
3. Inspect windows and mirrors. Look for broken glass and loose or missing parts. See that mirrors are clean and properly adjusted for maximum visibility.
4. Check the operation of every door and latches and locks.
5. Inspect the components of the cooling system. Check the level of the coolant. Inspect the cooling system hoses for leaks and cracks.
6. Check the level of the other vehicle fluids, including the engine oil and the brake, power, and steering fluids.

NOTE *Allow the engine to cool before removing any pressure caps.*

SCAN 34-1 • Inspecting the Ambulance

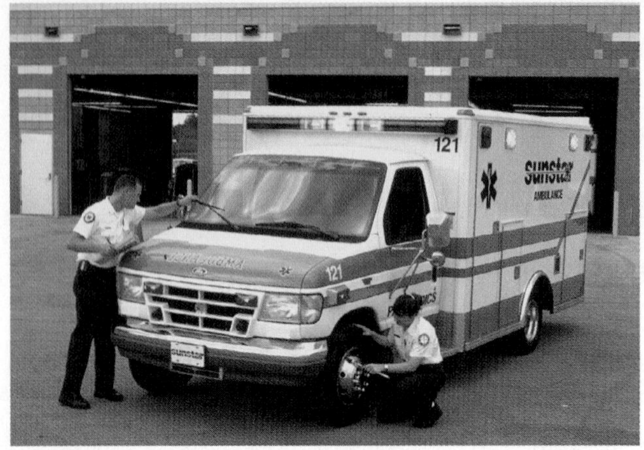

1. Check the ambulance body, wheels, tires, and windshield wipers.

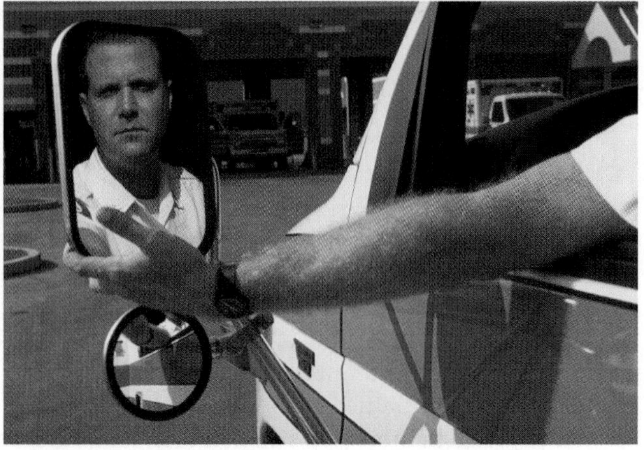

2. Check windows, doors, and mirrors.

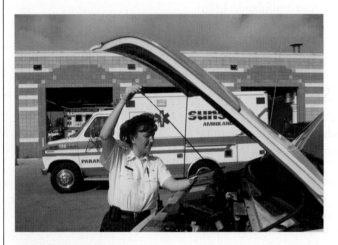

3. Check under the hood.

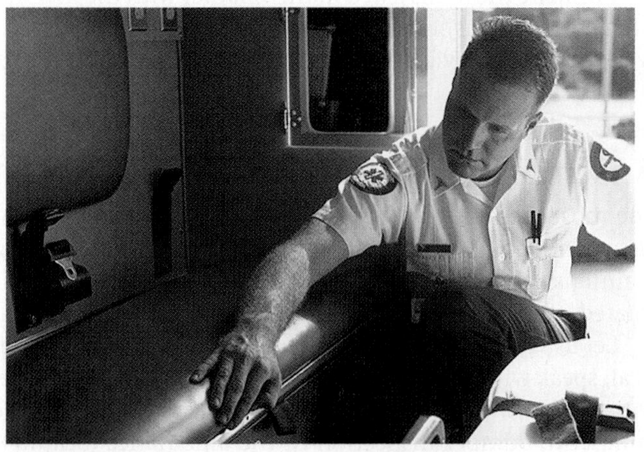

4. Check interior surfaces and upholstery.

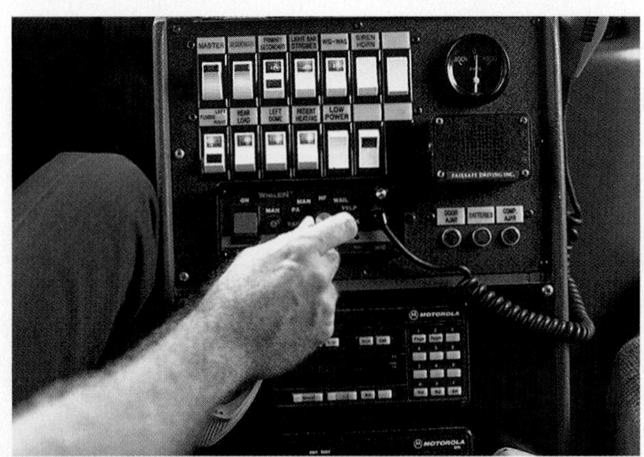

5. Check dash instruments and communications equipment.

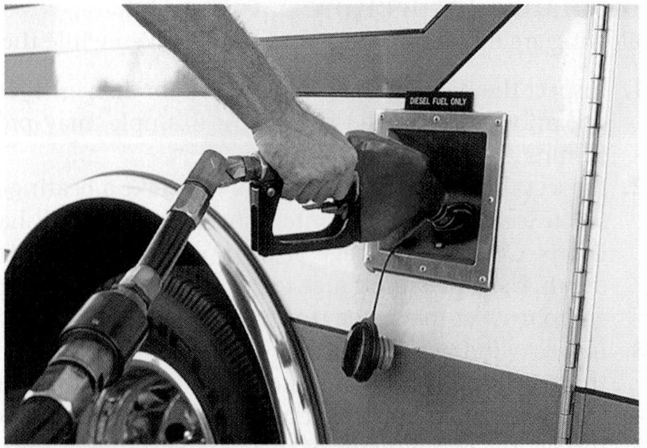

6. Check the fuel level and fill up.

7. Check the battery. If the battery has removable fill caps, check the level of the fluid. If the battery is the sealed type, determine its condition by checking the indicator port. Inspect the battery cable connections for tightness and signs of corrosion.
8. Inspect the interior surfaces and upholstery for damage and cleanliness.
9. Check the windows for operation. See that the interior surface of each window is clean.
10. Test the horn.
11. Test the siren for full range of operation.
12. Check the seat belts. Examine each belt to see that it is not damaged. Pull each belt from its storage spool to ensure that the retractor mechanisms work. Buckle each belt to ensure that latches work properly.
13. Adjust the driver's seat for comfort and optimum steering wheel and pedal operation.
14. Check the fuel level. Refuel after each call whenever practical.

Ambulance Inspection, Engine On

The next steps require you to start the engine. Pull the ambulance from quarters if engine exhaust fumes will be a problem. Set the parking brake, put the transmission in "park," and have your partner chock the wheels before undertaking the following steps:

1. Check the dash-mounted indicators to see if any light remains on to indicate a possible problem with oil pressure, engine temperature, or the vehicle's electrical system.
2. Check dash-mounted gauges for proper operation.
3. Depress the brake pedal. Note whether pedal travel seems correct or excessive. Check air pressure as needed.
4. Test the parking brake. Move the transmission level to a drive position. Replace the level to the "park" position as soon as you are sure that the parking brake is holding.
5. Turn the steering wheel from side to side.
6. Check the operation of the windshield wipers and washers. The glass should be wiped clean each time the blade moves.
7. Turn on the vehicle's warning lights. Have your partner walk around the ambulance and check each flashing and revolving light for operation. Turn off the warning lights.
8. Turn on the other vehicle lights. Have your partner walk around the ambulance again, this time checking the headlights (high and low beams), turn signals, four-way flashers, brake lights, side and rear scene illumination lights, and box marker lights.
9. Check the operation of the heating and air-conditioning equipment in both the driver's compartment and the patient compartment. This is also a good time to check the on-board suction if the engine is running.
10. Check transmission fluid.
11. Operate the communications equipment. Test portable as well as fixed radios and any radio-telephone communications.

Return the ambulance to quarters. While you are backing up, have your partner note whether the backup alarm is operating (if the vehicle is so equipped).

Inspection of Patient Compartment Supplies and Equipment

Shut off the engine and complete your inspection by checking the patient compartment and all exterior cabinets:

1. Check the interior of the patient compartment. Look for damage to the interior surfaces and upholstery. Be certain that any needed decontamination has been completed and that the compartment is clean.
2. Check treatment supplies and equipment and rescue equipment. Items should not only be identified, they should also be checked for completeness, condition, and

operation. Check the pressure of oxygen cylinders. Inflate air splints and examine them for leaks. Test oxygen and ventilation equipment for proper operation. Examine rescue tools for rust and dirt. Operate battery-powered devices to ensure that the batteries have a proper charge. Some equipment, such as the AED, may require additional testing. See that an item-by-item inspection of everything carried on the ambulance is done, with findings recorded on the inspection report.

3. When you are finished, complete the inspection report. Correct any deficiencies. Replace missing items. Make your supervisor aware of any deficiencies that cannot be immediately corrected.
4. Finally, clean the unit for infection control and appearance. Maintaining the ambulance's appearance enhances your organization's image in the public's eye. People who take pride in their work show it by taking pride in the appearance of their ambulance.

RECEIVING AND RESPONDING TO A CALL

In many areas of the country, a person needs only to dial 911 to access ambulance, fire, or police services 24 hours a day. A trained Emergency Medical Dispatcher (EMD) records information from callers, decides which service is needed, and alerts that service to respond. (Always say "nine-one-one" when talking to community or school groups. Children cannot find "eleven" on the phone dial or key pad.)

Role of the Emergency Medical Dispatcher

Many cities and communication centers train and certify Emergency Medical Dispatchers (EMDs) based on the medical priority card system, originated in 1979 through the leadership of Jeffrey Clawson, MD. An EMD is trained to perform the following tasks:

- Interrogate the caller and assign a priority to the call
- Provide prearrival medical instructions to callers and information to crews
- Dispatch and coordinate EMS resources
- Coordinate with other public safety agencies

When answering a call for help, the EMD must obtain as much information as possible about the situation that may help the responding crew. The questions the EMD should ask are:

1. *What is the exact location of the patient?* The EMD must ask for the house or building number and the apartment number, if any. It is important to ask the street name with the direction designator (e.g., North, East), the nearest cross street, the name of the development or subdivision, and the exact location of the emergency.
2. *What is your call-back number?* (Enhanced 911 will show the number.) "Stay on the line. Do not hang up until I (the EMD) tell you to." In life-threatening situations, the EMD will offer instruction to the caller, after the units have been dispatched, that the caller or others on the scene should follow until the units arrive. It is also important for the caller to stay on the line in case a question arises about the location that was given.
3. *What's the problem?* This will provide the chief complaint. It will help the EMD decide which line of questioning to follow and the priority of the response to send.
4. *How old is the patient?* Most ambulances are set up to respond to the scene with a pediatric kit if the patient is a child rather than an adult. If prearrival CPR instructions are given, it will be necessary to distinguish between an infant, a child, and an adult.
5. *What's the patient's sex?* (if not obvious from caller's voice or information)
6. *Is the patient conscious?* An unconscious patient is a higher response priority.
7. *Is the patient breathing?* If the patient is conscious and breathing, the EMD will often ask many additional questions relative to the chief complaint to determine the

appropriate level of response; for example, First Responders, EMT-Paramedics, or ambulance responding COLD (at normal speed—sometimes called Priority 3) or HOT (an emergency, lights-and-siren mode—sometimes called Priority 1). If the patient is not breathing, or the caller is not sure, the EMD will dispatch the maximum response and begin the appropriate prearrival instructions for a nonbreathing patient, which may also involve telephone CPR if the patient is pulseless.

If the call is for a traffic collision, a series of key questions must be asked to help determine the priority and amount of response. With good interrogation of the caller, it may be possible for the EMD to appropriately dispatch one unit HOT and backup units COLD, which in turn will help prevent emergency vehicle collisions.

1. *How many and what kinds of vehicles are involved?* The EMD should determine, if possible, how many vehicles are involved in the collision and if they are cars, trucks, or buses. Any injury resulting from a collision involving a bicycle, motorcycle, or pedestrian versus an automobile should receive the highest priority of response because of the mechanisms of injury involved. If the EMD learns that a truck is involved, he will try to determine if it is a vehicle that may be carrying a hazardous load.
2. *How many persons do you think are injured?* When the EMD learns from the caller that five people have been injured, he may send two or three ambulances at the same time. Time, and perhaps lives, may be saved by knowing the precise number of people injured in a collision.
3. *Do the victims appear trapped?* It may be necessary to dispatch a rescue unit also.
4. *What is the exact location of the collision?* You should be able to learn a street address or the name of the nearest cross street. If the collision has occurred in a rural or wilderness area, the EMD must try to pinpoint the location by asking questions about the nearest landmark visible from the caller's point of view (e.g., mile posts, water towers, large silos, or radio antennas). If the caller cannot pinpoint his location, the telephone company should be able to provide the location of the phone.

Next, the EMD should attempt to learn something about the scene. If the EMD learns that all lanes of a road leading to the collision scene are blocked, for example, operators can select alternative response routes.

1. Is traffic moving?
2. How many lanes are open?
3. How far is traffic backed up?
4. Are any of the vehicles on fire?
5. Are any of the vehicles leaking fuel?
6. Are any electrical wires down?
7. Do any of the vehicles appear unstable? Is any vehicle on its side or top?
8. Does a truck appear to be carrying a hazardous cargo?

This is how an EMD might dispatch an ambulance to the location of a sick person:

> MEDCOM to Ambulance 641 and Medic 640, respond priority one to a 60-year-old unconscious female with breathing difficulty. The location is the Boston Market on Route 9 with Kunker Road on the cross. Time now is 1745 hours.

The EMD will repeat the message to minimize any question as to its content and ensure the ambulance has received the call.

Operating the Ambulance

If you will be driving an ambulance even occasionally, you may be mandated to attend emergency vehicle operator training, which has both classroom and in-vehicle road sessions.

Being a Safe Ambulance Operator

To be a safe ambulance operator, you must:

- Be physically fit. You should not have any impairment that prevents you from operating the ambulance or any medical condition that might disable you while driving.
- Be mentally fit, with your emotions under control. The judgment of someone operating an ambulance should not be compromised by the excitement of lights and sirens.
- Be able to perform under stress.
- Have a positive attitude about your ability as a driver but not be an overly confident risk taker.
- Be tolerant of other drivers. Always keep in mind that people react differently when they see an emergency vehicle. Accept and tolerate the bad habits of other drivers without flying into a rage.

Some additional safety tips include:

- Never drive while under the influence of alcohol, illicit or "recreational" drugs such as marijuana or cocaine, medicines such as antihistamines, "pep pills," or tranquilizers.
- Never drive with a restricted license.
- Always wear your glasses or contact lenses if required for driving.
- Evaluate your ability to drive based on personal stress, illness, fatigue, or sleepiness.

Understanding the Law

Every state has statutes that regulate the operation of emergency vehicles. Emergency vehicle operators are generally granted certain exemptions with regard to speed, parking, passage through traffic signals, and direction of travel. However, the laws also state that if an emergency vehicle operator does not drive with due regard for the safety of others, he must be prepared to pay the consequences, such as tickets, lawsuits, or even time in jail.

Following are some points typically included in laws regulating ambulance operation:

- An ambulance operator must have a valid driver's license and may be required to complete a training program.
- Privileges granted under the law to the operators of ambulances apply when the vehicle is responding to an emergency or is involved in the emergency transport of a sick or injured person. When the ambulance is not on an emergency call, the laws that apply to the operation of nonemergency vehicles also apply to the ambulance.
- Even though certain privileges are granted during an emergency, the exemptions granted do not provide immunity to the operator in cases of reckless driving or disregard for the safety of others.
- Privileges granted during emergency situations apply only if the operator uses warning devices in the manner prescribed by law.

Most statutes allow emergency vehicle operators to:

- Park the vehicle anywhere if it does not damage personal property or endanger lives.
- Proceed past red stop signals, flashing red stop signals, and stop signs. Some states require that emergency vehicle operators come to a full stop, then proceed with caution. Other states require only that an operator slow down and proceed with caution.
- Exceed the posted speed limit as long as life and property are not endangered.
- Pass other vehicles in no-passing zones after properly signaling, ensuring that the way is clear, and taking precautions to avoid endangering life and prop-

erty. This does not include passing a school bus with its red lights blinking. Wait for the bus driver to clear the children and then turn off the red lights of the bus.

- With proper caution and signals, disregard regulations that govern direction of travel and turning in specific directions.

Should you ever become involved in an ambulance collision, the laws will be interpreted by the court based upon two key issues. (1) Did you use due regard for the safety of others? and (2) Was it a true emergency? The requirement of due regard actually sets a higher standard for drivers of emergency vehicles than for other drivers. This is why an investigation by the district attorney or grand jury, as well as your ambulance service, is not uncommon following a collision.

Most states reserve the emergency mode of operation for a true emergency, defined as one in which the best information available to you is that loss of life or limb is possible. When dispatched to a call, there is often not much information to go on, so a "collision" will get an emergency response. However, once you arrive and find that your patient is stable with no life-threatening injuries or conditions, it is no longer a true emergency. A lights-and-siren, high-speed response to the hospital in such a situation would be improper.

The exemptions described here are just examples of those often granted to ambulance operators. Do not assume that they are granted in your state. Obtain a copy of your state's rules and regulations and study them carefully.

Using the Warning Devices

Safe emergency vehicle operation can be achieved only when proper use of warning devices is coupled with sound emergency and defensive driving practices. Studies show that other drivers do not see or hear an ambulance until it is within 50 to 100 feet, so never let the lights and siren give you a false sense of security.

THE SIREN Although the siren is the most commonly used audible warning device, it is also the most misused. Consider the effects that sirens have on other motorists, patients in ambulances, and ambulance operators themselves:

- Continuous sound of a siren may cause a sick or injured person to suffer increased fear and anxiety, and his condition may worsen as stress builds up.
- Ambulance operators themselves are affected by the continuous sound of a siren. Tests have shown that inexperienced ambulance operators tend to increase their driving speeds from 10 to 15 miles per hour while continually sounding the siren. In some cases, operators using a siren were unable to negotiate curves that they could pass through easily when not sounding the siren. Sirens also affect hearing, especially if used for long periods with the siren speaker over the cab. The best placement for the speaker is in the vehicle grill.

Many states have laws that regulate the use of audible warning signals. Where there are no statutes, ambulance organizations usually create their own policies. If your organization does not, you may find the following suggestions helpful:

- Use the siren sparingly, and only when you must. Some states require use of the siren at all times when the ambulance is responding in the emergency mode. Others require it only when the operator is exercising any of the exemptions discussed earlier.
- Never assume that all motorists will hear your signal. Buildings, trees, and dense shrubbery may block siren sounds. Soundproofing keeps outside noises from entering vehicles, and radios or CD players also decrease the likelihood that an outside sound will be heard.
- Always assume that some motorists will hear your siren but ignore it.
- Be prepared for the erratic maneuvers of other drivers. Some drivers panic when they hear a siren.

- Do not pull up close to a vehicle and then sound your siren. This may cause the driver to jam on his brakes and you may be unable to stop in time. Use the horn when you are close to a vehicle ahead.
- Never use the siren indiscriminately, and never use it to scare someone.

THE HORN The horn is standard equipment on all ambulances. Experienced operators find that the judicious use of the horn often clears traffic as quickly as the siren. The guidelines for using a siren apply to the horn as well.

VISUAL WARNING DEVICES Whenever the ambulance is on the road, night or day, the headlights should be on. This increases the visibility of the vehicle to other drivers. In some states headlights are now required of all vehicles in low visibility conditions or whenever the windshield wipers are in use. Alternating flashing headlights should be used only if they are attached to secondary head lamps. In most states it is illegal to drive at night with one headlight out.

The large lights on the outermost corners of the box should blink in tandem, or unison, rather than wigwagging or alternating. This helps the vehicle that is approaching from a distance identify the full size of your vehicle. There are several types of lights on ambulances, including rotating lights, flashing lights, strobe lights, and the newer LED (light-emitting diode) lights. When planning the lighting package of an ambulance, check the research before making your decision. In general, it is wisest for the package to combine different types of lights in strategic places rather than just one type of lighting system.

Four-way flashers and directional signals should not be used as emergency lights. This is very confusing to the public, as well as being illegal in some states. Drivers expect a vehicle with four-way flashers on to be traveling at a very slow speed. Additionally, the flashers disrupt the function of the directional signals.

When the ambulance is in the emergency response mode, either en route to the scene or to the hospital with a high-priority patient, all the emergency lights should be used. The vehicle should be easily seen from 360 degrees.

In some communities, ambulances still follow an old tradition of using their emergency lights when returning to the station. However, this practice is very confusing to the public. Do not be surprised if other drivers do not pull over when you are on an emergency run if they constantly see your ambulance with emergency lights on. SAVE THE USE OF LIGHTS AND SIREN FOR LIFE- OR LIMB-THREATENING EMERGENCIES.

Speed and Safety

You are often told to drive slowly and carefully. At this point you may be inclined to say something like, "How will I ever get a seriously ill or injured person to a hospital if I poke along?" We are not suggesting that you "poke along." But do drive with these facts in mind:

- Excessive speed increases the probability of a collision.
- Speed increases stopping distance, reducing the chance of avoiding a hazardous situation.

Remember that the laws in most states excuse you from obeying certain traffic laws only in a true emergency and only with due regard for the safety of others. Except in these circumstances, obey speed limits, stoplights and signs, yield signs, and other laws and posted limits. Approach intersections with caution, avoid sudden turns, and always properly signal lane changes and turns. Be sure that the ambulance driver and all passengers wear seat belts whenever the ambulance is in motion.

Escorted or Multiple-Vehicle Responses

When the police provide an escort for an ambulance, there are additional hazards. Too often, the inexperienced ambulance operator follows the escort vehicle too closely and is unable to stop when the lead vehicle(s) make an emergency stop. Also, the inexperienced operator may assume that other drivers know his vehicle is following the escort. In fact, other drivers will often pull out in front of the ambulance just after the escort vehicle passes.

Because of the dangers involved with escorts, most EMS systems recommend no escorts unless the operator is not familiar with the location of the patient (or hospital) and must be given assistance from the police.

In multiple-vehicle responses, the dangers can be the same as those generated by escorted responses, especially when the responding vehicles travel in the same direction, close together. A great danger also exists when two vehicles approach the same intersection at the same time. Not only may they fail to yield for each other; other drivers may yield for the first vehicle but not the second. Obviously, great care must be used at intersections during multiple-vehicle responses.

Factors That Affect Response

Most ambulance collisions take place in seemingly safe conditions. In New York State, 18 years of ambulance-collision statistics show that the typical collision happens on a dry road (60 percent) with clear weather (55 percent) during daylight hours (67 percent) in an intersection (72 percent). During this period, there were 5,782 ambulance collisions, which involved 7,267 injuries and 48 fatalities! Additionally, an ambulance response can be affected by several factors:

- *Day of the week.* Weekdays usually have the heaviest traffic because people are commuting to and from work. In resort areas, weekend traffic may be heavier.
- *Time of day.* In major employment centers, traffic over major roads tends to be heavy in all directions during commuter hours.
- *Weather.* Adverse weather conditions reduce driving speeds and thus increase response times. A heavy snowfall can temporarily prevent any response at all. Be careful to lengthen your following distance whenever there is decreased road grip due to inclement weather.
- *Road maintenance and construction.* Traffic can be seriously impeded by road construction and maintenance activities. Be aware of area road construction and plan responses accordingly.
- *Railroads.* There are still more than a quarter-million grade crossings in the United States with traffic often blocked by long, slow freight trains. Some communities need a secondary response system on the other side of train tracks that split the town in half.
- *Bridges and tunnels.* Traffic over bridges and through tunnels slows during rush hours. Collisions—including ambulance collisions—tend to occur when drivers forget that bridges freeze before roadways.

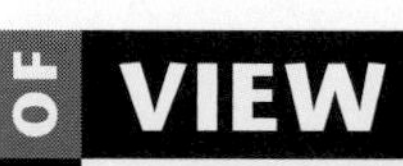

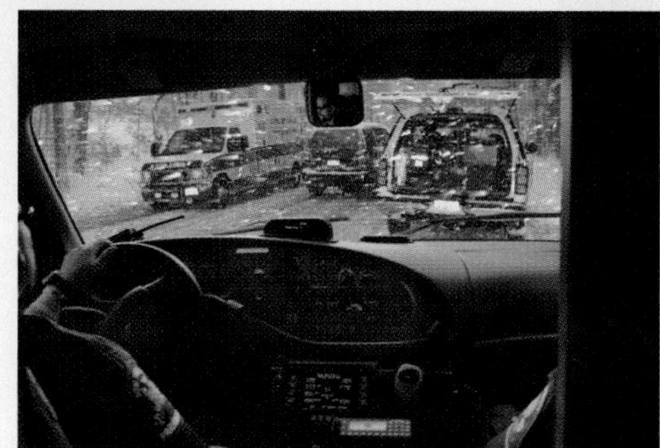
© Craig Jackson/In the Dark Photography

"I never realized when I started doing EMS that I'd have to drive in the same stuff that is causing all the crashes.

"We were called for a three-car collision on highway 17, a road on the outskirts of the city. With the snow that was building up it took us a good 15 white-knuckled minutes to get out there. We drove carefully, and most of the time at less than half the speed we would have used to get there on a clear day. People were sliding all over the road. We just had to tell ourselves we wouldn't do any good if we didn't get there.

"When we did get to the scene we had to be very careful parking so someone didn't hit us. A trooper and a fire engine were parked between our back door and the traffic. We were only at the scene for about 5 minutes when a car spun out of control and almost hit the trooper's car. Crazy.

"You don't have snow days in EMS like you had in school. That's for sure! C'mon spring."

- *Schools and school buses.* The reduced speed limits in force during school hours slow the flow of vehicles. An emergency vehicle should never pass a stopped school bus with its red lights flashing. Wait for the school bus driver to signal you to proceed by turning off the lights. In addition, emergency vehicles attract children, who often venture out into the street to see them. The operator of every emergency vehicle should slow down when approaching a school or playground. Obey the directions given by school crossing guards.

Selecting an Alternative Route

When it appears that an ambulance will be delayed in reaching a sick or injured person, the operator should consider taking an alternative route or requesting the response of another ambulance. Plan for times when changing conditions affect response. Obtain detailed maps of your service area. On the maps, indicate usually troublesome traffic spots such as schools, bridges, tunnels, railroad grade crossings, and heavily congested areas. Also indicate temporary problems such as road and building construction sites and long- and short-term detours. Using another color, indicate alternative routes, snow routes, and so on.

Hang one map in quarters and place another in the ambulance. Then when you encounter a problem area, you will be able to select an alternative route that will get you to your destination quickly and safely.

Positioning the Ambulance at the Scene of a Vehicle Collision

When responding to the scene of a vehicle collision, be sure to take all steps to size-up the scene—assessing scene safety and establishing a danger zone. Park at least 100 feet from the wreckage, upwind, and uphill (if possible) to avoid fire or any escaping hazardous liquids or fumes. If there is no fire or escaping liquids or fumes, park at least 50 feet from the wreckage.

Park in front of the wreckage if you are the first emergency vehicle on the scene so your warning lights can warn approaching motorists before flares and other signals can be placed. Remember that this will expose the back of your ambulance to traffic when you are taking out the stretcher and when you are loading the patient. If the scene has already been secured, park beyond the wreckage to prevent having your expensive ambulance struck by oncoming traffic. In either situation, use added caution on controlled-access (e.g., interstate) highways with high speed limits, where stopping distance is greatly increased. Keep in mind that on hills or around curves, drivers may not be able to see your ambulance in time to stop (Scan 34-2).

When backing up an ambulance, be aware that there are large blind spots in your mirrors and a danger of striking a pedestrian, object, or other vehicle. When possible, position someone at the rear of the ambulance to act as a spotter and guide the backing process (Figure 34-2).

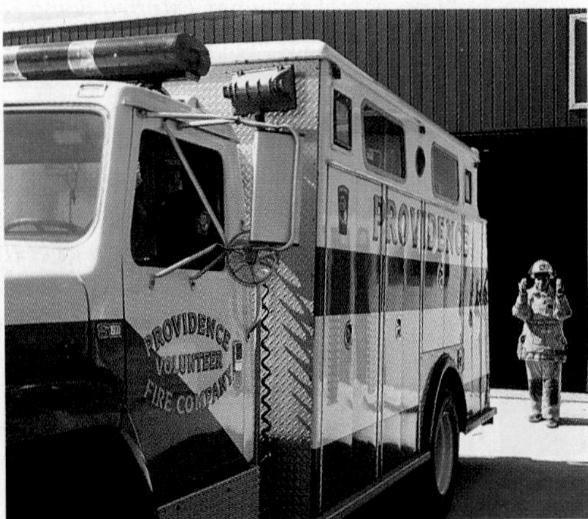

Figure 34-2 • Use a spotter to help guide the ambulance when backing up.

SCAN 34-2 • Parking the Ambulance

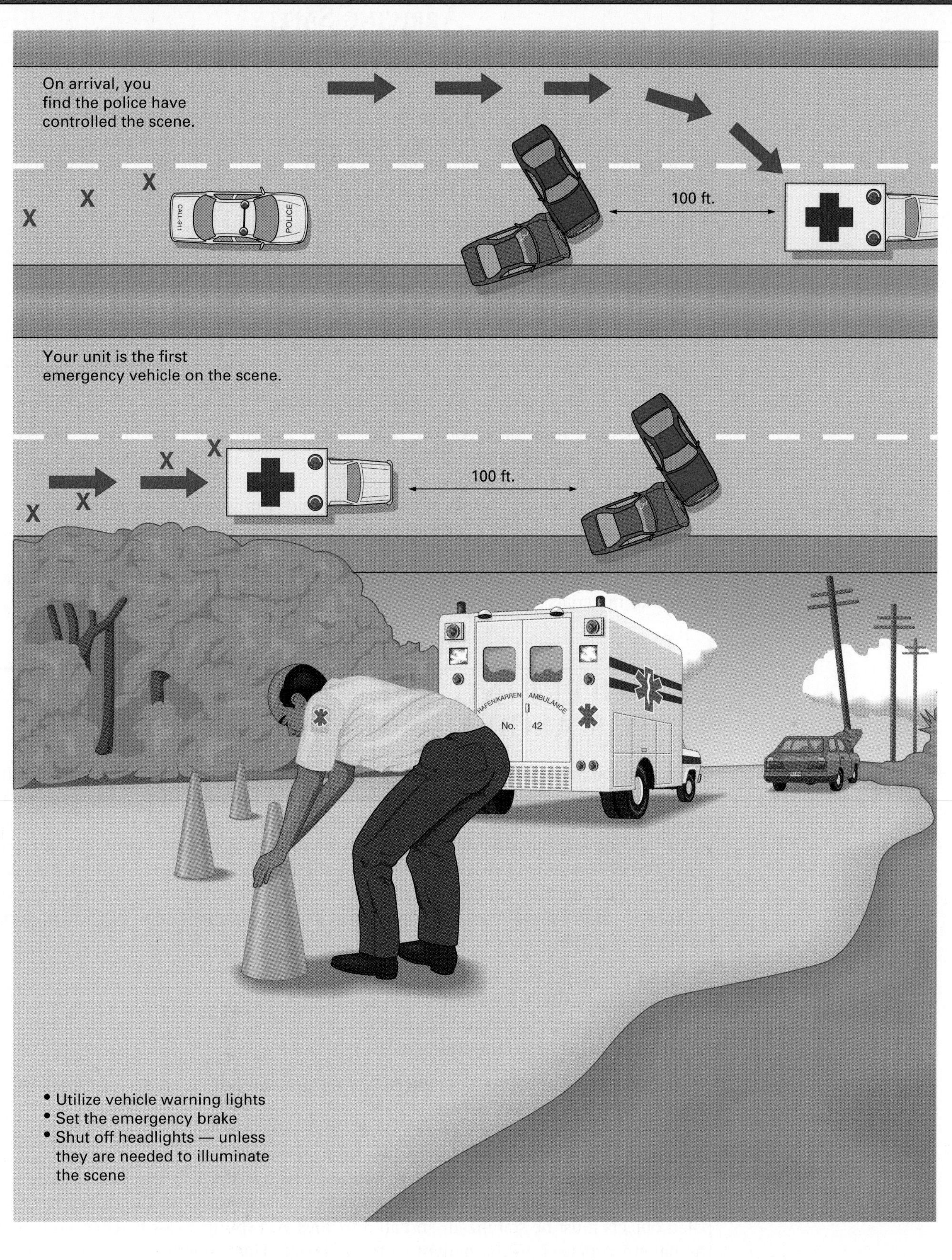

On arrival, you find the police have controlled the scene.
100 ft.
POLICE
Your unit is the first emergency vehicle on the scene.
100 ft.
HAFEN/KARREN AMBULANCE
No. 42
• Utilize vehicle warning lights
• Set the emergency brake
• Shut off headlights — unless they are needed to illuminate the scene

CRITICAL DECISION MAKING: ARRIVING SAFELY

While most of this text has discussed treating the patient at the scene, your response and vehicle placement is an important part of your responsibilities at a call. Proper vehicle placement ensures your safety and that of the vehicle, and its contents are available to you in a convenient location. For each of the following situations, explain where you would park the ambulance if you were first arriving.

1. You are called to a railroad car derailment.
2. You are called to a collision on the interstate. An engine company and trooper are parked at the scene, blocking oncoming traffic.
3. You are called to a scene involving domestic violence. Police are not yet on the scene.

Studies show that red revolving beacons attract drunk or tired drivers. Consider pulling off the road, turning off your headlights, and using just amber rear sealed beam blinkers that blink in tandem or unison to identify the size of your vehicle. Once the ambulance is parked, set its parking brake and firmly wedge wheel chocks under the tires in such a way that forward movement will be retarded if the ambulance is struck.

Be sure to perform a scene size-up and take all necessary Standard Precautions and hazardous materials precautions.

TRANSFERRING THE PATIENT TO THE AMBULANCE

On most ambulance runs you will be able to reach a sick or injured person without difficulty, assess his condition, carry out emergency care procedures where he lies, and then transfer him to the ambulance. At times, dangers at the scene or the priority of the patient will dictate moving the patient before assessment and emergency treatments can be completed. When a spinal injury is suspected, the patient's head must be manually stabilized, a cervical collar must be applied, and the patient must be immobilized on a spine board.

Transfer to the ambulance is accomplished in four steps, regardless of the complexity of the operation:

1. Select the proper patient-carrying device.
2. Package the patient for transfer.
3. Move the patient to the ambulance.
4. Load the patient into the ambulance.

The wheeled ambulance stretcher is the most commonly used device for transferring the patient to the ambulance.

The term *packaging* refers to the sequence of operations required to ready the patient to be moved and to combine the patient and the patient-carrying device into a unit ready for transfer. A sick or injured patient must be packaged so that his condition is not aggravated. Necessary care for wounds and other injuries should be completed, impaled objects must be stabilized, and all dressings and splints must be checked before the patient is placed on the patient-carrying device. The properly packaged patient is covered and secured to the patient-carrying device.

When packaging the severely ill or injured patient, packaging is a balance between expedience and function. The patient should be firmly secured to transport devices and backboards so he will not fall or worsen his current condition in any way. Yet the EMT recognizes that packaging must be done quickly and efficiently in order to get the patient to the hospital promptly as well as safely.

Covering a patient helps to maintain body temperature, prevents exposure to the elements, and helps ensure privacy (Figure 34-3). A single blanket or perhaps just a sheet may be all that is required in warm weather. A sheet and blankets should be used in cold weather. When practical, cuff the blankets under the patient's chin, with the top sheet outside. Do not leave sheets and blankets hanging loose. Tuck them under the mattress at the foot and sides of the stretcher. In wet weather, a plastic cover should be placed over the blankets during transfer. Remove it once you are in the ambulance to prevent overheating. In cold or wet weather cover the patient's head, leaving the face exposed.

A patient-carrying device should have a minimum of three straps for holding the patient securely. The first should be at the chest level, the second at hip or waist level, and the third on the lower extremities. Sometimes there is a fourth strap if two are crossed at the chest.

Newer stretchers have straps that act as a harness and restrain the upper body (Figure 34-4). By combining over-the-shoulder straps with encircling straps, the patient is more securely held on the stretcher in the event of a collision.

All patients, including those receiving CPR, must be secured to the patient-carrying device before transfer to the ambulance. If your patient is not on a carrying device such as a spine board but is just on the ambulance stretcher, some states, as a matter of policy, require shoulder harnesses that secure the patient to the stretcher to prevent him from sliding forward in case of a short stop.

While much has been said about protecting the patient from a possible ambulance collision, perhaps not enough has been said about protecting the EMT in the patient compartment, who is actually at greater risk. The patient is secured to the stretcher and obtains some safety benefit from that. Most of the time, the EMT is unsecured and vulnerable in the event of a collision. Remain seated, wearing a seat belt or harness when possible. While it isn't always possible to remain seated, avoid unnecessary movement during emergency response and transport.

Unsecured equipment turns into projectiles upon collision, threatening both patient and EMT. Always ensure that all equipment in the patient compartment (e.g., oxygen cylinders, kits) has been secured.

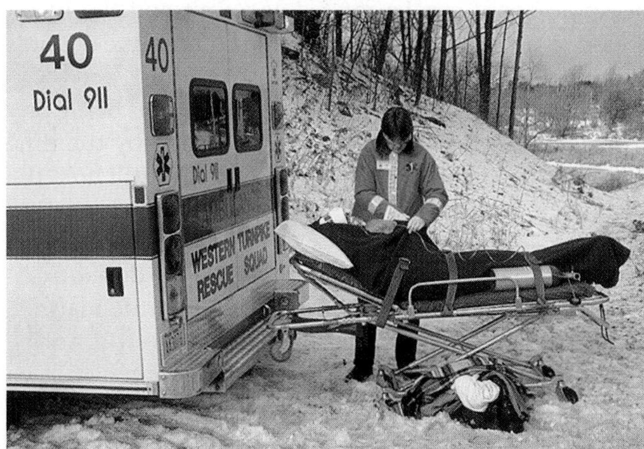

Figure 34-3 • A patient packaged for cold, wet conditions.

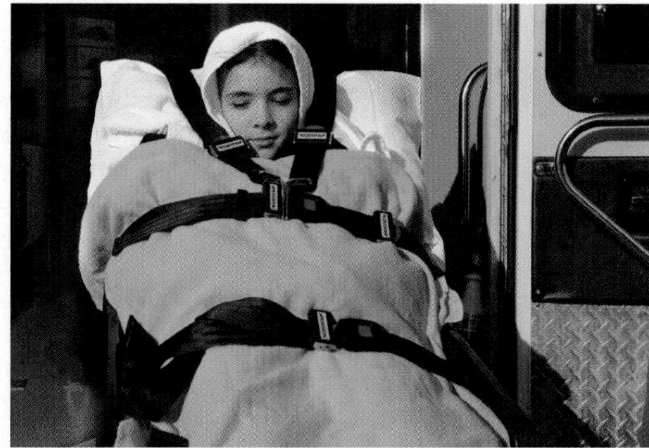

Figure 34-4 • Stretcher straps that act as a harness restrain the patient's upper body.

TRANSPORTING THE PATIENT TO THE HOSPITAL

Transport involves more than just driving to the hospital. A series of tasks must be undertaken from the time a patient is loaded into the ambulance until he is handed over to hospital personnel.

Preparing the Patient for Transport

The following activities may be required to prepare the patient for transport once he is in the ambulance:

- *Perform ongoing assessment.* Make sure that a conscious patient is breathing without difficulty once you have positioned him on the stretcher. If the patient is unconscious with an airway in place, make sure he has an adequate air exchange once you have moved him into position for transport.
- *Secure the stretcher in place in the ambulance.* Always ensure that the patient is safe during the trip to the hospital. Before closing the door, and certainly before signaling the ambulance operator to move, make sure that the cot is securely in place. Patient compartments are equipped with a locking device that prevents the wheeled stretcher from moving about while the ambulance is in motion. Failure to fully engage the locking device at both ends of the stretcher can have disastrous consequences once the ambulance is in motion.
- *Position and secure the patient.* During transfer to the ambulance, the patient must be firmly secured to a stretcher. This does not mean that he must be transported in that position. Positioning in the ambulance should be dictated by the nature of his illness or injury.
    - If he was not transferred to the ambulance in that position, shift an unconscious patient who has no potential spine injury, or one with an altered mental status, into the recovery position (on his side) that will promote maintenance of an open airway and the drainage of fluids.
    - Remember that the head and foot ends of the ambulance stretcher can be raised. A patient with breathing difficulty and no possibility of spinal injury may be more comfortable being transported in a sitting position. A patient in shock can be transported with the legs raised 8 to 12 inches.
    - A patient with potential spinal injury must remain immobilized on the long spine board, patient and board together being secured to the stretcher. If resuscitation is required, he must remain supine with constant monitoring of the airway and suctioning equipment ready. If resuscitation is not required, the unresponsive patient and spine board can be rotated as a unit and the board propped on the stretcher so that the patient is on his side for drainage of fluids and vomitus from the mouth.
    - Adjust the security straps. Security straps applied when a patient is being prepared for transfer to the ambulance may tighten unnecessarily by the time he is loaded into the patient compartment. Adjust straps so they still hold the patient safely in place but are not so tight that they interfere with circulation or respiration or cause pain.
- *Prepare for respiratory or cardiac complications.* If the patient is likely to develop cardiac arrest, position a short spine board or CPR board underneath the mattress prior to starting on the trip. Then, if he does go into arrest, time will not be wasted locating and positioning the board. Riding on a hard board may not be comfortable, but temporary discomfort is better than permanent injury or even death from delayed resuscitation.
- *Loosen constricting clothing.* Clothing may interfere with circulation and breathing. Loosen ties and belts and open any clothing around the neck. Straighten clothing that is bunched under safety straps. Remember that clothing bunched

at the crotch may be painful. Before you do anything to rearrange the patient's clothing, however, explain what you are going to do and why.

- *Check bandages.* Even properly applied bandages can loosen during transfer to the ambulance. Check each bandage to see that it is secure. Do not take a loosened bandage lightly. Severe bleeding can resume when pressure from a bandage is removed. If the wound site is covered with a sheet or blanket, bleeding may go unnoticed until the patient develops shock or is delivered to the hospital.
- *Check splints.* Immobilizing devices can also loosen during transfer to the ambulance. Inspect the bandages or cravats that hold board splints in place. Inspect traction devices to ensure that proper traction is still maintained. Check the splinted limb for distal pulses, motor function, and sensation. Remember that the safe adjustment of splinting devices is virtually impossible when an ambulance is pitching about during the trip to a hospital, so complete this step before the ambulance moves unless immediate transport is required.
- *Load a relative or friend who must accompany the patient.* Consider the following guidelines if your service does not prohibit the transportation of a relative or friend with a patient: First, encourage the person to seek alternative transportation, if available. If there is just no other way the relative or friend can get to the hospital, allow him to ride in the operator's compartment—not in the patient's compartment where he may interfere with patient care. Make certain the person buckles his seat belt. If an uninjured child must come along, bring the family's child car seat and use it.
- *Load personal effects.* If a purse, briefcase, overnight bag, or other personal item is to accompany the patient, make sure it is properly secured in the ambulance. If you load personal effects at the scene of a collision, be sure to tell a police officer what you are taking. Follow policies and fill out forms, if any, required by your local system for safeguarding personal effects.
- *Reassure the patient.* Apprehension often mounts in a sick or injured person after he is loaded in an ambulance. Not only is he held down by straps in a strange, confined space, but he may also be suddenly separated from family members and friends. Say a few kind words and offer a reassuring hand in a compassionate manner.

When you are satisfied that the patient is ready, signal the operator to begin the trip to the hospital. If this is a high-priority patient, most of the preparation steps—loosening clothing, checking bandages and splints, reassuring the patient, even vital signs—can be done en route rather than delaying transport.

Caring for the Patient en Route

At least one EMT in the patient compartment is minimum staffing for an ambulance, although two are preferred. Seldom will you be able to merely ride along with your patient. You may have to undertake a number of activities en route:

- *Notify the EMD.* Let them know that you are departing the scene.
- *Continue to provide emergency care as required.* If life-support efforts were initiated prior to loading the patient into the ambulance, they must be continued during

PEDIATRIC NOTE

Remember that a toy such as a teddy bear can do much to calm a frightened child. Many ambulance units carry a sanitized, soft or padded, brightly colored toy just for these occasions. It is difficult at best to get information from a young child whose parents may have been injured and transported in another ambulance. Small children do not, as a rule, carry identification. Don't forget, you are a complete stranger in a hostile environment.

The collision scene, confusion, noise, injuries, possible pain, disappearance of a parent, EMTs caring for injuries, and gathering information—all create a terrifying experience for a child. The presence of a female EMT or police officer may be helpful; sometimes young children feel more comfortable talking to a woman. A smile and a calm, reassuring tone of voice are things that cannot be learned from a textbook, yet they may be the most critical care needed by the frightened child.

transportation to the hospital. Maintain an open airway, resuscitate, administer to the patient's needs, provide emotional support, and do whatever else is required, including updating your findings from the initial patient assessment effort.

- *Compile additional patient information.* If the patient is conscious and emergency care efforts will not be compromised, record patient information. Compiling information during the trip to the hospital serves two purposes. First, it allows you to complete your report. Second, supplying information temporarily takes your patient's mind off his problems. Remember, however, that this is not an interrogation session. Ask your questions in an informal manner.
- *Perform ongoing assessment and monitor vital signs.* Keep in mind that vital sign changes indicate a change in a patient's condition. For example, an unexplained increase in pulse rate may signify deepening shock. Record vital signs and be prepared to report changes to an emergency department staff member as soon as you reach the medical facility. Reassess vital signs every 5 minutes for an unstable patient, every 15 minutes for a stable patient.
- *Notify the receiving facility.* Transmit patient assessment and management information and provide your estimated time of arrival.
- *Recheck bandages and splints.* Even though you checked bandages after loading the patient into the ambulance, check them again while in transit.
- *Collect vomitus if the patient becomes nauseated.* If he is not already in position, arrange the patient so that the chance of his aspirating vomitus is minimized. Be prepared to apply suction. Place an emesis basin or bag by his mouth. When he has finished vomiting, place a towel over the container and deliver it to emergency department personnel when you hand over the patient. Examination of the vomitus may be important to treatment, especially in cases of poisoning. Wear a mask, protective eyewear, and disposable gloves if your patient is vomiting.
- *Talk to the patient, but control your emotions.* Continued conversation is often soothing to a frightened patient.
- *Advise the ambulance operator of changing conditions.* No one likes a "back-seat driver." However, sometimes you will need to ask the ambulance operator to adjust his speed or alter his driving technique to suit the patient's needs. On the one hand, if what began as a routine transport develops into an emergency call, you may have to ask the operator to accelerate. On the other hand, if you think that swaying because of high speeds and uneven streets is detrimental to a patient's condition, have the operator slow down or take an alternative route.

  While the operator of an ambulance is responsible for his vehicle and passengers, it is your responsibility to care for sick and injured persons; thus, the operator should drive the ambulance according to your suggestions. The decision on use of lights and siren should always be made with the patient's medical condition in mind.
- *If cardiac arrest develops, have the operator stop the ambulance.* While he's doing that, apply and operate the AED. Signal the operator to start up again once you have completed the shock sequence or determined that the patient does not have a shockable rhythm. Make certain that the emergency department is made aware of the arrest. If you routinely position a rigid device between the back of high-risk patients and the cot mattress, you have only to drop the cot back to a horizontal position and start CPR. If not, you must position an object like a short spine board or CPR board so that chest compression efforts will be effective.
- *If the patient remains pulseless despite the AED, begin CPR.* Local protocols may mandate intercept by an Advanced Life Support (ALS) team. You may want the ambulance operator to assist you with CPR or AED while additional resources come to your aid. Use your judgment on this.

TRANSFERRING THE PATIENT TO THE EMERGENCY DEPARTMENT STAFF

You should take the following steps to ensure that the transfer of a patient to the care of emergency department personnel is accomplished smoothly and without incident. Brief as it may be, the transfer is a crucial step during which your primary concern must be the continuation of patient-care activities. The steps of the transfer are illustrated in Scan 34-3.

- *In a routine admissions situation or when an illness or injury is not life-threatening, check first to see what is to be done with the patient.* If emergency department activity is particularly hectic, it might be better to leave your patient in the relative security and comfort of the ambulance while your operator determines where he is to be taken. Otherwise the patient may be subjected to distressing sights and sounds and perhaps be in the way. (If you do this, make sure an EMT remains with the patient at all times.) UNDER NO CIRCUMSTANCES SHOULD YOU SIMPLY WHEEL A NON-EMERGENCY PATIENT INTO A HOSPITAL, PLACE HIM IN A BED, AND LEAVE HIM! This is an important point. Unless you transfer care of your patient directly to a member of the hospital staff, you may be open to a charge of abandonment.

  Staff members may be treating other seriously ill and injured persons, so suppress any urge to demand attention for your patient. Simply continue emergency care measures until someone can assume responsibility for the patient. When properly directed, transfer the patient to a hospital stretcher.
- *Assist emergency department staff as required and provide a verbal report.* Stress any changes in the condition of the patient that you have observed.
- *As soon as you are free from patient-care activities, prepare the prehospital care report.* Remember, the job is not over until the paperwork is complete. Find a quiet spot and complete your prehospital care report (PCR).
- *Transfer the patient's personal effects.* If a patient's valuables or other personal effects were entrusted to your care, transfer them to a responsible emergency department staff member. Some services have policies that involve obtaining a written receipt from emergency department personnel as protection from a charge of theft.
- *Obtain your release from the hospital.* This task is not as formal as it sounds. Simply ask the emergency department nurse or physician if your services are still needed. In rural areas where not all hospital services are available, it may be necessary to transfer a seriously ill or injured person to another medical facility. If you leave and have to be recalled, the patient will lose valuable time.

TERMINATING THE CALL

An ambulance run is not really over until the personnel and equipment that comprise the prehospital emergency care delivery system are ready for the next response. The functions of EMTs in this final phase of activity include more than just changing the stretcher linen and cleaning the ambulance. A number of tasks must be accomplished at the hospital, during the return to quarters, and after arrival at the station.

At the Hospital

While still at the hospital, the ambulance crew should begin making the ambulance ready to respond to another call. Time, equipment, and space limitations sometimes preclude vigorous cleaning of the ambulance while it is parked at the hospital.

SCAN 34-3 • Transferring the Patient

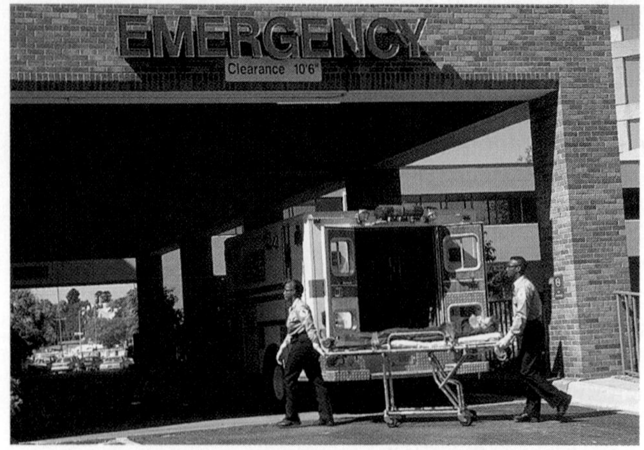

1. Transfer the patient as soon as possible. Stay with the patient until transfer is complete.

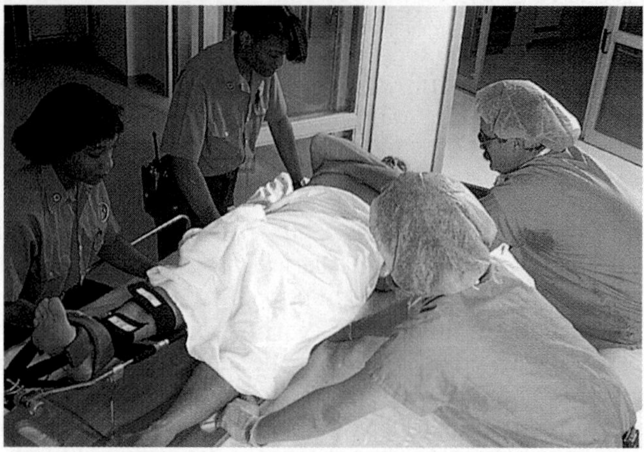

2. Assist the emergency department staff as required.

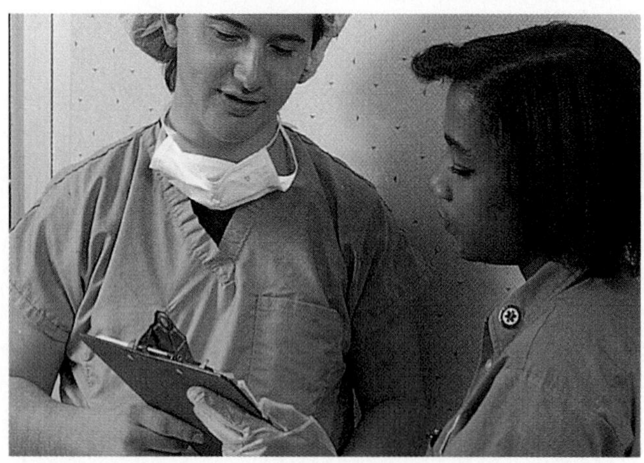

3. Transfer patient information as a verbal report and in a written prehospital care report.

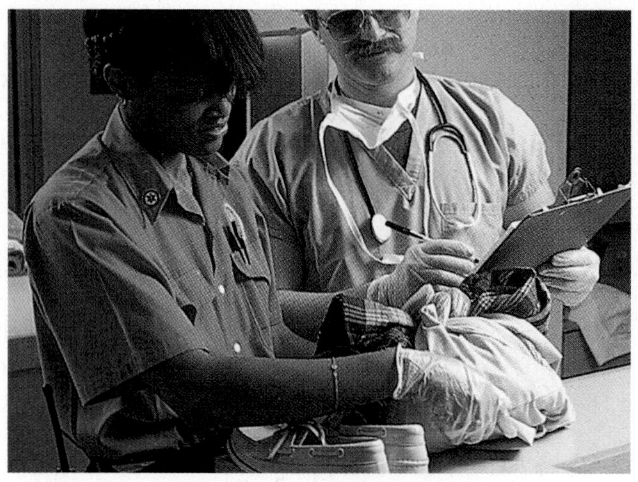

4. Transfer the patient's personal effects.

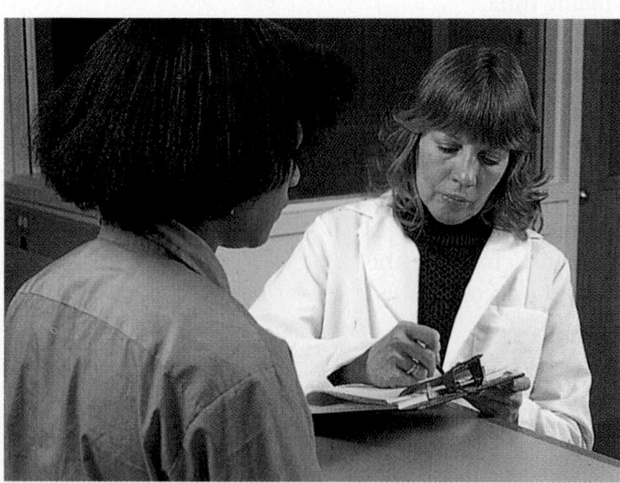

5. Obtain your release from the hospital.

However, you should make every effort to quickly prepare the vehicle for the next patient (Scan 34-4):

1. *Quickly clean the patient compartment* while wearing heavy duty, dishwashing-style gloves. Follow biohazard disposal procedures according to your agency's OSHA exposure control plan. Examples of biohazards are contaminated dressings and used suction catheters.
   - Clean up blood, vomitus, and other body fluids that may have soiled the floor. Wipe down any equipment that has been splashed. Place disposable towels used to clean up blood or body fluids directly in a red bag.
   - Remove and dispose of trash such as bandage wrappings, open but unused dressings, and similar items.
   - Sweep away caked dirt that may have been tracked into the patient compartment. When the weather is inclement, sponge up water and mud from the floor.
   - Bag dirty linens or blankets to be appropriately laundered.
   - Use a deodorizer to neutralize odors of vomit, urine, and feces. Various sprays and concentrates are available for this purpose.
2. *Prepare respiratory equipment for service:*
   - Clean and then properly disinfect nondisposable, used bag-valve-mask units and other reusable parts of respiratory-assist and inhalation-therapy devices to keep them from becoming reservoirs of infectious agents that can easily contaminate the next patient. Disinfect the suction unit.
   - Place used disposable items in a plastic bag and seal it. Replace the items with similar ones carried in the ambulance as spares.
3. *Replace expendable items:*
   - If you have a supply replacement agreement with the hospital, replace expendable items from hospital storerooms on a one-for-one basis—such as sterile dressings, bandaging materials, towels, disposable oxygen masks, disposable gloves, sterile water, and oral airways.
   - Do not abuse this exchange program. Keep in mind that the constant abuse of a supply-replacement program usually leads to its discontinuation. At the very least, abuse places a strain on ambulance-hospital relations.
4. *Exchange equipment according to your local policy:*
   - Exchange items such as splints and spine boards. Several benefits are associated with an equipment exchange program: There is no need to subject patients to injury-aggravating movements just to recover equipment, crews are not delayed at the hospital, and ambulances can return to quarters fully equipped for the next response.
   - When equipment is available for exchange, quickly inspect it for completeness and operability. Parts are sometimes lost or broken when an immobilizing device is removed from a patient.
   - If you do find that a piece of equipment is broken or incomplete, notify someone in authority so the device can be repaired or replaced.
5. *Make up the ambulance cot.* The following procedure is one of many that can be used to make up a wheeled ambulance stretcher:
   - Raise the stretcher to the high-level position, if possible; this makes the procedure easier. The stretcher should be flat with the side rails lowered and straps unfastened.
   - Remove unsoiled blankets and pillows, and place them on a clean surface.
   - Remove all soiled linen, and place it in the designated receptacle.
   - Clean the mattress surface with an appropriate EPA-approved, low-level disinfectant unless there is visible blood, which should be cleaned up using a 1:100 bleach/water solution.
   - Turn the mattress over; rotation adds to the life of the mattress.
   - Center the bottom sheet on the mattress and open it fully. If a full-sized bed sheet is used, first fold it lengthwise.

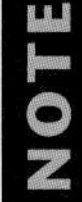

A neatly prepared stretcher inspires the patient's confidence. Do not use stained linen, even though it might be clean. Always make the presentation of your stretcher a matter of personal and professional pride.

SCAN 34-4 • Activities at the Hospital

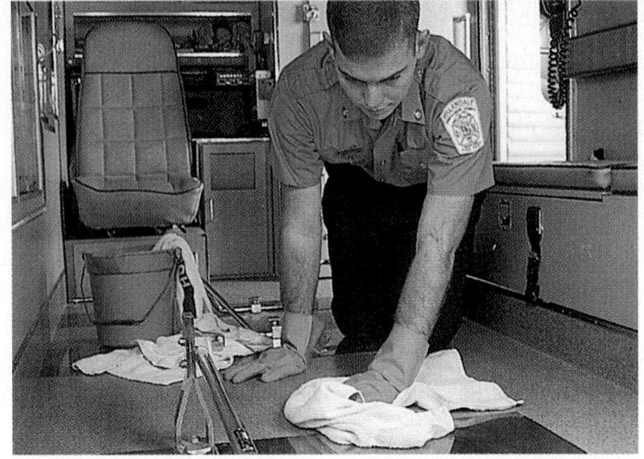

1. Clean the ambulance interior as required.

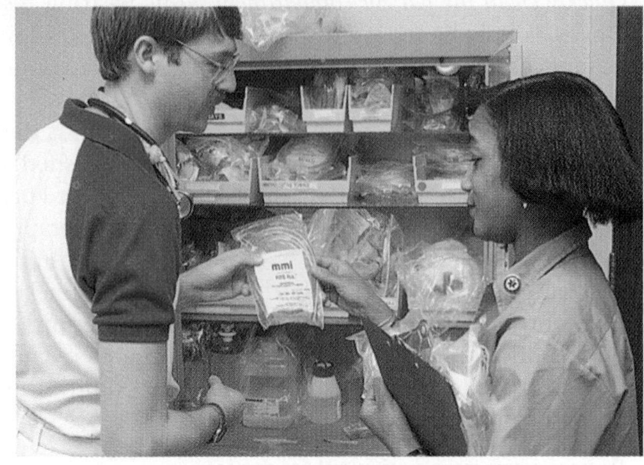

2. Replace respiratory equipment as required.

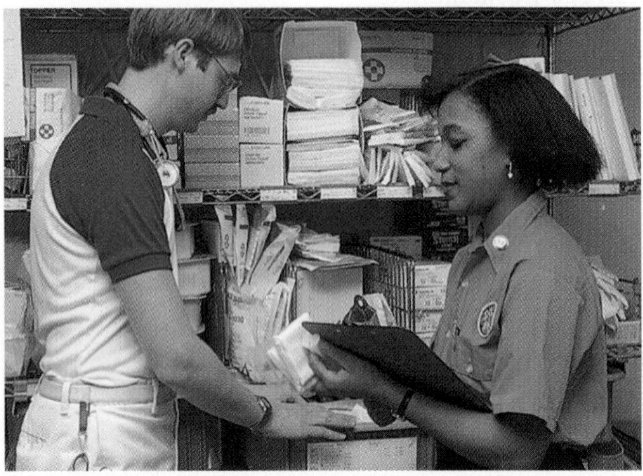

3. Replace expendable items per local policies.

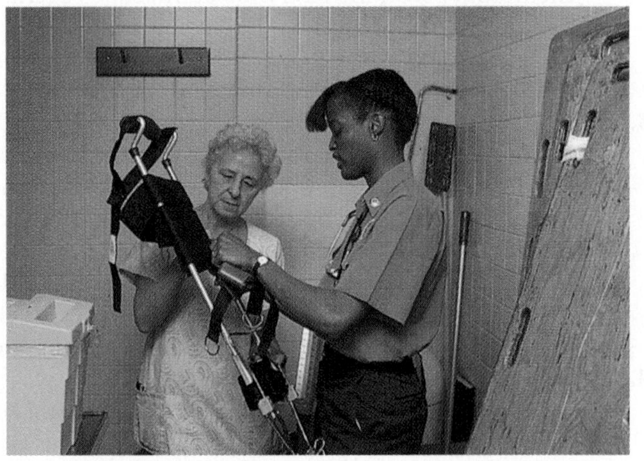

4. Exchange equipment per local policies.

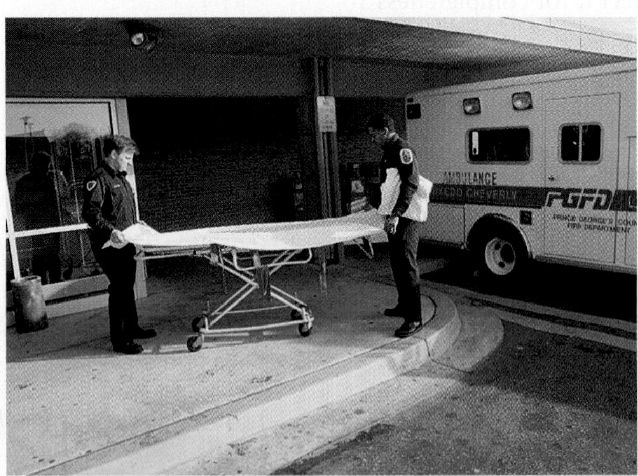

5. Make up the wheeled stretcher.

- Tuck the sheet under each end of the mattress; form square corners and then tuck under each side.
- Place a disposable pad, if one is used, on the center of the mattress.
- Fully open the blanket. If a second blanket is used, open it fully and match it to the first blanket. This task should be done with an EMT at each end of the stretcher.
- Open a top sheet in the same way, placing it on top of the blanket. Fold the blanket(s) and top sheet together lengthwise to match the width of the stretcher; fold one side first, then the other.
- Tuck the foot of the folded blanket(s) and sheet under the foot of the mattress.
- Tuck the head of the folded blanket(s) and sheet under the head of the mattress.
- Place the slip-covered pillow lengthwise at the head of the mattress and secure it with a strap.
- Buckle the safety straps and tuck in excess straps.
- Raise the side rails and foot rest.

The stretcher is now ready for the next patient. It must be re-emphasized that this is one of many techniques for preparing a wheeled ambulance stretcher for service. Whatever the method, it should meet the following objectives:

- Preparation for the next call should be done as soon and as quickly as possible.
- All linens, blankets, and pouches should be stored neatly on the stretcher.
- All linens and blankets should be folded or tucked so that they will be contained within the stretcher frame.
- The cot must be replaced in the ambulance.
- Any nondisposable patient-care items should be replaced.
- A check should be made for equipment left in the hospital.

En Route to Quarters

Emphasis should be on a safe return. An ambulance operator may practice every suggestion for safe vehicle operation while en route to the hospital and then totally disregard those suggestions during the return to quarters. Defensive driving must be a full-time effort. Do not forget that the driver and all passengers must wear seat belts.

1. *Radio the EMD.* Let him know that you are returning to quarters and that you are available (or not available) for service. Valuable time is lost if an EMD has to locate and alert a backup ambulance when he does not know that a ready-for-service unit is on the road. Be sure that you notify the EMD if you stop and leave the ambulance unattended for any reason during the return to quarters.
2. *Air the ambulance if necessary.* If the patient just delivered to the hospital has an airborne communicable disease, or if it was not possible to neutralize disagreeable odors while at the hospital, make the return trip with the windows of the patient compartment partially open, weather permitting. If the unit has sealed windows, use the air-conditioning or ventilating system (do not set on "recirculate") to air the patient compartment out.
3. *Refuel the ambulance.* Local policy usually dictates the frequency with which an ambulance is refueled. Some services require the operator to refuel after each call regardless of the distance traveled. In other services the policy is to refuel when the gauge reaches a certain level. At any rate, the fuel should be at such a level that the ambulance can respond to an emergency and then to the hospital without fear of running out.

In Quarters

When you return to quarters, a number of activities need to be completed before the ambulance can be placed in service and before it is ready for another call (Scan 34-5).

SCAN 34-5 • Terminating Activities in Quarters

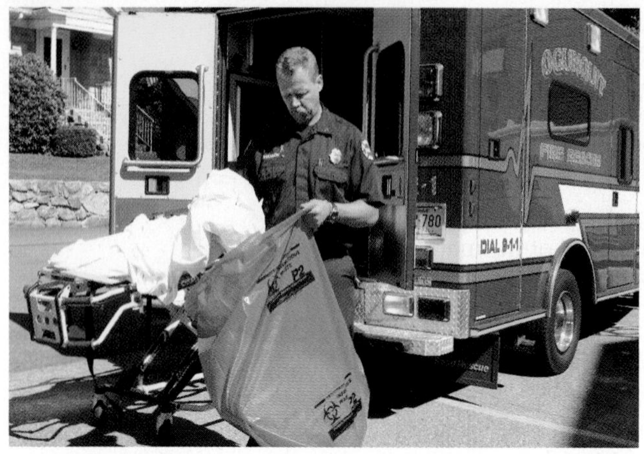

1. Place contaminated linens in a biohazard container, and noncontaminated linens in a regular hamper.

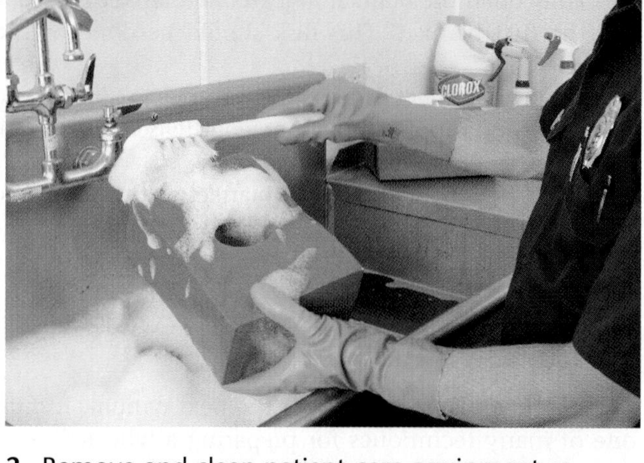

2. Remove and clean patient-care equipment as required.

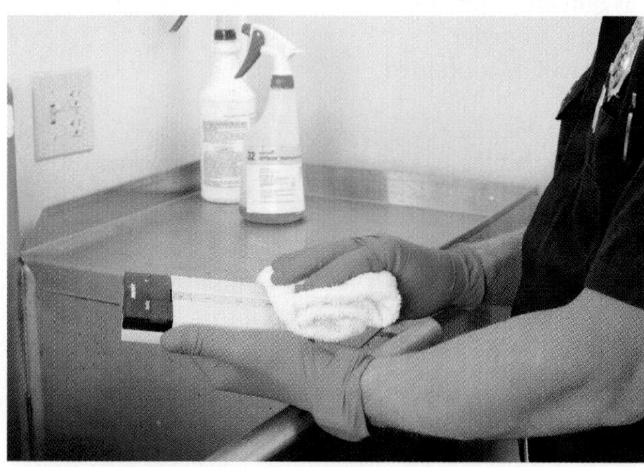

3. Clean and sanitize respiratory equipment as required.

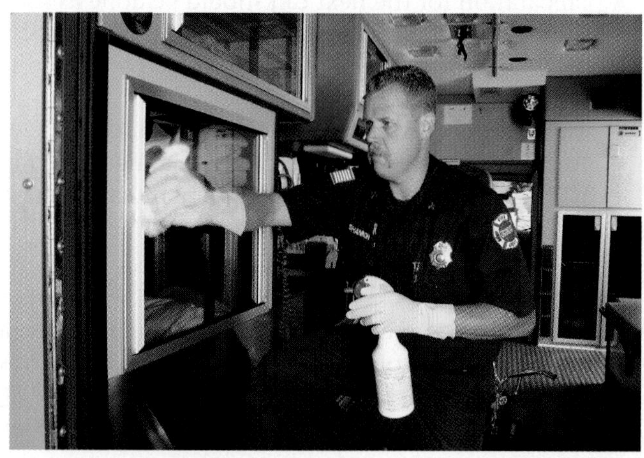

4. Clean and sanitize the ambulance interior as required. Use germicide on devices or surfaces that were in contact with blood or other body fluids.

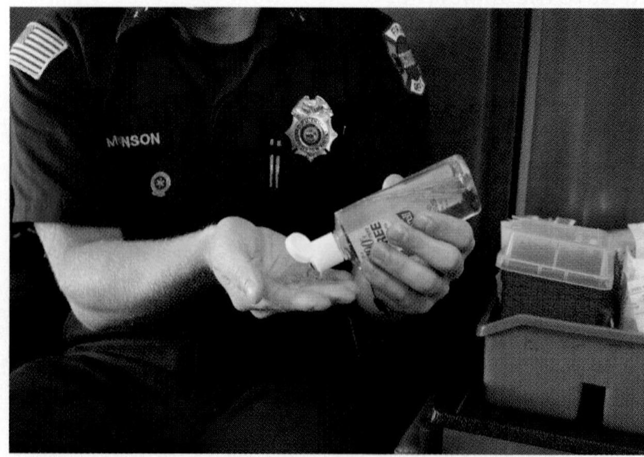

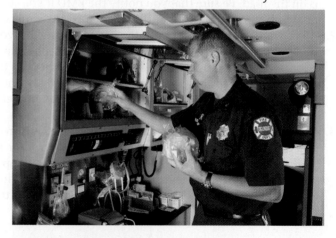

5. Wash hands thoroughly, and change soiled clothing. Do this first if exposed to a communicable disease.

6. Replace expendable items as required.

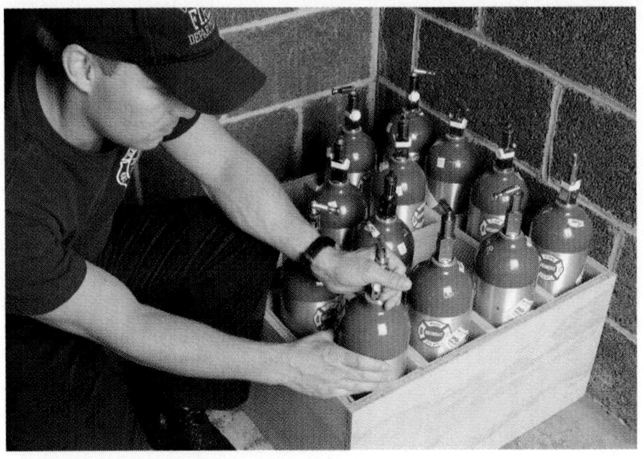

7. Replace oxygen cylinders as necessary.

8. Replace patient-care equipment as needed.

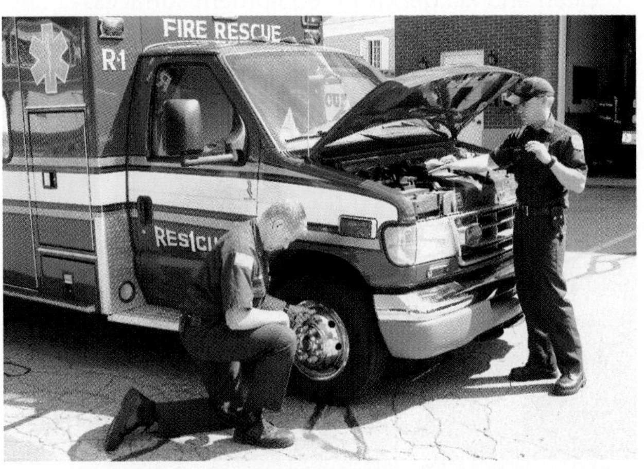

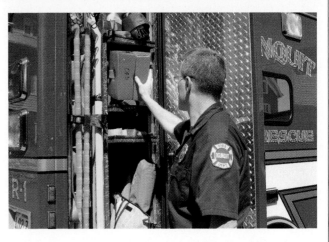

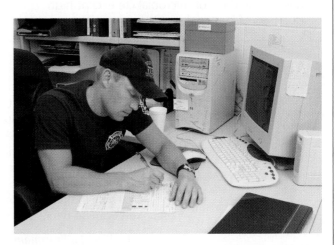

9. Maintain the ambulance as required. Report problems that will take the vehicle out of service.

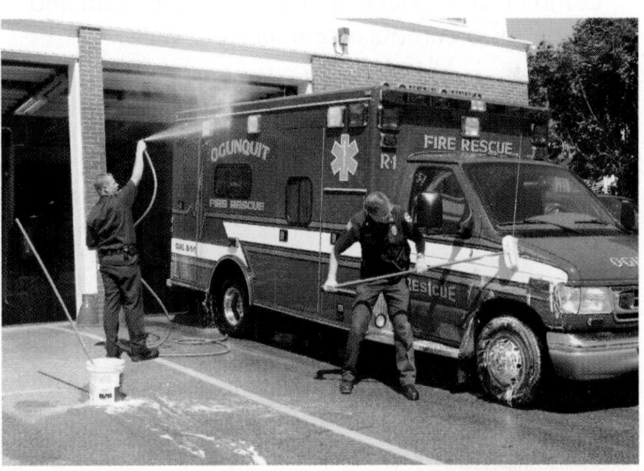

10. Clean the ambulance exterior as needed.

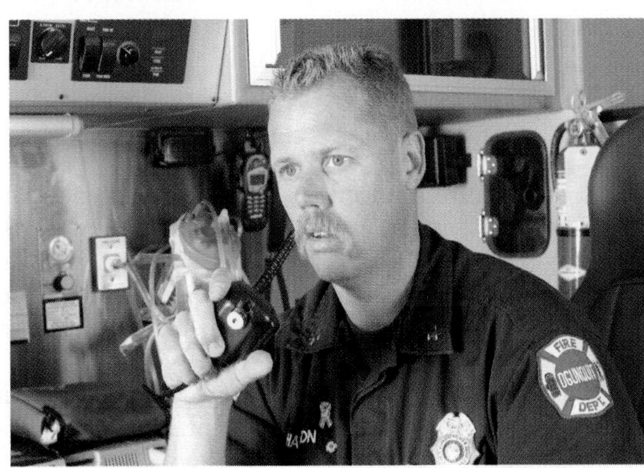

11. Report the unit ready for service.

12. Complete any unfinished report forms as soon as possible.

SCAN 34-6 • Cleaning and Disinfecting Equipment

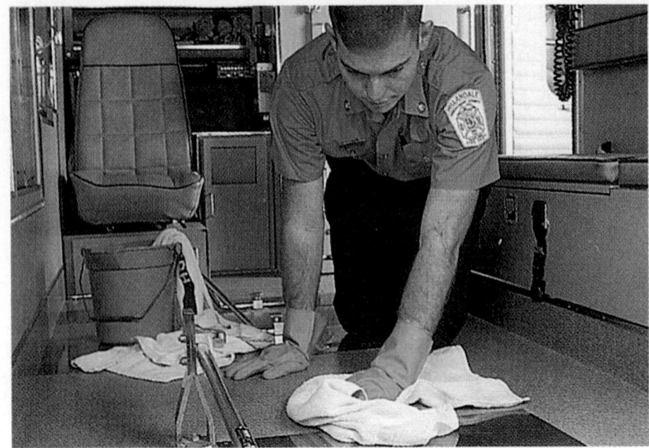

1. A low-level disinfectant approved by the U.S. Environmental Protection Agency (for example, a commercial product such as Lysol) will clean and kill germs on ambulance floors and walls.

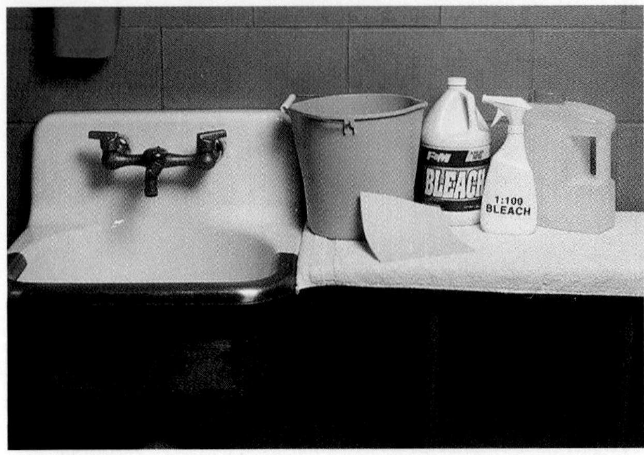

2. An intermediate-level disinfectant, such as a mixture of 1:100 bleach-to-water, can be used to clean and kill germs on equipment surfaces.

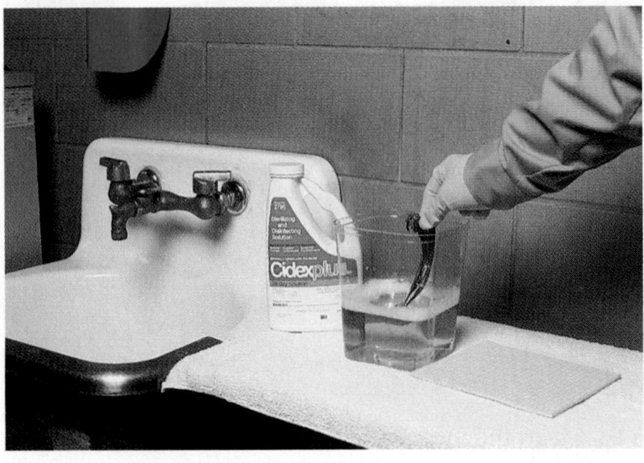

3. A high-level disinfectant, such as Cidex Plus, will destroy all forms of microbial life except high numbers of bacterial spores.

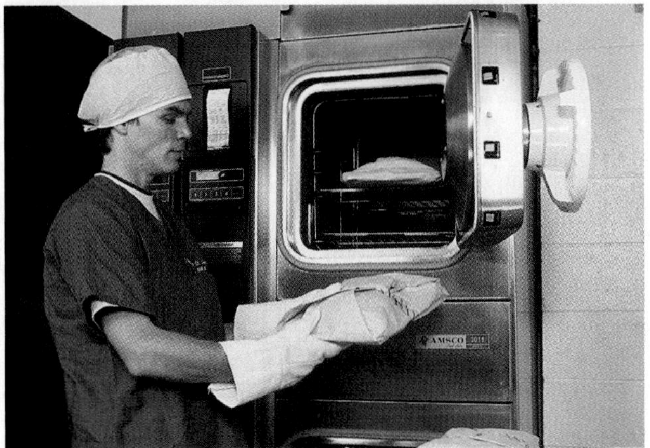

4. Sterilization is required to destroy all possible sources of infection on equipment that will be used invasively.

With the emphasis today on protection from infectious diseases, you need to take every precaution to protect yourself. It is essential that you follow your agency's OSHA exposure control plan. Always wear gloves when handling contaminated linen, cleaning the equipment, handling the respiratory equipment, and cleaning the ambulance interior (there may be many hidden nooks and crannies where the patient's blood or body fluids could be).

Once in quarters, you are ready to complete cleaning and disinfecting chores. Consult Scan 34-6 for the levels of reprocessing to be used for equipment.

1. *Place badly contaminated linens in a biohazard container, and noncontaminated linens in a regular hamper.*
2. *As necessary, clean any equipment that touched the patient.* Brush stretcher covers and other rubber, vinyl, and canvas materials clean, then wash them with soap and water.

3. *Clean and disinfect used nondisposable respiratory-assist and inhalation therapy equipment:*
   - Disassemble the equipment so that all surfaces are exposed.
   - Fill a large plastic container with the cleaning solution outlined in your service's infection control plan.
   - Clean the inner and outer surfaces with a suitable brush. Inner surfaces can be cleaned with a small bottle brush, while outer surfaces can be cleaned with a hand or nail brush. Make sure all encrusted matter is removed.
   - Rinse the items with tap water.
   - Soak the items in an EPA-approved germicidal solution. An inhalation therapist at a local hospital can suggest a germicide suitable for respiratory equipment. Follow directions for dilution, safe handling, and soaking time. Gloves are recommended when using some germicides.
   - After the prescribed soaking period, hang the equipment in a well-ventilated clean area and allow it to dry for 12 to 24 hours.
4. *Clean and sanitize the patient compartment.* Use an EPA-approved germicide to clean any fixed equipment or surfaces contacted by the patient's body fluids.
5. *Prepare yourself for service:*
   - Wash thoroughly, paying attention to the areas under your fingernails. Remember that contaminants can collect there and become a source of infection not only to you but also to the persons whom you touch.
   - Change soiled clothes. Clean contaminated clothing as soon as possible, especially if you were exposed to someone with a communicable disease. It is a good policy to bring a spare uniform to work, and each EMS agency should have a washer and dryer. It is against OSHA regulations for blood or body fluid soiled clothes to be taken home to be washed.
6. *Replace expendable items* with items from the unit's storeroom.
7. *Replace or refill oxygen cylinders* in accordance with your service's procedures.
8. *Replace patient-care equipment.*
9. *Carry out post-operation vehicle maintenance procedures as required.* If you find something wrong with the vehicle, correct the problem or make someone in authority aware of it.
10. Clean the vehicle. A clean exterior lends a professional appearance to an ambulance. Check for broken lights, glass and body damage, door operation, and other parts that may need repair or replacement.
11. Complete any unfinished report forms as soon as possible, and report the unit ready for service.

AIR RESCUE

In some circumstances, it is best for a patient to be transported by an air rescue helicopter (Figure 34-5) or fixed-wing aircraft. The following are some considerations for use of this kind of transport. Since geographic and other circumstances and the availability of such transport will vary in different localities, follow your local protocols.

When to Call for Air Rescue

Air rescue may be required for any of the following reasons:

- *Operational reasons.* Operational reasons for air rescue include: (1) to speed transport to a distant trauma center or other special facility, (2) when extrication of a high-priority patient is prolonged and air rescue can speed transport, or (3) when a patient must be rescued from a remote location that can only be reached by helicopter. Follow local protocols.

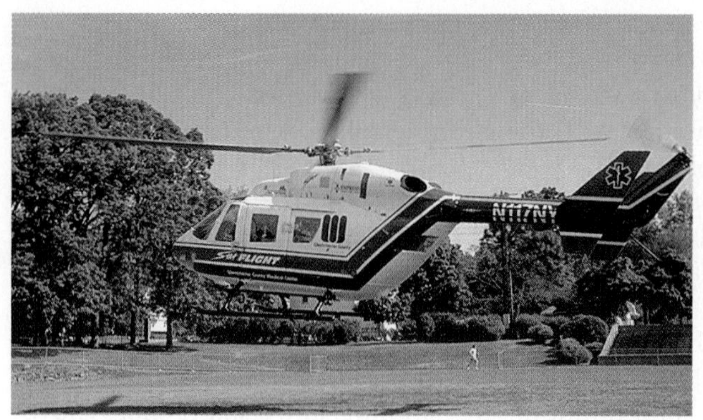

Figure 34-5 • Patients are sometimes transported by air rescue helicopter.

- *Medical reasons.* Medical reasons for air rescue include if the patient is high priority for rapid transport; for example, a patient in shock, a patient with a Glasgow Coma Scale total of less than 10, a patient who has a head injury with altered mental status, a patient with chest trauma and respiratory distress, a patient with penetrating injuries to the body cavity, a patient with an amputation proximal to the hand or foot, a patient with extensive burns, or a patient with a serious mechanism of injury.

  Patients with certain medical conditions may also be flown by helicopter. Cardiac patients requiring catheterization or surgery, stroke patients, and those patients requiring hyperbaric oxygen treatment (e.g., a carbon monoxide poisoning) are examples of medical patients who may also be flown by air. In many cases you will transport these patients to your local hospital for stabilization and the helicopter will transfer the patient from one hospital to another. Cardiac-arrest patients are usually not transported by air rescue unless they are hypothermic. Follow local protocols.

How to Call for Air Rescue

Air rescue may be called for by any law enforcement, fire, or EMS command officer at the scene of an incident, or you, as an EMT, may radio dispatch for advice if you think such a service is needed. When calling an air rescue service, give your name and call-back number, your agency name, the nature of the situation, the exact location including crossroads and major landmarks, and the exact location of a safe landing zone. Follow local protocols.

How to Set Up a Landing Zone

A helicopter requires a landing zone, or LZ, approximately 100-by-100 feet (approximately 30 large steps on each side) on ground with less than an 8-degree slope. The landing zone and approach/departure path should be clear of wires, towers, vehicles, people, and loose objects (Figure 34-6). The landing zone should be marked with one flare in an upwind position. During night operations, NEVER shine a light into the pi-

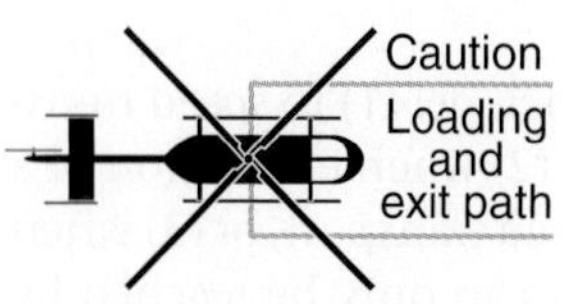

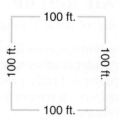

Figure 34-6 • Helicopter landing zone.

lot's eyes during landing or takeoff or while the aircraft is running on the ground. Keep emergency red lights on.

Describe the landing zone to the air rescue service:

- *Terrain.* "The landing zone is located on top of a hill." "The landing zone is located in a valley."
- *Major landmarks.* "There is a river (major highway, factory, water tower) to the north (or other direction) of the landing zone."
- *Estimated distance to nearest town.* "The landing zone is approximately 12 miles west of Centerville."
- *Other pertinent information.* "There are wires on the east side of the landing zone." "There is a deep ditch to the west." "Winds are out of the north-northeast at about 10 mph."

How to Approach a Helicopter

Do not approach a helicopter unless escorted by the flight personnel. Allow the helicopter crew to direct the loading on board of the patient. Stay clear of the tail rotor at all times. Keep all traffic and vehicles 100 feet or more distant from the helicopter. Do not smoke within 200 feet of the aircraft. Be aware of the danger areas around helicopters, as shown in Scan 34-7. NEVER walk around the tail rotor area.

SCAN 34-7 • Danger Areas Around Helicopters

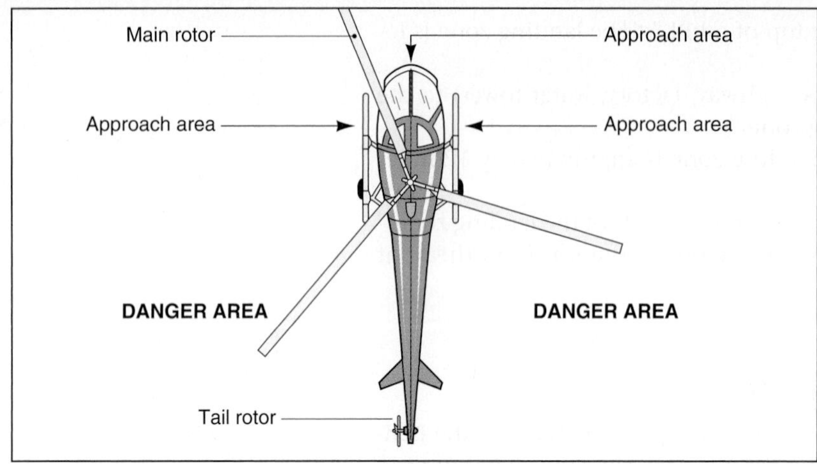

A. The area around the tail rotor is extremely dangerous. A spinning rotor cannot be seen.

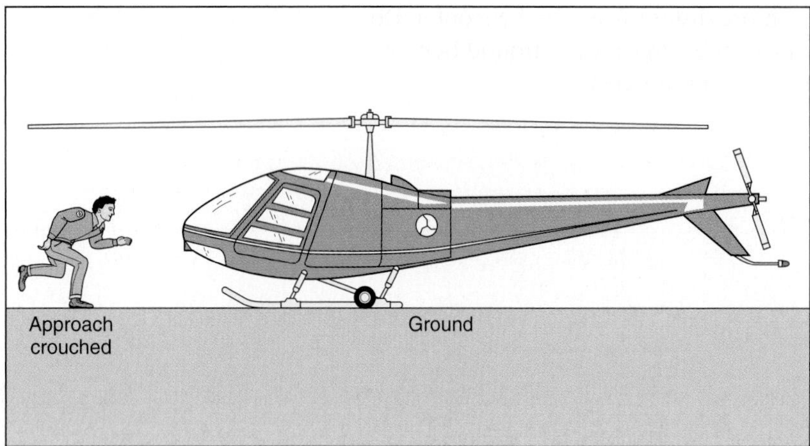

B. A sudden gust of wind can cause the main rotor of a helicopter to dip to a point as close as 4 feet from the ground. Always approach a helicopter in a crouch when the rotor is moving.

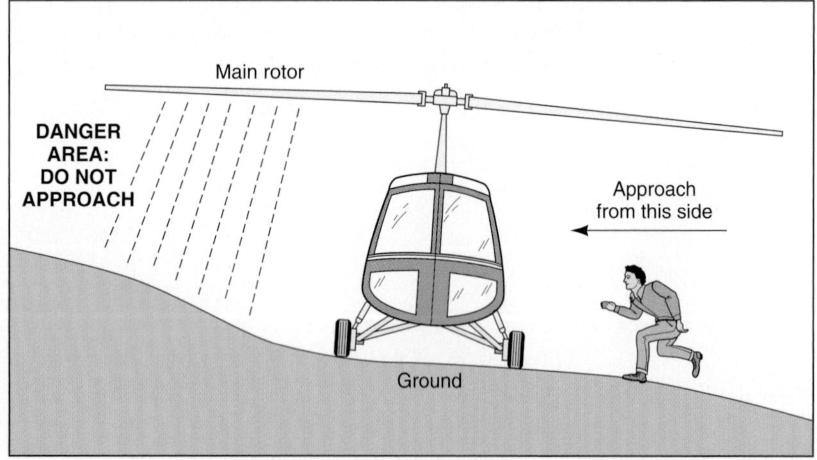

C. Approach the aircraft from the downhill side when a helicopter is parked on a hillside.

CHAPTER REVIEW

SUMMARY

There are five phases to ambulance operations:

1. *Preparing for the call.* Make sure that all required equipment and supplies are on board, in good repair or operating order, and properly stored. Inspect the ambulance itself to make sure that it is ready for service.
2. *Receiving and responding to the call.* Receive call information from the EMD (Emergency Medical Dispatcher). Operate the ambulance safely. Understand the laws of your state and locality with regard to operation in an emergency situation, and always operate the ambulance with due regard for the safety of others. Park the ambulance outside the danger zone at a vehicle collision site.
3. *Transferring the patient to the ambulance.* Select a patient-carrying device suitable for the patient's injuries or medical condition. Make sure that the patient is properly packaged and secured to the device. Ensure that the stretcher is secured within the ambulance before the ambulance begins to move.
4. *Transporting the patient to the hospital.* Perform and document ongoing assessment, needed treatments, and patient's condition. Notify dispatch, and transmit information to the receiving facility.
5. *Transferring the patient to the emergency department staff.* Do not leave the patient until emergency department personnel have taken over his care. Assist in transferring the patient to the hospital stretcher. Give a verbal report to emergency department personnel. Complete your prehospital care report. Transfer the patient's personal effects. Obtain your release from hospital personnel.

At the conclusion of the call, make up the ambulance stretcher, clean and restock the ambulance, and make sure that it is in good order for the next call.

On some occasions, your service may request that an air-rescue service transport the patient. Be aware of procedures for requesting this service, for setting up a landing zone, and for safety procedures around a helicopter.

REVIEW QUESTIONS

1. List five categories of equipment and supplies that should be carried on an ambulance. (pp. 902–907)
2. Describe the laws (those described in this chapter or your local or state laws) with regard to operation of an ambulance in an emergency. Describe considerations for safe operation of an ambulance in emergency and nonemergency situations. (pp. 911–917)
3. Describe the steps that must be followed in transferring a patient to an ambulance; for care of the patient en route; and for transferring a patient to emergency department personnel. (pp. 918–923)
4. Describe the steps that should be followed when air rescue is required. (pp. 931–933)

CRITICAL THINKING

- What equipment should you include in a kit that you carry to the scene? How should the equipment be positioned so that you can reach urgently needed items quickly? What special items, if any, should be in the kit to meet local needs?

Thinking and Linking

Think back to Chapter 1, "Introduction to Emergency Medical Care," where you read about the roles and responsibilities of the EMT.

- How do your daily roles and responsibilities as an EMT as described in Chapter 1 relate to the various phases of an ambulance call as described in this chapter?

Think back to Chapter 2, "The Well-Being of the EMT-Basic."

- If you didn't clean your ambulance properly and blood was left on the bench seat, what disease could be transmitted to you or another crew member?

MEDIA RESOURCES 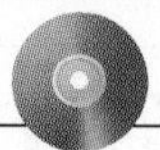

See the Student CD at the back of this book for quizzes, a case study activity, and other features related to this chapter. In particular, take a look at the Case Study regarding ambulance operations. Also, visit the Companion Website for *Emergency Care* at **www.prenhall.com/limmer**, where you will find additional reinforcement and links to other resources.

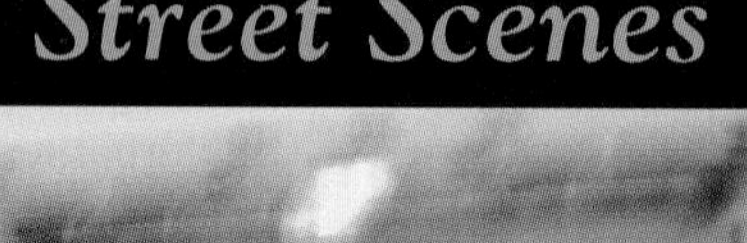

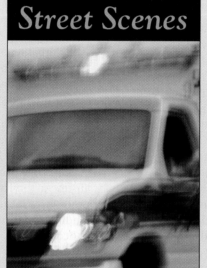

You receive a priority-1 call. "Ambulance 19, respond to 1901 Greentop Road for a report of a cardiac arrest." You acknowledge, get into the ambulance, and buckle up. Your partner does the same and turns on the red lights and siren. The dispatcher tells you that there is no additional information from the caller, and you will be the first unit to arrive. You know it will be a long response because the call is at the far end of your district, and you feel pressured to hurry. As you approach an intersection, your partner changes the siren from wail to yelp and goes through without slowing down. "That light was red," you tell him. He doesn't respond and keeps driving at the same speed. When he starts to weave through traffic, you suggest an alternative route to avoid the approaching rush-hour congestion.

Street Scene Questions

1. When operating an ambulance using the red lights and siren, what precautions do you need to take?
2. How can speed affect the safety of ambulance operation?
3. What driving techniques might be used to make driving to this scene safer?

All of a sudden, a car comes out of a driveway and into your path. Your partner hits the brakes, performs an evasive move, and just misses the other vehicle. You notice that a box of tissues and a stethoscope landed on the floor in the patient compartment. "What would have happened if I had been back there with a patient?" you ask. Your partner finally realizes he is driving too fast and slows down. At the next intersection, he slows down even more and makes sure that traffic has come to a stop before going through. During the rest of the response, you focus on preparing for your arrival on the scene.

You have decided to load all your equipment on the stretcher and wheel it to the front door as soon as the ambulance is parked. As you pull up to the scene, your partner finds a good spot to park where the ambulance will not create a hazard. He leaves the warning lights on for visibility.

Street Scene Questions

4. What should you do first for patient care?
5. What information should you provide to the dispatcher?

Your patient is in his bedroom, sitting on his bed, and greets you as you approach. You immediately ask him why EMS was called. "My wife called because I passed out. It's happened before, but my doctor isn't sure what causes it." Your partner radios dispatch that the patient is alert and that another unit is not needed. You assess the patient, obtain a patient history, and get a set of vital signs. The patient is alert and oriented, his pulse is 82 with a blood pressure of 130/82, respirations are 20, and skin is unremarkable. The patient says that he takes a medication because his cholesterol is "way up there." The patient's wife reports that he was sitting in a chair and slumped over. She did not see any seizure activity. He did not respond to verbal stimulus, so she moved him to the floor. He regained consciousness within 2 minutes.

The patient consents to transport to the hospital for further evaluation. You move him by stair chair from the bedroom to the stretcher. The patient is placed on the stretcher and all the safety straps are fastened. You place the stretcher into the ambulance compartment and, after it is in the bracket, you recheck to make sure it is secured properly. Your partner puts the stair chair away in its compartment and asks what the priority is to the hospital. "Priority 2," you answer. "Based on the assessment, there is no need to use the red light and siren."

Street Scenes Sample Documentation

PATIENT NAME: Faris Kazi **PATIENT AGE:** 66

CHIEF COMPLAINT

"I passed out"

PAST MEDICAL HISTORY

- [ ] None
- [ ] Allergy to
- [ ] Hypertension
- [ ] Stroke
- [ ] Seizures
- [ ] Diabetes
- [ ] COPD
- [ ] Cardiac
- [x] Other (List)
- [ ] Asthma

Syncope

Current Medications (List)

Pravachol

VITAL SIGNS

TIME	RESP	PULSE	B.P.	MENTAL STATUS	R PUPILS L	SKIN
1730	Rate: 20; [x] Regular [ ] Shallow [ ] Labored	Rate: 82; [x] Regular [ ] Irregular	130/82	[x] Alert [ ] Voice [ ] Pain [ ] Unresp.	Normal (R ✓, L ✓); Dilated; Constricted; Sluggish; No-Reaction	[x] Unremarkable [ ] Cool [ ] Pale [ ] Warm [ ] Cyanotic [ ] Moist [ ] Flushed [ ] Dry [ ] Jaundiced
1742	Rate: 18; [x] Regular [ ] Shallow [ ] Labored	Rate: 84; [x] Regular [ ] Irregular	130/80	[x] Alert [ ] Voice [ ] Pain [ ] Unresp.	Normal (R ✓, L ✓); Dilated; Constricted; Sluggish; No-Reaction	[x] Unremarkable [ ] Cool [ ] Pale [ ] Warm [ ] Cyanotic [ ] Moist [ ] Flushed [ ] Dry [ ] Jaundiced
	Rate: ; [ ] Regular [ ] Shallow [ ] Labored	Rate: ; [ ] Regular [ ] Irregular	/	[ ] Alert [ ] Voice [ ] Pain [ ] Unresp.	Normal; Dilated; Constricted; Sluggish; No-Reaction	[ ] Unremarkable [ ] Cool [ ] Pale [ ] Warm [ ] Cyanotic [ ] Moist [ ] Flushed [ ] Dry [ ] Jaundiced

NARRATIVE On arrival at a reported cardiac arrest, we are met by an alert male patient. His wife reports patient slumped over and "passed out" while sitting in a chair. She moved him to the floor, and he regained consciousness within 2 minutes. She did not observe any seizure activity. He appears to be in no obvious distress and denies complaint. He states a history of syncope, which is currently being assessed by his physician. Our patient assessment is unremarkable, and our plan is to transport patient for further evaluation of syncope.

CHAPTER 35

Gaining Access and Rescue Operations

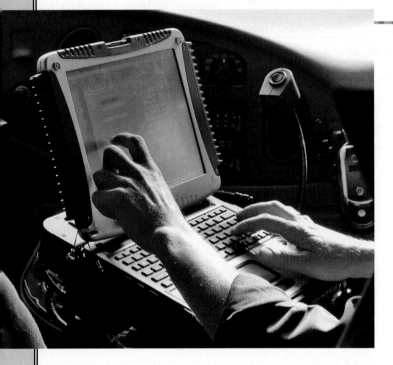

CORE CONCEPTS

The following are core concepts that will be addressed in this chapter:

- Extrication and the extrication process
- What personal protective equipment to wear at the rescue scene
- How to determine the need for an extrication
- The need for personal safety at rescue scenes

DOT OBJECTIVES

***KNOWLEDGE AND ATTITUDE**

7-2.1 Describe the purpose of extrication. (p. 939)

7-2.2 Discuss the role of the EMT in extrication. (pp. 939–940, 959)

7-2.3 Identify what equipment for personal safety is required for the EMT. (pp. 942–945)

7-2.4 Define the fundamental components of extrication. (pp. 939–959)

7-2.5 State the steps that should be taken to protect the patient during extrication. (p. 945)

7-2.6 Distinguish between simple and complex access. (pp. 955–956)

There are at least ten types of specialty rescue teams that may be available in various communities. Each specialty requires a significant amount of additional training over and above your EMT course. These specialties include vehicle rescue, water rescue, ice rescue, high-angle rescue, hazardous materials response, trench rescue, dive rescue, back country or wilderness rescue, farm rescue, and confined space rescue. Training that is available in each of these specialties often depends on the types of emergency responses that might be required in your community. If there is a gorge in the area, there often is a high-angle team. If there is a river with low-head dams running through your district, a water rescue team would be appropriate.

In this chapter, the focus is on the role of the EMT at a vehicle collision where extrication of the patient is required, since this is the most common type of rescue across the United States.

VEHICLE RESCUE

Extrication is the process by which entrapped patients are rescued from vehicles, buildings, tunnels, or other places. There are 10 phases of the extrication or rescue process that you, as an EMT, should understand:

1. Preparing for the rescue
2. Sizing up the situation
3. Recognizing and managing hazards
4. Stabilizing the vehicle prior to entering
5. Gaining access to the patient
6. Providing initial patient assessment and a rapid trauma exam
7. Disentangling the patient
8. Immobilizing and extricating the patient from the vehicle
9. Providing a detailed physical exam, ongoing assessment, treatment, and transport to the most appropriate hospital
10. Terminating the rescue

Every step of this process needs input from you, the EMT, acting as an advocate for the patient's medical needs. Attention to safety must be your highest priority—to help minimize the potential for injury to yourself, the other rescuers, or any additional injury to your patient. Although you may never personally perform disentanglement, since in many communities this is accomplished by a fire department rescue squad, it is important for you to understand the process so you can keep your patient informed and anticipate any dangerous steps in the extrication action plan.

You have already learned about some of the 10 phases of the extrication process (phases 2, 3, 6, 8, and 9) in the Assessment and Trauma modules, as well as in Chapter 34, "Ambulance Operations." You will learn about phases 1–5 and 7 in this chapter.

Preparing for the Rescue

Vehicle rescue prior to the mid-1960s is best described as crude. So-called "rescue" trucks were usually small walk-in step vans that carried more equipment for fire suppression and salvage than for rescue. The inventory of rescue equipment might have included some long prybars, a few lengths of utility rope, a minimal hand tool kit, shovels and brooms, and—if the rescue unit was progressive—a 4-ton hydraulic jack kit. Proper protective clothing and gear for rescue personnel were similarly lacking. Personnel were poorly trained for rescue and, more often than not, victims were simply pulled through openings created by the collision.

Modern rescue is a far more sophisticated process. It requires preparation that is a combination of training, practice, and the right protective gear and tools. As previously discussed, training and practice for specific types of rescue, including vehicle rescue, will be above and beyond your EMT course. Availability of such training will depend to a great extent on the kinds of rescues most likely to be required in your area. The kinds of protective gear and tools that should be available for vehicle rescue will be discussed throughout this chapter.

Sizing Up the Situation

As you arrive on the scene of a collision, it is important to have a keen eye, because the first thing you need to do is evaluate hazards and calculate the need for additional BLS (basic life support—EMT level) or ALS (advanced life support—EMT-Paramedic level) backup, police, fire, or specialty rescue response, or services such as a power company representative. Quickly determine how many patients are involved, their priority, and the mechanisms of injury. If you think additional ambulances will be needed, call for them right away. You can always cancel them if they are not actually needed.

An important part of scene size-up is determining the extent of the patient's entrapment and the most appropriate means of getting the patient out. As soon as possible, evaluate if the patient is high or low priority. During scene size-up, you must be able to "read" a collision vehicle and develop a plan of action based on your knowledge of rescue operations and your estimate of the patient's condition and priority. During all of this, you will keep in mind that the most seriously injured patients have, at a maximum, a "golden hour" from the time of the injury until surgery at the hospital to control internal bleeding and other life-threatening conditions. Beyond the golden hour, survival rates are believed to diminish drastically. As the patient advocate on the scene, you must plan how you can begin emergency care and initiate transport as rapidly as possible.

A low-priority patient can wait for rescue personnel to force open the doors, then remove the roof and/or displace the front end of the vehicle. For such a patient, there is time to do a short spine board or vest immobilization, then carefully transfer the patient to the stretcher using the long board. If the patient is a high priority, it may make more sense to use the rapid extrication technique, whether for a vertical removal through the opened roof or for a horizontal removal through a doorway. The principles

CRITICAL DECISION MAKING:
WHEN MINUTES COUNT, DECISIONS MATTER

Patient priority is an important consideration in rescue operations. More time is available to gain access to a stable patient than to an unstable one who needs quick transport. Scene decisions are based both on the type of entrapment and on the patient's condition. Your responsibility as an EMT is to represent the patient's needs in the rescue effort. For each patient described here, determine whether the extrication must be done quickly because the patient is unstable or if more time is available.

1. Your patient was involved in a head-on crash. The patient is unresponsive with a rapid pulse.
2. Your patient was driving a car that was rear-ended. She is alert and oriented. Her pulse is 80, respirations 16. The frame has shifted so none of the doors will open.
3. Your patient was a front-seat passenger who was thrown into the back seat. You can only reach the patient's upper body, but you find a rapid pulse and clammy skin. The patient is alert and talking with you.

of spinal immobilization remain the same whether the patient is low or high priority, but the requirements for speed of removal will dictate the specific technique you use.

During the scene size-up, check to see if the vehicle is equipped with air bags. A car with an air bag has a large, rectangular steering wheel hub. A passenger-side bag, if the car has one, would be located in the glove-compartment area. Special steps should be followed if the air bag or bags have not deployed. If an air bag has deployed, observers may have noticed "smoke" inside the vehicle during deployment. This actually is not smoke but dust from the cornstarch or talcum used to lubricate the bag, as well as from the seal and particles from within the bag. The powder may contain sodium hydroxide, which can irritate the skin. For this reason, it will be important to wear protective gloves and eyewear when you gain access to the passenger compartment. It also will be important to protect the patients from getting additional dust in their eyes or wounds. Experts recommend that the EMT lift a deployed bag and examine the steering wheel and dash, which may reveal if the patients struck any of these areas with enough energy to damage them.

Recognizing and Managing Hazards

In some rural areas, fire departments have no rescue capabilities, and ambulance services are called upon to carry out vehicle rescue on their own. In areas where rescue and fire units are available, the ambulance may nevertheless arrive at the scene first. In this situation, time and lives can be saved if EMTs—after sizing up the situation and calling for the appropriate additional help—are able to recognize and initiate hazard management, at least until personnel with more expertise arrive.

Hazards at a collision scene can range from nuisances—such as broken glass and debris, a slippery road, inclement weather, or darkness—to severe threats to safety—such as traffic, downed wires, spilled fuel, or fire. Also during scene size-up, watch out for loaded bumpers. Most cars are equipped with 5-mile-per-hour bumpers designed to absorb low-speed front and rear-end collision damage. If the bumpers were involved in the collision, you may notice that the bumper shock absorber system is compressed, or "loaded." Never stand in front of a loaded bumper. If it springs out and strikes your knees, it will likely break your legs. Some rescue teams are trained to unload or chain the shock absorber to prevent an uncontrolled release.

Traffic and spectators can become hazards if they are not controlled. A number of EMTs have been killed at the scenes of collisions by oncoming traffic when drivers were watching the collision and did not see the EMT.

As explained in the following sections, some collision-related hazards must be managed, if not eliminated, before any attempt is made to reach injured persons in damaged vehicles.

Safeguarding Yourself from Hazards

Collision sites can be dangerous workplaces. Jagged edges, flying glass, and fire are only a few of the hazards you may need to deal with. Remember that you are no good to your patient and crew if you become a patient yourself. It is vital that you take the time to properly protect yourself before engaging in any rescue activities. *The unsafe act that contributes most to collision scene injuries is failure to wear protective gear during rescue operations*. The following human factors can increase the potential for an EMT to be injured at a collision site:

- Careless attitude toward personal safety
- Lack of skill in tool use
- Physical problems that impede strenuous effort

Unsafe and improper acts and omissions also cause injuries:

- Failure to eliminate or control hazards
- Failure to select the proper tool for the task
- Using unsafe tools
- Failure to recognize mechanisms of injury and unsafe surroundings
- Lifting heavy objects improperly
- Deactivating safety devices designed to prevent injury
- Failure to wear highly visible outer clothing, especially when exposed to traffic (Figure 35-1)
- Failure to realize that hybrid vehicles may make no noise when running but not moving.

At a collision scene any personnel who are allowed to work in the "inner circle"—that is, the area immediately around and including the vehicle—should wear full protective gear to avoid being injured. Figure 35-2 shows an EMT dressed for a rescue operation with minimal hazards.

Learn the value of protective gear. Get your own if your service does not provide it (most states require it on ambulances), and use it! Consider reviewing the following National Fire Protection Association standards when purchasing protective gear and uniforms: NFPA 1972 (Helmets for Structural Firefighting), NFPA 1973 (Gloves for Structural Firefighting), and NFPA 1975 (Station/Work Uniforms).

Choosing the Correct Level of Protection

EMS personnel have a wide selection of personal protective equipment (PPE) available to them. Until recently, most PPE was designed for structural firefighting and not for rescue/EMS operations. Today, rescuers have a wide variety of compact lightweight helmets with integral eye protection. There are now PPE garments designed for urban search and rescue (USAR) operations that are ideal for EMS. They are lightweight, breathable, and provide protection from flame, fluids, and common chemicals. This is in stark contrast to firefighter PPE, which is designed with greater insulation to provide protection from heat/flame. As a result, firefighter PPE is much heavier and more bulky.

WORKING IN TRAFFIC A major hazard for the EMT is being struck by a vehicle while working in traffic. All highway workers are required to wear a high-visibility helmet and safety vest to comply with OSHA safety requirements. While rescuers have not typically been required to wear safety vests and helmets, they should wear them, too. Safety vests greatly enhance both day and night visibility, giving rescuers added protection because

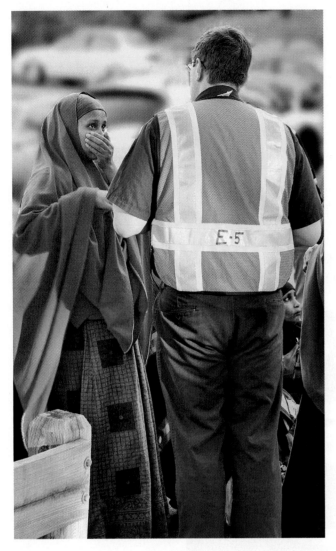

Figure 35-1 • An EMT wears a highly visible vest at a high-traffic scene.

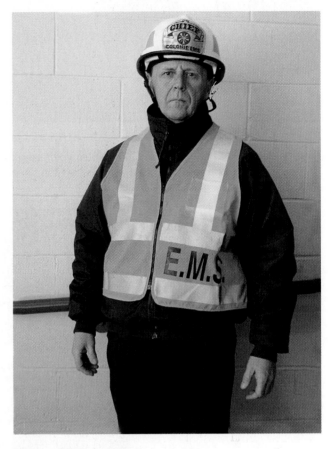

Figure 35-2 • An EMT dressed for rescue operations. *(© Jon Politis)*

motorists can see them. The best way to understand this is to study Figures 35-3A and 35-3B, which show clothing with reflective elements in daytime and nighttime settings.

DURING EXTRICATION OPERATIONS When extrication is in process at a motor-vehicle collision, the rescuer has an increased exposure to flame, glass, fluids, and sharp objects. The best practice is to wear EMS or firefighter turnout clothing, including a helmet and eye protection (Figure 35-4).

MATCHING THE LEVEL OTHERS ARE WEARING One of the easiest ways to determine the correct PPE is to look at what other workers are doing in the industry and "match" their level of PPE. A typical construction site is a "hard hat" job. In other words, workers there are required to wear a hard hat and safety glasses. So the rescuer should wear that level of PPE, too. On the highway it would be a hard hat and safety vest, and at an extrication it would be full turnouts.

Specific PPE

Following are descriptions of personal protective equipment that EMTs should use during rescue operations.

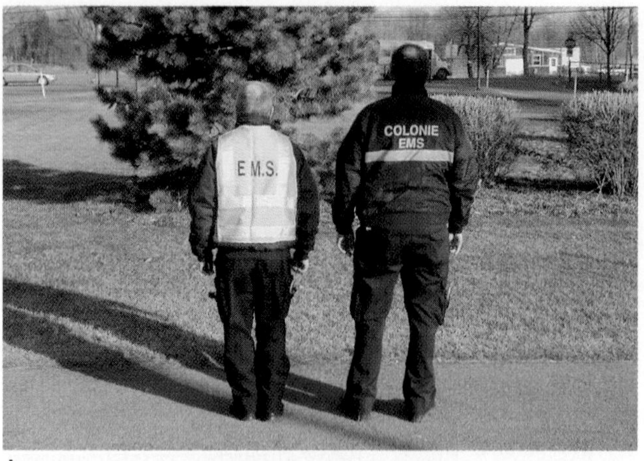

A

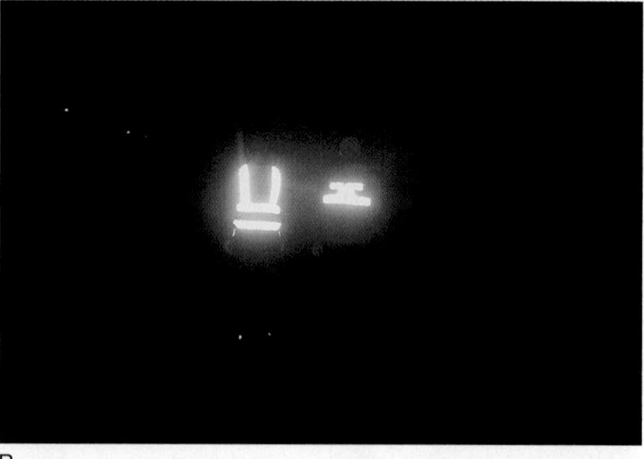
B

Figure 35-3 • EMTs working in traffic should be dressed for both daytime and nighttime visibility. Photo (A) shows EMTs dressed for daytime visibility. Photo (B) shows how the same clothing would appear in approaching headlights at night. *(Both: © Jon Politis)*

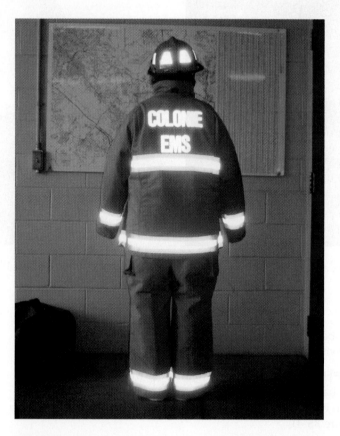

Figure 35-4 • Full turnout should be worn at an extrication. *(© Jon Politis)*

HEADGEAR Good head protection is essential. Trendy baseball caps, uniform hats, and wool watch caps do little except protect against sunlight, identify the wearer as a member of an emergency service, or keep the head warm. Plastic "bump caps" worn by butchers and warehouse workers also do not provide adequate protection.

One good piece of headgear that does offer adequate protection is the rescue helmet. The model shown in Figure 35-2 does not have the firefighter's helmet rear brim, which can be awkward in tight spaces, although many EMTs do prefer and use firefighters' helmets.

All helmets should be brightly colored with reflective stripes and lettering to make the wearer visible both day and night, and the Star of Life on each side to identify the wearer as an EMS provider. The level of training should also be indicated to make scene management easier when many EMS and rescue units are on hand.

EYE PROTECTION Eye protection is vital. Hinged plastic helmet shields do not provide adequate protection; flying particles can strike the eyes from underneath or from the side. Protection is best provided by safety goggles with a soft vinyl frame that conforms to the face and indirect venting to keep them fog-free, or safety glasses with large lenses and side shields.

HAND PROTECTION Because EMTs stick their hands into all sorts of unfriendly places, every EMT should have optimal hand protection. Good protection is afforded by wearing disposable vinyl or other synthetic gloves underneath either firefighter's gloves or leather gloves.

Firefighter's gloves will protect an EMT's hands from a variety of sharp, hot, cold, and dangerous surfaces. They are bulky, but can be worn in most rescue situations. If greater dexterity is needed, intermediate-weight leather gloves can be worn. Fabric garden or work gloves are too thin to offer adequate protection.

BODY PROTECTION An EMT will often protect head, eyes, and hands and leave the body virtually unprotected. Light shirts or nylon jackets should never be allowed inside the inner circle because they do little to protect from jagged metal, broken glass, or flash fires.

Good upper body protection is offered by wearing either a short or mid-length turnout coat that meets Occupational Safety and Health Administration (OSHA) requirements. A heavy duty EMS or rescue jacket can be used to protect you from weather and minor injury. As with helmets, bright colors and reflective material will help make your jacket more visible.

Good lower body protection can be provided by wearing either turnout pants with cuffs wide enough to pull over work shoes or fire-resistant trousers or jumpsuits. Serious consideration should be given to wearing high-top, steel toe work shoes with extended tops to protect the ankles.

Safeguarding Your Patient from Hazards

When your patients have been injured in a collision, it is your responsibility to see to it that further injuries are not inflicted during the rescue operation. You can minimize the chance of such additional injuries by shielding the patient and exercising care. The following items can be used to protect the patient from heat, cold, flying particles, and other hazards:

- *An aluminized rescue blanket* offers protection from weather and, to a degree, from flying particles. A paper blanket does not afford this protection; it merely hides the patient's view of the debris that is about to strike him.
- *A lightweight vinyl-coated paper tarpaulin* can protect from weather.
- *A wool blanket* should be used to protect from cold. Cover the wool blanket with an aluminized blanket or a salvage cover whenever glass must be broken near a patient, since glass particles are just about impossible to remove from wool blankets.
- *Short and long spine boards* can shield a patient from contact with tools and debris.
- *Hard hats, safety goggles, industrial hearing protectors, disposable dust masks, and thermal masks* (in cold weather—and unless the patient has airway or breathing problems or is on oxygen) will protect a patient's head, eyes, ears, and respiratory passages.

Managing Traffic Hazards

Collisions almost always produce traffic problems. Often the wreckage blocks lanes of traffic. Even if it does not, backups are caused when curious drivers slow down to "rubberneck," or stare at the scene. Rescuers, firefighters, and police usually handle traffic control. However, what if the ambulance EMTs are responding alone or ahead of other emergency service units?

Obviously, personal safety, rescue, and emergency care have priority. However, an ambulance crew should still initiate basic traffic control, channeling vehicles past the scene. Remember to be extremely watchful and careful when you work to control traffic to be sure that you are not struck by an approaching or passing vehicle.

Your ambulance with its warning lights will serve as the first form of traffic control. However, you should position other warning devices as soon as possible. Bad weather, darkness, vegetation, and curved or hilly roadways may keep approaching motorists from seeing your ambulance soon enough to stop safely.

Using Flares for Traffic Control

Although some argue that flares are unsafe, when used properly they are still a good device for warning motorists of dangerous conditions. Moreover, several dozen flares can be carried behind the front seat of an ambulance, while battery-powered flashing lights—an alternative to flares—take up valuable compartment space.

Scan 35-1 shows the proper positioning of flares at collision scenes, including a straight road, a curved road, and a hill. Keep in mind that the stopping distance for large trucks is much greater than for cars. When the road carries truck traffic, extend the flare strings beyond the distances shown.

Remember the following points when you place flares:

- Look for and avoid spilled fuel, dry vegetation, and other combustibles before you ignite and position flares, especially at a road edge.
- Do not throw flares out of moving vehicles.
- Position a few flares at the edge of the danger zone as soon as the ambulance is parked. They will supplement the ambulance warning lights.
- Take a handful of flares and walk (carefully) toward oncoming traffic.
- Position the flares every 10 feet, if possible, to channel vehicles into an unblocked lane. (Do not turn your back to traffic while placing flares.)
- If the collision has occurred on a two-lane road, position flares in both directions.
- Never use a flare as a traffic wand; flares can spew molten phosphorous, which can cause third-degree burns to the skin.

Controlling Spectators

Spectators do more than just create problems for passing motorists. If allowed to wander freely, they will close in on the wreckage just to get a better view. They may get so close that they interfere with rescue and emergency care efforts.

Rescue squads, police, and fire units have personnel and equipment for crowd control; ambulances usually do not. However, an EMT can usually initiate some crowd-control measures. If local policies permit it, ask for assistance from one or more responsible-looking bystanders. Ask the persons you recruit to keep the spectators away from the danger zone. Give them a roll of barricade tape if you have one. Be sure not to put the recruited personnel in unsafe positions such as near spilled fuel or an unstable vehicle.

Coping with Electrical Hazards

Electricity poses many dangers at vehicle-collision scenes. When there is an electrical hazard, establish a danger zone and a safe zone. The danger zone should only be entered by individuals responsible for controlling the hazard, such as power company personnel or specialty rescue. The safe zone should be sufficiently far away to ensure that an arcing or moving wire could not possibly injure any of the rescue personnel or bystanders.

Keep in mind the safety points in the following list. Many have to do with taking precautions around conductors. A conductor is a wire or any other object or material that will carry electricity.

SCAN 35-1 • Positioning Flares to Control Traffic

Posted speed (mph)	*Stopping distance for that speed*		*Posted speed (in feet)*		*Distance of the farthest warning device*
20 mph	50 feet	+	20 feet	=	70 feet
30 mph	75 feet	+	30 feet	=	105 feet
40 mph	125 feet	+	40 feet	=	165 feet
50 mph	175 feet	+	50 feet	=	225 feet
60 mph	275 feet	+	60 feet	=	335 feet
70 mph	375 feet	+	70 feet	=	445 feet

Flares are positioned according to a formula that includes the stopping distance for the posted speed plus a margin of safety.

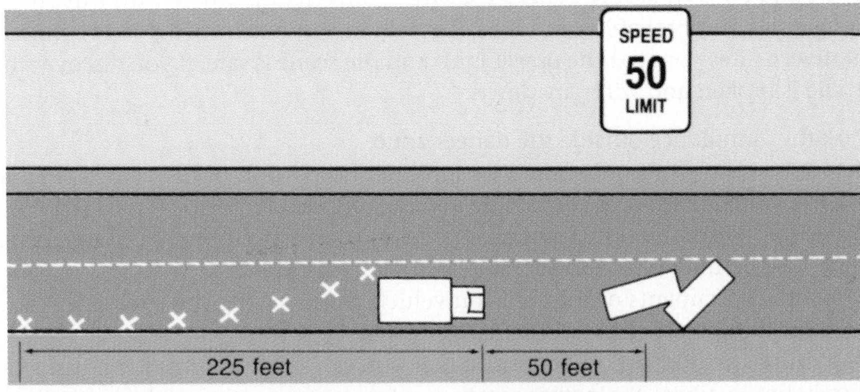

Flares positioned on a straight road. Approaching vehicles are moved into the correct lane before they reach the edge of the danger zone.

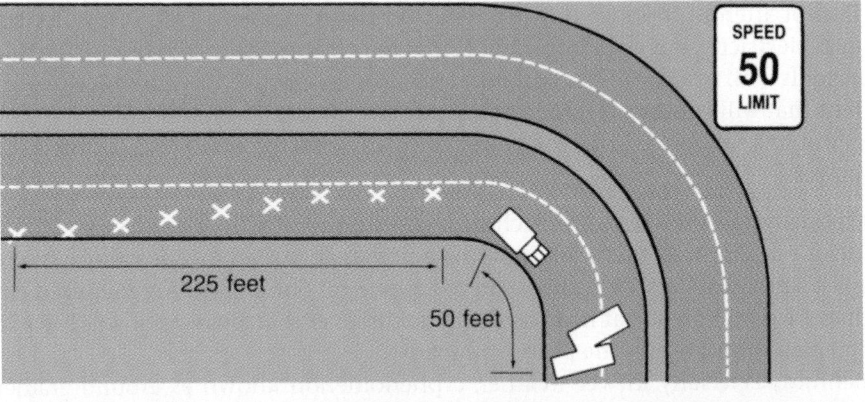

Flares positioned ahead of a curved section of road. The start of the curve is considered to be the edge of the danger zone.

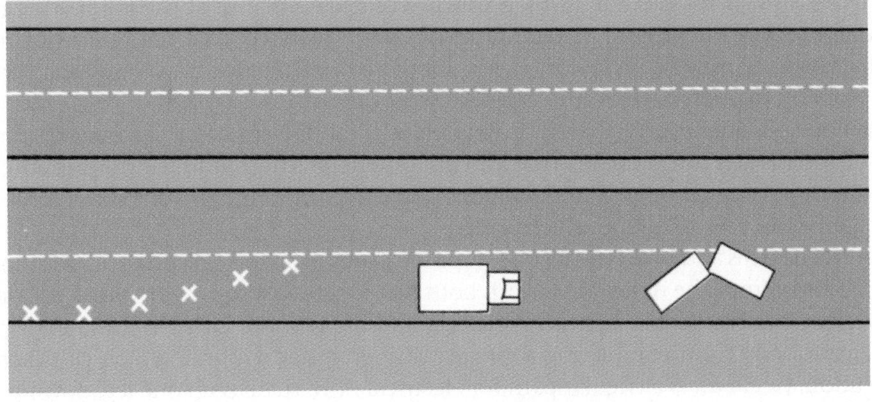

Flares positioned on a hill. The flares slow approaching vehicles and make them turn into the correct lane before they reach the top of the hill.

- High voltages are not as uncommon on roadside utility poles as people often think. In some areas, wood poles support conductors of as much as 500,000 volts.
- Assume that the entire area is extremely dangerous. Conductors may have touched and energized any part of the system, including electrical, telephone, cable TV, and other wires supported by the utility pole, guy wires, ground wires, the pole itself, the ground surrounding the pole, and nearby guard rails and fences. Assume that severed or displaced conductors may be touching and energizing every wire and conductor at the highest voltage present. Dead wires may be re-energized at any moment. Energized conductors may arc to the ground.
- Ordinary protective clothing does not protect against electrocution.

Remembering these points and the following procedures may keep you alive at the scene of a collision where unconfined electricity is a hazard.

BROKEN UTILITY POLE WITH WIRES DOWN A broken utility pole with wires down is very dangerous. You probably cannot work safely in the area until a power company representative assures you that the power is off and the scene is safe. If you discover that a utility pole is broken and wires are down:

- Park the ambulance outside the danger zone.
- Before you leave the ambulance, be sure that no portion of the vehicle, including the radio antenna, is contacting any sagging conductors.
- Order spectators and nonessential emergency service personnel from the danger zone. Use perimeter tape to set up a large safety zone.
- Discourage occupants of the collision vehicle from leaving the wreckage.
- Prohibit traffic flow through the danger zone.
- Determine the number of the nearest pole you can safely approach, and ask your dispatcher to advise the power company of the pole number and location.
- Do not attempt to move downed wires. Metal implements will, of course, conduct electricity, but even implements that may not appear to be conductive, such as tools with wood handles or natural fiber ropes, may have a high moisture content that will conduct electricity and may electrocute a well-intentioned rescuer.
- Stand in a safe place until the power company cuts the wires or disconnects the power.

Be especially careful when approaching a collision located in a dark area such as a rural roadside at night. As you walk from the ambulance, sweep the area ahead of you, to each side and overhead, with the beam of a powerful hand light. An energized conductor may be dangling just at head level. If you discover that a wire is down, leave the area immediately and notify the power company.

Sometimes, especially in wet weather, a phenomenon known as ground gradient may provide your first clue that a wire is down. Voltage is greatest at the point where a conductor touches the ground, then diminishes with distance from the point of contact. That distance may be several inches or many feet. Being able to recognize and respond properly to energized ground can save your life.

Stop your approach immediately if you feel a tingling sensation in your legs and lower torso. This sensation means that you are on energized ground. Current is entering one foot, passing through your lower body, and exiting through your other foot. If you continue on, you risk being electrocuted!

Turn 180 degrees and take one of two escape measures. Hop to a safe place on one foot. Or shuffle away from the danger area with both feet together, allowing no break in contact between your two feet or between your feet and the ground. Either technique helps prevent your body from completing a circuit with energized ground, which can cause electrocution. (A circuit is a circular path for electrical flow, such as up one leg, down the other, and through the ground. Hopping on one leg or keeping your feet together creates a straight path rather than a circular circuit, which may prevent electrocution.)

BROKEN UTILITY POLE WITH WIRES INTACT Even if wires are intact, a broken utility pole is still dangerous. Wires that are still holding up the pole can break at any time, dropping the pole and wires onto the scene. If you arrive to find such a situation:

- Park the ambulance outside the danger zone.
- Notify your dispatcher of the situation.
- Stay outside the danger zone until power company representatives can de-energize the conductors and stabilize the pole.
- Keep spectators and other emergency service personnel out of the danger zone.

DAMAGED PAD-MOUNTED TRANSFORMER When electrical cables run underground, the transformer may be mounted on a pad above ground (Figure 35-5). When an above-ground pad-mounted electrical transformer is struck and damaged, it poses a serious threat. In such a situation:

- Request an immediate power company response.
- Do not touch either the transformer case or a vehicle touching it, and warn other emergency service personnel not to touch it, either.
- Stand in a safe place until the power company de-energizes the transformer.
- Keep spectators out of the danger zone.

Coping with Vehicle Fires

When you find a vehicle on fire, always request the response of firefighting apparatus. Do not assume that someone else has called the fire department. In fact, an engine should always stand by at a vehicle rescue.

Extinguishing a vehicle fire is the responsibility of persons who are trained and equipped for the job: firefighters. Nonetheless, there are some measures that trained EMTs can take when they arrive before fire units (Scan 35-2).

For small fires, a 15- or 20-pound class A:B:C dry chemical fire extinguisher can extinguish virtually anything that may be burning in a vehicle, including upholstery, fuel, and electrical components. Only burning magnesium and other flammable metals cannot be extinguished by an A:B:C extinguisher. Before you try to put out a fire, always put on a full set of protective gear.

FIRE IN THE ENGINE COMPARTMENT If the hood is fully open, stand close to an A-post (front roof-supporting post) of the vehicle and, if possible, with your back to the wind to guard against the agent blowing back into your face or entering the passenger compartment. (Dry chemical extinguishing agents irritate respiratory passages and may contaminate open wounds.) Then sweep the extinguisher across the base of the fire with short bursts. Use no more than necessary to extinguish the fire. You will need what is left if there is a subsequent flare-up.

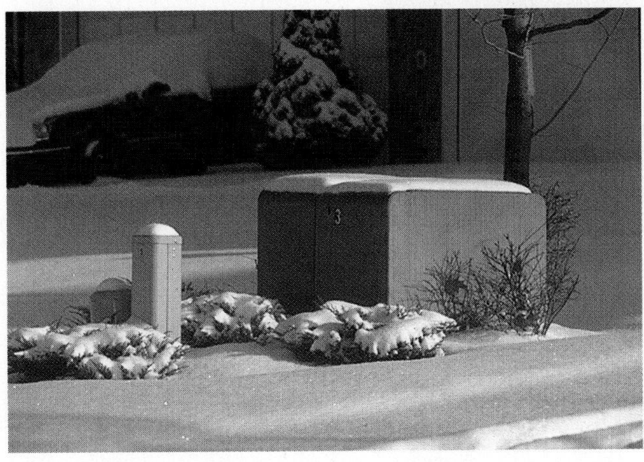

Figure 35-5 • A pad-mounted transformer, if damaged, poses a serious threat.

SCAN 35-2 • Extinguishing Fires in Collision Vehicles

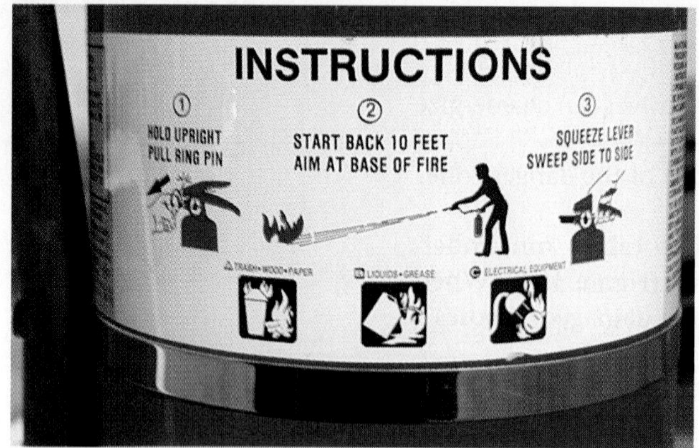

Markings that identify an extinguisher that can be used for Class A, B, and C fires.

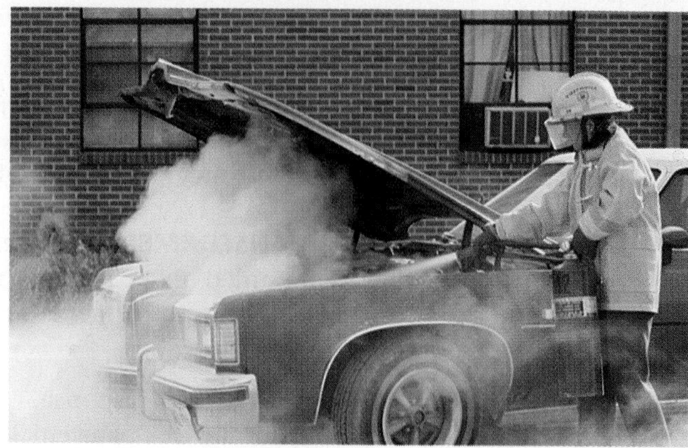

Extinguishing a fire in the engine compartment when the hood is fully open.

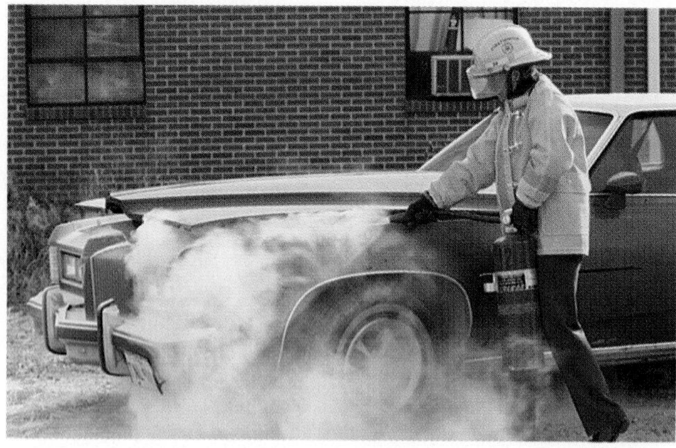

Extinguishing a fire in the engine compartment when the hood is partially open.

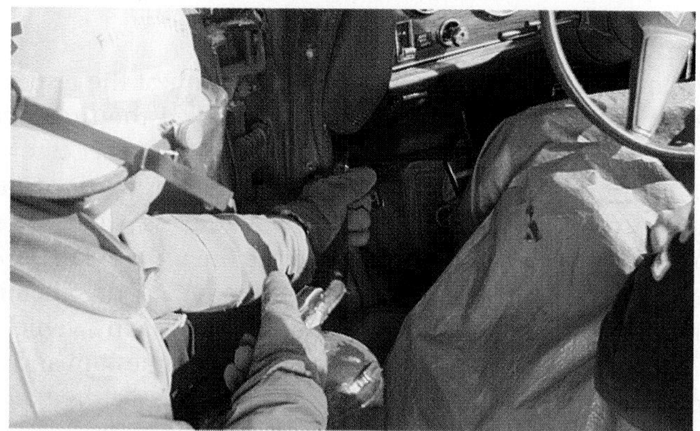

Extinguishing a fire under the dash. Care must be taken not to fill the vehicle's interior with a cloud of agent.

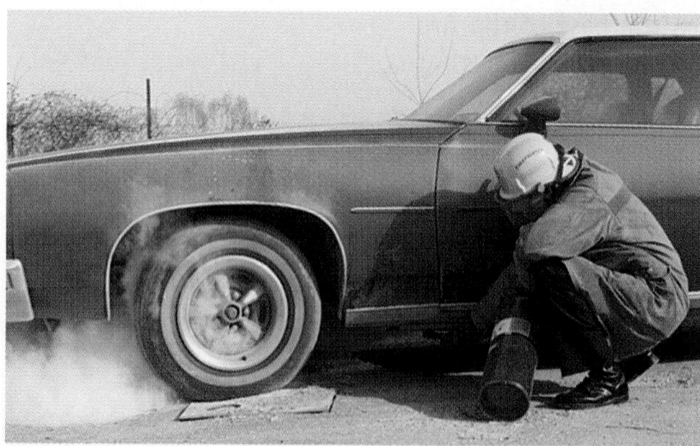

Extinguishing fuel burning under a vehicle. Flames are swept away from the vehicle.

If the hood is open to the safety latch, do not raise the hood farther—leave it where it is. This will help to restrict air flow and deprive the fire of oxygen. Then direct the agent through any opening to the engine compartment: between hood and fender, around the grill, under a wheel well, or through a broken head lamp assembly. Again, use no more agent than is needed.

If the hood is closed tight, let the fire burn under the closed hood, leaving its extinguishment to the fire department, and continue to get the patients out of the vehicle. The firewall should protect the passenger area long enough to get the patients out of the vehicle, using emergency moves.

FIRE IN THE PASSENGER COMPARTMENT OR TRUNK If the fire is under the dash or in upholstery or other combustibles, carefully apply the agent directly to the burning material. Apply sparingly to avoid creating a cloud of powder that may be harmful to occupants. If there is fire in the trunk, as with fire under a closed hood, leave extinguishment to the fire department and continue working to get patients out of the vehicle.

FIRE UNDER THE VEHICLE Using a portable unit to extinguish burning fuel under a vehicle may be an exercise in futility when the spill is large. But when people are trapped in the vehicle, you may feel you must try. Attempt to sweep the flames from under the passenger compartment as you apply the agent. If you do extinguish the fire, be sure that sources of ignition are then kept away. The vehicle's own catalytic converter (usually found in the area under the front passenger's feet) can be an ignition source since its temperature can reach over 1,200 degrees.

TRUCK FIRES An A:B:C extinguisher can also be used to combat truck fires. Be aware, however, that burning truck tires are especially dangerous. Flames can quickly spread to the body of the vehicle and its cargo, or the tires can blow apart when heated by fire. NEVER stand directly in front of a truck wheel when there is a fire; approach from a 45-degree angle.

NOTE *At times you will find that fuel is leaking from a damaged vehicle but is not on fire. If you discover that a fuel tank is leaking, call for fire department response. The decision to continue the rescue effort should be governed by your perception of the danger. You should not be expected to continue rescue operations if gasoline is pooled under the vehicle or flowing toward a source of ignition. Warn spectators away from flowing fuel. Do not use flares near spilled fuel or in the path of flowing fuel. Watch where you park your vehicle, as your ambulance's catalytic converter can easily ignite spilled fuel or other combustibles.*

Coping with a Vehicle's Electrical System

Many rescue units routinely disable the electrical system of every collision vehicle by cutting a battery cable. This was a reasonable practice years ago when vehicles had more combustible materials and when wiring did not have self-extinguishing insulation. Today, however, the situation is different. Unless gasoline is pooled under a vehicle or undeployed air bags need to be disabled, cutting the battery out of the electrical system may not only be a waste of time, it may actually hinder the rescue operation. Remember that many cars have electrically powered door locks, window operators, and seat adjustment mechanisms. Being able to lower a window rather than breaking it eliminates the likelihood of spraying occupants with glass. Being able to operate door locks may eliminate the need to force doors open. And being able to operate a powered seat will create space in front of an injured driver.

If there is reason to disrupt the electrical system, disconnect the ground cable from the battery. In this way, you will not be likely to produce a spark that can drop onto spilled fuel or ignite battery gases. Such a spark can be created when the positive cable is pulled away from the battery terminal, or when a tool touches a metal component while in contact with the positive terminal or cable.

Stabilizing a Vehicle

Unstable collision vehicles pose a hazard to rescuers and patients alike. Scan 35-3 shows methods for stabilizing a vehicle involved in a collision.

NOTE

Rescuers often fail to stabilize a collision vehicle because it appears to be stable. Rather than taking the chance of incorrectly "reading" a collision vehicle's stability—and having the vehicle move during rescue with disastrous results—you should consider any collision vehicle from which patients need to be extricated to be unstable and act accordingly.

If your ambulance is equipped with stabilization equipment, you should attend a formal vehicle rescue course that includes basic stabilization procedures taught by a qualified instructor. If the ambulance is not equipped for stabilization procedures, or if you are not trained, stand by until a rescue unit has stabilized the vehicle, even if roof posts are intact and the vehicle appears to be stable.

The information on vehicle stabilization that follows is intended only to help you, as an EMT, understand the process that trained personnel will be following. It is not a substitute for formal training in stabilization procedures.

Vehicle on Its Wheels

A collision vehicle that is upright on four inflated tires looks stable. However, it is easily rocked up and down, side to side, and back and forth on its suspension as rescuers climb into and over it. These motions can seriously aggravate occupants' injuries. First, if rescuers have access to the inside of the vehicle, they should make sure the engine is turned off, the vehicle is in park, the keys are removed from the ignition, and the parking brake is set. The best method of stabilizing a vehicle on its wheels is using three step chocks, one on each side and a third under the front or back of the vehicle.

Then—in situations where significant "tool work" must be done to extricate, such as door or roof removal—all the tires should be deflated. This can be accomplished by simply pulling the valve stems from their casing with pliers. (Slashing the tires is an inappropriate technique for deflating tires.) A police officer should be told the tires have been deflated so investigators will not think that the tires are flat as a result of the collision.

NOTE

Tires do not need to be deflated in all crashes—only in situations where significant "tool work," such as door or roof removal, must be done to extricate a patient or patients.

A listing of the equipment that can be carried to accomplish vehicle stabilization and gaining access is listed in Table 35-1. If the ambulance is not equipped with step chocks, a degree of stabilization can be accomplished by placing wheel chocks or 2″ × 4″ cribbing in front of and behind two tires on the same side.

If a car has rolled over several times and come to rest on its wheels, the roof may be crushed, which may preclude access through windows. The roof may need to be raised before doors can be opened or the roof can be removed.

Vehicle on Its Side

When a vehicle is on its side, spectators will often attempt to push it back onto its wheels. They fail to realize that this movement may injure, or more severely injure, occupants of the vehicle. Instead, the vehicle should be stabilized on its side. If the vehicle is on its side, do not attempt to gain access before it is stabilized using ropes, stabilization struts, and/or cribbing. While a car on its side may appear stable, simply climbing onto one side in an attempt to open a door may cause the vehicle to drop onto its roof or wheels. Moreover, you can be trapped under the vehicle when it topples.

NOTE

When placing cribbing, NEVER kneel on both knees. Always squat, so you can quickly move away from the vehicle if you have to. Once the vehicle is stabilized, if a door must be opened, tie it in the fully open position before you try to crawl inside.

A person who will act as a safety guide can be placed at each end of the vehicle to "feel" the movement of the vehicle and quickly warn the rescuers placing cribbing, struts, or ropes to get back if the vehicle begins to fall over. Some services will deploy two ropes looped around the same wheel in both directions so that personnel can temporarily hold the vehicle stable while struts and/or cribbing are placed. There are many

SCAN 35-3 • Stabilizing Vehicles Involved in a Collision

Stabilizing a car on its wheels with cribbing while patient contact is initiated.

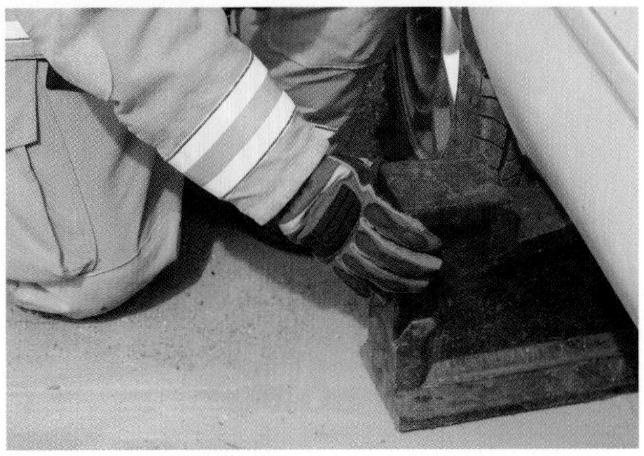

A vehicle on its side stabilized with cribbing.

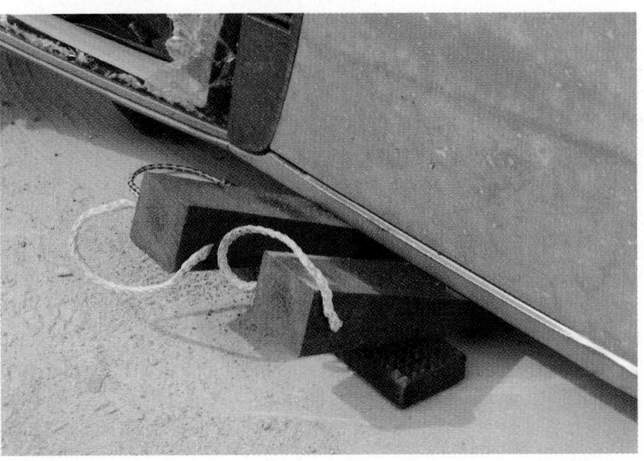

Placing a step chock. Keep hands clear of the vehicle while placing the chock.

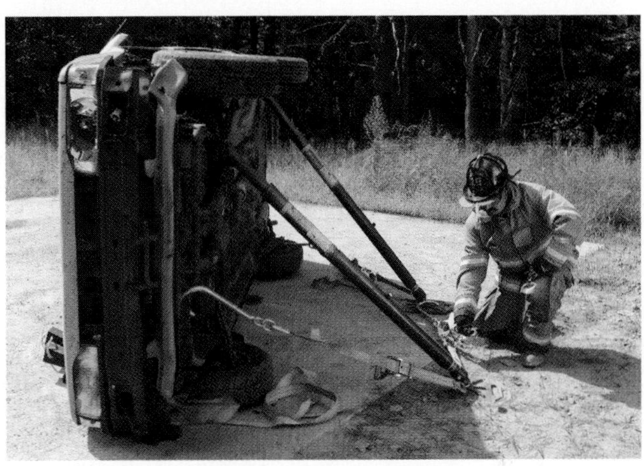

A vehicle on its side stabilized with struts.

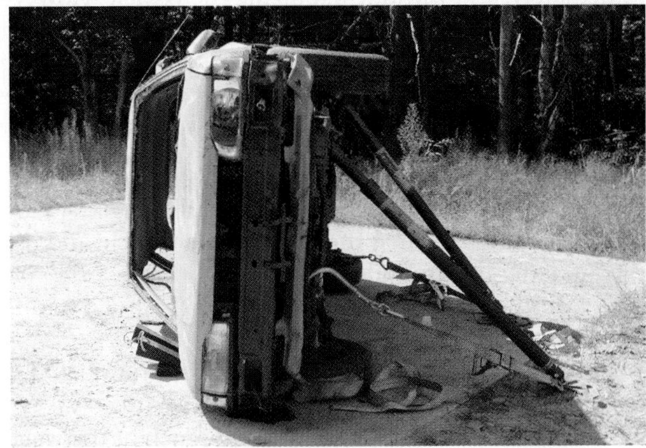

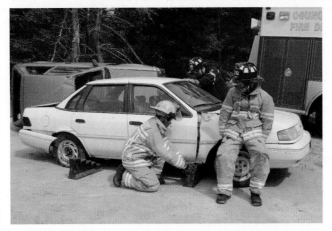

A vehicle on its side stabilized with cribbing and struts.

TABLE 35-1 • Supplies and Equipment for Vehicle Stabilization and Gaining Access

QUANTITY	ITEM	
10	2″ × 4″ × 8″ cribbing	
10	4″ × 4″ × 18″ cribbing	
4	Step chocks	
6	Wood wedges	
2	Vehicle wheel chocks	
100 feet	Nylon $^{1}/_{2}$″ utility rope	
2 sets	Struts	
1	"Door-and-window kit" with hand tools such as. . .	
	1	pair, battery pliers
	1	12″ adjustable wrench
	1	3- or 4-pound drilling hammer
	1	spring-loaded center punch
	2	hacksaws with spare blades
	1	10″ locking-type pliers
	1	10″ water-pump pliers
	Several	12″ to 15″ flat prybars
	1	8″ flat blade screwdriver
	1	12″ flat blade screwdriver
	1	spray container of power steering fluid as a lubricant
1	Flathead ax	
1	Glas-Master windshield saw	
1	Combination forcible entry tool such as a Halligan or Biel tool	
500 feet	Perimeter tape	

ways to stabilize a vehicle on its side, from using manpower alone to using hydraulic rams and pneumatic jacks. The objective is to increase the number of contacts with the ground to make the vehicle on its side more stable.

Vehicle on Its Roof

If the vehicle is resting on its roof, roof posts are intact, and the vehicle appears stable, it may be tempting to try to reach the vehicle's occupants by gaining access through window or door openings—immediately, and without stabilizing the vehicle. However, if the posts collapse, as is often the case when the windshield integrity has been broken, the vehicle may come crashing down and injure the EMT who is attempting to climb into the vehicle or who has an arm in a window opening. You must wait to gain access until the rescue crew has stabilized the vehicle. This is usually accomplished by building a box crib with 4 × 4s under the vehicle.

A vehicle on its roof is likely to be in one of four positions:

- Horizontal, with the roof crushed flat against the body of the vehicle and both the trunk lid and hood contacting the ground
- Horizontal, resting entirely on the roof, with space between the hood and the ground and space between the trunk lid and the ground
- Front end down, with the front edge of the hood contacting the ground and the rear of the car supported by the C-posts (rear posts)
- Front end up, with the trunk lid contacting the ground and much of the weight of the vehicle supported by the A-posts (front posts)

If the vehicle is tilted with the engine, which is the heaviest part of the vehicle, on the ground and the trunk in the air, it can often be stabilized by using two step chocks upside down under the trunk.

When the roof is crushed flat against the body, as when all the roof posts have collapsed, the car is essentially a steel box resting on the ground with the occupants completely trapped inside. Unless the vehicle is on a hill or perched precariously on debris or another vehicle, this is the one time when stabilization is unnecessary. The structure is rigid. In such a situation it may be impossible to gain access through a window, door, or the roof. However, it may be possible to cut through the floor pan and have an EMT either crawl inside, if the opening is big enough or the EMT small enough, or to reach through the opening to touch and offer emotional support to the occupants until rescue personnel can lift or open the vehicle.

If the vehicle is unstable and cannot be safely approached by an EMT, get as close as you safely can so you can talk or signal to the occupants to reassure them that help is on its way and begin getting an idea of their condition.

Remember that when the vehicle is found in any of the positions described previously, it should be considered unstable and must be stabilized by trained personnel prior to entry by an EMT.

Gaining Access

The National Highway Safety Act of 1966 required states to improve prehospital emergency care capabilities. It was recognized that EMS personnel could not do much for collision victims who could not be extricated from vehicles in time for life-saving efforts to be effective. Therefore, vehicle rescue training courses were developed, and bigger and better-equipped rescue units were placed in service.

Training courses began to prepare EMS personnel for a wide range of collision scene rescue activities aimed at gaining access to patients: unlocking and unlatching doors with commercially available and homemade tools, removing windshields intact, using hydraulic rescue tools to open vehicle doors one at a time, and so on.

Problems did not start to plague the rescue services until the mid-1980s. Suddenly extrications were taking longer, powerful rescue tools did not seem to be working properly, and procedures that had worked well for years were no longer successful. The reason for this apparent backslide? Improved vehicle construction.

For example, the Nader pin (named for Ralph Nader, the consumer advocate who lobbied for the device) is a case-hardened pin in an automobile door. In a collision, the cams in the door locks grasp the pin to keep the door from flying open. Prior to the Nader pin, rescue personnel could open a door with a crowbar. Subsequently, rescuers had to start using a hydraulic spreader to peel the cams off the pins. Safety features designed to keep occupants inside wrecked vehicles were keeping rescuers out! Each new safety improvement to vehicles created a new challenge to rescue personnel.

Vehicle rescue training was becoming a complicated business, and rescuers were being asked to learn dozens of techniques, some of which could be used only on certain models of cars. The need for effective but simplified procedures became evident. The next few pages will describe a procedure that has been developed to meet this need.

Simple Access

First remember that, as an EMT, your responsibility is not the rescue of the vehicle but the rescue of the patient. You will usually assume that an occupant or occupants of the vehicle have sustained life-threatening injuries, and that at least one EMT needs to gain quick access to the patient, even while rescuers are working to gain a more wide-open access, create exitways, and disentangle occupants.

After the vehicle is stable enough for you to approach it safely, check to see if a door can be opened or if an occupant of the vehicle can roll down a window or unlock a door. (Try Before You Pry!) Such ordinary ways of getting into the vehicle are known as simple access.

Complex Access

If simple access fails, you may need to use tools or special equipment to break a window and gain access even while the rescue crew is dismantling the vehicle for extrication of the occupants. When tools or equipment are used for this purpose, the process is known as complex access.

All automotive glass is one of two types: laminated or tempered. Windshields and some side and rear van and truck windows are laminated safety glass—two sheets of plate glass bonded to a sheet of tough plastic like a glass-and-plastic sandwich. Most passenger car side and rear windows are tempered glass. They are very resilient, but when they do break, rather than shattering into sharp fragments they break into small, rounded pieces.

You will usually try to gain access through a side or rear window as far as possible from the passengers. Use a spring-loaded center punch against a lower corner to break the glass (Figure 35-6). Punch out finger holds in the top of the window and use your gloved fingers to pull fragments away from the window.

A flathead ax is usually required to break through a windshield. This can also be done very quickly using a Glas-Master saw (Figure 35-7). A windshield is usually not broken to gain access, but the rescue squad may need to remove it if they plan to displace the dash or steering column or remove the roof. Before the windshield is broken, passengers should be covered with aluminized rescue blankets or tarps, if possible. Avoid the use of hospital-style blankets that will allow the tiny slivers of glass to pass through and come in contact with the patient.

Once an entry point is gained, at least one EMT, who is properly dressed, should crawl inside the vehicle and immediately begin the initial assessment and rapid trauma exam as well as manual cervical stabilization. Do not forget to explain what is going on and provide emotional support to the patient by talking and reassuring him that everything that can be done for him is being done. Access holes are usually small, so do not be tempted to pull a patient out of an access hole prior to spinal immobilization.

Disentanglement: A Three-Part Action Plan

In most instances, EMTs will not be directly involved in disentanglement other than acting as the patient's advocate and being the EMT inside the vehicle. However, it is helpful to understand the plan for complex access that may be used by rescue personnel to free the trapped patient.

Following is a description of a three-part procedure that can be accomplished by fire, rescue, and EMS personnel with the appropriate equipment. The procedure is not vehicle specific; that is, it can be used on virtually any car or truck. The procedure does not include a lot of techniques that require special equipment. Personnel can be trained in a short course. And, most important to EMS personnel, there is no need to fill several compartments of the ambulance with rescue equipment.

STEPS ONE AND TWO: GAIN ACCESS BY DISPOSING OF DOORS AND ROOF For more than 25 years, emergency service personnel have been trained to carry out a pro-

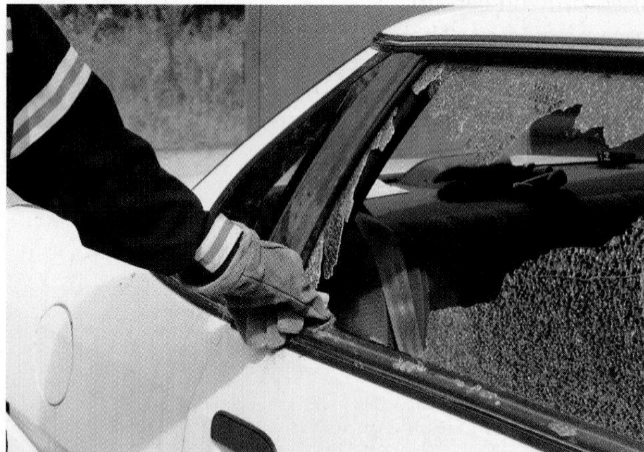

Figure 35-6 • Using a spring-loaded center punch to break the window glass.

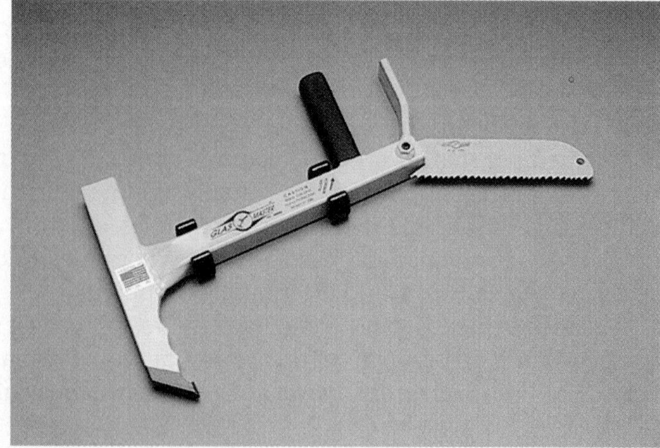

Figure 35-7 • A Glas-Master saw can aid in windshield removal.

gression of procedures to reach the occupants of a wrecked vehicle: first try the doors; if that fails, unlock and unlatch the doors by nondestructive or destructive means; when all else fails, gain access through window openings. This multipart procedure is time-consuming and requires a number of tools.

A quicker and far more efficient procedure is first to dispose of the doors and then to dispose of the roof as soon as hazards have been controlled and the vehicle is stable. Disposing of the doors and roof has three benefits:

- It makes the interior of the vehicle accessible. EMS personnel can stand beside or climb into the vehicle and pursue emergency care efforts while rescuers carry out disentanglement procedures.
- It creates a large exitway through which an occupant can be quickly removed when he has a life-threatening injury or when fire or another hazard is threatening the operation.
- It provides fresh air and helps cool off the patient when heat is a problem.

Scan 35-4 illustrates procedures for removing the doors and roof using hydraulic tools. If you don't have a hydraulic rescue tool, you can accomplish these procedures with ordinary hacksaws and a spray container of lubricant.

NOTE

After roof posts are cut and/or doors removed, ensure that all sharp edges are covered with appropriate protection to avoid injury to the rescuers and the patient.

STEP THREE: DISENTANGLE OCCUPANTS BY DISPLACING THE FRONT END Most vehicle rescue training courses include procedures for displacing or removing seats, dash assemblies, steering wheels, steering columns, and pedals. A quicker and more efficient way to disentangle an injured driver and/or passenger from these mechanisms of entrapment is to displace the entire front end of the vehicle. While the task sounds difficult, it is not. Scan 35-5 illustrates a procedure for displacing the front end of a passenger car with a hydraulic rescue tool. A dash displacement can also be accomplished with heavy duty jacks and hacksaws.

If the steering wheel hub is large and rectangular, the car probably has an air bag or bags (the passenger-side bag being in the glove compartment area). If the bags have not deployed, they are not likely to deploy now unless extrication involves displacing the dash or steering wheel. If such displacement is to be done, air bag manufacturers recommend following these guidelines:

- Avoid placing your body or objects against an air bag module or in its path of deployment.
- Disconnect the battery cables, starting with the negative terminal.

POINT OF VIEW

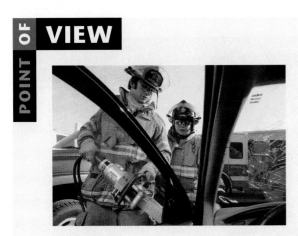

"I was driving along, minding my own business, when a truck pulled out from a side street in front of me. It was a horrible crash. I can still hear the loud crunch and breaking glass. I should say I can still feel *it. It was awful. My airbags went off. I was sitting in a cloud of dust.*

"I tried to get out and I couldn't. The door wouldn't open. Then I noticed that my ankle was killing me. My foot was wedged under the gas pedal.

"I was upset. OK, I was freaking out. In fact, I was pretty irrational when the ambulance got there. They tried to calm me down and told me the fire department was on the way to get me out. I was getting calmer until I saw and heard those giant whatchamacallits they were going to use to cut*—yes, cut—me out. Then they put a blanket over me so I'd be safe. I was never claustrophobic—until then. I don't mean to be a whiner, but that really shook me!*

"They got me out of the car on a board and into the ambulance, but by the time I got to the hospital I was shaking and spent. What an ordeal. I don't want to imply for a minute that the EMTs and firefighters were any less than professional. They were great. But let me tell you, that was a day I don't ever *want to live again.*

"Oh, no. I never thought about my car. I'll bet it's in pieces. Oh, no...."

SCAN 35-4 • Disposing of Doors and Roof

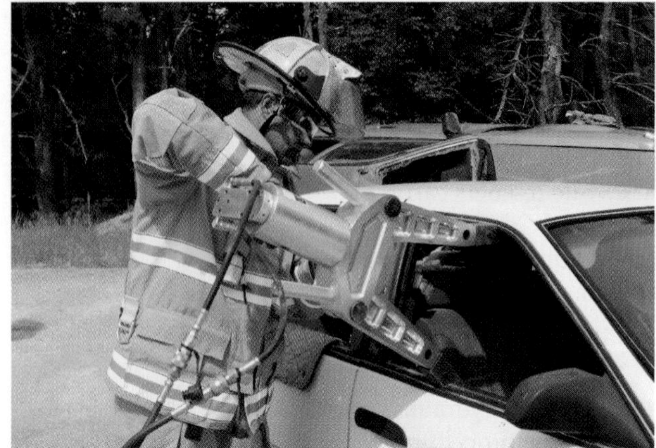

Displace the door to expose hinges and move the door away from the patient compartment.

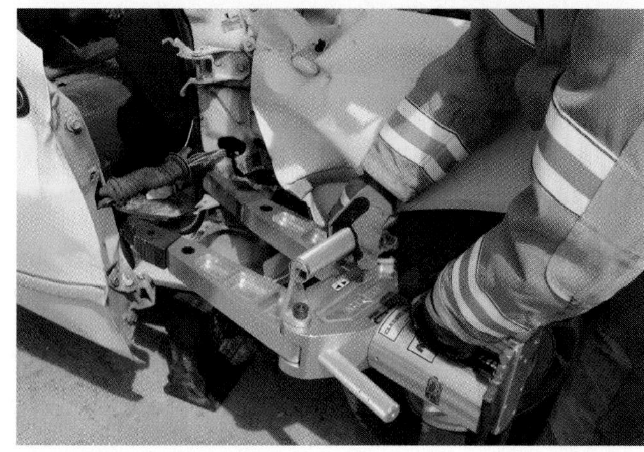

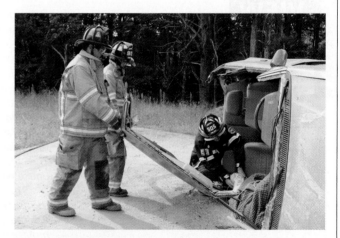

Remove the door.

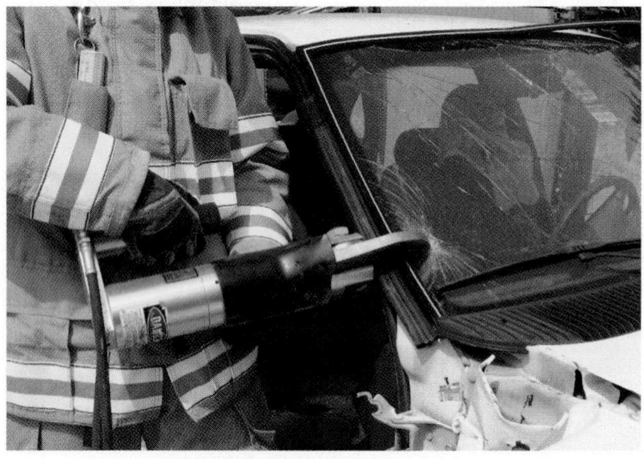

Cut the "A" post to begin roof removal.

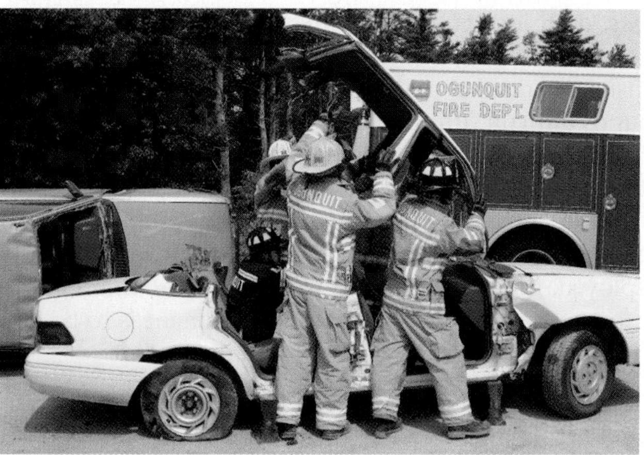

With "B" and "C" posts cut, roll the roof away while a rescuer enters the rear seat to stabilize the patient's head and neck.

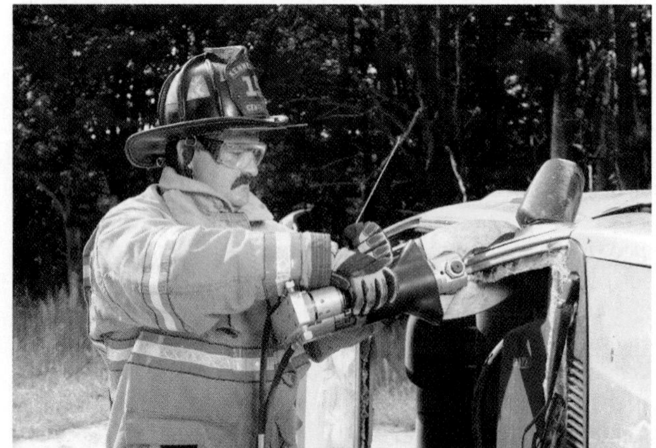

For a vehicle on its side, cut the posts.

Then remove the roof to expose and extricate the patient.

SCAN 35-5 • Displacing the Front End of a Car

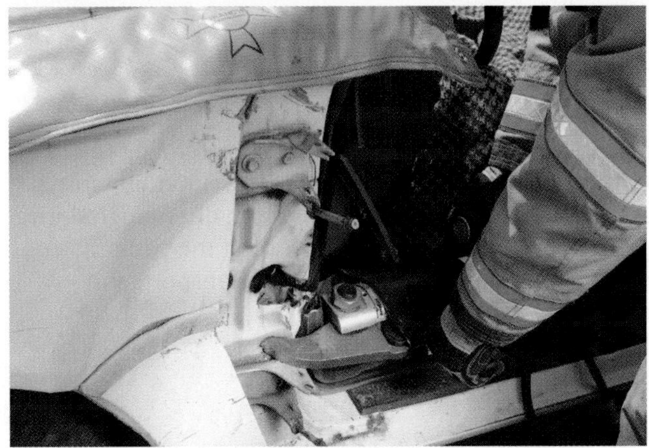

Make cuts for the spreader tool.

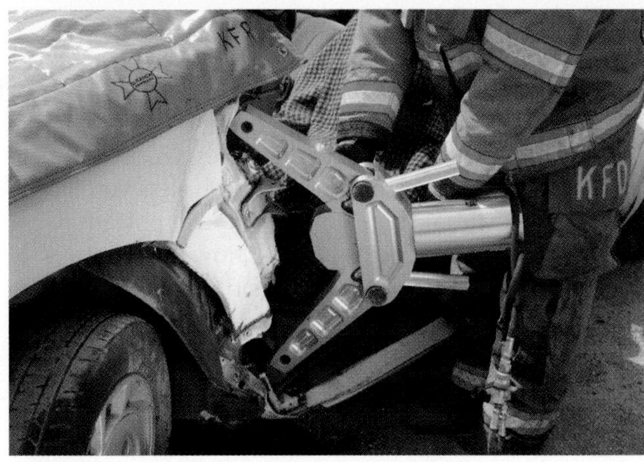

Use the spreader to roll back the dash.

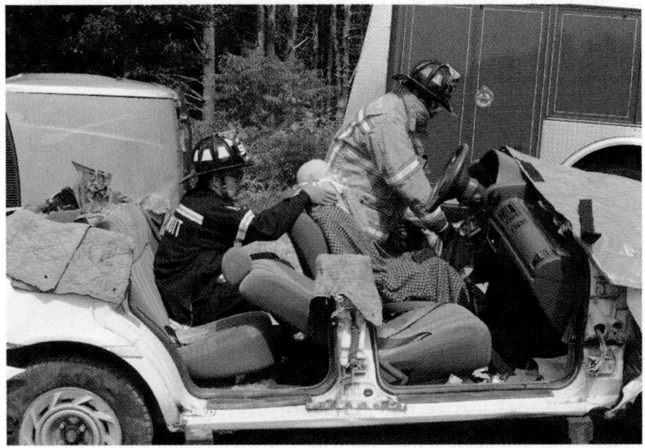

Displace the dashboard to gain access to the patient.

- Do not displace or cut the steering column until the system has been fully deactivated.
- Do not cut or drill into an air bag module.
- Do not apply heat in the area of the steering wheel hub.

Must the three-part procedure just described be used for all extrication operations? Must the three procedures always be accomplished in the same order? Must these procedures always be used? Not at all. In some cases, it may be necessary only to force a door open to reach a single patient and create an exitway for his removal. In other cases, it may be prudent to open doors before disposing of the roof or to dispose of the roof before displacing the doors. In still other situations, there may be no need to displace the front end of a collision vehicle.

The extent to which you, as an EMT, will participate in vehicle rescue procedures depends on the role your EMS unit plays in vehicle rescue and whether or not your ambulance arrives ahead of fire and rescue units. The main purpose for the EMT to know extrication procedures is to incorporate them into the patient care plan.

CHAPTER REVIEW

SUMMARY

As an EMT, you will not usually be responsible for vehicle or other kinds of rescue and extrication unless you undertake special training. However, it is important to understand how the process is done, how it may affect the patient, and how you can gain early access to the patient to begin care.

Vehicle extrication or rescue includes 10 phases: preparing for the rescue, sizing up the situation, recognizing and managing hazards, stabilizing the vehicle, gaining access to the patient, providing initial assessment and a rapid trauma exam, disentangling the patient, immobilizing and extricating the patient, providing ongoing assessment and transport, and terminating the rescue.

REVIEW QUESTIONS

1. Explain the role of the EMT in the size-up of a motor-vehicle collision. (pp. 940–941)
2. Discuss what the EMT should do upon arrival at a collision if a power pole is broken in half and the lines are down in the street. (p. 948)
3. Explain whom you should call for assistance in your community if, on size-up of a collision, you observe a truck turned on its side and leaking fuel. (p. 951)
4. Discuss ways to stabilize a vehicle that is resting on its wheels, a vehicle that is resting on its side, and a vehicle that is resting on its roof. (pp. 952–955)
5. Explain the difference between simple access and complex access to a patient in a vehicle. (pp. 955–956)

CRITICAL THINKING

- With knowledge of your own community, which of the ten types of rescue specialty teams are needed and who provides the service?
- After considering the safety of yourself and others, what should be your primary goal at the scene of a vehicle collision?

MEDIA RESOURCES

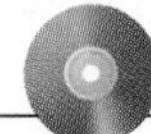

See the Student CD at the back of this book for quizzes, a case study activity, and other features related to this chapter. In particular, take a look at the Case Study regarding extrication and rescue operations. Also, visit the Companion Website for *Emergency Care* at **www.prenhall.com/limmer**, where you will find additional reinforcement and links to other resources.

Street Scenes

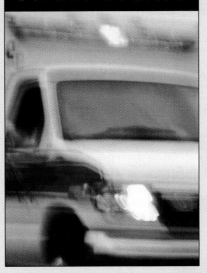

You're on the scene of a one-car crash into a telephone pole. You position the ambulance about 50 feet behind the crash site with warning lights on, and both you and your partner put on full turnout gear including helmet, gloves, eye protection, and a reflective vest.

To control traffic, your partner places flares over a 200-foot section leading to the scene. You look around to make sure that there are no wires in the area and none on the vehicle. The scene appears to be safe. You go to the patient, notice the passenger side is intruded 2 feet, and see only one passenger, the driver. Two wheels of the vehicle are up on the sidewalk and the car appears to be unstable. You identify yourself to the occupant but don't get a response. Next, you try to open the door, but it is jammed. The car must have spun around as you observe there is more damage on the driver's side of the vehicle. You advise dispatch that heavy rescue is needed.

Street Scene Questions

1. What are the scene safety issues that you need to address?
2. What techniques should you consider for extrication?

Heavy rescue has an ETA of 10 minutes. The patient isn't responding, so you and your partner agree that entry is needed now. First, you put blocks at the wheels to make sure the car doesn't shift. Next, you pick a spot on the window that seems to place the patient at lowest risk, use a punch, and start removing glass. Once inside, you observe that your patient is a male about 30 years old with snoring respirations. You perform an initial assessment and find he is only responsive to painful stimuli. The snoring respirations stop when you move his jaw forward and manually stabilize his head and neck, but his breathing remains irregular. You administer oxygen, and you suspect that you may need to start assisting respirations. At that moment, heavy rescue arrives and you report scene status and patient condition.

Street Scene Questions

3. Should rapid extrication be considered for this patient?
4. Describe assessment for this patient.

The lieutenant of heavy rescue tells you he will handle the battery disconnect and have his crew check to see if more cribbing is needed for vehicle stability. You maintain an airway and manual stabilization of the patient from inside the vehicle, while your partner applies a cervical collar and leaves to prepare the backboard. Rescue is able to pop a door open and allow full access to the patient. You are just about to say that the patient is clear when you see his foot is caught under a pedal. You tell the lieutenant from heavy rescue, and his crew sets up a small hydraulic jack. You make sure the patient is protected.

Once the foot is free, you and your partner decide that a rapid extrication is the best approach and move the patient to the board. When the patient is outside the vehicle, your partner is able to perform a rapid trauma assessment while you maintain manual stabilization. He checks the chest and it seems okay (the patient was wearing a seat belt).

The patient's respiration rate is about 28 and slightly irregular; ventilatory assistance is not needed yet. His pulse is 90 and regular. The patient is secured to the board and taken to the ambulance for further assessment and transport to the hospital. Considering the damage to the vehicle, the only injuries you find are a bump on the left side of the head and a swollen left ankle. By the time you get to the hospital, the patient is responding to verbal stimuli.

Later that day you are curious about this patient and call the hospital. The charge nurse tells you the patient suffered only a concussion and a bruised ankle and he will stay overnight for observation.

Street Scenes Sample Documentation

PATIENT NAME: *Malik Cooper* **PATIENT AGE:** *30*

CHIEF COMPLAINT

Unresponsiveness

PAST MEDICAL HISTORY

- [ ] None
- [ ] Allergy to
- [ ] Hypertension
- [ ] Stroke
- [ ] Seizures
- [ ] Diabetes
- [ ] COPD
- [ ] Cardiac
- [ ] Other (List)
- [ ] Asthma

Unknown

Current Medications (List)

Unknown

VITAL SIGNS

TIME	RESP	PULSE	B.P.	MENTAL STATUS	PUPILS (R / L)	SKIN
0010	Rate: 28 [ ] Regular [ ] Shallow [ ] Labored	Rate: 90 [X] Regular [ ] Irregular	120/76	[ ] Alert [ ] Voice [ ] Pain [✓] Unresp.	[✓] Normal [✓] [ ] Dilated [ ] [ ] Constricted [ ] [ ] Sluggish [ ] [ ] No-Reaction [ ]	[ ] Unremarkable [ ] Cool [ ] Pale [✓] Warm [ ] Cyanotic [ ] Moist [ ] Flushed [✓] Dry [ ] Jaundiced
0015	Rate: 28 [ ] Regular [ ] Shallow [X] Labored	Rate: 90 [X] Regular [ ] Irregular	124/76	[ ] Alert [✓] Voice [ ] Pain [ ] Unresp.	[✓] Normal [✓] [ ] Dilated [ ] [ ] Constricted [ ] [ ] Sluggish [ ] [ ] No-Reaction [ ]	[ ] Unremarkable [ ] Cool [ ] Pale [✓] Warm [ ] Cyanotic [ ] Moist [ ] Flushed [✓] Dry [ ] Jaundiced
	Rate: [ ] Regular [ ] Shallow [ ] Labored	Rate: [ ] Regular [ ] Irregular	/	[ ] Alert [ ] Voice [ ] Pain [ ] Unresp.	[ ] Normal [ ] [ ] Dilated [ ] [ ] Constricted [ ] [ ] Sluggish [ ] [ ] No-Reaction [ ]	[ ] Unremarkable [ ] Cool [ ] Pale [ ] Warm [ ] Cyanotic [ ] Moist [ ] Flushed [ ] Dry [ ] Jaundiced

NARRATIVE *Our patient is the victim of an apparent slow-moderate speed crash. He was restrained with a seatbelt. A witness reported the vehicle impacted on the driver's side door into a telephone pole. On our arrival, our patient is noted to be unresponsive with snoring respirations. Patient is accessed after forcible entry. We immediately maintained an airway, applied manual C-spine stabilization, and O_2 by nonrebreather mask. A rigid cervical collar is also applied prior to the arrival of heavy rescue. We determine this patient to be unstable. After a brief extrication, our patient is removed from the vehicle on a long backboard with appropriate manual stabilization. Patient has a bump on the left side of his head and a swollen left ankle, which was pinned down by the brake pedal. Once en route, we performed a quick reassessment. Patient's mental status improved to "verbal" during transport to the hospital.*

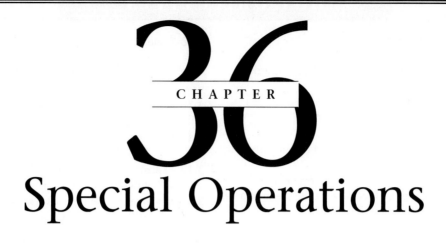

Special Operations

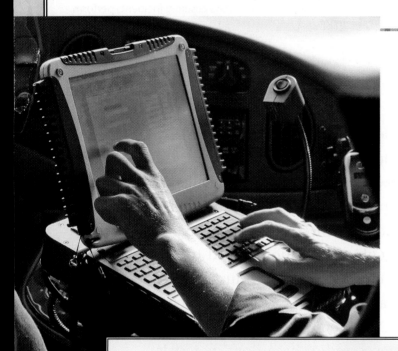

CORE CONCEPTS

The following are core concepts that will be addressed in this chapter:

- How to identify and take appropriate action in a hazardous-materials incident
- How to identify a multiple-casualty incident
- The role of an EMT at a multiple-casualty incident
- The incident command system

KEY TERMS

cold zone, p. 967
Command, p. 978
decontamination, p. 972
disaster plan, p. 977
hazardous material, p. 964
hot zone, p. 967
Incident Command, p. 978
Incident Command System (ICS), p. 977
multiple-casualty incident, p. 976
National Incident Management System (NIMS), p. 977
singular command, p. 978
staging area, p. 989
staging supervisor, p. 989
transportation supervisor, p. 990
treatment area, p. 987
treatment supervisor, p. 987
triage, p. 981
triage area, p. 987
triage supervisor, p. 981
triage tag, p. 987
unified command, p. 978
warm zone, p. 967

DOT OBJECTIVES

*KNOWLEDGE AND ATTITUDE

7-3.1 Explain the EMT's role during a call involving hazardous materials. (pp. 966–976)

7-3.2 Describe what the EMT should do if there is reason to believe that there is a hazard at the scene. (pp. 966–976)

7-3.3 Describe the actions that an EMT should take to ensure bystander safety. (pp. 966–967)

7-3.4 State the role that the EMT should perform until appropriately trained personnel arrive at the scene of a hazardous materials situation. (pp. 966–971)

7-3.5 Break down the steps to approaching a hazardous situation. (pp. 966–971)

7-3.6 Discuss the various environmental hazards that affect EMS. (pp. 966–971)

7-3.7 Describe the criteria for a multiple-casualty situation. (pp. 976–977)

7-3.8 Evaluate the role of the EMT in the multiple-casualty situation. (pp. 976–990)

7-3.9 Summarize the components of basic triage. (pp. 981, 983–989)

7-3.10 Define the role of the EMT in a disaster operation. (pp. 976–990)

7-3.11 Describe basic concepts of incident management. (pp. 977–981)

7-3.12 Explain the methods for preventing contamination of self, equipment, and facilities. (pp. 971–976)

7-3.13 Review the local mass casualty incident plan. (pp. 976–990)

*SKILLS

7-3.16 Given a scenario of a mass casualty incident, perform triage.

You have already learned how to deal with many situations in which an individual patient needs emergency care. However, you also need to know what to do if you are called to the scene of an explosion, an airline crash, a multiple vehicle pile-up, an earthquake, or other situation in which there may be many known or potential victims. Although you are not trained to deal with all the complexities of such emergencies, you must be able to recognize them and call for the appropriate assistance. This chapter offers the essentials that every EMT should know about special operations involving multiple patients and/or hazardous materials.

HAZARDOUS MATERIALS

Hazardous materials (hazmats) are everywhere, and EMS frequently responds to incidents involving them. Because many incidents begin as routine EMS calls, it will be up to you to recognize a hazmat early, be familiar with your local plan for management of a hazardous material incident, and understand your role in such an incident.

According to the U.S. Department of Transportation (DOT), a **hazardous material** is "any substance or material in a form which poses an unreasonable risk to health, safety, and property when transported in commerce." One of the undesirable aspects of our modern world is the growing number of such materials (Table 36-1). Hazardous materials are used for the manufacture of products and also can be the waste products of manufacturing. Even though safety procedures have been established and are followed for the most part, accidents involving hazardous materials do occur. Hazardous materials incidents are especially likely to take place at factories, along railroads, and on local, state, and federal highways.

hazardous material any substance or material in a form which poses an unreasonable risk to health, safety, and property when transported in commerce.

TABLE 36-1 • Examples of Hazardous Materials

MATERIAL	POSSIBLE HAZARD
Benzene (benzol)	Toxic vapors; can be absorbed through the skin; destroys bone marrow
Benzoyl peroxide	Fire and explosion
Carbon tetrachloride	Damages internal organs
Cyclohexane	Explosive; eye and throat irritant
Diethyl ether	Flammable and can be explosive; irritant to eyes and respiratory tract; can cause drowsiness or unconsciousness
Ethyl acetate	Irritates eyes and respiratory tract
Ethylene chloride	Damages eyes
Ethylene dichloride	Strong irritant
Heptane	Respiratory irritant
Hydrochloric acid	Respiratory irritant; exposure to high concentration of vapors can produce pulmonary edema; can damage skin and eyes
Hydrogen cyanide	Highly flammable; toxic through inhalation or absorption
Methyl isobutyl ketone	Irritates eyes and mucous membranes
Nitric acid	Produces a toxic gas (nitrogen dioxide); skin irritant; can cause self-ignition of cellulose products (e.g., sawdust)
Organochloride (Chlordane, DDT, Dieldrin, Lindane, Methoxyclor)	Irritates eyes and skin; fumes and smoke toxic
Perchloroethylene	Toxic if inhaled or swallowed
Silicon tetrachloride	Water-reactive to form toxic hydrogen chloride fumes
Tetrahydrofuran (THF)	Damages eyes and mucous membranes
Toluol (toluene)	Toxic vapors; can cause organ damage
Vinyl chloride	Flammable and explosive; listed as a carcinogen

As an EMT, you will be highly skilled in emergency care. However, without specialized training, you are still a layperson when it comes to hazardous materials. Special training is required to understand hazmats, to work at the scene of incidents involving these materials, and to render the scene safe. You cannot judge the state of a container or the probability of explosion without the benefit of such training. Do not believe that you can use safety equipment unless you are trained in the care, field testing, and use of the equipment. With hazmat incidents, you may be able to do nothing more than stay a safe distance away from the scene until expert help arrives.

Training Required by Law

Two federal agencies—the Occupational Safety and Health Administration (OSHA) and the Environmental Protection Agency (EPA)—have developed regulations to deal with the increasing frequency of hazmat emergencies. These regulations are meant to enhance the knowledge, skills, and safety of emergency response personnel, as well as to bring about a more effective response to hazmat emergencies. The regulations are described in the OSHA publication "29 CFR 1910.120—Hazardous Waste Operations and Emergency Response Standard."

According to the regulations, it is the responsibility of employers to determine, provide, and document the appropriate level of training for each employee. Training is required for "all employees who participate, or who are expected to participate, in emergency response to hazardous substance accidents."

The regulations identify four levels of training:

- *First Responder Awareness.* Rescuers at this level are likely to witness or discover a hazardous substance release. They are trained only to recognize the problem and initiate a response from the proper organizations. There are no minimum training hours required.
- *First Responder Operations.* This level of training is for those who initially respond to releases or potential releases of hazardous materials in order to protect people, property, and the environment. They stay at a safe distance, keep the incident from spreading, and protect others from any exposures. A minimum of 8 hours of training is required.
- *Hazardous Materials Technician.* This level is for rescuers who actually plug, patch, or stop the release of a hazardous material. A minimum of 24 hours of training is required.
- *Hazardous Materials Specialist.* This level of rescuer is expected to have advanced knowledge and skills and to command and support activities at the incident site. A minimum of 24 hours of additional training is required.

Most of the training levels outlined by OSHA have a fire-service focus. EMS responders should be trained to the awareness level and perhaps the operations level but in different skills. Responding to this difference, the National Fire Protection Association has published Standard #473, which deals with competencies for EMS personnel at hazardous materials incidents.

Regardless of agency affiliation, as an EMT you play an important role. You are usually among the first on the scene for all types of hazmat calls. Your initial decisions and actions lay crucial groundwork for the remainder of the incident.

Responsibilities of the EMT

Recognize a Hazmat Incident

Whether hazmat incidents are very obvious or very subtle, you must quickly recognize one for what it is. It helps to be aware of the locations where hazmats are likely. They include highway incidents involving common carriers, trucking terminals, chemical plants or places where chemicals are used, delivery trucks, agriculture and garden centers, railway incidents, and laboratories.

Every community has chemical hazards. Identification starts with awareness and knowledge of what exists in the community. Spend some time with local police and fire agencies. Learn about or develop preincident plans for common hazardous materials.

When you arrive at a potential incident, as an EMT you must restrain your natural impulse to take action. Never assume the scene is safe. After the initial patients, EMTs are the most likely to become injured or killed because they tend to react quickly. Therefore, assess the situation first. Take a command position and stay a safe distance from the site before you take action. Once a hazmat is recognized, only those personnel trained to the technician level and equipped with the proper personal protective equipment should enter the immediate site. All victims leaving the site of the incident should be considered contaminated until proven otherwise.

Control the Scene

As a responding EMT, you may be the first to recognize that a hazardous material situation exists. For example, you may answer a call to a business where four employees are ill after being in the warehouse. When there are multiple medical victims, "think hazmat."

Your primary concerns at the scene of a hazardous material incident are your safety and the safety of your crew, the patient, and the public. Should you arrive first at the scene of a hazardous material incident, establish a "danger zone" and a "safe zone." Keep all people out of the danger zone, and try to convince them to leave the immediate area. Stay in the safe zone until expert help arrives and makes other areas safe to enter.

The safe zone should be on the same level as, and upwind from, the hazardous material incident site. Avoid being downhill in case there are flowing liquids or gases that are burning or otherwise unsafe. Avoid low-lying areas in case fumes are escaping and hanging close to the ground. Avoid placing yourself higher than the accident scene so that you will not be in the path of escaping gases or heated air. Also be alert to the fact that a sewer system can rapidly spread hazardous materials over a large area.

Call for the help that you will need. The support services required at the scene of a hazardous material accident may include fire services, special rescue personnel, local or state hazardous materials experts, and law enforcement personnel for crowd control. If the incident has taken place at an industrial site or along a railway, the company experts in hazardous materials need to be notified. Much of this can be done by a single call to your dispatcher.

Implement your agency's Incident Management System. Establish and remain in command until you are relieved by someone higher in the chain of command.

The situation must be prevented from becoming worse. Establish a perimeter, evacuate people if necessary, and direct bystanders to a safe area. It cannot be overemphasized that EMTs should not risk personal safety by initiating rescue attempts.

While help is on the way, establish control zones. Isolate the **hot zone** (the area of contamination or the area of danger). Establish a decontamination corridor (area where patients will be decontaminated) in the **warm zone,** an area immediately adjacent to the hot zone. Equipment and other emergency rescuers should be staged in the next adjacent area—the **cold zone.** Station yourself in the cold zone.

hot zone
area immediately surrounding a hazmat incident; extends far enough to prevent adverse effects outside the zone.

warm zone
area where personnel and equipment decontamination and hot zone support take place; it includes control points for the access corridor and thus assists in reducing the spread of contamination.

cold zone
area where the Incident Command post and support functions are located.

Identify the Substance

An attempt must be made to identify the hazardous material and assess the severity of the situation. Until that is done, it will be difficult to determine the risk to the public, rescuers, patients, and the environment. You must try to find out what the substance is and what its properties and dangers might be; whether or not there is imminent danger of the contamination spreading; what you can hear, see, and smell; how many victims are involved; and if there is any danger of secondary contamination from the victims. (Secondary contamination occurs when a contaminated person makes contact with someone who previously was "clean.")

Because it is not safe to approach the scene, you must obtain information indirectly or from a distance. Ways of obtaining information safely may include the following:

- *Use binoculars to look for identifying signs, labels, or placards from a safe distance* (Figure 36-1). In many cases there will be a colored placard (Figure 36-2) on the storage container, vehicle, tank, or railroad car.

Do not approach the scene to obtain this information.

NOTE

Recent studies by the Office of Technology Assessment have shown that some states report 25 to 50 percent of identification placards have been found to be incorrect. These same studies indicate that many shipping documents also are inaccurate or incomplete.

- A commonly used placarding system is the National Fire Protection Association (NFPA) 704 System. It uses numerical and color coding to show the type and degree of health hazard, fire hazard, reactivity, and specific hazard contained within a fixed facility (Figure 36-3).

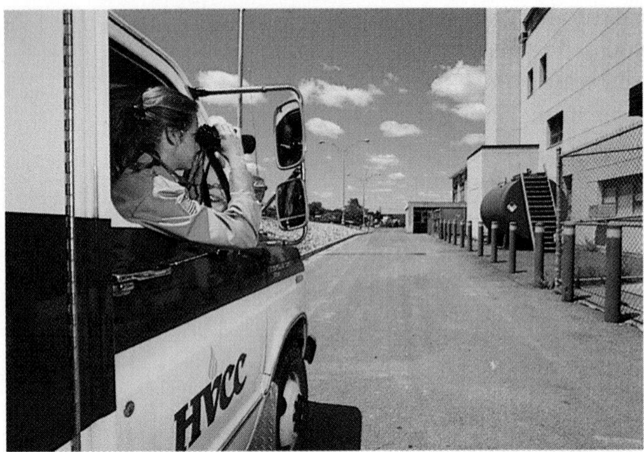

Figure 36-1 • Binoculars will allow a visual inspection of the hot zone from a safe distance.

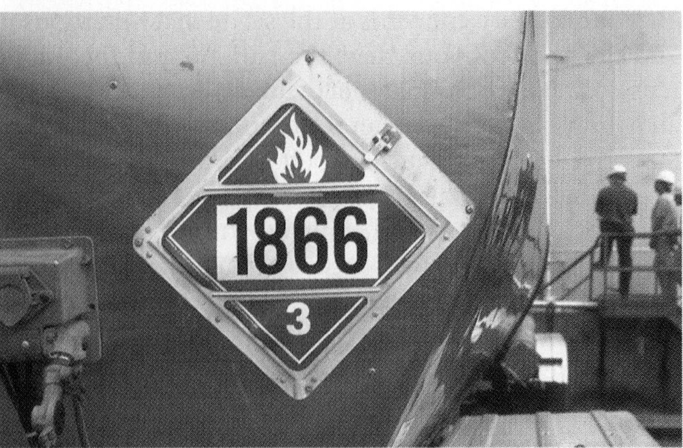

Figure 36-2 • Vehicles carrying hazardous materials are required to display placards that communicate the nature of their cargo.

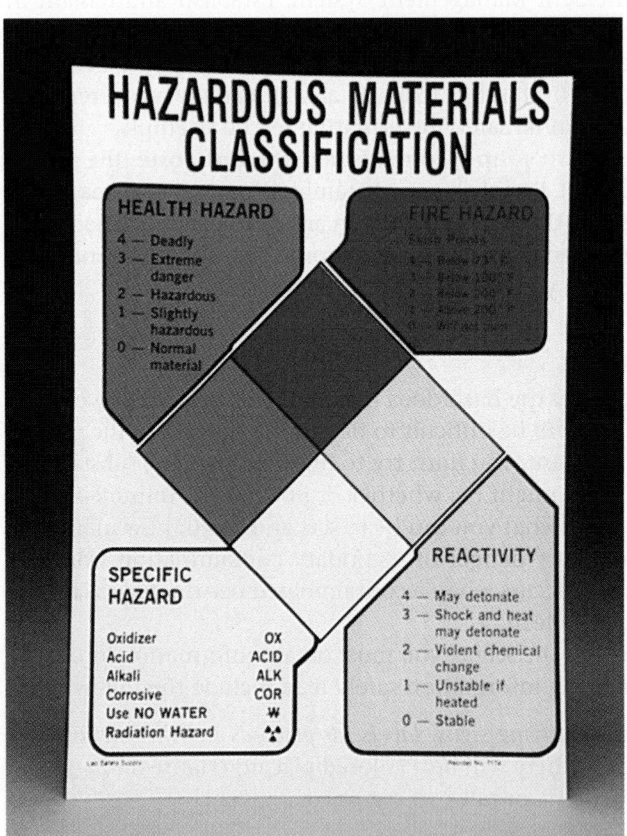

Figure 36-3 • This is the key to the National Fire Protection Association (NFPA) 704 System of numeric and color codes to hazardous materials.

- The U.S. Department of Transportation requires that packages, storage containers, and vehicles containing hazardous materials bear labels or placards with markings that identify the nature of the contents (Figure 36-4). Diamond-shaped placards used in the transportation of dangerous goods not only show the hazard class, such as "explosives," "flammable gas," "poison," or other, they also bear a division number which provides more specific information on the material, as shown in Table 36-2. In addition, a four-digit identification number may appear on the placard itself or on a panel near the placard.

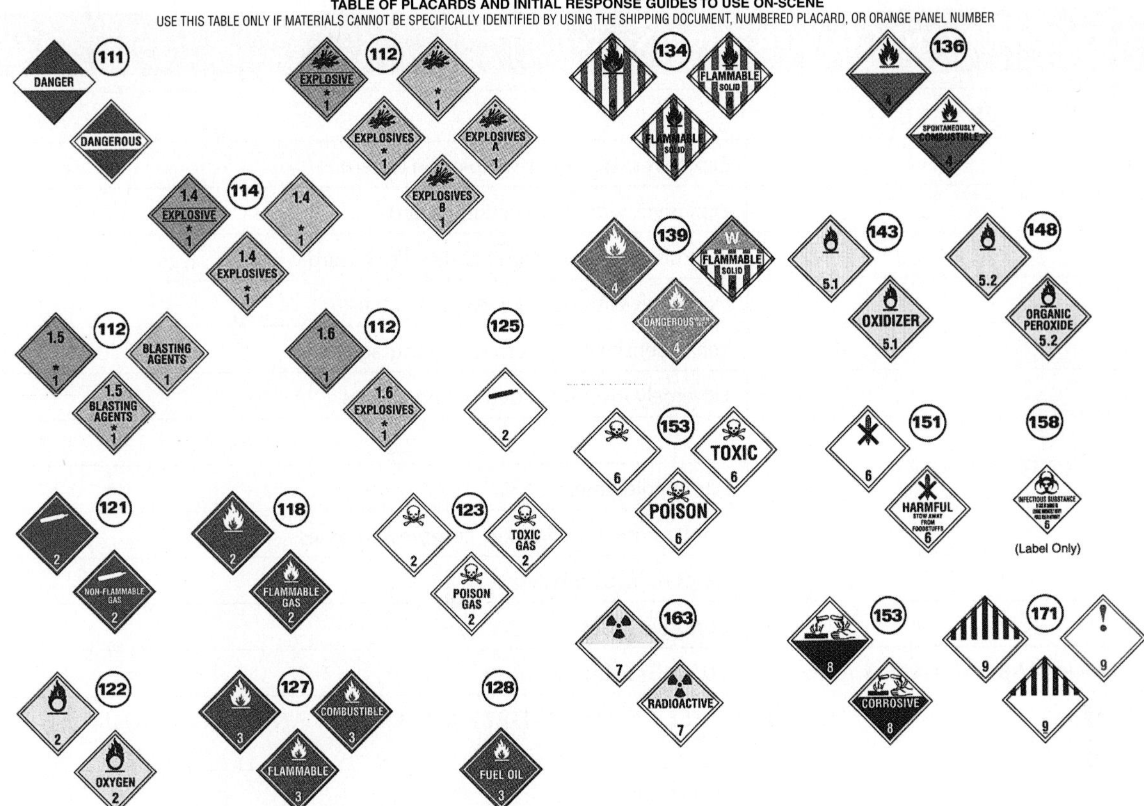

Figure 36-4 • The U.S. Department of Transportation (DOT) requires that hazard labels or placards be displayed on packages, storage containers, and vehicles containing hazardous materials.

Older placards are usually orange and have an identification number preceded by the letters UN or UA. Your dispatcher may have access to the name of the material through this identification number.

- *Invoices, bills of lading (trucks), and shipping manifests (trains).* If you can safely obtain them, these will identify the exact substance being transported, the exact quantity, its place of origin, and its destination.
- *Material Safety Data Sheets (MSDS).* MSDS are required to be provided on hazardous materials by all manufacturers. These sheets must be maintained at the work site by the employer and available to all employees on the grounds that employees working with hazardous materials have a right to know about them. If you can safely obtain these sheets, they generally name the substance, its physical properties, fire and explosion hazard information, health hazard information, and emergency first aid treatment.
- *Interview workers or others leaving the hot zone.* They may be good sources of information about the substance involved. Vehicle drivers, plant and railroad personnel, and perhaps even bystanders may be able to tell you the name of the hazardous material. Workers at a manufacturing site often understand very well what chemicals are used, the processes, and reactions. However, note that workers may identify a substance by its trade name and not realize that it is a mixture of many chemicals.

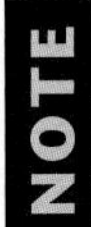

Do not take hasty action because you think you have identified the nature of the substance. Seek and follow expert advice. Do only what you have been trained to do.

EMTs are only expected to understand some of the common substance-identifying systems available and to make a preliminary identification based on this information. On the basis of this preliminary information, you can obtain advice about what initial

TABLE 36-2 • Hazard Classification System	
CLASS 1—EXPLOSIVES	
Division 1.1	Explosives with a mass explosion hazard
Division 1.2	Explosives with a projection hazard
Division 1.3	Explosives with predominantly a fire hazard
Division 1.4	Explosives with no significant blast hazard
Division 1.5	Very insensitive explosives; blasting agents
Division 1.6	Extremely insensitive detonating articles
CLASS 2—GASES	
Division 2.1	Flammable gases
Division 2.2	Nonflammable, nontoxic, compressed gases
Division 2.3	Gases toxic by inhalation
Division 2.4	Corrosive gases
CLASS 3—FLAMMABLE LIQUIDS AND COMBUSTIBLE LIQUIDS	
CLASS 4—FLAMMABLE SOLIDS; SPONTANEOUSLY COMBUSTIBLE MATERIALS; AND DANGEROUS-WHEN-WET MATERIALS	
Division 4.1	Flammable solids
Division 4.2	Spontaneously combustible materials
Division 4.3	Dangerous-when-wet materials
CLASS 5—OXIDIZERS AND ORGANIC PEROXIDES	
Division 5.1	Oxidizers
Division 5.2	Organic peroxides
CLASS 6—TOXIC MATERIALS AND INFECTIOUS SUBSTANCES	
Division 6.1	Toxic materials
Division 6.2	Infectious substances
CLASS 7—RADIOACTIVE MATERIALS	
CLASS 8—CORROSIVE MATERIALS	
CLASS 9—MISCELLANEOUS DANGEROUS GOODS	
Division 9.1	Miscellaneous dangerous goods
Division 9.2	Environmentally hazardous substances
Division 9.3	Dangerous wastes

actions should be taken at the scene from your dispatcher, a hazardous materials expert, or one of the following sources:

- *Emergency Response Guidebook* (ERG2008) (Figure 36-5). This essential booklet, published by the U.S. Department of Transportation, Transport Canada, and the Secretariat of Communications and Transportation of Mexico, provides the names of chemicals and concise but thorough descriptions of the actions that should be taken in case of a hazmat emergency. Be sure to have the latest edition in your vehicle at all times.

- *Chemical Transportation Emergency Center (CHEMTREC)* has been established in Washington, DC, as a service of the Chemical Manufacturers Association. They can provide your dispatcher or you with information about the hazardous material. They have a 24-hour toll-free telephone number for the United States and Canada, which is 800-424-9300. For calls originating elsewhere and for collect calls the number is 703-527-3887. When you call, keep the line open so that changes at the scene can be reported to CHEMTREC and the center can confirm that they have contacted the shipper or manufacturer. CHEMTREC will be able to direct you as to your initial course of action.
- *CHEM-TEL, Inc.* is an emergency response communication service that can be reached 24 hours a day at 800-255-3924 in the United States and Canada. For calls originating elsewhere or collect calls, use 813-979-0626.
- *A current list of state and federal radiation authorities* (who provide information and technical assistance on handling incidents involving radioactive materials) is maintained by both CHEMTREC and CHEM-TEL, Inc.
- *Regional poison control centers* are a source that is often overlooked during a hazardous material situation. Using their reference and medical resources, they can provide essential guidance in the decontamination and treatment of patients affected by hazardous materials.

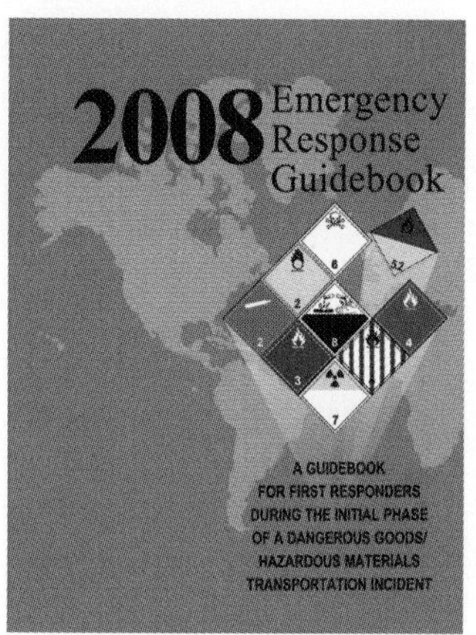

Figure 36-5 • Have the latest edition of the *Emergency Response Guidebook* in your vehicle at all times.

When you call one of the previously named sources for advice, do the following:

1. Give your name, call-back number, e-mail address, and FAX number.
2. Explain the nature and location of the problem.
3. Report the identification number(s) of the material(s) involved, if there is a safe way for you to obtain this information.
4. Give the name of the carrier, shipper, manufacturer, consignee, and point of origin.
5. Describe the container type and size.
6. Report if the container is on rail car, truck, open storage, or housed storage.
7. Estimate the quantity of material transported and released.
8. Report local conditions (e.g., the weather, terrain, and proximity to schools or hospitals).
9. Report injuries and exposures.
10. Report local emergency services that have been notified.
11. Keep line of communication open at all times.

If there is no identification number and no one knows what is being carried, you may have no other choice but to wait for experts to arrive at the scene. When a hazmat team arrives, they will identify and deal with unknown substances, using the necessary computer and textbook resources.

Establish a Treatment Area

All EMS personnel and equipment must be staged in the cold zone. EMS personnel have two responsibilities at a hazmat incident: to monitor and rehabilitate the hazmat team members and to take care of the injured.

Rehabilitation Operations

In order to safely enter the hot zone, the hazmat team members must wear chemical-protective clothing and breathing apparatus that both slows heat loss and prevents heat stress. Team members must be carefully monitored prior to, during, and after emergency operations. This is done to make sure that their condition does not deteriorate to a point where safety or the integrity of the operation is jeopardized. To address this need, an area of operations called rehabilitation (rehab) should be established. While the rehab area supervisor may not be an EMS provider, all rehab operations must include EMTs or advanced-level EMTs.

The characteristics of the rehab area must include the following:

- Located in the cold zone
- Protected from weather (shielded from rain or snow, a warm area in a cold environment, a cool area in a warm environment)
- Large enough to accommodate multiple rescue crews
- Easily accessible to EMS units
- Free from exhaust fumes
- Allows for rapid re-entry into the emergency operation

While suiting up in chemical-protective equipment, hazmat team members should have their baseline vital signs taken. When the hazmat team members show signs of fatigue or when they have had 45 minutes of work time, they are sent to rehab. As soon as possible after exit from the hot zone, reassess their vital signs. If heart rate exceeds 110 beats per minute, an oral temperature should be taken. If temperature exceeds 100.6°F, the rescuer must stay in rehab until his pulse slows and temperature returns to normal. Always follow local protocols and consult medical direction. All pre-entry and exit vitals should be tracked on a flow sheet.

In addition to medical monitoring, rehab should be set up for prehydration and hydration, rest, and in some cases nourishment of hazmat team members. Proper hydration is an important element in preventing heat stress and promoting optimal physical performance. Heat injury is usually caused by imbalances of water and electrolytes during periods of high heat stress and physical exertion. During physical exertion, at least one quart of water per hour should be consumed. For short-duration emergency operations, electrolyte sport drinks usually are not necessary. However, if they are used they should be diluted to half strength. Coffee and caffeinated beverages should be avoided because they promote dehydration.

When incidents will be of extended duration, some type of nourishment may be provided in rehab. Foods low in salt and saturated fats are ideal. Bananas, apples, oranges, and other fruits are excellent for fast nourishment. In cold environments, soups and stews are more easily eaten and digested than sandwiches.

Care of Injured and Contaminated Patients

Hazardous materials or terrorist incidents (see Chapter 37, "EMS Response to Terrorism") involve civilians and/or First Responders. Prompt, safe, and effective decontamination procedures are essential to protect against, or reduce the effects of, exposure to both victims and First Responders. Decontamination is performed to protect citizens, personnel, equipment, and the environment from the harmful effects of the contaminants.

decontamination a chemical and/or physical process that reduces or prevents the spread of contamination from persons or equipment; the removal of hazardous substances from employees and their equipment to the extent necessary to preclude foreseeable health effects.

The National Fire Protection Association (NFPA) defines **decontamination** as a chemical and/or physical process that reduces or prevents the spread of contamination from persons or equipment. According to the Occupational Safety and Health Administration (OSHA), decontamination is the removal of hazardous substances from employees and their equipment to the extent necessary to preclude foreseeable health effects.

EMTs must work with Incident Command and hazmat team members to determine the most appropriate course of action. The decision to stay at the scene and decontaminate or to begin evacuation must be made after careful consultation with CHEMTREC, the poison control center, and other reference sources.

In the decontamination (decon) corridor in the warm zone, the hazmat team will decontaminate hazmat team members and any patients rescued. EMS is responsible for setting up the medical treatment area in the cold zone to receive decontaminated patients. Unless EMS personnel are trained to the hazmat technician level, they must remain in the cold zone.

The field decon process is designed to remove contaminants and deliver a relatively "clean" patient to EMS personnel for care and transportation (Figure 36-6). However, there is a chance of secondary contamination from patients to EMS personnel. It is important that EMS personnel work closely with the decon officer and consult with medical direction on both treatment and appropriate protection during transportation.

The following points are important when treating and transporting hazmat patients:

- Field-decontaminated patients are not completely "clean." Chemicals that pose a risk of secondary contamination to rescuers sometimes settle in hard-to-clean areas of the body. These areas are typically the scalp/hair, groin, buttocks, between fingers and toes, and the armpits.
- Personal protective equipment or clothing (PPE/PPC) is needed to prevent secondary contamination of rescuers. EMS personnel need to wear PPE such as Tyvek coveralls and booties to prevent contamination and exposure. A double layer of gloves also may need to be worn. Often nitrile or neoprene is best, because these are more

9-Station Decontamination Procedure

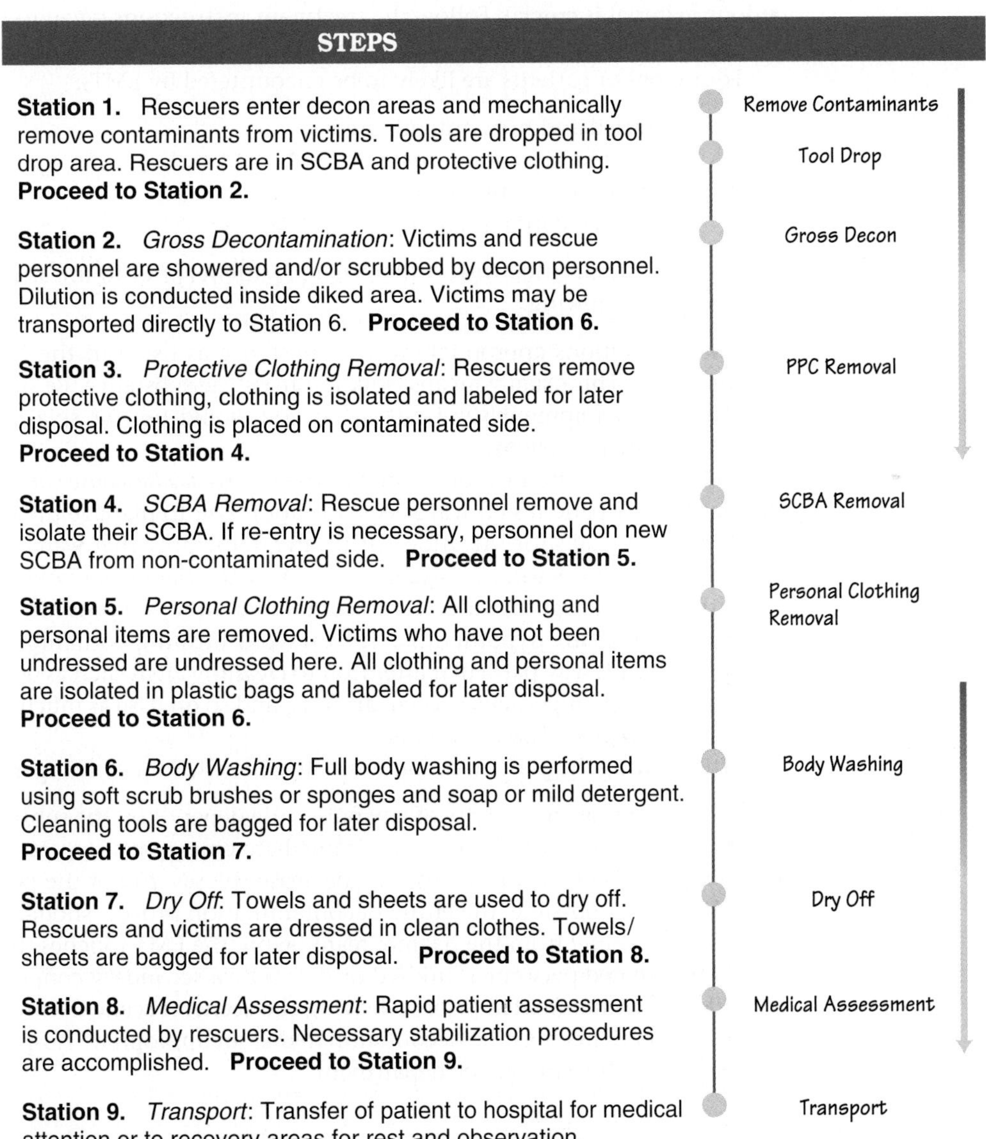

STEPS
Station 1. Rescuers enter decon areas and mechanically remove contaminants from victims. Tools are dropped in tool drop area. Rescuers are in SCBA and protective clothing. Proceed to Station 2.
Station 2. Gross Decontamination: Victims and rescue personnel are showered and/or scrubbed by decon personnel. Dilution is conducted inside diked area. Victims may be transported directly to Station 6. Proceed to Station 6.
Station 3. Protective Clothing Removal: Rescuers remove protective clothing, clothing is isolated and labeled for later disposal. Clothing is placed on contaminated side. Proceed to Station 4.
Station 4. SCBA Removal: Rescue personnel remove and isolate their SCBA. If re-entry is necessary, personnel don new SCBA from non-contaminated side. Proceed to Station 5.
Station 5. Personal Clothing Removal: All clothing and personal items are removed. Victims who have not been undressed are undressed here. All clothing and personal items are isolated in plastic bags and labeled for later disposal. Proceed to Station 6.
Station 6. Body Washing: Full body washing is performed using soft scrub brushes or sponges and soap or mild detergent. Cleaning tools are bagged for later disposal. Proceed to Station 7.
Station 7. Dry Off: Towels and sheets are used to dry off. Rescuers and victims are dressed in clean clothes. Towels/sheets are bagged for later disposal. Proceed to Station 8.
Station 8. Medical Assessment: Rapid patient assessment is conducted by rescuers. Necessary stabilization procedures are accomplished. Proceed to Station 9.
Station 9. Transport: Transfer of patient to hospital for medical attention or to recovery areas for rest and observation.
Remove Contaminants
Tool Drop
Gross Decon
PPC Removal
SCBA Removal
Personal Clothing Removal
Body Washing
Dry Off
Medical Assessment
Transport

Figure 36-6 • An example of a field decontamination process.

resistant to chemicals than standard latex or vinyl gloves. Consult with the decon officer to determine if your PPE is suitable or if they have more appropriate PPE.

- Protect vehicles from contamination. In the decon process, patients are washed and are usually dripping wet. Since they cannot be completely decontaminated in the field, some of their water runoff could contaminate an emergency vehicle. To prevent this, the water runoff must be contained by either placing the patient in a disposable decontamination pool or covering the inside of an ambulance vehicle with plastic.
- Consider used equipment as disposable. When an item such as a spine board, splint, blood-pressure cuff, or stethoscope is used, it may not be able to be decontaminated and may require disposal.
- Structural firefighting clothing is not designed or recommended for working in hazardous material environments. If personnel in firefighting gear encounter a hazardous chemical environment, they should take precautions to minimize the chance of contamination. A team in bunker gear can stand back and apply a fog stream to contaminated persons.

When treating a contaminated patient is unavoidable, identification of the hazardous material is crucial. Follow the treatment instructions given in the *Emergency Response Guidebook* or by the poison control center.

Four types of patients are likely to be encountered by EMTs:

- Uninjured and not contaminated
- Injured and not contaminated
- Uninjured and contaminated
- Injured and contaminated

If you are confronted with contaminated patients prior to the arrival of the hazmat team, do the following:

1. Take precautions appropriate to the substance as listed in the *Emergency Response Guidebook*. This usually means isolation from the substance. Be sure to use personal protective equipment similar to what you would use for splash protection from bloodborne pathogens.
2. Follow the first aid measures listed in the *Emergency Response Guidebook*.
3. Manage the patient's critical needs. Do not forget to manage the ABCs.
4. If treatment calls for irrigation with water, remember that water only dilutes most substances. It does not neutralize them. Cut the patient's clothing off and irrigate with large amounts of water. Try to contain the runoff. If possible, use tepid or warm water to prevent hypothermia. Try to avoid flushing contaminants directly into open wounds. Pay particular attention to cleaning areas such as dense body hair, ear canals, navel, fingernails, crotch, armpits, and so on. Use as much disposable equipment as possible. Discard it later.
5. After treating the patient, decontaminate yourself. Your clothing may need disposal.

Remember that the severity of any poisoning depends on the substance, route of entry, dosage, and duration of contact. Immediate emergency care measures as listed in the *Emergency Response Guidebook* may decrease the severity of the poisoning and save lives. Whenever possible, the entire decontamination process should be carried out by qualified personnel from the hazmat team before the EMT touches the patient.

Contaminated personnel (injured or not) pose a secondary contamination risk and should be decontaminated prior to leaving the scene. If scene decontamination is not performed, patients must be decontaminated at an appropriate hospital decon site before entry into the emergency department.

Phases of Decontamination

The two major phases of decontamination are gross decontamination and secondary decontamination. (There is usually a third or tertiary decontamination phase, but it generally occurs at a medical facility and may involve such processes as sterilization or debridement.)

Gross decontamination is the removal or chemical alteration of the majority of the contaminant. It must be assumed that some residual contaminant will always remain on the host after gross decontamination. This residual contamination can cause cross-contamination. *Secondary decontamination* is the alteration or removal of most of the residual product contamination. It provides a more thorough decontamination than the gross effort. However, some contaminant may still remain attached to the host.

Mechanisms for Decontamination

There are seven common mechanisms for performing decontamination. They are:

- *Emulsification.* The production of a suspension of ordinarily immiscible (unmixable)/insoluble materials using an emulsifying agent such as a surfactant, soap, or detergent.
- *Chemical reaction.* A process that neutralizes, degrades, or otherwise chemically alters the contaminant. Normally, a chemical reaction does not ensure that all hazards have been eliminated, and reaction procedures can be both difficult and dangerous to perform. Chemical reaction is therefore not recommended for use on living tissue.
- *Disinfection.* A process that removes the biological (etiological) contamination hazards as the disinfectant destroys microorganisms and their toxins.
- *Dilution.* A process that simply reduces the concentration of the contaminant. It is most commonly used for substances that are miscible (mixable)/soluble. Huge quantities of solvent may be required to dilute even small volumes of some solute contaminants.
- *Absorption and adsorption.* The penetration of a liquid or gas into another substance. An example is water into a sponge.
- *Removal.* The physical process of removing contaminants by pressure or vacuum. Most efforts involve the use of water, though solids can be removed with brushes and wipes; even air can be used.
- *Disposal.* The aseptic removal of a contaminated object from a host, after which the object is disposed of. (*Aseptic* means using sterile instruments and/or otherwise preventing the spread of the contaminant.)

Decontamination Procedures

The objectives of the responders assigned to decontamination are to:

- Determine the appropriate level of protective equipment based on materials and associated hazards
- Properly wear and operate in PPE
- Establish operating time log
- Set up and operate the decontamination line
- Prioritize the decontamination of victims according to a triage system
- Perform triage in PPE
- Be able to communicate while in PPE

A basic list of equipment required for decontamination is:

- Buckets
- Brushes
- Decontamination solution
- Decontamination tubs
- Dedicated water supply
- Tarps or plastic sheeting
- Containment vessel for water runoff
- Pump to transfer wastewater from decontamination tubs to containment vessel

- A-frame ladder (to reach the top of the responder's suit)
- Appropriate-level PPE for responders performing decontamination

DECONTAMINATION FOR VICTIMS WEARING PPE Take the following steps to decontaminate a victim who is wearing PPE:

1. Rinse, starting at the head and working down.
2. Scrub the suit with a brush, starting at the head and working down. Pay special attention to heavily contaminated areas (e.g., hands, feet, front of suit).
3. Rinse again, starting at the head and working down.
4. Assist responder in removing PPE.
5. Contain the runoff of hazardous wastewater.

DECONTAMINATION FOR VICTIMS NOT WEARING PPE The decontamination of victims not wearing PPE proceeds differently. As always, the first and foremost consideration is responder safety. If responders are incapacitated, they are unable to help others.

A public address system should be used to direct ambulatory victims to a decontamination line. This provides a rapid form of triage. Victims should be instructed to begin decontamination by removing their clothing. Shoes, socks, jewelry, watches, and other items that trap materials against the skin are removed. Contact lenses should be removed as soon as possible; double-bag clothing for disposal or decontamination later. Valuables and identification should be bagged and may (based on hazards) be carried by the victims.

Next, the victims should receive a 2- to 5-minute water rinse. Solid or particulate contaminants should be lightly brushed off (dry decontamination) as completely as possible prior to washing (wet decontamination). Viscous liquid contaminants (including vesicants, which are blistering agents) should be blotted off prior to washing. If the material is water reactive, it must be brushed off prior to the application of water. Rinsing is done as needed to flush remaining chemicals that may react with the moisture of the skin and eyes. An appropriate decontamination solution should also be used.

Washing and rinsing should start at the head to reduce contamination on or near the nose, mouth, ears, and eyes. If contact lenses have been removed, the eyes should be irrigated. Open wounds should be irrigated starting from the area nearest the body core and working outward. Plastic wrap may be used to isolate the wound once it has been cleaned. A low-water-pressure system should be used to avoid aggravating soft-tissue injuries and to avoid overspray and splashing. A low-pressure system will also help prevent the creation of an aerosol out of dry product.

During decontamination, victims should be given some type of cover for modesty and protection from the elements.

While not strictly a form of self-protection, "decon" is vital to prevent, reduce, and remove contamination for both responders and victims.

MULTIPLE-CASUALTY INCIDENTS

multiple-casualty incident (MCI) any medical or trauma incident involving multiple patients.

A **multiple-casualty incident (MCI)**—or in some areas, a multiple-casualty situation (MCS)—is an event that places a great demand on EMS equipment and personnel resources (Figure 36-7). The number of patients required before an MCI can be declared varies in practice. Some jurisdictions will declare an MCI for as few as three patients on the grounds that practice with smaller-scale incidents will help prepare for larger ones. Other jurisdictions reserve the MCI designation for five, seven, or more patients. The most common MCI is an automobile collision with three or more patients. You will likely respond to many incidents with 3 to 15 potential patients. Incidents with large-scale casualties are rare and apt to be "once in a career" events.

The important ingredient in defining an MCI is that, for whatever reason, the ability of the EMS system to respond to the situation is challenged or hampered by the sit-

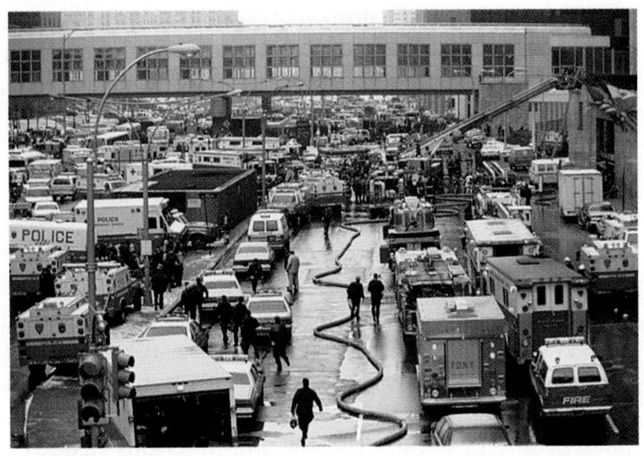

Figure 36-7 • A multiple-casualty incident. *(© Black Star)*

uation itself. For any MCI plan to be effective, it must be flexible and expandable enough to be used from small three-patient incidents to large-scale incidents of 15 or more patients. In other words, the plan for "the big one" should be a logical extension of the same plan used to manage smaller incidents.

Multiple-Casualty-Incident Operations

Though the principles of managing small- and large-scale MCIs are generally the same, large-scale MCIs unfold over a longer period of time and require greater support from outside agencies. Well-trained and practiced EMTs can usually cope with a small-scale MCI pretty well. However, experience has shown that even the best-trained EMTs have a difficult time managing an incident of greater magnitude.

One way to minimize the operating difficulties of a large-scale MCI is for every EMT to be familiar with the local **disaster plan.** A disaster plan is a predefined set of instructions that tells a community's various emergency responders what to do in specific emergencies. While no disaster plan can address every problem that could arise, there are several features common to every good disaster plan. The disaster plan should be:

disaster plan
a predefined set of instructions for a community's emergency responders.

- *Written to address the events that are conceivable for a particular location* (e.g., Kansas needs to plan for tornadoes, not hurricanes).
- *Well publicized.* Each emergency responder should be familiar with the plan and how it is to be put into operation.
- *Realistic.* The plan must be based on the actual availability of resources.
- *Rehearsed.* Experience has proven that the only way to get a plan to work correctly is to exercise it and, in so doing, work out the unforeseen "bugs."

It is beyond the scope of this text to teach you how to write a disaster plan or even to impart enough knowledge for you to be in charge of a disaster operation. However, it is important to introduce basic information about your potential roles in such an incident.

Incident Command System

By federal declaration the **National Incident Management System (NIMS)** is the management system used by federal, state, and local governments to manage emergencies in the United States. A subset of the NIMS system is also known as the **Incident Command System (ICS).** While not specifically a plan designed for MCI management, it provides a clear management framework for all types of large-scale incidents. In addition, it is mandated by law for the management of some types of incidents, such as those involving hazardous materials.

National Incident Management System (NIMS)
the management system used by federal, state, and local governments to manage emergencies in the United States.

Incident Command System (ICS)
a subset of the National Incident Management System (NIMS) designed specifically for management of multiple-casualty incidents.

ICS originated in California, where it was designed as a management plan to handle large-scale firefighting operations involving multiple agencies and jurisdictions. A flexible tool for managing people and resources, the system components include Command, Operations, Logistics, Planning, and Finance. The most commonly used components are Command and Operations.

Command

Command
The first on the scene to establish order and initiate the Incident Command System.

Command, which must be established at all incidents, is the person who assumes responsibility for incident management. This individual stays in command unless that function is transferred to another person or until the incident is brought to a conclusion.

IMS systems recognize that the manageable span of control is six people. As the MCI escalates and becomes more complex, the number of people and span of control become too large for one person to manage effectively. At this point, Command designates people to handle the specific functions needed to manage the operation. The basic elements of the incident management system—with sections such as Operations being subordinate to Command—are:

- Operations
- Planning
- Finance
- Logistics

Command assumes all incident management functions except those that Command may delegate to someone else. Unless an incident is very complex, the most common function designated is Operations.

singular command
command organization in which a single agency controls all resources and operations.

unified command
command organization in which several agencies work independently but cooperatively.

There are two methods of command—singular and unified. In **singular command,** a single agency controls all resources and operations. In many communities, for example, EMS is managed by fire services. Accordingly, singular command is often used at fire and rescue incidents. However, if police agencies have major involvement, if there is a separate EMS provider, or if other agencies are involved, unified command is more appropriate (Figure 36-8). In **unified command,** several agencies work independently but cooperatively rather than one agency exercising control over the others. In most communities unified command is the best way to manage resources. It recognizes that large-scale incidents tend to be complex and that the right agency must take the lead at the right time, with command officers from all agencies cooperating.

Command Functions

Incident Command
the person or persons who assume overall direction of a large-scale incident.

Initially, **Incident Command** is assumed by the most senior member of the first service on the scene. Very often this will be an EMS unit, and the senior EMS person may assume Incident Command. Depending on jurisdiction, laws, or protocols, Incident Command may be later transferred to another individual or may be continued by whoever established it.

Two modes or phases of action must then be undertaken: scene size-up/triage and organization/delegation. First, Command and the crew do an initial scene size-up, start the triage process, and call for backup. While waiting for help, initial triage is completed and Command gets ready for arriving resources.

When reinforcements arrive, there are two options for the person who initially assumed command: Continue to be in command or transfer command to someone of higher rank. In a unified system, Incident Command would be assumed cooperatively by the Command of each service. Command is positioned at a location close enough to allow observation of the scene but secure enough to permit management of incoming resources and communication with others. In a unified command system, EMS, Police, and Fire Command establish one field command post together and stay there. Some plans call for the field command vehicle or command post to be designated by placing two traffic cones on top of the vehicle being used. In a singular command

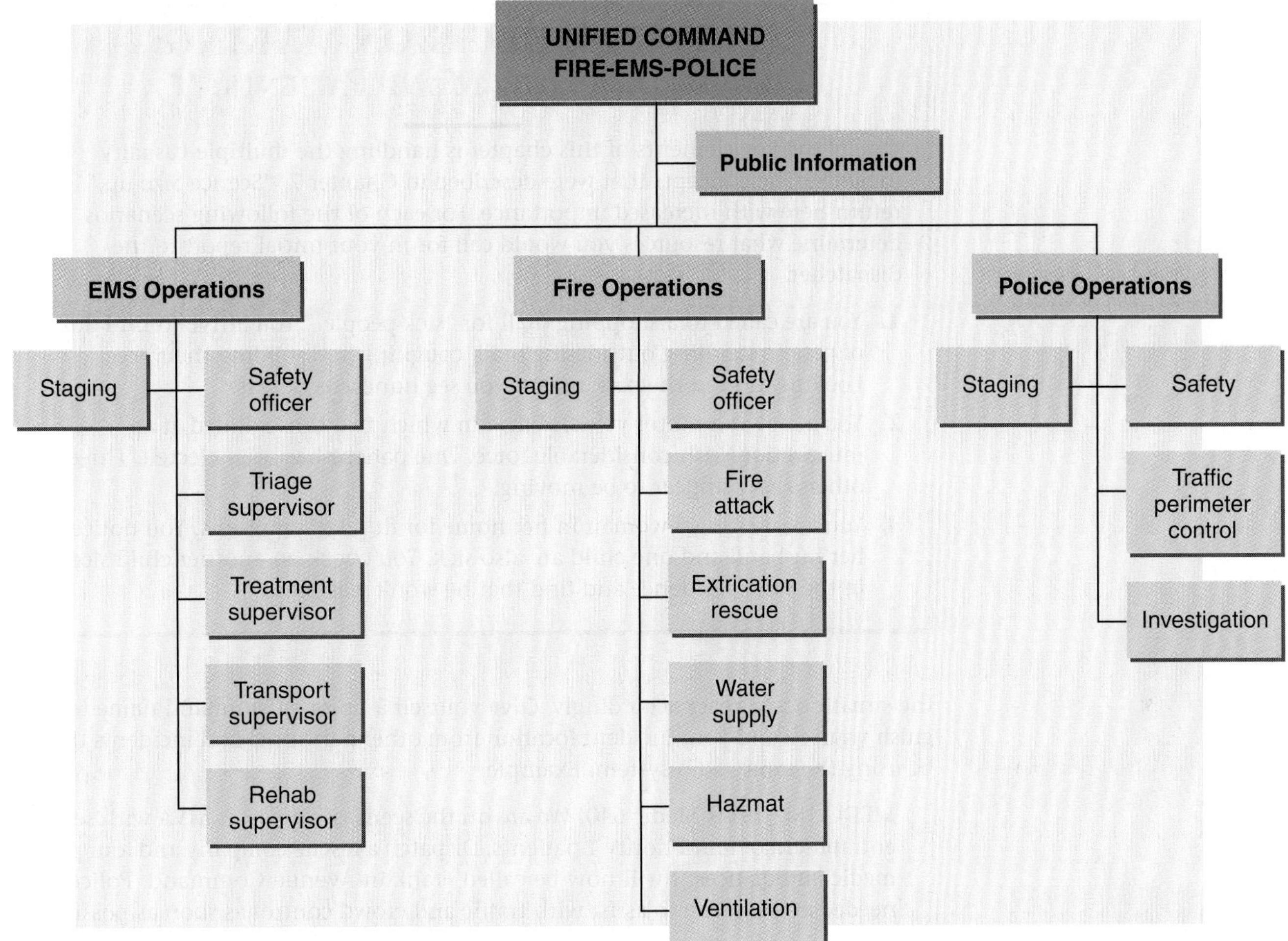

Figure 36-8 • A unified command organization.

mode, one person acts as Command, and EMS would typically be a group under the Operations section.

Scene Size-Up

Size-up the scene by making a sweep to determine what needs must be met:

1. Arrive at the scene and establish Incident Command. Put on the proper identification.
2. Do a quick walk through the scene (or, if it is a hazmat scene, observe from a safe distance) and assess the number of patients, hazards, and degree of entrapment. Identify the number of patients, including the "walking wounded," apparent priority of care, need for extrication, number of ambulances needed, other factors affecting the scene and corresponding resources needed to address them, and areas where resources can be staged.
3. Get as calm and composed as possible to radio in an initial scene report and call for additional resources.

Communications

Once scene size-up has been done, an initial scene report should be made to the communications center. Keep the report short and to the point, but give enough information for the communications center and other responders to understand the severity of

CRITICAL DECISION MAKING: We Have *How Many* Patients???

One of the key elements of this chapter is handling the multiple-casualty incident. The concepts that were described in Chapter 7, "Scence Size-up," return here with increased importance. For each of the following scenarios, determine what resources you would call for in your initial report to the dispatcher.

1. You are called to a shopping mall for "sick people." You arrive to find dozens of people standing outside the mall, coughing and rubbing their eyes. Looking around the parking lot, you see hundreds of cars.
2. You arrive at a motor vehicle crash in which two cars collided at an intersection with considerable force. One patient has been ejected. Three others don't appear to be moving.
3. You are treating a woman in her home for flu-like symptoms. You notice that her husband and one child are also sick. You check on another child sleeping in the same residence and find that he won't wake up.

the situation and react accordingly. Give yourself a unique Command name to distinguish yourself and your incident location from other personnel and incidents that may be using the same radio system. Example:

> MEDCOM, this is Medic 640. We are on the scene of a two-car MVA with severe entrapment of four Priority 1 patients. Dispatch a rescue company and four paramedic ambulances. I will now be called Franklin Avenue Command. Police are needed at the scene to assist with traffic and crowd control as soon as possible.

If the disaster plan is to be put into operation, it is critical that other responding units be informed of this fact. Your communications may also include telling other units what equipment to bring, what they should plan on doing once they arrive, how best to access the scene, and where to park.

As help begins to arrive, control of on-scene communication is important. Once units arrive, as much face-to-face communication as possible should be used, especially between Command and Command's direct subordinates. This will help to reduce radio channel crowding. If you feel you are getting too tied up in radio communications, designate a radio aide.

Basically, the flow of communications at the scene should correspond to the organizational chart being used. Accordingly, the only unit talking to the communications center and requesting resources is Command. The only ones who talk to Command are those directly subordinate to Command. All others talk only to the officer or supervisor they are assigned to.

Organization

Getting organized early and aggressively is very important. You must have a plan to deploy resources when they arrive. You must have decided what subordinate officers will be needed and where resources will be placed. A common mistake is to underestimate the resources that will be needed. Somehow new patients not found during size-up have a way of appearing. Think big. Order big. Put resources in the staging area if they are not needed right away. In urban/suburban incidents, backup can be fast and overwhelming. Think about supply and staging areas early or you take the chance of being overrun.

It is important to prevent "freelancing." Freelancing is uncoordinated or undirected activity at the scene. Given the opportunity, most rescuers will arrive on the scene and begin setting their own priorities. Command can prevent this problem. When established early, people and crews are assigned to tasks as they arrive.

Often it is helpful to have some personal tools to help get organized. For example, many organizations have distilled the major points of their plans into a "tactical worksheet" they can use in the field. With enough use, the plan can become committed to memory. (See Figure 36-9.)

Scene Management

The senior person on the first arriving EMS unit, who will likely have assumed Incident Command, will be known simply as Command and will establish a command post to oversee the medical aspects of the incident and the safety of all personnel, to designate area supervisors, and to work closely with the fire and police commanders. On larger incidents, Command may have an aide to assist with communications as well as a public information officer and a safety officer.

It is important to keep uninjured people from becoming injured. This will probably require restricting access to the scene to only those personnel performing triage (explained later), extrication from wreckage, and patient care. As resources arrive at the scene, police officers or safety officers may take over this function.

EMS Branch Functions

Under NIMS, in a very large and complex multiple-casualty incident, EMS will function as a branch under the Operations section. For smaller MCIs, the EMS person who has assumed Incident Command may be able to handle all aspects of management without delegating tasks to others. However, as an incident increases in size and complexity, additional staff and area supervisors will be needed (Figures 36-10 through 36-12). EMS operations generally include the following:

- Mobile command center
- Extrication (in cases of entrapment)
- Staging area
- Triage area
- Treatment area
- Transportation area
- Rehabilitation area

Individuals and agencies on the scene will be assigned particular roles in one or more areas. Most systems use brightly colored reflective vests that can be worn over protective clothing to make each incident sector officer easy to identify. Any EMT arriving at the scene at this time would be expected to report to an area supervisor for assignment of specific duties. Once assigned a specific task, the EMT should complete the task and report back to the area supervisor.

Once organization has been established, the next task is to quickly assess all the patients and assign each a priority for receiving emergency care or transportation to definitive care. This process is called **triage,** which comes from a French word meaning "to sort." The most knowledgeable EMS provider becomes the **triage supervisor.** The triage supervisor calls for additional help if needed, assigns available personnel and equipment to patients, and remains at the scene to assign and coordinate personnel, supplies, and vehicles.

triage
the process of quickly assessing patients at a multiple-casualty incident and assigning each a priority for receiving treatment; from a French word meaning "to sort."

triage supervisor
the person responsible for overseeing triage at a multiple-casualty incident.

Primary Triage

When faced with more than one patient, your goal must be to afford the greatest number of people the greatest chance of survival. To accomplish this goal, you must provide care to patients according to the seriousness of illness or injury while keeping in mind that spending a lot of time trying to save one life may prevent a number of other patients from receiving the treatment they need.

COLONIE EMS *Incident Tactical Worksheet*

Location ______
Med. Command ______

_____ Establish unified command with fire & police
_____ Place 2 cones on command vehicle
_____ Put bib on
_____ Designate triage officer
_____ Advise inbound units where to stage
_____ Advise crews to stay with units until given instructions
_____ Advise units to switch to EMS Admin., 265 or 715

LEVEL 1 (3-10 Patients)
- ___ Declare MCI
- ___ EMS All Call
- ___ Request # of Units Needed
- ___ Cover Town/Sr. Medic Act 615
- ___ Roll Call Hospitals
- ___ Transport Officer?

(2-5 Amb. Needed)

LEVEL 2 (11-25 Patients)
- ___ Declare MCI
- ___ EMS All Call
- ___ Request # of Units Needed
- ___ Cover Town/Sr. Medic Act 615
- ___ Roll Call Hospitals
- ___ Get Mutual Aid Units
- ___ Designate Treatment Officer
- ___ Designate Transport Officer
- ___ Designate Staging Officer
- ___ REMO MD to Scene
- ___ Consider Rehab & CISD

(6-13 Amb. Needed)

LEVEL 3 (over 25 Patients)
- ___ Declare MCI
- ___ EMS All Call
- ___ Request # of Units Needed
- ___ Cover Town/Sr. Medic Act 615
- ___ Roll Call Hospitals
- ___ Get Mutual Aid Units
- ___ Designate Treatment Officer
- ___ Designate Transport Officer
- ___ Designate Staging Officer
- ___ REMO MD to Scene
- ___ Request Bus to Scene

(over 13 Amb. Needed)

FIRE
- ___ Assess # of Units Needed
- ___ EMS All Call Req. 619
- ___ Designate Triage
- ___ Set up Rehab at Air Bank
- ___ Use 619 as ALS Unit

RESCUE
- ___ Establish Perimeter
- ___ Request Speciality Units
- ___ Triage Officer Handles Inner Circle

HAZ-MAT
- ___ Req. # of Units Needed
- ___ EMS All Call
- ___ Est. Command in Cold Zone
- ___ Designate Triage
- ___ Identify Agent
- ___ Research Decontamination
- ___ Research Med.
- ___ Medical Baseline Assessment of Team
- ___ Don Protective Barriers
- ___ Assist With Decontamination
- ___ Rehabilitate

HOSPITAL ROLL CALL	AMCH	St. PETERS	MEMORIAL	VA	ELLIS	St. CLARE'S	LEONARD	St. MARY'S	SAMARITAN
CAN TAKE									
# PATIENTS SENT									

 # OF PATIENTS BY PRIORITY

1 (Red)	2 (Yellow)	3 (Green)	0 (Black)	TOTALS

UNITS RESPONDING

620 621 622 ______ ______
630 631 632 ______ ______
640 641 642 ______ ______
650 651 652 ______ ______
610 611 605 ______ ______
TSU-1 TSU-2 ______ ______
619 ___ ___ ______ ______
Guild. ___ ___ ______ ______
CPHM ___ ___ ______ ______
Albany ___ ___ ______ ______
Mohawk ___ ___ ______ ______
Empire ___ ___ ______ ______

UNITS IN STAGING

620 621 622 ______ ______
630 631 632 ______ ______
640 641 642 ______ ______
650 651 652 ______ ______
610 611 605 ______ ______
TSU-1 TSU-2 ______ ______
619 ___ ___ ______ ______
Guild. ___ ___ ______ ______
CPHM ___ ___ ______ ______
Albany ___ ___ ______ ______
Mohawk ___ ___ ______ ______
Empire ___ ___ ______ ______

Figure 36-9 • An example of an incident tactical worksheet.

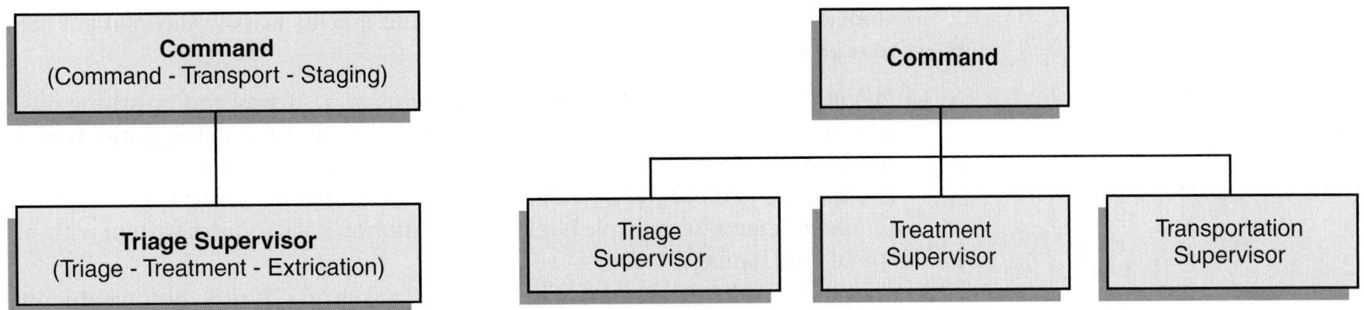

Figure 36-10 • An organization for a smaller incident.

Figure 36-11 • An organization for a medium-size incident.

- **Command** (Site or Command Post)
  - **Site Operations** (Site)
    - **Staging** Officer
    - **Safety** Officer
    - **Transportation** Supervisor
      - Radio Comm. Aide
    - **Treatment** Supervisor
      - P-1 Tx Leader
      - P-2 Tx Leader
      - P-3 Tx Leader
      - Supply Aide
    - **Triage** Supervisor
      - Triage Aides
    - **Rehab.** Supervisor

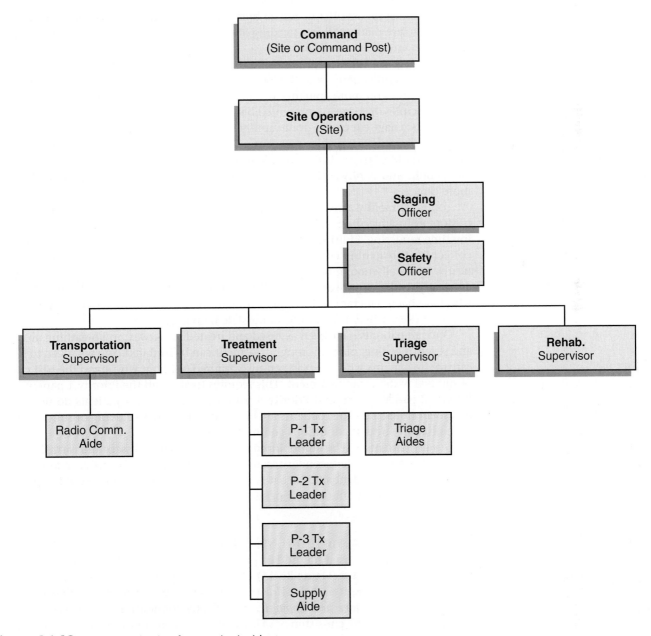

Figure 36-12 • An organization for a major incident.

To properly triage a group of patients, you should quickly classify each patient into one of four groups:

- *Priority 1: Treatable Life-Threatening Illness or Injuries.* Airway and breathing difficulties; uncontrolled or severe bleeding; decreased mental status; patients with severe medical problems; shock (hypoperfusion); severe burns
- *Priority 2: Serious But Not Life-Threatening Illness or Injuries.* Burns without airway problems; major or multiple bone or joint injuries; back injuries with or without spinal cord damage
- *Priority 3: "Walking Wounded."* Minor musculoskeletal injuries; minor soft-tissue injuries
- *Priority 4 (sometimes called Priority 0): Dead or Fatally Injured.* Examples include exposed brain matter, cardiac arrest (no pulse for over 20 minutes except with cold-water drowning or severe hypothermia), decapitation, severed trunk, and incineration.

Patients in arrest are considered Priority 4 (or 0) when resources are limited. The time that must be devoted to rescue breathing or CPR for one person is not justified when there are many patients needing attention. Once ample resources are available, patients in arrest become Priority 1.

How triage is performed depends on the number of injuries, the immediate hazards to personnel and patients, and the location of backup resources. Local operating procedures will give you more guidance on the exact method of triage for a given situation. Basic principles of triage are presented here.

The first triage cut can be done rapidly by using a bullhorn, PA system, or loud voice to direct all patients capable of walking (Priority 3) to move to a particular area. This has a two-fold purpose. It quickly identifies the individuals who have an airway and circulation, and it physically separates them from patients who will generally need more care.

You must rapidly assess each remaining patient, stopping only to secure an airway or stop profuse bleeding. It is important that you not develop "tunnel vision"—spending time rendering additional care to any one patient and thus failing to identify and correct life-threatening conditions of the remaining patients. If Priority 3 patients are nearby and well enough to help, they may be employed to assist you by maintaining an airway or direct pressure on bleeding wounds of other patients. Priority 3 patients who have been reluctant to leave ill or injured friends or relatives may be permitted to stay near them where they can be of possible help later.

Once all patients have been assessed and treated for airway and breathing problems and severe bleeding, more thorough treatment can be initiated. You will need to render care to the patients who are most seriously injured or ill but who stand the best chance of survival with proper treatment. This requires treating all the Priority 1 patients first, Priority 2 patients next, and Priority 3 patients last. Priority 4 patients do not receive treatment unless no other patients are believed to be at risk of dying or suffering long-term disability if their conditions go unattended.

Usually patients will be immobilized on backboards if necessary and carried by "runners" to the appropriate secondary sector (as described later). Extensive treatment does not occur at the incident site since it is in a hazard zone and since it could impede rescue and initial treatment of other patients.

START Triage: A National Standard for Rapid Primary Triage

The most commonly used method of prioritizing patients in the United States is the START method of triage (Figure 36-13). It was developed by the Newport Beach, California, Fire Department and the Hoag Hospital in Newport Beach California. *START* stands for *Simple Triage and Rapid Treatment.* The foundation of the system is the speed, simplicity, and consistency of its application. It relies on some simple com-

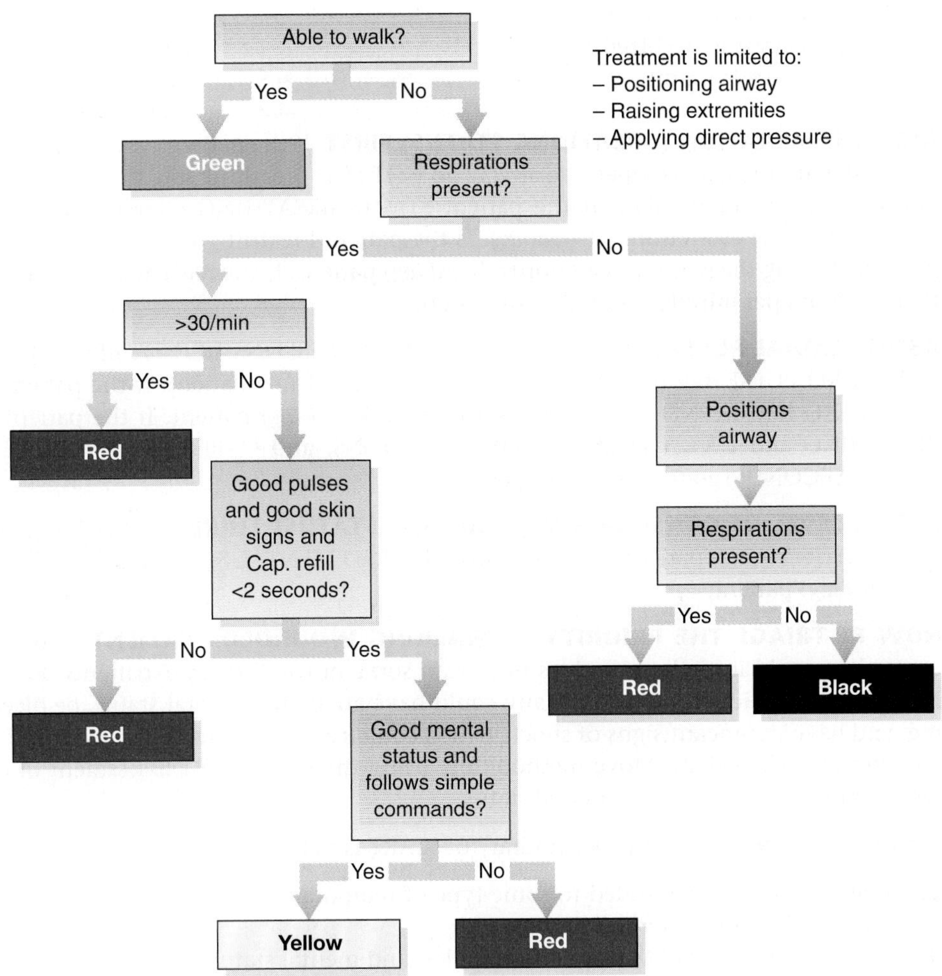

Figure 36-13 • START triage.

mands and the following physiologic parameters that can be remembered by the mnemonic *RPM*:

Respiration
Pulse
Mental Status

START triage is intended to be completed in about 30 seconds per patient.

Begin by asking all patients who can walk to get up and go to a collection point such as an ambulance or a building. Since those who can do this are . . .

- Conscious
- Able to follow commands
- Able to walk

. . . they obviously are perfusing their brain, are breathing, have a pulse, and have a nervous system that is working for now. All of these patients are considered to be Priority 3 (*green tag*) patients for right now. (They are often called the "walking wounded.") This also leaves people at the site who are unable to hear, walk, or follow commands and are the Priority 0, 1, or 2 patients. Now you must focus your attention on those among these patients who are likely to be of higher priority.

Start making your triage sweep methodically, avoiding patients who are obviously conscious. The only three treatments provided during START triage are to:

- Open an airway and insert an OPA
- Apply pressure to bleeding
- Elevate an extremity

ASSESS RESPIRATION (BREATHING STATUS) FIRST If the patient is NOT BREATHING and your attempts to open the airway do NOT start breathing, tag the patient as a Priority 0 (*black tag*) patient. If the patient STARTS BREATHING after the airway is opened, then tag as a Priority 1 (*red tag*). Is the patient breathing more than 30 times per minute? Tag the patient as a Priority 1 (*red tag*) patient. Is the patient breathing less than 30 times per minute? Go to the next step.

ASSESS RADIAL PULSE SECOND If the patient is UNRESPONSIVE, NOT BREATHING, and has NO PULSE, tag the patient as a Priority 0 (*black tag*) patient. If the patient is BREATHING but has NO PULSE, tag as a Priority 1 (*red tag*) patient. If the patient is BREATHING and HAS A PULSE, GOOD SKIN SIGNS, and CAPILLARY REFILL LESS THAN 2 SECONDS, go to the next step.

ASSESS LEVEL OF CONSCIOUSNESS (MENTAL STATUS) THIRD If ALERT, tag as a Priority 2 (*yellow tag*) patient. If there is any ALTERED MENTAL STATUS, tag as a Priority 1 (*red tag*) patient.

NOW RE-TRIAGE THE PRIORITY 3 "WALKING WOUNDED" PATIENTS Just because they could initially walk does not mean some of the Priority 3 patients do not have serious medical conditions! Many could have an altered mental status, be bleeding, and have significant signs of shock, which could cause them to be recategorized as a higher priority patient. Move methodically using the same START assessment of (1) respiration, (2) pulse, and (3) mental status.

A START SUMMARY A quick summary of START is as follows:

1. Order the walking wounded to some type of temporary collection point. They are considered Priority 3 (*green*) for now.
2. Assess all others for RPM (respiration, pulse, and mental status) and tag as follows:

   Priority 1 (red) are patients who have:
   - Altered mental status, or . . .
   - Absent radial pulse, or . . .
   - Respirations of greater than 30/minute

   Priority 2 (yellow) are patients who:
   - Are alert, and . . .
   - Have radial pulses present, and . . .
   - Have respirations less than 30/minute

   Priority 0 (black) are patients who:
   - Are not breathing (after an attempt to open the airway), or . . .
   - Have no pulse and are not breathing
3. Re-triage all walking wounded.

Patient Identification

By now it should be clear that a system will be required to group and identify patients by treatment priority. A widely used system is to color-code patients according to their priority. The START system, discussed previously, is one example of a color-coding system. Other systems' color codes may differ slightly. For example, Priority 1 might be red; Priority 2, yellow; Priority 3, green; and Priority 4 (if a separate category) might be black or gray.

Since different localities have different systems, it is important that you know and understand the system used in your area. It is equally important that different services in the same region use the same coding system. This is because many MCIs are multiple-agency events. If each agency were to use a different system, there would be no way to correctly coordinate the order in which patients are to receive care.

As you move among patients to conduct initial triage, you should affix a **triage tag** to each patient, indicating the priority group to which that patient has been assigned. Triage tags are color-coded and may have space in which limited medical information can be recorded (Figures 36-14, 36-15, and 36-16).

triage tag
color-coded tag indicating the priority group to which a patient has been assigned.

There are some local variations of the triage tag. Some use adhesive-backed colored shipping labels. Others use colored surveyor's tape or duct tape to classify patients. Surveyor's tape can be quickly tied on as an arm band. Duct tape will stick to just about anything in any kind of weather. For this reason it is particularly useful in an MCI setting. It is also useful to have a laundry marker or wax pencil handy for wet conditions when a standard pen or pencil will not write well.

Whatever system you use, it is vital that the color coding be easily located and identified. Properly done, this allows a later EMT to quickly identify which treatment group patients belong to and to institute treatment accordingly.

triage area
the area where secondary triage takes place at a multiple-casualty incident.

treatment area
the area in which patients are treated at a multiple-casualty incident.

treatment supervisor
person responsible for overseeing treatment of patients who have been triaged at a multiple-casualty incident.

Secondary Triage and Treatment

As more personnel arrive at the incident scene, they should be directed to assist with the completion of initial triage. If triage has been completed, these EMTs can initiate treatment.

Secondary triage is generally performed at a patient collection point or **triage area** from which patients are assigned to a treatment group.

Patients are physically separated into treatment groups based on their priority level as designated by a triage tag. Some systems call for vehicles to carry red, yellow, and green tarps, which are used to designate these areas. An area to which triaged patients are removed is referred to as a **treatment area.** Each treatment area should have its own **treatment supervisor,** an EMT responsible for overseeing the triage and treatment

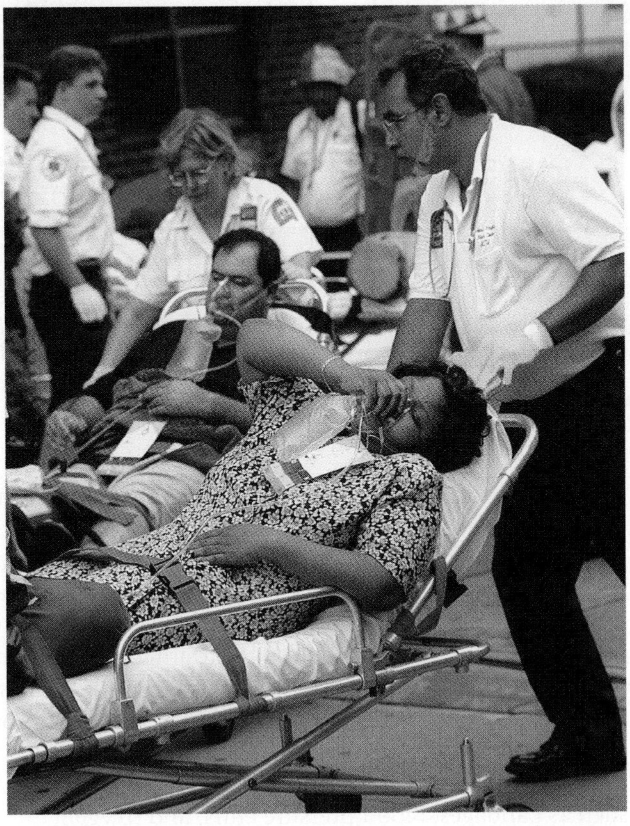

Figure 36-14 • The triage tag indicates the priority group to which that patient has been assigned. *(© Black Star)*

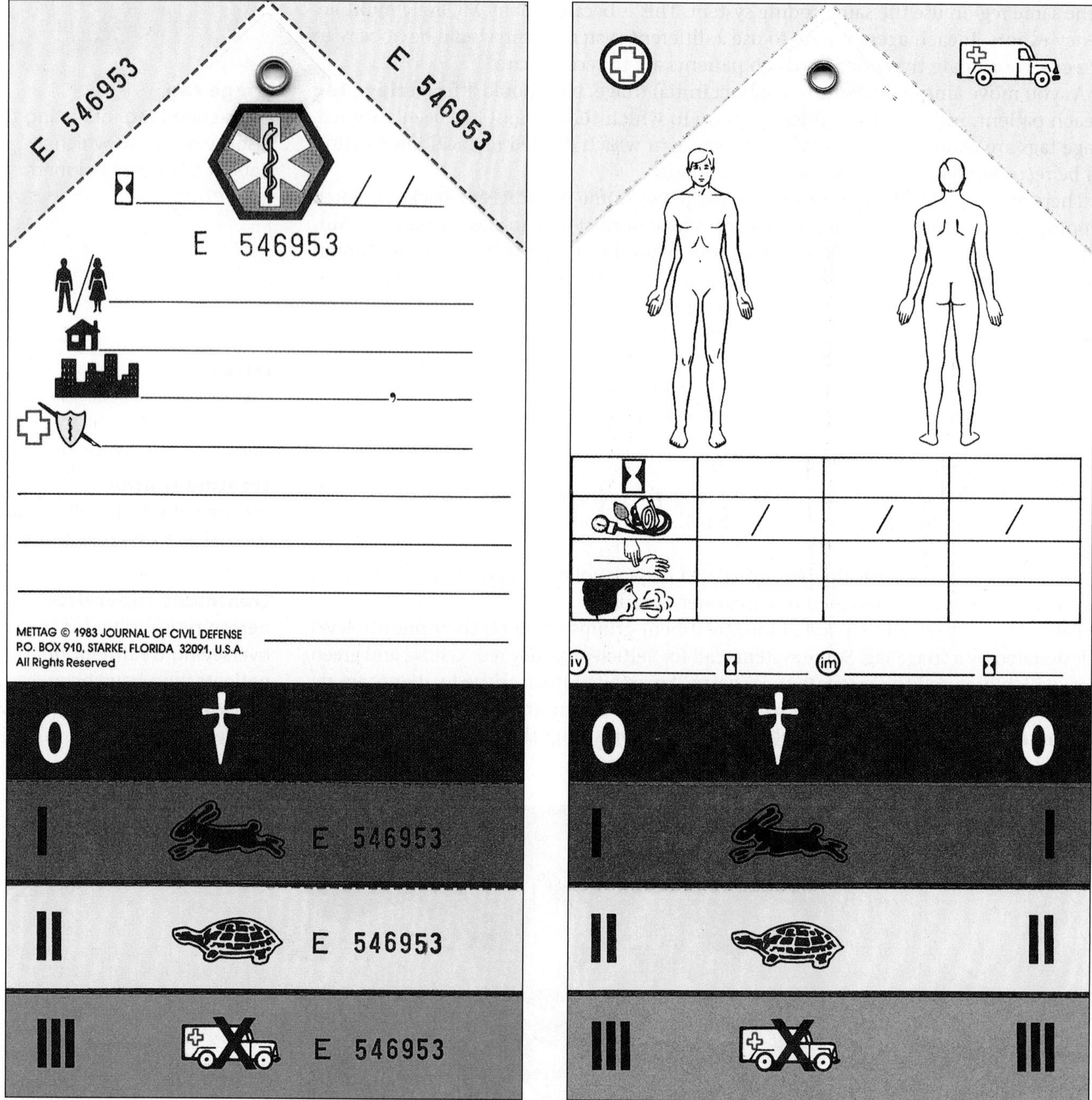

Figure 36-15 • Triage tag (front and back) used to identify Priority 1, 2, 3, and 0 patients.

within that area. The treatment supervisor should re-triage the patients in that area to determine the order in which they will receive treatment. Secondary triage is important to ensure that patients are treated and transported according to their priority.

During secondary triage, it may be necessary to re-categorize a patient whose condition has deteriorated or improved or who was incorrectly triaged to a higher or lower priority group than was medically warranted. This will necessitate moving the patient to the proper treatment area as resources permit. Some systems use a different disaster tag during secondary triage on which more detailed information about the patient can be recorded (Figure 36-16).

The treatment area EMTs will need supplies and equipment from the ambulances such as bandages, blood pressure cuffs, and oxygen.

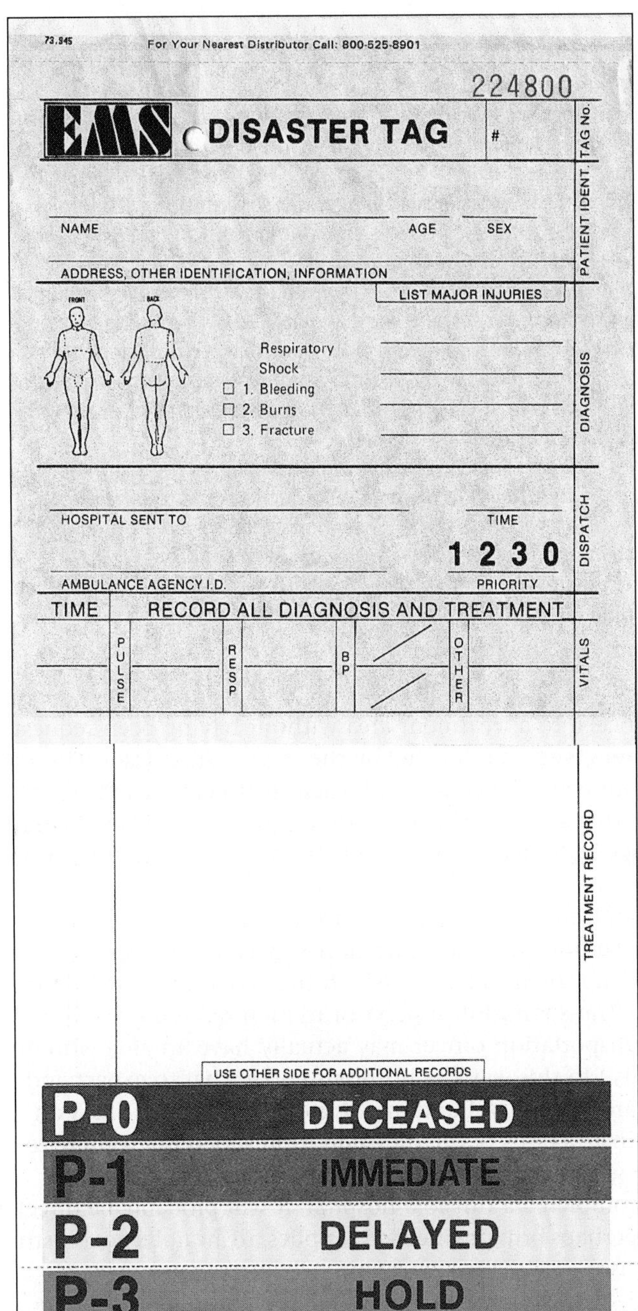
73.545 For Your Nearest Distributor Call: 800-525-8901

224800

EMS DISASTER TAG #

TAG No.

NAME AGE SEX

ADDRESS, OTHER IDENTIFICATION, INFORMATION

PATIENT IDENT.

LIST MAJOR INJURIES

Respiratory
Shock
☐ 1. Bleeding
☐ 2. Burns
☐ 3. Fracture

DIAGNOSIS

HOSPITAL SENT TO TIME

1 2 3 0

AMBULANCE AGENCY I.D. PRIORITY

DISPATCH

TIME | RECORD ALL DIAGNOSIS AND TREATMENT

PULSE RESP BP OTHER

VITALS

TREATMENT RECORD

USE OTHER SIDE FOR ADDITIONAL RECORDS

P-0 DECEASED
P-1 IMMEDIATE
P-2 DELAYED
P-3 HOLD

TREATMENT RECORD

TIME	RECORD ALL DIAGNOSIS AND TREATMENT

P-0	DECEASED	Expired Non-survivor
P-1	IMMEDIATE	Airway-respiratory, cardiac problems uncontrolled hemorrhage, open chest-abdomen severe head injury, shock, burns or medical.
P-2	DELAYED	Spinal cord injury, multiple-major fractures moderate burns, uncomplicated head injury.
P-3	HOLD	All minor & uncomplicated fractures, wounds, other injuries, burns & psychological problems.

Figure 36-16 • EMS disaster tag (front and back).

Transportation and Staging Logistics

Once patients have been properly assessed and triaged, and once treatment for the patients has been initiated according to their priority, consideration must be given to the order in which the patients will be transported to a hospital. Again, this is done according to triage priority.

It is advisable to have a **staging area** from which ambulances can be called to transport patients. The staging area will be the responsibility of the **staging supervisor.** This person must keep track of the ambulance vehicles and personnel. In large-scale incidents, the staging supervisor may need to arrange to meet human needs, such as rest rooms, meals, and rotation of crews.

staging area
the area where ambulances are parked and other resources are held until needed.

staging supervisor
person responsible for overseeing ambulances and ambulance personnel at a multiple-casualty incident.

POINT OF VIEW

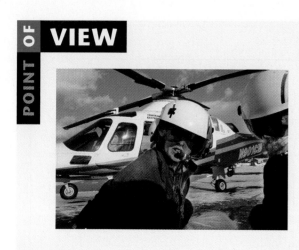

"You know how you figure if you ever get into a car crash it'll be a fender bender? Not me. I had to do it big. Real big.

"I was on the freeway, coming over the crest of a hill. Fortunately, I was going slow enough so I was able to stop just before a big wreck on the other side. There must've been 10 or 12 cars all over the road. Sounds like I did good, right? Nope. The tractor-trailer behind me couldn't stop fast enough. He hit me so hard he pushed me into the car in front of me and then into three others. Squished my little car like an accordion.

"While that was really the pits, I never realized that there would be injured people all over the place. I mean this road was littered with crashed cars and injured people. When the rescue people finally got to my car, they tied a red ribbon around my wrist and put a red sticker on my windshield. I was starting to feel bad. I asked an EMT what the red meant. He smiled at me very nicely and said, 'You'll be heading out first.'

"OK, great, I thought. Things were getting a little fuzzy. Then I saw spacemen heading my way. They had helmets on. They took me to a helicopter. I couldn't believe it. I thought maybe I was hallucinating, but sure enough, they loaded me in and flew me to the gosh-darned hospital.

"Too bad I couldn't have flown that helicopter to work and missed that whole crash thing. I'd probably still have my spleen!"

transportation supervisor person responsible for communicating with sector officers and hospitals to manage transportation of patients to hospitals from a multiple-casualty incident.

No ambulance should proceed to a treatment area without having been requested by the **transportation supervisor** and directed by the staging supervisor. The staging supervisor is responsible for communicating with each treatment area the number and priority of the patients in that area. This information can then be used by the transportation supervisor to arrange for transport of patients from the scene to the hospital in the most efficient way.

It is vital that no ambulance transport any patient without the approval of the transportation supervisor. This is because the transportation supervisor is responsible for maintaining a list of patients and the hospitals to which they are transported. This information is relayed from the transportation supervisor to each receiving hospital. (In a large-scale incident, the transportation officer may actually have an aide who does nothing but speak to hospitals.) In this way the hospitals know what to expect and receive only the patients they are capable of handling. It is critical that the EMTs on the ambulance comply with the instructions of the transportation supervisor. Failure to do so may result in patients being transported to the wrong facilities.

Once an ambulance has completed a run to a hospital, it will probably be directed to return to the staging area, perhaps bringing needed supplies, to await its next instructions from the staging supervisor.

Communicating with Hospitals

It is important that receiving hospitals be alerted to the nature of the MCI or disaster as soon as the magnitude of the incident is known. This allows the hospitals to call in additional personnel or to clear beds as necessary to accept the anticipated number of patients.

Because radio communication channels will be heavily used, the transportation officer, not individual EMTs, should communicate with the hospitals. This will keep unnecessary radio usage to a minimum. It will also ensure that the proper information is recorded at both ends of the ambulance ride. In large-scale MCIs, it is not necessary to give a patient report for each patient. This is because the treating and transporting EMTs will most likely be different and because there will generally be too many patients to allow EMTs to give a good patient radio report under the circumstances. In these instances, the hospital may be told only that they are receiving a Priority 1 patient with respiratory problems, for example.

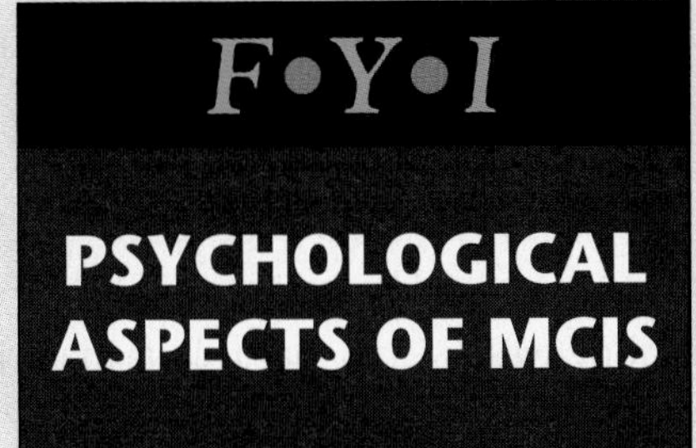

During MCIs, EMTs often encounter another, frequently overlooked condition: psychologically stressed patients. While they may outwardly exhibit few signs of injury or emotional stress, people involved in MCIs have been subjected to devastating circumstances with which they are normally unprepared to cope. Proper early management of the psychologically stressed patient can support later treatment and help ensure a faster recovery.

Adequately managing a patient during an MCI may require you to administer "psychological first aid." This may take the form of talking with a terrified parent, child, or witness. You should not attempt to engage in psychoanalysis and should not say things that are untrue in an attempt to calm a patient. However, a caring honest demeanor can reassure a patient, as will listening to the patient and acknowledging his fears and problems. Often this is all the patient will need.

Patients are not the only ones subject to emotional stress during a multiple-casualty incident; emergency responders are as well. It is very important that you understand that large-scale or horrific MCIs (Figures 36-17 and 36-18) may affect rescuers as much as, if not more than, non-rescuers.

EMTs who become emotionally incapacitated should be treated as patients and removed to an area where they can rest without viewing the scene. These patients must be monitored by an EMS provider until a clinically competent provider can take over. These EMTs should not be allowed to return to duty without first being evaluated by someone professionally trained to do so. ■

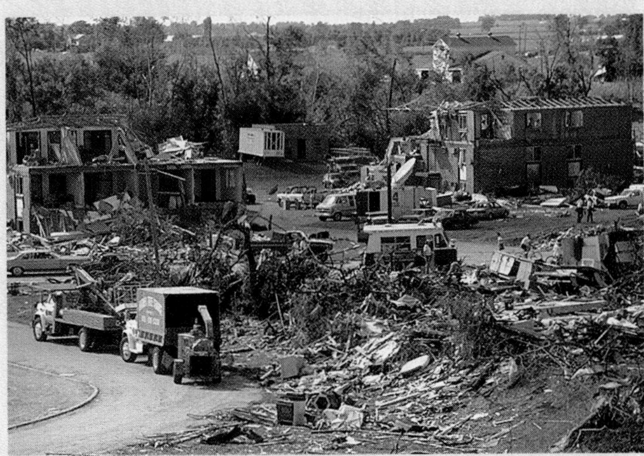

Figure 36-17 • A tornado can cause great devastation. *(© Steve Leonard/Black Star)*

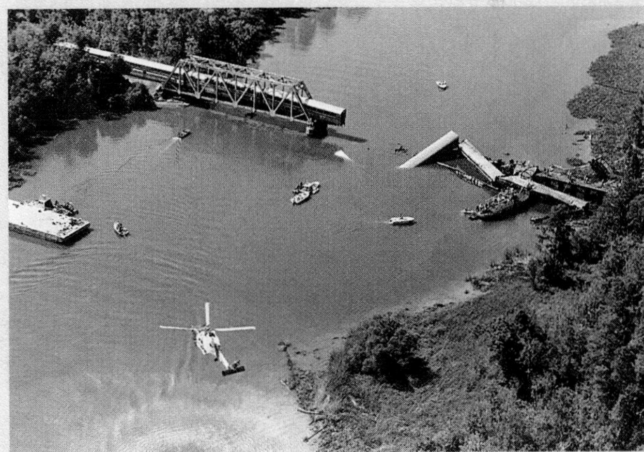

Figure 36-18 • A train wreck can cause multiple casualties. *(© Black Star)*

CHAPTER REVIEW

SUMMARY

Become familiar with your local plans for dealing with hazardous materials and multiple-casualty incidents. Practice every chance you get. Understand the management systems and triage systems used in your area, and be prepared to do your part. Also remember that hazardous materials incidents require specialized training beyond your expertise. However, you can learn to recognize them quickly, call for the appropriate assistance, and help to ensure the safety of rescuers, patients, and bystanders.

KEY TERMS

cold zone area where the Incident Command post and support functions are located.

Command the first on the scene to establish order and initiate the Incident Command System.

decontamination a chemical and/or physical process that reduces or prevents the spread of contamination from persons or equipment; the removal of hazardous substances from employees and their equipment to the extent necessary to preclude foreseeable health effects.

disaster plan a predefined set of instructions for a community's emergency responders.

hazardous material any substance or material in a form which poses an unreasonable risk to health, safety, and property when transported in commerce.

hot zone area immediately surrounding a hazmat incident; extends far enough to prevent adverse effects outside the zone.

Incident Command the person who assumes overall direction of an incident.

Incident Command System (ICS) a subset of the National Incident Management System (NIMS).

multiple-casualty incident (MCI) any medical or trauma incident involving multiple patients.

National Incident Management System (NIMS) the management system used by federal, state, and local governments to manage emergencies in the United States.

singular command command organization in which a single agency controls all resources and operations.

staging area the area where ambulances are parked and other resources are held until needed.

staging supervisor person responsible for overseeing ambulances and ambulance personnel at a multiple-casualty incident.

transportation supervisor person responsible for communicating with sector officers and hospitals to manage transportation of patients to hospitals from a multiple-casualty incident.

treatment area the area in which patients are treated at a multiple-casualty incident.

treatment supervisor person responsible for overseeing treatment of patients who have been triaged at a multiple-casualty incident.

triage the process of quickly assessing patients at a multiple-casualty incident and assigning each a priority for receiving treatment; from a French word meaning "to sort."

triage area the area where secondary triage takes place at a multiple-casualty incident.

triage supervisor the person responsible for overseeing triage at a multiple-casualty incident.

triage tag color-coded tag indicating the priority group to which a patient has been assigned.

unified command command organization in which several agencies work independently but cooperatively.

warm zone area where personnel and equipment decontamination and hot zone support take place; it includes control points for the access corridor and thus assists in reducing the spread of contamination.

REVIEW QUESTIONS

1. List the information in an initial report of a hazardous material incident. (p. 971)
2. Explain how to identify a hazardous material and how to obtain information about that material. (pp. 967–971)
3. Describe the general assessment and emergency care of a patient with a hazardous material injury. (pp. 971–976)
4. Describe the major components and benefits of an incident management system. (pp. 977–978)

5. Define the basic role of the EMT at a multiple-casualty incident. (pp. 976–990)
6. Explain why patients are assigned priorities during triage. (p. 981)
7. Identify four priority categories of triage. (p. 984)

CRITICAL THINKING

- Your call is to a motor-vehicle collision with an unknown number of injuries. As your unit approaches the scene, you see that three cars and downed wires are involved. You get a whiff of gasoline as you pass by. The drivers are visible in each vehicle—one appears to be conscious and the other two are bent forward or slumped back. There are passengers visible in two vehicles, one or more of whom may need extrication. How should you proceed?

MEDIA RESOURCES

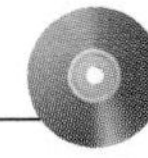

See the Student CD at the back of this book for quizzes, a case study activity, and other features related to this chapter. In particular, take a look at the Case Study regarding START triage and MCI management. Also, visit the Companion Website for *Emergency Care* at **www.prenhall.com/limmer,** where you will find additional reinforcement and links to other resources.

Street Scenes

It's raining hard and there's a loud noise on the station PA system with the dispatcher saying: "Ambulances Alpha 2, Alpha 5, Bravo 1, and Charlie 10, respond to a three-car motor-vehicle crash at the intersection of Avenues A and B. Unknown how many occupants. Timeout of 1933 hours." You turn to your partner and say, "This call is only about 10 blocks away. We should be the first on scene." As you head toward the scene, you are notified by dispatch that the police are on scene and report a total of nine occupants. Additional ambulances are being dispatched.

You and your partner agree that you will establish Incident Command and he will do triage. "Dispatch, Bravo 1 is on scene and establishing Incident Command." The first thing you do is put on the Command bib for identification. Your partner puts on the triage bib and takes triage tags to check on the occupants. You briefly tell the police officer you are Incident Command and he informs you that his captain is responding and has three units handling traffic control. He has also requested heavy rescue from the fire department in case extrication is needed.

With flashlight in hand and trying to keep the rain out of your eyes, you perform a scene size-up. You realize that you need a place to stage the other ambulances for easy access and so they don't get blocked in. You see a location and quickly share your idea with the police officer. He agrees. He will tell his units to make sure that area is accessible for the ambulances. You call dispatch on the radio using the identifier "Incident Command" and ask that they instruct all responding ambulances to stage in the parking lot of the insurance company.

Street Scene Questions

1. As Incident Command, what are some of the things you need to do?
2. What information do you expect first from the triage officer?
3. How will you decide what patients go to what hospitals?

Your partner advises you that three patients are Priority 1, five are Priority 2, and one is Priority 3. You radio dispatch with this information. You are told that a canvass of local hospitals has already been done and the trauma center can handle all Priority 1 patients and the other patients can be divided between the other three area hospitals. You ask that they call the trauma center back and confirm that they will be getting three patients and the other hospitals will be getting two each.

You then ask dispatch to tell you how many ambulances have been dispatched. You are informed there is a total of five. Remembering that one of the ambulances is yours, you request two more ambulances. Two ambulances are on-scene and parked in the staging area. You tell them to each take a Priority 1 patient. The next ambulance is assigned to the last Priority 1 patient. You ask the triage officer if some of the Priority 2 or 3 patients can be doubled up, which seems appropriate for four of the patients.

Street Scene Questions

4. Is there a need for a safety officer on this scene?
5. How should patient information be transmitted to the hospitals?
6. What information should you be sharing with Police Command and Fire Command?

The fire captain tells you that his crew has disconnected the batteries of all the vehicles and will stand by to assist with extrication. Access has been gained to all patients using hand tools. You ask if his safety officer can continue in that role until all the patients are off the scene.

The first ambulance is loaded and en route to the trauma center. The second will be en route shortly. You advise these crews to notify the hospital directly but tell them to keep the transmission short.

The last Priority 1 patient is out of the car, and you tell the triage supervisor that the other hospitals get two patients each. He should coordinate this with crews and tell them to call the patient information to the hospital directly.

Within 30 minutes of the call notification, every patient is en route to a hospital. You let Police and Fire Command know. Your partner looks at you and says, "Not bad for someone who looks like a drowned rat."

Street Scenes Sample Documentation

SPECIAL INCIDENT REPORT *On arrival during a heavy rainstorm, we noticed 3-car motor-vehicle crash with a total of 9 patients. We activated our agency's MCI plan. I assumed EMS command, and my partner became the triage officer. I maintained unified command with police and fire command. As requested by triage, additional units were requested and staged as needed. We transported a total of 3 priority-one patients, 5 priority-two patients, and 1 priority-three. Total scene time was 30 minutes. We returned to service after restocking.*

CHAPTER 37

EMS Response to Terrorism

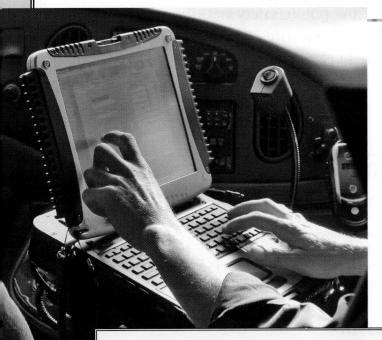

CORE CONCEPTS

The following are core concepts that will be addressed in this chapter:

- Types of terrorist events
- How to identify a terrorist event
- How to respond to and deal with harms from a terrorist event
- Characteristics of weaponizable agents

KEY TERMS

contamination, p. 1004
dissemination, p. 1006
domestic terrorism, p. 996
exposure, p. 1003
international terrorism, p. 997
permeation, p. 1004
rem, p. 1019
routes of entry, p. 1003
secondary devices, p. 998
strategies, p. 1020
tactics, p. 1020
terrorism, p. 996
weaponization, p. 1008
weapons of mass destruction (WMD), p. 997
zoonotic, p. 1014

NOTE *There are no objectives in the National Standard Curriculum that pertain to the material in this chapter.*

Terrorism is nothing new on the planet. Its history dates back hundreds of years to the dark ages. Even just since the early 1900s, there have been thousands of bombings and incendiary devices used for terrorist purposes. Of course, EMS has had a prominent part in responding to violent acts since its inception in the early 1970s.

Since the terrorist attacks of September 11, 2001, however, the role of emergency responders has been redefined. Emergency services provided by EMS, fire rescue, and law enforcement are now defined by the U.S. government as one of five parts of the National Critical Infrastructure—the infrastructure considered to be critical to the continued operation of our nation.

EMS is a key part of the public safety net, the support network that ensures the safety and health of our citizens (Figure 37-1). Thus, the evolution of EMS involves not only improvements in emergency medical care but a constant refinement of the response mission as well.

terrorism the unlawful use of force or violence against persons or property to intimidate or coerce a government, the civilian population, or any segment thereof, in furtherance of political or social objectives. (U.S. Department of Justice, FBI, definition)

domestic terrorism terrorism directed against the government or population without foreign direction.

DEFINING TERRORISM

The U.S. Department of Justice, Federal Bureau of Investigation (FBI), defines **terrorism** as "the unlawful use of force or violence against persons or property to intimidate or coerce a government, the civilian population or any segment thereof, in furtherance of political or social objectives."

The Federal Bureau of Investigation further defines two types of terrorism that occur in the United States: domestic terrorism and international terrorism.

Domestic Terrorism

Domestic terrorism involves groups or individuals whose terrorist activities are directed at the government or population, without foreign direction. Domestic terrorism

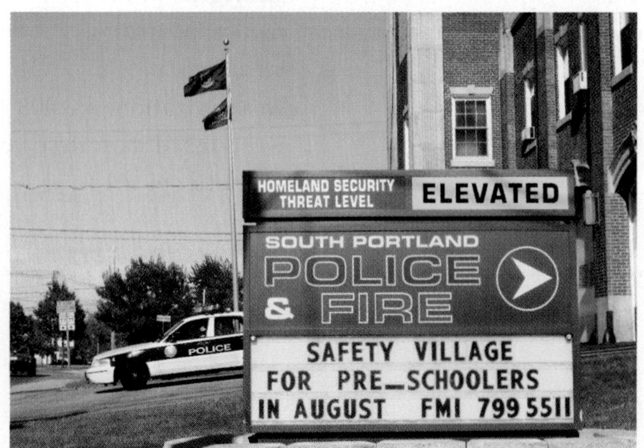

Figure 37-1 • Soon after September 11, 2001 terrorist attacks, this sign outside the South Portland, Maine, Police and Fire building indicated a yellow, or elevated, terrorism threat level. As advised by the U.S. Department of Homeland Security, threat levels may be red (severe), orange (high), yellow (elevated), blue (guarded), or green (low).

is changing, moving away from structured organizations to a fragmented, leaderless phenomenon in which individuals or small groups act independently.

Domestic terrorist groups or individuals can be fueled by a range of motivations. A wide variety of domestic terrorist groups and individuals have been identified, including environmental terrorists, survivalists, militias, racial-hate groups, and groups with extreme political, religious, or other philosophies or beliefs.

International Terrorism

International terrorism involves groups or individuals whose terrorist activities are foreign-based and/or directed by countries or groups outside the targeted country or whose activities cross national boundaries. One trend in international terrorism is the shift from well-organized, state-sponsored localized groups to loosely organized, international networks of terrorists. The Al Qaeda network is an example.

international terrorism terrorism that is foreign-based or directed.

These loosely networked individuals and groups have increasingly turned to a variety of sources of funding, including private sponsorship, drug trafficking, crime, and illegal trade. Concurrently, there is a growing trend away from terrorism that is politically motivated to terrorism that is religiously or ideologically motivated.

Types of Terrorism Incidents

In addition to armed attacks, incidents of terrorism may involve what are often called the CBRNE agents:

Chemical
Biological
Radiological
Nuclear
Explosive

The CBRNE agents are considered to be technological hazardous agents—a broad field of which hazmats (the types of hazardous materials that were discussed in Chapter 36, "Special Operations") are a subcategory. The CBRNE agents are often called **weapons of mass destruction (WMD),** which are weapons intended to cause widespread harm and/or fear among a population.

weapons of mass destruction (WMD) weapons, devices, or agents intended to cause widespread harm and/or fear among a population.

Terrorism incidents can also encompass criminal activities. In such acts as arson, environmental crime, and industrial sabotage, criminal and technological incidents overlap.

Of course, terrorism can also be committed by conventional or unanticipated means, such as flying an airplane into a building.

While the Department of Justice, as noted earlier, uses a narrow definition of terrorism, EMS has responsibilities for violent incidents that go well beyond that limited scope. This chapter will cover principally terrorism involving CBRNE agents.

TERRORISM AND EMS

First Responders as Targets

First Responders are often principal targets of a terrorist attack, as will be discussed in more detail later. Responders must stay alert and never assume the incident scene is safe until this is verified by appropriate agencies or authorities. Responders must weigh the threat or risk of their actions against the benefit of their actions. This is true at all emergency scenes, of course, but even more true at the scene of a terrorist attack.

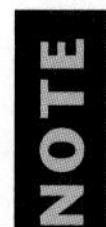

Always remember: The safety of the EMS provider is the most important consideration when responding to a potential terrorist incident. The responder who gets hurt cannot help others.

POINT OF VIEW

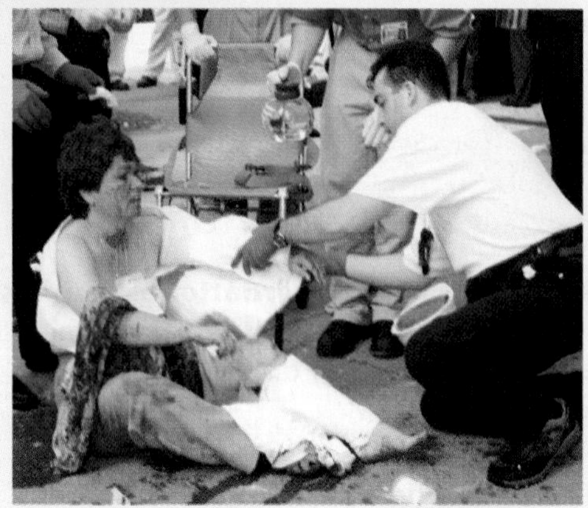
© Ciniglio Lorenzo/Corbis Sygma

"When you take your EMT class you learn about a lot of things. You even learn about what to do at multiple-casualty incidents.

"I had some minor MCIs in my early days. Car crashes with 5 patients, a fire with a lot of smoke inhalation. But nothing could prepare me—no class and no experience—for the real "big one." A terrorist incident.

"I'm not going to tell stories. All I can say is that sometimes things are of a magnitude that you can't even conceive until you are there. You are a small cog in a big wheel. You feel like you are both so small in a big incident, and yet so important for being there. The injuries and specific things you see actually become secondary to the hugeness of it all.

"It was tough. It was enormous. It was mass humanity and mass confusion at the same time. It'll happen again somewhere. It may happen to you. It will be tough, but you'll be glad you were there to do your job. Someone has to."

Identify the Threat Posed by the Event

EMS response to a terrorist event is complicated. You may be dealing with a hazardous materials or mass casualty incident, using recognized protocols, such as the hazmat procedures and Incident Command System discussed in Chapter 36, "Special Operations." A terrorist incident, however, may involve two additional factors that all responders will have to take into account: deliberate targeting of responders and crime scene considerations.

secondary devices destructive devices, such as bombs, placed to be activated after an initial attack and timed to injure emergency responders and others who rush in to help care for those targeted by an initial attack.

Terrorists have a history of utilizing **secondary devices** and/or booby traps to target emergency responders. In January 1997, a bomb went off outside an Atlanta family-planning clinic. One hour after the initial detonation, a second bomb went off close to the point where the Incident Command post had been established, which resulted in several injuries to responders and could have caused deaths.

If the incident is a potential act of terrorism, it is also a crime scene. While there will be similarities between terrorist events and non-terrorist mass-casualty incidents (such as major transportation collisions and hazmat incidents), crime scene considerations, such as the need to preserve evidence and the need to guard against further criminal activity, will complicate responder operations.

Regardless of the mechanism or motive behind an incident, responders should remain focused on reducing the impact of the event as efficiently and safely as possible. Whether dealing with a terrorist or a non-terrorist event, all responders should follow their agency's established operating guidelines. All responders on the scene should operate under an Incident Command System and utilize some type of personnel accountability system that is compatible with those used by all participating agencies.

Recognizing suspicious incidents may be difficult, but being alert to clues, surroundings, and events will greatly assist in identification. Clues such as the OTTO signs, discussed in the following list, will help with this process:

Occupancy or location
Type of event
Timing of the event
On-scene warning signs

Occupancy or Location

Clues provided by the occupancy or location of the event include the following:

- *Symbolic and historical targets* include those that represent some organization or event that is particularly offensive in the minds of an extremist individual or group. Examples might include Bureau of Alcohol, Tobacco, and Firearms (BATF) offices for those who oppose all forms of gun control; Internal Revenue Service (IRS) offices for tax resisters; or a national monument such as the Statue of Liberty for anti-Americans. The World Trade Center (Figure 37-2A), with its great height and location at the financial hub of New York City, became such a target twice, in 1993 and on September 11, 2001. The Pentagon (Figure 37-2B) was also targeted on September 11, 2001, as a strike at the U.S. military.

- *Public buildings or assembly areas* provide the opportunity for attention-getting mass casualties. Some of these public buildings are also symbolic targets, so the terrorist can cause massive casualties and link the owner/operator of the building or assembly area with danger in the minds of the public. Examples of these would include shopping malls, convention centers, entertainment venues, and tourist destinations.
- *Controversial businesses* are usually those that have a history of attracting the enmity of extremist groups. Family planning clinics, nuclear facilities, and furriers all fall into this category.
- *Infrastructure systems* include those operations that are necessary for the continued functioning of our society. Major cities are full of targets such as bridges, power plants, phone companies, water treatment plants, mass transit, and hospitals. Attacks on any of these have the potential to disrupt entire regions and cost hundreds of millions of dollars to correct.

Type of Event

Certain types of events should raise your awareness of possible terrorist involvement. In general, they can be categorized as follows:

- *Explosions and/or incendiaries* are among the favorite weapons of terrorists. Any bombing or suspicious fire may raise suspicions of terrorist involvement, especially when combined with location or occupancy factors as previously listed.
- *Incidents involving firearms* are always treated as suspicious. If they occur in conjunction with other indicating factors, terrorism is a definite possibility.
- *Nontrauma mass casualty incidents* have occurred as the arsenal of terrorism increases in sophistication. When large numbers of victims are generated without obvious (physical) injury, but with symptoms of illness, you may suspect terrorist involvement.

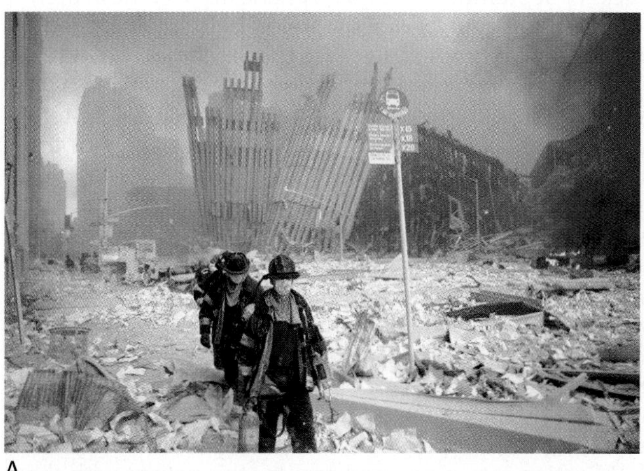

A

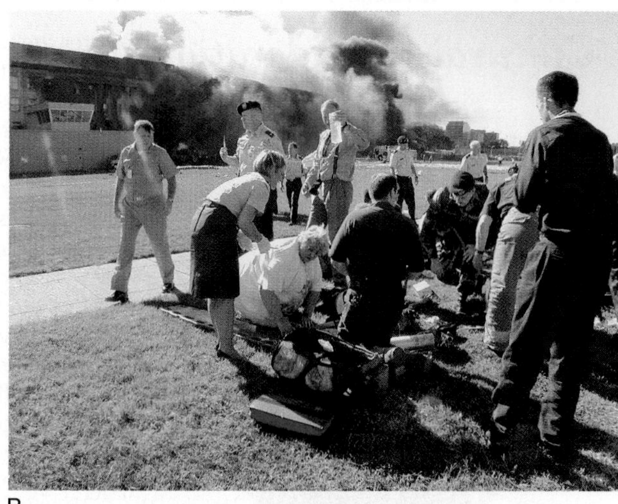

B

Figure 37-2 • (A) The Twin Towers of the World Trade Center in New York City were destroyed and thousands were killed on September 11, 2001, when terrorists flew hijacked jetliners into those famous skyscrapers. *(© Corbis/Sygma)* (B) The Pentagon was also the target of a hijacked jetliner on September 11, 2001. *(© AP Images/US Navy, Journalist First Class Mark D. Farram)*

Timing of the Event

For many years to come, April 19 will be a day around which government facilities operate at a heightened state of security awareness. It is the anniversary of both the fire at the Branch Davidian compound in Waco, Texas, and the bombing of the Alfred P. Murrah building in Oklahoma City, and so has become a rallying point for anti-government extremists. National holidays are also possible target dates.

Aside from significant anniversaries and holidays, events that occur on specific days of the week and times of day are worth treating with suspicion. A fire at a government building during the weekend or during a time when few people are likely to be present, for example, may indicate terrorism or other criminal activity.

On-Scene Warning Signs

When you arrive on the scene, you should always watch for signs that you are dealing with a suspicious incident. Unexplained patterns of illness or deaths can be attributed to chemical, radiological, or biological agents. Some of these substances have recognizable odors and/or tastes. Unexplained signs and symptoms of skin, eye, or airway irritation may be linked to chemical contamination, as may unexplained vapor clouds, mists, and plumes.

Always remain on the lookout for chemical containers, spray devices, or lab equipment in unusual locations. Watch for items or containers that appear out of place at unusual incidents, which might contain a secondary device. Fires, spot fires, and fires of unusual behavior may also arouse suspicion, as can anything that appears abnormal for a given incident scene.

Recognize the Harms Posed by the Threat

To implement self-protection measures, you must first understand the types of harm to which you can be exposed. These types of harm—Thermal, Radiological, Asphyxiation, Chemical, Etiological, Mechanical, and Psychological—can be categorized utilizing the acronym TRACEM-P.

The TRACEM-P Harms

- *Thermal harm* refers to harm caused by either extreme heat, such as that generated by burning liquids or metals, or extreme cold from cryogenic materials such

Cultural Considerations

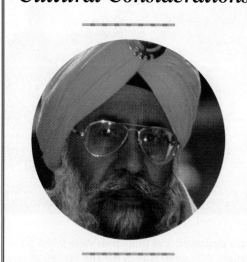

After the terrorist attacks of September 11, 2001, Americans became acutely aware that persons from foreign countries or of foreign birth might be plotting terrorist acts within our own borders. Because the September 11th terrorists were Middle Easterners, we tended to become wary of anyone who was—or even looked sort of like he might be—a person of Middle Eastern origin. The man pictured here could be from South Asia, probably not the Middle East, but because he has brown skin and wears a turban, he may well have become a target of suspicion among some of his neighbors.

We know, of course, that most persons of foreign birth are not terrorists—yet at the same time we have been asked to be vigilant, on the lookout for odd behavior or other clues to possible terrorist plots.

So how should you behave when your patient is a person of foreign birth with a "different" look or accent? Of course you will be alert to any clues such as evidence of a chemical lab or the presence of weapons or explosives—this is part of your scene size-up, no matter the background of the patient—but it is not your job to decide where your patient is from, and you will always be aware that your first obligation is to assess and care for this patient with the same warmth and professionalism as with any other patient.

as liquid oxygen. Radiant heat can melt protective clothing and other equipment if an individual is too near the heat source.

- *Radiological harm* refers to danger from alpha particles, beta particles, or gamma rays, generally produced by sources such as nuclear fuels, by-products of nuclear power production, or nuclear bombs. Figure 37-3 shows the relative penetrating power of the three types of radiation.
- *Asphyxiation* is caused by a lack of oxygen in the atmosphere. One common cause of this is heavier-than-air gases such as argon, carbon dioxide, or chemical vapors in a confined space. Extremely dusty situations such as the site of the World Trade Center towers collapse create additional problems. An oxygen level of 19.5 percent is required for normal breathing.
- *Chemical harm* is posed by toxic or corrosive materials. These can include acids such as sulfuric, caustics such as lye, and chemical toxins ranging from cyanides to nerve agents.
- *Etiological harm—etiology* concerns the causes of disease—comes from either disease-causing organisms such as bacteria and viruses or toxins derived from living organisms.
- *Mechanical harm* is any sort of physical trauma such as gunshot wounds, slip-trip-and-fall injuries, and injury from bomb fragments or shrapnel.
- *Psychological harm* can, of course, result from any violent or traumatic event. Terrorist events are designed to create fear, invoke panic, reduce faith in government, and (as the name indicates) cause terror. In fact, this is generally the purpose of a terrorist attack. Responders and victims will be subject to post-traumatic stress and survival guilt. These effects may occur during or right after the event or may manifest themselves at a much later time.

Professional counseling is available to responders in many local communities.

TIME/DISTANCE/SHIELDING

Protection of the First Responder is based on avoiding or minimizing exposure through the principles of time, distance, and shielding.

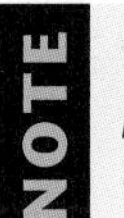

Remember: All forms of protection can be defined in terms of time, distance, and shielding.

- *Time.* Minimize your time at a dangerous scene, such as a crime scene or a hazmat scene. Spend the shortest amount of time possible in the dangerous area or exposed to a hazardous material, a biological agent, or radiation. An example of utilizing time constraints would be executing rapid entries to perform reconnaissance or rescue. The less time you spend in the affected area, the less likely you are to become injured. Minimizing the time you spend in the affected area will also reduce the chance of contaminating a crime scene.
- *Distance.* Maximize your distance from the hazard area or the projected hazard area. One example of utilizing distance would be avoiding contact by following the recommended guidelines regarding hazardous materials in the current

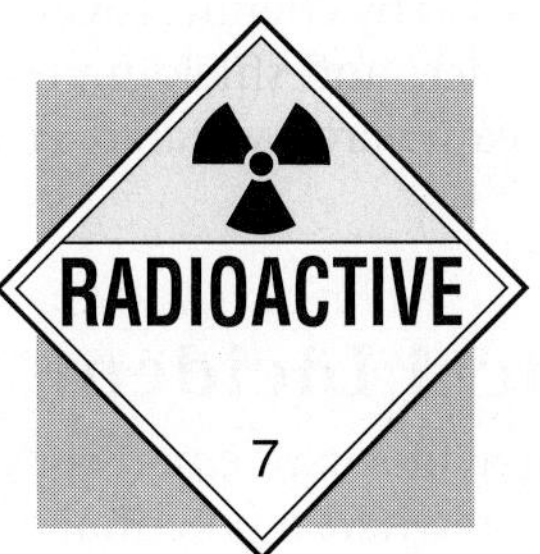

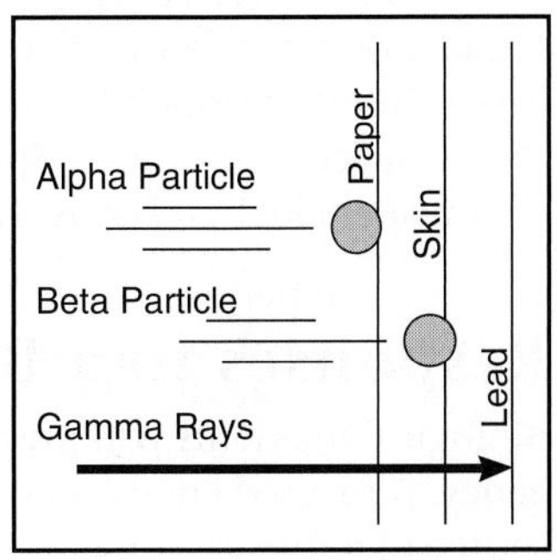

Figure 37-3 • The relative penetrating power of alpha, beta, and gamma radiation.

edition of the *Emergency Response Guidebook*. You can determine the safe distances from vehicles suspected of containing explosives from the recommendations in *Vehicle Bomb Explosion Hazard and Evacuation Distance Tables* obtainable from the Bureau of Alcohol, Tobacco, and Firearms.
- *Shielding*. Use appropriate shielding to address specific hazards. Shielding can consist of vehicles, buildings, fire-protection clothing, hazmat suits, positive-pressure self-contained breathing apparatus, and personal protective equipment (PPE). Also consider the vaccinations recommended by your service to provide immunization against specific diseases.

Responders should use all three forms of protection whenever possible. Just because you feel properly shielded does not mean that you can spend excessive time in close proximity to a contaminated site.

RESPONSES TO TERRORISM

The following sections will cover the TRACEM-P harms for the CBRNE terrorism categories. For each category, the primary harm will appear in bold type. The others listed will be secondary harms. The TRACEM-P harms that are not listed are not relevant to the CBRNE category (chemical, biological, radiological/nuclear, explosive) that is being discussed.

Responses to a Chemical Incident

Chemical incidents can include many classes of hazardous materials. Materials can be inhaled, ingested, absorbed, or injected. The materials can include industrial chemical or warfare-type agents.

Types of Harm from Chemical Incidents

The following types of harm can result from chemical incidents:

- *Thermal harm* is a secondary harm since many chemical reactions create heat. Also the chemicals involved may be flammable.
- *Asphyxiation* is a secondary harm and is possible because some chemical reactions may deplete oxygen or create gases that displace oxygen.
- *Chemical harms* are the primary harm and include a wide variety of effects such as corrosivity and reactivity. They may also have a variety of systemic effects that may attack the central nervous system, cardiovascular system, respiratory system, and other body systems.
- *Mechanical harm* is a secondary harm that must be taken into account because corrosive chemicals like strong acids can weaken structural elements.
- *Psychological harm* is a secondary harm because many individuals will react emotionally to a possible chemical exposure.

Self-Protection Measures at a Chemical Incident

Because of the wide variety of hazards posed by chemical agents, responders should take care to use the principles of time, distance, and shielding to minimize exposure risks under all circumstances. Specialized teams are available in most areas to deal with chemical incidents (Figure 37-4).

Responses to a Biological Incident

Biological incidents will present as either a focused emergency or a public health emergency. A focused emergency is a situation where a potential or actual point of origin or source of a disease is located (such as a single case or a small and localized number of

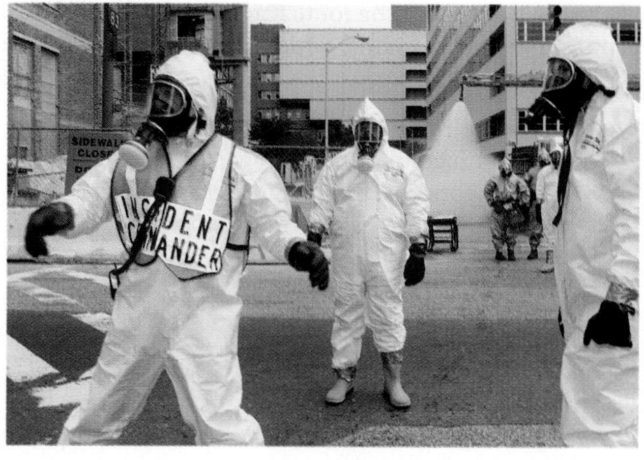

Figure 37-4 • In Baltimore, a specialized team trains to handle a bioterror incident. *(© AP Images/Alex Dorgan-Ross)*

cases of a disease) and attempts are made to prevent or minimize damage and spread. A public health emergency manifests itself as a sudden demand upon the public health infrastructure with no apparent explanation for the occurrence. Causative agents may be bacteria, viruses, or toxins. These agents may cause harm by being inhaled or ingested into the body.

- *Bacteria* are single-celled organisms that can grow in a variety of environments. Dangers to humans come from two directions: disease-causing bacteria growing in the human body, and bacteria that grow outside of the body but produce toxins that may pose a danger. (*Rickettsia* are sometimes classified as a genus of bacteria, sometimes as organisms that share characteristics of both bacteria and viruses. Like bacteria, they can be destroyed by antibiotics. Like viruses, they can only live and multiply inside cells. They cause diseases such as Q fever and typhus. In the remainder of this chapter, rickettsia will be grouped with bacteria.)
- *Viruses* are the smallest known entity capable of reproduction. They only grow inside of living cells and cause those cells to produce additional viruses.
- *Toxins* are poisons produced by living organisms. The organisms may be bacteria, fungi, flowering plants, insects, fish, reptiles, or mammals.

Critical Information About Biological Incidents

WHAT IS AN EXPOSURE? **Exposure** equals the *dose* or the *concentration* of the agent multiplied by *time* (the duration of the exposure).

exposure
the dose or concentration of an agent multiplied by the time, or duration.

- *Chemical doses* are generally measured in milligrams per kilograms of body weight. *Biological doses* are measured in fractions of micrograms per kilograms of body weight.
- *Concentration* of an agent is measured in parts per million.

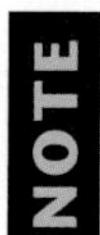

Remember that if you reduce the dose, concentration, or time near the agent, you will reduce the exposure.

Remember that infectious dose data are standardized. They are typically based on a 70-kg or 150-pound male in good health. Individuals who fall below these parameters may become infected at lower doses. Examples include the elderly, who are often in poor health, and young children, whose body weight is less than 150 pounds.

FOUR MAJOR ROUTES OF ENTRY **Routes of entry** are critical concepts that must be understood prior to studying individual WMD agents. Exposures occur through "routes" or pathways into the body. Biological agents can enter the body through four routes:

routes of entry
pathways into the body, generally by absorption, ingestion, injection, or inhalation.

- Absorption (skin contact)
- Ingestion (mouth)
- Injection (needles or projectiles)
- Inhalation (breathing)

The skin is seldom the route through which biological agents enter the body. The exception is T2 mycotoxins, which can be absorbed through the skin. Items that affect skin absorption are:

- Injury to the skin
- Skin temperature/blood flow
- Higher concentration = greater exposure
- Area with more hair = more exposure
- Length of exposure
- Type of agent

Ingestion is a common route to infection. Ingestion includes swallowing biological agents in food or drink or accidentally swallowing the agent by itself. One highly likely way to become infected is to eat or drink before completing decontamination procedures.

Injection or puncturing can be accidental or purposeful. Vectors (such as mosquitoes or fleas) can carry biological agents from one host to another. Personnel can become infected with biological agents by accidentally injecting themselves through improper handling of a needle or puncturing themselves with a jagged piece of debris. Common infection routes for biological infection are:

- Vector (a disease-carrying organism)
- Jagged glass or metal
- Syringes
- High-pressure devices

Inhalation has the potential to cause more biological agent infection than any other route of exposure, provided the particle is small enough to reach the lower respiratory tract. The degree of infection is based on:

- Rate of breathing
- Depth of breathing

Decontamination after inhalation is only psychologically beneficial.

contamination
contact with or presence of a material (contaminant) that is present where it does not belong and that is somehow harmful to persons, animals, or the environment.

WHAT IS CONTAMINATION? Contamination is caused by contact with or presence of a *contaminant*, which is material that is present where it does not belong and that is somehow harmful to persons, animals, or the environment. As contaminants, biological agents may be in the solid, liquid, or aerosol form. Dealing with each of these requires a different set of skills and operations.

Things that can be contaminated include:

- Hard and soft surfaces
- Skin and hair
- Clothing

EXPOSURE VERSUS CONTAMINATION Exposure occurs when a substance is taken into the body through one of the routes of exposure. Contamination occurs when a substance clings to surface areas of the body or clothing.

permeation
the movement of a substance through a surface or, on a molecular level, through intact materials; penetration, or spreading.

Clothing and other materials can become *permeated* with a contaminant. (**Permeation** is the movement of a substance through a surface or, on a molecular level, through intact materials. In general, it means penetration, or spreading.) However, biological agents can usually be washed out of clothing. In most cases, clothing and personal protective equipment (PPE) can be reused after decontamination.

Types of Harm from Biological Incidents

The following types of harm can result from biological incidents:

- *Chemical harm* could be a secondary hazard, for example at the scene of a clandestine laboratory.

- *Etiological harm* is the primary type of harm. These materials are classified as Class 6 Hazardous Materials (Poison) by the U.S. Department of Transportation.
- *Mechanical harm* is a possible secondary hazard where explosives have been used to disperse the agent.
- *Psychological harm* is a secondary harm. Just the thought of possible exposure to or contamination by a biological agent can cause stress, even if the person has not actually come in contact with the agent.

Self-Protection Measures at a Biological Incident

Take care to limit exposure and contamination if a biological incident is suspected. Personal protective equipment provides a shield to isolate a person from the hazards that can be encountered at an incident. Such equipment includes both personal protective clothing and respiratory protection. Adequate personal protection equipment should protect the respiratory system, skin, face, hands, feet, head, and body.

Limiting exposure and contamination can be accomplished by responders prioritizing protective measures at any incident. The order of protection priorities should be:

- Self-protection (Always protect yourself first. You don't need more patients at the scene.)
- Using the buddy system
- Availability of Rapid Intervention Teams
- Civilian protection (Moving civilians to an area of refuge may be their best protection.)

Responses to a Radiological/Nuclear Incident

Intelligence sources report that the use of an actual nuclear device to cause a nuclear detonation is highly unlikely, if not nearly impossible, for terrorists to accomplish. Instead, radiological or nuclear terrorist incidents would most likely involve the use of a conventional explosive device or other means to spread radioactive materials. Spreading of radioactive materials might also be accomplished through sabotage at or an attack on a nuclear power facility.

Identifying a nuclear incident may be difficult because radiation cannot be detected by the senses and symptoms of radiological exposure are generally delayed for hours or days.

Types of Harm from Radiological/Nuclear Incidents

The following types of harm can result from radiological/nuclear incidents:

- *Thermal harm* would be a primary harm from a nuclear explosion.
- *Radiological harm* is the primary danger from radiological materials. Because of the nature of the materials, this will represent an ongoing hazard, the scope of which will only be determined when the amount and identity of the substance involved is ascertained.
- *Chemical harm* is a secondary harm and is a concern because of the fact that many radiological substances are also chemical hazards. This is an area often overlooked by responders concentrating on radiation effects.
- *Mechanical harm* would be a primary harm from a nuclear explosion.
- *Psychological harm* is a secondary harm. As in all terrorist incidents, a sudden traumatic occurrence can cause immediate or delayed emotional or psychological reactions.

Self-Protection Measures at a Radiological/Nuclear Incident

Time, distance, and shielding are the mainstays of self-protection at a radiological incident. The use of radiological detection equipment is the best method of determining whether your self-protection measures are appropriate and effective.

As noted in the following section, *all* explosive incidents should be treated as potential disseminations of radiological (or biological or chemical) materials. This will ensure taking the appropriate protective measures, even before the nature of the explosion can be ascertained. Additionally, review the information on decontamination procedures in Chapter 36, "Special Operations."

Responses to an Explosive Incident

NOTE

Because of the frequent practice of suicide bombing, always keep in mind that one of the bomb victims may be the bomber. For this reason, always search all patients at the scene for weapons prior to transport.

Explosive incidents can involve a wide variety of devices, from small pipe bombs to large vehicle bombs. The incident may involve an attack against a fixed target or against a group of people such as emergency responders. The incident may be an isolated event or may involve secondary devices, booby traps, or suicide bombers.

Materials involved will always include some form of explosives. However, as noted earlier, the detonation may also be designed to disperse biological, chemical, or radiological materials. The type of explosive may be improvised or commercially manufactured. The bomb itself may be equipped with switches or controls that can be activated by light, pressure, movement, or radio transmission. For this reason, untrained personnel should never attempt to neutralize an unexploded device.

Bombs are the most frequent weapons currently used by terrorists.

Types of Harm from Explosive Incidents

The following types of harm can result from explosive incidents:

- *Thermal harm* is a primary hazard to those exposed to the heat generated by the detonation. It is usually not an ongoing risk unless unexploded materials are present.
- *Asphyxiation* is a potential secondary harm because of the possibility of extremely dusty conditions.
- *Radiological harm* is a possibility if the device was designed for the purpose of dispersing radiological contamination or was detonated in an area containing radiological materials. In this case, the hazard can persist for long periods of time.
- *Chemical hazards* can come from products created as a result of the explosive reaction either from chemicals already present at the detonation site or if chemicals have been included in the device for dispersal.
- *Etiological harm* may be a risk if the device is used as a dispersion mechanism for biological agents. Otherwise, it may be a secondary risk resulting from mechanical trauma.
- *Mechanical harm* is another primary harm typically seen at bombing incidents. It can result from blast overpressure, shock waves, and fragmentation.
- *Psychological harm* would result as in any violent incident. A stunned response could last seconds or minutes, causing individuals to "freeze" and be temporarily unable to think or act. Delayed reaction shows up later in the form of post-traumatic stress.

Self-Protection Measures at an Explosive Incident

With explosive incidents, the responder needs both preblast and postblast protection. Preblast is defined as that portion of operations that occurs after a written or verbal warning is received but before an explosion takes place. Postblast refers to operations occurring after at least one detonation has occurred.

DISSEMINATION AND WEAPONIZATION

dissemination spreading.

It is important to be familiar with the potential methods for **dissemination** of CBRNE materials, particularly chemical, biological, and radiological/nuclear agents (Figure 37-5). Responders also must not forget that many industrial materials can be used just as effectively as military agents.

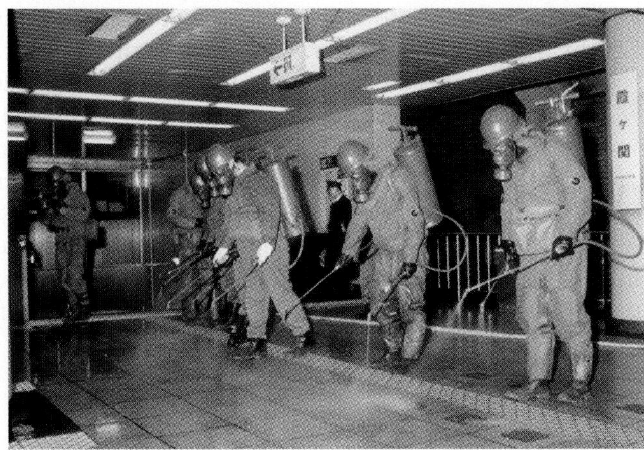

Figure 37-5 • CBRNE agents can be weaponized and disseminated in an enormous variety of ways. In 1995, as an example, members of Aum Shinrikyo, a Japanese religious cult, released sarin, a deadly nerve agent, into the Tokyo subway system, killing 12 people and sending thousands to the hospital. Their purpose, according to experts, was to hasten the end of the world. They transported liquid sarin in tightly sealed packages made to look like lunch boxes or bottled drinks, then punctured the packages with umbrellas and left them in subway cars and stations where the volatile substance escaped and permeated the atmosphere as a gas. Its quick dispersal in the atmosphere meant fewer deaths than the perpetrators probably intended. The photo shows a clean-up crew at work in the subway. *(© Neville Elder/Corbis Sygma)*

The Respiratory Route

The most effective and most common means of dissemination is to enable the material to enter through the respiratory tract. As you have learned in the respiratory care sections of this text, the respiratory tract has a vast and delicate surface area that is exposed to the outside environment through respiration. The deeper into the passageways of the lungs that a terrorist can "place" a harmful material, and the longer the material remains there, the more effective it will be.

The passageways of the respiratory system become smaller and smaller the deeper they progress into the lungs. Particulates, gases, and vapors will be trapped and held at various levels based upon factors such as the size of the particles, the depth and rate of respiration, and whether or not the material is water or lipid (nonwater) soluble.

Other routes of exposure, as discussed in the following text, can be harmful or lethal, but remember that the most effective means of achieving mass casualties is to have the materials enter the body through respiration.

Other Routes

Other means of dissemination depend upon the agent used. For example, effectiveness of the ingestion, or alimentary, route of exposure depends on whether the agent can survive the stomach's acidic environment. Many bacteria cannot live in low pH conditions, but others can. An example would be anthrax, a bacterium that can survive for long periods of time and in harsh environments as dormant spores. (Anthrax can infect a person through contact with the skin, ingestion, or inhalation—inhalation being the most lethal route.)

Some have raised concerns over a terrorist's ability to contaminate a domestic water supply as an ingestion route of exposure. Processes such as dilution, filtration, and chlorination greatly reduce this potential threat. Additionally, the fact that only 1 percent of a domestic water supply is consumed through ingestion further reduces the potential effectiveness of this means of dissemination.

The dermal, or percutaneous, route of exposure (through the skin) is very effective with the blister agents, or vesicants, but less effective with many of the biological agents. Only a few biological materials are dermally active, because healthy, intact skin provides an excellent barrier. The use of vectors such as fleas to disseminate biological agents (e.g., bubonic plague) would present significant logistical difficulties to the terrorist and is therefore not likely to be a readily selected means of dissemination.

Some bacterial and many viral agents can be disseminated effectively by human-to-human contact. With such agents, especially when there is a delayed incubation period, it is possible to infect a large population prior to detection. These factors are of particular concern with smallpox, pneumonic plague, and viral hemorrhagic fevers, to name a few.

Weaponization

weaponization packaging or producing a material, such as chemical, biological, or radiological agent, so that it can be used as a weapon; for example, by dissemination in a bomb detonation or as an aerosol sprayed over an area or introduced into a ventilation system.

In summary, **weaponization** of *most* of the agents we will discuss is most effective when targeted through the inhalation route. If the terrorist can get the materials into a respirable form—that is to say, in particles no more than approximately 3 to 5 microns in diameter—the greatest number of casualties can be achieved. Such airborne dissemination can be created by applying various forms of energy to the material. Energy such as heat would cause a liquid to evaporate faster, resulting in a higher airborne concentration, and explosives or sprayers could also be used to aerosolize and disseminate the materials.

CHARACTERISTICS OF CBRNE AGENTS

Characteristics of the various CBRNE agents (chemical, biological, radiological/nuclear, and explosive) are discussed in the following sections.

Chemical Agents

Chemical Agent Considerations

PHYSICAL CONSIDERATIONS Known agents cover the whole range of physical properties. Under various ambient conditions, their physical state may be gaseous, liquid, or solid. Their vapor pressures vary from high to negligible. Their vapor densities vary from slightly lighter than air to considerably heavier. The range of odors varies from none to highly pungent or characteristic. They may be soluble or insoluble in water. These varied physical properties affect the behavior of the agent in the field with respect to such considerations as vapor hazard, persistency, and possible means of decontamination.

VOLATILITY CONSIDERATIONS Agents that have a low boiling point and high vapor pressure tend to be nonpersistent; that is, they will evaporate more readily. Evaporation presents good news and bad news. The bad news is that the more volatile (easily evaporable) a material, the greater the airborne concentration that will be released. The good news is that the more volatile a material, the less time it will remain on a surface area. Agents that have a high boiling point (therefore, a lower vapor pressure) tend to be more persistent.

CHEMICAL CONSIDERATIONS The only general characteristic of the known chemical agents is that they are sufficiently stable to survive dissemination and transport to the site of their action. However, their inherent reactivity and stability can vary widely. Some chemically reactive agents naturally denature rapidly, whereas other, less-reactive agents require, for example, bleach solutions to inactivate them. Solid adsorbents (e.g., Fuller's earth) are also very effective decontaminants.

TOXICOLOGICAL CONSIDERATIONS Keep in mind that not all individuals of a species react in the same way to a given amount of agent. Some are more or less sensitive as a result of various factors, including genetic background, race, and age. The route of entry can also influence the effect. Toxicological studies estimate the potential biological effects of chemical agents by different routes of entry. The physical properties of the materials may alter the toxicological effects and the response of the affected system.

Classifications of Chemical Agents

Chemical weapons can be classified broadly in the following manner:

- *Choking agents* are predominately respiratory irritants and can be found not only as weaponized materials but also as commonly encountered industrial chemicals.
- *Vesicating agents (blister agents)* cause chemical changes in the cells of exposed tissues almost immediately on contact. However, in many cases, the effects are not felt or realized until hours after the exposure.
- *Cyanides,* formerly referred to as "blood agents," actually have no impact on the blood. They work by preventing the use of oxygen within the cells of the body.
- *Nerve agents* inhibit an enzyme that is critical to proper nerve transmission, allowing the parasympathetic nervous system to run out of control. Many agencies carry nerve agent antidote kits for their emergency response personnel (Figure 37-6).
- *Riot control agents* include irritating materials and lacrimators (tear-flow increasers). Effects of these materials seldom last more than several minutes after exposure has ended.

Biological Agents

Biological agents are defined as microorganisms or toxins that can cause disease processes. Most commonly, the biological agents are bacteria, viruses, or toxins, and a wide variety of biological agents are of concern as possible agents of terrorism. Virtually any biological material can be weaponized and disseminated; some are just more effective than others.

It is important to understand the differences between a bacterium, a virus, and a toxin. The differences can influence the ease of manufacture as well as the availability of antidotes and, to some extent, their effectiveness. Some characteristics of the three were noted earlier in the chapter. Additional characteristics are discussed in the following text.

A *bacterium* is a small, free-living microorganism. "Free-living" means that it can live outside of a host cell. If provided the proper environment (temperature, moisture, food), these organisms can survive on their own and reproduce by simple cellular division. Many bacteriological agents respond to antibiotic therapies and, for the most part, are treatable conditions if detected early enough.

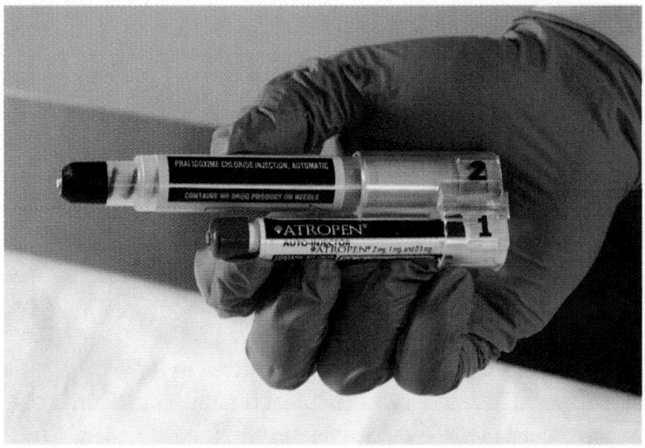

Figure 37-6 • Many emergency response agencies provide nerve agent antidote kits to their personnel.

A *virus* is an organism that requires a host cell inside which to live and reproduce; thus, it is intimately dependent upon the cell that it infects. The diseases that viruses produce generally do not respond to antibiotics, which cannot reach them inside their host cells, but some may be responsive to the few antiviral compounds that exist.

In contrast to bacteria and viruses, *toxins* are not living organisms. Simply put, a toxin is a poisonous chemical compound that is produced by or derived from a living organism. The producing organism could be plant, an animal, or a microorganism. Examples include ricin, which is derived from the castor bean; mycotoxins, which are produced by fungi; or the botulinum toxin, which is produced by the bacterium *Clostridium botulinum*.

Other types of biological agents exist, but bacteria, viruses, and toxins are the most common.

Biological Agent Considerations

The biological weapons of greatest concern are listed in Table 37-1, a biological quick reference table. As you review this table, note that the primary concern for all of the biological agents would be personal protection if the agent is transmitted from human to human. The role of EMS in patient care and treatment will be primarily supportive in nature.

TABLE 37-1 • Biological Agent Quick Reference Guide

DISEASE (CLASS)	ROUTE OF INFECTION	INCUBATION PERIOD/ ONSET TIME	HUMAN-TO-HUMAN TRANSMISSION
		BACTERIA	
Anthrax (Bacterium)	S, D, R	1 to 6 days	No, except for cutaneous infection
Cholera (Bacterium)	D, DC	1 to 5 days	Rare
Plague, Bubonic (Bacterium)	V, R	2 to 10 days	High
Plague, Pneumonic (Bacterium)	V, R	2 to 3 days	High
Q Fever (Bacterium)	V, R	2 to 10 days	Rare
Tularemia (Bacterium)	V, R, D	2 to 10 days	No

V = vector, R = respiratory, D = digestive, DC = direct human-to-human contact, S = skin

Regardless of whether the agent is a bacterium, a virus, or a toxin, there are certain features that influence their potential for use as weapons. They are:

- Infectivity
- Virulence
- Toxicity
- Incubation period
- Transmissibility
- Lethality
- Stability

Unique to many of these biological agents, and distinct from their chemical counterparts, is the ability to multiply over time and actually increase their effect. Therefore, biological material that can replicate itself readily has a greater potential to be transmitted from person to person. The potential epidemiological impacts of such a biological weapon are obvious.

The factors listed are discussed in more detail below.

- *Infectivity.* The infectivity of an agent reflects the relative ease with which the microorganisms involved establish themselves in a host species. Pathogens with

SIGNS AND SYMPTOMS	DECONTAMINATION OR INFECTION CONTROL PROCEDURES	PREHOSPITAL CARE
	BACTERIA	
Fever, malaise, and mild chest discomfort, followed by severe respiratory distress with difficulty breathing, sweating, stridor (harsh breathing sounds), and cyanosis (bluish skin color); shock and death within 24 to 36 hours of severe symptoms.	Universal body decontamination with low-pressure, soap and water wash, then 0.5 percent hypochlorite solution, then second soap and water wash.	Supportive according to local protocol.
Range of no symptoms to severe symptoms with sudden onset, vomiting, abdominal distension, and pain with little or no fever followed rapidly by diarrhea. Fluid loss can exceed 5 to 10 liters per day.	Enteric precautions, soap and water washes, and a hypochlorite solution for equipment. Personal contact rarely causes infection.	Supportive care directed at rapid fluid replacement.
High fever, chills, malaise, tender lymph nodes (buboes), may progress to infection throughout the bloodstream, with spread to the central nervous system, lungs, and elsewhere.	Isolation precautions, secretion, and lesion (open sore or skin infection) precautions. Use of soap and water for personnel decon; use heat, UV rays, or disinfectants for equipment.	Supportive care and respiratory and circulatory support.
High fever, chills, headache, coughing up blood, and blood poisoning, with rapid progression to breathing difficulty, stridor (harsh breathing sounds), and cyanosis (bluish skin color); death is due to respiratory failure, circulatory collapse.	Strict isolation precautions. Use of soap and water for personnel decon, heat, UV rays, and disinfectants for equipment.	Supportive care and respiratory and circulatory support.
Fever, cough, and sharp chest pain.	Use of soap and water or a weak 0.5 percent hypochlorite solution.	Supportive care.
Local ulcer and regionally enlarged lymph nodes that may develop into abscesses, fever, chills, headache, and malaise. Fever, headache, malaise, discomfort behind the breastbone, weight loss, nonproductive cough.	Secretion and lesion precautions, strict isolation not required, use of heat or disinfectants renders organism harmless.	Supportive care.

continued

TABLE 37-1 • (Continued)

DISEASE (CLASS)	ROUTE OF INFECTION	INCUBATION PERIOD/ ONSET TIME	HUMAN-TO-HUMAN TRANSMISSION
		TOXINS	
Botulinum (Toxin)	D, R	24 hours to several days	No
Ricin (Toxin)	D, R	24 to 72 hours	No
Staphylococcal Enterotoxin B (SEB) (Toxin)	D, R	4 to 6 hours	No
Trichothecene Mycotoxins (T2) (Toxin)	R, S, DC, D	Minutes to hours	Yes
		VIRUSES	
Smallpox (Virus)	R, S, DC	10 to 12 days	High
Venezuelan Equine Encephalitis (VEE) (Virus)	R, V	2 to 6 days	Low
Viral Hemorrhagic Fevers (VHFs) (Virus)	DC, V, R	3 to 21 days	Moderate

V = vector, R = respiratory, D = digestive, DC = direct human-to-human contact, S = skin

high infectivity cause disease with relatively few organisms, whereas those with low infectivity require a larger number. High infectivity does not necessarily mean that the symptoms and signs appear more quickly nor that the illness will be more severe, simply that it takes only a small number of organisms to produce symptoms, regardless of timing or severity.

- *Virulence.* The virulence of an agent reflects the relative severity of disease produced by a microorganism. Different strains of the same microorganism may cause diseases of different severity.
- *Toxicity.* The toxicity of an agent reflects the relative severity of illness or incapacitation produced by a toxin.
- *Incubation period.* A sufficient number of microorganisms or a sufficient quantity of toxin must penetrate the body to produce infection (the infective dose), or intoxica-

SIGNS AND SYMPTOMS	DECONTAMINATION OR INFECTION CONTROL PROCEDURES	PREHOSPITAL CARE
	TOXINS	
Drooping eyelids, weakness, dizziness, dry mouth and throat, blurred vision and double vision, impaired speech, hoarseness, difficulty swallowing, followed by symmetrical descending paralysis and respiratory failure.	0.5 percent hypochlorite solution and/or soap and water.	Aggressive respiratory support, and supportive care for other symptoms.
Weakness, fever, cough, and fluid in the lungs 18 to 24 hours post-exposure, followed by severe respiratory distress and death from lack of blood oxygen in 36 to 72 hours.	0.5 percent hypochlorite solution and/or soap and water.	Supportive care with aggressive airway management. Volume replacement of gastrointestinal fluid loss.
Sudden onset, with fever, chills, headache, muscle pain, and nonproductive cough. Some may develop respiratory distress and pain behind the breastbone. If ingested, nausea, vomiting, and diarrhea.	0.5 percent hypochlorite solution and/or soap and water.	Supportive care directed at respiratory support.
Skin pain, itching, redness, blisters, tissue death; nose and throat pain, nasal discharge, sneezing, cough, breathing difficulty, wheezing, chest pain; and coughing up blood; lack of muscle coordination, shock, and death.	Soap and water, after clothing has been removed. Eye exposure—copious saline irrigation.	Supportive care directed at respiratory and circulatory support.
VIRUSES		
Malaise, fever, chills, vomiting, headache, backache; 2 to 3 days later, sores which develop into pus-filled blisters, more abundant on face and extremities.	Strict quarantine with respiratory isolation for a minimum of 16 to 17 days following exposure for all contacts. Patients are infectious until all scabs heal.	Supportive care.
Sudden onset, with malaise, spiking fever, chills, severe headache, intolerance of light, and muscle pains. Nausea, vomiting, cough, sore throat, and diarrhea may follow.	Standard Precautions; infectious through mosquito bites.	Pain relievers for headache and muscle pain, anticonvulsants and respiratory support.
Fever, easy bleeding, purplish beneath-the-skin hemorrhage spots, low blood pressure, shock, swelling, malaise, muscle pain, headache, vomiting, and diarrhea	Decontamination with hypochlorite or phenolic disinfectants. Standard Precautions.	Supportive care directed at respiratory and circulatory support.

tion (the intoxicating dose). Infectious agents then must multiply (replicate) to produce disease. The time between exposure and the appearance of symptoms is known as the incubation period. This is governed by many variables, including the initial dose, virulence, route of entry, rate of replication, and host immunological factors.

- *Transmissibility.* Some biological agents can be transmitted directly from person to person. Indirect transmission (for example, via vectors, such as insects) may be a significant means of spread as well. In the context of biological warfare casualty management, the relative ease with which an agent is passed from person to person (its transmissibility) constitutes the principal concern.
- *Lethality.* Lethality reflects the relative ease with which an agent causes death in a susceptible population. We can quantify the relative lethality of a material by determining its "lethal dose" or "lethal concentration" (LD or LC).

- *Stability.* The viability of a biological agent is affected by various environmental factors, including temperature, relative humidity, atmospheric pollution, ultraviolet light, and sunlight. A quantitative measure of stability is an agent's decay rate (e.g., "aerosol decay rate").

Additional factors that may influence the suitability of a microorganism or toxin as a biological weapon include ease of production, stability when stored or transported, and ease of dissemination.

Bacteria

As noted earlier, bacteria are single-celled organisms that can grow in a variety of environments. Like the cells of the human body, they have an internal cytoplasm surrounded by a rigid cell wall. Unlike human body cells, they lack an organized nucleus and other intracellular structures. They can reproduce independently, but they require a host to provide food and other support. To obtain this, they bind to the outsides of host cells in the body.

For purposes of weaponization, bacteria are relatively easy to grow, reproduce, and spread.

zoonotic
able to move through the animal-human barrier; transmissible from animals to humans.

ANTHRAX Anthrax is a naturally occurring **zoonotic** disease (a disease that can move through the animal-human barrier) found commonly in livestock. As carriers of anthrax, cattle, sheep, and horses can infect humans naturally, particularly those who handle hair, wool, hides, or excrement of infected animals.

The most common human form of anthrax seen in natural cases is the cutaneous form of anthrax, which is also known as *woolsorter's disease*. This condition is found in those persons who have had open sores or lacerations contaminated with anthrax spores during the handling of hides or shearing of wool.

Anthrax also can be transmitted by contaminated meat. However, this is extremely rare because cooking the meat will destroy the anthrax. If transmitted in this way, the gastrointestinal form of anthrax would be seen.

As noted earlier, anthrax can survive the acids of the stomach when so many other biological agents will not readily survive the ingestion route of exposure. Anthrax is a *sporulating bacterium*. Simply put, sporulating (spore-producing) bacteria create a hard seed-like shell over themselves that makes them very resistant to breakdown by UV light and other insults. Therefore, areas contaminated by anthrax can remain contaminated for long periods of time. This is why special sporucidal soaps are best used as decontamination materials.

The form of anthrax that is of greatest concern is the inhalational form. If anthrax can be aerosolized in small enough particles (3 to 5 microns in diameter) so that they can be inhaled and retained in the deeper portions of the respiratory tract, then this form of anthrax can be transmitted by the respiratory route. This form of anthrax is very lethal.

With all forms of anthrax, antibiotic therapy works well to counteract the effects, provided that antibiotics are given early enough in the disease process. The problem with inhalational anthrax, however, is that it commonly presents with nonspecific respiratory symptoms and may not be recognized as anthrax. Therefore, the start of antibiotics may be delayed and, if they are not started before the "anthrax eclipse," such therapy may have little benefit. The eclipse is a brief, 12- to 37-hour period during the disease process in which recovery seems to be occurring and the patient feels much better. However, shortly after the eclipse, the symptoms return and death follows in 2 to 3 days.

CHOLERA Outbreaks of cholera typically are seen in developing nations, particularly those without effective sanitary systems. This gastroenteritic agent is more incapacitating than it is lethal if proper care is rendered.

Essentially, cholera is a diarrheal disease caused by the bacterium *Vibrio cholera*. This bacterium readily multiplies within the small intestines and releases an enterotoxin that causes the intestines to release large volumes of fluids. This results in severe diarrhea and a characteristic "rice water" stool. Death generally occurs from the secondary effects of severe dehydration and electrolyte imbalances.

Proper supportive care aimed at correcting these dehydration-related problems and the use of antibiotics is generally very effective. From a personal protection standpoint, responders should avoid direct contact with bodily fluid and excrement. Otherwise, human-to-human transmission is low.

PLAGUE We know it best as the "Black Death" of the Middle Ages, which was a naturally occurring form of the plague. The plague bacterium (*Yersinia pestis*) is a zoonotic bacterium carried by rats and ground squirrels. The bacterium is transmitted to humans by fleas.

In such a naturally occurring infection of the human, the plague begins as the bubonic form (*bubo-* referring to a swollen or enlarged lymph node), primarily in the legs. With lack of treatment, it progresses to the systemic form, which develops into the highly contagious pneumonic plague. Pneumonic plague would be the primary syndrome seen if plague were aerosolized and inhaled, whereas bubonic plague would be seen first in natural occurrences or if weaponized via vectors such as fleas.

The incubation period for plague is 2 to 10 days, depending upon the form. The pneumonic form has an incubation period of as little as 2 to 3 days. As with many aerosolized biological weapons, the initial symptoms would be fever, weakness, and nonspecific respiratory symptoms. As the pneumonia progresses rapidly, bloody sputum, severe dsypnea (breathing difficulty), and cyanosis (bluish skin color) would be found. Definitive diagnosis can only be made by laboratory tests and is impossible in the field.

Since the pneumonic form is highly transmissible human-to-human by aerosolized droplets generated by coughing, respiratory precautions would be indicated. Field care would consist of self-protection and supportive treatment of the patient. Again, antibiotics will be required and are most effective if started within 24 hours of the onset of the pneumonic form.

Q FEVER Q fever is a zoonotic rickettsial disease caused by *Coxiella burnetii.* The natural disease results from exposure to domestic livestock. Q fever in spore form can withstand harsh environments and remain viable for months. Q fever as a biological weapons agent is similar to anthrax.

The incubation period for Q fever is about 10 to 20 days with uneventful recovery as a rule. It has multiple symptoms including fever, chills, and headache. Q fever pneumonia is a frequent complication. Other symptoms can include sweating, malaise, fatigue, loss of appetite, and weight loss. The fatality rate is low.

Q fever is diagnosed through serology testing. Other laboratory findings may not be helpful due to the difficulty in isolating rickettsia. Treatment consists of antibiotics and support therapy.

TULAREMIA Tularemia is a zoonotic disease caused by *Francisella tularensis* (gram negative bacillus). It is also known as rabbit fever or deer fly fever. Natural exposure to tularemia is usually from the bites of infected animals, deer flies, ticks, or mosquitoes. Tularemia has been weaponized in aerosol form.

The symptoms of tularemia include fever, headache, and weight loss. A patient may have respiratory symptoms, substernal discomfort, and a nonproductive cough. Pneumonia may also be present. Natural tularemia has a mortality rate of 5 to 10 percent.

Tularemia is diagnosed by laboratory serology. The treatment of tularemia is antibiotics with appropriate support therapy. Isolation is not required.

Toxins

As discussed earlier, toxins are not living organisms but rather chemical compounds produced by living organisms. Toxins, including botulinum toxin, shiga toxin, shellfish toxin, and ricin, are some of the most deadly compounds known.

Toxins are not volatile; that is, they do not vaporize or aerosolize without the application of energy such as an explosive. In addition, most toxins are not dermally active, so intact skin provides an effective barrier. (An exception is the T2 mycotoxin, which is derived from a fungus.) Since toxins do not replicate themselves, they are not human-to-human transmissible. The best method of weaponization varies with the particular toxin. As examples, botulinum is best disseminated through ingestion, whereas the T2 mycotoxin is most effective when aerosolized.

BOTULINUM The botulinum toxin is one of the deadliest compounds known. It has an LD(50) (lethal dose for 50 percent of the test population) of 0.001 mcg/kg or 0.1 mcg for a 220-pound human. By weight, botulinum is 15,000 to 100,000 times more toxic than the nerve agents.

RICIN Ricin is a potent protein toxin that is derived from the beans of the castor plant. Ricin has gained a lot of attention in recent years because some groups in the United States have manufactured the material with the specific intent of killing law enforcement officers and public officials. In addition, the recipe for ricin has been published (along with others) on the Internet and in various books. Around the world, assassinations, as well as nonterrorist murder attempts, have occurred using ricin.

The major effect of ricin is to interrupt the body's protein manufacturing process at the cellular level by altering the RNA needed for proper proteins. This results in cellular death and necrosis, or tissue death. It is readily available and easily made. It is very effective by any route of exposure and is most effective through inhalation. The patient will present with symptoms characteristic of the route of exposure. Treatment is supportive, depending upon the route of exposure.

STAPHYLOCOCCAL ENTEROTOXIN B (SEB) SEB is a toxin that most commonly affects the gastrointestinal tract, when ingested, to produce a form of food poisoning. After aerosolization and inhalation, SEB produces a potentially deadly syndrome.

As with most of the biological toxins, the respiratory form normally would present in the early stages with fever, general weakness, and nonspecific respiratory symptoms. Later, fevers ranging from 103°F to 106°F (39°C to 41°C), retrosternal chest pain (pain behind the breast bone), and pulmonary edema (fluid in the lungs) may be seen. Severe cases can be fatal, but more often SEB, especially after ingestion, is incapacitating in nature. Treatment is supportive and no specific antitoxin is available.

TRICHOTHECENE MYCOTOXINS (T2) Trichothecene mycotoxins (T2) are produced from fungal metabolism (usually molds). T2 is soluble in water and heat resistant and can penetrate intact skin. Natural trichothecene has caused moldy corn toxicosis in animals. There is suspicion that T2 has been weaponized.

The symptoms of T2 exposure include weight loss, vomiting, diarrhea, weakness, dizziness, hypotension, and shock. The onset of illness occurs within hours of exposure, and death occurs within 12 hours. There is currently no vaccine for T2 exposure. Skin decontamination is recommended using soap and water or hypochlorite. These solutions remove the toxin, but do not neutralize it.

The treatment for T2 exposure is based on the symptoms. Absorbic acid has been proposed to reduce lethality. Dexamethasone has also been shown to reduce lethality. Superactive activated charcoal will adsorb remaining toxin and reduce lethality for ingested T2 poisons.

Viruses

Viruses are the simplest microorganisms and are obligatory intracellular parasites; that is, they replicate only inside host cells. In contrast to human body cells—which contain a nucleus, the nucleic acids DNA and RNA, and various structures necessary for life and reproduction—a virus contains only one nucleic acid, either DNA or RNA.

A virus replicates by attaching itself to a host cell and then penetrating the cell with its own genetic code, DNA or RNA. The viral genetic code then instructs the host cell to produce the necessary components to allow the virus to replicate. During this process, the host cell might then release the virus or might be destroyed.

Since the replication of a virus depends on a complicated process using host cells, it is not easy to manufacture viruses in large quantities. A terrorist organization trying to grow them would have to meet significant logistical demands. The organization would need to have well-educated personnel and be very well financed compared to those attempting to make weapons using either bacteria or biological toxins. Therefore, although possible, the weaponized use of a virus is less likely than the weaponization of a bacterium or toxin.

SMALLPOX In 1980, the World Health Organization (WHO) declared the smallpox virus to have been eradicated worldwide through immunization efforts. The last eight cases of smallpox occurred in the United States in 1949. The last documented case of smallpox anywhere in the world occurred in 1978 in Birmingham, England, when the virus accidentally escaped its containment and infected and killed an unimmunized medical photographer. The director of the laboratory from which the escape occurred later committed suicide.

Today, there are only two known repositories of the virus, the Centers for Disease Control and Prevention (CDC) in Atlanta, Georgia, and the Russian equivalent, Vector, in Novizbresk, Russia. However, clandestine stockpiles may exist in other parts of the world. If they exist, we do not know their extent or location.

Immunization against smallpox in the United States stopped in the 1970s and those immunizations given had an effective duration estimated at only 10 years. Therefore, the majority of U.S. citizens today have no immunity to the virus.

Smallpox is a highly contagious disease with an incubation period that averages 12 days. Early signs and symptoms include acute-onset fever, weakness, headache, backache, and vomiting. This is followed in 2 to 3 days by the development of a rash and chickenpox-like blisters starting in the area of the mouth, throat, and face, and spreading to the hands and forearms. Although the blisters also form on the trunk of the body, they are more predominant on the face and extremities than are the blisters found in chickenpox (an important diagnostic distinction). The patient should be considered contagious until all of the scabs separate from the skin. The mortality rate for smallpox in the unvaccinated patient is 30 percent.

Transmission of smallpox occurs by respiratory droplets, therefore requiring respiratory isolation. Furthermore, a strict 17-day quarantine is required for any person in contact with a smallpox patient.

ENCEPHALITIS Encephalitis (inflammation of the brain) has numerous forms: eastern, western, St. Louis, and others. The weaponization concern is the Venezuelan Equine Encephalitis, or VEE. This zoonotic disease is, as the name indicates, endemic to the geographical region of Venezuela. An outbreak of this form of encephalitis must be scrutinized closely.

Naturally occurring encephalitis is a disease found in birds and wild animals and is transmitted to horses and humans by mosquitoes. Thus, any naturally occurring VEE outbreak should be associated with an outbreak in animals. If humans only were infected with VEE without the corresponding effects on indigenous animals, then the potential for an unnatural occurrence should be investigated.

Since encephalitis causes swelling of the brain, the patient will present with neurological symptoms. VEE onset is sudden with fever and the profound central nervous system effects of headache, photophobia (intolerance of light), and altered consciousness.

It is estimated that 90 to 100 percent of persons exposed to VEE would be susceptible to its effects. However, because the fatality rate is 1 percent or less, VEE is far more likely to be incapacitating than lethal. Human-to-human transmission is possible, so appropriate body substance precautions should be taken, including respiratory protection (HEPA or N-95 respirator) in the case of any patient with a productive cough.

THE VIRAL HEMORRHAGIC FEVERS (VHFS) Names of these diseases are commonly heard and, in the public's perception, are associated with deadly diseases. In fact, VHF is a classification of a group of diseases that includes ebola, dengue fever, yellow fever, lassa fever, and many more. What these diseases have in common are their effects.

Caused by viruses, they change the clotting characteristics of the blood and the permeability of the capillaries. This results in systemic hemorrhage and liquefaction of solid organs, all in association with a fever (hence the name *viral hemorrhagic fevers*).

These highly contagious and highly lethal diseases present with a rapid onset of fever, weakness, and easy bruising and bleeding. Many times the effects can be seen first in the sclera of the eyes (the fibrous tissue covering the "whites" of the eyes). In this area, bleeding and leaking of the capillaries may be easily observed. This is then followed by the involvement of all mucous membranes.

The method of transmission to humans varies as much as the number of diseases included in the classification of viral hemorrhagic fevers. Definitely, contact with blood and other secretions is a mode. The respiratory portal of entry is even more likely. Therefore, Standard Precautions and aggressive respiratory precautions must be taken. With few exceptions, there are no vaccines and no cures, and the use of antiviral therapies has met with only limited success. The field treatment of patients will be directed to preventing the spread of the disease and providing supportive care and treatment for hypovolemia (decreased blood pressure caused by capillary permeability and hemorrhage). Depending upon the disease, the mortality rate will range between 5 and 90 percent.

Radioactive/Nuclear Devices

Potential Scenarios

When considering the possibility of a terrorist organization using a nuclear weapon, four potential scenarios should be evaluated: (1) the use of a military nuclear weapon; (2) the use of an improvised nuclear weapon; (3) the use of a "dirty bomb," or radiological dispersal device; and (4) the sabotage of a nuclear facility.

MILITARY NUCLEAR DEVICES Although not unheard of, it is highly unlikely that any terrorist organization could both (1) successfully obtain a military nuclear device, and (2) successfully deploy and activate the device without detection by intelligence-gathering agencies. In addition, the potential of a retaliatory response by the United States (or any other nation with nuclear weapons) is a powerful deterrent.

IMPROVISED NUCLEAR DEVICE Everyone has heard that the basic information needed to construct a nuclear device is easily obtained. This might very well be the case. However, knowing how to construct the device to the exacting specifications necessary to make it work is another issue. In addition, the physical act of assembling the weapon—that is, placing the radioactive material into the device without the proper shielding—would expose the individual to unsurvivable levels of radiation. Even if all of these obstacles could be overcome, the intelligence community more than likely would detect the acquisition of the prerequisite materials and information before the device could be constructed.

RADIOLOGICAL DISPERSAL DEVICE (RDD) OR "DIRTY BOMB" An RDD is simply any means used to disseminate a radioactive material; for example, a conventional bomb that would spread a radioactive substance upon exploding. This is a more likely scenario than the first two possibilities, which would involve using an actual atom-splitting nuclear bomb. However, an RDD poses many of the same logistical problems in getting the radioactive material out of its containment and into the device without killing oneself. And, if we as emergency responders learn to regard all explosive incidents as a potential dissemination means for radioactive materials (as well as for chemical and biological materials), we can use very readily available detection equipment to confirm or rule out the presence of radioactive materials.

SABOTAGE From the standpoint of nuclear terrorism, the most likely scenario is the sabotage of an existing facility. However, nuclear power plants within the United States are highly hardened facilities. With close regulation, the security at these facilities can

TABLE 37-2 • Systemic Effects of Rem Dosages

STARTING DOSE	SYSTEM AFFECTED	EFFECTS
150 rem*	Blood	• Suppression of the blood-forming characteristics of the bone marrow. • Opportunistic diseases after the white blood cells die and are not replaced (7 days). • Anemia as red blood cells die off (in approximately 30 days). • Clotting difficulties as platelets are not replaced (30–60 days).
500 rem	Gastrointestinal system	• Death of the tissues of the gastrointestinal (GI) tract. • Nausea and vomiting with profound fluid loss. • Hypovolemia (fluid loss) and shock. • Prognosis is poor if symptom onset is within 2 hours of the exposure.
1,000 rem	Central nervous system	• Damage to the vascular bed of the central nervous system (CNS). • Results in cerebral edema (swelling of the brain) and profound CNS effects (headaches, blurred vision, stroke-like symptoms, and death). • Prognosis is poor for radiological exposures with CNS effects.

*rem = roentgen equivalent (in) man; a measure of radiation dosage

be tightened significantly if intelligence-gathering activities indicate credible threats. Furthermore, the checks and balances and redundant safety measures used at such plants would make it very difficult for an act of sabotage to occur without being detected in advance. The more likely target would be the less hardened, small-scale facilities such as those found in universities.

None of this is to say that there is no potential for an act of nuclear terrorism. However, the possibility of success is limited.

Effects of Radiation

If a radiological material were to be used, three body systems would be most severely affected: the blood-forming system (specifically the bone marrow), the gastrointestinal system, and the central nervous system. These effects and the **rem** dose necessary to produce them are summarized in Table 37-2.

rem
roentgen equivalent (in) man; a measure of radiation dosage.

Incendiary Devices

The use of incendiary devices by terrorists is more plausible than the use of nuclear devices. Obviously, it is not hard either to obtain or to initiate items like Molotov cocktails, propane bombs, or even small, shaped charges on existing storage containers of flammable gases or liquids. In addition, the terrorist may elect to initiate the weapon with complicated chemical, electronic, or mechanical initiation devices. In these cases, the impacts of the initiation items themselves must be considered (chemicals, the use of radios, and so on).

Specialized teams are generally available to deal with incendiary devices.These teams are often affiliated with the military or with law enforcement agencies (Figure 37-7). Since even seemingly small devices can cause considerable damage, know how to contact the agency that is responsible for dealing with incendiary devices in your area.

The treatment for patients who incur thermal and blast injuries from these weapons would not differ from those for any other thermal or blast injury, and local protocols must be followed. As appropriate, your system's hazmat and multiple-casualty incident procedures, as discussed in Chapter 36, "Special Operations," should be followed.

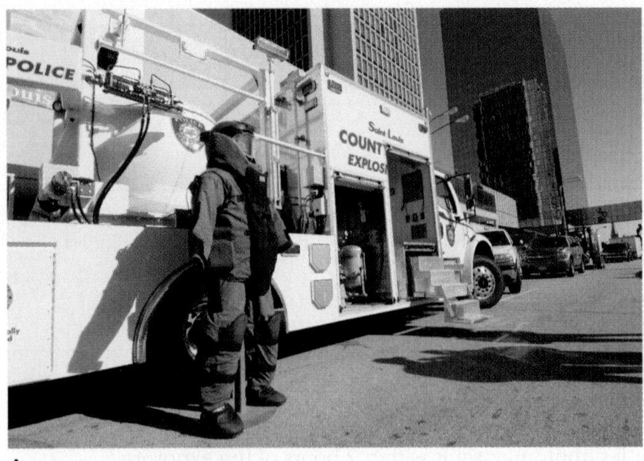

A

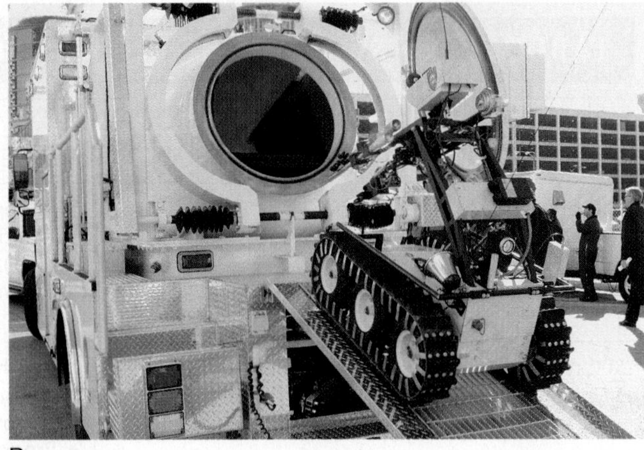
B

Figure 37-7 • (A) A specialized truck contains equipment for handling explosives, including (B) a robot that can be rolled out to deactivate an explosive device, allowing crew members to remain at a safe distance. *(Both: © Ray Kemp/911 Imaging)*

STRATEGY AND TACTICS

EMS responders should understand how to apply tactical considerations to isolate the incident site, notify the appropriate authorities, identify agent indicators, and protect critical assets. Use of an Incident Command System was discussed in Chapter 36, "Special Operations."

Priorities for responders are:

- Life safety
- Incident stabilization
- Protection of property

Additional critical asset considerations include:

- Responders
- Responders' equipment
- Organizational function continuity

strategies broad general plans designed to achieve desired outcomes.

tactics specific operational actions to accomplish assigned tasks.

Strategies are broad general plans designed to achieve desired outcomes. **Tactics** are specific operational actions responders take to accomplish their assigned tasks. This section will discuss tactics for:

- Isolation
- Notification
- Identification
- Protection

Isolation

Initial Considerations

Approaching an act of terrorism (which is also a criminal event) presents unique challenges to the EMS responder. To effectively implement scene control and ensure public safety, emergency responders must quickly and accurately evaluate the incident area and determine the severity of danger. Once the magnitude of the incident is realized, attempts to isolate the danger can begin. Establishing control (work) zones early will enhance public protection and facilitate medical treatment.

Initially, when response resources are limited, isolating the hazard area and controlling a mass exodus of panicked and contaminated people will likely overwhelm the best efforts of first-arriving responders (Figure 37-8). Responders must use any and all available resources effectively and efficiently to prepare the scene for ongoing operations.

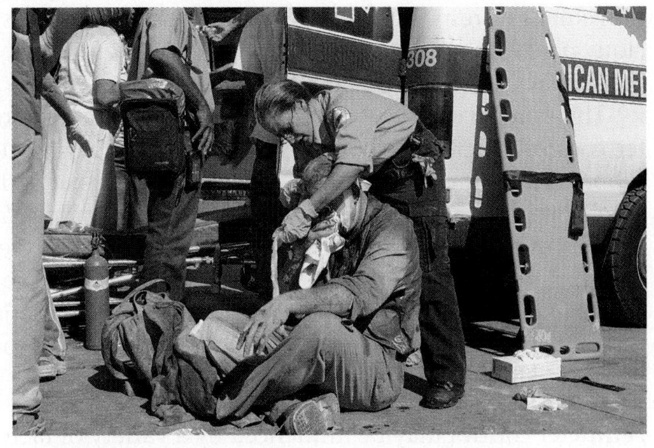

Figure 37-8 • Panicked, contaminated people can overwhelm the best efforts of first-arriving responders when response resources are limited. *(© AP Images/Amy Sancetta)*

Responders must be aware that terrorists may still be lurking nearby, waiting for responders to arrive. In fact, as noted earlier, the responders could be the actual targets. Terrorists may also be among the injured. If this is suspected, initial scene control will likely be delayed and dictated by law enforcement activities.

As in all hazardous situations, self-protection is a top priority. A responder who becomes a patient only adds to the burden on available resources. Responders must anticipate the potential for multiple hazard locations.

Responders may have to define outer and inner operational perimeters. There may be several hazards within the outer perimeter that must be isolated, especially when victims are scattered throughout the boundaries of the incident or when there have been multiple targets that contain dangers.

Controlling the scene, isolating hazards, and attempting to conduct controlled evacuations will be resource intensive and require law enforcement personnel. Inordinate security may be needed for the event, so responders should request additional assistance early.

After a bombing, access to the scene may be limited due to rubble or debris. Police activity may also interfere with establishing access and exit avenues for EMS operations. Another problem may involve large numbers of contaminated victims and would-be rescuers moving in and out of the exclusion zone in an uncontrolled manner. In chemical, biological, and radiological/nuclear incidents, secondary contamination is a major risk.

Establishing Perimeter Control

Law enforcement agencies should establish perimeter control at terrorist incidents by following recognized methods or standard operating procedures. Maintaining control of the perimeter may be difficult due to the design of the terrorist or panic among the patients.

Responders need to recognize and evaluate dangers critical to implementing perimeter control. Adequate evaluation of potential harm will guide decisions and considerations for setting stand-off distances or establishing work zones. In order to perform this task efficiently and effectively, responders should first take time to perform an adequate size-up of the situation.

When initially determining your operating perimeter, it is better to overestimate the size of the perimeter than to underestimate. Once you establish a perimeter, it is often easier to reduce than to increase the perimeter after operations are set up. Depending on the size and complexity of the incident, you may need to divide the boundaries or identify them as having outer and inner perimeters.

The *outer perimeter* is the most distant control point or boundary of the incident. It is used to restrict all public access to the incident. For example, the outer perimeter established after the bombing of the Alfred P. Murrah Federal Building in Oklahoma City enclosed 20 square blocks. The World Trade Center footprint was over 16 acres with the perimeter encompassing all of lower Manhattan. The *inner perimeter* (or hot zone) isolates known hazards within the outer perimeter. It is often used to control movement of responders. Inner perimeters would be established when several suspicious parcels are sighted. The locations of these items would be isolated until such time as specialists have rendered the area safe.

There are several types of terrorist incidents that may require outer and inner perimeter controls. Incidents involving improvised explosive devices should always have responders thinking about secondary devices. Use inner perimeters to control access to any suspicious area. In cases involving chemical or biological dispersion devices, you may need to use inner perimeters to isolate areas highly suspected of contamination as well as of possible secondary devices. In cases of radioactive contamination, inner perimeters may be necessary to isolate possible areas of contamination until specialists with radiation meters have determined the actual level of danger to responders.

Perimeter Control Factors

Perimeter control may be influenced by a variety of factors. They should all be considered and weighed in relation to each other when attempting to determine the next course of action.

The amount and type of resources on hand will provide a rough estimate of what it is possible to accomplish. The capability of available resources must also be considered. People should not attempt actions beyond their training. The ability of the resources to self-protect is a related factor. No matter how well trained personnel are, if they are unable to properly protect themselves, they cannot function in a hazardous environment. The size and configuration of the incident, as well as the stability of the incident, will also come into play.

NOTE

Never lose sight of the fact that the behavior of a material is not determined by whether the release was accidental or deliberate.

These factors are the same whether you are dealing with a noncriminal hazardous materials incident or a terrorist attack.

Notification

In a terrorism event, it is critical that appropriate response and support agencies (at local/state/federal levels) be notified. Notification is usually required by established directives, procedures, or statutes. The appropriate agencies and points of contact should be noted in local EMS or emergency management plans.

It is not the responsibility of an on-scene EMT to perform notification functions. Notification is usually done by a dispatch center or emergency operations center. However, an initial radio report by an EMT is often the "trigger event" that starts the notification process. For example, notification that a possible improvised explosive device (IED) is involved generates a notification of federal law enforcement agencies.

Identification

Identify any indicators of a particular agent (Figures 37-9 A to D). Note the presence of any chemical containers or lab materials, for example, especially those that seem out of place at the site or for which hazardous materials data sheets or shipping manifests are missing. Observe placards and labels on storage tanks or vehicles from a safe distance with binoculars. Obtain the correct spelling of a chemical or biological agent. Consult your current edition of the *Emergency Response Guidebook*. Contact a poison control center or a CHEMTREC or CHEMTEL hotline, as appropriate, to help identify and deal with the substance. (Review Chapter 36, "Special Operations," with regard to hazardous materials incidents.)

If there is an unusual pattern or incidence of illness, document the numbers of patients involved, their signs and symptoms, and any other relevant information, including pertinent negatives (for example, the absence of an obvious cause for the outbreak). Transmit this information to the appropriate authorities.

Protection

Protection of critical assets is an important function in terrorism or other criminal incidents. EMS critical assets include people, vehicles, and equipment/supplies. An appli-

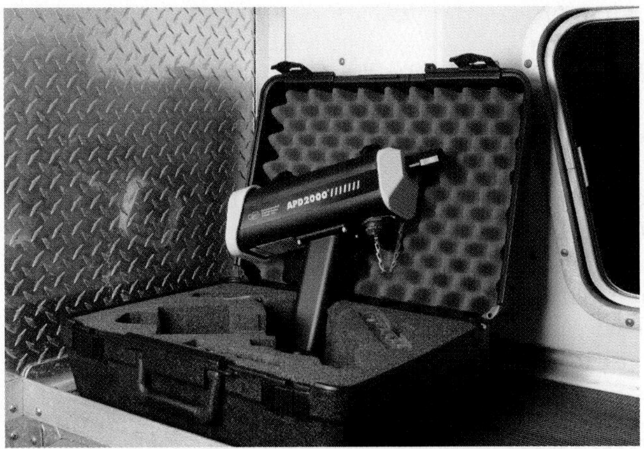

A

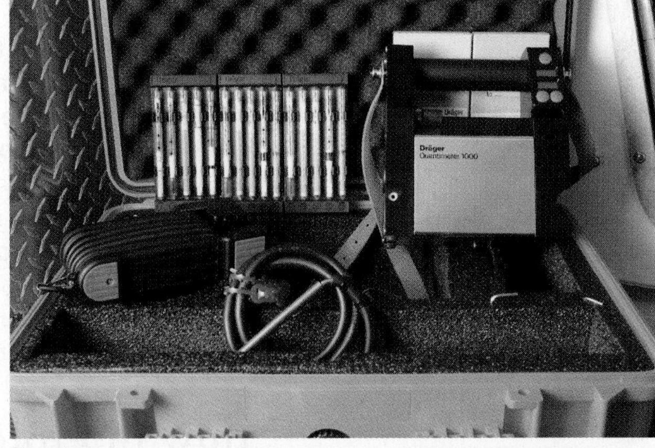

B

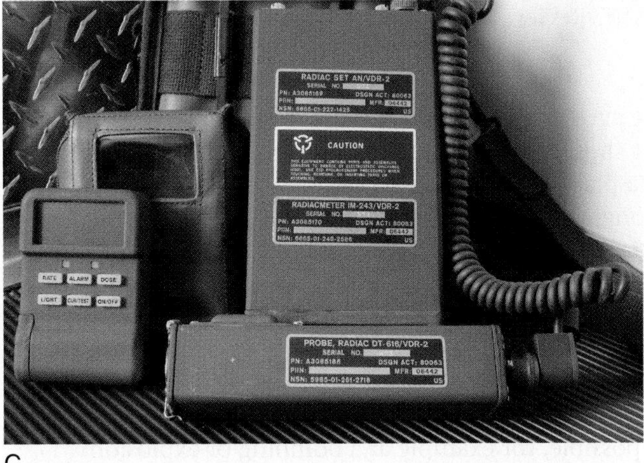

C

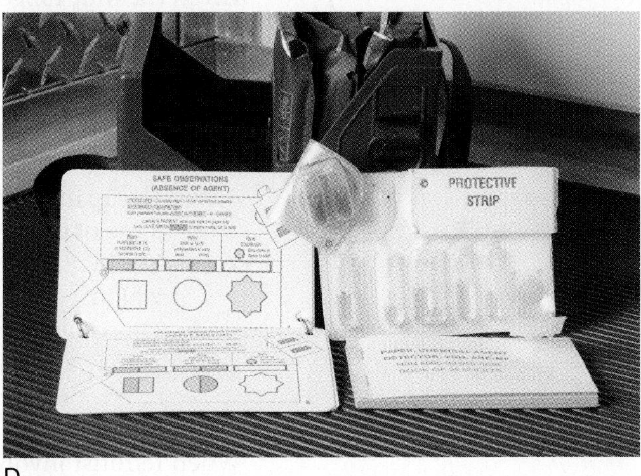

D

Figure 37-9 • Some emergency and rescue services carry detectors to help identify the presence of various CBRNE agents. Examples include: (A) a chemical agent monitor; (B) a detector kit for gases, vapors, and aerosols; (C) a radiation detector; and (D) a detector kit for multiple agents including nerve agents, blister agents, and blood agents. *(© Pearson Education, courtesy of Ogunquit, Maine, Fire-Rescue)*

cable military term is *force protection.* Force protection means that EMS forces are protected to ensure mission accomplishment.

Effective protection requires a partnership between EMS responders and security agencies (e.g., law enforcement, private security, and National Guard units). Security agencies provide protection through perimeter protection, entry control, and traffic control.

EMTs are not armed or trained in security protection; they do not directly engage in security operations. As an EMT, your protection responsibilities include the following:

- Make an initial scene size-up to determine security threats.
- Request protection (read security) via radio as soon as practical.
- Establish vehicle staging and triage/treatment areas in protected locations.
- Advise EMS Command about protection/security concerns.
- Immediately report suspicious people or activities.

SELF-PROTECTION AT A TERRORIST INCIDENT

At this point, it is a good idea to review and reinforce what you have learned about protecting yourself in the event that you are called to respond to a terrorist incident.

Protect Yourself First

As always, remember that if you, the EMT, are injured, you cannot help anyone else. For self-protection, you can rely mostly on what you already know about multiple-casualty incidents, the incident management system, personal protective equipment (PPE), crime scenes, hazardous materials incidents, and decontamination procedures.

A few elements may be involved in a terrorist incident that would not necessarily be involved in the usual range of EMS calls. These include the fact that First Responders are often targets of a terrorist attack . . . that an unusual incidence or pattern of illness may result from a deliberately disseminated biological agent that cannot immediately be identified . . . and that an explosive device may have been detonated not only for the purpose of causing physical damage but also to spread a chemical, biological, or radiological agent.

How to Protect Yourself

Given the wide range of possible agents and devices that can be used in terrorist attacks, how can you best protect yourself? Review the following guidelines, summarized from the text of this chapter.

Recognize a Possible Terrorist Event

Remember the OTTO clues that should arouse suspicion of terrorist involvement:

- Occupancy or location (a place or business that terrorist groups might target)
- Type of event (perhaps one with large crowds)
- Timing (a national holiday or an anniversary date important to terrorist organizations)
- On-scene clues (chemical containers or other out-of-place items, an unexplained pattern of illness)

Don't Rush In!

When terrorist involvement is possible, for example at a bombing or explosion:

- Wait until the appropriate authority says the scene is safe to enter.
- Follow your Incident Command protocols.
- Wear appropriate personal protective equipment (PPE).
- Beware of possible secondary explosive devices or booby traps.
- Search all patients for explosives or weapons—or wait for police to do so—since a suicide bomber may be one of the patients.

Understand the TRACEM-P Harms

Understand what kind of harm is most likely to result from any given type of terrorist weapon or agent and focus your self-protective measures accordingly. The TRACEM-P harms are:

- Thermal
- Radiological
- Asphyxiation
- Chemical
- Etiological (disease-causing)
- Mechanical
- Psychological

Time, Distance, Shielding

These three elements can be put to use to reduce exposure to every type of terrorist agent. Don't forget to use all three, when possible.

The following paragraphs will summarize the likely TRACEM-P harms, as well as appropriate time/distance/shielding measures, for each type of CBRNE (chemical, biological, radiological/nuclear, explosive) agent.

At a Chemical Incident

Chemical harm is the primary potential harm. Keep exposure *time* to a minimum (for example, rotate teams for short periods; decontaminate yourself as quickly as possible). Remain at a *distance*, outside the contaminated area, unless trained and equipped to enter it. *Shield* yourself by wearing protective clothing and respiratory protection such as self-contained breathing apparatus (SCBA).

At a Biological Incident

Etiological harm is the primary potential harm—that is, the possibility of contracting the disease yourself. Limit exposure and contamination. Keep exposure *time* at a minimum, except as needed to assess and treat patients. Promptly take recommended decontamination measures (review Table 37-1). Stay at a *distance* from contaminated areas as much as possible. *Shield* yourself by keeping recommended vaccinations and inoculations up-to-date and by wearing clothing and equipment that protects your skin, face, hands, feet, head, body, and respiratory system (for example, a HEPA or N-95 mask).

At a Radiological/Nuclear Incident

Radiological harm is the primary potential harm, with potential *thermal harm* and *mechanical harm* if an explosive device was involved. Limit your *time* in the contaminated area. Local protocols should define exact time limits for exposure. Follow your local decontamination procedures promptly after any exposure. Remain at a *distance* from the contaminated area unless you are trained and equipped to enter it. *Shield* yourself behind structures or materials that are impervious to penetration by alpha, beta, and gamma radiation (review Figure 37-3).

At an Explosive Incident

Thermal and *mechanical harms* are the primary potential harms at an explosive incident. *Etiological harm* is possible if the device was used to disperse biological agents; *chemical harm* if used to disperse chemical agents. If an explosion has already occurred, limit the *time* you spend in the hazardous area, given the possibility of secondary explosions or attacks on First Responders. For the same reasons, remain at a *distance* from the scene until authorities declare it safe to enter. *Shield* yourself by wearing proper turnout gear, including hard hat, protective gloves, fire-protection clothing—or as necessary for a scene where structural collapse has occurred or may occur. Also wear PPE appropriate for a chemical, biological, or radiological incident if there is any possibility that the explosive device was used to disperse such agents.

CRITICAL DECISION MAKING:
It Could Happen to You . . .

Terrorism can come from many sources and on many scales—from local to nationwide. Your safety from a number of hazards is vital. In each situation explain what hazards you may suspect and how to keep yourself safe. It is the most important decision you can make.

1. You are called to respond with the police and fire department to an office complex where a worker opened an envelope containing white powder.
2. There was an explosion in a downtown office complex. You respond with the police and fire department to treat victims from the blast.

CHAPTER REVIEW

SUMMARY

The EMS responder has entered a new era of violence in society. The possibility of terrorism occurring in your area is increasing and complicates the job of the EMT. In the first decade of EMS (the 1970s), EMTs commonly raced into dangerous scenes without considering the possibility of being harmed. They would commonly immerse themselves in blood and body fluids without understanding the dangers. Those days are gone, and new challenges exposing EMS to great danger have replaced them. The EMT's safety is the most important aspect of any response. Vigilance and awareness are the best approaches to safety in the modern response world.

KEY TERMS

contamination contact with or presence of a material (contaminant) that is present where it does not belong and that is somehow harmful to persons, animals, or the environment.

dissemination spreading.

domestic terrorism terrorism directed against the government or population without foreign direction. *See also* terrorism; international terrorism.

exposure the dose or concentration of an agent multiplied by the time, or duration.

international terrorism terrorism that is foreign-based or directed. *See also* terrorism, domestic terrorism.

permeation the movement of a substance through a surface or, on a molecular level, through intact materials; penetration, or spreading.

rem roentgen equivalent (in) man; a measure of radiation dosage.

routes of entry pathways into the body, generally by absorption, ingestion, injection, or inhalation.

secondary devices destructive devices, such as bombs, placed to be activated after an initial attack and timed to injure emergency responders and others who rush in to help care for those targeted by an initial attack.

strategies broad general plans designed to achieve desired outcomes.

tactics specific operational actions to accomplish assigned tasks.

terrorism the unlawful use of force or violence against persons or property to intimidate or coerce a government, the civilian population, or any segment thereof, in furtherance of political or social objectives. (U.S. Department of Justice, FBI, definition)

weaponization packaging or producing a material, such as chemical, biological, or radiological agent, so that it can be used as a weapon; for example, by dissemination in a bomb detonation or as an aerosol sprayed over an area or introduced into a ventilation system.

weapons of mass destruction (WMD) weapons, devices, or agents intended to cause widespread harm and/or fear among a population.

zoonotic able to move through the animal-human barrier; transmissible from animals to humans.

REVIEW QUESTIONS

1. List and briefly describe the five most common types of terrorism incidents. (pp. 997, 1002–1006, 1008–1019)
2. What is a secondary device? What precautions should be taken by an EMT regarding secondary devices? (pp. 998, 1023–1025)
3. List several types of events that should trigger an EMT's suspicion of possible terrorism involvement. (pp. 998–1000, 1024)
4. List the seven types of harm that result from a terrorism incident—and the seven-letter acronym for these types of harm. (pp. 1000–1001, 1024–1025)
5. Briefly discuss the concept of time, distance, and shielding. (pp. 1001–1002, 1024–1025)
6. Discuss several self-protection measures for biological incidents. (pp. 1005, 1025)
7. Discuss the tactics for isolation, notification, identification, and protection. (pp. 1020–1023)

CRITICAL THINKING

Thinking and Linking

Think back to Chapter 36, "Special Operations." Link the information on multiple-casualty incidents, hazmats, and decontamination from that chapter with information in this chapter as you consider the following situation:

- Multiple medic units are called to a "possible mass casualty incident" at the main airport terminal. The first arriving unit reports that there is a mass exodus of people from the terminal. Many of the victims have some type of fluid on their clothing with an unusual odor. They are clearly contaminated with an unknown substance. What immediate actions should be taken? What protection measures are critical? What decontamination procedures should be implemented?

MEDIA RESOURCES

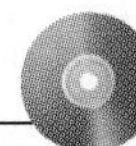

See the Student CD at the back of this book for quizzes, a case study activity, and other features related to this chapter. In particular, take a look at the Case Study regarding EMS response to a scene where a number of people are suffering from the sudden onset of similar symptoms—a possible instance of biological terror. Also, visit the Companion Website for *Emergency Care* at **www.prenhall.com/limmer**, where you will find additional reinforcement and links to other resources.

Street Scenes

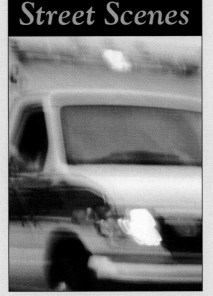

So far, it's been a slow Wednesday afternoon for your unit, Medic 15. At 14:45 things change. The dispatcher announces, "Medic 15, Engine 11, respond to 5565 Baypoint Boulevard at the Conference Center construction site, worker down from unknown injuries." You and your partner suspect some type of construction injury. One minute later, the dispatcher states, "Medic 15, Engine 11, additional information, two more workers are down; we are now receiving multiple calls."

Your partner reminds you that the Conference Center project was vehemently opposed by the Environmental Life Movement (ELM) because the site was on previously protected wetlands.

On arrival, you are met by the construction manager. He is extremely emotional and says, "There's guys collapsing all over the place. We noticed a funny smell; then it got hard to breathe."

Street Scene Questions

1. What are the indicators that this may be a suspicious incident?
2. What steps should be taken to isolate the area?
3. What steps should be taken to identify a possible mechanism of injury?
4. Identify the critical personal protection issues on this scene.

You follow your service's hazmat and multiple-casualty incident procedures and wait in the cold zone while a rescue team with hazmat suits and self-contained breathing apparatus brings the construction workers out from the toxic environment and the decon team conducts decontamination procedures. With proper personal protection in place, you then perform assessment/triage, treatment, and transport.

Officials suspect that the cause of the incident was a deliberate—rather than an accidental—release of a toxic agent, but the exact substance involved and its source are still under investigation.

Street Scenes

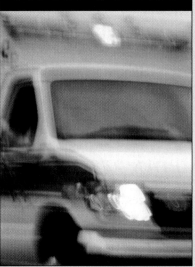

At 03:30, your medic unit responds to a "car fire with possible injuries." The dispatcher reminds you that the location is near the headquarters of Stop American Imperialism, an organization that opposes America's involvement in the Middle East and other parts of the world. A group called Patriots United is suspected of recently vandalizing the storefront from which Stop American Imperialism operates.

You and Engine 15 arrive simultaneously. There is a car on fire in a dead-end alley. You can't see a patient or a bystander, so you stand by while the engine pulls a line into the alley. Suddenly, the engine crew stops and retreats. The Lieutenant states, "We see some type of wire stretched across the alley!"

Street Scene Questions

1. What are the indicators that this is a suspicious incident?
2. What protection precautions should be initiated—and by whom?
3. Discuss the proper notification procedures. What support agencies are required on this scene?

The incident turns out to be not a simple car fire or collision but, instead, a bombing. The alley where the car was bombed runs directly behind the Stop American Imperialism storefront, and the bombed-out car is registered to one of that organization's leaders. Neither he nor anyone else was in the car when it was bombed, so officials believe the bombing was intended to lure emergency responders to the scene where they would be killed or injured by the secondary device, a trip-wired booby trap. Investigators are following various clues at the scene, including components of the bomb device, to track down the perpetrators.

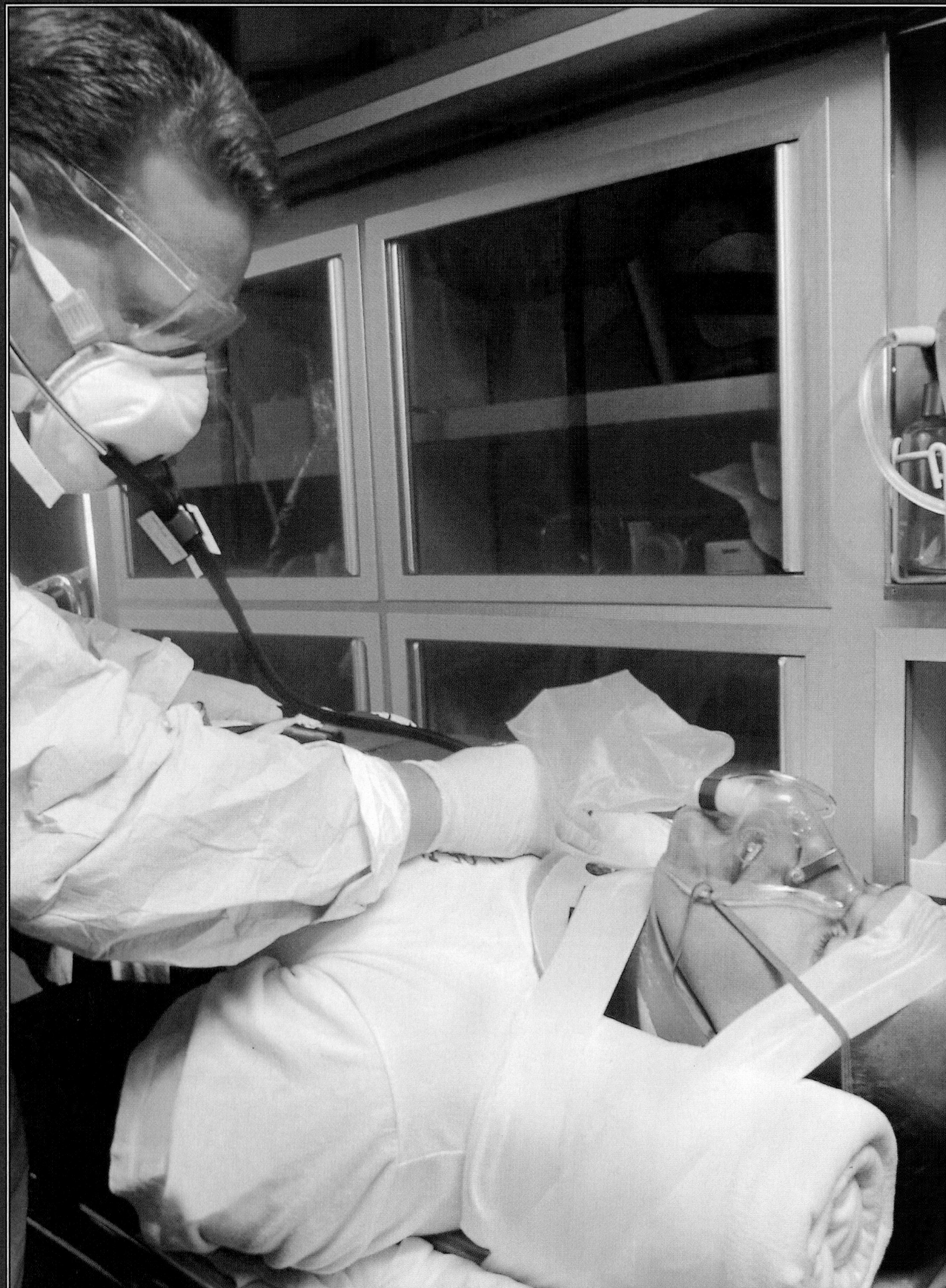

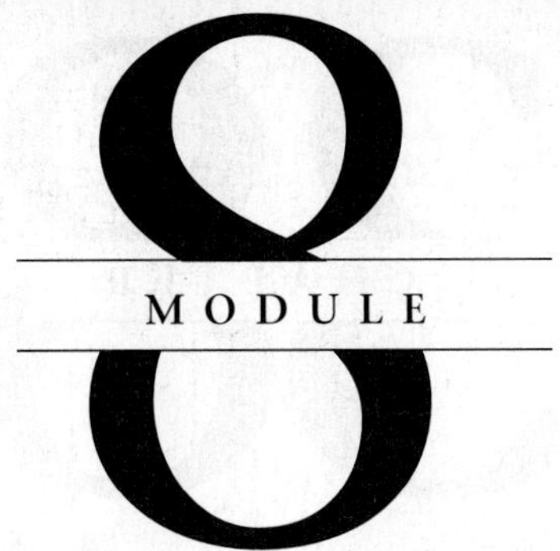

MODULE

Advanced Airway Management

This module (Chapter 38) focuses on two major advanced airway techniques: orotracheal intubation and insertion of a nasogastric tube in children. Orotracheal intubation consists of inserting an endotracheal tube through the mouth into the trachea and inflating a cuff to seal off the airway. This greatly reduces the chance that the patient will aspirate stomach contents, blood, or foreign matter into the lungs. Ventilation can be accomplished through the tube. Alternative devices such as the Combitube®, the laryngeal mask airway (LMA™), and the King LT® airway can also offer airway protection during ventilation.

In stressful situations, children often swallow air, which distends the stomach, crowding the lungs and inhibiting respiration. Inserting a nasogastric tube through the child's nose into the stomach can relieve the distention and allow adequate ventilation to take place.

Advanced Airway Management

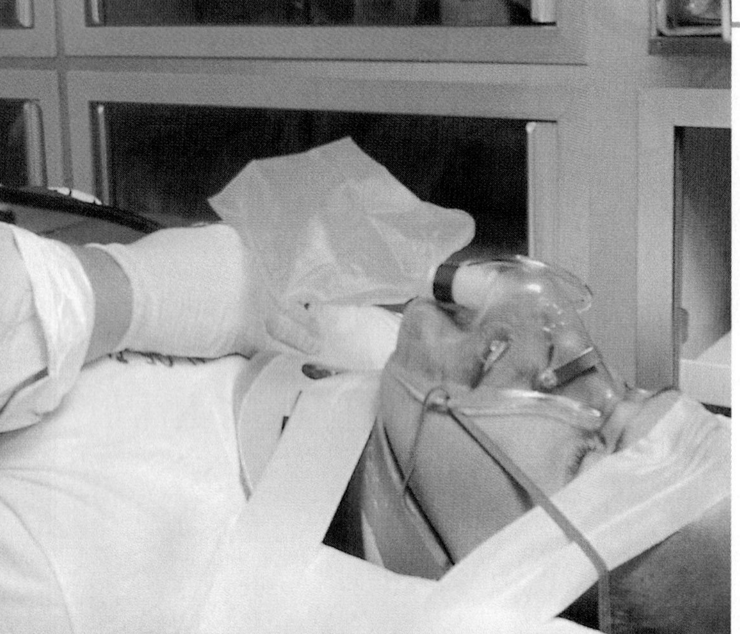

CORE CONCEPTS

The following are core concepts that will be addressed in this chapter:

- The purpose and procedures for orotracheal intubation
- How to perform cricoid pressure
- The purpose and procedures for gastric tube insertion in children

KEY TERMS

alveoli, p. 1035
bronchioles, p. 1035
capnometry, p. 1049
carina, p. 1034
cricoid cartilage, p. 1034
cricoid pressure, p. 1047
endotracheal tube, p. 1038
epiglottis, p. 1034
esophageal detector device (EDD), p. 1049
esophagus, p. 1034
glottic opening, p. 1039
hypopharynx, p. 1034
hypoxia, p. 1038
intubation, p. 1038
laryngoscope, p. 1038
larynx, p. 1034
mainstem bronchi, p. 1034
nasogastric tube (NG tube), p. 1055
nasopharynx, p. 1034
oropharynx, p. 1034
orotracheal intubation, p. 1038
stylet, p. 1042
trachea, p. 1034
vallecula, p. 1034
vocal cords, p. 1034

DOT OBJECTIVES

*KNOWLEDGE AND ATTITUDE

8-1.1 Identify and describe the airway anatomy in the infant, child, and adult. (pp. 1034–1037)

8-1.2 Differentiate between the airway anatomy in the infant, child, and adult. (pp. 1034–1037)

8-1.3 Explain the pathophysiology of airway compromise. (pp. 1034–1037)

8-1.4 Describe the proper use of airway adjuncts. (p. 1037)

8-1.5 Review the use of oxygen therapy in airway management. (p. 1037)

8-1.6 Describe the indications, contraindications, and technique for insertion of nasal gastric tubes. (pp. 1055, 1057) (Scan 38-2, p. 1056)

8-1.7 Describe how to perform cricoid pressure. (pp. 1047–1048)

8-1.8 Describe the indications for advanced airway management. (pp. 1034–1037, 1043, 1052, 1055, 1057)

8-1.9 List the equipment required for orotracheal intubation. (pp. 1039–1043)

8-1.10 Describe the proper use of the curved blade for orotracheal intubation. (pp. 1039, 1041, 1047) (Scan 38-1, pp. 1044–1046)

8-1.11 Describe the proper use of the straight blade for orotracheal intubation. (pp. 1034, 1041, 1047) (Scan 38-1, pp. 1044–1046)

8-1.12 State the reasons for and proper use of the stylet in orotracheal intubation. (p. 1042) (Scan 38-1, pp. 1044–1046)

8-1.13 Describe the methods of choosing the appropriate size endotracheal tube in an adult patient. (pp. 1041–1042)

8-1.14 State the formula for sizing an infant or child endotracheal tube. (pp. 1052–1053)

8-1.15 List complications associated with advanced airway management. (pp. 1038–1039)

8-1.16 Define the various alternative methods for sizing the infant and child endotracheal tube. (pp. 1052–1053)

8-1.17 Describe the skill of orotracheal intubation in the adult patient. (pp. 1043, 1046–1051) (Scan 38-1, pp. 1044–1046)

8-1.18 Describe the skill of orotracheal intubation in the infant and child patient. (pp. 1051–1055)

8-1.19 Describe the skill of confirming endotracheal tube placement in the adult, infant, and child patient. (pp. 1048–1051, 1054)

8-1.20 State the consequence of and the need to recognize unintentional esophageal intubation. (pp. 1048–1051, 1054)

8-1.21 Describe the skill of securing the endotracheal tube in the adult, infant, and child patient. (pp. 1051, 1054)

8-1.22 Recognize and respect the feelings of the patient and family during advanced airway procedures. (p. 1046)

8-1.23 Explain the value of performing advanced airway procedures. (pp. 1034, 1037)

8-1.24 Defend the need for the EMT to perform advanced airway procedures. (pp. 1034, 1037)

8-1.25 Explain the rationale for the use of a stylet. (p. 1042)

8-1.26 Explain the rationale for having a suction unit immediately available during intubation attempts. (pp. 1057, 1059) (Scan 38-3, p. 1058)

8-1.27 Explain the rationale for confirming breath sounds. (pp. 1048–1051, 1054)

8-1.28 Explain the rationale for securing the endotracheal tube. (pp. 1051, 1054)

*SKILLS

8-1.29 Demonstrate how to perform cricoid pressure.

8-1.30 Demonstrate the skill of orotracheal intubation in the adult patient.

8-1.31 Demonstrate the skill of orotracheal intubation in the infant and child patient.

8-1.32 Demonstrate the skill of confirming endotracheal tube placement in the adult patient.

8-1.33 Demonstrate the skill of confirming endotracheal tube placement in the infant and child patient.

8-1.34 Demonstrate the skill of securing the endotracheal tube in the adult patient.

8-1.35 Demonstrate the skill of securing the endotracheal tube in the infant and child patient.

Airway control is the highest priority in managing any critically ill or injured patient, because without an adequate airway the patient will die no matter what other care you provide. Advanced airway management can only be effective and successful if you have already mastered the basic airway techniques discussed in Chapter 6, "Airway Management."

ANATOMY AND PHYSIOLOGY

nasopharynx (NAY-zo-FAIR-inks) the area directly posterior to the nose.

oropharynx (OR-o-FAIR-inks) the area directly posterior to the mouth.

hypopharynx (HI-po-FAIR-inks) the area directly above the openings of both the trachea and the esophagus.

trachea (TRAY-ke-uh) the "windpipe"; the structure that connects the pharynx to the lungs.

esophagus (eh-SOF-uh-gus) the tube that leads from the pharynx to the stomach.

epiglottis (EP-i-GLOT-is) a leaf-shaped structure that prevents food and foreign matter from entering the trachea.

vallecula (val-EK-yuh-luh) a groove-like structure anterior to the epiglottis.

larynx (LAIR-inks) the voice box.

vocal cords two thin folds of tissue within the larynx that vibrate as air passes between them, producing sounds.

cricoid (KRIK-oid) **cartilage** the ring-shaped structure that circles the trachea at the lower edge of the larynx.

mainstem bronchi (BRONG-ki) the two large sets of branches that come off the trachea and enter the lungs. There are right and left mainstem bronchi. The singular is bronchus.

carina (kah-RI-nah) the fork at the lower end of the trachea where the two mainstem bronchi branch.

The anatomy and physiology of the respiratory system have already been discussed at length in Chapter 4, "The Human Body;" Chapter 6, "Airway Management;" and Chapter 16, "Respiratory Emergencies." There are, however, specific aspects of both airway anatomy and physiology that the EMT who performs advanced airway skills must understand in greater depth in order to optimize the effectiveness and success of these advanced skills.

Anatomy

Air initially enters the respiratory tract via the nose and the mouth. Air that enters through the nose then passes through the **nasopharynx** and air that enters through the mouth passes through the **oropharynx**. The **hypopharynx** is the area directly above the openings of both the **trachea** (windpipe) and the **esophagus** (the tube to the stomach). The **epiglottis** is a leaf-shaped structure that acts as a covering to the opening of the trachea. The epiglottis protects the airway by covering the entrance to the trachea when food or liquids are being swallowed. Anterior to the epiglottis is a groove-like structure called the **vallecula.**

The epiglottis allows air to pass into the opening of the trachea and through the **larynx,** or voice box. The larynx contains the two **vocal cords.**

Giving support to the larynx and trachea are several rigid pieces of cartilage. The thyroid cartilage is a shield-shaped structure that is at the anterior of the larynx. Multiple horseshoe-shaped cartilages give support to the trachea. The **cricoid cartilage** is a cartilage at the lower portion of the larynx. It is unique in that it is the only tracheal cartilage that completely surrounds the windpipe.

Once air has passed through the larynx, it proceeds through the trachea until the trachea bifurcates, or splits, into the two **mainstem bronchi** at the level of the carina. The right mainstem bronchus splits off the **carina** at less of an angle than the left mainstem bronchus. Because of the angle of the right mainstem bronchus, objects that pass all the way down the trachea (such as aspirated food) tend to lodge in the right rather than the left mainstem bronchus. The bronchi subsequently divide into smaller air passages called **bronchioles** until reaching the level of the **alveoli** where the exchange of oxygen and carbon dioxide takes place.

When trying to study and memorize the anatomy of the airway, remember that the majority of the time when you are managing a critical airway problem the patient will be supine, or lying flat. For this reason it is important to visualize the anatomy in both the traditional upright "anatomical position" (Figure 38-1) and in the supine position (Figure 38-2).

Physiology

The most important aspect of respiratory physiology for the EMT who uses advanced airways is an understanding of what can cause the respiratory system to fail so severely that an advanced airway is necessary. When the respiratory system functions properly, adequate breathing is the result of many factors including the following:

- Functioning brainstem where the brain's centers of respiratory control are located
- Open airway
- Intact chest wall
- Ability of gas exchange to take place at the alveoli

Injuries or illnesses that affect any of these components can result in inadequate breathing and respiratory failure. For example, a massive head injury could result in both brainstem injury and an airway obstructed by blood and broken teeth. Similarly, a pa-

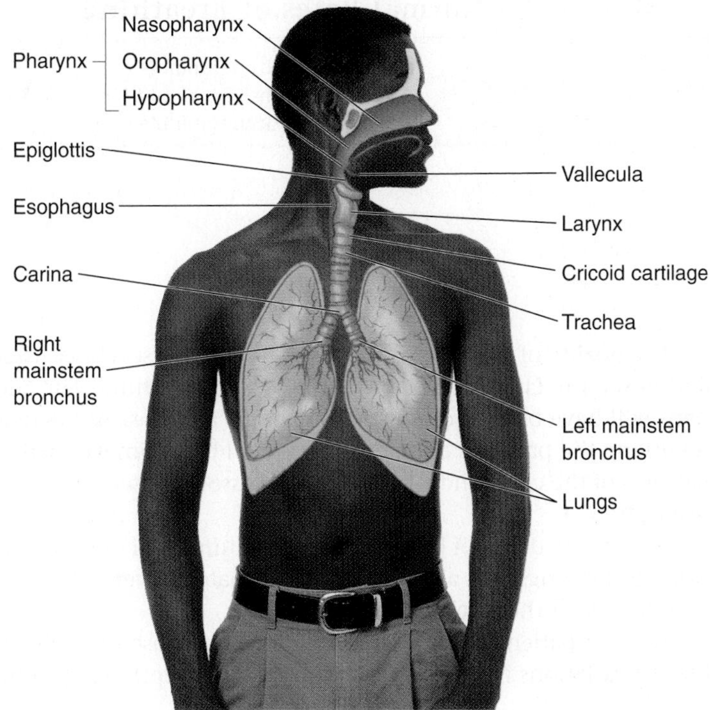

Figure 38-1 • The airway.

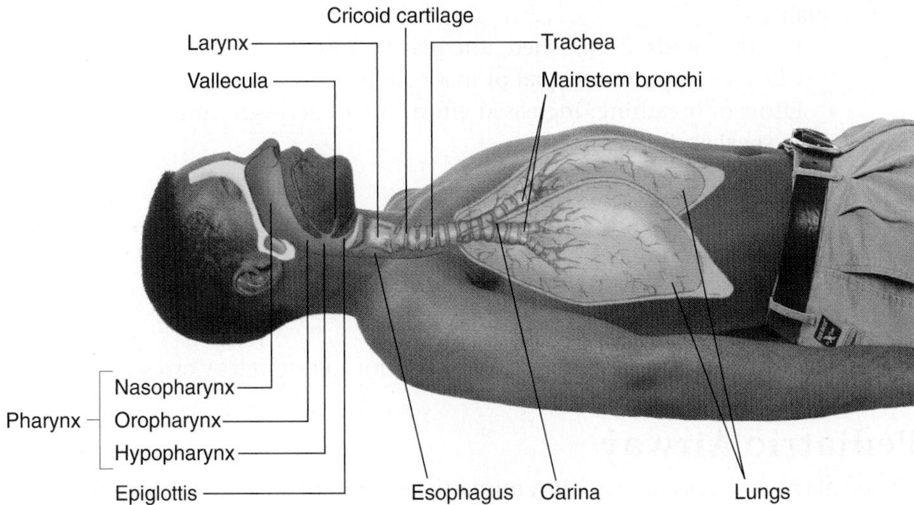

Figure 38-2 • The airway, supine position.

tient with massive pulmonary edema from congestive heart failure can go into respiratory failure because edema prevents adequate gas exchange at the level of the alveoli.

Assessing the adequacy of a patient's breathing is an essential skill when making decisions about what basic and advanced airway management is indicated. A patient's respiratory status can range anywhere from normal, unlabored breathing to complete cessation of breathing or respiratory arrest. Recognition of adequate breathing or respiratory arrest is rarely a diagnostic challenge for the EMT. Rather, it is essential for the EMT to recognize the more subtle signs and symptoms of inadequate breathing. Review the discussion of inadequate breathing in Chapter 6, "Airway Management."

In general, when assessing the adequacy of breathing you should carefully observe the rate, rhythm, quality, and depth of the patient's respirations. The normal rate of breathing is dependent on the patient's age (Table 38-1). An adequately breathing patient will normally be breathing in a regular rather than an irregular rhythm.

bronchioles (BRONG-kee-olz) smaller branches of the bronchi.

alveoli (al-VE-o-li) the microscopic sacs of the lungs where gas exchange with the bloodstream takes place.

TABLE 38-1 • Normal Rates of Breathing	
Adult	12 to 20 breaths per minute
Child	15 to 30 breaths per minute
Infant	25 to 50 breaths per minute

The quality of a patient's breathing should be assessed by listening for breath sounds and observing chest expansion and effort of breathing. The adequately breathing patient will have breath sounds that are equal and present bilaterally. In addition, when observing the patient's chest during normal breathing you will note equal and full expansion of the chest and a lack of any accessory muscle use in the chest or neck during inspiration.

Finally, the depth of breathing (tidal volume) will normally be sufficient not only to expand the lungs, but also to ensure adequate delivery of oxygen and removal of carbon dioxide at the level of the alveoli.

When a patient is in respiratory distress because of inadequate breathing, the following variations in rate, rhythm, quality, and depth will be noted:

- Rate—outside the normal range: either too fast or too slow
- Rhythm—irregular pattern of breathing
- Quality—
  - Breath sounds: diminished, unequal, or absent
  - Chest expansion: unequal or inadequate
  - Effort of breathing: increased effort, use of accessory muscles, and inability to speak in full sentences
- Depth—shallow

In addition, you may also note the following signs and symptoms in the patient with inadequate breathing:

- Cyanosis in the lips, nailbeds, and fingertips
- Cool and clammy skin
- Agonal breathing (gasping breaths just prior to respiratory arrest)

Pediatric Airway

The pediatric airway is not simply a miniature version of an adult airway. The anatomy and physiology of infants' and children's respiratory systems differ in important respects from those of adults (Figure 38-3). Not surprisingly, these younger patients may also have different signs and symptoms of respiratory failure than adults.

Features that are unique to the anatomy and physiology of the infant and child versus the adult include the following:

- All structures in the mouth and nose are smaller in the child and can be more easily obstructed.
- Tongue is proportionately larger, occupying more of the mouth and pharynx.
- Trachea is softer and more flexible, allowing the airway to be closed off if the neck is too far extended when opening the airway.
- Trachea is narrower, allowing the airway to become more easily obstructed if swelling occurs.
- Narrowest area in the airway is at the level of the cricoid cartilage.
- Because the chest wall is softer, the diaphragm is relied on heavily for the work of breathing.

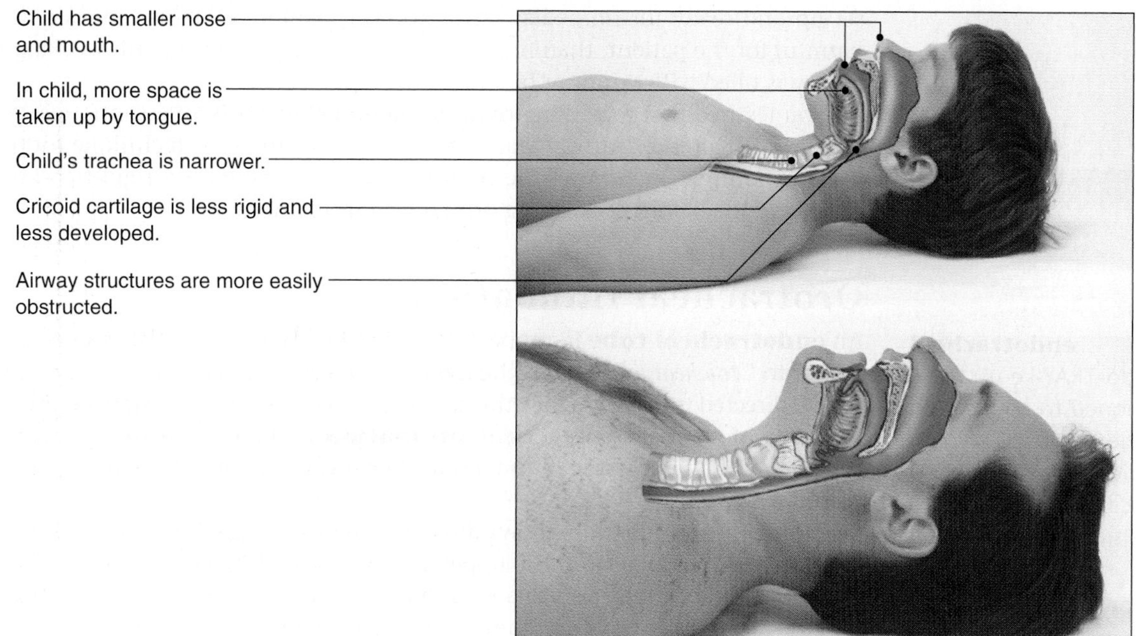
Child has smaller nose and mouth.
In child, more space is taken up by tongue.
Child's trachea is narrower.
Cricoid cartilage is less rigid and less developed.
Airway structures are more easily obstructed.

Figure 38-3 • Comparison of child and adult respiratory passages.

Although infants and children may manifest inadequate breathing with the signs and symptoms already discussed for adults, they also frequently show respiratory distress in other ways, including:

- Slower than normal heart rate
- Weak or absent peripheral pulses
- Retractions between and below the ribs, above the clavicles, and at the sternal notch
- Nasal flaring, in which the nostrils "flare" open with inhalation
- So-called "seesaw" breathing, in which the chest and abdomen move in opposite directions during breathing

Recognition of respiratory distress and inadequate breathing is especially critical in infants and children, since respiratory failure is the leading cause of cardiac arrest in this age group.

MANAGEMENT OF THE AIRWAY

Although this chapter is about advanced airway management, it cannot be overemphasized that the primary management of any airway is with basic airway techniques such as opening and suctioning the airway, administering supplemental oxygen, and using oro- and nasopharyngeal airways. You should review these skills (as taught in Chapter 6, "Airway Management") prior to learning the techniques of advanced airway management.

Oropharyngeal Suctioning

The goal of airway management is keeping the airway open and free of obstructions. If the airway is obstructed with secretions, blood, or foreign materials, the airway will have to be suctioned. Suction equipment should always be within easy reach when managing any critically ill patient. If the patient is being managed outside the ambulance, either an electrical or a hand-operated suction device should be brought to the patient's side. If the patient is in the ambulance, the on-board suction system should be set up and ready for immediate use. Nothing is more embarrassing for the EMT, or harmful for the patient, than fumbling around to get a suction unit working when the airway is filled with vomit or blood.

You learned that a working rigid-tip suction catheter is an essential piece of equipment. In Chapter 6, "Airway Management," you learned the technique for oropharyngeal suctioning—suctioning the mouth and pharynx—with a rigid-tip catheter. This must be done before performing orotracheal intubation.

Orotracheal Intubation

endotracheal (EN-do-TRAY-ke-ul) **tube** a tube designed to be inserted into the trachea. Oxygen, medication, or a suction catheter can be directed into the trachea through an endotracheal tube.

intubation (IN-tu-BAY-shun) insertion of a tube.

orotracheal (OR-o-TRAY-ke-ul) **intubation** placement of an endotracheal tube through the mouth and into the trachea.

laryngoscope (lair-ING-uh-skope) an illuminating instrument that is inserted into the pharynx to permit visualization of the pharynx and larynx.

An **endotracheal tube** is a tube designed to be inserted into the trachea (*endo* meaning "into," *tracheal* referring to the trachea). Oxygen, medication, or a suction catheter can be directed into the trachea through the endotracheal tube. **Intubation** means the insertion of a tube. **Orotracheal intubation** is the placement of an endotracheal tube orally; that is, by way of the mouth (*oro* means "mouth"), then through the vocal cords and into the trachea.

Orotracheal intubation allows direct ventilation of the lungs through the endotracheal tube, bypassing the entire upper airway. The endotracheal tube is placed through the vocal cords with direct visualization of the process (that is, seeing what you are doing). A **laryngoscope** is an illuminating instrument that is inserted into the pharynx and allows you to visualize the pharynx and larynx.

The advantages of orotracheal intubation of the apneic (nonbreathing) patient include:

- Complete control of the airway (the tube going directly into the trachea prevents the tongue, blood, or debris that may be present in the upper airway from interfering with the passage of air into the trachea and lungs)
- Minimizes the risk of aspiration (the tube blocks vomitus or foreign matter from being aspirated, or breathed into the lungs)
- Allows for better oxygen delivery (oxygen is fed directly to the lungs via the trachea)
- Allows for deeper suctioning of the airway (a flexible suction catheter can be passed through the endotracheal tube to suction the trachea to the level of the carina)

Complications

Although orotracheal intubation is frequently a life-saving procedure, it has many potential complications. Orotracheal intubation is considered an "invasive" technique because it requires placement of equipment inside the body cavity. Whenever you perform an invasive procedure, you must be aware of the potential complications and be prepared to recognize and treat them should they arise. These concerns about invasive procedures are never more critical than in orotracheal intubation, since improper placement of the endotracheal tube in the apneic patient can rapidly result in the patient's death if it is not immediately detected and corrected.

Specific complications of orotracheal intubation include:

- *Slowing of the heart rate.* Stimulation of the airway with the laryngoscope and the endotracheal tube can lead to a slowing of the heart. The patient's heart rate should be monitored throughout the intubation.
- *Soft-tissue trauma.* This may occur to the teeth, lips, tongue, gums, and airway structures.
- *Hypoxia.* Prolonged attempts at intubation may lead to inadequate oxygenation, or oxygen starvation, known as **hypoxia.** To prevent this, you should ventilate the patient with high-concentration oxygen (ventilations provided at the normal rate, or 12 ventilations per minute) prior to intubation. Any attempts to insert the endotracheal tube (during which ventilations cannot be provided) should be limited to no more than 30 seconds.

hypoxia (hi-POK-se-uh) inadequate oxygenation, or oxygen starvation.

- *Vomiting.* Stimulation of the airway may cause the patient to gag and vomit.
- *Right mainstem intubation.* The endotracheal tube has to remain superior to the carina (before the point where the right and left mainstem bronchi branch off) in order to send air into both lungs. If the tube is advanced too far, the tube is likely to go down the steep right mainstem bronchus. Mainstem intubation results in only one lung being ventilated and the development of hypoxia.
- *Esophageal intubation.* This is the most serious complication. The unrecognized placement of the tube in the esophagus rather than the trachea prevents any ventilation of the lungs and will rapidly result in death.
- *Accidental extubation.* Even if the endotracheal tube is properly placed initially, the tube can become dislodged while moving the patient, or by the patient himself if he regains consciousness. Reassess chest wall movement and breath sounds after every major move with the intubated patient, such as down the stairs or from the floor to the stretcher.

Equipment

Orotracheal intubation requires specialized equipment.

STANDARD PRECAUTIONS Because of the high risk of splattering of sputum or blood during intubation, it is essential that Standard Precautions be taken. This means that a mask and goggles or other protective eyewear be worn in addition to gloves. This is mandatory since your face will be in direct line with the path of secretions, blood, and vomit coming from the mouth while you attempt to visualize the airway.

LARYNGOSCOPE A laryngoscope is made up of two components: the handle that contains the batteries, and the blade that is inserted in the airway and illuminates the airway. In most laryngoscopes, the handle and the blades are two separate pieces that need to be assembled with each use. In these devices, the blade is placed parallel to the handle and the notch at the base of the blade is attached to the bar on the handle.

The blade is then lifted to a 90-degree angle with the handle and, as the blade locks into place, the light at the tip of the blade illuminates (Figure 38-4). Always check the light at the end of the blade to ensure that it illuminates with a bright white color and that the bulb is tightly secured to the blade. It should be noted that some disposable laryngoscopes are preassembled with the handle and blade as a single fixed unit.

No matter what type of laryngoscope you use, it is essential that you conduct a daily check of the device to ensure that it is working properly. Spare batteries and bulbs should always be stored with the laryngoscope.

Laryngoscope blades are specifically designed to fit into the anatomy of the airway, providing optimal illumination of the vocal cords to enable you to pass the endotracheal tube between them. Most commercially available blades are designed with the light on the right side of the blade. This requires that the handle of the scope be held in the left hand to provide optimal illumination of the airway.

There are two general types of blades: straight and curved. Both types of blades come in assorted sizes ranging from the smallest size, 0, to the largest size, 4. The size of the blade used depends on the size of the patient. Most adult patients can be intubated using a size 2 or 3 straight blade or a size 3 curved blade. (Pediatric blade sizes will be discussed later in this chapter.) The decision as to whether to use a straight or curved blade depends on individual preference; however, straight blades are preferred for pediatric orotracheal intubations.

Each blade type is designed to enable you to visualize the cords by taking advantage of different anatomical mechanisms. The straight blade is designed so that the tip of the blade is placed under the epiglottis to lift the epiglottis upward and bring the **glottic opening** (the opening to the trachea) and the vocal cords into view (Figure 38-5). The curved blade is designed so that the tip of the blade is inserted into the vallecula so that lifting the laryngoscope handle upward brings the glottic opening and the vocal cords into view (Figure 38-6).

glottic opening
the opening to the trachea.

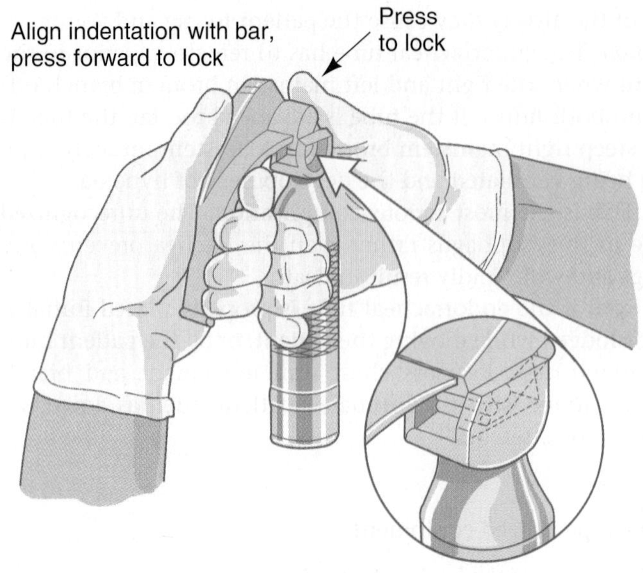
Align indentation with bar,
press forward to lock
Press
to lock
A

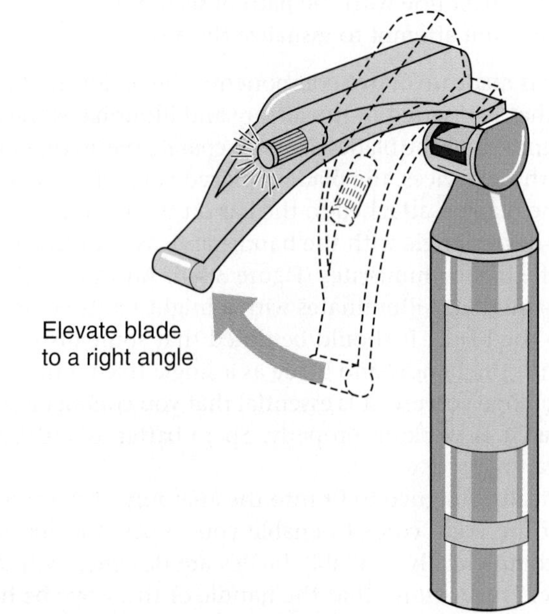
Elevate blade
to a right angle
B

Figure 38-4 • (A) Affix the laryngoscope blade and (B) then elevate it.

ENDOTRACHEAL TUBE The endotracheal tube (Figure 38-7) consists of a single lumen tube through which air and supplemental oxygen are delivered. At the end of the tube that will remain outside the patient is a standard 15-millimeter adapter for connection to the bag-valve unit.

The distal end of the tube (the end that will go into the patient) has a cuff. It is designed to be inflated after the tube is placed to prevent leakage of air and fluid around the tip of the tube. Usually 8 to 10 cc of air will result in an adequate seal.

The cuff is filled with a 10-cc syringe at the inflation valve. Just below the inflation valve is the pilot balloon, which fills when the cuff is inflated. Since the cuff is inside the trachea, you will not be able to see if it is inflated, but the inflation of the pilot balloon will verify that there is air in the cuff. If the pilot balloon does not hold air, then you must assume that the cuff at the end of the tube has also failed.

Endotracheal tubes used on infants and children less than 8 years old may or may not have a cuff (see Orotracheal Intubation of an Infant or Child later in this chapter).

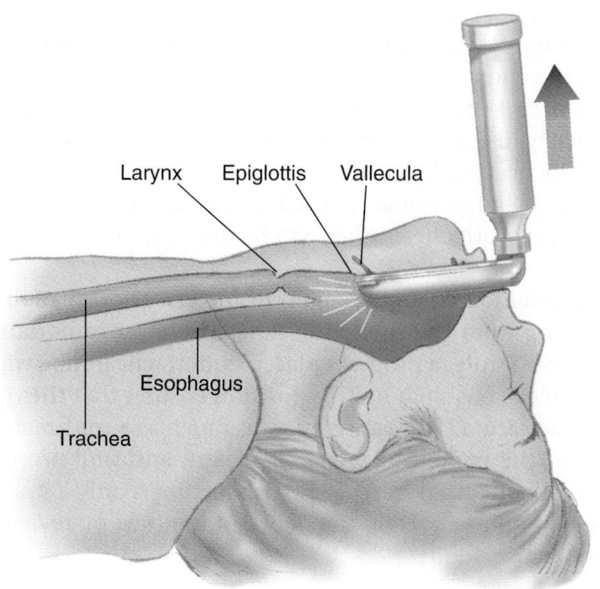

Figure 38-5 • The straight blade lifts the epiglottis.

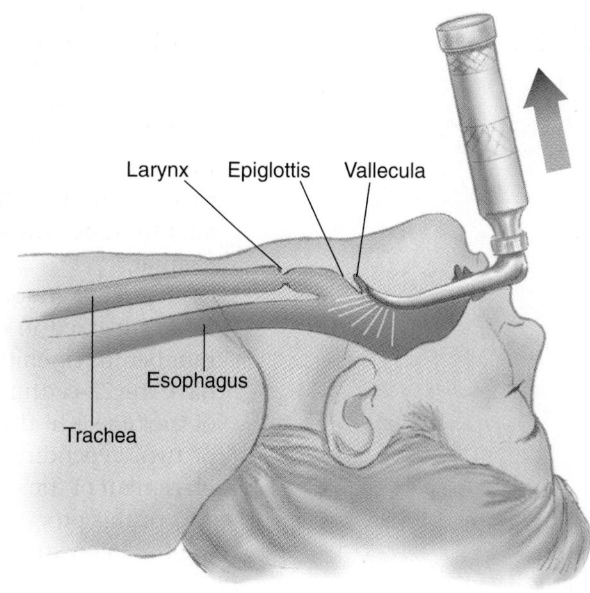

Figure 38-6 • The curved blade lifts the vallecula.

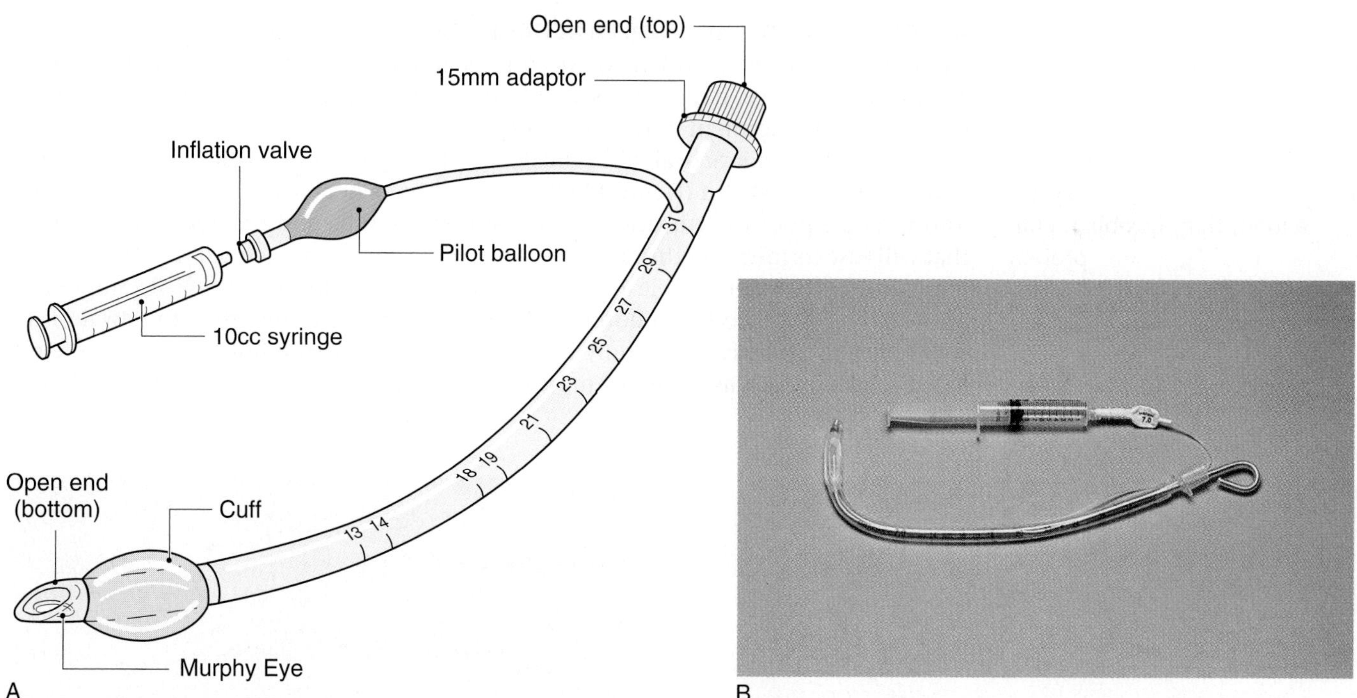

Figure 38-7 • (A) The endotracheal tube and (B) endotracheal tube with stylet in place.

Many endotracheal tubes have a small hole on the left side of the tube opposite the bevel, known as a Murphy eye. This feature is designed to lessen the chances of tube obstruction.

Endotracheal tubes come in various diameters, from 2.0 millimeters (used on premature infants) to 10.0 millimeters (used on very large adults). The diameter measured is the distance from one side of the internal wall of the tube to the other, called the internal diameter or "i.d." No matter what the internal diameter of the tube, the standard 15-millimeter adapter is affixed to the end of the tube.

When determining the proper size of the endotracheal tube for the adult patient, the rule of thumb is: In an emergency, use a 7.5-mm tube. For more precise sizing of the endotracheal tube, it is generally accepted that the adult male should receive either an 8.0- or an 8.5-mm tube and the adult female should receive from a 7.0- to an 8.0-mm tube. The sizing of pediatric endotracheal tubes will be discussed later in this chapter.

The adult endotracheal tube has a standard length of 33 centimeters. The side of the tube is marked in centimeters starting from the tip of the tube. The most important number to remember is that, as a general rule, a properly placed endotracheal tube will have the 22-centimeter mark at the teeth of an adult. This position ensures that the tip of the tube is in the trachea above the carina. This can vary by as much as a centimeter or two, depending on the height of the patient. (As you will learn, ensuring proper placement of the tube is a critical skill, and checking the length marking is only a small part of this procedure.) It may be helpful to envision the depth of the tube by reviewing the following distances in the average adult:

- 15 centimeters from the teeth to the vocal cords
- 20 centimeters from the teeth to the suprasternal notch
- 25 centimeters from the teeth to the carina

As you can see, there is very little room for error when placing the endotracheal tube, since only a few centimeters can mean the difference between proper placement and the tube being past the carina into the right mainstem bronchus.

ACCESSORIES TO THE ENDOTRACHEAL TUBE There are several accessories to the endotracheal tube with which you need to be familiar. These include the stylet, lubricant, a 10-cc syringe, devices for securing the tube once it is placed, devices for ensuring the proper placement of the tube, and a suction device.

stylet
a long, thin, flexible metal probe.

Because the endotracheal tube is made of relatively flexible plastic, it is generally recommended that a **stylet** (Figure 38-8)—a long, thin, bendable metal probe—be inserted into the tube prior to intubation to help stiffen the tube and provide it with a shape that will ease its insertion through the vocal cords. It is recommended that the stylet be lubricated with water-soluble lubricant, such as K-Y® jelly, Lubrifax®, or Surgilube®, prior to insertion into the endotracheal tube to allow for a smooth withdrawal of the stylet once the tube is successfully placed. (A silicone-based lubricant or a petroleum-based lubricant such as Vaseline® must not be used.)

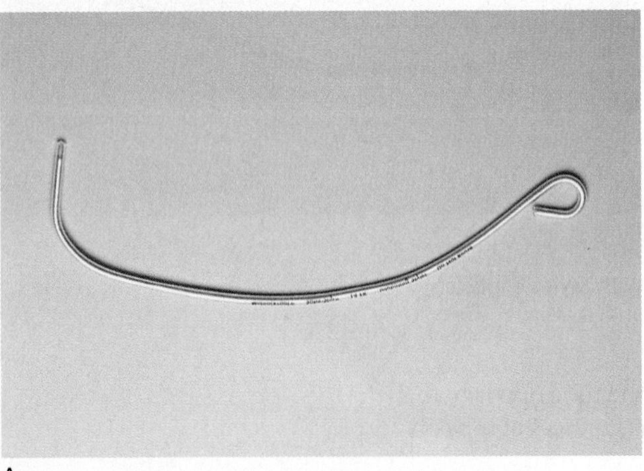

A

B

Figure 38-8 • (A) Stylet and (B) stylet in place.

Once the lubricated stylet is inserted, the endotracheal tube should be shaped into a "hockey stick" configuration. To avoid trauma to the airway, do not insert the stylet past the tip of the tube. Since the stylet is longer than the endotracheal tube, it is easy to inadvertently allow the tip to extend beyond the end of the tube. Such an error, however, could cause a puncture of the trachea. To avoid this complication, the tip of the stylet should not be inserted beyond the proximal end of the Murphy eye and the excess length should be bent over the 15-mm adapter.

When performing orotracheal intubation, it is often a problem that excessive oral secretions obstruct an adequate view of the vocal cords. Paradoxically, airways are sometimes very dry, thus making insertion of the tube difficult because of friction between the end of the tube and the patient's pharynx and glottis. For these reasons, it is important both that a wide bore suction device be operational and within easy reach during intubation attempts and that water-soluble lubricant be applied to the outside of the distal portion of the tube. The suction device should be turned on and placed by your right hand (since your left hand will be holding the laryngoscope). In general, you can use half a small packet of lubricant on the stylet and the other half of the packet on the outside of the tube.

Another piece of essential equipment for use with the endotracheal tube is a 10-cc syringe. As mentioned earlier, the syringe is used to inflate the cuff through the inflation valve. The syringe should also be used to test that the cuff is intact and holds air prior to inserting the tube. Once the integrity of the cuff has been ensured, the air should be withdrawn, but the syringe should remain attached to the tube so that it is easily found when it is time to reinflate the cuff after the patient is intubated. It should be noted that, following final inflation of the cuff, the 10-cc syringe should be detached from the inflation valve to prevent any subsequent leakage of air out of the cuff and back into the syringe.

One of the final steps in orotracheal intubation is securing the tube to the patient so that it does not move or become dislodged. This is especially important in the prehospital setting where the tube can easily be dislodged during patient movement. Prior to securing the endotracheal tube, an oral airway or similar device should be inserted as a bite block in case the patient becomes responsive and gnaws at the tube. There are a number of methods for securing endotracheal tubes. The preferred method is to use one of the commercially available devices manufactured for this purpose. Cloth tape is acceptable but less desirable. The manner in which tubes are secured is usually determined by the medical direction of the EMS system you work in. Whatever method you use to secure the tube, make sure the tube is firmly secured in place and able to withstand the tugs and pulls that are routine during moves of critically ill patients.

Indications

When properly performed, orotracheal intubation is clearly a life-saving technique. It is essential, however, that you know under what conditions a patient needs to be intubated. The following is a list of indications:

- Inability to ventilate the apneic patient
- Patient is without a gag reflex or cough
- Patient is unresponsive to any painful stimuli
- Cardiac arrest

Technique of Insertion—Adult Patient

Orotracheal intubation is the most complicated and difficult procedure the EMT is expected to perform. Properly performed, it is truly a life-saving procedure. Incorrectly performed, the EMT's actions can easily result in the patient's death. Because many EMTs will only rarely perform orotracheal intubation, it is essential that you not only learn and practice the technique extensively during your training but also practice the technique on a regular basis once you are a certified EMT.

The following is a step-by-step guide to orotracheal intubation of the adult patient (Scan 38-1).

SCAN 38-1 • Orotracheal Intubation—Adult Patient

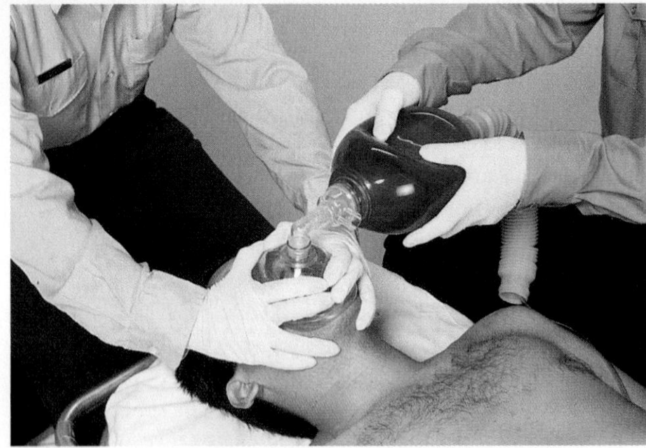

Step 1: Ventilate the patient.

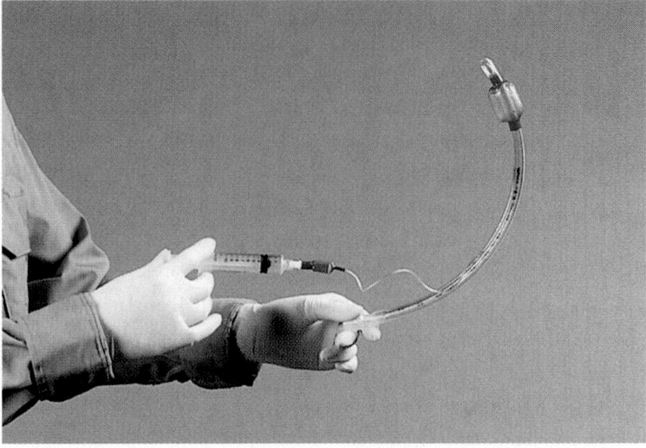

Step 2: Assemble, prepare, and test all equipment.

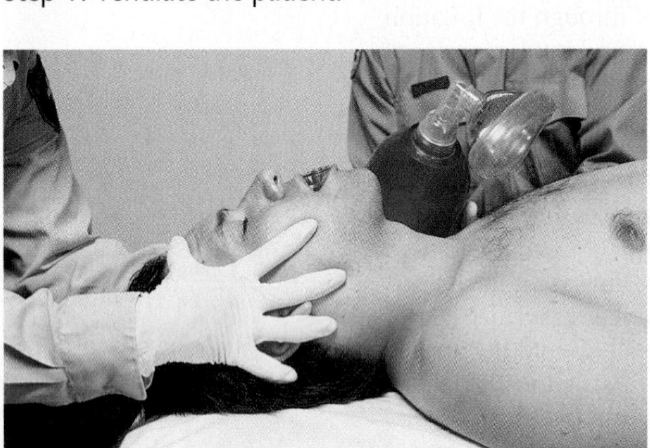

Step 3: Position the patient's head.

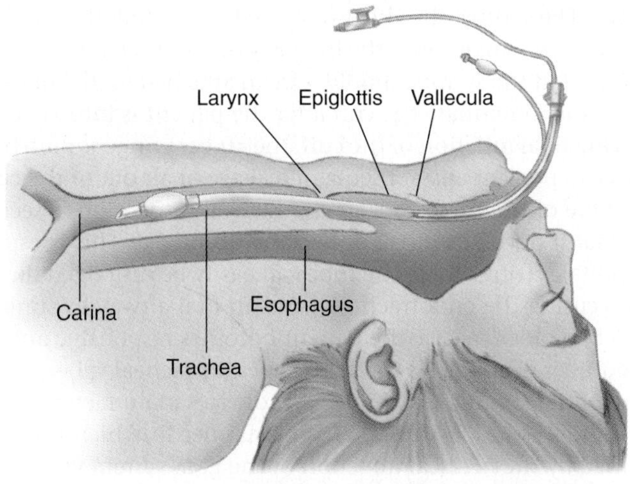

Step 4: Make sure the airway is aligned. (If trauma is suspected, keep the patient's head and neck in a neutral position. Endotracheal tube is shown already in place.)

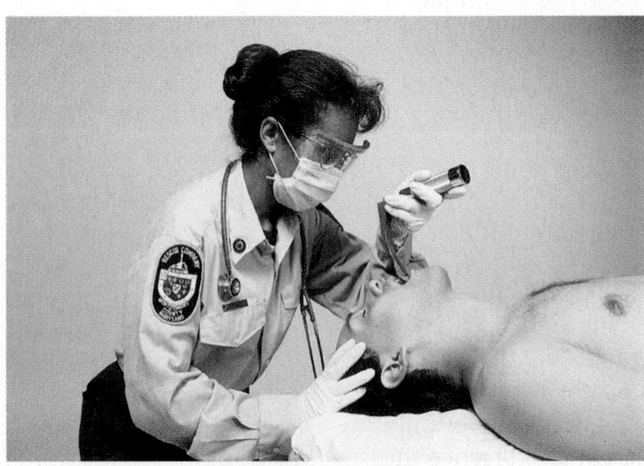

Step 5: Prepare to insert the laryngoscope blade.

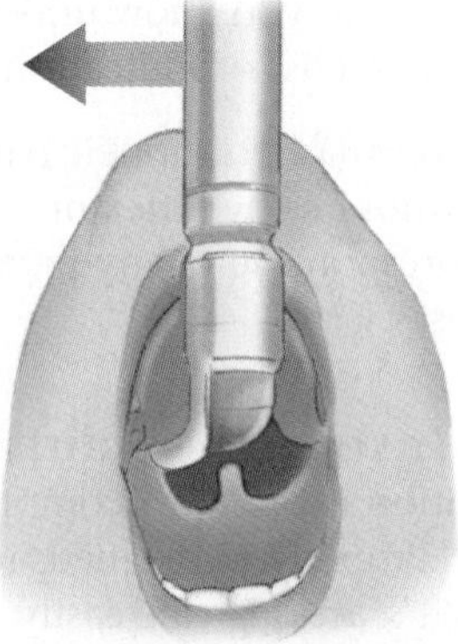

Step 6: Lift the tongue out of the way.

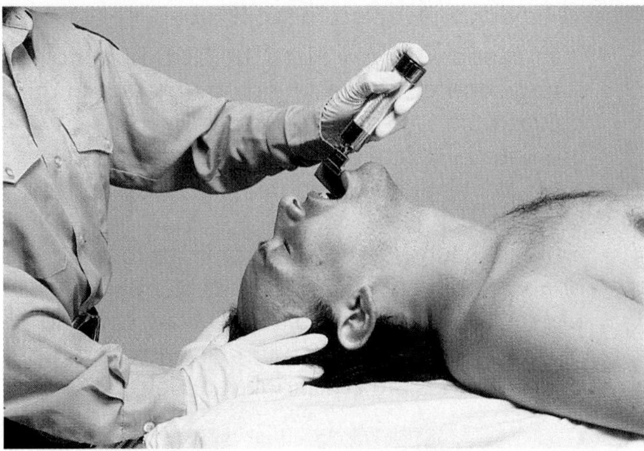

Step 7: Insert the blade (curved blade into vallecula; straight blade under epiglottis) and lift to bring glottic opening into view.

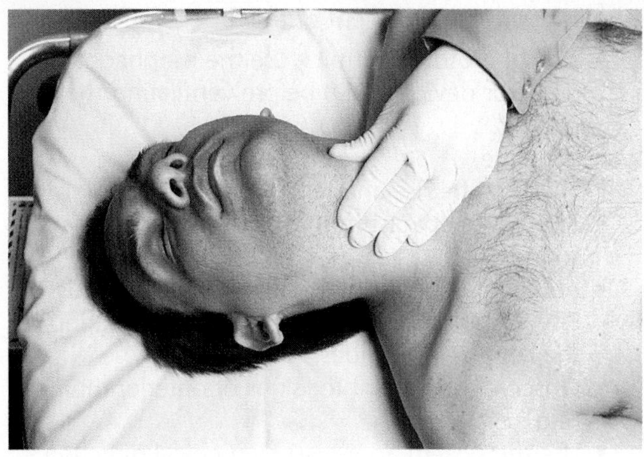

Step 8: A second rescuer may perform cricoid pressure during intubation to suppress vomiting and aid visualization.

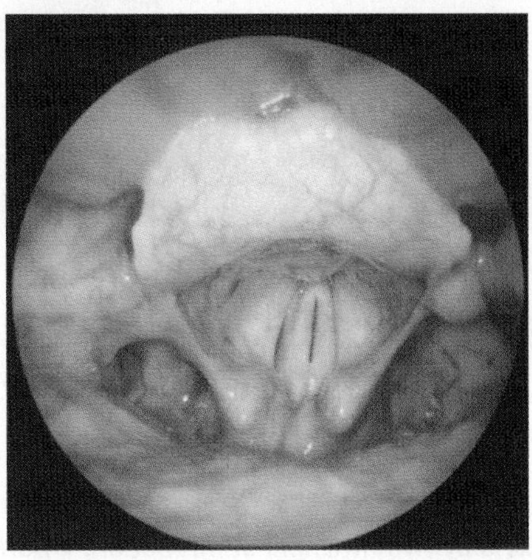

Step 9: Visualize the glottic opening. *(Phototake, New York)*

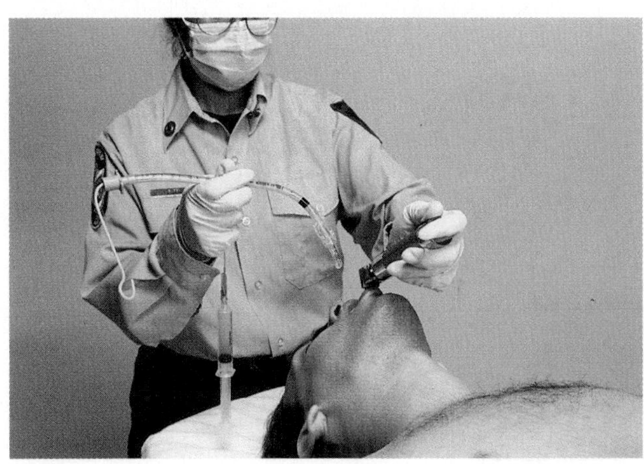

Step 10: Insert endotracheal tube with stylet.

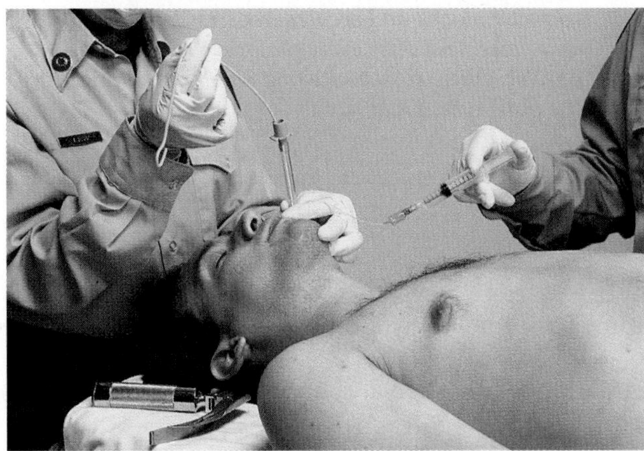

Step 11: Remove laryngoscope and stylet. Inflate the cuff with 5 to 10 cc of air.

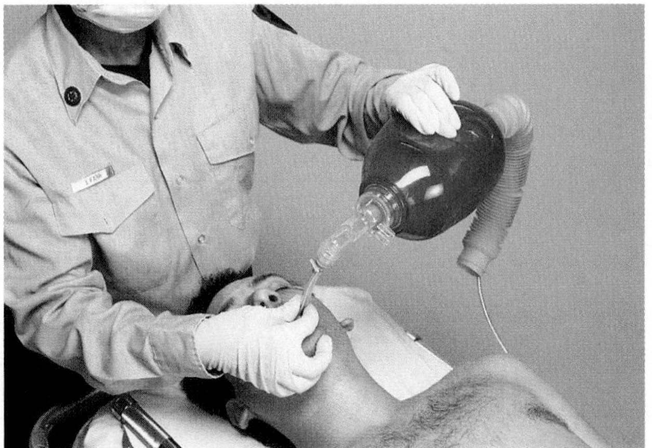

Step 12: Attach a bag-valve unit or other ventilation device to the tube.

continued

SCAN 38-1 • (Continued)

Confirm correct placement of the tube:

- If local protocol permits, use the esophageal detector device (EDD) before ventilating the patient.
- Ventilate.
- Observe the rise and fall of the chest.
- Auscultate epigastrium for absence of breath sounds.
- Auscultate over both lungs for breath sounds. The sounds should be equal when comparing the left and right sides.
- Observe the patient for signs of deterioration, (e.g., cyanosis).
- Use the system approved by medical direction to confirm correct placement. This might include use of an end-tidal CO_2 detector or, in a patient who is perfusing, a pulse oximeter.

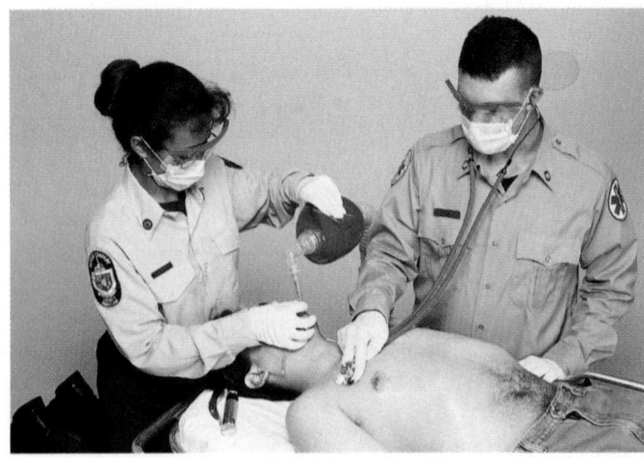

Step 13: Auscultate lung and epigastrium areas to confirm correct placement.

Correct any incorrect placement of tube:

- If air cannot be drawn into the EIDD bulb or syringe and/or breath sounds are present in the epigastrium—the esophagus has been intubated. Deflate the cuff and withdraw the tube. Ventilate for 1 minute before another attempt.
- If breath sounds are present on right, diminished or absent on left—the right mainstem bronchus has probably been intubated. Deflate cuff and gently withdraw tube (continue ventilation) until breath sounds are equal right and left.

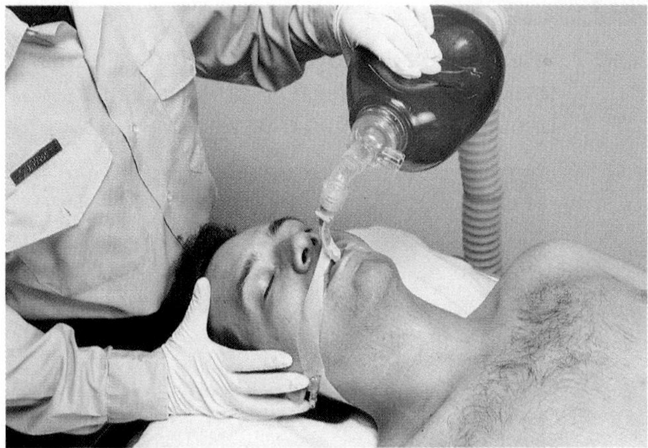

Step 14: If correct placement is confirmed, secure the tube in place.

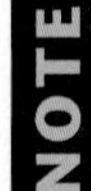

Make only two attempts at intubation. If both attempts fail, insert an oral airway and continue to ventilate with a pocket mask or bag-valve mask. Aggressively suction the airway. If the tube has been correctly placed and secured, reassess breath sounds and placement after every major move with the patient. Offer reassurance and emotional support to the patient and family.

Preparation

1. Ensure Standard Precautions. This should include gloves, goggles or other protective eyewear, and a mask.
2. Ensure that adequate ventilation with a bag-valve mask and high-concentration oxygen is being performed.
3. Ventilate the patient at a rate of 12 breaths per minute prior to any intubation attempts.
4. Assemble, prepare, and test all equipment including:
   - A suction unit with a large bore rigid tip (It should be functional and positioned so that it is within easy reach of the intubator's right hand should it be needed.)

- The cuff on the endotracheal tube (It should be tested and then deflated, with the 10-cc syringe left attached to the inflation valve.)
- The laryngoscope (Assemble and ensure that the light is bright and constant.)
- The stylet (Insert the stylet into the tube and form the tube into a hockey-stick shape.)
- The device that will be used to secure the tube after successful intubation

5. Position yourself at the patient's head so that, during intubation, left and right are your left and right as well as the patient's left and right.

Visualizing the Glottic Opening and Vocal Cords

6. Position the patient's head to ensure good visualization of the vocal cords. Remove the oral airway.
7. Hold the laryngoscope in your left hand and insert the laryngoscope into the right corner of the patient's mouth.
8. Use a sweeping motion to lift the tongue upward and to the left, out of the way, to enable visualization of the glottis.
9. Insert the blade into the proper anatomical location:
   - Curved blade fits into the vallecula.
   - Straight blade lifts the epiglottis.
10. Lift the scope up and away from the patient:
    - If trauma is not suspected, tilt the head, lift the chin, and attempt visualization of the cords. If the cords cannot be seen, raise the patient's shoulders approximately 1 inch by placing a towel beneath them and attempt visualization again.
    - If trauma is suspected, the patient will have to be intubated with the head and neck in a neutral position with a second rescuer maintaining in-line stabilization of the neck and head.
11. Avoid using the teeth as a fulcrum.
12. Application of **cricoid pressure** during intubation attempts may be beneficial. Cricoid pressure is performed by a second rescuer who uses his index finger and thumb to exert direct pressure on the patient's cricoid cartilage (Figures 38-9 and 38-10). Since the cricoid cartilage is the only cartilage in the neck that completely encircles the trachea, direct pressure helps to compress the esophagus, which is posterior to the trachea, reducing the risk of vomiting. In addition, the pressure often brings the vocal cords into better view. Cricoid pressure should be maintained until the patient is intubated.
13. Visualize the glottic opening and vocal cords. Once the cords come into view do not lose sight of them!

cricoid pressure
pressure applied to the cricoid cartilage to suppress vomiting and bring the vocal cords into view.

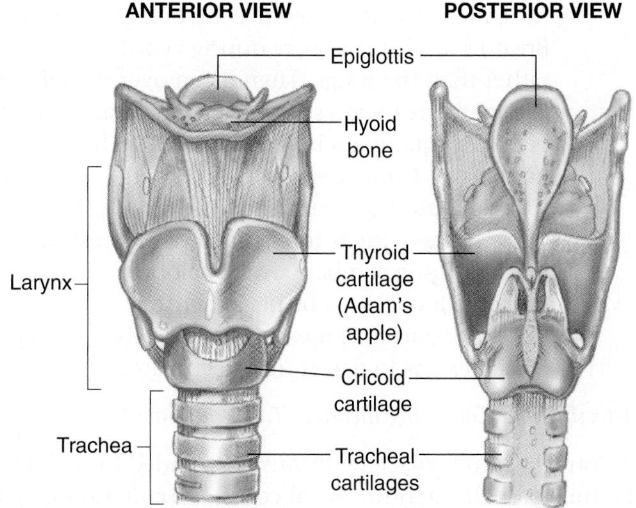

Figure 38-9 • The tracheal cartilages are C-shaped, open at the posterior side next to the esophagus. The cricoid cartilage at the lower end of the larynx is the only cartilage that completely encircles the trachea.

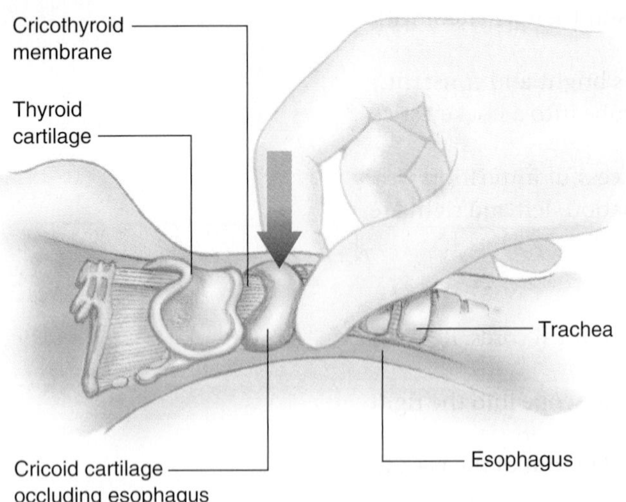

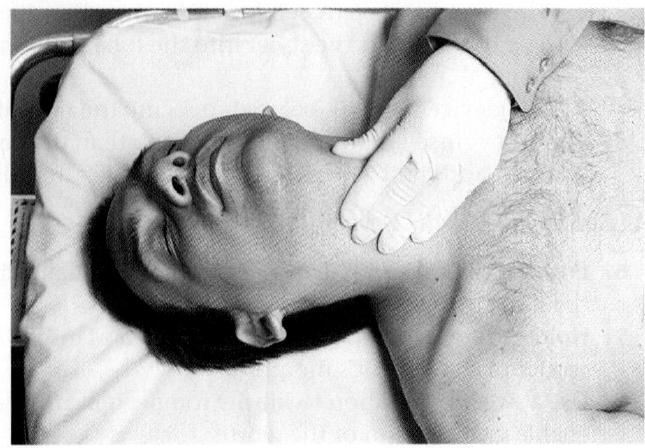

Figure 38-10 • In cricoid pressure, pressure is placed on the cricoid cartilage, pushing it posteriorly against the esophagus. By closing off the esophagus, vomiting is suppressed. The maneuver also helps bring the vocal cords into view.

Inserting the Endotracheal Tube

14. With the right hand, carefully insert the endotracheal tube through the vocal cords. The tube should be inserted just deep enough so that the cuff is past the cords. Verify that the endotracheal tube is at about 22 cm at the gums and teeth.

15. Remove the laryngoscope and extinguish the lamp.

16. While holding the tube securely, remove the stylet, if used.

17. Inflate the cuff with 5 to 10 cc of air and remove the syringe.

18. Continue to hold onto the endotracheal tube. Never let go of the endotracheal tube until it is secured in place.

19. Place a capnometry device or sensor between the tube and the bag-valve mask (BVM) or use an esophageal detector device to verify tube placement. (See Detecting and Correcting Incorrect Tube Placements, Steps 22 and 23.)

20. Have a partner attach the bag valve to the endotracheal tube and deliver artificial ventilations.

Ensuring Correct Tube Placement

21. The single most accurate way of ensuring proper tube placement in the trachea (Figure 38-11) is visualizing the endotracheal tube as it passes through the vocal cords. All the following methods are for verification of tube placement:

- Observe the patient's chest rise and fall with each ventilation.
- Auscultate for the presence of breath sounds. Begin over the epigastrium. Breath sounds heard here during ventilations indicate air entering the stomach rather than the lungs. Then listen over the left apex (top of the left lung area). Compare the breath sounds with those at the right apex. Breath sounds should be heard equally on both sides. Finally, listen over the left base (bottom of the lung area). Compare the breath sounds with those at the right base. Breath sounds should be heard equally on both sides.
- Observe the patient for signs of deterioration after tube placement; for example, becoming combative or developing cyanosis. Both are signs of hypoxia and probable incorrect tube placement.
- Use other objective measures as described in Steps 22 and 23 to confirm correct placement or to detect incorrect placement.

Detecting and Correcting Incorrect Tube Placements

Endotracheal tube placement must be verified by at least two methods after observing the tube pass through the vocal cords. Auscultation is one verification technique. The

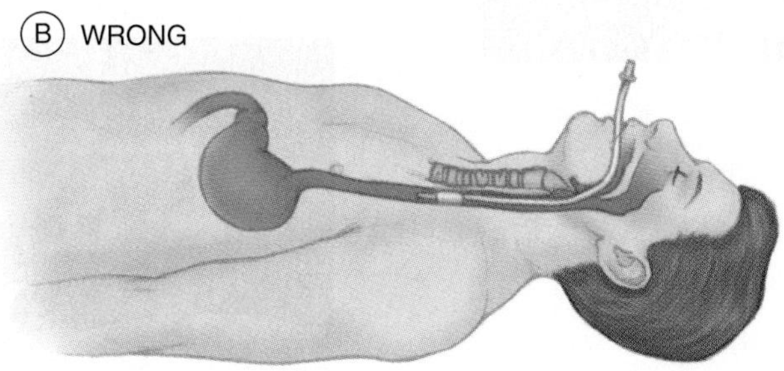

Figure 38-11 • (A) The endotracheal tube is correctly placed in the trachea. (B) The endotracheal tube is incorrectly placed in the esophagus—a life-threatening error.

second verification is accomplished by the use of an esophageal detector device (Figure 38-12A and 38-12B) or by capnometry (Figure 38-12C).

22. Auscultate for breath sounds:
   - If breath sounds are diminished or absent on the left but present on the right, it is likely the tube has advanced beyond the carina and intubated the right mainstem bronchus. If this occurs, deflate the cuff and gently withdraw the tube while artificially ventilating and while auscultating over the left apex of the chest. Take care not to completely remove the endotracheal tube. When the breath sounds become equal at both the left and right apex, reinflate the cuff.
   - If breath sounds are only present in the epigastrium, the esophagus has been intubated and air is being sent into the stomach instead of the lungs (review Figure 38-11). Since esophageal intubation is a fatal occurrence, immediately deflate the cuff and withdraw the tube. Ventilate for 1 minute prior to your second attempt to intubate.

23. Use an esophageal detector device or capnometry to detect or measure exhaled carbon dioxide:
   - The **esophageal detector device (EDD)** may be used to detect incorrect placement (or to verify correct placement). The EDD is a disposable bulb (review Figure 38-12A) or syringe (review Figure 38-12B). After the endotracheal tube has been placed and before any ventilation attempts, attach the EDD to the endotracheal tube and squeeze the bulb or push in the syringe. If the tube is in the esophagus, its soft, unsupported walls will collapse around the end of the tube. This will prevent air from being drawn into the EDD. If it is a bulb device, the bulb will remain collapsed and will not refill; if it is a syringe device, you will not be able to draw the plunger out of the syringe reservoir. By contrast, if the tube is in the trachea, the rigid trachea remains patent, allowing an EDD bulb to refill or the plunger of an EDD syringe to be easily withdrawn from the syringe reservoir.
   - **Capnometry** is the measurement of exhaled carbon dioxide. Capnometry can be used to confirm a properly placed endotracheal tube (by indicating adequate exhaled carbon dioxide), or it can indicate that a tube has been improperly placed initially or that a properly placed tube has become displaced at any time during the call.

NOTE

Displaced endotracheal tubes are a frequent problem because of the patient movement that can occur during assessment and transport. Displaced tubes are also a serious source of liability for EMS providers who intubate.

esophageal detector device (EDD)
a device that uses a bulb or syringe to attempt to withdraw air from an endotracheal tube to determine correct placement in the trachea (from which air can easily be withdrawn) or incorrect placement in the esophagus (in which the soft esophagus will collapse and prevent air from being withdrawn).

capnometry
(kap-NOM-uh-tree)
the measurement of exhaled carbon dioxide. A graphic recording or display of capnometric measurement is called *capnography*.

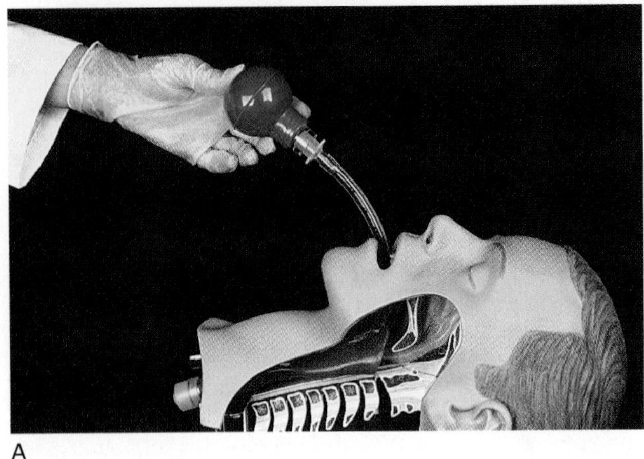

A

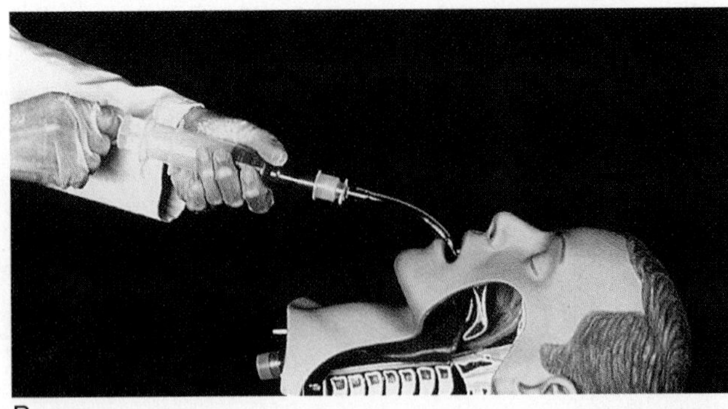

B

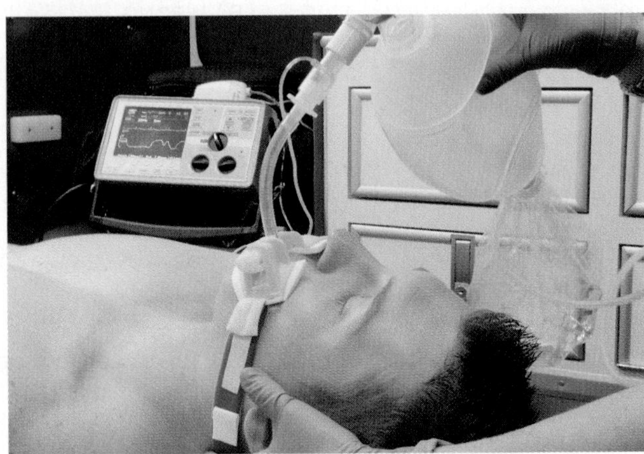

C

Figure 38-12 • (A) Esophageal intubation detector device, bulb style. (B) An esophageal intubation detector device—syringe style. (C) Waveform capnometry on an intubated patient. *(Photo C: © Ray Kemp/911 Imaging)*

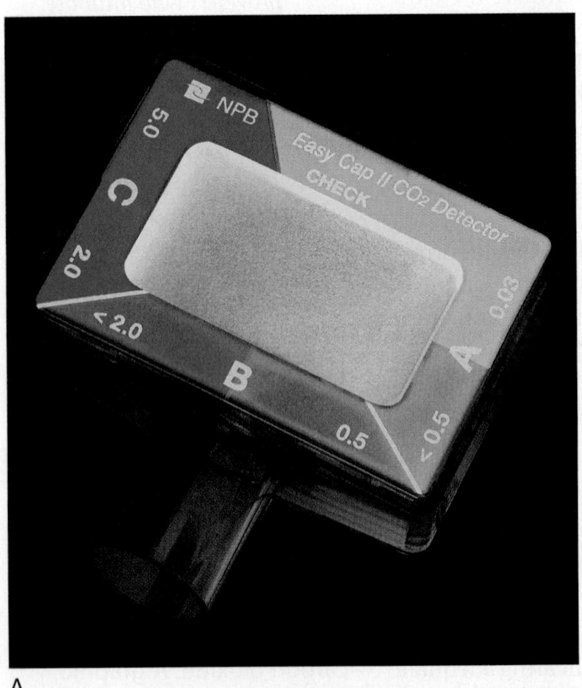

A

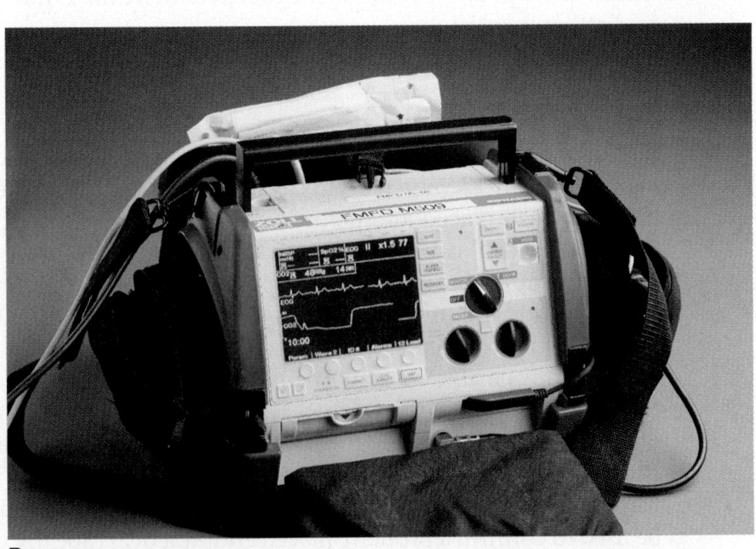

B

Figure 38-13 • (A) Colorimetric capnometry. *(Reprinted by permission of Nellcor Puritan Bennett LLC, Pleasanton, California)* (B) Waveform capnometry. *(© Scott Metcalfe)*

After intubating, but before applying the BVM to the tube, an in-line sensor is applied to the 15/22-mm adapter at the proximal end of the tube. There are two types of devices: colorimetric and waveform. The colorimetric device (Figure 38-13A) attaches between the tube and the BVM and changes color during the ventilatory cycle, indicating changes in the levels of carbon dioxide. Use caution as vomitus or medications in the tube may cause the device to read improperly or not at all.

The waveform device (Figure 38-13B), like the colorimetric device, is connected between the tube and BVM. The waveform device is then connected to a cardiac monitor with capnography capabilities or to a stand-alone capnometer. The capnometer provides a continuous reading, called a waveform, that displays the levels of carbon dioxide present in the lungs during different stages of ventilation. Observing the expected changes in carbon dioxide levels in the lungs during ventilation and CPR, through the waveform, indicates that the endotracheal tube is properly placed not only initially but throughout resuscitation and the entire call.

Frequently monitor the waveform reading as well as reauscultating the lungs after patient movement or if changes are noted in the patient's condition.

NOTE

Colorimetric capnometric devices do not provide a lasting record as most waveform capnometric devices do.

NOTE

The EMT should make only two attempts at orotracheal intubation. If both attempts fail, insert an oral airway; continue to ventilate the patient with high-concentration oxygen via bag-valve mask; and aggressively suction the airway.

Securing the Tube

24. If breath sounds are heard bilaterally and no sounds are heard over the epigastrium, the endotracheal tube should be secured in place using the system that is approved by your Medical Director. An oral airway may be inserted as a bite block to protect the tube. Note the depth of the tube at the teeth both before and after securing it to ensure that the tube has not been dislodged during the procedure.

Ongoing Assessment

25. Be sure to assess and reassess the breath sounds following every major move with the patient.

NOTE

Although the complications of orotracheal intubation have already been discussed, it cannot be overemphasized that inadvertent esophageal intubation will likely result in the patient's death. Because of the magnitude of this complication, if at any time—despite your efforts to properly assess tube placement—you are in doubt of proper tube placement, immediately withdraw the tube and manage the airway with basic airway adjuncts.

Orotracheal Intubation of an Infant or Child

Although the goal of orotracheal intubation is identical in both adult and pediatric patients, intubation of the infant and child requires special training because of various considerations of anatomy, physiology, and size. The specific anatomy and physiology of the pediatric airway has been discussed earlier. The importance of these factors as they relate to orotracheal intubation are as follows:

- In an infant or child, it is often difficult to create a single clear visual plane from the mouth through the pharynx and into the glottis for orotracheal intubation because of such factors as the relatively large size of the tongue.
- Because of size differences among infants and children as well as the fact that the narrowest portion of the airway is at the level of the cricoid ring, the proper sizing of the endotracheal tube is crucial.
- Because infants and children tend to develop hypoxia and bradycardia (slowed heartbeat) easily during intubation attempts, pediatric intubations require careful monitoring coupled with swift and accurate technique.

POINT OF VIEW

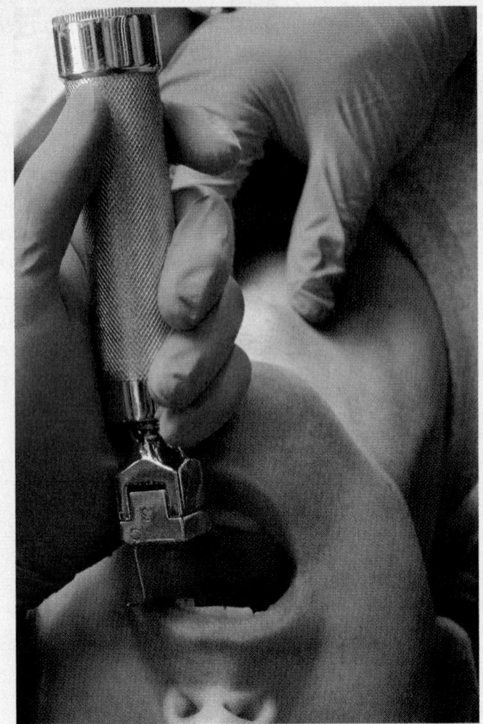

"I remember in class how our instructor told us intubation wasn't easy. She told us if we screwed up it could cost a patient his life. So when I got to my first call where I'd be doing it solo, I was terrified. Making it worse was that it was a young person—an overdose.

"I found I just had to focus—to follow and remember the steps. The patient was well oxygenated. I had one of the other crew members put some pressure on the cricoid. In my head I did everything I had done on the mannequin in class. Our instructor made us practice until we could do it in our sleep. Well, now I know why.

"When you mix in a little vomit and look at a patient's real airway—not an airway on an old plastic mannequin—it looks different. But I did it. I did it. And I was excited, but I knew we couldn't let our guard down. By the time we got the patient on the stretcher and to the rig there would be a dozen chances for the tube to get displaced. I'd gotten it in and I didn't want to lose it!

"We hooked up capnometry just to be sure. It worked. The tube stayed in place, and the patient made it to the hospital, and, we learned later, she survived.

"Phew. What a call."

The indications for orotracheal intubation of the infant and child are similar to those for the adult patient as follows:

- When prolonged artificial ventilation is required
- When adequate artificial ventilation cannot be achieved by other means
- To ventilate the clearly apneic patient
- To ventilate the cardiac arrest patient
- To control the airway of an unresponsive patient without a cough or gag reflex

The laryngoscope blades and the endotracheal tubes necessary for the orotracheal intubation of infants and children must be carefully sized to the patient. In general the straight blade, usually a size 1, is preferred in infants and small children because it provides for greater displacement of the tongue and better visualization of the glottis. As in adults, the blade lifts the epiglottis, bringing the vocal cords into view. In older children the curved blade is often preferred because the blade's broad base displaces the tongue better, allowing better visualization of the vocal cords once the blade is placed into the vallecula and lifted.

Assorted sizes of endotracheal tubes should always be stocked in the pediatric airway kit. As previously mentioned, the proper sizing of the tube is essential in children. Ideally a chart should be placed in the airway kit to assist the EMT in determining what size tube is generally used for a specific age patient. As an alternative a Broselow™ tape can be used to estimate tube size based on the height of the patient (Figure 38-14).

A formula—(patient's age in years + 16) ÷ 4 = tube size—can also be used to estimate the proper size. Finally, a less accurate method is to use the diameter of the patient's little finger or the diameter of the nasal opening to estimate correct tube size.

Because infants are often the pediatric patients who require orotracheal intubation, it is helpful to simply memorize that newborns and small infants generally require a 3.0 to a 3.5 tube, and a 4.0 tube can be used for older infants up to the age of 1 year. No

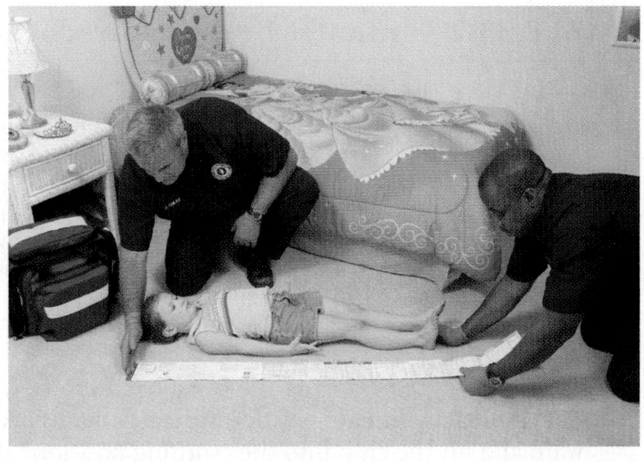

Figure 38-14 • A Broselow™ tape can be used to estimate the tube size based on the height of a pediatric patient.

matter what system you use in determining tube size, it is always prudent to have one half-size larger tube and one half-size smaller tube on stand-by, since the size of the glottic structure does vary in infants and children.

Endotracheal tubes come in both cuffed and uncuffed versions. Cuffed tubes are always used in adult patients. In the pediatric population, either cuffed or uncuffed tubes may be used. For younger children and infants, uncuffed tubes are sometimes used since the narrowing at the level of the cricoid cartilage serves as a functional cuff, snugging the tube in the airway. Uncuffed tubes (Figure 38-15) should display a vocal cord marker to ensure proper placement of the tube. This marker is designed so that the vocal cords are at the level of the translucent marker in the tube. A cuffed tube should be inserted, like the adult tube, just deep enough that the cuff material is inferior to the cords.

Proper depth of tube placement can also be approximated by age (Table 38-2). However, direct visualization of the tube being placed at the proper depth is the best measure of tube depth.

The step-by-step procedure for orotracheal intubation of infants and children is very similar to the procedure outlined for adults (earlier and Scan 38-1). There are, however, some important differences that you must keep in mind when performing a pediatric intubation:

1. The rate of ventilation both before and after intubation must be adjusted to the patient's age.
2. In the patient who has a pulse, the heart rate must be continuously monitored during intubation attempts, since mechanical stimulation of the airway and hypoxia can both slow the heart rate. If the heart rate is noted to slow during intubation, the blade should immediately be withdrawn and the infant or child reventilated with high-concentration oxygen.

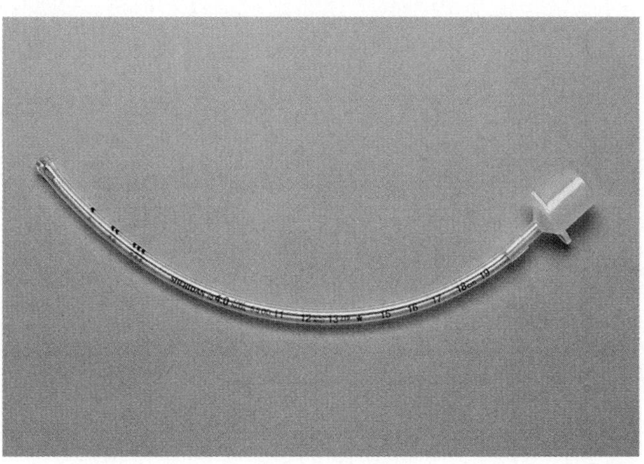

Figure 38-15 • An uncuffed endotracheal tube is used for patients under 8 years of age.

TABLE 38-2 • Infant/Child Endotracheal Tubes	
MEASUREMENT OF ENDOTRACHEAL TUBE AT THE TEETH	
6 months to 1 year	12 cm teeth to mid-trachea
2 years	14 cm teeth to mid-trachea
4 to 6 years	16 cm teeth to mid-trachea
6 to 10 years	18 cm teeth to mid-trachea
10 to 12 years	20 cm teeth to mid-trachea

3. The optimal manner of positioning the patient's head is to gently tilt the head forward and lift the chin into the "sniffing position" (Figure 38-16).
4. Very little force is needed to intubate the infant or child. Gentle finesse is the rule, not the exception.
5. Cricoid pressure is also often beneficial, but the landmarks may be difficult to locate in the infant and child. In addition, excessive pressure on the relatively soft cartilage may cause tracheal obstruction.
6. When using a straight blade, realize that the epiglottis in infants and children is not as stiff as in adults and may partially obscure a clear view of the vocal cords.
7. Since distances in the infant and child are small, be certain to hold onto the tube until you are ensured that it is well secured. As with adults, reassess tube placement every time you move the patient.
8. In infants and children, the best indicator of tube placement is symmetrical rise and fall of the chest during ventilation.
9. Breath sounds in infants and children can often be misleading since the chest is small and sounds are easily transmitted from one area to another.
10. Observe the patient for increase in heart rate and improving color after intubation. An infant or child who becomes dusky in color and slows his heart rate after intubation is likely not to be properly intubated.
11. Once tube placement is confirmed, the patient should be secured to an appropriate device to prevent any head movement from dislodging the tube.
12. If the tube is properly placed but there is inadequate chest expansion, seek out one of the following causes:
    - The tube is too small and there is an air leak around the tube at the glottic opening. This is detected by auscultating over the neck. The tube should be replaced by a larger tube.

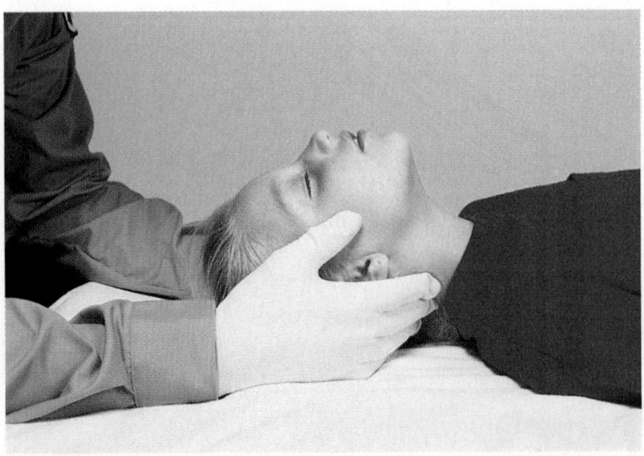

Figure 38-16 • Place the pediatric patient's head in the "sniffing" position for intubation.

- The pop-off valve on the bag-valve device has not been deactivated.
- There is a leak in the bag-valve device.
- The ventilator is delivering an inadequate volume of air/oxygen.
- The tube is blocked with secretions. This can be treated initially with endotracheal suctioning (see later in this chapter). If suctioning fails, the tube should be removed.

13. Infants and children are at risk for the same complications of orotracheal intubation as adult patients. Inadvertent esophageal intubation is perhaps even more rapidly fatal in infants and children than adults. In addition, barotrauma from overinflation of the lungs can result in collapse of the lung, which can further compromise your ability to ventilate the patient.

Nasogastric Intubation of an Infant or Child

An additional procedure the EMT may have to master in conjunction with orotracheal intubation of an infant or child is the placement of a **nasogastric tube (NG tube).** A nasogastric tube is inserted through the nose into the infant's or child's stomach. The most common use of the NG tube in regard to advanced airway management is to decompress the stomach and proximal bowel of air. In infants and children, air frequently fills the stomach and bowel after overly aggressive artificial ventilation or as a result of air swallowing. The NG tube provides a route for escape of the excess air. The NG tube can also be used to drain the stomach of blood or other substances. In the hospital setting, NG tubes can be used to give medication and provide a route for nutrition as well.

nasogastric (NAY-zo-GAS-trik) **tube (NG tube)**
a tube designed to be passed through the nose, nasopharynx, and esophagus. It is used to relieve distention of the stomach in an infant or child patient.

The indications for insertion of the NG tube in pediatric patients are as follows:

- Inability to adequately ventilate the patient because of distention of the stomach
- Unresponsive patient with gastric distention

Many experts believe that the NG tube should only be inserted after the trachea has been secured with an endotracheal tube to prevent incorrectly placing the NG tube into the trachea instead of the esophagus. Other possible complications of NG intubation include trauma to the nose, triggering vomiting, and—in very rare cases—passing the tube into the cranium through a basilar skull fracture. *Because of the risk of cranial intubation with the NG tube, the presence of major facial trauma or head trauma is considered a contraindication to the nasogastric tube.* In such cases, the insertion of the tube through the mouth (orogastric technique) is preferred.

The equipment required for nasogastric tube insertion is listed in Table 38-3. The procedure for insertion of the nasogastric tube as illustrated in Scan 38-2 is:

1. Prepare and assemble all equipment.
2. Ensure that the patient is well oxygenated prior to the procedure.

TABLE 38-3 • Nasogastric Intubation Equipment

Nasogastric tubes of various sizes:	
Newborn/infant:	8.0 French
Toddler/preschool:	10.0 French
School age:	12.0 French
Adolescent:	14.0 to 16.0 French
20-cc syringe	
Water-soluble lubricant	
Emesis basin	
Tape	
Stethoscope	
Suction unit with connecting tube	

SCAN 38-2 • Nasogastric Intubation— Infant or Child

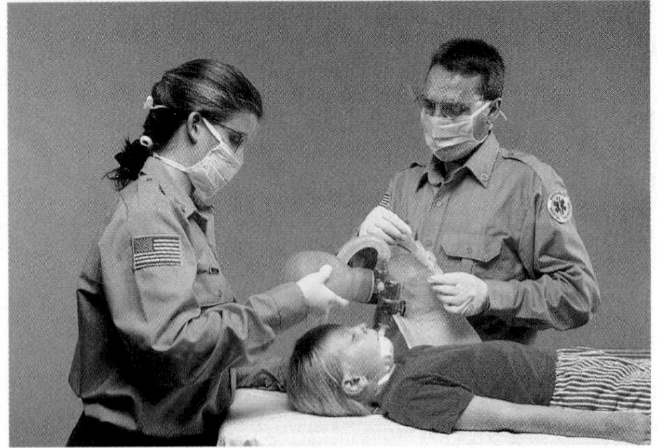

Step 1: Oxygenate the patient.

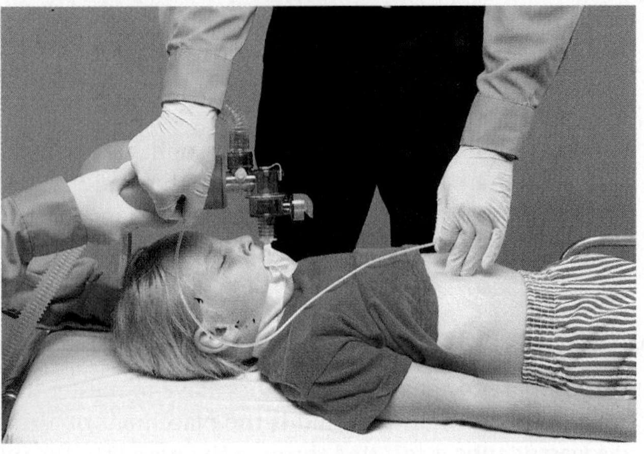

Step 2: Measure the tube from the tip of the nose, over the ear, to below the xiphoid process.

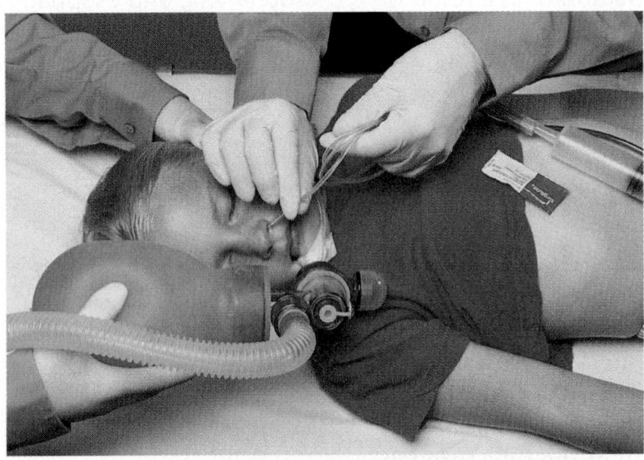

Step 3: Pass the lubricated tube gently downward along the nasal floor to the stomach.

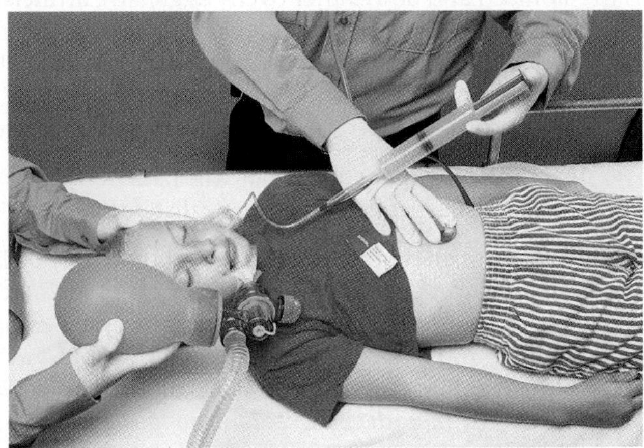

Step 4: To confirm correct placement, auscultate over the epigastrium. Listen for bubbling while injecting 10 to 20 cc of air into the tube.

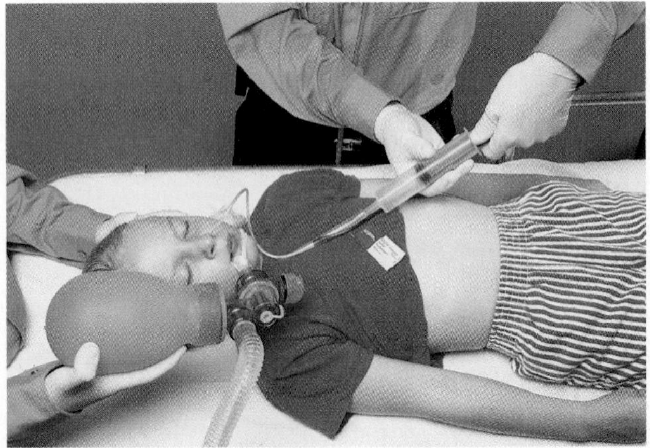

Step 5: Use suction to aspirate stomach contents.

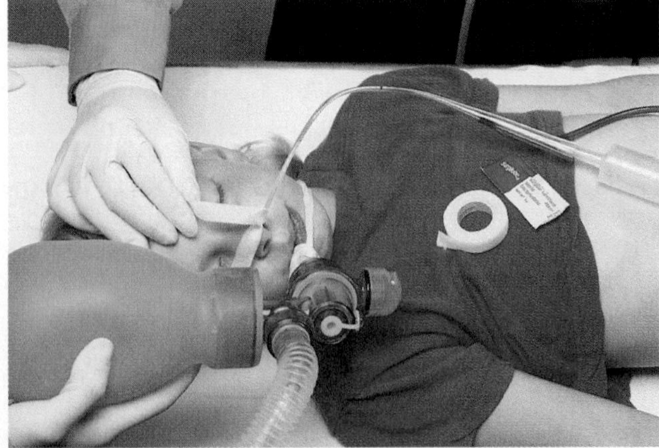

Step 6: Secure the tube in place.

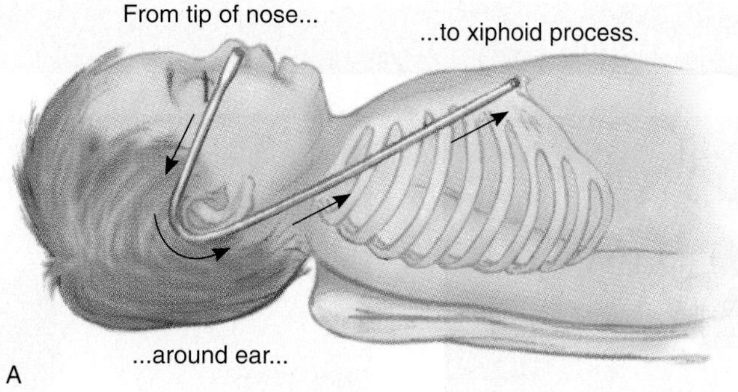

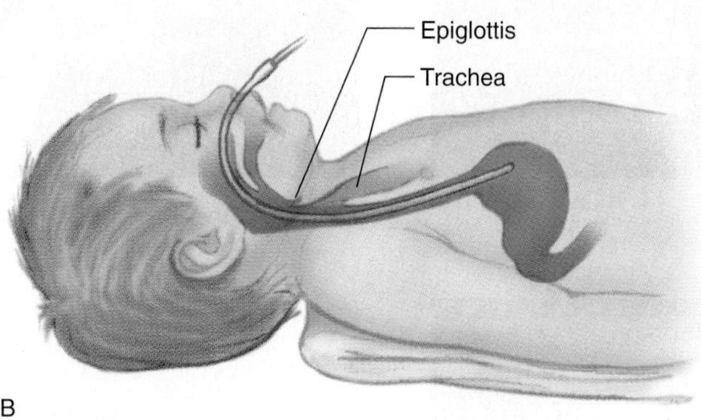

Figure 38-17 • (A) Measure the nasogastric tube from the tip of the nose around the ear, to below the xiphoid process. (B) The nasogastric tube in position, ready to attach to suction.

3. Measure the tube from the tip of the nose and around the ear to below the xiphoid process. (If the tube will be inserted by the orogastric technique, measure from the lips.) This length will determine the depth the tube will be inserted (Figure 38-17).
4. Lubricate the end of the tube.
5. Pass the tube gently downward along the nasal floor.
6. Confirm that the tube is in the stomach by:
   - Aspirating stomach contents
   - Auscultating a rush of air over the epigastrium while injecting 10–20 cc of air into the tube
7. Aspirate gastric contents.
8. Secure the tube in place with tape.

Orotracheal Suctioning

In conjunction with your training in advanced airway management, you may also be trained in the techniques of orotracheal suctioning. For this procedure, a flexible soft suction catheter is used to suction the trachea, usually down to the level of the carina in the artificially ventilated patient. This procedure is sometimes referred to as "deep suctioning" to set it apart from the basic airway management procedure, suctioning of the oropharynx, in which suctioning does not advance as far as the trachea.

The indications for orotracheal suctioning are as follows:

- *Obvious secretions in the airway.* This may be detected by either moist bubbling sounds during ventilation with the bag-valve mask or by visible secretions inside the endotracheal tube after the patient has been intubated.
- *Poor compliance with bag-valve-mask ventilation.* Resistance to ventilation may be caused by secretions below the level of the larynx in the trachea.

The technique for orotracheal suctioning is shown in Scan 38-3. (*Note:* Although orotracheal suctioning can be performed on an unintubated patient, the procedure is

SCAN 38-3 • Orotracheal Suctioning

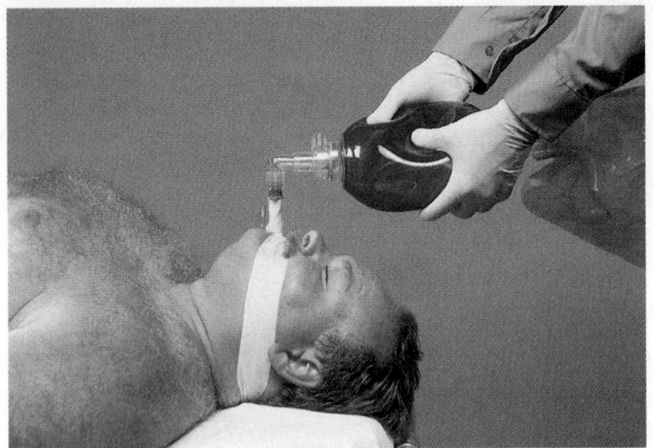

Step 1: Preoxygenate the patient.

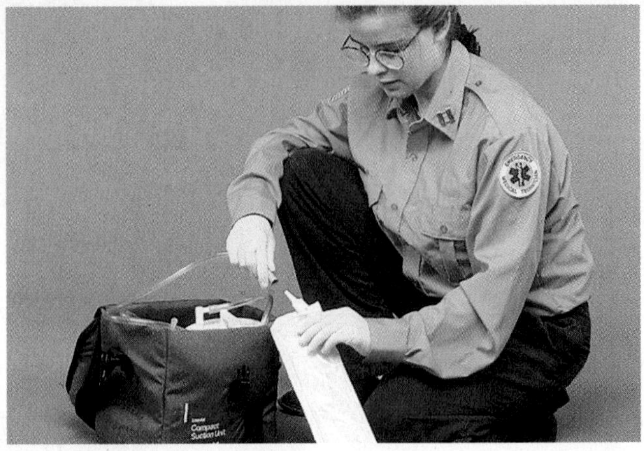

Step 2: Carefully check equipment.

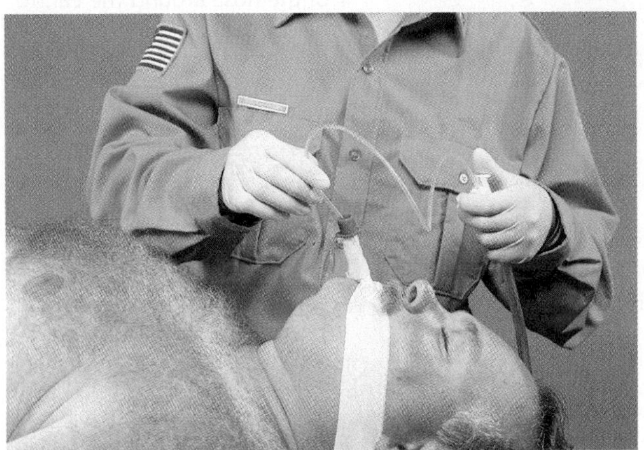

Step 3: Insert the catheter without applying suction.

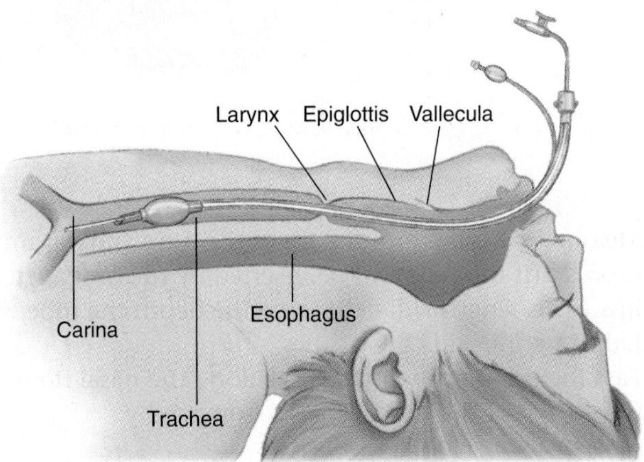

Step 4: Advance the catheter to the desired level, which may be as far as the carina.

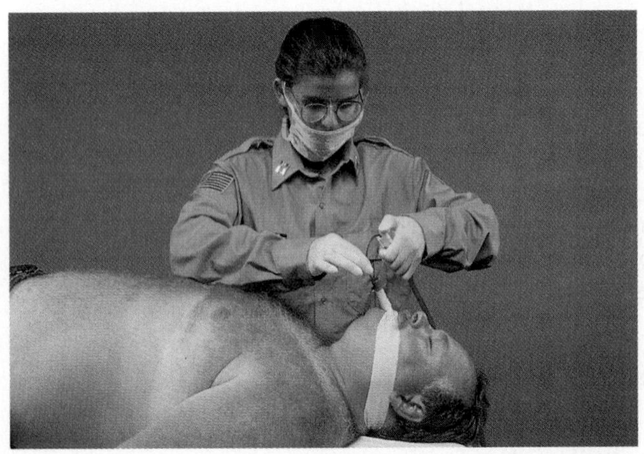

Step 5: Then apply suction and withdraw the catheter with a twisting motion.

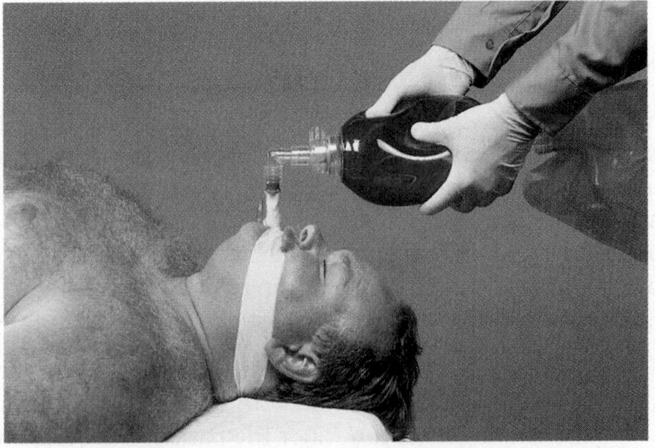

Step 6: Resume ventilation. Suctioning procedure should interrupt ventilation for no more than 15 seconds.

by far most commonly performed through an endotracheal tube.) Specific steps in the procedure include:

1. Preoxygenate the patient with high-concentration oxygen prior to attempting suction.
2. Check that all equipment is operating correctly.
3. Use sterile technique.
4. Observe Standard Precautions. Be especially mindful to have eye protection, as splattering during deep suctioning is common.
5. Approximate the desired length of the catheter to be inserted by measuring from the lips to the ear to the nipple line. This will approximate the level of the carina.
6. Advance the catheter to the desired location.
7. Apply suction and withdraw the catheter in a twisting motion.
8. Resume ventilations.
9. Attempts at deep suctioning should not exceed 15 seconds to prevent hypoxia.

Deep suctioning is not without potential complications. Most of the serious complications relate to the fact that the ventilated patient is deprived of oxygen during suctioning. Preoxygenation prior to suctioning, careful technique, and limiting suctioning to 15 seconds can help prevent the following complications of deep suctioning:

- Cardiac dysrhythmias
- Hypoxia
- Coughing
- Damage to the lining (mucosa) of the airway
- Spasm of the bronchioles (bronchospasm) if catheter extends past the carina
- Spasm of the vocal cords (laryngospasm) during orotracheal suctioning

Alternative Airways

In some EMS systems medical direction may elect to allow the EMT to use alternative airways such as the Combitube®, the laryngeal mask airway (LMA™), or the King LT® airway. Although these devices do not provide the definitive airway control of an endotracheal tube, when properly used they provide superior ventilation of the apneic patient as compared with a simple oral airway adjunct.

Esophageal Tracheal Combitube®

The esophageal tracheal combitube or, more commonly, "Combitube®" (Figure 38-18), is a double lumen airway where the two lumens are separated by a partition wall. In other words, it is just like two tubes joined together into one larger tube.

When the EMT inserts the Combitube®, it usually goes into the esophagus. The person managing the airway initially ventilates through tube #1, the blue tube, which has a closed end but has perforations between the two cuffs. These holes are very close to the larynx. Since there is a cuff above and a cuff below these perforations, when the tube is in the esophagus the oxygen forced into tube #1 goes into the larynx and trachea.

If ventilating through tube #1 does not result in ventilation, the tube is probably in the trachea. In this case, the EMT ventilates through tube #2, which has an open end that allows oxygen to go into the trachea. This is the same way a patient with an endotracheal tube is ventilated.

When the trachea is sealed, the cuff prevents stomach contents from being aspirated, but it does not prevent ventilations from entering the trachea via the tube that passes through the cuff.

The Combitube® is intended for use on unconscious patients over 5 feet (152 cm) tall. There is also a smaller device, the Combitube® SA (SA stands for small adult), for use on unconscious patients between 4 and 5½ feet (122 cm to 168 cm) tall.

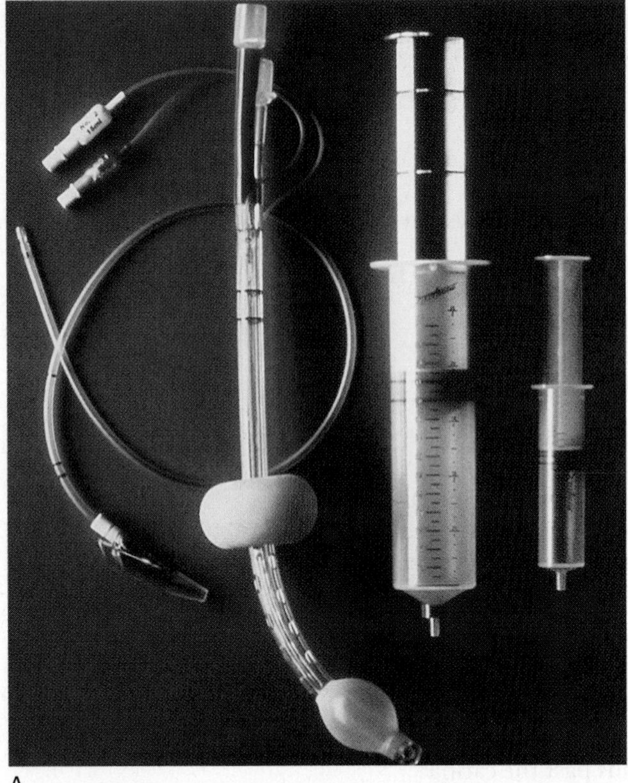

A

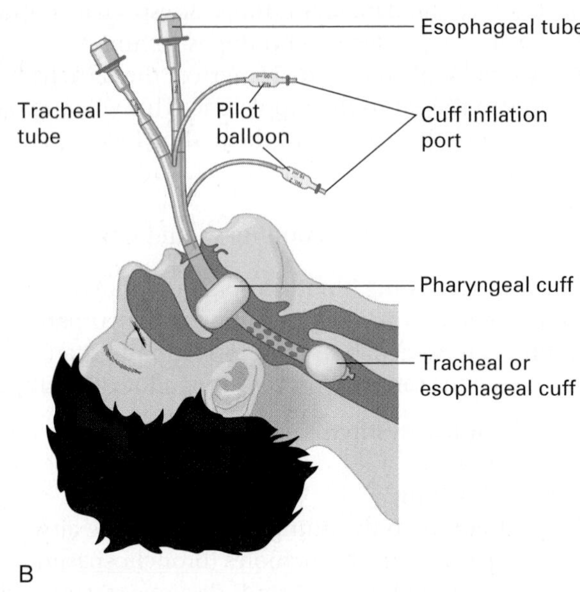

B

Figure 38-18 • (A) The esophageal tracheal Combitube® and (B) the Combitube® in place.

The Combitube® should not be used on:

- Conscious patient or one with a gag reflex
- Patient under 5 feet (152 cm) tall
- Patient under the age of 16
- Patient who has swallowed a corrosive substance
- Patient with a known esophageal disease

Follow these steps to insert the Combitube® after ensuring the patient is receiving adequate ventilations and checking the integrity of the cuffs (Scan 38-4):

NOTE *Whenever a Combitube® is inserted or extubated, gloves, mask, and protective eyewear should be worn to protect the EMT from the potential spraying of body fluids.*

1. After lubricating the cuffs generously with water-soluble lubricant, insert the device blindly, advancing it down the center of the mouth and throat while following the natural curve of the throat. Use a tongue-jaw lift to open the airway for insertion. Watch for the two black rings on the Combitube® that are used for measuring the depth of insertion. Stop advancing the tube when the teeth, or their bony cavities if the teeth are missing, are positioned between these rings. Do not use excessive force to advance the tube.
2. Use the large syringe on the inflation valve marked #1 to inflate the pharyngeal cuff with 100 cc of air (85 cc for the Combitube® SA). On inflation, the device will seat itself in the posterior pharynx behind the hard palate.
3. Use the smaller syringe on the inflation valve marked #2 to fill the smaller cuff with 15 cc of air (12 cc for the Combitube® SA).
4. Usually the tube will have been placed in the esophagus. On this assumption, ventilate through the esophageal connector. It is the external tube that is the longer of the two and is marked #1. You must listen for the presence of breath sounds in the lungs and the absence of sounds from the epigastrium in order to be sure that the tube is, in fact, placed in the esophagus.

SCAN 38-4 • Ventilating with the Combitube®

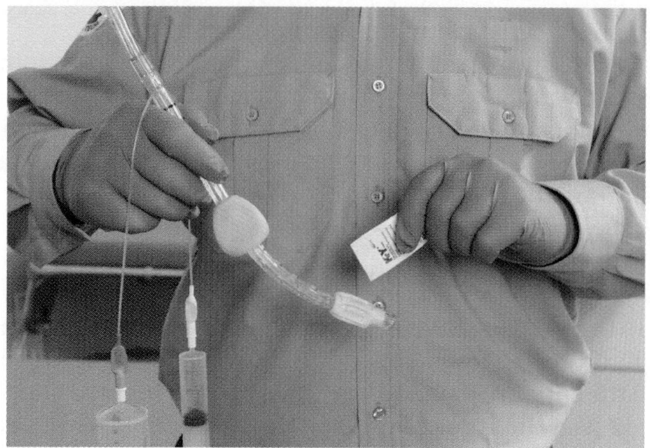

Step 1: Lubricate the tube generously with water-soluble lubricant.

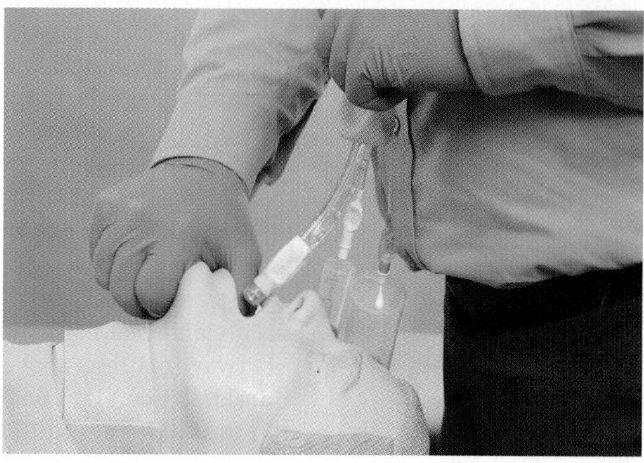

Step 2: Insert the tube, advancing it down the center and along the natural curve of the mouth and throat. Use a tongue-jaw lift to open the airway for insertion. Stop when the teeth are between the two black rings. Do not use excessive force. Inflate the cuffs.

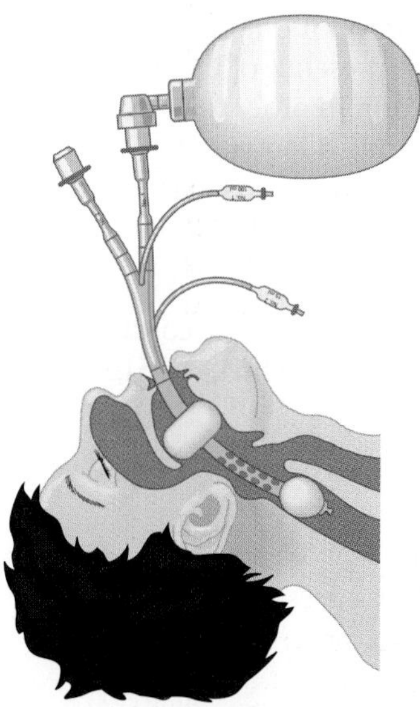

Step 3: Usually the tube will have been placed in the esophagus. On this assumption, ventilate through tube #1. Listen for the presence of breath sounds in the lungs and the absence of sounds from the epigastrium.

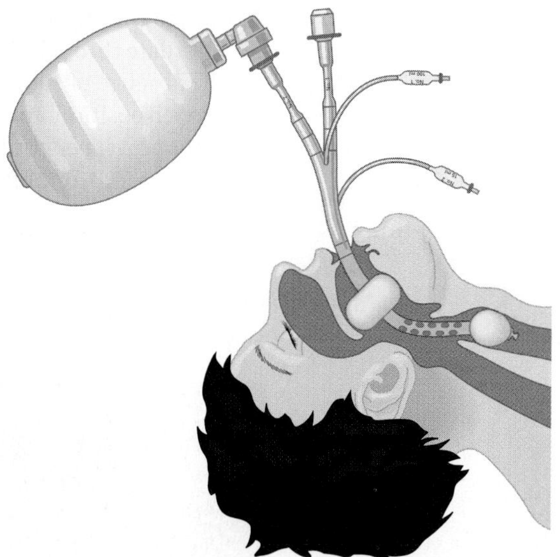

Step 4: If there is an absence of lung sounds and presence of sounds in the epigastrium, the tube has been placed in the trachea. In this case, ventilate through tube #2. Listen again to be sure of proper placement.

5. If there is an absence of lung sounds and presence of sounds in the epigastrium, the tube has been placed in the trachea. In this case, change the ventilator to the shorter tracheal connector, which is marked #2. Listen again to be sure of proper placement of the tube.

The biggest advantage of the Combitube® is that rapid intubation is possible independent of the position of the patient, which is helpful for trauma patients requiring limited cervical spine movement.

If the patient becomes conscious, you must remove the tube. Remember that extubation is likely to be followed by vomiting. Follow these guidelines for removing the Combitube®:

- Always have the suction unit with a rigid Yankauer tip standing by.
- Do not deflate the cuffs until the patient has resumed breathing or an endotracheal tube has been inserted and its cuff is inflated in the trachea.
- Provided there is no possibility of a spinal injury, or if the patient is secured to a spine board, turn the patient on his side, insert the syringe into the one-way valve, and withdraw air from the cuffs.
- Carefully remove the tube, staying alert for vomiting.

Laryngeal Mask Airway (LMA™)

The laryngeal mask airway (LMA™) (Figure 38-19) is a supraglottic airway, that is, an airway that rests above the glottis. At the lower end of it is a small oval mask with an inflatable cuff that fits around the entrance to the larynx. The LMA™ is inserted blindly into the throat until it seats itself in the correct position. There are a number of sizes available to make this easier.

Follow these steps to insert the LMA™ (Figure 38-20) after ensuring the patient is receiving adequate ventilations and checking the integrity of the cuff:

1. Lubricate the posterior side of the cuff with water-soluble lubricant. After putting the patient's head into the "sniffing position" (if no cervical spine injury is suspected), insert the tube, advancing it with the open side facing anteriorly. Stop advancing the tube when you feel resistance.
2. Inflate the cuff by injecting the proper amount of air.
3. Ventilate through the tube. Listen for the presence of breath sounds in the lungs and the absence of sounds from the epigastrium in order to be sure that the cuff is in the proper position and that you are ventilating adequately.
4. After you have confirmed ventilation, insert an oropharyngeal airway (to prevent the patient from biting through the tube if he wakes up) and secure the tube.

There are several different models of LMA™, so be sure to familiarize yourself with the one used by your EMS agency. All of them are latex-free, according to the manufacturer. Although you should be able to ventilate the patient who has an LMA™ in place relatively

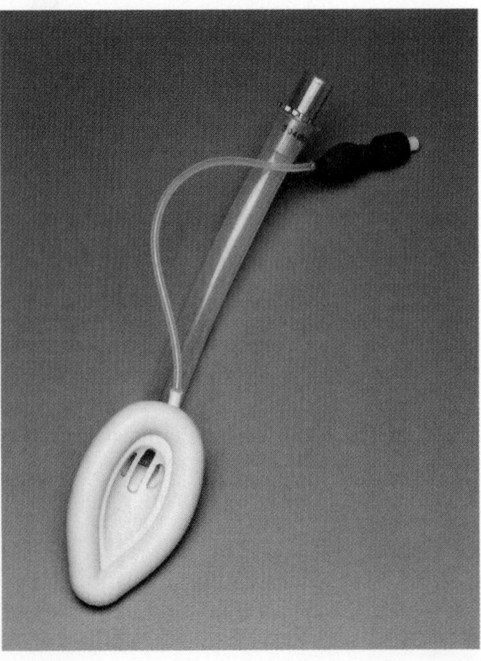

Figure 38-19 • The laryngeal mask airway (LMA™). *(© LMA North American, Inc.)*

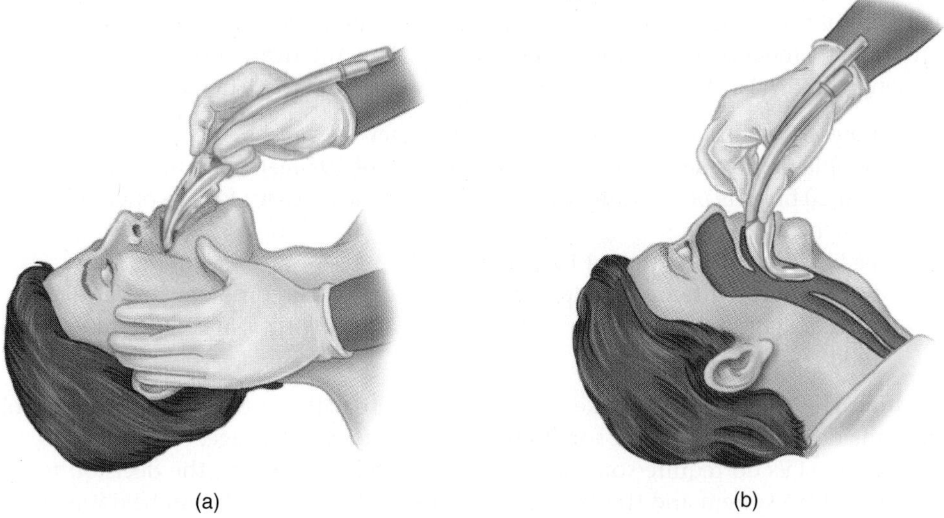

Figure 38-20 • (A) Inserting the laryngeal mask airway. (B) The laryngeal mask airway in place.

easily, keep in mind that the cuff on the LMA™ does not protect the patient's lungs from aspiration. Vomitus and other materials can still get past the cuff and into the lungs.

King LT® Airway

The King LT® airway is a supraglottic airway designed to be used either for positive pressure ventilation or for oxygenation of a spontaneously breathing patient. It has a large cuff that disperses pressure over a wide area, which stabilizes the airway at the base of the tongue and minimizes the risk of injury to the vocal cords and trachea. It is easy and quick to insert. It can be cleaned, sterilized, and reused.

A disposable latex-free model, the King LT-D™, which is available in pediatric and adult sizes, is recommended for prehospital use. An additional model, the King LTS-D™, allows for gastric access through a second channel, which permits passage of a gastric tube or provides a channel for regurgitation or a "vent" to relieve gastric pressure while the patient is being ventilated or oxygenated through the primary channel.

Automatic Transport Ventilators

Automatic transport ventilators (ATVs) have been used extensively in Europe for a number of years (Figure 38-21). The devices are rapidly gaining popularity in the United States as recent studies have demonstrated them to be superior in some respects to manual ventilation with the bag-valve mask.

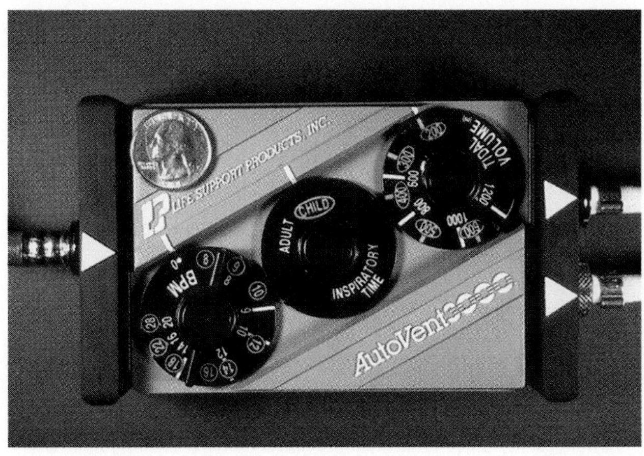

Figure 38-21 • The automatic transport ventilator (ATV). The coin is shown for scale. *(© Edward T. Dickinson, MD)*

ATVs are compact devices that have controls that set both the rate of ventilation and the tidal volume. Tidal volumes are determined by the patient's weight. A number of different ATV models are commercially available. The American Heart Association recommends that ATVs should meet certain minimum standards. They should:

- Have the ability to deliver 100 percent oxygen
- Be able to provide default rates of ventilation of 10 breaths per minute for adults and 20 breaths per minute for children, with the capacity for the operator to adjust the rate
- Be lightweight (less than 4 kg) and rugged
- Be equipped with an audible alarm to alert the user to problems in ventilation
- Have a standard 15/22-mm coupling to connect with a mask or endotracheal tube

Although some units are marketed for pediatric use with controls for lower tidal volumes, the device is not suitable for children less than 5 years of age.

Because ATVs do require some additional training for safe use, the decision to use ATVs in an EMS system and the establishment of ATV protocols should be done by the Medical Director.

CRITICAL DECISION MAKING: BACK TO BASICS

It is only fitting that the last decision-making feature brings the airway concept full circle. The best *advanced* airway care is based on a foundation of solid *basic* airway care. For each patient described here, decide what additional information you would need to determine adequacy of breathing and whether advanced airway care would be necessary.

1. Your 64-year-old male patient is experiencing chest pain. He is pale and sweaty. He is breathing at 22 breaths per minute. His pulse is 92 weak and regular; blood pressure is 102/58. He is alert but anxious.
2. Your 57-year-old patient is found on the floor with shallow, gasping respirations at 6/minute. He complained of a headache before falling to the floor.
3. You find an adolescent patient at the edge of a swimming pool with CPR being done by bystanders. The teenage male had been drinking and hadn't been seen for about 20 minutes when he was found floating in the pool. Compressions bring up copious amounts of vomit.

CHAPTER REVIEW

SUMMARY

Airway control is the highest priority in managing any critically ill or injured patient, because without an adequate airway the patient will die no matter what other care you provide. Control of a patient's airway is recognized as so crucial a skill that advanced airway skills are now included as an elective in the EMT curriculum.

Advanced airway management centers on the skill of orotracheal intubation, the placement of an endotracheal tube through the mouth and into the patient's trachea. This permits complete control of the airway, minimizes the risk of aspiration, allows for better oxygen delivery, and allows for deep suctioning of the trachea.

Endotracheal intubation of infants and children is similar to the procedure for adults with these exceptions: All structures in the mouth and nose are smaller; the tongue is proportionately larger; the trachea is softer, more flexible, and narrower; the airway is especially narrow at the cricoid cartilage; and the chest wall is softer.

These differences result in the airways of infants and children being more easily obstructed, in the optional use of uncuffed endotracheal tubes under the age of 8 because the narrow cricoid can act as a cuff, and in distinctive breathing patterns. Infants and children are more susceptible to damage from incorrect placement of a tube and to interruptions of the supply of oxygen and must be monitored especially carefully during intubation and suctioning procedures.

Nasogastric intubation is performed on infants and children to relieve the pressure of swallowed air in the stomach.

Endotracheal suctioning is performed by inserting a suction catheter—usually through an endotracheal tube—to the level of the carina.

KEY TERMS

alveoli (al-VE-o-li) the microscopic sacs of the lungs where gas exchange with the bloodstream takes place.

bronchioles (BRONG-kee-olz) smaller branches of the bronchi.

capnometry (kap-NOM-uh-tree) the measurement of exhaled carbon dioxide. A graphic recording or display of capnometric measurement is called *capnography*.

carina (kah-RI-nah) the fork at the lower end of the trachea where the two mainstem bronchi branch.

cricoid (KRIK-oid) **cartilage** the ring-shaped structure that circles the trachea at the lower edge of the larynx.

cricoid pressure pressure applied to the cricoid cartilage to suppress vomiting and bring the vocal cords into view.

endotracheal (EN-do-TRAY-ke-ul) **tube** a tube designed to be inserted into the trachea. Oxygen, medication, or a suction catheter can be directed into the trachea through an endotracheal tube.

epiglottis (EP-i-GLOT-is) a leaf-shaped structure that prevents food and foreign matter from entering the trachea.

esophageal detector device (EDD) a device that uses a bulb or syringe to attempt to withdraw air from an endotracheal tube to determine correct placement in the trachea (from which air can easily be withdrawn) or incorrect placement in the esophagus (in which the soft esophagus will collapse and prevent air from being withdrawn).

esophagus (eh-SOF-uh-gus) the tube that leads from the pharynx to the stomach.

glottic opening the opening to the trachea.

hypopharynx (HI-po-FAIR-inks) the area directly above the openings of both the trachea and the esophagus.

hypoxia (hi-POK-se-uh) inadequate oxygenation, or oxygen starvation.

intubation (IN-tu-BAY-shun) insertion of a tube.

laryngoscope (lair-ING-uh-skope) an illuminating instrument that is inserted into the pharynx to permit visualization of the pharynx and larynx.

larynx (LAIR-inks) the voice box.

mainstem bronchi (BRONG-ki) the two large sets of branches that come off the trachea and enter the lungs. There are right and left mainstem bronchi. The singular is bronchus.

nasogastric (NAY-zo-GAS-trik) **tube (NG tube)** a tube designed to be passed through the nose, nasopharynx, and esophagus. It is used to relieve distention of the stomach in an infant or child patient.

nasopharynx (NAY-zo-FAIR-inks) the area directly posterior to the nose.

oropharynx (OR-o-FAIR-inks) the area directly posterior to the mouth.

orotracheal (OR-o-TRAY-ke-ul) **intubation** placement of an endotracheal tube through the mouth and into the trachea.

stylet a long, thin, flexible metal probe.

trachea (TRAY-ke-uh) the "windpipe"; the structure that connects the pharynx to the lungs.

vallecula (val-EK-yuh-luh) a groove-like structure anterior to the epiglottis.

vocal cords two thin folds of tissue within the larynx that vibrate as air passes between them, producing sounds.

REVIEW QUESTIONS

1. Explain why it is important for EMTs to be able to perform orotracheal intubation. (pp. 1034–1037)
2. List and explain the errors in intubation that can lead to a patient's death. (pp. 1038–1039)
3. Explain the procedures for ensuring correct placement of an endotracheal tube. (pp. 1048–1051, 1054)
4. Explain reasons and describe the procedure for insertion of a nasogastric tube in an infant or child. (pp. 1055–1057)
5. Explain how orotracheal suctioning differs from oropharyngeal suctioning. Explain reasons why orotracheal suctioning may be advisable. (pp. 1057–1059)

CRITICAL THINKING

- You have successfully intubated a nonbreathing patient and transferred him to the ambulance. During your ongoing assessment you auscultate the chest and find that there are breath sounds on the right, but not the left. What does this indicate? What should you do in this situation?

Thinking and Linking

Think back to Chapter 6, "Airway Management," as well as to Basic Cardiac Life Support training that was a prerequisite to your EMT training (reviewed in Appendix C, "The Future of EMS Education"). Link information on basic airway management with information from this chapter, "Advanced Airway Management," as you consider the following situation:

- You are looking into your patient's airway with a laryngoscope when your patient starts to regurgitate. What basic airway management steps should you have taken before undertaking laryngoscopy on this patient, and what basic airway management equipment should you have ready to deal with the current situation?

MEDIA RESOURCES

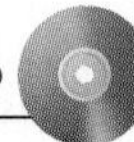

See the Student CD at the back of this book for quizzes, a case study activity, animations, videos, and other features related to this chapter. In particular, take a look at the Virtual Airway Tour and the animations and videos on the respiratory system and endotracheal intubation. Also, visit the Companion Website for *Emergency Care* at **www.prenhall.com/limmer**, where you will find additional reinforcement and links to other resources.

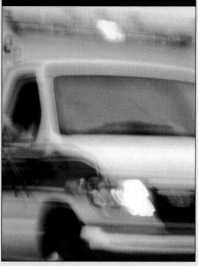

You and your partner are asked to stand by for your community's annual Memorial Day parade. As the first floats and bands begin passing the reviewing stand, you hear a lady scream for help. Turning to your left, you see three people standing over a man lying on the ground. You grab your medical gear and hurry to the patient. Someone identifying himself as a doctor states the man does not have a pulse.

Street Scene Questions

1. What priority would you assign this patient?
2. What definitive treatment do pulseless patients require?

While taking Standard Precautions, your general impression is of an unconscious elderly male. Jan, your partner, performs an initial assessment, verifies pulselessness, and calls for the AED. You proceed to the head of the patient to manage his airway, while Jan opens the AED and applies the pads. The patient has a patent airway, with no signs of foreign objects or fluids. You grab an oropharyngeal airway, size it, and insert it into the patient's oropharynx. Simultaneously, the doctor hands you the bag-valve mask, which he has already hooked up to your oxygen bottle. You begin ventilating the patient while Jan finishes applying the AED.

Jan clears the patient and presses "analyze." The AED advises "shock." After one shock, reassessment verifies the patient has a pulse. However, he is not breathing. You also now observe secretions in the patient's oropharynx. Jan hands you the portable suction with the rigid catheter attached. Slipping your protective eyewear over your eyes, you insert the catheter into the patient's oropharynx. After clearing the patient's airway, the patient is still in respiratory arrest.

Street Scene Questions

3. What alternatives for managing the airway might you consider?
4. What assessment procedures should be performed at this time?

Since your EMS system allows you to use advanced airway maneuvers, the decision is made to orally intubate the patient. While you prepare your equipment, it is determined the patient has a pulse of 80 and regular with a blood pressure of 80/46. The patient is loaded into the ambulance on a backboard as he is being ventilated.

Grabbing a curved laryngoscope blade and an 8.0 endotracheal tube, you ensure that the lighted blade is functioning. Jan places the patient's head into a sniffing position, and you insert the blade into the vallecula and lift to visualize the glottic opening. While you do this, Jan presses downward on the cricoid cartilage, which helps you better visualize the opening. You insert the endotracheal tube with a stylet and observe it pass through the vocal cords. Removing the laryngoscope and stylet, you inflate the cuff and attach the bag-valve mask. Jan listens to the lungs and epigastrium, and tells you that the tube is placed correctly. You double-check with an esophageal intubation detector device.

Street Scene Question

5. How often should this patient be reassessed?

Securing the tube, you quickly reassess vitals and then recheck the tube in case it has become misplaced. You inform medical direction of your actions, and tell them you will be at their facility in 3 minutes. En route, you continually assess lung sounds. You observe the patient's eyes open, and he responds to your commands to keep his hands away from the tube. At the hospital, you quickly transfer the patient to a bed in the emergency department.

Later that day, you learn that the patient is doing well. He had suffered a myocardial infarction.

Street Scenes Sample Documentation

PATIENT NAME: Rafael Gomez **PATIENT AGE:** 67

CHIEF COMPLAINT

Cardiac arrest

PAST MEDICAL HISTORY

- [ ] None
- [ ] Allergy to
- [ ] Hypertension
- [ ] Stroke
- [ ] Seizures
- [ ] Diabetes
- [ ] COPD
- [ ] Cardiac
- [ ] Other (List)
- [ ] Asthma

Unknown

Current Medications (List)

Unknown

VITAL SIGNS

TIME	RESP	PULSE	B.P.	MENTAL STATUS	R PUPILS L	SKIN
1005	Rate: 0; [ ] Regular [ ] Shallow [ ] Labored	Rate: 0; [ ] Regular [ ] Irregular	0/0	[ ] Alert [ ] Voice [ ] Pain [x] Unresp.	Normal: R [x] L [x]; Dilated: R [ ] L [ ]; Constricted: R [ ] L [ ]; Sluggish: R [ ] L [ ]; No-Reaction: R [ ] L [ ]	[ ] Unremarkable [ ] Cool [ ] Pale [ ] Warm [ ] Cyanotic [ ] Moist [ ] Flushed [ ] Dry [ ] Jaundiced
1010	Rate: 0; [ ] Regular [ ] Shallow [ ] Labored	Rate: 80; [x] Regular [ ] Irregular	80/46	[ ] Alert [ ] Voice [ ] Pain [x] Unresp.	Normal: R [x] L [x]; Dilated: R [ ] L [ ]; Constricted: R [ ] L [ ]; Sluggish: R [ ] L [ ]; No-Reaction: R [ ] L [ ]	[ ] Unremarkable [ ] Cool [ ] Pale [ ] Warm [ ] Cyanotic [ ] Moist [ ] Flushed [ ] Dry [ ] Jaundiced
	Rate: ; [ ] Regular [ ] Shallow [ ] Labored	Rate: ; [ ] Regular [ ] Irregular	/	[ ] Alert [ ] Voice [ ] Pain [ ] Unresp.	Normal: R [ ] L [ ]; Dilated: R [ ] L [ ]; Constricted: R [ ] L [ ]; Sluggish: R [ ] L [ ]; No-Reaction: R [ ] L [ ]	[ ] Unremarkable [ ] Cool [ ] Pale [ ] Warm [ ] Cyanotic [ ] Moist [ ] Flushed [ ] Dry [ ] Jaundiced

NARRATIVE Patient was a bystander-witnessed cardiac arrest. Physician on scene stated patient had no pulse; verified by EMS crew. CPR ongoing while AED attached and detected shockable rhythm (see AED printout attached). One shock delivered with patient's pulse returning. No respirations; airway secretions noted. Patient suctioned with rigid catheter and decision to intubate with #8.0 ET tube x 1 attempt = successful. Prior to intubation, patient oxygenated with BVM and OPA. Lung sounds equal bilaterally and negative findings over epigastric area. Patient reassessed throughout with no changes noted other than patient seemed to respond to verbal stimuli as we neared the hospital. On-line medical direction established.

APPENDIX A

ALS ASSIST SKILLS

Local protocol may require you to assist more highly trained EMS personnel in the administration of advanced life support (ALS) procedures. There are several new skills you can learn to enhance your capability as a "team player" on such calls. Your instructor will discuss the skills that are authorized by your Medical Director. However, the most common are:

- Assisting in the endotracheal intubation of a patient
- Applying ECG electrodes
- Assisting in intravenous (IV) fluid therapy
- Assisting with continuous positive airway pressure (CPAP) and bi-level positive airway pressure (BiPAP)

NOTE

The information in this Appendix is intended as a summary of ALS assist skills. More detailed information and additional in-service training may be required. Consult with your instructor on local protocols.

ASSISTING WITH ENDOTRACHEAL INTUBATION

Among the highest priorities of patient care is to assure a patent airway and to prevent aspiration. The "gold standard" for airway care is the endotracheal tube. This is because the endotracheal tube is directly inserted into the trachea, forming an open pathway for air, oxygen, or medications to be blown into the lungs. In addition, adult sizes have an inflatable cuff that seals off the trachea to prevent aspiration. (In an infant or young child, the narrow trachea creates a seal.) Other airway devices, such as the Combitube®, are used when endotracheal intubation is unsuccessful and by those who have been trained in the device but not in endotracheal intubation.

Patients who typically need to have an endotracheal tube inserted are those in pulmonary or cardiopulmonary arrest, trauma patients in need of airway control or supplemental oxygen, and those in respiratory distress or failure due to overdose, fluid in the lungs, asthma, asphyxia, or allergic reaction.

In some areas, EMTs will be trained to perform endotracheal intubation of a patient. (The skill is taught as an elective in Chapter 38, "Advanced Airway Management.") In other areas, only EMT-Intermediates or EMT-Paramedics will perform endotracheal intubation, but EMTs may be asked to assist with the procedure. The skills of assisting with endotracheal intubation are presented in the following sections.

Preparing the Patient for Intubation

Before the paramedic inserts the endotracheal tube, you may be asked to give the patient extra oxygen. This can easily be accomplished by ventilating with a bag-valve-mask device that is connected to oxygen and includes a reservoir. Then the paramedic will position the patient's head to align the mouth, pharynx, and trachea. The paramedic will remove the oral airway and pass the endotracheal tube through the mouth (sometimes through the nose) into the throat past the vocal cords and into the trachea. This procedure usually requires a laryngoscope to move the tongue and other obstructions out of the way.

In order to maneuver the tube past the vocal cords correctly, the paramedic will need to see them. You may be asked to gently press on the throat to push the vocal cords into the paramedic's view. You will do this by pressing your thumb and index finger just to either side of the throat over the cricoid cartilage, the ring-shaped cartilage just below the thyroid cartilage, or Adam's apple. This procedure is known as cricoid pressure (Figure A-1).

Once the tube is properly placed, the cuff is inflated with air from a 10-cc syringe. While holding the tube, the paramedic assures proper tube placement by using at least two methods, including auscultation of both lungs and the epigastrium and using an esophageal intubation detector device or end-tidal CO_2 detector (Figure A-2). If the tube has been correctly placed, there will be sounds of air entering the lungs but no sounds of air in the epigastrium. Air sounds in the epigastrium indicate that the tube has been incorrectly placed in the esophagus instead of the trachea so that air is entering the stomach instead of the lungs. The tube position must be corrected immediately by removing the tube, reoxygenating the patient, and repeating the process of intubation.

NOTE

Be especially careful not to disturb the endotracheal tube. Movement of the patient to a backboard, down stairs, and into the ambulance can easily cause displacement of the tube. If the tube comes out of the trachea, the patient receives no oxygen and will certainly die.

The correctly positioned tube is anchored in place with tape or a commercially made tube restraint. The entire procedure—including the last ventilation, passing the tube, and the next ventilation—should take less than 30 seconds.

You might be asked to assist the advanced providers by monitoring the lung and epigastric sounds throughout the call. Many systems now use continuous end-tidal carbon dioxide detection when an endotracheal tube is in place as one method of monitoring tube placement.

If the tube is pushed in too far, it will most likely enter the right mainstem bronchus, preventing oxygen from entering the patient's left lung. (You can identify this by noting breath sounds on the right side with no sounds over the left or the epigastrium.)

If the tube is pulled out, it can easily slip into the esophagus and send all the ventilations directly to the stomach, denying the patient oxygen (indicated by breath sounds over the epigastrium). Tube displacement is a fatal complication if it goes unnoticed.

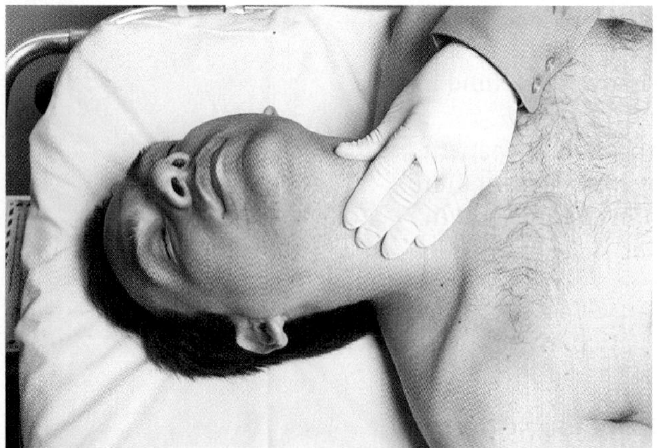

Figure A-1 • In cricoid pressure, press your thumb and index finger on either side of the medial throat over the cricoid cartilage.

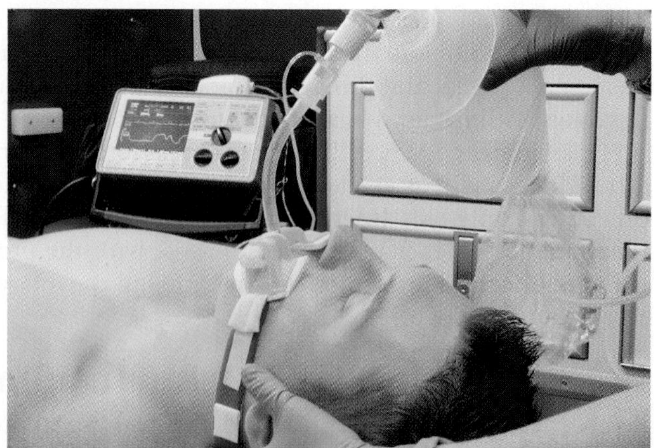

Figure A-2 • An end-tidal CO_2 detector can ensure proper placement of the endotracheal tube. *(© Ray Kemp/911 Imaging)*

NOTE RE CAPNOMETRY

As noted in Chapter 38, "Advanced Airway Management," more and more EMS systems are using end-tidal CO_2 measurement or capnometry to assist in confirming endotracheal tube placement. While some sort of capnometry has been in use to verify ET tube position for some time, various forms of capnometry are also being used on patients who are not intubated to measure respiratory function and to add valuable information when diagnosing some respiratory and metabolic conditions.

By using a special nasal cannula (Figure A-3), sometimes called a sidestream or sampling cannula, a small sample of the patient's exhaled carbon dioxide is obtained for analysis. This analysis is presented in a numeric reading as well as a waveform, which provides important diagnostic information.

To assist in the use of capnometry with a sidestream device, you will connect the cannula to an oxygen cylinder as described in Chapter 6, "Airway Management." You will also connect another (generally the smaller) tube to the capnometer, which is usually part of the cardiac monitor. You should explain to your patient about the prongs that will rest in the nose as well as the single prong that will rest over the upper lip.

Ventilating the Tubed Patient

When you are asked to ventilate a tubed patient, keep in mind that even very little movement can displace the tube. Look at the gradations on the side of the tube. In the typical adult male, for example, the 22-cm mark will be at the teeth when the tube is properly placed. If the tube moves, report this to the paramedic immediately.

Hold the tube against the patient's teeth with two fingers of one hand (Figure A-4). Use the other hand to work the bag-valve-mask unit. A patient with an endotracheal tube offers less resistance to ventilations, so you may not need two hands to work the bag. If you are ventilating a breathing patient, be sure to provide ventilations that are

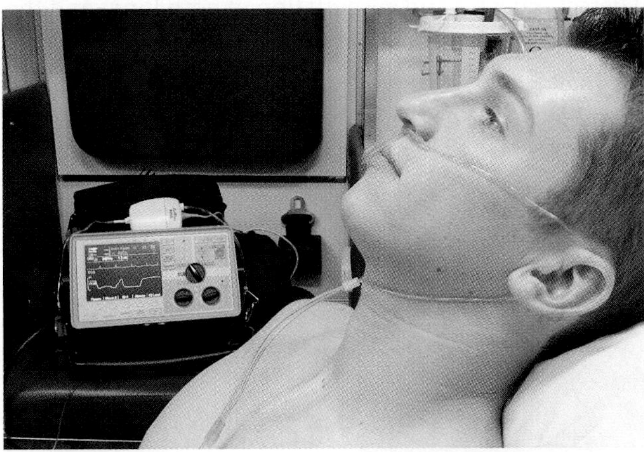

Figure A-3 • A special nasal cannula, sometimes called a sidestream or sampling cannula, obtains a small sample of exhaled CO_2 for analysis. *(© Ray Kemp/911 Imaging)*

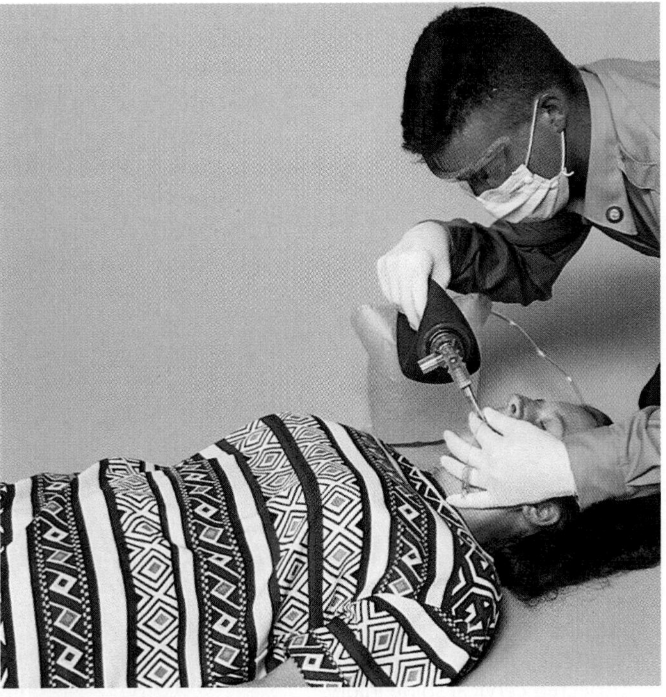

Figure A-4 • Make sure the endotracheal tube does not move. Hold it with two fingers against the patient's teeth.

timed with the respiratory effort as much as possible so the patient can take full breaths. It is also possible to help the patient increase respiratory rate, if needed, by interposing extra ventilations. Remember these cautions:

- Pay close attention to what the ventilations feel like. Report any change in resistance. Increased resistance when ventilating with the bag-valve mask is one of the first signs of air escaping through a hole in the lungs and filling the space around the lungs, which is an extremely serious problem. A change in resistance can also indicate that the tube has slipped into the esophagus.
- With each defibrillation attempt, carefully remove the bag from the tube. If you do not, the weight of the unsupported bag may accidentally displace the tube.
- Watch for any change in the patient's mental status. A patient who becomes more alert may need to be restrained from pulling out the tube. In addition, an oral airway generally is used as a bite block (a device that prevents the patient from biting the endotracheal tube). If the patient's gag reflex returns along with increased consciousness, you may need to pull the bite block out a bit.

Finally, during a cardiac arrest in the absence of an IV line for administering medications, you may be asked to stop ventilating and remove the BVM. The paramedic may then inject a medication such as epinephrine down the tube. To increase the rate at which medication enters the bloodstream through the respiratory system, you then may be asked to ventilate the patient for a few minutes (give ventilations at a faster-than-normal rate).

Assisting with a Trauma Intubation

Occasionally you will be asked to assist in the endotracheal intubation of a patient with a suspected cervical spine injury. Since using the "sniffing position," which involves elevating the neck, risks worsening cervical spine injury, some modifications are necessary. Your role will change as well. You may be required to provide manual in-line stabilization during the whole procedure.

To accomplish this, the paramedic will hold manual stabilization while you apply a cervical collar. In some EMS systems, the patient may be intubated without a cervical collar in place but with attention to manual stabilization during and after intubation. Since the paramedic must stay at the patient's head, it will be necessary for you to stabilize the head and neck from the patient's side (Figure A-5). Once you are in position, the paramedic will lean back and use the laryngoscope, which will bring the vocal cords into view. The patient can then be tubed.

After intubation, you will hold the tube against the teeth until placement is confirmed with both an esophageal detector device and auscultation of both lungs and the epigastrium. Then the tube is anchored. At that time you can change your position to

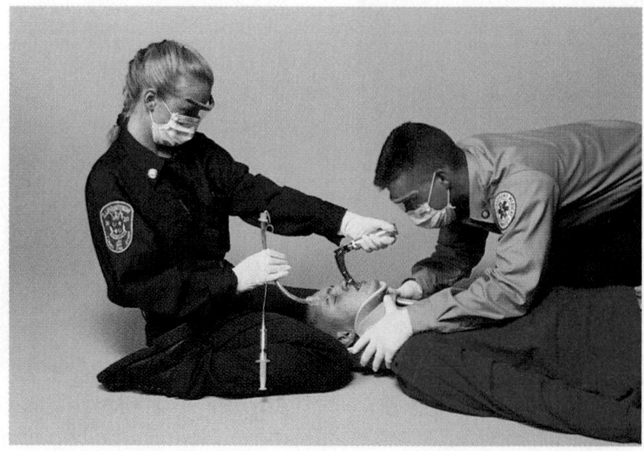

Figure A-5 • To assist in the intubation of a patient with suspected cervical spine injury, maintain manual stabilization throughout the procedure.

a more comfortable one. However, until the patient is immobilized on a long backboard, it will be necessary to assign another EMS worker to maintain manual stabilization while you ventilate the patient. Never assume that a collar provides adequate immobilization by itself. Manual stabilization must be used in addition to a collar until the head is taped in place on the backboard.

APPLYING ECG ELECTRODES

An electrocardiogram (ECG) provides data on the heart's electrical activity. In the field, it is used to alert EMS personnel to life-threatening rhythm disturbances. Interpretation of an ECG has traditionally been a paramedic skill. However, to save time on calls you may be asked to assist. Make sure that you review the ECG equipment (Figure A-6). You should know how to turn on the monitor, how to record an ECG strip, how to change the battery, and how to change the roll of ECG paper. (These are the things that most often need to be done while the paramedic is involved with the patient.)

You also may be asked to carry out four steps in the process of applying the electrodes:

1. Turn on the ECG monitor.
2. Plug in the monitoring cables or "leads."
3. Attach the monitoring cables to the electrodes.
4. Apply the electrodes to the patient's body.

Become familiar with the electrodes used by the paramedics with whom you work. There are two types: monitoring electrodes (with smaller pads) and combination monitoring/defibrillator electrodes (with larger pads). The one most commonly used by paramedics is the monitoring electrode.

If you are asked to apply monitoring electrodes to the patient's body, you will need three or four (depending on the device)—each one giving a different "view" of the heart's electrical activity. First prepare the patient's skin. The best connection is on dry, bare skin, so it may be necessary to shave excessive hair and dry the area. Use a wash cloth to remove oil from the skin and consider using an antiperspirant on patients with very sweaty skin. Become familiar with the monitoring configuration (where to place the electrodes) used by ALS personnel in your system. The most common setup is placing the negative (white) electrode under the center of the right clavicle, the positive (red) electrode on the left lower chest, and the ground (black or green) electrode under the center of the left clavicle or the right lower chest (Figure A-7A).

The abbreviations on the cables that attach to the electrodes have the initials LA, RA, LL, and RL for left arm, right arm, left leg, and right leg. Some ALS providers prefer

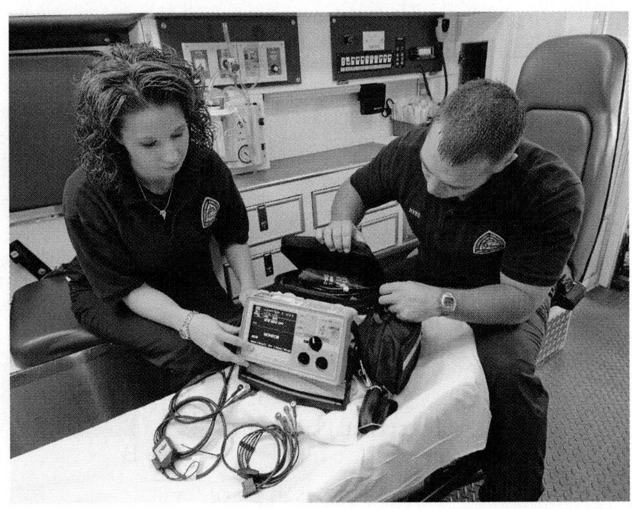

Figure A-6 • Check the ECG monitor/defibrillator. *(© Ray Kemp/911 Imaging)*

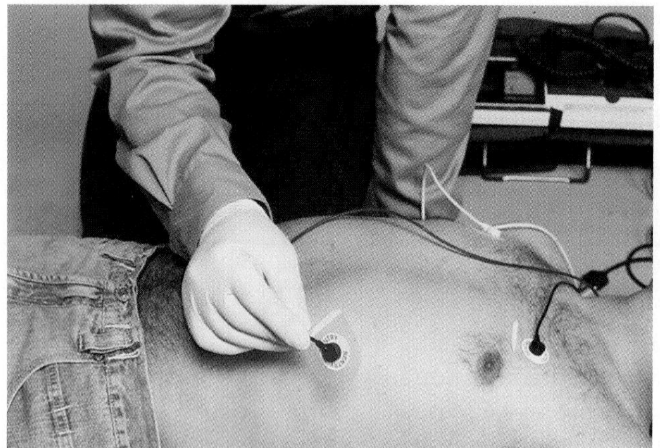

Figure A-7A • The most common positioning of electrodes for an ECG is shown here. Become familiar with the monitoring configuration used by ALS personnel in your system.

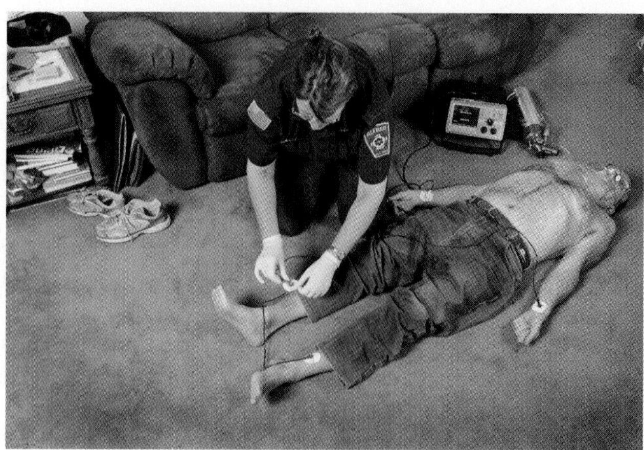

Figure A-7B • Some ALS providers prefer placing electrodes on the extremities.

the electrodes to be placed on the actual extremities (Figure A-7B) rather than on the corresponding portion of the torso as shown in Figure A-7A. Procedures for this vary, so follow the directions from the ALS provider you are assisting or the protocols of your EMS system.

Some ALS systems have moved toward the routine use of a 12-lead ECG in the field. These machines usually provide a computerized interpretation of the patient's cardiogram that can easily be transmitted to the emergency department via cellular phone. A 12-lead ECG is used to assist in the diagnosis of an acute myocardial infarction (AMI). In the case of an AMI, "time is muscle." As the clock ticks, more and more heart muscle becomes dysfunctional and finally dies in the absence of oxygenated blood. With field diagnosis of AMI made possible by the 12-lead ECG, the time from AMI to hospital treatment with drugs or procedures to break up the clots causing the AMI can be reduced.

If 12-lead ECG monitors are used in your system, ask the paramedics to review the lead placement with you as this is slightly more complex than the simple three electrodes you may be used to. Figure A-8 demonstrates lead placement for the 12-lead ECG, and shows the 12-lead electrodes in place.

Lead V_1 The electrode is at the fourth intercostal space just to the right of the sternum.
Lead V_2 The electrode is at the fourth intercostal space just to the left of the sternum.
Lead V_3 The electrode is at the line midway between leads V_2 and V_4.
Lead V_4 The electrode is at the midclavicular line in the fifth interspace.
Lead V_5 The electrode is at the anterior axillary line at the same level as lead V_4.
Lead V_6 The electrode is at the midaxillary line at the same level as lead V_4.

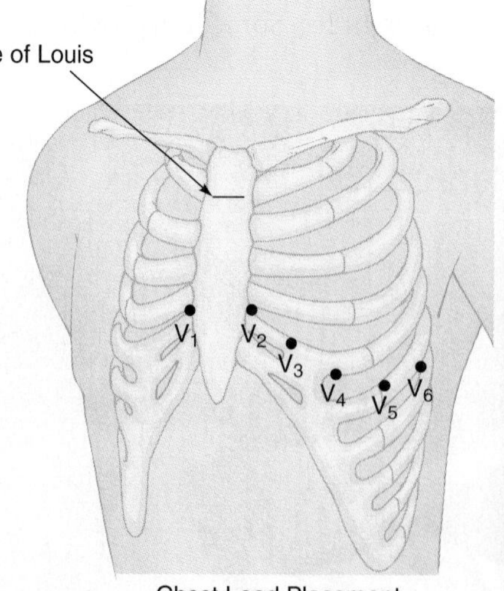

A

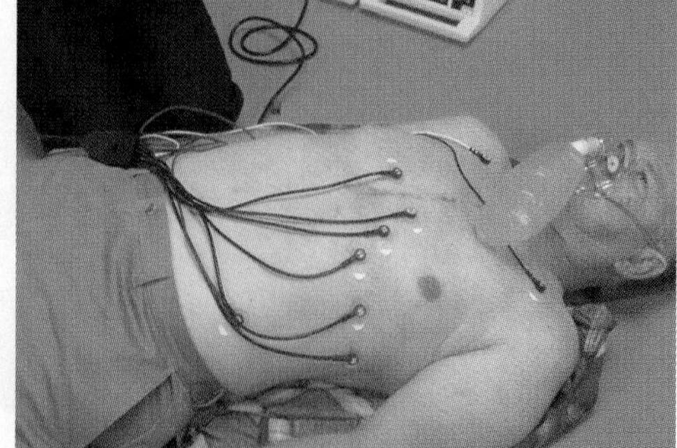

B

Figure A-8 • (A) 12-lead ECG lead placement (B) 12-lead electrodes in place.

ASSISTING IN IV THERAPY

Setting Up an IV Fluid Administration Set

IV therapy is an advanced life support procedure. An intravenous (IV) line is inserted into a vein so that blood, fluids, or medications can be administered directly into the patient's circulation. A blood transfusion is almost always given at the hospital. An infusion of other fluids or medications can usually be done in the field.

The bag of fluid that feeds the IV is usually a clear plastic bag that collapses as it empties. The administration set is the clear plastic tubing that connects the fluid bag to the needle, or catheter. There are three important parts to this tubing:

- The *drip chamber* is near the fluid bag. There are two basic types: the mini drip and the macro drip. The mini drip is used when minimal flow of fluid is needed (with children, for example). Sixty small drops from the tiny metal barrel in the drip chamber equal 1 cubic centimeter (cc) or 1 milliliter (mL). The macro drip is used when a higher flow of fluid is needed (for a multitrauma patient in shock, for example). There is no little barrel in the drip chamber of the macro drip, and just 10 to 15 large drops equal 1 cc or 1 mL.
- The *flow regulator* is located below the drip chamber. It is a device that can be pushed up or down to start, stop, or control the rate of flow (Figure A-9).
- The *drug or needle port* is below the flow regulator. The paramedic can inject medication into this opening.

An extension set includes an extra length of tubing, which can make it easier to carry or disrobe the patient without accidentally pulling out the IV. Extension sets are

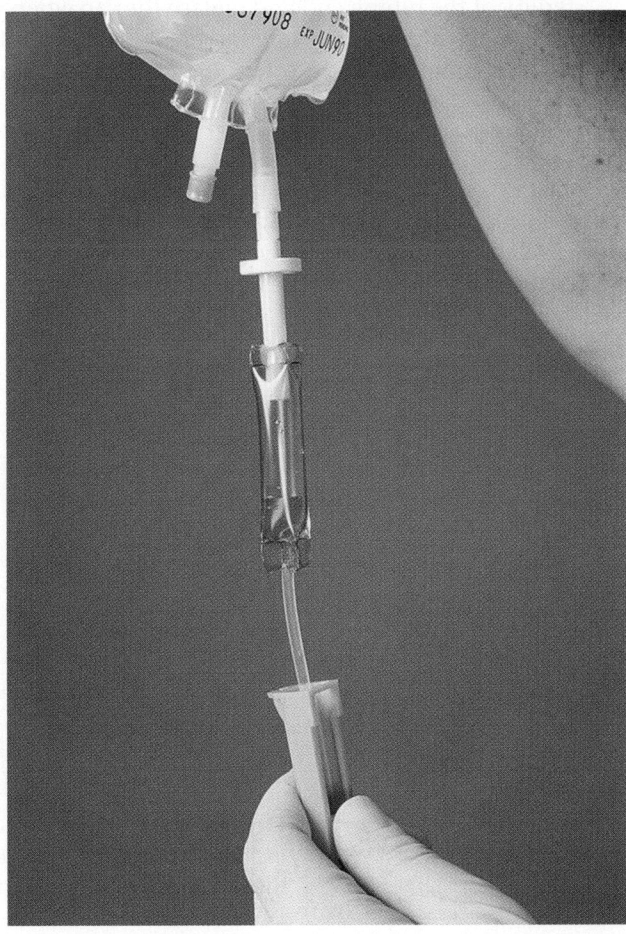

Figure A-9 • Located below the drip chamber, the flow regulator is a stopcock that can be pushed up or down to start, stop, or control the rate of flow.

sometimes not used with the macro drip set because lengthening tubing reduces the flow rate.

In most cases, a paramedic will insert the IV into the patient's vein. However, you may be enlisted to help set up the IV administration set. You will need to:

1. Take out and inspect the fluid bag. The bags come in a protective wrapping to keep them clean. If you are setting up the IV, you must remove the wrapper, then inspect the bag to be sure it contains the fluid that has been ordered. Check the expiration date to make sure the fluid is usable, and look to see that the fluid is clear and free of particles. Squeeze the bag to check for leaks. Occasionally, the fluid comes in a bottle. If so, be sure it is free of cracks. If anything is wrong, report the problem and inspect another bag or bottle (Figure A-10).
2. Select the proper administration set. Uncoil the tubing, and do not let the ends touch the ground.
3. Connect the extension set to the administration set, if an extension set is to be used.
4. Make sure the flow regulator is closed. To do this, roll the stopcock away from the fluid bag.
5. Remove the protective covering from the port of the fluid bag and the protective covering from the spiked end of the tubing (Figure A-11). Insert the spiked end of the tubing into the fluid bag with a quick twist. Do this carefully. Maintain sterility. If these parts touch the ground, they must not be used. Running germs or dirt directly into a patient's bloodstream can be extremely serious, even fatal.
6. Hold the fluid bag higher than the drip chamber. Squeeze the drip chamber a time or two to start the flow. Fill the chamber to the marker line (approximately one-third full).
7. Open the flow regulator and allow the fluid to flush all the air from the tubing. You may need to loosen the cap at the lower end to get the fluid to flow. Maintain the sterility of the tubing end and replace the cap when you are finished. Most sets can be flushed without removing the cap. Be sure that all air bubbles have been flushed from the tubing to avoid introducing a dangerous air embolism into the patient's vein.
8. Turn off the flow.

Make certain that the setup stays clean until the paramedic removes the needle and connects the IV tubing to the catheter inside the patient's vein. Occasionally, the paramedic will draw blood from the vein to obtain samples before inserting the IV. You may be asked to assist by placing the blood in sample tubes and labeling the tubes with the

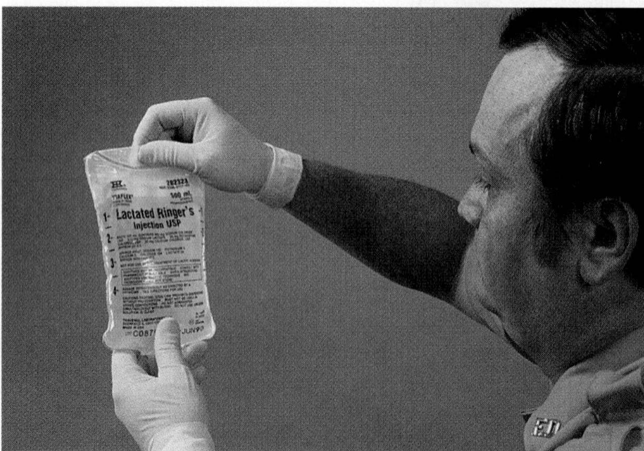

Figure A-10 • Inspect the IV bag to be sure it contains the solution that was ordered, for clarity, leaks, and to be sure it has not expired.

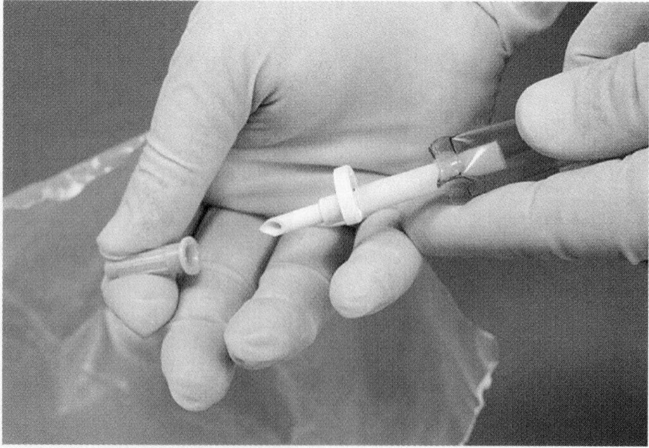

Figure A-11 • Setting up the IV administration set includes removing the protective coverings from the port of the fluid bag and the spiked end of the tubing.

patient's name and any other information that your hospital requires. Remember that they are potential carriers of pathogens. Be sure to take Standard Precautions. Carry the blood tubes to a safe place where they will not be in danger of breaking.

Do not be surprised if you are asked to hold up the patient's arm for a few minutes during a cardiac arrest. During cardiac arrest, medications can be more effective if the arm is temporarily raised after a drug is injected into the IV.

Maintaining an IV

An IV must continue to flow at the proper rate once it has been inserted into the patient's vein. However, a number of things may interrupt the flow. If you are charged with maintaining an IV, be sure to check for and correct the following problems:

- Flow regulator may be closed.
- Clamp may be closed on the tubing.
- Tubing may kink.
- Tubing may get caught under the patient or the backboard.
- Constricting band used to raise the vein for insertion of the needle may have been mistakenly left on the patient's arm, perhaps covered by a sleeve.

The position of the IV or of the patient's arm also may need to be adjusted. Some IVs only flow when the patient's arm or IV site is in a certain position. Adjusting or even splinting the arm may be helpful as long as the splint is not too tight. Since the IV flow usually depends on gravity, be sure that the bag is held well above the IV site and the patient's heart.

Insufficient flow can cause blood to clot in the catheter. This can be prevented by adjusting the flow to an adequate "keep the vein open" or KVO rate. The KVO rate varies, but it is usually about 30 drops per minute for a micro drip and 10 drops per minute for a macro drip set. If the drip chamber is overfilled, clamp the tubing, invert the drip chamber, and pump some fluid back into the bag.

An IV with a flow rate that is too fast is called a "runaway IV." It can rapidly overload the patient with fluid and cause serious problems, especially in an infant or child.

An infiltrated IV is one where the needle has either punctured the vein and exited the other side or has pulled out of the vein. In either case, the fluid is flowing into the surrounding tissues instead of into the vein. An unnoticed infiltrated IV can be very dangerous. Certain high-concentration medications (such as 50 percent dextrose) can cause the death of the surrounding tissue. In addition to complaining of pain, the patient will show swelling at the site (noticeable in all but some obese patients). The person in charge of maintaining the IV must stop the flow and discontinue the IV according to local protocol. If you are not authorized to do this, report the problem immediately to the paramedic or medical direction.

If you learn how to help advanced life support personnel start an IV, run through an administration set, label blood tubes, and maintain an IV, valuable time can be saved at the scene and during transport.

CONTINUOUS POSITIVE AIRWAY PRESSURE (CPAP) AND BI-LEVEL POSITIVE AIRWAY PRESSURE (BIPAP)

Continuous positive airway pressure—commonly called *CPAP*—is a method of treating patients with certain respiratory diseases. Used commonly in the hospital, CPAP units can now be found in the field.

When a patient is ventilated with a BVM or FROPVD, oxygen is introduced into the patient and then is totally exhaled. With CPAP (Figure A-12), a measured amount of oxygen (or an air/oxygen combination) remains in the patient's lungs. This is called *positive end-expiratory pressure* or *PEEP*. It is measured in centimeters of water pressure, noted as cmH_2O. This remaining positive pressure in the lungs helps to expand collapsed alveoli—as in chronic obstructive pulmonary diseases (COPD)—or helps move fluid from the lungs—as in congestive heart failure. Another device you may hear about is *BiPAP—bi-level positive airway pressure*. BiPAP consists of two different levels of pressure, which change during the respiratory cycle. BiPAP is available in some EMS systems.

There are many different brands and types of such devices. Common in most CPAP devices are high-pressure oxygen connectors, which require a different connection than you would use for a nasal cannula or nonrebreather mask.

CPAP in the field is administered through a face mask (Figure A-13). If administered early enough, the patient may not need bag-valve-mask ventilation and intubation. Masks for CPAP must fit to the face with a tight and complete seal. Since patients are experiencing difficulty breathing and may be anxious, achieving this mask seal may be difficult as it will cause anxiety to the patient. Remember that the CPAP device is not a ventilator. When the patient's respiratory efforts become inadequate or absent, discontinue CPAP and begin pocket mask or BVM ventilations.

Assisting with CPAP Devices

To assist with a CPAP device:

1. Assist the ALS provider in assessment of the patient. Apply oxygen by nonrebreather mask while assessing the patient. Take vitals and apply an ECG monitor. At some point, start an IV.
2. When it is determined that CPAP is necessary, prepare the equipment as specified by the manufacturer. This usually involves connecting CPAP to a high-pressure oxygen hose and connecting the hose to an oxygen source. CPAP can use considerable amounts of oxygen.
3. Remove the nonrebreather mask. Place the CPAP mask on the patient's face and secure it. Many CPAP masks have head straps.
4. A valve will be attached to the mask. Either by the valve or by another adjustment, the ALS provider will adjust the oxygen levels and pressure. Remember that a firm and complete mask seal must be maintained.

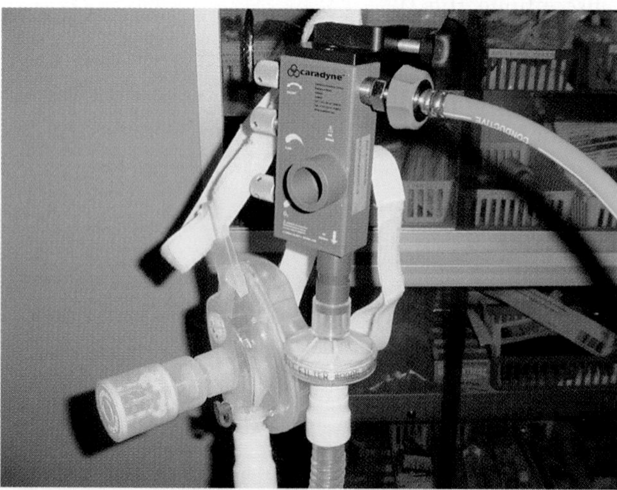

Figure A-12 • Continuous positive airway pressure (CPAP). *(© Dan Hartlestadt, Courtesy: Caradyn Corporation)*

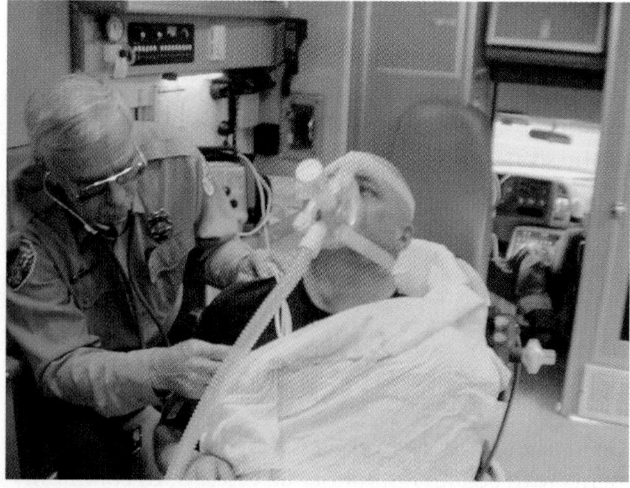

Figure A-13 • CPAP in the field is administered through a face mask. *(© Dan Hartlestadt, Courtesy: Caradyn Corporation)*

5. Monitor the patient. Reassess vital signs frequently. If the patient deteriorates and/or if the patient's respirations become inadequate or absent, CPAP will be discontinued and bag-valve-mask or pocket-face-mask ventilation must begin.

CPAP is a valuable tool for prehospital providers in treating patients with serious pulmonary conditions. Early identification of the problem and application of a CPAP device can prevent deterioration of the patient that might otherwise result in respiratory and cardiac arrest.

APPENDIX B

BASIC CARDIAC LIFE SUPPORT REVIEW

Before beginning your EMT-Basic course, you are required to have completed a course in cardiopulmonary resuscitation (CPR). The elements of CPR are reviewed here.

BEFORE BEGINNING RESUSCITATION

When a patient's breathing and heartbeat stop, *clinical death* occurs. This condition may be reversible through CPR and other treatments. However, when the brain cells die, *biological death* occurs. This usually happens within 10 minutes of clinical death, and it is not reversible. In fact, brain cells will begin to die after 4 to 6 minutes without fresh oxygen supplied by circulating blood from air breathed in and carried to the brain. *Cardiopulmonary resuscitation (CPR)* consists of the actions you take to revive a person—or at least temporarily prevent biological death—by keeping the person's heart and lungs working.

Before you begin resuscitation (rescue breathing or CPR), you must take certain steps, including assessing the patient, activating EMS, positioning the patient, and ensuring an open airway. These first steps are listed in Table B-1.

Assessing the Patient

Patient assessment is crucial. Never initiate resuscitation without first establishing that the patient needs it. The required assessments are often described as determining un-

TABLE B-1 • Basic Life Support Sequence

ABCs	ASSESSMENT	ACTIONS	SPECIAL CONSIDERATIONS
	Determine unresponsiveness ("Are you okay?")	*If unresponsive:* • Activate EMS. • Position patient.	*For child/infant:* Activate EMS after 5 cycles (2 minutes) of resuscitation.
Airway	**Airway open?**	*If unresponsive, assume airway is or may become compromised.* • Open the airway.	*If no trauma, use head-tilt, chin-lift.* *If trauma is suspected, use jaw thrust.*
Breathing	**Determine breathlessness** (Look, listen, feel)	*If no breathing:* • Provide 2 ventilations.	*If breathing is present:* Continue care as necessary. *If first ventilation is unsuccessful:* Reposition head and try again. *If ventilations are still unsuccessful:* Follow airway obstruction clearance procedures.
Circulation	**Determine pulselessness** (Carotid pulse) Check for pulse	*If no pulse:* • Begin chest compressions (CPR).	*In an infant:* Feel for brachial pulse. *If pulse is present but breathing is absent:* Continue rescue breathing. *In infants and children with pulse less than 60/min.: Begin chest compressions.*

responsiveness, breathlessness, and pulselessness—or the ABCs (airway, breathing, and circulation). As Table B-1 shows, these categories overlap.

Determining Unresponsiveness

When you encounter a patient who has collapsed, your first action is to determine unresponsiveness. Tap or gently shake the patient (being careful not to move a patient with possible spinal injury) and shout, "Are you okay?" The patient who is able to respond does not require resuscitation.

If the patient is unresponsive, immediately activate EMS ("phone first") unless the patient's condition is likely caused by a problem other than heart disease (e.g., submersion, injury, or drug overdose). If the patient is a child or an infant, activate EMS after 2 minutes of resuscitation ("phone fast") unless you have reason to think the patient's condition is caused by heart disease. Then position the patient and open the airway with the head-tilt, chin-lift or the jaw-thrust maneuver.

Determining Breathlessness

Determine breathlessness by the look-listen-feel method. Place your ear beside the patient's nose and mouth with your face turned toward the patient's chest. Look for chest rise and fall. Listen and feel for escape of air from the mouth or nose. The patient who is breathing adequately does not require resuscitation.

If the patient is not breathing, provide two ventilations (as explained later).

Determining Pulselessness

Determine pulselessness by feeling for the carotid artery in an adult or a child, or feeling for the brachial artery in an infant. The adult patient who has a pulse does not require chest compressions. If an infant or child has a pulse slower than 60 beats per minute, begin CPR (ventilations and chest compressions).

If the patient has a pulse but is not breathing, provide rescue breathing (artificial ventilations). If the adult patient is pulseless, begin CPR (ventilations and chest compressions).

Assessing the ABCs

Assessments of the ABCs are included in the previously described steps. Keep the ABCs in mind throughout every patient encounter, whether or not resuscitation is underway. If the answer to any of the ABC questions is no, take the appropriate steps to correct the situation:

Is the patient's airway open?
Is the patient breathing?
Does the patient have circulation of blood (a pulse)?

Activating EMS

If you have assistance, the other person should call 911 or otherwise activate the EMS system as soon as a patient collapses or is discovered in collapse. The quicker a defibrillator can reach the patient, the greater the patient's chances of survival.

If you are alone, and the patient is an adult, first determine unresponsiveness (as described earlier) and then activate EMS before returning to the patient to initiate the next steps. If the patient is a child or an infant, perform 2 minutes of resuscitation before activating EMS.

The reason for the difference in timing of EMS activation is that cardiac arrest in an adult is likely to be the result of a disturbance of the heart's electrical activity that will require defibrillation; so getting defibrillation equipment to the patient takes precedence over starting CPR. When cardiac arrest is probably not the result of a disturbance of the heart's electrical activity, however (e.g., submersion, injury, or drug overdose), it is more important to perform rescue breathing, so you perform CPR briefly before activating EMS.

Children and infants generally have healthy hearts, and cardiac arrest is likely to have resulted from respiratory arrest. In this situation, rescue breathing is more likely to be helpful in a child than in an adult, and defibrillation will not help. When the child has heart disease, however, cardiac arrest is more like that of an adult, so calling for a defibrillator is more important than performing rescue breathing.

So, in most cases, 2 minutes of resuscitation before activating EMS is recommended for children and infants, but immediate activation of EMS is recommended for adults.

NOTE: ACTIVATING EMS

"Phone first." If an adult is unresponsive, *activate EMS immediately* (unless the condition is likely caused by a problem other than heart disease)

"Phone fast." If a child is unresponsive, *perform 2 minutes of resuscitation (approximately 5 cycles of compressions and ventilations) before activating EMS* (unless the condition is likely caused by heart disease).

Positioning the Patient

As soon as you have determined unresponsiveness and activated EMS, make sure that the patient is lying supine (on his back) before attempting to open the airway and assess breathing and circulation. If you find the patient in some other position, help him to the floor or stretcher. If the patient is already lying on the floor, move him onto his back. If you suspect that the patient may have been injured, you or a helper must support the patient's neck and hold the head still and in line with his spine while you are moving, assessing, and caring for him.

Opening the Airway

Most airway problems are caused by the tongue. As the head tips forward, especially when the patient is lying on his back, the tongue may slide into the airway. When the patient is unconscious, the risk of airway problems is worsened because unconsciousness causes the tongue to lose muscle tone and the muscles of the lower jaw (to which the tongue is attached) to relax.

Two procedures can help to correct the position of the tongue and thus open the airway. These procedures are the head-tilt, chin-lift maneuver and the jaw-thrust maneuver.

Head-Tilt, Chin-Lift Maneuver

The head-tilt, chin-lift maneuver (Figure B-1) provides for maximum opening of the airway. It is useful on all patients who need assistance in maintaining an airway or breathing. It is one of the best methods for correcting obstructions caused by the tongue. However, since it involves changing the position of the head, the head-tilt, chin-lift maneuver should be used only on a patient who you can be quite sure has not suffered a spinal injury.

Follow these steps to perform the head-tilt, chin-lift maneuver:

1. Once the patient is supine, place one hand on the forehead and the fingertips of the other hand under the bony area at the center of the patient's lower jaw.
2. Tilt the head by applying gentle pressure to the patient's forehead.
3. Use your fingertips to lift the chin and support the lower jaw. Move the jaw forward to a point where the lower teeth are almost touching the upper teeth. Do not compress the soft tissues under the lower jaw, which can press and close off the airway.
4. Do not allow the patient's mouth to close. To provide an adequate opening at the mouth, you may need to use the thumb of the hand supporting the chin to pull back the patient's lower lip. For your own safety (to prevent being bitten), do not insert your thumb into the patient's mouth.

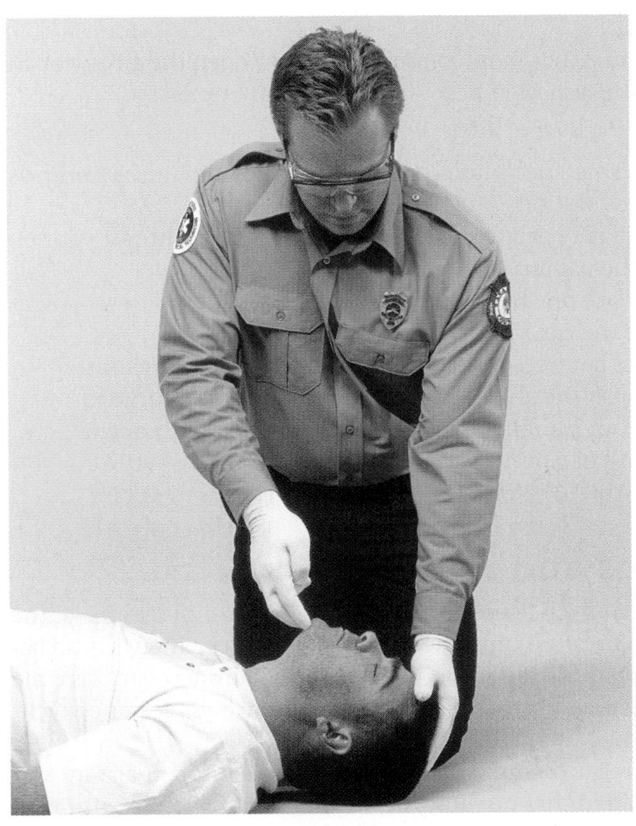

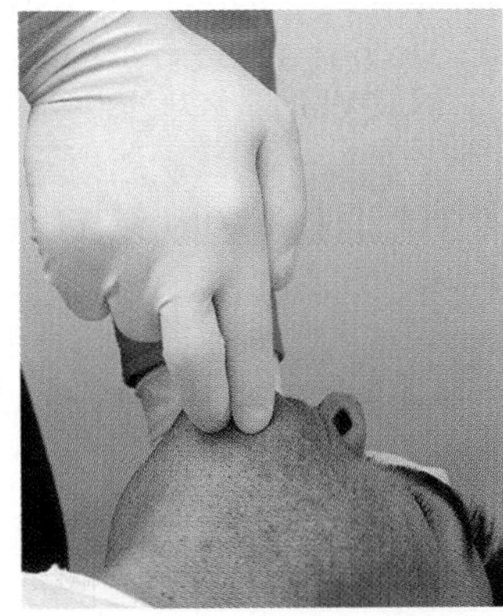

Figure B-1 • The head-tilt, chin-lift maneuver, side view. Insert shows the EMT's fingertips under the bony area at the center of the patient's lower jaw.

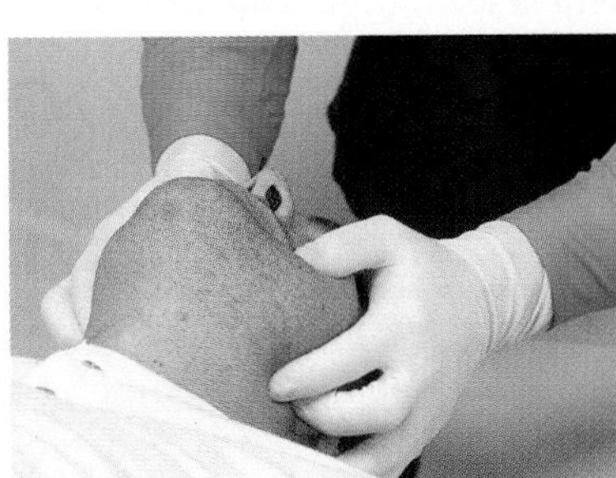

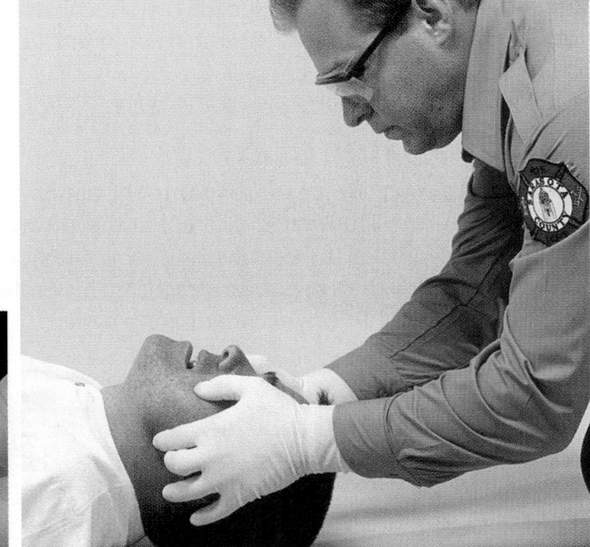

Figure B-2 • The jaw-thrust maneuver, side view. Insert shows the EMT's finger position at the angle of the jaw just below the ears.

NOTE

The jaw-thrust maneuver is the only widely recommended procedure for use on patients with possible head, neck, or spinal injuries.

Jaw-Thrust Maneuver

The jaw-thrust maneuver (Figure B-2) is most commonly used to open the airway of an unconscious patient or one with suspected head, neck, or spinal injuries.

Follow these steps to perform the jaw-thrust maneuver:

1. Carefully keep the patient's head, neck, and spine aligned, moving him as a unit, as you place him in the supine position.
2. Kneel at the top of the patient's head. For greater comfort, you might rest your elbows on the same surface the patient is lying on.
3. Reach forward and gently place one hand on each side of the patient's lower jaw, at the angles of the jaw below the ears.
4. You can help to stabilize the patient's head by using your wrists or forearms.
5. Using your index fingers, push the angles of the patient's lower jaw forward.
6. Retract the lower lip with your thumb if necessary to keep the mouth open.
7. Do not tilt or rotate the patient's head. THE PURPOSE OF THE JAW-THRUST MANEUVER IS TO OPEN THE AIRWAY WITHOUT MOVING THE HEAD OR NECK.

Initial Ventilations and Pulse Check

Deliver 2 breaths, each delivered over 1 second and of sufficient volume to make the chest rise (Table B-2). If the first breath is unsuccessful, reposition the patient's head before attempting the second breath. If the second ventilation is unsuccessful, assume that there is a foreign-body airway obstruction and perform airway clearance techniques (as described later).

If the initial ventilations are successful, you have confirmed an open airway and should feel for a pulse. If the patient has no pulse, begin chest compressions with ventilations (as described later under CPR). If the patient has a pulse but breathing is absent or inadequate, perform rescue breathing.

RESCUE BREATHING

Mouth-to-Mask Ventilation

Mouth-to-mask ventilation is performed using a pocket face mask with a one-way valve. The pocket face mask is made of soft, collapsible material and can be carried in your pocket, jacket, or purse. The steps of mouth-to-mask ventilation are summarized in Table B-2 and illustrated in Scan B-1.

Gastric Distention

Rescue breathing can force some air into the patient's stomach, causing the stomach to become distended. This may indicate that the airway is blocked, that there is improper head position, or that the ventilations being provided are too large or too quick to be accommodated by the lungs or the trachea. This problem is seen more frequently in infants and children but can occur with any patient.

TABLE B-2 • Rescue Breathing

	ADULT	CHILD	INFANT
Age	Puberty and older	1 yr to puberty	Birth to 1 yr
Ventilation duration	1 sec.	1 sec.	1 sec.
Ventilation rate	10–12 breaths/min.	12–20 breaths/min.	12–20 breaths/min.

SCAN B-1 • Mouth-to-Mask Ventilation

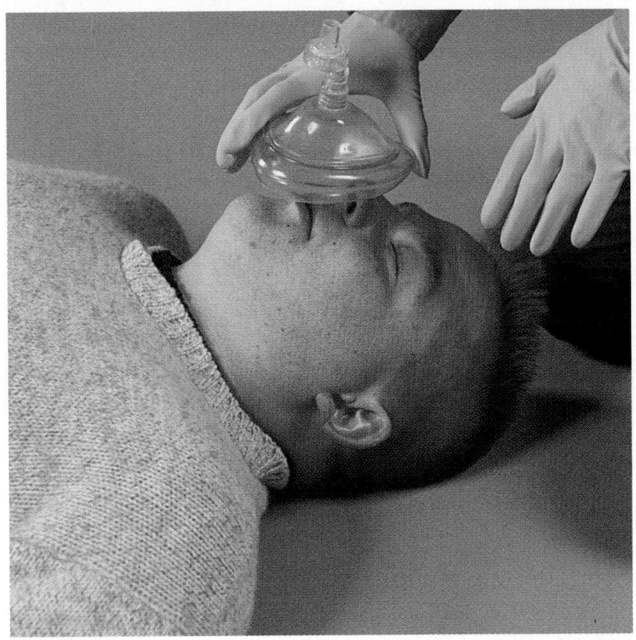

Step 1: Position the patient and prepare to place the mask.

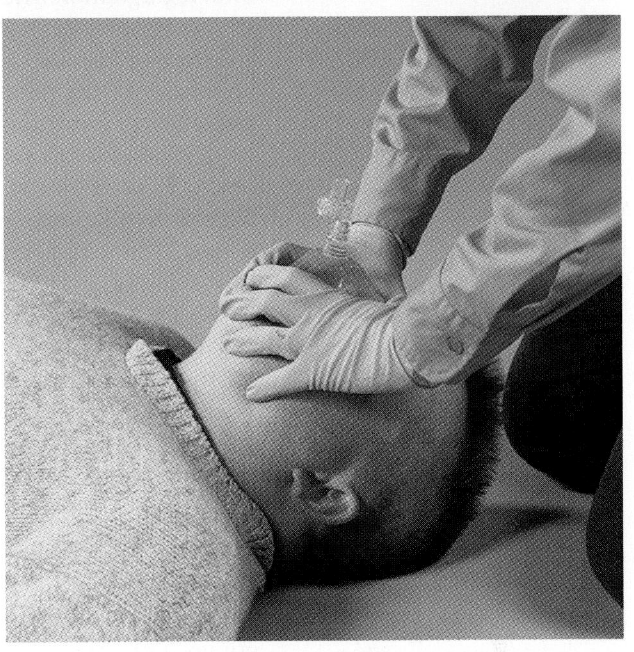

Step 2: Seat the mask firmly on the patient's face.

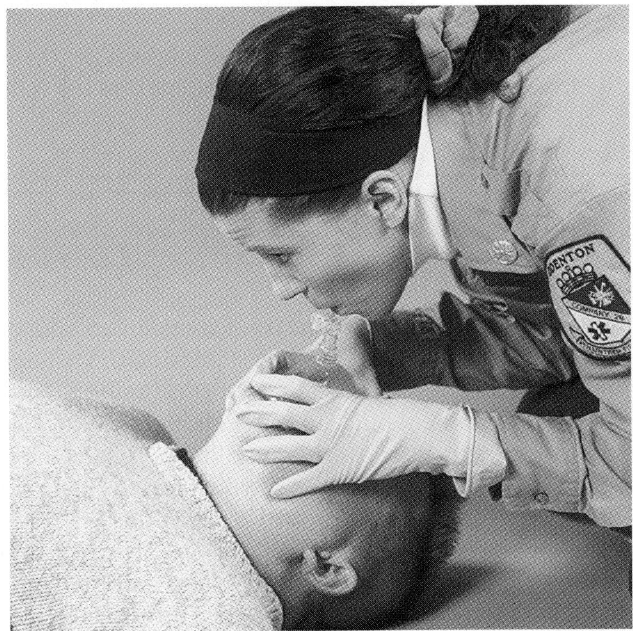

Step 3: Open the patient's airway and watch the chest rise as you ventilate through the one-way valve.

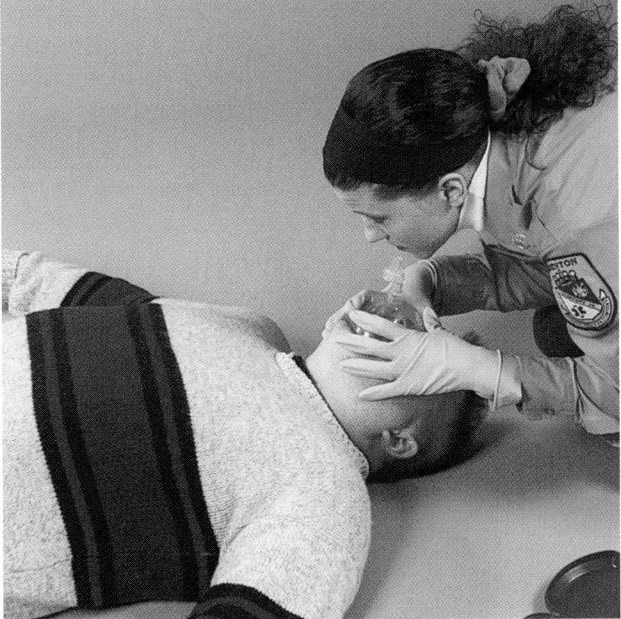

Step 4: Watch the patient's chest fall during exhalation. Ventilate the adult patient 10 to 12 times a minute, a child or infant 12 to 20 times a minute. If the pocket mask has an oxygen inlet, provide supplemental oxygen.

A slight bulge is of little worry, but major distention can cause two serious problems. First, the air-filled stomach reduces lung volume by forcing the diaphragm upward. Second, regurgitation (the passive expulsion of fluids and partially digested foods from the stomach into the throat) or vomiting (the forceful expulsion of the stomach's contents) is a strong possibility. This could lead to additional airway obstruction or aspiration of vomitus into the patient's lungs. When this happens, lung damage can occur and a lethal form of pneumonia may develop.

The best way to avoid gastric distention, or to avoid making it worse once it develops, is to position the patient's head properly, avoid too forceful and too quickly delivered ventilations, and limit the volume of ventilations delivered. The volume delivered should be limited to the size breath that causes the chest to rise. This is why it is so important to watch the patient's chest rise as each ventilation is delivered and to feel for resistance to your breaths.

When gastric distention is present, be prepared for vomiting. If the patient does vomit, roll the entire patient onto his side. (Turning just the head may allow for aspiration of vomitus as well as aggravation of any possible neck injury.) Manually stabilize the patient's head and neck as you roll him. Be prepared to clear the patient's mouth and throat of vomitus with gauze and gloved fingers. Apply suction if you are trained and equipped to do so.

Recovery Position

Patients who resume adequate breathing and pulse after rescue breathing or CPR, and who do not require immobilization for possible spinal injury, are placed in the recovery position. The recovery position allows for drainage from the mouth and prevents the tongue from falling backward and causing an airway obstruction.

The patient should be rolled onto his side. This should be done moving the patient as a unit, not twisting the head, shoulders, or torso. The patient may be rolled onto either side; however, it is preferable to have the patient facing you so that monitoring and suctioning may be more easily performed.

If the patient does not have respirations that are sufficient to support life, the recovery position must not be used. The patient should be placed supine and his ventilations assisted.

CPR

Checking for Circulation

Before beginning CPR, you must confirm that the patient is pulseless. In an adult or child (not infant), check the carotid pulse (Figure B-3). While stabilizing the patient's head and maintaining the proper head tilt, use your hand that is closest to the patient's neck to locate his "Adam's apple" (the prominent bulge in the front of the neck). Place the tips of your index and middle fingers directly over the midline of this structure. Slide your fingertips to the side of the patient's neck closest to you. Keep the palm side of your fingertips against the patient's neck. Feel for a groove between the Adam's apple and the muscles located along the side of the neck. Very little pressure needs to be applied to the neck to feel the carotid pulse. Keep in mind that laypeople are taught not to check for a pulse, but to look for signs of circulation: normal breathing, coughing, or movement. In an infant, check for a brachial pulse (Figure B-4). If the adult patient is pulseless, begin CPR. If an infant or child has a pulse slower than 60 beats per minute, begin CPR (ventilations and chest compressions).

To provide chest compressions, place the patient supine on a hard surface and compress the chest by applying downward pressure with your hands. This action causes an increase of pressure inside the chest and possible actual compression of the heart itself, one or both of which force the blood out of the heart and into circulation. When pressure is released, the heart refills with blood. The next compression sends this fresh blood into circulation and the cycle continues.

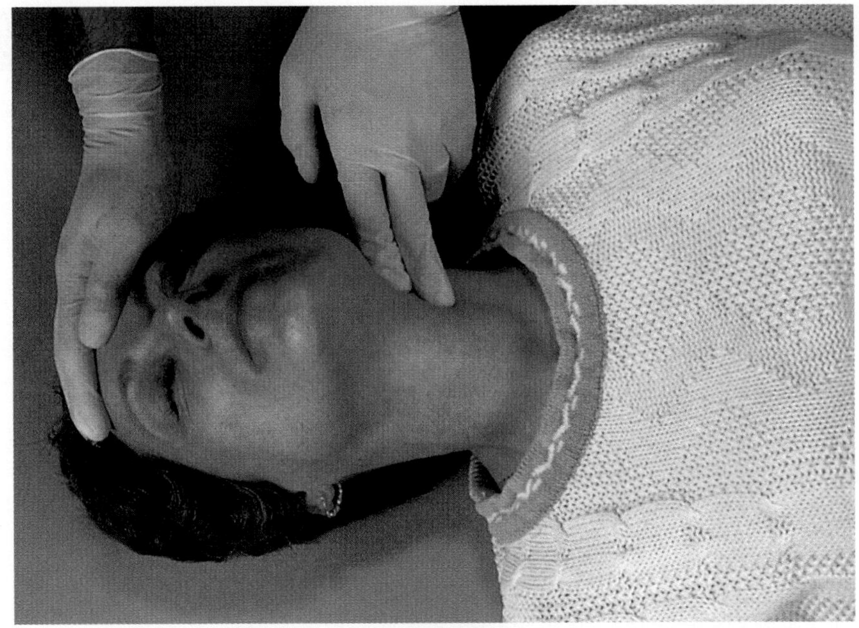

Figure B-3 • Check the carotid pulse to confirm circulation.

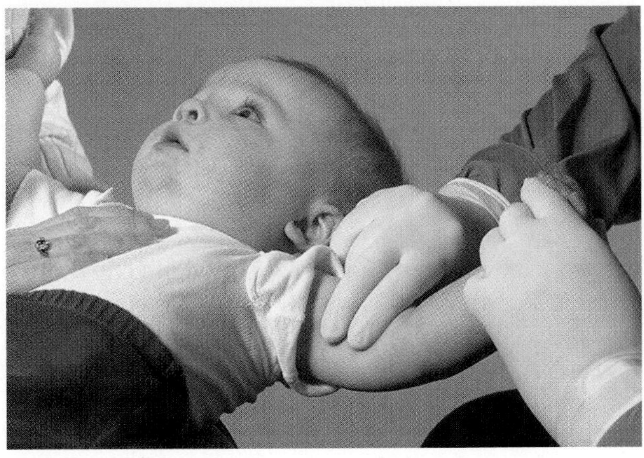

Figure B-4 • For infants, determine circulation by feeling for a brachial pulse.

NOTE
Do not initiate CPR on any adult who has a pulse.

How to Perform CPR

CPR is a method of artificial breathing and circulation. When natural heart action and breathing have stopped, we must provide an artificial means to oxygenate the blood and keep it in circulation. This is accomplished by providing chest compressions and ventilations.

CPR can be done by one or by two rescuers. All of the information under Providing Chest Compressions and Providing Ventilations applies to both one-rescuer and two-rescuer CPR. Specific information about each type of CPR follows under One-Rescuer CPR and Two-Rescuer CPR. Scans B-2 and B-3 can help you follow and review these procedures as they are described in the following text. These procedures are for an adult patient. Procedures for infants and children will be described later.

Providing Chest Compressions

After you have placed the patient supine on a hard surface and your hands are properly positioned on the CPR compression site:

1. Straighten your arms and lock your elbows. You must not bend the elbows when delivering or releasing compressions.

SCAN B-2 • Locating the CPR Compression Sited

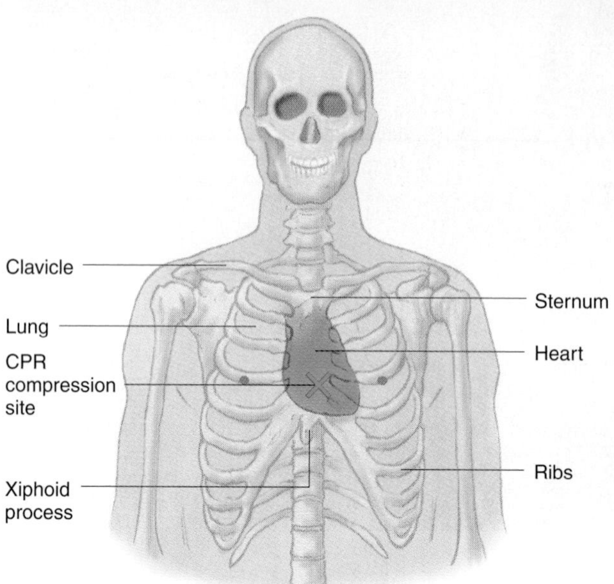

Locate the compression site for CPR by placing the heel of the hand on the sternum between the nipples. This correlates with the lower half of the sternum.

2. Make certain that your shoulders are directly over your hands (directly over the patient's sternum). This will allow you to deliver compressions straight down onto the site. Keep both of your knees on the ground or floor.
3. Deliver compressions STRAIGHT DOWN, with enough force to depress the sternum of a typical adult $1\frac{1}{2}$ to 2 inches.
4. Fully release pressure on the patient's sternum, but *do not* bend your elbows and *do not* lift your hands from the sternum, which can cause you to lose correct positioning of your hands. Your movement should be from your hips. Compressions should be delivered in a rhythmic, not a "jabbing," fashion. THE AMOUNT OF TIME YOU SPEND COMPRESSING SHOULD BE THE SAME AS THE TIME FOR THE RELEASE. This is known as the 50:50 rule: 50 percent compression, 50 percent release.

Providing Ventilations

Ventilations are given between sets of compressions. The mouth-to-mask techniques described earlier for rescue breathing are used.

One-Rescuer and Two-Rescuer CPR

Scan B-3 shows the techniques of one-rescuer CPR and two-rescuer CPR for the adult patient and describes compression rates and ratios for CPR on adults, children, and infants.

How to Join CPR in Progress

If CPR has been started by someone who is trained to perform CPR but is not part of the EMS system, and you join this person to perform CPR:

1. Identify yourself as someone who knows CPR and ask to help.
2. Ensure that EMS has been activated.

SCAN B-3 • CPR Summary—Adult Patient

<table>
<tr><th>ONE RESCUER</th><th colspan="2">FUNCTIONS</th><th>TWO RESCUERS</th></tr>
<tr><td></td><td colspan="2">• Establish unresponsiveness
• If there's no response, call 911
• Position patient
• Open airway
• Look, listen, and feel
(no more than 10 seconds)</td><td></td></tr>
<tr><td></td><td colspan="2">• Deliver 2 breaths (1 sec/ventilation).
If unsuccessful, reposition head and try again. Clear airway if necessary.</td><td></td></tr>
<tr><td></td><td colspan="2">• Check carotid pulse . . .
(5–10 seconds)

If no pulse . . .
• Begin chest compressions</td><td></td></tr>
<tr><td></td><td colspan="2">DELIVER COMPRESSIONS

1½–2 inches
100/min.</td><td></td></tr>
<tr><td></td><td colspan="2">DELIVER VENTILATIONS
10–12 breaths/min.
Compression: Ventilation ratio

30:2</td><td></td></tr>
<tr><td></td><td>• Do 5 cycles

• Check pulse</td><td>• Ventilator checks effectiveness</td><td></td></tr>
<tr><td></td><td colspan="2">CONTINUE PERIODIC ASSESSMENT</td><td></td></tr>
</table>

NOTE: Wear gloves and use either a pocket mask with one-way valve or bag-valve mask

3. Allow the first rescuer to complete a cycle of 30 compressions and 2 ventilations.
4. Check for a pulse. If there is no pulse, start one-rescuer CPR. If you tire before EMS arrives, let the other rescuer perform CPR. Alternate until EMS arrives.

If you wish to join another member of the EMS system who has initiated CPR, you should:

1. Identify yourself and your training, and state that you are ready to perform two-rescuer CPR.
2. While the first rescuer is providing compressions, spend 5 seconds checking for a carotid pulse produced by each compression. This is to determine if the compressions being delivered are effective. Inform the first rescuer if there is or is not a pulse

being produced. (If the first rescuer cannot deliver effective compressions, you will have to take over for him when CPR is resumed.)

3. You should say, "Stop compressions," and check for spontaneous pulse and breathing. This should take only a few seconds.
4. If there is no pulse, you should state, "No pulse. Continue CPR."
5. The first rescuer resumes compressions, and the second rescuer provides two ventilations during a pause after every fifteenth compression. If desired, the second rescuer can start compressions and allow the first rescuer to provide the ventilations.

CPR Techniques for Children and Infants

The techniques of CPR for children and infants are essentially the same as those used for adults. However, some procedures and rates differ when the patient is a child or an infant. (If younger than 1 year of age, the patient is considered an infant. Between 1 year and puberty, the patient is considered a child. Over the age of puberty, adult procedures apply to the patient. Keep in mind that the size of the patient can also be an important factor. A very small 9-year-old may have to be treated as a child.)

The techniques of CPR for an infant are shown in Scan B-4. For a child, CPR is conducted as for an adult, the chief difference in procedure being the hand position—using the heel of one or two hands—for chest compressions (Figure B-5). To compare adult, child, and infant CPR, see Table B-3.

When CPR must be performed, adults, children, and infants are placed on their backs on a hard surface. For an infant, the hard surface can be the rescuer's hand or forearm. For an infant or a child, use the head-tilt, chin-lift or the jaw-thrust maneuver, but apply only a slight tilt for an infant. Too great a tilt may close off the infant's airway;

SCAN B-4 • Infant CPR

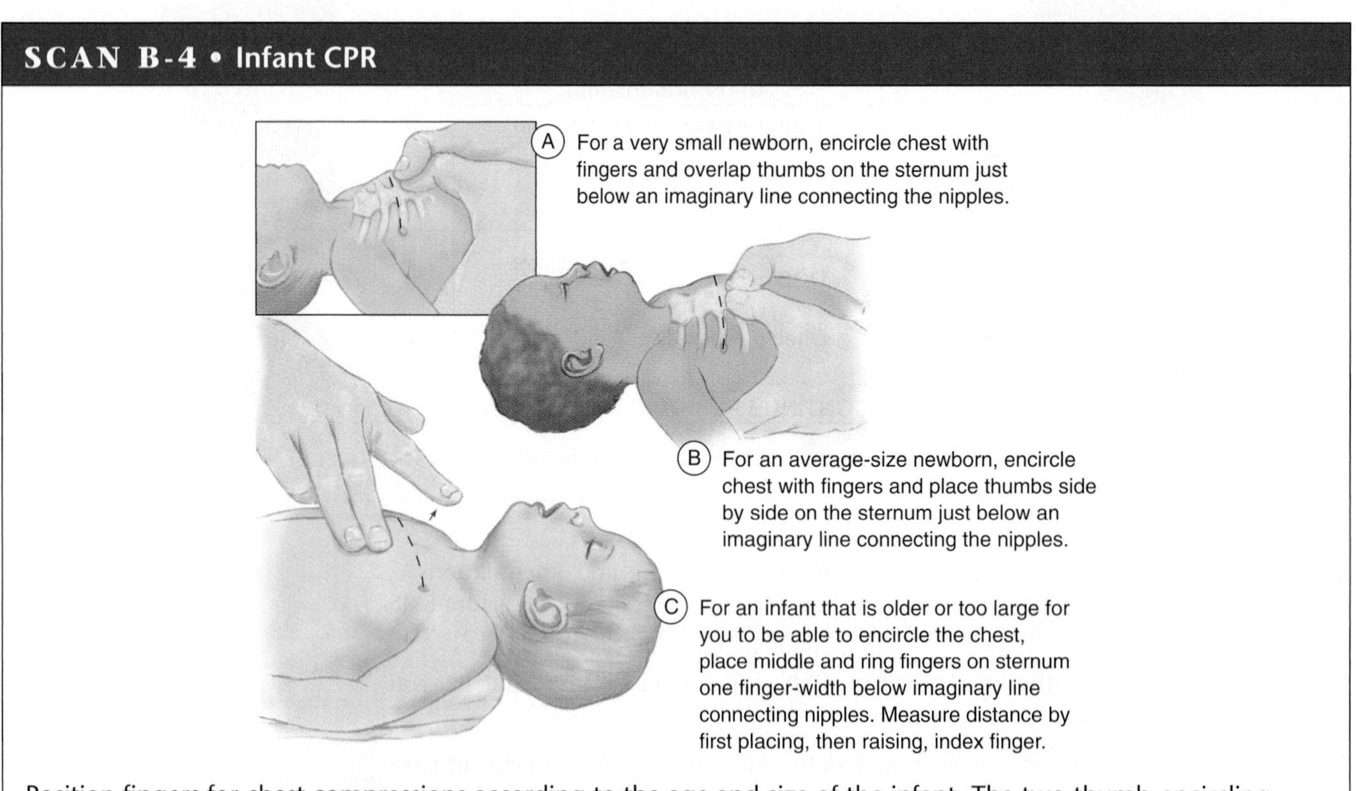

A For a very small newborn, encircle chest with fingers and overlap thumbs on the sternum just below an imaginary line connecting the nipples.
B For an average-size newborn, encircle chest with fingers and place thumbs side by side on the sternum just below an imaginary line connecting the nipples.
C For an infant that is older or too large for you to be able to encircle the chest, place middle and ring fingers on sternum one finger-width below imaginary line connecting nipples. Measure distance by first placing, then raising, index finger.

Position fingers for chest compressions according to the age and size of the infant. The two thumb-encircling hands method is preferred when two rescuers are present.

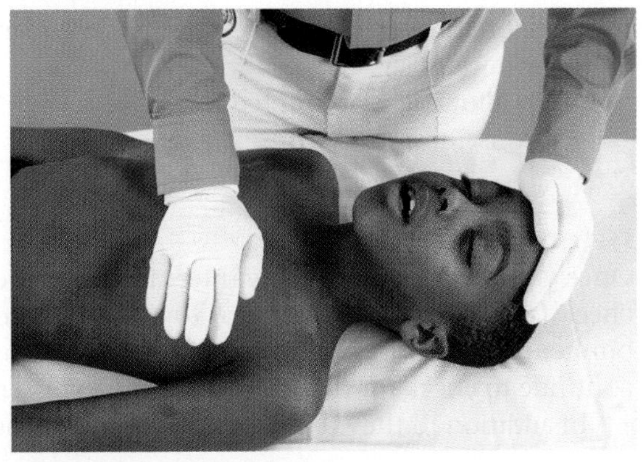

Figure B-5 • Performing chest compressions on a child.

TABLE B-3 • CPR for Adults, Children, and Infants

	ADULT	CHILD	INFANT
Age	Puberty and older	1 yr to puberty	Birth to 1 yr
Compression depth	1½ to 2 inches	⅓ to ½ depth of chest	⅓ to ½ depth of chest
Compression rate	100/min.	100/min.	100/min. (newborn 120/min.)
Each ventilation	1 second	1 second	1 second
Pulse check location	Carotid artery (throat)	Carotid artery (throat)	Brachial artery (upper arm)
One-rescuer CPR compressions-to-ventilations ratio	30:2	30:2 (alone) 15:2 (2 rescuers)	30:2 (alone) 15:2 (2 rescuers) 3:1 (newborn)
When working alone: Call 911 or emergency dispatcher	After establishing unresponsiveness—before beginning resuscitation unless submersion, injury, or overdose	After establishing unresponsiveness and 2 minutes of resuscitation unless heart disease present	After establishing unresponsiveness and 2 minutes of resuscitation unless heart disease present

however, make certain that the opening is adequate (note chest rise during ventilation). Always be sure to support an infant's head. Take these steps to establish a pulse in an infant or a child:

- *For an infant,* you should use the brachial pulse.
- *For a child,* determine circulation in the same manner as for an adult.

Special Considerations in CPR

How to Know If CPR Is Effective

To determine if CPR is effective, *if possible have someone else feel for a carotid pulse* during compressions and watch to see the patient's chest rise during ventilations. *Listen for exhalation of air,* either naturally or during compressions, as additional verification that air has entered the lungs.

In addition, any of the following indications of effective CPR may be noticed:

- Pupils constrict.
- Skin color improves.
- Heartbeat returns spontaneously.

- Spontaneous, gasping respirations are made.
- Arms and legs move.
- Swallowing is attempted.
- Consciousness returns.

Interrupting CPR

Once you begin CPR, you may interrupt the process for no more than a few seconds to check for pulse and breathing or to reposition yourself and the patient. The first recommended pulse and breathing check is after the first 2 minutes of CPR. You should continue to check for these vital signs every few minutes.

In addition to these built-in interruptions, you may interrupt CPR to:

- Move a patient onto a stretcher.
- Move a patient down a flight of stairs or through a narrow doorway or hallway.
- Move a patient on or off the ambulance.
- Suction to clear vomitus or airway obstructions.
- Allow for defibrillation or advanced cardiac life support measures to be initiated.

When CPR is resumed, begin with chest compressions rather than with ventilations.

When Not to Begin or to Terminate CPR

As discussed earlier in this chapter, CPR should not be initiated when you find that the patient—even though unresponsive and perhaps not breathing—does have a pulse. Usually, of course, you will perform CPR when the patient has no pulse. *However, there are special circumstances in which CPR should not be initiated even though the patient has no pulse:*

- *Obvious mortal wounds.* These include decapitation, incineration, a severed body, and injuries that are so extensive that CPR cannot be effectively performed (e.g., severe crush injuries to the head, neck, and chest).
- *Rigor mortis.* This is the stiffening of the body and its limbs that occurs after death, usually within 4 to 10 hours.
- *Obvious decomposition.*
- *A line of lividity.* Lividity is a red or purple skin discoloration that occurs when gravity causes the blood to sink to the lowest parts of the body and collect there. Lividity usually indicates that the patient has been dead for more than 15 minutes unless the patient has been exposed to cold temperatures. Using lividity as a sign requires special training.
- *Stillbirth.* CPR should not be initiated for a stillborn infant who has died hours prior to birth. This infant may be recognized by blisters on the skin, a very soft head, and a strong disagreeable odor.

In all cases, if you are in doubt, seek a physician's advice. Once you have started CPR, you must continue to provide CPR until:

- Spontaneous circulation occurs . . . then provide rescue breathing as needed.
- Spontaneous circulation and breathing occur.
- Another trained rescuer can take over for you.
- You turn care of the patient over to a person with a higher level of training.
- You are too exhausted to continue.
- You receive a "no CPR" order from a physician or other authority per local protocols.

If you turn the patient over to another rescuer, this person must be trained in basic cardiac life support.

CLEARING AIRWAY OBSTRUCTIONS

Not every airway problem is caused by the tongue (the situation in which you would use the head-tilt, chin-lift maneuver or the jaw-thrust maneuver, described earlier, to open the airway). The airway can also be blocked by foreign objects or materials. These can include pieces of food, ice, toys, or vomitus. This problem is often seen with children and with patients who have abused alcohol or other drugs. It also happens when an injured person's airway becomes blocked by blood, broken teeth, dentures, or when a person chokes on food.

Airway obstructions are either partial or complete. Partial and complete obstructions have different characteristics that may be noted during assessment, and each type has a different procedure of care. It is important to understand the differences between partial and complete obstruction and the correct care for each.

Mild Airway Obstruction

A conscious patient trying to indicate an airway problem will usually point to his mouth or hold his neck. Many do this even when a partial obstruction does not prevent speech. Ask the patient if he is choking, or ask if he can speak or cough. If he can, then the obstruction is mild.

Have the conscious patient with an apparent mild airway obstruction cough. A strong and forceful cough indicates he is exchanging enough air. Continue to encourage the patient to cough in the hope that such action will dislodge and expel the foreign object. *Do not* interfere with the patient's efforts to clear the obstruction by means of forceful coughing.

In cases where the patient has an apparent mild airway obstruction but he cannot cough or has a very weak cough, or the patient is blue or gray or shows other signs of poor air exchange, treat the patient as if there is a severe airway obstruction, as described in the following section.

Severe Airway Obstruction

Be alert for signs of a severe airway obstruction in the conscious or unconscious patient:

- *The conscious patient* with a severe airway obstruction will try to speak but will not be able to. He will also not be able to breathe or cough. Usually, he will display the distress signal for choking by clutching the neck between thumb and fingers.
- *The unconscious patient* with a severe airway obstruction will be in respiratory arrest. When ventilation attempts are unsuccessful, it becomes apparent that there is an obstruction.

Conscious Adult or Child

For the conscious adult or child (not infant), use abdominal thrusts to clear a foreign body as follows:

Abdominal Thrusts

1. Make a fist, and place the thumb side of this fist against the midline of the patient's abdomen between waist and rib cage. Avoid touching the chest, especially the area immediately below the sternum.
2. Grasp your properly positioned fist with your other hand and apply pressure inward and up toward the patient's head in a smooth, quick movement. Deliver 5 rapid thrusts.

Chest thrusts are used in place of abdominal thrusts when the patient is in the late stages of pregnancy, or when the patient is too obese for abdominal thrusts to be effective. For the conscious adult who is standing or sitting perform chest thrusts as follows:

Chest Thrusts

1. Position yourself behind the patient and slide your arms under his armpits, so that you encircle his chest.
2. Form a fist with one hand, and place the thumb side of this fist on the midline of the sternum about two to three finger widths above the xiphoid process. This places your fist on the lower half of the sternum but not in contact with the edge of the rib cage.
3. Grasp the fist with your other hand and deliver 5 chest thrusts directly backward toward the spine.

Unconscious Adult or Child

For the unconscious adult or child (not infant) or for a conscious patient who cannot sit or stand, or if you are too short to reach around the patient to deliver thrusts, proceed as follows:

CPR

1. Place the patient in a supine position.
2. Perform CPR. Every time you open the airway, look in the mouth for an object. If, and only if, you see an object, remove it by sweeping your fingers in the patient's mouth from one side to the other.

If the obstruction is not relieved after a series of 5 thrusts, reassess your position and the patient's airway (if the patient is unconscious, also attempt finger sweeps to try to remove the obstruction). Attempt to ventilate the patient and, if unsuccessful, repeat the series of thrusts. Repeat the sequence until the obstruction is relieved.

Airway Clearance Sequences

Table B-4 lists sequences of procedures to use in the event of a severe airway obstruction or a mild airway obstruction. Note that for an adult, as discussed earlier, you should activate the EMS system as soon as unresponsiveness is determined, before carrying out the remainder of the airway clearance procedures.

Airway clearance procedures are considered to have been effective if any of the following happens:

- Patient re-establishes good air exchange or spontaneous breathing.
- Foreign object is expelled from the mouth.
- Foreign object is expelled into the mouth where it can be removed by the rescuer.
- Unconscious patient regains consciousness.
- Patient's skin color improves.

If a person has only a mild airway obstruction and is still able to speak and cough forcefully, do not interfere with his attempts to expel the foreign body. Carefully watch him, however, so that you can immediately provide help if this partial obstruction becomes a complete one.

Procedures for a Child or Infant

The procedure for clearing a foreign body from the airway of a child is very similar to that used for an adult. The airway clearance procedure for an infant uses a combination of back blows and chest compressions as shown in Scan B-5.

TABLE B-4 • Airway Clearance Sequences

AGE	ADULT	CHILD	INFANT
Conscious	Puberty and older Ask, "Are you choking?" Abdominal thrusts until obstruction is relieved or patient loses consciousness.	1 yr–puberty Ask, "Are you choking?" Abdominal thrusts until obstruction is relieved or patient loses consciousness.	Birth–1 yr Observe signs of choking (small objects or food, wheezing, agitation, blue color, not breathing). Series of: 5 back blows and 5 chest thrusts.
Unconscious	Establish unresponsiveness. If alone, call for help. Then open airway. Attempt to ventilate. If unsuccessful, reposition head and attempt to ventilate again. If unsuccessful, perform CPR. Remove objects from the mouth if they become visible.	Establish unresponsiveness. Open airway. Attempt to ventilate. If unsuccessful, reposition head and attempt to ventilate again. If unsuccessful, perform CPR. Remove visible objects (NO blind sweeps). After 2 minutes, call for help if alone.	Establish unresponsiveness. Open airway. Attempt to ventilate. If unsuccessful, reposition head and attempt to ventilate again. If unsuccessful, perform CPR. Remove visible objects (NO blind sweeps). After 2 minutes, call for help if alone.

For both a child and an infant, a major difference from adult procedures is:

- If the child or infant becomes unconscious, send someone else to activate the EMS system. If no one else is available, wait until you have either relieved the obstruction or you have attempted the airway obstruction sequence for 2 minutes.

NOTE

As an EMT-Basic you will be trained as a "professional rescuer" in CPR. The training you will receive will be more in-depth than a lay rescuer or bystander would receive. The course for people who wish to learn CPR and have no medical background differs from the training you receive in the following ways:

- Lay rescuers are not trained to check for a pulse before beginning compressions in CPR. If the patient is not breathing and does not otherwise respond (breathing, cough, or movement), the lay rescuer is supposed to begin compressions.
- As an EMT you will be taught additional techniques that are not taught to lay rescuers, such as the two-thumbs-encircling-hands technique for two-rescuer compression in infants.
- Lay rescuers may be reluctant to do rescue breathing, especially on a stranger. In this case, you may find a lay rescuer performing chest compressions without rescue breathing. While not ideal, if it's a choice between compressions without respirations and nothing at all, compressions without respirations is acceptable for the lay rescuer.

It is possible for you to come upon a bystander performing CPR and see some of these differences in practice. If you ask the bystander, "Does the patient have a pulse?" he might not have checked, nor was he required to do so.

Remember that performing CPR is quite stressful for the bystander. In many cases this CPR will be performed by one family member on another. It is important to be supportive and use a nonjudgmental tone about the efforts taken by the bystander.

SCAN B-5 • Clearing the Airway—Infant

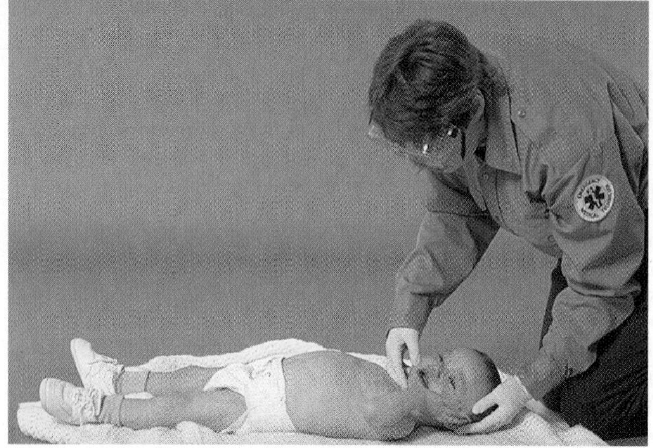

Step 1: Recognize and assess for choking. Look for breathing difficulty, ineffective cough, and lack of strong cry.

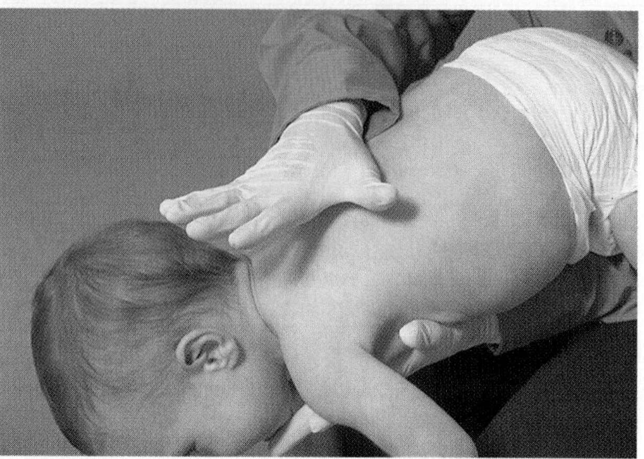

Step 2: Give up to 5 back blows and . . .

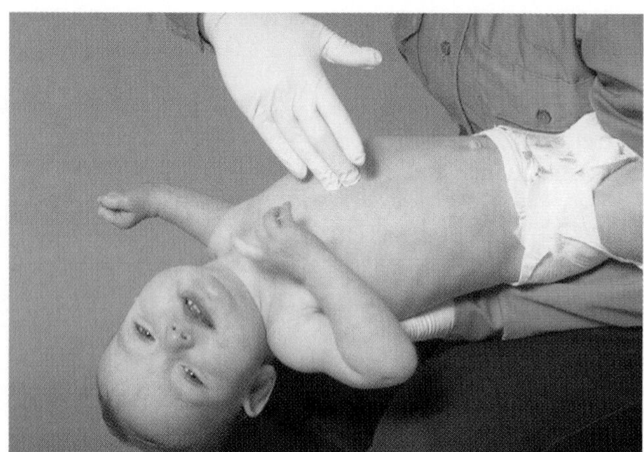

Step 3: 5 chest thrusts.

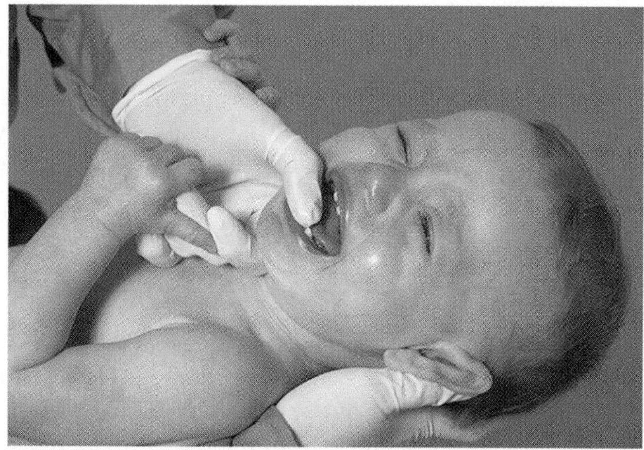

Step 4: If the infant becomes unresponsive, open the airway and look for a foreign body. If you see one, use a finger sweep to remove it. (Never do blind finger sweeps.) Attempt to ventilate. If this fails, reposition the head and try again. If you are not successful, start CPR. If you are working alone, after 2 minutes activate the EMS system and continue airway clearance and ventilation efforts. Transport as quickly as possible.

NOTE

For realism, this photo sequence shows airway clearance procedures being performed on a real baby. The baby is awake. In practice, of course, a baby with an airway obstruction is likely to be unresponsive.

THE FUTURE OF EMS EDUCATION

Emergency medical services is a very young field when compared to other health care professions. Medicine has been recognized as a healing profession since the time of Hippocrates more than 2,000 years ago. Nursing started as a group of volunteers who transformed themselves into professional health care providers over the course of a century. Although ambulance service has been available in some areas since the nineteenth century, EMS has been recognized as a separate field worthy of attention for only a few decades.

EMS has been experiencing growing pains, especially over the last 10 years. What does the future hold for EMS and, in particular, EMS education? To understand the future, one must first look to the past and see the path EMS has taken in its short existence.

EMS EDUCATION IN THE PAST

In the 1950s and 1960s, before there was such a thing as an EMT, "ambulance drivers" often had no training—and didn't need any since they didn't usually provide care beyond transport with lights and siren. Some took first aid courses offered by the American Red Cross or other organizations, but they were the exception.

The first EMT-Ambulance classes, as they were called then, took place around 1970. Often taught by physicians who had an interest in ambulance work, the courses emphasized trauma management because of an important paper that had been released by the National Academy of Sciences in 1967. "Accidental Death and Disability: The Neglected Disease of Modern Society" described how thousands of people were dying on the highways from motor-vehicle trauma, often with injuries that did not have to be fatal if appropriate treatment had been instituted promptly at the scene or en route to a hospital.

Because of this emphasis on trauma, EMS at the federal level became the responsibility of the agency that came to be called the National Highway Traffic Safety Administration (NHTSA) within the United States Department of Transportation (US DOT).

In 1984, DOT recognized the need to update the EMT-A curriculum and awarded a contract to revise the program. This 81-hour course included new material on the pneumatic anti-shock garment (PASG), among other things. In 1990, DOT awarded a contract to revise the EMT-A curriculum again. This time, the revision process encountered a number of obstacles and challenges.

According to the contract, the length of the course was capped at 110 hours. Consequently, the curriculum developers had to cut some material to prevent the course from being too long. CPR was removed from the course and became a prerequisite. Clinical time was removed and replaced not with a fixed number of hours, but with a specified number of patient contacts in a supervised clinical setting. The curriculum developers had to face the problem of not just *how* to teach EMTs, but also *what* to teach EMTs. The EMS community, and in particular some segments of it, was very vocal about what should be included in the course and what should be excluded from the course. Because of these and other issues, the contract that was awarded in 1990 was not completed until 1994.

While the curriculum was being revised, the National Registry of EMTs took a leadership role in implementing a solution. Representatives of the Registry, the National Council of State EMS Training Coordinators, the National Association of State EMS Directors, the National Association of EMS Physicians, and NHTSA met and drafted a document called the "National EMS Education and Practice Blueprint" (Figure C-1). The EMS community, through representatives of major EMS organizations, met to review the draft and made suggestions for improvement. After incorporating these suggestions, the document was released in 1993.

The "Blueprint" was the first attempt to plan EMS education in a way that allowed for advancement in an organized manner. There was now a clear progression of knowledge and skills from the First Responder to the EMT-Basic to the EMT-Intermediate to the EMT-Paramedic.

Within a few years, the need to revise the EMS Education and Practice Blueprint became apparent. When representatives of the EMS community met, they quickly decided that rather than revise the Blueprint, the group should take a broader view. Thus, they drafted the "EMS Education Agenda: A Systems Approach."

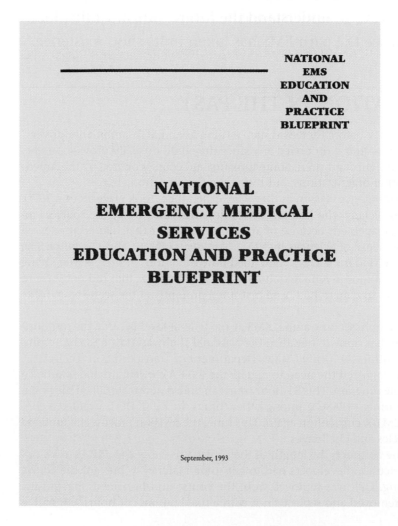
NATIONAL EMS EDUCATION AND PRACTICE BLUEPRINT

NATIONAL EMERGENCY MEDICAL SERVICES EDUCATION AND PRACTICE BLUEPRINT

September, 1993

Figure C-1 • The National EMS Education and Practice Blueprint was released in 1993.

The Education Agenda took a comprehensive view of the subject and called for a system with five interdependent components: *core content, a scope of practice model, education standards, national testing and certification,* and finally *national accreditation of education institutions* (Figure C-2). No single component of the system can stand alone. For EMS education to improve in a systematic manner, all five components must be present.

Core content, simply put, is a list of the topics and skills an EMS provider at some level might be responsible for. The core content does not describe which level should include any particular topic or skill. Interventions that are not included in the core content are not authorized for any level of EMS provider. For example, the EMS Core Content specifically excludes field amputation from any level of EMS provider's responsibilities.

The *scope of practice model* takes the interventions listed in the Core Content and arranges them according to the levels of EMS providers. The National EMS Scope of Practice Model (Figure C-3) calls for four provider levels: Emergency Medical Responder (EMR), Emergency Medical Technician (EMT), Advanced EMT (AEMT), and Paramedic.

Each state has the right and responsibility to regulate licensed professionals in the manner it sees fit. Although no state is obligated to follow the model, the model provides a uniform approach to describing the levels of EMS providers, describes nationally recognized levels for the purpose of certification testing, and makes it easier for states to recognize the training an EMS provider brings from another state.

The *National EMS Education Standards* replace the former DOT national standard curricula. Instead of having a detailed outline with specific learning objectives, education institutions and instructors now have been provided more general statements about the competencies providers should have. Because EMS has not used education standards before, abbreviated content outlines are included with the standards. There are no lesson plans or even suggestions for the order in which topics should be taught.

National testing and certification constitute the fourth element of the Education Agenda. If you graduate from nursing school or medical school, before you can practice you must pass a national exam. The Education Agenda calls for this same approach

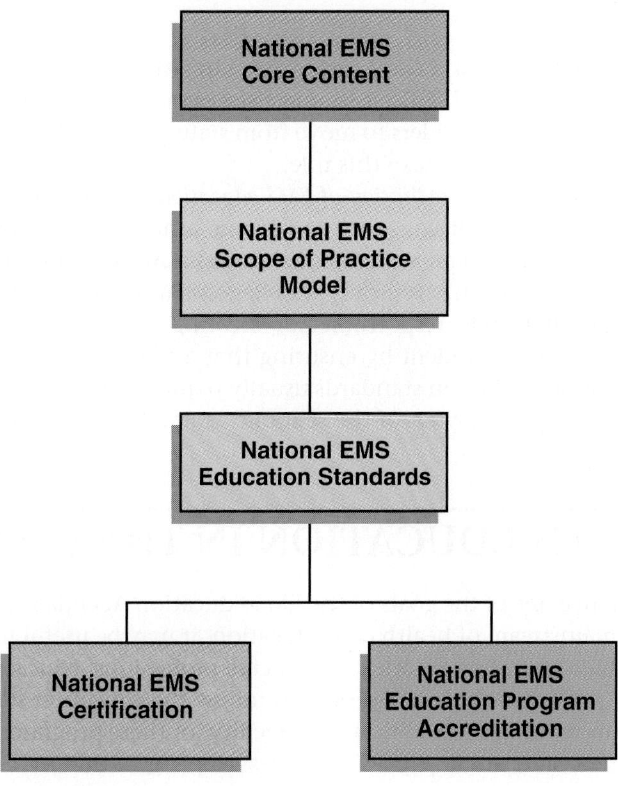

Figure C-2 • The EMS Education Agenda calls for a system of five interdependent components.

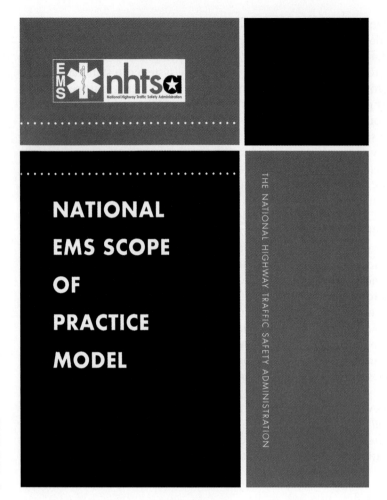

Figure C-3 • The National EMS Scope of Practice Model calls for four provider levels: EMR, EMT, AEMT, and Paramedic.

to national testing and certification in EMS. This should lead to a national standard for knowledge and skills. It should also promote reciprocity between states and make it easier for EMS providers to move from state to state. The National Registry of EMTs has positioned itself to take this role.

National accreditation of EMS education institutions is the last element of the Education Agenda. If you want to become a nurse, respiratory therapist, or physician, you must enroll in an accredited institution. Accreditation in this respect refers to an institute of learning, typically a college or university, that meets the standards set by a national body responsible for creating these standards. Accreditation protects the prospective student by ensuring that a school meets certain requirements. For example, accreditation standards usually require that a school's faculty be qualified and that the physical layout of the school be suitable for education.

EMS EDUCATION IN THE PRESENT

Since one of the goals of the EMS Education Agenda is to bring EMS education into the mainstream of health care education, it may be useful to compare the status of current EMS education to other health care professions' education systems (Table C-1).

Other health care programs follow the education standards and guidelines of their accrediting bodies. Individual faculty for these programs, who almost always have master's or doctoral degrees, create lesson plans based on the standards of their field of care.

TABLE C-1 • Education in EMS Compared to Other Health Care Fields

	EMS	OTHER HEALTH CARE FIELDS
Source of content for instructors to teach	National standard curricula	Education standards
Location of education programs	FR, EMT-B, EMT-I: typically stand-alone Paramedic: often, but not always, affiliated with college or university	Accredited college or university
Qualifications of instructors	Licensed or certified at level being taught High school diploma May or may not have degree	Licensed or certified at level being taught Master's or doctoral degree
Examination for certification or licensure	EMT-B and paramedic: mostly National Registry exam FR and EMT-I: many state-developed exams	National board exam
Interstate recognition	If applicant has NREMT card, usually quick and easy; if not, often must take state exam	Since applicant must have national certification, no additional exam necessary
Student selection process	FR and EMT: must be at least 18 years old (usually); preadmission testing rare; very few applicants turned away; some courses canceled because not enough applicants EMT-I: variable Paramedic: often tested for academic ability; positions sometimes competitive	Formal testing of academic ability; always more applicants than positions; highest performers admitted, others turned away
Education infrastructure (classrooms, equipment, supplies, clinical opportunities, library, counseling, financial aid, etc.)	FR and EMT-B: very limited; depends on time, talents, and resources of instructor EMT-I: variable Paramedic: if accredited program, access to all resources of college	Access to all resources of college
Student outcomes	FR and EMT-B: few instructors fail students, leaving certification exam to filter out incompetent providers; 50 percent never practice in EMS EMT-I: variable EMT-P: variable unless program accredited; majority find employment in field	Stringent academic standards; achievement at less than required level leads to expulsion from program Overwhelming majority find employment in field

EMS instructors typically have associates or bachelor's degrees rather than more advanced graduate degrees. They have usually completed an instructor course approved by their state EMS office. They must write lesson plans from scratch, based on the U.S. DOT national standard curricula, which include specific learning objectives and detailed content outlines. Many busy instructors use lesson plans developed by others, often the publishers of EMS textbooks.

Teaching other health care programs is usually a full-time position. Teaching EMT courses is typically something EMS instructors do in addition to their regular jobs, which limits the time they have for writing lesson plans and making other course preparations. Unless the EMS instructor teaches at a college or university, he or she often has little in the way of resources to draw on.

According to the State of EMS Education Research Project, conducted by the National Association of EMS Educators, many EMT-Basic (EMT-B) instructors are basically one-person operations. Although a few people may help teach skill labs, the EMT-B instructor takes care of not only teaching but also photocopying, maintaining equipment, performing clerical tasks, counseling students, and just about anything else an instructor might be called upon to do. Perhaps the most surprising result of these challenges is that EMS instructors manage to teach EMT classes that produce good, and often excellent, EMTs.

Students in other health care programs have to fill out extensive applications in order to be accepted as a student, and the programs select students who have demonstrated ability and achievement. Many applicants are denied entrance to such a program, either because they are not qualified or because there are not enough open spots in the program to accommodate all qualified applicants. In EMS, however there are few prerequisites for entrance into First Responder and EMT courses. Sometimes, especially in sparsely populated rural areas, courses are canceled for lack of sufficient students.

When a student in another health care profession enrolls in that profession's education program, he or she knows that the academic standards are rigorous and that, without significant effort, there is a real risk of failing the program and not being allowed to take the national board examination. When a student completes an EMS course, even if he or she has performed poorly (or even failed the course), many instructors nonetheless allow the student to take the certification or licensure exam. This is particularly true at the First Responder and EMT-B levels. Accredited paramedic courses, however, follow an approach very much like that of other health care professions' education programs.

The national board examination that other health care students take is the single certification exam that all students, nationwide, must pass before they can apply for state licensure. EMS does not have a nationally recognized certification exam, but the National Registry of EMTs has been working toward this and has made significant progress, especially at the EMT-B and paramedic levels.

After health care students graduate, pass the board examination, and get licensed in a state, they typically find employment in their field—except in EMS. According to the Longitudinal EMT Attribute and Demographic Study (LEADS), 50 percent of EMT-Bs never practice in EMS. At the paramedic level, this is much less common, probably because of the greater investment the student must make in terms of time and money.

States currently recognize more than 40 levels of EMS personnel. All states recognize EMT-Bs as having fairly similar scopes of practice. The same is true of paramedics. This is not the case with other levels. Many states license First Responders, with some modest variations on what they can do. Most states have at least one level between EMT and paramedic, but some states have none and some have two or more. These levels have widely varying scopes of practice. A First Responder, EMT, or paramedic who moves from one state to another can usually gain recognition of his or her previous EMS education without having to take the course again. An EMT-Intermediate, or any person with a licensure level between EMT-B and paramedic, often has a much more difficult time.

One of the areas in which EMS has made some progress is in accreditation. The Commission on Accreditation of Allied Health Education Programs accredits more than 200 paramedic programs through the Committee on Accreditation of Educational Programs for the EMS Professions (CoAEMSP). There are no accreditation programs for First Responder and EMT-B courses. Accredited paramedic programs must demonstrate they have the resources necessary to provide a quality education, including qualified faculty, adequate physical plant, sufficient equipment and supplies, effective evaluations of both students and the program itself, appropriate clinical sites, and responsiveness to the needs of the community, to name just a few.

EMS EDUCATION IN THE FUTURE

Predicting the future is always a risky business, but the planning the EMS community has done over the last five years will soon pay off. The most significant changes in EMS education will most likely be a result of the EMS Education Agenda. The system of five components that the Agenda calls for (review Figure C-2) will affect virtually every aspect of how a student becomes an EMS professional.

Most states will probably adopt the four levels of EMS personnel called for by the Agenda. The Emergency Medical Responder (EMR) will replace the First Responder, EMT will replace EMT-Basic, Advanced EMT will replace EMT-Intermediate, and Paramedic will replace EMT-Paramedic.

When states actually make these changes will depend on a number of factors. For the transition to be orderly, there will need to be close coordination among states, the National Registry, and publishers, among others. A state cannot implement a new level until a certification exam is ready. At the same time, if the exam is ready long before the states are, there will be significant confusion. Instructors cannot teach courses unless they have textbooks and support materials available. Fortunately, the National Association of State EMS Officials has recognized these challenges and has been coordinating with the different groups to ensure that there will be a smooth transition. The National Registry has already discussed with state EMS offices when a good time would be to change from the existing exams to the new exams. Because of the potential for great confusion during this change, the Registry plans to discontinue an exam when its replacement is available. In other words, unlike the last time the national standard curricula were revised, there is no plan for an overlap in availability of old and new exams for any particular level.

All three of these groups (states, National Registry, publishers) are implementing plans to ease the EMS community through the transition. State EMS offices are reviewing necessary changes to laws, rules, regulations, and protocols. They are also looking at how to update instructors. The National Registry is expanding its item bank so that it will have enough exam questions for its computer-based test. Publishers are revising their textbooks and also considering how to assist instructors. For example, since the education standards will not have specific learning objectives or detailed content outlines, publishers are looking at how to create lesson plans that cover these standards.

No state is obligated to follow the EMS Education Agenda. Although doing so would improve coordination and ease reciprocity, it is ultimately up to each state to determine how best to provide its citizens and visitors with quality prehospital care. There are advantages to implementing the Agenda, but it is possible that some states may decide they are not able or not willing to do so. One of the effects of such a decision would be to make it more difficult for EMS personnel licensed in one state to gain licensure in another state.

Nevertheless, it is expected that the vast majority of states will adopt the Agenda and participate in a system of EMS education that should result in more consistent education and evaluation.

How EMS education will be delivered may see some changes. It remains to be seen what the appropriate role of distance education is in EMS initial education. Distance programs in continuing education, however, have grown significantly over a relatively short period of time. As simulation mannequins, computer simulations, and similar devices (Figures C-4 and C-5) become better, less expensive, and more available, they may play a strong role in providing EMS students with consistent, controlled educational experiences.

When states begin using the new personnel levels, there will be some changes to the scope of practice for each level. For example, at the EMT level, students will learn how to use pulse oximetry. This is a skill most EMT-Bs already use, but it is not included in the EMT-B national standard curriculum. Other additions include EMT administration of aspirin; humidifiers, partial rebreather masks, and Venturi masks in oxygen administration; automated transport ventilators for ventilating patients at consistent rates with appropriate pressures; automated blood pressure monitors; assisting a patient in administering his or her own prescribed medications (including, but not limited to, auto-injectors); and mechanical devices for compressions and ventilations in CPR (Table C-2).

The Emergency Medical Responder (EMR), who will replace the First Responder of today, will learn how to administer unit-dose auto-injectors for care of oneself or one's peer (e.g., MARK I), take a manual blood pressure, ventilate with a bag-valve mask, and administer oxygen by means of a nasal cannula and nonrebreather mask (Table C-3).

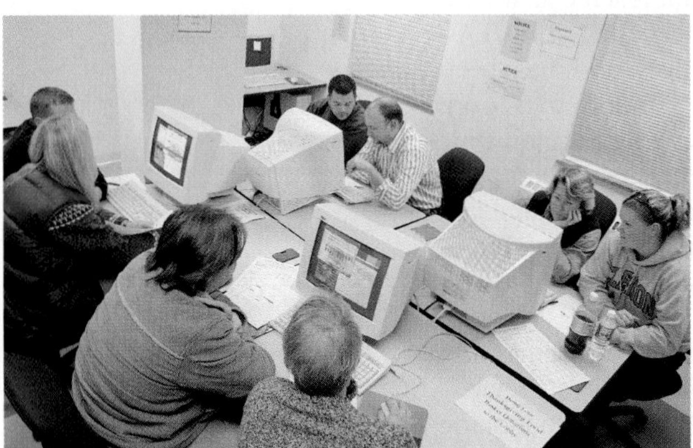

Figure C-4 • EMS education of the future will make more and more use of technical aids such as computer simulations.

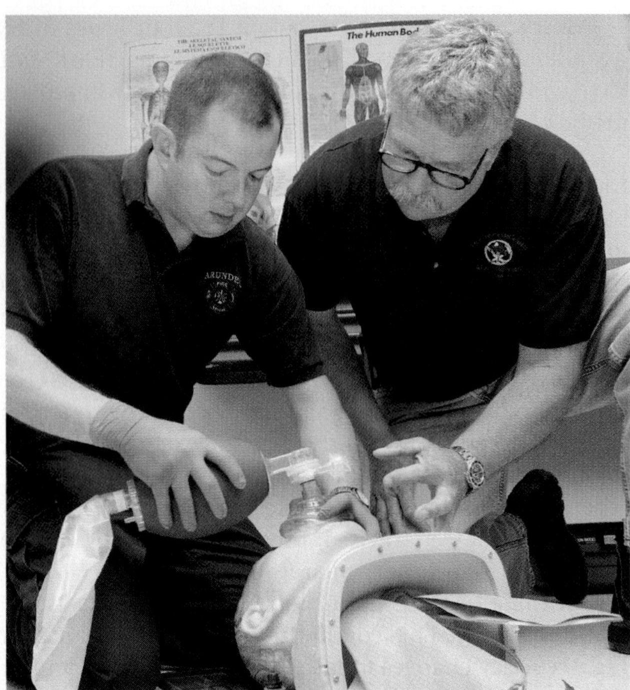

Figure C-5 • Simulation mannequins help students practice skills such as airway maintenance and ventilation.

TABLE C-2 • Additions to EMT Scope of Practice
Pulse oximetry
Aspirin
Humidifiers
Partial rebreather masks
Venturi mask
Automatic Transport Ventilator (ATV)
Automated BP
Assisting a patient in administering his/her own prescribed medications (including auto-injection)
Mechanical CPR devices

TABLE C-3 • Additions to First Responder Scope of Practice to Reach EMR Level
Unit dose auto-injectors for self or peer care (MARK I)
Manual BP
BVM
Oxygen therapy, including nasal cannula and nonrebreather face mask

The Advanced EMT (AEMT), who will replace the EMT-Intermediate, will have a number of skills beyond the EMT level, including: multilumen airways (e.g., Combitube) and supraglottic airways (e.g., LMA and King LT); blood glucose monitoring; insertion of peripheral intravenous lines; intraosseous access (insertion of a needle into a bone to gain vascular access) in children; nitroglycerin for chest pain of suspected ischemic origin; subcutaneous or intramuscular injection of epinephrine for anaphylaxis; intramuscular glucagon and intravenous dextrose for hypoglycemia; inhaled beta agonist (e.g., albuterol) for shortness of breath with wheezing; narcotic antagonist (antidote) for narcotic overdose; and inhaled nitrous oxide for relief of pain (Table C-4).

TABLE C-4 • Interventions in the AEMT Scope of Practice beyond EMT Level
Multilumen and supraglottic airways
Blood glucose monitoring
Peripheral IV lines
Pediatric intraosseous (IO) access
Nitroglycerin for chest pain of suspected ischemic origin
Epinephrine for anaphylaxis
Glucagon and IV dextrose for hypoglycemia
Inhaled beta agonist for dyspnea and wheezing
Narcotic antagonist
Nitrous oxide for pain relief

TABLE C-5 • Interventions in the Paramedic Scope of Practice beyond AEMT Level
Endotracheal intubation
Percutaneous cricothyrotomy
Decompress the pleural space
Gastric decompression
Enteral and parenteral administration of approved prescription medications
Access indwelling catheters and implanted central IV ports for fluid and medication administration
Administer medications by IV infusion
Maintain an infusion of blood or blood products

The paramedic level will see the addition of a few skills, but it is probably easier to understand what a paramedic can do if we look at the paramedic skills that will be beyond the AEMT level. These include endotracheal intubation, percutaneous cricothyrotomy (i.e., creating an airway with a needle into the trachea, but not a scalpel), decompression of the pleural space (insertion of a needle between the ribs to relieve a tension pneumothorax), gastric decompression (insertion of a tube down the esophagus into the stomach to relieve gastric distention), administration of approved prescription medications, accessing indwelling catheters and implanted central IV ports for fluid and medication administration, administration of medications by IV infusion, and maintaining an infusion of blood or blood products (but not starting such an infusion) (Table C-5).

One change we can be sure of is that states will have some kind of organized system for bringing EMT-Bs up-to-date on the changes in the EMT scope of practice. In many states, this will probably take the form of a short transition course. In others, the same thing may be accomplished by a requirement for continuing education of a specific type. Still other states may have other means of achieving the same goal.

What other changes are in store for EMS education? It is difficult to say. A new group, the National EMS Advisory Council, will make some suggestions. However, since this group was taking shape just as this book went to press, it is not possible to say what kinds of changes they may recommend to the Department of Transportation. There are a number of possibilities.

Considering the continuing pressure on hospitals to discharge patients earlier, it is likely that more patients will be sent home with high tech equipment. EMS personnel will need to adapt to these changes and have at least a basic understanding of how to intervene when a potential problem occurs.

The threat of terrorist acts affecting public health has made many state health departments and EMS offices consider how EMS personnel might be employed during a public health emergency. Such an expanded role would not necessarily be limited to terrorist acts. If pandemic influenza strikes, there may be significant changes to EMS functions and operations.

Between 20 and 30 years ago, EMS began transporting trauma patients directly to trauma centers instead of other hospitals under certain circumstances. These patients were not that common. Now, there are movements to use the same kind of approach for patients with certain cardiac problems and strokes, problems that EMS sees every day. Frequent extended transports may mean big changes for EMS, although these will probably involve more operational than educational changes.

The question of which patients should receive spine immobilization in the field and who should make that decision is receiving more and more attention. As data accumulate, we may be able to make defensible, evidence-based decisions about being selective with this intervention.

Continuing strain on the health care system may, of course, lead to completely unexpected and unpredictable changes. Perhaps an advanced paramedic practitioner will significantly expand the scope of interventions available to EMS. Perhaps personnel at existing levels will see their responsibilities and scopes of practice change in response to different pressures.

One change that is very unlikely to occur on a routine basis is EMS personnel making decisions about which patients do and don't need transport. The evidence to date suggests strongly that EMS personnel are not able to make these decisions accurately today. Providing sufficient additional clinical expertise to allow for this would be a significant challenge, particularly in today's health care environment where it is becoming progressively more difficult for EMS students to gain access to clinical sites. Similarly, it is unlikely that there will be significant expansion of EMS scopes of practice within a short time. Suggestions for such changes will very probably go through the system advocated by the EMS Education Agenda, where the EMS community considers the benefits, risks, and other effects on the EMS system and its patients before adopting such changes.

One thing we can be sure of: States and regions will continue to experiment with different interventions. These research projects are the best way for the EMS system to grow in a responsible manner so that patients will receive the best prehospital care possible.

ANSWER KEY

The following are text questions and answers/discussion suggestions for Critical Decision Making, a feature within the narrative, and for end-of-chapter Review Questions, Critical Thinking Questions, and Street Scene Questions.

CHAPTER 1 INTRODUCTION TO EMERGENCY MEDICAL CARE

Critical Decision Making: A Key Concept

Critical decision making essentially means that an EMT takes in information from the scene, the patient assessment, and other sources and makes appropriate decisions after synthesizing—or interpreting all of—the information. . . . Some examples of critical decision making:

Q1: *Deciding which hospital to transport someone to.* Should you take your patient to the closest hospital or to a more distant specialty hospital?

Q2: *Deciding whether you should administer a medication to a patient.* Will it help the patient's current condition? Could it make the condition worse?

For discussion: What information would you gather to help you make decisions like these? (Responses will vary.)

Review Questions

Q1: What are the components of the Emergency Medical Services system?
A1: *The components are 911 and emergency medical dispatchers, First Responders, EMTs (all levels) and ambulances, emergency department, and other hospital units.*

Q2: What are some of the special designations that hospitals may have? List them. Then name the special centers you have in your region.
A2: *Trauma center, burn center, pediatric care center, poison control center, cardiac center, and stroke center. (Responses will vary for your area.)*

Q3: What are the four national levels of EMS training and certification?
A3: *First Responder, EMT, EMT-Intermediate, EMT-Paramedic.*

Q4: What are the roles and responsibilities of the EMT?
A4: *Safety of the crew, patient, and bystanders; patient assessment; patient care; lifting and moving; transport; transfer of care; and patient advocacy.*

Q5: What are desirable personal and physical attributes of the EMT?
A5: *Be in good health and able to lift and carry up to 125 pounds; good eyesight and hearing; able to clearly communicate in written and oral form; pleasant; sincere; cooperative; resourceful; a self-starter; emotionally stable; able to lead; and neat and clean. (Students might offer additional desirable attributes from the textbook.)*

Q6: What is the definition of the term *quality improvement*?
A6: *A process of continuous self-review with the purpose of identifying and correcting aspects of the system that require improvement.*

Q7: What is the difference between on-line and off-line medical direction?
A7: *In on-line medical direction, the on-duty physician gives orders directly to the EMT by telephone or radio. In off-line medical direction, the EMT carries out written standing orders from the Medical Director.*

Critical Thinking

Q1: What qualities would you like to see in an EMT who is caring for you? How can you come closer to being this kind of EMT?
A1: *Responses will vary.*

Q2: You are devoting a considerable amount of time to becoming an EMT. How do you plan to refresh your knowledge and stay current once you are out of the classroom?
A2: *By taking advantage of conferences, seminars, lectures, classes, videotapes, and demonstrations.*

Street Scenes

Q1: What would have been a more appropriate action for Chuck when the shift started?
A1: *Students should understand that Chuck Hartley has a professional responsibility to set a good example for the new EMT. He should arrive in a well-kept uniform and involve the new EMT in all aspects of the job. For example, a new EMT should help check the ambulance and equipment at the start of the shift. An explanation of operating procedures should also be provided. In other words, a new EMT needs to know what is expected of him or her.*

Q2: What behavior characteristics of Chuck's would be considered unprofessional?
A2: *Chuck Hartley exhibits numerous unprofessional behavior characteristics. They include: an unkempt uniform, telling the new EMT to sit until he or she is needed, failure to introduce himself to the patient, referring to the patient as "Hon," loudly criticizing the new EMT, and dismissal of patient concerns (instructing her to tell the doctor).*

Q3: What would you expect from someone providing initial field training?
A3: *Ask students to brainstorm a list of their expectations. That is, what characteristics would they hope to find in the EMTs who will train them? Answers might include the following:*

- *Good communication skills.*
- *Neat and well-kept appearance.*
- *Polite and courteous behavior, both with other EMTs and with patients.*
- *Willingness to explain the job.*
- *Understanding of the needs of a new EMT (empathy).*
- *Good patient skills.*
- *Willingness to act as a team player.*

Q4: What did Susan Miller do that was appropriate and professional?
A4: *Susan Miller came to work in a well-pressed uniform. She expressed an obvious interest and memory of the new EMT and communicated job expectations in a clear manner. She set an example by providing an orientation to the ambulance, equipment, and agency procedures. She made the new intern a part of the call and provided numerous examples of professional patient care. She monitored actions taken by the new EMT, making every effort not to belittle the person. When the call was completed, Susan took time to critique the run, reinforcing the skills needed to become a good EMT.*

Q5: How was Susan's behavior beneficial to you as a new EMT?

A5: *Answers will vary, but most students will note the points mentioned in the preceding question. The basic concept is this: Susan set a good professional standard and served as a role model for the EMT to follow.*

Q6: What personal traits are the professional standards for EMTs?

A6: *Ask students to brainstorm a list of personal traits that they hope to develop as professional EMTs. Students might use descriptive adjectives or phrases such as "pleasant," "sincere," "cooperative," "neat," "respectful," "good listener," "sense of initiative," and so on.*

CHAPTER 2 THE WELL-BEING OF THE EMT

Critical Decision Making: Standard Precautions

Some of the most important decisions you will make have to do with routine things such as Standard Precautions. Many decisions about the level of precautions will be taken during the scene size-up. Others are taken throughout the call. Examples include:

Q1: When called to a motor vehicle collision where you observe broken glass, you should expect broken skin and the potential for contact with blood—even if you don't see wounds. Vinyl gloves to protect you from blood as well as heavy-duty gloves to protect you from the broken glass are prudent.

Q2: When called to a nursing home for an interfacility transfer, you must reach under the patient to move the person to your stretcher. Because of the possibility of contact with urine, feces, or bed sores, you should wear vinyl gloves.

Q3: You are called to a patient with a sprained ankle. There are no open wounds. Guidelines indicate that no precautions are necessary, although many routinely wear gloves on all calls.

Q4: You are working with an advanced life support crew treating a patient with chest pain. While there are no open wounds, the paramedic started an IV and some blood is present on the patient's forearm from the IV start and a small amount is seen on the IV tubing. Gloves are required.

Q5: You are treating a patient with chest pain who suddenly becomes unresponsive. The patient requires suction. In addition to the gloves you may already be wearing you will now need to protect your face from spatter encountered in airway and suction procedures.

For discussion: What similar situations would call for these or other Standard Precautions? (Answers will vary.)

Review Questions

Q1: Name some of the causes of stress for an EMT and explain some ways the EMT can alleviate job-related stress.

A1: *Causes of stress may include multiple-casualty incidents, injuries to infants and children, severe injuries, abuse and neglect, the death of a coworker, or personal situations.*

Ways to reduce job-related stress include developing more healthful and positive dietary habits, exercising, relaxing, and changing the shift you are working or area to which you are assigned. Seek professional assistance if necessary.

Q2: Describe the purpose and process of a critical incident stress debriefing (CISD).

A2: *The purpose of CISD is to assist emergency care workers in dealing with the stress that is related to a major incident. It is held within 24 to 72 hours after an incident and is an open discussion of the feelings experienced during and after the call. All information is confidential. Follow-up is provided by a peer member of the team within 24 hours after the CISD.*

Q3: What are the stages of grief? How should the EMT deal with these emotions?
A3: *Denial—The patient denies the fact that he or she is dying.*
Anger—The patient becomes angry.
Bargaining—The patient tries to postpone death, even if only briefly.
Depression—The patient is sad or in despair over things left undone.
Acceptance—The patient is ready to die.
Understanding what the families and the patients go through can help an EMT deal with the stress they feel as well as his or her own emotions.

Q4: List the types of personal protective equipment used in Standard Precautions. Identify a condition or patient with which each one should be used.
A4: *Protective gloves—Used with controlled bleeding, suctioning, artificial ventilation, CPR.*
Eye protection—Used with splashing, spattering, or spraying body fluids.
Masks—Used with infections spread by airborne droplets (measles).
Gowns—Used with arterial bleeding, childbirth.

Critical Thinking

Q: You are called to an unknown emergency at a tavern. As you approach the scene, you see a man lying supine in the parking lot, apparently bleeding profusely. Two other men are scuffling, and one seems to have a gun. What actions must you take?
A: *Unless you stay safe, you will not be able to help your patient and you may suffer serious injury—or die. Retreat to a safe place and call for a response by law enforcement. Approach the patient only when they inform you that the scene is safe.*

Street Scenes

Q1: Why wear protective gloves on this type of call?
A1: *The patient has bad facial injuries that may bring the EMT into contact with blood and other body fluids. As emphasized in the text, gloves help minimize possible exposure to bloodborne pathogens. Intact skin can offer some protection in case of accidental exposure. In this case, however, the EMT is aware of a partially healed cut on his hand, making the potential risk of exposure even greater if no gloves are worn.*

Q2: What is the impact of an occupational exposure on you, your family, and your fellow EMS workers?
A2: *Answers will vary. However, students should understand the devastating effects of occupational exposure, especially the possibility of transferring the disease to family members and/or fellow EMS workers. In addition, occupational exposure can cause considerable anxiety as an EMT waits to determine if he or she has actually gotten the disease. Some students may also note the side effects of prescribed medications to treat the disease.*

Q3: What can you expect after exposure?
A3: *Students should understand the importance of notifying their supervisor. Ask them to brainstorm what they think will occur next. Compare their responses against the actions listed in the two paragraphs following Question 3—occupational evaluation at the emergency department, physical examination, baseline blood tests, and so on.*

Q4: How will stress be a factor in your life for the next few months?
A4: *Answers will vary, but most students will note the anxiety of awaiting test results. They may also indicate strained marital relationships and the tension created by an inability to talk to coworkers, out of either fear or embarrassment.*

Q5: How important is hand washing?
A5: *Answers should reflect information in the text, noting the importance of hand washing as a first-line defense against infection.*

Q6: What type of Standard Precautions should EMTs always be ready to use on all EMS calls?

A6: *At a minimum, all EMTs should have gloves and eye protection immediately available. Students might mention gowns and other protective gear as well.*

CHAPTER 3 MEDICAL/LEGAL AND ETHICAL ISSUES

Critical Decision Making: Ethical Dilemmas

Not all critical or difficult decisions you make will be clinical in nature. You may be faced with an ethical dilemma that will test your decision-making skills. For each of the situations listed below describe how you would handle the situation.

Q1: You are driving the ambulance to the hospital and listening to the conversation in the back between a paramedic and an EMT. You hear the paramedic say, "Oh, no! I can't believe I just did that. I gave her 10 times the dose I was supposed to." You hear the paramedic ask the EMT not to tell anyone. What do you do?

A1: *You have an ethical responsibility to tell the truth about what you heard. If this event isn't reported, harm could come to the patient. While reporting fellow EMTs is not popular, it might be possible to talk to the provider who made the mistake and encourage him to tell the truth.*

Q2: You are on the way home from a sporting event. While there you had two drinks. You come across a crash with injury. What do you do?

A2: *Providing care while you are intoxicated is a recipe for disaster. Considering how large the drinks were and how long ago you had them would help to determine if you were intoxicated. Some recommend not stopping if you have consumed any alcohol. How would you feel as a patient if you smelled alcohol on the breath of an EMT treating you?*

Q3: A patient tells you that he received the injury you are treating while climbing a fence after being involved in a break-in at a local business. The patient swears he was just the lookout, and if anyone knows he told he may be killed. What do you do?

A3: *Unfortunately you have no way of knowing if the patient is even telling the truth. Most would recommend reporting this to the police. Follow your local guidelines and protocols.*

Review Questions

Q1: Define *scope of practice, negligence, duty to act, abandonment,* and *confidentiality.*

A1: *Scope of Practice—a set of regulations and ethical considerations that define the scope, or extent and limits, of the EMT's job.*
Negligence—a finding of failure to act properly in a situation in which there was a duty to act, needed care as would reasonably be expected of the EMT was not provided, and harm was caused to the patient as a result.
Duty to Act—an obligation to provide care to a patient.
Abandonment—leaving a patient after care has been initiated and before the patient has been transferred to someone with equal or greater medical training.
Confidentiality—the obligation not to reveal information obtained about a patient except to other health care professionals involved in the patient's care, or under subpoena, or in a court of law, or when the patient has signed a release of confidentiality.

Q2: List several steps that must be taken when a patient refuses care or transportation.

A2:
1) *The patient must be mentally competent and oriented.*
2) *The patient must be fully informed and understand the risks associated with refusing treatment and/or transport.*
3) *The patient must sign a "release" form.*

Q3: List several types of evidence and ways you may act to preserve it at a crime scene.

A3: *Types of evidence include the condition of the scene, the condition of the patient, fingerprints and footprints, and microscopic evidence.*

You can help to preserve evidence by remembering what you touch, minimizing your impact on the scene, and working with the police.

Critical Thinking

Q: You are called to the scene of a motor-vehicle collision. An 8-year-old child has been struck by a vehicle and fortunately has sustained only slight injuries. Who can give consent for her care? How might you obtain consent?

A: *Her parents, guardians, or caretakers can give it. If these individuals are not on the scene, ask the child how to contact them. If contact is not immediately possible, their consent to treat the child is implied.*

Street Scenes

Q1: Was it appropriate not to include the information that the patient has AIDS during the radio report to the hospital?

A1: *As explained in the text, EMTs should consider all patient information as confidential. Radio transmissions can be monitored. Therefore, the EMT should share only data directly related to immediate care. In this particular situation, the presence of AIDS has no direct bearing on the care steps initiated in the field. As a result, hospital staff does not need to know about the presence of AIDS at this time. (Note to Instructor: Reinforce the devastating consequences of any breach of patient confidentiality.)*

Q2: What is the obligation of these EMTs concerning the confidentiality of patient information?

A2: *Answers will vary, but should reflect the ideas stated in the chapter. New EMTs must understand that all patient information should be treated as confidential and should not be released except with written permission or upon request by legal subpoena.*

Q3: Would you have handled the transfer of information differently?

A3: *Answers will vary. (Note to Instructor: This question is intended to stimulate discussion. Students may offer various approaches, but each one should be geared at protecting the patient's confidentiality.)*

Q4: Would it be appropriate to tell all the hospital staff so they would know to take infection control precautions?

A4: *No. This information is not relevant to providing immediate patient care. Infection control precautions should be the standard in any medical institution and should not rely upon information supplied by the EMT.*

Q5: Should the information that this patient has AIDS be shared with other EMS providers in case they get a call for this patient?

A5: *No. Again, this would be a breach of patient confidentiality. Not only is this action inappropriate, sharing information may carry some legal consequences, especially if it has a negative impact on the patient. (For example, the patient's medical history might become public knowledge or even affect the willingness of some individuals to treat the patient.)*

Q6: What are the principles for confidentiality that EMTs should always maintain?

A6: *Answers should reflect the ideas in the chapter. (Note to Instructor: If a situation arises in which an EMT is asked to share information [e.g., releasing a patient care report], he or she might consult at attorney concerning local, state, and federal requirements/laws related to patient confidentiality. Also, you might encourage students to explore local protocols on this matter.)*

CHAPTER 4 THE HUMAN BODY

Critical Decision Making: Identifying Possible Areas of Injury

For each of the following patients identify what organ or body system may be involved in that patient's complaint.

Q1: Your patient falls in an icy parking lot. She tries to catch herself and breaks the bones of the arm just above the wrist. What are these bones called?
A1: *Radius and ulna.*

Q2: Your patient was the driver of a car that was hit in a "T-bone," or side impact, crash. He was the driver. He complains of pain in the left upper abdominal quadrant. What organ is located in this area that can cause severe internal bleeding?
A2: *The spleen.*

Q3: Your patient was riding a motorcycle and was thrown over the handlebars in a crash. She has broken the large bone in her right thigh. What bone is this, and would you expect blood loss from the fracture?
A3: *The femur. Yes, blood loss can exceed 1 liter.*

Review Questions

Q1: Define the following anatomical terms: *medial, anterior, mid-clavicular, lateral, posterior, distal.*
A1: *Medial—toward the vertical midline of the body.*
Anterior—the front of the body or body part.
Mid-clavicular—the center of each clavicle.
Lateral—to the side, away from the vertical midline of the body.
Posterior—the back of the body or body part.
Distal—farther away from the torso.

Q2: List the three functions of the musculoskeletal system.
A2: *1) To give the body shape.*
2) To protect vital internal organs.
3) To provide for body movement.

Q3: Name the five divisions of the spine and describe the location of each.
A3: *Cervical—neck.*
Thoracic—upper back.
Lumbar—lower back.
Sacral—back wall of pelvis.
Coccyx—tailbone.

Q4: Describe the physical processes of inhalation and exhalation.
A4: *Inhalation is an active process. The intercostal (rib) muscles and the diaphragm contract. The diaphragm lowers and the ribs move upward and outward. This expands the size of the chest cavity, causing air to flow into the lungs.*
Exhalation is a passive process during which the intercostal muscles and the diaphragm relax. The ribs move downward and inward, while the diaphragm rises. This movement causes the chest cavity to decrease in size and forces air from the lungs.

Q5: List four places a peripheral pulse may be felt.
A5: *1) The thumb side of the wrist.*
2) The inside of the arm between the elbow and shoulder.
3) The back of the inside part of the ankle.
4) The top of the foot.

Q6: Describe the central nervous system and peripheral nervous system.
A6: *The central nervous system is comprised of the brain and spinal cord. The peripheral nervous system consists of two types of nerves: sensory and motor.*

Q7: List three functions of the skin.
A7: *Three functions are 1. protection; 2. temperature regulation; 3. sensation.*
[Note: Students may list other functions that are covered in the chapter but not the lecture.]

Critical Thinking

Q: As an EMT, you are called to respond to a teenage boy who has taken a hard fall from his dirt bike. He has a deep gash on the outside of his left arm about halfway between the shoulder and the elbow and another on the inside of his right arm just above the wrist. His left leg is bent at a funny angle about halfway between hip and knee, and when you cut away his pants leg, you see a bone sticking out of a wound on the front side. You take the necessary on-scene assessment and care steps and are on the way to the hospital in the ambulance. How do you describe the patient's injuries over the radio to the hospital staff?
A: *Sample Response: The patient has a deep laceration on the posterior surface of his left arm and a deep laceration on the interior surface of his right forearm, proximal to the wrist. The patient's left thigh is painful, swollen, and deformed with bone ends protruding through the anterior surface.*

Street Scenes

Q1: As you assess your young patient, how does his anatomy impact on the process?
A1: *Answers will vary. However, students should understand that knowledge of the patient's anatomy is key to effective assessment and care. Use of anatomical terms and landmarks also provides a "common language" for communication among EMS personnel and other members of the medical community, such as hospital staff. In this particular case, knowledge of the relationship between the tongue and the mandible helped the EMT to decide upon the correct airway maneuvers—manual stabilization of the head and neck, movement of the jaw forward, and movement of the tongue in the direction of the mandible.*

Q2: What should you be alert to when examining the abdomen?
A2: *In examining the abdomen, the EMT should inspect for discoloration, guarding, or tenderness. If the patient experiences pain, the EMT should also try to identify the quadrant in which the pain is located. The location of pain, coupled with other anatomical knowledge, can help identify possible internal injury. In this scenario, pain in the upper left quadrant and a bruise, possibly from the lap portion of the seat belt, lead the EMT to suspect injury to the spleen.*

Q3: What are the significant findings based on the assessment and your knowledge of the human body?
A3: *The initial findings indicate that there may be abdominal injury, possibly to the spleen. Because the spleen is vascular, there could be a significant amount of blood loss (hence the concern with changing vital signs). The EMT is also concerned with possible spinal injury, confirmed by the patient's reaction to touch. (<u>Note to Instructor:</u> Reinforce that the abdomen is less protected in the pediatric patient than in the adult patient. As a result, internal injury to a child such as the one in the scenario can be quite severe.)*

Q4: Do you have any concerns about additional injuries to this patient? If so, what are they?
A4: *As noted in Question 3, the EMT should suspect the possibility of cervical spine injury in the lower back (lumbar region). Relevant reasons include the patient's age, the force of the crash, and the patient's reaction when touched in the lumbar region of the spine.*

CHAPTER 5 LIFTING AND MOVING PATIENTS

Critical Decision Making: Choosing a Patient-Carrying Device

For each of the following patients, choose a carrying device to get the patient from the scene to the ambulance stretcher:

Q1: A patient complaining of severe respiratory distress who is in an upstairs back bedroom.
A1: *Use a stair chair unless his injury is so severe he can't sit up or requires ventilation. Then a Reeves-type stretcher is a better option.*

Q2: A patient thrown from an ATV several hundred yards into the woods.
A2: *Place a backboard (long spine board) in a Stokes (wire frame) basket for transport out of the woods.*

Q3: A patient who fell down several stairs from the back deck to the concrete landing. He complains of neck and back pain.
A3: *Place the patient on a backboard (long spine board).*

Q4: An unresponsive medical patient found down a narrow hallway on the first floor.
A4: *Using a Reeves-type device would allow two EMTs to carry the patient out of the hallway to the stretcher.*

Review Questions

Q1: Define the term *body mechanics*. Then describe several principles of body mechanics related to safe lifting and moving.
A1: *Body mechanics is the proper use of the body to facilitate lifting and moving. Principles of body mechanics include:*

- *Position your feet properly, shoulder-width apart.*
- *When lifting, use your legs, not your back, to do the lifting.*
- *When lifting, never twist or attempt to make any moves other than the lift.*
- *When lifting with one hand, do not compensate.*
- *Keep the weight as close to your body as possible.*
- *When carrying a patient on stairs, use a stair chair instead of a stretcher when possible.*

Q2: List several situations that may require an emergency move of a patient.
A2: *The scene is hazardous; care of life-threatening conditions requires repositioning; or other patients must be reached.*

Q3: Describe several lifts and drags.
A3: *Lifts include the extremity lift; the direct ground lift, the draw-sheet method; and the direct carry method. Drags include the shoulder drag, the foot drag, the "fireman's drag," the incline drag, the clothes drag, and the blanket drag.*

Q4: Define a long-axis drag and explain its importance.
A4: *A long-axis drag is a drag from the shoulders of the patient that causes the remainder of the body to fall into its natural anatomical position, with the spine and all limbs in normal alignment. This emergency move minimizes or prevents aggravation of a spinal injury.*

Critical Thinking

Q: For each of the following patients, use the knowledge gained in this chapter to identify the appropriate procedure or device for lifting and moving that patient:

a. A patient who has fallen 18 feet and has suspected spinal injuries.

b. A patient with chest pain (with no spinal injury) who lives on the fifth floor of a building with no elevator.
c. A patient who is found in an environment with a risk of immediate explosion.

A: **a.** *A spine board.*
b. *A stair chair.*
c. *Shoulder drag.*

Street Scenes

Q1: What device should be used to remove the patient from the vehicle?
A1: *The EMT should apply a cervical collar and a short immobilization device. After conducting the necessary neuro exams, the patient should be rotated onto a long board.*

Q2: What patient-care issues are important when using an extrication device?
A2: *Sample patient-care issues include negative impact on the airway or breathing and patient discomfort. Point out that the cervical collar should not be applied too tightly and that the short board straps should not restrict respirations. When rotating the patient onto the long board, the leg straps of the short immobilization device may need to be loosened to prevent patient discomfort.*

Q3: What is the next thing to consider when actually moving the patient from the vehicle?
A3: *The key to moving any patient is a well-coordinated team effort. The EMT who is providing head stabilization needs to announce all the moves. For example, he or she might say, "Slide the patient onto the long board on the count of three." The crew must continually monitor the patient, especially the ABCs and any change in the level of consciousness. A quick neuro exam should be done both before and after the move.*

Q4: What emergency-care equipment was used for this patient? Why?
A4: *Equipment included a cervical collar, short immobilization device (vest-type extrication device), long board, straps, head immobilizer, stretcher, and stretcher locking device. The equipment was selected based on local protocols for the mechanism of injury and for maximum patient safety (i.e., to protect against possible neck or spinal injury).*

Q5: What is the next step before moving this patient again?
A5: *The EMT should continue talking to the patient to make sure her level of responsiveness has not changed and no breathing difficulty has developed. A member of the crew should also perform another quick neuro exam, with the patient having pulses, movement, and sensation in all four extremities. Some students may also say that the EMTs should check straps to make sure that the patient is secured to the long board and that everyone knows what he or she should do to secure a smooth move.*

Q6: What other safety considerations should be considered when moving the long board to the wheeled stretcher?
A6: *Sample responses: Make sure the wheeled cot is held so that it does not move. Ensure that personnel carrying the backboard face in the same direction. If somebody needs to back up while placing the board on the stretcher, the person should be guided by placing a hand at his or her back. There should be sufficient personnel carrying the long board, and each person should keep a firm grip on the board until placed completely on the stretcher. The straps of the wheeled cot must be secured before the patient is moved.*

CHAPTER 6 AIRWAY MANAGEMENT

Critical Decision Making: Oxygen or Ventilation?

For each of the following patients, decide whether you would administer oxygen or ventilate the patient.

Q1: A patient who was found on the floor by a relative. He has no pulse or respirations.
A1: *Ventilate.*

Q2: A 14-year-old patient who has a broken femur. She is alert; pulse 110 strong and regular; respirations 28, rapid and deep.
A2: *Administer oxygen.*

Q3: A 64-year-old male with chest pain. He is alert; pulse 56; respirations 18 and normal.
A3: *Administer oxygen.*

Q4: A 78-year-old patient with COPD. He has had increasing difficulty breathing over the past few days. He responds verbally but is not oriented. His pulse is 124; respirations 36 and shallow.
A4: *Ventilate.*

Review Questions

Q1: Name the main structures of the airway.
A1: *Nose, mouth, pharynx, larynx, trachea, bronchi, and lungs.*

Q2: Explain why care for the airway is the first priority of emergency care.
A2: *Simply stated, patients without an adequate airway die.*

Q3: Name the signs of adequate breathing and of inadequate breathing.
A3: *Signs of adequate breathing include: adequate and equal expansion of both sides of the chest with inhalation; air entering and leaving the nose, mouth, and chest; breath sounds present and equal on both sides of the chest; sound from the mouth and nose should be typically free of gurgling, gasping, crowing, and wheezing; no blue or gray coloration of the skin; normal rate, rhythm, quality, depth of breathing typical for a person at rest.*

Signs of inadequate breathing include: Chest movements are absent, minimal, or uneven; movements associated with breathing are limited to the abdomen; no air can be felt or heard at the nose or mouth, or exchange is below normal; breath sounds are diminished or absent; noises such as wheezing, snoring, gurgling, or gasping are heard during breathing; the rate of breathing is too rapid or too slow; breathing is very shallow, very deep, or appears labored; the patient's skin, lips, tongue, earlobes, or nail beds are blue or gray; inspirations or expirations are prolonged; the patient has difficulty speaking; in children, there may be a pulling in of the muscles above the clavicles and between and below the ribs; nasal flaring may be present (especially in infants and children).

Q4: Explain when the head-tilt, chin-lift maneuver should be used and when the jaw-thrust maneuver should be used to open the airway—and why.
A4: *The head-tilt, chin-lift should be used in patients who do not have the possibility of a head, neck, or spinal injury. The jaw-thrust maneuver should be used whenever there is a possibility of head, neck, or spinal injury; this will help to prevent aggravating an injury to the central nervous system.*

Q5: Name the techniques of artificial ventilation in the recommended order of preference.
A5: *1. Mouth-to-mask; 2. two-person, bag-valve mask; 3. flow-restricted, oxygen-powered ventilation device; 4. one-person, bag-valve mask.*

Q6: Explain how airway adjuncts and suctioning help in airway management and artificial ventilation.
A6: *The main function of airway adjuncts (of the type covered in this chapter) is to keep the tongue from blocking the airway. Suctioning keeps the airway clear of foreign materials, blood, vomitus, and other secretions.*

Q7: Name patient problems that would benefit from administration of oxygen and explain how to decide whether a nonrebreather mask, nasal cannula, or Venturi mask should be used to deliver oxygen to a patient.

A7: *Patient problems that would benefit from oxygen include: respiratory or cardiac arrest; heart attacks and stroke; shock; blood loss; lung diseases; broken bones; head injuries; and any other serious illness or injury. Whenever possible, a nonrebreather mask should be used because it provides a higher concentration of oxygen than a nasal cannula or Venturi mask. A nasal cannula should only be used when a patient feels "suffocated" by a mask and refuses to wear one. A Venturi mask should be used when a specific concentration of oxygen is required.*

Critical Thinking

Q: On arrival at the emergency scene, you find an adult female patient with gurgling sounds in the throat and inadequate breathing slowing to almost nothing. How do you proceed to protect the airway and support the patient's breathing?

A: *Open the airway, suction, insert an airway adjunct, and ventilate using oxygen at 15 liters per minute.*

Street Scenes

Q1: What is your first priority when starting to assess this patient?

A1: *After a rapid check for responsiveness, the airway becomes the first and most important patient priority. (Note to Instructor: You might review and reinforce anatomical differences between the respiratory passages of an adult and a child.)*

Q2: What type of emergency care should you be prepared to give?

A2: *Because the child is about 2 years old, abdominal thrusts should be used. (Note to Instructor: You might point out that if the foreign body had not been expelled after the appropriate number of thrusts, the next step would have been to check the airway. If ALS is available, the EMTs should have already summoned support.)*

Q3: What equipment should you have taken into the house to make sure you are properly prepared for this call?

A3: *Stress that airway equipment, including suction, should be taken to the side of every patient. In this case, equipment should include appropriately sized pediatric masks, BVM, OPAs, and oxygen tubing.*

Q4: What is the best way to determine if the ventilations are adequate?

A4: *Chest rise is the best way to determine if the ventilations are adequate. Additional indicators include skin color and an increase in pulse rate. (Note to Instructor: A pulse oximeter can also be used, but time should never be taken away from providing ventilatory assistance in order to hook it up. Pulse oximetry will be covered at the end of Chapter 9, "Vital Signs and SAMPLE History.")*

Q5: What additional assessment should be done on this patient?

A5: *Additional assessment might include: observation of ventilations and respiratory effort and listening for sounds of noisy respirations. The goal is to support ventilations with a BVM and blow-by oxygen until the heart rate improves and the child is able to breathe on his own. Stress that the EMTs should monitor the patient even after ventilatory support is stopped.*

CHAPTER 7 SCENE SIZE-UP

Critical Decision Making: Determining Areas of Concern at the Scene

For each of the following scenes, determine a few areas of concern you would want to check before proceeding to the patient.

Q1: An 18-wheeler with an enclosed trailer slid off the road into a ditch in an ice storm. The vehicle is in the ditch, leaning to the right.

A1: *The possibility that the truck is carrying hazardous materials and the stability of the truck are initial concerns. Safety from traffic at the scene is a major concern. After determining if it is safe to approach, you should assess the number of patients (make sure no other vehicles are involved or under the truck) and determine if extrication is needed.*

Q2: A van and a passenger car collided on an interstate highway.

A2: *Do not walk in or along the highway until you are safe from traffic. Look for leaking gas and other safety hazards. Determine the number of patients and if extrication is needed.*

Q3: You arrive at an office building and see people running out the front and side doors in a panic. One person appears bloody and is running toward your ambulance.

A3: *There are multiple safety concerns here. The mass exodus from the building could be caused by anything from a person who is shooting to an explosion of some sort. In this case you may be too close to the scene. Plan for an extended multiple-casualty incident.*

Q4: You respond to a residence with the fire department and arrive on scene first. A resident meets you at the end of the driveway and tells you there is a strong smell of natural gas in his house.

A4: *Maintain a safe distance from the residence. Do not enter the house for any reason due to the risk of explosion. Determine if the man believes there is anyone in the residence and report it to incoming fire units. Request the gas company if it hasn't already been done.*

Q5: You respond to a construction site for a fall.

A5: *Watch for unstable construction equipment or buildings. Determine the number of patients and if any special rescue teams will be necessary to access the patient.*

Review Questions

Q1: For each of the following dangers, describe actions that must be taken to remain safe at a collision scene:

- Leaking gasoline
- Toxic or hazardous material spill
- Vehicle on fire
- Downed power lines

A1: *In the case of leaking gasoline or a vehicle fire, consider the danger zone to be 100 feet in all directions from the wreckage. Park outside the danger zone, upwind, and uphill if possible. Avoid gutters, ditches, and gullies that can carry fuel to the ambulance. Do not use flares. Use orange traffic cones during daylight and reflective triangles at night.*

In the case of hazardous materials, check with a hazardous materials reference to determine the danger zone. In all cases, park upwind. Park uphill if liquid is flowing, but on the same level if there are gases that may arise. Park behind a natural or an artificial barrier.

In the case of downed power lines, consider the danger zone as the area in which people or vehicles might be contacted by energized wires if the wires pivot around their points of attachment.

Q2: List several indicators of violence or potential violence at an emergency scene.

A2: *Indicators include fighting or loud voices, weapons visible or in use, signs of alcohol or drug use, unusual silence, knowledge of prior violence.*

Q3: Describe several situations where it is appropriate to wear disposable gloves. Describe situations where you would additionally wear protective eyewear and mask. Describe situations where you would wear an N-95 or HEPA respirator.

A3: *Protective gloves—controlled bleeding, suctioning, artificial ventilation, CPR. Eye protection—splashing, spattering, or spraying body fluids. Masks—infections spread by airborne droplets. N-95 or HEPA respirator—disease spread by airborne particles.*

Q4: Describe common mechanism-of-injury patterns.
A4: *Injuries to bones and joints are common to falls and vehicle collisions. Burns are common to fires and explosions. Penetrating soft-tissue injuries can be associated with gunshot wounds.*

Q5: List sources of information about the nature of a patient's illness.
A5: *Sources include the patient, family members or bystanders, the scene.*

Q6: List several medical and trauma situations where you may require additional assistance.
A6: *Responses will vary.*

Critical Thinking

Q: You are called to the scene of a shooting at a fast food restaurant. En route, you plan your scene size-up strategy. What actions do you anticipate taking on arrival?
A: *First you will make certain the police have secured the scene before you enter it. If you fail to do so, you might easily find yourself and your partner hostages or shooting victims. Once the scene is secure, you will proceed with normal scene size-up steps: Take Standard Precautions. Confirm the mechanism of injury (reported to be a gunshot in this case). Establish the number of patients (there might be several shooting victims or persons injured by falls or in other ways or even a person suffering a heart attack from the stress of the event). Decide if more resources are needed to handle the call.*

Street Scenes

Q1: What other scene size-up issues are left to consider?
A1: *Issues might include a quick check for the number of patients, identification of the mechanism of injury, rapid assessment to determine the severity of injuries, need for additional resources, and so on. The placard on the side of the truck also needs to be identified to determine the contents of the truck and the potential need for a special hazmat team. (Note to Instructor: More information on hazardous materials can be found in Chapter 36, "Special Operations." You might want to refer students to some of the placards found in this chapter.)*

Q2: Is the scene now safe or do other precautions need to be taken?
A2: *Although the crew has donned protective gear and made efforts to limit traffic hazards, they must wait until the vehicles are stabilized and the placard identified before safely approaching the patients.*

Q3: What Standard Precautions should be considered?
A3: *Standard Precautions should include, at a minimum, disposable gloves and eye shields—especially because of the high probability of cuts and open wounds from this type of collision.*

Q4: When the second ambulance arrives, where should it be located in relation to the collision scene?
A4: *Student answers should take into account information in Scan 7-2 in the chapter. Sample response: The second ambulance should be parked in a staging area that is upwind from the scene and at a safe distance. Safeguards should also be taken so that the ambulance is away from moving traffic and has an easy means of egress after the patient is loaded.*

Q5: What precautions should you take to protect the patients from any further harm while they are being extricated from the vehicle?

A5: *The patients need to be properly covered and protected during the extrication process. Also, a member of the crew should remain with the patients to calm their fears, answer questions, and monitor their status.*

Q6: How should you plan to make sure that you can safely get the patient from the scene to the ambulance?

A6: *Encourage students to recall the information already learned about lifting and moving patients in Chapter 5. They should also consider, as the scenario does, whether the ambulance should be moved closer to the patient to facilitate loading.*

CHAPTER 8 THE INITIAL ASSESSMENT

Critical Decision Making: Determining Priority

For each patient described here, determine whether that patient should be classified as a high or lower priority at the end of the initial assessment.

Q1: A responsive patient who is sitting up and having difficulty breathing.
A1: *High priority*

Q2: A man who "passed out" at a wedding and is still unresponsive.
A2: *High priority*

Q3: A responsive child who got his foot caught in bike spokes and may have broken the foot.
A3: *Lower priority*

Q4: A responsive patient who describes severe pain in his abdomen.
A4: *High priority*

Q5: A patient who only moans (doesn't respond with words or actions) and appears to have ingested alcohol.
A5: *High priority*

Review Questions

Q1: List factors you will take into account in forming a general impression of a patient.
A1: *Medical or trauma; if injured, identify mechanisms of injury; age; sex.*

Q2: Explain how to assess a patient's mental status with regard to the AVPU levels of consciousness.
A2: *Alert—The patient is awake if he can answer your questions. The patient is oriented to person if he can tell you his name. The patient is oriented to place if he can tell where he is. The patient is oriented to time if he can tell you the day, date, and time.*
Verbal—If the patient appears to have a depressed level of consciousness, determine if the patient responds to verbal stimuli like talking or shouting.
Painful—If the patient does not respond to verbal stimuli, determine if he responds to painful stimuli by rubbing your knuckles across his sternum or by pinching his toe.
Unresponsive—The patient will not respond to verbal or painful stimuli.

Q3: Explain how to assess airway, breathing, and circulation during the initial assessment. Explain the interventions you will take for possible problems with airway, breathing, and circulation.
A3: *Airway—If the patient is talking or crying, the airway is open. If the airway is not open or the patient is not alert or is breathing noisily, open the airway by using the jaw thrust for trauma patients and head-tilt, chin-lift for medical patients. Suction the airway and insert an airway adjunct. If the airway is blocked, perform the Heimlich maneuver, or back blows and chest thrusts, as appropriate.*

Breathing—If the patient is not alert, use the technique you learned in CPR class to listen, look, and feel for breath. Perform rescue breathing if necessary. If the patient is breathing, count the breathing rate. If a conscious patient is breathing at a rate of less than 8 breaths per minute or more than 24 breaths per minute, administer oxygen using a nonrebreather mask.

Circulation—Take the patient's pulse. Start with the radial pulse in adults and the brachial pulse in infants. If you cannot feel these peripheral pulses, check the carotid pulse. If the pulse is absent, administer CPR and apply an automated external defibrillator. (The AED should not be used on patients under 12 years of age or trauma patients.) Check for bleeding and control any major bleeding. Check the skin for temperature, moisture, and color. Warm, pink, dry skin indicates good circulation. Pale, cool, and moist skin indicates poor circulation.

Q4: Explain what is meant by the term *priority decision.*

A4: *Determining whether a patient has a life-threatening condition that requires immediate transport to the hospital.*

Q5: Explain what special interventions are required

- if a patient has suffered trauma
- if a patient is unresponsive

A5: *Trauma patients need manual stabilization of the head and spine during the initial assessment. To further protect the spine, a jaw-thrust maneuver should be used to open the airway rather than the head-tilt, chin-lift maneuver.*

Unresponsive patients—A level of responsiveness below that of Alert may indicate the possibility of a life-threatening problem. Provide high-concentration oxygen by nonrebreather mask and transport as a high-priority patient.

Critical Thinking

Q: Your patient, injured in a car crash, is breathing at 6/minute. Would you administer oxygen by nonrebreather mask or provide artificial ventilations? Describe the technique you would use.

A: *A patient whose breathing rate is slower than 8/minute should receive positive pressure ventilations with 100% oxygen. You will be assisting, rather than replacing, the patient's own ventilations. If the patient is alert, he will probably find this intimidating, so explain what you are doing and offer reassurance, such as "I'm going to help you breathe." Seal a pocket face of BVM over the patient's mouth and nose and synchronize ventilations with the patient's by watching for the start of chest rise. Squeeze the bag every time you see the patient's chest start to rise. This patient is breathing only 6 times per minute, so add an extra artificial ventilation between every breath the patient takes on his own to achieve a rate of approximately 12 per minute with adequate minute volume. (Review this technique of assisting ventilations as described in Chapter 6.)*

Street Scenes

Q1: What should be done immediately upon contact with an unconscious patient who has fallen?

A1: *While rapidly determining responsiveness, the EMT should perform axial in-line stabilization on the spine followed by an assessment of the ABCs.*

Q2: What are some considerations when opening the airway of an unconscious patient?

A2: *In order to maintain c-spine stabilization, the jaw-thrust maneuver is the most appropriate method for securing the airway. It accomplishes two objectives—opening the airway by bringing the tongue and jaw forward while at the same time maintaining in-line stabilization of the spine (in case the spine has been injured).*

Q3: Using the AVPU scale, what is the level of responsiveness of a patient who responds to you calling out his name?
A3: *The level of responsiveness is VERBAL because the patient is responding to a verbal stimulus.*

Q4: Would knowing the cause of Joey's seizures change how you perform his initial assessment?
A4: *Initial assessment should always follow the same general steps: form a general impression, assess mental status, assess airway, assess breathing, assess circulation, and determine priority. The cause of Joey's seizures might confirm whether or not he has a medical condition, but the EMTs must still identify any immediate life-threatening conditions, correct them, and then decide on the patient's priority for immediate transport or further on-scene interventions. (Note to Instructor: Stress that if the steps in initial assessment are not followed consistently and systematically, it is very possible to overlook and neglect to manage a life-threatening situation.)*

Q5: For Joey, what is the best position to prevent airway problems from occurring?
A5: *The patient should be positioned on his side (sometimes referred to as the coma position) if there is no possibility of spinal injury. This will allow for drainage. If cervical-spine trauma is suspected, then the patient should be frequently suctioned. The EMT should only rotate the patient if these conditions are met: full immobilization to a backboard, placement of a cervical collar, and application of the necessary head immobilization devices. (Note to Instructor: For more on seizures in children, see Chapter 31, "Infants and Children.")*

Q6: How did Joey's priority change during this call?
A6: *It was downgraded because of his improved mental status.*

Q7: What is the value of following a systematic method of assessment for threats to life?
A7: *See the answer to Question 4.*

Q8: How much more assessment is appropriate before you transport this patient?
A8: *Because the patient is high priority (compromised breathing and diminished circulation), students should understand that the EMT would need to spend as little time on the scene as possible. If they have not already done so, the EMTs should radio for ALS intervention. A SAMPLE history can be completed en route.*

CHAPTER 9 VITAL SIGNS AND SAMPLE HISTORY

Critical Decision Making: Solving Assessment Problems

An accurate history and set of vital signs are an important foundation for critical decision making. For each of the common EMS situations that follow, describe how you would solve the problem you are faced with. In some cases, you may think of more than one potential solution.

Q1: You are trying to count the respiratory rate of a very talkative middle-aged male. Every time you think you're beginning to get an accurate count, he starts talking again.
A1: *First, observe the ease with which the patient speaks. If he speaks long (six-plus-word) sentences without having to catch his breath the patient is experiencing minimal distress. You can wait a short time for him to stop talking or tell him you'll need him to be quiet so you can listen to his lungs (or heart) while you are really counting respirations through the stethoscope. If patients are aware you are counting their breaths the results may not be accurate.*

Q2: You are about to put a blood pressure cuff on a 40-year-old male when he says that you can't put the cuff on that arm. He is a kidney dialysis patient and says he has a "shunt" in that arm. Because of the small room he is in, you can't get over to his other side.

A2: *Obtain the blood pressure once you move the patient to a transportation device and into a more open area. Remember you will have other indicators including mental status, pulse, respirations, and skin color which are a significant part of the patient picture.*

Q3: An 80-year-old male is complaining of mild abdominal pain. When you ask him if he has any medical problems, he says no. On the kitchen table you can easily see at least half a dozen prescription bottles.

A3: *Ask the patient if he takes any medications. If he says no, ask specifically about the medications you see. They may not belong to him, but if they do seeing them may jog his memory. It is common to have to ask questions more than one way. Any patient may forget important conditions because of the stress of an emergency.*

Q4: The patient is an unconscious 32-year-old female who was thrown from a car when it flipped over. When you attempt to check the pulse at the patient's wrist, you search and search but can't find it.

A4: *In a patient with a serious mechanism of injury you should next go to the carotid artery to check the pulse. Look for other signs of life including moving, moaning, or respiratory effort. If a patient had been responsive and you couldn't feel a pulse, you should check the pulse at her other wrist.*

Review Questions

Q1: Name the vital signs.

A1: *Respiration; pulse; skin color, temperature, and condition (plus capillary refill in infants and children); pupils; and blood pressure.*

Q2: Explain why vital signs should be taken more than once.

A2: *The patient's condition may change while in your care. You should repeat vital signs on stable patients every 15 minutes. You should repeat vital signs on unstable patients every 5 minutes. You should also repeat vital signs after every medical intervention.*

Q3: Explain the meaning of the letters S-A-M-P-L-E in patient assessment.

A3: *Signs/Symptoms*
Allergies
Medications
Pertinent past history
Last oral intake
Events leading to the injury or illness

Critical Thinking

Q: How might the EMT get a SAMPLE history when a patient is unconscious?

A: *Ask family members, friends, or coworkers. Look for the medical alert bracelets, medallions, or wallet cards. Look for the patient's medications.*

Street Scenes

Q1: What is your primary concern for this patient?

A1: *After determining scene safety, the EMT's primary concern is assessment of the ABCs. In the case of Ms. Alvarez, the airway is patent, but her breathing is a little rapid. This finding warrants further assessment and at least high-concentration oxygen.*

Q2: What vital signs should be taken even if a no transport decision is being considered?

A2: *Vital signs include: number of respirations per minute (including quality), pulse rate per minute (including quality), blood pressure, skin color, and temperature, and an evaluation of the pupils.*

Q3: Ideally, what should the patient history include?
A3: *At a minimum, the EMT should try to include the information in a SAMPLE history. Because Ms. Alvarez is complaining of abdominal pain, questions during the patient interview should be aimed at determining the quality and severity of the pain, the length of time the patient has experienced the pain, what the pain "feels like," and what, if anything, brought on the pain. (Note to Instructor: You might explain to students the signs and symptoms are suggestive of abdominal bleeding, pointing out the seriousness of this condition.)*

Q4: What other patient history information should be obtained?
A4: *Sample response: If the patient's pain has already been evaluated, the EMT might ask if Ms. Alvarez has had previous episodes of the condition, whether she has seen a doctor, and if so, what the doctor has said. The EMT should also inquire about any medications that the patient might be taking for the abdominal pain or for any other medical conditions.*

Q5: Should you take another set of vital signs?
A5: *Yes. A patient with rapid respirations and signs and symptoms suggesting possible abdominal bleeding should have vital signs taken approximately every 10 minutes or according to state or local protocols.*

Q6: How might you get the patient to rethink her decision not to be transported?
A6: *Sample response: In a calm manner, the EMT should give the patient an honest appraisal of the vital signs and assessment. The EMT should also point out possible consequences of refusing transport. If the patient still expresses an unwillingness to go to the hospital, the EMT should contact medical direction and perhaps request the patient's permission to contact her personal physician. Also, if one EMT has been unable to convince the patient to go to the hospital, another member of the crew might try to convince her to change her mind. (Note to Instructor: You might have students review information on consent from Chapter 3, "Medical/Legal and Ethical Issues.")*

CHAPTER 10 ASSESSMENT OF THE TRAUMA PATIENT

Critical Decision Making: Rapid Trauma or Focused Exam?

For each of the following patients determine if you should perform a rapid trauma exam or a focused examination.

Q1: Your patient was found ejected from a vehicle in a rollover collision.
A1: *This patient should receive a rapid trauma exam—even if he appears to have minor injuries—due to the mechanism of injury.*

Q2: Your patient tripped and believes he broke his wrist. He complains of no other injuries.
A2: *This patient will receive a focused exam as long as the mechanism of injury doesn't indicate that additional injury is likely (e.g., hitting his head during the fall).*

Q3: Your patient only complains of minor neck pain after a frontal impact accident in which there was considerable damage and airbag deployment.
A3: *This patient will receive a rapid trauma exam due to the significant mechanism of injury.*

Q4: Your patient fell about 6 feet from a tree and believes he broke his ankle. Bystanders tell you he briefly lost consciousness.
A4: *This was intentionally designed as a borderline situation. While 6 feet may not match standards for significant mechanism of injury in an adult, the loss of consciousness should alert you to potentially serious problems and cause you to be cautious and complete a rapid trauma exam. You can always slow down if the patient is found to be stable.*

Review Questions

Q1: Explain why it is important to reconsider the mechanism of injury at the beginning of the focused history and physical exam of a trauma patient.

A1: *When you first arrive at the scene and must take in so much information at once, it is easy to miss things.*

Q2: Explain how the focused history and physical exam of a trauma patient with a significant mechanism of injury differs from that of a trauma patient with no significant mechanism of injury.

A2: *For the patient without a significant mechanism of injury, it is not necessary to perform a rapid trauma assessment. Instead, you can focus your assessment just on the areas that the patient tells you are painful or that you suspect may be injured. Baseline vital signs and a SAMPLE history must be obtained on all patients. (Table 10-1)*

Q3: Name the signs and symptoms for which the letters DCAP-BTLS stand.

A3: *Deformities*
Contusions
Abrasions
Punctures/penetrations
Burns
Tenderness
Lacerations
Swelling

Q4: List the steps of the rapid trauma assessment and describe the kind of patient for whom the rapid trauma assessment is appropriate.

A4: *The steps are: head, neck, chest, abdomen, pelvis, extremities, and posterior. A patient with a significant mechanism of injury needs a rapid trauma assessment.*

Q5: What are the additional areas that you assess in the detailed physical exam that you did not evaluate in the rapid trauma assessment?

A5: *The scalp and cranium, face, ears, nose, and mouth.*

Q6: List the areas covered in the detailed physical exam. What do you look and feel for as you assess each of these areas?

A6: *Refer to Table 10-5 in the chapter.*

Critical Thinking

As an EMT, how would you balance the need for appropriate on-scene assessment and treatment with the need for speed in getting the patient to the hospital in each of the following situations?

Q1: You arrive at the residence to find a patient who explains that he has accidentally cut his finger with a kitchen knife. The cut is bleeding profusely.

A1: *Although the cut is bleeding profusely, the cut to a finger is not a significant mechanism of injury. Unless you are unable to control the bleeding with direct pressure and other normal methods, you can complete on-scene assessment and care before transporting the patient.*

Q2: You arrive at a schoolyard to find a girl who bystanders say was shot by a rival gang member. She is lying in a pool of blood but is able to speak to you.

A2: *This is a significant mechanism of injury with significant blood loss that has already taken place and unknown internal injuries to the patient. Because she is able to speak, assume that her airway and breathing are adequate, at least for the moment. Immediately apply direct pressure to control the bleeding, administer oxygen by nonrebreather mask, provide manual stabilization of the head and neck, apply a cervical collar, immobilize the patient to a backboard, and transport her expeditiously, providing ongoing monitoring and any needed additional care en route.*

Q3: You are called to respond to a man who has been found unconscious on a sidewalk next to an apartment building in the middle of the night. There were no witnesses to explain what may have happened to him.

A3: *There is no way to know the cause of this patient's condition. Quickly ensure adequate airway and breathing, provide oxygenation or ventilation as needed, provide manual stabilization of the head and neck, apply a cervical collar, immobilize the patient to a backboard, and transport without spending additional time at the scene, monitoring the patient's condition en route.*

Street Scenes

Q1: What is the priority of this patient?

A1: *The patient is suffering from multi-trauma. The ABCs are the first priority, while protecting the cervical spine. The first treatment priority is securing the airway and assuring adequate respirations (breathing). Due to facial injuries, the EMTs must make sure that mucus, blood, and/or teeth are not causing airway obstructions. After applying a cervical collar and placing the patient on a backboard, the EMTs should suction as needed and, if necessary, turn the patient on his side to allow for drainage. Next, the EMTs should apply occlusive dressing over the stab wound. They should also provide the patient with high-concentration oxygen and, if necessary, assist ventilation. (Note to Instructor: Stress to students that in this scenario the EMTs should remain alert to the possibility of tension pneumothorax throughout the call. Explain this condition and/or refer students to the appropriate information and diagrams in Chapter 27, "Soft-Tissue Injuries.")*

Q2: What should be done next?

A2: *The patient requires rapid transport to a trauma center. After managing the airway and breathing, and controlling any external bleeding, the EMTs should package the patient for immediate transport.*

Q3: When should vital signs be taken?

A3: *A baseline set of vital signs should be taken as soon as possible. Because the patient has a serious mechanism of injury, vitals should be retaken every 5–10 minutes.*

Q4: What should you do next?

A4: *The patient seems to have developed difficulty breathing until the EMT lifts part of the occlusive dressing and allows some air to escape. Point out that this is suggestive of tension pneumothorax (see Question 1). In this situation, a corner of the occlusive dressing should be raised, which provides some relief. If this is successful, the EMTs should then continue to monitor the patient. They should remain prepared to assist ventilations and, if time allows, consider requesting ALS intercept. (Note to Instructor: Intercept, however, should not delay transport time significantly.)*

Q5: What should be done for the detailed physical exam, if there is time before reaching the trauma center?

A5: *The ABCs remain the first priority. However, as time and patient conditions permit, the detailed assessment should include the head-to-toe survey suggested in the chapter. In the case of this scenario, you might stress these points: 1. If the EMTs did not check the posterior when they backboarded the patient, they should do so now. 2. They should also pay special attention to facial injuries and parts of the body that made contact with the ground when the patient was first thrown down.*

Q6: How will DCAP-BTLS help with the assessment?

A6: *Deformities—injuries from being thrown on the ground or beaten;*
Contusions—facial cuts/wounds;
Abrasions from mugging or from falling;
Penetrations— the EMTs would have already identified the penetrating knife wound;
Burns— unlikely;
Tenderness— areas hit or impacted with great force (from mugging or from hitting the ground);

Lacerations— may be evident from causes already mentioned;
Swelling— should be anticipated to any part of the body that received an injury due to great force.

CHAPTER 11 ASSESSMENT OF THE MEDICAL PATIENT

Critical Decision Making: Challenges in History Gathering

Some patients are easier to get a history from than others. Consider what you might say and do to improve your history gathering in the following circumstances:

Q1: A 79-year-old female keeps talking, saying a lot about things that have nothing to do with the problem you are there for.

A1: *Listening is important, but you will eventually need to focus the history or transport will be delayed. Redirecting the patient politely with phrases such as, "I see, but I need to focus on why you called today. Can you tell me about. . ." may help.*

Q2: A 16-year-old female is surrounded by her family. She has abdominal pain that you suspect may be from a pregnancy, but you have not yet asked her if she might be pregnant.

A2: *You can ask the question while the parents aren't in the room or when bringing the patient out to the ambulance. It may be possible to have a parent leave the room to get something (medications or the patient's coat) so you can ask the question privately.*

Q3: A 32-year-old male with diabetes, according to his family, has not eaten lately. He is sometimes combative, sometimes quiet. When you ask him questions, he gives you a vacant stare and says nothing.

A3: *In this case the patient's behavior may be due to his medical condition. His family may be the best source of information. If he can answer he may do so very slowly so giving a little time (but not so much as to cause delay in treatment) may help.*

Q4: A 22-year-old male college student, his roommate tells you, has been acting strange the last few weeks. The patient is now sitting on his bed with his knees drawn up against his chest, rocking back and forth saying things that don't make sense to you.

A4: *While ensuring your safety, get down to the patient's level and attempt to establish rapport. Talk slowly and quietly. Ask questions that are easy to answer (e.g., ask the patient's name) to see if the patient is oriented enough to respond.*

Review Questions

Q1: Explain how and why the focused history and physical exam for a medical patient differs from the focused history and physical exam for a trauma patient.

A1: *In medical patients, unlike trauma patients, there are not many external sources of information about what is wrong with the patient. For medical emergencies, the most important source of information about the problem is usually what the patient can tell you. So, when the patient is awake and responsive, obtaining the patient's history comes first.*

Q2: Explain how and why the focused history and physical exam for a responsive medical patient differs from the focused history and physical exam for an unresponsive medical patient.

A2: *For the responsive medical patient, the first step of your focused history and physical exam would be talking with the patient to obtain the history of his or her present illness and the SAMPLE history, followed by performing the physical exam and gathering the* *vital signs. In the unresponsive medical patient, the process is turned around. Because you cannot obtain a history from the patient, you will begin with a rapid physical assessment and collection of baseline vital signs. After these procedures, you will gather as much of the patient's history as you can from any bystanders or family members who may be present.*

Critical Thinking

Q: As an EMT, how would you deal with the following situations?

a. What questions would you ask to get a history of the present illness from a patient with a chief complaint of chest pain?

b. You are trying to get information from the very upset son of an unresponsive man. He is the only available family member. He is so upset that he is having difficulty talking to you. How can you quickly get him to calm down and give you his father's medical history?

c. You are interviewing a very pleasant older man. Unfortunately, your assessment is taking a long time because he does not answer your questions and instead starts talking about other things. He lives alone and appears to be lonely. How should you handle this?

A: **a.** *Onset—What were you doing when the pain started?*
Provokes—Can you think of anything that might have triggered this pain?
Quality—Can you describe the pain for me?
Radiation—Where exactly is the pain? Does it seem to spread anywhere or does it stay right here?
Severity—How bad is the pain?
Time—When did the pain start? Has it changed at all since it started?

b. *Put your hand on his shoulder and say: "I know you are concerned about your father. You can help him by trying to calm down and answer a few questions for me about his medical history. Take a few deep breaths. Good. You look calmer. Are you ready to answer my questions?"*

c. *Continue to talk to him for a few minutes about unrelated matters, then say, "Sir, I'm really enjoying our conversation. However, I need to get back into service as soon as possible so that I can take care of other patients. So, I need you to answer a few questions for me related to the problem you're having today. Okay?"*

Street Scenes

Q1: What priority is this patient?

A1: *As always, the first priority is protection of the airway and breathing. In the scenario, the airway appears clear, but the breathing is rapid and mildly labored. Some students might mention the administration of high-concentration oxygen by a nonrebreather mask. (Note to Instructor: Stress that this equipment should be close at hand and ready for immediate use.)*

Q2: What are the next steps in the management of this patient?

A2: *The EMTs should take a baseline set of vitals, as indicated in the opening part of the scenario. After eliminating any immediate life threats, the EMTs should begin to gather a history of the present illness (OPQRST), focusing on questions that pertain to the condition cited by the patient. If they have not yet administered oxygen (see Question 1), they should begin to do so now. The EMTs should also monitor the patient to see if the oxygen helps. (Note to Instructor: Depending upon local protocols, some students may suggest the use of a pulse oximeter to monitor the patient.)*

Q3: What part of the focused history and physical exam should follow next?

A3: *The EMTs should complete any of the OPQRST questions and then ask specific questions for the SAMPLE history. Of particular importance is the use of an inhaler or other* *medications commonly prescribed to asthma patients. Students might also mention aspects of the focused physical exam that relate to the patient's condition, repeat of vital signs, and so on.*

Q4: What signs or symptoms would you look for to determine if the patient was getting better or worse?

A4: *Some signs and symptoms of a worsening condition might include: an increase in the level of consciousness, more labored breathing, use of accessory muscles, tripoding, increased difficulty talking (e.g., one-word answers), a respiratory rate that is either too fast or too slow, increased patient anxiety, and so on. Some signs and symptoms of an improving condition might include: a "normal" respiration rate (e.g., little or no distress), the ability to talk in complete sentences, an alert mental state, absence of cyanosis, the high oxygen saturation reading on the pulse oximeter, and so on.*

CHAPTER 12 ONGOING ASSESSMENT

Critical Decision Making: Trending Vital Signs

Observing a trend in vital signs is more valuable than getting an individual set of vitals. Observing trends is essential for making accurate decisions such as transport destination and whether ALS may be necessary. Look at the following sets of vital signs for three patients and determine the trend for each patient.

Q1: A 32-year-old male fell about 15 feet from a roof and has multiple injuries. His vital signs have been:

Time	Pulse	BP	Resp	Skin
2140	88	120/90	20, shallow	Pale but dry
2155	84	100/80	18, shallow	Pale but dry
2200	80	90/60	16, full	Pale but dry

How would you describe the trend of his vital signs: deteriorating, essentially unchanged, returning to normal, or not possible to determine?

A1: *Deteriorating*

Q2: A 64-year-old female fell to the floor and is complaining of hip pain. Her vital signs have been:

Time	Pulse	BP	Resp	Skin
1330	108	160/90	24, shallow	Pale but dry
1345	112	150/90	20, shallow	Pale but dry
1350	96	140/80	20, full	Pale but dry

How would you describe the trend of her vital signs: deteriorating, essentially unchanged, returning to normal, or not possible to determine?

A2: *Returning to normal*

Q3: A 19-year-old female injured her left ankle and lower leg in a soccer game. Her vital signs have been:

Time	Pulse	BP	Resp	Skin
1922	108	126/96	20, shallow	Pale and sweaty
1930	116	110/80	22, shallow	Pale and sweaty
1935	124	90/70	22, full	Pale and sweaty

How would you describe the trend of her vital signs: deteriorating, essentially unchanged, returning to normal, or not possible to determine?

A3: *Deteriorating*

Review Questions

Q1: Name the four steps of the ongoing assessment and list what assessment you will make during each step.

A1:
1) *Repeat the initial assessment—Reassess mental status. Maintain open airway. Monitor breathing for rate and quality. Reassess pulse for rate and quality. Monitor skin color and temperature. Reestablish patient priorities.*
2) *Repeat and record the vital signs.*
3) *Repeat the focused history and physical exam—chief complaints and injuries.*
4) *Check interventions—Assure adequacy of oxygen delivery and artificial ventilation. Assure management of bleeding.*

Q2: Explain the value of recording, or documenting, your assessment findings, and explain the meaning of the term *trending.*

A2: *By documenting findings, the EMT can note any changes in the patient's condition, adjust treatment, or begin new treatment. Trending is evaluating and recording changes in a patient's condition, such as slowing respirations or rising pulse rate, that may show improvement or deterioration, and that can be shown by documenting repeated assessments.*

Critical Thinking

Q: What do you need to do if your ongoing assessment turns up one of these findings?

a. Gurgling respirations
b. Bag on nonrebreather mask collapses completely when the patient inhales
c. Snoring respirations

A: **a.** *Suction patient.*
b. *Increase oxygen.*
c. *Open airway.*

Street Scenes

Q1: How does the patient's mental status affect the way you maintain the patient's airway?

A1: *Patients who are less than alert (responding to verbal or painful stimuli) may have difficulty maintaining their airways. These patients may position themselves in such a manner as to occlude their airways through a partial blockage by the tongue—a condition that can be resolved by repositioning. Also, with less-than-alert patients, EMTs need to be prepared for suctioning. They may also need to move these patients into a position that will facilitate drainage. (Note to Instructor: Point out that when a patient is unresponsive, he or she must be monitored constantly. EMTs should be prepared to reposition the patient as needed, to insert an OPA [if no gag reflex is present], and to apply suctioning. Patients with an altered mental status require constant assessment of the airway and immediate availability of the necessary equipment to correct any problems that may develop.)*

Q2: What questions should you ask the patient and her husband?

A2: *Explain that at this point the EMTs should have completed a SAMPLE survey. Questions might include the following: Has the patient had a similar condition in the past? Is the patient taking any blood pressure medication? If so, what is the medication? Is the patient compliant in taking it? In specifically questioning the husband, the EMTs might ask: "When was the last time you saw your wife?" "Was she manifesting any of* *the current signs or symptoms at that point, such as trouble walking, slurred speech, or obvious facial drooping?" In specifically questioning the patient, the EMTs might ask: "Are you having any trouble breathing?" "Are you in any pain?" (Note to Instructor: You might choose to introduce the topic of a stroke at this point and/or refer students to examine the signs and symptoms listed in Chapter 19, "Diabetic Emergencies and Altered Mental Status," of the textbook.)*

Q3: How should you perform an ongoing assessment on this patient?

A3: *Student answers should reflect the steps listed in the chapter. For example, the EMTs should monitor the patient's airway, breathing, and any changes in her level of consciousness. They should periodically reassess the patient's speech and observe facial drooping. The EMTs should reassess the patient's pupils and vital signs approximately every 10 minutes. They should also periodically reevaluate changes in movement, strength, and sensation in all extremities.*

CHAPTER 13 COMMUNICATIONS

Critical Decision Making: Communications Challenges

Communication may take various forms in EMS: for example, written, face-to-face verbal, or by radio. Make your decisions based on the scenarios below:

Q1: You are en route to a call of unknown nature for an elderly patient. First Responders arrived at the scene about five minutes ago and you are still ten minutes from the scene. Dispatch has not called you on the radio with an update on the patient's condition. What are some of the reasons why this might be the case? How should you proceed?

A1: *The First Responders may be busy with a critical patient, they may have forgotten, they could be in danger, or their radio may not work. Call on the radio and ask for an update.*

Q2: A 17-year-old male drank a large amount of alcohol and then "passed out," according to his friends, who called 911. When you arrive, you find the patient initially unresponsive to painful stimuli, then a few minutes later able to slur some words when you ask him questions. A few minutes after that, he withdraws when you apply a painful stimulus. How should you describe his mental status to the hospital while you are en route?

A2: *Advise the hospital that the patient has apparently ingested a large quantity of alcohol. (Never assume this is the only problem.) Advise of his current level of responsiveness (painful stimuli) and note that it has varied. Recontact the hospital if the patient's condition worsens so they can prepare.*

Q3: You are at the scene of a two-car motor vehicle collision and would like to give the local hospital some warning that you will be transporting a severely injured patient in a few minutes. Unfortunately, when you try to call the hospital on the radio, they are unable to understand what you are saying. How should you proceed?

A3: *Depending on time and resources you could step away from the chaotic scene to eliminate background noise and try again. Be sure you are talking slowly and clearly. If it appears to be a radio problem ask the dispatcher if they heard the transmission. If so, they could advise the hospital by radio or phone for you.*

Q4: You have just arrived at the scene of a 34-year-old diabetic male who is "out of it," according to what the caller told dispatch. One of his friends, trying to be helpful, tells you that he thinks the patient is "conscious but unresponsive." Confused as to what this might mean, you proceed to the patient and find him sitting in a chair, staring straight ahead, not saying anything. When you ask him a question, he doesn't answer and doesn't even look at you. When you pinch his arm, he looks down at his arm but doesn't respond in any other way. How can you describe this patient's mental status in a way that will give the hospital an accurate impression of what is going on? Hint: Describe what you observe instead of trying to attach labels to this patient.

A4: *By stating "The patient is nonverbal but his eyes are open and he localizes pain by looking where painful stimulus is applied," you have painted a picture of the patient's mental status.*

Review Questions

Q1: List several guidelines for proper use of the EMS radio system.

A1: *Refer to Table 13-1 in the chapter.*

Q2: List the steps of a medical radio report and describe the communication that may be necessary during each part.

A2:
1) *Unit identification and level of provider ("Memorial Hospital, this is Community BLS Ambulance 6 en route to your location?. . .")*
2) *Estimated time of arrival (". . . with a 15-minute ETA.")*
3) *Patient's age and sex ("We are transporting a 68-year-old male patient...")*
4) *Chief complaint (". . .who complains of pain in his abdomen.")*
5) *Brief, pertinent history of the present illness ("Onset of pain was two hours ago and is accompanied by slight nausea.")*
6) *Major past illnesses ("The patient has a history of high blood pressure and arthritis.")*
7) *Mental status ("He is alert and oriented, never lost consciousness.")*
8) *Baseline vital signs ("His vital signs are pulse 88 regular and full, respirations 20 and unlabored, skin normal, and blood pressure 134 over 88.")*
9) *Pertinent findings of the physical exam ("Our exam revealed tenderness in both upper abdominal quadrants. They did not appear rigid.")*
10) *Emergency medical care given ("For care, we have placed him in a position of comfort.")*
11) *Response to emergency medical care ("The level of pain has not changed during our care. Mental status has remained unchanged. Vital signs are basically unchanged.")*
12) *If your system requires, or if you have questions, contact medical direction. ("Does medical direction have any orders?")*

Q3: List several guidelines for effective interpersonal communication with patients.

A3: *Use eye contact.*
Be aware of your position and body language.
Use language the patient can understand.
Be honest.
Use the patient's proper name.
Listen.

Critical Thinking

Q: The following information, describing a patient, is in random order. Organize the information and present a medical radio report as if you were radioing the hospital.

A: *The correct sequence for a medical radio report is indicated by the numbers in parentheses that precede the information items:*
(5) Chest pain radiating to the shoulder
(3) 56 years old
(13) Oxygen applied at 15 liters per minute via nonrebreather
(9) Alert and oriented
(4) Female

(7) Came on 20 minutes ago while mowing the lawn
(8) History of high blood pressure and diabetes
(2) ETA 20 minutes
(10) Pulse 86, respirations 22, skin cool and moist, blood pressure 110/66, SpO_2 *96%*
(14) Oxygen relieved the pain slightly
(6) Denies difficulty breathing
(15) You are requesting orders from medical direction
(1) You are on Community BLS Ambulance 4
(11) Lung sounds equal on both sides
(12) Placed in a position of comfort

Street Scenes

Q1: What type of scene safety information do you want to know from the sheriff's deputy?

A1: *While answers may vary, stress that EMTs should never take scene safety for granted—even when other response units have already arrived on scene. At this time, the crew still needs specific details such as the presence of gas leaks and/or fire, whether or not the vehicle has been stabilized, the condition of traffic, and so on. The EMTs also need to know the best means to access the scene, the location of a staging area for the ambulance, the status of additional rescue units, and so on. (Note to Instructor: You might want to introduce the concept of the Incident Command System and/or refer students to information on this topic in Chapter 36, "Special Operations," of the textbook.)*

Q2: Should you contact the First Responders or wait until they contact you?

A2: *Answers will vary. The responding EMTs can benefit from information provided by the First Responders. Yet, these units/individuals need time to do a scene size-up and a quick patient assessment. If the First Responders have been on scene for a "reasonable amount of time" (often a judgment call), then a radio transmission might be made to the scene. (Note to Instructor: If you have introduced the Incident Command System in Question 1, you might want to point out the benefit of centralizing communication through one person (the incident commander or some other officer) assigned this duty at the scene. In this scenario, much of the information from the First Responders is relayed through the dispatcher.)*

Q3: What patient information would be helpful to know?

A3: *Sample responses: Patient information should start with the level of responsiveness (i.e., is the patient still unresponsive and what is the status of his ABCs?). The EMTs also need to know if the airway can be maintained and if ventilations need to be assisted. Answers to these two questions will significantly impact the tasks assigned to EMS personnel. Based on the mechanism of injury, the EMTs might assume the need for c-spine precautions, in-line stabilization, and extrication. However, this information should be confirmed either by the dispatcher or direct request from the EMTs themselves. If time permits (as it does in this scenario), the EMTs should seek vital signs for a fuller patient "picture" and regular progress reports on changes while en route to the scene.*

Q4: What information should be provided to the incident commander upon arrival?

A4: *The EMTs should inform the incident commander, in this case the fire captain, of the level of care that their unit is able to provide. The EMTs then need to coordinate care steps with the First Responders already on scene. They should confirm the information received thus far and seek relevant updated information. The EMTs should then take over the appropriate tasks, such as those mentioned in the scenario.*

Q5: What type of coordinated effort between Ambulance 40 and Fire Rescue 8 should be done to ensure the best care?

A5: *Sample responses: In the scenario, the two units decide such issues as the use of rapid extrication and the use of personnel to perform assessments, communication with the helicopter crew, stabilization of the patient's head and neck, rotation of the patient onto a backboard, and so on. The key to success on this run is teamwork. The units must* *work together, through a team leader (incident commander), to develop a plan and to coordinate the extrication effort. This is not the place to debate command. There must be someone in charge of extrication as well as someone responsible for providing care—this may or may not be the same person. (Note to Instructor: Encourage students to find out about local protocols at incidents involving multiple units in your community.)*

Q6: What information about both the patient's condition and the landing zone needs to be relayed to the helicopter?

A6: *Sample responses: The flight crew should be provided with current patient information, particularly the ABCs. The EMT communicating with the helicopter should transmit the most recent set of vital signs, any significant changes that have occurred in the patient's condition, and progress in extricating the patient. If a SAMPLE history is known, the EMT can also radio this information to the flight crew. Finally, the flight crew needs to know the exact location of the landing zone (LZ) and any obstructions that they may encounter. (Note to Instructor: You might introduce the topic of air rescue and/or refer students to information on helicopter transport in Chapter 34, "Ambulance Operations." Of particular use is the section on "How to Set Up a Landing Zone.")*

CHAPTER 14 DOCUMENTATION

Critical Decision Making: Choosing How and What to Document

The documentation you produce may be looked at years later in criminal and civil cases—as well as being reviewed by your QI committee. You will need to make decisions about how and what you document . . . as you will see in the questions that follow.

Q1: After the police secure the scene, you treat a man and woman who apparently had a dispute. Neither sustained any life-threatening injuries, so you have time to gather more information at the scene. Even though you and your partner evaluate them in different rooms, they are still angry and trading insults. The boyfriend claims she is a two-timing slut who has syphilis and chlamydia. The girlfriend claims he is an alcoholic and a drug addict. How much of this should you document on the PCR? How should you phrase any information you obtained in this way?

A1: *Only information that is relevant medically should be documented. For example, if the patient is a drug addict it may be pertinent to note whether the patient admitted to or denied alcohol or drug use prior to this incident. Alcohol or drug use may also make a patient incapable of providing consent or making an informed patient refusal. Use objective (factual) statements rather than subjective (opinion) statements in your documentation. Use terms like* patient stated *before noting subjective information so anyone reading the report will know the source.*

Q2: Three years from now, you receive a notice to appear for a deposition regarding a call you had a long time ago. So much time has passed that you don't remember the call. Are you allowed to look at the PCR before you go? Why or why not?

A2: *Yes. You are allowed to look at the call report or PCR before you go. This is a legal document that records your observations and actions at the call. It will refresh your memory and not cause bias or interference with the legal proceedings.*

Q3: When you treat a 3-year-old girl for an arm injury, you suspect she has been abused. How do the privacy rules of HIPAA affect what you may and should do with regard to reporting this situation to the authorities?

A3: *Cases such as child, elder, and sexual abuse exempt providers from any HIPAA privacy requirements associated with a report to appropriate authorities and relevant health care providers. As a matter of fact, many states specifically provide immunity from lawsuits for those who report these suspected incidents in good faith.*

Review Questions

Q1: Explain the term *minimum data set* and why it is important.
A1: *These are minimum data elements that the U.S. Department of Transportation recommends be included in all prehospital care reports nationwide. This will aid in research.*

Q2: Explain what is meant by "objective" and "subjective" information in the narrative portion of the prehospital care report. Explain what is meant by "a pertinent negative."
A2: *Subjective information is that which is from an individual point of view—the patient, bystanders, even the EMT (e.g., Patient says, "I feel like I've got the flu."). Objective information is that which is observable, measurable, and verifiable (e.g., vital signs). A pertinent negative is something that is not true but that is important to note (e.g., "The patient states that her chest pain does not radiate.").*

Q3: Explain how spelling and the use of codes, abbreviations, and medical terms relate to writing a clear and accurate narrative report.
A3: *Written reports that cannot be read by others may cause harmful errors in patient care. They also make it hard for the quality improvement team to conduct reviews and research.*

Q4: List some important steps to take and information to include when documenting a patient refusal.
A4: *1) Try again to persuade the patient to go to a hospital.*
2) Ensure the patient is able to make a rational, informed decision (e.g., not under the influence of alcohol or other drugs, or illness/injury effects).
3) Inform the patient why he should go and what may happen to him if he does not.
4) Consult medical direction as directed by local protocol.
5) If the patient still refuses, document any assessment findings and emergency medical care given, then have the patient sign a refusal form.
6) Have a family member, police officer, or bystander sign the form as a witness. If the patient refuses to sign the refusal form, have a family member, police officer, or bystander sign the form verifying that the patient refused to sign.

Q5: Describe some possible consequences of falsifying information on a prehospital care report.
A5: *Poor patient care; suspension or revocation of your EMT certificate or license.*

Q6: Describe how to properly correct an error in a prehospital care report.
A6: *Draw a single line through an error, initial it, and write the correct information beside it.*

Critical Thinking

Q: Write a narrative report for a call you have been on. If you have not yet been on an ambulance, write one that describes an injury or illness that has happened to you or a family member. If a prehospital care report form is available, complete the whole form, including the check-off or fill-in boxes as well as the narrative portion.
A: *Answers will vary.*

Street Scenes

Q1: What information is important to include in the prehospital care report?
A1: *The following information should be included in a prehospital care report: run data (agency name, unit number, date, times, run call number, names and certification levels of crew members); patient data (nature of call, mechanism of injury, location of patient, treatment, signs and symptoms, baseline vitals, level of consciousness, SAMPLE history, care administered and the effects of each care step, changes in the patient's condition*

throughout the call, insurance and billing information); narrative (objective and pertinent subjective information, pertinent negatives).

Q2: What is the importance of doing an accurate and thorough prehospital care report?

A2: *Answers may vary somewhat, but students should stress the functions of the prehospital care report mentioned in the chapter (i.e., inclusion of the report in the patient's hospital record, potential use as a legal document in civil and criminal cases, and use of data for administrative purposes, education, or quality improvement).*

Q3: Should you have your partner read and comment on the prehospital care report before considering it complete?

A3: *Yes, because of the teamwork involved in EMS calls. (Note to Instructor: Stress that it is always possible to overlook information or to see situations from a personal perspective. Point out that many EMS services expect the PCRs to be written by a single author. Therefore, any changes or modifications should be made by the person who wrote the report in the first place.)*

Q4: What are the ramifications of having a prehospital care report in the hospital record that is different from the original copy on file with your EMS agency?

A4: *Most students will pick up on the point in the scenario, stressing the legal implications of alterations should a patient decide to file a suit at a later time.*

CHAPTER 15 GENERAL PHARMACOLOGY

Critical Decision Making: How or Whether to Assist with Medications

Your decisions on how, or whether, to assist patients with their medications are a critical part of your practice as an EMT. The following questions will test your knowledge and decision making in this vital area.

Q1: You are treating a patient who has chest pain. He tells you his wife has nitroglycerin. He asks if he should take her pills. What should you tell him?

A1: *You are not allowed to assist a patient with anything other than his own medication. Using another's medication may be dangerous. You should tell him "no."*

Q2: You are treating a patient who is diabetic. She appears very sleepy and only responds to loud verbal stimulus by briefly opening her eyes. The patient's sister says, "Give her some sugar!" Should you? Why or why not?

A2: *While the patient may have a diabetic condition, her level of consciousness rules out the use of oral glucose. The patient should be promptly transported to the hospital. If advanced life support is available, they would be able to give glucose by IV, which may benefit the patient.*

Q3: Your COPD patient is breathing 48 times per minute shallowly. His wife believes his "lung problems" have been acting up. Would the patient's inhaler help him?

A3: *No. The patient is breathing inadequately. He would not be able to take a deep enough breath to get the medication from the inhaler into his lungs and provide a benefit. This patient needs to be ventilated.*

Review Questions

Q1: Name the drugs that are carried on the ambulance and may be administered by the EMT under certain circumstances.

A1: *Activated charcoal, oral glucose, oxygen.*

Q2: Name the drugs that the EMT may assist the patient in taking if they have been prescribed for him and with approval by medical direction.
A2: *Prescribed inhaler, nitroglycerin, epinephrine auto-injector.*

Q3: Medications may take the form of tablets. Name several other forms that medications may have.
A3: *Liquids, gels, suspensions, fine powder for inhalation, gases, sublingual spray, liquid/vaporized fixed-dose nebulizers.*

Q4: Name the four "rights" you must check before administering a medication.
A4: *1. Right patient? 2. Right medication? 3. Right dose? 4. Right route of administration?*

Q5: Name several routes by which medications may be administered.
A5: *Oral, intramuscular, intravenous, subcutaneous, sublingual, endotracheal, inhaled.*

Critical Thinking

Q: A patient is complaining of chest pain. "Here's some nitroglycerin," says a family member. "Give him that." What do you do?
A: *Determine if the patient has a prescription for the nitro. Determine when the patient last took nitro, how much was taken, and what effect it had on the chest pain. Consult medical direction.*

Street Scenes

Q1: What additional patient history should you obtain?
A1: *The EMT should find out if the patient has a prescription for nitroglycerin. If so, the EMT should ask questions such as the following: "Do you have the nitro with you now?" "Have you taken any nitro since the onset of pain?" If the patient has taken any nitro, the EMT should ask these questions. "When did you take the nitro?" "What, if any, effect did the nitro have on the pain?" The EMT should also inquire about previous episodes of chest pain, pertinent medical history, activities immediately preceding this episode, and so on.*

Q2: Should you let the patient take nitroglycerin? Why, or why not?
A2: *If the patient has his own prescription, the EMT should allow him to take it. (Note to Instructor: Discuss any local protocols that might limit the administration of nitroglycerin. For example, most protocols have parameters for minimum blood pressure and/or pulse that serve as criteria for the administration of nitro.)*

Q3: Are vital signs important if nitroglycerin is going to be taken by the patient?
A3: *As indicated in Question 2, vital signs must be taken before nitro is administered to the patient. Thereafter, the EMT should retake vital signs every 5–10 minutes. All vital signs must be documented. (Refer students to the sample documentation in the chapter.)*

Q4: What information do you want to know about the nitroglycerin?
A4: *Answers should center on the "four rights": Is this the right patient? (Does the patient's name match the name on the bottle or spray?) Is this the right medication? (Is the name of the medication on the container? If so, is it nitroglycerin or an appropriate trade name?) Is this the right dose for the patient? (Usually, that means one tablet or one spray.) Is this the correct route of administration? (Usually, nitro is administered via a sublingual route—i.e., under the tongue.)*

Q5: How should the nitroglycerin be administered?
A5: *One tablet should be placed under the patient's tongue until it dissolves. The tablet should not be chewed or swallowed.*

Q6: When should vital signs be taken again?
A6: *Vital signs should be taken every 5–10 minutes after administration of nitro or in accordance with local/regional protocols.*

CHAPTER 16 RESPIRATORY EMERGENCIES

Critical Decision Making: Assisting with a Prescribed Inhaler

As an EMT you may be allowed to assist a patient in using his prescribed inhaler. Certain inhalers deliver a medication that relaxes narrowed airways and provides tremendous benefit to the patient when they are used properly. For each of the situations that follows, decide whether you should or should not assist the patient with the inhaler.

Q1: You are called to a 14-year-old patient who complains of difficulty breathing. He tells you he has a history of asthma. The patient's pulse is 104 strong and regular, respirations 28 with audible wheezes, blood pressure 130/84, skin warm and dry. The patient's parents are present. The inhaler is prescribed to the patient.

A1: *This patient would benefit from the use of an inhaler. Always follow local protocols and medical direction for use of medications.*

Q2: You are called to a 67-year-old patient who complains of difficulty breathing. The patient tells you she has a history of breathing problems but doesn't know specifically which ones. Her vital signs are pulse 122 strong and regular, respirations 28 with audible wheezes, blood pressure 104/64, skin cool and dry. The patient's daughter presents an inhaler, saying, "This is mine, but it's what I use when I'm wheezing."

A2: *Do not use the inhaler because it isn't prescribed to the patient. Additionally, wheezes may be present in conditions other than asthma. Nothing says the wheezes in the patient are from the same disease as the wheezes experienced by the daughter.*

Q3: You are called to a 24-year-old female who was exercising when she developed difficulty breathing. She has a history of asthma. You find her looking tired and weak. Her vital signs are pulse 142, respirations 42 and shallow, blood pressure 96/56, skin cool and moist. You do not hear any wheezes. A friend ran and got the patient's inhaler from her car.

A3: *While the inhaler is indicated for the patient's asthma, it won't do much good here because the patient isn't breathing adequately. The reason you don't hear wheezes is that she isn't breathing enough to move air through the constricted airways. The medication in the inhaler won't get deep into the lungs where it is needed. Ventilate the patient with a BVM connected to oxygen, transport promptly, and request an ALS intercept if available in your area.*

Review Questions

Q1: List the normal rates of breathing for adults, children, and infants. List the other signs of adequate breathing.

A1: *Normal rates: adults, 12–20 breaths per minute; children, 15–30 breaths per minute; and infants, 25–50 breaths per minute.*

Q2: List the signs of inadequate breathing.

A2: *Refer to Table 16-1.*

Q3: Explain the treatment you will give, as an EMT, when a patient's breathing is inadequate.

A3: *Provide artificial ventilation with supplemental oxygen.*

Q4: List the signs and symptoms of breathing difficulty.

A4: *Refer to Figure 16-2.*

Q5: Explain the treatment you may give, as an EMT, for breathing difficulty when breathing is adequate.

A5: *Provide oxygen at 15 liters per minute using a nonrebreather mask. Seek permission from medical direction to use an inhaler if one has been prescribed for the patient.*

Q6: Explain the steps to follow before, during, and after helping a patient use a prescribed inhaler.

A6: *Refer to Scans 16-1 and 16-2.*

Q7: List some differences between adult and infant/child respiratory systems.

A7: *Mouth and nose—in general, all structures are smaller and more easily obstructed than in adults.*

Pharynx—infants' and children's tongues take up proportionally more space in the mouth than do adults'.

Trachea—narrower and obstructed more easily by swelling; softer and more flexible. Like other cartilage in the infant and child, the cricoid cartilage is less developed and less rigid.

Diaphragm—chest wall is softer; infants and children tend to depend more heavily on the diaphragm for breathing.

Q8: List some special considerations in the assessment and treatment of infants and children with respiratory problems.

A8: *Retractions are more commonly seen in children than adults. Cyanosis (blue-gray) is a late finding in children. Very frequent coughing may be present rather than wheezing in some children. A low pulse is a sign of respiratory trouble and an indication to recheck ventilations. Check head position; insert airway; suction fluids as necessary.*

It is important to distinguish between an upper airway obstruction and a lower airway disease, since with the latter, probing the airway can set off spasms.

Critical Thinking

Q: For each of the following patients, state whether the patient's breathing seems adequate or inadequate—and explain your reasoning:

a. A 45-year-old male patient experiencing severe difficulty in breathing. His respirations are 36/minute and very shallow. He has minimal chest expansion and can barely speak.

b. A 65-year-old female who tells you that she has trouble breathing. Her respirations are 20/minute and slightly labored. Her respirations are regular and there appears to be good chest expansion.

c. A 3-year-old patient who has had a respiratory infection recently. Her parents called because she is having difficulty breathing. You observe retractions of the muscles between the ribs and above the collarbones as well as nasal flaring. The child seems drowsy. Respirations are 40/minute.

A: a. *Inadequate—Rapid rate of respiration; shallow breaths; minimal chest expansion; difficulty speaking.*

b. *Inadequate—Rapid rate of respiration; labored breathing.*

c. *Inadequate—Retractions; nasal flaring; rapid rate of respiration.*

Street Scenes

Q1: What is the first thing you should do for this patient?

A1: *As with any patient, the EMT should protect the airway and evaluate breathing. He or she should make sure that the airway is clear and then provide ventilations as necessary. (See Question 4.) (Note to Instructor: Point out that although the patient is speaking, the tongue or secretions could still be a potential problem.)*

Q2: What questions should you ask the husband? The neighbor?

A2: *The husband should be asked the questions in the SAMPLE history, except for "E" (event). That part of the history should be elicited from the neighbor. Examples of questions the EMT might ask the neighbor include: "What type of activity was*

Mrs. Bartolone performing at the onset of her breathing problem?" "When did you first observe the episode?" "What posture was the patient in at that time?" "Was her breathing fast or slow?" "Could she speak in complete sentences?" "Was she working to breathe?" "Was her breathing noisy?" "Did you notice any peculiar skin color—especially around the lips?"

Q3: What is the significance of the medical history provided by the husband?
A3: *The medical history reveals that Mrs. Bartolone had to be intubated and placed on a ventilator during an episode 6 months earlier. This information, coupled with the patient's long smoking history, indicates that the EMT should consider her a high medical emergency.*

Q4: How much oxygen should the patient receive?
A4: *The patient should receive high-concentration oxygen, since her normal 2 liters per minute are obviously insufficient in this situation.*

Q5: Is the patient a good candidate for an inhaler?
A5: *No. Signs and symptoms in the scenario indicate that the patient is in immediate need of oxygen. Also, as later paragraphs indicate, local protocols require that a patient be alert to receive help with a ventilator. Mrs. Bartolone, however, demonstrates signs of drowsiness.*

Q6: Should this patient be considered a high priority with red light and siren for transport to the hospital?
A6: *Probably. Everything in the case study points toward rapid transport. In most systems, this usually means use of a red light and siren.*

CHAPTER 17 CARDIAC EMERGENCIES

Critical Decision Making: Meeting Sublingual Nitroglycerin Criteria

You are treating a patient with chest pain. For each scenario provided, decide whether this patient meets the general criteria for sublingual nitroglycerin administration. Each of the patients has nitroglycerin prescribed to him by his cardiologist.

Q1: You are treating a patient with chest pain. He is 84 years old. His wife tells you that he began having a sensation in his chest he thought was indigestion about 2 hours ago. The patient is very pale and sweaty and appears sleepy. His pulse is 104 slightly irregular, respirations 28 and adequate, blood pressure 94/66.
A1: *This patient does not meet the criteria because his blood pressure is too low. Even if your protocol allowed nitroglycerin administration at 90 mmHg systolic, his rapid pulse and pale, sweaty skin should be additional indicators that he could crash after nitroglycerin administration.*

Q2: You are treating a 68-year-old male patient who has a history of angina pectoris. He tells you that he began having chest discomfort just after eating dinner. The discomfort is in the center of his chest and is described as a heavy feeling. It feels like the last time he had a heart problem. His vital signs are pulse 92 strong and regular, respirations 20 and adequate, blood pressure 138/92, skin warm and moist.
A2: *This patient meets the criteria for nitroglycerin administration in that he has suspected cardiac chest pain and his vitals are within acceptable limits. Determine if he has taken any nitroglycerin yet and ask about use of erectile dysfunction medications before you administer any nitroglycerin.*

Q3: You are treating a 49-year-old male patient complaining of pain in his "stomach." He states the pain is below his diaphragm and radiates to the left side. He has taken one nitroglycerin spray without relief. The patient states this pain is not like his one heart attack. His vital signs are pulse 68 strong and regular, respirations 18 and adequate, blood pressure 112/68, skin warm and dry.

A3: *This patient is trickier than the first two. The confounding factor is that the pain is atypical (especially when compared to prior conditions) but could still be cardiac in nature. His first nitroglycerin spray didn't work. His vital signs are still within acceptable limits. Get a more detailed history and contact medical direction for additional advice.*

Review Questions

Q1: What position is best for the patient with:

a. Difficulty breathing and a blood pressure of 100/70?

b. Chest pain and blood pressure of 180/90?

A1: *Patients who are having difficulty breathing typically are more comfortable sitting up. Patients with chest pain generally are more comfortable sitting up unless they are hypotensive.*

If in doubt, ask the patient in which position he feels better.

Q2: What is the best way to transfer a patient with difficulty breathing, chest pressure, and a blood pressure of 160/100 down a flight of stairs?

A2: *Stair chair. (Chapter 5)*

Q3: Describe how to "clear" a patient before administering a shock.

A3: *State "Clear!" and be sure no one is touching the patient before delivering a shock.*

Q4: List three safety measures to keep in mind when using an AED.

A4: *1) Do not defibrillate a soaking-wet patient.*

2) Do not defibrillate the patient if he is touching anything metallic that other people are also touching.

3) If you see a nitroglycerin patch on the patient's chest, remove it carefully before defibrillating.

Q5: List the steps in the application of an AED.

A5: *Refer to Scan 17-4. Some students may also cite information from their textbooks.*

Critical Thinking

Q: Evaluate the system you work or live in with respect to the chain of survival. Which links are strong and which need work? How successful is your system in resuscitating patients from cardiac arrest?

A: *Responses will vary.*

Street Scenes

Q1: What type of emergency equipment needs to be taken to the side of every potential cardiac patient?

A1: *Equipment includes: nonrebreather mask, oxygen, a nasal cannula (in the event the patient will not accept the nonrebreather), a suction unit, equipment to take vital signs, a defibrillator (AED) in case of cardiac arrest, bag-valve mask with oxygen reservoir. (Note to Instructor: Some students may note a stair chair if, as in the case study, the patient must be carried down stairs.)*

Q2: What are the treatment priorities for this patient?

A2: *As with any other patient treatment priorities, include the ABCs. At present, the patient's airway is open, but if she becomes unconscious or vomits, the EMT should become immediately concerned. The EMT should continually monitor the patient for rate of respirations* *and quality of breathing. If needed, respirations can be supported with a BVM and supplemental oxygen. (Note to Instructor: Although cardiac patients are usually most comfortable sitting up to breathe, this may affect circulation if the patient is in cardiogenic shock. Remind students that it is not appropriate to lay a patient flat if it impairs breathing and/or makes the patient anxious. Stress the importance of continually monitoring the patient for changes in pain, level of consciousness, breathing, and vital signs.)*

Q3: What assessment information do you need to obtain next?

A3: *The EMT needs to obtain a set of vital signs and a SAMPLE history. Data solicited by the EMT should include: any relevant medical history, current treatment by a physician, prescribed medications (particularly nitroglycerin), presence of an implanted device (pacemaker or defibrillator), and so on. Additionally, the patient should be asked about the signs and symptoms that led her to summon EMS. Using the OPQRST model, the EMT might ask these questions:*

- ***O**nset: When did the signs and symptoms begin?*
- ***P**rovocation: What was the patient doing when the symptoms started? Does anything cause the pain to lessen or intensify?*
- ***Q**uality: Can the patient describe what the pain feels like?*
- ***R**adiation: Where is the pain felt, and does it radiate to other parts of the body such as the neck or arms?*
- ***S**everity: How would the patient rate the pain on a scale of 1 to 10? Has the severity of the pain changed after the administration of nitroglycerin and/or oxygen?*
- ***T**ime: How long has the patient had these particular signs and symptoms?*

Q4: What should you do next?

A4: *The EMT should immediately connect the patient to the AED. While this is being done, the other crew member should ventilate the patient with a BMV and supplemental oxygen. Once the AED is connected, the EMT should push the "analyze" button and follow the instructions issued by the device. (Note to Instructor: Some students may go on to list the care steps described in the case study.)*

CHAPTER 18 ACUTE ABDOMINAL EMERGENCIES

Critical Decision Making: Assessing a Patient with Abdominal Pain

Each patient with abdominal pain will receive a history and physical examination. In the patient presentations below determine what part or parts of the history or physical examination are missing.

Q1: A 26-year-old female patient complains of pain in her lower left abdominal quadrant. The pain radiates from left to right lower quadrants. She denies allergies or medications. The pain came on while she was sitting at her desk earlier in the day. Her vital signs are pulse 104 and slightly irregular, respirations 22, blood pressure 128/90, skin warm and dry.

A1: *For all patients with abdominal pain you should get a history of oral intake as well as a history of recent vomiting, urination, and bowel movements. Females should also be asked about obstetric and gynecologic history and possibility of pregnancy. You will also perform a physical examination including palpation of the abdominal quadrants.*

Q2: A 14-year-old boy complains of abdominal pain. It began slowly over a day or two and has gradually become more severe. His parents are present. The patient denies medical history, allergies, or meds. He hasn't eaten since yesterday because of the pain. His vital signs are pulse 96 strong and regular, respirations 20 and adequate, blood pressure 104/72, skin warm and dry.

A2: *You have the oral intake history, but ask specifically about recent bowel and bladder activity. Palpate the abdomen. Ask about vomiting and fever.*

Q3: A 56-year-old man complains of severe pain in both lower quadrants of his abdomen which developed suddenly and without apparent provocation. The pain is intermittent and comes in waves. He has a history of high blood pressure and high cholesterol and takes medications for both. His pulse is 88 strong and regular, respirations 18 and adequate, blood pressure 158/104, skin cool and moist.

A3: *As with the first two questions, ask about vomiting and recent bowel and bladder activity. Determine oral intake. Palpate the abdomen.*

Review Questions

Q1: List five signs and symptoms of abdominal distress.

A1: *Five signs and symptoms seen with abdominal distress are visceral pain (which is dull and persistent and usually originates from the hollow organs), parietal pain (which is sharp and localized), tearing pain as seen with AAA, referred pain (which is felt somewhere other than where it originates), and pain from a heart attack (which may be described by the patient as abdominal pain).*

Q2: Describe the difference between visceral and parietal pain and describe a condition that may be responsible for each.

A2: *Visceral pain is described as being dull and persistent and usually originates from the hollow organs; parietal pain is sharp and localized and may change with body position. Visceral pain may be symptomatic of a person who has a kidney stone, and parietal pain is seen with patients having internal abdominal bleeding.*

Q3: Describe the emergency care for a patient experiencing abdominal pain or distress.

A3: *Treat the ABCs, administer 15 lpm of oxygen by nonrebreather mask, place the patient in a position of comfort, and transport promptly. As part of the ongoing assessment, vital signs should be monitored during transport.*

Q4: Name the four abdominal quadrants and explain how the quadrants are determined.

A4: *The quadrants are determined by dividing the abdomen into quadrants with imaginary lines drawn both vertically and horizontally through the umbilicus (the navel). The right and left sides of the quadrants are the patient's right and left.*

Critical Thinking

Q: You are called to a patient with abdominal pain. You arrive to find him sitting on the couch, doubled over with pain. He describes the pain as severe and says it began as "on and off" over the past several days. It became severe within the hour. What additional SAMPLE questions would you ask the patient? What position would he likely be most comfortable in?

A: *As part of the "S" (Signs and Symptoms) in SAMPLE, the patient has already supplied some of the OPQRST information about his pain (Onset; Severity, and Time). Ask questions about the other OPQRST factors (Provocation/Palliation—What makes the pain better or worse? Quality—Can you describe what the pain is like? Region/Radiation—Can you point to where you feel the pain?) Then continue questioning the patient about the rest of the SAMPLE history (Allergies, Medications, Pertinent Past History, Last Oral Intake, and Events Leading to the Emergency). If the patient were female, you would also ask questions about the patient's menstrual cycle, possible vaginal bleeding, and other questions that might indicate a possible ectopic pregnancy.*

Street Scenes

Q1: What is your initial impression of this patient?

A1: *Sample response: This patient seems to be showing signs of a medical emergency. Her skin color is pale and sweaty, she is breathing rapidly, and the pulse is fast. This patient* *should be considered unstable based on this information, and rapid intervention and transport considered.*

Q2: What is the significance of the patient's initial presentation?

A2: *The symptoms reportedly came on suddenly. The rapid breathing, fast pulse, and pale/sweaty skin are initial "clues" that this patient has a potential medical emergency. Consider requesting ALS intervention unless transporting directly to the hospital will take less time.*

Q3: Why would you want to see the trash can?

A3: *The vomit can provide a number of important pieces of information for the hospital. Some of the helpful information is quantity, contents, blood/blood clots, coffee ground–looking material, color, and consistency.*

Q4: Why would you request advanced life support?

A4: *This patient may require IV therapy in order to replace the fluid and possible blood loss. Also, if she has a breathing emergency that requires a protected airway (and you do not do endotracheal intubation) then ALS will be able to protect the airway, if necessary, and prevent aspiration if the patient vomits again.*

Q5: Do you agree with the transport priority? Why or why not?

A5: *Yes, this patient seems to be having a potentially life-threatening event that requires definitive care, possibly surgery, and/or blood replacement. The need to get her to a hospital rapidly is important.*

Q6: Do you believe this patient is in shock? Explain your reasoning.

A6: *Yes, the patient seems to be in compensated shock at present and possibly deteriorating into decompensated shock. She has a rapid pulse, pale and sweaty skin, her breathing is becoming rapid, and her blood pressure may be dropping [don't know her baseline normal with the medication she is taking], which is a late sign of shock.*

Q7: What effect might her history have on her current condition?

A7: *It is always important to take notice of something as significant as a "ministroke." The other issue is that she is on blood pressure medication, which may be the reason for the low blood pressure and not the result of her presenting problem. The aspirin she is taking may also be responsible for abdominal bleeding.*

Q8: What position should the patient be placed in?

A8: *She should be placed in a position of comfort. Pain will most importantly cause discomfort to the patient and aggravate her to the point where vital signs are affected and the ability to do an ongoing assessment is also affected.*

CHAPTER 19 DIABETIC EMERGENCIES AND ALTERED MENTAL STATUS

Critical Decision Making: The Taste of Sweet Success

For each patient below determine if the general criteria are met for you to administer glucose to the patient. Oral glucose is carried on your ambulance. For the purposes of this exercise, assume that your blood glucose monitor isn't available. (It is sometimes important to make decisions independent of devices.)

Q1: Your patient is confused. She doesn't know what day it is and is talking but not making any sense. Her nurse's aide tells you the patient is diabetic and has been having trouble with managing her blood sugar levels. She will occasionally take insulin but not eat and vice versa.

A1: *This patient appears to be responsive and able to protect her airway. Her altered mental status and diabetic history round out the facts needed to decide glucose would be appropriate at this time.*

Q2: At a facility for disabled youth, a 19-year-old man recovering from a head injury was seizing prior to your arrival, but the seizure has stopped. He responds to loud verbal stimulus. The patient has a history of diabetes.

A2: *While this patient has a diabetic history, there is nothing that says his seizure is related to his diabetes (as opposed to his head injury). Additionally, his mental status isn't alert enough to administer an oral medication. If he comes out of his seizure and becomes alert, you can obtain a further history.*

Q3: You respond to a motor vehicle collision and find one patient sitting behind the wheel of his car, rocking back and forth, muttering incoherently. The accident was low-speed with a very minor impact. You observe a medical identification bracelet that indicates the patient is diabetic.

A3: *Although this patient was involved in a collision, it could have been a diabetic emergency that caused it. His altered mental status and diabetic history is enough to administer the glucose. Ensure that he is able to control his own airway before administering the medication.*

Review Questions

Q1: List the chief signs and symptoms of a diabetic emergency.

A1: *Rapid onset of altered mental status; taking prescribed insulin after missing a regular meal; vomiting a meal after taking prescribed insulin; an unusual amount of work or physical exercise; intoxicated appearance, staggering, slurred speech, unconsciousness; elevated heart rate; cold, clammy skin; hunger; seizures; insulin found on scene; uncharacteristic behavior; anxiety; combativeness.*

Q2: Explain how you can determine a medical history of diabetes.

A2: *Question the patient or bystanders. Look for medications and blood- or urine-glucose-testing materials. Look for a medical identification device.*

Q3: Explain what treatment may be given by an EMT for a diabetic emergency and the criteria for giving it.

A3: *Give oral glucose in accordance with local protocol if all three of the following criteria are present: 1. The patient has a history of diabetes. 2. The patient's mental status is altered. 3. The patient is awake enough to swallow.*

Q4: Tell whether treatment of a diabetic emergency should be given before or after baseline vital signs are taken. (Answer according to your local protocol.)

A4: *Answers will vary according to your local protocol.*

Q5: Explain the care that should be given to a patient who has had a seizure.

A5: *Protect the airway. If the patient is cyanotic, assure an open airway and provide artificial ventilations with supplemental oxygen. Treat any injuries the patient may have sustained during the convulsion, or rule out trauma. Transport to the medical facility, monitoring vital signs and respirations closely.*

Q6: Explain the care that should be given to a conscious and to an unconscious patient with suspected stroke.

A6: *Conscious patient: Try to calm and reassure the patient. Then protect the airway and administer oxygen. Transport the patient in a semi-sitting position.*

Unconscious patient: Maintain an open airway and provide high-concentration oxygen. Transport the patient lying on his or her side.

Q7: Explain the care that should be given to a patient who has experienced dizziness or syncope.

A7: *Administer high-concentration oxygen. Loosen any tight clothing around the neck. Get the patient flat if there is no reason not to do so. Call ALS if it is available in your area. Treat any injuries associated with a fall. Transport the patient in a position of comfort.*

Critical Thinking

Q: You are dispatched to a "man behaving oddly" at a train station. When you arrive, you find that the man is unconscious. "He's drunk," a bystander tells you. "He was staggering and slurring his words." As you assess the patient, you find a medical identification bracelet that tells you he is a diabetic. Do you administer oral glucose? How do you proceed?

A: *This patient is not a candidate for oral glucose. Although he has a history of diabetes and an altered mental status, he is not alert enough to swallow. Treat him like any other patient with an altered mental status: Secure the airway, place him supine and provide artificial ventilations if necessary, if he does not need ventilations place him in the recovery position, and transport. Request ALS intercept if available.*

Street Scenes

Q1: Does this patient need a thorough assessment?

A1: *All patients should receive a thorough assessment. (Note to Instructor: Stress that numerous medical conditions can account for drunken behavior. Emphasize that it is dangerous and irresponsible for an EMT to assume that a patient is drunk on the basis of appearance. [See Question 3.] Even if a person has been drinking, a full assessment should be done. Remind students of the dangers and potential legal liabilities that EMS providers assume when they quickly dismiss a patient as intoxicated.)*

Q2: What is the first concern when starting to assess this patient?

A2: *The first concern is scene safety. Before approaching the patient, the EMTs must decide whether they need additional police assistance. Once the scene is secured and the patient contained as needed, the EMTs should focus on the ABCs. (Note to Instructor: Questions the EMTs might ask include: "Is the airway open?" "Is there a danger that an altered mental status may prevent the patient from maintaining his own airway without assistance?" "Is breathing adequate and is the patient moving an adequate amount of air?" "Are there signs of external or internal hemorrhage?")*

Q3: What types of underlying medical problems might make a patient appear to be drunk?

A3: *Sample underlying medical problems include: head injury, seizure disorder, meningitis, diabetic emergency, heat stroke, internal bleeding, reaction to medication, poisoning, stroke (brain attack), psychiatric disorder, and so on.*

Q4: Does your assessment plan change at this point?

A4: *Yes. The presence of a medical alert bracelet indicates that the patient has diabetes. Because a diabetic emergency can be a life-threatening situation, the EMTs should take a full set of vital signs, obtain a SAMPLE history, and request ALS support (for providing IV glucose). (Note to Instructor: Point out that the oral administration of food or a sugar substance may not be advisable due to the patient's level of consciousness and ability to maintain his airway.)*

Q5: How will you get a SAMPLE history if the patient is alone?

A5: *Sample responses: Although the patient may be able to answer some questions, an altered mental status may affect the accuracy of responses. The medical alert bracelet—or a card in the patient's wallet—might provide additional information about a medical history and possible information on allergies. The patient may also have insulin or an insulin pump. EMT might question bystanders. Questions might include: "Did you see anyone with the patient?" "How rapidly did the condition seem to come on?" "Did the patient act combative?" As the focused physical exam continues, the EMTs should evaluate the patient for cold, clammy skin; an elevated heart rate; and so on. If the patient has vomited or vomits during assessment, a true diabetic emergency may exist.*

Q6: What is the priority level of this patient? Is there a need to call for ALS assistance?

A6: *As indicated in Question 4, the EMTs should summon ALS. This patient is potentially unstable and needs glucose. Although many EMS systems allow EMTs to administer oral glucose, they may do so only if there are no potential airway problems or if there is no potential for decreased mental status. An ALS unit may be needed to administer IV glucose or to test blood sugar levels.*

CHAPTER 20 ALLERGIC REACTIONS

Critical Decision Making: Is Your Patient Overreacting?

The purpose of this exercise will be to determine the difference between an allergic reaction and anaphylaxis and to determine whether epinephrine should be administered.

Q1: Your 24-year-old patient ate a meal that he believes contained shellfish. He is allergic to shrimp. While the kitchen staff rushes to determine if shrimp was used in or near the preparation of the patient's meal, you perform an examination. The patient is sweating and nervous. He appears to be breathing adequately. You do not note any wheezing or stridor. His face is slightly red. His pulse is 88 strong and regular, respirations 24, blood pressure 108/74, and skin warm and moist.

A1: *This patient does not have respiratory or circulatory compromise but they may be on the way. His vital signs and adequate breathing indicate this is not the time to give epinephrine. However, the nature of shellfish allergies is that they may become severe. This would be one to report to medical direction for advice.*

Q2: You are called to a 50-year-old woman who received a narcotic pain reliever after minor dental surgery. She believes she is allergic to some pain medication but can't remember which one. She has vomited twice. One time she believes she saw blood in her vomit. Her vital signs are pulse 92 strong and regular, respirations 22 and adequate without wheezes or stridor, blood pressure 148/86, skin warm and dry, pupils equal and reactive to light.

A2: *This is not an anaphylactic reaction. Epinephrine would not be appropriate at this time. Transport the patient and observe her for signs of allergic reaction.*

Q3: Your patient is a parent who came into his daughter's kindergarten class as a helper. After eating a cookie he developed a funny feeling in his tongue, which progressed to swelling. He is anxious and sweaty when you see him. His pulse is 126 and regular, respirations 32 and slightly labored, blood pressure 96/58, skin cool and moist, pupils equal and react to light.

A3: *This is a prime candidate for the epinephrine auto-injector. He has signs of airway compromise and shock. Follow local protocols to give the medication.*

Review Questions

Q1: What are the indications for administration of an epinephrine auto-injector?

A1: *Patient exhibits the signs of an allergic reaction; medication is prescribed for this patient by a physician; medical direction authorizes use for this patient.*

Q2: List some of the more common causes of allergic reactions.

A2: *Insect bites/stings—bees, wasps, and so on.*
Food—nuts, crustaceans, peanuts, and so on.
Plants—poison ivy, plant pollen, and so on.
Medications—penicillin.
Others—dust, chemicals, soaps, makeup, and so on.

Q3: List signs or symptoms of an anaphylactic reaction associated with each of the following: skin, respiratory system, and cardiovascular system.

A3: *Skin—itching; hives; red skin; swelling of the face; warm, tingling feeling in the face, mouth, chest, feet, and hands.*
Respiratory system—tightness in throat or chest; cough; rapid breathing; labored, noisy breathing; hoarseness, muffled voice, or loss of voice; stridor; wheezing.
Cardiovascular system—increased heart rate, decreased blood pressure.

Critical Thinking

Q: Your patient is a 60-year-old who used his friend's EpiPen and is now complaining of chest pain. He thought he might have been stung and, although he wasn't sure, his friend had said "Here, I can help you with that," handed him the EpiPen, and helped him inject himself with epinephrine. You know that one action of epinephrine is making the heart beat more strongly. Could this be causing the patient's chest pain? How? And how should you now proceed to assess and care for this patient?

A: *The epinephrine could be causing the patient's chest pain, especially if he has an underlying cardiac condition. Treat him as you would any patient with chest pain. Take a history, especially determining if he has a history of angina or heart disease and if he may have prescribed nitroglycerin. Place him in a position of comfort, administer high-concentration oxygen by nonrebreather mask, and transport him immediately. If he has prescribed nitroglycerin, contact medical direction to report the patient's history and that he has been injected with epinephrine, and request advice from the medical direction physician regarding administering the prescribed nitroglycerin.*

Street Scenes

Q1: What is your impression of Mr. Meeker's condition?

A1: *Sample response: Mr. Meeker is showing signs and symptoms of an anaphylactic reaction. He is using accessory muscles to breathe, and his face and neck look flushed. In addition, he cannot speak in complete sentences. He seems potentially unstable and needs to be monitored closely for what may be a life-threatening condition.*

Q2: What do you think might be happening to him?

A2: *In addition to some of the points mentioned in Question 1, students may note the possibility of more severe respiratory distress as well as cardiovascular involvement, particularly with an increased heart rate and decreased blood pressure. If ALS is delayed, rapid transport would be advised.*

Q3: What do you suspect is beginning to happen to your patient?

A3: *From the information gathered thus far, it would appear that Mr. Meeker is going into severe respiratory distress, which could in turn lead to respiratory arrest. Even if the patient does get definitive care (injection of epinephrine), he will probably need ventilatory support and supplemental oxygen.*

Q4: What further treatment should you render?

A4: *Students will probably offer information from the case study (i.e., provide high-concentration oxygen via a bag-valve mask). (Note to Instructor: Stress the need to monitor the patient for shock and quick ALS intercept or rapid transport to the nearest hospital.)*

CHAPTER 21 POISONING AND OVERDOSE EMERGENCIES

Critical Decision Making: Find the Clues

In each of the following scenarios decide what information you will need to gather—and where to obtain it—to ensure proper treatment for the patient.

Q1: Your patient states he has taken an overdose of prescription medications.
A1: *Look for prescription bottles and nonprescription meds. Look throughout the house, including kitchen, bedroom, and bath. Check garbage cans for empty containers. Look for loose pills anywhere in the house. Of course ask the patient what he took and what medications he knows of around the house.*

Q2: Your patient is found in a closed garage with the car running.
A2: *After ensuring your safety and getting the patient extricated from the hazardous environment, you should attempt to determine how long the patient had been in the garage with the car running. You may get this from the patient (if he is conscious) or from family or neighbors.*

Q3: Your patient is found in the garden, confused and drooling.
A3: *Look for any chemicals the patient may have been using in the garden. Do not become overcome by the same thing that overcame the patient. Look around the garden, in garages or sheds, and even in garbage cans for chemical containers.*

Review Questions

Q1: What are four ways in which a poison can be taken into the body?
A1: *Ingested, inhaled, absorbed, and injected.*

Q2: What is the sequence of assessment steps in cases of poisoning?
A2: *Detect and treat immediately life-threatening problems in the initial assessment. Perform a focused history and physical exam including a SAMPLE history. Assess baseline vital signs. Consult medical direction. Transport the patient with all containers and labels from the substance. Perform ongoing assessment en route.*

Q3: What information must you gather in a case of poisoning before contacting medical direction?
A3: *1) What substance was involved?*
2) When did the exposure occur?
3) How much was ingested?
4) Over how long a period did the ingestion occur?
5) What interventions have the patient, family, or well-meaning bystanders taken?
6) What is the patient's estimated weight?
7) What effects is the patient experiencing from the ingestion?

Q4: What are the emergency care steps for ingested poisoning?
A4: *Refer to Scan 21-1.*

Q5: What are the emergency care steps for inhaled poisoning? For absorbed poisoning?
A5: *Refer to Scan 21-3 and Scan 21-4.*

Critical Thinking

Q: A local farmer calls 911, concerned because one of his farm hands has tried to clean up some spilled pesticide powder with his hands. On arrival, you find that the patient insists he has brushed all the powder off, feels fine, and doesn't need to go to the hospital. As he talks, he continues to make brushing motions at his jeans on which you can see the marks of a powdery residue. How do you manage the situation?
A: *Prevent the patient from brushing at his jeans. Making sure that you are wearing protective gloves, brush off as much of the powder that remains on his hands and other body areas as possible. Do not try to rinse contaminated areas with water or any other "neutralizing" substance. Remove the patient's jeans and any other clothing or jewelry that might be contaminated with the pesticide. Transport him immediately, bringing along the pesticide container and its labels.*

Street Scenes

Q1: What questions would you ask the patient's mother next?

A1: *Sample questions might include: "Do you have the original container?" "Do you know how much oil was previously in the lamp?" "Did you see your child drink the oil?" "What clues convinced you that she had actually swallowed the oil?" "When do you think your daughter might have drunk the oil?" "Have you provided any treatment for your daughter?" "Has your daughter vomited?" "How much did she vomit?" "Did you save the vomit?"*

Q2: What signs or symptoms should you inquire about?

A2: *Signs and symptoms for this substance can vary depending upon a number of factors such as the weight of the patient, amount ingested, stomach contents, and whether or not the patient has vomited. The EMTs should determine the level of consciousness and establish a baseline set of vitals. They should also observe skin color and temperature. As with any patient, the EMTs must ensure that the child can maintain her own airway and breathing. They must also monitor for changes that will alert them to the seriousness of the poisoning. (Note to Instructor: Stress the need to check pupils to determine whether they are equal and reactive. Explain that some poisons cause the pupils to constrict or dilate. The pupils may or may not react to light. Emphasize that seizure activity can also occur with an ingested poison.)*

Q3: What treatments would you initiate?

A3: *As implied in Question 2, most of the care should be focused on the ABCs. The EMTs should consider the need for immediate transport. Depending upon local or state protocols, they can contact poison control en route to the hospital. Because the ingested substance is a petroleum-based product, the use of both activated charcoal and syrup of ipecac is contraindicated. The lamp, or at least some of the oil, should be transported to the hospital along with the patient.*

Q4: Should you contact someone for advice? If yes, then who?

A4: *Answers will depend upon state, regional, and/or local protocols. As previously indicated, the EMTs might consider contacting poison control. In addition, they should also discuss supportive care with medical direction. (Note to Instructor: Tell students that as EMTs they should weigh use of a residential telephone against any delays in transport. If their unit does not possess a mobile phone, they might ask the dispatcher to contact poison control and then relay information to the ambulance while in transit.)*

CHAPTER 22 ENVIRONMENTAL EMERGENCIES

Critical Decision Making: Safety First

Consider the following situations and identify the safety hazards.

Q1: You are taking a walk while on vacation. You hear a sound from the water and see that several hundred feet out in the water a person is struggling to stay afloat.

A1: *This is a long distance to swim. Even if you could swim out there, the patient could inadvertently pull you under. Call for help and look for a way to safely rescue the swimmer.*

Q2: You are ice skating with the family and hear screaming. Someone has fallen through the ice. A group of people have gathered around the hole, peering downward.

A2: *The obvious risk is the one you should be worried about: you and the others falling in. Clear the ice. Call for help. Look for devices such as ropes or sticks that could be used for a rescue.*

Q3: You are on a hiking path and hear screaming. A hiker has been bitten by a snake. He is in pain and holding his leg. He is sitting by an outcropping of rocks.

A3: *The snake (or other snakes) could still be around—especially around the rocks. The patient should be moved to a clearing where both you and the patient will have less chance of further bites.*

Review Questions

Q1: Describe when it is appropriate to treat a cold emergency with active rewarming and when you should perform passive rewarming.

A1: *Passive rewarming is always permitted. Active rewarming may be permitted if the patient is alert and responsive, medical direction orders it, and transport time will be great.*

Q2: List five situations in which a patient may be suffering from hypothermia along with another, more obvious medical condition or injury.

A2: *Alcohol ingestion, underlying illness, overdose or poisoning, major trauma, outdoor resuscitation, decreased ambient temperature.*

Q3: Name the signs and symptoms of a late or deep localized cold injury.

A3: *Initially, the skin of the affected area appears white and waxy. As the condition progresses to actual freezing, the skin turns mottled or blotchy, the color turns from white to grayish-yellow, and finally to grayish-blue. Swelling and blistering may occur.*

Q4: Describe the management of a patient suffering from heat emergency who has moist, pale, and cool skin.

A4: *1. Remove the patient to a cooler environment. 2. Administer oxygen. 3. Remove clothing and cool patient by fanning. 4. Put patient in shock position. 5. Give patient water if responsive and not nauseated. 6. Apply moist towels over muscle cramps. 7. Transport.*

Q5: Describe the management of a patient suffering from a heat emergency who has hot, dry skin.

A5: *1. Remove the patient to the ambulance with air conditioner on high. 2. Remove clothing, apply cool packs to neck, groin, and armpits. Fan aggressively. 3. Administer oxygen. 4. Transport immediately.*

Q6: Describe the proper care for a patient suffering from snakebite.

A6: *1. Call medical direction. 2. Treat for shock and conserve body heat. Keep the patient calm. 3. Clean fang marks with soap and water. 4. Remove jewelry on the bitten extremity. 5. Immobilize the bitten extremity. 6. Apply light constricting bands above and below bite if ordered to do so by medical direction. 7. Transport.*

Critical Thinking

Q1: You respond to a snakebite. There, you find a patient and witnesses who describe a snake to you in great detail. Where would you find information on what type of snake this was, if it was poisonous, and how to treat the patient? What would you do if the snake was still present?

A1: *As an EMT, it is not your job to identify the snake. If the snake is dead and present at the scene, place it in a sealed jar so you can transport it with the patient. Call medical direction for advice. Treat the patient for shock and keep him calm. Clean the site of the fang marks with soap and water. Remove any rings, bracelets, or other constricting items on the bitten extremity. Immobilize the bitten extremity with a splint. If possible, keep the bitten extremity at or below the level of the heart. If ordered by medical direction, apply light constricting bands above and below the wound. Transport the patient, monitoring his vital signs en route.*

Q2: You have a patient who is experiencing hypothermia, is half a mile into the woods, and is not accessible by ambulance. Do you have clothing available that would protect you and your crew/team from hypothermia during the trip in and out? If you will be an EMT in a warm climate, change the situation. It is hot and humid. A hiker has experienced a heat emergency. Can you and your crew/team get the patient out without experiencing a heat emergency yourselves? In either case, what transport device(s) and resources would you use to remove the patient from the woods?

A2: *For the hypothermic patient, be sure you are wearing warm clothing as you proceed to the patient's location. Bring along blankets for the patient. For the hyperthermic patient, wear clothing that will allow your body to remain as cool as possible while still being protective. For the patient, bring along cool packs to apply to neck, groin, and armpits if the patient is extremely hot (with skin that is hot and either moist or dry). Bring water to moisten the patient's skin and something to fan the patient with. In either case, administer oxygen by nonrebreather mask and remove the patient to the ambulance (patient compartment warm for the hypothermic patient, air conditioned for the hyperthermic patient). In either case, bring along an appropriate transport device, such as a basket stretcher, to remove the patient from the remote area to the ambulance.*

Street Scenes

Q1: What concerns might you have for this patient?

A1: *Besides the obvious (ABCs, etc.), the EMTs should suspect hypothermia as well as other underlying problems such as malnutrition or untreated medical conditions. Because of the patient's situation, he is at risk of pneumonia and respiratory infections as well as medical conditions suggested by the signs and symptoms (stroke, trauma from a fall, and so on).*

Q2: What assessment needs to be performed?

A2: *Sample response: Basically, the patient needs complete focused and detailed assessments. As with all patients, the EMTs must assess the ABCs, make sure the patient's minute volume for breathing is adequate, and consider the use of supplemental oxygen. Once the EMTs complete the initial assessment and initiate immediate care, they should take a complete set of baseline vital signs. Because the patient was found outside on a cold night, he needs to be assessed for hypothermia. The EMTs should determine, if possible, orientation to time and place and other items in a SAMPLE history. A detailed head-to-toe survey should be utilized to determine whether the patient has other medical problems or has sustained a traumatic fall.*

Q3: Should you rewarm this patient? If so, when should you start?

A3: *Active rewarming in the field is not recommended. However, the EMTs might initiate passive rewarming. For example, the EMTs should remove all wet clothing and wrap the patient in one or more blankets. They may also consider a thermal (space) blanket as an outer shell. The patient's head should be covered to prevent additional heat loss. Unless recommended by medical direction and/or local protocols, the EMTs should NOT apply hot packs or administer warm fluids in a prehospital setting. The exceptions include rare cases of long or delayed transport time and then only with approval from medical direction. The EMTs should reassess the patient frequently. Stress that even with passive warming, an unresponsive patient or patient suffering from extreme hypothermia can downgrade rapidly.*

Q4: How often should you take vital signs?

A4: *Vital signs should be taken as often as every 5–10 minutes. (Note to Instructor: The more hypothermic the patient, the harder it is to take vital signs—i.e., signs can be depressed. Heart rate and respirations can fall "below normal," but the patient may still sustain the rate/respirations and survive. Stress that hypothermic patients should not be considered dead until they are warm and dead. When a person becomes hypothermic, he or she can sometimes survive neurologically intact for a significant period of time after vital signs have become depressed.)*

Q5: When moving the patient out of the ambulance and onto the hospital stretcher, what precautions should be taken?

A5: *Hypothermic patients should be handled gently. "Rough" handling can result in ventricular fibrillation. (Note to Instructor: Stress the need to keep a defibrillator (AED) close to the patient throughout transport.)*

CHAPTER 23 BEHAVIORAL EMERGENCIES

Critical Decision Making: Psych Condition . . . or Hidden Medical Condition?

For each of these patients describe how your assessment would determine if the patient was suffering from a medical problem or a psychiatric problem.

Q1: Your patient is a 56-year-old man who was found to be "talking to God" and generally mumbling at the grocery store.

A1: *In this case, a stroke or diabetes could cause similar symptoms. Obtain a history from the patient and observe for medical alert identification. If you have the ability to perform blood glucose measurement, do so. A stroke scale may be helpful if the patient is cooperative. A history of head injury or other cause of altered mental status should be explored.*

Q2: Your patient is a 21-year-old student who was found on the outskirts of his campus, acting strangely with a slight smell of alcohol on his breath.

A2: *Alcohol may have caused the emergency, but it isn't the only potential cause. As in the first case, perform a thorough history and a blood glucose measurement. Stroke isn't as likely in a 21-year-old. Consider drug use in addition to alcohol. Also look for evidence of head injury or seizure history.*

Q3: Your patient is an 84-year-old woman who is in a nursing home. She has a history of depression and cardiac problems. This morning she became agitated and angry with the staff.

A3: *Depression won't normally cause aggressive behavior. Dementia or Alzheimer's may. Look for a history of this as well as compliance with her medications. Look for evidence of seizure, head injury, or diabetes. You may not be able to perform a stroke scale, but observe for signs of asymmetry in speech or for movement that is new to the patient.*

Review Questions

Q1: Name several conditions that can alter a person's mental status and behavior.

A1: *Low blood sugar; lack of oxygen; inadequate blood to the brain or stroke; head trauma; mind-altering substances; excessive cold; excessive heat; psychological conditions.*

Q2: List several methods that can help calm the patient suffering a behavioral or psychiatric emergency.

A2: *Speak slowly and calmly. Use a calm and reassuring tone. Listen to the patient and make him aware of this. Do not be judgmental. Show compassion, not pity. Use positive body language; avoid crossing one's arms or looking disinterested. Acknowledge the patient's feelings. Do not enter the patient's personal space, staying at least 3 feet away.*

Q3: Describe the signs and symptoms of a behavioral or psychiatric emergency.

A3: *Panic or anxiety; unusual appearance, disordered clothing, poor hygiene; agitated or unusual activity; unusual speech patterns or inability to carry on a coherent conversation.*

Q4: Describe what you can do when scene size-up reveals that it is too dangerous to approach the patient.

A4: *Call for the police and wait for them. Do not leave the patient alone. Try to talk to the patient from a safe distance.*

Q5: List several factors that can help you assess the patient's risk for suicide.
A5: *Threats of suicide; depression; high current or recent stress levels; previous attempts or suicide threats; a suicide plan; recent emotional trauma; age (15–25 and over 40 at greater risk); alcohol and drug abuse; sudden improvement from depression.*

Q6: Research your state law. Then describe the circumstances that must exist for you to treat and transport a behavioral emergency patient without consent.
A6: *Answers will vary.*

Critical Thinking

Q: You are called to respond to an intoxicated minor who is physically aggressive, threatens suicide, and whose parents permit you to treat but not transport. How would you manage this patient?
A: *Be aware of your state laws regarding involuntary restraint and transport of a minor. Most states have laws that allow a patient to be transported against his will if he is a danger to himself or others. If the parents to do not give permission to transport the patient, it will be helpful to call for a law enforcement response for the safety of yourself, the patient, and the parents, and to help avoid liability problems if you attempt transport on your own.*

Street Scenes

Q1: What is your first and most important concern?
A1: *The first and foremost concern for the EMT is scene safety. If the scene is known to be unsafe or if the patient is believed to have violent tendencies, EMS personnel should not even get close to the scene until law enforcement officials have secured it. (Note to Instructor: Stress that EMS personnel cannot provide care if they become hurt. In fact, if EMS personnel become injured in this type of situation, the event is compounded by the need to summon other units. Tell students: Be safe! Be cautious!)*

Q2: How should you handle the matter of scene safety?
A2: *In this case, scene safety should be handled by the appropriate law enforcement agency. Police officers are trained and equipped to handle these situations. As indicated in the scenario, the EMTs should make sure that all EMS personnel and bystanders are in a safe area in case the patient exits the building prior to the arrival of police officers. They should then await and follow law enforcement directives.*

Q3: When should you approach the patient?
A3: *The EMT should approach the patient after police declare the scene safe. In addition, a police officer might need to remain in the area until everybody is confident that the patient will not attempt to harm himself or others. In this scenario, the EMT decides to approach without a partner to minimize patient agitation. However, a police officer remains in the area. (Note to Instructor: In some cases, a police officer might accompany EMS personnel to the hospital. As emphasized in the chapter, physical restraints are used cautiously and only in select situations.)*

Q4: How should the patient be approached?
A4: *Answers should reflect the guidelines in the chapter. Rules for approaching a patient with a behavior disorder include: 1. Identify yourself. 2. Speak slowly and clearly. 3. Listen to the patient. 4. Do not be judgmental. 5. Use positive body language. 6. Acknowledge the patient's feelings. 7. Do not enter the patient's personal space. 8. Be alert to the patient's emotional status.*

Q5: What are the safety concerns when working with an agitated patient?
A5: *Answers should reflect guidelines in the chapter. Guidelines for dealing with agitated patients include: 1. Be alert and remain concerned with scene safety. 2. Treat life-threatening problems during the initial survey. 3. Remember that some medical or traumatic injuries may mimic behavioral emergencies. 4. Be prepared to spend time talking with the patient.*

5. Encourage the patient to discuss the problem; then listen. 6. Never play along with visual or auditory hallucinations. 7. If it appears that it might help, involve a family member or friend. 8. Only consider physical restraints as a last resort. If used, make every attempt not to cause additional harm to the patient. Pay very close attention to airway and breathing throughout the entire transport to the hospital.

Q6: Does this patient need a medical assessment?

A6: *Yes. All patients need to be assessed. In cases of behavioral emergencies, EMTs should never assume the absence of an underlying medical or trauma-related condition. If behavioral patients will cooperate, EMS personnel have an ethical and legal responsibility to take a full set of vital signs and to conduct a focused and/or detailed assessment. (Note to Instructor: Be sure to emphasize the importance of communication skills in the management of behavioral emergencies. In fact, you might want to have students role-play this situation, questioning and listening to the responses of the patient.)*

CHAPTER 24 OBSTETRICS AND GYNECOLOGICAL EMERGENCIES

Critical Decision Making: My Baby Won't Wait!

Being able to determine whether birth is imminent is an important skill for an EMT. For each of the scenarios presented, determine if you should stay and prepare for delivery or should transport the patient to the hospital.

Q1: Your patient states contractions are severe, about 30 seconds apart. She feels the need to push and suspects she has accidentally moved her bowels. There is significant bulging, and you can see the baby's head crowning. This is her fourth child.

A1: *This baby is coming—and quickly. Prepare for delivery at the scene.*

Q2: Your patient reports contractions are about 5–10 minutes apart but feel strong. This is her first child. You do not observe any crowning or bulging. She is not sure if her water has broken.

A2: *This baby will likely wait. Ask about feeling the need to push and if she feels like she must move her bowels. In the absence of either of these, you should make it to the hospital.*

Q3: Your patient reports contractions that are about 2 minutes apart. They have been this way for about 8 hours. Her water broke when the contractions started. She doesn't feel she is progressing through labor and is concerned for her baby.

A3: *Transport this patient. Since there has been no significant change over 8 hours and there are no signs of imminent delivery, transport is the correct decision.*

Review Questions

Q1: Name and describe the anatomical structures of a woman's body that are associated with pregnancy.

A1: *Uterus (womb)—organ in which a fetus grows, responsible for labor and expulsion of infant.*
Cervix—the neck of the uterus.
Vagina—lower part of the birth canal.
Perineum—skin area between vagina and anus, commonly torn during delivery.

Q2: Describe the three stages of labor.

A2: *First stage—starts with regular contractions and the thinning and gradual dilation of cervix and ends when the cervix is fully dilated.*

Second stage—the time from when the baby enters the birth canal until it is born.
Third stage—begins when the baby is born until the afterbirth (placenta, umbilical cord, some tissues for the amniotic sac, and the lining of the uterus) is delivered.

Q3: Explain how to evaluate and to prepare the mother for delivery.
A3: *Ask the patient's name, age, and expected due date.*
Ask if this is her first pregnancy.
Ask her how long she has been having labor pains, how often she is having the pains, if her "bag of waters" has broken, and if she has had any bleeding or "bloody show."
Ask her if she is straining as though she needs to move her bowels.
Examine the mother for crowning.
Feel for uterine contractions.
Take vital signs.
Control the scene so the mother will have privacy.
Put on surgical gloves, gowns, caps, face masks, and eye protection.
Place the mother on a bed, sturdy table, or the ambulance stretcher.
Remove any of the patient's clothing or underclothing that obstructs your view of the vaginal opening.
Position your assistant at the mother's head.
Position the obstetric kit on a table or chair with all items within easy reach.

Q4: Name, in the order of the inverted pyramid, the steps that may be taken to resuscitate a newborn infant.
A4: *Clear the baby's airway.*
Keep the baby on the side with the head slightly lower than the body and again suction the mouth, then the nose.
Establish that the baby is breathing. If not, stimulate breathing. If this is unsuccessful, provide artificial ventilations.
Assess the infant's heart rate. Initiate artificial ventilation and chest compressions if necessary.
Provide supplemental oxygen if necessary.

Q5: Name and describe several possible complications of delivery.
A5: *Breech presentation—breech presentation occurs when the buttocks or lower extremities are low in the uterus and will be the first part of the fetus delivered.*
Prolapsed umbilical cord—condition where the cord presents through the birth canal before delivery of the head; presents a serious emergency that endangers the life of the unborn fetus.
Limb presentation—occurs when a limb of the infant protrudes from the birth canal.
Multiple births.
Meconium—amniotic fluid that is greenish or brownish-yellow rather than clear; an indication of possible fetal or maternal distress during labor.
Premature birth.
Stillbirth and death.

Q6: Name and describe several possible predelivery emergencies.
A6: *Vaginal bleeding, seizures, ectopic pregnancy, miscarriage and abortion, trauma during pregnancy.*

Critical Thinking

Q: You are called to respond to a pregnant woman who is in labor. During your evaluation, you find that this is the woman's first pregnancy, the baby's head is not yet crowning, and contractions are 10 minutes apart. You ask the mother if she feels she needs to move her bowels, and she says she does not. Do you prepare for delivery at the scene? Or do you transport the mother to the hospital? Explain your reasoning.

A: *Transport the mother to the hospital. The duration between labor pains (10 minutes) indicates that it will be some time before the baby is born. Because the mother does not feel the need to move her bowels, the baby is not yet in the birth canal. Also, first deliveries often take longer than subsequent deliveries.*

Street Scenes

Q1: What should be the first priority when entering the scene?

A1: *EMTs should always consider scene safety whenever they approach any call, regardless of its nature. They also need to take appropriate Standard Precautions. Any childbirth scenario carries a high potential for exposure to bodily fluids. In addition to gloves, the EMTs should don a gown and splash protector for the face. (Note to Instructor: Emphasize some of the factors that should be taken into account during the scene size-up, such as the general appearance of the mother, the amount of space available for delivery and care, the stage of labor, and so on.)*

Q2: Should ALS assistance be requested?

A2: *Yes. Although the delivery might be uneventful, there is always the possibility of complications, especially in a premature birth. For example, if the mother experiences significant blood loss, she might require an IV. The newborn might need advanced airway maneuvers, particularly if meconium is present. If the delivery is uneventful, ALS can always be cancelled. If ALS will be delayed, the EMTs should consider rapid transport. Sometimes the quickest access to ALS may be arrival at the nearest hospital.*

Q3: What questions should you ask the mother or the father?

A3: *Sample questions to the mother might include: "What is your name and age?" "When was your expected due date?" "Do you feel like moving your bowels?" Sample questions to either parent might include: "Did the doctor alert you to any potential problems?" "Is this your first child?" "Has the water broken?" "When did the labor pains start?"*

Q4: What immediate care should be provided to the newly born child?

A4: *The umbilical cord must be removed from around the baby's neck. The EMTs can either gently free the cord (as in the scenario) or cut it. Otherwise, the EMTs should follow the relevant care steps in Scan 24-1 and the steps discussed under "The Newly Born Child" in the chapter. (Note to Instructor: You might want to advise students on the steps involved in cutting an umbilical cord from around a baby's neck. Stress that it is preferable to free the cord. However, if the cord must be cut, the EMT should place two clamps—one a few inches from where the cord exits the vagina and the other a few inches from the baby's belly button. Every effort must be made not to harm either the baby or the mother. The cord may be tough, so the EMT should angle the cut away from both patients.)*

Q5: What care should your partner be giving to the mother?

A5: *The EMT should administer oxygen to the mother and keep her warm. (Note to Instructor: Tell students that the placenta can take up to 30 minutes or longer to deliver. It is usually recommended that EMS personnel wait 20 minutes for the placenta to deliver and then transport the patient. However, this guideline can vary, depending upon state or local protocols. If the placenta delivers in the field, it should be taken to the hospital for examination. If there is excess bleeding, then one of the EMTs should place sanitary napkins over the mother's vaginal opening. The EMT should then tell the mother to lower her legs and place them together without squeezing. The EMTs should allow the mother to nurse the baby if she wants. They should also provide the necessary psychological support.)*

CHAPTER 25 PUTTING IT ALL TOGETHER FOR THE MEDICAL PATIENT

Critical Decision Making: Problems, Problems

Each brief patient presentation below details a patient with dual problems—or two potential causes for the same problem. You will be asked how to differentiate one from the other. (Note: Solutions for these questions are drawn from material throughout the *Medical Emergencies* module.)

Q1: You are treating a patient who is experiencing difficulty breathing. The patient has a history of COPD and congestive heart failure. He has a prescribed inhaler and wants to know if he should use it.

A1: *This is challenging—and medical direction can help, if necessary. If the patient believes it is his COPD and has increased sputum production, a history of recent infection, and so on, it may be prudent to give the medication. If he has fluid buildup, swollen ankles, or has to sleep on more pillows or in a chair recently, it may be the CHF. This is a difficult call.*

Q2: You are called by a wife who reports her husband suddenly became confused. He has a history of diabetes and recently had a stroke. He is alert enough to receive sugar, but how can you tell the difference between this possible diabetic condition and stroke?

A2: *Use a stroke scale and blood glucose monitor. This case is more clear cut. You can always make a call to the on-line physician.*

Q3: A patient who has a history of heart problems calls because he has had a feeling of indigestion for several hours. He also has a history of acid reflux—which he thought this was—but his medication wasn't working. He wants to know if you think he should go to the hospital.

A3: *This isn't about medication—it is about whether he should go to the hospital. The answer is yes. It is difficult to distinguish between some digestive conditions and heart attack—even in the hospital. He should go for the ride and let the physicians check him out.*

Review Questions

Q1: What are the decisions an EMT must make for a medical patient with regard to interventions?

A1: *The decisions that an EMT must make center on questions related to airway, breathing, circulation, priority, and interventions.*

Q2: What steps should the EMT follow when a patient seems to require two interventions?

A2: *Sample response: When faced with this kind of situation, an EMT should assess the patient as usual. He or she should then determine if the patient meets the criteria for one or more of the interventions available to EMTs. If there is any reason to believe a particular intervention may harm the patient or if unusual circumstances make it difficult to assess the effect of intervention, the EMT should consult with medical direction (even if not required by local protocols).*

Q3: What are the advantages to consulting on-line medical direction in a difficult medical case?

A3: *Medical direction can indicate what, if any, interventions the EMT might employ.*

Q4: How can an EMT learn more about a patient's complaint that is not covered in the EMT curriculum?

A4: *Sample responses: 1. Ask the patient to describe the condition; 2. Contact a higher level of EMS provider, such as a paramedic; 3. Contact medical direction. [Stress the limits of* *medical references—such as the effect on a family seeing an EMT flip through the pages, the complicated level of information in most references, and so on.]*

Q5: What is an appropriate response on the part of an EMT when a patient tells him she has Crohn's disease?

A5: *Sample response: The EMT should be honest with the patient and admit being unfamiliar with the disease. The EMT might then take some of the steps suggested in Question 4.*

Critical Thinking

Q: You are treating a 65-year-old male for carbon monoxide poisoning. He is responsive only to pain, and he is tolerating a nasal airway well. He is breathing adequately, so you apply high-concentration oxygen by nonrebreather mask. His wife tells you that he is not supposed to get any more than 2 liters per minute of oxygen because he has emphysema. What should you do? Explain your answer.

A: *Sample response: The EMT is faced with a dilemma. The patient's wife says that the intervention might harm the patient. However, the patient is in need of oxygen, and a basic rule of EMS is never to deprive a patient of oxygen if he or she needs it. Although it is unlikely that the administration of high-concentration oxygen will affect the patient's breathing problems in the short term, the EMT must be prepared to assist ventilations with a bag-valve mask (BMV) with an oxygen reservoir. The EMT should provide an explanation to the wife as time and the patient's conditions permit. The EMT should also confer with medical direction—an important step in this situation.*

Street Scenes

Q1: What pertinent signs or symptoms should you inquire about?

A1: *Immediate signs and symptoms focus on the ABCs. Once this information has been solicited and immediate care provided (if needed), the patient can be asked about any pain and for information to prepare a SAMPLE history. Particularly important might be the patient's past medical history and further description of his illness.*

Q2: What further patient assessment should you perform?

A2: *Additional patient assessment would include a baseline set of vitals and completion of the SAMPLE history if this hasn't already been done. If the patient has a number of medications, the EMTs might also check these medications and question the patient about compliancy. Part of the assessment might also involve contacting medical direction for advice.*

Q3: What treatment should you provide to Mr. Jones at this time?

A3: *Sample response: On the return call, the EMTs should follow the ABC assessment. They should determine if the patient has a patent airway and evaluate his level of responsiveness. The EMTs should provide the necessary interventions to protect the patient's airway and to ensure adequate respirations. They should assess and reassess vital signs, every 5–10 minutes. Transport to the hospital, as indicated in the scenario, is in order.*

CHAPTER 26 BLEEDING AND SHOCK

Critical Decision Making: No Pressure, No Problem

In the following patients, use material you learned in this chapter to determine if your early decision-making would lead you to expedite the call because you suspected shock or if, instead, you believe the patient will likely be stable. You will not be provided a blood pressure—but in each patient you will find enough information to make a proper early decision without a blood pressure reading.

Q1: Your patient was working on scaffolding that collapsed, causing him to fall one story (about 10 feet). He is conscious, alert but anxious, and complains of pain to the right side of his chest. His pulse is 102 and regular, respirations 26, skin cool and moist, pupils equal and reactive to light.
A1: *Expedite because of the potential for internal (chest, lung) injury. His vitals are elevated. This could be serious.*

Q2: Your patient is found sitting in a bathroom stall at an upscale restaurant. He is pale, sweaty, and leaning against the wall. He tells you he has had a problem with bleeding hemorrhoids recently. There is bright red blood in the toilet bowl. When you stand the patient up to move him to the stretcher, he feels like he is going to pass out.
A2: *Just because the bleeding is from hemorrhoids doesn't mean he isn't in shock. His appearance screams shock. His feeling when he stands up confirms it (orthostatic hypotension). Move it!*

Q3: You are called to an assault. A 26-year-old man was struck in the head by his girlfriend. She used a telephone to strike him once in the nose and again in the forehead. The police called you to evaluate a nosebleed. The patient's shirt has blood streaked down it. His nose is oozing blood now. He is alert and oriented. His pulse is 78 strong and regular, respirations 14, skin warm and dry.
A3: *He hasn't lost enough blood to have shock. Your bigger concerns would be if he couldn't maintain his airway because of blood flow or if the head injury were a concern. Right now there doesn't seem to be a big rush, but he needs transport.*

Review Questions

Q1: Name the three main types of blood vessels and describe the type of bleeding you would expect to see from each one.
A1: *Arteries: Arterial bleeding is often rapid, spurting with each heartbeat, profuse, and bright red. Veins: Venous blood is usually a steady flow, can be quite heavy, and is usually dark red or maroon in color. Capillaries: Capillary bleeding is usually slow, oozing, and red (though not as bright as arterial blood).*

Q2: List the patient care steps in external bleeding control.
A2: *Refer to Scan 26-1.*

Q3: Define perfusion and hypoperfusion.
A3: *Perfusion: When blood reaches and fills the capillaries, supplying oxygen and nutrients to the cells and tissues.*

Hypoperfusion: Inadequate perfusion of the body's tissues and organs (shock).

Q4: List the signs and symptoms of shock. Which would you expect to see early? Which are late signs? Explain what causes each of them.
A4: *Refer to Table 26-1, Figure 26-12, and information in the chapter.*

Q5: List the three major types of shock and what causes each.
A5: *Hypovolemic (hemorrhagic) shock—caused by uncontrolled bleeding; cardiogenic shock—caused by inadequate pumping of blood by the heart; neurogenic shock—caused by uncontrolled dilation of blood vessels due to nerve paralysis from spinal cord injury.*

Q6: List the emergency care steps for treating a patient in shock.
A6: *Refer to Scan 26-2.*

Q7: In gauging the optimal time between injury and definitive care, when does the clock start running and when does the clock stop running?
A7: *The clock starts running at the time of injury and stops running in the operating room.*

Critical Thinking

Q: A patient has been involved in a motor-vehicle crash. There is considerable damage to his vehicle. The steering column and wheel are badly deformed. The patient complains of a "sore chest." You note no external bleeding. The patient's vital signs are pulse 116, respirations 20, and blood pressure 106/70. How would you proceed to assess and care for this patient?

A: *The mechanism of injury suggests the possibility of internal bleeding. Vitals indicate that shock may be starting. Treating for shock—maintaining airway; providing high-concentration oxygen and assisting with ventilations if necessary; controlling any external bleeding; applying and inflating the PASG if approved by medical direction; keeping the patient warm; providing immediate transport—is prudent.*

Street Scenes

Q1: What is the priority for this patient? Does an initial assessment still need to be done?

A1: *The fact that the patient has sustained some type of traumatic injury makes him a candidate for high-priority treatment. Even so, the First Responders still need to perform some kind of initial assessment to determine such information as level of responsiveness, breathing, and signs of internal bleeding—always a possibility with trauma.*

Q2: What assessment information do you want to receive from Squad 31?

A2: *In addition to the mechanism of injury, the EMTs would want assessment information such as vital signs (respiration rate, pulse, blood pressure, and skin color). They might also ask about bruising or discoloration over the injured area. These are important signs of possible internal bleeding.*

Q3: Is the mechanism of injury important information about this patient?

A3: *Yes. In the case of a trauma patient, the mechanism of injury can help determine the location and type of injuries sustained by a patient. (Note to Instructor: You might ask students to suggest some of the conditions that the mechanism of injury reported by Squad 31 might indicate—e.g., broken ribs, a flailed segment [which could affect breathing and/or account for hemothorax or pneumothorax], or injury to internal organs either through bruising or bleeding.)*

Q4: What is the treatment priority for this patient?

A4: *Treatment priorities depend upon the ABCs. Because the EMTs suspect internal bleeding, rapid transport is indicated. The EMTs should consider administration of high-concentration oxygen by nonrebreather mask. They should also attempt to keep the patient warm and remain alert to signs of shock.*

Q5: How often should you get a new set of vital signs?

A5: *Vital signs should be taken every 5–10 minutes to determine changes in the patient's condition. In cases of internal bleeding, the EMTs can expect that the pulse rate will increase and become more thready. They can also expect the respiratory rate to become more rapid and increasingly labored. The patient's skin will grow paler and become more moist. As the signs and symptoms of shock (hypoperfusion) intensify, the EMTs can expect dilated pupils, delayed capillary refill time (although not always a reliable indicator), and cyanosis around the lips and nail beds. The detailed assessment may reveal tenderness in the left upper abdominal quadrant.*

CHAPTER 27 SOFT-TISSUE INJURIES

Critical Decision Making: Burns—By the Numbers

For each of the following patients, determine the approximate body surface area burned and the degree of the burn.

Q1: Your patient fell asleep by the pool and was sunburned over the backs of both legs, his back, and the backs of both arms. The skin is bright red.
A1: *45 percent superficial.*

Q2: Your patient works at a fast food restaurant. She was by the fryer when someone threw in an ice cube as a joke to scare her. Hot grease splashed up and covered the anterior portion of her left forearm and her entire right hand. The skin is red and blistered.
A2: *Approximately 3.25 percent partial thickness.*

Q3: Your patient fell asleep while smoking. He has circumferential burns on both legs and has burned the entire right arm. The legs are red and blistered. The patient's right arm is severely charred and peeling.
A3: *36 percent partial thickness (legs) 9 percent full thickness (arm).*

Review Questions

Q1: List three types of closed soft-tissue injuries.
A1: *Contusions, hematomas, crush injuries.*

Q2: List four types of open soft-tissue injury.
A2: *Abrasions, lacerations, punctures, avulsions, amputations, crush injuries.*

Q3: Describe the care for an open wound to the chest.
A3: *Maintain an open airway. Provide basic life support if necessary. Seal the open chest wound as quickly as possible, with your gloved hand if necessary. Apply an occlusive dressing (depending on local protocols, sealed on all four sides or with a flutter valve). Administer high-concentration oxygen. Care for shock. Transport as soon as possible.*

Q4: Describe the care for impaled objects in the eye.
A4: *Place a roll of 3-inch gauze bandage or folded 4 × 4s on either side of the object, along the vertical axis of the head. Fit a disposable paper cup over the impaled object and allow it to come to rest on the dressing rolls. Have another rescuer stabilize the dressings and cup while you secure them in place with self-adherent roller bandage or with a wrapping of gauze. The uninjured eye should be dressed and bandaged to reduce eye movements. Provide oxygen and care for shock. Continue to reassure the patient and provide emotional support.*

Q5: Explain when you would remove an object impaled in the cheek and when you would, instead, stabilize an object impaled in the cheek.
A5: *An object impaled in the cheek should only be removed if it has already gone through the inside surface of the cheek and can be easily pulled out in the same direction that it entered. If this cannot be done, the object should be stabilized in place.*

Q6: Describe the three classifications (depths) of burns.
A6: *Superficial burn—a burn that involves only the epidermis. Partial thickness burn—a burn in which the epidermis is burned through and the dermis is damaged. Full thickness burn—a burn in which all the layers of the skin are damaged.*

Q7: Differentiate between a dressing and a bandage.
A7: *A dressing is placed directly on a wound. A bandage holds a dressing in place.*

Q8: List the qualities and purpose of an effective bandage. How could you tell if a bandage were improperly applied?
A8: *The bandage should hold the dressing snugly in place and cover all four of its edges, but not restrict blood supply.*

Critical Thinking

Q: You have been caring for a patient who shot himself in the chest with a nail gun. You applied an occlusive dressing around the wound. The patient is now suddenly beginning to deteriorate. He is having extreme difficulty breathing and his color has worsened. Breath sounds have become almost totally absent on the side with the impaled nail. What complication might you suspect is causing his worsening condition? How could this be corrected?

A: *Absent breath sounds on the side of the injury may indicate a collapsed lung. The nail may also have damaged a major blood vessel or the heart itself. If the occlusive dressing you applied is sealed on all four sides, air building up in the chest cavity will have no way to escape and can cause lung collapse and increase pressure on the heart. An open chest wound is a TRUE EMERGENCY. Maintain an open airway. Administer oxygen, care for shock, and transport as quickly as possible. Provide basic life support if necessary (ventilations or CPR). Request ALS intercept if available and if it will not delay arrival at the hospital.*

Street Scenes

Q1: What is your general impression of this patient?

A1: *Sample response: The patient seems alert and appears to have walked to the present location after her injury. She has an open airway and is breathing without any obvious distress. Judging from the blood-soaked towel, the immediate focus of care is on "C," or circulation.*

Q2: What priority would you assign to her?

A2: *Until further assessment, the patient might be assigned low-priority transport. However, she has the potential to lose a significant amount of blood, and the EMTs should be ready to upgrade the patient's priority as necessary.*

Q3: What interventions are appropriate at this time?

A3: *The bleeding must be controlled. The EMTs might apply direct pressure with a sterile dressing, or they might leave the towel in place if the bleeding is being controlled. If necessary, they can use a pressure point to make sure the bleeding is stopped. (Note to Instructor: Point out that, based on information in the scenario, it would be inappropriate to apply a tourniquet. Once the bleeding is controlled, the EMTs should assess pulses, motor ability, and sensation in the injured arm. They might also administer high-concentration oxygen and observe for signs of shock.)*

Q4: Would you change the priority of transport of this patient based on what you now know? Why or why not?

A4: *A suspicion of alcohol consumption should not interfere with assessment and treatment. A set of vitals and a SAMPLE history must be obtained. Based on the pool of blood on the patio and the lack of motion in several of the patient's fingers, the patient appears to have the potential to become unstable. The EMTs should consider upgrading her priority from "low" to "high" because of their findings.*

Q5: What interventions are appropriate for this patient?

A5: *Sample response: The bleeding must be monitored and the patient's arm stabilized with some type of splinting device or sling. Vital signs should be taken every 5–10 minutes and compared with the baseline set of vitals. Motor function and sensation should be reassessed as well. Because of the potential for shock, the patient should be kept warm and perhaps placed on the cot with her legs elevated.*

CHAPTER 28 MUSCULOSKELETAL INJURIES

Critical Decision Making: Sticks and Stones May Break My Bones, but Trauma Centers Save Me

For each of these patients, determine whether you would stay and splint or, as a higher priority, consider transport to a trauma center, using a backboard as the main splinting device.

Q1: You are called to a patient who tripped and tried to catch himself with an outstretched arm. He believes he broke his wrist and hit his head when he fell. He is alert and oriented. His vital signs are pulse 88 strong and regular, respirations 16, blood pressure 140/84, skin warm and dry, pupils equal and reactive to light.

A1: *A local hospital for this patient is acceptable as long as the head injury isn't more severe than the suspected fracture. If his mental status and vitals stay within normal limits, a trauma center may not be necessary. When in doubt, radio the hospital for medical direction.*

Q2: You are called to an industrial complex where a large spool pinned a man by the legs. The workers are able to move the spool for you to safely access the patient. The patient is in extreme pain. Your physical examination reveals deformity in both thighs and the patient's left lower leg. The patient is agitated. His pulse is 112 and regular, respirations 24 and adequate, blood pressure 108/64, pupils equal and reactive to light.

A2: *Backboard and transport to a trauma center. He has multiple fractures with an altered mental status and vitals which indicate shock.*

Q3: Your patient was ejected from a vehicle and found about 20 feet away. He complains only of a broken arm. Your physical assessment doesn't reveal any other injuries. The patient is alert and oriented. His pulse is 130 and weak, respirations 28 and adequate, blood pressure 88/56, skin cool and moist, pupils equal and reactive to light.

A3: *He doesn't have major complaints but his mechanism of injury and vital signs scream trauma center. Backboard your patient and go there promptly.*

Review Questions

Q1: Describe the basic anatomy of bone and its purposes.

A1: *Bones are hard, flexible, complex structures composed of calcium and protein fibers. Bones are covered by a strong, white fibrous material called periosteum through which the blood vessels and nerves pass as they enter and leave the bone. They are the body's framework, providing support and protection for the internal organs. They store salts and metabolic materials and are a site of red blood cell production. With the muscles, ligaments, and tendons, they play a major part in the body's ability to move.*

Q2: Identify the signs and symptoms of musculoskeletal injury.

A2: *Pain and tenderness; deformity or angulation; grating, or crepitus; swelling; bruising; exposed bone ends; joints locked into position; nerve and blood vessel compromise.*

Q3: Describe basic emergency care for painful, swollen, deformed extremities, including general guidelines for splinting long bones and joints.

A3: *Take and maintain all Standard Precautions. Perform the initial assessment. After life-threatening conditions have been addressed, all patients with a painful, swollen, or deformed extremity must be splinted. For a low-priority (stable) patient, splint before transport. For a high-priority (unstable) patient, immobilize the whole body on a long spine board, then load and go. If appropriate, cover open wounds with sterile dressings, elevate the extremity, and apply a cold pack to the area to help reduce swelling.*

Injured long bones should be realigned using manual traction and then splinted. Injured joints should be splinted in the position found unless the distal extremity is cyanotic or lacks pulses. See Scans 28-1 and 28-2.

Q4: Explain why angulated deformed injuries to the long bones should be realigned to anatomical position.

A4: *This is done to restore effective circulation to the affected extremity and to fit it into a splint.*

Q5: List the basic principles of splinting.

A5: *Expose area and control bleeding before splinting. Assess PMS function before and after splinting. Align long-bone injuries with gentle traction if there is severe deformation.*

Splint to immobilize injury site and adjacent joints. Splint patients before moving. Pad splints for patient comfort. Choose splinting method based on severity of patient's condition and priority decision. If patient is unstable, don't waste time splinting.

Q6: Describe the hazards of splinting.

A6: *Neglecting life-threatening conditions; applying the splint so tightly that soft tissues are compressed and injury is caused to nerves, blood vessels, and muscles; applying the splint so loosely or inappropriately that further soft-tissue injury occurs.*

Q7: Describe the basic types of splints carried on ambulances.

A7: *Rigid, formable, and traction.*

Critical Thinking

Q: A hiker drives his boot under an old tree root and is tossed head over heels down the slope of a small hill. When he finally comes to rest, his left leg is bent below the knee at an unusual angle. Your initial assessment shows an alert adult male, guarding a grossly deformed left leg. He hasn't lost consciousness and has no other pain. You find he has a strong radial pulse, normal skin, and no bleeding. How should you proceed?

A: *Care for potential development of shock, administering a high concentration of oxygen. Check distal PMS function. Align the extremity. Splint using an air-inflated splint, the two-splint method, or single-splint with an ankle hitch. Recheck distal PMS function.*

Street Scenes

Q1: What priority would you assign to this patient? Why?

A1: *Because the patient appears stable, the EMTs would probably assign a low priority. (Note to Instructor: You might point out that this priority could change after a complete assessment. It is always possible that the patient may have some internal bleeding at the injury location.)*

Q2: How would you continue your assessment?

A2: *The EMTs should perform a focused history and physical examination. They should ask the patient about allergies, medications, her last meal, and so on. They should also take a baseline set of vitals.*

Q3: What signs and symptoms might you expect to find with a broken long bone?

A3: *Signs and symptoms include: pain and tenderness, deformity or angulation, grating (crepitus), swelling, bruising, exposed bone ends, joints locked in one position, and nerve and/or blood-vessel compromise. (Note to Instructor: When assessing a patient with a possible musculoskeletal injury, the EMTs might also consider assessing the five p's: pain, pale skin, pulses diminished, paresthesia [a tingling sensation], and paralysis [an inability to move].)*

Q4: What are your major concerns with possible broken bones in the extremities?

A4: *The major concern with this type of injury is possible nerve, vessel, or muscle damage below the injury. As part of the assessment, the EMTs should take the following steps: evaluate pedal pulses, look at skin color, feel for temperature, check capillary refill in the foot, ask the patient to move her foot and toes, see if the patient can feel one of them touch her toes and foot.*

Q5: What interventions are appropriate for this patient?

A5: *After assessing the patient, the EMTs should splint the patient, making sure that the procedure is done with as little movement as possible. The entire leg should be secured to provide immobilization in the joint above and below the injury site. The EMTs might apply padding as appropriate and then reassess vitals as well as pulses, motor function, and sensation below the injury site.*

CHAPTER 29 INJURIES TO THE HEAD AND SPINE

Critical Decision Making: More than a Pain in the Neck

Which patients do you immobilize and which do not require immobilization? (*Note:* Use the general concepts from this chapter to make your determination. Your protocols in the field may vary.)

Q1: Your patient was the driver of a vehicle that was struck in the rear end while stopped at a light. The patient denies pain, but you observe her rubbing her neck and looking like she may have some pain.

A1: *If the patient appears to have pain (even if she denies it) and she consents to care, she should be immobilized. Sometimes the shock of the crash masks the pain temporarily.*

Q2: Your patient was in the back seat of a car that was hit broadside (T-bone). She doesn't complain of neck pain, but her head was knocked into the side of the car during the collision. She has a large hematoma on the right side of her head from the impact.

A2: *The head injury and significant mechanism of injury indicate that immobilization is necessary here.*

Q3: Your patient was a passenger in a car that was struck in the driver's side in a minor collision. She denies all injury and isn't sure she wants to go to the hospital.

A3: *Without a significant mechanism of injury, complaint of pain, or distracting condition evident, she doesn't require immobilization.*

Review Questions

Q1: Name the two components of the nervous system and discuss their functions.

A1: *Brain—Messages from all over the body are received by the brain, which decides how to respond to changing conditions both inside and outside the body.*
Spinal cord—Relay between most of the body and the brain.

Q2: List five signs of a brain injury and explain why mechanism of injury is important in determining possible brain injury.

A2: *Visible skull fragments; altered mental status; deep laceration or severe bruise to the head; depression or deformity of the skull; severe pain at the site of a head injury; Battle's sign; raccoon eyes; one eye appears sunken; bleeding or clear fluid from ears or nose; personality change; Cushing's syndrome; irregular breathing patterns; temperature increase; blurred or multiple image vision; impaired hearing or ringing in the ears; equilibrium problems; forceful vomiting; posturing; paralysis on one side of body; seizure activity; deteriorating vital signs.*

Determining possible skull or brain injury can be very difficult. Therefore, you should always assume skull or brain injury when indicated by mechanism of injury.

Q3: Describe the appropriate emergency treatment of a patient with possible head or brain injury.

A3: *Take Standard Precautions. Use the jaw-thrust maneuver to open and maintain the airway. Monitor changes in breathing. Apply a rigid collar and immobilize the neck and spine. Administer high-concentration oxygen and artificially ventilate if necessary. Control bleeding. Keep the patient at rest. Monitor vital signs every 5 minutes. Talk to the conscious patient, providing emotional support. Dress and bandage open wounds. Manage the patient for shock. Transport promptly.*

Q4: List five mechanisms of injury that would support suspicion of a spine injury.

A4: *If a patient: was involved in a motor-vehicle or motorcycle collision, was struck by a vehicle, fell to the ground from a height, received blunt trauma to the spine or above the clavicles, sustained penetrating trauma to the head, neck, or torso, was involved in a diving accident, was found hanging by the neck, was found unconscious due to trauma.*

Q5: Describe the appropriate emergency care for a patient with a possible spine injury.

A5: *Provide manual in-line stabilization for the head and neck. Assess ABCs. Assess the head and the neck. Apply a rigid cervical collar and maintain manual stabilization. Apply the appropriate immobilization device at the appropriate speed. Administer high-concentration oxygen and evaluate the need for artificial ventilation. Reassess sensory and motor function in all four extremities.*

Critical Thinking

Q: You are called to the scene of a motor-vehicle collision. After assuring scene safety and taking Standard Precautions, you approach the car, which has struck a bridge abutment, and note a deformed steering wheel. The driver's side door is open and out; in the middle of the bridge, you see a person you presume to be the driver wandering erratically toward the opposite side of the bridge. How should you proceed?

A: *Go to the patient. Identify yourself. Seek consent for treatment. Due to the mechanism of injury, assume the possibility of injuries to the head and spine. Provide manual in-line stabilization for the head and neck. Assess ABCs. Quickly assess sensory and motor function in all four extremities. Assess the head and the neck. Apply a rigid collar and maintain manual stabilization. Apply the appropriate immobilization device at the appropriate speed. Administer high-concentration oxygen and reevaluate the need for artificial ventilation. Reassess sensory and motor function in all four extremities. Control bleeding. Dress and bandage open wounds. Keep the patient at rest. Manage the patient for shock, even if shock is not present. Reassure the patient. Monitor vital signs every 5 minutes.*

Street Scenes

Q1: What is your general impression of this patient?

A1: *The patient appears to be unconscious with a head and possible spine injury. The oozing from the head seems to be from an abrasion but merits closer assessment in case it is an indication of a more significant injury, such as an open skull fracture. Because of the mechanism of injury and the patient's lack of consciousness, the teenager should probably be considered a high priority for transport.*

Q2: What immediate treatment should be provided?

A2: *Assessment and protection of the ABCs are always the priority. In order to accomplish these tasks, manual in-line stabilization of the head and neck must be applied. After confirming the source of bleeding (from an abrasion), the EMTs should focus on the patient's level of consciousness. They should take a baseline set of vitals and elicit a SAMPLE history from the patient, bystanders, and mother (when she arrives). (Note to Instructor: Encourage students to mention specific care steps, such as the following: Control of bleeding from the head wound and application of a dressing. [Keep pressure to a minimum if a skull fracture is suspected.] Administration of high-concentration oxygen and application of a cervical collar. Placement of the patient on a backboard, securing the torso first and then the head. Use of head blocks and the appropriate immobilization device to secure the head in place. Reassessment of the patient's vital signs, level of responsiveness, and so on.)*

Q3: How should you monitor changing levels of responsiveness in a patient with a head injury?

A3: *A good way of monitoring changes in the level of responsiveness is to ask the patient to repeat the number that he was previously told. If he can't remember the number, repeat it and ask him to recall it a minute or two later. Another method might be to ask the patient age-appropriate questions, such as his birthday, name, and so on. The purpose is to ascertain the level of alertness and any changes for the better or worse. (Note to Instructor: It is important that EMTs become familiar with the neurological assessment method used in your area and that local hospitals understand this tool. For example, if EMS systems use the Glasgow Coma Scale (GCS), then EMTs need to ensure that the receiving hospitals understand the "scoring" system. The same holds true for AVPU. Evaluation tools have limited effectiveness if they can't be used to communicate information on the patient's neurological status.)*

CHAPTER 30 PUTTING IT ALL TOGETHER FOR THE TRAUMA PATIENT

Critical Decision Making: Falling for Your Attention

Assume you have a local hospital 15 minutes away and a trauma center 25 minutes away. Determine which patients should be transported to the trauma center and which could be transported to the local hospital—and explain why.

Q1: Your 30-year-old patient fell 4 feet from a ladder and got his lower leg caught in a rung. He believes he broke his lower left leg. His pulse is 96 strong and regular, respirations 18 and adequate, blood pressure 126/86, pupils equal and reactive to light, skin warm and dry. He is alert. There are distal pulses in the extremity.

A1: *Local hospital is likely OK as long as the patient remains stable en route.*

Q2: Your patient is an 8-year-old male who fell 8–10 feet from a tree to the ground. He is holding his right wrist and says it hurts. As you talk with him and his parents, you note that he appears confused. As you move him to the ambulance, you believe his mental status is decreasing. Pulse 82 strong and regular, respirations 24, blood pressure 122/86, pupils equal and sluggishly reactive to light, mental status as noted above.

A2: *The mental status is the most alarming issue. The potential for head injury should point you in the direction of prompt transport to the trauma center.*

Q3: Your patient is a 32-year-old female who is 30 weeks pregnant and fell down a flight of stairs. She struck her head and has pain in her left shoulder. Her main concern is the brisk vaginal bleeding that began since the fall.

A3: *This woman has trauma to her extremities—and possibly to her uterus. This is a serious condition. The trauma center would be the prudent choice, but consult medical direction. The obstetric surgery capabilities at the local hospital may be warranted.*

Review Questions

Q1: What considerations must the EMT weigh when considering whether to perform an intervention at the scene?

A1: *Life-threatening injuries related to the ABCs of initial assessment must be taken care of immediately. Basically, the EMT must perform those interventions that, if not done at once, could impact upon patient outcome (e.g., permanent disability or death). Such interventions usually include any procedure required to open the airway (such as suctioning), support ventilations, or control bleeding. In addition, the EMT should perform in-line stabilization of the cervical spine.*

Q2: What are the interventions that should generally be performed for a critical trauma patient at the scene?
A2: *Students should name the procedures listed in Chapter 30 of the textbook.*

Q3: When might it be appropriate for EMTs to bypass a closer hospital for a trauma center?
A3: *The decision to bypass a closer hospital in favor of a more distant trauma center is based upon local, regional, or state protocols. Specialized trauma centers can usually provide the definitive treatment required by the patient with multiple injuries. They usually have surgical specialists available 24 hours a day and can provide life-saving interventions upon the patient's immediate arrival.*

Q4: What are the three "Ts" of multiple trauma patient management?
A4: *Teamwork, timing, and transport.*

Q5: When might it be appropriate not to apply a traction splint in the field to an obviously fractured femur?
A5: *Although a fractured femur is a severe injury, it becomes a lesser priority if the patient does not have a patent airway or needs ventilatory support. Life-threatening conditions related to the ABCs must come first. In addition, if application of a traction splint would result in a "significant" delay in transport and if the patient is a high priority, then splinting might be postponed so that the patient can receive definitive care at a trauma center or hospital. The EMT must remember to treat the whole patient and avoid distraction by a single injury—even if the injury is as serious as a fractured femur. In other words, interventions must be prioritized while keeping in mind the importance of the "golden hour."*

Critical Thinking

Q: A controversy exists regarding whether patients with penetrating trauma, such as stab and gunshot wounds, should have spinal immobilization before transport. What factors would have to be considered in this type of case? What do your local protocols say about the topic?
A: *Factors that affect the decision to immobilize patients with penetrating trauma include: mechanism of injury, location of the injury, report by patient and/or bystander on what occurred, and information yielded by the patient assessment. Student answers will vary, depending upon local protocols.*

Street Scenes

Q1: What is your initial impression of the crash?
A1: *Sample response: It appears to be a high-impact crash involving two vehicles—a full-size pickup truck and a compact car. At least two patients are slumped over inside the smaller vehicle and fluid is draining from under the engine. The scene must be secured for a number of reasons—a potentially unstable vehicle, an unknown (and possibly hazardous) fluid leak, high-speed traffic, curious onlookers, and so on. Heavy extrication equipment may be required, and the patients might be high priority, based upon the mechanism of injury (high-speed collision).*

Q2: What additional resources will be necessary on scene?
A2: *Additional resources might include: police units to control the traffic, heavy rescue for extrication, a fire department crew to handle the leaking fluid, and additional ambulances (depending upon the severity of the injuries and the final number of patients).*

Q3: Which patient should be transported first?
A3: *The passenger should be transported before the driver if necessary. Unlike the driver, who was found conscious but "dazed," the passenger appears motionless at first. Although responsive to verbal stimuli, she is highly agitated, suggesting possible head in-*

jury. Her airway is clear, but she exhibits slightly labored and shallow breathing. Patient complaints of right arm pain point to a possible fracture. The patient's radial pulse (strong and rapid) and skin (warm and dry) suggest that her body may be compensating for some blood loss (although the signs do not yet point to a critical situation). The patient is also unrestrained, which means easier removal than the fully restrained driver. (Some students may also discount the driver of the pickup truck, who is ambulatory and reports no immediate life threats.)

Q4: What is your critical decision regarding the female patient?

A4: *Given the mechanism of injury and the initial assessment findings listed in the preceding answer, the EMTs might conclude that the passenger has sustained multiple-system trauma and requires rapid transport to the nearest trauma center and/or hospital. This decision would necessitate rapid extrication, as described in the scenario.*

Q5: What critical interventions should you perform on-scene?

A5: *Sample critical interventions include: in-line stabilization with a jaw-thrust maneuver to ensure an open airway, application of a cervical collar, rapid extrication based on local protocols, a rapid neurological assessment (for pain, sensation, and movement) both before and after extrication, placement and immobilization on a backboard (with proper use of head immobilizers), careful monitoring of the airway, suctioning and application of high-concentration oxygen as necessary, provision for possible ventilatory support (bag-valve mask with an oxygen reservoir), immobilization of right arm (possibly en route to the hospital), ongoing assessment (vitals every 5–10 minutes).*

Q6: What further information would you like to attain about the female patient?

A6: *Sample response: If the EMTs have not already taken a baseline set of vitals, they should do so now (to monitor changes in the patient's condition). Although the patient is only alert to verbal stimuli, the EMTs can put together a partial SAMPLE history. For example, they might question the husband or driver of the pickup truck, take down information on the patient's medic alert bracelet, and so on. They should also perform a focused head-to-toe assessment, paying close attention to lung sounds, pain upon palpation, and signs/symptoms of head trauma (fluid from the nose and ears, deformity, sluggish/nonreactive pupils), and so on. The EMTs might also try to elicit information pertinent to the pregnancy, which should be communicated to medical direction and the receiving hospital as soon as possible.*

Q7: To what type of receiving facility should your patient be transported?

A7: *Local, regional, or state protocols usually establish guidelines for transport to a trauma center or hospital. Medical direction, if available, can advise on the most appropriate action. As previously stated, assessment findings would indicate rapid transport to a trauma center, if available, within an appropriate time frame.*

CHAPTER 31 INFANTS AND CHILDREN

Critical Decision Making: The Little Ones Make Us Nervous

The decision making in this section will involve your "from-the-doorway" pediatric assessment. With the information provided, determine if the patient is in a serious or a less serious condition.

Q1: You are met at the door by an upset mother who is holding a limp 13-month-old child in her arms.

A1: *Serious. The patient's limpness is an immediate flag that something is wrong. This is called poor muscle tone and is a serious finding. The upset mother is also a piece in the puzzle.*

Q2: A 3-year-old child is reported as having a croupy cough and difficulty breathing. She is screaming and clinging to her mother as you approach.

A2: *Less serious. The fact that the little girl is "screaming" means that she can move air in and out. Clinging to her mother indicates muscle tone and an appropriate mental status.*

Q3: A child has fallen from a high sliding board. You arrive to find the child holding his left forearm against his body while quietly clinging to his mother.

A3: *Serious (until more info can be obtained). The fact that the child is holding his injured arm and clinging to his mother is good. Look for his mental status and why he is quiet before making a final determination. If you approach him and he turns shyly into his mother, you may upgrade this to less serious.*

Review Questions

Q1: Name one psychological/social characteristic that you would be likely to find in a patient of each of the following ages and explain how you would tailor your actions as an EMT to accommodate this characteristic: 2-year-old, 6-year-old, and 15-year-old.

Q2: Describe how each of the differences you named for question 1, above, will affect your assessment of the infant or child patient.

A1 and 2: *Answers will vary according to student choices. Refer to Table 31-1.*

Q3: Describe key differences in the anatomy and physiology of infants and children with regard to the following:

- head
- airway and respiratory system
- chest
- abdomen
- body surface
- blood volume

A3: *Head: Larger and heavier than an adult's until age 4; infants up to 1 year or 18 months have a "soft spot" or fontanelle in the skull. Airway and respiratory system: Immature neck muscles; airway structures narrower and less rigid than an adult's; smaller nose and mouth, more space taken up by tongue, narrower trachea, cricoid cartilage less rigid; airway structures more easily blocked; chest wall softer. Chest and abdomen: Chest structures less developed and more elastic; musculoskeletal structures of chest and abdomen less well developed; vital organs not as well protected. Body surface: Larger in proportion to body mass, hence more prone to heat loss through the skin; head, body, and extremities differently proportioned than an adults, affecting estimates of extent of burns. Blood volume: Less blood volume, hence bleeding that would be moderate in an adult may be life-threatening in an infant or child.*

Q4: Describe ways of calming and interacting effectively with the infant or child patient and with the parent or caregiver.

A4: *Take into account the child's age and psychology (see Table 31-1). Identify yourself, let the young child hold a familiar toy; position yourself at child's eye level, smile; explain what you are doing in terms the child can understand; let the child see your face and make eye contact; stop occasionally to make sure the child understands what is happening; never lie to the child but let the child know you are there to help.*

Q5: Explain some of the elements of a general impression of the infant or child patient that you can obtain "from the doorway"—before you approach the patient.

A5: *The "from the doorway" elements of the Pediatric Assessment Triangle are appearance, work of breathing, and circulation to the skin, as explained in the chapter and illustrated in Figure 31-6.*

Q6: Explain how to differentiate between an upper airway obstruction and a lower airway disease or disorder. Explain how and why the two should be treated differently.

A6: *Airway obstruction usually occurs in the upper airway, roughly the larynx and above, where foreign body obstruction may be the cause of difficulty. Airway diseases (for example, croup or epiglottitis) are more likely to affect the lower airway, the larynx and below. If there are clear signs of foreign body obstruction perform abdominal thrusts to force the object out of the airway. Perform finger sweeps to remove the object only if it is clearly visible. If there are signs of respiratory distress without a clear indication of foreign body obstruction, put nothing in the child's mouth, administer oxygen or assisted ventilations as needed, and transport the patient immediately and continue to reassess en route.*

Q7: Explain the main steps of emergency treatment for any infant or child trauma patient.

A7: *Ensure an open airway using the jaw-thrust maneuver; suction as necessary with a rigid suction catheter, provide high-concentration oxygen, ventilate with a pediatric pocket mask or bag-valve mask as needed; provide spinal immobilization; transport immediately and continue to reassess en route.*

Q8: Explain how suspicion of child abuse should or should not affect the care you provide for an infant or child patient. Explain the reporting requirements regarding child abuse and neglect in your state or locality.

A8: *Provide care for any injuries as you would for any patient. Do not confront the child or caregiver as to whether abuse has taken place. Report any suspicions of child abuse to the hospital staff and in accordance with local policies.*

Critical Thinking

Q: You are called to the scene of a collision between a vehicle and a 5-year-old on a bicycle. The child is lying near the curb surrounded by anxious adults and looking very scared. Based on what you know about the developmental characteristics of children as well as common injury patterns in children, explain some of the special elements you should take into consideration as you proceed to assess and care for this patient.

A: *At this age, children don't like being separated from parents—keep them nearby. Assure the child, if necessary, that the accident was not a punishment for being bad. Don't lie to the patient; explain what you are doing honestly and be reassuring. Because patients this age are modest, try to provide privacy from onlookers (except parents) during assessment and care. The mechanism of injury in this case suggests a strong possibility of head injury, abdominal injury with internal bleeding, and lower extremity injury (possibly a femur fracture).*

Street Scenes

Q1: What is your assessment plan for this patient?

A1: *With pediatric patients, the focus is on the initial assessment—particularly ensuring an open airway and adequate breathing. Based on the limited information provided by the dispatcher, the EMTs need to approach the patient while doing a scene size-up and making sure they have taken all Standard Precautions. They will need to determine quickly whether the airway is open and whether the child needs repositioning and/or suctioning. Once the airway is secure, the EMTs must evaluate breathing, check the quality of respirations, decide upon the need for oxygen therapy, and check for any circulation compromise or bleeding.*

Q2: What equipment should be brought into the house?

A2: *The pediatric bag should contain the basic airway equipment, including suction, nonrebreather mask, BVM with oxygen tank, and oral pharyngeal airways in a variety of sizes. (Note to Instructor: Depending upon medical direction and/or local protocols, the EMTs might also bring equipment for endotracheal intubation.)*

Q3: Should ALS be dispatched to the scene prior to your arrival?

A3: *Yes. This is a true medical emergency. In infants and children, respiratory arrest can lead to cardiac arrest (as a result of hypoxia). Therefore, the patient may need endotracheal intubation, which is usually an ALS skill. An ALS team can intubate the child and provide drug therapy if necessary. Also, an extra set of trained hands and additional support can be beneficial in these types of cases.*

Q4: What care should be provided next?

A4: *After performing a head-tilt, chin-lift maneuver and suctioning the mucus, the EMTs should administer oxygen therapy. Because pediatric patients are reluctant to have a nonbreather mask placed over their mouths—even with a decreased level of responsiveness—the EMTs should use the "blow-by" method.*

Q5: What additional assessment needs to be done?

A5: *Once the child is breathing, the EMTs should obtain a full set of baseline vital signs, including level of responsiveness and skin color and temperature. They should also begin to question the mother to obtain information for a SAMPLE history. (Note to Instructor: Encourage students to explain how the mother should be involved with the patient at this point. Compare their answers to actions taken in the scenario and suggested in the chapter.)*

Q6: What information needs to be relayed to the ALS unit?

A6: *Sample response: initial presentation of the patient, level of responsiveness, vital signs, pertinent data from the SAMPLE history, and any changes in the patient's condition.*

CHAPTER 32 PATIENTS WITH SPECIAL NEEDS

Critical Decision Making: EMTs Need to Know

Patients with special needs can pose challenges for EMS providers. For each of the following situations, explain how you would handle it and where you might turn for help or advice.

Q1: You are treating an unresponsive diabetic patient when you notice he has an insulin pump. You believe you should turn it off but are not sure how.

A1: *The patient's family would be the first place to look for answers. You may also contact medical direction for advice. Many devices have an obvious switch to turn it off.*

Q2: You are treating a patient who had just performed peritoneal dialysis at home. She complains of excruciating pain with even the least little movement.

A2: *In this case the patient may be the best source of information. While you should be considerate of the pain she is in, she will be able to answer your questions about how the dialysis works and also give you information on how best to move her with minimal pain.*

Q3: You are called for a possible respiratory infection in a child. You arrive to find the patient has a trach and a ventilator. You are not sure how to transport the ventilator.

A3: *The parents or visiting health care workers are the best source of information. Since health care workers aren't always present, parents are trained in operation and troubleshooting the devices. If the ventilator can't be transported, transport the patient without the ventilator and ventilate the patient through the trach tube en route. Be sure to alert the hospital that you are about to arrive with a patient who needs a ventilator.*

Review Questions

Q1: List several advanced medical devices you might find when responding to patients with special needs at home.

A1: *The following are advanced medical devices that may be found in homes of special needs patients:*

- *Respiratory devices*
  - *Continuous positive airway pressure (CPAP)*
  - *Tracheostomy tube*
  - *Home ventilator*
- *Cardiac devices*
  - *Implanted pacemaker*
  - *Automatic implanted cardiac defibrillator (AICD)*
  - *Left ventricular assist device*
- *Gastro-urinary devices*
  - *Nasogastric tubes (NG tube)*
  - *Gastric tube (G-tube)*
  - *Urinary catheters*
  - *Ostomy bags*
  - *Peritoneal dialysis*
- *Central IV Catheters*
  - *Peripherally inserted central catheters (PICC) lines*
  - *Central venous lines (Groshong®, Hickman®, Broviac®)*
  - *Implanted port (Port-a-Cath® and Mediport®)*
- *Devices to assist physical impairment*
  - *TDD/TYY phone*
  - *Computer that speaks words*
  - *Cane, walker, or brace*
  - *Wheelchair*

Q2: Differentiate congenital from acquired diseases or conditions.

A2: *A congenital disease or condition is one that is present at birth such as congenital heart disease. An acquired disease or condition is one that occurs after birth and may be the result of exposure to a virus or bacteria or may be the result of another medical condition or trauma. Examples of acquired diseases include COPD or AIDS.*

Q3: If a tracheostomy tube is blocked and your protocols allow, describe a method of clearing the blockage.

A3: *To clear a blockage, carefully insert a whistle-tip suction catheter into the stoma. Determine the correct depth of insertion by measuring the suction tubing against the length of the obturator, which is the same length as the trach tube itself. If you can't locate the obturator for measurement, stop insertion of the suction catheter when you feel resis-tance. Suction as the catheter is being withdrawn, using a twisting motion as it is slowly removed. If the patient requires further suctioning (indicated by visible or audible mucus), insert the suction tip into a container of sterile water to remove any mucus left in the catheter, and then repeat. If the patient is on a ventilator, he may need to be ventilated by a BVM between suctionings.*

Q4: If a ventilator that a patient relies on to breathe malfunctions, what life support care should you perform?

A4: *In the case of a mechanical failure, or during transport of the patient, a bag-valve-mask device can take over the function of the ventilator. During this procedure, the EMT should adjust the rate, volume, and pressure of the BVM to the patient's comfort level. This can be done with guidance from the patient. If the patient can't provide guidance, observe for adequate chest rise and improving skin color. (NOTE: If the BVM does not fit the tube attachment, use the face mask from the BVM to cover the stoma and secure the mask to provide a good seal against the neck, then ventilate as normal.)*

Q5: If a patient's pacemaker or AICD malfunctions, in addition to transport to the hospital, what care should you provide?

A5: *Malfunctions can be caused by patient's coming into close proximity to electronic anti-theft device (usually found in the doorways of businesses), metal detectors, stereo speakers, cellular phones, electric motors (as in power tools), and gas-powered tools (such as chainsaws and snow blowers). So, patients with pacemakers or AICDs who are found close to any of these devices should be moved away as soon as practically possible. Also, depending on the relative distance the EMT should consider an ALS transport. Individuals with these devices are high-risk cardiac patients and should be treated as such with high-concentration oxygen and frequent assessment. If the patient goes into cardiac arrest, CPR and an AED should be used as indicated.*

Q6: If a patient cannot hear or cannot speak, describe several methods, that might facilitate communication with the patient.

A6: *The first thing that should be done when approaching the patient is to determine his ability to hear and/or speak. If a hearing loss patient can read lips, then use this approach. If not, then communicate by writing questions and actions that will be written on a piece of paper. TDD/TTY phones, if available can be used to relay information. These approaches will also work for patients who are unable to speak. In addition, some patients who are aphasic (unable to speak) may have a computer that speaks words they type into the device and this can be used to help communicate.*

Critical Thinking

Q. You are called to respond to a patient who has an arteriovenous (AV) fistula that is used during his triweekly visits to the dialysis center. The patient presents as pale, sweaty, anxious, and almost incoherent. Could the cause of his condition be related to the AV fistula? How might you determine if this is the case? What actions should you take?

A. *The fistula may have ruptured, causing significant blood loss, which would be indicated by swelling at the site. Apply direct pressure and do not release it until advised by a physician to do so.*

Street Scenes

Q1: What priority is this patient?

Q2: What additional information do you need to treat the patient?

A1 and 2: *Next to Amber you see several small soft suction catheters. You remove one from the package, attach it to your suction device, measure the length to insert by comparing it to the obturator on the table next to the patient, and suction some mucus out of her trach tube. Amber's color begins to improve. Your partner tells you the patient's pulse is 128 and her respiratory rate is 44.*

Q3: How should you reassess the patient?

Q4: What equipment should you take to the hospital with Amber?

A3 and 4: *You listen to Amber's breathing through her trach tube and no longer hear the gurgling sounds that were initially audible. She is moving air well. Although her color is better than when you found her, she appears pale and still in some respiratory distress, although less than before you suctioned her. Amber's pulse oximeter reading has increased from 85 percent to 91 percent. You gather Amber's "Ready-To-Go" bag with her medical records and Emergency Information Form as you prepare her for transport. You administer high-concentration oxygen and suction her trach tube a few more times on the trip to the Emergency Department.*

CHAPTER 33 GERIATRIC PATIENTS

Critical Decision Making: Changes with Age

Geriatric patients differ from those in other age groups. This exercise asks you to apply your understanding of these differences to your assessment and decision making.

Q1: You are treating a geriatric patient who, you suspect, has fractured her hip. The patient is pale and is breathing rapidly. You suspect shock, but her pulse is 84. She is a diabetic, has a cardiac history and hypertension, and takes several medications. If she is in shock, why isn't her pulse more rapid?

A1: *The patient may be taking medications that lower her heart rate. Beta blockers and calcium channel blockers may be the culprits here.*

Q2: Your geriatric patient hasn't felt well for the past several days. She complains of a cough and flu-like symptoms. She has become increasingly weak. Her family suspects the flu, but she doesn't have a fever. Why?

A2: *Temperature regulation and response in the elderly is diminished. The elderly patient with flu may not spike a fever as would a younger patient with a similar condition.*

Q3: You are called to an assisted living facility for a man who is "just not right." He was fine last night. The man complains of suddenly feeling very weak and is having a little difficulty breathing. The nurse wants him sent to the hospital in case he is having a heart attack. Why would she think this?

A3: *The elderly don't perceive pain the same as younger adults and children. It is more common than not for an elderly patient to have a silent (without chest pain) heart attack.*

Review Questions

Q1: Describe how to approach an elderly patient who has vision and hearing impairments.

A1: *Place yourself where the patient can see you. Try to be at the same level as the patient, even if it means crouching or kneeling. Speak loudly, slowly, clearly, and distinctly. Ask just one question at a time. Give the patient plenty of time to respond to your questions.*

Q2: What question should you ask to determine if an elderly patient's condition is normal or a change from baseline?

A2: *Ask how the patient is different compared to a week ago.*

Q3: Name some of the most common medical conditions that cause EMS to be called for elderly patients. Name the most common mechanism of injury to elderly patients.

A3: *The most common medical conditions include cardiac and respiratory problems and neurological problems like stroke. Falls are the most common mechanism of injury.*

Q4: Name the two most common mechanisms of injury to patients over age 65.

A4: *Falls and motor vehicle collisions.*

Critical Thinking

Q: You respond to an elderly woman who has fallen and injured her hip. When you arrive, you find a 90-year-old woman lying on the kitchen floor, alert and oriented, complaining of hip pain. She is somewhat hard of hearing. Her 91-year-old husband is very upset over what happened and blaming himself for her fall. How should you approach your assessment of the patient? How should you deal with her husband?

A: *Assess and care for the patient as you would any patient with a suspected hip fracture. (Review patient care for a hip fracture in Chapter 28.) Immobilize the patient to a backboard, taking care to pad the board to accommodate any skeletal abnormalities. Handle the patient carefully to avoid causing any further skeletal injuries. Administer high-concentration oxygen. Reassure the patient's husband, explaining that falls happen and there was probably nothing he could have done to prevent it. Let him ride along with his wife to the hospital and offer to call any family members or neighbors he would like to notify and to make sure he has a ride home from the hospital and someone to look in on him while is wife is hospitalized.*

Street Scenes

Q1: What is your initial priority for providing care to this patient?

A1: *The ABCs are the first concern in regard to care and treatment for the EMT. This patient is showing signs and symptoms of respiratory distress. The first priority is to ensure that the patient has a patent airway. Although the patient is talking there may be problems with position, mucous blockage, and dentures. Therefore, the airway must be checked and monitored (take vital signs frequently) with corrective action taken as required. In regard to breathing the patient needs oxygen immediately; be prepared to assist with ventilations. If ALS is not immediately available then consider prompt transport.*

Q2: After the initial assessment is completed, what assessment information should be obtained next?

A2: *After the initial exam, perform the history and physical exam. Ask the patient the SAMPLE history questions. Considering that he is having trouble talking this may not work well and the EMT may need to see if there is information written down somewhere, a relative who can be called, or a neighbor who may have information. It is important to remember that either diverting attention from this "sick" patient or delaying transport too long is probably not in the patient's best interest and the remainder of the SAMPLE history needs to be obtained at the hospital. The remainder of the physical examination is to make sure that the patient doesn't have any other presenting problems that require care by EMS. Continued monitoring of vital signs needs to occur during this part of the assessment. If needed, a detailed assessment can be done.*

Q3: Why is the condition of the apartment significant?

A3: *The fact that the apartment is messy may indicate that this patient may not be taking very good care of his own medical needs, such as diet and medication compliance. In addition, the messiness may mean that it is not regularly cleaned, which could trigger asthma episodes. This information is important to pass on to the hospital to help in making decisions about discharge planning when they decide to send this patient home, as he may need some type of support services.*

Q4: Based on the assessment, would you expect this patient's condition to worsen? How should you be prepared if it does?

A4: *The assessment indicates that this patient may worsen; providing ventilatory assistance with a bag-valve mask (BVM) with supplemental oxygen will need to be done. The vital signs and level of consciousness need to be monitored closely and the BVM prepared so ventilatory assistance can be started immediately, if indicated. Prepare the patient for immediate transport. Monitor closely so you know when the nonrebreather mask is no longer adequate and the BVM must be used.*

Q5: What additional assessment should be done en route to the hospital? How often should the vital signs be taken?

A5: *In addition to vital signs (respiratory rate, skin color, etc.), see if the patient is talking better (longer sentences between breaths). If the patient seems to be more alert and is able to talk better then try to get a better SAMPLE history. As part of the SAMPLE history ask the patient if he has pain or discomfort anywhere and other significant complaints besides the difficulty breathing. This is done so the EMT doesn't overlook other significant problems that require immediate care and treatment. Vital signs should be taken every 5 minutes because the patient is unstable.*

Q6: What information about the patient's living situation seems significant enough to provide the hospital staff?

A6: *As previously mentioned, the fact that the apartment is messy may indicate that the patient lacks social supports and is unable to take care of himself adequately (he appears to live alone) without assistance. Make sure that you share this information with the appropriate people in the emergency department so they can plan properly for this patient's discharge.*

CHAPTER 34 AMBULANCE OPERATIONS

Critical Decision Making: Arriving Safely

For each of the following situations, explain where you would park the ambulance if you were first arriving.

Q1: You are called to a railroad car derailment.

A1: *Park uphill and upwind to potential chemical incidents. You must also be aware of the risk of explosion (e.g., a propane car) and park a significant distance away until the hazards are dealt with. Patients may be brought to you in a safe zone.*

Q2: You are called to a collision on the interstate. An engine company and trooper are parked at the scene, blocking oncoming traffic.

A2: *Park past the collision. On an interstate scene you should have a blocking vehicle (e.g., a fire engine or highway department barricade truck) between you and oncoming traffic. By parking past the scene, you will be able to load the patient with the safety of the blocking vehicles behind you.*

Q3: You are called to a scene involving domestic violence. Police are not yet on the scene.

A3: *Stage out of sight from the residence and far enough away so any dangerous persons won't come from the scene to you. Drive to the scene only when advised the police have secured it.*

Review Questions

Q1: List five categories of equipment and supplies that should be carried on an ambulance.

A1: *Ambulances should carry basic supplies of infection control, and patient comfort and protection; initial and focused assessment equipment; equipment for transfer of patients; equipment for airway maintenance, ventilation, and resuscitation; oxygen therapy and suction equipment; equipment for assisting with cardiac resuscitation; supplies and equipment for the immobilization of suspected bone injuries; supplies for wound care and treatment of shock; supplies for childbirth; supplies, equipment, and medication for the treatment of acute poisoning, snakebite, chemical burns, and diabetic emergencies; miscellaneous and safety equipment.*

Q2: Describe the laws (those described in this chapter or your local and state laws) with regard to operation of an ambulance in an emergency. Describe considerations for safe operation of an ambulance in emergency and nonemergency situations.

A2: *Most state laws: Require an ambulance operator to have a valid driver's license and may require completion of a training program. Grant privileges during emergency operation of an ambulance that usually do not apply during nonemergency operation. Do not grant immunity from charges of reckless driving and disregard for the safety of others. Allow privileges only if the operator uses warning devices as prescribed by law. Allow an ambulance to be parked anywhere as long as it does not damage personal property or* *endanger lives. Allow an ambulance operator to proceed past red stop signals, flashing red stop signals, and stop signs after slowing or stopping. Allow an ambulance operator to exceed the posted speed limit as long as life and property are not endangered. Allow an ambulance operator to pass another vehicle in no-passing zones. Allow an ambulance operator to disregard regulations that govern direction of travel and turning in specific directions.*

(Responses will vary depending on your state and local laws.)

The driver and all passengers should wear safety belts. Become familiar with the characteristics of your vehicle. Be alert to changes in weather and road conditions. Exercise caution in the use of red lights and siren. Select an appropriate route. Maintain a safe following distance. Drive with due regard for the safety of others. Know appropriateness of using lights and sirens. Headlights are the most visible warning device on an emergency vehicle.

Q3: Describe the steps that must be followed in transferring a patient to an ambulance; for care of the patient en route; and for transferring a patient to emergency department personnel.

A3: *Transferring a patient to an ambulance: Ensure an open airway and adequate air exchange. Secure the stretcher in place in the ambulance. Position and secure the patient. Prepare for respiratory and cardiac complications. Loosen constrictive clothing. Check bandages. Check splints. Assess and record vital signs. Load a relative or friend who must accompany the patient. Load personal effects. Reassure the patient.*

Care of the patient en route: Notify the EMD that you are departing the scene. Continue to provide emergency care as required. Compile additional patient information. Perform ongoing assessment and continue monitoring vitals. Notify the receiving facility. Recheck bandages and splints. Collect vomitus if the patient becomes nauseated. Talk to the patient. Control your emotions. Advise the ambulance driver of changing conditions. If cardiac arrest develops, have the operator stop the ambulance while you initiate CPR.

Transferring a patient to emergency department personnel: In a routine admissions situation or when an illness or injury is not life-threatening, check first to see what is to be done with the patient. Assist emergency department staff as required and provide a verbal report. As soon as you are free from patient-care activities, prepare the prehospital care report. Transfer the patient's personal effects. Obtain your release from the hospital.

Q4: Describe the steps that should be taken when air rescue is required.

A4: *Give your name and callback number, your agency name, the nature of the situation, the exact location including crossroads and major landmarks, and the exact location of a safe landing zone. Describe the safe landing zone to the air rescue service.*

Critical Thinking

Q: What equipment should you include in a kit that you carry to the scene? How should the equipment be positioned so that you can reach urgently needed items quickly? What special items, if any, should be in the kit to meet local needs?

A: *The kit you carry to the scene should have all the equipment you need for the initial assessment and the focused medical or trauma exam on patients of all ages. This includes the following: airway, suctioning device and catheters, infection control equipment, orotracheal and nasotracheal equipment (if permitted by local protocol for EMTs), stethoscope, pocket mask with one-way valve, bag-valve masks, oxygen, oxygen delivery devices, blood pressure cuffs, bandages and dressing, occlusive dressings, pneumatic anti-shock garment (if permitted by local protocol for EMTs), automated external defibrillator, set of rigid cervical collars, backboards and straps, scissors, blankets, disposable thermometer and hypothermia thermometer, and pen light.*

Street Scenes

Q1: When operating an ambulance using the red lights and siren, what precautions do you need to take?

A1: *Even though operating with red lights and siren, an ambulance driver still must exercise caution in regard to speed, passing other vehicles, going through intersections, obeying stop signs or stop lights, and so on. The driver is responsible for the crew's safety, the safety of other motorists and pedestrians, and for his or her own safety. (Note to Instructor: Point out that a collision en route means delayed delivery of patient care and the removal of an ambulance and/or crew from EMS service. Provide the following safety guidelines to students: 1. Use the siren sparingly. 2. Never assume that motorists will see the warning lights or hear the siren. 3. Always assume that some motorists will hear the siren or see the lights and ignore them anyway. 4. Expect erratic maneuvers from drivers who may panic or become confused as you approach or pass. 5. Do not pull close to a vehicle and then activate the siren. 6. Never use lights or siren indiscriminately.)*

Q2: How can speed affect the safety of ambulance operation?

A2: *Speed is a significant factor in placing EMS personnel and other people at risk. Excessive speed increases the possibility of collisions. Speed also increases stopping distance and makes it more difficult to avoid hazardous situations. (Note to Instructor: Stress that speed can be a contributing factor in crashes involving emergency vehicles even when they are using lights and siren. Point out that most states will excuse ambulance drivers from certain traffic laws only in a true emergency and only with due regard for the safety of others.)*

Q3: What driving techniques might be used to make driving to this scene safer?

A3: *Answers should take into account preceding comments. Specific to this scenario would be: careful review of the use of lights and siren, extreme care in going through the intersection and red light (instead of "blowing through"), and selection of an alternate route (instead of dangerously weaving through traffic).*

Q4: What should you do first for patient care?

A4: *After parking and positioning the ambulance safely, the EMTs should follow the standard approach for all patients—observe for scene safety, take all necessary Standard Precautions, ascertain the reason for the call, determine the patient's level of responsiveness, evaluate the ABCs, and so on.*

Q5: What information should you provide to the dispatcher?

A5: *The EMTs should advise the dispatcher of the patient's level of consciousness, the status of airway and breathing, baseline vital signs, and whether any additional units (such as ALS) are needed. They should also indicate the patient priority, expected arrival time at an emergency facility, and so on.*

CHAPTER 35 GAINING ACCESS AND RESCUE OPERATIONS

Critical Decision Making: When Minutes Count, Decisions Matter

For each patient described here, determine whether the extrication must be done quickly because the patient is unstable or if more time is available.

Q1: Your patient was involved in a head-on crash. The patient is unresponsive with a rapid pulse.

A1: *Unstable patient—quick extrication.*

Q2: Your patient was driving a car that was rear-ended. She is alert and oriented. Her pulse is 80, respirations 16. The frame has shifted so none of the doors will open.

A2: *Stable patient—time may be available.*

Q3: Your patient was a front-seat passenger who was thrown into the back seat. You can only reach the patient's upper body, but you find a rapid pulse and clammy skin. The patient is alert and talking with you.

A3: *Unstable patient—quick extrication.*

Review Questions

Q1: Explain the role of the EMT in the size-up of a motor-vehicle collision.

A1: *Upon arrival on the scene of a collision, it is important for the EMT to evaluate hazards and calculate the need for additional BLS or ALS backup, police, fire, or specialty rescue response, or services (such as the power company).*

Q2: Discuss what the EMT should do upon arrival at a collision if a power pole is broken in half and the lines are down in the street.

A2: *Park the ambulance outside the danger zone. Before you leave the ambulance, be sure that no portion of the vehicle, including the radio antenna, is contacting any sagging conductors. Order spectators and nonessential emergency service personnel from the danger zone. Use perimeter tape to set off a large safety zone. Discourage occupants of the collision vehicle from leaving the wreckage. Prohibit traffic flow through the danger zone. Determine the number of the nearest pole you can safely approach, and ask your dispatcher to advise the power company of the pole number and location. Do not attempt to move downed wire. Stand in a safe place until the power company cuts the wires or disconnects the power.*

Q3: Explain whom you should call for assistance in your community if, on size-up of a collision, you observe a truck turned on its side and leaking fuel.

A3: *Responses will vary depending on your local area.*

Q4: Discuss ways to stabilize a vehicle that is resting on its wheels, a vehicle that is resting on its side, and a vehicle that is resting on its roof.

A4: *Resting on its wheels: Make sure the engine is off, the transmission is in park, the keys are removed from the ignition, and the parking brake is set. Place cribbing on each side and either the front or back. Deflate all tires.*

Resting on its side: Use ropes, hi-lift jacks, and cribbing.

Resting on its roof: Use 4 × 4s to build a box crib under the vehicle.

Q5: Explain the difference between simple access and complex access to a patient in a vehicle.

A5: *Simple access includes ordinary ways of getting into a vehicle—such as opening the door or having the patient roll down the window. Complex access is when tools or equipment are needed to gain entry into the vehicle.*

Critical Thinking

Q1: With knowledge of your own community, which of the 10 types of rescue specialty teams are needed and who provides the service?

A1: *Responses will vary depending on your local situation.*

Q2: After considering the safety of yourself and others, what should be your primary goal at the scene of a vehicle collision?

A2: *Care of the patient—planning how you can begin emergency care and initiate transport as rapidly as possible.*

Street Scenes

Q1: What are the scene safety issues that you need to address?

A1: *Scene safety issues deal with both seen and unseen hazards. While vehicle instability is an obvious safety issue for both the patient and the rescuers, the EMTs should suspect* *possible gasoline leaks and/or problems with the vehicle's electrical system. (Note to Instructor: You might provide students with the following list of hazards that rescuers should consider when dealing with motor-vehicle crashes with at least one entrapped patient: 1. Vehicle instability. 2. Possible injury of patient or rescuers during disentanglement. 3. Potential for vehicle fire. 4. Adverse environmental conditions. 5. Downed electrical wires. 6. Use of incorrect tools. 7. Improper stabilization and/or movement of the vehicle. 8. Lack of proper traffic or spectator control [particularly as the rescue scene expands]. 9. Absence of proper protective gear. 10. Careless attitudes.)*

Q2: What techniques should you consider for extrication?

A2: *The first and foremost concerns are checking for any leaking fluids, particularly gasoline, and stabilizing the vehicle. The EMTs might also consider disconnecting the battery. Once the vehicle is stabilized, the EMTs should look for the safest way of accessing the patient, safeguarding both themselves and the injured driver. (Note to Instructor: Explain to students that it is possible to overlook the obvious in a stressful situation. For example, before breaking a window, the EMTs should ensure that the door on the less damaged side of the vehicle cannot be opened. If a window must be broken, the EMTs should make every effort to protect the patient from shards of glass, perhaps using padding or insulating material for protection.)*

Q3: Should rapid extrication be considered for this patient?

A3: *Yes. Based upon the initial assessment of snoring respirations and level of responsiveness (response only to painful stimuli), the patient appears to be unstable. There is every indication for the need of respiratory assistance. The use of rapid extrication, of course, depends upon the ETA of the rescue team and advice from medical direction.*

Q4: Describe assessment for this patient.

A4: *Sample response: The assessment follows in ABC order. The snoring respirations must be corrected. In most cases, this will require a jaw-thrust maneuver (in a trauma patient) to move the tongue forward, while a second EMT applies a cervical collar. Next, the EMTs should evaluate respirations. At the very least, this patient should receive high-concentration oxygen by nonrebreather mask. The EMTs should also be prepared to assist ventilations with a bag-valve mask and an oxygen reservoir. Next, the EMTs should check circulation for external hemorrhage and overt signs and symptoms of internal bleeding. Because this is a trauma patient, the EMTs should then initiate a head-to-toe neurological assessment. Once this is completed, they should obtain a set of vital signs. A SAMPLE history can be taken if the patient regains consciousness. When these steps are completed, they can conduct a focused and detailed assessment as indicated by patient conditions.*

CHAPTER 36 SPECIAL OPERATIONS

Critical Decision Making: We Have *How Many* Patients???

For each of the following scenarios, determine what resources you would call for in your initial report to the dispatcher.

Q1: You are called to a shopping mall for "sick people." You arrive to find dozens of people standing outside the mall, coughing and rubbing their eyes. Looking around the parking lot, you see hundreds of cars.

A1: *Activate your MCI plan. Based on the fact that you see "dozens" of people, you may be looking at 25+ patients and more may still be inside. This is a large-scale multiple-casualty incident and must be treated as such. It is bigger than calling for additional ambulances. This will require prolonged operations and resources. Be sure the hazmat team is activated.*

Q2: You arrive at a motor-vehicle collision in which two cars collided at an intersection with considerable force. One patient has been ejected. Three others don't appear to be moving.

A2: *Assume that you will need an ambulance and crew for each of the four critical patients. You may also need to call for fire department response for extrication or personnel assistance.*

Q3: You are treating a woman in her home for flu-like symptoms. You notice that her husband and one child are also sick. You check on another child sleeping in the same residence and find that he won't wake up.

A3: *This may be a carbon monoxide situation. Assume that there are four patients—and you and your crew may now also fall into the patient category. Exit the building, taking the patients with you. Immediately call for additional ambulances and the fire department.*

Review Questions

Q1: List the information in an initial report of a hazardous materials incident.

A1: *Alert the dispatcher to the fact that you are dealing with a hazmat incident and request appropriate support services. Try to identify the hazardous material by using binoculars to look for identifying signs, labels, or placards. If they can be obtained safely, you can also identify the materials through invoices, bills of lading, shipping manifests, and MSDSs or through interviews with people leaving the scene of the incident. You should be able to tell the dispatcher and/or a source of information on hazardous materials as much of the following as can safely be determined: your name and callback number; the nature and location of the problems; the identification number of the materials involved; the name of the carrier, shipper, manufacturer, consignee, and point of origin of the material; type of container and size; quantity of material transported and released; local conditions; emergency services that have been notified.*

Q2: Explain how to identify a hazardous material and how to obtain information about that material.

A2: *Vehicle drivers, plant and railroad personnel, and even bystanders may be able to tell you the name of a hazardous material. In many cases, there will be a colored placard on the vehicle, tank, or railroad car. There may also be an invoice, shipping manifest, bill of lading, or MSDS. Consulting the Emergency Response Guidebook or calling CHEMTREC or CHEM-TEL can provide you with information about the hazardous material.*

Q3: Describe the general assessment and emergency care of a patient with a hazardous materials injury.

A3: *Move the patient(s) to the safe zone as quickly as possible if there is no risk to you. Provide basic life support. Administer high-concentration oxygen. Immediately flush with water the skin, clothing, and eyes of anyone who has come in contact with the hazardous material. Remove the jewelry of any exposed person and continue flushing with water for 20 minutes. Remove protective gear according to local guidelines. Transport the patient as soon as possible.*

Q4: Describe the major components and benefits of an incident management system.

A4: *An incident management system provides a single, orderly means of communicating for decision making among all agencies involved in the incident. (Refer to Figures 36-8, 36-10, 36-11, and 36-12 for the major components of an incident management system.)*

Q5: Define the basic role of an EMT at a multiple-casualty incident.

A5: *If you are the first EMT on the scene, determine whether your area's incident management system needs to be initiated. Give a radio report on the nature of the emergency, its exact location, and the best estimate of the number of patients. Take command of the situation until relieved. After an incident manager has been determined, fulfill the EMS role to which you are assigned (including that of EMS command). Quickly assess all pa-*

tients and assign each a priority for receiving emergency care or transportation for definitive care.

Q6: Explain why patients are assigned priorities during triage.
A6: *This is done to allow the greatest number of people the greatest chance of survival.*

Q7: Identify four priority categories of triage.
A7: *Priority 1: Treatable life-threatening illness or injury.*
Priority 2: Serious but not life-threatening illness or injury.
Priority 3: Walking wounded.
Priority 4 (or 0): Dead or fatally injured.

Critical Thinking

Q: Your call is to a motor-vehicle collision with an unknown number of injuries. As your unit approaches the scene, you see that three cars and downed wires are involved. You get a whiff of gasoline as you pass by. The drivers are visible in each vehicle—one appears to be conscious and the other two are bent forward or slumped back. There are passengers in two vehicles, one or more of whom may need extrication. How would you proceed?
A: *Establish a danger zone and a safe zone. Keep all people out of the danger zone, and try to convince them to leave the immediate area. The safe zone should be on the same level as, and upwind from, the accident site. Call for the help that you will need. Give a radio report on the nature of the emergency, its exact location, hazardous materials, and the best estimate of the number of patients. Take command of the situation until relieved. After an incident manager has been determined, fulfill the EMS role to which you are assigned (including that of EMS command). When it is safe to enter the danger zone, quickly assess all patients and assign each a priority for receiving emergency care or transportation for definitive care.*

Street Scenes

Q1: As EMS command, what are some of the things you need to do?
A1: *When establishing EMS command, the size of the incident dictates tasks. For the incident described in the scenario, the following tasks might be handled by the EMT who established command: 1. Perform a scene size-up (with a quick walk through the scene). 2. Identify special extrication situations and/or hazardous conditions that may impact on patient care and safety. 3. Locate a staging area. 4. Communicate with other on-scene agencies (in this case, the police). 5. Delegate triage. 6. Determine the need for back-up units. 7. Alert dispatch to the number of patients and the severity of their injuries. 8. Ask dispatch to identify the number/location of hospitals able to handle these patients. 9. Request additional resources required for transport (if needed). 10. Develop a plan for deploying resources. 11. Assign a safety officer.*

Q2: What information do you expect first from the triage officer?
A2: *The triage officer will provide EMS command with the total number of patients and their priorities. Priorities should be assigned in accordance with the local or regional standard so that everyone understands the classifications.*

Q3: How will you decide what patients go to what hospitals?
A3: *As indicated in the scenario, dispatch will contact hospitals with the triage information to determine the number and/or kinds of patients that they can handle. The EMT who has established command must then decide whether there are enough resources to route patients to these sites.*

Q4: Is there a need for a safety officer on this scene?
A4: *Yes. A safety officer performs an important role in multiple-casualty incidents. This person can monitor the "big picture" to ensure that no unsafe actions are taken that would endanger either the patients or rescue personnel. This "extra pair of eyes" can identify*

problems that may have been missed or overlooked as a result of the stressful situation or because of environmental conditions such as darkness or high levels of noise.

Q5: How should patient information be transmitted to the hospitals?

A5: *There are a number of ways this can be accomplished. For example, each crew might notify the hospital directly. In this case, the EMS command should encourage crews to keep their transmissions short and concise due to the congested "air space." As an alternative, the EMS command (or incident command) might assign a communication officer to handle the transmission of all information.*

Q6: What information should you be sharing with police command and fire command?

A6: *The EMS command should inform police command of the number of patients, the location of a staging area, estimated times involved in extrication and transport, the number of ambulances responding to the scene (for traffic control), and so on. The EMS command should tell fire command about any hazardous situations (gasoline leaks, downed wires, etc.) and about extrications that may require specialized tools and/or skills.*

CHAPTER 37 EMS RESPONSE TO TERRORISM

Critical Decision Making: It Could Happen to You . . .

In each situation, explain what hazards you may suspect and how to keep yourself safe. This is the most important decision you can make.

Q1: You are called to respond with the police and fire department to an office complex where a worker opened an envelope containing white powder.

A1: *Do not enter the area. The hazmat team should bring decontaminated patients to you. Do not allow contaminated patients or rescuers into your ambulance nor take contaminated patients to the hospital.*

Q2: There was an explosion in a downtown office complex. You respond with the police and fire department to treat victims from the blast.

A2: *Do not enter the area until the area has been secured for stability and additional undetonated explosive devices. Terrorists may place secondary devices designed to harm rescuers.*

Review Questions

Q1: List and briefly describe the five most common types of terrorism incidents.

A1: *The five most common types of terrorist incidents are chemical, biological, radiological, nuclear, and explosive. A chemical event is usually a gaseous material that is released into the atmosphere and this substance has properties that are very toxic or potentially fatal when inhaled. A biological substance is a bacteria, virus, or toxin that can cause immediate illness or death or a substance that can take time making people sick. Radiological event is when radiological material is released into the atmosphere, and depending on a number of factors such as proximity, quantity of the material, and potency, can have immediate or long-range impact to human or animals. Nuclear can be very similar to radiological but may have the added potential of incendiary potential that could do immediate harm to a large area depending on its size. An explosive device, such as a bomb, can cause injury from the initial explosion and the damage which this causes and the percussion of a large device. Also, these devices sometimes contain material (e.g., nails) that is shot into the area of the explosion that can also cause harm.*

Q2: What is a secondary device? What precautions should be taken by an EMT regarding secondary devices?

A2: *A secondary device is one that goes off after the first device. For example, a device that is set off inside a building and another device is set to explode in an area where people might congregate after exiting the building. EMS responders need to be alert to the fact that in a terrorist event there may be more than one device and scene safety including being alert to this fact are a priority. Responders must try to stay clear from the area until it is deemed safe and when establishing staging and triage areas make sure these areas have been secured and, if necessary, guarded during the entire event.*

Q3: List several types of events that should trigger an EMT's suspicion of possible terrorism involvement.

A3: *Some of the types of events that should trigger the EMT to be suspicious are: symbolic and historical targets, public building or places of assembly, controversial businesses, and infrastructure systems.*

Q4: List the seven types of harm that result from a terrorism incident—and the seven-letter acronym for these types of harm.

A4: *The seven types of harm from an incendiary system are: thermal, radiological, asphyxiation, chemical, etiological, mechanical, and psychological. The acronym for these is TRACEM-P.*

Q5: Briefly discuss the concept of time, distance, and shielding.

A5: *Minimize the time that you are in the area of possible risk at a dangerous scene, maximize the distance from the hazardous area, and use as much shielding as possible whether it be a vehicle, structure, or use of specialized protective clothing and protective breathing apparatus. The more shielding the better, so more than one method should be used when available.*

Q6: Discuss several self-protection measures for biological incidents.

A6: *Distance can be helpful. The farther away from the immediate area of danger the better (also pay attention to wind direction). Use of appropriate protective equipment is potentially another effective protection technique, particularly if a responder intends to get near or within the contaminated area. This may include specialized protective breathing equipment. Limiting the time in the contaminated area should also be a consideration.*

Q7: Discuss the tactics of isolation, notification, identification, and protection.

A7: *Isolation can take on many forms at an incident where terrorism is suspected. Make sure that emergency responders and civilians don't get hurt by a secondary device; only permit those that have a need to be there and wearing proper protective gear to enter inside the perimeter. This also allows for control in an area that is apt to be very chaotic. Notification is alerting the appropriate agencies that there is an event. Many times EMS is one of the first to arrive at an act of terrorism and notifying additional resources and specialized response units needs to occur quickly. Identification refers to the agent or material that might be involved. This is important information for protecting responders and making decisions on the types of protective equipment and barriers that are required. In addition, knowing the agent will help in determining how to handle decontamination. Therefore, determining what agents are involved needs to be a priority. Protection is done to shield critical assets from additional harm and damage. Responders must first ensure that they are protected and once that is done try to protect vehicles, equipment, and supplies.*

Critical Thinking

Q: Multiple medic units are called to a "possible mass casualty incident" at the main airport terminal. The first arriving unit reports that there is a mass exodus of people from the terminal. Many of the victims have some type of fluid on their clothing with an unusual odor. They are clearly contaminated with an unknown substance. What immediate actions should be taken? What protection measures are critical? What decontamination procedures should be implemented?

A: *The first-in unit should initiate the local multiple-casualty-incident (MCI) plan, establish control of the scene, attempt to identify the possible hazardous substance by such measures as interviewing those exiting the scene of the incident, consulting the Emergency Response Guidebook, and calling CHEMTREC or another source of hazardous materials information. Decontamination and treatment areas should be established. (Review procedures for hazmat incidents and multiple-casualty incidents in Chapter 36.)*

Street Scenes (#1)

Ask a student to volunteer to read aloud to the class the case study from the chapter. Discuss answers to the questions at appropriate points within the scenario.

Q1: Make an initial scene survey to determine security threats.

A1: *There are multiple casualties, a "funny smell," and a radical group has opposed construction.*

Q2: What steps should be taken to isolate the area?

A2: *The area should immediately have a parameter established, for which law enforcement usually takes the primary responsibility. This process should also include determining an inner and outer perimeter. Notify other responding units of the danger in the area and not to enter.*

Q3: What steps should be taken to identify a possible mechanism of injury?

A3: *Attempt to determine what is the mechanism of injury by starting with the initial clues of the smell, numerous victims, and symptoms of the victims. Ask if there is any construction material that might cause these symptoms when talking with the construction manager. See if there is a container that may have markings that can be called in to CHEMTREC for possible identification of the substance. If no container can be identified, then study the signs/symptoms of the ill/injured for possible clues that can be provided to Poison Control, which is a good resource for identification and specific case.*

Q4: Identify the personal protection issues on the scene.

A4: *Those who need to be in the inner perimeter (hot zone) need to have full protective equipment (specifically rated for HAZMAT), which includes proper protective breathing apparatus. Until the substance is identified and specific hazards and risks known, nobody should enter without proper personal protective equipment (PPE).*

Street Scenes (#2)

Ask a student to volunteer to read aloud to the class the case study from the chapter. Discuss answers to the questions at appropriate points within the scenario.

Q1: What are the indicators that this is a suspicious incident?

A1: *The first indicator that this is a suspicious event is the location of the incident (headquarters of a militant group), the next is that the fire is in a dead-end of an alley, and another is the wire that is observed stretched across the alley.*

Q2: What protection precautions should be initiated?

A2: *Everyone should retreat from the immediate area to a safe distance and shield. Until the possible secondary device (wire across the alley) is deactivated by experts the scene remains dangerous and unsafe. The other possible issue is the possibility there may be an explosive device in the car.*

Q3: Discuss the proper notification procedures. What support agencies are required on the scene?

A3: *The first is the police to establish a perimeter and protect civilians and responders. Then experts in explosive devices who can deactivate the device(s). Certain federal law enforcement agencies may also be needed to investigate.*

CHAPTER 38 ADVANCED AIRWAY MANAGEMENT

Critical Decision Making: Back to Basics

For each patient described here, decide what additional information you would need to determine adequacy of breathing and whether advanced airway care would be necessary.

Q1: Your 64-year-old male patient is experiencing chest pain. He is pale and sweaty. He is breathing at 22 breaths per minute. His pulse is 92 weak and regular; blood pressure is 102/58. He is alert but anxious.

A1: *The rate of 22 may be adequate, but you must determine depth to know if the breathing is truly adequate. His anxiety, vitals, and skin color all indicate hypoxia. Even if the patient's breathing is currently adequate, it may deteriorate later in the call. Monitor the patient's breathing carefully.*

Q2: Your 57-year-old patient is found on the floor with shallow, gasping respirations at 6/minute. He complained of a headache before falling to the floor.

A2: *This patient is breathing inadequately. He should be ventilated with a BVM or pocket face mask and supplemental oxygen. The use of an advanced airway will depend on his gag reflex.*

Q3: You find an adolescent patient at the edge of a swimming pool with CPR being done by bystanders. The teenage male had been drinking and hadn't been seen for about 20 minutes when he was found floating in the pool. Compressions bring up copious amounts of vomit.

A3: *The patient requires ventilation and CPR—although you should check the patient status for yourself when you take over from lay rescuers. Advanced airways would be used if you are trained and authorized to use them. The benefit of inserting an advanced airway would be to offer some protection against aspiration of vomitus.*

Review Questions

Q1: Explain why it is important for EMTs to be able to perform orotracheal intubation.

A1: *It provides complete control of the airway. It minimizes the risk of aspiration. It allows for better oxygen delivery. It allows for deeper suctioning of the airway.*

Q2: List and explain the errors of intubation that can lead to a patient's death.

A2: *Failure to hyperventilate the patient before intubation, or taking too long to perform the intubation, can result in hypoxia. Intubating the right bronchus can result in hypoxia. Unrecognized intubation in the esophagus will result in rapid death from hypoxia.*

Q3: Explain the procedures for assuring correct placement of an endotracheal tube.

A3: *Refer to Scan 38-1, steps 9, 13, and 14.*

Q4: Explain reasons and describe the procedure for insertion of a nasogastric (NG) tube in an infant or a child.

A4: *An NG tube is used in pediatric patients to decompress the stomach and proximal bowel of air, thus improving the effectiveness of artificial ventilation. Refer to Scan 38-2 for insertion procedures.*

Q5: Explain how orotracheal suctioning differs from oropharyngeal suctioning. Explain reasons why orotracheal suctioning may be advisable.

A5: *Orotracheal suctioning is "deep suctioning" that goes beyond the upper airway into the lower airway; it may be necessary if there are obvious secretions in the airway or there is resistance to artificial ventilation. Refer to Scan 38-3 for orotracheal suctioning procedures.*

Critical Thinking

Q: You have successfully intubated a nonbreathing patient and transferred him to the ambulance. During your ongoing assessment, you auscultate the chest and find that there are breath sounds on the right, but not the left. What does this indicate? What should you do in this situation?

A: *This condition indicates that the endotracheal tube has advanced beyond the carina, intubating the right mainstem bronchus (possibly when the patient was moved during transfer to the ambulance). Deflate the cuff and withdraw the tube while artificially ventilating and while auscultating over the left apex of the chest. Don't remove the tube completely, but when the breath sounds become equal bilaterally, reinflate the cuff and secure the tube.*

Street Scenes

Q1: What priority would you assign the patient?

A1: *The patient would be assigned a high priority. As indicated, a person who claimed to be a doctor stated that the patient did not have a pulse. The EMTs should nonetheless assess the ABCs and level of responsiveness to verify the patient's condition, especially the absence of a pulse.*

Q2: What definitive treatment do pulseless patient require?

A2: *A pulseless patient requires cardiopulmonary resuscitation. To the EMT, this means that once the airway is established (perhaps through use of suctioning and an oropharyngeal airway), rescue breathing should commence. The EMTs should administer high-concentration oxygen via a BVM, followed by assessment of a pulse. In the absence of a pulse, they should perform cardiac compressions. The patient should be connected to a defibrillator as soon as possible, with shocks delivered as indicated.*

Q3: What alternatives for managing the airway might you consider?

A3: *While numerous airway adjuncts exist, the most effective method for protecting the airway and ventilating a nonbreathing patient is endotracheal intubation. If trained and authorized by medical direction, the EMTs should perform this procedure as soon as time and personnel permit.*

Q4: What assessment procedures should be performed at this time?

A4: *The initial assessment of endotracheal intubation is direct cord visualization—that is, making sure the tube has passed through the cords. Once this is done, then an esophageal intubation detector device should be used. If the device indicates that the tube is in the trachea (and NOT in the esophagus), the cuff should be inflated according to protocol. Then both the lungs and epigastrium should be auscultated while ventilating with a BVM. The EMTs should secure the tube. If available and if approved by local protocols, they might also consider additional assessment tools such as pulse oximetry and/or capnometry.*

Q5: How often should this patient be reassessed?

A5: *The patient should be frequently assessed for a number of reasons. First, he could become pulseless again and require CPR or another defibrillation. Second, endotracheal tubes can become dislodged from the trachea because of the frequent movement patients must endure during treatment, packaging, and transport. At a minimum, assessments should be done with each patient move. (Note to Instructor: For intubated patients in post-cardiac arrest, lung sounds and pulses should be assessed every minute or two.)*

REFERENCE SECTION

MUSCULOSKELETAL SYSTEM

Skeleton

The skeleton is a living framework made by the joining of bones. It serves to provide support, body movement powered by muscular contractions, protection for the vital organs and other soft structures, blood cell production, and storage for essential minerals. There are 206 bones in the adult body, forming the two divisions of the skeletal system. The axial skeleton is comprised of skull, vertebrae, rib cage, and sternum. The upper and lower extremities and the shoulder and pelvic girdles form the appendicular skeleton.

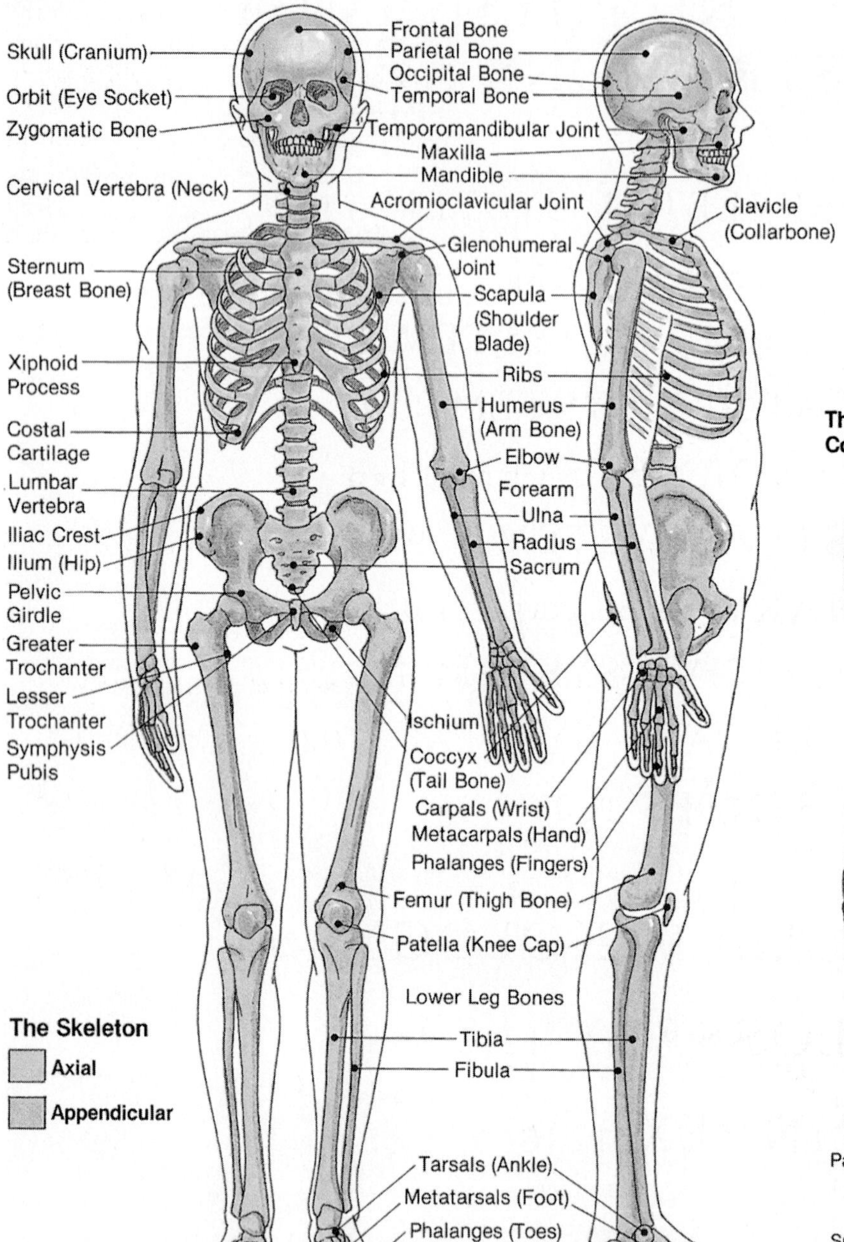

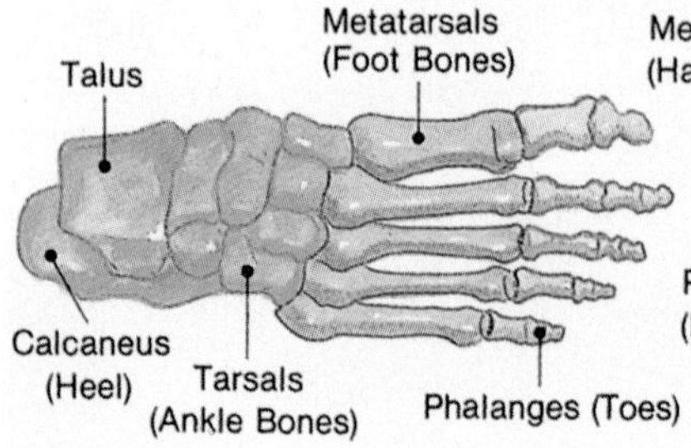

Skull (Cranium)
Frontal Bone
Parietal Bone
Occipital Bone
Temporal Bone
Orbit (Eye Socket)
Zygomatic Bone
Temporomandibular Joint
Maxilla
Mandible
Cervical Vertebra (Neck)
Acromioclavicular Joint
Clavicle (Collarbone)
Glenohumeral Joint
Sternum (Breast Bone)
Scapula (Shoulder Blade)
Xiphoid Process
Ribs
Humerus (Arm Bone)
Costal Cartilage
Elbow
Lumbar Vertebra
Forearm
Ulna
Radius
Iliac Crest
Ilium (Hip)
Sacrum
Pelvic Girdle
Greater Trochanter
Lesser Trochanter
Symphysis Pubis
Ischium
Coccyx (Tail Bone)
Carpals (Wrist)
Metacarpals (Hand)
Phalanges (Fingers)
Femur (Thigh Bone)
Patella (Knee Cap)
Lower Leg Bones
Tibia
Fibula
Tarsals (Ankle)
Metatarsals (Foot)
Phalanges (Toes)
Calcaneus (Heel)

The Skeleton

Axial

Appendicular

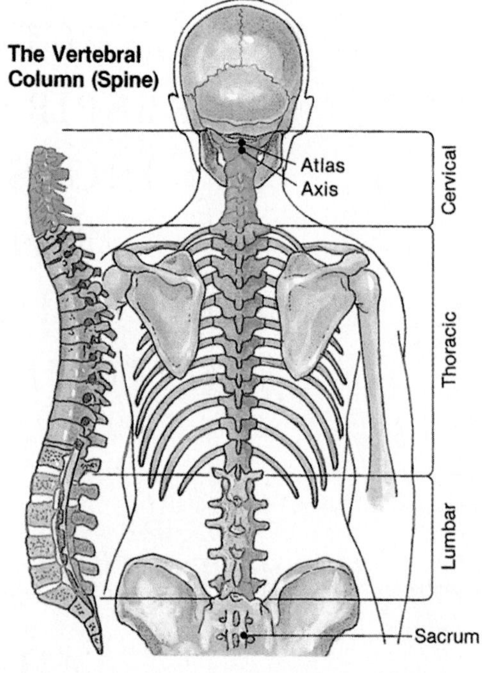

Talus
Metatarsals (Foot Bones)
Calcaneus (Heel)
Tarsals (Ankle Bones)
Phalanges (Toes)

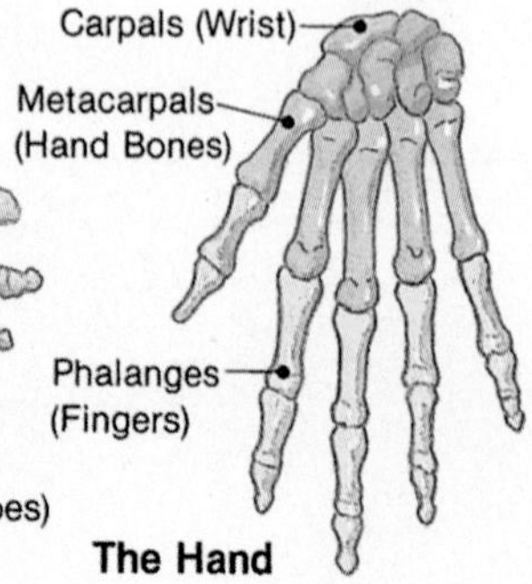

Carpals (Wrist)
Metacarpals (Hand Bones)
Phalanges (Fingers)

The Hand

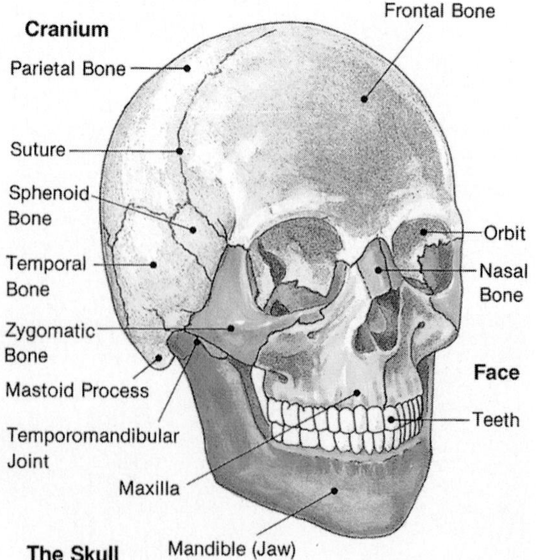

MUSCULOSKELETAL SYSTEM

Muscles

The tissues of the muscular system comprise 40 percent to 50 percent of the body's weight. The skeletal muscles of the body are voluntary muscles, subject to conscious control. They exhibit the properties of excitability; that is, they will react to nerve stimulus. Once stimulated, skeleton muscles are quick to contract and can relax and very quickly be ready for another contraction. There are 501 separate skeletal muscles that provide contractions for movement, coordinated support for posture, and heat production. Muscles connect to bones by way of tendons.

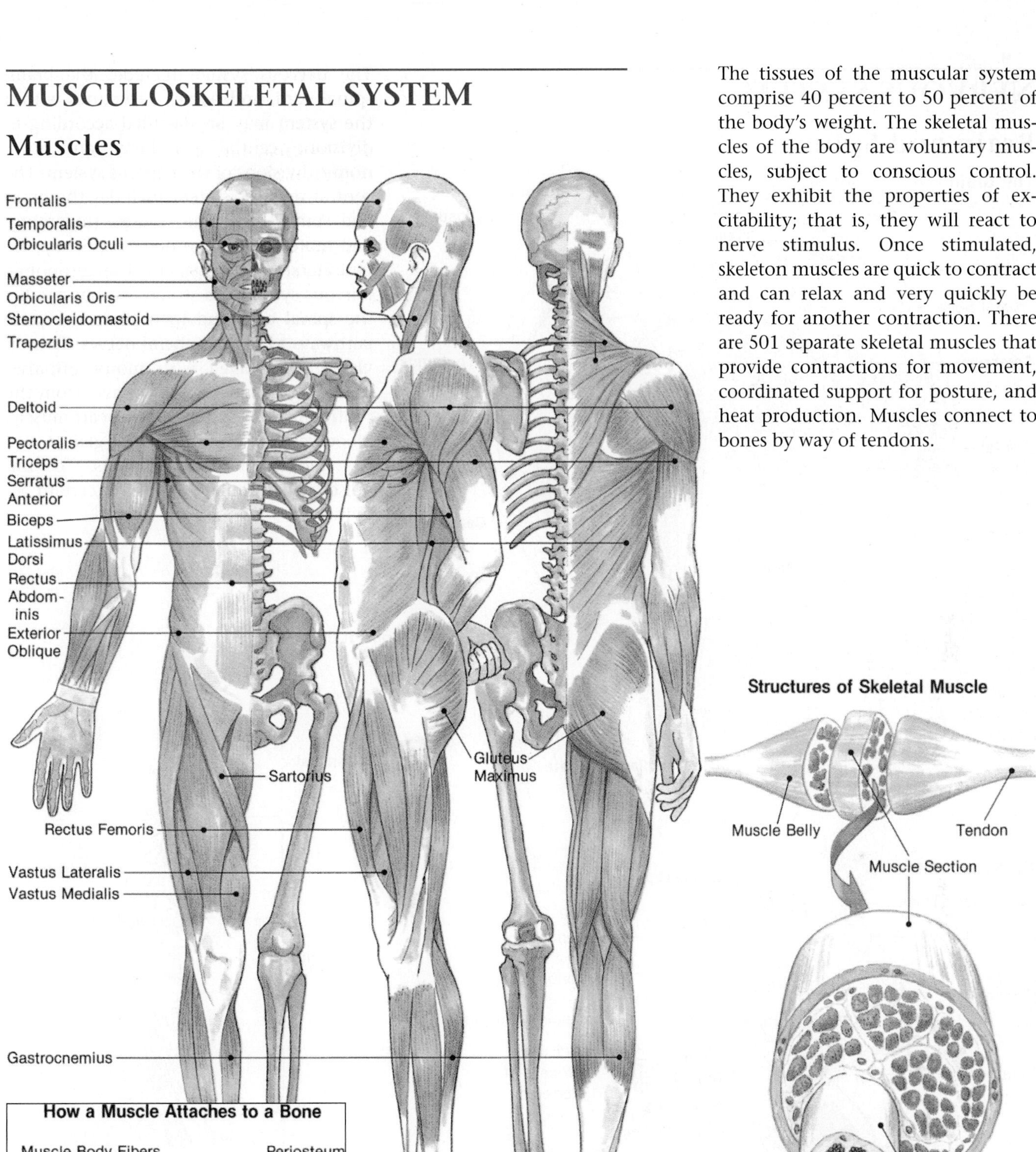

NERVOUS SYSTEM

Brain and Spine

The nervous system includes the brain, spinal cord, and nerves. Structures within the system may be classified according to divisions: central, peripheral, and autonomic divisions of the nervous system. The central nervous system includes the brain and spinal cord. The sensory (incoming) and motor (outgoing) nerves make up the peripheral nervous system. The autonomic nervous system has structures that parallel the spinal cord and then share the same pathways as the peripheral nerves. This division is involved with motor impulses (outgoing commands) that travel from the central nervous system to the heart muscle, blood vessels, secreting cells of glands, and the smooth muscles of organs. The impulses will stimulate or inhibit certain activities.

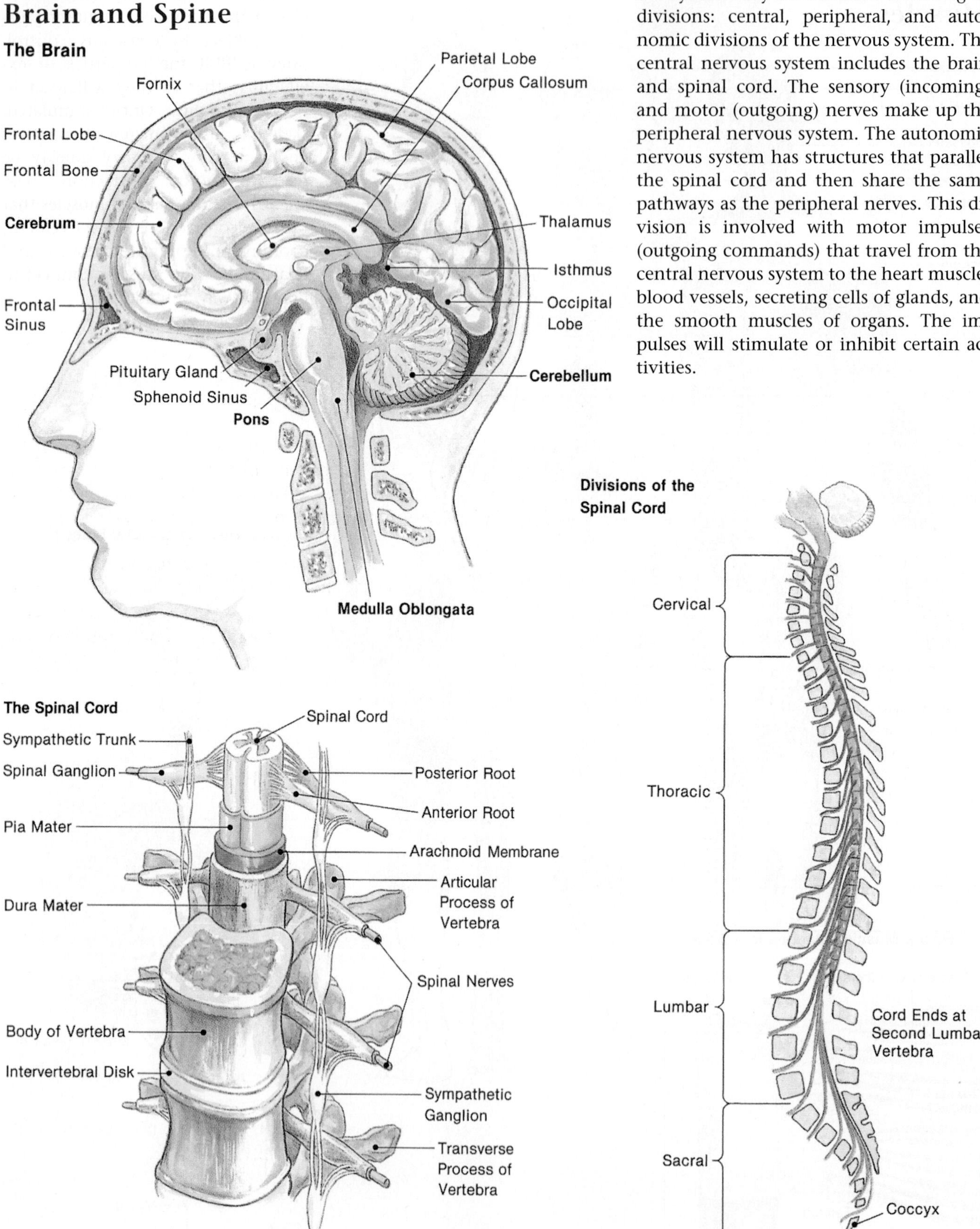

NERVOUS SYSTEM

Nerves

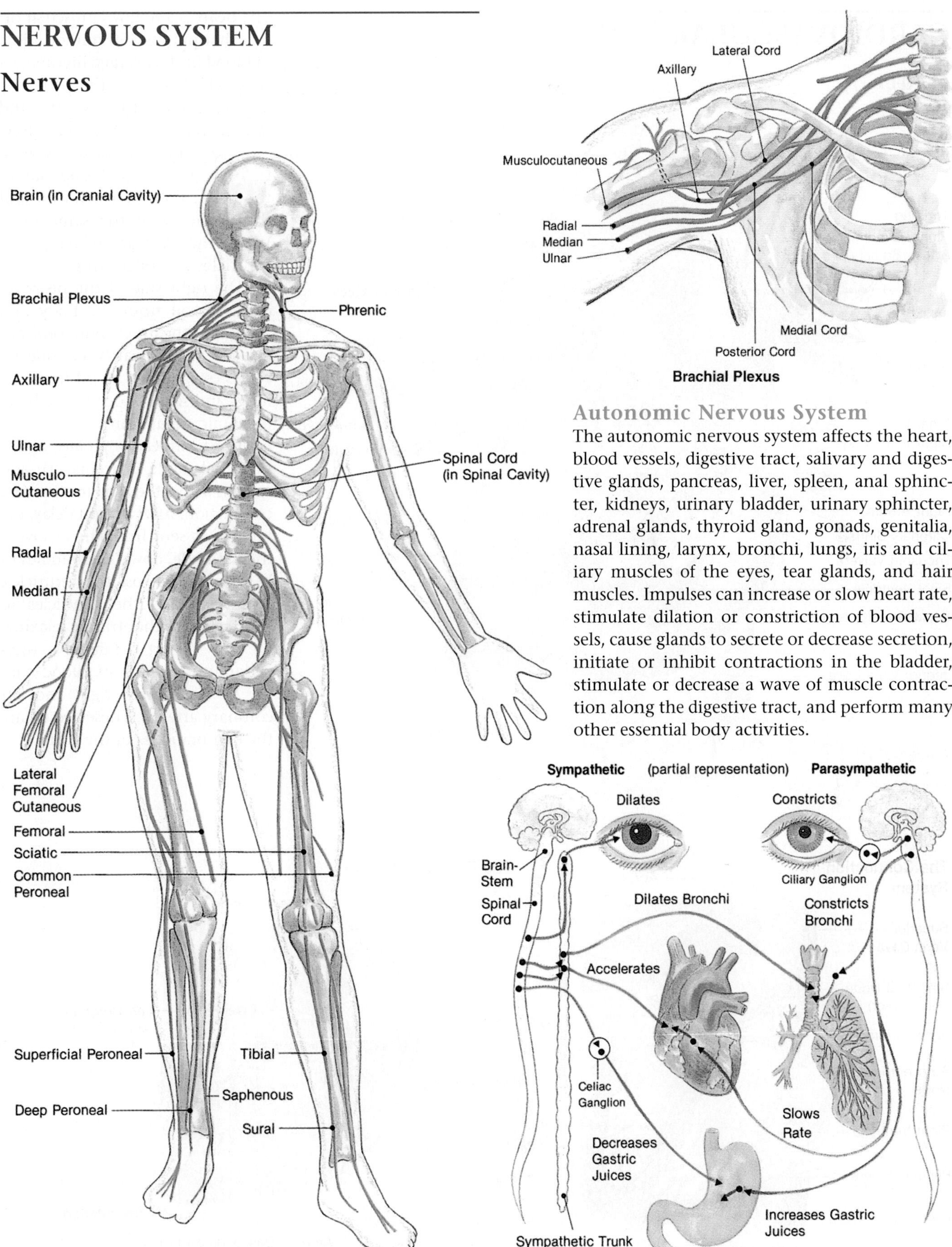

Autonomic Nervous System

The autonomic nervous system affects the heart, blood vessels, digestive tract, salivary and digestive glands, pancreas, liver, spleen, anal sphincter, kidneys, urinary bladder, urinary sphincter, adrenal glands, thyroid gland, gonads, genitalia, nasal lining, larynx, bronchi, lungs, iris and ciliary muscles of the eyes, tear glands, and hair muscles. Impulses can increase or slow heart rate, stimulate dilation or constriction of blood vessels, cause glands to secrete or decrease secretion, initiate or inhibit contractions in the bladder, stimulate or decrease a wave of muscle contraction along the digestive tract, and perform many other essential body activities.

CARDIOVASCULAR SYSTEM

Heart

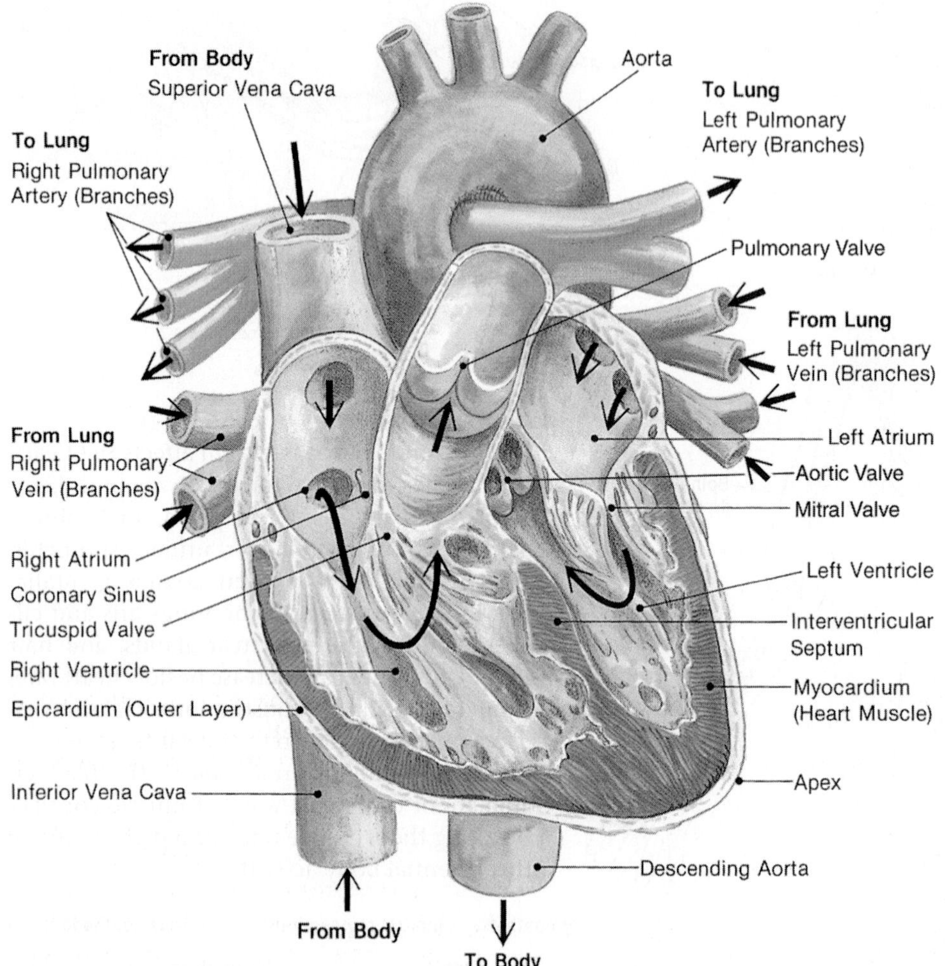

The heart is a hollow, muscular organ that pumps 450 million pints of blood in the average lifetime. Its superior chambers, the atria, receive blood. Both atria fill and then contract at the same time. The inferior chambers are the ventricles. They pump blood out of the heart. Both ventricles fill and then contract at the same time. When the atria are relaxing, the ventricles are contracting.

The right side of the heart receives blood from the body and sends it to the lungs (pulmonic circulation). The heart's left side receives oxygenated blood from the lungs and sends it out to the body (systemic circulation).

The heartbeat originates at the sinoatrial node (pacemaker) and spreads across the atria to stimulate contraction. After a slight delay, the impulse is sent from the atrioventricular node, down the bundles of His, and out across the ventricles. This stimulates the ventricles to contract while the atria are relaxing.

The heart muscle (myocardium) receives its blood supply by way of the right and left coronary arteries. These vessels are the first branches of the aorta.

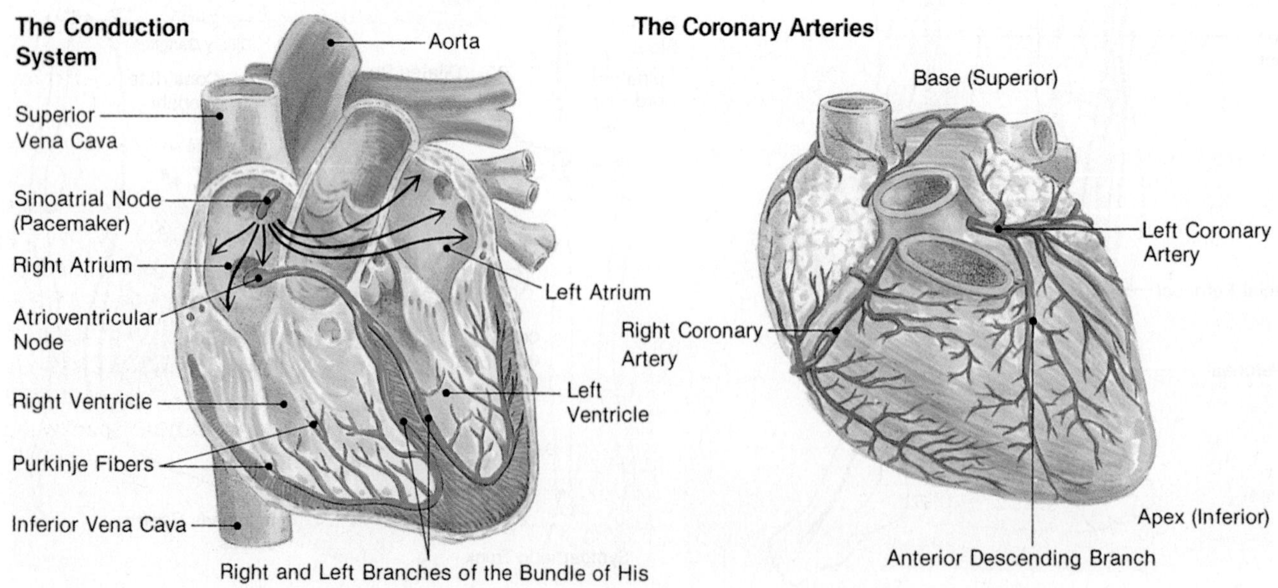

CIRCULATORY SYSTEM

Blood Vessels

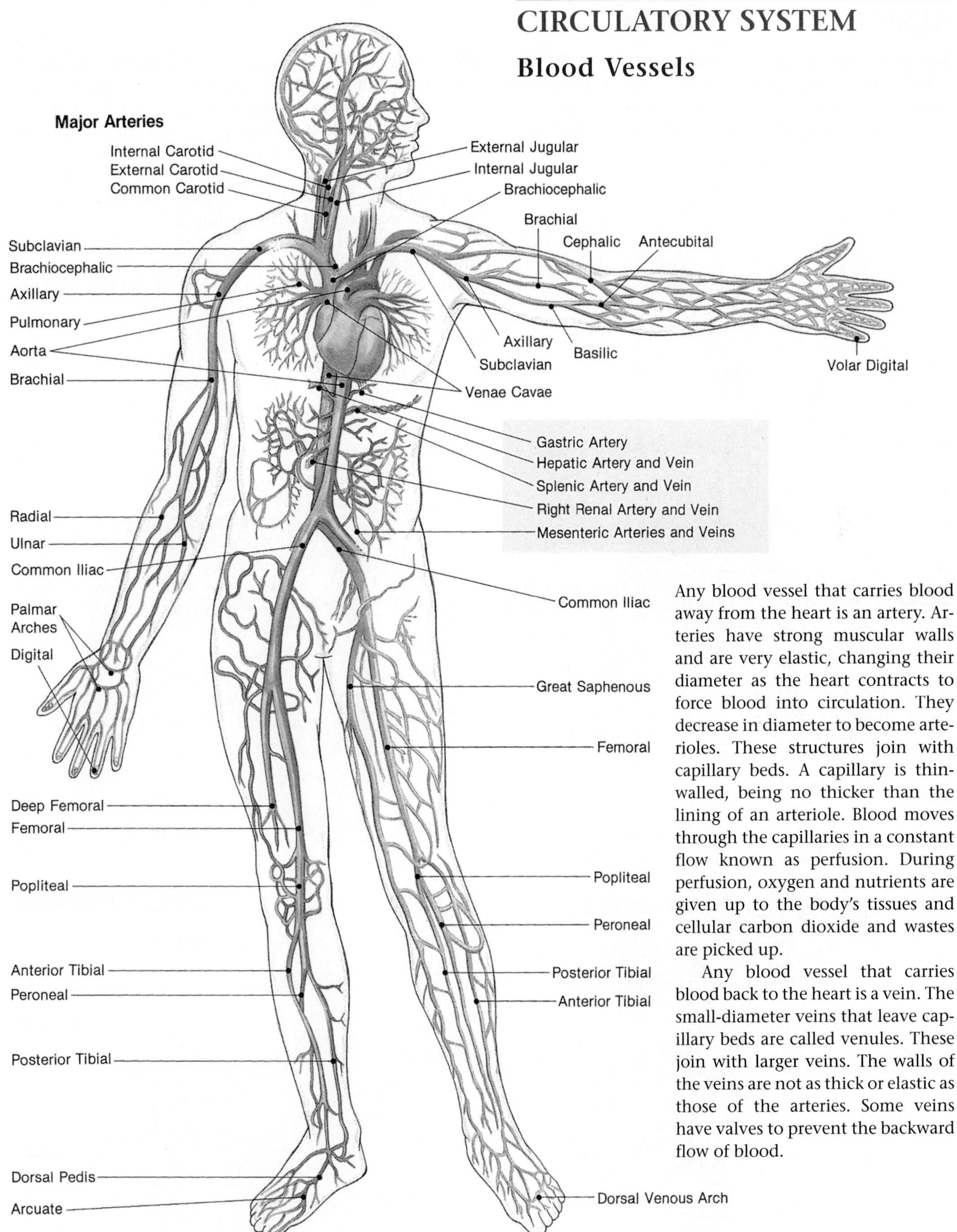

Any blood vessel that carries blood away from the heart is an artery. Arteries have strong muscular walls and are very elastic, changing their diameter as the heart contracts to force blood into circulation. They decrease in diameter to become arterioles. These structures join with capillary beds. A capillary is thin-walled, being no thicker than the lining of an arteriole. Blood moves through the capillaries in a constant flow known as perfusion. During perfusion, oxygen and nutrients are given up to the body's tissues and cellular carbon dioxide and wastes are picked up.

Any blood vessel that carries blood back to the heart is a vein. The small-diameter veins that leave capillary beds are called venules. These join with larger veins. The walls of the veins are not as thick or elastic as those of the arteries. Some veins have valves to prevent the backward flow of blood.

RESPIRATORY SYSTEM

The airway consists of structures involved with the conduction and exchange of air. Conduction is the movement of air to and from the exchange levels of the lungs. Air enters through the nose (primary) and mouth (secondary) and travels down the pharynx to enter the larynx. After passing through the larynx, air enters the trachea. At its distal end, the trachea branches into the left and right primary bronchi. These bronchi branch into secondary bronchi, which then branch into the bronchioles. Some of the bronchioles end as closed tubes. Air movement in them helps the lungs expand. The rest of the bronchioles carry the air to the exchange levels of the lungs.

The respiratory bronchioles turn into alveolar ducts. These form alveolar sacs that are made up of the alveoli. Gas exchange takes place between the alveoli and the capillaries in the lungs.

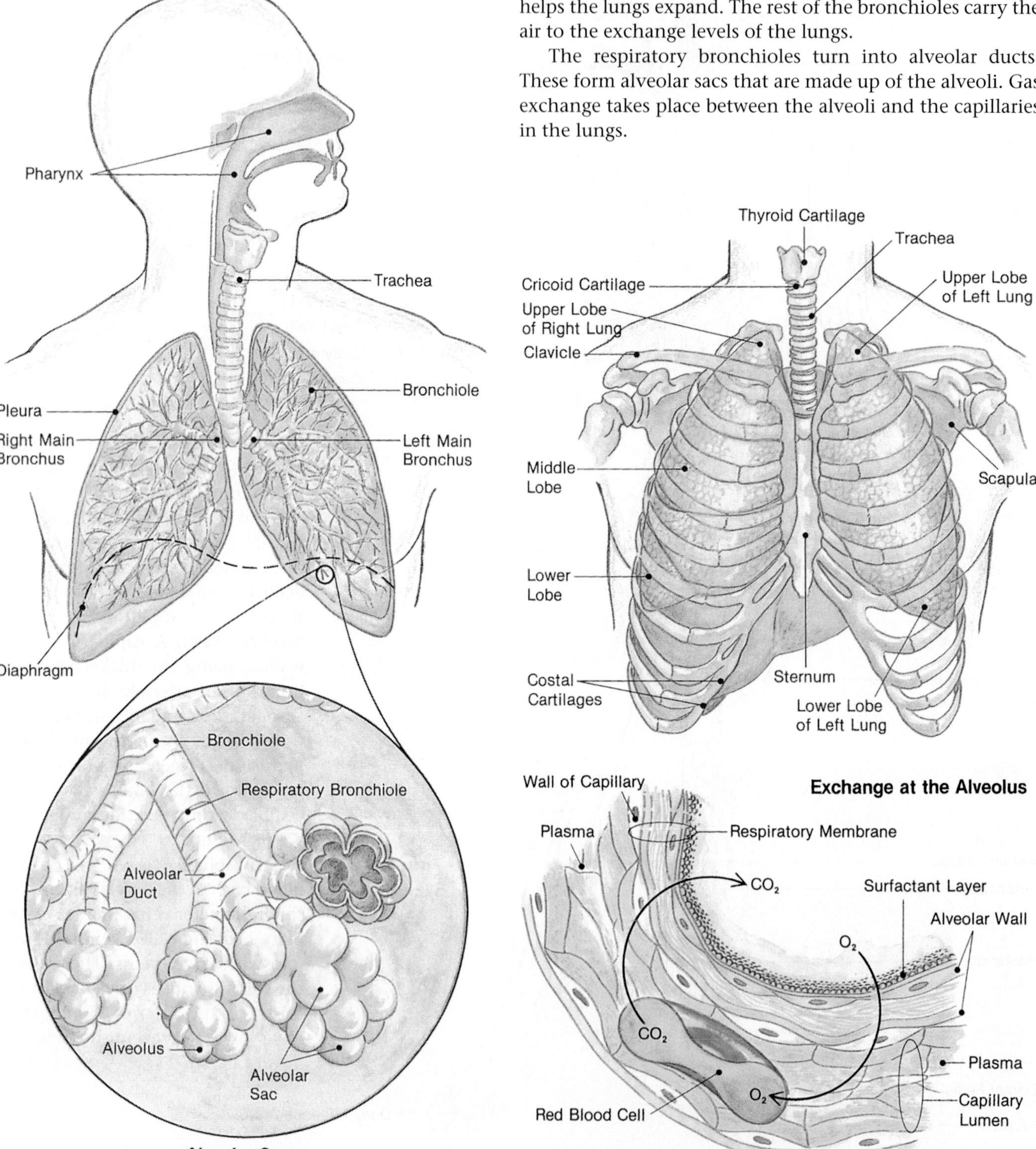

DIGESTIVE SYSTEM

The digestive system includes the digestive tract and various supportive structures and accessory glands. The tract begins at the oral cavity with the teeth and tongue. The salivary glands release saliva into the mouth to moisten food for swallowing. The tract continues down the throat to the esophagus, through the cardiac sphincter, and into the stomach. Acid and digestive enzymes are added to the food to produce chyme. The chyme passes through the pyloric sphincter to enter the small intestine. Digestive enzymes from the pancreas and bile from the liver are added to the chyme. The processes of digestion and absorption are completed in the small intestine. Wastes are carried through the ileocecal valve into the large intestine. The wastes are moved to the rectum, from where they can be expelled through the anus.

Liver, Stomach, and Pancreas

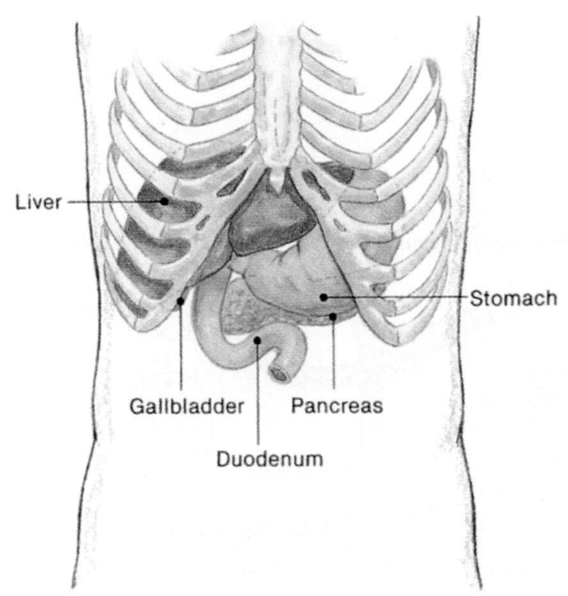

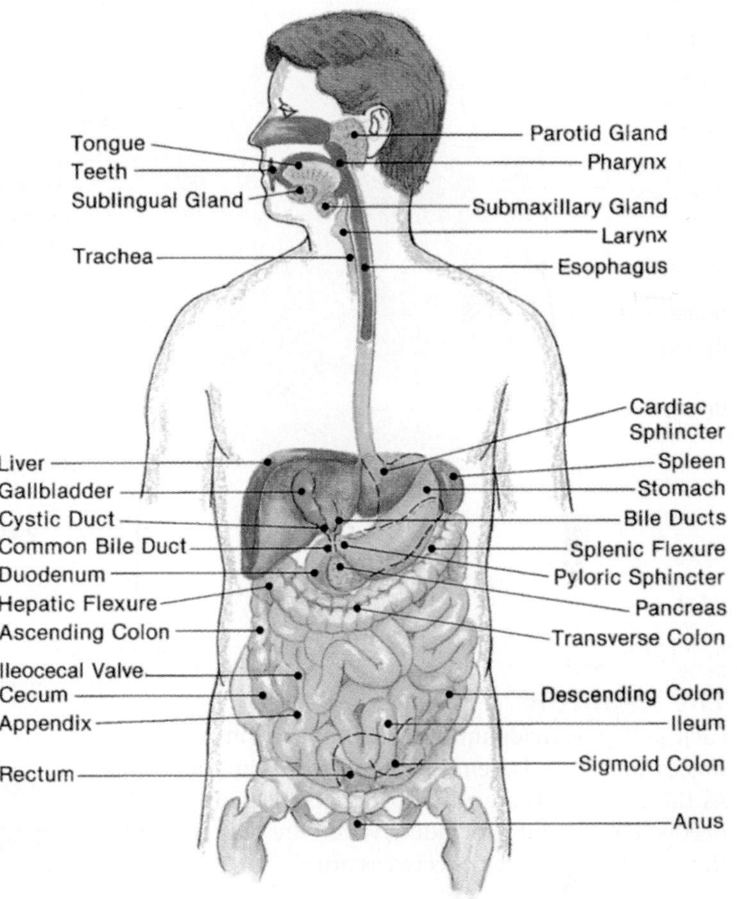

Organs of the Digestive System

Small Intestine

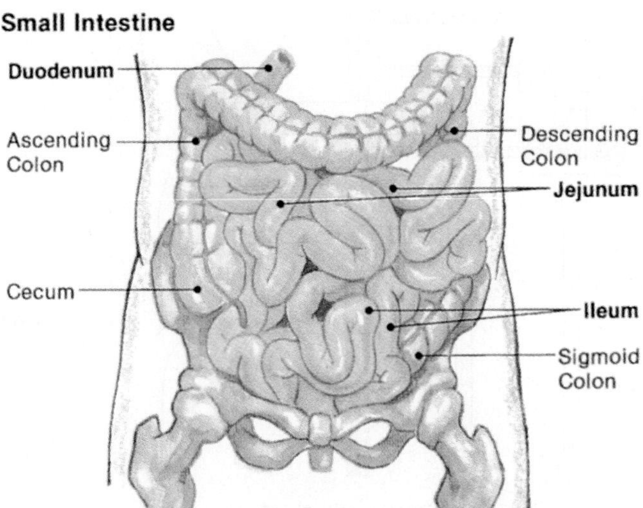

Large Intestine

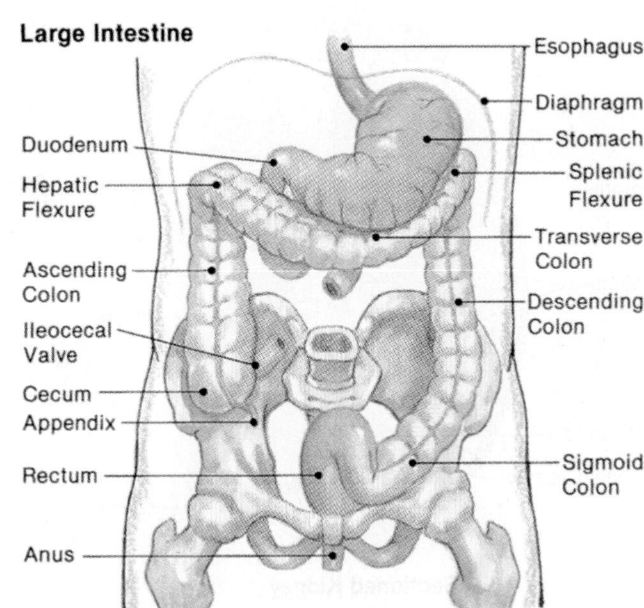

URINARY SYSTEM

The urinary system is part of the body's excretory structures (urinary system, lungs, sweat glands, and intestine). The kidneys remove the wastes of chemical activities (metabolism) in the body. These wastes are removed from the blood to produce urine. At the same time, the kidneys remove certain excess compounds, regulate the blood pH (acid-base balance), and as well as the concentration of sodium, potassium, chlorine, glucose, and other important chemicals.

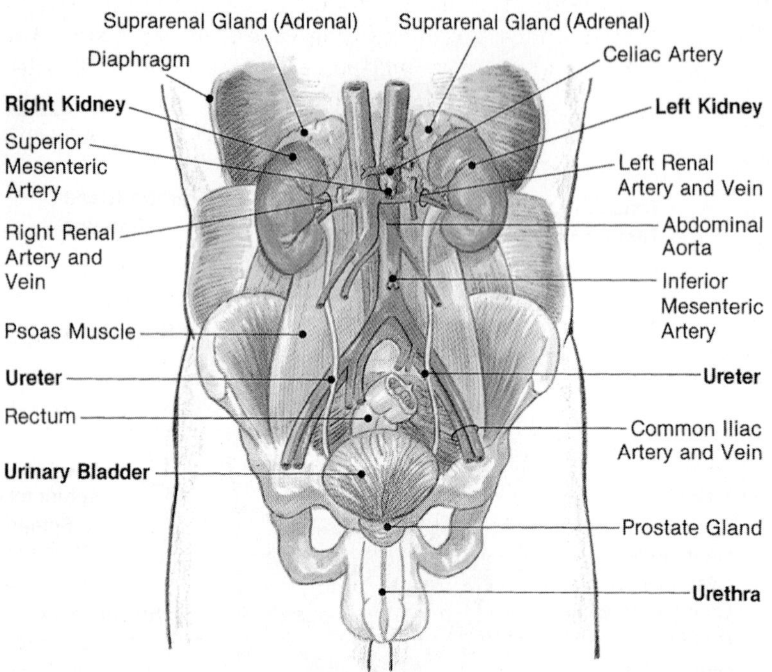

The Nephron

Each kidney is made up of microscopic nephrons. Both wastes and needed chemicals are filtered from the blood. As these materials are passed through the nephron, the needed compounds (including water) are sent back into the blood. Wastes are collected as urine.

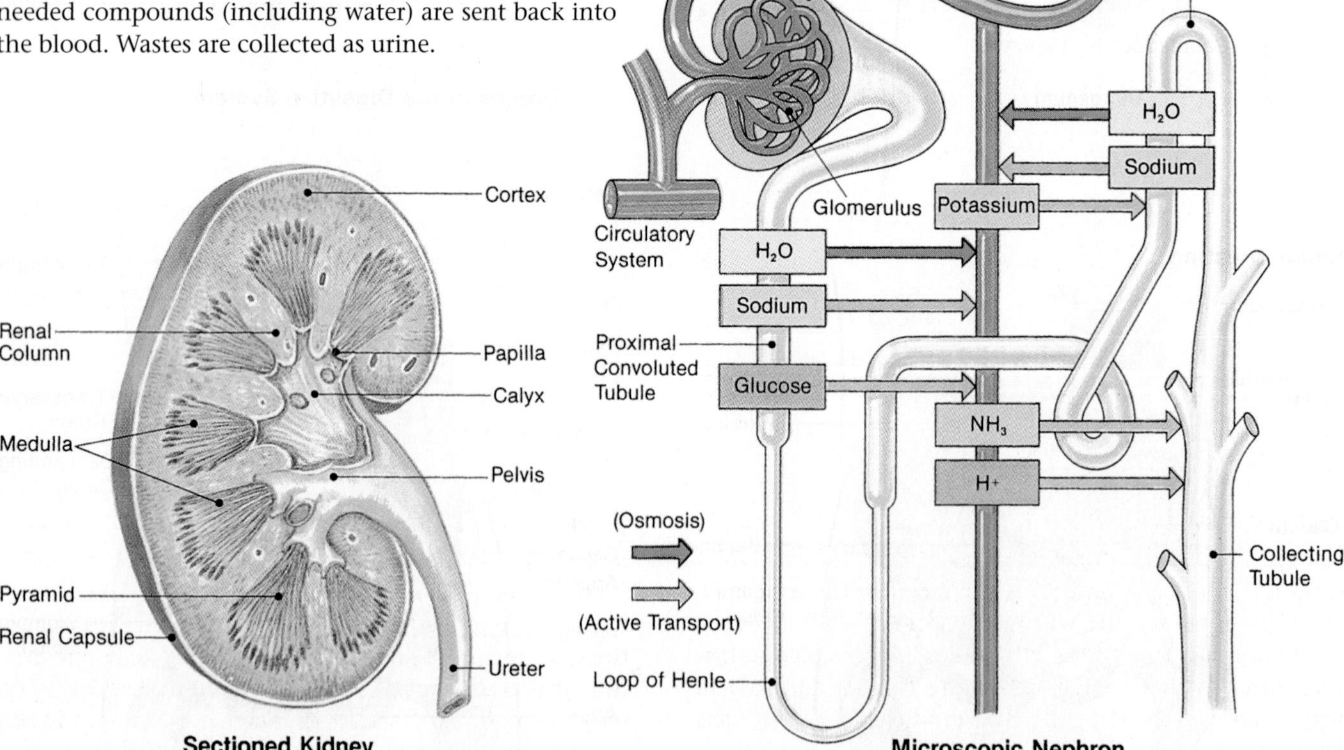

REPRODUCTIVE SYSTEM

The reproductive system consists of the organs, glands, and supportive structures that are involved with human sexuality and procreation. In the male, spermatozoa and the hormone testosterone are produced in the testes. The female produces ova (eggs) and the hormones estrogen and progesterone in her ovaries. The union of ovum and sperm produce a single cell called a zygote. Through growth, cell division, and cellular differentiation (the formulation of specialized cells) the new individual develops and matures.

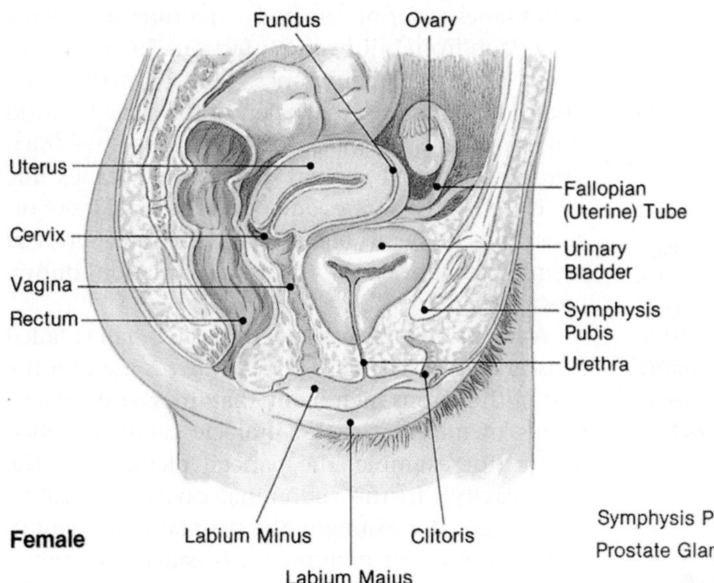

Female

Labium Minus (singular), Labia Minora (plural)
Lablum Majus (singular), Labia Majora (plural)

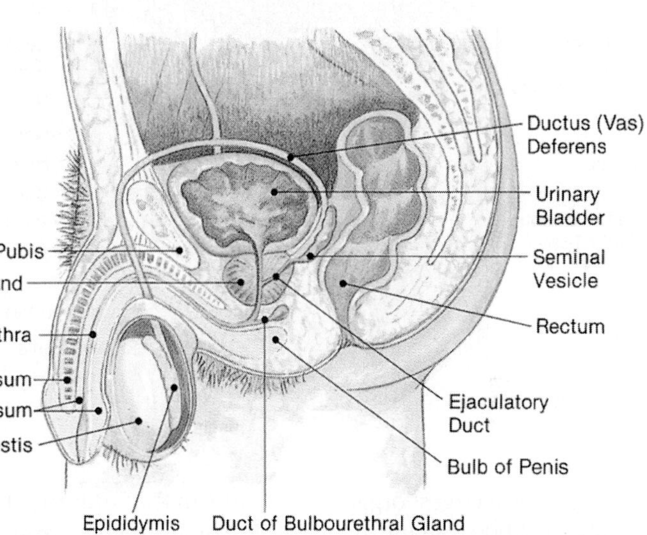

Male

The Ovary

Suspensory Ligament of Ovary
End of Fallopian Tube
Released Ovum
Mature Follicle
Maturing Follicle
Primary Follicle (Ovum and Single Layer of Follicle Cells)
Ovum
Ovarian Ligament
Corpus Luteum (Produces Estrogen and Progesterone)
Egg Nest
Corpus Albicans

The Breast

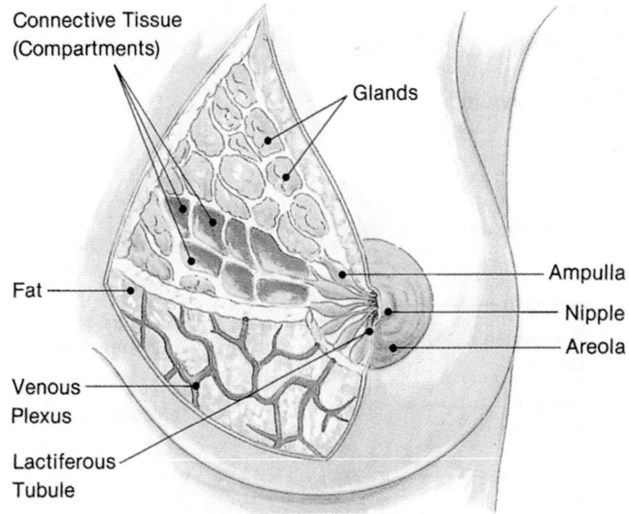

The developing ovum and its supportive cells are called a follicle. Each month, follicle-stimulating hormone (FSH) from the pituitary gland starts the growth of several follicles. Usually, only one will mature and release an ovum (ovulation). During its growth, the follicle produces estrogen. After ovulation, the remaining cells of the follicle form a specialized structure that produces both estrogen and progesterone.

The breasts contain the mammary glands that produce milk (lactation). A mammary gland is a highly modified form of sweat gland. Estrogen stimulates the growth of the ducts, while progesterone stimulates the development of the secreting (milk-producing) cells. Lactic hormone from the pituitary stimulates milk production. Another pituitary hormone, oxytocin, stimulates the milk-producing cells to eject their milk into the ducts.

INTEGUMENTARY SYSTEM

The Skin

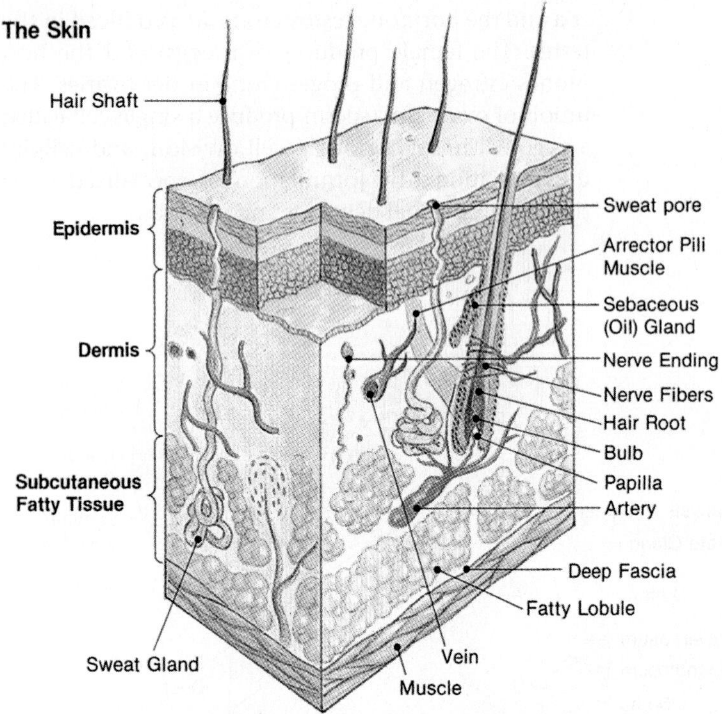

The skin is the largest organ of the body. In the adult the skin covers about 3,000 square inches (1.75 square meters) and weighs about 6 pounds. It is involved with protection, insulation, thermal regulation, excretion, and the production of vitamin D.

The Peritoneum

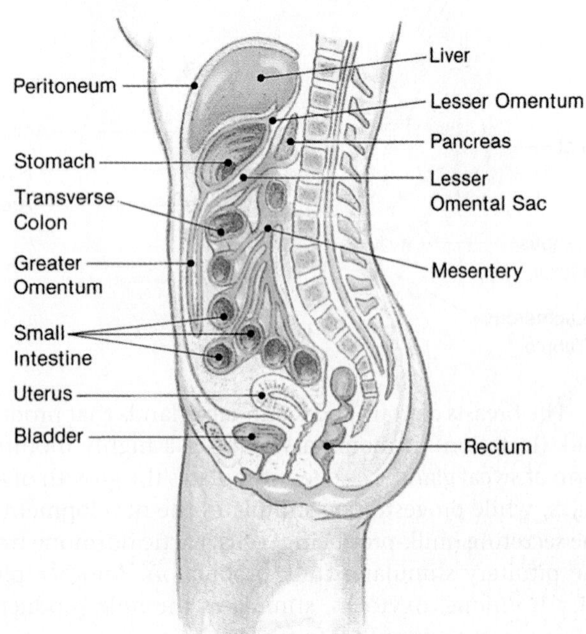

Membranes

Membranes

Membranes cover or line body structures to provide protection from injury and infection. There are four major classes of membranes. Mucous membranes line those structures that open to the outside world (for example, the mouth, the airway, digestive tract, urinary tract, and vagina). Serous membranes line the closed body cavities and cover the outsides of organs. The cutaneous membrane is the skin. Synovial membranes line joints to reduce friction during movement.

A serous membrane that covers an organ is called a visceral layer. The term *parietal layer* is used for the part of the serous membrane that lines a cavity. The serous membrane in the thoracic cavity is called pleura (for example, the parietal pleura lines the chest cavity). In the abdominal cavity, it is called peritoneum (for example, the parietal peritoneum). A double layer of peritoneum is called mesentery. The membrane that lines the sac surrounding the heart is pericardium.

Synovial Joint

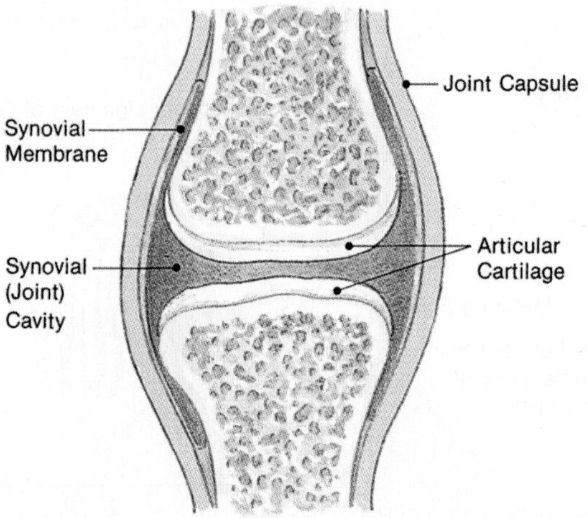

The Pleura

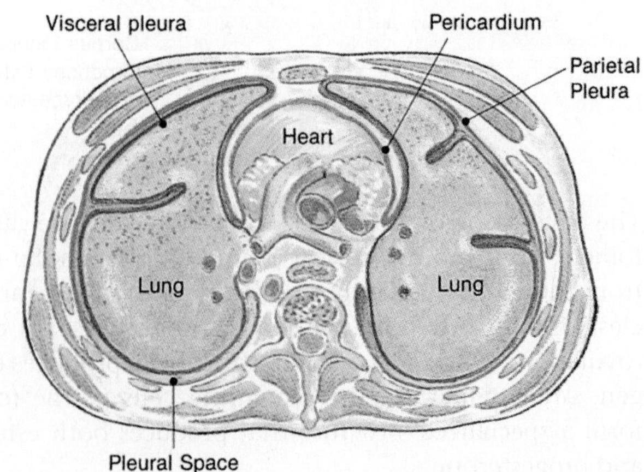

SENSES

Eye and Ear

The body has the sense of vision, hearing, balance and equilibrium, touch, pain, heat, cold, pressure, taste, and smell.

The eye can receive and focus light and then convert this energy into nerve impulses to be sent to the brain. The nerve impulses originate from the retina. Visual receptors in the retina called rods can work in low intensity light. They have no color function. The visual receptors called cones operate in high intensity light and do receive colors.

The Eye

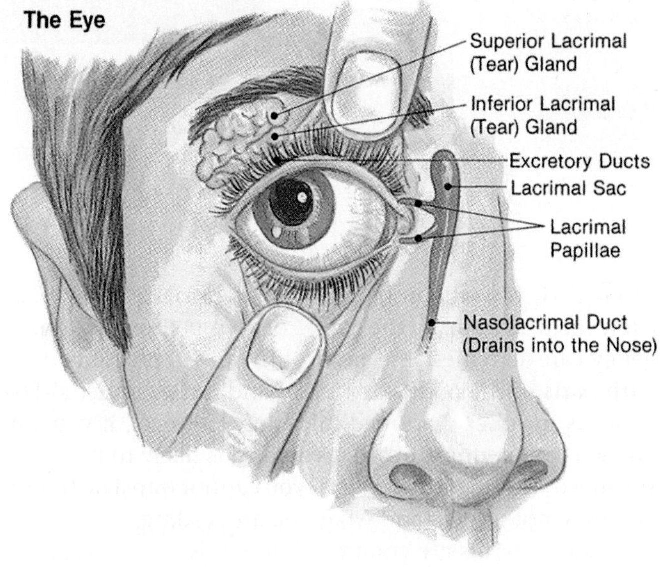

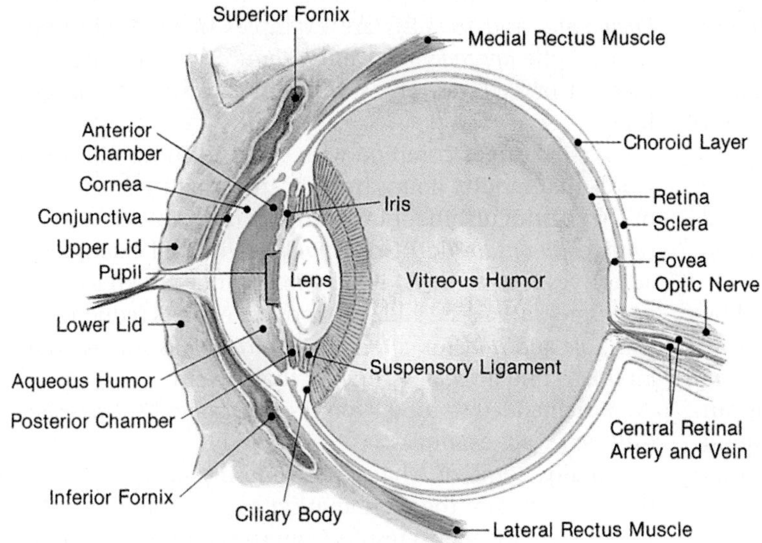

The ear's functions include hearing, static equilibrium (balance while standing still), and dynamic equilibrium (balance when moving). The outer and middle ear are responsible for sound gathering and its transmission. The inner ear has the nerve endings for hearing and equilibrium.

The Ear

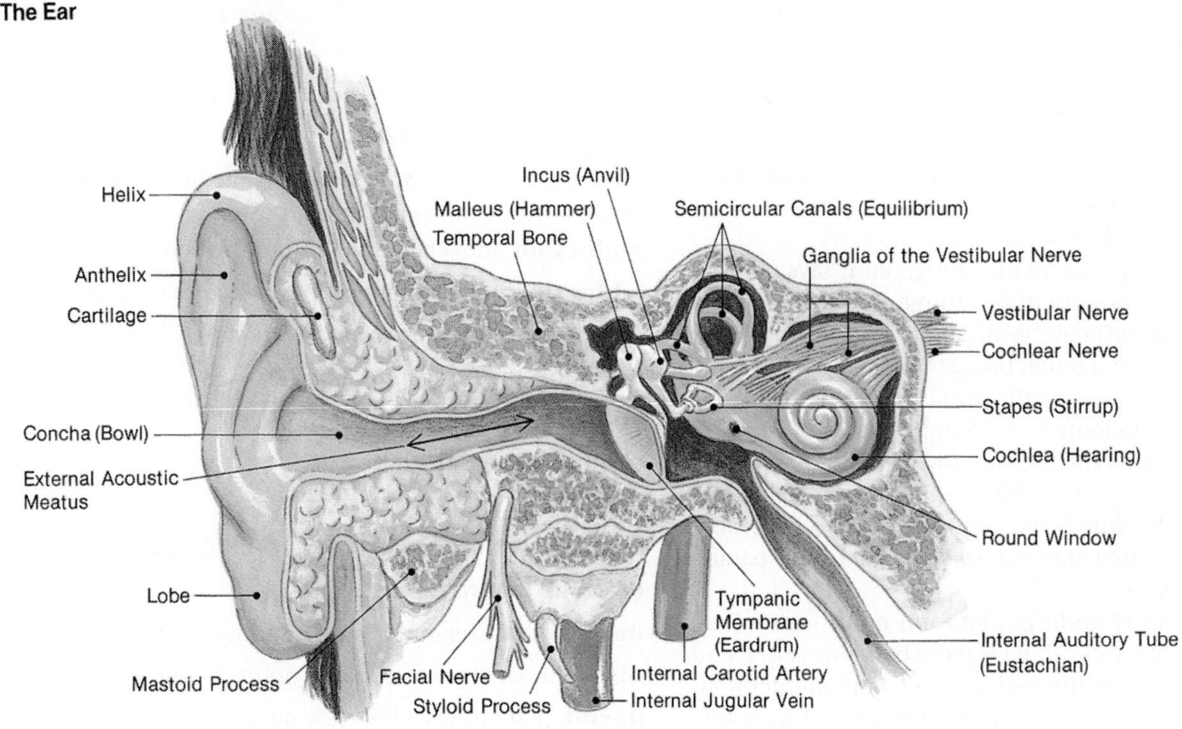

As an EMT, you will probably never have to use more than a few medical terms in the course of your prehospital emergency care activities, and most of them will probably deal with parts of the body. Physicians and nurses prefer EMTs to speak in other than medical terms. However, if you are an avid reader, much of what you read is likely to be freely sprinkled with medical terms; if you cannot translate them, you may not understand what you are reading.

Medical terms are comprised of words, roots, combining forms, prefixes, and suffixes—all little words, if you will, and each with its own definition.

Sometimes medical terms are made up of two whole words. For example, the word *small* is joined with the word *pox* to form the medical term *smallpox*, the name of a disease. If only it were always so simple!

Roots are the foundations of words and are not used by themselves. *Therm* is a root that means heat; to use it alone would make no sense. But when a vowel is added to the end of the root to make it the *combining form therm/o*, it can be joined with other words or roots to form a compound term. *Therm/o* and *meter* (an instrument for measuring) combine to form *thermometer*, an instrument for measuring heat or temperature.

More than one root or combining form can be joined to form medical terms; *electrocardiogram* is a good example. The combining forms *electr/o* (electric) and *cardi/o* (heart) are joined to the suffix *-gram* (a written record) to form the term that means a written record of the heart's electrical activity.

Prefixes are used to modify or qualify the meanings of roots. They usually tell the reader what kind of, where (or in what direction), or how many.

The root *-pnea* relates to breathing, but it says nothing about the quality or kind of breathing. Adding the prefix *dys-* qualifies it as difficult breathing.

Abdominal pain is a rather broad term; it gives the reader no clue as to exactly where the pain is located either inside or outside the abdomen. Adding the prefix *intra-* to *abdominal* pinpoints the location of the pain, for *intra-abdominal pain* means pain within the abdomen. *-Plegia* refers to paralysis of the limbs. The prefix *quadri-* tells the reader how many limbs are paralyzed. *Quadriplegia* means paralysis of all four limbs.

Suffixes are word endings that form nouns, adjectives, or verbs. Medical terms can have more than one suffix, and a suffix can appear in the middle of a compound term affixed to a combining form. A number of suffixes have specialized meanings. *-Itis* means inflammation; thus *arthritis* means inflammation of a joint. *-Iac* forms a noun indicating a person afflicted with a certain disease, as for example, *hemophiliac*.

Some suffixes are joined to roots to form terms that indicate a state, quality, condition, procedure, or process. *Pneumonia* and *psoriasis* are examples of medical conditions, while *appendectomy* and *arthroscopy* are examples of medical procedures. The suffixes in each case are underlined.

Some suffixes combine with roots to form adjectives, words that modify nouns by indicating quality or quantity or by distinguishing one thing from another. *Gastric*, *cardiac*, *fibrous*, *arthritic*, and *diaphoretic* are all examples of adjectives formed by adding suffixes (underlined) to roots.

Some suffixes are added to roots to express reduction in size, *-ole* and *-ule*, for example. An *arteriole* is smaller than an *artery*, and a *venule* is smaller than a vein.

When added to roots, *-e* and *-ize* form verbs. *Excise* and *Catheterize* are examples.

Finally, some of what are commonly accepted as suffixes are actually the combination of a root and a suffix. *-Megaly* (enlargement) results from the combination of the root *megal* (large) and the suffix *-y* (which forms the term into a noun). *Cardiomegaly* means enlargement of the heart.

Standard Terms

The following terms are used to denote direction of movement, position, and anatomical posture.

abduction movement away from the body's midline.

adduction movement toward the body's midline.

afferent conducting toward a structure.

anterior the front surface of the body.

anterior to in front of.

caudad toward the tail.

cephalad toward the head.

circumduction circular movement of a part.

craniad toward the cranium.

deep situated remote from the surface.

distal situated away from the point of origin.

dorsal pertaining to the back surface of the body.

dorsiflexion bending backward.

efferent conducting away from a structure.

elevation raising a body part.

extension stretching, or moving jointed parts into or toward a straight condition.

external situated outside.

flexion bending, or moving jointed parts closer together.

inferior situated below.

internal situated inside.

laterad toward the side of the body.

lateral situated away from the body's midline.

lateral rotation rotating outward away from the body's midline.

left lateral recumbent lying horizontal on the left side.

mediad toward the midline of the body.

medial situated toward the body's midline.

medial rotation rotating inward toward the body's midline.

palmar concerning the inner surface of the hand.

peripheral away from a central structure.

plantar concerning the sole of the foot.

posterior pertaining to the back surface of the body.

posterior to situated behind.

pronation lying face downward or turning the hand so the palm faces downward or backward.

prone lying horizontal, face down and flat.

protraction a pushing forward, as the mandible.

proximal situated nearest the point of origin.

recumbent lying horizontal, generally speaking.

retraction a drawing back, as the tongue.

right lateral recumbent lying horizontal on the right side.

rotation turning around an axis.

superficial situated near the surface.

superior situated above.

supination lying face upward or turning the hand so the palm faces forward or upward.

supine lying horizontal, flat on the back and face up.

ventral the front surface of the body.

Planes

A plane is an imaginary flat surface that divides the body into sections.

coronal or frontal plane an imaginary plane that passes through the body from side to side and divides it into front and back sections.

midsagittal plane an imaginary plane that passes through the body from front to back and divides it into right and left halves.

sagittal plane an imaginary plane parallel to the median plane. It passes through the body from front to back and divides the body into right and left sections.

transverse plane an imaginary plane that passes through the body and divides it into upper and lower sections.

Word Parts

Prefixes are generally identified by a following dash (*ambi-*). Combining forms have a slash and a vowel following the root (*arthr/o*). Suffixes are generally identified by a preceding dash (*-emia*).

a- (not, without, lacking, deficient) *afebrile*, without fever.

ab- (away from) *abduct*, to draw away from the midline.

abdomin/o (abdomen) *abdominal*, pertaining to the abdomen.

-able, -ible (capable of) *reducible*, capable of being reduced (as a fracture).

ac- (to) *acclimate*, to become accustomed to.

acou (hear) *acoustic*, pertaining to sound or hearing.

acr/o (extremity, top, peak) *acrodermatitis*, inflammation of the skin of the extremities.

acu (needle) *acupuncture*, the Chinese practice of piercing specific peripheral nerves with needles to relieve the discomfort associated with painful disorders.

ad- (to, toward) *adduct*, to draw toward the midline.

aden/o (gland) *adenitis*, inflammation of a gland.

adip/o (fat) *adipose*, fatty; fat (in size).

aer/o (air) *aerobic*, requiring the presence of oxygen to live and grow.

af- (to) *afferent*, conveying toward.

ag- (to) *aggregate*, to crowd or cluster together.

-algesia (painful) *hyperalgesia*, overly sensitive to pain.

-algia (painful condition) *neuralgia*, pain that extends along the course of one or more nerves.

ambi- (both sides) *ambidextrous*, able to perform manual skills with both hands.

ambl/y (dim, dull, lazy) *amblyopia*, lazy eye.

amphi-, ampho- (on both sides, around both) *amphigonadism*, having both testicular and ovarian tissues.

amyl/o (starch) *amyloid*, starchlike.

an- (without) *anemia*, a reduced volume of blood cells.

ana- (upward, again, backward, excess) *anaphylaxis*, an unusual or exaggerated reaction of an organism to a substance to which it becomes sensitized.

andr/o (man, male) *android*, resembling a man.

angi/o (blood vessel, duct) *angioplasty*, surgery of blood vessels.

ankyl/o (stiff) *ankylosis*, stiffness.

ant-, anti- (against, opposed to, preventing, relieving) *antidote*, a substance for counteracting a poison.

ante- (before, forward) *antecubital*, situated in front of the elbow.

antero- (front) *anterolateral*, situated in front and to one side.

ap- (to) *approximate*, to bring together; to place close to.

apo- (separation, derivation from) *apoplexy*, sudden neurologic impairment due to a cardiovascular disorder.

-arium, -orium (place for something) *solarium*, a place for the sun.

arteri/o (artery) *arteriosclerosis*, thickening of the walls of the smaller arteries.

arthrio (joint, articulation) *arthritis*, inflammation of a joint or joints.

articul/o (joint) *articulated*, united by joints.

as- (to) *assimilate*, to take into.

at- (to) *attract*, to draw toward.

audi/o (hearing) *audiometer*, an instrument to test the power of hearing.

aur/o (ear) *auricle*, the flap of the ear.

aut/o (self) *autistic*, self-centered

bi- (two, twice, double, both) *bilateral*, having two sides; pertaining to two sides.

bi/o (life) *biology*, the study of life.

blephario (eyelid) *blepharitis*, inflammation of the eyelid.

brachi/o (upper arm) *brachialgia*, pain in the upper arm.

brady- (slow) *bradycardia*, an abnormally slow heart rate.

bronch/o (larger air passages of the lungs) *bronchitis*, inflammation of the larger air passages of the lungs.

bucc/o (cheek) *buccal*, pertaining to the cheek.

cac/o (bad) *cacosmis*, a bad odor.

calc/o (bad) *calculus*, an abnormal hard inorganic mass such as a gallstone.

calcane/o (heel) *calcaneus*, the heel bone.

calor/o (heat) *caloric*, pertaining to heat.

cancr/o (cancer) *cancroid*, resembling cancer.

capit/o (head) *capitate*, head-shaped.

caps/o (container) *capsulation*, enclosed in a capsule or container.

carcin/o (cancer) *carcinogen*, a substance that causes cancer.

cardi/o (heart) *cardiogenic*, originating in the heart.

carp/o (wrist bone) *carpal*, pertaining to the wrist bone.

cat-, cata- (down, lower, under, against, along with) *catabasis*, the stage of decline of a disease.

-cele (tumor, hernia) *hydrocele*, a confined collection of water.

celi/o (abdomen) *celiomyalgia*, a pain in the muscles of the abdomen.

-centesis (perforation or tapping, as with a needle) *abdominocentesis*, surgical puncture of the abdominal cavity.

cephal/o (head) *electroencephalogram*, a recording of the electrical activity of the brain.

cerebr/o (cerebrum) *cerebrospinal*, pertaining to the brain and spinal fluid.

cervic/o (neck, cervix) *cervical*, pertaining to the neck (or cervix).

cheil/o, chil/o (lip) *cheilitis*, inflammation of the lips.

cheirio, chir/o (hand) *cheiralgia*, pain in the hand.

chlor/o (green) *chloroma*, green cancer, a greenish tumor associated with myelogenous leukemia.

chol/e (bile, gall) *choledochitis*, inflammation of the common bile duct.

chondr/o (cartilage) *chondrodynia*, pain in a cartilage.

chrom/o, chromat/o (color) *monochromatic*, being of one color.

chron/o (time) *chronic*, persisting for a long time.

-cid- (cut, kill, fall) *insecticide*, an agent that kills insects.

circum- (around) *circumscribed*, confined to a limited space.

-cis- (cut, kill, fall) *excise*, to cut out.

-clysis (irrigation) *enteroclysis*, irrigation of the small intestine.

co- (with) *cohesion*, the force that causes various particles to unite.

col- (with) *collateral*, secondary or accessory; a small side branch such as a blood vessel or nerve.

col/o (colon, large intestine) *colitis*, inflammation of the colon.

colp/o (vagina) *colporrhagia*, bleeding from the vagina.

com- (with) *comminuted*, broken or crushed into small pieces.

con- (with) *congenital*, existing from the time of birth.

contra- (against, opposite) *contraindicated*, inadvisable.

cor/e, core/o (pupil) *corectopia*, abnormal location of the pupil of the eye.

cost/o (rib) *intercostal*, between the ribs.

crani/o (skull) *cranial*, pertaining to the skull.

cry/o (eold) *cryogenic*, that which produces low temperature.

crypt/o (hide, cover, conceal) *cryptogenic*, of doubtful origin.

cyan/o (blue) *cyanosis*, bluish discoloration of the skin and mucous membranes.

cyst/o (urinary bladder, cyst, sac of fluid) *cystitis*, inflammation of the bladder.

-cyte (cell) *leukocyte*, white cell.

cyt/o (cell) *cytoma*, tumor of the cell.

dacry/o (tear) *dacryorrhea*, excessive flow of tears.

dactyl/o (finger, toe) *dactylomegaly*, abnormally large fingers or toes.

de- (down) *descending*, coming down from.

dent/o (tooth) *dental*, pertaining to the teeth.

derm/o, dermat/o (skin) *dermatitis*, inflammation of the skin.

dextr/o (right) *dextrad*, toward the right side.

di- (twice, double) *diplegia*, paralysis affecting like parts on both sides of the body.

dia- (through, across, apart) *diaphragm*, the partition that separates the abdominal and thoracic cavities.

dipl/o (double, twin, twice) *diplopia*, double vision.

dips/o (thirst) *dipsomania*, alcoholism.

dis- (to free, to undo) *dissect*, to cut apart.

dors/o (back) *dorsal*, pertaining to the back.

-dynia (painful condition) *cephalodynia*, headache.

dys- (bad, difficult, abnormal, incomplete) *dyspnea*, labored breathing.

-ectasia (dilation or enlargement of an organ or part) *gastrectasia*, dilation (stretching) of the stomach.

ecto- (outer, outside of) *ectopic*, located away from the normal position.

-ectomy (the surgical removal of an organ or part) *appendectomy*, surgical removal of the appendix.

electr/o (electric) *electrocardiogram*, the written record of the heart's electrical activity.

-emia (condition of the blood) *anemia*, a deficiency of red blood cells.

en- (in, into, within) *encapsulate*, to enclose within a container.

encephal/o (brain) *encephalitis*, inflammation of the brain.

end-, endo- (within) *endotracheal*, within the trachea.

ent-, ento- (within, inner) *entopic*, occurring in the proper place.

enter/o (small intestine) *enteritis*, inflammation of the intestine.

ep-, epi- (over, on, upon) *epidermis*, the outermost layer of skin.

erythr/o (red) *erythrocyte*, a red blood cell.

esthesia (feeling) *anesthesia*, without feeling.

eu (good, well, normal, healthy) *euphoria*, an abnormal or exaggerated feeling of well-being.

ex- (out of, away from) *excrement*, waste material discharged from the body.

exo- (outside, outward) *exophytic*, to grow outward or on the surface.

extra- (on the outside, beyond, in addition to) *extracorporeal*, outside the body.

faci/o (face, surface) *facial*, pertaining to the face.

febr/i (fever) *febrile*, feverish.

-ferent (bear, carry) *efferent*, carrying away from a center.

fibr/o (fiber, filament) *fibrillation*, muscular contractions due to the activity of muscle fibers.

-form (shape) *deformed*, abnormally shaped.

-fugal (moving away) *centrifugal*, moving away from a center.

galact/o (milk) *galactopyria*, milk fever.

gangli/o (knot) *ganglion*, a knotlike mass.

gastr/o (stomach) *gastritis*, inflammation of the stomach.

gen/o (come into being, originate) *genetic*, inherited.

-genesis (production or origin) *pathogenesis*, the development of a disease.

-genic (giving rise to, originating in) *cardiogenic*, originating in the heart.

gloss/o (tongue) *glossal*, pertaining to the tongue.

glyc/o (sweet) *glycemia*, the presence of sugar in the blood.

gnath/o (jaw) *gnathitis*, inflammation of the jaw.

gnos/o (knowledge) *prognosis*, a prediction of the outcome of a disease.

-gram (drawing, written record) *electrocardiogram*, a recording of the heart's electrical activity.

-graph (an instrument for recording the activity of an organ) *electrocardiograph*, an instrument for measuring the heart's electrical activity.

-graphy (the recording of the activity of an organ) *electrocardiography*, the method of recording the heart's electrical activity.

gynec/o (woman) *gynecologist*, a specialist in diseases of the female genital tract.

hem/a, hem/o, hemat/o (blood) *hematoma*, a localized collection of blood.

hemi- (one-half) *hemiplegia*, paralysis of one side of the body.

hepat/o (liver) *hepatitis*, inflammation of the liver.

heter/o (other) *heterogeneous*, from a different source.

hidr/o, hidrot/o (sweat) *hidrosis*, excessive sweating.

hist/o (tissue) *histodialysis*, the breaking down of tissue.

hom/o, home/o (same, similar, unchanging, constant) *homeostasis*, stability in an organism's normal physiological states.

hyal/o (glass) *hyaline*, glassy, transparent.

hydr/o (water, fluid) *hydrocephalus*, an accumulation of cerebrospinal fluid in the skull with resulting enlargement of the head.

hyper- (beyond normal, excessive) *hypertension*, abnormally high blood pressure.

hypn/o (sleep) *hypnotic*, that which induces sleep.

hypo- (below normal, deficient, under, beneath) *hypotension*, abnormally low blood pressure.

hyster/o (uterus, womb) *hysterectomy*, surgical removal of the uterus.

-iasis (condition) *psoriasis*, a chronic skin condition characterized by lesions.

iatr/o (healer, physician) *pediatrician*, a physician that specializes in children's disorders.

-id (in a state, condition of) *gravid*, pregnant.

idio (peculiar, separate, distinct) *idiopathic*, occurring without a known cause.

il- (negative prefix) *illegible*, cannot be read.

ile/o (ileum) *ileitis*, inflammation of the ileum.

ili/o (ilium) *iliac*, pertaining to the ilium.

im- (negative prefix) *immature*, not mature.

in- (in, into, within) *incise*, to cut into.

infra- (beneath, below) *infracostal*, below a rib, or below the ribs.

inter- (between) *intercostal*, between two ribs.

intra- (within) *intraoral*, within the mouth.

intro- (within, into) *introspection*, the contemplation of one's own thoughts and feelings; self-analysis.

ir/o, irid/o (iris) *iridotomy*, incision of the iris.

ischi/o (ischium) *ischialgia*, pain in the ischium.

-ismus (abnormal condition) *strabismus*, deviation of the eye that a person cannot overcome.

iso- (same, equal, alike) *isometric*, of equal dimensions.

-itis (inflammation) *endocarditis*, inflammation within the heart.

kerat/o (cornea) *keratitis*, inflammation of the cornea.

kinesi/o (movement) *kinesialgia*, pain upon movement.

labi/o (lip) *labiodental*, pertaining to the lip and teeth.

lact/o (milk) *lactation*, the secretion of milk.

lal/o (talk) *lalopathy*, any speech disorder.

lapar/o (flank, abdomen, abdominal wall) *laparotomy*, an incision through the abdominal wall.

laryng/o (larynx) *laryngoscope*, an instrument for examining the larynx.

lept/o (thin) *leptodactylous*, having slender fingers.

leuc/o, leuk/o (white) *leukemia*, a malignant disease characterized by the increased development of white blood cells.

lingu/o (tongue) *sublingual*, under the tongue.

lip/o (fat) *lipoma*, fatty tumor.

lith/o (stone) *lithotriptor*, an instrument for crushing stones in the bladder.

-logist (a person who studies) *pathologist*, a person who studies diseases.

log/o (speak, give an account) *logospasms*, spasmodic speech.

-logy (study of) *pathology*, the study of disease.

lumb/o (loin) *lumbago*, pain in the lumbar region.

lymph/o (lymph) *lymphoduct*, a vessel of the lymph system.

-lysis (destruction) *electrolysis*, destruction (of hair, for example) by passage of an electric current.

macr/o (large, long) *macrocephalous*, having an abnormally large head.

malac/o (a softening) *malacia*, the morbid softening of a body part or tissue.

mamm/o (breast) *mammary*, pertaining to the breast.

-mania (mental aberration) *kleptomania*, the compulsion to steal.

mast/o (breast) *mastectomy*, surgical removal of the breast.

medi/o (middle) *mediastinum*, middle partition of the thoracic cavity.

mega- (large) *megacolon*, an abnormally large colon.

megal/o (large) *megalomaniac*, a person impressed with his own greatness.

-megaly (an enlargement) *cardiomegaly*, enlargement of the heart.

melan/o (dark, black) *melanoma*, a tumor comprised of darkly pigmented cells.

men/o (month) *menopause*, cessation of menstruation.

mes/o (middle) *mesiad*, toward the center.

meta- (change, transformation, exchange) *metabolism*, the sum of the physical and chemical processes by which an organism survives.

metr/o (uterus) *metralgia*, pain in the uterus.

micr/o (small) *microscope*, an instrument for magnifying small objects.

mon/o (single, only, sole) *monoplegia*, paralysis of a single part.

morph/o (form) *morphology*, the study of form and shape.

multi- (many, much) *multipara*, a woman who has given two or more live births.

myc/o, mycet/o (fungus) *mycosis*, any disease caused by a fungus.

my/o (muscle) *myasthenia*, muscular weakness.

myel/o (marrow, also often refers to spinal cord) *myelocele*, protrusion of the spinal cord through a defect in the spinal column.

myx/o (mucous, slimelike) *myxoid*, resembling mucus.

narc/o (stupor, numbness) *narcotic*, an agent that induces sleep.

nas/o (nose) *oronasal*, pertaining to the nose and mouth.

ne/o (new) *neonate*, a newborn infant.

necr/o (corpse) *necrotic*, dead (when referring to tissue).

nephr/o (kidney) *nephralgia*, pain in the kidneys.

neur/o (nerve) *neuritis*, inflammation of nerve pathways.

noct/i (night) *noctambulism*, sleep walking.

norm/o (rule, order, normal) *normotension*, normal blood pressure.

null/i (none) *nullipara*, a woman who has never given birth to a child.

nyct/o (night) *nycturia*, excessive urination at night.

ob- (against, in front of, toward) *obturator*, a device that closes an opening.

oc- (against, in front of, toward) *occlude*, to obstruct.

ocul/o (eye) *ocular*, pertaining to the eye.

odont/o (tooth) *odontalgia*, toothache.

-oid (shape, form, resemblance) *ovoid*, egg-shaped.

olig/o (few, deficient, scanty) *oligemia*, lacking in blood volume.

-oma (tumor, swelling) *adenoma*, tumor of a gland.

o/o- (egg) *ooblast*, a primitive cell from which an ovum develops.

onych/o (nail) *onychoma*, tumor of a nail or nail bed.

oophor/o (ovary) *oophorectomy*, a surgical removal of one or both ovaries.

-opsy (a viewing) *autopsy*, postmortem examination of a body.

opthalm/o (eye) *opthalmic*, pertaining to the eyes.

opt/o, optic/o (sight, vision) *optometrist*, a specialist in adapting lenses for the correcting of visual defects.

or/o (mouth) *oral*, pertaining to the mouth.

orch/o, orchid/o (testicle) *orchitis*, inflammation of the testicles.

orth/o (straight, upright) *orthopedic*, pertaining to the correction of skeletal defects.

-osis (process, an abnormal condition) *dermatosis*, any skin condition.

oste/o (bone) *osteomyelitis*, inflammation of bone or bone marrow.

ot/o (ear) *otalgia*, earache.

ovari/o (ovary) *ovariocele*, hernia of an ovary.

ov/i, ov/o (egg) *oviduct*, a passage through which an egg passes.

pachy- (thicken) *pachyderma*, abnormal thickening of the skin.

palat/o (palate) *palatitis*, inflammation of the palate.

pan- (all, entire, every) *panacea*, a remedy for all diseases, a "cure-all."

para- (beside, beyond, accessory to, apart from, against) *paranormal*, beyond the natural or normal.

path/o (disease) *pathogen*, any disease-producing agent.

-pathy (disease of a part) *osteopathy*, disease of a bone.

-penia (an abnormal reduction) *leukopenia*, deficiency in white blood cells.

peps/o, pept/o (digestion) *dyspepsia*, poor digestion.

per- (throughout, completely, extremely) *perfusion*, the passage of fluid through the vessels of an organ.

peri- (around, surrounding) *pericardium*, the sac that surrounds the heart and the roots of the great vessels.

-pexy (fixation) *splendopexy*, surgical fixation of the spleen.

phag/o (eat) *phagomania*, an insatiable craving for food.

pharyng/o (throat) *pharyngospasms*, spasms of the muscles of the pharynx.

phas/o (speech) *aphasic*, unable to speak.

phil/o (like, have an affinity for) *necrophilia*, an abnormal interest in death.

phleb/o (vein) *phlebotomy*, surgical incision of a vein.

-phobia (fear, dread) *claustrophobia*, a fear of closed spaces.

phon/o (sound) *phonetic*, pertaining to the voice.

phor/o (bear, carry) *diaphoresis*, profuse sweating.

phot/o (light) *photosensitivity*, abnormal reactivity of the skin to sunlight.

phren/o (diaphragm) *phrenic nerve*, a nerve that carries messages to the diaphragm.

physi/o (nature) *physiology*, the science that studies the function of living things.

pil/o (hair) *pilose*, hairy.

-plasia (development, formation) *dysplasia*, poor or abnormal formation.

-plasty (surgical repair) *arthroplasty*, surgical repair of a joint.

-plegia (paralysis) *paraplegia*, paralysis of the lower body, including the legs.

pleur/o (rib, side, pleura) *pleurisy*, inflammation of the pleura.

-pnea (breath, breathing) *orthopnea*, difficult breathing except in an upright position.

pneum/o, pneumat/o (air, breath) *pneumatic*, pertaining to the air.

pneum/o, pneumon/o (lung) *pneumonia*, inflammation of the lungs with the escape of fluid.

pod/o (foot) *podiatrist*, a specialist in the care of feet.

-poiesis (formation) *hematopoiesis*, formation of blood.

poly- (much, many) *polychromatic*, multicolored.

post- (after, behind) *postmortem*, after death.

pre- (before) *premature*, occurring before the proper time.

pro- (before, in front of) *prolapse*, the falling down, or sinking of a part.

proct/o (anus) *proctitis*, inflammation of the rectum.

pseud/o (false) *pseudoplegia*, hysterical paralysis.

psych/o (mind, soul) *psychopath*, one who displays aggressive antisocial behavior.

-ptosis (abnormal dropping or sagging of a part) *hysteroptosis*, sagging of the uterus.

pulmon/o (lung) *pulmonary*, pertaining to the lungs.

py/o (pus) *pyorrhea*, copious discharge of pus.

pyel/o (renal pelvis) *pyelitis*, inflammation of the renal pelvis.

pyr/o (fire, fever) *pyromaniac*, compulsive fire setter.

quadri- (four) *quadriplegia*, paralysis of all four limbs.

rach/i (spine) *rachialgia*, pain in the spine.

radi/o (ray, radiation) *radiology*, the use of ionizing radiation in diagnosis and treatment.

re- (back, against, contrary) *recurrence*, the return of symptoms after remission.

rect/o (rectum) *rectal*, pertaining to the rectum.

ren/o (the kidneys) *renal*, pertaining to the kidneys.

retro- (located behind, backward) *retroperineal*, behind the perineum.

rhin/o (nose) *rhinitis*, inflammation of the mucous membranes of the nose.

-rrhage (abnormal discharge) *hemorrhage*, abnormal discharge of blood.

-rrhagia (hemorrhage from an organ or body part) *menorrhea*, excessive uterine bleeding.

-rrhea (flowing or discharge) *diarrhea*, abnormal frequency and liquidity of fecal discharges.

sanguin/o (blood) *exsanguinate*, to lose a large volume of blood either internally or externally.

sarc/o (flesh) *sarcoma*, a malignant tumor.

schiz/o (split) *schizophrenia*, any of a group of emotional disorders characterized by bizarre behavior (erroneously called split personality).

scler/o (hardening) *scleroderma*, hardening of connective tissues of the body, including the skin.

-sclerosis (hardened condition) *arteriosclerosis*, hardening of the arteries.

scoli/o (twisted, crooked) *scoliosis*, sideward deviation of the spine.

-scope (an instrument for observing) *endoscope*, an instrument for the examination of a hollow body, such as the bladder.

-sect (cut) *transsect*, to cut across.

semi- (one-half, partly) *semisupine*, partly, but not completely, supine.

sept/o, seps/o (infection) *aseptic*, free from infection.

somat/o (body) *psychosomatic*, both psychological and physiological.

son/o (sound) *sonogram*, a recording produced by the passage of sound waves through the body.

spermat/o (sperm, semen) *spermacide*, an agent that kills sperm.

sphygm/o (pulse) *sphygmomanometer*, a device for measuring blood pressure in the arteries.

splen/o (spleen) *splenectomy*, surgical removal of the spleen.

-stasis (stopping, controlling) *hemostasis*, the control of bleeding.

sten/o (narrow) *stenosis*, a narrowing of a passage or opening.

stere/o (solid, three-dimensional) *stereoscopic*, a three-dimensional appearance.

steth/o (chest) *stethoscope*, an instrument for listening to chest sounds.

sthen/o (strength) *myasthenia*, muscular weakness.

-stomy (surgically creating a new opening) *colostomy*, surgical creation of an opening between the colon and the surface of the body.

sub- (under, near, almost, moderately) *subclavian*, situated under the clavicle.

super- (above, excess) *superficial*, lying on or near the surface.

supra- (above, over) *suprapubic*, situated above the pubic arch.

sym-, syn- (joined together, with) *syndrome*, a set of symptoms that occur together.

tachy- (fast) *tachycardia*, a very fast heart rate.

-therapy (treatment) *hydrotherapy*, treatment with water.

therm/o (heat) *thermogenesis*, the production of heat.

thorac/o (chest cavity) *thoracic*, pertaining to the chest.

thromb/o (clot, lump) *thrombophlebitis*, inflammation of a vein.

-tome (a surgical instrument for cutting) *microtome*, an instrument for cutting thin slices of tissue.

-tomy (a surgical operation on an organ or body part) *thoracotomy*, surgical incision of the chest wall.

top/o (place) *topographic*, pertaining to special regions (of the body).

trache/o (trachea) *tracheostomy*, an opening in the neck that passes to the trachea.

trans- (through, across, beyond) *transfusion*, the introduction of whole blood or blood components directly into the bloodstream.

tri- (three) *trimester*, a period of 3 months.

trich/o (hair) *trichosis*, any disease of the hair.

-tripsy (surgical crushing) *lithotripsy*, surgical crushing of stones.

troph/o (nourish) *hypertrophic*, enlargement of an organ or body part due to the increase in the size of cells.

ultra- (beyond, excess) *ultrasonic*, beyond the audible range.

uni- (one) *unilateral*, affecting one side.

ur/o (urine) *urinalysis*, examination of urine.

ureter/o (ureter) *ureteritis*, inflammation of a ureter.

urethr/o (urethra) *urethritis*, inflammation of the urethra.

vas/o (vessel, duct) *vasodilator*, an agent that causes dilation of blood vessels.

ven/o (vein) *venipuncture*, surgical puncture of a vein.

ventr/o (belly, cavity) *ventral*, relating to the belly or abdomen.

vesic/o (blister, bladder) *vesicle*, a small fluid-filled blister.

viscer/o (internal organ) *visceral*, pertaining to the viscera (abdominal organs).

xanth/o (yellow) *xanthroma*, a yellow nodule in the skin.

xen/o (stranger) *xenophobia*, abnormal fear of strangers.

xer/o (dry) *xerosis*, abnormal dryness (as of the mouth or eyes).

zo/o (animal life) *zoogenous*, acquired from an animal.

abandonment leaving a patient after care has been initiated and before the patient has been transferred to someone with equal or greater medical training.

ABCs airway, breathing, and circulation.

abdominal quadrants four divisions of the abdomen used to pinpoint the location of a pain or injury: the right upper quadrant (RUQ), the left upper quadrant (LUQ), the right lower quadrant (RLQ), and the left lower quadrant (LLQ).

abortion spontaneous (miscarriage) or induced termination of pregnancy.

abrasion (ab-RAY-zhun) a scratch or scrape.

abruptio placentae (ab-RUPT-si-o plah-SENT-ta) a condition in which the placenta separates from the uterine wall; a cause of prebirth bleeding.

absorbed poisons poisons that are taken into the body through unbroken skin.

acetabulum (AS-uh-TAB-yuh-lum) the pelvic socket into which the ball at the proximal end of the femur fits to form the hip joint.

acquired disease/condition a disease or condition that occurs after birth.

acromioclavicular (ah-KRO-me-o-klav-IK-yuh-ler) **joint** the joint where the acromion and the clavicle meet.

acromion (ah-KRO-me-on) **process** the highest portion of the shoulder.

activated charcoal a substance that absorbs many poisons and prevents them from being absorbed by the body.

active rewarming application of an external heat source to rewarm the body of a hypothermic patient.

acute myocardial infarction (AMI) (ah-KUTE MY-o-KARD-e-ul in-FARK-shun) the condition in which a portion of the myocardium dies as a result of oxygen starvation; often called a heart attack by laypersons.

advance directive a DNR order.

afterbirth the placenta, membranes of the amniotic sac, part of the umbilical cord, and some tissues from the lining of the uterus that are delivered after the birth of the baby.

air embolism gas bubble in the bloodstream. The plural is *air emboli*. The more accurate term is *arterial gas embolism (AGE)*.

airway the passageway by which air enters or leaves the body. The structures of the airway are the nose, mouth, pharynx, larynx, trachea, bronchi, and lungs. *See also* patent airway.

allergen something that causes an allergic reaction.

allergic reaction an exaggerated immune response.

alveoli (al-VE-o-li) the microscopic sacs of the lungs where gas exchange with the bloodstream takes place.

amniotic (am-ne-OT-ik) **sac** the "bag of waters" that surrounds the developing fetus.

amputation (am-pyu-TAY-shun) the surgical removal or traumatic severing of a body part, usually an extremity.

anaphylaxis (an-ah-fi-LAK-sis) a severe or life-threatening allergic reaction in which the blood vessels dilate, causing a drop in blood pressure, and the tissues lining the respiratory system swell, interfering with the airway. Also called *anaphylactic shock*.

anatomical position the standard reference position for the body in the study of anatomy. In this position, the body is standing erect, facing the observer, with arms down at the sides and the palms of the hands forward.

anatomy the study of body structure.

aneurysm (AN-u-rizm) the dilation, or ballooning, of a weakened section of the wall of an artery.

angina pectoris (AN-ji-nah [or an-JI-nah] PEK-to-ris) pain in the chest, occurring when blood supply to the heart is reduced and a portion of the heart muscle is not receiving enough oxygen.

anterior the front of the body or body part.

antidote a substance that will neutralize the poison or its effects.

aorta (ay-OR-tah) the largest artery in the body. It transports blood from the left ventricle to begin systemic circulation.

apnea (ap-ne-ah) no breathing.

appendix a small tube located near the junction of the small and large intestines in the right lower quadrant of the abdomen, the function of which is not well understood. Its inflammation, called appendicitis, is a common cause of abdominal pain.

arterial bleeding bleeding from an artery, which is characterized by bright red blood and as rapid, profuse, and difficult to control.

arteriole (ar-TE-re-ol) the smallest kind of artery.

artery any blood vessel carrying blood away from the heart.

artificial ventilation forcing air or oxygen into the lungs when a patient has stopped breathing or has inadequate breathing. Also called *positive pressure ventilation.*

asystole (ay-SIS-to-le) a condition in which the heart has ceased generating electrical impulses.

atria (AY-tree-ah) the two upper chambers of the heart. There is a right atrium (which receives unoxygenated blood returning from the body) and a left atrium (which receives oxygenated blood returning from the lungs).

auscultation (os-kul-TAY-shun) listening. A stethoscope is used to auscultate for characteristic sounds.

auto-injector a syringe preloaded with medication that has a spring-loaded device which pushes the needle through the skin when the tip of the device is pressed firmly against the body.

automatic implanted cardiac defibrillator (AICD) a device implanted under the skin that can detect a life-threatening cardiac dysrhythmia and respond by delivering one or more shocks to correct the rhythm.

automatic transport ventilator (ATV) a device that provides positive pressure ventilations. It includes settings designed to adjust ventilation rate and volume, and is portable and easily carried on an ambulance.

automaticity (AW-to-muh-TISS-it-e) the ability of the heart to generate and conduct electrical impulses on its own.

autonomic (AW-to-NOM-ik) **nervous system** the division of the peripheral nervous system that controls involuntary motor functions.

AVPU a memory aid for classifying a patient's level of responsiveness, or mental status. The letters stand for alert, verbal response, painful response, unresponsive.

avulsion (ah-VUL-shun) the tearing away or tearing off of a piece or flap of skin or other soft tissue. This term also may be used for an eye pulled from its socket or a tooth dislodged from its socket.

bag-valve mask (BVM) a handheld device with a face mask and self-refilling bag that can be squeezed to provide artificial ventilations to a patient. It can deliver air from the atmosphere or oxygen from a supplemental oxygen supply system.

bandage any material used to hold a dressing in place.

base station a two-way radio at a fixed site such as a hospital or dispatch center.

behavior the manner in which a person acts.

behavioral emergency when a patient's behavior is not typical for the situation; when the patient's behavior is unacceptable or intolerable to the patient, his family, or the community; or when the patient may harm himself or others.

bilateral on both sides.

blood pressure the pressure caused by blood exerting force against the walls of blood vessels. Usually arterial blood pressure (the pressure in an artery) is measured. See also diastolic blood pressure and systolic blood pressure.

blood pressure monitor machine that automatically inflates a blood pressure cuff and measures blood pressure.

blunt-force trauma injury caused by a blow that does not penetrate the skin or other body tissues.

body mechanics the proper use of the body to facilitate lifting and moving and prevent injury.

bones hard but flexible living structures that provide support for the body and protection to vital organs. Types of bones are long, short, flat, and irregular. The typical long bone has a cylindrical shaft and a rounded end or head, which is connected to the shaft by the neck.

brachial (BRAY-ke-ul) **artery** artery of the upper arm; the site of the pulse checked during infant CPR.

brachial pulse the pulse felt in the upper arm.

bradycardia (BRAY-duh-KAR-de-uh) slow pulse; any pulse rate below 60 beats per minute.

breech presentation when the baby appears buttocks or both legs first during birth.

bronchi (BRONG-ki) the two large sets of branches that come off the trachea and enter the lungs. There are right and left bronchi. *Singular* bronchus.

bronchioles (BRONG-kee-olz) smaller branches of the bronchi.

bronchoconstriction constriction, or blockage, of the bronchi that lead from the trachea to the lungs.

calcaneus (kal-KAY-ne-us) the heel bone.

capillary (KAP-i-lair-e) a thin-walled, microscopic blood vessel where the oxygen/carbon dioxide and nutrient/waste exchange with the body's cells takes place.

capillary bleeding bleeding from capillaries, which is characterized by a slow, oozing flow of blood.

capnometry (kap-NOM-uh-tree) the measurement of exhaled carbon dioxide. A graphic recording or display of capnometric measurement is called *capnography.*

cardiac compromise a blanket term that refers to a heart problem with a rapid onset.

cardiac conduction system a system of specialized muscle tissues which conduct electrical impulses that stimulate the heart to beat.

cardiac muscle specialized involuntary muscle found only in the heart.

cardiogenic shock shock, or lack of perfusion, brought on not by blood loss, but by inadequate pumping action of the heart. It is often the result of a heart attack or congestive heart failure.

cardiovascular (KAR-de-o-VAS-kyu-ler) **system** the system made up of the heart (cardio) and the blood vessels (vascular); the circulatory system.

carina (kah-RI-nah) the fork at the lower end of the trachea where the two mainstem bronchi branch.

carotid (kah-ROT-id) **arteries** the large neck arteries, one on each side of the neck, that carry blood from the heart to the head.

carotid pulse the pulse felt along the large carotid artery on either side of the neck.

carpals (KAR-pulz) the wrist bones.

cartilage tough tissue that covers the joint ends of bones and helps to form certain body parts such as the ear.

cell phone a phone that transmits through the air instead of over wires so that the phone can be transported and used over a wide area.

central IV catheter a catheter surgically inserted for long-term delivery of medications or fluids into the central circulation.

central nervous system (CNS) the brain and spinal cord.

central pulses the carotid and femoral pulses, which can be felt in the central part of the body.

central rewarming application of heat to the lateral chest, neck, armpits, and groin of a hypothermic patient.

cephalic (se-FAL-ik) **presentation** when the baby appears head first during birth. This is the normal presentation.

cerebrospinal (suh-RE-bro-SPI-nal) **fluid (CSF)** the fluid that surrounds the brain and spinal cord.

cervix (SUR-viks) the neck of the uterus at the entrance to the birth canal.

chief complaint in emergency medicine, the reason EMS was called, usually in the patient's own words.

circulatory system *see* cardiovascular system.

clavicle (KLAV-i-kul) the collarbone.

closed extremity injury an injury to an extremity with no associated opening in the skin.

closed wound an internal injury with no open pathway from the outside.

cold zone area where the Incident Command post and support functions are located.

colostomy (ko-LOS-to-me) similar to an ileostomy, a surgical opening in the wall of the abdomen with a bag in place to collect excretions from the digestive system.

Command the first on the scene to establish order and initiate the Incident Command System.

compensated shock when the patient is developing shock but the body is still able to maintain perfusion. *See* shock.

concussion mild closed head injury without detectable damage to the brain. Complete recovery is usually expected.

conduction the transfer of heat from one material to another through direct contact.

confidentiality the obligation not to reveal information obtained about a patient except to other health care professionals involved in the patient's care, or under subpoena, or in a court of law, or when the patient has signed a release of confidentiality.

congenital disease/condition a disease or condition that is present at birth.

congestive heart failure (CHF) the failure of the heart to pump efficiently, leading to excessive blood or fluids in the lungs, the body, or both.

consent permission from the patient for care or other action by the EMT.

constrict (kon-STRIKT) get smaller.

contamination contact with or presence of a material (contaminant) that is present where it does not belong and that is somehow harmful to persons, animals, or the environment; the introduction of dangerous chemicals, disease, or infectious materials.

continuous positive airway pressure (CPAP) a device that exerts constant pressure through a tube and mask worn by a patient to keep airway passages from collapsing at the end of a breath.

contraindications (KON-truh-in-duh-KAY-shunz) specific signs or circumstances under which it is not appropriate and may be harmful to administer a drug to a patient.

contusion (kun-TU-zhun) a bruise; in brain injuries, a bruised brain caused when the force of a blow to the head is great enough to rupture blood vessels.

convection carrying away of heat by currents of air or water or other gases or liquids.

coronary (KOR-o-nar-e) **arteries** blood vessels that supply the muscle of the heart (myocardium).

coronary artery disease (CAD) diseases that affect the arteries of the heart.

cranium (KRAY-ne-um) the bony structure making up the forehead, top, back, and upper sides of the skull.

crepitation (krep-uh-TAY-shun) the grating sound or feeling of broken bones rubbing together. Also called *crepitus* (KREP-uh-tus).

cricoid (KRIK-oid) **cartilage** the ring-shaped structure that circles the trachea at the lower edge of the larynx.

cricoid pressure pressure applied to the cricoid cartilage to suppress vomiting and bring the vocal cords into view.

crime scene the location where a crime has been committed or any place that evidence relating to a crime may be found.

critical incident stress management (CISM) a comprehensive system that includes education and resources to both prevent stress and to deal with stress appropriately when it occurs.

crowning when part of the baby is visible through the vaginal opening.

crush injury an injury caused when force is transmitted from the body's exterior to its internal structures. Bones can be broken; muscles, nerves, and tissues damaged; and internal organs ruptured, causing internal bleeding.

cyanosis (SIGH-uh-NO-sis) a blue or gray color resulting from lack of oxygen in the body.

danger zone the area around the wreckage of a vehicle collision or other incident within which special safety precautions should be taken.

DCAP-BTLS a memory aid to remember deformities, contusions, abrasions, puncture/penetrations, burns, tenderness, lacerations, and swelling—symptoms of injury found by inspection or palpation during patient assessment.

dead space areas of the lungs outside the alveoli where gas exchange with the blood does not take place.

decompensated shock occurs when the body can no longer compensate for low blood volume or lack of perfusion. Late signs such as decreasing blood pressure become evident. *See* shock.

decompression sickness a condition resulting from nitrogen trapped in the body's tissues caused by coming up too quickly from a deep, prolonged dive. A symptom of decompression sickness is "the bends," or deep pain in the muscles and joints.

decontamination a chemical and/or physical process that reduces or prevents the spread of contamination from persons or equipment; the removal of hazardous substances from employees and their equipment to the extent necessary to preclude foreseeable health effects.

delirium tremens (duh-LEER-e-um TREM-uns) **(DTs)** a severe reaction that can be part of alcohol withdrawal, characterized by sweating, trembling, anxiety, and hallucinations. Severe alcohol withdrawal with the DTs can lead to death if untreated.

dermis (DER-mis) the inner (second) layer of skin, rich in blood vessels and nerves, found beneath the epidermis.

designated agent an EMT or other person authorized by a Medical Director to give medications and provide emergency care. The transfer of such authorization to a designated agent is an extension of the Medical Director's license to practice medicine.

detailed physical exam an assessment of the head, neck, chest, abdomen, pelvis, extremities, and posterior of the body to detect signs and symptoms of injury. It differs from the rapid trauma assessment only in that it also includes examination of the face, ears, eyes, nose, and mouth during the examination of the head; it may be done less rapidly; and it may be done en route to the hospital after earlier on-scene assessments and interventions are completed.

diabetes mellitus (di-ah-BEE-tez MEL-i-tus) also called *sugar diabetes* or just *diabetes*, the condition brought about by decreased insulin production or the inability of the body cells to use insulin properly. The person with this condition is a diabetic.

dialysis the process of filtering the blood to remove toxic or unwanted wastes and fluids.

diaphragm (DI-uh-fram) the muscular structure that divides the chest cavity from the abdominal cavity. It is a major muscle of respiration.

diastolic (di-as-TOL-ik) **blood pressure** the pressure remaining in the arteries when the left ventricle of the heart is relaxed and refilling.

digestive system system by which food travels through the body and is digested, or broken down into absorbable forms.

dilate (DI-late) get larger.

dilution (di-LU-shun) thinning down or weakening by mixing with something else. Ingested poisons are sometimes diluted by drinking water or milk.

direct carry a method of transferring a patient from bed to stretcher, during which two or more rescuers curl the patient to their chests, then reverse the process to lower the patient to the stretcher.

direct ground lift a method of lifting and carrying a patient from ground level to a stretcher in which two or more rescuers kneel, curl the patient to their chests, stand, then reverse the process to lower the patient to the stretcher.

disaster plan a predefined set of instructions for a community's emergency responders.

dislocation the disruption or "coming apart" of a joint.

dissemination spreading.

distal farther away from the torso. *See also* proximal.

distention (dis-TEN-shun) a condition of being stretched, inflated, or larger than normal.

do not resuscitate (DNR) order a legal document, usually signed by the patient and his physician, which states that the patient has a terminal illness and does not wish to prolong life through resuscitative efforts.

domestic terrorism terrorism directed against the government or population without foreign direction. *See also* terrorism; international terrorism.

dorsal referring to the back of the body or the back of the hand or foot. This is a synonym for posterior.

dorsalis pedis (dor-SAL-is PEED-is) **artery** artery supplying the foot, lateral to the large tendon of the big toe.

downers depressants, such as barbiturates, that depress the central nervous system. They are often used to bring on a more relaxed state of mind.

draw-sheet method a method of transferring a patient from bed to stretcher by grasping and pulling the loosened bottom sheet of the bed.

dressing any material (preferably sterile) used to cover a wound that will help control bleeding and help prevent additional contamination.

drowning the process of experiencing respiratory impairment from submersion/immersion in liquid, which may result in death, morbidity (illness or other adverse effects), or no morbidity.

duty to act an obligation to provide care to a patient.

dyspnea (DISP-ne-ah) shortness of breath; labored or difficult breathing.

dysrhythmia (dis-RITH-me-ah) a disturbance in heart rate and rhythm.

eclampsia (e-KLAMP-se-ah) a severe complication of pregnancy that produces seizures and coma.

ectopic (ek-TOP-ik) **pregnancy** when implantation of the fertilized egg is not in the body of the uterus, occurring instead in the oviduct (fallopian tube), cervix, or abdominopelvic cavity.

edema (eh-DEEM-uh) swelling resulting from a buildup of fluid in the tissues.

embolism (EM-bo-lizm) blockage of a vessel by a clot or foreign material brought to the site by the blood current.

endocrine (EN-do-krin) **system** system of glands that produce chemicals called hormones that help to regulate many body activities and functions.

endotracheal (EN-do-TRAY-ke-ul) **tube** a tube designed to be inserted into the trachea. Oxygen, medication, or a suction catheter can be directed into the trachea through an endotracheal tube.

epidermis (ep-i-DER-mis) the outer layer of the skin.

epiglottis (EP-i-GLOT-is) a leaf-shaped structure that prevents food and foreign matter from entering the trachea.

epilepsy (EP-uh-lep-see) a medical condition that causes seizures. With proper medication, many epileptic patients will no longer have seizures.

epinephrine (EP-uh-NEF-rin) a hormone produced by the body. As a medication, it dilates respiratory passages and is used to relieve severe allergic reactions.

esophageal detector device (EDD) a device that uses a bulb or syringe to attempt to withdraw air from an endotracheal tube to determine correct placement in the trachea (from which air can easily be withdrawn) or incorrect placement in the esophagus (in which the soft esophagus will collapse and prevent air from being withdrawn).

esophagus (eh-SOF-uh-gus) the tube that leads from the pharynx to the stomach.

evaporation the change from liquid to gas. When the body perspires or gets wet, evaporation of the perspiration or other liquid into the air has a cooling effect on the body.

evisceration (e-vis-er-AY-shun) an intestine or other internal organ protruding through a wound in the abdomen.

exhalation (EX-huh-LAY-shun) a passive process in which the intercostal (rib) muscles and the diaphragm relax, causing the chest cavity to decrease in size and air to flow out of the lungs. Also called *expiration*.

expiration (EK-spuh-RAY-shun) *see* exhalation.

exposure the dose or concentration of an agent multiplied by the time, or duration.

expressed consent consent given by adults who are of legal age and mentally competent to make a rational decision in regard to their medical well-being.

extremities (ex-TREM-i-teez) the portions of the skeleton that include the clavicles, scapulae, arms, wrists, and hands (upper extremities) and the pelvis, thighs, legs, ankles, and feet (lower extremities).

extremity lift a method of lifting and carrying a patient during which one rescuer slips hands under the patient's armpits and grasps the wrists, while another rescuer grasps the patient's knees.

feeding tube a tube used to provide delivery of nutrients to the stomach. A nasogastric feeding tube is inserted through the nose and into the stomach; a gastric feeding tube is surgically implanted through the abdominal wall and into the stomach.

femoral (FEM-or-al) **artery** the major artery supplying the thigh.

femur (FEE-mer) the large bone of the thigh.

fetus (FE-tus) the baby as he develops in the womb.

fibula (FIB-yuh-luh) the lateral and smaller bone of the lower leg.

flail chest fracture of two or more adjacent ribs in two or more places that allows for free movement of the fractured segment.

flowmeter a valve that indicates the flow of oxygen in liters per minute.

flow-restricted, oxygen-powered ventilation device (FROPVD) a device that uses oxygen under pressure to deliver artificial ventilations. Its trigger is placed so that the rescuer can operate it while still using both hands to maintain a seal on the face mask. It has automatic flow restriction to prevent overdelivery of oxygen to the patient.

focused history and physical exam the step of patient assessment that follows the initial assessment.

Fowler's position a sitting position.

fracture (FRAK-cher) any break in a bone.

full thickness burn a burn in which all the layers of the skin are damaged. There are usually areas that are charred black or areas that are dry and white. Also called *third-degree burn.*

gag reflex vomiting or retching that results when something is placed in the back of the pharynx. This is tied to the swallow reflex.

gallbladder a sac on the underside of the liver that stores bile produced by the liver.

general impression impression of the patient's condition that is formed on first approaching the patient, based on the patient's environment, chief complaint, and appearance.

glottic opening the opening to the trachea.

glucose (GLU-kos) a form of sugar, the body's basic source of energy.

Good Samaritan laws a series of laws, varying in each state, designed to provide limited legal protection for citizens and some health care personnel when they are administering emergency care.

hallucinogens (huh-LOO-sin-uh-jens) mind-affecting or mind-altering drugs that act on the central nervous system to produce excitement and distortion of perceptions.

hazardous material any substance or material in a form which poses an unreasonable risk to health, safety, and property when transported in commerce.

hazardous-material incident the release of a harmful substance into the environment.

head-tilt, chin-lift maneuver a means of correcting blockage of the airway by the tongue by tilting the head back and lifting the chin. It is used when no trauma, or injury, is suspected.

hematoma (hem-ah-TO-mah) a swelling caused by the collection of blood under the skin or in damaged tissues as a result of an injured or broken blood vessel; in a head injury, a collection of blood within the skull or brain.

hemorrhage (HEM-o-rej) bleeding, especially severe bleeding.

hemorrhagic (HEM-or-AJ-ik) **shock** shock resulting from blood loss.

HIPAA The Health Insurance Portability and Accountability Act, a federal law protecting the privacy of patient-specific health care information and providing the patient with control over how this information is used and distributed.

hives red, itchy, possibly raised blotches on the skin that often result from allergic reactions.

hot zone area immediately surrounding a hazmat incident; extends far enough to prevent adverse effects outside the zone.

humerus (HYU-mer-us) the bone of the upper arm, between the shoulder and the elbow.

humidifier a device connected to the flowmeter to add moisture to the dry oxygen coming from an oxygen cylinder.

hyperglycemia (HI-per-gli-SEE-me-ah) high blood sugar.

hyperthermia (HI-per-THURM-e-ah) an increase in body temperature above normal, which is life-threatening in its extreme.

hypoglycemia (HI-po-gli-SEE-me-ah) low blood sugar.

hypoperfusion (HI-po-per-FEW-zhun) inability of the body to adequately circulate blood to the body's cells to supply them with oxygen and nutrients. *See also* shock.

hypopharynx (HI-po-FAIR-inks) the area directly above the openings of both the trachea and the esophagus.

hypothermia (HI-po-THURM-e-ah) generalized cooling that reduces body temperature below normal, which is life-threatening in its extreme.

hypovolemic (HI-po-vo-LE-mik) **shock** shock resulting from blood or fluid loss.

hypoxia (hi-POK-se-uh) an insufficiency of oxygen in the body's tissues.

ileostomy (il-e-OS-to-me) *see* colostomy.

ilium (IL-e-um) the superior and widest portion of the pelvis.

implied consent the consent it is presumed a patient or patient's parent or guardian would give if they could, such as for an unconscious patient or a parent who cannot be contacted when care is needed.

Incident Command the person who assumes overall direction of an incident.

Incident Command System (ICS) a subset of the National Incident Management System (NIMS).

index of suspicion awareness that there may be injuries.

indications specific signs or circumstances under which it is appropriate to administer a drug to a patient.

induced abortion expulsion of a fetus as a result of deliberate actions taken to stop the pregnancy.

inferior away from the head; usually compared with another structure that is closer to the head (e.g., the lips are inferior to the nose).

ingested poisons poisons that are swallowed.

inhalation (IN-huh-LAY-shun) an active process in which the intercostal (rib) muscles and the diaphragm contract, expanding the size of the chest cavity and causing air to flow into the lungs. Also called *inspiration.*

inhaled poisons poisons that are breathed in.

inhaler a spray device with a mouthpiece that contains an aerosol form of a medication that a patient can spray into his airway.

initial assessment the first element in assessment of a patient; steps taken for the purpose of discovering and dealing with any life-threatening problems. The six parts of initial assessment are: forming a general impression, assessing mental status, assessing airway, assessing breathing, assessing circulation, and determining the priority of the patient for treatment and transport to the hospital. Also called *primary assessment* or *primary survey.*

injected poisons poisons that are inserted through the skin; for example, by needle, snake fangs, or insect stinger.

inspiration (IN-spuh-RAY-shun) *see* inhalation.

insulin (IN-suh-lin) a hormone produced by the pancreas or taken as a medication by many diabetics.

international terrorism terrorism that is foreign-based or directed. *See also* terrorism, domestic terrorism.

interventions actions taken to correct a patient's problems.

intubation (IN-tu-BAY-shun) insertion of a tube.

involuntary muscle muscle that responds automatically to brain signals but cannot be consciously controlled.

irreversible shock when the body has lost the battle to maintain perfusion to vital organs. Even if adequate vital signs return, the patient may die days later due to organ failure.

ischium (ISH-e-um) the lower, posterior portions of the pelvis.

jaw-thrust maneuver a means of correcting blockage of the airway by moving the jaw forward without tilting the head or neck. Used when trauma, or injury, is suspected to open the airway without causing further injury to the spinal cord in the neck.

joint the point where two bones come together.

jugular (JUG-yuh-ler) **vein distention (JVD)** bulging of the neck veins.

labor the three stages of the delivery of a baby that begin with the contractions of the uterus and end with the expulsion of the placenta.

laceration (las-er-AY-shun) a cut; in brain injuries, a cut to the brain.

large intestine the muscular tube that removes water from waste products received from the small intestine and removes anything not absorbed by the body toward excretion from the body.

laryngoscope (lair-ING-uh-skope) an illuminating instrument that is inserted into the pharynx to permit visualization of the pharynx and larynx.

larynx (LAIR-inks) the voice box.

lateral to the side, away from the midline of the body.

left ventricular assist device (LVAD) a battery-powered mechanical pump implanted in the body to assist a failing left ventricle in pumping blood to the body.

liability being held legally responsible.

ligament tissue that connects bone to bone.

limb presentation when an infant's limb protrudes from the vagina before the appearance of any other body part.

liver the largest internal organ of the body, produces bile to assist in breakdown of fats and assists in the metabolism of various substances in the body.

local cooling cooling or freezing of particular (local) parts of the body.

lungs the organs where exchange of atmospheric oxygen and waste carbon dioxide take place.

mainstem bronchi (BRONG-ki) the two large sets of branches that come off the trachea and enter the lungs. There are right and left mainstem bronchi. *Singular* bronchus.

malar (MAY-lar) the cheek bone, also called the *zygomatic bone*.

malleolus (mal-E-o-lus) protrusion on the side of the ankle. The lateral malleolus, at the lower end of the fibula, is seen on the outer ankle; the medial malleolus, at the lower end of the tibia, is seen on the inner ankle.

mandible (MAN-di-bul) the lower jaw bone.

manual traction the process of applying tension to straighten and realign a fractured limb before splinting. Also called *tension*.

manubrium (man-OO-bre-um) the superior portion of the sternum.

maxillae (mak-SIL-e) the two fused bones forming the upper jaw.

mechanism of injury a force or forces that may have caused injury.

meconium staining amniotic fluid that is greenish or brownish-yellow rather than clear as a result of fetal defecation; an indication of possible maternal or fetal distress during labor.

medial toward the midline of the body.

medical direction oversight of the patient-care aspects of an EMS system by the Medical Director. *Off-line medical direction* consists of standing orders issued by the Medical Director that allow EMTs to give certain medications or perform certain procedures without speaking to the Medical Director or another physician. *On-line medical direction* consists of orders from the on-duty physician given directly to an EMT in the field by radio or telephone.

Medical Director a physician who assumes ultimate responsibility for the patient care aspects of the EMS system.

medical patient a patient suffering from one or more medical diseases or conditions.

mental status level of responsiveness.

metacarpals (MET-uh-KAR-pulz) the hand bones.

metatarsals (MET-uh-TAR-sulz) the foot bones.

mid-axillary (mid-AX-uh-lair-e) **line** a line drawn vertically from the middle of the armpit to the ankle.

mid-clavicular (mid-clah-VIK-yuh-ler) **line** the line through the center of each clavicle.

midline an imaginary line drawn down the center of the body, dividing it into right and left halves.

minute volume the amount of air breathed in during each respiration multiplied by the number of breaths per minute.

miscarriage spontaneous abortion.

mobile radio a two-way radio that is used or affixed in a vehicle.

multiple birth when more than one baby is born during a single delivery.

multiple-casualty incident (MCI) an emergency involving multiple patients.

muscle tissue that can contract to allow movement of a body part.

musculoskeletal (MUS-kyu-lo-SKEL-e-tal) **system** the system of bones and skeletal muscles that support and protect the body and permit movement.

narcotics a class of drugs that affect the nervous system and change many normal body activities. Their legal use is for the relief of pain. Illicit use is to produce an intense state of relaxation.

nasal (NAY-zul) **bones** the bones that form the upper third, or bridge, of the nose.

nasal cannula (NAY-zul KAN-yuh-luh) a device that delivers low concentrations of oxygen through two prongs that rest in the patient's nostrils.

nasogastric (NAY-zo-GAS-trik) **tube (NG tube)** a tube designed to be passed through the nose, nasopharynx, and esophagus. It is used to relieve distention of the stomach in an infant or child patient.

nasopharyngeal (NAY-zo-fah-RIN-jul) **airway** a flexible breathing tube inserted through the patient's nose into the pharynx to help maintain an open airway.

nasopharynx (NAY-zo-FAIR-inks) the area directly posterior to the nose.

National Incident Management System (NIMS) the management system used by federal, state, and local governments to manage emergencies in the United States.

nature of the illness what is medically wrong with a patient.

negligence a finding of failure to act properly in a situation in which there was a duty to act, that needed care as would reasonably be expected of the EMT was not provided, and that harm was caused to the patient as a result.

nervous system the system of brain, spinal cord, and nerves that govern sensation, movement, and thought.

neurogenic shock hypoperfusion due to nerve paralysis (sometimes caused by spinal cord injuries) resulting in the dilation of blood vessels that increases the volume of the circulatory system beyond the point where it can be filled.

911 system a system for telephone access to report emergencies. A dispatcher takes the information and alerts EMS or the fire or police departments as needed. *Enhanced 911* has the additional capability of automatically identifying the caller's phone number and location.

nitroglycerin (NYE-tro-GLIS-uh-rin) **(NTG)** a drug that helps to dilate the coronary vessels that supply the heart muscle with blood.

nonrebreather mask a face mask and reservoir bag device that delivers high concentrations of oxygen. The patient's exhaled air escapes through a valve and is not rebreathed.

occlusion (uh-KLU-zhun) blockage, as of an artery by fatty deposits.

occlusive dressing any dressing that forms an airtight seal.

ongoing assessment a procedure for detecting changes in a patient's condition. It involves four steps: repeating the initial assessment, repeating and recording vital signs, repeating the focused assessment, and checking interventions.

open extremity injury an extremity injury in which the skin has been broken or torn through from the inside by an injured bone or from the outside by something that has caused a penetrating wound with associated injury to the bone.

open wound an injury in which the skin is interrupted, exposing the tissue beneath.

OPQRST a memory device for the questions asked to get a description of the present illness: Onset, Provokes, Quality, Radiation, Severity, Time.

oral glucose (GLU-kos) a form of glucose (a kind of sugar) given by mouth to treat an awake patient (who is able to swallow) with an altered mental status and a history of diabetes.

orbits the bony structures around the eyes; the eye sockets.

organ donor a person who has completed a legal document that allows for donation of organs and tissues in the event of death.

oropharyngeal (OR-o-fah-RIN-jul) **airway** a curved device inserted through the patient's mouth into the pharynx to help maintain an open airway.

oropharynx (OR-o-FAIR-inks) the area directly posterior to the mouth.

orotracheal (OR-o-TRAY-ke-ul) **intubation** placement of an endotracheal tube through the mouth and into the trachea.

ostomy bag an external pouch that collects fecal matter diverted from the colon or ileum through a surgical opening (colostomy or ileostomy) in the abdominal wall.

oviduct fallopian tube; tube that carries eggs from an ovary to the uterus.

oxygen a gas commonly found in the atmosphere. Pure oxygen is used as a drug to treat any patients whose medical or traumatic condition may cause them to be hypoxic, or low in oxygen.

oxygen cylinder a cylinder filled with oxygen under pressure.

oxygen saturation (SpO_2) the ratio of the amount of oxygen present in the blood to the amount that could be carried, expressed as a percentage.

pacemaker a device that uses electrical impulses to regulate rhythms of the heart, usually implanted under the skin.

palmar referring to the palm of the hand.

palpation touching or feeling. A pulse or blood pressure may be palpated with the fingertips.

pancreas a gland located behind the stomach that produces insulin and juices that assist in digestion of food in the duodenum of the small intestine.

paradoxical (pair-uh-DOCK-si-kal) **motion** movement of a section of ribs that is opposite to the direction of movement of the rest of the chest during respiration.

parietal pain a localized, intense pain that arises from the parietal peritoneum, the lining of the abdominal cavity.

partial thickness burn a burn in which the epidermis (first layer of skin) is burned through and the dermis (second layer) is damaged. Burns of this type cause reddening, blistering, and a mottled appearance. Also called *second-degree burn.*

passive rewarming covering a hypothermic patient and taking other steps to prevent further heat loss and help the body rewarm itself.

patella (pah-TEL-uh) the kneecap.

patent airway an airway (passage from nose or mouth to lungs) that is open and clear and will remain open and clear, without interference to the passage of air into and out of the body.

pathogens the organisms that cause infection, such as viruses and bacteria.

pedal edema accumulation of fluid in the feet or ankles.

pelvis the basin-shaped bony structure that supports the spine and is the point of proximal attachment for the lower extremities.

penetrating trauma injury caused by an object that passes through the skin or other body tissues.

perfusion the supply of oxygen to and removal of wastes from the cells and tissues of the body as a result of the flow of blood through the capillaries.

perineum (per-i-NE-um) the surface area between the vagina and anus.

peripheral nervous system (PNS) the nerves that enter and leave the spinal cord and travel between the brain and organs without passing through the spinal cord.

peripheral pulses the radial, brachial, posterior tibial, and dorsalis pedis pulses, which can be felt at peripheral (outlying) points of the body.

peritoneum the membrane that lines the abdominal cavity (the *parietal peritoneum*) and covers the organs within it (the *visceral peritoneum*).

permeation the movement of a substance through a surface or, on a molecular level, through intact materials; penetration, or spreading.

personal protective equipment (PPE) equipment that protects the EMS worker from infection and/or exposure to the dangers of rescue operations.

phalanges (fuh-LAN-jiz) the toe bones and finger bones.

pharmacology (FARM-uh-KOL-uh-je) the study of drugs, their sources, characteristics, and effects.

pharynx (FAIR-inks) the area directly posterior to the mouth and nose. It is made up of the oropharynx and the nasopharynx.

physiology the study of body function.

placenta (plah-SEN-tah) the organ of pregnancy where exchange of oxygen, nutrients, and wastes occurs between a mother and fetus.

placenta previa (plah-SEN-tah PRE-vi-ah) a condition in which the placenta is formed in an abnormal location (low in the uterus and close to or over the cervical opening) that will not allow for a normal delivery of the fetus; a cause of excessive prebirth bleeding.

plane a flat surface formed when slicing through a solid object.

plantar referring to the sole of the foot.

plasma (PLAZ-mah) the fluid portion of the blood.

platelets components of the blood; membrane-enclosed fragments of specialized cells.

pneumothorax air in the chest cavity.

pocket face mask a device, usually with a one-way valve, to aid in artificial ventilation. A rescuer breathes through the valve when the mask is placed over the patient's face. It also acts as a barrier to prevent contact with a patient's breath or body fluids. It can be used with supplemental oxygen when fitted with an oxygen inlet.

poison any substance that can harm the body by altering cell structure or functions.

portable radio a handheld two-way radio.

positional asphyxia death of a person due to a body position that restricts breathing for a prolonged time.

positive pressure ventilation *see* artificial ventilation.

posterior the back of the body or body part.

posterior tibial (TIB-ee-ul) **artery** artery supplying the foot, behind the medial ankle.

power grip gripping with as much hand surface as possible in contact with the object being lifted, all fingers bent at the same angle, hands at least 10 inches apart.

power lift a lift from a squatting position with weight to be lifted close to the body, feet apart and flat on the ground, body weight on or just behind balls of feet, back locked in. The upper body is raised before the hips. Also called the *squat-lift position.*

preeclampsia (pre-e-KLAMP-se-ah) a complication of pregnancy where the woman retains large amounts of fluid and has hypertension. She may also experience seizures and/or coma during birth, which is very dangerous to the infant.

premature infant any newborn weighing less than $5\frac{1}{2}$ pounds or born before the 37th week of pregnancy.

pressure dressing a bulky dressing held in position with a tightly wrapped bandage that applies pressure to help control bleeding.

pressure point a site where a main artery lies near the surface of the body and directly over a bone. Pressure on such a point can stop distal bleeding.

pressure regulator a device connected to an oxygen cylinder to reduce cylinder pressure to a safe pressure for delivery of oxygen to a patient.

priapism (PRY-ah-pizm) persistent erection of the penis that may result from spinal injury and some medical problems.

priority the decision regarding the need for immediate transport of the patient vs. further assessment and care at the scene.

prolapsed umbilical cord when the umbilical cord presents first and is squeezed between the vaginal wall and the baby's head.

prone lying face down.

protocols lists of steps, such as assessments and interventions, to be taken in different situations. Protocols are developed by the Medical Director of an EMS system.

proximal closer to the torso. *See also* distal.

pubis (PYOO-bis) the medial anterior portion of the pelvis.

pulmonary arteries the vessels that carry blood from the right ventricle of the heart to the lungs.

pulmonary edema accumulation of fluid in the lungs.

pulmonary veins the vessels that carry oxygenated blood from the lungs to the left atrium of the heart.

pulse the rhythmic beats caused by the beating heart as waves of blood move through and expand the arteries.

pulse oximeter an electronic device for determining the amount of oxygen carried in the blood, known as the oxygen saturation or SpO_2.

pulse quality the rhythm (regular or irregular) and force (strong or weak) of the pulse.

pulse rate the number of pulse beats per minute.

pulseless electrical activity (PEA) a condition in which the heart's electrical rhythm remains relatively normal, yet the mechanical pumping activity fails to follow the electrical activity, causing cardiac arrest.

puncture wound an open wound that tears through the skin and destroys underlying tissues. A *penetrating puncture wound* can be shallow or deep. A *perforating puncture wound* has both an entrance and an exit wound.

pupil the black center of the eye.

quality improvement a process of continuous self-review with the purpose of identifying and correcting aspects of the system that require improvement.

radial artery artery of the lower arm. It is felt when taking the pulse at the wrist.

radial pulse the pulse felt at the wrist.

radiation sending out energy, such as heat, in waves into space.

radius the lateral bone of the forearm.

rapid trauma assessment a rapid assessment of the head, neck, chest, abdomen, pelvis, extremities, and posterior of the body to detect signs and symptoms of injury.

reactivity (re-ak-TIV-uh-te) in the pupils of the eyes, reacting to light by changing size.

recovery position lying on the side. Also called *lateral recumbent position.*

red blood cells components of the blood. They carry oxygen to and carbon dioxide away from the cells.

referred pain pain that is felt in a location other than where the pain originates.

rem roentgen equivalent (in) man; a measure of radiation dosage.

repeater a device that picks up signals from lower-power radio units, such as mobile and portable radios, and retransmits them at a higher power. It allows low-power radio signals to be transmitted over longer distances.

respiration (RES-pir-AY-shun) breathing.

respiratory arrest when breathing completely stops.

respiratory distress increased work of breathing; a sensation of shortness of breath.

respiratory failure the reduction of breathing to the point where oxygen intake is not sufficient to support life.

respiratory quality the normal or abnormal (shallow, labored, or noisy) character of breathing.

respiratory rate the number of breaths taken in 1 minute.

respiratory rhythm the regular or irregular spacing of breaths.

respiratory system the system of nose, mouth, throat, lungs, and muscles that brings oxygen into the body and expels carbon dioxide.

routes of entry pathways into the body, generally by absorption, ingestion, injection, or inhalation.

rule of nines a method for estimating the extent of a burn. For an adult, each of the following areas represents 9 percent of the body surface: the head and neck, each upper extremity, the chest, the abdomen, the upper back, the lower back and buttocks, the front of each lower extremity, and the back of each lower extremity. The remaining 1 percent is assigned to the genital region. For an infant or child the percentages are modified so that 18 percent is assigned to the head, 14 percent to each lower extremity.

rule of palm a method for estimating the extent of a burn. The palm of the patient's hand, which equals about 1 percent of the body's surface area, is compared with the patient's burn to estimate its size.

SAMPLE history the present and past medical history of a patient, so called because the elements of the history begin with the letters of the word *sample*: signs/symptoms, allergies, medications, pertinent past history, last oral intake, events leading to the injury or illness.

scapula (SKAP-yuh-luh) the shoulder blade.

scene size-up steps taken by an ambulance crew when approaching the scene of an emergency call: checking scene safety, taking Standard Precautions, noting the mechanism of injury or nature of the patient's illness, determining the number of patients, and deciding what, if any, additional resources to call for.

scope of practice a set of regulations and ethical considerations that define the scope, or extent and limits, of the EMT's job.

secondary devices destructive devices, such as bombs, placed to be activated after an initial attack and timed to injure emergency responders and others who rush in to help care for those targeted by an initial attack.

seizure (SEE-zher) a sudden change in sensation, behavior, or movement. The most severe form of seizure produces violent muscle contractions called convulsions.

shock the inability of the body to adequately circulate blood to the body's cells to supply them with oxygen and nutrients. This is a life-threatening condition. Also known as *hypoperfusion.*

side effect any action of a drug other than the desired action.

sign an indication of a patient's condition that is objective, or can be observed by another person; an indication that can be seen, heard, smelled, or felt by the EMT or others.

singular command command organization in which a single agency controls all resources and operations.

skeleton the bones of the body.

skin the layer of tissue between the body and the external environment.

skull the bony structure of the head.

small intestine the muscular tube between the stomach and the large intestine, divided into the duodenum, the jejunum, and the ileum, which receives partially digested food from the stomach and continues digestion. Nutrients are absorbed by the body through its walls.

sphygmomanometer (SFIG-mo-mah-NOM-uh-ter) the cuff and gauge used to measure blood pressure.

spinous (SPI-nus) **process** the bony bump on a vertebra.

spleen an organ located in the left upper quadrant of the abdomen that acts as a blood filtration system and a reservoir for reserves of blood.

spontaneous abortion when the fetus and placenta deliver before the 28th week of pregnancy; commonly called a miscarriage.

sprain the stretching and tearing of ligaments.

staging area the area where ambulances are parked and other resources are held until needed.

staging supervisor person responsible for overseeing ambulances and ambulance personnel at a multiple-casualty incident.

Standard Precautions a strict form of infection control that is based on the assumption that all blood and other body fluids are infectious.

standing orders a policy or protocol issued by a Medical Director that authorizes EMTs and others to perform particular skills in certain situations.

status epilepticus (STAY-tus or STAT-us ep-i-LEP-ti-kus) a prolonged seizure or when a person suffers two or more convulsive seizures without regaining full consciousness.

sternum (STER-num) the breastbone.

stillborn born dead.

stoma (STO-ma) a permanent surgical opening in the neck through which the patient breathes; a surgically created opening into the body, as with a tracheostomy, colonostomy, or ileostomy.

stomach muscular sac between the esophagus and the small intestine where digestion of food begins.

strain muscle injury resulting from overstretching or overexertion of the muscle.

strategies broad general plans designed to achieve desired outcomes.

stress a state of physical and/or psychological arousal to a stimulus.

stroke a condition of altered function caused when an artery in the brain is blocked or ruptured, disrupting the supply of oxygenated blood or causing bleeding into the brain.

stylet a long, thin, flexible metal probe.

subcutaneous (SUB-ku-TAY-ne-us) **layers** the layers of fat and soft tissues found below the dermis.

sucking chest wound an open chest wound in which air is "sucked" into the chest cavity.

suctioning (SUK-shun-ing) use of a vacuum device to remove blood, vomitus, and other secretions or foreign materials from the airway.

sudden death a cardiac arrest that occurs within 2 hours of the onset of symptoms. The patient may have no prior symptoms of coronary artery disease.

superficial burn a burn that involves only the epidermis, the outer layer of the skin. It is characterized by reddening of the skin and perhaps some swelling. An example is a sunburn. Also called *first-degree burn.*

superior toward the head (e.g., the chest is superior to the abdomen).

supine lying on the back.

supine hypotensive syndrome dizziness and a drop in blood pressure caused when the mother is in a supine position and the weight of the uterus, infant, placenta, and amniotic fluid compress the inferior vena cava, reducing return of blood to the heart and cardiac output.

symptom an indication of a patient's condition that cannot be observed by another person but rather is subjective, or felt and reported by the patient.

syncope (SIN-ko-pee) fainting.

systolic (sis-TOL-ik) blood pressure the pressure created in the arteries when the left ventricle contracts and forces blood out into circulation.

tachycardia (TAK-uh-KAR-de-uh) rapid pulse; any pulse rate above 100 beats per minute.

tactics specific operational actions to accomplish assigned tasks.

tarsals (TAR-sulz) the ankle bones.

tearing pain sharp pain that feels as if body tissues are being torn apart.

temporal (TEM-po-ral) **bone** bone that forms part of the side of the skull and floor of the cranial cavity. There is a right and a left temporal bone.

temporomandibular (TEM-po-ro-man-DIB-yuh-lar) **joint** the movable joint formed between the mandible and the temporal bone, also called the TMJ.

tendon tissue that connects muscle to bone.

tension pneumothorax a type of pneumothorax in which air that enters the chest cavity is prevented from escaping.

terrorism the unlawful use of force or violence against persons or property to intimidate or coerce a government, the civilian population or any segment thereof, in furtherance of political or social objectives. (U.S. Department of Justice, FBI, definition)

thorax (THOR-ax) the chest.

thrombus (THROM-bus) a clot formed of blood and plaque attached to the inner wall of an artery or vein.

tibia (TIB-e-uh) the medial and larger bone of the lower leg.

torso the trunk of the body; the body without the head and the extremities.

tourniquet (TURN-i-ket) a device used for bleeding control that constricts all blood flow to and from an extremity.

toxin a poisonous substance secreted by bacteria, plants, or animals.

trachea (TRAY-ke-uh) the "windpipe"; the structure that connects the pharynx to the lungs.

tracheostomy (tray-ke-OS-to-me) a surgical incision held open by a metal or plastic tube.

traction splint a splint that applies constant pull along the length of a lower extremity to help stabilize the fractured bone and to reduce muscle spasm in the limb. Traction splints are used primarily on femoral shaft fractures.

transportation supervisor person responsible for communicating with sector officers and hospitals to manage transportation of patients to hospitals from a multiple-casualty incident.

trauma patient a patient suffering from one or more physical injuries.

treatment area the area in which patients are treated at a multiple-casualty incident.

treatment supervisor person responsible for overseeing treatment of patients who have been triaged at a multiple-casualty incident.

Trendelenburg (trend-EL-un-berg) **position** a position in which the patient's feet and legs are higher than the head. Also called *shock position.*

trending changes in a patient's condition over time, such as slowing respirations or rising pulse rate, that may show improvement or deterioration, and that can be shown by documenting repeated assessments.

triage the process of quickly assessing patients at a multiple-casualty incident and assigning each a priority for receiving treatment; from a French word meaning "to sort."

triage area the area where secondary triage takes place at a multiple-casualty incident.

triage supervisor the person responsible for overseeing triage at a multiple-casualty incident.

triage tag color-coded tag indicating the priority group to which a patient has been assigned.

ulna (UL-nah) the medial bone of the forearm.

umbilical (um-BIL-i-kal) **cord** the fetal structure containing the blood vessels that carry blood to and from the placenta.

unified command command organization in which several agencies work independently but cooperatively.

universal dressing a bulky dressing.

uppers stimulants such as amphetamines that affect the central nervous system to excite the user.

urinary catheter a tube inserted into the bladder through the urethra to drain urine from the bladder.

uterus (U-ter-us) the muscular abdominal organ where the fetus develops; the womb.

vagina (vah-JI-nah) the birth canal.

vallecula (val-EK-yuh-luh) a groove-like structure anterior to the epiglottis.

valve a structure that opens and closes to permit the flow of a fluid in only one direction.

vein any blood vessel returning blood to the heart.

venae cavae (VE-ne KA-ve) the superior vena cava and the inferior vena cava. These two major veins return blood from the body to the right atrium. (Venae cavae is plural, vena cava singular.)

venom a toxin (poison) produced by certain animals such as snakes, spiders, and some marine life forms.

venous bleeding bleeding from a vein, which is characterized by dark red or maroon blood and as a steady flow, easy to control.

ventilation the breathing in of air or oxygen or providing breaths artificially.

ventilator a device that breathes for a patient.

ventral referring to the front of the body; a synonym for anterior.

ventricles (VEN-tri-kulz) the two lower chambers of the heart. There is a right ventricle (which sends oxygen-poor blood to the lungs) and a left ventricle (which sends oxygen-rich blood to the body).

ventricular fibrillation (VF) (ven-TRIK-u-ler fib-ri-LAY-shun) a condition in which the heart's electrical impulses are disorganized, preventing the heart muscle from contracting normally.

ventricular tachycardia (V-Tach) (ven-TRIK-u-ler tak-i-KAR-de-uh) a condition in which the heartbeat is quite rapid; if rapid enough, ventricular tachycardia will not allow the heart's chambers to fill with enough blood between beats to produce blood flow sufficient to meet the body's needs.

Venturi mask a face mask and reservoir bag device that delivers specific concentrations of oxygen by mixing oxygen with inhaled air.

venule (VEN-yul) the smallest kind of vein.

vertebrae (VER-tuh-bray) the 33 bones of the spinal column. *Singular* vertebra.

visceral pain a poorly localized, dull or diffuse pain that arises from the abdominal organs, or viscera.

vital signs outward signs of what is going on inside the body, including respiration; pulse; skin color, temperature, and condition (plus capillary refill in infants and children); pupils; and blood pressure.

vocal cords two thin folds of tissue within the larynx that vibrate as air passes between them, producing sounds.

volatile chemicals vaporizing compounds, such as cleaning fluid, that are breathed in by the abuser to produce a "high."

voluntary muscle muscle that can be consciously controlled.

warm zone area where personnel and equipment decontamination and hot zone support take place; it includes control points for the access corridor and thus assists in reducing the spread of contamination.

water chill chilling caused by conduction of heat from the body when the body or clothing is wet.

watt the unit of measurement of the output power of a radio.

weaponization packaging or producing a material, such as chemical, biological, or radiological agent, so that it can be used as a weapon; for example, by dissemination in a bomb detonation or as an aerosol sprayed over an area or introduced into a ventilation system.

weapons of mass destruction (WMD) weapons, devices, or agents intended to cause widespread harm and/or fear among a population.

white blood cells components of the blood. They produce substances that help the body fight infection.

wind chill chilling caused by convection of heat from the body in the presence of air currents.

withdrawal referring to alcohol or drug withdrawal in which the patient's body reacts severely when deprived of the abused substance.

xiphoid (ZI-foid) **process** the inferior portion of the sternum.

zoonotic (ZO-uh-NOT-ik) able to move through the animal-human barrier; transmissible from animals to humans.

zygomatic (ZI-go-MAT-ik) **arches** form the structure of the cheeks.

INDEX

Page numbers followed by f indicate figures; those followed by t indicate tables.

A

B

C

D

E

F

G

H

I

J

K

L

M

N

O

P

Q

R

S

T

U

V

W

X

Z

Pearson Education, Inc.

YOU SHOULD CAREFULLY READ THE TERMS AND CONDITIONS BEFORE USING THE CD-ROM PACKAGE. USING THIS CD-ROM PACKAGE INDICATES YOUR ACCEPTANCE OF THESE TERMS AND CONDITIONS.

Pearson Education, Inc. provides this program and licenses its use. You assume responsibility for the selection of the program to achieve your intended results, and for the installation, use, and results obtained from the program. This license extends only to use of the program in the United States or countries in which the program is marketed by authorized distributors.

LICENSE GRANT

You hereby accept a nonexclusive, nontransferable, permanent license to install and use the program ON A SINGLE COMPUTER at any given time. You may copy the program solely for backup or archival purposes in support of your use of the program on the single computer. You may not modify, translate, disassemble, decompile, or reverse engineer the program, in whole or in part.

TERM

The License is effective until terminated. Pearson Education, Inc. reserves the right to terminate this License automatically if any provision of the License is violated. You may terminate the License at any time. To terminate this License, you must return the program, including documentation, along with a written warranty stating that all copies in your possession have been returned or destroyed.

LIMITED WARRANTY

THE PROGRAM IS PROVIDED "AS IS" WITHOUT WARRANTY OF ANY KIND, EITHER EXPRESSED OR IMPLIED, INCLUDING, BUT NOT LIMITED TO, THE IMPLIED WARRANTIES OR MERCHANTABILITY AND FITNESS FOR A PARTICULAR PURPOSE. THE ENTIRE RISK AS TO THE QUALITY AND PERFORMANCE OF THE PROGRAM IS WITH YOU. SHOULD THE PROGRAM PROVE DEFECTIVE, YOU (AND NOT PRENTICE-HALL, INC. OR ANY AUTHORIZED DEALER) ASSUME THE ENTIRE COST OF ALL NECESSARY SERVICING, REPAIR, OR CORRECTION. NO ORAL OR WRITTEN INFORMATION OR ADVICE GIVEN BY PRENTICE-HALL, INC., ITS DEALERS, DISTRIBUTORS, OR AGENTS SHALL CREATE A WARRANTY OR INCREASE THE SCOPE OF THIS WARRANTY.

SOME STATES DO NOT ALLOW THE EXCLUSION OF IMPLIED WARRANTIES, SO THE ABOVE EXCLUSION MAY NOT APPLY TO YOU. THIS WARRANTY GIVES YOU SPECIFIC LEGAL RIGHTS AND YOU MAY ALSO HAVE OTHER LEGAL RIGHTS THAT VARY FROM STATE TO STATE.

Pearson Education, Inc. does not warrant that the functions contained in the program will meet your requirements or that the operation of the program will be uninterrupted or error-free.

However, Pearson Education, Inc. warrants the diskette(s) or CD-ROM(s) on which the program is furnished to be free from defects in material and workmanship under normal use for a period of ninety (90) days from the date of delivery to you as evidenced by a copy of your receipt.

The program should not be relied on as the sole basis to solve a problem whose incorrect solution could result in injury to person or property. If the program is employed in such a manner, it is at the user's own risk and Pearson Education, Inc. explicitly disclaims all liability for such misuse.

LIMITATION OF REMEDIES

Pearson Education, Inc.'s entire liability and your exclusive remedy shall be:

1. the replacement of any diskette(s) or CD-ROM(s) not meeting Pearson Education, Inc.'s "LIMITED WARRANTY" and that is returned to Pearson Education, or

2. if Pearson Education is unable to deliver a replacement diskette(s) or CD-ROM(s) that is free of defects in materials or workmanship, you may terminate this agreement by returning the program.

IN NO EVENT WILL PRENTICE-HALL, INC. BE LIABLE TO YOU FOR ANY DAMAGES, INCLUDING ANY LOST PROFITS, LOST SAVINGS, OR OTHER INCIDENTAL OR CONSEQUENTIAL DAMAGES ARISING OUT OF THE USE OR INABILITY TO USE SUCH PROGRAM EVEN IF PRENTICE-HALL, INC. OR AN AUTHORIZED DISTRIBUTOR HAS BEEN ADVISED OF THE POSSIBILITY OF SUCH DAMAGES, OR FOR ANY CLAIM BY ANY OTHER PARTY.

SOME STATES DO NOT ALLOW FOR THE LIMITATION OR EXCLUSION OF LIABILITY FOR INCIDENTAL OR CONSEQUENTIAL DAMAGES, SO THE ABOVE LIMITATION OR EXCLUSION MAY NOT APPLY TO YOU.

GENERAL

You may not sublicense, assign, or transfer the license of the program. Any attempt to sublicense, assign or transfer any of the rights, duties, or obligations hereunder is void.

This Agreement will be governed by the laws of the State of New York.

Should you have any questions concerning this Agreement, you may contact Pearson Education, Inc. by writing to:

Director of New Media
Higher Education Division
Pearson Education, Inc.
One Lake Street
Upper Saddle River, NJ 07458

Should you have any questions concerning technical support, you may contact:

Product Support Department: Monday–Friday 8:00 A.M. –8:00 P.M. and Sunday 5:00 P.M.-12:00 A.M. (All times listed are Eastern). 1-800-677-6337

You can also get support by filling out the web form located at http://247.prenhall.com

YOU ACKNOWLEDGE THAT YOU HAVE READ THIS AGREEMENT, UNDERSTAND IT, AND AGREE TO BE BOUND BY ITS TERMS AND CONDITIONS. YOU FURTHER AGREE THAT IT IS THE COMPLETE AND EXCLUSIVE STATEMENT OF THE AGREEMENT BETWEEN US THAT SUPERSEDES ANY PROPOSAL OR PRIOR AGREEMENT, ORAL OR WRITTEN, AND ANY OTHER COMMUNICATIONS BETWEEN US RELATING TO THE SUBJECT MATTER OF THIS AGREEMENT.